PRINCIPLES OF

RUBIN'S Pathology

Seventh Edition

PRINCIPLES OF RUBIN'S Pathology

Seventh Edition

Emanuel Rubin, MD

Distinguished Professor of Pathology, Anatomy and Cell Biology
Kimmel Medical College
Thomas Jefferson University
Philadelphia, Pennsylvania
American Medical Writer's Award: Best Medical Textbook of the Year, 1989
Tom Kent Award of Group for Research in Pathology Education (GRIPE): Excellence in Pathology Education, 2001
Association of Pathology Chairs: Distinguished Service Award, 2006
American Society for Investigative Pathology: Robbins Distinguished Educator Award, 2017

Howard M. Reisner, PhD

Professor of Pathology and Laboratory Medicine
Department of Pathology and Laboratory Medicine
The University of North Carolina at Chapel Hill School of Medicine
Chapel Hill, North Carolina
Professor of Pathology
Jerry M. Wallace School of Osteopathic Medicine
Campbell University
Buies Creek, North Carolina

Illustrations by Dimitri Karetnikov, George Barile, and Kathy Jaeger.

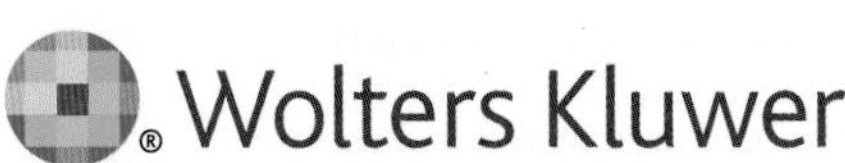

Philadelphia • Baltimore • New York • London
Buenos Aires • Hong Kong • Sydney • Tokyo

Acquisitions Editor: Crystal Taylor
Product Development Editor (Freelance): Andrew Hall
Product Development Editor (In-House): Andrea Vosburgh
Editorial Coordinator: Katherine Burland
Marketing Manager: Michael McMahon
Senior Production Project Manager: Alicia Jackson
Team Lead, Design: Stephen Druding
Manufacturing Coordinator: Margie Orzech
Prepress Vendor: S4Carlisle Publishing Services

Seventh edition

9 8 7 6 5 4 3 2 1

Printed in China

Library of Congress Cataloging-in-Publication Data

Names: Rubin, Emanuel, 1928- editor. | Reisner, Howard M., editor.
Title: Principles of Rubin's pathology / [edited by] Emanuel Rubin, MD, Distinguished Professor of Pathology, Anatomy and Cell Biology, Kimmel Medical College, Thomas Jefferson University, Philadelphia, Pennsylvania, American Medical Writer's Award: Best Medical Textbook of the Year, 1989, Tom Kent Award of Group for Research in Pathology Education (GRIPE): Excellence in Pathology Education, 2001, Association of Pathology Chairs: Distinguished Service Award, 2006, American Society for Investigative Pathology: Robbins Distinguished Educator Award, 2017, Howard M. Reisner, PhD, Professor of Pathology and Laboratory Medicine Department of Pathology and Laboratory Medicine, The University of North Carolina at Chapel Hill School of Medicine, Chapel Hill, North Carolina, Professor of Pathology, Jerry M. Wallace School of Osteopathic Medicine, Campbell University, Buies Creek, North Carolina ; illustrations by Dimitri Karetnikov, George Barile, and Kathy Jaeger.
Other titles: Essentials of Rubin's pathology.
Description: Seventh edition. | Philadelphia : Wolters Kluwer Health, [2019] | Revision of: Essentials of Rubin's pathology / editors, Emanuel Rubin, MD, Howard M. Reisner, PhD. 2014. 6th ed. | Includes index.
Identifiers: LCCN 2018031336 | ISBN 9781496350329
Subjects: LCSH: Pathology.
Classification: LCC RB111 .E856 2019 | DDC 616.07—dc23
LC record available at https://lccn.loc.gov/2018031336

LWW.com

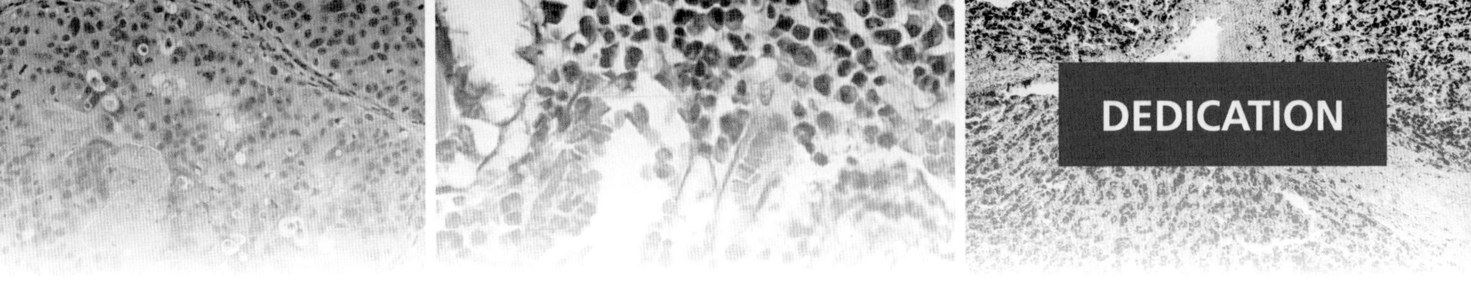

DEDICATION

We dedicate this book to our wives and families, whose love and support throughout this endeavor sustained us; to our colleagues, from whom we have learned so much; and to students everywhere, upon whose curiosity and energy the future of medical science depends.

Profound thanks to my teachers and colleagues, to whom I owe many things, especially an enduring curiosity related to medical science. They taught me to eat from the Tree of Knowledge and persuaded me that surface simplicity derives from hidden depths.

Emanuel Rubin, MD

Cui dono lepidum novum libellum
Arido modo pumice expolitum?
Emily, tibi atque etiam do

Howard M. Reisner, PhD

We dedicate this book to our wives and families, whose love and support throughout this endeavor sustained us; to our colleagues, from whom we have learned so much; and to students everywhere, upon whose curiosity and energy the future of medical science depends.

ABOUT THE AUTHORS

Emanuel Rubin, MD

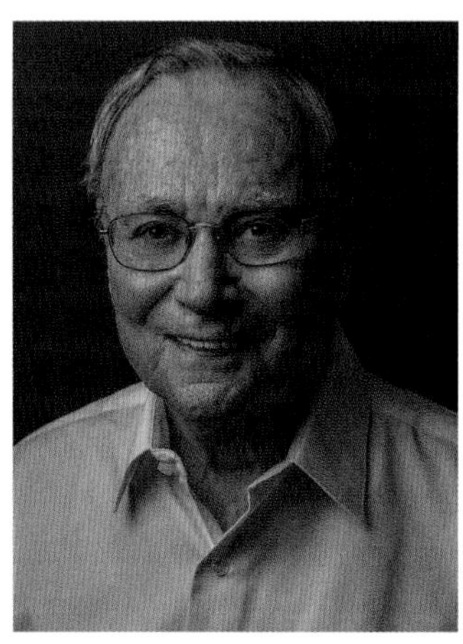

Dr. Rubin, who was born in Brookylyn, NY, and reared in Atlantic City, NJ, attended Harvard Medical School and trained in pathology at Mount Sinai Hospital in New York. He served as Chairman of Pathology at Mt. Sinai, Drexel, and Thomas Jefferson medical schools, and as Adjunct Professor of Biochemistry and Biophysics at the University of Pennsylvania School of Medicine. He is currently Distinguished Professor of Pathology, Anatomy and Cell Biology at Kimmel Medical College of Thomas Jefferson University in Philadelphia.

Dr. Rubin's research interests, which have been continuously funded by the National Institutes of Health (NIH), have spanned clinical studies, cell biology and biochemistry of the liver and heart, together with the clinical and experimental effects of alcohol. His bibliography lists more than 300 scientific and educational publications. His achievements have been recognized by major research and education awards of the principal pathology societies (including the American Society for Investigative Pathology, the US-Canadian Academy of Pathology, the International Academy of Pathology, and the Group for Research in Pathology Education), honorary degrees from prominent European universities, and the MERIT Award of the NIH.

Rubin's Pathology, which was founded more than 30 years ago, pioneered the use of graphic design, color photographs, and systematic icons in a textbook of pathology. The text has been translated into numerous languages, including Spanish, Portuguese, Italian, Japanese, and Korean.

Dr. Rubin's most profound regret is his inability to continue a lifetime participation in tennis and golf, owing to osteoarthritis of the shoulders.

Howard M. Reisner, PhD

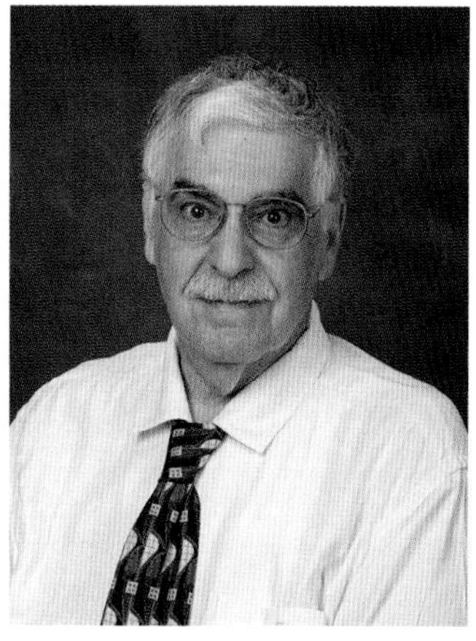

Although Howard Reisner was born in Brooklyn and raised in New York City, he has lived in Durham for over 40 years and counts himself as having near-native status in North Carolina. He is a 1967 graduate of City University of New York and earned his PhD from Case Western Reserve University in 1971 in biology, specializing in immunology and human genetics. He has been at The University of North Carolina ever since, starting as a Post-Doctoral Fellow (in Medicine) and, after moving to the Department of Pathology and Clinical Laboratory Medicine, working his way toward his current appointment as Professor.

Dr. Reisner trained in the area of hemostasis (and particularly in the immunogenetics of F.VIII and F.IX defects, which are expressed as hemophilia a and hemophilia b, respectively). His initial work occurred during a sojourn in Paris, where he kept his wife company during her tenure as an invited scientist in the laboratory of the late Dr. Jean Dausset (a subsequent Nobel Prize recipient). This was a fortunate happenstance because Dr. Reisner was able to fill a position in the hemostasis group in pathology on his return.

Dr. Reisner's research involves the use of immunotechnology both in hemostasis and drug discovery (working with diamidine-like antiparasitic agents under development). More recently, he has been involved in the use of digital image analysis in the analysis of surgical biopsies. Dr. Reisner has an extensive teaching background and was elected to the UNC Academy of Educators and has won several teaching awards. He currently teaches general pathology at multiple venues, including the Osteopathic School of Medicine at Campbell University and the Medical and Dental Schools of UNC, besides, occasionally, undergraduates at UNC. He likes cats and cooking, and has been known to read an occasional fantasy novel when not working on textbook editing.

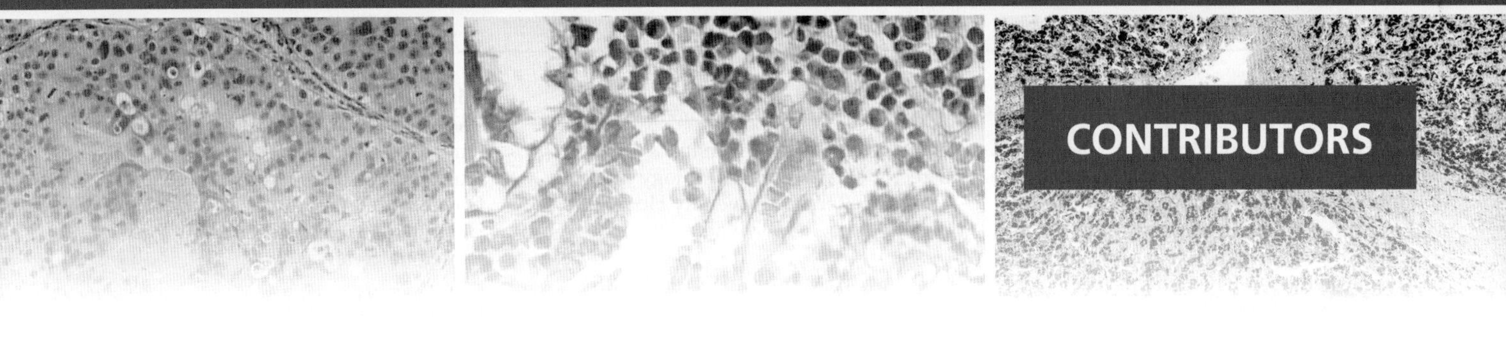

CONTRIBUTORS

Ronnie M. Abraham, MD
Clinical Assistant Professor
Departments of Pathology and Dermatology
University of Illinois College of Medicine
Peoria, Illinois

Michael F. Allard, MD
Professor of Pathology and Laboratory Medicine
University of British Columbia
Cardiovascular Pathologist
Department of Pathology and Laboratory Medicine
The iCAPTURE Centre
St. Paul's Hospital
Vancouver, British Columbia, Canada

Mary Beth Beasley, MD
Professor of Pathology
Mount Sinai Medical Center
New York, New York

Thomas W. Bouldin, MD
Professor of Pathology and Laboratory Medicine
Department of Pathology and Laboratory Medicine
University of North Carolina Hospitals
Chapel Hill, North Carolina

Linda A. Cannizzaro, PhD
Professor of Pathology
Albert Einstein College of Medicine
Director of Clinical and Molecular Cytogenetics
Montefiore Medical Center
Bronx, New York

Diane L. Carlson, MD
Assistant Attending
Department of Pathology
Memorial Sloan Kettering Cancer Center
New York, New York

Emily Y. Chu, MD, PhD
Department of Dermatology
Hospital of the University of Pennsylvania
Perelman Center for Advanced Medicine
Philadelphia, Pennsylvania

Philip L. Cohen, MD
Assistant Professor of Dermatology
Temple University School of Medicine
Chief, Section of Rheumatology
Temple University Hospital
Philadelphia, Pennsylvania

Ivan Damjanov, Peter A. McCue, MD, PhD
Professor of Pathology
The University of Kansas School of Medicine
Pathologist
Department of Pathology
University of Kansas Medical Center
Kansas City, Kansas

Jeffrey M. Davidson, PhD
Professor of Pathology
Vanderbilt University School of Medicine
Senior Research Career Scientist
Medical Research Service
Veterans Affairs Tennessee Valley Healthcare System
Nashville, Tennessee

Elizabeth G. Demicco, MD, PhD
Assistant Professor of Pathology
Icahn School of Medicine at Mount Sinai
Pathologist
Mount Sinai Hospital
New York, New York

David E. Elder, MD, ChB, FRCPA
Professor of Pathology and Laboratory Medicine
University of Pennsylvania School of Medicine
Director of Anatomic Pathology
Hospital of the University of Pennsylvania
Philadelphia, Pennsylvania

Alina Dulau Florea, MD
Medical Officer
National Institute of Health Clinical Center
Bethesda, Maryland

Gregory N. Fuller, MD, PhD
Professor of Pathology
Chief of Neuropathology
The University of Texas M.D. Anderson Cancer Center
Houston, Texas

Roberto A. Garcia, MD
Assistant Professor of Pathology
Mount Sinai School of Medicine
Chief of Orthopaedic and Soft Tissue Pathology
Mount Sinai Hospital
New York, New York

J. Clay Goodman, MD
Professor of Pathology and Neurology
Walter Henrick Moursund Chair in Neuropathology
Associate Dean of Undergraduate Medical Education
Baylor College of Medicine
Houston, Texas

Avrum I. Gotlieb, MD, CM, FRCP
Professor of Laboratory Medicine and Pathology
University of Toronto
Staff Pathologist
Laboratory Medicine Program
University Health Network
Toronto, Ontario, Canada

Leana Guerin, MD
Anatomic and Clinical Pathology
Lawrence Memorial Hospital
Lawrence, Kansas

Philip Hawkins, PhD, FRCP, FRCPath, FMedSci
Professor of Medicine
Centre for Amyloidosis and Acute Phase Proteins
University College London Medical School
Head, National Amyloidosis Centre
Royal Free Hospital
London, England

Kendra Iskander, MD
General Surgery
St. Joseph Health Medical Group
Eureka, California

J. Charles Jennette, MD
Brinkhous Distinguished Professor
Chair of Pathology and Laboratory Medicine
University of North Carolina, School of Medicine
Chief of Service
Department of Pathology and Laboratory Medicine
University of North Carolina Hospitals
Chapel Hill, North Carolina

Sergio A. Jimenez, MD
Professor and Co-Director
Jefferson Institute of Molecular Medicine
Director of Connective Tissue Diseases
Director of Scleroderma Center
Department of Dermatology and Cutaneous Biology
Thomas Jefferson University
Philadelphia, Pennsylvania

Lawrence C. Kenyon, MD, PhD
Associate Professor of Pathology, Anatomy and Cell Biology
Thomas Jefferson University
Pathologist and Neuropathologist
Department of Pathology, Anatomy and Cell Biology
Thomas Jefferson University Hospital
Philadelphia, Pennsylvania

Michael J. Klein, MD
Professor of Pathology and Laboratory Medicine
Weill Medical College of Cornell University
Pathologist-in-Chief and Director of Pathology and Laboratory Medicine
Hospital for Special Surgery
New York, New York

David S. Klimstra, MD
Chief of Surgical Pathology
Department of Pathology
Memorial Sloan Kettering Cancer Center
New York, New York

Gordon K. Klintworth, MD, PhD
Professor of Pathology
Joseph A.C. Wadsworth Research Professor of Ophthalmology
Duke University
Durham, North Carolina

Shauying Li, MD
Assistant Professor
Department of Pathology, Microbiology and Immunology
Vanderbilt University Medical Center
Nashville, Tennessee

Amber Chang Liu, MSc
Harvard Medical School
Resident Physician
Department of Anesthesiology, Critical Care and Pain Medicine
Massachusetts General Hospital
Boston, Massachusetts

David Lombard, MD, PhD
Assistant Professor of Pathology
Department of Pathology and Institute of Gerontology
Staff Pathologist
Department of Pathology
University of Michigan
Ann Arbor, Michigan

Peter A. McCue, MD
Professor of Pathology
Thomas Jefferson University
Director of Anatomic Pathology
Thomas Jefferson University Hospital
Philadelphia, Pennsylvania

Bruce M. McManus, MD, PhD, FRSC
Professor of Pathology and Laboratory Medicine
University of British Columbia
Director, Providence Heart and Lung Institute
St. Paul's Hospital
Vancouver, British Columbia, Canada

Maria J. Merino, MD
Chief of Translational Pathology
Department of Pathology
National Cancer Institute
Bethesda, Maryland

Marc S. Micozzi, MD, PhD
Private Practice, Forensic Medicine
Policy Institute for Integrative Medicine
Bethesda, Maryland

Frank Mitros, MD
Frederic W. Stamler Professor
Department of Pathology
University of Iowa
Iowa City, Iowa

Anna Marie Mulligan, MB, MSc, FRCPath
Assistant Professor of Laboratory Medicine and Pathobiology
University of Toronto
Anatomic Pathologist
Department of Laboratory Medicine
St. Michael's Hospital
Toronto, Ontario, Canada

Hedwig S. Murphy, MD, PhD
Associate Professor of Pathology
University of Michigan
Staff Pathologist
Department of Pathology and Laboratory Medicine
Veterans Affairs Ann Arbor Health System
Ann Arbor, Michigan

George L. Mutter, MD
Associate Professor of Pathology
Harvard Medical School
Pathologist
Department of Pathology
Brigham and Women's Hospital
Boston, Massachusetts

Frances P. O'Malley, MB, FRCPC
Professor of Laboratory Medicine and Pathobiology
University of Toronto
Staff Pathologist
Department of Pathology and Laboratory Medicine
Mount Sinai Hospital
Toronto, Ontario, Canada

Jaime Prat, MD, PhD, FRCPath
Professor of Pathology
Director of Pathology
Autonomous University of Barcelona
Director of Pathology
Hospital de la Santa Creu i Sant Pau
Barcelona, Spain

Daniel G. Remick, MD
Chair and Professor
Department of Pathology and Laboratory Medicine
Boston University School of Medicine
Chief of Pathology
Department of Pathology and Laboratory Medicine
Boston Medical Center
Boston, Massachusetts

Emanuel Rubin, MD
Distinguished Professor of Pathology, Anatomy and Cell Biology
Kimmel Medical College
Thomas Jefferson University
Philadelphia, Pennsylvania

Jeffrey E. Saffitz, MD, PhD
Mallinckrodt Professor of Medicine
Harvard Medical School
Chairman
Department of Pathology
Beth Israel Deaconess Medical Center
Boston, Massachusetts

Alan L. Schiller, MD
Professor and Chairman
Department of Pathology
John A. Burns School of Medicine
University of Hawaii
Honolulu, Hawaii

David A. Schwartz, MD, MSHyg, FCAP
Clinical Professor of Pathology
Department of Pathology
Augusta University
Augusta, Georgia

Gregory C. Sephel, PhD
Associate Professor of Pathology
Departments of Pathology, Microbiology and Immunology
Vanderbilt University School of Medicine
Nashville, Tennessee

Elias S. Siraj, MD
Associate Professor of Medicine
Section of Endocrinology
Temple University School of Medicine
Program Director, Endocrinology Fellowship
Temple University Hospital
Philadelphia, Pennsylvania

Edward B. Stelow, MD
Associate Professor of Pathology
University of Virginia
Charlottesville, Virginia

David S. Strayer, MD, PhD
Professor of Pathology
Department of Pathology and Cell Biology
Jefferson Medical College of Thomas Jefferson University
Philadelphia, Pennsylvania

Arief A. Suriawinata, MD
Associate Professor of Pathology
Geisel School of Medicine at Dartmouth
Hanover, New Hampshire
Section Chief of Anatomic Pathology
Dartmouth-Hitchcock Medical Center
Lebanon, New Hampshire

Swan N. Thung, MD
Professor of Pathology
Mount Sinai School of Medicine
Director
Division of Liver Pathology
Mount Sinai Medical Center
New York, New York

William D. Travis, MD
Professor of Pathology
Weill Medical College of Cornell University
Attending Thoracic Pathologist
Memorial Sloan Kettering Cancer Center
New York, New York

Riccardo Valdez, MD
Assistant Professor of Pathology
Section Head, Hematopathology
Department of Laboratory Medicine and Pathology
Mayo Clinic
Scottsdale, Arizona

Jeffrey S. Warren, MD
Aldred S. Warthin Endowed Professor of Pathology
Director
Division of Clinical Pathology
University of Michigan Medical School
University of Michigan Hospitals
Ann Arbor, Michigan

Kevin Jon Williams, MD
Professor of Medicine
Chief
Section of Endocrinology, Diabetes and Metabolism
Temple University School of Medicine
Philadelphia, Pennsylvania

Robert Yanagawa, MD, PhD
Assistant Professor
Division of Cardiac Surgery
University of Toronto, Faculty of Medicine
Toronto, Ontario, Canada

Mary M. Zutter, MD
Professor of Pathology and Cancer Biology
Vanderbilt University
Director of Hematopathology
Vanderbilt University Medical Center
Nashville, Tennessee

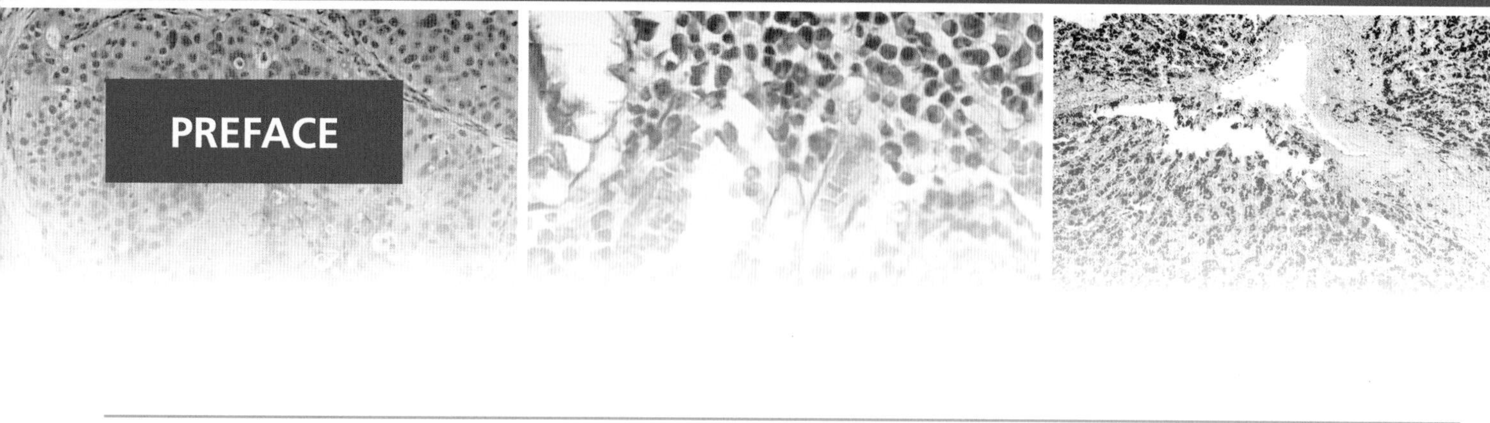

PREFACE

An honest tale speeds best being plainly told
(Shakespeare, Richard III)

Pathology is the medical science that deals with all aspects of disease, but with special reference to the essential nature, the causes, and the development of abnormal conditions. In this sense, literacy in pathology is the bedrock of practice and research for the student of medicine.

The organization of a textbook should reflect its incorporation into the curriculum for which it is intended. The current trend toward an integrated curriculum, which emphasizes the combination of basic science and clinical information in separate sections devoted to individual organ systems, requires a similar approach in a textbook dedicated to the study of pathology. In this context, chapters concerned with principles of general pathology (Chapters 1 to 6) are applicable to all or most organ systems, whereas those that pertain to organs or systemic disease include pathologic descriptions, epidemiology, molecular biology, clinical features, and so on. "Success is directly proportional to the degree of positive adaptation to change" (Chavan).

Particular attention is paid throughout to the impact of molecular genetics on our insights into the causes and manifestations of disease, including the correlation between genotype and phenotypic expression. For reference purposes, we have identified many of the relevant gene mutations and their chromosomal locations.

In his treatise *On the Natural Faculties*, Galen wrote, "The chief merit of language is clearness, and we know that nothing detracts from this as do unfamiliar terms." We have kept this admonition in mind in editing the text and graphic material. Separate sections of epidemiology, pathogenesis, pathology, and clinical features are each identified by unique icons. Attention is often directed to the key points by the use of bulleted lists and boldface type.

To aid the student in understanding and retaining complex and detailed information, we have placed emphasis on graphic representation of the pathogenesis of disease, the complications of various disorders, and the sequence of pathologic alterations. Because graphic images utilize pattern recognition, one of the most fundamental characteristics of the human brain, they powerfully communicate abstract and complex material. At the same time, we have been guided by Einstein's concept that "everything should be made as simple as possible, but not simpler." Each chapter is headed by a list of questions that the student should be able to answer in a coherent manner.

Sadly, attempting to edit a comprehensive textbook of pathology without missing any errors is like trying to live without sin—worth the effort, but probably impossible. As Isaac Newton observed (1703), "To explain all nature is too difficult a task for any one man or even for any one age. Tis much better to do a little with certainty & leave the rest for others that come after you." However, the inevitability of human mistakes has not deterred us from including new and still controversial concepts. Some of these will stand the test of time; the others will be corrected in subsequent editions.

Emanuel Rubin
Howard Reisner

ACKNOWLEDGMENTS

The seventh edition of *Principles of Rubin's Pathology* is based on the hard work and insights of all those who made the seventh edition of *Rubin's Pathology* possible. In addition, the editors would like to thank the managing and editorial staff at Wolters Kluwer, in particular Shannon Magee and Crystal Taylor. We would also like to thank Elizabeth Shamblin for her work designing the animations that accompany the book.

The editors also acknowledge the contributions made by our colleagues who participated in writing previous editions and those who offered suggestions and ideas for the current edition.

Stuart A. Aaronson
Mohammad Alomari
Adam Bagg
Karoly Balogh
Sue Bartow
Douglas P. Bennett
Marluce Bibbo
Hugh Bonner
Patrick J. Buckley
Stephen W. Chensue
Daniel H. Connor
Jeffrey Cossman
John E. Craighead
Mary Cunnane
Giulia DeFalco
Hormuz Ehya
Joseph C. Fantone
John L. Farber
Kevin Furlong
Antonio Giordano
Barry J. Goldstein
Stanley R. Hamiliton
Terrence J. Harrist
Arthur P. Hays
Steven K. Herrine
Serge Jabbour
Robert B. Jennings
Kent J. Johnson
Anthony A. Killeen
Robert Kisilevsky
William D. Kocher
Robert J. Kurman
Ernest A. Lack
Antonio Martinez-Hernandez
Steven McKenzie
Wolfgang J. Mergner
Victor J. Navarro
Adebeye O. Osunkoya
Juan Palazzo
Stephen Peiper
Robert O. Peterson
Roger J. Pomerantz
Martha Quezado
Timothy R. Quinn
Stanley J. Robboy
Brian Schapiro
Roland Schwarting
Stephen M. Schwartz
Benjamin H. Spargo
Charles Steenbergen, Jr.
Craig A. Storm
Steven L. Teitelbaum
Ann D. Thor
John Q. Trojanowski
Benjamin F. Trump
Beverly Y. Wang
Jianzhou Wang
Bruce M. Wenig

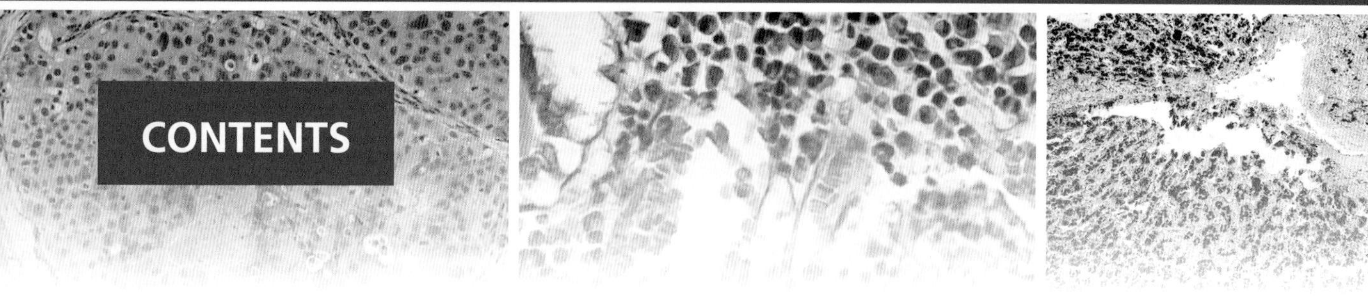

CONTENTS

1 Cell Adaptation, Injury, Death, and Aging

David S. Strayer[1] ▪ Emanuel Rubin[1] ▪ David Lombard[2]

LEARNING OBJECTIVES

- Describe adaptive cellular responses to stress, including atrophy, hypertrophy, hyperplasia, metaplasia, and dysplasia.
- What are the molecular mechanisms associated with atrophy and hypertrophy?
- Provide examples of metaplasia that occur as a response to cellular injury.
- List the cellular changes associated with dysplasia and provide several examples.
- Explain the metabolic and cellular changes associated with hydropic swelling.
- Provide a timeline for the biochemical and cellular changes associated with ischemic cell injury.
- Describe the mechanisms that provoke the production of reactive oxygen species.
- List four reactive oxygen species important in cell injury and describe the mechanism resulting in their toxicity.
- Describe cellular antioxidant defenses and the mechanisms by which they function.
- Explain the generation of reactive oxygen species in reperfusion injury.
- List cellular constituents that may accumulate as a result of cell stress and injury.
- Define and describe the cellular appearance and localization of "wear and tear" pigment.
- Why may abnormal iron storage occur? What is the mechanism by which such accumulation results in organ damage?
- Differentiate between dystrophic and metastatic calcification.
- List and define several mechanisms of cell death.
- What are the histologically defined forms of cell death? What specific etiologies are associated with each?
- Provide a sequence of important events in the production of ischemic cell death.
- Define and describe the cellular changes associated with apoptosis. Provide examples of the role of apoptosis in development, normal physiology, and disease.
- Describe and differentiate major apoptotic signaling pathways.
- Describe the role of mitochondria in provoking apoptosis.
- Discuss the role of telomere shortening in cellular senescence and longevity.
- Provide a hypothesis for the role of dietary restriction in longevity.
- Define the term progeria and describe two progeric diseases.
- Provide a hypothesis for the role of dietary restriction affecting longevity.

***Pathology** is the study of structural and functional abnormalities that are expressed as diseases of organs and systems. Although classic theories attributed diseases to imbalances or noxious effects of humors on specific organs, in the 19th century Virchow proposed that injury to the smallest living unit of the body, the cell, was the basis of all diseases. To this day, clinical and experimental pathology remains rooted in this concept, which is now extended by an increased understanding of the molecular nature of many disease processes.*

A living cell must maintain the ability to produce energy, much of which is spent in establishing a barrier between the internal milieu of the cell and a hostile environment. The plasma membrane, associated ion pumps, and receptor molecules serve this purpose. A cell must also be able to adapt to adverse environmental conditions, for example, changes in temperature, solute concentrations, oxygen supply, or the presence of noxious agents. If an injury exceeds the adaptive capacity of the stressed cell, the cell dies. From this perspective, pathology is the study of cell injury and the expression of a cell's preexisting capacity to adapt to such injury.

The mechanisms of cellular stress that eventuate in cell injury and cell death are central to understanding the mechanisms of disease and the inevitable process of aging. The cellular, biochemical, and molecular consequences of these events represent the science of pathology, but are also critical in the clinical practice of pathology.

[1] Cell Adaptation, Injury, and Death
[2] Aging

REACTIONS TO PERSISTENT STRESS AND CELL INJURY

Persistent cellular stress leads to a number of adaptive responses, although in some settings, neoplasia or cell death may follow such effects.

Atrophy

Atrophy is a decrease in size or function of cells or organs. It occurs in both pathologic and physiologic settings. Importantly, atrophy is an active response rather than a passive shutdown of cellular processes. For example, atrophy may result from disuse of skeletal muscle or from loss of hormonal signals following menopause. However, most commonly, atrophy reflects harmful processes, especially those involved in certain chronic diseases and biologic aging.

Atrophy of an organ differs from cellular atrophy. Reduction in an organ's size may be caused either by reversible cell shrinkage or by irreversible loss of cells. For example, renewing physical activity of a disused limb may cause atrophic muscle cells to resume their usual size and function. By contrast, atrophy of the brain in Alzheimer disease reflects extensive cell death; the size of the organ cannot be restored (Fig. 1-1). See Table 1-1 for conditions leading to atrophy.

Table 1-1

Conditions Associated With Atrophy

Disease or Condition	Examples of Conditions in Which Atrophy Occurs
Aging	Most organs that do not continuously turn over; most common setting for atrophy to occur
Chronic disease	Prototype for atrophy occurring in chronic-disease is cancer; also seen in congestive heart failure, chronic obstructive pulmonary disease, cirrhosis of the liver, and AIDS
Ischemia	Hypoxia, decreased nutrient availability, and renal artery stenosis
Malnutrition	Generalized atrophy
Decreased functional demand	Limb immobilization, as in a fracture
Interruption of trophic signals	Denervation atrophy following nerve injury; menopause effect on the endometrium and other organs
Increased pressure	Decubitus ulcers, passive congestion of the liver

Hypertrophy

Hypertrophy is an increase in cell or organ size and functional capacity. When trophic signals or functional demands increase, adaptive changes to satisfy these needs lead to larger cells (hypertrophy) and, in some cases, increased cell number (hyperplasia). In several organs (e.g., heart, skeletal muscle), such adaptive responses are achieved mainly by increased cell size, which leads to increased organ mass (Fig. 1-2). In other organs (e.g., kidney), cell numbers and cell size may both increase. The situations that are associated with increased cell and organ mass are in many, but not all, cases the converse of those that lead to atrophy. See Table 1-2 for conditions leading to hypertrophy.

Mechanisms of Cellular Hypertrophy

Whether the stimulus to enlarge is increased workload or response to endocrine or neuroendocrine mediators, there are certain processes that usually contribute to generating cellular hypertrophy. Some proteins that are not involved in hypertrophy are removed, even as production of proteins that promote hypertrophy increases. Signals that elicit hypertrophic responses vary, depending on cell type and circumstances. The example of skeletal muscle hypertrophy is often used to illustrate some critical general principles that

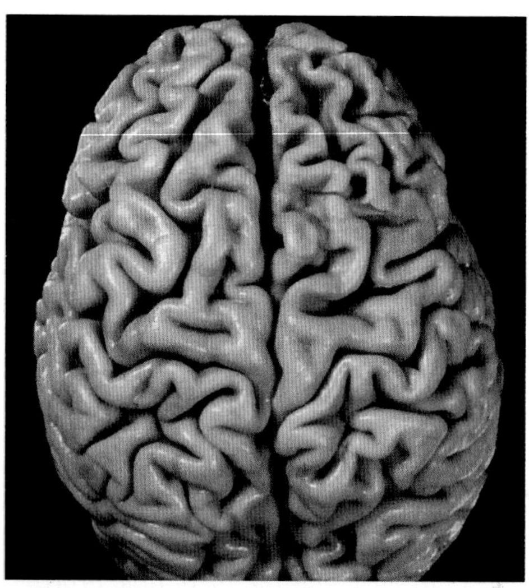

FIGURE 1-1. Atrophy of the brain. Marked atrophy of the frontal lobe is characterized by thinned gyri and widened sulci. (Courtesy of Dr. F. Stephen Vogel, Duke University.)

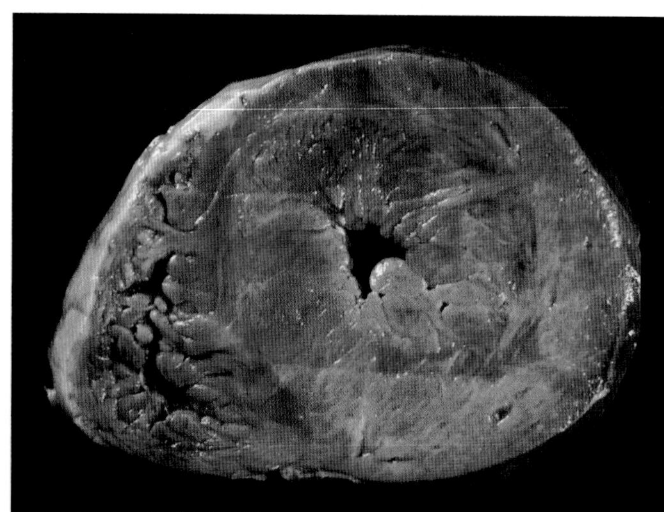

FIGURE 1-2. Myocardial hypertrophy. Cross section of the heart of a patient with long-standing hypertension shows pronounced, concentric left ventricular hypertrophy.

Table 1-2

Conditions Associated With Hypertrophy

Condition	Examples of Conditions in Which Hypertrophy Occurs
Puberty	Surge in androgens and growth hormone increases downstream mediators increasing mass of muscle and other tissue
Increased trophic signaling	Cells and organs responsive to soluble-mediators such as the thyroid or breast undergo hypertrophy when levels of trophic hormones (thyroid-stimulating hormone and estrogen/progesterone) increase
Increased-functional demand	Exercise under heavy loads such as-weightlifting leads to hypertrophy of type II (fast twitch) fibers

apply to many cell types. However, each tissue responds to different signals. Table 1-3 provides examples of important signaling mechanisms in the hypertrophic response. Whatever mechanisms initiate signaling to stimulate hypertrophy, there are a limited number of downstream pathways that mediate the effects of such signaling. Increased gene expression, particularly of growth-promoting transcription factors, such as Fos and Myc, and concomitant increases in protein translation are important. These are associated with augmentation of translational initiators and elongation factors and are critical for hypertrophy. Moreover, during hypertrophy, cell death is inhibited. For example, stimulation of specific receptors activates several enzymes (e.g., Akt, PI3K) that promote cell survival, largely by inhibiting programmed cell death.

Molecular Mechanisms in Atrophy and Hypertrophy

Atrophy and hypertrophy, although phenotypically presenting as polar opposites, affect the same molecular intermediates. The protein kinase Akt controls the balance between atrophy and hypertrophy. The two processes have been extensively studied in skeletal muscle, which responds rapidly to changes in demand for energy storage and contractile force. In skeletal muscle, when the muscle is immobilized, the need for contraction decreases (unloading), and myocytes activate adaptive mechanisms. Muscle disuse increases extracellular myostatin, a protein in the transforming growth factor-β (TGF-β) family. Myostatin binding activates its receptor, which inhibits Akt. A transcription factor, FOXO, which is normally inhibited by Akt, is thereby released from that suppression. Ultimately, FOXO activity results in degradation of muscle protein and fiber atrophy.

In contrast to disease, resistance training leads to increased synthesis of extracellular IGF-I. When IGF-I binds to its cell membrane receptor on type II muscle fibers, it initiates a signaling cascade that promotes Akt activation. This event stimulates mTOR (mammalian target of rapamycin), which upregulates protein synthesis. Akt-independent mechanisms are also important in muscle hypertrophy (and prevention of atrophy). Depletion of ATP stimulates AMP kinase, thereby

Table 1-3

Signaling Mechanisms in Hypertrophy

Mechanism	Example
Growth factor stimulation	Insulin-like growth factor-I on muscle
Neuroendocrine stimulation	Adrenergic signaling in the heart
Ion channels	Calcium channel activity in the heart stimulates downstream enzymes (e.g., calcineurin) to produce hypertrophy
Chemical mediators	Nitric oxide, angiotensin II, and bradykinin support hypertrophy in some tissues
Oxygen supply	Increased functional demand resulting in oxygen deficit stimulates angiogenesis, which is a key component in adaptive hypertrophy
Hypertrophy antagonists	Some chemical mediators such as atrial natriuretic factor either prevent or slow adaptive hypertrophy

increasing transcription of mitochondrial DNA and the number of mitochondria. As a result, increasing oxidative metabolism produces additional ATP. Further details of the molecular mechanisms of atrophy and hypertrophy are outlined in Figure 1-3.

Adaptive Responses: Hyperplasia, Metaplasia, and Dysplasia

Atrophy and hypertrophy are both expressed at the organ level, although they are ultimately the result of changes in cell size or number, or both. Other adaptive processes are expressed predominantly at the level of cells and tissues and reflect cellular adaptations. For example, a description of ductal hyperplasia (as might be found in a breast) refers to an increase in the number of cells lining the duct. A cervix demonstrating dysplasia has cells that microscopically demonstrate disordered growth. In gross appearance, the cervix may well appear normal.

Hyperplasia

Stimuli that induce hyperplasia and the mechanisms by which they act vary greatly from one tissue and cell type to the next. This process may occur as a response to an altered endocrine milieu, increased functional demand, or chronic injury.

Increased Functional Demand

Increased physiologic requirements may result in hyperplasia. For example, at high altitudes, low atmospheric oxygen tension causes compensatory hyperplasia of erythroid precursors in the bone marrow and thus increased blood erythrocytes (Fig. 1-4). In this fashion, a greater number of cells compensates for the decreased oxygen carried by each erythrocyte. Similarly, chronic blood loss, as in excessive menstrual bleeding or colon cancer, also causes hyperplasia of erythrocytic elements in the marrow.

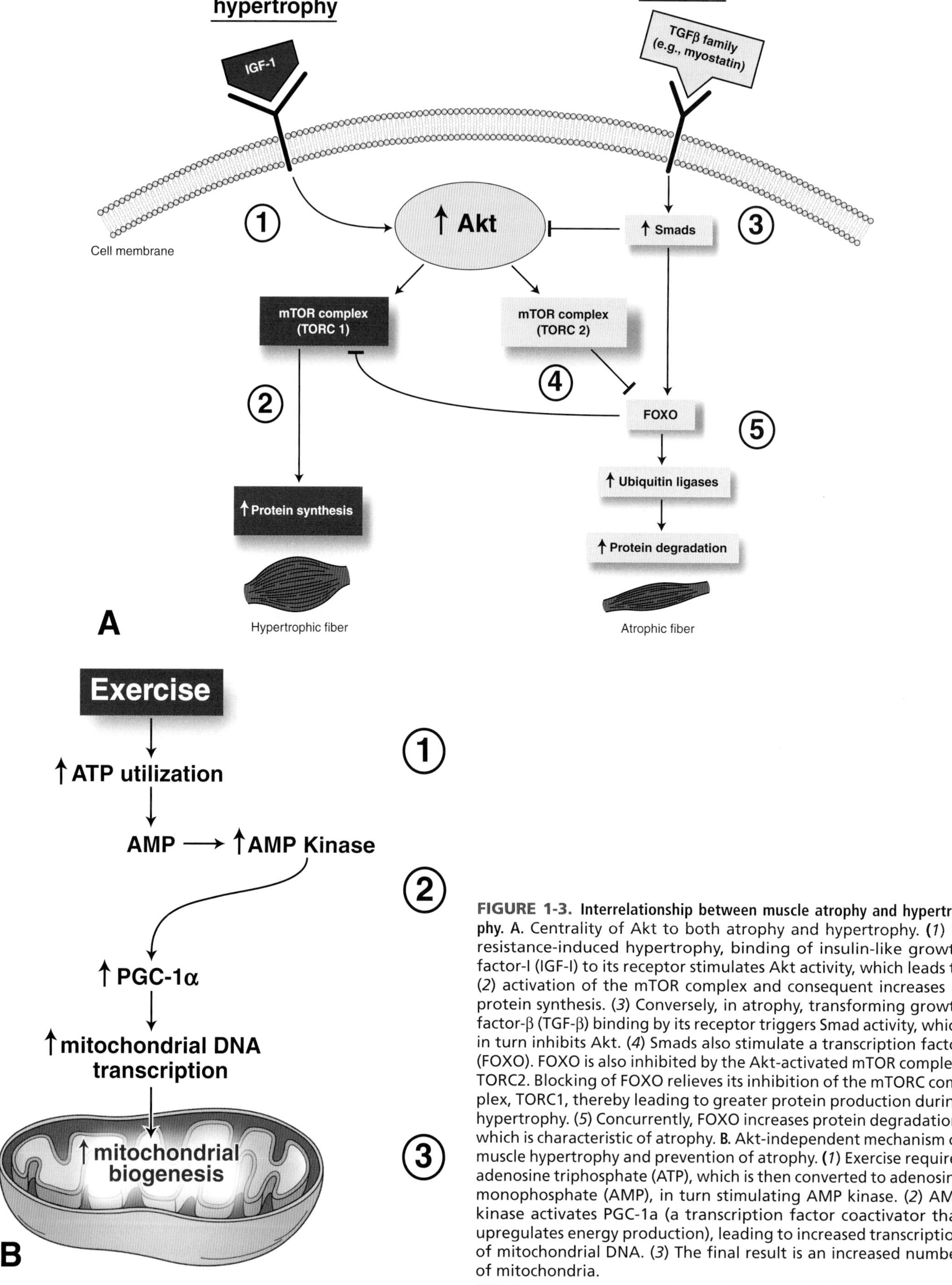

FIGURE 1-3. Interrelationship between muscle atrophy and hypertrophy. A. Centrality of Akt to both atrophy and hypertrophy. (*1*) In resistance-induced hypertrophy, binding of insulin-like growth factor-I (IGF-I) to its receptor stimulates Akt activity, which leads to (*2*) activation of the mTOR complex and consequent increases in protein synthesis. (*3*) Conversely, in atrophy, transforming growth factor-β (TGF-β) binding by its receptor triggers Smad activity, which in turn inhibits Akt. (*4*) Smads also stimulate a transcription factor (FOXO). FOXO is also inhibited by the Akt-activated mTOR complex, TORC2. Blocking of FOXO relieves its inhibition of the mTORC complex, TORC1, thereby leading to greater protein production during hypertrophy. (*5*) Concurrently, FOXO increases protein degradation, which is characteristic of atrophy. **B.** Akt-independent mechanism of muscle hypertrophy and prevention of atrophy. (*1*) Exercise requires adenosine triphosphate (ATP), which is then converted to adenosine monophosphate (AMP), in turn stimulating AMP kinase. (*2*) AMP kinase activates PGC-1a (a transcription factor coactivator that upregulates energy production), leading to increased transcription of mitochondrial DNA. (*3*) The final result is an increased number of mitochondria.

Hormonal Stimulation

Changes in hormone concentrations can elicit proliferation of responsive cells. These changes may reflect developmental, pharmacologic, or pathologic influences. For example, the normal increase in estrogens at puberty or early in the menstrual cycle leads to hyperplasia of endometrial and uterine stromal cells. Estrogen administration to postmenopausal women has the same effect. Enlargement of the male breast, called gynecomastia, may occur in men with excess estrogens. For example, estrogen therapy for prostate cancer at one time produced gynecomastia. Similarly, chronic liver failure results in an inability to metabolize estrogens and subsequent gynecomastia results. Ectopic hormone production may be a tumor's first presenting symptom as demonstrated by hyperplasia of erythrocytes in the bone marrow secondary to erythropoietin secretion by renal tumors.

Chronic Injury

Persistent injury may result in hyperplasia. Long-standing inflammation or chronic physical or chemical injury is often accompanied by a hyperplastic response. For instance, pressure from ill-fitting shoes causes hyperplasia of the skin of the foot, so-called corns or calluses. Resultant thickening of the skin protects it from the continued pressure. Chronic inflammation of the bladder (chronic cystitis) often produces hyperplasia of the bladder epithelium. Inappropriate hyperplasia can itself be harmful, as characterized by conspicuous hyperplasia of the skin that occurs in psoriasis (Fig. 1-4D).

The variety of cellular and molecular mechanisms responsible for the increased mitotic activity that characterizes hyperplastic responses clearly relates to altered control of cell proliferation. These topics are discussed in Chapters 2 and 4.

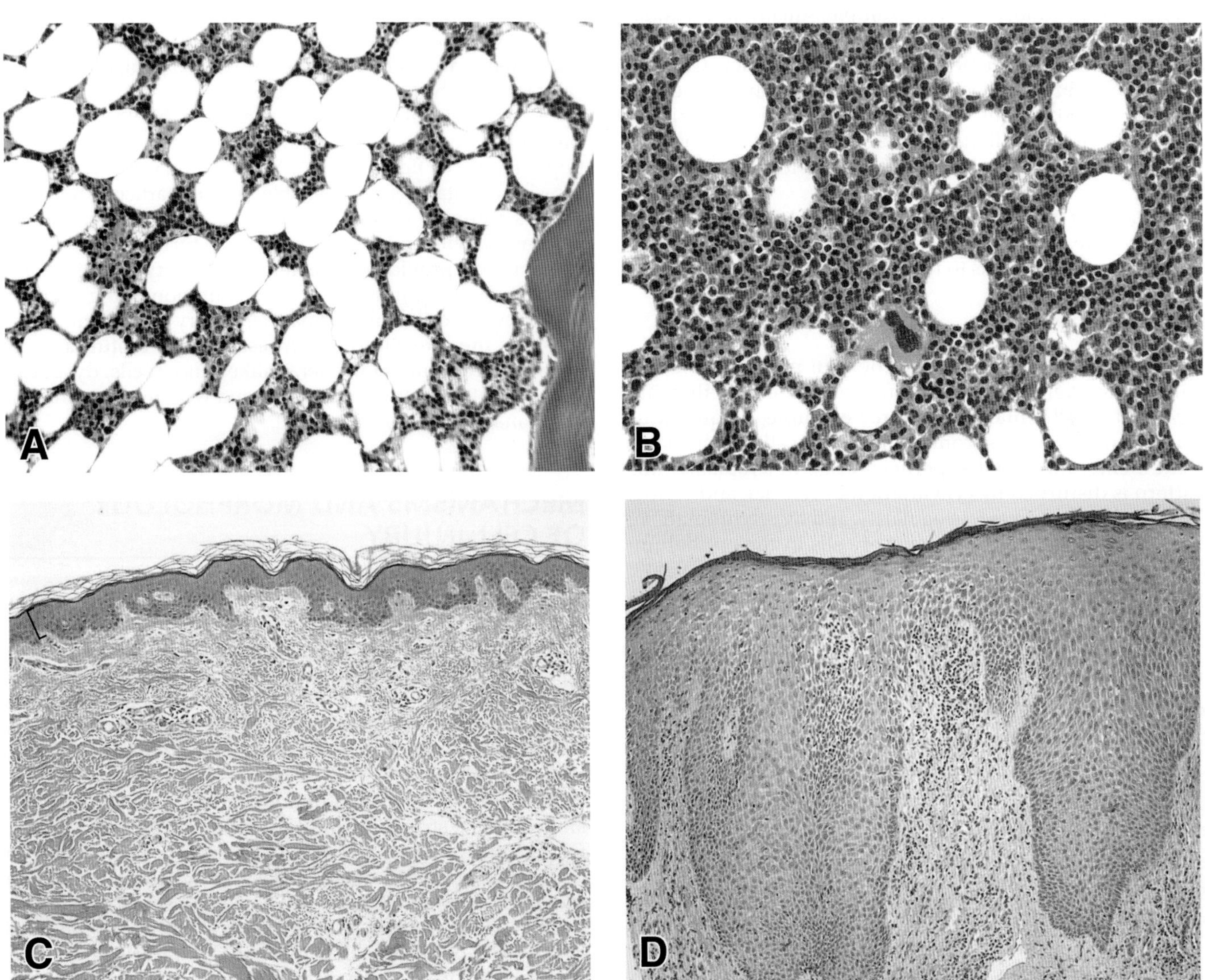

FIGURE 1-4. Hyperplasia. A. Normal adult bone marrow. Normocellular bone marrow shows the usual ratio of fat to hematopoietic cells. **B.** Hyperplasia of the bone marrow. Cellularity is increased; fat is relatively decreased. **C.** Normal epidermis. Epidermal thickness is modest (*bracket*) compared to the dermis (below). **D.** Epidermal hyperplasia in psoriasis is shown at the same magnification as in **C.** The epidermis is thickened owing to an increase in the number of squamous cells.

Metaplasia

Metaplasia is usually an adaptive response to persistent injury. A tissue will assume a phenotype that protects it best from the insult. Most often, glandular epithelium is replaced by squamous epithelium. Columnar or cuboidal lining cells that are committed to mucus production may not be adequately resistant to the effects of chronic irritation or a pernicious chemical. For example, prolonged exposure of bronchial epithelium to tobacco smoke gives rise to squamous metaplasia. A similar response is associated with chronic infection in the glandular epithelium of the endocervix (Fig. 1-5).

The process is not restricted to squamous differentiation. When highly acidic gastric contents reflux chronically into the lower esophagus, the squamous epithelium of the esophagus may be replaced by glandular mucosa (**Barrett esophagus**). This effect can be thought of as an adaptation to protect the esophagus from injury by gastric acid and pepsin, to which the glandular mucosa is more resistant.

Although metaplasia may be thought of as adaptive, it is not necessarily innocuous. For example, squamous metaplasia may protect a bronchus from tobacco smoke, but it also impairs mucus production and ciliary clearance. Cancers may develop in metaplastic epithelium; malignancies of the lung, cervix, esophagus, stomach, and bladder often arise in such areas. However, if the chronic injury ceases, there is little stimulus for cells to proliferate, and the epithelium does not become cancerous.

Metaplasia is often fully reversible. If the noxious stimulus is removed (e.g., when one stops smoking), the metaplastic epithelium often returns to normal.

Dysplasia

The cells that comprise an epithelium normally exhibit uniformity of size, shape, and nuclei. Moreover, they are arranged in a regular fashion; for example, a squamous epithelium progresses from plump basal cells on the basement membrane to flat superficial cells. In dysplasia, this pattern is disturbed by (1) variation in cell size and shape; (2) nuclear enlargement, irregularity, and hyperchromatism; and (3) disorderly arrangement of cells in the epithelium (Fig. 1-6). Dysplasia occurs most often in hyperplastic squamous epithelium, as in epidermal actinic keratosis (caused by sunlight), and in areas of squamous metaplasia, such as in the bronchus or the cervix. It is not, however, exclusive to squamous epithelium. For example, dysplastic changes occur in the columnar mucosal cells of the colon in ulcerative colitis, in metaplastic epithelium of Barrett esophagus (see Chapter 11), in glands of prostatic intraepithelial neoplasia, and in the urothelium of the bladder (see above and Chapter 15).

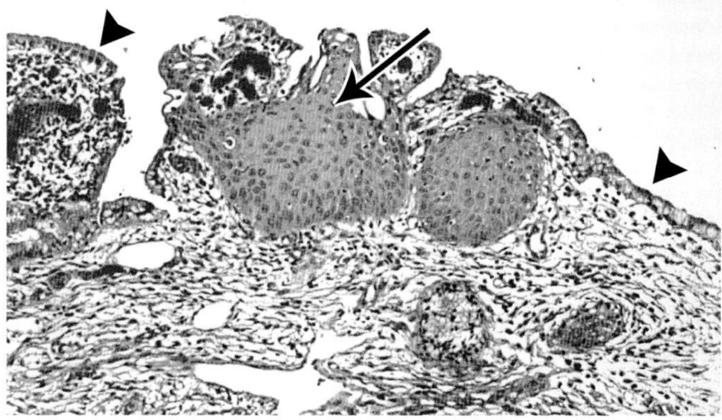

FIGURE 1-5. Squamous metaplasia. A section of endocervix shows the normal columnar epithelium at both margins (*arrowheads*) and a focus of squamous metaplasia in the center (*arrow*).

Similar to metaplasia, dysplasia is a response to persistent injury and often regresses. For example, if smoking ceases or if human papilloma virus disappears from the cervix, cells return to normal. However, dysplasia shares many cytologic features with cancer, and the line between the two may be very fine indeed. It may be difficult to distinguish severe dysplasia from early cancer of the cervix by gross or microscopic appearance.

Dysplasia is a preneoplastic lesion, in that it is a necessary stage in the multistep cellular evolution to cancer. In fact, dysplasia is included in morphologic classifications of the stages of intraepithelial neoplasia in several organs (e.g., cervix, prostate, bladder). Severe dysplasia is considered an indication for aggressive preventive therapy to (1) cure the underlying cause, (2) eliminate a noxious agent, or (3) surgically remove the offending tissue.

As in the development of cancer (see Chapter 4), dysplasia results from sequential mutations in a proliferating cell population. The fidelity of DNA replication is imperfect, and occasional mutations are inevitable. When a particular mutation confers a growth or survival advantage, the progeny of the mutant cell will tend to predominate. In turn, their continued proliferation provides a greater opportunity for additional mutations. Accumulation of such mutations progressively distances the cell from normal regulatory constraints. **Dysplasia is the morphologic expression of a disturbance in growth regulation.** However, unlike cancer cells, dysplastic cells are not entirely autonomous, and with intervention, the tissue may still revert to normal.

MECHANISMS AND MORPHOLOGY OF CELL INJURY

All cells have efficient mechanisms to deal with shifts in environmental conditions. When environmental changes exceed the cell's capacity to maintain normal homeostasis, acute cell injury occurs. Mechanisms involved in the responses to stress include cell swelling, adaptation to decreased blood flow, reaction to oxidative stress, reperfusion injury, and increased cell storage. These changes are reversible if stress is removed early enough.

If the stress is relieved in time, the damage is reversible, and complete structural and functional integrity is restored. For example, when circulation to the heart is interrupted for less than 30 minutes, all structural and functional alterations prove to be reversible. The cell can also be exposed to persistent sublethal stress, as in mechanical irritation of the skin or exposure of the bronchial mucosa to tobacco smoke. Cells have time to adapt to reversible injury in a number of ways, each of which has a morphologic counterpart. On the other hand, if the stress is sufficiently severe, irreversible injury proceeds to cell death. The moment when reversible injury becomes irreversible injury, the "point of no return," is not known at present.

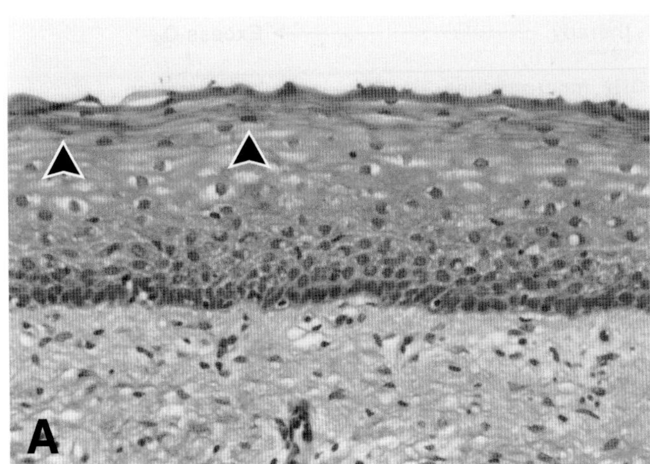

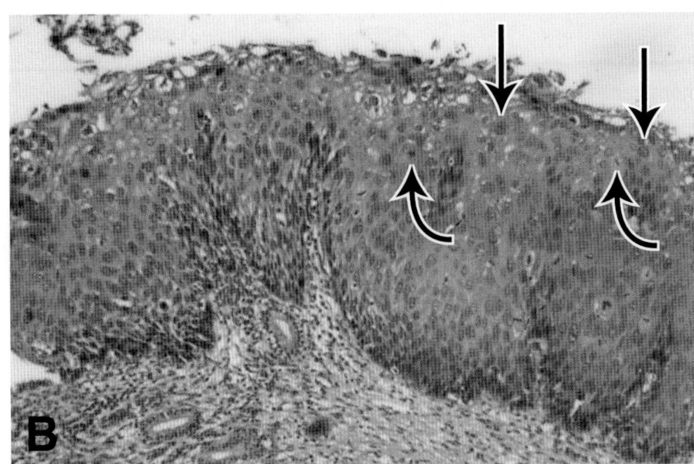

FIGURE 1-6. Dysplasia. A. Nondysplastic cervical epithelium. Normal cervix shows no mitotic activity above the most basal layers, but rather shows epithelial maturation, with flattening of the cells and progressive diminution of nuclei (*arrowheads*). **B.** At the same magnification, dysplastic epithelium of the uterine cervix lacks normal polarity, and individual cells show hyperchromatic nuclei and a greater than normal nucleus-to-cytoplasm ratio. Compare, for example, the size and hyperchromaticity of nuclei in the dysplastic cells (*straight arrows*) with the characteristics of normal counterparts at comparable height in the normal cervix. In contrast to normal cervix, cellular arrangement in dysplastic epithelium is disorderly, largely lacking appropriate histologic maturation, from the basal layers to the surface. Mitotic figures far above the basal layers (*curved arrows*) are common.

Hydropic Swelling

Hydropic swelling is characterized by a large, pale cytoplasm and a normally located nucleus. The greater volume is caused by increased water content and reflects acute, reversible cell injury. It may result from such varied causes as chemical and biologic toxins, viral or bacterial infections, ischemia, excessive heat or cold, and so on (Fig. 1-7).

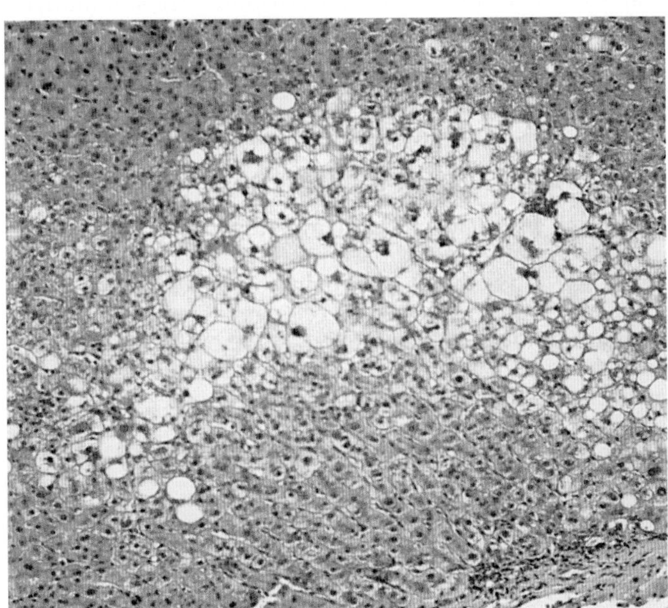

FIGURE 1-7. Hydropic swelling. The liver of a patient with toxic hepatic injury shows severe hydropic swelling in the centrilobular zone. Affected hepatocytes exhibit central nuclei and cytoplasm distended by excess fluid.

Hydropic swelling results from impairment of cellular volume regulation, a process that controls ionic concentrations in the cytoplasm. This regulation, particularly for sodium, involves three components: (1) the plasma membrane, (2) the plasma membrane sodium (Na^+) pump, and (3) adenosine triphosphate (ATP). The plasma membrane prevents two gradient-driven ion flows: the flow of Na^+ from the extracellular fluid into the cell and the flow of K^+ out of the cell. The barrier to sodium is imperfect and its relative leakiness permits some passive entry of sodium into the cell. To compensate for this intrusion, the energy-dependent, plasma membrane sodium pump (Na^+/K^+-ATPase), which is fueled by ATP, extrudes sodium from the cell. Noxious agents may interfere with this membrane-regulated process by (1) increasing plasma membrane permeability to Na^+, thereby exceeding the capacity of the pump to extrude the ion; (2) damaging the pump directly; or (3) interfering with ATP synthesis, and so depriving the pump of its fuel. In any event, accumulation of sodium in the cell leads to increased intracellular water to maintain isosmotic conditions. The cell then swells. The subcellular changes in cell organelles are reflected in functional derangements (e.g., reduced protein synthesis, impaired energy production) (Fig. 1-8). **After withdrawal of the stress that caused the reversible cell injury, by definition, the cell returns to its normal state.**

Ischemic Cell Injury

Ischemia refers to the interruption of blood flow, such as occurs in heart attacks and strokes. Loss of blood flow results in decreased O_2 and key nutrients, such as glucose, and increased CO_2 in cells. When tissues are deprived of oxygen by ischemia, ATP cannot be produced by aerobic metabolism and is instead made inefficiently by anaerobic metabolism. A series of chemical and pH imbalances is initiated, which

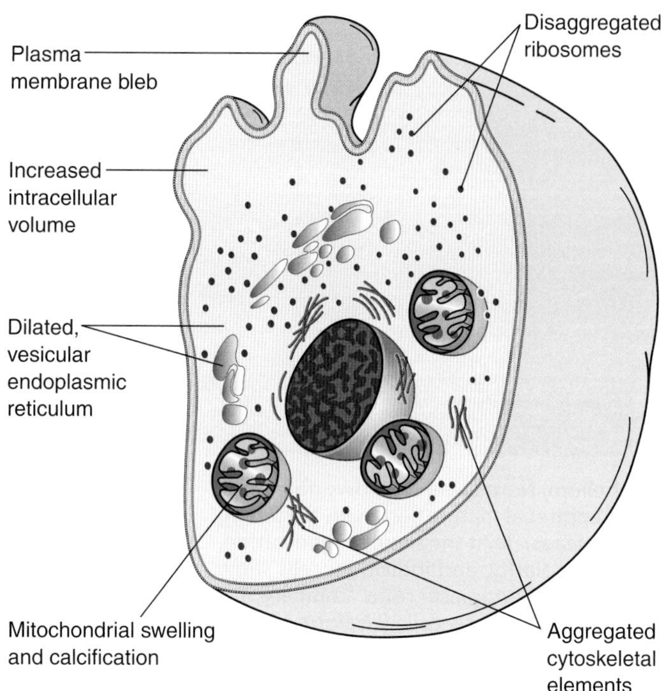

FIGURE 1-8. Ultrastructural features of reversible cell injury.

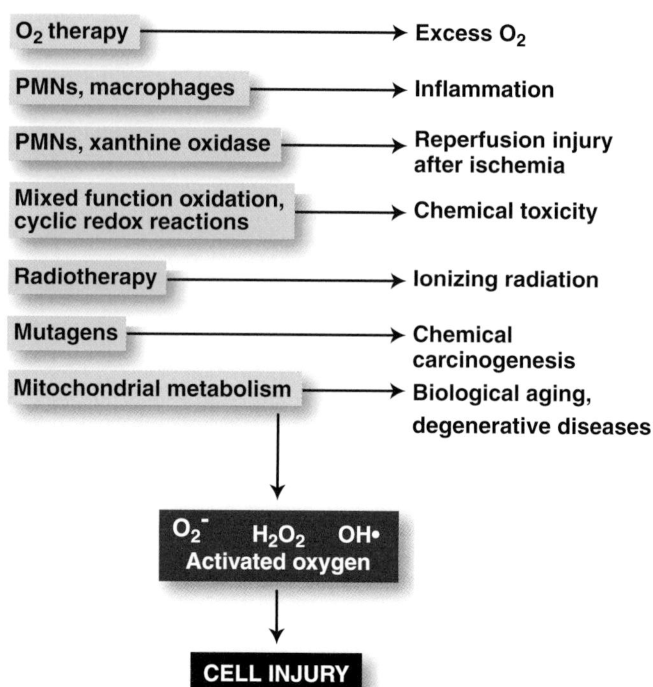

FIGURE 1-9. The role of activated oxygen species in cell injury. H_2O_2, hydrogen peroxide; O_2, oxygen; O_2^-, superoxide; OH•, hydroxyl radical; PMNs, polymorphonuclear neutrophils.

are accompanied by multiple deleterious events, including acidosis, increased generation of reactive oxygen species (ROS) and free radicals, loss of glycogen stores, disruption of intracellular Ca^{2+} homeostasis, increased intracellular Ca^{2+}, mitochondrial injury, and DNA damage. The damage produced by short periods of ischemia tends to be reversible if circulation is restored. However, long periods of ischemia are associated with irreversible cell injury and death, as described below. Tissue damage related to ischemic injury is termed an infarct. Hence, a heart attack is a myocardial infarct (MI).

Oxidative Stress

A major component of ischemic damage and many other modes of cell injury result from the generation of highly reactive chemical compounds, namely, reactive oxygen species (ROS) and free radicals. Such compounds may be generated by intrinsic cellular processes such as "leaks" in mitochondrial electron transport or produced by neutrophils as part of the acute inflammatory response (see Chapter 2). Many exogenous components of the environment also contain reactive oxygen species (ROS). Whatever the source, such agents can react with and damage virtually any molecule within the cell.

Reactive Oxygen Species

Reactive oxygen species (ROS) cause cell and tissue injury in many settings (Fig. 1-9). Oxygen (O_2), as the terminal electron acceptor in mitochondria, is reduced from O_2 to H_2O. The resultant energy is harnessed as an electrochemical potential across the mitochondrial inner membrane.

Conversion of O_2 to H_2O entails transfer of four electrons. Three partially reduced species represent transfers of varying numbers of electrons and are intermediate between O_2 and H_2O (Fig. 1-10). These are O_2^-, superoxide (one electron); H_2O_2, hydrogen peroxide (two electrons); and OH•, the hydroxyl radical (three electrons). Under physiologic conditions, these ROS come from several sources, including leaks in mitochondrial electron transport and mixed-function oxygenases (P450). In addition, physiologic ROS are important cellular signaling intermediates. The major forms of ROS and their attributes are summarized in Table 1-4. Importantly, excessive ROS levels both cause and aggravate many disorders.

Superoxide

The superoxide anion (O_2^-) is produced mainly by leaks in mitochondrial electron transport or as part of inflammatory responses. In phagocytic inflammatory cells, activation of a plasma membrane oxidase produces O_2^-, which is then converted to H_2O_2 and eventually to other ROS (Fig. 1-11). These ROS are key effectors of cellular defenses that destroy pathogens, fragments of necrotic cells, or other phagocytosed material (see Chapter 2). ROS, acting as signaling intermediates, elicit the release of proteolytic and other degradative enzymes, which are critical effectors of neutrophil-mediated destruction of bacteria and other foreign materials.

Hydrogen Peroxide

Superoxide anions are converted by superoxide dismutase (SOD) to H_2O_2. Hydrogen peroxide is also produced directly by a number of oxidases in cytoplasmic peroxisomes (Fig. 1-10). By itself, H_2O_2 is not particularly injurious, and it is largely metabolized to H_2O by catalase. However, when produced in excess, it is converted to highly reactive OH•. In neutrophils, myeloperoxidase transforms H_2O_2

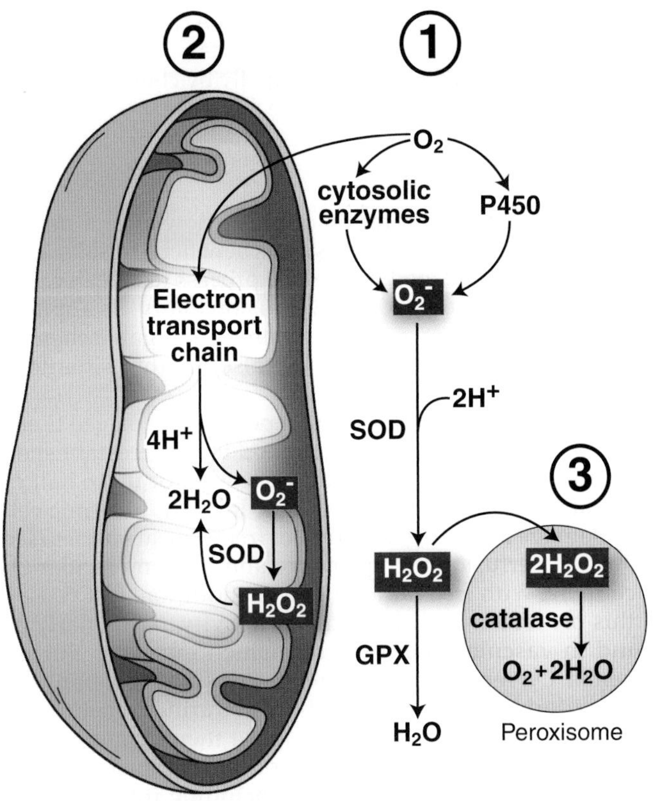

FIGURE 1-10. Mechanisms by which reactive oxygen radicals are generated from molecular oxygen and then detoxified by cellular enzymes. Circulating oxygen delivered to the cell may follow one of three paths: (*1*) Molecular O_2 is converted to O_2^- in the cytosol. O_2^- is reduced to H_2O_2 by cytosolic SOD (Cu/Zn SOD), and finally to water. (*2*) O_2 enters the mitochondria, where inefficiencies in electron transport result in conversion of O_2 to O_2^-. This superoxide is rendered less reactive by further reduction to H_2O_2, via mitochondrial SOD (MnSOD). This H_2O_2 is then converted to H_2O by GPX. (*3*) Cytosolic H_2O_2 enters peroxisomes where it is detoxified to H_2O by catalase. CoQ, coenzyme Q; GPX, glutathione peroxidase; H^+, hydrogen ion; H_2O, water; H_2O_2, hydrogen peroxide; O_2, oxygen; O_2^-, superoxide; SOD, superoxide dismutase.

to a potent radical, hypochlorite (OCl^-), which is lethal for microorganisms. Moreover, if released extracellularly, OCl^- can kill cells.

Most cells have efficient mechanisms for removing H_2O_2. Two different enzymes reduce H_2O_2 to water: (1) catalase within peroxisomes and (2) glutathione peroxidase (GPX) in both the cytosol and mitochondria (Fig. 1-10). GPX uses reduced glutathione (GSH) as a cofactor in a reaction yielding oxidized glutathione (GSSG). Because it is membrane permeable, H_2O_2 generated in mitochondria affects the oxidant balance, not only in mitochondria but also in other cellular compartments.

Hydroxyl Radical

Hydroxyl radicals (OH•) are formed by (1) radiolysis of water, (2) reaction of H_2O_2 with ferrous iron (Fe^{2+}) or cuprous copper (Cu^{1+}) (Fenton reaction), and (3) reaction of O_2^- with H_2O_2 (Haber–Weiss reaction). **The hydroxyl radical, the most reactive of all ROS, can damage macromolecules by several mechanisms**. By virtue of the Fenton reaction, iron is often an active participant in oxidative damage to cells. In a number of different cell types, H_2O_2 stimulates iron uptake and so increases production of hydroxyl radicals. Figure 1-12 summarizes the mechanisms of cell injury by ROS.

Table 1-4

Reactive Oxygen Species

Molecule	Attributes
Hydrogen peroxide (H_2O_2)	Forms free radicals via Fe^{2+}-catalyzed Fenton reaction Diffuses widely within the cell
Superoxide anion (O_2^-)	Generated by leaks in the electron transport chain and some cytosolic reactions Produces other ROS Does not readily diffuse far from its origin
Hydroxyl radical (OH•)	Generated from H_2O_2 by Fe^{2+}-catalyzed Fenton reaction The intracellular radical most responsible for attack on macromolecules
Peroxynitrite (ONOO•)	Formed from the reaction of nitric oxide (NO) with O_2^- Damages macromolecules
Lipid peroxide radicals (RCOO•)	Organic radicals produced during lipid peroxidation
Hypochlorous acid (HOCl)	Produced by macrophages and-neutrophils during respiratory burst that accompanies phagocytosis Dissociates to yield hypochlorite-radical (OCl^-)

Fe^{2+}, ferrous iron; ROS, reactive oxygen species.

Nitric Oxide and Peroxynitrite

Nitric oxide (NO) is a reactive nitrogen molecule that is found in many cells and has a half-life measured in seconds. It is the product of nitric oxide synthase (NOS), a ubiquitous enzyme that comes in two forms: inducible NOS (iNOS) and constitutive NOS, which are found in several tissues. NO has diverse signaling properties and may be harmful or protective to cells, depending on the circumstances. As a free radical, NOF096 reacts with many molecular targets and activates or inhibits numerous cell functions. Additionally, when NO reacts with oxygen, it forms the highly destructive peroxynitrite ion ($ONOO^-$).

Antioxidant Defenses

Cells possess potent antioxidant defenses, including detoxifying enzymes and exogenous free-radical scavengers (e.g., vitamins). The major enzymes that convert ROS to less reactive molecules are superoxide dismutase (SOD), catalase, and GPX.

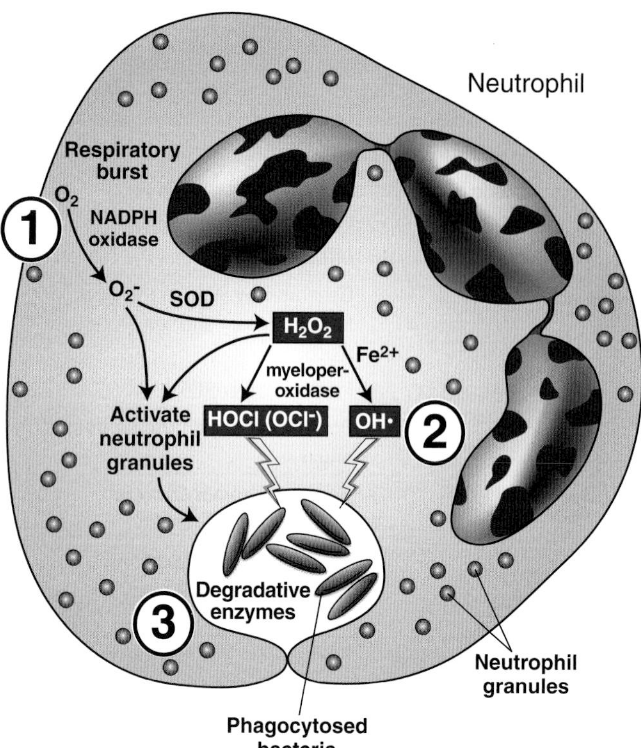

FIGURE 1-11. Generation of reactive oxygen species (ROS) in neutrophils as a result of phagocytosis of bacteria. (*1*) The respiratory burst in neutrophils begins with reduction of O_2 to O_2^- by NADPH oxidase. In turn, O_2^- is converted to H_2O_2 by SOD. (*2*) ROS (HOCl, OH•) are produced from H_2O_2 by myeloperoxidase. Concurrently, O_2^- and H_2O_2 activate neutrophil granules to release degradative enzymes. (*3*) Bacteria are engulfed by neutrophils, where they are destroyed by ROS and degradative enzymes. Fe^{2+}, ferrous iron; H_2O_2, hydrogen peroxide; HOCl, hypochlorous acid; NADPH, reduced nicotinamide adenine dinucleotide phosphate; OCl^-, hypochlorite radical; OH•, hydroxyl radical; SOD, superoxide dismutase.

Detoxifying Enzymes

- **SOD** is the first line of defense against O_2^-, converting it to H_2O_2 ($O_2^- + 2H^+ \rightarrow H_2O_2$).
- **Catalase**, mainly located in peroxisomes, is one of two enzymes that complete the detoxification of O_2^- by converting H_2O_2 to water, thereby, preventing its conversion to OH• ($2H_2O_2 \rightarrow 2H_2O + O_2$).
- **GPX** catalyzes the reduction of H_2O_2 and lipid peroxides in mitochondria and the cytosol ($H_2O_2 + 2GSH \rightarrow 2H_2O + GSSG$).

Scavengers of ROS

- **Vitamin E (α-tocopherol)** is a terminal electron acceptor that aborts free-radical chain reactions. As it is fat soluble, α-tocopherol protects membranes from lipid peroxidation.
- **Vitamin C (ascorbate)** is water soluble and reacts directly with O_2 and OH•, and some products of lipid peroxidation. It also serves to regenerate the reduced form of vitamin E.
- **Retinoids**, the precursors of vitamin A, are lipid soluble and act as chain-breaking antioxidants.
- **NO•** may scavenge ROS, principally by chelation of iron and combination with other free radicals.

Reperfusion Injury

Reperfusion is the restoration of blood flow after a period of ischemia. Although reperfusion is beneficial in salvaging cells that have remained viable, the process itself can cause damage, to which the term "reperfusion injury" is applied. Such harm occurs most often in settings of organ ischemia, such as myocardial infarction, but also in other situations (e.g., organ transplantation).

Reperfusion injury reflects the exposure of damaged tissue to the oxygen that arrives when blood flow is reestablished (reperfusion). In the heart, it may account for up to half of the final size of myocardial infarcts. Initially, ischemic cellular damage leads to generation of free-radical species (see above). Reperfusion then provides abundant molecular O_2 to combine with free radicals to form additional ROS. Key to this process is xanthine oxidase activity, particularly as found in vascular endothelium, which increases during ischemia. On reperfusion, oxygen returns and the abundant purines derived from ATP catabolism during ischemia become substrates for xanthine oxidase thereby generating a sudden rise in ROS. The evolution of reperfusion injury also involves many other factors, including inflammatory mediators, platelet-activating factor (PAF), NOS and NO•, intercellular adhesion molecules, dysregulation of Ca^{2+} homeostasis, and many more.

Intracellular Storage

The accumulation of normal or abnormal substances within a cell may be a sign of cellular stress or injury, whether the accumulated substances are innocuous or harmful. This material within the cell may be from either endogenous or exogenous sources (Fig. 1-13).

Fat

Abnormal accumulation of fat is most conspicuous in the liver (see Chapter 12). Briefly, hepatocytes always contain some fat, because they take up free fatty acids released from adipose tissue and convert them to triglycerides. Most such newly synthesized triglycerides are secreted by the liver as lipoproteins. If delivery of free fatty acids to the liver increases, as in diabetes, or intrahepatic lipid metabolism is disturbed, as in alcoholism, triglycerides accumulate in liver cells. Fatty liver is visualized as lipid globules in the cytoplasm (Fig. 1-13B). Other organs, including the heart, kidney, and skeletal muscle, also store fat. **Fat storage is always reversible, and there is no evidence that excess fat in the cytoplasm *per se* interferes with cell function.**

Glycogen

Glycogen is degraded in steps by a series of enzymes, any of which may be deficient because of an inborn error of metabolism. Regardless of the specific enzyme deficiency, the result is a glycogen storage disease (see Chapter 5). These inherited disorders affect the liver, heart, and skeletal muscle,

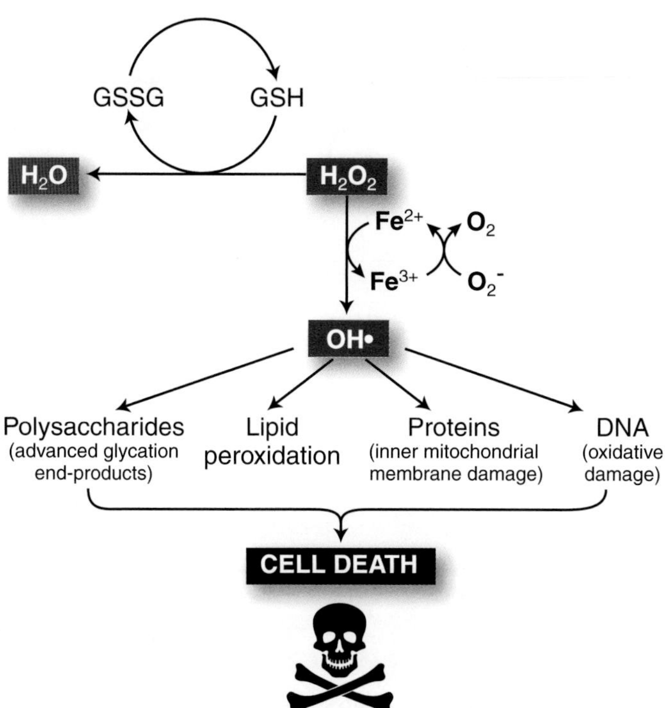

FIGURE 1-12. Mechanisms of cell injury by activated oxygen species. Fe^{2+}, ferrous iron; Fe^{3+}, ferric iron; GSH, glutathione; GSSG, oxidized glutathione; H_2O_2, hydrogen peroxide; O_2, oxygen; O_2^-, superoxide anion; OH•, hydroxyl radical.

and range from mild and asymptomatic conditions to those that are inexorably progressive and fatal.

Inherited Lysosomal Storage Diseases

As with glycogen, catabolism of certain complex lipids and mucopolysaccharides (glycosaminoglycans) takes place by a sequence of enzymatic steps. Since these enzymes are located in the lysosomes, their absence results in lysosomal storage of incompletely degraded lipids, such as cerebrosides (Gaucher disease) and gangliosides (Tay–Sachs disease) or products of mucopolysaccharide catabolism (Hurler and Hunter syndromes). (See Chapter 5 for the metabolic bases of these disorders and those chapters on specific organ systems affected.)

Cholesterol

Cholesterol is a critical component of all plasma membranes. When stored in excess, it is closely associated with atherosclerosis and cardiovascular disease, which is the leading cause of death in the Western world (see Chapter 8) (Fig. 1-13A).

In some disorders characterized by elevated blood levels of cholesterol (e.g., familial hypercholesterolemia), macrophages store cholesterol. If clusters of these cells in subcutaneous tissues are grossly visible, they are called **xanthomas**.

Lipofuscin

Lipofuscin is a mixture of lipids and proteins that appears as a golden-brown pigment and has been termed "wear and tear" pigment. It tends to accumulate by accretion of peroxidized unsaturated lipids and oxidized, cross-linked proteins. Lipofuscin appears mainly in postmitotic cells (e.g., neurons, cardiac myocytes) or in cells that cycle infrequently (e.g., hepatocytes) and increases with age. It is often more conspicuous in conditions associated with atrophy of an organ (Fig. 1-13C).

Melanin

Melanin is an insoluble, brown-black pigment found principally in epidermal cells of the skin, but also in the eye and other organs (Fig. 1-13D). It is located in intracellular organelles known as **melanosomes** and results from polymerization of certain oxidation products of tyrosine. The amount of melanin is responsible for the differences in skin color among the various races, as well as the color of the eyes. It serves a protective function owing to its ability to absorb ultraviolet light. In white persons, exposure to sunlight increases melanin formation (tanning) as protection against the damaging effects of solar radiation. The hereditary inability to produce melanin is known as **albinism**. The presence of melanin is also a marker of cancers that arise from melanocytes (**melanoma**). Melanin is discussed in detail in Chapter 20.

Exogenous Pigments

Anthracosis refers to storage of carbon particles in the lung and regional lymph nodes (Fig. 1-13E). Virtually, all urban dwellers inhale particulates of organic carbon generated by the burning of fossil fuels. This material accumulates in alveolar macrophages and is also transported to hilar and mediastinal lymph nodes, where the indigestible material is stored indefinitely within macrophages. Although the gross appearance of the lungs of persons with anthracosis may be alarming, the condition is innocuous.

Tattoos refers to the introduction of insoluble metallic and vegetable pigments into the skin, where they are principally engulfed by dermal macrophages and persist for a lifetime.

Iron and Other Metals

Iron

About 25% of the body's total iron content is in an intracellular storage pool composed of the iron-storage proteins **ferritin** and **hemosiderin**. The liver and bone marrow are particularly rich in ferritin, although it is present in virtually all cells. Hemosiderin is a partially denatured form of ferritin that aggregates easily and is recognized microscopically as yellow-brown granules in the cytoplasm. Normally, hemosiderin is found mainly in the spleen, bone marrow, and liver.

Total body iron may be increased by enhanced intestinal iron absorption, as in some anemias, or by repeated blood transfusions, which deliver iron-containing erythrocytes. Increasing the body's total iron content leads to progressive accumulation of hemosiderin, which is called **hemosiderosis**. In this case, iron is present throughout the body, including the skin, pancreas, heart, kidneys, liver, and endocrine organs. However, intracellular accumulation of iron in hemosiderosis does not injure cells.

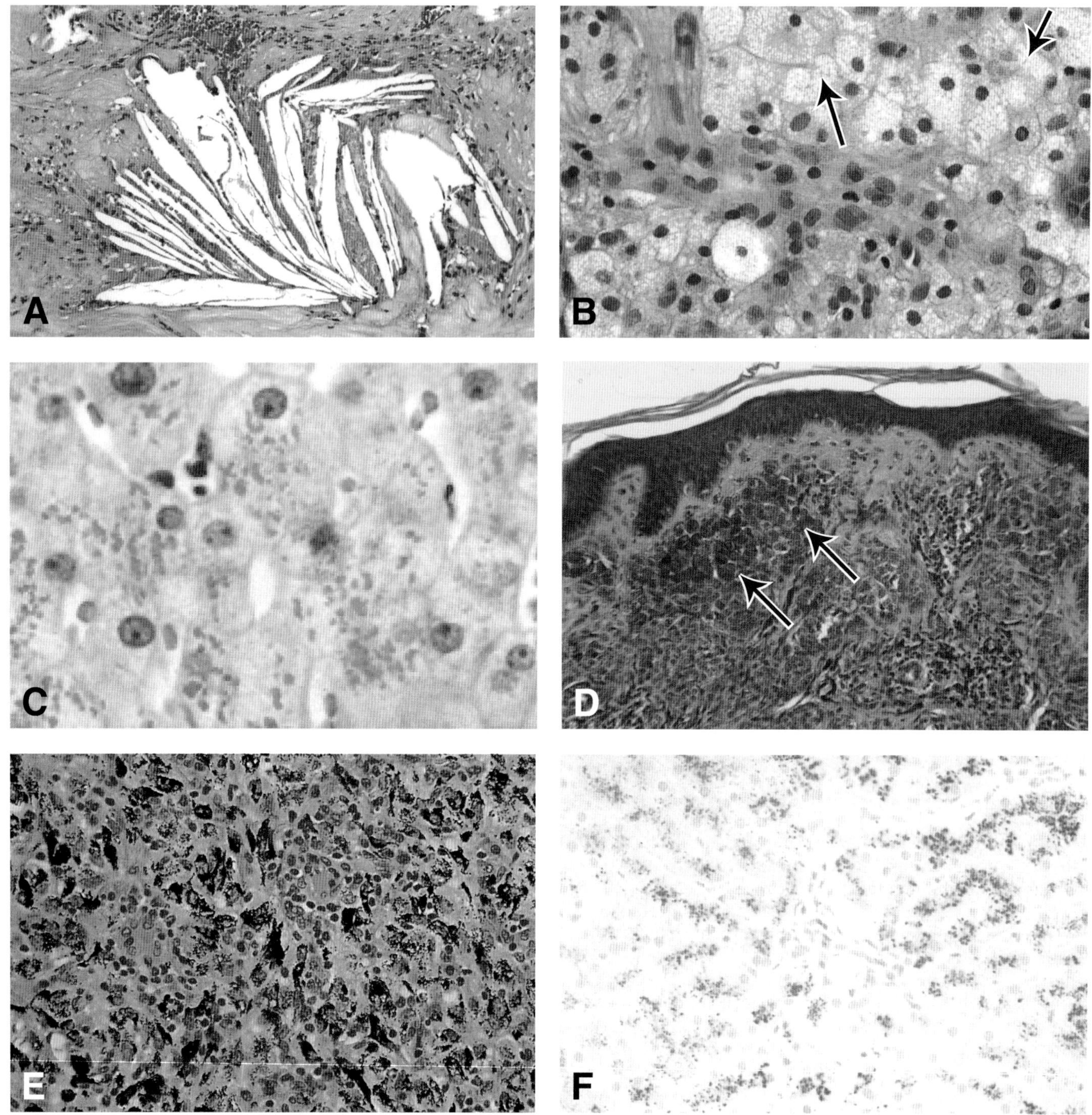

FIGURE 1-13. Abnormal intracellular storage. A. Abnormal cholesterol accumulation is characterized by transparent clefts, shown here in an atherosclerotic plaque. **B.** Lipid is stored in macrophages (*arrows*) in a cutaneous xanthoma. **C.** Lipofuscin in the liver from an 80-year-old man appears as golden cytoplasmic granules in lysosomes. **D.** Melanin (*arrows*) is stored in the cells of an intradermal nevus. **E.** Carbon pigment storage. A mediastinal lymph node, which drains the lungs, exhibits numerous macrophages that contain black anthracotic (carbon) pigment. This material was inhaled and originally deposited in the lungs. **F.** Iron storage in hereditary hemochromatosis. Prussian blue stain of the liver reveals large deposits of iron within hepatocellular lysosomes.

If, contrariwise, the increase in total body iron is extreme, it damages vital organs including the liver, heart, testes, and pancreas. Iron overload can result from a genetic abnormality in iron absorption, namely, **hereditary hemochromatosis (HH)** (see Chapter 12; Fig. 1-13F). Tissue injury in HH most likely reflects iron-generated oxidative stress, as described above.

Other Metals

Excess accumulation of lead, particularly in children, causes mental retardation and anemia. The storage of other metals also presents dangers. In Wilson disease (see Chapter 12), a hereditary disorder of copper metabolism, storage of excess copper in the liver and brain results into severe chronic disease of those organs.

Retention of Calcium

Calcium enters dead or dying cells because they cannot maintain a steep calcium gradient (see below). This cellular calcification is not ordinarily visible except by electron microscopy as inclusions within mitochondria.

In "dystrophic" calcification, macroscopic calcium salt deposits occur in injured tissues. This process does not simply represent accumulation of calcium derived from the bodies of dead cells but is rather caused by extracellular deposition of calcium from the circulation or interstitial fluid. Dystrophic calcification is often visible to the naked eye and ranges from gritty, sand-like grains to firm, rock-hard material. Often, calcification has no functional consequences. However, dystrophic calcification that occurs in crucial locations (e.g., such as the mitral or aortic valves) gives rise to obstruction of blood flow by making valve leaflets rigid and narrowing valve orifices (mitral and aortic stenosis). Dystrophic calcification in atherosclerotic coronary arteries contributes to narrowing of those vessels.

Unlike dystrophic calcification, which has its origin in cell injury, "metastatic" calcification reflects deranged calcium metabolism and is associated with increased serum calcium concentrations **(hypercalcemia)**. In general, almost any disorder that increases blood calcium levels can lead to calcification in inappropriate locations, such as pulmonary alveolar septa, renal tubules, and blood vessels. Metastatic calcification is seen in various disorders, including chronic renal failure, vitamin D intoxication, and hyperparathyroidism.

CELL DEATH

Cell death may be the result of environmental stress or may be preprogrammed and necessary for the development and survival of the organism. In some cases, cell death represents the consequences of unregulated injury and is termed *necrosis*, but in other instances, complex intracellular molecular pathways respond to external and internal triggers to cause the cell's demise. *Apoptosis* is the best-characterized example. Programmed cell death manages the size and diversity of many tissue compartments by eliminating obsolescent cells, as in the gastrointestinal tract, skin, and hematopoietic system. Not all such mechanisms eliminate only older, senescent cells; in some cases, cells such as autoreactive lymphocyte clones or those with irreparable DNA lesions may be targeted for destruction.

Historically, cell death was referred to as necrosis, but now apoptosis and autophagy are also well-characterized mechanisms. These processes had formerly been viewed as separate, nonintersecting roads. Necrosis was defined as an accidental form of cell death caused by a hostile environment to which a cell could not adapt effectively; it was seen as a passive process. By contrast, apoptosis is a form of cellular suicide in which the cell participates actively in its own demise. It is a mechanism by which individual cells activate their own signaling systems to sacrifice themselves for the preservation of the organism. Because the principal pathways of cell death may overlap, it is important to understand how the processes manifest morphologically.

In addition to apoptosis, diverse suicide programs have been identified: autophagic cell death, necroptosis, NETosis, and so forth. For example, autophagy is also an active signaling process that is elicited when a stressful environment requires autodigestion of a portion of the cell's macromolecular constituents. To further complicate matters, many of these programmed pathways interrelate extensively so that clear-cut distinctions are not always possible.

Necrosis

Necrosis occurs when hostile external forces overwhelm the cell's adaptive abilities. Diverse insults can cause necrotic cell death, which typically affects geographically localized groups of cells. The response to this process is usually acute inflammation, which itself may generate further cell injury (see Chapter 2). The stimuli that initiate pathways leading to necrosis are highly variable and produce diverse and recognizable histologic and cytologic patterns.

Coagulative Necrosis

Coagulative necrosis refers to specific light microscopic appearances of dead or dying cells (Fig. 1-14). Shortly after a cell's death, its outline is maintained. When stained with the usual combination of hematoxylin and eosin, the cytoplasm of a necrotic cell is more deeply eosinophilic (red) than usual. Nuclear chromatin (blue) is initially clumped and then redistributes along the nuclear membrane. Three morphologic changes are as follows:

- **Pyknosis:** The nucleus becomes smaller and stains deeply basophilic as chromatin clumping continues.
- **Karyorrhexis:** The pyknotic nucleus breaks up into many smaller fragments scattered about the cytoplasm.
- **Karyolysis:** The pyknotic nucleus may be extruded from the cell or it may progressively lose chromatin staining.

Early ultrastructural changes in a dying or dead cell reflect an extension of alterations associated with reversible cell injury. In addition to the nuclear changes described above, the dead cell features dilated endoplasmic reticulum, disaggregated ribosomes, swollen and calcified mitochondria, aggregated cytoskeletal elements, and plasma membrane blebs.

After a variable time, depending on the tissue and circumstances, the lytic activity of intracellular and extracellular enzymes causes the cell to disintegrate. This is particularly the case when necrotic cells have elicited an acute inflammatory response.

The appearance of necrotic tissue has traditionally been described as **coagulative necrosis** because it resembles the coagulation of proteins that occurs upon heating. This term, although based on obsolete concepts, remains useful as a morphologic descriptor.

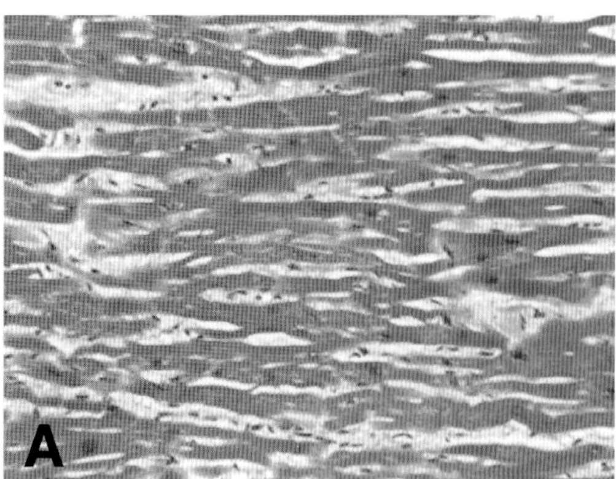

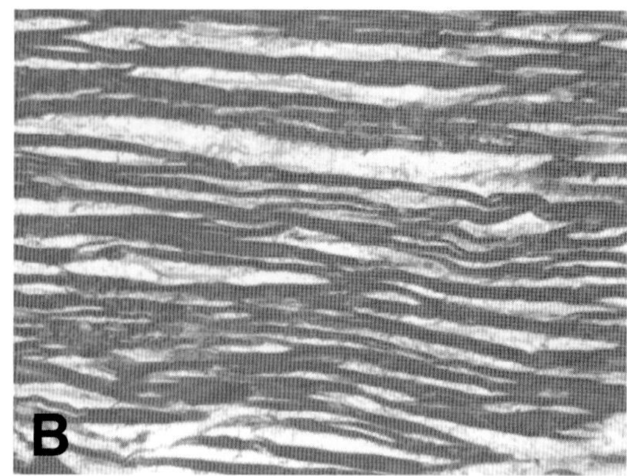

FIGURE 1-14. Coagulative necrosis. A. Normal heart. All myocytes are nucleated, and striations are clear. **B.** Myocardial infarction. The heart from a patient following acute myocardial infarction. The necrotic cells are deeply eosinophilic and most have lost their nuclei.

Liquefactive Necrosis

When the rate at which necrotic cells dissolve greatly exceeds the rate of repair, the resulting appearance is termed **liquefactive necrosis** (Fig. 1-15). Polymorphonuclear leukocytes of the acute inflammatory reaction contain potent hydrolases capable of digesting dead cells. A sharply localized collection of these acute inflammatory cells, generally in response to bacterial infection, produces rapid cell death and tissue dissolution. The result is often an **abscess**, a cavity formed by liquefactive necrosis in a solid tissue. In time, the abscess is walled off by a fibrous capsule that contains its contents.

Coagulative necrosis of the brain may occur after cerebral artery occlusion and is often followed by rapid dissolution—liquefactive necrosis—of the dead tissue by a mechanism that cannot be attributed to the action of an acute inflammatory response. It is not clear why coagulative necrosis in the brain and not elsewhere is followed by the disappearance of necrotic cells, but the abundant lysosomal enzymes, or different hydrolases specific to cells of the central nervous system (CNS), may be responsible. Liquefactive necrosis of large areas of the CNS can lead to a cavity or cyst that persists for life of the person.

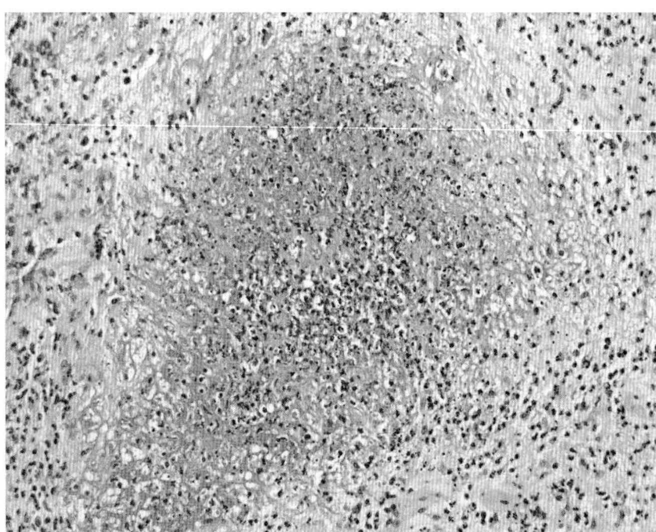

FIGURE 1-15. Liquefactive necrosis in an abscess of the skin. The abscess cavity is filled with polymorphonuclear leukocytes.

Fat Necrosis

Fat necrosis specifically affects adipose tissue and most commonly results from pancreatitis or trauma. The unique feature determining this type of necrosis is the presence of triglycerides in adipose tissue. In the peripancreatic fat, for example, the process begins when digestive enzymes that are normally found only in the pancreatic duct and small intestine lumen are released from injured pancreatic acinar cells and ducts into extracellular spaces. On extracellular activation, these enzymes digest both the pancreas itself and surrounding tissues, including adipocytes (Fig 1-16).

1. Phospholipases and proteases attack plasma membranes of adipocytes, releasing their stored triglycerides.
2. Pancreatic lipase hydrolyzes the triglycerides, an effect that produces free fatty acids.
3. Free fatty acids bind Ca^{2+} and precipitate as soaps. These appear as amorphous, basophilic deposits at the edges of irregular islands of necrotic adipocytes.

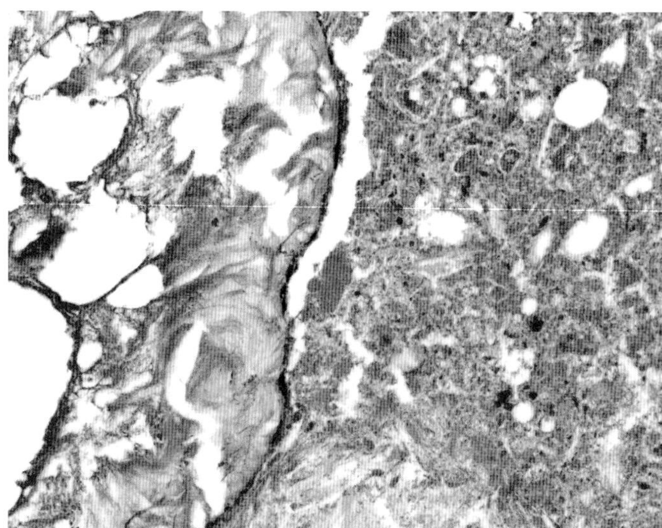

FIGURE 1-16. Fat necrosis. Peripancreatic adipose tissue from a patient with acute pancreatitis shows fatty acids precipitated as calcium soaps, which appear as amorphous, basophilic deposits (*left*). These appear at the periphery of the irregular island of necrotic adipocytes (*right*).

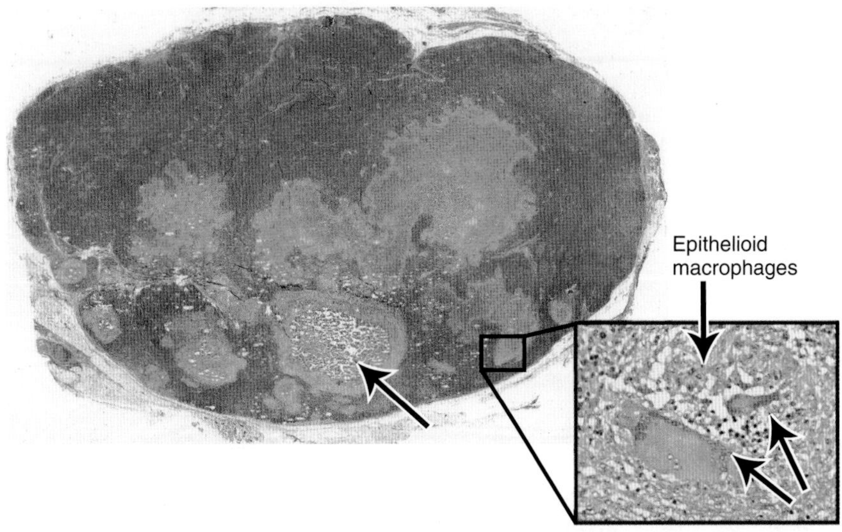

FIGURE 1-17. Caseous necrosis in a tuberculous lymph node. Hilar lymph node from a patient with active tuberculosis. Irregular pink areas of caseous necrosis (*arrow*) are evident against a background of lymphocytes. (*Inset*) Granulomas on the periphery of necrotic areas show epithelioid macrophages and multinucleated giant (Langhans) cells (*arrows*).

Grossly, fat necrosis appears as an irregular, chalky white area embedded in otherwise normal adipose tissue. In the case of traumatic fat necrosis, triglycerides and lipases are released from the injured adipocytes. In the breast, fat necrosis due to trauma is common and may mimic a tumor, particularly if calcification has occurred.

Caseous Necrosis

Caseous necrosis is characteristic of tuberculosis and is seen, less often, in other settings as well. The lesions of tuberculosis are granulomas, or tubercles. In the center of such granulomas, the accumulated mononuclear cells that mediate a chronic inflammatory reaction to the offending mycobacteria are killed. Unlike coagulative necrosis, the necrotic cells in granulomas lose their cellular outlines. They do not disappear by lysis, however, as in liquefactive necrosis. Rather, the dead cells persist indefinitely as amorphous, coarsely granular, eosinophilic debris. Grossly, this material is grayish white, soft, and friable. It resembles clumpy cheese, hence the name **caseous necrosis** (Fig. 1-17). This distinctive type of necrosis is generally attributed to the toxic effects of mycobacterial cell walls, which contain complex waxes (peptidoglycolipids) that exert potent biologic effects.

Fibrinoid Necrosis

Fibrinoid necrosis is an alteration of injured blood vessels, in which insudation and accumulation of plasma proteins cause the wall to stain intensely with eosin. The term is a misnomer; however, as the eosinophilia of the accumulated plasma proteins obscures the underlying alterations in the blood vessel, making it difficult, if not impossible, to determine whether there truly is necrosis in the vascular wall (Fig. 1-18).

Ischemic Cell Death

Myocardial infarcts and stroke together represent the most common cause of mortality in the Western world and are both due to ischemic cell death. Selective ion permeability of the cell membrane maintains intracellular concentrations of Na^+ and Ca^{2+} orders of magnitude less than extracellular levels. The opposite holds for K^+. Whatever the lethal insult, cell necrosis is heralded by loss of the plasma membrane's permeability barrier function. If ischemia is incomplete or if the episode of ischemia is brief, normal ionic equilibrium can be reestablished without tissue damage. However, if ionic balance cannot be restored, the resulting disturbance is thought to represent the "point of no return" for the injured cell. Thus, ischemic cell injury and death share the same pathophysiologic spectrum. Many crucial cell functions are exquisitely regulated by minute fluctuations in cytosolic-free calcium concentration ($[Ca^{2+}]_i$). **In this way, massive influx of Ca^{2+} through a damaged plasma membrane is the key to ischemic cell damage** and may ensure

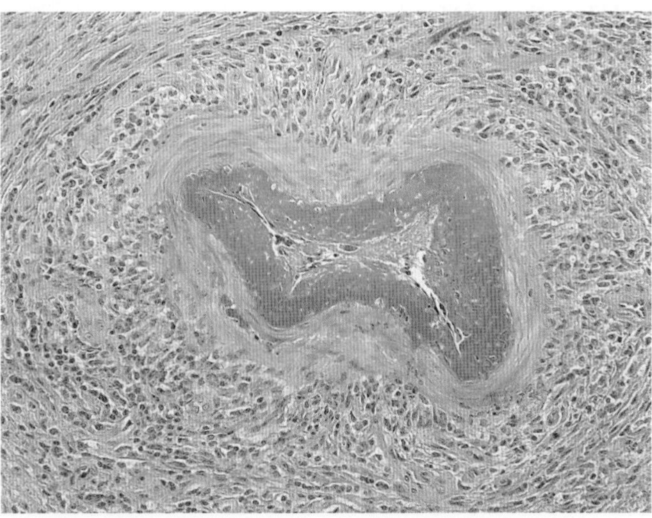

FIGURE 1-18. Fibrinoid necrosis. An inflamed muscular artery in a patient with systemic arteritis shows a sharply demarcated, homogeneous, deeply eosinophilic zone of necrosis.

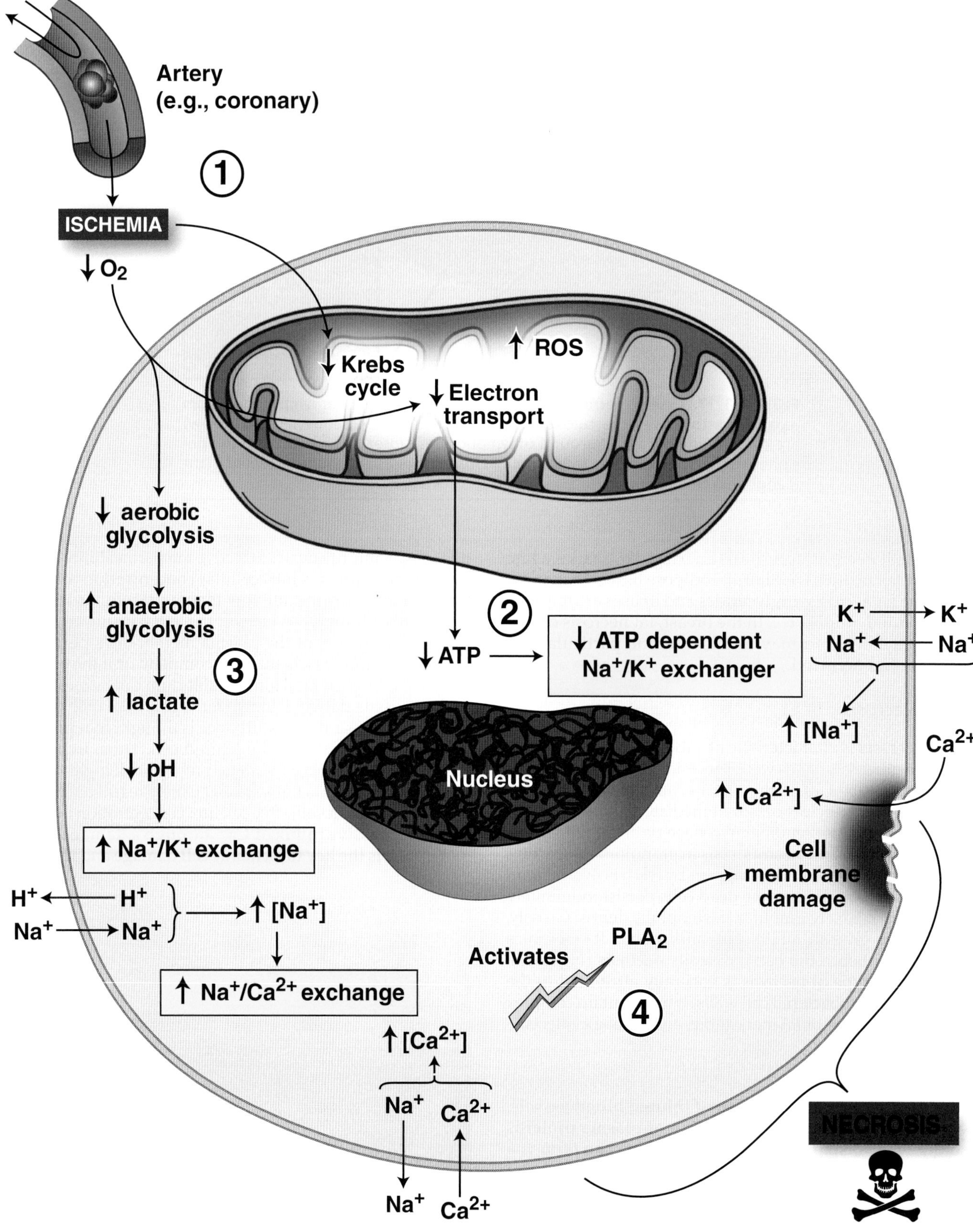

FIGURE 1-19. Mechanisms by which ischemia leads to cellular death by necrosis. (*1*) Loss of oxygen due to vascular occlusion impairs mitochondrial function, resulting in decreased energy (adenosine triphosphate [ATP]) production by aerobic processes. (*2*) Decreased ATP impairs ATP-dependent ion exchangers. (*3*) The loss of aerobic processes causes anaerobic glycolysis to predominate, with consequent intracellular acidosis, eventually leading to increased cytosolic (Ca^{2+}). (*4*) Ca^{2+}-dependent phospholipases are then activated, causing loss of cell membrane integrity and necrosis. PLA_2, phospholipase A_2; ROS, reactive oxygen specie.

loss of viability. The major events by which ischemia leads to cell death are summarized below (Fig. 1-19). Some of these events may occur simultaneously; others may be sequential.

1. **Interruption of blood supply decreases delivery of O_2 and glucose.** For most cells, but especially for cardiac myocytes and neurons, which do not store much energy, this combined insult is formidable.
2. **Distortion of the activities of pumps in the plasma membrane skews the ionic balance of the cell.** Na^+ accumulates because lack of ATP impairs the Na^+/K^+ ion exchanger. This effect leads to activation of the Na^+/H^+ ion exchanger. This pump is normally quiescent, but when intracellular acidosis threatens, it pumps H^+ out of the cell in exchange for Na^+ to maintain proper intracellular pH. The resulting increase in intracellular sodium activates the Na^+/Ca^{2+} ion exchanger, which increases calcium entry. Ordinarily, excess intracellular Ca^{2+} is extruded by an ATP-dependent calcium pump. However, with ATP in very short supply, Ca^{2+} accumulates in the cell.
3. **Anaerobic glycolysis leads to overproduction of lactate and decreased intracellular pH.** The lack of O_2 during myocardial ischemia blocks ATP production and inhibits mitochondrial oxidation of pyruvate. Instead of entering the citric acid cycle, pyruvate is reduced to lactate in the cytosol, a process called anaerobic glycolysis. Lactate accumulation lowers cytosolic pH (acidification), thereby initiating a spiral of events that propels the cell downward toward disaster.
4. **Activation of phospholipase A_2 (PLA_2) and proteases disrupts the plasma membrane and cytoskeleton.** Elevated $[Ca^{2+}]_i$ in an ischemic cell activates PLA_2, accelerating degradation of membrane phospholipids and consequent release of free fatty acids and lysophospholipids. The latter act as detergents that solubilize cell membranes. Both fatty acids and lysophospholipids are also potent mediators of inflammation (see Chapter 2), effects that may further disrupt the integrity of the already compromised cell.
5. **Calcium also activates a series of proteases that attack the cytoskeleton and its attachments to the cell membrane.** As cohesion between cytoskeletal proteins and the plasma membrane is disrupted, membrane blebs form and cause the cell's shape to change. The combination of electrolyte imbalance and increased cell membrane permeability induces the cell swelling, often a morphologic prelude to its dissolution.
6. **Lack of O_2 impairs mitochondrial electron transport, thereby decreasing ATP synthesis and facilitating production of ROS.** Normally, 1% to 3% of O_2 entering mitochondria is converted to ROS because of inefficiencies in the electron transport chain. During ischemia, generation of ROS increases because of damage to ROS detoxification mechanisms and impaired processing of reactive oxygen intermediates. Oxidative damage inhibits the function of the electron transport chain and decreases its ability to produce ATP.
7. **Mitochondrial damage promotes release of cytochrome c (Cyt c) to the cytosol.** Resulting loss of Cyt c from the electron transport chain further diminishes ATP synthesis and may also trigger apoptotic cell death (see below).
8. **The cell dies.** When a cell can no longer maintain itself as a metabolic unit, it dies. The line between reversible and irreversible cell injury (i.e., the "point of no return") is not precisely defined.

PROGRAMMED CELL DEATH

Programmed cell death (PCD) refers to processes that are lethal to individual cells and are regulated by preexisting signaling pathways within those cells. When first observed, PCD was thought to represent a passive form of cell death. However, we now recognize various forms of PCD that entail activation of cellular signaling cascades.

Apoptosis

Morphology of Apoptosis

Apoptosis is a pattern of cell death that is triggered by a variety of extracellular and intracellular stimuli and is carried to its conclusion by organized cellular signaling cascades. Apoptotic cells are recognized by nuclear fragmentation and pyknosis, generally against a background of viable cells. Importantly, apoptosis occurs in single cells or small groups of cells, whereas necrosis characteristically involves larger geographic areas of cell death. Histologic features of apoptotic cells include (1) nuclear condensation and fragmentation, (2) segregation of cytoplasmic organelles into distinct regions, (3) blebs of the plasma membrane, and (4) membrane-bound cellular fragments, which often lack nuclei (Fig. 1-20).

Removal of Apoptotic Cells

Once apoptosis has led a cell to DNA fragmentation and cytoskeletal dissolution, the final phase, the ***apoptotic body***, remains. Apoptotic bodies are phagocytosed by tissue macrophages.

Phosphatidylserine (PS), a phospholipid that is normally on the interior aspect of the cell membrane, is externalized in cells undergoing apoptosis. PS is recognized by macrophages and activates ingestion of an apoptotic cell's remains without release of intracellular constituents, thus avoiding an inflammatory reaction (Fig. 1-21). Mononuclear phagocytes ingest the debris from apoptotic cells, but recruitment of neutrophils or lymphocytes is rare. This situation is unlike that of cells that undergo necrotic cell death, which tends to elicit acute inflammatory responses (see Chapter 2).

Caspase Cascade Mechanism for Apoptosis

Apoptosis is a highly conserved cell death process that depends on a family of cysteine proteases (caspases) as crucial signaling intermediates and as executioners.

Apoptosis in Development and Physiology

Apoptosis plays a critical role in development by effecting the alteration and regression of structures during embryogenesis. For example, apoptosis mediates the disappearance of interdigital tissues to yield discrete fingers and toes, converts solid primordia to hollow tubes (e.g., gastrointestinal tract), produces the four-chamber heart, and mediates other body-sculpting activities. Lymphocyte clones that recognize self-antigens are deleted by apoptosis, thereby avoiding potentially dangerous autoimmune disease. Physiologic apoptosis principally affects progeny of stem cells that are constantly dividing (e.g., stem cells of the hematopoietic system, gastrointestinal mucosa and epidermis). Apoptosis of mature cells in these organs prevents overpopulation of the respective cell compartments

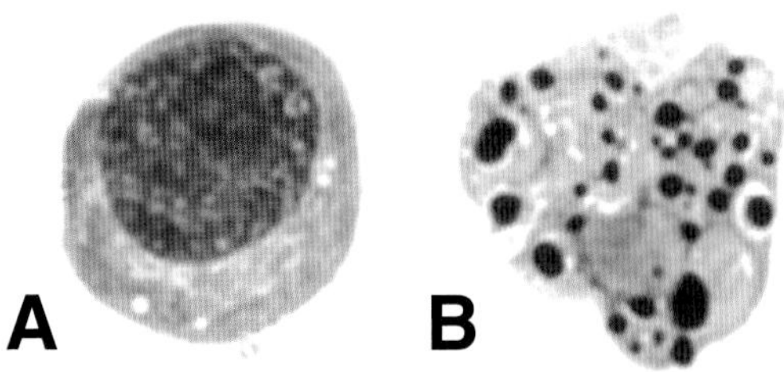

FIGURE 1-20. Apoptosis. A viable cell **(A)** contrasts with an apoptotic cell **(B)** in which the nucleus has undergone condensation and fragmentation.

by removing excess cells. Thus, normal organ size and architecture are maintained.

Apoptosis and Obsolescent Cells

Cell turnover is essential to maintaining the size and function of many organs. For example, as cells are continuously supplied to the circulating blood, older and less functional white blood cells must be eliminated to maintain the normal complement of the cells. Indeed, pathologic accumulation of polymorphonuclear leukocytes in chronic myeloid leukemia results from a mutation that inhibits apoptosis and so allows these cells to persist. In the small intestinal mucosa, cells migrate from the depths of the crypts to the tips of the villi, where they undergo apoptosis and are sloughed into the lumen.

Apoptosis also maintains the balance of cellularity in organs that respond to trophic stimuli, such as hormones, as in the regression of lactational hyperplasia of the breast in women who have stopped nursing their infants. Later in life, postmenopausal atrophy of the endometrium follows loss of hormonal support.

Apoptosis and Mutant Cells

The integrity of an organism requires that damaged cells be eliminated. There is a finite, albeit low, error rate in DNA replication, owing to the imperfect fidelity of DNA polymerases. Environmental stresses such as ultraviolet (UV) light, ionizing radiation, and DNA-binding chemicals may also alter DNA structure. There are several means, the most important of which probably involves p53, by which cells recognize genomic abnormalities and "assess" whether or not they can be repaired. If the DNA damage is too severe to be repaired, a cascade of events leads to apoptosis. This process protects an organism from the consequences of a nonfunctional cell or one that cannot control its own proliferation (e.g., a cancer cell). However, cancer cells often evolve mechanisms to circumvent apoptosis that might otherwise eliminate them (see Chapter 4).

Apoptosis as a Defense against Dissemination of Infection

When a cell "detects" nonchromosomal DNA replication, as in a viral infection, it tends to initiate apoptosis. In destroying infected cells, the body limits the spread of the virus. Many viruses have evolved mechanisms that manipulate cellular apoptosis via genes whose products inhibit apoptosis. Some of these viral proteins bind and inactivate cellular proteins (e.g., p53) that are important in triggering apoptosis. Others may interfere with the signaling pathways that activate apoptosis.

Mechanisms of Apoptosis

The various apoptosis signaling pathways include the following:

- In ***extrinsic apoptosis***, certain plasma membrane receptors are activated by their ligands.
- The ***intrinsic pathway*** is initiated by diverse intracellular stresses and is characterized by a central role for mitochondria.
- ***p53-activated apoptosis*** occurs in response to cellular stress or DNA damage.
- The ***perforin/granzyme pathway*** is triggered when cytotoxic T cells attack their cellular targets, with transfer of granzyme B from the killer cell to its intended victim.

A family of cysteine proteases, called caspases, is central to apoptosis. Sequential activation of these enzymes, which entails conversion from proenzyme forms to catalytically

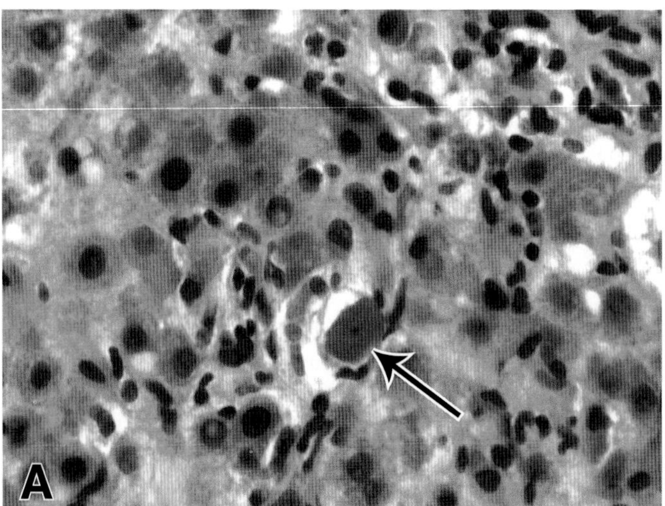

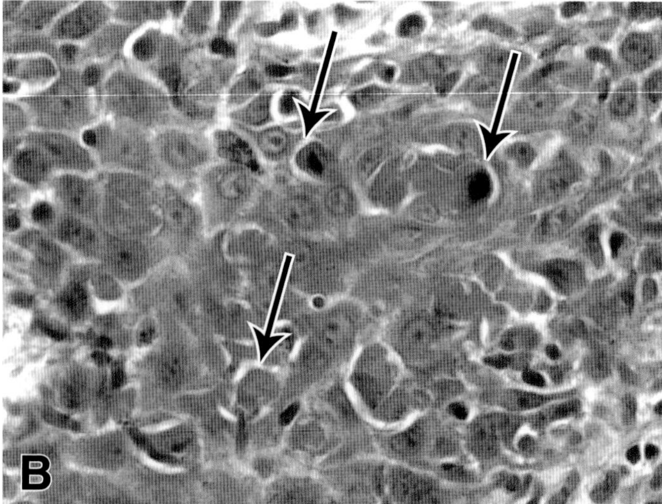

FIGURE 1-21. Apoptotic cells. Apoptotic cells are indicated by arrows in the case of apoptosis in the liver in viral hepatitis **(A)** and in the skin in erythema multiforme **(B)**.

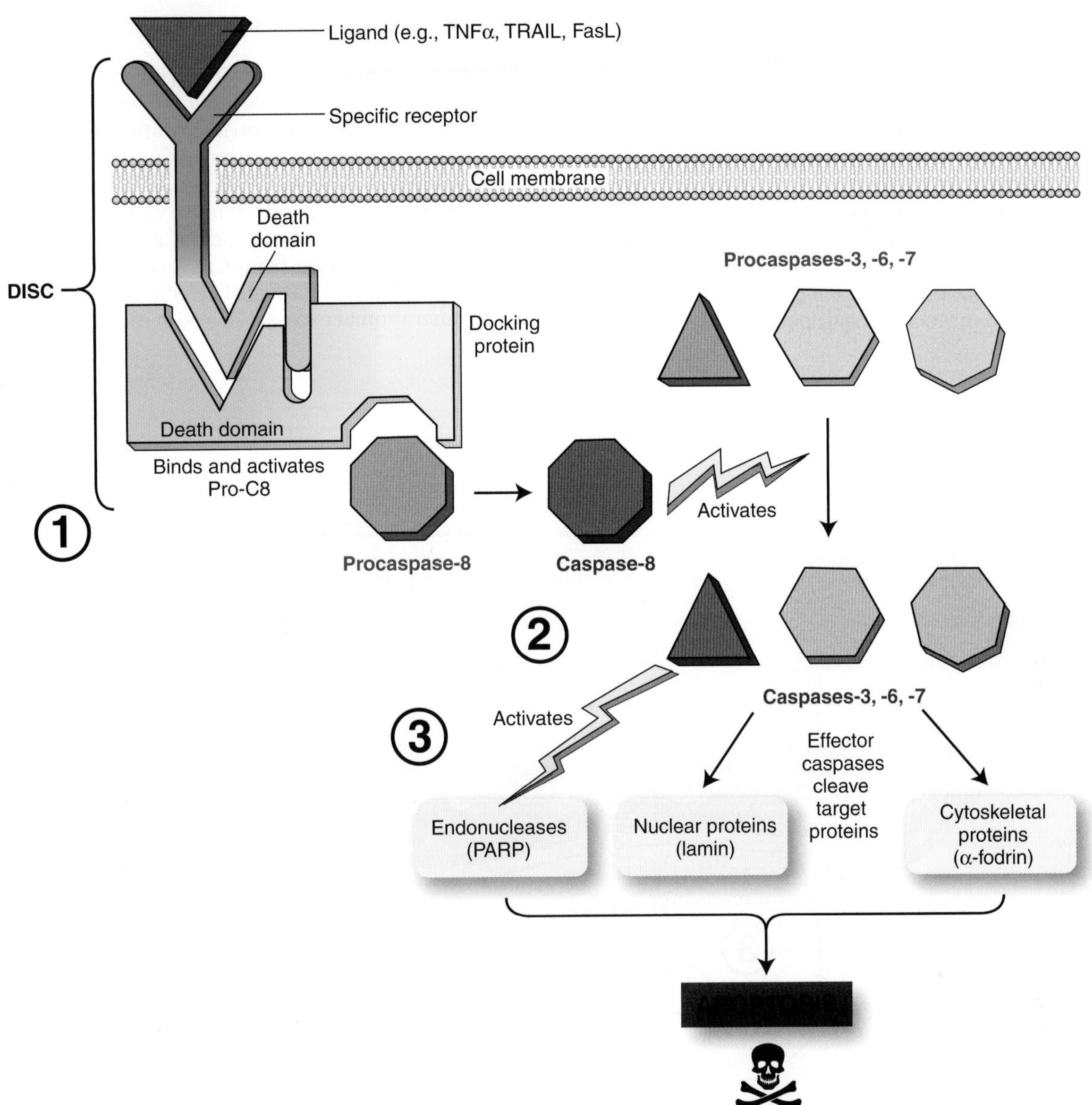

FIGURE 1-22. Extrinsic pathway of apoptosis. Ligand–receptor interactions that lead to caspase activation. (*1*) A number of ligands bind to their respective cell membrane receptors. As a result, the cytoplasmic tails of these receptors bind to the "death domains" of docking proteins, to form a death-inducing signaling complex (DISC). In turn, these proteins activate procaspase-8. (*2*) The conversion of procaspase-8 to activated caspase-8 then convertsprocaspases-3, -6, and -7 to their respective active forms. (*3*) Caspases-3, -6, and -7, especially caspase-3, are executioners that cleave target proteins, which leads to apoptosis. TNF, tumor necrosis factor; TRAIL, TNF-related apoptosis-inducing ligand; PARP, poly-ADP-ribosylpolymerase.

active enzymes, is central to apoptotic pathways. Some 14 caspases are now known, of which about half are important participants in apoptotic signaling.

Although the various pathways to apoptosis may start differently and signal via different members of this enzyme family, these diverse roads all generally lead to the killer enzymes, namely, caspases -3, -6, and -7.

Extrinsic Apoptosis

Prominent examples of initiation of apoptosis at the cell membrane are the binding of TNF-α to its receptor (TNFR) and the recognition of Fas ligand (FasL) by its receptor, Fas. TNF-α is a soluble cytokine, whereas FasL is found in the plasma membrane of certain cells, such as cytotoxic effector lymphocytes.

At the cell surface, TNFR and Fas become activated upon binding to their ligands. Specific amino acid sequences in the cytoplasmic tails of these transmembrane receptors, called death domains, act as docking sites for the corresponding death domains of other proteins (Fig. 1-22). After binding to the ligand-activated receptors, the docking proteins stimulate downstream signaling molecules, especially procaspases-8 and -10, which are converted to their active forms, caspases-8 and -10. In turn, these caspases activate further downstream caspases in the apoptosis pathway.

The ultimate caspases in this process are "effector," or "executioner," caspases-3, -6, and -7. Caspase-3, the most commonly activated effector caspase, stimulates enzymes that cause nuclear fragmentation (e.g., caspase-activated DNase [CAD], which degrades chromosomal DNA). Caspase-3 also destabilizes the cytoskeleton as the cell begins to fragment into apoptotic bodies.

The extrinsic (death receptor) pathway of apoptosis intersects the intrinsic (mitochondrial) pathway via caspase-8, which cleaves a cytoplasmic protein, Bid. Truncated Bid (tBid) translocates to mitochondria, where it can activate apoptosis through the intrinsic (mitochondrial) pathway (see below).

Mitochondrial Intrinsic Pathway of Apoptosis

Disturbance of mitochondrial integrity and specifically failure of the normally impermeable inner mitochondrial membrane is key to the initiation of the intrinsic pathway of apoptosis. The mitochondrial permeability transition pore (MPTP) within this inner membrane is normally closed, effectively separating the contents of the mitochondrial matrix from the space between the inner and outer mitochondrial membrane. Injury to the mitochondria resulting from Ca^{2+} accumulation, decrease of mitochondrial pH, or damage to electron transport with subsequent generation of excess ROS result in opening of the MPTP.

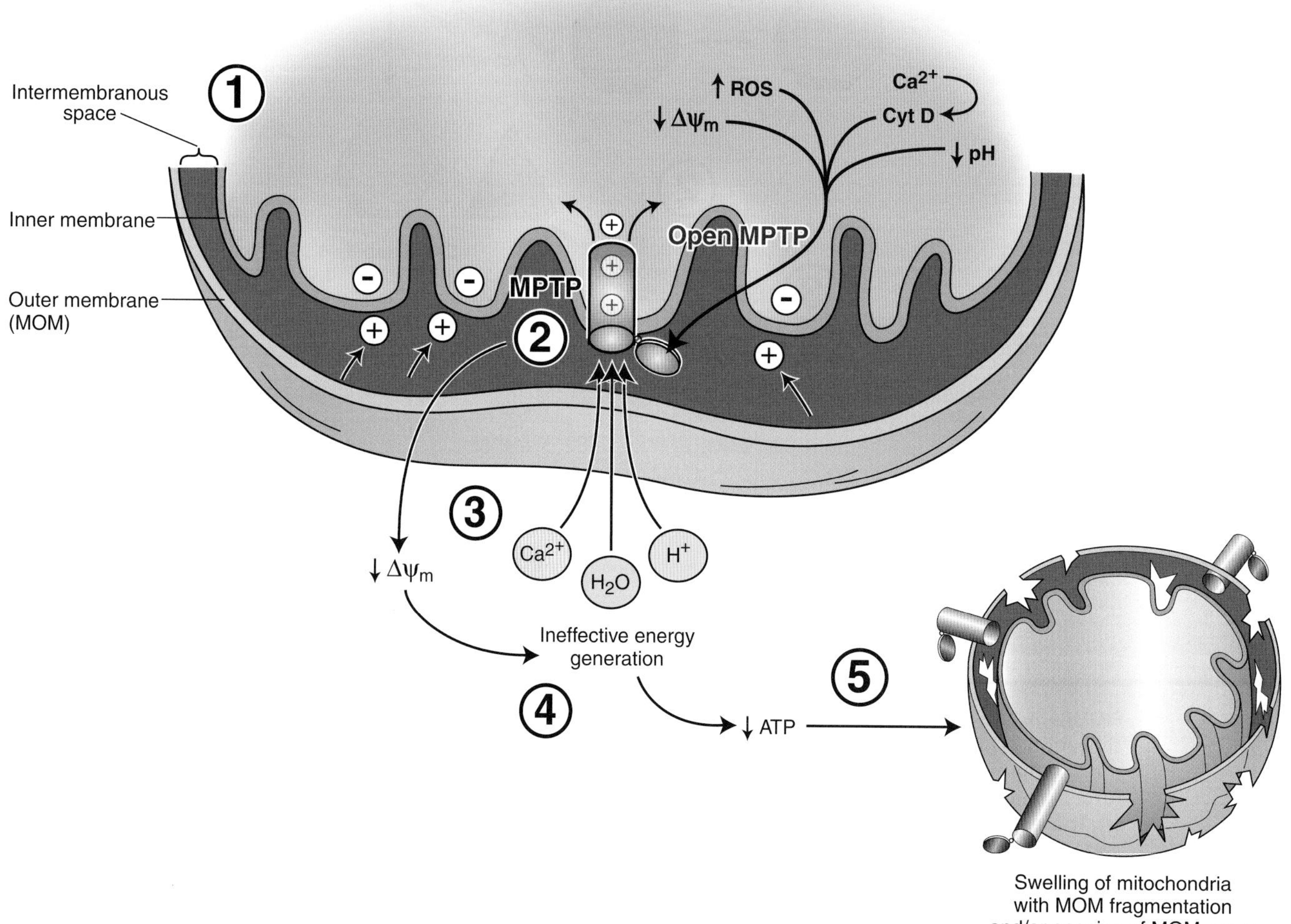

FIGURE 1-23. The intrinsic pathway of apoptosis. A. Causes and consequences of mitochondrial permeability transition pore (MPTP) activation. (*1*) A variety of stresses, including altered mitochondrial membrane potential ($\Delta\psi_m$), increased reactive oxygen species (ROS) and Ca^{2+}, and decreased pH differential, affect the mitochondrial matrix. (*2*) As a result, the MPTP opens. (*3*) The high colloid oncotic pressure of the mitochondrial matrix drives an influx of water and accompanying solutes through the MPTP into the mitochondrial matrix. Concomitant cation influx neutralizes the cross-membrane $\Delta\psi_m$ and pH differential. (*4*) This disrupts energy production, which further impairs the mitochondrion's ability to rectify the imbalance. (*5*) Water influx leads to swelling of the organelle and fragmentation of the mitochondrial outer membrane (MOM). **B.** The MOM in the intrinsic pathway of apoptosis. (*1*) Molecules—Smac/diablo, cytochrome c (Cyt c), apoptosis-inducing factor (AIF)—that are attached to the inner membrane, or free in the intermembranous space, become detached. (*2*) They then exit through outer membrane pores or holes and activate cytosolic effectors of apoptosis. ATP, adenosine triphosphate.

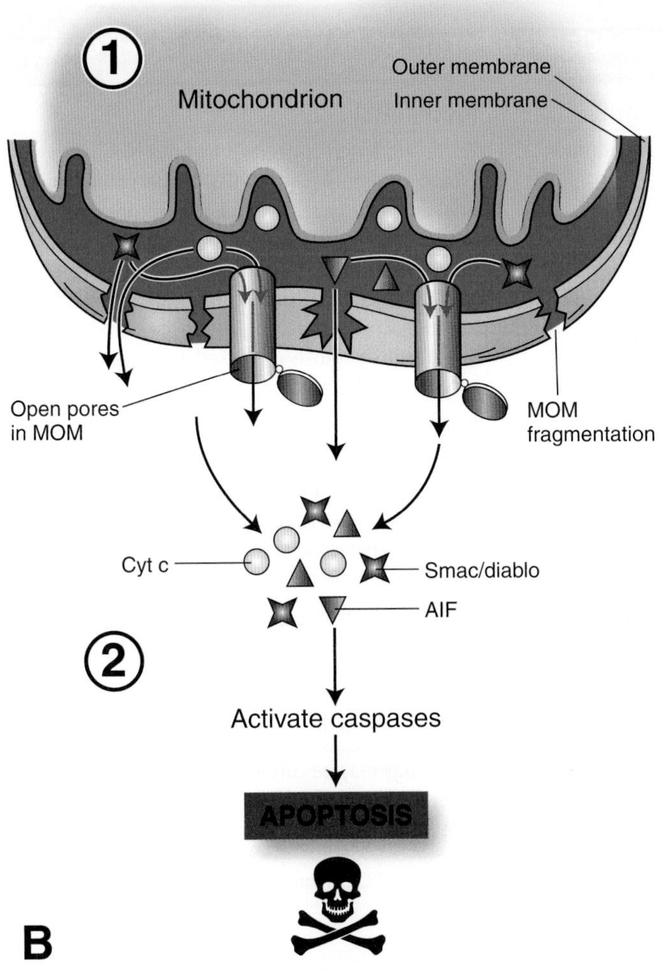

FIGURE 1-23. *(Continued)*

This opening has several consequences. Water, protons (H^+), and salts enter the mitochondrial matrix resulting in mitochondrial swelling, collapse of the electrochemical potential across the inner membrane, and failure of ATP production. Damage to the outer mitochondrial membrane allows inner membrane proteins (including Cyt c, Smac/diablo, and apoptosis-inducing factor [AIF]) to exit the mitochondria into the cytosol, where they activate the next phase of intrinsic apoptosis. Details of the process are found in Figure 1-23.

Mechanisms That Control the Intrinsic Pathway

The Normal Mitochondrion

Among other proteins, Cyt c and Smac/diablo are attached to the outer surface of the inner mitochondrial membrane, facing the intermembranous space. Opposite these, and attached to the outer membrane, are complexes of Bax and/or Bak bound to antiapoptotic Bcl-2 family members. In equilibrium, Bcl-2 (Bcl-xL, Mcl-1, etc.) inhibits proapoptotic functions of Bax/Bak, and the mitochondrial default setting is prosurvival.

The Bcl-2 Family of Proteins

Many intracellular agents, often involved in stress or injury, act via members of the Bcl-2 family termed BH3-only. Such may include increasing concentrations of some BH3-only proteins (e.g., by activating transcription), altering their conformations from quiescent to active, modifying enzymes, and so forth. The now-active BH3-only molecules may interpose themselves into Bcl-2 (Bcl-xL, etc.) complexes with Bak and Bax. This process dissociates these complexes, thereby liberating Bax and Bak to form channels in the outer mitochondrial membrane. These passages, called mitochondrial apoptosis-induced channels (MACs), allow release of toxic mitochondrial proteins (Cyt c, Smac/diablo, etc.) into the cytosol-free Bax can also be directly activated by BH3-only proteins to form MACs (Fig. 1-24).

Apoptosis Activated by p53

Within the nucleus, p53 is both a transcriptional activator and a repressor, depending on the target gene. Triggering of p53 (such as might occur with irreparable genomic damage) stimulates transcription of many proapoptotic proteins, such as Bad, Bax, NOXA, PUMA, and others. Simultaneously, it represses transcription of prosurvival proteins, including Bcl-2, Bcl-xL, and Mcl-1, resulting in cell death. p53 also regulates cell cycle, metabolism, and many other cell functions (see Chapter 4).

Apoptosis Activated by Granzymes

Activation of caspase signaling occurs when cytotoxic T lymphocytes (CTLs) and natural killer (NK) cells recognize a cell as foreign. These lymphocytes release two major molecular species, namely, perforin and granzymes. Perforin, as its name suggests, punches a hole in the plasma membrane of a target cell through which proteins from the lymphocyte enter. Granzymes belong to a family of serine proteases, among which the best understood is granzyme B. This protease activates cytosolic Bid, a BH3-only protein, by cleaving it to tBid (Fig. 1-25). In turn, tBid increases mitochondrial release of Cyt c and other cell death effector proteins. It also converts several procaspases (notably procaspase-3) to active caspases. Granzyme A is also released by NK cells and CTLs into target cells. Granzymes A and B together induce cell death by caspase-independent mechanisms. They activate the DNA nicking enzyme, CAD (see above), which degrades genomic DNA.

Special Forms of Programmed Cell Death

Additional forms of PCD, which may act independently of apoptosis or interact with apoptotic processes under special circumstances, are outlined in Table 1-5.

BIOLOGIC AGING

Aging *refers to a process characterized by progressive dysfunction, frailty and increasing mortality.* Biologic aging is distinct from disease, in that, the latter represents an abnormal and unpredictable pathologic condition, whereas aging is both universal and inevitable. Yet, aging and disease are intimately related; aging represents a key risk factor—and in many cases, the dominant risk factor—for many of the diseases described elsewhere in this volume.

Environmental and Genetic Influences

Considerable evidence shows that aging is subject to strong genetic and environmental influences. For example, it is now possible to achieve dramatic life span extension (up to 65%)

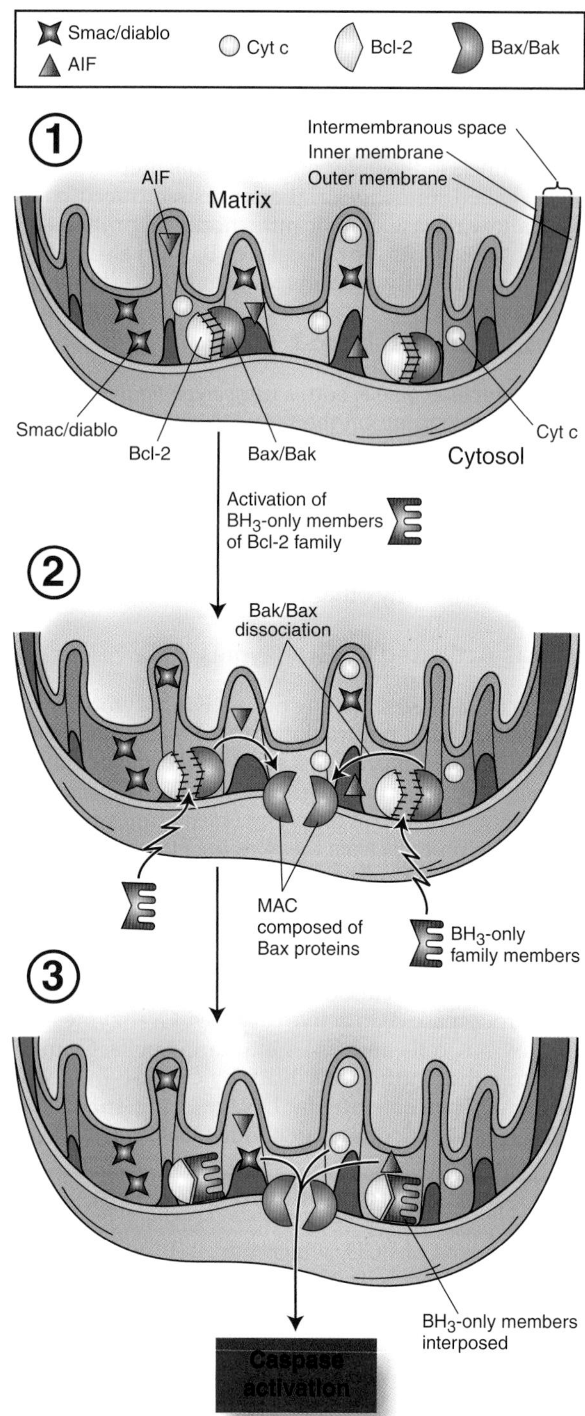

FIGURE 1-24. Formation of pores in the outer mitochondrial membrane during activation of the intrinsic pathway of apoptosis. (*1*) At equilibrium, Cyt c, Smac/diablo, and apoptosis-inducing factor (AIF) either are attached to the mitochondrial inner membrane or float in the intermembranous space. The complex of oligomeric Bak/Bax with antiapoptotic Bcl-2 family cousins resides at the outer membrane. (*2*) When BH3-only members of the Bcl-2 clan are activated, they interpose themselves between their prosurvival relatives and Bak/Bax, thereby freeing Bak/Bax proteins. The latter then form a pore (MAC) in the outer mitochondrial membrane. (*3*) Proapoptotic proteins Cyt c, Smac/diablo, AIF, and others exit from the mitochondrion via the MAC pore. Once in the cytosol, these proteins facilitate activation of the caspase cascade and so cause apoptosis. Cyt c, cytochrome c; MAC, mitochondrial apoptosis-induced channel.

Table 1-5

Specialized Forms of Programmed Cell Death

Form	Mechanism
Necroptosis	Fas ligand or tumor necrosis factor-α binding to "death receptors" (RIP1, RIP3) triggers mitochondrial damage, decrease in adenosine triphosphate production and increased intracellular Ca^{2+} resulting in activation of calcium dependent degradative enzymes (calpains). Increases in intracellular iron promotes reactive oxygen species production. When apoptosis is blocked, necroptosis may serve as an alternative.
Anoikosis	A form of apoptosis triggered by loss of epithelial cell–cell contacts. May inhibit cancer metastases.
Pyroptosis	Caspase-1 dependent PCD, which is triggered by activation of pattern recognition receptors stimulating inflammasomes as discussed in Chapter 2. Important in inflammation and host-defense against pathogens.
NETosis	NETs are masses of chromatin released by predominantly by neutrophils as part of a necrosis-like form of death. The NETs serve as traps for bacteria and other pathogens.
Autophagy	Autophagy may be considered either as an independent form of PCD or part of the process of apoptosis.

NETs, neutrophil extracellular traps; PCD, programmed cell death.

in rodent models through single-gene mutations in specific signaling pathways, or even by administering certain small molecules. Reduced food intake without malnutrition (dietary restriction [DR]) promotes longevity in many species, from budding yeast to rodents and perhaps even nonhuman primates.

Relative to our forebears, those who live in advanced industrialized societies already benefit from a greatly increased life span. The dramatic increase in life span stems mostly from reduced child mortality and improved public health measures, as well as advances in medical care. If current trends hold, life expectancy at birth in developed countries may reach 100 years by the mid-21st century. The **maximum** documented life span for any human is 122 years, and few people live to be much older than 100.

CELLULAR SENESCENCE AND ORGANISMAL AGING

When human fibroblasts are passaged serially in culture, they do not replicate indefinitely. Instead (like yeast), after many passages, they enter a nondividing state called **replicative senescence**. During this time, they remain postmitotic but are viable for an extended period. Senescent cells are characterized by (1) an enlarged, flattened appearance; (2) absence of molecular markers of proliferation; (3) persistent foci of unrepaired DNA damage; and (4) expression of senescence-associated β-galactosidase and $p16^{Ink4a}$ protein.

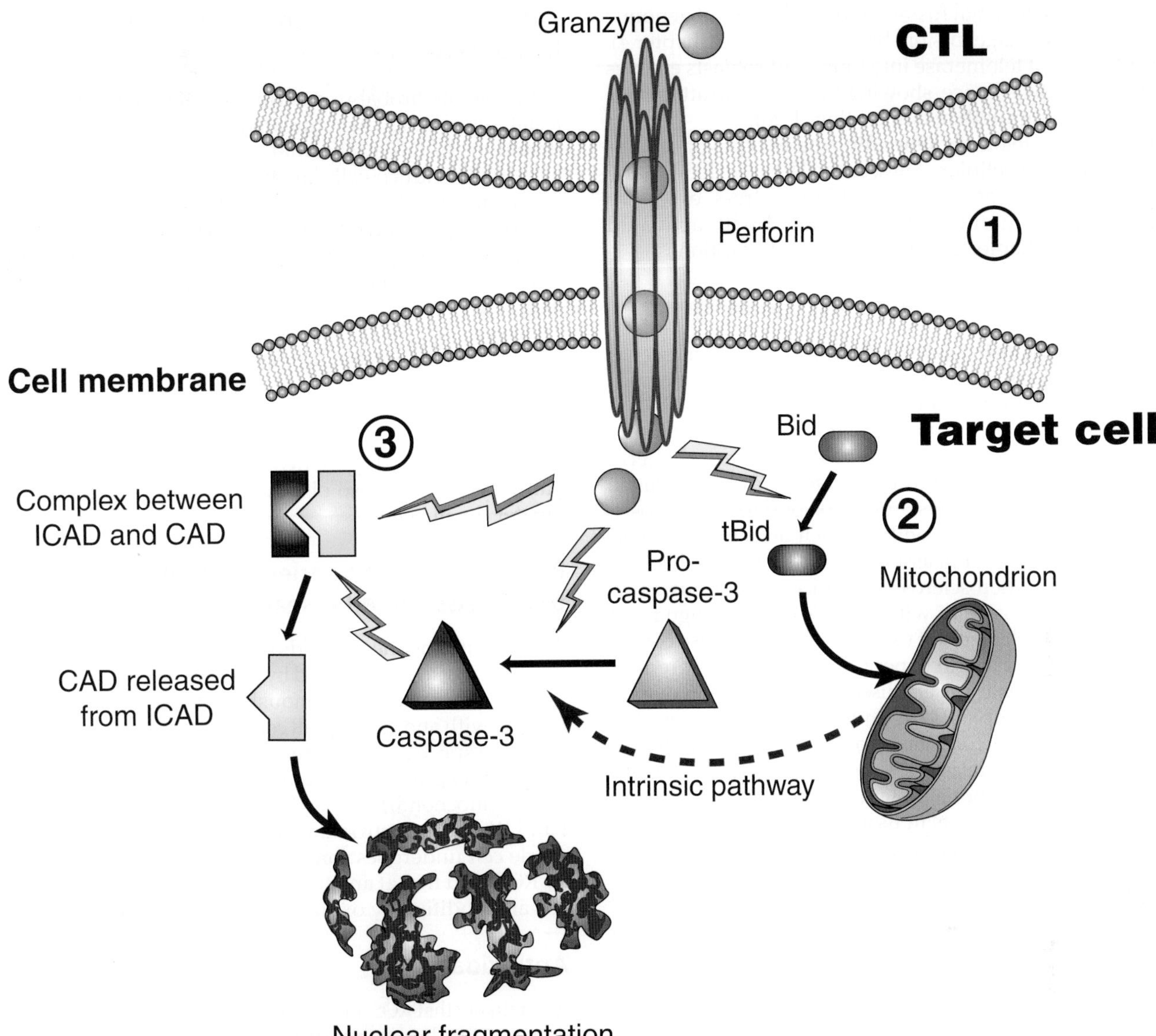

FIGURE 1-25. Cell death caused by CTLs. (*1*) Granzyme and perforin are two molecules made, mainly, by CTLs and natural killer cells. After a CTL binds its cellular victim, perforin molecules combine to create an intercellular channel through which granzyme enters the target cell. (*2*) Granzyme cleaves cytoplasmic Bid to its active form, tBid, which translocates into mitochondria and triggers the intrinsic pathway of apoptosis. It also activates procaspase-3 to caspase-3, via which apoptosis may proceed. (*3*) Granzyme may also disrupt the complex between CAD and its inhibitor, ICAD. This effect releases the DNase (CAD) to elicit a caspase-independent form of apoptosis. The CAD–ICAD complex may also be cleaved by caspase-3. CAD, caspase-activated DNase; CTL, cytotoxic T lymphocyte; ICAD, inhibitor of CAD.

Telomere Shortening Promotes Replicative Senescence

In human cells, replicative senescence is largely due to attrition of **telomeres**, which are a series of short repetitive nucleotide sequences (TTAGGG in vertebrates) at the 3′ ends of chromosomes (see below and 4). DNA polymerase, the enzyme that replicates DNA, begins at the 5′ and works toward the 3′ end. It cannot copy linear chromosomes all the way to their distal ends, so telomeres tend to shorten with each cell division. Telomeres protect the genes that are near chromosomal ends from being lost with repeated cell divisions. Certain crucial cell types, such as stem cell populations, express an enzyme, **telomerase**, that restores sequences lost during replication and thus stabilizes the length of their telomeres. By contrast, most human somatic cells, such as fibroblasts, do not express significant levels of telomerase. Consequently, their telomeres shorten with each cell division, thereby representing a "mitotic clock" that counts DNA replication events. Some types of cellular injury, such as oxidative stress, can directly damage telomeres, independent of replication.

Telomeres are normally protected by a protein complex termed **shelterin**. When telomeres shorten beyond a critical point, the release of shelterin exposes telomeres, which triggers a DNA damage response that can cause irreversible cell cycle arrest or apoptosis. Telomere attrition can also lead to end-to-end chromosomal fusions and other types of genomic instability via breakage–fusion–bridge cycles (see Chapter 4). Reintroduction of telomerase into human fibroblasts enables them to bypass senescence, showing that telomere attrition is limiting for their growth in culture (Fig. 1-26).

In addition to telomere shortening, other types of cellular injury also induce cellular senescence. These include many DNA-damaging agents, such as oxidative stress, excessive mitogenic stimulation like that associated with activated oncogenes (see Chapter 4), and chromatin disruption.

The Role of Telomere Maintenance in Longevity

During aging, progressive cellular dysfunction and senescence is attributed to telomere erosion. However, laboratory mice have very long telomeres, and yet these animals age, so that (at least in mice) telomere attrition may not be needed for aging to occur. In humans, rare mutations in telomerase or shelterin components give rise to shortened telomeres and aplastic anemia, skin and nail defects, infertility, pulmonary fibrosis, and cancer. Even in people without such defects, shortened telomeres are also found in association with human diseases such as cirrhosis, atherosclerosis, and ulcerative colitis. Such associations are consistent with histories of prolonged cell proliferation or high levels of oxidative stress in these conditions. Short telomere length in peripheral blood cells predicts susceptibility to coronary artery disease, neoplasia, and overall mortality in older people. These findings suggest that eroded telomeres can indeed contribute to age-associated pathologies, if not necessarily to aging *per se*. Genetically engineered mouse strains that cannot maintain telomeres show reduced longevity, as well as defects in tissues that require rapid cell proliferation and stem and progenitor cell activity, principally, bone marrow, skin, gut, and testes. Altogether, these studies demonstrate that telomere maintenance contributes to cellular and organismal homeostasis, its role in human longevity is less clear.

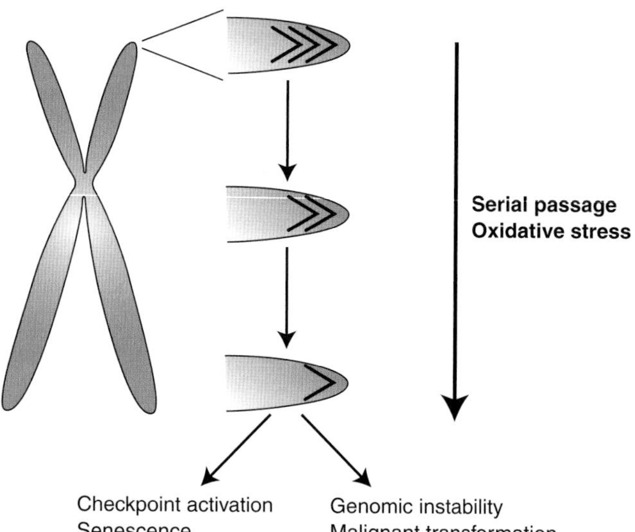

FIGURE 1-26. Deleterious consequences of telomere shortening in mammalian cells.

Precise Molecular Mechanisms of Aging Remain Obscure

Many factors probably contribute to the degenerative manifestations of aging. Accumulated unrepaired macromolecular damage—to DNA, chromatin, proteins, and lipids—may eventually induce cellular dysfunction, manifesting at the organismal level as aging. To counter the effects of such damage, cells have evolved elaborate, well-regulated mechanisms to repair many types of macromolecular lesions. Alternatively, cells with certain types of severe damage, such as to mitochondria and nuclear DNA, can also be removed by apoptosis (as previously noted). This damage-based model of aging predicts that mutant organisms with increased longevity should also show more robust resistance to damage-inducing stressors. This is in fact typically—though not always—observed. The model also predicts that cellular repair systems should be intimately related, genetically speaking, to prolongevity pathways. This is also observed empirically, as outlined in greater detail below.

Reactive Oxygen Species Contribute to Age-Associated Disease

A long-standing theory holds that macromolecular damage in the context of aging is caused by **reactive oxygen species (ROS)**, mostly generated endogenously in mitochondria. ROS can interact with and damage all cellular macromolecules, causing a diverse spectrum of lesions in nucleic acids, modifying and inactivating proteins, and damaging lipids. Most ROS generation in mitochondria occurs because of "leakage" at complexes I and III of the electron transport chain. It is estimated that a single cell undergoes some 100,000 attacks on DNA per day by ROS, and that at any time, 10% of protein molecules in the cell are modified by oxidative carbonyl adducts.

Antioxidants

It is unlikely that ROS are the single major driver of age-associated damage. Studies in hundreds of thousands of people given supraphysiologic doses of antioxidant dietary supplements have not found any significant benefit on life span, disease development, or general health; indeed, adding certain antioxidants is associated with *increased* mortality.

Stem Cell Function Declines with Aging

Adult stem cells in many mammalian tissues are critical for proper organ function and for repair following injury. These stem cells may lose functionality with age, thus impairing tissue homeostasis and contributing to degenerative disease. This notion has been best evaluated in the context of hematopoietic stem cells (HSCs), which give rise to all mature cell types in the blood. Aging is not characterized by fewer HSCs, but it is associated with impaired HSC function. Clinically, it has long been known that HSC transplants from young donors are more likely to be successful than those from older donors. In aged people, HSCs increasingly follow myeloid, rather than lymphoid, differentiation. There are progressive defects in HSC mobilization and homing, and aged HSCs also accumulate unrepaired oxidative damage to DNA.

As mentioned previously, expression of the tumor suppressor $p16^{Ink4a}$ is induced in senescent cells. Genetic studies in humans have linked polymorphisms near the $p16^{Ink4a}$ locus to diverse age-associated pathologies (e.g., coronary atherosclerosis, type 2 diabetes, and frailty). These data suggest that p16^{Ink4a} or a closely linked gene product can regulate aging in humans in important ways, via effects on stem cells or other cell types.

Genetic Diseases Resembling Premature Aging

There are rare diseases that seem to resemble accelerated aging **(progerias)**. The two best-studied such conditions are **Werner syndrome** (WS) and **Hutchinson–Gilford progeria syndrome** (HGPS).

Werner Syndrome

WS is caused by recessive mutations in the *WRN* gene, which encodes a DNA helicase involved in many aspects of DNA metabolism, including replication, repair, and telomere maintenance. Patients with mutations in *WRN* show poor growth in adolescence, premature hair graying, thinning of the skin, cataracts, diabetes, and atherosclerosis. They also have a tendency to develop cancer, specifically sarcomas, leukemias, and other malignancies. WS patients typically succumb to myocardial infarction or cancer by their 40s or 50s (Fig. 1-27).

Despite the apparent similarities of WS to normal aging, this disease is by no means a perfect mimic of the aging process. For example, some disorders commonly associated with physiologic aging, such as Alzheimer disease, are not observed in WS. Thus, WS is an example of a **segmental progeria**—that is, a syndrome that recapitulates some, but not all, aspects of accelerated aging. Cultured WS fibroblasts show chromosomal instability, sensitivity to DNA cross-linking agents, and a reduced replicative life span. This last observation has been used to argue for the validity of cellular senescence as a model system to study aging.

Hutchinson–Gilford Progeria Syndrome

HGPS is caused by autosomal dominant mutations in the *LMNA* gene, whose product is a protein, **lamin A**. These children show reduced growth, hair loss, scleroderma-like skin changes, and atherosclerosis (Fig. 1-28). Patients with HGPS die at an average age of 13 years, typically from myocardial infarction or stroke. The most common mutation associated with HGPS causes missplicing of the LMNA transcript, leading to accumulation of **progerin**, a defective precursor of lamin A protein. Normally, lamin A is a key part of the nuclear lamina that provides structural integrity to the nucleus in differentiated cells. By contrast, progerin accumulates in the nucleus, resulting in a distorted nuclear outline and nuclear blebbing. The buildup of progerin interferes with chromatin organization, impairing gene expression and DNA repair. HGPS is at the severe end of a spectrum of disorders associated with mutations in the *LMNA* gene, collectively termed "laminopathies." These diseases are associated with defects in muscle, adipose tissue, and peripheral nerves.

It is unclear whether the study of WS, HGPS, and related disorders improves understanding of the biology of aging. These conditions may represent disease phenotypes whose pathogenesis is unrelated to physiologic aging.

Defects in DNA Repair Cause Degenerative Phenotypes

On the basis of the progerias, it is suggested that DNA is an important target, perhaps the principal target, of age-associated damage. In this respect, ROS are thought to represent one major source of aging-associated DNA damage (see above). This is an intuitively appealing notion; unlike other cellular macromolecules such as proteins and lipids, damaged nuclear DNA cannot simply be replaced, but instead must be repaired. Consistent with this notion, increased levels of chromosomal aberrations, as well as more subtle mutations, occur in peripheral blood leukocytes and other mammalian tissues with advancing age. Cells have evolved numerous systems to repair distinct DNA lesions (see Chapter 4). Unrepaired DNA damage activates cellular checkpoint responses, resulting in cell cycle arrest, apoptosis, or senescence. Although defects in DNA repair systems cause dramatic harmful effects, that fact does not prove that DNA damage is at the root of physiologic aging. At this time, a connection between DNA repair and aging remains an attractive, but unproven hypothesis.

Reduced Caloric Intake and Longevity

Dietary restriction (DR) promotes increased longevity in the large majority of organisms in which it has been tested, from budding yeast to rodents. In mice, reducing caloric intake by 30% to 50% routinely extends life span by 25% to 40%. Perhaps even more striking than its prolongevity effects, DR delays or prevents the onset of many age-associated conditions, including cancers, cardiovascular disease, neurodegeneration, diabetes, sarcopenia, and many others. However, DR is not a "free ride"; in rodents, it impairs certain immune responses and delays wound healing. In humans, DR has been associated with reduced bone density and muscle mass, and with depression.

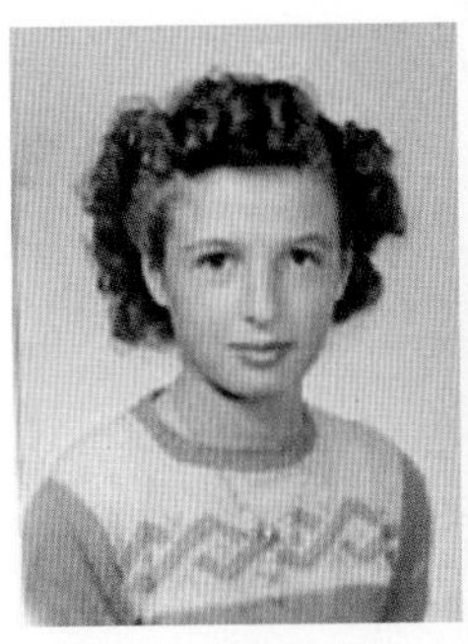

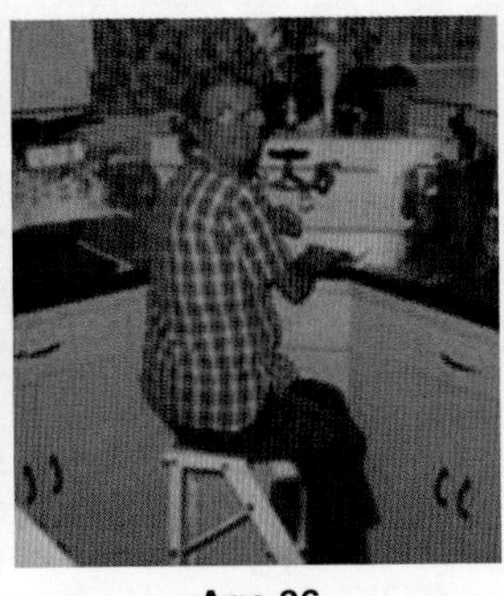

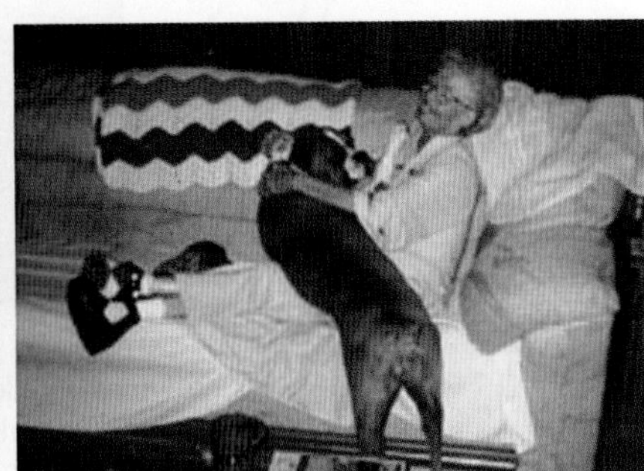

Age 8 Age 21 Age 36 Age 56

FIGURE 1-27. Werner syndrome. The premature appearance of aging phenotypes is evident. Used with permission from Hisama FM, Bohr VA, Oshima J. WRN's tenth anniversary. *Sci Aging Knowledge Environ*. 2006;2006(10):e18.

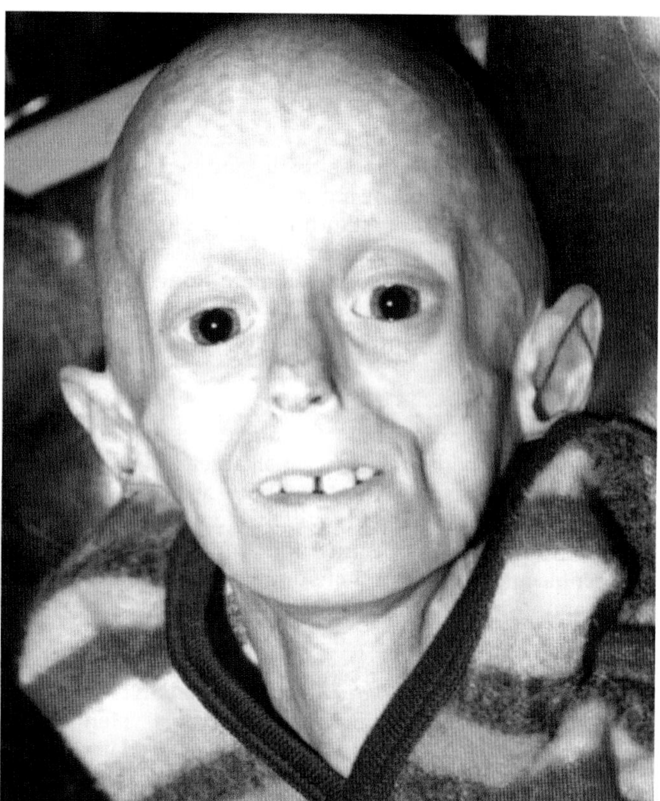

FIGURE 1-28. Hutchinson–Gilford progeria syndrome. A 10-year-old girl shows typical features of this disease.

Dietary Restriction

Can DR extend life span in humans? Persons who voluntarily limit their dietary intake experience improved serum lipid parameters, increased insulin sensitivity, reduced blood pressure and protection against obesity, type 2 diabetes, inflammation, carotid artery intimal hyperplasia, and left ventricular diastolic dysfunction. Thus, DR in humans does indeed confer dramatic protection against cardiovascular risk factors. However, the overall lowest mortality rate in humans is associated with a body mass index (BMI) of roughly 25, corresponding to a normal to slightly overweight status; both lower and higher BMIs are associated with decreased longevity. Thus, the low BMIs associated with DR in humans may have unforeseen negative consequences. In sum, DR can certainly extend health and likely life span. The molecular mechanisms underlying this effect are only beginning to be elucidated, but are likely to be complex.

Insulin and IGF-I Signaling

Insulin/IGF-I-like signaling (IIS) diminishes longevity. IIS is initiated when insulin or IGF family members bind their cognate cell surface receptors which encode tyrosine kinases (Fig. 1-29). These interactions activate the Akt kinase, which phosphorylates downstream proteins to regulate diverse processes, including cell survival, growth, cell cycle, metabolism, and stress resistance. The FOXO transcription factors are key targets of Akt; when IIS is active, Akt phosphorylation sequesters FOXO in the cytoplasm, where it is inactive. Increased FOXO

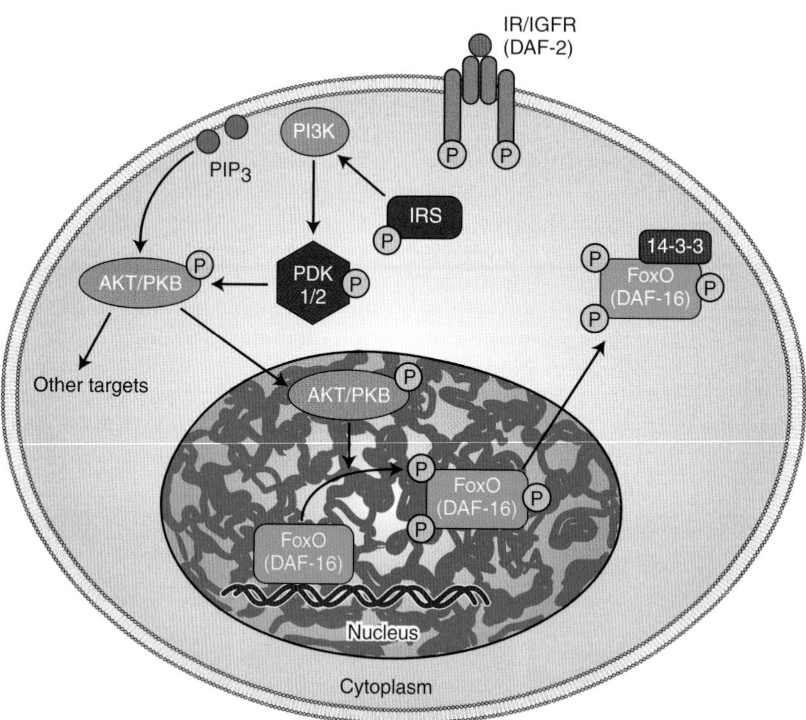

FIGURE 1-29. Insulin/insulin-like growth factor-I (IGF-I)-like signaling pathway. IIS begins when insulin or IGF-I binds to its cell surface receptors, which are tyrosine kinases. This initiates an intracellular signaling cascade involving generation of phosphatidylinositol triphosphate by phosphatidylinositol-3-kinase (PI3K), in turn, leading to activation of the downstream kinases PDK1 and Akt. FOXO transcription factors are key targets of this signaling pathway; in *Caenorhabditis elegans*, FOXO is termed DAF-16. IR/IRS, insulin receptor/insulin-like growth factor receptor; IRS, insulin receptor substrate; PDK, phosphoinositide-dependent kinase; PIP$_3$, Phosphatidylinositol (3,4,5)-trisphosphate.

activity is a key element in longevity driven by reduced IIS. Surprisingly, detailed studies have revealed that increased FOXO activity in only a subset of tissues is sufficient to confer extended life span.

Two naturally occurring mouse mutants, the Snell and Ames dwarf lines, have pituitary defects that reduce growth hormone (GH) and IGF-I levels, along with greatly extended longevity and delayed onset of age-associated disease. Remarkably, these mice also show preserved cognition in old age. Although they have reduced levels of several pituitary-derived hormones, it is their GH deficiency that is critical for their long life span. Thus, these data point to a role for IIS in limiting mammalian life span.

Could reduced IIS contribute to longevity in humans as well? Because insulin *resistance* in humans is typically a pathologic condition associated with disease states (obesity, atherosclerosis, dyslipidemia, etc.), the intuitive response to this question might be no. However, polymorphisms in the IGF-I receptor (IGFR), Akt, and FOXO genes have been identified in centenarians. In the case of IGFR, these polymorphisms are associated with reduced IGF-I signaling. Overall, there is solid evidence that chronically reduced IGF-I signaling in humans protects against disease and potentially promotes longevity.

mTOR Signaling

mTOR is a protein kinase that participates in conserved roles in limiting longevity in widely divergent species (Fig. 1-30). Through complex signaling pathways, mTOR phosphorylates many targets in the cell. In a broad sense, mTOR activates protein synthesis in response to availability of nutrients. Its inactivation occurs with nutrient deficiency leading toward recycling of cellular components. Hence, mTOR may also play a role in DR-mediated life span extension. Remarkably, the mTOR inhibitor, rapamycin, robustly extends mouse life span, even when treatment is initiated in older adults. Rapamycin also suppresses neoplasia and several other phenotypes of aging in treated animals. Overall, these data indicate that positive mTOR signaling limits longevity in a manner that is conserved in many different organisms.

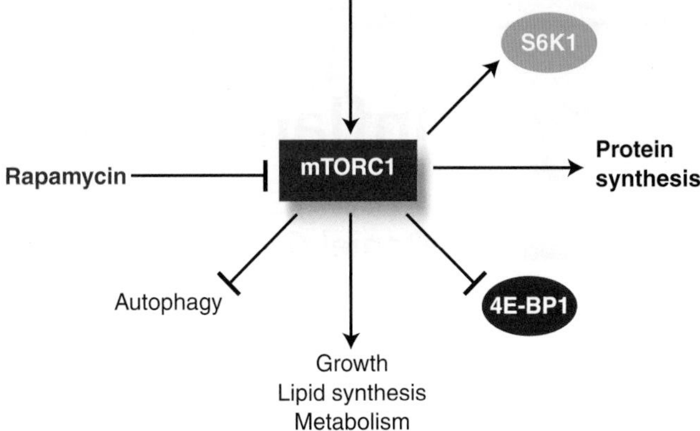

FIGURE 1-30. Mammalian target of rapamycin (mTOR) signaling. The mTOR kinase participates in two major complexes, termed mTORC1 and mTORC2. mTORC1 has been most closely linked to longevity. Multiple stimuli activate mTORC1. Two key downstream targets of mTORC1 are S6K1 and 4EBP1, through which mTORC1 promotes protein synthesis. Rapamycin acutely inhibits mTORC1 in a substrate-specific manner, but chronically can also inhibit mTORC2.

Sirtuins

Sirtuins are a family of enzymes whose best-characterized biochemical function is NAD^+-dependent **deacetylation** of target proteins. Intracellular NAD^+ levels rise with nutrient deprivation and stress; hence, sirtuin activity is a means by which cells sense and respond to their environments, akin to IIS and mTOR signaling.

Most research on mammalian sirtuins has focused on SIRT1. This protein deacetylates dozens of cellular proteins, including histones, p53, FOXO transcription factors, and many others, thus regulating key aspects of cell biology. SIRT1 attenuates many diseases associated with aging, including cardiac hypertrophy, neoplasia, glucose intolerance, neurodegeneration, and others. SIRT1 overexpression in the hypothalamus increases the mouse life span. Work in murine models suggests that several other sirtuins (SIRT3 and SIRT 6) participate in the protective effect of dietary restriction.

2 Inflammation and Repair

Hedwig S. Murphy[1] ▪ Kendra Iskander[2] ▪ David S. Strayer[2] ▪ Daniel G. Remick[2] ▪ Gregory C. Sephel[3] ▪ Jeffrey M. Davidson[3]

LEARNING OBJECTIVES

- Correlate the four cardinal signs of inflammation with pathophysiologic events that characterize acute inflammation.
- Distinguish between the inflammatory cells of acute and chronic inflammation.
- Distinguish between innate and adaptive immunity.
- Define the terms "DAMP," "PAMP," and "PRR."
- Discuss the role of toll-like receptors in innate immunity.
- Define the three major gene activation pathways activated by PRRs.
- Outline the temporal sequence of events following the initiation of acute inflammation.
- What is the Starling principle? How does it explain the production of inflammatory and noninflammatory edema?
- What is the "triple response" of acute inflammation? What are the pathophysiologic changes associated with it?
- Describe the changes in the endothelium mediated by (1) vasoactive mediators and (2) direct injury.
- List the major plasma-derived mediators of inflammation and describe their generation/activation.
- Contrast the three pathways of complement activation.
- Distinguish between the biologic activities of complement components.
- What are the potential effects of deficiencies in various complement components?
- List the major cell-derived mediators of inflammation and describe their generation/activation.
- Distinguish between the generation and activities of leukotrienes and lipoxins.
- Define the terms "autocrine, "paracrine," and "endocrine."
- List major cytokines produced by macrophages.
- What are the major roles of chemokines?
- List the cells most directly involved in inflammation and briefly define their major roles.
- Provide a temporal scheme for the recruitment of PMNs from the vasculature to the site of tissue injury.
- Define the adhesion molecules important in leukocyte recruitment.
- Differentiate between paracellular and transcellular diapedesis.
- List major chemotactic molecules and describe their source.
- Provide a temporal scheme for microorganism phagocytosis. Describe the processes of opsonization and internalization.
- List major factors important in oxidative and nonoxidative killing by inflammatory cells.
- Distinguish between the three types of neutrophil granules.
- Describe the steps that occur in the production of hypochlorous acid in neutrophils.
- List several important negative regulators of acute inflammation.
- Discuss important factors furthering chronic inflammation.
- Describe the role of the major cell types involved in chronic inflammation.
- Distinguish between granulomas and granulation tissue.
- Define the acute phase response.
- Define "provisional matrix" and describe its role in tissue repair.
- What are the major enzymes involved in tissue remodeling?
- Differentiate between the roles of factor XIII and tissue transglutaminase in wound repair.
- What are the major components of granulation tissue?
- Distinguish between the roles of fibroblasts and myofibroblasts in wound repair.
- Describe the process of angiogenesis in wound repair.
- Distinguish between primary and secondary healing in skin wounds.
- Distinguish between fibrosis and scarring.
- Distinguish between keloids and hypertrophic scars.
- Provide examples of labile, stabile, and permanent cell populations.
- Distinguish between the following: embryonic stem cell, adult stem cells, multipotential stem cells, induced pluripotential stem cells, and progenitor cells.
- Define the terms totipotent, pluripotent, multipotent, and unipotent.

[1] Inflammation
[2] Sepsis
[3] Repair, Regeneration and Fibrosis

OVERVIEW OF INFLAMMATION

Inflammation is a systemic and local reaction of tissues and microcirculation to a pathogenic insult. It is characterized by elaboration of inflammatory mediators and movement of fluid and leukocytes from the blood into extravascular tissues. This response localizes and eliminates altered cells, foreign particles, microorganisms, and antigens thereby allowing tissue repair to take place. Specific cells (1) attack and destroy injurious agents (e.g., infectious organisms, toxins, or foreign material), (2) enzymatically digest and remove them, or (3) wall them off. In the process, damaged cells and tissues are allowed repair. Responses to many damaging agents are immediate and stereotypic. The character of the inflammatory response is "modulated," depending on several factors, including (1) the nature of the offending agent, (2) duration of the insult, (3) extent of tissue damage, and (4) microenvironment.

The clinical signs of inflammation were described in the first century AD, by the Roman encyclopedist Aulus Celsus as **rubor** (redness), **calor** (heat), **tumor** (swelling), and **dolor** (pain). These *four cardinal signs of inflammation* correspond to inflammatory events of vasodilation, edema, and tissue damage

Inflammation usually defends the body but may also be harmful. Acute inflammatory responses may be exaggerated or sustained, with or without clearance of the offending agent. Tissue damage results; witness the ravages of bacterial pneumonia due to acute inflammation or joint destruction in septic arthritis. Continuing (chronic) inflammation may also damage tissue and cause scarring and loss of function, and is the basis for many degenerative diseases. Weak inflammatory responses lead to uncontrolled infection, as occurs in immunocompromised hosts.

Stages of Inflammation

- **Initiation** of an inflammatory response results in activation of soluble mediators and recruitment of inflammatory cells to the area. Molecules released from the offending agent, damaged cells, and extracellular matrix alter the permeability of nearby blood vessels to plasma, soluble molecules, and circulating inflammatory cells. This stereotypic immediate response leads to rapid flooding of injured tissues with fluid, coagulation factors, cytokines, chemokines, platelets, and inflammatory cells, neutrophils in particular (Figs. 2-1 and 2-2). This overall process is referred to as **acute inflammation**.
- **Amplification**, depending on the extent of injury, includes activation of mediators such as kinins and complement components. Additional leukocytes and macrophages are recruited to the area.
- **Destruction** of the damaging agent involves enzymatic digestion and phagocytosis of the foreign material or infectious organisms. At the same time, damaged tissue components are also removed, debris is cleared, and the repair process begins.
- **Termination** of the inflammatory response is mediated by intrinsic anti-inflammatory mechanisms that limit tissue damage and allow repair and a return to normal physiologic function. Alternatively, depending on the nature of the injury and specific inflammatory and repair responses, a scar may develop in place of normal tissue.
- **Chronic inflammation** is a persistent response. Some types of injury trigger sustained immune and inflammatory responses, in which injured tissue and foreign agents are not cleared. Chronic inflammatory infiltrates are largely lymphocytes, plasma cells, and macrophages (Fig. 2-3). Acute and chronic inflammatory infiltrates often coexist.

INITIATION OF INFLAMMATION

Infectious agents or damaged cells trigger signaling pathways, thereby provoking an innate or adaptive immune response. **Innate immunity** refers to the broad set of rapid host responses to injury that do not involve gene products or cells that employ variable regions. **Adaptive immunity** utilizes immunoglobulin molecules and T and B cells, which rely on variable regions of genes to generate immune specificity and is discussed in chapter 3. Inflammation involves a specific subset of humoral and cellular host defense mechanisms, which is central to the innate immune response.

In the setting of infection, **pathogen-associated microbial patterns** (PAMPs) of microorganisms are recognized by membrane-bound or endosomal families of **pattern-recognition receptors** (PRRs). **Danger (damage)-associated molecular patterns** (DAMPs) derived from damaged cells are released extracellularly after tissue injury and are also recognized by PRRs located on cell surfaces and intracellularly. Together, they activate intracellular cascades to drive a coordinated immune response (Figs. 2-4 and 2-5). With activation, the multifaceted inflammatory response commences and is amplified by (1) release of cytokines and chemokines, (2) activation of coagulation and complement cascades, and (3) release of free radical products (Fig. 2-5).

Pattern-Recognition Receptors

Four families of PRRs are found on inflammatory and immune cells: (1) toll-like receptors, (2) nucleotide oligomerization domain leucine-rich repeat proteins (NOD-like receptors), (3) cytoplasmic caspase activation and recruitment domain helicases, and (4) C-type lectin receptors.

Toll-Like Receptors

TLRs are a major class of PRRs found on immune, inflammatory, and tissue cells, including macrophages, endothelial cells, and epithelial cells (Table 2-1). TLRs on the cell surface recognize bacterial cell wall components and viruses. Specific TLRs recognize lipid and carbohydrates on gram-positive bacteria, fungi, lipopolysaccharides of gram-negative bacteria, and viral RNA. Although TLR engagement activates intracellular pathways to defend against microbial organisms, it may lead to excessive activation of cytokine cascades, notably contributing to septic shock.

NOD-Like Receptors

These intracellular soluble proteins are sensors for microbes (PAMPs) and cell injury (DAMPs). They form large molecular complexes, termed **inflammasomes**, that are linked to the proteolytic activation of pro-inflammatory cytokines.

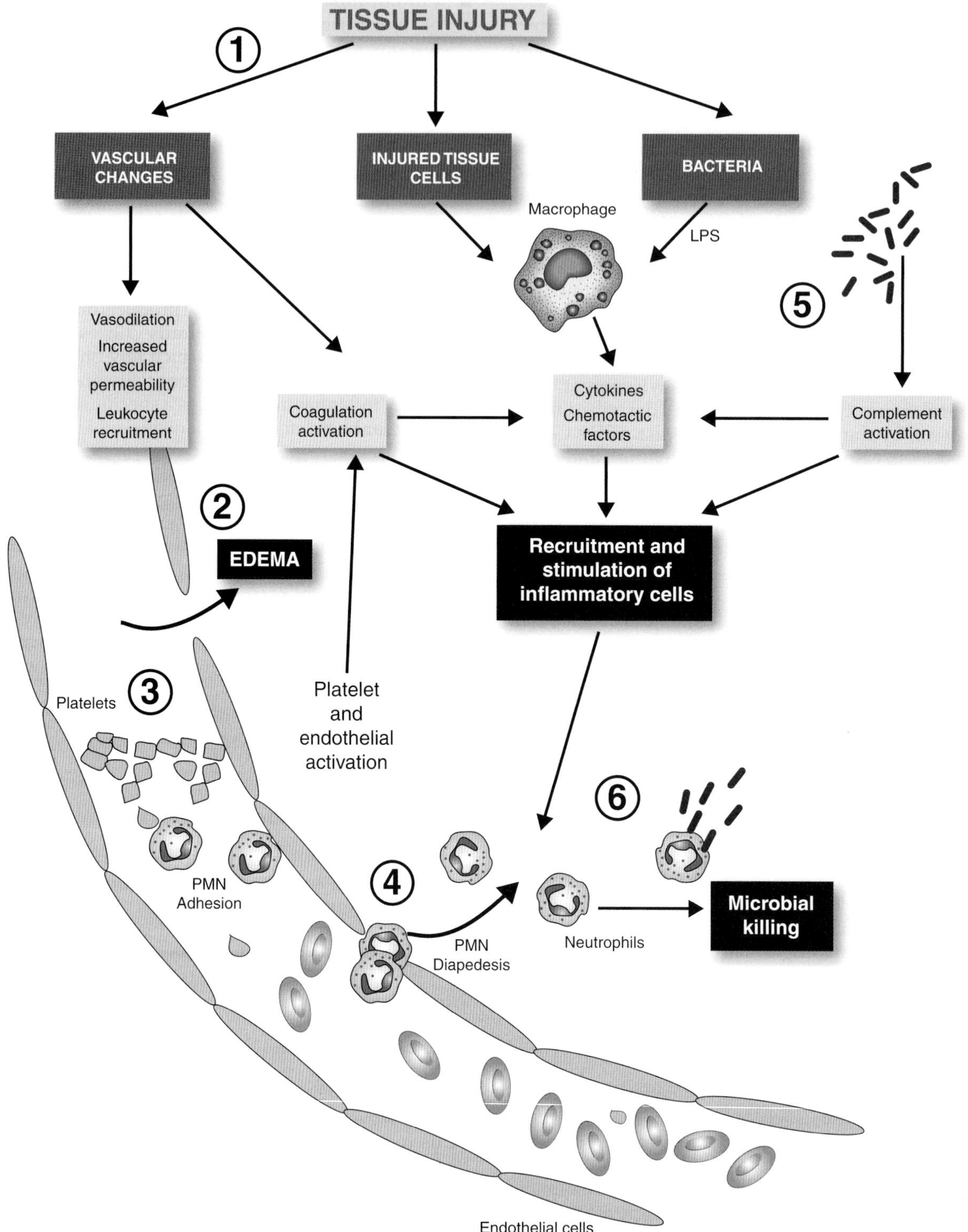

FIGURE 2-1. **The inflammatory response to injury.** (*1*) Tissue injury results in immediate and prolonged vascular changes. Chemical mediators and damaged tissue cells stimulate vasodilation and vascular injury, leading to (*2*) leakage of fluid into tissues (edema). (*3*) Platelets are activated to initiate clot formation and hemostasis and to increase vascular permeability via histamine release. (*4*) Vascular endothelial cells contribute to clot formation, anchor circulating neutrophils via their upregulated adhesion molecules, and retract to allow increased vascular permeability to plasma and to inflammatory cells. At the same time, microbes (*red rods*) (*5*) initiate activation of the complement cascade, which, along with soluble mediators from macrophages, (*6*) recruits neutrophils to the site of tissue injury. Neutrophils and macrophages eliminate microbes and remove damaged tissue so that repair can begin. LPS, lipopolysaccharides; PMN, polymorphonuclear neutrophils.

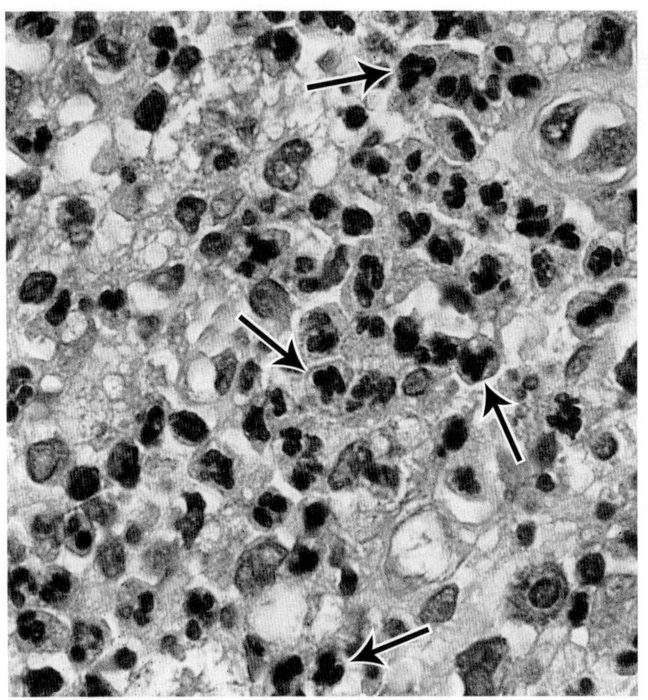

FIGURE 2-2. Acute inflammation. Densely packed polymorphonuclear leukocytes (PMNs) with multilobed nuclei (*arrows*).

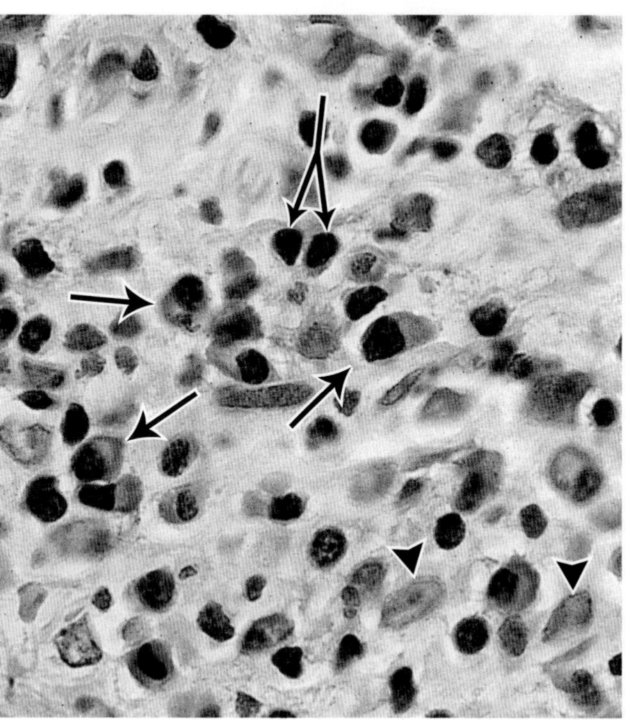

FIGURE 2-3. Chronic inflammation. Lymphocytes (*double-headed arrow*), plasma cells (*arrows*), and a few macrophages (*arrowheads*) are present.

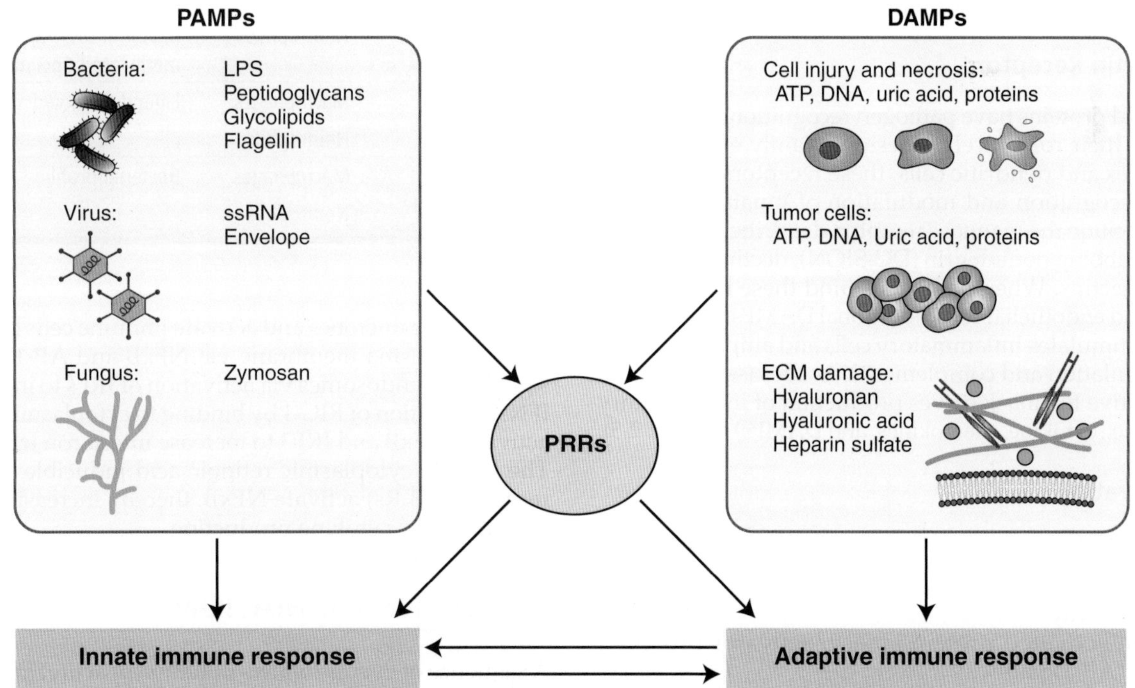

FIGURE 2-4. Pathogen-associated molecular pattern (PAMP) molecules and damage-associated molecular pattern (DAMP) molecules initiate adaptive and innate immune responses. Microbes release PAMPs. Damaged cells and tissue release DAMPs. Binding to receptors belonging to the family of pattern-recognition receptors (PRRs) mediates innate and adaptive immune responses. ATP, adenosine triphosphate; ECM, extracellular matrix; LPS, lipopolysaccharides.

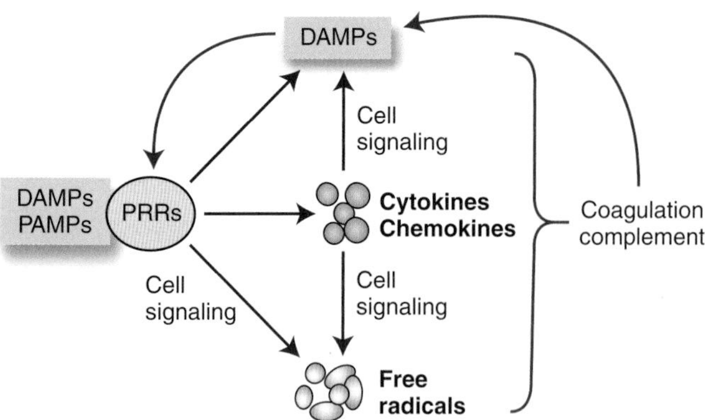

FIGURE 2-5. Damage-associated molecular pattern (DAMP) molecules and pathogen-associated molecular pattern (PAMP) molecules drive the multifaceted inflammatory response. Interaction of PAMP and DAMPs with pattern-recognition receptors (PRRs) initiates cell signaling, leading to enhanced activation of inflammatory mediators. These inflammatory signals can lead to further release of DAMPs and maintenance of the inflammatory response.

Cytoplasmic Caspase Activation and Recruitment Domain Helicases

This large family includes receptors such as retinoic acid inducible gene-1–like receptors (RIG-1–like receptors) expressed by macrophages, dendritic cells, and fibroblasts. They are cytoplasmic RNA helicases (molecules that bind to and modify RNA-protein complexes) that survey for microbes and recognize viral RNA in the cytoplasm.

C-Type Lectin Receptors

Glycosylated proteins have pathogen recognition functions in addition to their role in cell adhesion. Mainly expressed on macrophages and dendritic cells, these receptors participate in fungal recognition and modulation of innate immunity. Members include the mannose receptor, dendritic cell–specific ICAM-3–grabbing nonintegrin (DC-SIGN), dectin-1, dectin-2, and the collectins. When pathogens bind these receptors on epithelial and endothelial cells, additional DAMPs are released. This effect stimulates inflammatory cells and amplifies activation of coagulation and complement cascades (see below). In turn, a positive feedback drives production of inflammatory mediators (i.e., cytokine, chemokines, and DAMPs) (see Fig. 2-5).

Gene Activation

Pattern-recognition receptors activate three major signaling pathways:

- NFκB pathway
- Mitogen-activated protein kinase/activator protein-1 (MAPK/AP-1) pathway
- Interferon regulatory factor (IRF) pathway

Activation of NFκB promotes induction of pro-inflammatory cytokines. MAPK activates AP-1, which induces pro-inflammatory cytokines. IRFs activate type 1 interferons (IFNs) and pro-inflammatory mediators. Via these signal transduction pathways, microbial recognition activates transcription factors, which in turn bind specific sequences in gene promoters.

Table 2-1

Pathogen Recognition Receptors

Toll-Like Receptor	Cell Expression	Pathogen Recognized
TLR1	Macrophages Neutrophils	Lipid and carbohydrates from gram-positive bacteria
TLR2	Macrophages Basophils Neutrophils	Lipid and carbohydrates from gram-positive bacteria Fungal organisms
TLR3	Macrophages	Nucleic acid and derivatives Double-stranded RNA (viral DNA)
TLR4	Macrophages Basophils Neutrophils	Lipopolysaccharide from gram-negative bacteria
TLR5	Macrophages Neutrophils	Bacterial flagellin
TLR6	Macrophages Neutrophils	Lipid and carbohydrates from gram-positive bacteria
TLR7	Macrophages Neutrophils	Nucleic acid and derivatives (viral DNA)
TLR8	Macrophages Neutrophils	Nucleic acid and derivatives (viral DNA)
TLR9	Macrophages Neutrophils	Nucleic acid and derivatives Bacterial DNA containing unmethylated CpG motifs
TLR10	Macrophages Neutrophils	Ligand unknown
TLR11 (pseudogene)	Macrophages Neutrophils	Bacterial profilin

TLRs engage microbes and activate immune cells by signaling from the plasma membrane via NFκB and AP-1. TLRs also signal from endosomes via activation of IRFs to induce type 1 IFNs. Activation of RIG-1 by binding to cytoplasmic viral RNA activates NFκB and IRF3 to increase interferon transcription. The soluble cytoplasmic retinoic acid inducible gene-1–like receptors (RLRs) activate NFκB, thereby increasing IFN and inflammatory cytokine production.

ACUTE INFLAMMATION

A sequence of events follows initiation of acute inflammation:

1. ***As the immediate response to injury or insult, blood vessels rapidly and transiently constrict and then dilate.*** Under the influence of nitric oxide (NO), histamine, and other soluble agents, vasodilation allows increased blood flow and expansion of the capillary bed.
2. ***Increased vascular permeability enables fluid and plasma components to accumulate in affected tissues.*** Endothelial

cells are connected to each other by tight junctions and separated from the tissue by a limiting basement membrane (Fig. 2-6A). Thus, the endothelium is a permeability barrier as fluid moves between intravascular and extravascular spaces. ***Disruption of this barrier function is a hallmark of acute inflammation.*** Shortly after tissue injury, specific inflammatory mediators are produced at the site of injury, thereby directly increasing permeability of capillaries and postcapillary venules. Vascular leakage reflects endothelial cell contraction, endothelial cell retraction, and alterations in transcytosis. Endothelial cells are also damaged, either by direct injury to the cells or indirectly by leukocytes. Thus, there may be extensive loss of the permeability barrier, so that fluid and cells leak into the extravascular space, a condition called **edema** (Fig. 2-6B and C).

3. ***Soluble mediators stimulate intravascular platelets and inflammatory cells.*** These factors include kinins and complement. Components of the coagulation cascade are activated (Figs. 2-1 and 2-7), causing more vascular permeability and edema.
4. ***Neutrophils are recruited to the injured site.*** All these vascular changes, vasodilation, and edema increase the concentration of red blood cells and leukocytes within the capillary network. Chemotactic factors then recruit leukocytes, especially neutrophils, from the vascular compartment into the injured tissue (see Figs. 2-1 and 2-2). Once in tissues, these leukocytes start attacking offending agents, so damaged components can be removed and tissue repair can commence. These cells secrete additional mediators, which either enhance or inhibit the inflammatory response.

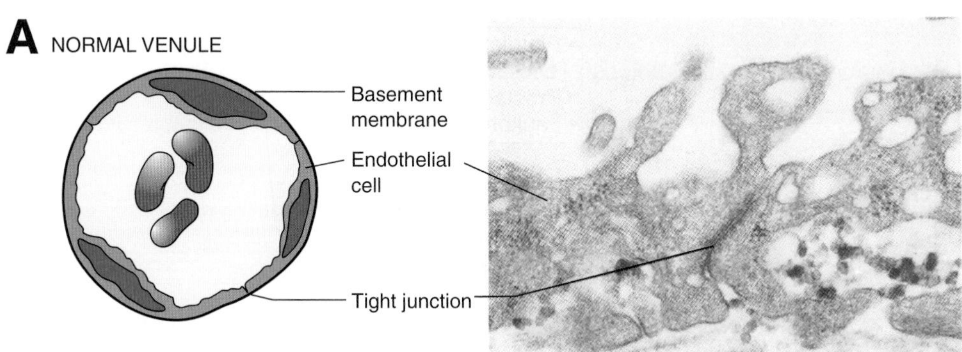

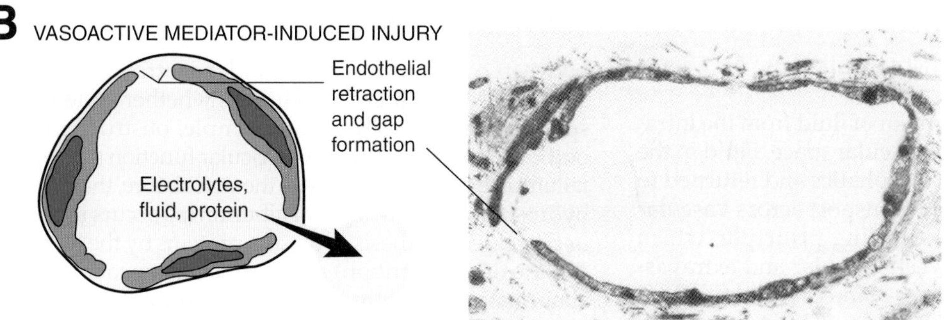

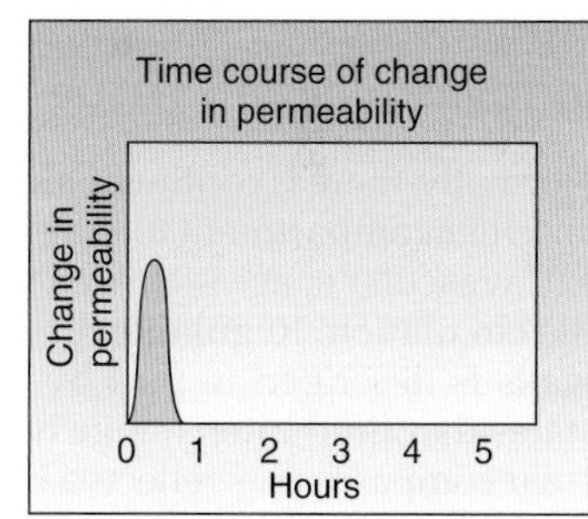

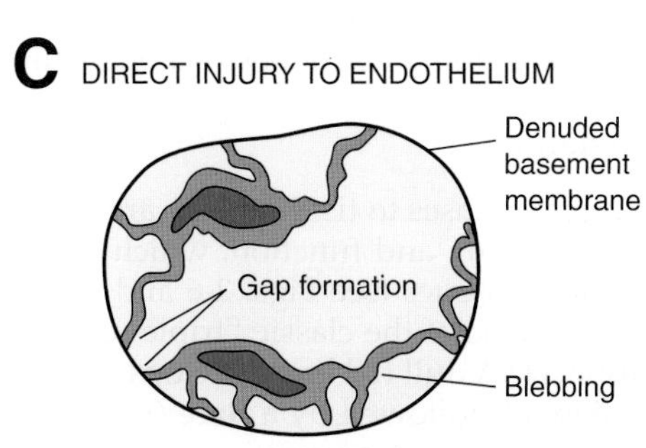

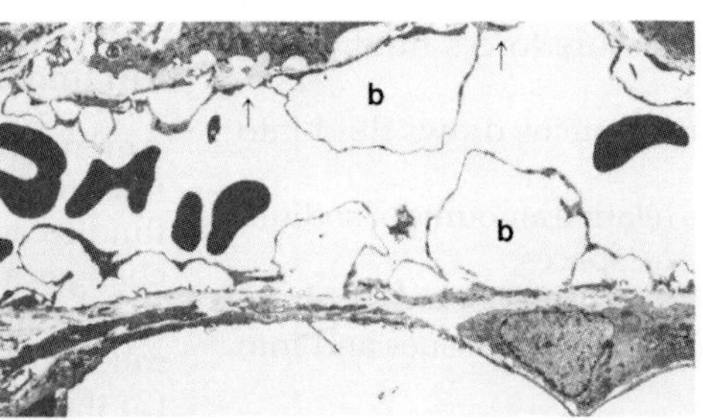

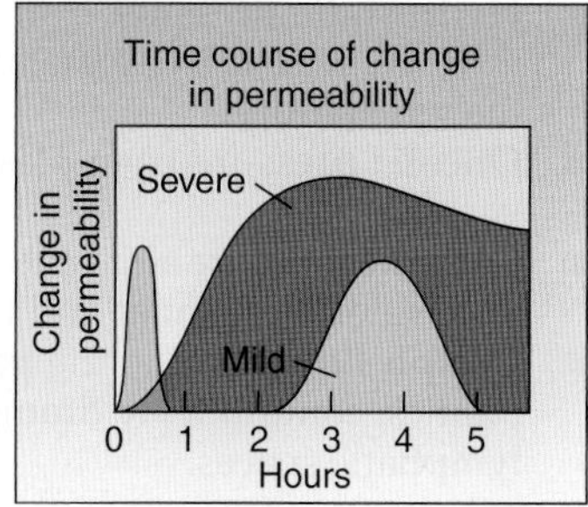

FIGURE 2-6. Responses of the microvasculature to injury. A. The wall of the normal venule is sealed by tight junctions between adjacent endothelial cells. **B.** During mild vasoactive mediator-induced injury, the endothelial cells separate and permit the passage of the fluid constituents of the blood. **C.** With severe direct injury, the endothelial cells form blebs (*b*) and separate from the underlying basement membrane. Areas of denuded basement membrane (*arrows*) allow a prolonged escape of fluid elements from the microvasculature.

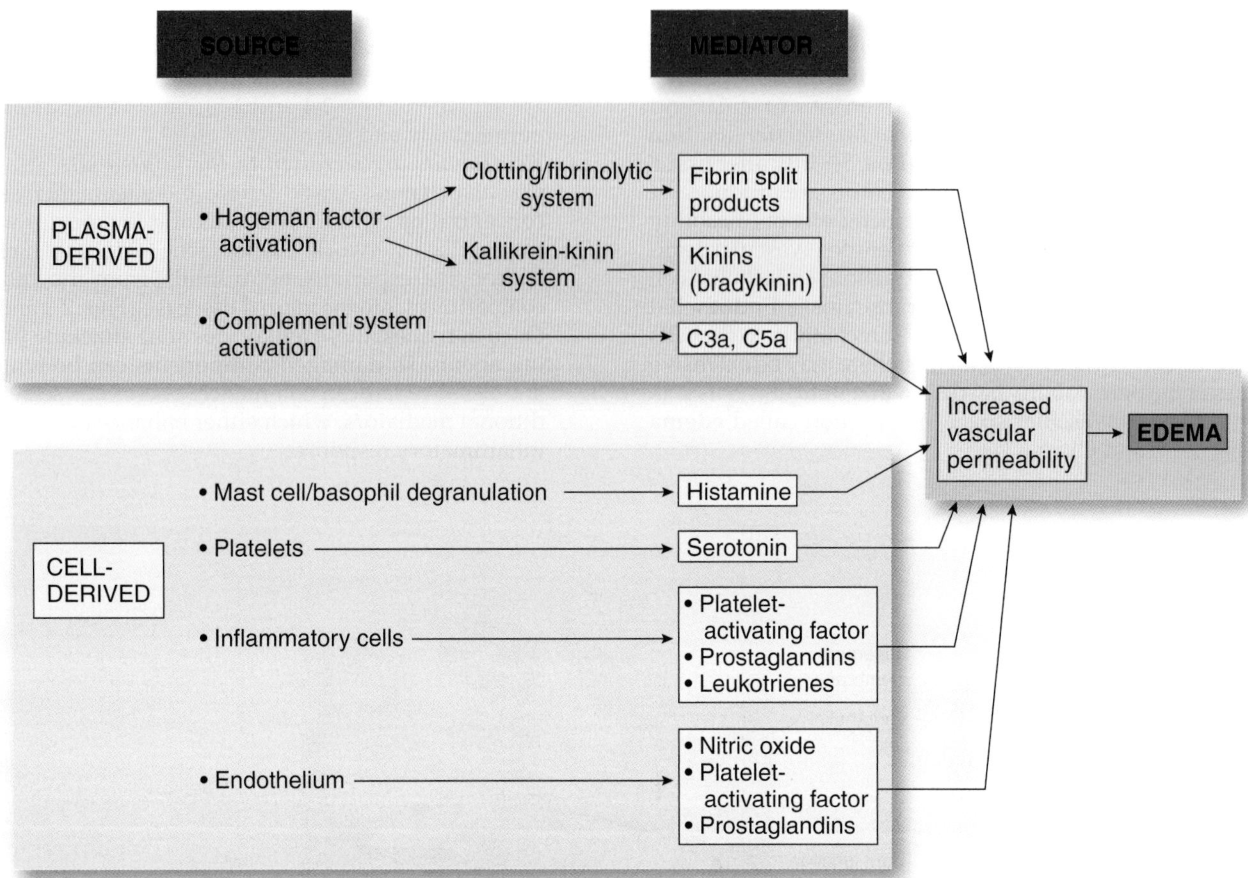

FIGURE 2-7. Inflammatory mediators of increased vascular permeability. Plasma and cell-derived products generate potent vasoactive mediators.

Intravascular and Tissue Fluid Levels

Normally, there is continual movement of fluid from the intravascular compartment to the extravascular space. Fluid in the extravascular space is cleared via lymphatics and returned to the circulation. Regulation of fluid transport across vascular walls is described in part by the **Starling principle**, which states that fluid interchange between vascular and extravascular compartments reflects a balance of forces that draw fluid into vascular spaces or out into tissues (see Chapter 8). These forces include the following:

- **Hydrostatic pressure** from blood flow and plasma volume. Increased hydrostatic pressure forces fluid out of the vasculature.
- **Oncotic pressure** from plasma proteins draws fluid into vessels.
- **Osmotic pressure** also reflects relative amounts of sodium and water in vascular and tissue spaces.
- **Lymph flow**, that is, the passage of fluid through lymphatics, continuously drains fluid out of tissues and into lymphatic spaces.

Noninflammatory Edema

If the balance of forces controlling fluid transport is altered, flow into the extravascular compartment or clearance through lymphatics is disrupted. The net result is fluid accumulation in interstitial spaces **(edema)**. This excess fluid expands spaces between cells and the extracellular matrix and causes tissue swelling. Many clinical conditions, whether systemic or organ specific, lead to edema. For example, obstruction of venous outflow or decreased right ventricular function (congestive heart failure) causes back pressure in the vasculature, thereby increasing hydrostatic pressure. Loss of albumin (as occurs in renal disease or decreased synthesis of plasma proteins by the liver in hepatic disease or malnutrition) reduces plasma oncotic pressure. Any abnormality of sodium or water retention alters osmotic pressure and the balance of fluid forces. Finally, **lymphedema** may result from obstruction to lymphatic flow, most often due to surgical removal of lymph nodes, radiation, or obstruction by tumor.

Inflammatory Edema

Among the earliest responses to tissue injury are changes in microvasculature anatomy and function, which may allow fluid to accumulate in tissues (see Figs. 2-6 and 2-7). These changes are characteristic of the classic "triple response" of acute inflammation. (1) A dull red line develops at the site of mild trauma to skin, (2) followed by a **flare** (red halo), and (3) then a **wheal** (swelling). A vasoactive mediator causes vasodilation and increased vascular permeability at the site of injury. The triple response can be explained as follows:

1. **Transient vasoconstriction of arterioles** at a site of insult is the earliest vascular response to mild skin injury. This process is caused by neurogenic and chemical mediator systems and usually resolves within seconds to minutes.

2. **Vasodilation of precapillary arterioles** then increases blood flow to the tissue (**hyperemia)**. This effect is caused by release of specific mediators and is responsible for redness and warmth at sites of tissue injury.
3. **An increase in endothelial cell barrier permeability** results in edema. Fluid passes from intravascular compartments as blood passes through capillaries and venules where it produces local stasis and plugging of dilated small vessels with erythrocytes. These changes are reversible after mild injury; within several minutes to hours, extravascular fluid is cleared via lymphatics.

The vascular response to injury is a dynamic event, with sequential physiologic and pathologic changes. **Vasoactive mediators**, originating from plasma and cells, are generated at sites of tissue injury (Fig. 2-7). These molecules bind specific receptors on vascular endothelial and smooth muscle cells, resulting in vasoconstriction or vasodilation. Vasodilation of arterioles increases blood flow and exacerbates fluid leakage into the tissue. Vasoconstriction of postcapillary venules increases capillary bed hydrostatic pressure, further stimulating edema formation.

After injury, vasoactive mediators bind specific receptors on endothelial cells, causing reversible endothelial cell contraction and gap formation (Fig. 2-6B). This discontinuity in the endothelial barrier gives rise to extravasation (leakage) of intravascular fluids into the extravascular space. Mild direct endothelial injury causes a biphasic response: an early change in permeability within 30 minutes of injury, followed by a second increase in vascular permeability after 3 to 5 hours. With severe damage, fluid progressively moves into the extravascular compartment, peaking 3 to 4 hours after injury.

Severe direct injury to the endothelium, such as injury caused by burns or caustic chemicals, may produce irreversible damage. In such cases, the vascular endothelium separates from the basement membrane, promoting cell blebbing (blisters or bubbles between the endothelium and basement membrane). This leaves areas of basement membrane naked (Fig. 2-6C), disrupting the barrier between intravascular and extravascular spaces.

Specialized terminology used in describing the consequences of inflammation is summarized in Table 2-2.

PLASMA-DERIVED MEDIATORS IN THE INFLAMMATORY RESPONSE

Plasma-Derived Mediators of Inflammation

Chemical mediators help to trigger, amplify, and terminate inflammatory processes (Fig. 2-8). Cell- and plasma-derived mediators work in concert to activate cells by binding specific receptors, activating cells, recruiting cells to sites of injury, and stimulating release of additional soluble mediators. These mediators themselves are short-lived or are inhibited by intrinsic mechanisms, effectively turning off the response and allowing the process to resolve. This effect acts as "on" and "off" control mechanisms of inflammation.

Plasma contains the elements of three major enzyme cascades, each composed of a series of proteases. Sequential activation of proteases results in release of important chemical mediators. These interrelated systems include (1) the **coagulation cascade**, (2) **kinins**, and (3) the **complement system** (Figs. 2-9 and 2-10). The coagulation cascade is discussed in Chapter 18; the kinin and complement systems are presented here.

Table 2-2

Definitions

Term	Definition
Edema	Accumulation of fluid in the extravascular space and interstitial tissues
Effusion	Excess fluid in body cavities (e.g., peritoneum or pleura)
Transudate	Edema fluid with a low protein content (specific gravity <1.015)
Exudate	Edema fluid with a high protein concentration (specific gravity >1.015), which frequently contains inflammatory cells
Serous exudate, or effusion	The absence of a prominent cellular response and has a yellow, straw-like color
Serosanguineous exudate	A serous exudate, or effusion, that contains red blood cells and has a reddish tinge
Fibrinous exudate	Large amounts of fibrin, owing to activation of the coagulation system. When a fibrinous exudate occurs on a serosal surface, such as the pleura or pericardium, it is termed "fibrinous pleuritis" or "fibrinous pericarditis."
Purulent exudate or effusion	Contains prominent cellular components. Purulent exudates and effusions are often associated with pathologic conditions, such as pyogenic bacterial infections, in which polymorphonuclear neutrophils predominate.
Suppurative inflammation	A purulent exudate is accompanied by significant liquefactive necrosis; the equivalent of pus.

Kinins and the Inflammatory Response

Kinins are potent inflammatory agents formed in plasma and tissue by the action of serine protease kallikreins on specific plasma glycoproteins, called **kininogens**. Bradykinin and related peptides regulate multiple physiologic processes, including blood pressure, contraction and relaxation of smooth muscle, plasma extravasation, cell migration, inflammatory cell activation, and inflammatory-mediated pain responses. The immediate effects of kinins are mediated by B_1 and B_2 receptors. The former are induced by inflammatory mediators and selectively activated by bradykinin metabolites. The latter are expressed constitutively and widely.

Kinins act quickly and then are rapidly inactivated by kininases. Perhaps the most significant function of kinins is their ability to amplify inflammatory responses by stimulating local tissue cells and inflammatory cells to generate additional mediators, such as prostanoids, cytokines (e.g., tumor necrosis factor-α [TNF-α] and interleukins), NO, and tachykinins.

Hageman factor (clotting factor XII) plays a major role in the production of kinins. The factor is present within the plasma and is activated by exposure to negatively charged surfaces,

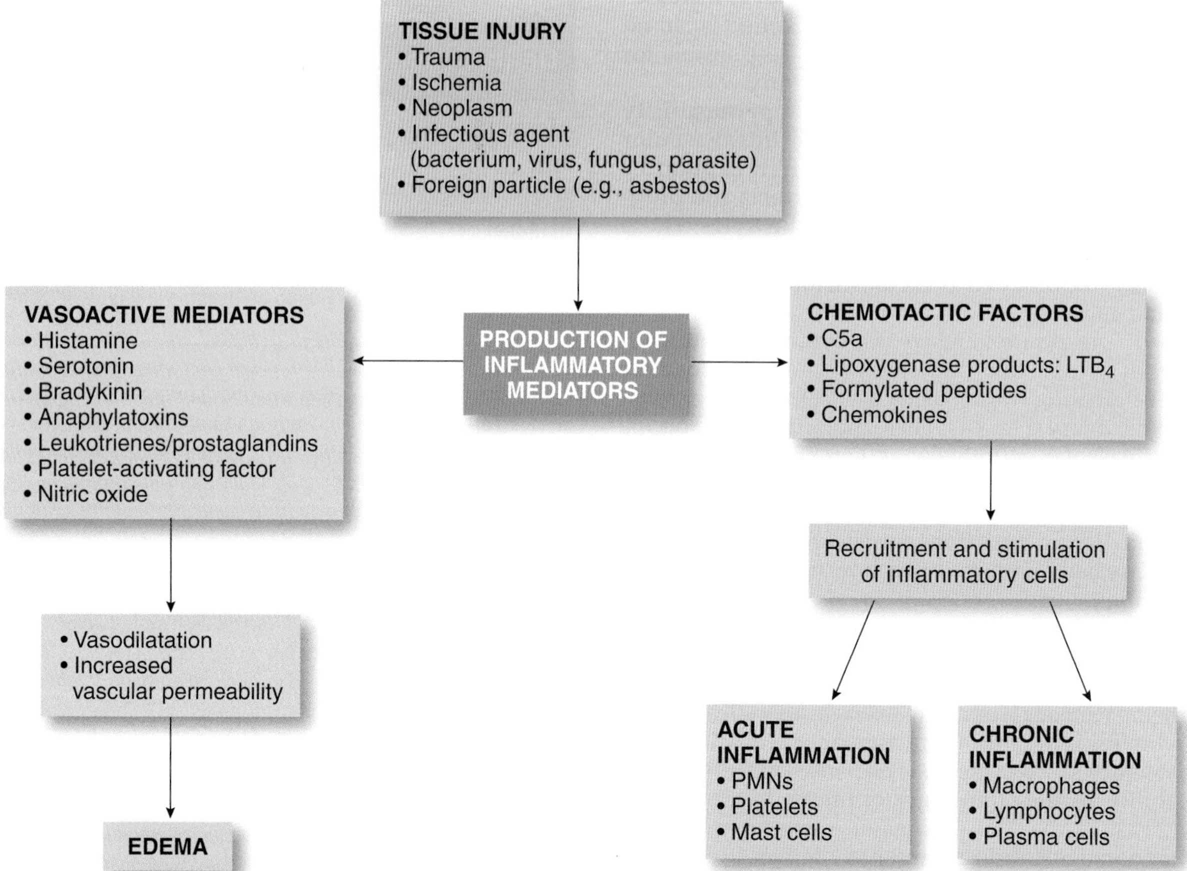

FIGURE 2-8. Mediators of the inflammatory response. Tissue injury stimulates the production of inflammatory mediators in plasma and released into the circulation. Additional factors are generated by tissue cells and inflammatory cells. These vasoactive and chemotactic mediators promote edema and recruit inflammatory cells to the site of injury. LTB^4, leukotriene B_4; PMNs, polymorphonuclear leukocytes.

such as basement membranes, proteolytic enzymes, bacterial lipopolysaccharides, and foreign materials. It triggers activation of additional plasma proteases (Fig. 2-9), leading to the following:

- **Conversion of plasminogen to plasmin:** Plasmin generated by activated Hageman factor induces clot dissolution (fibrinolysis). Products of fibrin degradation (fibrin split products) increase vascular permeability in the skin and lung. Plasmin also cleaves complement components, generating biologically active products, such as anaphylatoxins, C3a, and C5a.
- **Conversion of prekallikrein to kallikrein:** Plasma kallikrein, also generated by activated factor XII, cleaves high–molecular-weight kininogen to produce several vasoactive low–molecular-weight peptides, collectively called **kinins**.
- **Activation of the alternative complement pathway.**
- **Activation of the coagulation system** (see Chapter 18).

Role of Complement in the Immune Response

The complement system is a group of proteins found in plasma and on cell surfaces. Its main function is defense against microbes. The complement system has over 30 proteins, including plasma enzymes, regulatory proteins, and cell lytic proteins. They are mainly made in the liver and are activated in sequence.

Physiologic activities of the complement system include (1) defense against pyogenic bacterial infection by opsonization, chemotaxis, activation of leukocytes, and lysis of bacteria and cells; (2) bridging innate and adaptive immunity to defend against microbial agents by augmenting antibody responses and enhancing immune memory; and (3) disposal of immune products and products of inflammatory injury by clearing immune complexes from tissues and removing apoptotic cells. Certain complement components, namely **anaphylatoxins**, are vasoactive mediators. Others fix opsonins to cell surfaces. Still others lyse cells by generating a lytic complex, termed C5b-9 **(membrane attack complex [MAC])**. Proteins that activate complement are themselves activated by three convergent routes: the **classical**, **mannose-binding lectin (MBL)**, and **alternative** pathways.

The Classical Complement Pathway

Activators of the classical pathway include antigen–antibody (Ag–Ab) complexes, products of bacteria and viruses, proteases, urate crystals, apoptotic cells, and polyanions (polynucleotides). This pathway includes C1 through C9, the nomenclature following historical order of discovery. Following C1q binding, active C1s initiates the cascade by

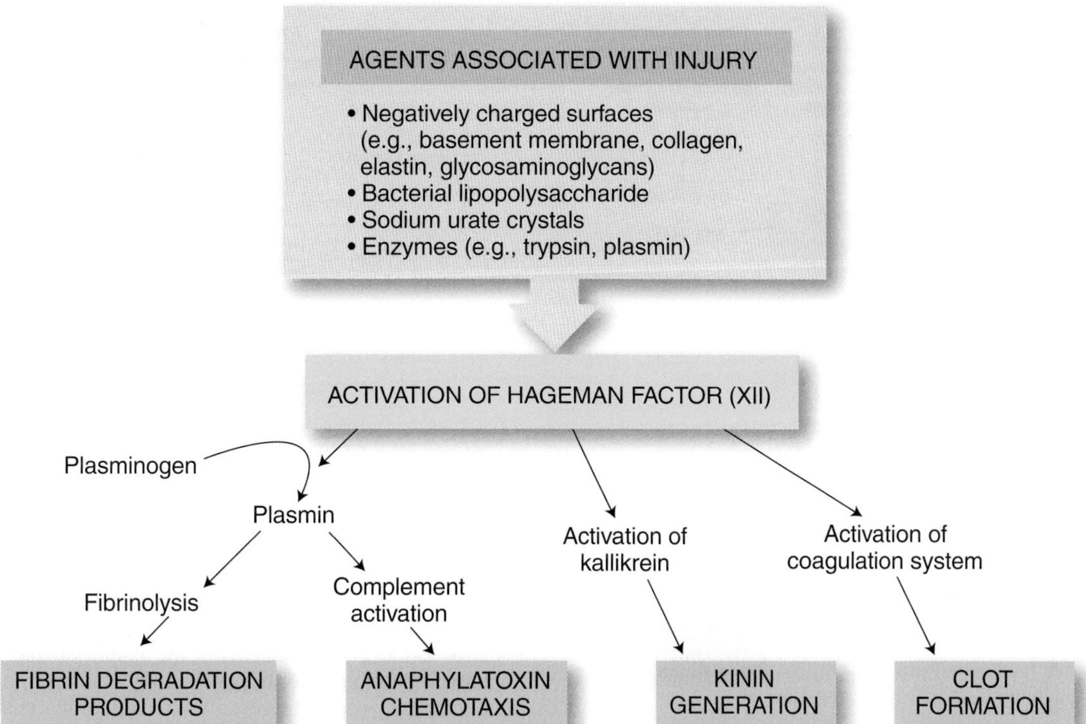

FIGURE 2-9. Hageman factor activation and inflammatory mediator production. Hageman factor activation is a key event leading to conversion of plasminogen to plasmin, resulting in generation of fibrin split products and active complement products. Activation of kallikrein produces kinins, and activation of the coagulation system results in clot formation.

cleaving C4. This triggers a cascade that leads to formation of the MAC (Fig. 2-10).

The Mannose-Binding Pathway

The mannose- or lectin-binding pathway shares some elements with the classical pathway. It begins when microbes with terminal mannose groups bind **mannose binding lectin (MBL)**, one of the family of calcium-dependent lectins, or **collectins**. This multifunctional acute phase protein resembles immunoglobulin M (IgM) in binding many oligosaccharide structures. It is similar to IgG by interacting with phagocytic receptors and C1q. This last property enables it to interact with C1r–C1s or with a serine protease called MASP (*M*BL-*a*ssociated *s*erine *p*rotease) to activate complement (see Fig. 2-10).

The Alternative Pathway

This pathway is initiated by derivative products of microorganisms, like endotoxin (from bacterial cell surfaces), zymosan (yeast cell walls), polysaccharides, cobra venom factor, viruses, tumor cells, and foreign materials. Alternative pathway members are "factors," followed by a letter (see Fig. 2-10). The alternate pathway is triggered by the binding of spontaneously formed C3b to an initiating substance such as bacterial surface carbohydrate or protein. In the presence of factors B and D, an alternative pathway C3 convertase is formed, which ultimately leads to the activation of C5 and assembly of MAC. The alternate pathway also serves to amplify complement components activated by the classical and mannose-binding pathways.

The Complement System

Biologic Activities of Complement Components

The endpoint of complement activation is MAC formation and cell lysis. Cleavage products generated at each step both catalyze the next step in the cascade and have supporting roles as important inflammatory molecules (Fig. 2-11):

- **Anaphylatoxins** (C3a, C4a, C5a): These pro-inflammatory molecules mediate smooth muscle contraction and increase vascular permeability.
- **Opsonins** (C3b, iC3b): In bacterial opsonization, a specific molecule (e.g., IgG or C3b) binds the surface of a bacterium. The process enhances phagocytosis by allowing receptors on phagocytic cell membranes (e.g., Fc receptor or C3b receptor) to recognize and bind the opsonized bacterium.
- **Pro-inflammatory molecules** (MAC, C5a): These chemotactic factors also activate leukocytes and tissue cells to generate oxidants and cytokines and induce mast cell and basophil degranulation.
- **Lysis** (MAC): C5b binds C6 and C7, and subsequently C8 to the target cell; C9 polymerization is catalyzed to lyse the cell membrane.

Regulation of the Complement System

Proteins in serum and on cell surfaces protect the host from indiscriminate injury by regulating complement activation. Four major mechanisms mediate this effect:

- **Spontaneous decay:** C4b2a and C3bBb and their cleavage products, C3b and C4b, decrease by decay.

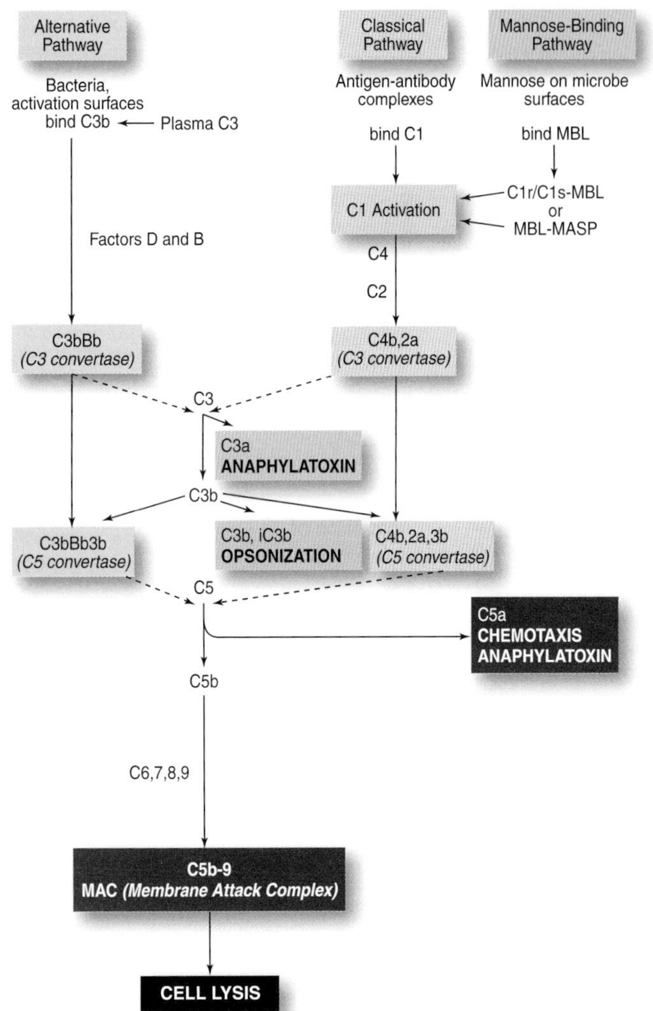

FIGURE 2-10. Complement activation. The alternative, classical, and mannose-binding pathways lead to generation of the complement cascade of inflammatory mediators and to cell lysis by the MAC. MBL, mannose-binding lectin; MBL-MASP, MBL-associated serine protease.

- **Proteolytic inactivation:** Plasma inhibitors include factor I (an inhibitor of C3b and C4b) and serum carboxypeptidase N (SCPN). SCPN removes a carboxy-terminal arginine from anaphylatoxins C4a, C3a, and C5a. Deleting this single amino acid markedly decreases their biologic activities.
- **Binding active components:** C1 esterase inhibitor (C1 INA) binds C1r and C1s to form an irreversibly inactive complex. Other binding proteins in the plasma include factor H- and C4b-binding protein. These complex with C3b and C4b, respectively, increasing their susceptibility to proteolytic cleavage by factor I.
- **Cell membrane–associated molecules:** Two proteins linked to the cell membrane by glycophosphoinositol (GPI) anchors are decay-accelerating factor (DAF, CD55) and protectin (CD59). CD 59 prevents the association of C8 and C9 preventing the formation of MAC. DAF binds membrane-associated C3b and C4b, preventing the conversion of C2 to C2a and also blocking formation of the alternative pathway C3b convertase. Hence, DAF also indirectly blocks the formation of MAC.

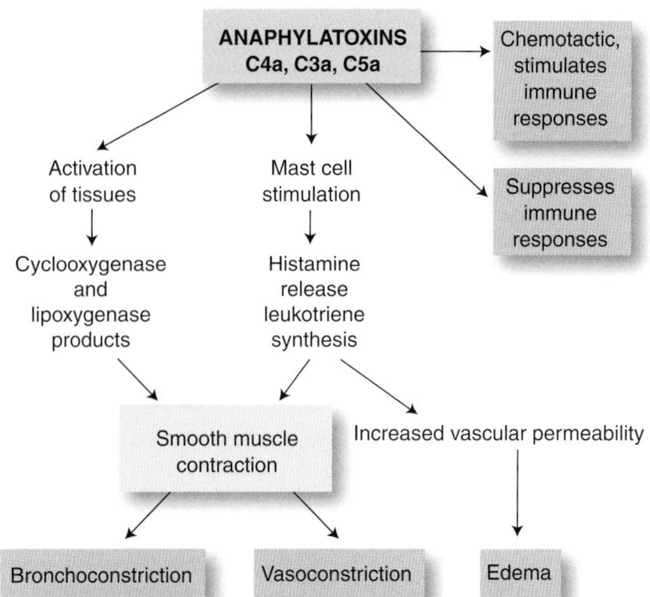

FIGURE 2-11. Biologic activity of the anaphylatoxins. Complement activation products, generated during activation of the complement cascade, regulate vascular permeability, cell recruitment, and smooth muscle contraction.

The Complement System and Microorganisms

When the mechanisms regulating this balance malfunction or are deficient because of mutation, resulting imbalances in complement activity can cause tissue injury. Uncontrolled systemic activation of complement may occur in sepsis, playing a central role in the development of septic shock (see below).

Immune Complexes

Immune complexes (Ag–Ab complexes) form on bacterial surfaces and associate with C1q, activating the classical pathway. Complement then promotes physiologic clearance of circulating immune complexes. However, if these complexes are made continuously and in excess (e.g., in chronic immune responses), relentless activation consumes, and therefore, depletes complement. Failure of complement function, whether due to complement depletion, deficient complement binding, or defects in complement activation, results in immune deposition and inflammation, which in turn may trigger autoimmunity.

Infectious Disease

Defense against infection is a key role of complement. If the system functions poorly, the person is overly susceptible to infection.

- Defects in antibody production, complement proteins, or phagocyte function increase susceptibility to pyogenic infections with organisms such as *Haemophilus influenzae* and *Streptococcus pneumoniae.*
- Deficiencies in MAC formation lead to increased infections, particularly with meningococci.
- Deficiency of complement MBL results in recurrent infections in young children.

Thick capsules may protect some bacteria from lysis by complement. Some bacterial enzymes can also inhibit the effects of complement components, especially C5a. Or, they can also increase catabolism of components, such as C3b, thereby reducing formation of C3 convertase. Some bacteria and viruses, on the other hand, may use cell-bound components and receptors to facilitate cell entry. *Mycobacterium tuberculosis*, Epstein–Barr virus, measles virus, picornaviruses, HIV, and flaviviruses use complement components to target inflammatory or epithelial cells.

Inflammation and Necrosis

The complement system amplifies the inflammatory response. Anaphylatoxins C5a and C3a activate leukocytes, and C5a and MAC stimulate endothelial cells. These effects induce excess generation of oxidants and cytokines that injure tissues (see Chapter 1). After which nonviable or damaged tissues cannot regulate complement normally.

Complement Deficiencies

The importance of an intact and appropriately regulated complement system is exemplified in people with acquired or congenital deficiencies of specific complement components or regulatory proteins (Table 2-3). The most common congenital defect is a C2 deficiency, inherited as an autosomal recessive trait.

Acquired deficiencies of early complement components occur in patients with some autoimmune diseases, especially those associated with circulating immune complexes. These include certain forms of membranous glomerulonephritis and systemic lupus erythematosus. Deficiencies in early components of complement (e.g., C1q, C1r, C1s, C4) are strongly associated with susceptibility to lupus.

Patients lacking the middle (C3, C5) components are prone to recurrent pyogenic infections, membranoproliferative glomerulonephritis, and rashes. Those who lack terminal complement components (C6, C7, or C8) are vulnerable to infections with *Neisseria* species. Such differences in susceptibility underscore the roles of individual complement components in protecting from specific bacteria. Congenital defects in proteins that regulate the complement system (e.g., C1 inhibitor, serum carboxypeptidase) lead to chronic complement activation. Lack of C1 inhibitor is associated with hereditary angioedema.

Table 2-3

Hereditary Complement Deficiencies

Complement Deficiency	Clinical Association
C3b, iC3b, C5, MBL	Pyogenic bacterial infections Membranoproliferative glomerulonephritis
C3, properdin, MAC proteins	Neisserial infection
C1 inhibitor	Hereditary angioedema
CD59	Hemolysis, thrombosis
C1q, C1r and C1s, C4, C2	Systemic lupus erythematosus
Factors H and I	Hemolytic–uremic syndrome Membranoproliferative glomerulonephritis

MAC, membrane attack complex; MBL, mannose-binding lectin.

ROLE OF CELL-DERIVED MEDIATORS

Platelets, basophils, PMNs, endothelial cells, monocyte/macrophages, tissue mast cells, and the injured tissue itself may all potentially generate vasoactive and inflammatory mediators. Derivation of these molecules is as follows:

1. Metabolism of phospholipids and arachidonic acid (e.g., prostaglandins, thromboxanes, leukotrienes, lipoxins, platelet-activating factor [PAF])
2. Low–molecular-weight proteins secreted by activated cells notably macrophages termed cytokines
3. Preformed and stored in cytoplasmic granules (e.g., histamine, serotonin, lysosomal hydrolases) (see section on "Cells of Inflammation")
4. Derived from altered production of normal regulators of vascular function (e.g., nitric oxide and neurokinins)

Prostanoids, Leukotrienes, and Lipoxins

Phospholipids and fatty acid derivatives released from plasma membranes are metabolized into mediators and homeostatic regulators by inflammatory cells and injured tissues. As part of a complex regulatory network, prostanoids, leukotrienes, and lipoxins, which are derivatives of arachidonic acid, both promote and inhibit inflammation (Table 2-4). The net impact depends on several factors, including levels and profiles of prostanoid production, both of which change during an inflammatory response.

Table 2-4

Biologic Activities of Arachidonic Acid Metabolites

Metabolite	Biologic Activity
PGE_2, PGD_2	Induce vasodilation, bronchodilation; inhibit inflammatory cell function
PGI_2	Induces vasodilation, bronchodilation; inhibits inflammatory cell function
PGF_{2a}	Induces vasodilation, bronchoconstriction
TXA_2	Induces vasoconstriction, bronchoconstriction; enhances inflammatory cell functions (esp. platelets)
LTB_4	Chemotactic for phagocytic cells; stimulates phagocytic cell adherence; enhances microvascular permeability
LTC_4, LTD_4, LTE_4	Induce smooth muscle contraction; constrict pulmonary airways; increase microvascular permeability

LT. . ., leukotriene; PG. . ., prostaglandin; TXA_2, thromboxane A_2.

Prostanoids

Depending on the specific inflammatory cell and nature of the stimulus, activated cells generate arachidonic acid predominantly (1) from the glycerol of cell membrane phospholipids (in particular, phosphatidylcholine), (2) by stimulus-induced activation of phospholipase A_2 (PLA_2), and (3) by increased synthesis of secretory PLA_2 IIA in the presence of pro-inflammatory cytokines. Arachidonic acid is further metabolized by cyclooxygenases 1 and 2 (COX-1, COX-2) to generate prostanoids (Fig. 2-12). **COX-1** is constitutively expressed by most cells and increases upon cell activation. It is a key enzyme in the synthesis of prostaglandins, which in turn (1) protect the gut mucosa, (2) regulate water/electrolyte balance, (3) stimulate platelet aggregation to maintain normal hemostasis, and (4) maintain resistance to thrombosis on vascular endothelial cell surfaces. **COX-2** expression is generally low or undetectable but increases substantially upon stimulation to yield metabolites that are important in inducing pain and inflammation.

During inflammation, COX-2 becomes the major source of prostanoids. Both COX isoforms generate prostaglandin H_2 (PGH_2), which is the substrate for production of prostacyclin (PGI_2), PGD_2, PGE_2, $PGF_{2\alpha}$, and TXA_2 (thromboxane). The quantity and variety of prostaglandins produced during inflammation depend in part on the cells present and their state of activation. Thus, mast cells make mostly PGD_2; macrophages generate PGE_2 and TXA_2; platelets are the major source of TXA_2; and endothelial cells secrete PGI_2.

Inhibition of COX is one mechanism by which nonsteroidal anti-inflammatory drugs (NSAIDs), including aspirin, indomethacin, and ibuprofen, exert potent analgesic and anti-inflammatory effects. NSAIDs block COX-2–induced formation of prostaglandins, and so mitigate pain and inflammation. However, they also affect COX-1, decreasing homeostatic functions and affecting the stomach and kidneys adversely. This complication has led to the development of COX-2–specific inhibitors.

Leukotrienes

Leukotrienes are the second major family of derivatives of arachidonic acid (see Fig. 2-12). The enzyme 5-lipoxygenase (5-LOX) promotes the synthesis of 5-hydroperoxyeicosatetraenoic acid (5-HpETE) and leukotriene A_4 (LTA_4) from arachidonic acid. LTA_4 is metabolized to LTB_4, a potent chemotactic agent for neutrophils, monocytes, and macrophages. In other cells, especially mast cells, basophils, and macrophages, LTA_4 is converted to LTC_4 and thence to LTD_4 and LTE_4. These three cysteinyl leukotrienes (1) stimulate smooth muscle contraction, (2) enhance vascular permeability, and (3) are responsible for many of the clinical symptoms associated with allergic-type reactions. Thus, they play a pivotal role in the development of asthma. Leukotrienes exert their action through high-affinity specific receptors, which are important targets of drug therapy.

Lipoxins

Lipoxins, the third class of arachidonic acid products, are made in the vascular lumen by cell–cell interactions (see Fig. 2-12). They are pro-inflammatory and generated during inflammation, atherosclerosis, and thrombosis. Aspirin initiates the production of 15-epi-LXs, which are anti-inflammatory lipid mediators. Thus, this is another pathway in which aspirin exerts a beneficial effect.

Cytokines

Many different cytokines, including interleukins, growth factors, colony-stimulating factors, interferons, and chemokines, are produced at sites of inflammation (Fig. 2-13).

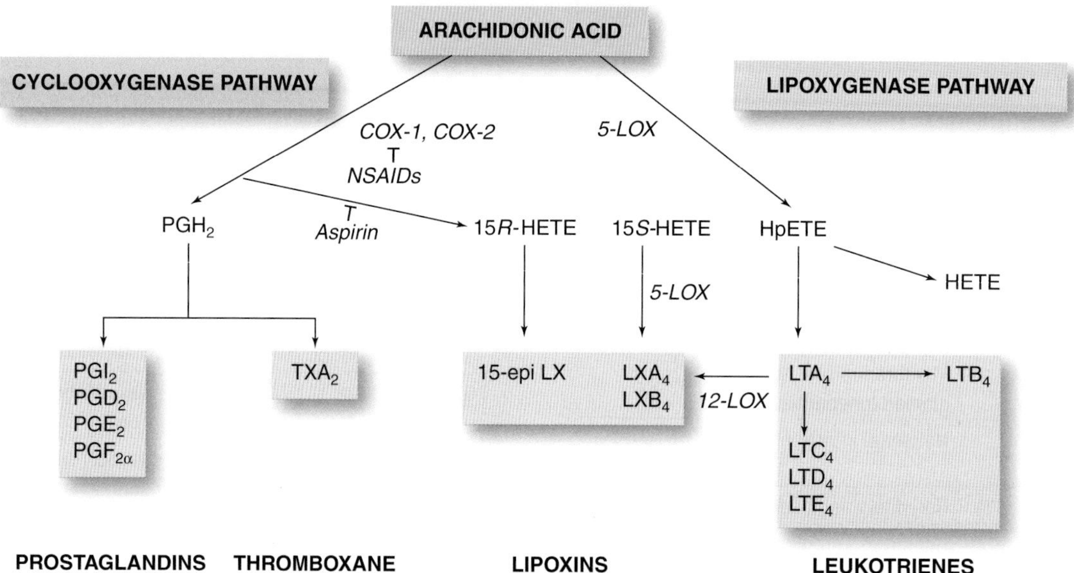

FIGURE 2-12. Biologically active arachidonic acid metabolites. The cyclooxygenase (COX) pathway of arachidonic acid metabolism generates prostaglandins (PG. . .) and thromboxane (TXA_2). The lipoxygenase (LOX) pathway forms lipoxins (LX. . .) and leukotrienes (LT. . .). Aspirin (acetylsalicylic acid) blocks the formation of 5-HETE (hydroxyeicosatetraenoic acid). nonsteroidal anti-inflammatory drugs (NSAIDs) block COX-1 and COX-2. HpETE, 5-hydroperoxyeicosatetraenoic acid.

Interleukins	Growth Factors	Chemokines	Interferons	Pro-Inflammatory Cytokines
IL-1 IL-6 IL-8 IL-13 IL-10	GM-CSF M-CSF	CC CXC XC CX3C	IFNα IFNβ IFNγ	TNFα
• Inflammatory cell activation	• Macrophage • Bactericidal activity • NK and dendritic cell function	• Leukocyte chemotaxis • Leukocyte activation	• Antiviral • Leukocyte activation	• Fever • Anorexia • Shock • Cytotoxicity • Cytokine induction • Activation of endothelial cells and tissue cells

FIGURE 2-13. Cytokines important in inflammation. GM-CSF, granulocyte–macrophage colony-stimulating factor; IFN, interferon; IL, interleukin; M-CSF, macrophage colony-stimulating factor; NK, natural killer; TNF, tumor necrosis factor.

Cytokines are low–molecular-weight proteins secreted by activated cells. They are produced at sites of tissue injury and regulate inflammatory responses from initial changes in vascular permeability to resolution and restoration of tissue integrity. Cytokines are inflammatory hormones that act in several modes: **autocrine**, affecting cells that make them; **paracrine**, affecting neighboring cells; and **endocrine**, acting via the bloodstream on distant cells. Although most cells produce cytokines, they differ in their cytokine repertoires.

Macrophages orchestrate tissue inflammatory responses via cytokine production. **Lipopolysaccharide (LPS)**, a constituent of gram-negative bacterial outer membranes, is a highly potent activator of macrophages, as well as of endothelial cells and leukocytes (Fig. 2-14). It triggers macrophage synthesis of TNF-α and interleukins (IL-1, IL-6, IL-8, IL-12, and others). Macrophage-derived cytokines (1) modulate endothelial cell–leukocyte adhesion (TNF-α), (2) leukocyte recruitment (IL-8), (3) acute phase responses (IL-6, IL-1), and (4) immune functions (IL-1, IL-6, IL-12).

IL-1 and TNF-α, produced by macrophages and other cells, are central to development and amplification of inflammatory responses. These cytokines activate endothelial cells to express adhesion molecules and then release cytokines, chemokines, and reactive oxygen species (ROS). TNF-α causes priming and aggregation of neutrophils. IL-1 and TNF-α are also among the mediators of fever, catabolism of muscle, shifts in protein synthesis, and hemodynamic effects associated with inflammatory states (Fig. 2-14).

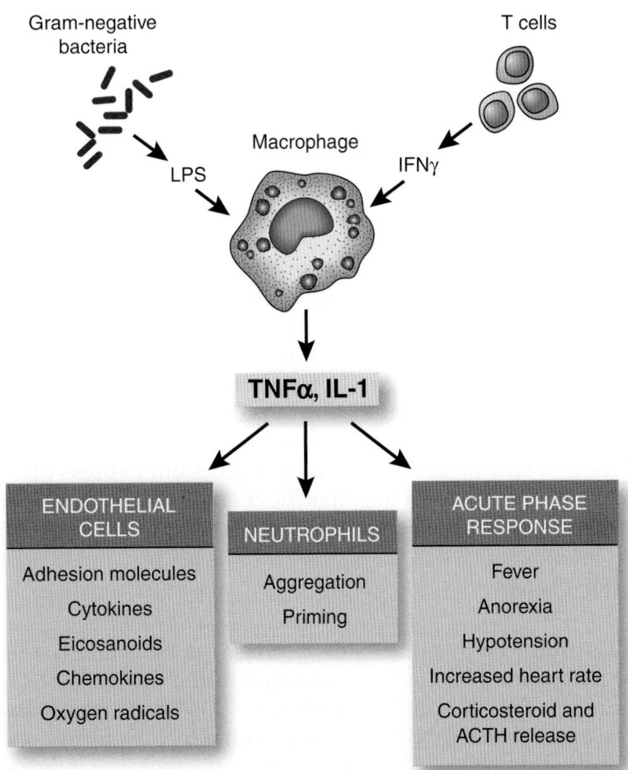

FIGURE 2-14. Central role of interleukin (IL)-1 and tumor necrosis factor (TNF)-α in inflammation. Lipopolysaccharide (LPS) and interferon-γ (IFN-γ) activate macrophages to release inflammatory cytokines, principally IL-1 and TNF-α, responsible for directing local and systemic inflammatory responses. ACTH, adrenocorticotrophic hormone.

Chemokines

There are more than 50 known chemokines that participate in inflammation and immunity. Chemotactic cytokines, or chemokines, stimulate cell activation, hematopoiesis, angiogenesis, and chemotaxis. They are small secreted molecules that bind G-protein–coupled receptors on target cells. Chemokines are produced by a variety of cell types, either constitutively or after induction, and differ widely in biologic action. This diversity is based on specific cell types targeted, specific receptor activation, and differences in intracellular signaling.

There are two functional classes of chemokines: **inflammatory chemokines** and **homing chemokines**. Inflammatory chemokines are elicited by bacterial toxins and inflammatory cytokines (especially IL-1, TNF-α, and IFN-γ) by a variety of tissue cells and by leukocytes themselves. They recruit leukocytes during host inflammatory responses. Homing chemokines are constitutively expressed and upregulated in disease.

Chemokines may be either immobilized or soluble molecules, controlling leukocyte motility and localization within extravascular tissues by establishing a chemotactic gradient. They generate this gradient by binding proteoglycans of the extracellular matrix or cell surfaces. As a result, high concentrations of chemokines persist at sites of tissue injury. Specific receptors on the surface of migrating leukocytes recognize matrix-bound chemokines and associated adhesion molecules, triggering cells to move along the chemotactic gradient to a site of injury.

Anchoring and Activity of Chemokines

Chemokines, which may be either immobilized or soluble molecules, control leukocyte motility and localization within extravascular tissues by establishing a chemotactic gradient. Specific receptors on the surface of migrating leukocytes recognize matrix-bound chemokines and associated adhesion molecules, causing cells to move along the chemotactic gradient to a site of injury. The process of responding to matrix-bound chemoattractants is **haptotaxis**. During this migration, the cell extends a pseudopod toward increasing chemokine concentrations. At the leading front of the pseudopod, marked changes in levels of intracellular calcium are associated with assembly and contraction of cytoskeleton proteins. As a result, the cell is pulled along the chemical gradient. Chemokines are also displayed on cytokine-activated vascular endothelial cells. This process can augment integrin-dependent adhesion of leukocytes, resulting in their firm arrest (see below). The variety and combinations of chemokine receptors on cells allow for diverse biologic functions. Neutrophils, monocytes, eosinophils, and basophils share some receptors but express other receptors exclusively. Thus, specific chemokine combinations can recruit selective cell populations.

Nitric Oxide

NO is produced by nitric oxide synthase (NOS), which oxides the guanidino nitrogen of L-arginine in the presence of O_2. There are three main NOS isoforms: (1) constitutively expressed **neuronal** (nNOS), (2) **endothelial** (eNOS) forms, and (3) **inducible NOS** (iNOS). Inflammatory cytokines increase the expression of iNOS, generating intracellular and extracellular NO, which has many roles in vascular physiology and pathophysiology:

- NO generated by eNOS is **endothelium-derived relaxing factor** (EDRF), mediating vascular smooth muscle relaxation.
- NO prevents platelet adherence and aggregation at sites of vascular injury, reduces leukocyte recruitment, and scavenges oxygen radicals.

Neurokinins

The neurokinin family of peptides includes substance P (SP) and neurokinins A (NKA) and B (NKB). These peptides are distributed throughout the central and peripheral nervous systems and link the endocrine, nervous, and immune systems. Diverse biologic processes are associated with these peptides, including extravasation of plasma proteins and edema, vasodilation, smooth muscle contraction and relaxation, salivary secretion, airway contraction, and transmission of nociceptive responses. ***Injury to nerve terminals during inflammation evokes an increase in neurokinins, which in turn stimulate production of inflammatory mediators, such as histamine, NO, and kinins.***

CELLS OF INFLAMMATION

Leukocytes are the major cellular participants in inflammation and include neutrophils, T and B lymphocytes, monocytes, macrophages, eosinophils, mast cells, and basophils. Each cell type has specific functions, but they overlap and change as inflammation progresses. ***Inflammatory cells and resident tissue cells interact with each other in a continuous response during inflammation.***

Neutrophils

PMNs predominate in acute inflammation. They are stored in bone marrow, circulate in the blood, and rapidly accumulate at sites of injury or infection (Figs. 2-15A and 2-16). PMNs have granulated cytoplasm and a 2- to 4-lobed nucleus. Neutrophil receptors recognize (1) the Fc portion of IgG and IgM; (2) complement components C5a, C3b, and iC3b; (3) arachidonic acid metabolites; (4) chemotactic factors; and (5) cytokines. In tissues, PMNs phagocytose invading microbes and dead tissue, and then undergo apoptosis, largely during the resolution phase of acute inflammation. In addition to microbicidal and proinflammatory properties, PMNs interact with dendritic cells, T cells, and macrophages.

Endothelial Cells

Endothelial cells line blood vessels as a monolayer and help separate intravascular and extravascular spaces. They produce antiplatelet and antithrombotic agents that maintain blood vessel patency and secrete vasodilators and vasoconstrictors that regulate vascular tone. Injury to a vessel wall interrupts the endothelial barrier and exposes local procoagulant signals (Fig. 2-15B).

Endothelial cells are gatekeepers in inflammatory cell recruitment; they may promote or inhibit tissue perfusion and influx of inflammatory cell. Inflammatory agents such as bradykinin and histamine, endotoxins, and cytokines induce endothelial cells to display adhesion molecules that anchor and activate leukocytes, causing them to present major histocompatibility complex (MHC) class I and II molecules, and generate key vasoactive and inflammatory mediators.

Primary granule
Secondary granule
Granules (lysosomes)

A

POLYMORPHONUCLEAR LEUKOCYTE

CHARACTERISTICS AND FUNCTIONS
- Central to acute inflammation
- Phagocytosis of microorganisms and tissue debris
- Mediates tissue injury

PRIMARY INFLAMMATORY MEDIATORS
- Reactive oxygen metabolites
- Lysosomal granule contents

Primary granules	**Secondary granules**
Myeloperoxidase	Lysozyme
Lysozyme	Lactoferrin
Defensins	Collagenase
Bactericidal/permeability increasing protein	Complement activator
Elastase	Phospholipase A_2
Cathepsins protease 3	CD11b/CD18
Glucuronidase	CD11c/CD18
Mannosidase	Laminin
Phospholipase A_2	
	Tertiary granules
	Gelatinase
	Plasminogen activator
	Cathepsins
	Glucuronidase
	Mannosidase

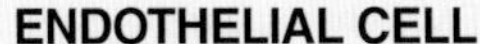

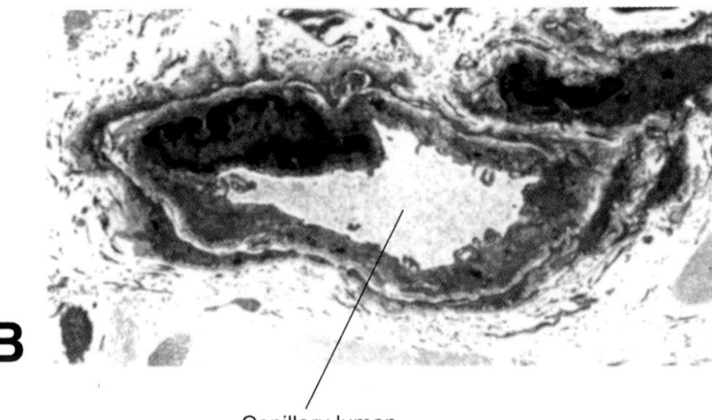

B

ENDOTHELIAL CELL

CHARACTERISTICS AND FUNCTIONS
- Maintains vascular integrity
- Regulates platelet aggregation
- Regulates vascular contraction and relaxation
- Mediates leukocyte recruitment in inflammation

PRIMARY INFLAMMATORY MEDIATORS
- von Willebrand factor
- Nitric oxide
- Endothelins
- Prostanoids

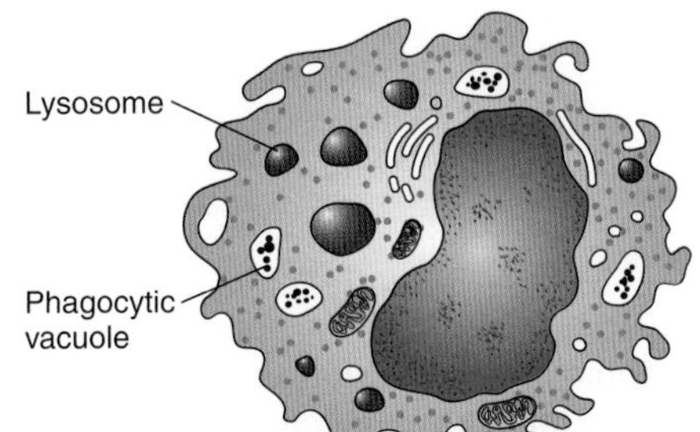

C

MONOCYTE/MACROPHAGE

CHARACTERISTICS AND FUNCTIONS
- Regulates acute and chronic inflammatory response
- Regulates coagulation/fibrinolytic pathway
- Regulates immune response (see Chapter 4)

PRIMARY INFLAMMATORY MEDIATORS
- Enzymes
- Proteins
- Complement proteins
- Chemokines
- Cytokines
- Reactive oxygen species
- Antioxidants
- Coagulation factors
- Bioactive lipids

FIGURE 2-15. Cells of inflammation: morphology and function. A. Neutrophil. **B.** Endothelial cell. **C.** Monocyte/macrophage.

Monocyte/Macrophages

Circulating monocytes (Fig. 2-15C) are bone marrow–derived cells that have a single lobed or kidney-shaped nucleus. They may exit the circulation to migrate into tissue and become resident macrophages, which accumulate at sites of acute inflammation and clear pathogens, cell debris, and apoptotic cells. Monocytes/macrophages produce potent mediators, thereby influencing initiation, progression, and resolution of acute inflammatory responses. They also have a central role in regulating progression to, and maintenance of, chronic inflammation. Macrophages respond to inflammatory stimuli by (1) phagocytosis of cell debris and microorganisms, (2) chemotaxis, (3) antigen processing and presentation, and (4) secretion of immunomodulatory factors. A large repertoire of surface receptors mediates these various macrophage functions; some immune receptors are macrophage specific, but others are shared with PMNs and lymphocytes.

Classically activated macrophages (Figs. 2-17 and 2-18) are driven by IFN-γ, TNF-α, and LPS to promote pro-inflammatory responses and release ROS and immune defense cytokines. Alternatively, activated macrophages respond to IL-4 and IL-13

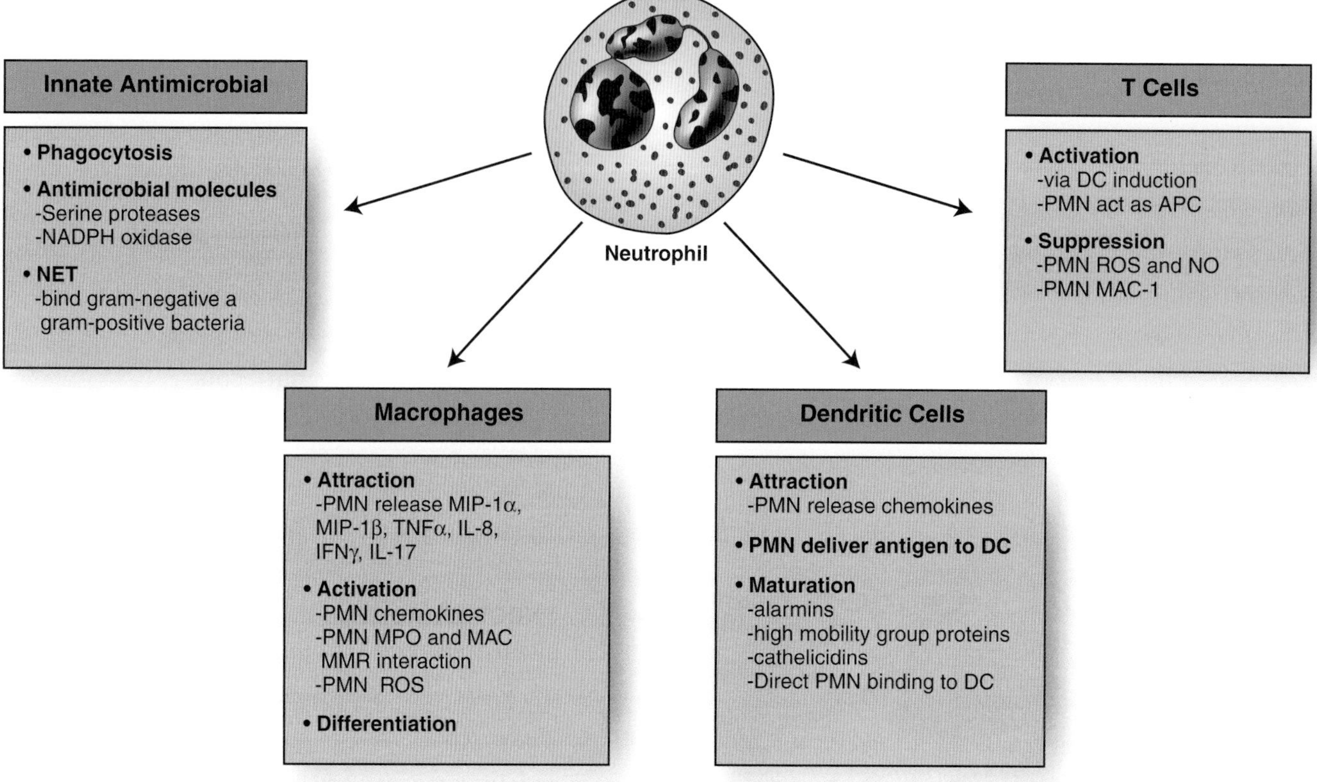

FIGURE 2-16. Effector functions of neutrophils. APC, antigen-presenting cell; DC, dendritic cell; IFN, interferon; IL, interleukin; MAC, membrane attack complex; MIP, macrophage inflammatory protein; MMR, macrophage mannose receptor; MPO, myeloperoxidase; NADPH, nicotinamide adenine dinucleotide phosphate; NO, nitric oxide; PMN, polymorphonuclear leukocyte; ROS, reactive oxygen species; TNF, tumor necrosis factor.

to help clear parasitic infections. Macrophages also respond to cytokines such as IL-10 and TGF-β to promote resolution of inflammation or switch acute to chronic inflammatory responses.

Like PMNs, macrophages are phagocytes and, similar to dendritic cells, are crucial in antigen processing and presentation. Members of this mononuclear phagocyte system are functionally diverse and include bone marrow macrophages, alveolar macrophages (lung), Kupffer cells (liver), microglial cells (CNS), Langerhans cells (skin), mesangial cells (kidney), and tissue macrophages throughout the body.

Mast Cells and Basophils

Basophils (Fig. 2-19A), the least common leukocyte in the blood, can migrate into tissue to participate in inflammatory responses. Similar mast cells are long-lived and permanently reside in all supporting tissues. They are important in regulating vascular permeability and bronchial smooth muscle tone, especially in hypersensitivity reactions (see Chapter 3). Mast cells are seen in connective tissues and particularly on lung and gastrointestinal mucosal surfaces, in the dermis and in the microvasculature.

Granulated mast cells and basophils have cell surface receptors for IgE. When IgE-sensitized mast cells or basophils are stimulated by antigens, physical agonists (cold, trauma), or cationic proteins, inflammatory mediators in dense cytoplasmic granules are secreted into extracellular tissues. These granules contain (1) acid mucopolysaccharides (including heparin), (2) serine proteases, (3) chemotactic mediators for neutrophils and eosinophils, and (4) notably, histamine, a primary mediator of early increased vascular permeability. Stimulation of mast cells and basophils also leads to the release of products of arachidonic acid metabolism (LTC_4, LTD_4, and LTE_4) and cytokines, such as TNF-α and IL-4.

Eosinophils

Eosinophils (Fig. 2-19B) circulate in the blood and are recruited to tissue in a manner similar to that of PMNs. They are often seen in settings of IgE-mediated reactions, such as allergy and asthma. Eosinophils contain leukotrienes and platelet-activating factor (PAF), acid phosphatase, and peroxidase. They express IgA receptors and exhibit large granules that contain eosinophil major basic protein, both of which are involved in defense against parasites.

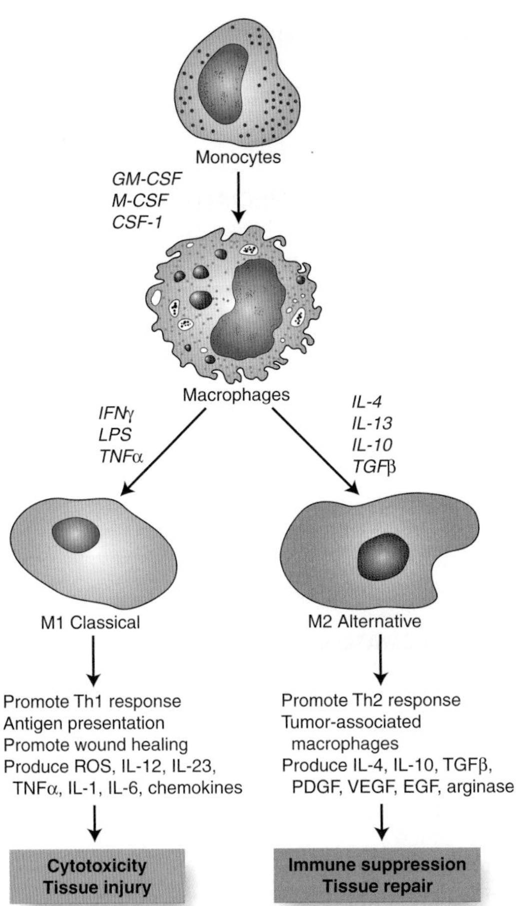

FIGURE 2-17. Macrophage activation states. CSF-1, colony-stimulating factor-1; EGF, epidermal growth factor; GM-CSF, granulocyte–macrophage colony-stimulating factor; IFN, interferon; IL, interleukin; LPS, lipopolysaccharides; M-CSF, macrophage colony-stimulating factor; PDGF, platelet-derived growth factor; ROS, reactive oxygen species; TGF, transforming growth factor; TNF, tumor necrosis factor; VEGF, vascular endothelial growth factor.

Platelets

Platelets (Fig. 2-19C) play a primary role in normal homeostasis and in initiating and regulating clotting (see Chapter 18). They produce inflammatory mediators, such as potent vasoactive substances and growth factors that modulate mesenchymal cell proliferation. Platelets are small (about 2 mm), lack nuclei, and have three types of inclusions: (1) **dense granules**, rich in serotonin, histamine, calcium, and ADP; (2) **α-granules**, containing fibrinogen, coagulation proteins, platelet-derived growth factor (PDGF), and other peptides and proteins; and (3) **lysosomes**, which sequester acid hydrolases.

Platelets adhere, aggregate, and degranulate when they contact fibrillar collagen (e.g., after vascular injury that exposes interstitial matrix proteins) or thrombin (after activation of the coagulation system) (Fig. 2-20). Degranulation releases serotonin (5-hydroxytryptamine), which, like histamine, directly increases vascular permeability. In addition, platelet TXA_2 an arachidonic acid metabolite plays a key role in platelet aggregation and mediates smooth muscle contraction. On activation, platelets, as well as phagocytic cells, secrete cationic proteins that neutralize the negative charges on endothelium and promote increased permeability.

LEUKOCYTE RECRUITMENT

An essential feature of inflammation is the accumulation of leukocytes, especially PMNs, in affected tissues. Swift recruitment requires a response orchestrated by chemoattractants that induce directed cell migration. A variety of inflammatory stimuli, including pro-inflammatory cytokines, bacterial endotoxins, and viral proteins, stimulate endothelial cells, resulting in loss of barrier function and recruitment of leukocytes. Leukocytes adhere to activated endothelium and are themselves activated in the process. They then flatten and migrate from the vascular space through the vessel wall

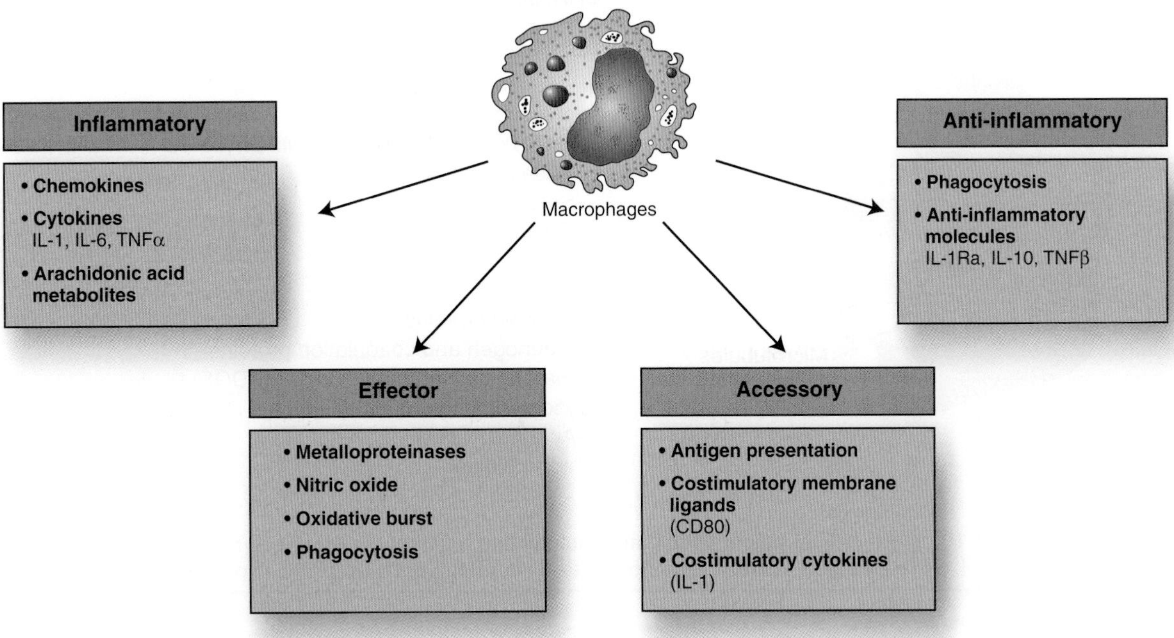

FIGURE 2-18. Effector functions of macrophages. IL, interleukin; TNF, tumor necrosis factor.

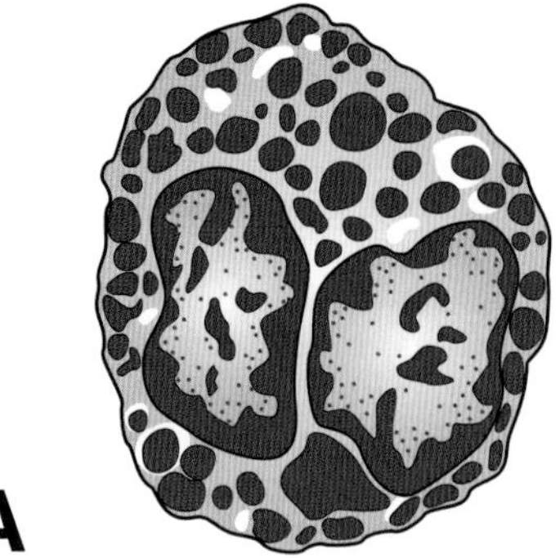

MAST CELL (BASOPHIL)

CHARACTERISTICS AND FUNCTIONS
- Binds IgE molecules
- Contains electron-dense granules

PRIMARY INFLAMMATORY MEDIATORS
- Histamine
- Leukotrienes (LTC, LTD, LTE)
- Platelet-activating factor
- Eosinophil chemotactic factors
- Cytokines (e.g., TNF-α, IL-4)

EOSINOPHIL

CHARACTERISTICS AND FUNCTIONS
- Associated with:
  -Allergic reactions
  -Parasite-associated inflammatory reactions
  -Chronic inflammation
- Modulates mast cell-mediated reactions

PRIMARY INFLAMMATORY MEDIATORS
- Reactive oxygen metabolites
- Lysosomal granule enzymes (primary crystalloid granules)
  -Major basic protein
  -Eosinophil cationic protein
  -Eosinophil peroxidase
  -Acid phosphatase
  -β-Glucuronidase
  -Arylsulfatase B
  -Histaminase
- Phospholipase D
- Prostaglandins of E series
- Cytokines

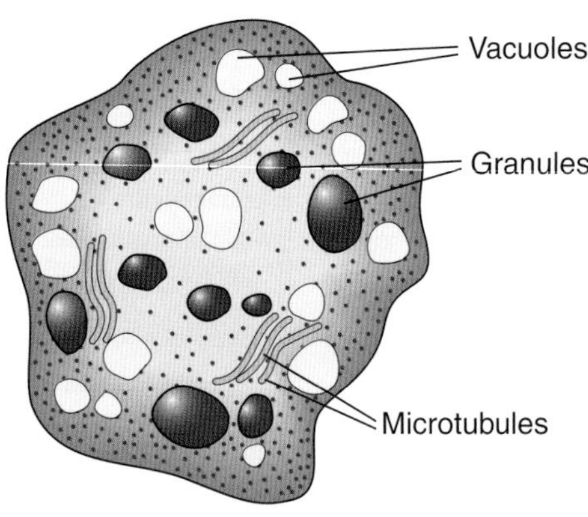

PLATELET

CHARACTERISTICS AND FUNCTIONS
- Thrombosis; promotes clot formation
- Regulates permeability
- Regulates proliferative response of mesenchymal cells

PRIMARY INFLAMMATORY MEDIATORS
- Dense granules
  -Serotonin
  -Ca^{2+}
  -ADP
- α-Granules
  -Cationic proteins
  -Fibrinogen and coagulation proteins
  -Platelet-derived growth factor (PDGF)
- Lysosomes
  -Acid hydrolases
- Thromboxane A_2

FIGURE 2-19. More cells of inflammation: morphology and function. A. Mast cell/basophil. **B.** Eosinophil. **C.** Platelet. ADP, adenosine diphosphate; IL, interleukin; TNF, tumor necrosis factor.

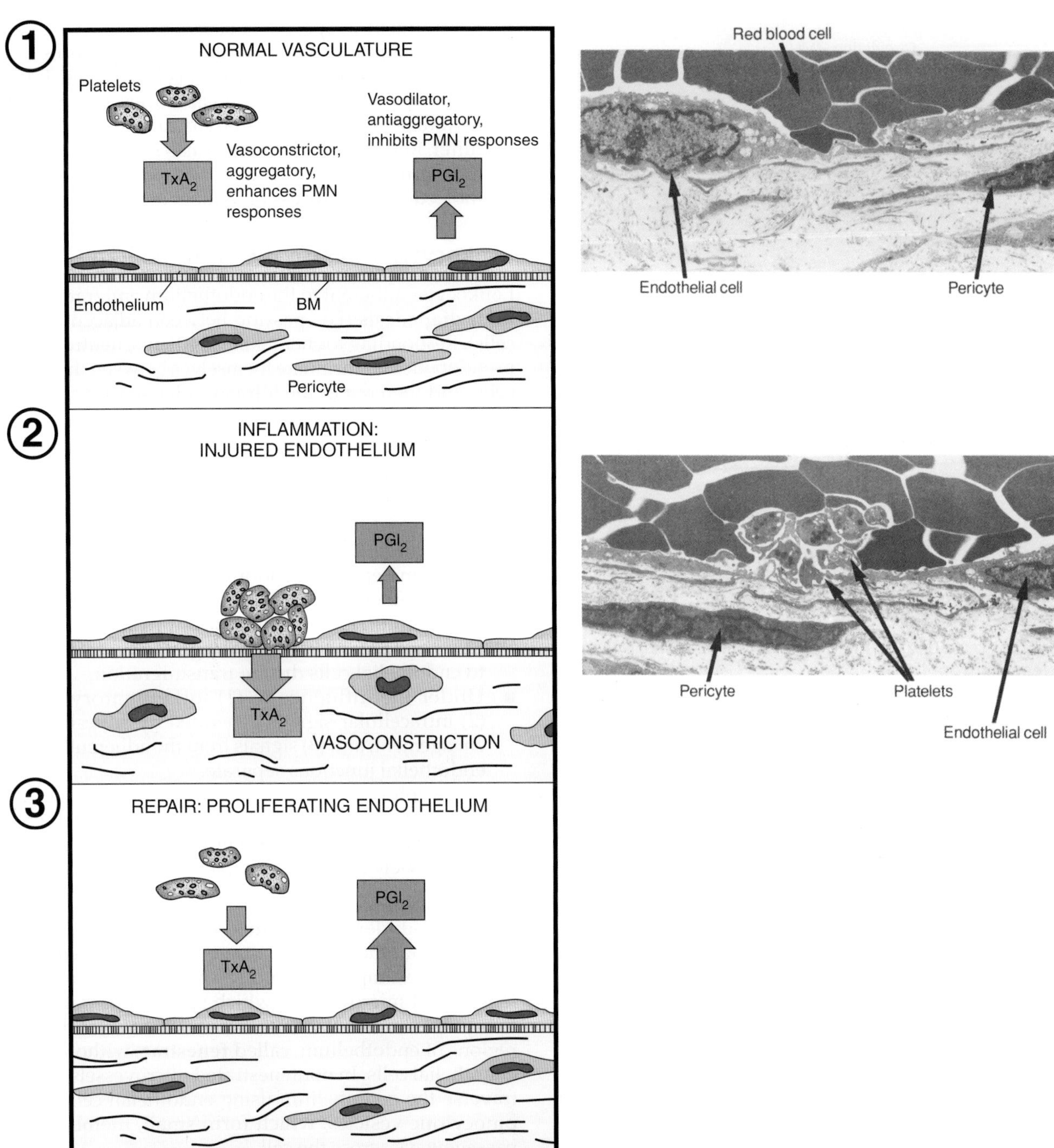

FIGURE 2-20. Regulation of platelet and endothelial cell interactions by thromboxane A_2 (TXA_2) and prostaglandin I_2 (PGI_2). (*1*) Platelet-derived TXA_2 and endothelial-derived PGI_2 maintain vasodilation and vasoconstriction in balance. (*2*) During inflammation, the normal balance is shifted to vasoconstriction, increased vascular permeability, platelet aggregation, and polymorphonuclear neutrophil (PMN) responses. (*3*) During repair, the prostaglandin effects predominate, inhibiting PMN responses and promoting normal blood flow. BM, basement membrane.

and into surrounding tissue. **Chemotaxis** is a dynamic and energy-dependent process of directed cell migration in which leukocytes migrate from the endothelium toward the target tissue. They travel down a gradient of one chemoattractant in response to a second, more distal chemoattractant. In the extravascular tissue, PMNs ingest foreign material, microbes, and dead tissue (Fig. 2-21).

Tethering, Rolling, and Firm Adhesion

Leukocyte recruitment begins in postcapillary venules and is a multistep sequential process, which involves the interplay of adhesion molecules on both the endothelium and neutrophil (Fig 2-22):

- Of initial importance is the altered expression of a class of adhesion molecules termed **selectins**. The selectin family

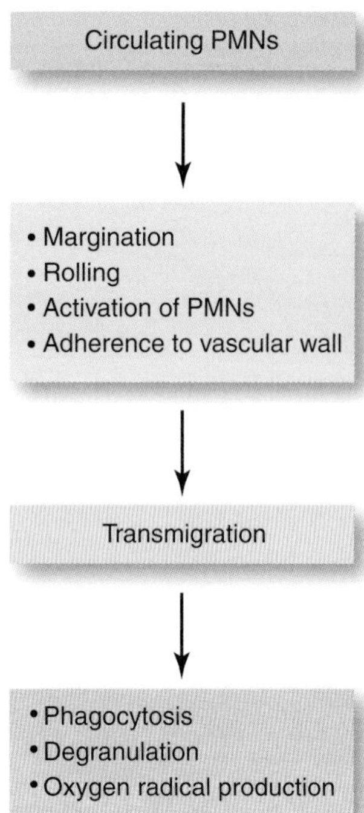

FIGURE 2-21. Leukocyte recruitment and activation. PMNs, polymorphonuclear neutrophils.

includes P-selectin, E-selectin, and L-selectin. These molecules share a similar structure, a chain of transmembrane glycoproteins with an extracellular lectin-binding domain. The selectins bind to the sialyl-Lewis X moiety, on **addressins**, which allows for rapid cell attachment and rolling.

- **P-selectin** is preformed and stored in Weibel–Palade bodies within the endothelium. It rapidly moves to the endothelial surface upon stimulation with histamine, thrombin, or other inflammatory mediators. Cytokines and bacterial LPS stimulate the synthesis of **E-selectin** on the endothelial surface. Both newly expressed endothelial selectins bind to the constitutively expressed sialyl-Lewis X moiety of the PSGL-1 addressin, which is on the neutrophil surface. This initial interaction, termed **tethering**, slows the neutrophils and allows them to interact with endothelial cells. A breaking and reforming of the adhesive connections occurs, which result in neutrophil **rolling** on the endothelial surface (Fig. 2-22).
- The close proximity of neutrophil and endothelial cells allows for additional interactions promoted by a variety of mediators (notably the chemokine CXCL-8, IL-8 stored in, and released from, the Weibel–Palade body). Such interactions further the firm adhesion that promotes **leukocyte arrest**. Critical to this increase in adhesion is the class of molecules termed **integrins**, which bind to **Ig superfamily ligands** on endothelial cells.
- Integrins have transmembrane α- and β-chains arranged as heterodimers. Very late activation (VLA) molecules include VLA-4 ($\alpha_4\beta_1$) on leukocytes and lymphocytes, which bind vascular cell adhesion molecule-1 (VCAM-1) on endothelial cells. The β_2 integrins bind ICAM-1 and ICAM-2 (Fig. 2-22). Leukocyte integrins exist in a low-affinity state but are converted to a high-affinity state via a G-protein–mediated conformational change, which occurs when the neutrophils are activated. In addition, neutrophil L-selectin is upregulated. The net result is a transition from leukocyte rolling to firm adhesion.
- Recruitment of specific subsets of leukocytes to areas of inflammation results from the unique patterns or densities of adhesion molecules on cell surfaces. Leukocyte adherence to arterioles and capillaries also has different requirements because hydrodynamic forces in these vessels differ. Regional recruitment is also influenced by vascular flow conditions, which alter the expression of adhesion molecules and process of leukocyte transmigration.

Leukocytes Traverse the Endothelium

Leukocytes adherent to the endothelium emigrate by **paracellular diapedesis** (i.e., passing between adjacent endothelial cells). Responding to chemokine gradients, neutrophils extend pseudopods and insinuate themselves between the endothelial cells, and then out of the intravascular space.

- Adhesion molecules, which are expressed intercellularly, contribute to tight adhesion between endothelial cells. However, they may also release during leukocyte transmigration or redistribute to cell surfaces to facilitate leukocyte recruitment (Fig. 2-23). These molecules include JAMs, CD99, and PECAM-1 (CD31, platelet endothelial cell adhesion molecule) on endothelial cell surfaces, which bind to each other to keep cells together. JAMs are proteins of the immunoglobulin superfamily. JAMs and particularly CD99 and PECAM are also integral to neutrophil adhesion to endothelial cells during transmigration.
- Under the influence of (1) inflammatory mediators, (2) intracellular signals generated by adhesion molecule engagement, and (3) signals from the adherent neutrophils, endothelial junctions separate.
- Neutrophils mobilize elastase to their pseudopod membranes, inducing endothelial cells to retract and separate at the advancing edge of the neutrophil, a process facilitated by PMN-elicited increases in endothelial cell intracellular calcium.

A little-understood method of migration of neutrophils through endothelial cells is **transcellular diapedesis**. Some tissues, for example, gut mucosa and secretory glands, contain fenestrated microvessels, which serve as passages through the cytoplasm. PMNs may traverse such routes through thin regions of endothelium, called **fenestrae**, without damaging endothelial cells. In nonfenestrated microvessels, PMNs may traverse the endothelium using endothelial cell caveolae or pinocytotic vesicles, which form small, membrane-bound passageways across the cell.

Chemotactic Molecules

Leukocytes must be accurately positioned at sites of inflammatory injury to function correctly. For the right subsets of leukocytes to arrive in a timely fashion, they must receive specific directions. ***Leukocytes are guided through vascular and extravascular spaces by a complex interaction of attractants, repellants, and adhesion molecules.***

The most important neutrophil chemotactic factors are (1) C5a, (2) bacterial and mitochondrial products (particularly low–molecular-weight N-formylated peptides such as FMLP), (3) products of arachidonic acid metabolism (especially LTB_4), (4) products of matrix degradation, and (5) chemokines. Chemokines represent a key mechanism of leukocyte recruitment because they generate a chemotactic gradient by binding to matrix proteoglycans. As a result, high concentrations of

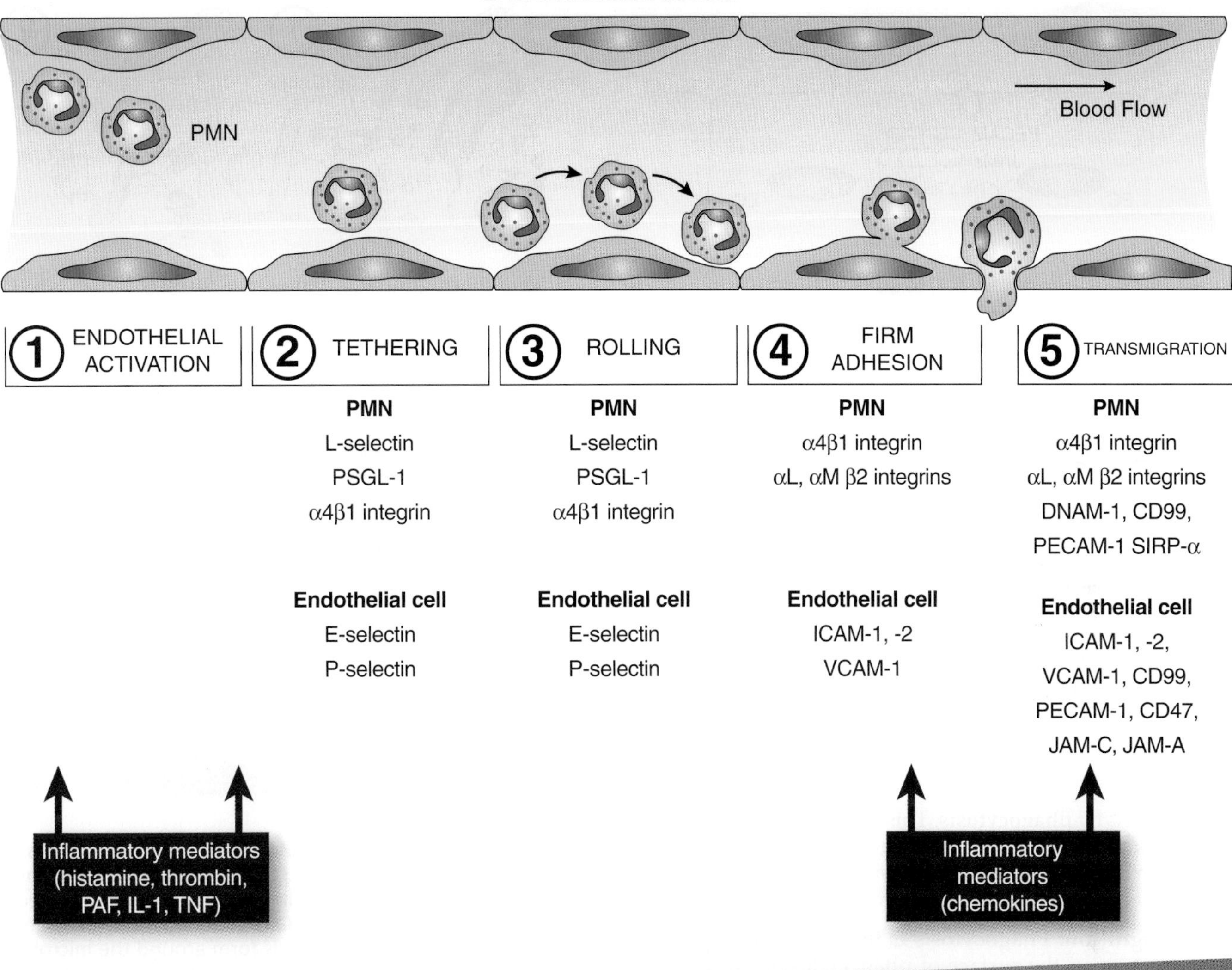

FIGURE 2-22. Neutrophil adhesion and extravasation. (*1*) Inflammatory mediators activate endothelial cells to increase expression of adhesion molecules. Sialyl-Lewis X on neutrophil P-selectin glycoprotein-1 (PSGL-1) and E-selectin ligand binds to P- and E-selectins to facilitate (*2*) tethering and (*3*) rolling of neutrophils. Increased integrins on activated neutrophils bind to intercellular adhesion molecule-1 (ICAM-1) on endothelial cells to form (*4*) a firm attachment. (*5*) Endothelial cell attachments to one another are released and neutrophils then pass between separated cells to enter the tissue. IL, interleukin; JAMs, junctional adhesion molecules; PAF, platelet-activating factor; PECAM, platelet endothelial cell adhesion molecule; PMN, polymorphonuclear neutrophil; TNF, tumor necrosis factor; VCAM, vascular cell adhesion molecule.

chemokines persist at sites of tissue injury. In turn, specific receptors on migrating leukocytes bind matrix-bound chemokines, moving cells along the chemotactic gradient to the site of injury.

The cocktail of chemokines within a tissue largely determines the types of leukocytes that come to the site. Chemotactic factors for lymphocytes, basophils, and eosinophils are also produced at sites of tissue injury and may be secreted by activated endothelial cells, tissue parenchymal cells, or other inflammatory cells.

INFLAMMATORY CELL FUNCTIONS IN ACUTE INFLAMMATION

Phagocytosis of Microorganisms and Tissue Debris

Many inflammatory cells are **phagocytes**. Neutrophils, monocytes, tissue macrophages, and dendritic cells recognize, internalize, and digest foreign material, microorganisms, or

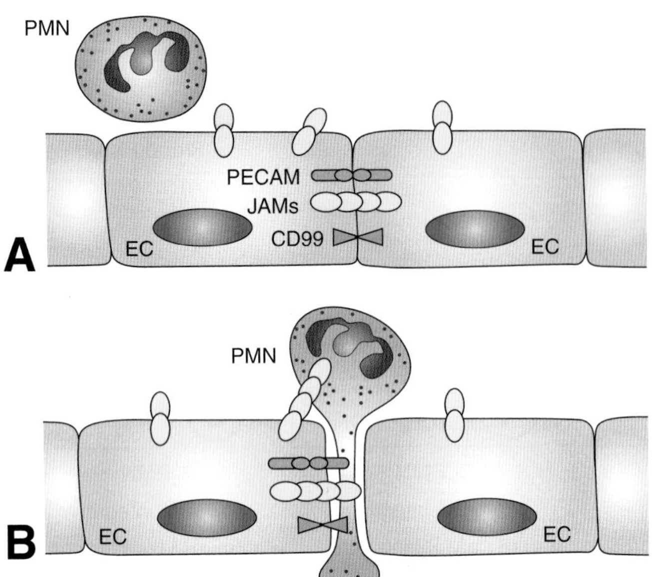

FIGURE 2-23. Endothelial cell junctional molecules participate in leukocyte recruitment. A. Junctional molecules contribute to cell–cell adhesion and maintenance of endothelial barrier function. **B.** These same molecules regulate paracellular transmigration of leukocytes. EC, endothelial cell; JAMs, junctional adhesion molecules; PECAM, platelet endothelial cell adhesion molecule; PMN, polymorphonuclear neutrophil.

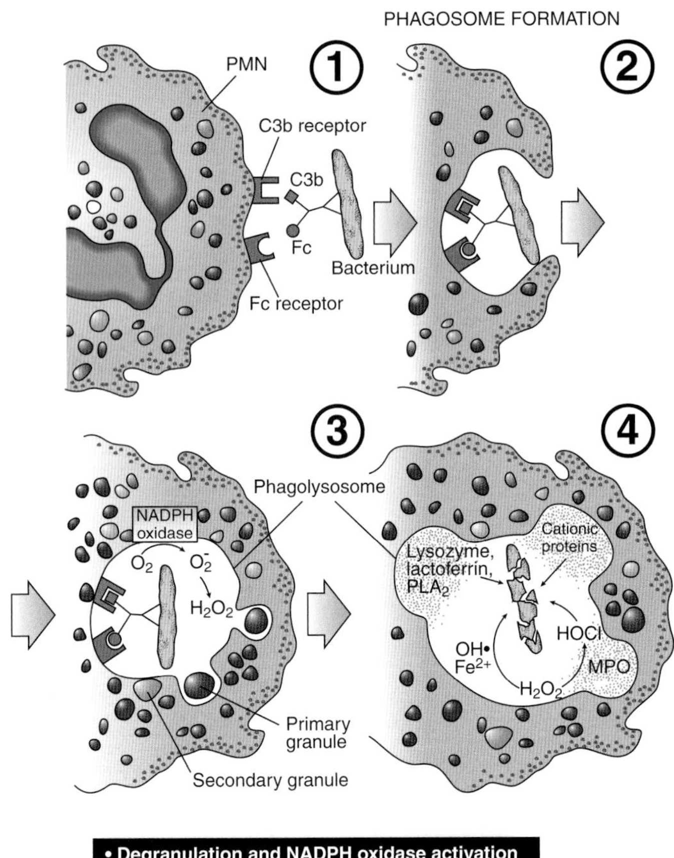

FIGURE 2-24. Mechanisms of neutrophil bacterial phagocytosis and cell killing. (*1*) Opsonins such as C3b coat the surface of microbes, allowing recognition by the neutrophil C3b receptor. (*2*) Receptor clustering triggers intracellular signaling and actin assembly within the neutrophil. Pseudopods form around the microbe to enclose it within a phagosome. (*3*) Lysosomal granules fuse with the phagosome to form a phagolysosome, into which the lysosomal enzymes and oxygen radicals are released to (*4*) kill and degrade the microbe. Fe^{2+}, ferrous iron; HOCl, hypochlorous acid; MPO, myeloperoxidase; NADPH, nicotinamide adenine dinucleotide phosphate; PLA_2, phospholipase A_2; PMN, polymorphonuclear neutrophil.

cellular debris by **phagocytosis**. This term is defined as ingestion by eukaryotic cells of large (usually >0.5 μm) insoluble particles and microorganisms. The complex process involves a sequence of transmembrane and intracellular signaling events:

1. **Recognition:** Phagocytosis is initiated when specific receptors on the surface of phagocytic cells recognize their targets (Fig. 2-24). Phagocytosis of most biologic agents is enhanced by, if not dependent on, their coating (**opsonization**) with plasma components **(opsonins)**, particularly immunoglobulins or C3b. Phagocytic cells have specific opsonic receptors, including those for Ig Fcγ (FcRs) and complement components. Many pathogens have evolved mechanisms to evade phagocytosis by leukocytes. Polysaccharide capsules, protein A, protein M, or peptidoglycans around bacteria can prevent complement deposition or antigen recognition and receptor binding.
2. **Signaling:** Clumping of opsonins at bacterial surfaces causes phagocyte plasma membrane Fcγ receptors to cluster. This process triggers intracellular signaling via tyrosine kinases that associate with the Fcγ receptor.
3. **Internalization:** Actin assembly occurs directly under the receptor bound target to be phagocytized. Polymerized actin filaments push the plasma membrane forward. The plasma membrane remodels to increase surface area and to form pseudopods surrounding the foreign material. The resulting phagocytic cup engulfs the foreign agent. The membrane then "zippers" around the opsonized particle to enclose it in a vacuole called a **phagosome** (Fig. 2-24).
4. **Digestion:** The phagosome with the foreign material fuses to cytoplasmic lysosomes to form a **phagolysosome,** into which lysosomal enzymes are released. The acid pH in the phagolysosome activates these hydrolytic enzymes, which then degrade the phagocytosed material. Some microorganisms have evolved mechanisms for evading killing by neutrophils by preventing lysosomal degranulation or inhibiting neutrophil enzymes.

Inflammatory Cell Enzymes

PMNs and macrophages are critical for degrading microbes and cell debris but may also cause tissue injury (Fig. 2-25). Although debridement of damaged tissue by proteolytic breakdown facilitates tissue repair, degradative enzymes can damage endothelial and epithelial cells and degrade connective tissue.

Inflammatory cells possess an array of enzymes used to degrade microbes and tissue. Neutrophil primary, secondary,

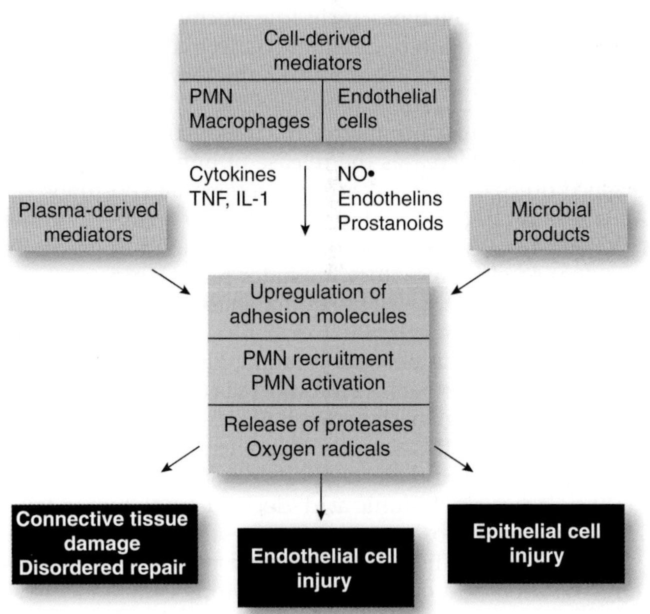

FIGURE 2-25. Mechanisms of cell and tissue damage. IL, interleukin; NO•, nitric oxide; PMN, polymorphonuclear neutrophil; TNF, tumor necrosis factor.

and tertiary granules are morphologically and biochemically distinct; each has unique activities (see Fig. 2-15).

- **Primary granules (azurophilic granules):** Antimicrobial and proteinase activity of these granules can directly activate other inflammatory cells. Potent acid hydrolases and neutral serine proteases digest diverse macromolecules. Lysozyme and PLA_2 degrade bacterial cell walls and biologic membranes and are important in killing bacteria. Myeloperoxidase, a key enzyme in the metabolism of hydrogen peroxide, generates toxic ROS.
- **Secondary granules (specific granules):** These contain PLA_2, lysozyme, and proteins that initiate killing of specific cells. In addition, their contents include the cationic lactoferrin, a vitamin B_{12}–binding protein and matrix metalloproteinase (collagenase) specific for type IV collagen.
- **Tertiary granules (small storage granules, C granules):** These are released at the leading front of neutrophils during chemotaxis. They are the source of enzymes that promote migration of cells through basement membranes and tissues, including proteinases, cathepsin, gelatinase, and urokinase-type plasminogen activator (u-PA).

In the macrophage, the specific array of agents released varies, depending on the role of the macrophage as pro- or anti-inflammatory (see Figs. 2-15C and 2-18).

Inflammatory Cells, ROS- and Non-ROS-Mediated Mechanisms

Bacterial Killing by Reactive Oxygen Species

Phagocytosis is accompanied by metabolic reactions in inflammatory cells that lead to production of oxygen metabolites (see Chapter 1). These ROS are more reactive than oxygen itself and contribute to the killing of ingested bacteria (see Fig. 2-24).

- **Superoxide anion (O_2^-):** Phagocytosis activates an NADPH oxidase in PMN cell membranes. This enzyme is a multicomponent electron transport complex that reduces molecular oxygen to O_2^-. Activation of NADPH oxidase is enhanced by prior exposure of cells to a chemotactic stimulus or LPS. NADPH oxidase increases oxygen consumption and stimulates the hexose monophosphate shunt. Together, these cell responses are the **respiratory burst**.
- **Hydrogen peroxide (H_2O_2):** O_2^- is rapidly converted to H_2O_2 at the cell surface and in phagolysosomes by superoxide dismutase (SOD). H_2O_2 is stable and is a source for generating additional reactive oxidants.
- **Hypochlorous acid (HOCl):** Myeloperoxidase (MPO), a neutrophil product with a very strong cationic charge, is secreted from granules during exocytosis. In the presence of a halide, usually chlorine, MPO catalyzes the conversion of H_2O_2 to HOCl. This powerful oxidant is a major bactericidal agent made by phagocytic cells. It also helps activate neutrophil-derived collagenase and gelatinase, both of which are secreted as latent enzymes.
- **Hydroxyl radical (OH•):** Reduction of H_2O_2 via the Haber–Weiss reaction forms the highly reactive OH•. This occurs slowly at physiologic pH, but if ferrous iron (Fe^{2+}) is present, the Fenton reaction rapidly converts H_2O_2 to OH•, which is a potent bactericidal agent. Further reduction of OH• yields H_2O (see Chapter 1).
- **Nitric oxide (NO•):** Phagocytes and endothelial cells produce NO• and its derivatives, which have many physiologic and nonphysiologic effects. NO• and other free radicals interact with one another to balance their cytotoxic and cytoprotective effects. NO• can react with oxygen radicals to form toxic molecules such as peroxynitrite and *S*-nitrosothiols, or it can scavenge O_2^-, thereby reducing the amount of toxic radicals.

Monocytes, macrophages, and eosinophils also make oxygen radicals, depending on their state of activation and the stimulus to which they are exposed. Defective phagocytic cell function occurs in several congenital diseases. The importance of oxygen-dependent bacterial killing is exemplified in **chronic granulomatous disease** of childhood, a hereditary deficiency of NADPH oxidase. Affected patients fail to produce O_2^- and H_2O_2 during phagocytosis and so are prone to recurrent infections, especially with gram-positive cocci. Patients with a related genetic deficiency in MPO cannot produce HOCl and are excessively susceptible to fungal infections with *Candida* (Table 2-5).

Nonoxidative Bacterial Killing

Phagocytes, particularly PMNs and monocytes/macrophages, have substantial oxygen-independent antimicrobial activity. This activity mainly involves bactericidal proteins in cytoplasmic granules, such as lysosomal acid hydrolases and specialized noncatalytic proteins unique to inflammatory cells.

Defects in Leukocyte Function

The importance of acute inflammatory cells in protection from infection is underscored by the frequency and severity of infections when PMNs are depleted or defective. ***The most common such deficit is iatrogenic neutropenia secondary to cancer chemotherapy.*** Functional impairment of phagocytes may occur at any step in the sequence: adherence, emigration, chemotaxis, phagocytosis, or killing. These disorders may be acquired or congenital. Acquired diseases, such as leukemia,

Table 2-5

Congenital Diseases of Defective Phagocytic Cell Function Characterized by Recurrent Bacterial Infections

Disease	Defect
Leukocyte adhesion deficiency (LAD)	LAD-1 (defective β_2-integrin expression or function [CD11/CD18])
	LAD-2 (defective fucosylation, selectin binding)
Hyper-IgE-recurrent infection, (Job) syndrome	Poor chemotaxis
Chediak–Higashi syndrome	Defective lysosomal granules, poor chemotaxis
Neutrophil-specific granule deficiency	Absent neutrophil granules
Chronic granulomatous disease	Deficient NADPH oxidase, with absent H_2O_2 production
Myeloperoxidase deficiency	Deficient HOCl production

H_2O_2, hydrogen peroxide; HOCl, hypochlorous acid; Ig, immunoglobulin; NADPH, nicotinamide adenine dinucleotide phosphate.

diabetes, malnutrition, viral infections, and sepsis, often entail defects in inflammatory cell function. Table 2-5 shows representative examples of congenital diseases linked to defective phagocytic function.

NEGATIVE REGULATORS OF ACUTE INFLAMMATION

The natural resolution of acute inflammation involves removal of the initial stimulus and subsequent apoptosis of inflammatory cells. Decreased pro-inflammatory mediators and increased anti-inflammatory mediators brake the process. Removal of damaged tissue and cell debris allows proper healing to take place.

The response to injury is, however, variable. Genetics and the sex and age of a patient determine the response to injury, extent of healing, and especially, progression to chronic inflammatory disease. Negative regulators of inflammation include the following:

- **Gene silencing and reprogramming:** Inflammation is associated with gene reprogramming, which (1) silences acute pro-inflammatory gene expression, (2) increases anti-inflammatory gene expression, and (3) allows the inflammatory process to start to resolve. Notably, TNF-α, IL-1β, and other pro-inflammatory genes are repressed. At the same time, expression of anti-inflammatory factors, such as IL-1 receptor antagonist (IL-1RA), TNF-α receptors, IL-6, and IL-10, increases.
- **Cytokines:** Several interleukins (IL-6, IL10 to IL13) limit inflammation by reducing production of TNF-α. This may occur by preserving IκB, thus blocking cell activation and release of inflammatory mediators.
- **Protease inhibitors:** Secretory leukocyte proteinase inhibitor (SLPI) and TIMP-2 are important in reducing the responses of a variety of cell types, including macrophages and endothelial cells, and in decreasing connective tissue damage.
- **Lipoxins:** Lipoxins are anti-inflammatory lipid mediators that inhibit leukotriene biosynthesis.
- **Glucocorticoids:** Stimulating the hypothalamic–pituitary–adrenal axis increases the release of immunosuppressive glucocorticoids. These have transcriptional and posttranscriptional suppressive effects on inflammatory response genes.
- **Kininases:** Kininases in plasma and blood degrade the potent pro-inflammatory mediator bradykinin.
- **Phosphatases:** A signal transduction mechanism that commonly regulates inflammatory cell signaling is rapid and reversible protein phosphorylation. Phosphatases and associated proteins balance the effect via dephosphorylation.
- **Transforming growth factor-β (TGF-β):** Apoptotic cells, particularly PMNs, induce TGF-β expression. TGF-β (1) suppresses pro-inflammatory cytokines and chemokines, (2) switches arachidonic acid–derived mediators to favor production of lipoxin and resolvin (resolution phase interaction products; omega-3 unsaturated fatty acid), (3) causes recognition and clearance of apoptotic cells and debris by macrophages, and (4) stimulates anti-inflammatory cytokines and fibrosis.

OUTCOMES OF ACUTE INFLAMMATION

A combination of regulatory activities and the short life span of neutrophils limit the duration of acute inflammatory reactions. As the source of tissue injury is eliminated, inflammation recedes and normal tissue architecture and physiologic function are restored. How the inflammation ends depends on the balance between cell recruitment, cell division, cell emigration, and cell death. If a tissue is to return to normal, the inflammatory process must be reversed: (1) the stimulus to injury must be removed, (2) pro-inflammatory signals turned off, (3) acute inflammatory cell influx ended, (4) tissue fluid balance restored, (5) cell and tissue debris removed, (6) normal vascular function restored, (7) epithelial barriers repaired, and (8) the extracellular matrix regenerated. As signals for acute inflammation wane, apoptosis of PMNs limits the immune response and resolution begins.

However, inflammatory responses can lead to other outcomes (Fig. 2-26):

- **Scar:** Although the body may eliminate the offending agent, if a tissue is irreversibly injured, normal architecture is often replaced by a scar.
- **Abscess:** If the area of acute inflammation is walled off by inflammatory cells and fibrosis, PMN products destroy the tissue, leaving an abscess (see Chapter 1).
- **Lymphadenitis:** Localized acute and chronic inflammation may cause secondary inflammation of lymphatic channels **(lymphangitis)** and lymph nodes **(lymphadenitis)**. These inflamed lymphatic channels appear as red streaks, and lymph nodes are enlarged and painful. Affected lymph nodes show lymphoid follicle hyperplasia and proliferation of mononuclear phagocytes in the sinuses **(sinus histiocytosis)**.
- **Persistent inflammation:** If an insulting agent persists or resolution is incomplete, inflammation may persist. This may be a prolonged acute response, with continued influx of neutrophils and tissue destruction, or, more commonly, chronic inflammation.

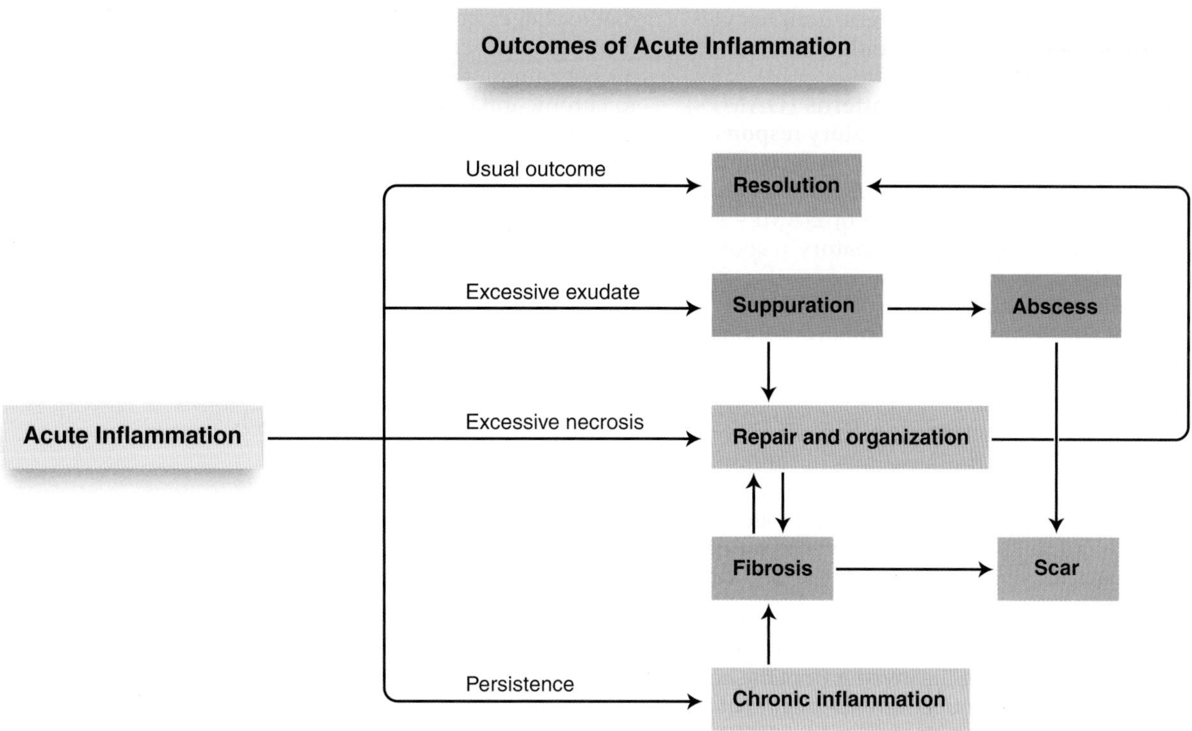

FIGURE 2-26. Outcomes of acute inflammation.

CHRONIC INFLAMMATION

In chronic inflammation, inflammatory cells persist, the stroma becomes hyperplastic, and tissue destruction and scarring may lead to organ dysfunction. The process may be localized, but it often progresses to disabling diseases, such as chronic lung disease, rheumatoid arthritis, ulcerative colitis, granulomatous diseases, autoimmune diseases, and chronic dermatitis. Acute and chronic inflammation are ends of a dynamic continuum with overlapping morphologies: (1) inflammation that features continued recruitment of chronic inflammatory cells is followed by (2) tissue injury due to a prolonged inflammatory response, and (3) an often-disordered attempt to restore tissue integrity. Macrophages are key determinants of the outcome (Fig. 2-27).

The events leading to amplified inflammatory responses resemble those of acute inflammation in several ways:

- **Specific triggers**, microbial products or injury, initiate the response.
- **Chemical mediators** direct recruitment, activation, and interaction of inflammatory cells. Activation of coagulation and complement generates small peptides that act to prolong the inflammatory response. Cytokines, specifically IL-6 and RANTES (CCL5), regulate a switch in chemokines, so that mononuclear cells are directed to the site. Other cytokines (e.g., IFN-γ) then promote macrophage proliferation and activation.
- **Inflammatory cells** enter from the blood. Interactions between lymphocytes, macrophages, dendritic cells, and fibroblasts generate antigen-specific responses. Macrophages have a central, controlling role, producing inflammatory

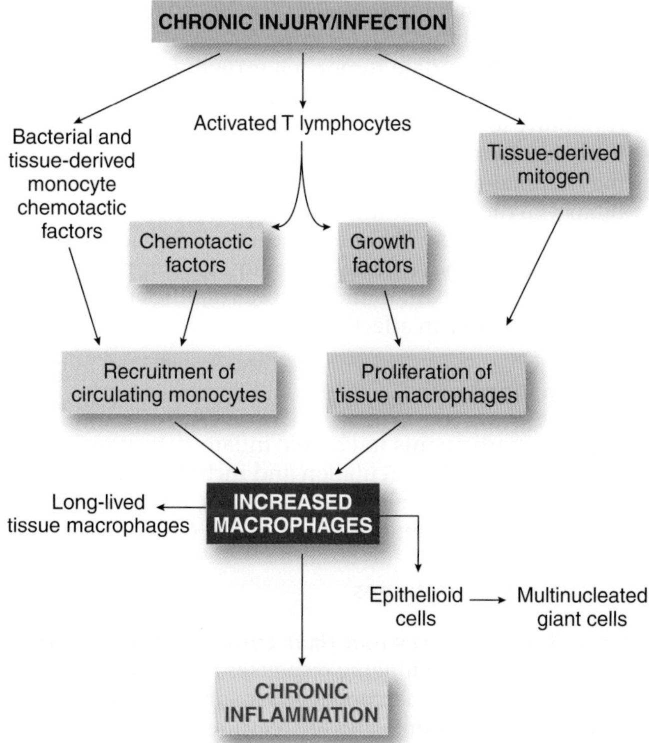

FIGURE 2-27. Accumulation of macrophages is central to development of chronic inflammation.

mediators that activate other macrophages, lymphocytes, and tissue fibroblasts (see Fig. 2-27) either to promote resolution or to perpetuate injury.

- **Damage and pathogen associated patterns (DAMPs) and PAMPs drive multifaceted inflammatory responses.** Interaction of PAMPs, DAMPs, and pattern recognition receptors (PRRs) increases activation of inflammatory mediators. This can cause more release of DAMPs and subsequent maintenance of the inflammatory response, even after the initial inciting event has passed (see Fig. 2-5).
- **Stromal cell activation and extracellular matrix (ECM)** remodeling occur, both of which affect cellular immune responses. Variable fibrosis may result, depending on the extent of tissue injury and the persistence of injury and inflammation.

Chronic inflammation is not synonymous with chronic infection, but if an inflammatory response does not eliminate an injurious agent, infection may persist. Chronic inflammation does not necessarily require infection; it may follow an acute inflammatory or immune response to a foreign antigen. Signals that lead to an extended response include the following:

- **Bacteria, viruses, and parasites:** These agents can provide signals to support persistent inflammatory responses, which may be directed toward isolating the invader from the host.
- **Apoptosis:** As apoptotic PMNs induce an anti-inflammatory reaction, defects in recognizing or responding to PMN remnants may lead to chronic inflammation.
- **Defective gene silencing:** Delayed or persistent expression of late pro-inflammatory genes helps to perpetuate the inflammatory environment. In this case, a gene-silencing phase does not occur, cytokine onslaught persists, and pathologic inflammation develops.
- **Trauma:** Extensive tissue damage releases mediators that prolong the inflammatory environment.
- **Cancer:** Chronic inflammatory cells, especially macrophages and T lymphocytes, may be recruited by tumors to feed and stimulate tumor cell growth (see Chapter 4). Chemotherapy may limit inflammation and increase susceptibility to infection.
- **Immune factors:** In many autoimmune diseases, including rheumatoid arthritis, chronic thyroiditis, and primary biliary cirrhosis, chronic inflammatory responses occur in affected tissues. There may be associated activation of antibody-dependent and cell-mediated immunity (see Chapter 3). Such autoimmune abnormalities may lead to persistent injury in affected organs.

Mononuclear Cells

The cellular participants in chronic inflammatory responses are recruited from the circulation and include macrophages, lymphocytes, plasma cells, dendritic cells, and eosinophils. Affected tissues contribute fibroblasts and endothelial cells.

Monocytes/Macrophages

Activated macrophages and their cytokines are central to inflammation and prolonging responses that lead to chronic inflammation. Tissue macrophages are stimulated and proliferate as circulating monocytes are recruited and differentiate into tissue macrophages (see Fig. 2-27). Under the influence of the microenvironment, resident tissue macrophages become phenotypically polarized into classically activated M1 macrophages and alternatively activated M2 macrophages (see Figs. 2-17 and 2-18). These cells produce inflammatory and immunologic mediators and regulate reactions leading to chronic inflammation. They also regulate lymphocyte responses to antigens and secrete other mediators that modulate the proliferation and activation of fibroblasts and endothelial cell proliferation and their activities.

When monocytes enter tissue and differentiate into macrophages, they acquire the ability to make additional matrix metalloproteinases and cysteine proteinases but lose the capacity to produce serine proteinases. The activities of these enzymes are central to tissue destruction that may occur in chronic inflammation. ***Other macrophage products include oxygen metabolites, chemotactic factors, cytokines, and growth factors*** (see Fig. 2-15C).

Lymphocytes

T cells regulate macrophage activation and recruitment; (1) they secrete specific mediators (lymphokines), (2) modulate antibody production and cell-mediated cytotoxicity, and (3) maintain immunologic memory (Fig. 2-28A). NK cells, as well as other lymphocyte subtypes, help defend against viral and bacterial infections.

Plasma Cells

Plasma cells are rich in rough endoplasmic reticulum and are the primary source of antibodies (Fig. 2-28B). Production of antibody to specific antigens at sites of chronic inflammation is important in antigen neutralization, clearance of foreign antigens and particles, and antibody-dependent cell-mediated cytotoxicity (see Chapter 3).

Fibroblasts

Fibroblasts are long-lived, ubiquitous cells, whose chief function is the production of components of the ECM (Fig. 2-28C). They are derived from mesoderm or neural crest and can differentiate into other connective tissue cells (e.g., chondrocytes, adipocytes, osteocytes, and smooth muscle cells). Fibroblasts are the construction workers of tissue, rebuilding the scaffolding of the ECM upon which tissue is reestablished.

Activated fibroblasts produce cytokines, chemokines, and prostanoids, creating a tissue microenvironment that further regulates the behavior of inflammatory cells in the damaged tissue. This process results in resolution and subsequent wound healing or chronic persistent inflammation.

Injury and Repair in Chronic Inflammation

Chronic inflammation is mediated by immunologic and nonimmunologic mechanisms and often occurs with reparative responses, namely, granulation tissue and fibrosis.

Extended Inflammatory Responses

The primary role of PMNs in inflammation is host defense and debridement of damaged tissue. The neutrophil response, however, is both yin and yang. PMN products protect the host from foreign invaders and help debride damaged tissues, but if they are not well regulated, these same products may prolong tissue damage and promote chronic inflammation.

A

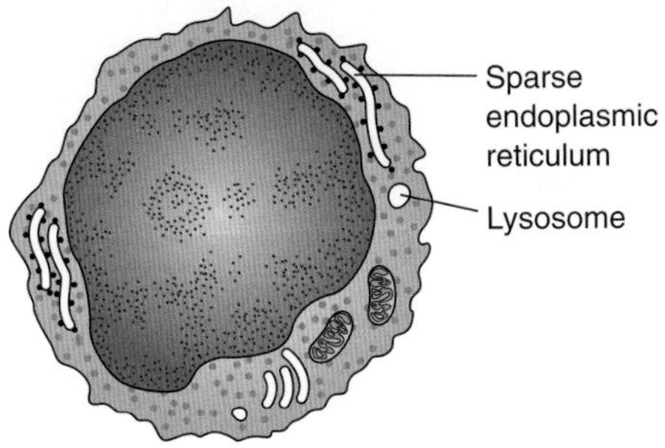

Sparse endoplasmic reticulum

Lysosome

LYMPHOCYTE

CHARACTERISTICS AND FUNCTIONS
- Associated with chronic inflammation
- Key cells in humoral and cell-mediated immune responses
- Cytokine production
- Multiple subtypes:

B cell → Plasma cell → Antibody production

T cell → Effector cells → Delayed hypersensitivity / Mixed lymphocyte reactivity / Cytotoxic "killer" cells (K cells)

T cell → Regulatory cells → Helper T cells / Suppressor T cells

Cytotoxic natural killer (NK) cell
Null cell

B

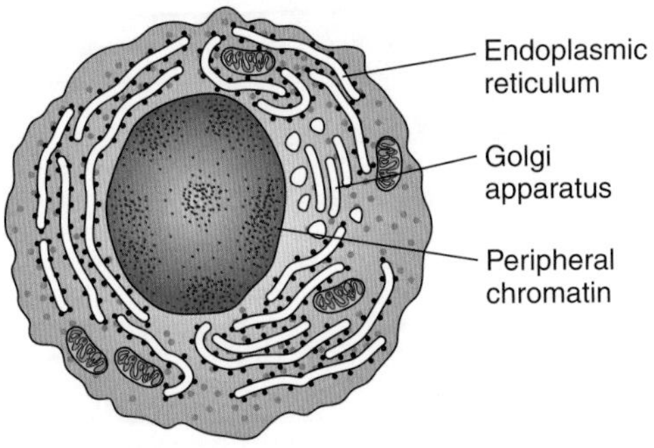

Endoplasmic reticulum

Golgi apparatus

Peripheral chromatin

PLASMA CELL

CHARACTERISTICS AND FUNCTIONS
- Associated with:
  - -Antibody synthesis and secretion
  - -Chronic inflammation
- Derived from B lymphocytes

C

FIBROBLAST

CHARACTERISTICS AND FUNCTIONS
- Produces extracellular matrix proteins
- Mediates chronic inflammation and wound healing

PRIMARY INFLAMMATORY MEDIATORS
- IL-6
- IL-8
- Cyclooxygenase-2
- Hyaluronan
- PGE_2
- CD40 expression
- Matricellular proteins
- Extracellular proteins

FIGURE 2-28. More cells of inflammation: morphology and function. A. Lymphocyte. **B.** Plasma cell. **C.** Fibroblast. IL, interleukin; PGE, prostaglandin E.

PMN enzymes are beneficial when they digest phagocytosed organisms intracellularly, they be destructive if they are released extracellularly. Thus, when PMNs accumulate, connective tissue may be digested by their enzymes.

Persistent tissue injury due to inflammatory cells is important in the pathogenesis of several diseases (e.g., emphysema, rheumatoid arthritis, some immune complex diseases, gout and acute respiratory distress syndrome). Phagocytic cell adherence, escape of ROS, and release of lysosomal enzymes together enhance cytotoxicity and tissue degradation. Proteinase activity is significantly elevated in chronic wounds, creating a proteolytic environment that prevents healing.

Granulomatous Inflammation

PMNs ordinarily remove agents that incite acute inflammatory responses. However, sometimes these cells cannot digest those substances. Such a situation is potentially dangerous, because it can lead to a vicious circle of (1) phagocytosis, (2) failure of digestion, (3) death of the PMN, (4) release of undigested provoking agents, and (5) repeated phagocytosis by a newly recruited PMN (Fig. 2-29). ***Granuloma formation is a protective response to chronic infection (e.g., some fungi, tuberculosis) or the presence of foreign material (e.g., suture or talc). It isolates a persistent offending agent, preventing it from disseminating and by restricting inflammation, protecting the host.*** In some granulomatous disorders, such as sarcoidosis, no inciting agent has yet been identified.

The principal cells involved in granulomatous inflammation are macrophages and lymphocytes (Fig. 2-30). Macrophages are mobile cells that continuously migrate through extravascular connective tissues. After amassing substances, they cannot digest, macrophages lose their motility and accumulate at the site of injury to form nodular collections of pale, epithelioid cells, termed **granulomas**.

Multinucleated giant cells are formed by cytoplasmic fusion of macrophages. The nuclei of such giant cells are often arranged around the periphery of the cytoplasm in a horseshoe pattern, in which case the cell is called a **Langhans giant cell** (Fig. 2-30B). **Foreign body giant cells** contain an undigested foreign material such as suture remnants (Fig. 2-30C). Granulomas are further classified by the presence or absence of necrosis. Certain infectious agents, notably

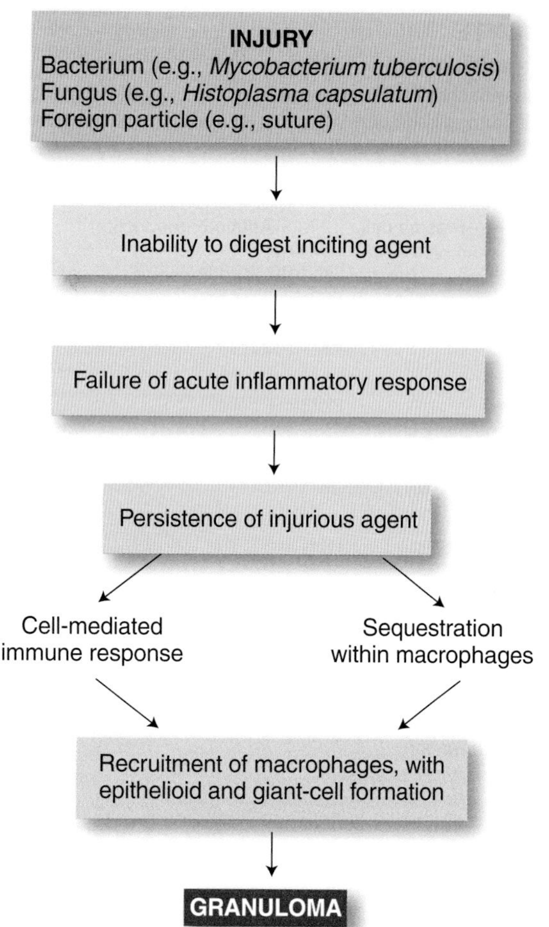

FIGURE 2-29. **Mechanism of granuloma formation.**

M. tuberculosis, characteristically produce necrotizing or **caseating granulomas**, the centers of which are filled with an amorphous mixture of debris and dead microorganisms and cells. In other diseases, such as sarcoidosis, granulomas characteristically lack necrosis.

CHRONIC INFLAMMATION AND TUMORIGENESIS

Several chronic infectious diseases are associated with development of cancer. For example, schistosomiasis in the urinary bladder leads to squamous cell carcinoma of that organ. Inflammation that is not specifically linked to infection may also be a risk factor for cancer. Patients with reflux esophagitis or ulcerative colitis are at higher risk for adenocarcinoma in those organs. An environment created by chronic inflammation promotes malignant transformation by several mechanisms (see Chapter 4):

- **Increased cell proliferation:** Chronically stimulated cell division increases the likelihood of transforming mutations in proliferating cells.
- **Oxygen and NO• metabolites:** Inflammatory metabolites, such as nitrosamines, may cause genomic damage (see Chapter 4).

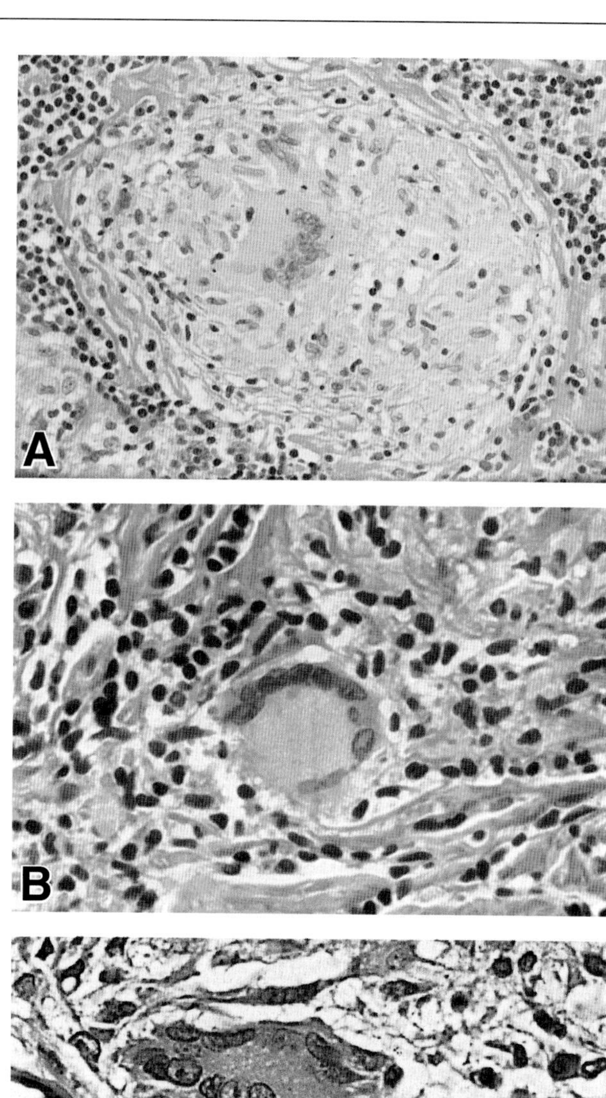

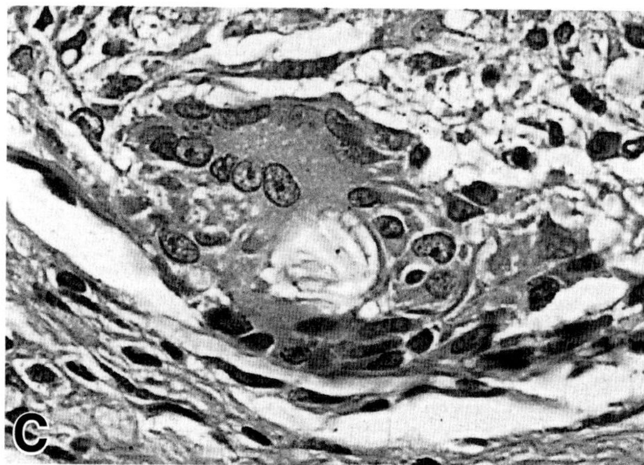

FIGURE 2-30. **Types of granulomas. A.** Granuloma with a multinucleated giant cell amid numerous pale epithelioid cells. **B.** Langhans giant cell shows nuclei arranged on the periphery of an abundant cytoplasm. **C.** Foreign body giant cell with numerous nuclei randomly arranged in the cytoplasm and foreign material in the center.

- **Chronic immune activation:** Chronic antigen exposure alters the cytokine milieu by suppressing cell-mediated immune responses. This creates a more permissive environment for malignant growth.
- **Angiogenesis:** Growth of new vessels is associated with inflammation and wound healing and is important in sustaining cancers.
- **Inhibition of apoptosis:** Chronic inflammation suppresses apoptosis. Increased cell division and decreased apoptosis favor survival and expansion of mutated cell populations.

SYSTEMIC MANIFESTATIONS OF INFLAMMATION

The symptoms associated with inflammation, including fever, myalgia, arthralgia, anorexia, and somnolence, are attributable to a number of cytokines, including IL-1, IL-6, and TNF-α. The most prominent systemic manifestations of inflammation are as follows:

- **Release of anti-inflammatory glucocorticoids** from the adrenal cortex
- **Leukocytosis** is most commonly associated with bacterial infections and tissue injury and is caused by release of specific mediators from macrophages and perhaps other cells.
- **Acute phase response** is a regulated physiologic reaction that occurs in inflammatory conditions. It is characterized clinically by fever, leukocytosis, decreased appetite, and altered sleep patterns, and chemically by changes in plasma levels of acute phase proteins. These molecules (Table 2-6) are synthesized primarily by the liver and released in large quantities into the circulation in response to an acute inflammatory challenge.
- **Fever:** The release of **pyrogens** by bacteria, viruses, or injured cells directly affects hypothalamic activity by stimulating production of cytokines (IL-1α, -1β and -6, and TNF-α) and interferons. IL-1 stimulates prostaglandin synthesis in hypothalamic thermoregulatory centers, thereby altering the "thermostat" that controls body temperature.
- **Shock:** With massive tissue injury or sepsis, the large quantities of cytokines, especially TNF-α, poured into the circulation affect the heart and peripheral vascular system by causing (1) generalized vasodilation, (2) increasing vascular permeability, (3) intravascular volume loss and ultimately myocardial depression, and (4) decreasing cardiac output. The condition is collectively termed the **systemic inflammatory response syndrome (SIRS)**. Sepsis may be defined as SIRS in the setting of infection.

TRIGGERS OF SEPSIS

Sepsis and Initial Site of Infection

The most common site of sepsis-related infection is the lungs. More than 40% of septic patients have a respiratory source of infection such as pneumonia. Fig. 12-2 shows the typical histopathology of bacterial pneumonia. Abdominal infections are the second most frequent cause of sepsis. These occur in many circumstances, including ruptured appendicitis, penetrating injuries to the bowel, and postsurgical anastomotic leaks. Urinary tract infections are the third most common starting point for sepsis. Additional causes of sepsis are attributable to soft tissue infections, primary bacteremia, meningitis, encephalitis, endocarditis, and others. Infections that precipitate sepsis may be acquired in the community or during the course of hospitalization (i.e., nosocomial infections). Patients who develop sepsis as a result of nosocomial infections have higher mortality rates than those with community-acquired pathogens.

Table 2-6

Acute Phase Proteins

Protein	Function
Mannose-binding protein	Opsonization/complement activation
C-reactive protein	Opsonization
α_1-Antitrypsin	Serine protease inhibitor
Haptoglobin	Binds hemoglobin
Ceruloplasmin	Antioxidant, binds copper
Fibrinogen	Coagulation
Serum amyloid A protein	Apolipoprotein
α_2-Macroglobulin	Antiprotease
Cysteine protease inhibitor	Antiprotease

Factors That Influence the Risk of Sepsis

Sepsis occurs more often in those who are at the extremes of life: the aged and very young children. Males are more likely to develop sepsis than are females, and blacks are more susceptible than are whites. People with chronic illnesses, especially if their immune systems are compromised, are particularly at risk. AIDS, iatrogenic immunosuppression (e.g., postchemotherapy), long-standing respiratory or circulatory insufficiency, and so forth, predispose patients to sepsis.

Influence of Pathogens

Infections with diverse types of pathogens may lead to sepsis, depending on the host response to the infectious insult. The nature of the infectious organisms that precipitate sepsis has shifted over time. Gram-positive bacteria are now responsible for more cases than are gram-negative organisms. A single bacterial species is responsible in over 85% of cases, with the remainder being due to polymicrobial bacterial infections or infections with fungi, anaerobes, viruses, or parasites. The incidence of fungal sepsis has increased sharply in recent years, but fungi still provoke only about 5% to 10% of cases overall.

Bacteremia (i.e., microbial infection of the bloodstream) may occur during sepsis, but it is not an essential component because local infections can lead to distant tissue damage and organ dysfunction. Blood cultures are positive in only 20% to 40% of patients with severe sepsis and 40% to 70% of those with septic shock. Clinical suspicion for sepsis should remain high particularly if an infection is suspected but not detectable.

E. coli is the most common cause of enteric gram-negative sepsis, but other gram-negative rods, including *Pseudomonas*, *Klebsiella*, and *Enterobacter* species, produce identical disease. The discussion that follows relates to gram-negative sepsis in general.

The presence of *E. coli* in the bloodstream causes septic shock through the effects of TNF (among other factors), whose release from macrophages is stimulated by bacterial endotoxin.

COURSE OF SEPSIS

Sepsis is part of a systemic overreaction that begins with inflammatory responses to infection. These responses reflect host recognition of pathogen-associated molecular patterns (PAMPs) that are present on invading microorganisms. PAMPs are perceived via pattern response receptors (PRRs), such as Toll-like receptors (TLRs) and C-type lectin receptors (CLRs) on dendritic cells (Fig. 12-3).

Endocytosis of these pathogens triggers major intracellular receptors of several types. Transmembrane TLR receptor binding to these mediators also activates NFκB within monocytes and stimulates production of pro-inflammatory cytokines, such as TNF-α and IL-6, chemokines like IL-8, intracellular adhesion molecule-1 ICAM-1, and NO (see Chapter 1).

Tissue necrosis releases damage-associated molecular pattern molecules (DAMPs or alarmins). DAMPs are recognized by pattern recognition receptors in cells of the innate immune system. In turn the interaction between DAMPs and PRRs drives those cells to produce more pro-inflammatory mediators. Following this proinflammation stimulatory process, the body is flooded with factors that induce, potentiate, and sustain uncontrolled inflammation.

Pro- and Anti-Inflammatory Activities in Sepsis

Just as pro-inflammatory influences protect the host against invading pathogens, anti-inflammatory circuits tend to protect the host from potentially injurious inflammatory activity. In sepsis, pro-inflammatory influences overwhelm counterregulatory braking mechanisms and lead to tissue necrosis beyond what is elicited by pathogens or what is necessary to contain the infection.

When anti-inflammatory influences in sepsis finally occur, they act not so much to rein in inflammation that can damage tissues but rather to suppress immune responses and render the host susceptible to subsequent secondary or other infections (Fig. 12-7). In so doing, they magnify the impact of the initial infection and simultaneously evoke more inflammation.

Circulation and Coagulation Are Abnormal in Sepsis

Disseminated intravascular coagulation (DIC) and dysfunctional patterns of circulation are characteristic of sepsis. PAMPs trigger the expression of tissue factor (TF) by endothelial and other cells, particularly monocytes. TF activates the coagulation cascade (see Chapter 18) via factor VI, resulting in intravascular microthrombus formation. Pathogen-activated neutrophils release neutrophil extracellular traps (NETs; see Chapter 1), which also precipitate coagulation (Fig. 12-8).

Under normal circumstances, clot formation activates fibrinolytic pathways, which should limit the extent of clotting. However, in sepsis, mediators of fibrinolysis (tissue factor inhibitor, antithrombin, plasminogen activator, and others) are impaired or inhibited.

As a result, unimpeded formation of intravascular thrombi (DIC) limits blood flow and thus hinders adequate oxygen delivery to organs.

At the same time, endothelial cells activate inducible nitric oxide synthase (iNOS). NO stimulates vasodilation, increases vascular permeability, and causes leakage of plasma from the vascular system into tissue spaces.

These diverse dysfunctions increase the severity of sepsis. Invading pathogens, in the context of host and environmental factors that limit host modulatory activities, trigger excessive inflammatory responses and DIC. Both of these effects create a cycle of tissue death, circulatory insufficiency, and poor oxygen delivery to tissues. Anti-inflammatory activities make matters worse because they limit the ability of the adaptive immune system to respond to invading pathogens. Anti-inflammatory regulators, therefore, set the stage for subsequent secondary infection with additional pathogens (Fig. 12-9).

THE BASIC PROCESSES OF HEALING

From scarring to regeneration, damaged tissue heals in ways that ensure the immediate survival of the organism. The study of wound healing now encompasses a variety of cells, matrix proteins, growth factors, and cytokines, which regulate and modulate the repair process. Nearly every stage in the repair process is redundantly controlled, and there is no single rate-limiting factor, except for uncontrolled infection. **Successful healing, which maintains tissue function and repairs tissue barriers, prevents blood loss and infection, and is usually accomplished through collagen deposition or scarring (fibrosis).** Advances in our understanding of critical factors—growth factors, extracellular matrix, and stem cell biology—are improving healing, offering the possibility of restoring injured tissues to their normal architecture. Successful repair relies on a crucial balance between tissue formation and tissue remodeling.

Many of the basic cellular and molecular mechanisms required for wound healing participate in other processes that involve dynamic tissue changes, such as development and tumor growth. Three key cellular mechanisms are necessary for wound healing once hemostasis is achieved:

- **Cellular migration**
- **Extracellular matrix organization and remodeling**
- **Cell proliferation**

Migration of Cells

Migration of cells into a wound and activation of local cells are initiated by changes in the mechanical environment and mediators. The latter are either expressed de novo by resident cells or released from preformed reserves stored in granules of **platelets** and **basophils**. These granules contain cytokines, chemoattractants, proteases, and mediators of inflammation, which together control vascular supply, degrade damaged tissue, and initiate the repair cascade. Platelets are activated when bound to collagen exposed at sites of endothelial damage. Activated platelets release platelet-derived growth factor (PDGF) and many other molecules that facilitate adhesion, coagulation, vasoconstriction, cell proliferation, and clot resorption. Cellularity of wound sites increases through proliferation and recruitment to sites of injury (Fig. 2-31). ***Cell types of unique importance in skin wounds include the following:***

- **Monocytes/macrophages** maintain a basal resident population in tissues; they are recruited transiently in larger numbers from bone marrow and spleen shortly after neutrophil entry. During their more extended residence time in wounds, macrophages phagocytose debris and orchestrate the developing granulation tissue and healing by releasing cytokines and chemoattractants.
- **Fibroblasts, myofibroblasts, pericytes, and smooth muscle cells** represent a spectrum of mesenchymal cells that are recruited locally and are also populated from mesenchymal progenitors in bone marrow. They migrate and propagate via signals from growth factors and matrix degradation products, populating a skin wound by day 3 or 4. These cells mediate the synthesis of connective tissue (fibroplasia), tissue remodeling, vascular integrity, wound contraction, and wound strength.
- **Endothelial cells** sprout from existing postcapillary venules and are also seeded by circulating bone marrow progenitors. Nascent capillaries form in response to growth factors and are visible in wound granulation tissue, together with fibroblasts, beyond day 3. Development of capillaries is critical for gas exchange, delivery of nutrients, and influx of inflammatory cells.
- **Epidermal cells** move across the surface of a skin wound (Fig. 2-31(5)). Reepithelialization is delayed if the migrating epithelial cells must reconstitute a damaged basement

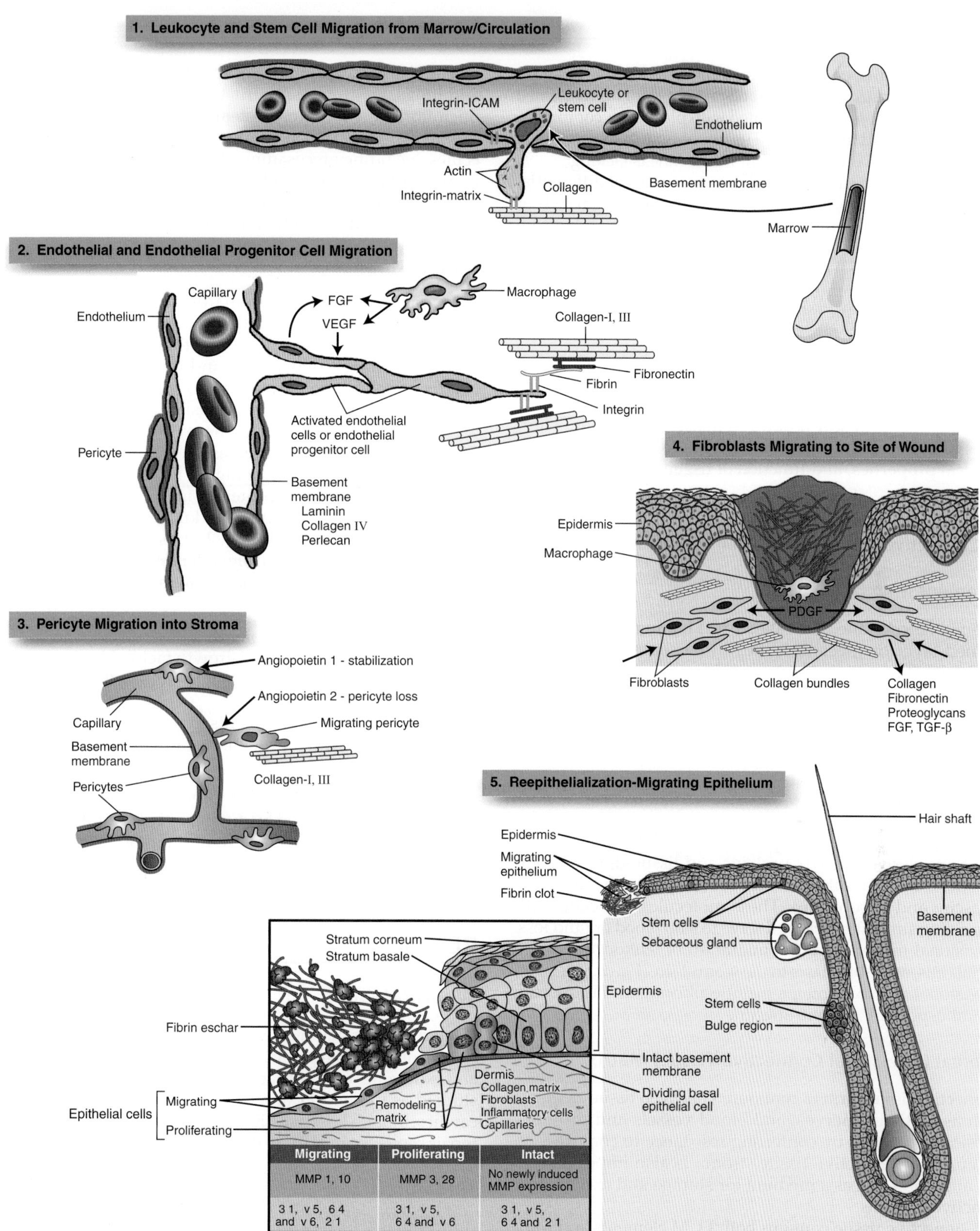

Migrating	Proliferating	Intact
MMP 1, 10	MMP 3, 28	No newly induced MMP expression
3 1, v 5, 6 4 and v 6, 2 1	3 1, v 5, 6 4 and v 6	3 1, v 5, 6 4 and 2 1

FIGURE 2-31. Resident and migrating cells initiate repair and regeneration. (*1*) After cytokine activation of capillary endothelium, leukocytes and bone marrow–derived circulating stem cells attach to, and migrate between, capillary endothelial cells; penetrate the basement membrane; and enter the interstitial matrix in response to chemotactic signals. (*2*) Under the influence of locally released angiogenic factors, capillary endothelial cells lose their connection with the basement membrane and extend through the provisional matrix to form new capillaries. Pericytes and basement membranes are required to stabilize new and existing capillary structures. (*3*) Pericytes detach from capillary endothelial cells and their basement membranes to migrate into the matrix. (*4*) Under the influence of growth factors, such as platelet-derived growth factor (PDGF), fibroblasts become bipolar and migrate through the matrix to the site of injury where transforming growth factor-β (TGF-β) can cause differentiation into smooth muscle actin-containing myofibroblasts. These then become bipolar and migrate through the matrix to the site of injury. (*5*) During reepithelialization, groups of basal keratinocytes at the wound edge release from underlying basement membrane, take on a migratory behavior and penetrate between the fibrin eschar (if present) and the granulation tissue that generates wound dermis. Migrating cells switch to a different display of integrin matrix receptors that recognize provisional matrix and stromal collagen (type I) and to different metalloproteinases that favor migration and matrix remodeling. FGF, fibroblast growth factor; MMP, matrix metalloproteinase; VEGF, vascular endothelial growth factor.

membrane. In open wounds, keratinocytes migrate between provisional matrix (see below) and preexisting or newly formed stromal collagen, which is coated with plasma glycoproteins, fibrinogen, and fibronectin. The phenotype of the epithelial layer is altered if the basement membrane is lacking.

- **Stem cells** from the bone marrow are capable of differentiation, proliferation, and migration. In the skin, stem cells or **progenitor cells** are present in the hair follicle and within the basal epidermal layer, where they provide renewable sources of epidermal and dermal cells. Stem cells for epidermal regeneration reside in the bulge region of the hair follicle and the interfollicular epidermis (Fig. 2-31(5)).

Extracellular Matrix

ECM is critical for repair and regeneration by providing the key components of scar tissue and the stem cell niche. Three types of extracellular matrix contribute to the organization, physical properties, and function of tissue:

- **Basement membrane**
- **Provisional matrix**
- **Connective tissue (interstitial matrix or stroma)**

Basement Membrane

Basement membrane, also called **basal lamina**, is a thin, well-defined layer of specialized ECM that separates cells that synthesize it from adjacent interstitial connective tissue. It is a supportive and biologic boundary important in development, healing, and regeneration. It also provides key signals for cell differentiation and polarity and contributes to tissue organization.

Provisional Matrix

Provisional matrix is the temporary extracellular organization of plasma-derived matrix proteins and tissue-derived components that accumulate at sites of injury (e.g., hyaluronan, tenascin, and fibronectin). These molecules associate with preexisting stromal matrix and serve to stop blood or fluid loss. Provisional matrix supports migration of leukocytes, endothelial cells, and fibroblasts to the wound site. Plasma-derived provisional matrix proteins include fibrinogen, fibronectin, thrombospondin, and vitronectin.

Stromal (Interstitial Connective Tissue) Matrix

Connective tissue forms a continuum between tissue elements such as epithelia, nerves, and blood vessels and provides physical protection by conferring resistance to compression or tension. Connective tissue stroma is also important for cell migration and as a medium for storage and exchange of bioactive proteins.

Connective tissue contains both ECM elements and individual cells that synthesize the matrix. The cells are primarily of mesenchymal origin and include fibroblasts, myofibroblasts, adipocytes, chondrocytes, osteocytes, and endothelial cells. Bone marrow–derived cells (e.g., mast cells, macrophages, transient leukocytes) are also present.

The ECM of connective tissue, also called **stroma** or **interstitium**, is defined by fibers formed from a large family of collagen molecules (Table 2-7). Of the fibrillar collagens, type I collagen is the major constituent of bone. Types I and III collagens are prominent in skin; type II collagen is predominant in cartilage. Elastic fibers, which impart elasticity to skin, large blood vessels, and lungs, are composite structures consisting of elastin and microfibrillar scaffolding proteins, such as fibrillin and fibulin. The so-called **ground substance** represents a number of molecules, including glycosaminoglycans (GAGs), proteoglycans, matricellular proteins, and fibronectin. These components are important in many biologic functions of connective tissue and in the support and modulation of cell attachment.

Remodeling

As repair proceeds, inflammatory cells become fewer in number and capillary formation is completed. In remodeling, fibroblast numbers rapidly rise and then fall as an equilibrium between collagen deposition, and degradation is restored. Matrix metalloproteinases (MMPs) are the main remodeling enzymes, but neutrophil cathepsins and serine proteases are also present at the early phase of wound debridement. MMP and ADAM are proteinases with zinc at the catalytic site (metzincins); they have highly localized protease activity. The activity of these proteases is controlled, in part, by a family of tissue-based molecules known as tissue inhibitors of metalloproteinases (TIMPs). ***The list of molecules needed for wound healing is indistinguishable from the list of MMP substrates.*** These include the following:

- Clotting factors
- Extracellular matrix proteins
- Latent growth factors and growth factor–binding proteins
- Receptors for matrix molecules and cell–cell adhesion molecules
- Immune system components
- Other MMPs, other proteinases, and proteinase inhibitors
- Chemotactic molecules

Once secreted, MMPs act largely near the cell surface, their activities controlled by diffusion/sequestration, reduced activation, substrate specificity, and peptide inhibitors. The family of TIMPs and the plasma-derived proteinase inhibitor, α_2-macroglobulin, are important regulators.

REPAIR

Wound Healing

Wound healing that results in scar formation remains the predominant mode of repair in adults. Given that wounds in the skin and extremities are easily accessible, they have been extensively studied as models. Healing within hollow viscera and body cavities, though less accessible for study, generally parallels the repair sequence in skin, as illustrated in Figures 2-32 and 2-33.

Thrombosis

A thrombus (clot)—a **scab** or **eschar** after it dries atop a surface wound—forms a barrier on wounded skin to invading microorganisms. The formation of the fibrin clot is essential to prevent loss of plasma and tissue fluid. Although the clot/thrombus is predominantly plasma fibrin, it is also rich in the adhesive protein fibronectin. The thrombus also contains contracting platelets, whose aggregation produces an initial burst of stored growth factors. At the site of injury, fibrin is bound to fibronectin and is progressively cross-linked by factor XIII (FXIII), a transglutaminase. Transglutaminase 2 (tissue transglutaminase) fosters cell adhesion, cell migration,

Table 2-7

Collagen Molecular Composition and Structure

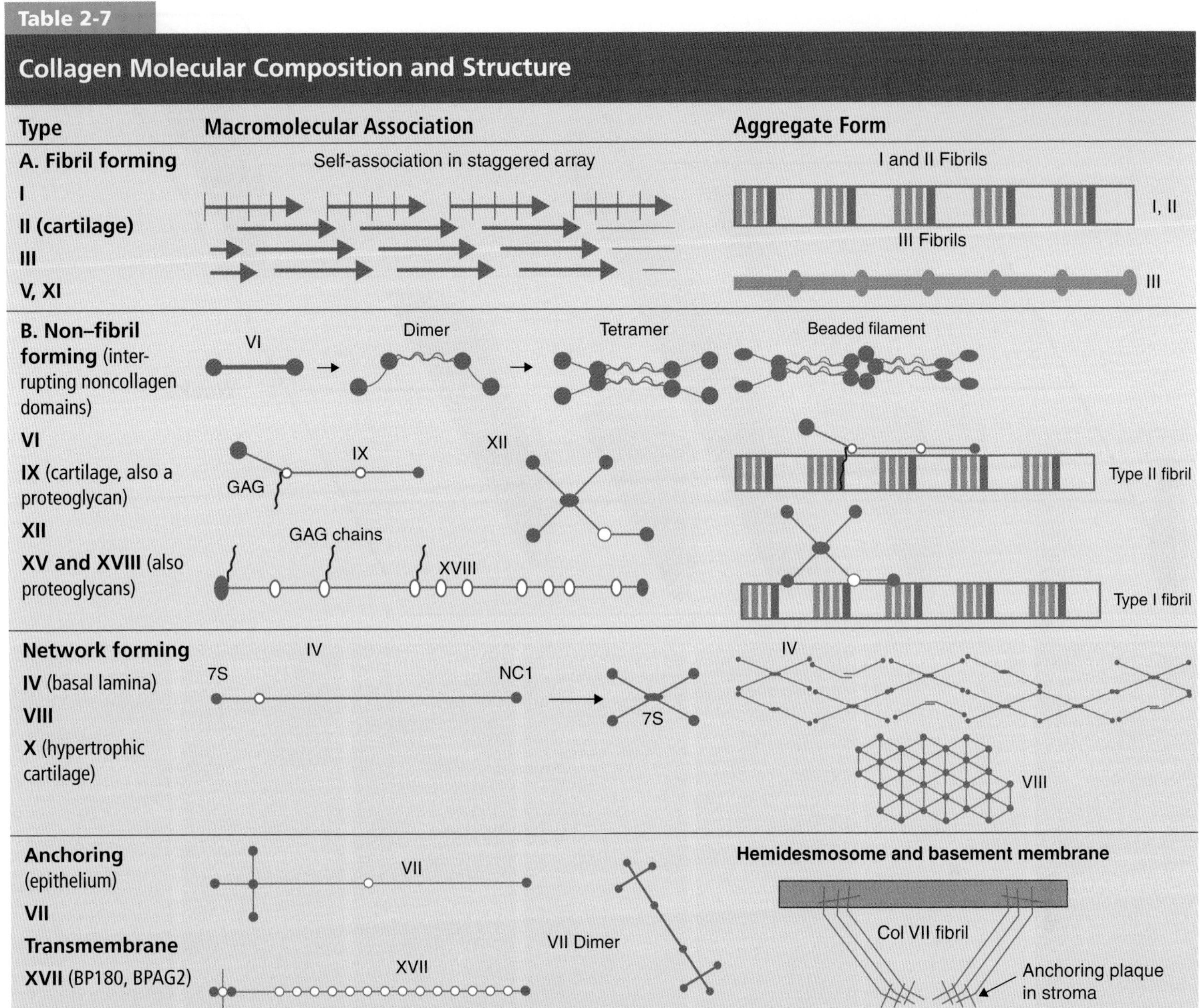

Type	Macromolecular Association	Aggregate Form
A. Fibril forming I **II (cartilage)** III V, XI	Self-association in staggered array	I and II Fibrils I, II III Fibrils III
B. Non–fibril forming (interrupting noncollagen domains) **VI** **IX** (cartilage, also a proteoglycan) **XII** **XV and XVIII** (also proteoglycans)	VI Dimer Tetramer IX GAG XII GAG chains XVIII	Beaded filament Type II fibril Type I fibril
Network forming **IV** (basal lamina) **VIII** **X** (hypertrophic cartilage)	IV 7S NC1 7S	IV VIII
Anchoring (epithelium) **VII** **Transmembrane** **XVII** (BP180, BPAG2)	VII VII Dimer XVII	**Hemidesmosome and basement membrane** Col VII fibril Anchoring plaque in stroma Anchoring fibril in papillary dermis

GAG, glycosaminoglycan.

and organization of wound extracellular matrix. It acts by (1) interlinking matrix proteins such as fibrinogen, fibronectin, collagen, and vitronectin; (2) providing local tensile strength; and (3) maintaining closure during the evolution of new extracellular matrix. The internal (nondesiccated) portion of the provisional matrix (see above) is transformed into granulation tissue by invasion of mononuclear cells, connective tissue, and vascular cells. At the same time, the outer portion (eschar) is a temporary repository for spent neutrophils and killed bacteria. As the granulation tissue is partitioned from the eschar by migrating epidermis, the portion of thrombus that is not repopulated by new tissue is digested. The scab then detaches.

Granulation Tissue

Granulation tissue is the transient, specialized organ of repair, which replaces the provisional matrix (Fig. 2-34). Microscopically, a mixture of fibroblasts, mononuclear cells, and red blood cells first invades the provisional matrix. This is followed by the development of extracellular matrix and patent capillaries, which are surrounded by pericytes and provide a blood supply to fibroblasts and inflammatory cells.

A key step in the process is recruitment of monocytes to the site of injury by chemokines and fragments of damaged matrix. Later, plasma cells are conspicuous, even predominant. Activated macrophages progressively shift from a proinflammatory M1 phenotype to the more constructive M2 phenotype. The latter release growth factors and cytokines (Table 2-8 and see below) that direct angiogenesis, activate fibroblasts to form new stroma, and continue the degradation and removal of the provisional matrix.

Granulation tissue is fluid rich, and its cellular constituents supply immunoglobulins, antibacterial peptides **(defensins)**, and growth factors. It is highly resistant to bacterial infection, allowing the surgeon to create anastomoses at such nonsterile sites as the colon.

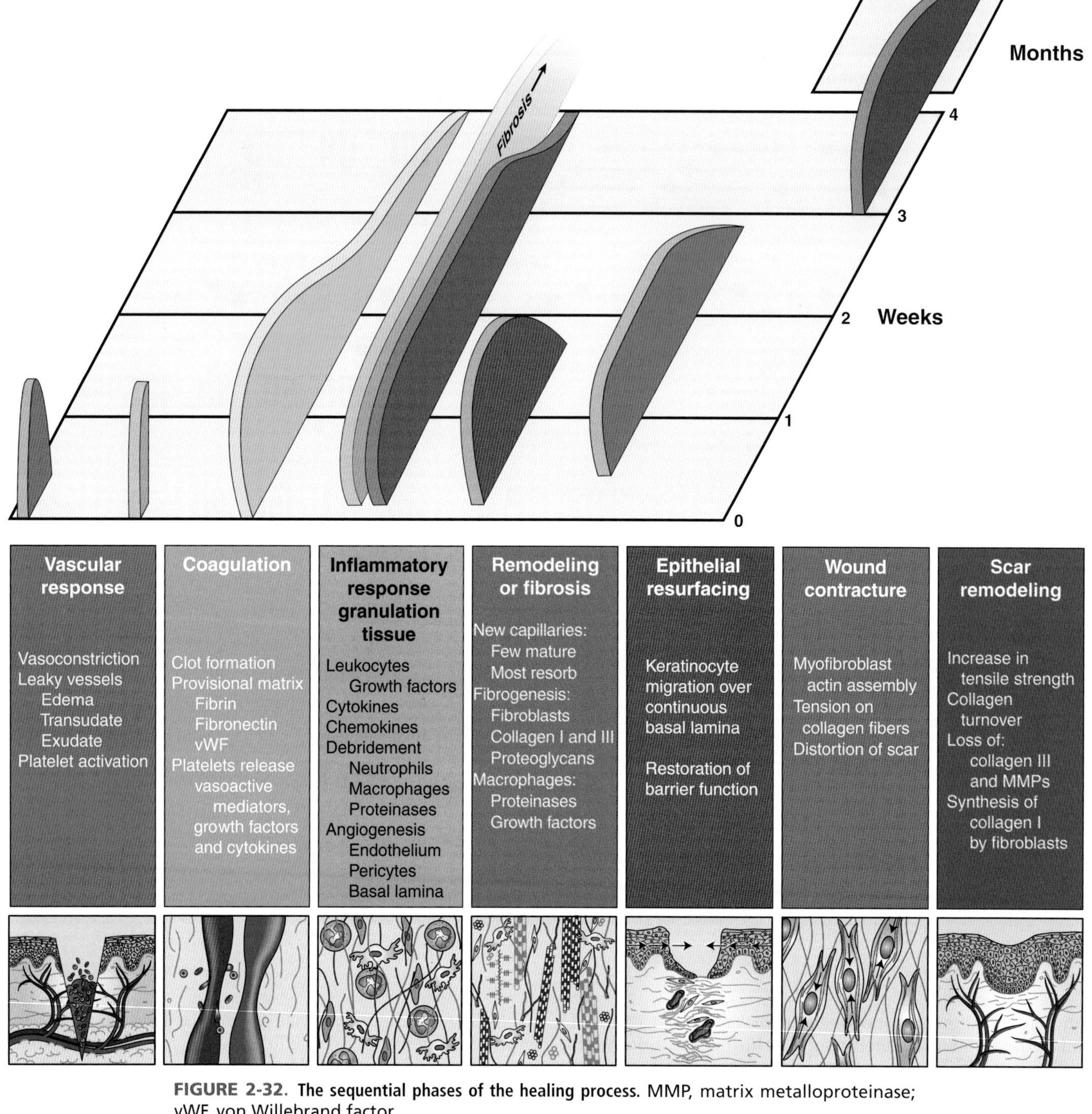

FIGURE 2-32. The sequential phases of the healing process. MMP, matrix metalloproteinase; vWF, von Willebrand factor.

Fibroblast Proliferation and Matrix Accumulation

Early granulation tissue matrix contains hyaluronan, proteoglycans, glycoproteins, and fine collagen fibers that predominantly consists of type III collagen (Figs. 2-32 and 2-33). Cytokines released by cells in the damaged area cause vascular leakage and attract both inflammatory cells and vascular endothelial cells. About 2 to 3 days after injury, activated fibroblasts and capillary sprouts are seen. Fibroblasts in the wound change from oval to bipolar, as they begin to produce collagen and other matrix proteins, such as fibronectin, and develop contractile properties. Secretion of type III collagen is rapidly overwhelmed by type I collagen, which promotes the assembly of larger-diameter fibrils with greater tensile strength. Eventually, the matrix resumes its original composition of predominantly type I collagen and 15% to 20% type III collagen.

The rate of matrix accumulation peaks at 5 to 7 days, depending on the tissue. This process is strongly influenced by the production of TGF-β, which increases the synthesis

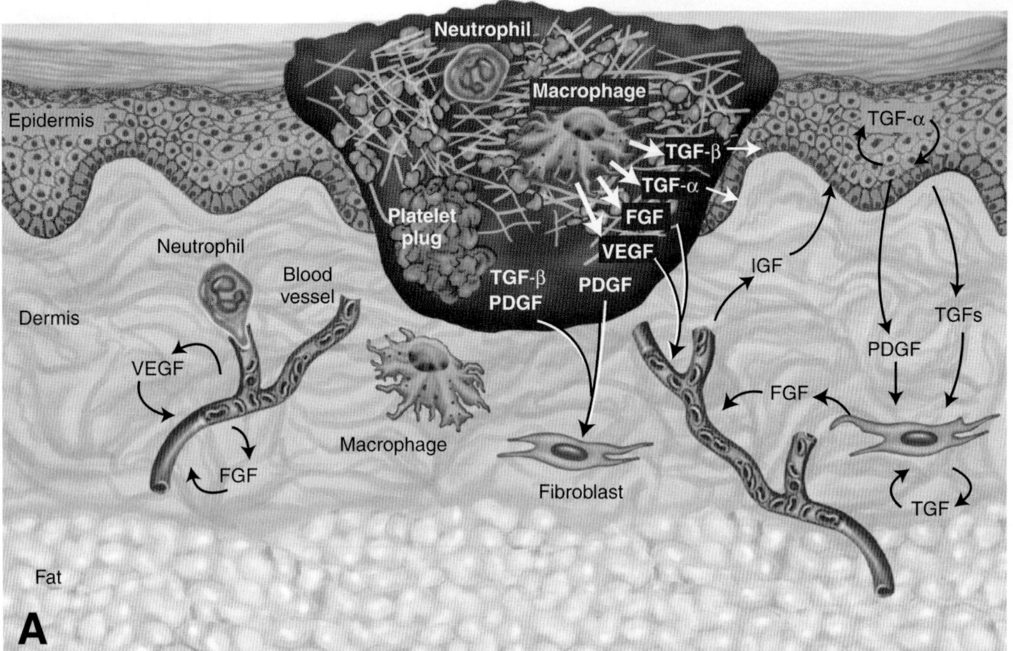

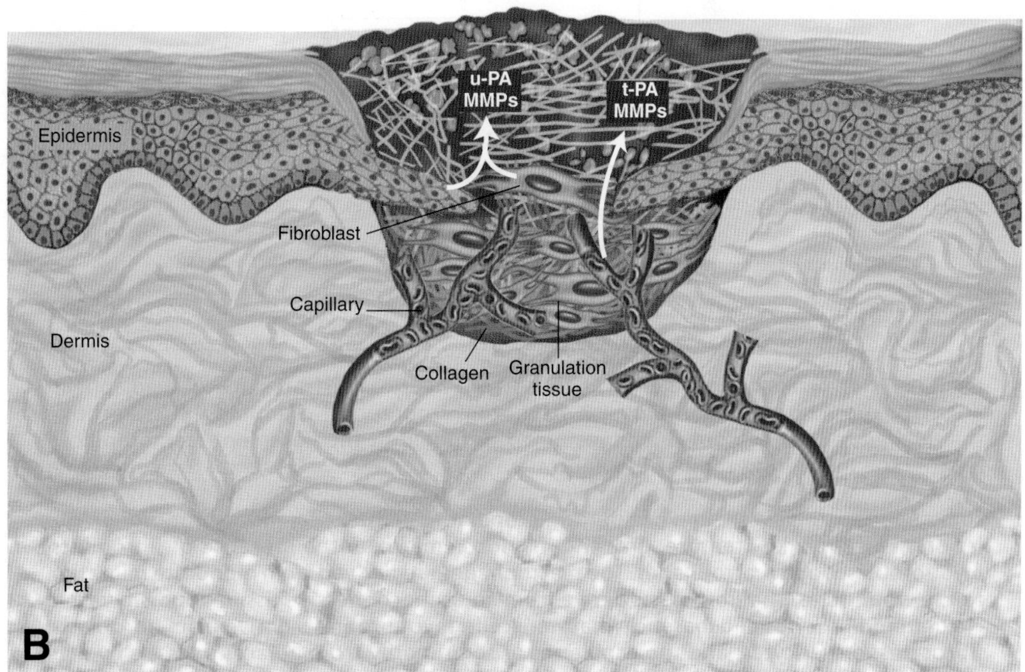

FIGURE 2-33. Cutaneous wound healing. A. 2–4 days. Growth factors controlling migration of cells are illustrated. Extensive redundancy is present, and no single growth factor is rate limiting. Most factors have multiple effects, as listed in Table 2-9. Growth factor signals first arise from degranulating platelets, but activated macrophages, resident tissue cells, injured epidermis, and the matrix itself release a complex interplay of interacting signals. **B. 4–8 days.** Capillary blood vessels invade and proliferate within the provisional matrix, and the epidermal keratinocytes advance along the granulation tissue below the thrombus. The upper, acellular portion of the wound site will become an eschar or scab. Fibroblasts deposit a collagen-rich matrix. FGF, fibroblast growth factor; IGF, insulin-like growth factor; MMPs, matrix metalloproteinases; PDGF, platelet-derived growth factor; TGF-β, transforming growth factor-β; t-PA, tissue plasminogen activator; u-PA, urokinase-type plasminogen activator; VEGF, vascular endothelial growth factor.

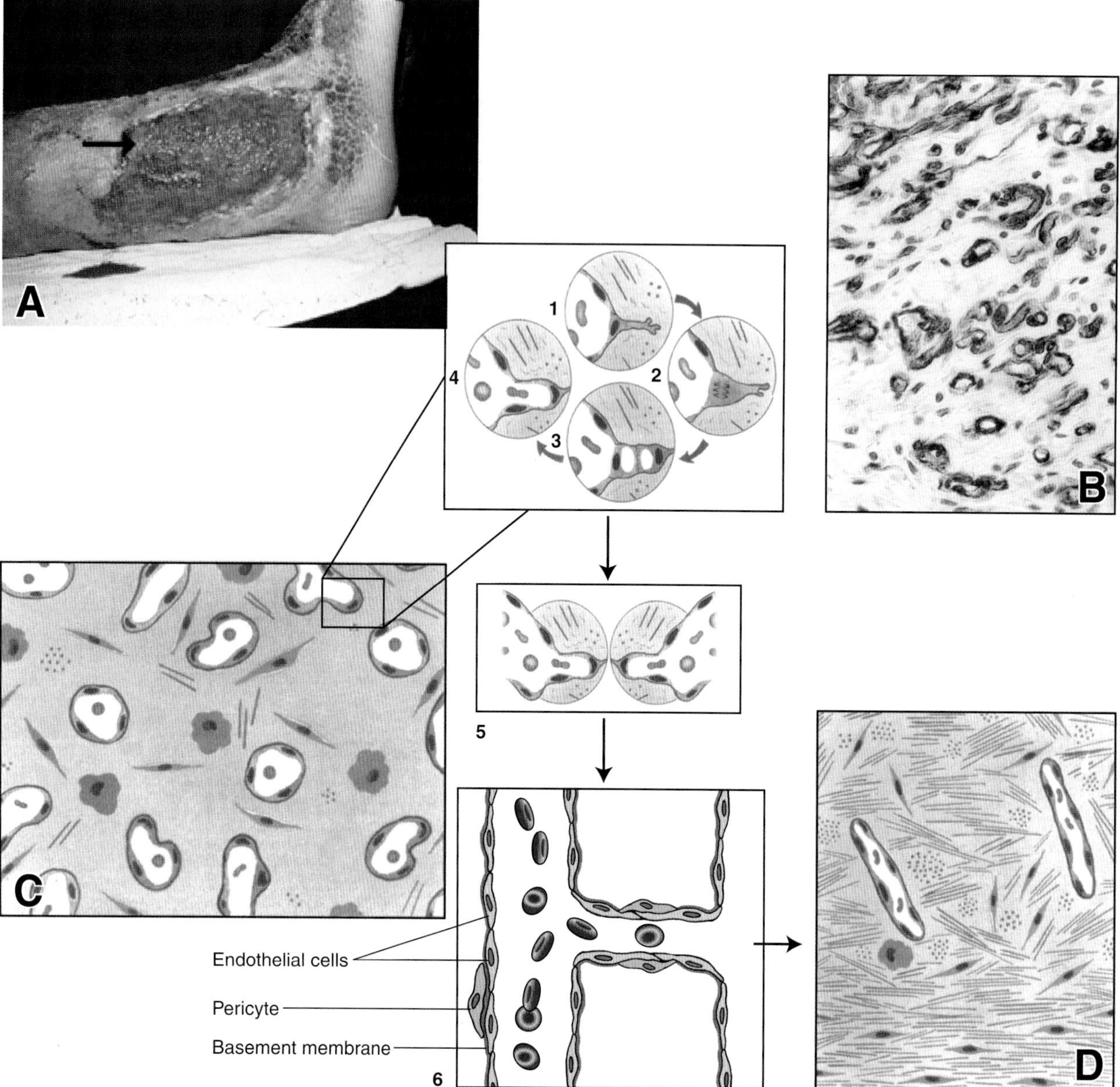

FIGURE 2-34. Granulation tissue. A. A venous stasis leg ulcer illustrates the cobbled appearance of exposed granulation tissue. **B.** A photomicrograph of granulation tissue shows thin-walled capillary sprouts immunostained to highlight the basement membrane collagens. The infiltrating capillaries penetrate a loose connective tissue matrix containing mesenchymal cells and occasional inflammatory cells. **C.** Granulation tissue has two major components: stromal cells and proliferating capillaries. Initially, capillary sprouts of granulation tissue are a key feature, growing in a loose matrix in the presence of fibroblasts, myofibroblasts, and macrophages. The macrophages are derived from monocyte migration to the wound site. The fibroblasts derive from adjacent connective tissue or possibly from circulating fibrocytes and mesenchymal stem cells; myofibroblasts derive from fibroblasts, fibrocytes, or pericytes; and the capillaries arise primarily from adjacent vessels by division of the lining endothelial cells (steps 1–6), in a process termed . Endothelial cells put out cell extensions, called *pseudopodia*, that grow toward the wound site. Cytoplasmic flow enlarges the pseudopodia, and eventually the cells divide. Vacuoles formed in the daughter cells eventually fuse to create a new lumen. The entire process continues until the sprout encounters another capillary sprout, with which it will connect. At its peak, granulation tissue is the most richly vascularized tissue in the body. **D.** Once repair has been achieved, most of the newly formed capillaries undergo apoptosis, leaving a pale, avascular scar rich in collagen.

Table 2-8

Extracellular Signals in Wound Repair

Phase	Factor(s)	Source	Effects
Coagulation	XIIIa	Plasma	Cross-linking of fibrin thrombus
	TGF-α, TGF-β, PDGF, ECGF, FGF	Platelets	Chemoattraction and activation of subsequent cells
Inflammation	TGF-β, chemokines TNF-α, IL-1, IL-6, CXCL12, CX3CL1, PDGF	Neutrophil, M1 macrophages, endothelial cells	Attract monocytes and fibroblasts; differentiate fibroblasts and stem cells
Granulation tissue formation	FGF-2, TGF-β, HGF	Keratinocytes, monocytes then fibroblasts	Various factors are bound to proteoglycan matrix
Angiogenesis	VEGFs, FGFs, HGF, angioprotein-1/-2 PDGF	Monocytes, macrophages, fibroblasts, endothelial cells	Development of blood vessels Pericyte growth
Contraction	TGF-β1, β2	Macrophages, fibroblasts, keratinocytes	Myofibroblasts differentiate, bind to each other and to collagen and contract
Reepithelialization	KGF (FGF-7), HGF, EGF, HB-EGF, TGF-α, activin, TGF-β3, CXCL10, CXCL11	Macrophages, platelets, fibroblasts, keratinocytes, endothelial cells	Epithelial proliferation, migration, and differentiation
Maturation, fibroplasia, arrest of proliferation	TGF-β1, PDGF, CTGF, IL-27, IL-4, CX3CL1, thrombospondin	M2 macrophages, fibroblasts, keratinocytes	Accumulation of ECM, fibrosis, tensile strength
	HSPG	Endothelium Secretory fibroblasts	HSPG: Capture of TGF-β, VEGF, and basic FGF in basement membrane
	Decorin proteoglycan		Decorin: Capture of TGF-β, stabilization of collagen structure, downregulation of migration, proliferation
	Interferon, CXCL10, CXCL11	Plasma monocytes	Suppresses proliferation of fibroblasts and endothelial cells and accumulation of collagen
	Increased local oxygen, decreased mechanotransduction	Repair process	Suppression of release of cytokines
Resolution and remodeling	PDGF, FGF, TGF-β, interleukins	Platelets, fibroblasts, keratinocytes, macrophages	Regulation of MMPs and TIMPs Remodeling by restructuring of ECM (e.g., collagen III replaced by collagen I)
	MMPs, t-PAs, u-PAs	Sprouted capillaries, epithelial cells, fibroblasts	
	Tissue inhibitors of MMPs	Local, not further defined	Balance the effects of MMPs in the evolving repair site
	Signals for arrest: CXCL11 or IP-9, CXCL10 or IP-10	Basal keratinocytes Neovascular endothelium	Reduce cellularity CXCR3 signals Reduced migration and proliferation of fibroblasts, endothelial cells, increased migration of keratinocytes

CTGF, connective tissue growth factor; CXCL10 and 11, chemokine CXC-type ligand 10 and 11; IP, interferon-γ–induced protein; ECGF, endothelial cell growth factor; ECM, extracellular matrix; EGF, epidermal growth factor; FGF, fibroblast growth factor; HB-EGF, heparin-binding EGF; HGF, hepatocyte growth factor; HSPG, heparan sulfate proteoglycan; IL, interleukin; KGF, keratinocyte growth factor (FGF-7); MMPs, matrix metalloproteinases; PDGF, platelet-derived growth factor; SDF-1, stromal cell–derived factor-1; TIMP, tissue inhibitor of metalloproteinase; TGF, transforming growth factor; TNF, tumor necrosis factor; t-PA, tissue plasminogen activator; u-PA, urokinase-type plasminogen activator; VEGF, vascular endothelial growth factor.

of collagen, fibronectin, TIMPs, and other matrix proteins, while decreasing MMP transcription and matrix degradation. Extracellular cross-linking of newly synthesized collagen progressively increases wound strength.

Epidermal growth factor (EGF) and at least 20 other growth factors have helped define the signaling mechanisms that rapidly change the course of repair and restoration. Growth factors expressed or mobilized early in wound responses include VEGF, FGF, PDGF, EGF, keratinocyte growth factor [KGF, FGF7], and others. They support migration, recruitment, and proliferation of cells involved in fibroplasia, reepithelialization, and angiogenesis. Growth factors that peak later (TGF-β, insulin-like growth factor-I [IGF-I]) sustain the maturation phase, growth, and remodeling of granulation tissue. The interactions among growth factors, other cytokines, and MMPs are illustrated in Tables 2-9 and 2-10.

Angiogenesis

The Growth of Capillaries

At its peak, granulation tissue has more capillaries per unit volume than any other tissue. New capillaries form by angiogenesis (i.e., sprouting of endothelial cells from preexisting capillary venules) (Fig. 2-34) and create the granular appearance for which the tissue is named. Angiogenesis is initiated by hypoxia and other cytokines, growth factors and various lipids, which stimulate or regulate VEGF. Hypoxia-inducible factor (HIF), whose stability is exquisitely regulated by tissue oxygen tension, is the main trigger for VEGF expression.

Quiescent capillary endothelial cells are activated by loss of basement membrane and local release of cytokines and growth factors. Disruption or paucity of basement membranes surrounding endothelial cells and pericytes predicts sites of endothelial cells sprouting into the provisional matrix. Endothelial passage through the matrix is an invasive process that requires the cooperation of plasminogen activators, matrix MMPs, and integrin receptors. The growth of new capillaries is supported by proliferation and assembly of endothelial cells (Fig. 2-34). There is also a possible contribution of limited numbers of mononuclear, bone marrow–derived endothelial progenitor cells; these are recruited, at least transiently, to support growing vessels.

Once capillary endothelial cells are immobilized, cell–cell contacts form, and an organized basement membrane develops on the exterior of the nascent capillary. An interplay between endothelial cells and pericytes occurs during angiogenesis. New capillaries that have not matured are leaky, create hemorrhage or edema, and may undergo apoptosis. Endothelial association with pericytes and signals from angiopoietin I, TGF-β, and PDGF is essential to establish a mature vessel phenotype of nonleaky capillaries.

Table 2-10

Growth Factors, Enzymes, and Other Factors Regulate Progression of Repair and Fibrosis

Secretion of Collagenase	PDGF, EGF, IL-1, TNF, Proteases
Movement of surface and stromal cells	t-PA (tissue plasminogen activator) u-PA (urokinase-type plasminogen activator) Elastase MMPs (matrix metalloproteinases) MMP-1 (collagenase 1) MMP-2 (gelatinase A) MMP-3 (stromelysin 1) MMP-8 (collagenase 2) MMP-9 (gelatinase B) MMP-13 (collagenase 3) MT1-MMP (MMP-14; membrane bound) MMP-19
Maturation or stabilization of blood vessels	Angiopoietins (Ang1, Ang2); PDGF; HIF-1
Inhibition of collagenase production	TGF-β
Increase of TIMP production	
Reduction in collagen production and turnover	Reduction in mechanotransduction feedback and release/activation of latent TGF-β
Collagen cross-linking and maturation	Lysyl oxidase, integrin receptors, fibronectin polymers, small proteoglycans

EGF, epidermal growth factor; HIF-1, hypoxia-inducible factor 1; IL, interleukin; MT1, membrane type-1; PDGF, platelet-derived growth factor; TGF, transforming growth factor; TIMP, tissue inhibitor of metalloproteinases; TNF, tumor necrosis factor.

Table 2-9

Growth Factors Control Various Stages in Repair

Attraction of monocytes/macrophages	PDGFs, FGFs, TGF-β, MCP-1 (CCL2)
Attraction of fibroblasts	PDGFs, FGFs, TGF-β, CTGF, EGFs, SDF-1
Proliferation of fibroblasts	PDGFs, FGFs, EGFs, IGF, CTGF
Angiogenesis	VEGFs, FGFs, HGF
Collagen synthesis	TGF-β, PDGFs, IGF, CTGF
Collagen secretion	PDGFs, FGFs, CTGF
Epithelial migration and proliferation	KGF, TGF-α, HGF, IGF of epithelium–epidermis
Resolution of repair	IP-9 (CXCL11), IP-10 (CXCL10)

CCL2, C-type chemokine ligand 2; CXCL 10 and 11, CXC-type chemokine ligand 10 and 11; CTGF, connective tissue growth factor; EGF, epidermal growth factor; FGF, fibroblast growth factor; HGF, hepatocyte growth factor; IGF, insulin-like growth factor; IP-9/10, interferon-γ–inducible protein 9/10; KGF, keratinocyte growth factor; MCP-1, macrophage chemotactic protein-1; PDGF, platelet-derived growth factor; SDF-1, stromal cell–derived factor-1; TGF, transforming growth factor; VEGF, vascular endothelial growth factor.

Reepithelialization

The epidermis constantly renews itself by the mitosis of keratinocyte stem cells in the basal layer. The squamous cells then cornify or keratinize as they mature, move toward the surface, and are shed a few days later. Maturation requires an intact layer of basal cells that are in direct contact with one another and with the basement membrane (Fig. 2-31(5)). If cell–cell contact is disrupted, basal epidermal cells migrate laterally and divide to reestablish contact with other basal cells. In partial-thickness skin wounds, where the epidermis is destroyed, specialized progenitor cells in the hair follicle become a primary source of regenerating epithelium (Fig. 2-31(5)). Once reestablished, the epidermal barrier demarcates the scab from the newly formed granulation tissue. When epithelial continuity is reestablished, the epidermis resumes its normal cycle of maturation and shedding. Epidermal integrity protects against infection and fluid loss.

Wound Contraction

Open wounds contract and deform as they heal, depending on the degree of attachment to underlying connective tissue structures. Wound contraction and fibrosis in particular involve a specialized cell of granulation tissue, the **myofibroblast** (Fig. 2-35), a cell that looks like a fibroblast but behaves like a smooth muscle cell. Myofibroblasts contain abundant actin stress fibers (often α-smooth muscle actin), desmin, vimentin, and a particular fibronectin splice variant that forms polymerized cellular fibronectin. Myofibroblasts respond to physical or mechanical forces and agents that cause smooth muscle cells to contract or relax.

Together with fibroblasts, myofibroblasts contribute to normal wound contraction and become more prevalent in deforming wound contracture. Myofibroblasts usually appear about the third day of wound healing, in parallel with the sudden appearance of contractile forces, which then diminish over the next several weeks. These cells are associated with an increase in type I collagen and are prevalent in fibrosis and hypertrophic scars.

Wound Strength

Skin incisions and surgical anastomoses in hollow viscera ultimately develop 75% of the strength of the unwounded site. Despite a rapid increase in tensile strength at 7 to 14 days, by the end of 2 weeks the wound still has a high proportion of type III collagen and has only about 20% of its ultimate strength. Most of the strength of the healed wound results from synthesis and intermolecular cross-linking of type I collagen during the remodeling phase. A 2-month-old incision, although healed, is still obvious. Incision lines and suture marks are distinct, vascular, and red. By 1 year, the incision is white and avascular, but usually still identifiable. As the scar fades further, it changes into an irregular line by stresses in the skin.

Conditions That Modify Repair

Location of the Wound

In addition to its size and shape, the location of a wound also affects healing. In sites where scant tissue separates skin and bone (e.g., over the anterior tibia), a wound in the skin cannot contract. Skin lesions in such areas, particularly burns, often require skin grafts because their edges cannot be apposed.

Nature of the Wound

The specialized terms primary and secondary healing describe the nature of healing in wounds with apposed or gaping margins (Fig 2-36).

Primary healing occurs when the surgeon closely approximates the edges of a wound. The actions of myofibroblasts are minimized, owing to the lack of mechanical strain. Regeneration of the epidermis is optimal, since epidermal cells need migrate only a minimal distance. **Secondary healing** proceeds when a large area of hemorrhage and necrosis cannot be totally corrected surgically. In this situation, myofibroblasts contract the wound and reinforce healing with extensive ECM. The resultant scarring repairs the defect.

Blood Supply

Wounds of the lower extremity in diabetics often heal poorly or may even require amputation because advanced atherosclerosis in the legs (peripheral vascular disease) and defective angiogenesis compromise blood supply and impede repair. Varicose veins of the legs, owing to failure of the venous valves to ensure venous return, can cause edema, formation of thick (fibrin) cuffs around microvessels, ulceration, and nonhealing (venous stasis ulcers). Bed/pressure sores (decubitus ulcers) result from prolonged, localized, dependent pressure, which diminishes both arterial and venous blood flow and results in intermittent ischemia.

Systemic Factors

No specific effect of age alone on repair has been found, although there is evidence that stem cell reserves (see later) are reduced with aging.

Coagulation defects, thrombocytopenia, and anemia impede repair. Exogenous corticosteroids retard wound repair by inhibiting collagen and protein synthesis and by suppressing both destructive and constructive aspects of inflammation. Complications or other treatments, for example, infection, obesity, diabetes, chemotherapy, or ionizing radiation, also slow repair processes.

Fibrosis and Scarring Contrasted

Successful wound repair that leads to localized transient scarring promotes rapid resolution of local injury. Scars reflect altered deposition of ECM compared to normal, surrounding tissue. Scarring is a typical response to tissue ischemia or infarction, where resident cells cannot be replaced. However, ***fibrosis, the continued and excessive deposition of ECM particularly collagen, is the pathologic consequence of persistent injury and causes loss of function.*** In many chronic diseases of skin and parenchymal organs, including many autoimmune diseases (e.g., scleroderma), the inflammation persists and is followed by progression to diffuse fibrosis. Thus, fibrosis is often the final common result of diverse diseases or injuries, the causes of which cannot be ascertained from the end result. ***Scarring, however, is often beneficial; it restores structural (if not necessarily functional) integrity to the injured area.***

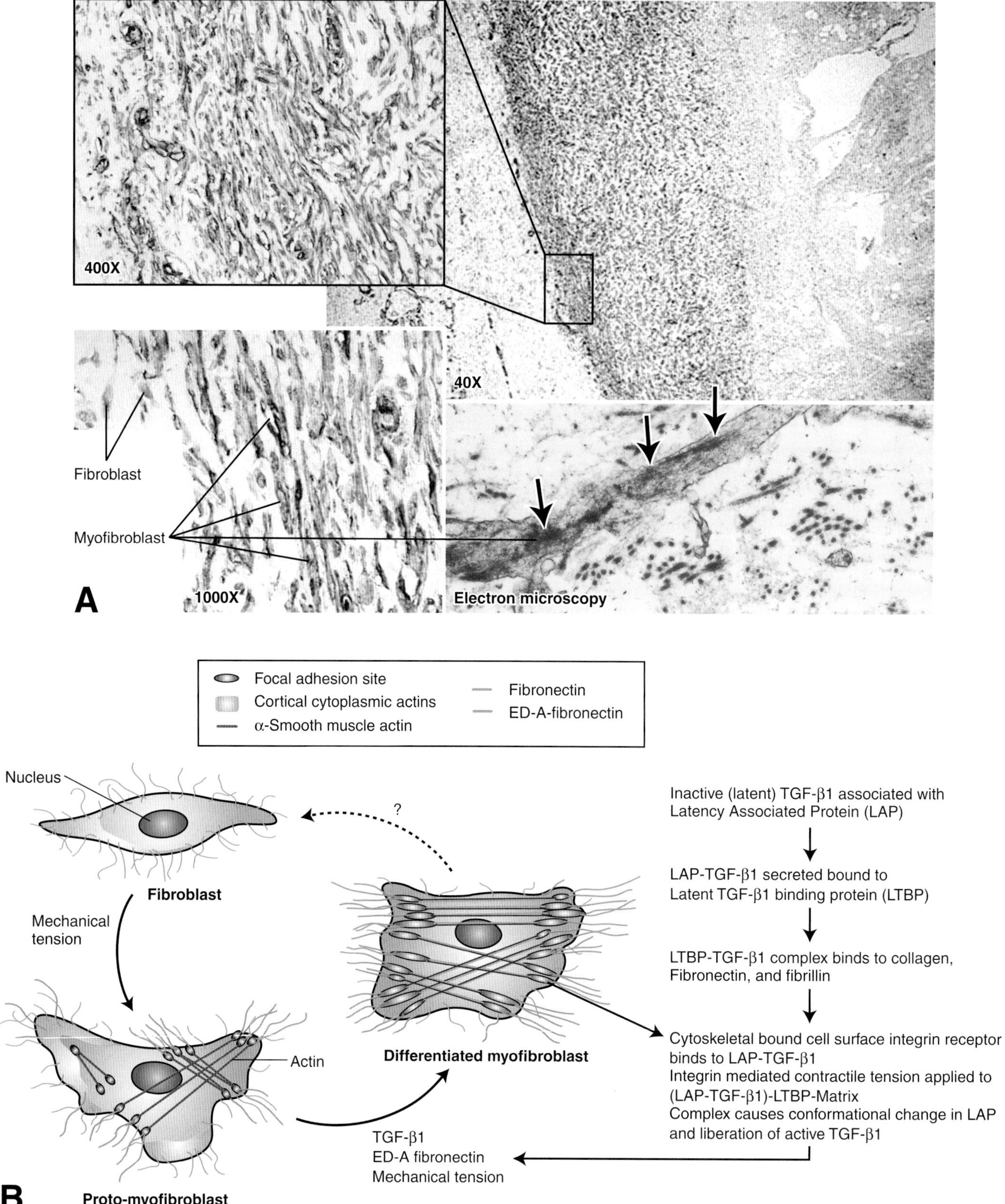

FIGURE 2-35. Myofibroblasts. Myofibroblasts have an important role in the repair reaction. These cells derive from pericytes or fibroblasts, with features intermediate between those of smooth muscle cells and fibroblasts, and they are characterized by the presence of discrete bundles of α-smooth muscle actin in the cytoplasm (*arrows*). Their clustered integrin receptors adhere tightly to and aid in formation of insoluble fibrils of cellular fibronectin, which align the cytoskeleton and bind collagen fibers, generating contractile forces important in wound contraction. **A. Myofibroblasts stained with anti–smooth muscle actin** can be viewed by light microscope at different magnifications. A band of cells (nuclei stain blue, α-smooth muscle actin stains brown) are stained in the papillary dermis of an ulcerated skin wound. Pericytes that surround capillaries also contain α-smooth muscle actin. α-Smooth muscle actin is seen in dense bundles by electron microscopy (*arrows*). **B. Development of myofibroblasts** from fibroblast and a model involving increased matrix production and matrix stiffness, leading to increased cytoskeletal contractility that activates matrix-bound latent transforming growth factor-β (TGF-β), hence creating a positive feedback system that magnifies matrix deposition and contractility. It is thought that this loop is normally interrupted by the phenomenon of tensional homeostasis, a biochemical set point.

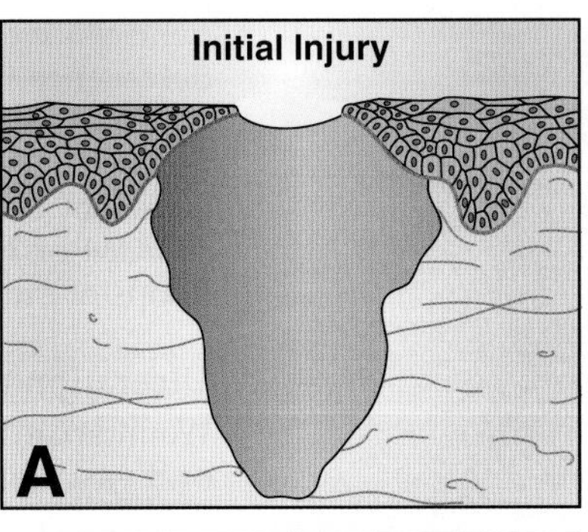

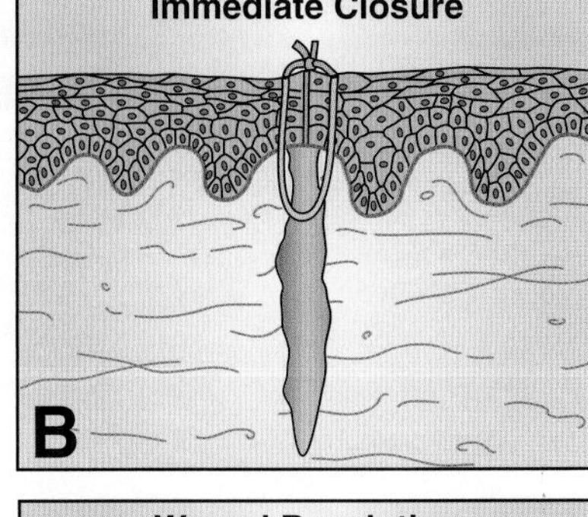

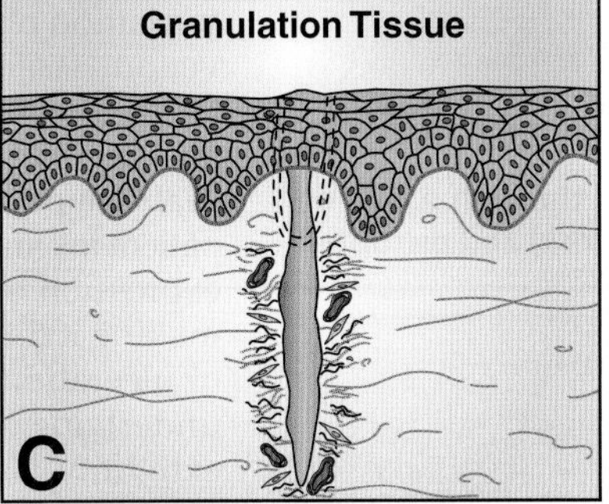

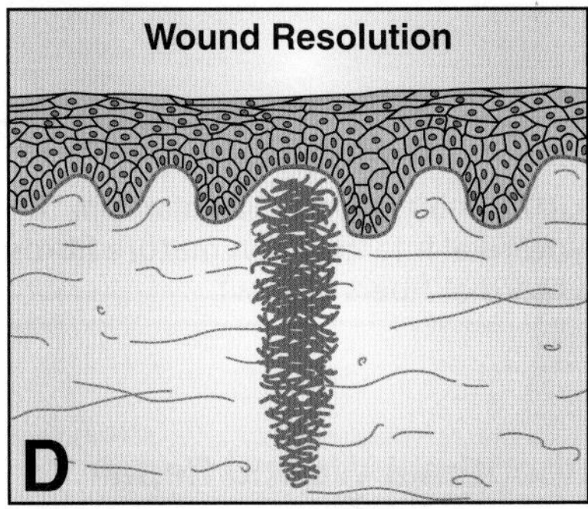

HEALING BY PRIMARY INTENTION (WOUNDS WITH APPOSED EDGES)

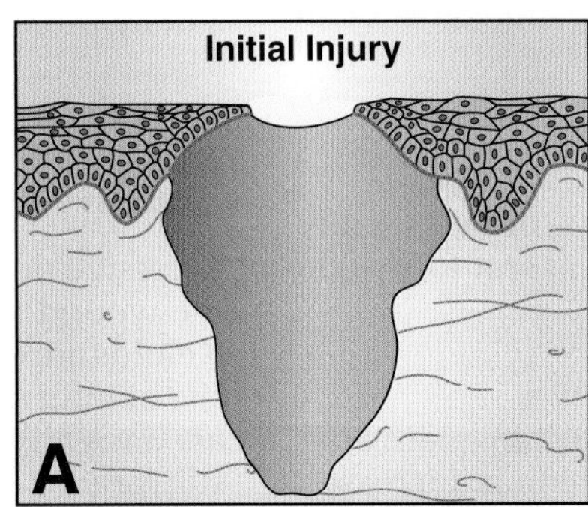

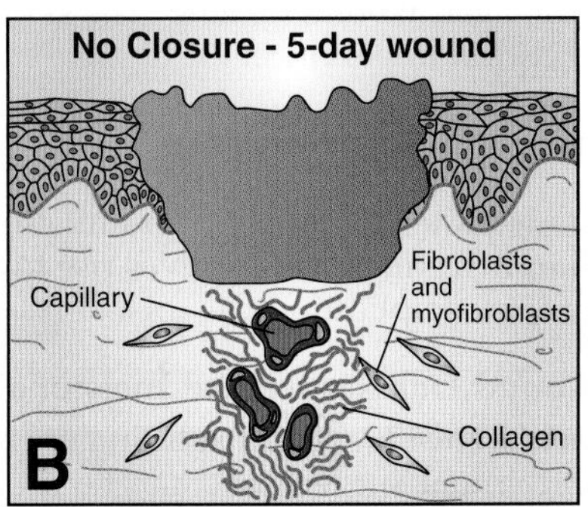

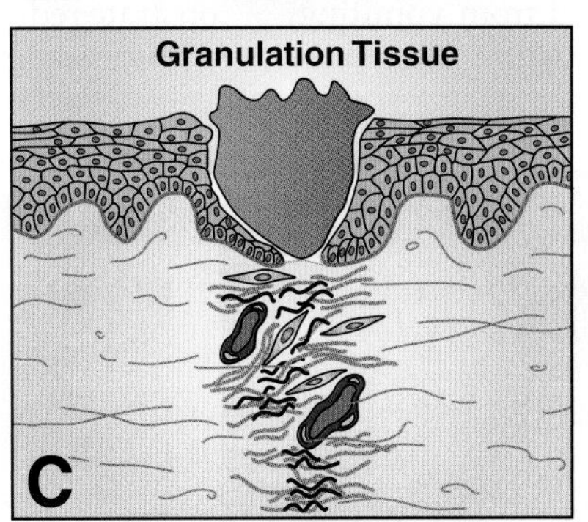

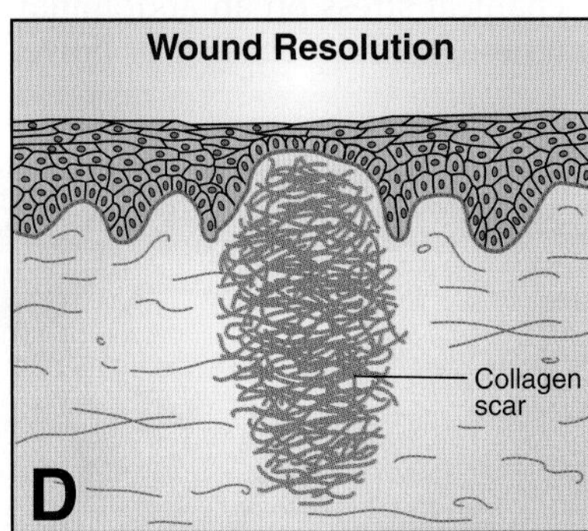

HEALING BY SECONDARY INTENTION (WOUNDS WITH SEPARATED EDGES)

FIGURE 2-36. *Top.* **Healing by primary intention. A.** An initial open, incised wound **(B)** with closely apposed wound edges is held together with a suture, leading to minimal tissue gaping or loss. **C.** There is decreased granulation tissue. Such a wound requires only minimal cell proliferation and neovascularization to heal. **D.** The result is a narrow, linear scar. *Bottom.* **Healing by secondary intention. A.** A gouged wound that remains or is left to remain open. The edges remain far apart, and there is substantial tissue loss. **B.** The healing process requires wound contraction (mechanical strain), extensive cell proliferation, matrix accumulation, and neovascularization (granulation tissue) to heal. **C.** The wound is reepithelialized from the margins, and collagen fibers are deposited throughout the granulation tissue. **D.** Granulation tissue is eventually resorbed, leaving a large collagenous scar that is functionally and esthetically imperfect.

Effects of Scarring

Scarring in parenchymal organs modifies their complex structure and never improves their function. For example, in the heart, the scar of a myocardial infarct serves to prevent rupture of the heart, but it reduces the amount of contractile tissue (Fig 2-37). If extensive enough, it may cause congestive heart failure or lead to a ventricular aneurysm (see Chapter 9). Pulmonary alveolar fibrosis causes respiratory failure. Infection in the peritoneum or even surgical exploration may create adhesions and intestinal obstruction. Scarring in the skin after burns or surgery produces unsatisfactory cosmetic results and may severely limit mobility. Hence, an important goal of therapeutic intervention is to create optimum conditions for "constructive" scarring and prevent pathologic "overshoot" of this process.

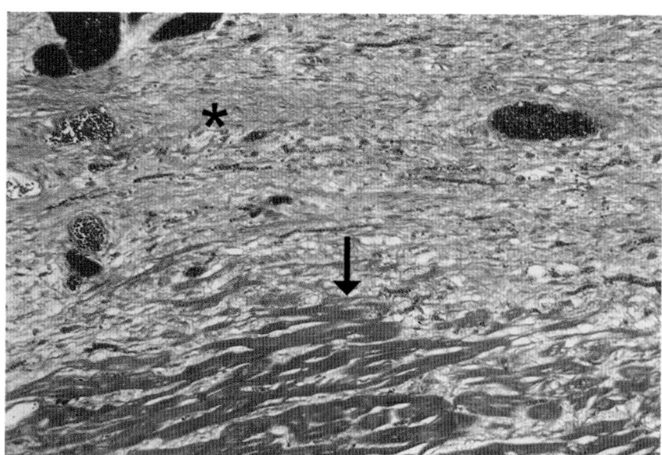

FIGURE 2-37. Myocardial infarction. A section through a healed myocardial infarct shows mature fibrosis (*asterisk*) and disrupted myocardial fibers (*arrow*).

Suboptimal Wound Repair

Abnormalities in any of the three healing processes—repair, contraction, and regeneration—result in unsuccessful or prolonged wound healing. The skill of the surgeon is often of critical importance.

Deficient Scar Formation

Inadequate formation of granulation tissue or an inability to form a suitable ECM gives rise to deficient scar formation and its complications.

Wound Dehiscence and Incisional Hernias

Dehiscence (a wound splitting open) is most frequent after abdominal surgery and can be life-threatening. Increased mechanical stress on an abdominal wound from vomiting, coughing, morbid obesity, or bowel obstruction may cause dehiscence of that wound. Systemic factors predisposing to dehiscence include metabolic deficiency, hypoproteinemia, and the general inanition that often accompanies metastatic cancer. **Incisional hernias** of the abdominal wall are defects caused by weak surgical scars, owing to insufficient deposition of ECM or inadequate cross-linking in the collagen matrix. Loops of intestine may be trapped within incisional hernias.

Ulceration

Wounds can ulcerate if an intrinsic blood supply is inadequate or if vascularization is insufficient during healing. Failure of the venous valves in the lower leg leads to tissue edema, the formation of pericapillary fibrin cuffs, and the generation of venous stasis ulcers, often on the inner aspect of the lower leg. Diabetic foot ulcers reflect a combination of poor arterial and capillary blood supply, which may be accompanied by a **diabetic peripheral neuropathy,** a disorder that renders the patient insensitive to the progressing ulcer. Diabetes also reduces expression of and cellular responsiveness to growth factors, making it difficult to stimulate the healing process. This form of ulceration, if left unchecked, proceeds to infection of the underlying bone (**osteomyelitis**) and progressive loss of the extremity. Nonhealing wounds also develop in areas devoid of sensation because of trauma or pressure. Such **decubitus ulcers** are commonly seen in patients who are immobilized in beds or wheelchairs. Constant pressure on the skin over a bony process can produce a local infarct in as little as 2 to 3 hours. These ulcers can be both broad and deep, with infection penetrating deep into connective tissue.

Excessive Scar Formation in the Skin

Excessive deposition of ECM, mostly excessive collagen, at the wound site results in hypertrophic scars and keloids. **Keloids** are exuberant scars that tend to progress beyond the site of initial injury and recur after excision (Fig. 2-38). They are unsightly, and attempts at surgical repair often result in a still larger keloid. Unlike normal scars, keloids do not demonstrate reduction in collagen synthesis if glucocorticoids are administered.

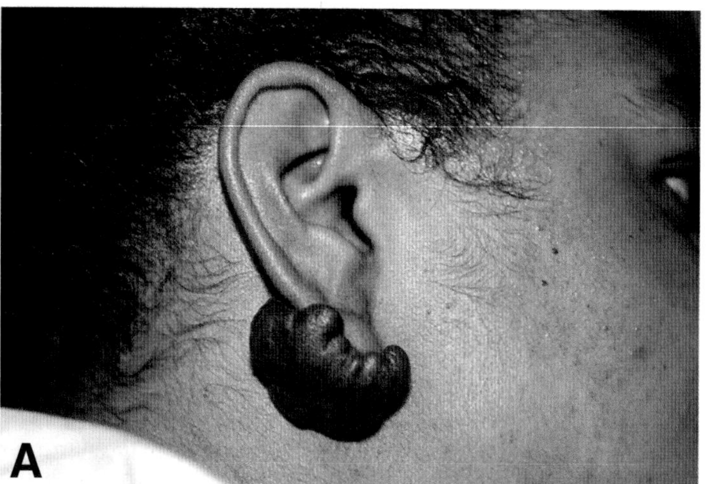

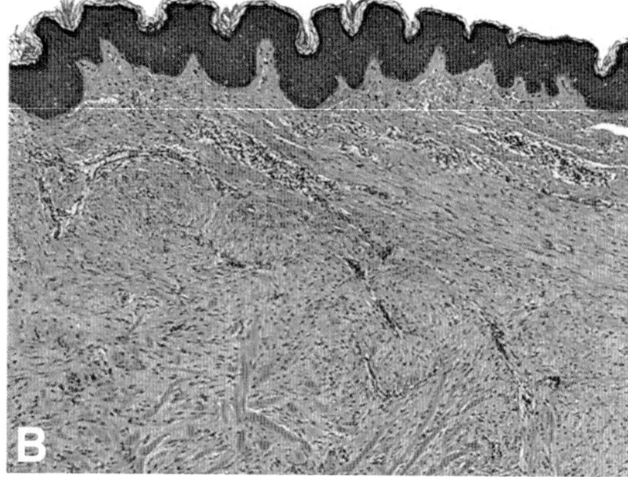

FIGURE 2-38. Keloid. A. A light-skinned black woman developed a keloid as a reaction to having her earlobe pierced. **B.** Microscopically, the dermis is markedly thickened by the presence of collagen bundles with random orientation and abundant cells.

By contrast, **hypertrophic scars** are confined within the wound margins, and the development of the scar is often associated with unrelieved mechanical stress. Hypertrophic scars often have a reddened appearance indicative of hypervascularity; tend to be pruritic, which suggests activation of mast cells producing histamine. Histologically, both keloids and hypertrophic scars exhibit broad and irregular collagen bundles. The rate of collagen synthesis and number of reducible cross-links remain high, suggesting a "maturation arrest" or block in the healing process.

Excessive Contraction

A decrease in the size of a wound depends on the presence of fibroblasts and myofibroblasts, development of cell–cell contacts, and sustained cell contraction. An exaggeration of these processes is termed **contracture** and results in severe deformity of a wound and surrounding tissues. Regions that normally show minimal wound contraction (e.g., the palms, soles, and anterior aspect of the thorax) are often prone to this complication. Contractures are particularly conspicuous when serious burns heal, and they can be severe enough to compromise the movement of joints. In the alimentary tract, a contracture (stricture) can obstruct the passage of food in the esophagus or block the flow of intestinal contents.

Several diseases are characterized by contracture and irreversible fibrosis of the superficial fascia, including **Dupuytren** contracture (palmar contracture), **Lederhosen disease** (plantar contracture), and **Peyronie** disease (contracture of the cavernous tissues of the penis). In these diseases, there is no known precipitating injury, even though the basic process is similar to contracture in wound healing.

Proliferative Potential of Cells

Cell populations divide at different rates. Some mature cells do not divide at all, while others cycle repeatedly.

- **Labile cells:** Labile cells are found in tissues that are in a constant state of renewal. Tissues in which more than 1.5% of the cells are in mitosis at any one time are composed of labile cells. Labile epithelial tissues that typically form physical barriers between the body and the external environment self-renew constantly. Examples include epithelia of the gut, skin, cornea, respiratory tract, reproductive tract, and urinary tract. Hematopoietic cells of the bone marrow and lymphoid organs involved in immune defense are also labile. PMNs and red blood cells are terminally differentiated cells that are rapidly renewed. ***Under appropriate conditions, tissues composed of labile cells regenerate after injury, provided enough stem cells remain.***
- **Stable cells:** Stable cells populate tissues that normally are renewed very slowly but are populated with progenitor cells capable of more rapid renewal after tissue loss. Liver, bone, and proximal renal tubules are examples of stable cell populations. Stable cells populate tissues in which less than 1.5% of cells are in mitosis. Stable tissues (e.g., endocrine glands, endothelium, and liver) do not have conspicuous stem cells. Rather, their cells require an appropriate stimulus to divide. ***The potential to replicate, not the actual number of steady state mitoses, determines the ability of an organ to regenerate.*** For example, the liver, a stable tissue with less than one mitosis for every 15, 000 cells, rapidly recovers through hepatocyte hyperplasia after loss of up to 75% of its mass.
- **Permanent cells:** Permanent cells are terminally differentiated, have lost all capacity for regeneration, and do not enter the cell cycle. Traditionally, neurons, chondrocytes, cardiac myocytes, and cells of the lens were considered permanent cells. It is thought that if lost, cardiac myocytes and neurons may be replaced from progenitors, but not from division of existing cardiac myocytes or mature neurons. Permanent cells do not divide, but do renew their organelles.

REGENERATION

Regeneration returns an injured tissue or lost appendage to its original state. Both regeneration and tissue maintenance require a population of stem or progenitor cells that can replicate and differentiate. The power to replenish or regenerate tissue is derived from a small number of long-lived, unspecialized **stem cells**, unique in their slow replication rate, capacity for self-renewal, and production of clonal progeny that rapidly divide and differentiate into more specialized cell types. Stem cells in most tissues, including bone marrow, epidermis, intestine, and liver, maintain sufficient developmental plasticity to orchestrate tissue-specific regeneration.

Embryonic and Adult Stem Cells

Embryonic stem cells (ESCs), up to the stage of the preimplantation blastocyst, can differentiate into all cells of the adult organism *and* preserve small populations of more restricted stem cells. Hence, these cells are **pluripotent**. Postnatal progenitor/stem cells, which are able to divide indefinitely without terminally differentiating, inhabit many adult tissues, and they have been identified even in tissues not known to regenerate. These **adult stem cells** may inhabit a specific tissue or be recruited to sites of injury from circulating cells of bone marrow origin. Either way, the recently appreciated presence of stem cells in many tissues underscores the importance of a permissive and supportive environment for stem cell–driven regeneration (Table 2-11). Multipotential stem cells of adult tissues have a more restricted range of cell differentiation than ESCs cells and can be isolated from autologous tissue, reducing concerns of immunologic rejection after implantation. More recently, regulators of transcription patterns active in embryonic stem cells have been used to restore pluripotency in differentiated cells of adult tissues (induced pluripotential stem [iPS] cell).

Stem cells are defined by common properties:

- Ability to divide without limit, avoid senescence, and maintain genomic integrity
- Capacity to intermittently undergo division or to remain quiescent
- Ability to propagate by self-renewal and differentiation of daughter cells
- Absence of lineage markers
- In some cases, specific anatomic localization
- Shared presence of growth and transcription markers common to uncommitted cells

Table 2-11

Adult Stem Cells Described in Mammals

Cell Type	Cell Source and Stability	Tissue Stem Cell and Role
Bone marrow–derived stem cells	Hematopoietic stem cells (HSCs)	HSC—Hematopoiesis, formation of all blood system cells
	Mesenchymal stem cells (MSCs)	MSC—Replenish non-blood cells of bone and bone marrow, provide HSC niche and potential source of progenitor cells for certain other tissues
Adult tissue stem cells except connective tissue (some may be bone marrow derived)[a]	Constantly renewing (labile) cells	Epidermis: unipotent basal keratinocyte basal stem cell and multipotent stem cells of hair follicle bulge and sebaceous gland
	• Epithelial and epithelial-like cells of epidermis and gut (ectoderm or endoderm derived)	Gut: multipotent columnar cells of small and large intestine crypt base
		Cornea: corneal epithelial stem cells are located in the basal layer of the limbus between the cornea and the conjunctiva (corneal stromal stem cells are similarly located but beneath the epithelial basement membrane)
	Persistent (stable) cells in tissues with less turnover • Epithelial, parenchyma, neural (endoderm or ectoderm derived)	Liver: compensatory hepatocyte hyperplasia for maintenance, for regeneration and in response to surgical resection (other liver cells also divide); hepatic stem cells, DNA markers in label retention studies are seen in cells in the canals of Hering, intralobular bile duct cells, peribiliary null cells and peribiliary hepatocytes
		Lung: putative lung bronchioalveolar progenitor or stem cells that form bronchiolar Clara cells and possibly alveolar cells. Some evidence for alveolar epithelial type II progenitor cells
		Ear: mammalian cochlea is not known to regenerate sensory hair cells, though some nonmammalian vertebrates do. Human MSCs have been differentiated to hair cells and auditory neurons in vitro
		Neural stem cells: multipotent, thought to be ependymal cells or astrocytes; subventricular zone of the lateral ventricle (possibly inactive in adult humans); subgranular zone of dentate gyrus of the hippocampus. Other potential sites are the olfactory bulb and subcallosal zone under the corpus callosum.
Connective tissue or MSCs outside bone marrow	Mesoderm derived	Skeletal: satellite cells—between sarcolemma and overlying basement membrane of myofiber—also derived from pericytes or bone marrow MSCs
	Progenitors of connective tissue cells; isolated from several tissues, although bone marrow origin cannot be excluded	Adipose: fat is a rich source of multipotential mesenchymal cells.
	Muscle cells	Kidney: there are findings supportive of kidney renal tubular and parietal epithelial podocyte (Bowman capsule) stem/progenitor cells. Cells of the kidney are of mesodermal origin, with the possible exception of the endothelial cell.
		Cardiac: cardiac progenitor or stem cells—multipotent cardiomyocytes capable of maintaining homeostasis, limited differentiation and proliferation after ischemic injury; bone marrow MSCs

[a]These may be the same as multipotent adult progenitor cells, which represent bone marrow stromal cells whose differentiation is influenced by in vitro growth conditions. These cells are capable of seeding tissues outside the bone marrow by one or more several possible processes: (a) specific progenitors or multipotent progenitors, (b) transdifferentiation, (c) cell fusion, and (d) dedifferentiation.

Self-Renewal

Self-renewal is the defining property of adult stem cells and of early ESCs in vivo. The definition of a stem cell depends on the ability of the cell to differentiate into multiple cell types, in vitro or in vivo. Stem cells achieve self-renewal by asymmetric cell division, which produces a new stem cell and a daughter cell that is able to proliferate transiently and to differentiate. In contrast to stem cells, these **progenitor** cells (transit amplifying cells) have little or no capability for self-renewal.

Stem Cell Differentiation Potential

The ability of ESCs to differentiate into all lineages diminishes as the embryo develops. Cells from the zygote and the first few divisions of the fertilized egg are **totipotent**; they can form any of approximately 200 different cell types in the adult body and the placenta. ESCs that are derived from the inner cell mass of the blastocyst are **pluripotent**, meaning they may differentiate into nearly all cell lineages within any of the three germ layers. Pluripotent stem cells of the postfertilization zygote, such as neural crest cells, may differentiate into many cell types, but they are not totipotent. Those adult cells that must self-renew throughout the lifetime of the organism are generally **multipotent** or able to differentiate into several cell types within one lineage or one of the germ layers. Hematopoietic stem cells, for example, are lineage restricted; they can form all the cells found in blood (Table 2-11). Marrow stromal cells (also known as mesenchymal stem cells [MSCs]) are multipotent stem cells within bone marrow that can mobilize into the bloodstream and be recruited to (injured) organs. MSCs can be induced to differentiate into multiple cell types in vitro (adipocytes, chondrocytes, osteoblasts, myoblasts, fibroblasts) derived from a single cell lineage, the mesoderm germ layer.

Tissue-specific cells support renewal as multipotent stem cells or as progenitor cells. Progenitor cells are **stable cells** that are distinguished from stem cells by their incapacity for self-renewal; however, they maintain the potential for differentiation and rapid proliferation. They are sometimes referred to as **unipotent** stem cells, as exemplified by the interfollicular basal keratinocyte of skin, although other skin cells may be multipotent or oligopotent.

Bone marrow contains hematopoietic, mesenchymal, and endothelial stem cells, providing a multifaceted regenerative capacity. Bone marrow stem cells, which are set aside during embryonic development, replenish the bone marrow mesenchyme and hematopoietic population. Endothelial progenitor cells from bone marrow have been implicated in tissue angiogenesis and may supplement endothelial hyperplasia during regeneration of blood vessels. Likewise, bone marrow–derived mesenchymal stem cells can populate repairing tissues in many distant sites (Table 2-11).

Pluripotency

Cell differentiation involves controlled regulation of gene expression within an existing DNA sequence. This occurs via (1) **epigenetic modification** to DNA without changing or rearranging the sequence; (2) reduced expression of pluripotency-limiting genes, including the polycomb group proteins; and (3) increased expression of lineage development genes. Epigenetic modifications include nucleic acid modifications within the DNA sequence, such as methylation, expression of microRNAs, and remodeling of chromatin organization by chromatin-associated proteins and modification of histone proteins (see Chapter 4). As noted above, it has proven possible to restore pluripotency in differentiated cells of adult tissues (induced pluripotential stem [iPS] cell) by manipulation of the expression of a limited number of genes.

Epigenetic modifiers stabilize and restrict transcriptional states as necessary for cell differentiation. They are heritable by their progeny (monoallelic epigenetic alteration inherited from egg or sperm is called **imprinting**). An interplay between epigenetic modifiers and lineage-determining transcription factors is necessary for the progressive differentiation states in a cell lineage. Differentiation is controlled at many levels, and it may involve cell–cell contact and extracellular signals. However, coactivation and coregulation of transcription factors associated with potency or lineage and epigenetic modifications are also key to the final state of a cell.

3 Immunopathology

Jeffrey S. Warren ▪ David S. Strayer ▪ Philip L. Cohen ▪ Sergio A. Jimenez

LEARNING OBJECTIVES

- Define the term hypersensitivity as related to immune diseases.
- Provide an overview of the classification system for immune hypersensitive reactions.
- Describe the role of the mast cell in type I hypersensitivity.
- Describe the clinical consequences of type I hypersensitivity in different sites of the body.
- List the various mechanisms of mast cell activation.
- Distinguish between the immediate and delayed phases of type I hypersensitivity in terms of the inflammatory mediators involved.
- Describe common mechanisms of immune-mediated damage in type II hypersensitivity.
- Describe the mechanism of tissue damage in type III hypersensitivity.
- Give common clinical examples of type III–mediated disease.
- Describe serum sickness and the Arthus reaction as models of type III hypersensitivity.
- Elucidate the mechanism of type IV hypersensitivity using poison ivy sensitivity as a model.
- Summarize the clinical findings and mode of inheritance of common forms of humoral immunodeficiency.
- Summarize the clinical findings and mode of inheritance of common forms of cellular and combined immunodeficiency.
- Distinguish between central and peripheral tolerance.
- Describe several current theories regarding the generation of autoimmune disease and cite supporting clinical examples.
- Provide examples of autoimmune diseases resulting from defects in innate immunity.
- Define the term antinuclear antibodies and explain their role in the etiology and pathogenesis of systemic lupus erythematosus (SLE).
- What is the role of immune factors in the pathogenesis of SLE?
- What are the most common sites of organ involvement in SLE?
- Distinguish between discoid and systemic lupus.
- What autoantibodies are associated with Sjögren syndrome?
- Distinguish between limited cutaneous, diffuse cutaneous, and fulminant forms of systemic sclerosis.
- Define CREST syndrome.
- What autoantibodies are associated with systemic sclerosis?
- Outline the pathophysiology and resultant tissue injury found in systemic sclerosis.
- Distinguish between hyperacute, acute, and chronic rejection using the kidney as an example.
- Briefly describe the nature of diseases associated with HIV/AIDS.
- Describe common modes of transmission of HIV-1.
- Discuss the mechanisms by which HIV-1 kills T lymphocytes.
- Describe the time course of HIV infection in terms of $CD4^+$ and $CD8^+$ counts, HIV viral load, and anti-HIV antibody.
- Define the term "acute retroviral syndrome."
- What is the role of CCR5 in the pathogenesis of AIDS?
- Describe neoplastic diseases associated with HIV/AIDS.
- Define immune reconstitution inflammatory syndrome (IRIS) and describe the pathophysiology of the syndrome.

IMMUNOLOGICALLY MEDIATED TISSUE INJURY

There are many diseases in which an immunologically triggered inflammatory response attacks the body's own tissues. A variety of foreign substances (e.g., dust, pollen, viruses, and bacteria) provoke protective responses. In certain situations, the protective effects of an immune response lead to harmful consequences, which can range from temporary discomfort to substantial injury. For example, in the process of ingesting and destroying bacteria, phagocytic cells (neutrophils and macrophages) often cause injury to surrounding tissue. An immune response that produces tissue injury is broadly called a **hypersensitivity** reaction. Many diseases are categorized as immune disorders or immunologically mediated conditions, in which an immune response to a foreign or self-antigen causes injury. Immune- or hypersensitivity-mediated diseases are common and include hives (urticaria), asthma, hay fever, hepatitis, glomerulonephritis, and other disorders.

Hypersensitivity reactions are classified according to the type of immune mechanism (Table 3-1). Types I, II, and III hypersensitivity reactions all involve antibodies specific for exogenous (foreign) or endogenous (self) antigens. Type IV hypersensitivity is T-lymphocyte mediated. The antibody isotype influences the mechanism of tissue injury.

- **Type I, or immediate-type hypersensitivity, reactions:** IgE antibody is formed and binds high-affinity receptors on mast cells and basophils via its Fc domain. Subsequent antigen binding and cross-linking of IgE trigger rapid (immediate) release of products from these cells, leading to the characteristic manifestations of urticaria, asthma, atopic allergies, and anaphylaxis.
- **Type II hypersensitivity reactions:** IgM or IgG antibody is formed against an antigen, often a cell surface protein. Less commonly, the antigen is an intrinsic structural component of the extracellular matrix (e.g., basement membrane). Such antigen–antibody coupling activates complement, which, in turn, lyses the cell (cytotoxicity) or damages the extracellular matrix. In some type II reactions, other antibody-mediated effects are operative.
- **Type III hypersensitivity reactions:** The antibody responsible for tissue injury is also usually IgM or IgG, but the mechanism of tissue injury differs. Antigen circulates in the vascular compartment until it is bound by antibody. The resulting immune complexes deposit in tissue where complement activation prompts the recruitment of leukocytes, which mediate tissue injury. In some type III reactions, antigen is bound by antibody in situ.
- **Type IV, cell-mediated** or **delayed-type, hypersensitivity reactions:** Antigen activation of T lymphocytes, usually with the help of macrophages, causes release of products by these cells, thereby generating tissue injury.

Many immunologic diseases are mediated by more than one type of hypersensitivity reaction. For example, in hypersensitivity pneumonitis, lung injury from inhaled fungal antigens involves types I, III, and IV reactions.

Immunoglobulin E-Mediated Hypersensitivity Reactions (Type I)

Immediate-type hypersensitivity entails localized or generalized reactions that occur immediately (within minutes) after exposure to an antigen or "allergen" to which the person has been previously sensitized. Clinical manifestations depend on the site of antigen exposure and the extent of sensitization. For example, when a reaction involves the skin, the characteristic localized reaction is a "wheal and flare," or urticaria. When the conjunctiva and upper respiratory tract are involved, sneezing and conjunctivitis result and we speak of hay fever (allergic rhinitis). In its generalized and most severe form, immediate hypersensitivity reactions are associated with bronchoconstriction, airway obstruction, and circulatory collapse, as seen in anaphylactic shock. There is a high degree of genetically determined variability in susceptibility to type I hypersensitivity reactions, and susceptible individuals are said to be "atopic."

Type I reactions usually feature IgE antibodies formed by a $CD4^+$, Th2, T-cell–dependent mechanism that bind avidly to Fcε receptors on mast cells and basophils. The high avidity ($K_d = 10^{-15}$ M) of IgE binding accounts for the term **cytophilic** antibody. Once exposed to a specific allergen that elicits IgE, a person is sensitized; subsequent exposures to that allergen or a cross-reacting epitope induce immediate hypersensitivity reactions. Once IgE is elicited, repeat exposure to antigen typically induces additional IgE antibody, rather than antibodies of other classes.

Bound to Fcε receptors on mast cells and basophils, IgE can persist for years. Upon re-exposure, recognition of the soluble antigen or allergen by IgE coupled to its surface Fcε receptor activates the mast cell or basophil. Released inflammatory mediators cause type I hypersensitivity reactions. As shown in Figure 3-1, the antigen (allergen) binds the Fab region of the IgE antibody. To activate the cell, antigen must cross-link at least two adjacent IgE antibody molecules.

Mast cells and basophils can also be activated by agents other than antibodies. For example, some persons develop urticaria after exposure to an ice cube (physical urticaria)

Table 3-1

Modified Cell and Coombs Classification of Hypersensitivity Reactions

Type	Mechanism	Examples
Type I (anaphylactic type): immediate hypersensitivity	IgE antibody–mediated mast cell activation and degranulation Non–Ig mediated	Hay fever, asthma, hives, anaphylaxis Physical urticarias
Type II (cytotoxic type): cytotoxic antibodies	Cytotoxic (IgG, IgM) antibodies formed against cell surface antigens; complement usually involved Noncytotoxic antibodies against cell surface receptors	Autoimmune hemolytic anemias, Goodpasture disease Graves disease
Type III (immune complex type): immune complex disease	Antibodies (IgG, IgM, IgA) formed against exogenous or endogenous antigens; complement and leukocytes (neutrophils, macrophages) often involved	Autoimmune diseases (SLE, rheumatoid arthritis), many types of glomerulonephritis
Type IV (cell-mediated type): delayed-type hypersensitivity	Mononuclear cells (T lymphocytes, macrophages) with interleukin and lymphokine production	Granulomatous disease (tuberculosis), delayed skin reactions (poison ivy)

Ig, immunoglobulin; SLE, systemic lupus erythematosus.

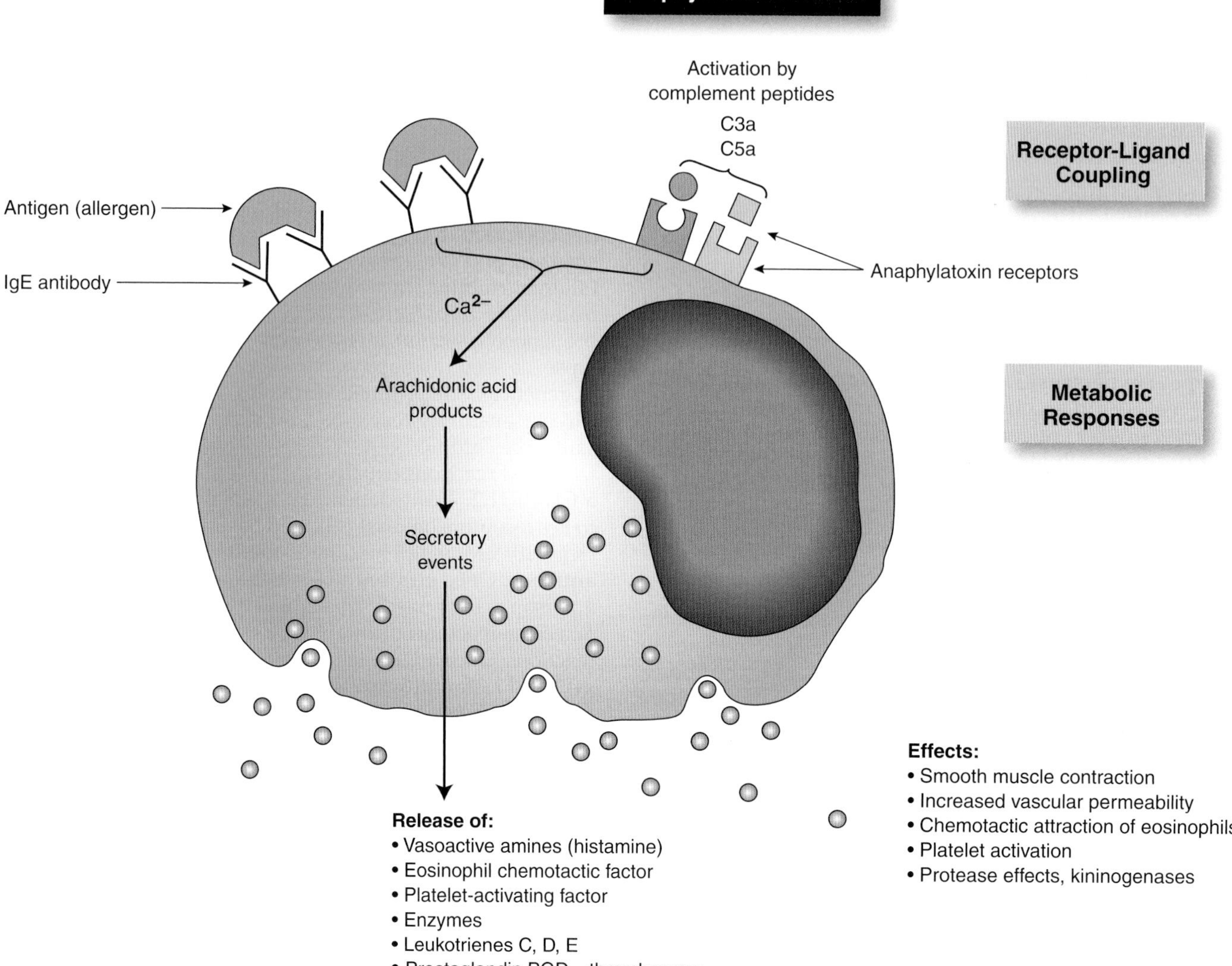

FIGURE 3-1. In a type I hypersensitivity reaction, antigen (allergen) binds to cytophilic surface IgE antibody on a mast cell or basophil and triggers cell activation and the release of a cascade of proinflammatory mediators. Mast cells and basophils can also be activated by anaphylatoxins such as C3a and C5a, as well as some physical stimuli (e.g., cold). These mediators are responsible for smooth muscle contraction, edema formation, and the recruitment of eosinophils. Ca^{2+}, calcium ion; Ig, immunoglobulin; PGD_2, prostaglandin D_2.

or pressure (dermographism). The complement-derived anaphylatoxic peptides, C3a and C5a, can directly stimulate mast cells by a different receptor-mediated process (Fig. 3-1). These cell-activating events trigger the release of stored granule constituents and the rapid synthesis and release of other mediators. Some compounds, such as melittin (from bee venom), and occasional drugs (e.g., morphine) activate mast cells directly.

Regardless of how mast cell activation is initiated, a rise in cytosolic-free calcium triggers (1) an increase in cAMP, (2) activation of several metabolic pathways within the mast cell, and (3) subsequent secretion of both preformed and newly synthesized products. Stored in granules, mediators are released within minutes and act rapidly. Of the granule constituents listed in Figure 3-1, histamine is particularly important. It induces constriction of vascular and nonvascular smooth muscle, causes microvascular dilation, and increases venule permeability. These effects are largely mediated through H_1 histamine receptors. Histamine also increases gastric acid secretion through H_2 histamine receptors and provokes the cutaneous wheal-and-flare reaction. In the lungs, it causes the early manifestations of immediate hypersensitivity, including bronchospasm, vascular congestion, and edema. Other preformed products released from mast cell granules include heparin, a series of neutral proteases (trypsin, chymotrypsin carboxypeptidase, and acid hydrolases), and both neutrophil and eosinophil chemotactic factors. The last is responsible for the accumulation of eosinophils, a characteristic finding in immediate hypersensitivity. The synthesis and secretion of cytokines by mast cells, by other recruited inflammatory cells, and even by indigenous cells (e.g., epithelium) are important in the so-called "late-phase" reaction of immediate hypersensitivity. Late-phase responses (1) typically last 2 to 24 hours, (2) are marked by a mixed inflammatory infiltrate, and (3) are mediated by many cytokines, including IL-1, IL-3, IL-4, IL-5, IL-6, TNF, granulocyte-macrophage colony-stimulating factor (GM-CSF), and macrophage inflammatory protein (MIP)-1α and MIP-1β.

Mast cell activation also increases the synthesis of arachidonic acid pathway products formed after activation of phospholipase A_2. Products of cyclooxygenase (prostaglandins D_2, E_2, and F_2 and thromboxane) and lipoxygenase (leukotrienes B_4, C_4, D_4, and E_4) are also produced. Arachidonic acid derivatives, generated by a variety of cell types, induce smooth muscle contraction, vasodilation, and edema. Leukotrienes C_4, D_4, and E_4, previously known as "slow-reacting substances of anaphylaxis," (SRS-As), are important in the delayed bronchoconstriction phase of anaphylaxis. Leukotriene B_4 is a potent chemotactic factor for neutrophils, macrophages, and eosinophils.

Another inflammatory mediator synthesized by mast cells is **platelet-activating factor** (PAF), a lipid derived from membrane phospholipids. PAF is a potent inducer of platelet aggregation and release of vasoactive amines, as well as a potent neutrophil chemotaxin. PAF can activate all types of phagocytic cells.

Activated T cells, specifically Th2 cells, produce cytokines that have important roles in allergic responses. This subset releases IL-4, IL-5, and IL-13, leading to IgE production and increased numbers of mast cells and eosinophils. In allergy-prone people, a similar response occurs via T cells that produce IL-4, IL-6, and IL-2, concentrations of which are also increased in allergic individuals. These patients also have reduced levels of IFN-γ, which suppresses the development of Th2 cells and subsequent production of IgE.

In summary, type I (immediate) hypersensitivity reactions are characterized by specific cytophilic antibody (IgE) that binds to high-affinity Fcε receptors on basophils and mast cells and reacts with a specific antigen (allergen). Activated mast cells and basophils release preformed (granule) products and synthesize mediators that cause the classic manifestations of immediate hypersensitivity and the late-phase reaction.

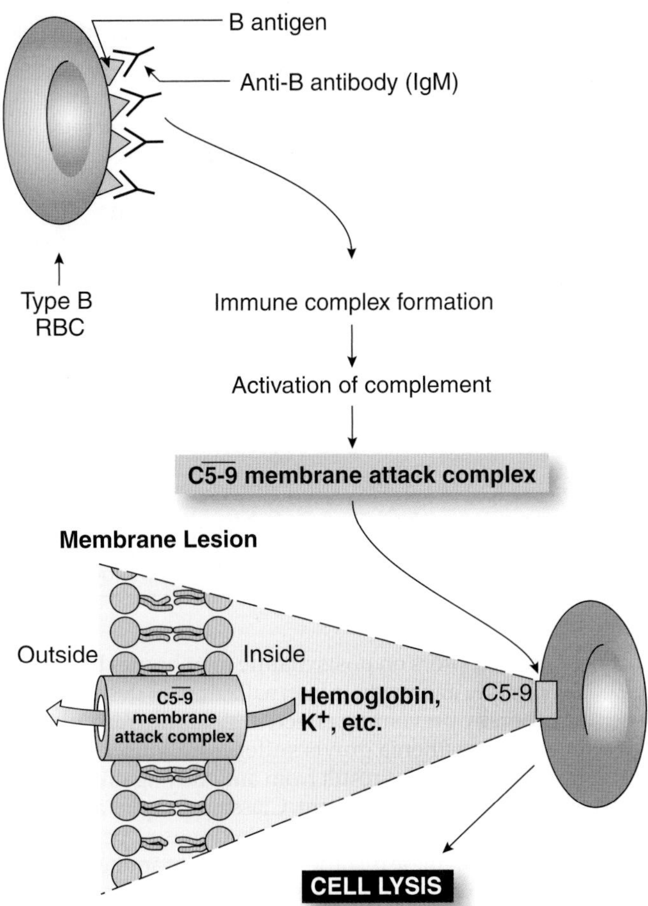

FIGURE 3-2. In a type II hypersensitivity reaction, binding of IgG or IgM antibody to an immobilized antigen promotes complement fixation. Activation of complement leads to amplification of the inflammatory response and membrane attack complex–mediated cell lysis. Ig, immunoglobulin, K^+, potassium ion; RBC, red blood cell.

Non–Immunoglobulin E Antibody-Mediated Hypersensitivity Reactions (Type II)

IgM and IgG mediate most type II reactions. These Ig isotypes activate complement via their Fc domains. There are several antibody-dependent mechanisms of tissue injury. Prototypic antibody-mediated erythrocyte cytotoxicity is illustrated in Figure 3-2. IgM or IgG antibody binds an antigen on the erythrocyte membrane. At sufficient density, bound Ig fixes complement via C1q and the classic pathway (see Chapter 2). Activated complement can destroy target cells directly, via C5b-9 complexes (Fig. 3-2). The C5b-9 **membrane attack complex** inserts like the staves of a barrel into the plasma membrane and forms holes or ion channels, destroying the permeability barrier and inducing cell lysis. This type of cell lysis is exemplified by certain autoimmune hemolytic anemias that result from antibodies against erythrocyte blood group antigens. In some transfusion reactions that reflect major blood group incompatibilities, intravascular hemolysis occurs through activation of complement.

Complement and antibody molecules can also destroy target cells by **opsonization**. Target cells that are coated (opsonized) with immunoglobulin and C3b molecules are bound by phagocytes that express Fc or C3b receptors. Complement activation near a target cell surface promotes formation and covalent bonding of C3b (Fig. 3-3). Many phagocytic cells, including neutrophils and macrophages, express cell membrane Fc and C3b receptors. By binding to these receptors, Ig or C3b bridges the target and effector (phagocytic) cells, thereby enhancing phagocytosis and subsequent intracellular destruction of the antibody- or complement-coated cell.

Some transfusion reactions, autoimmune hemolytic anemias, and drug reactions occur via antibody- and complement-mediated opsonization.

Antibody-dependent cell-mediated cytotoxicity (ADCC) does not require complement, but rather involves cytolytic leukocytes that attack antibody-coated target cells after binding via Fc receptors. Phagocytic cells and natural killer (NK) cells can act as effector cells in ADCC. Such cells synthesize homologs of terminal complement proteins (e.g., perforins), which participate in cytotoxic events. *Only rarely is antibody alone directly cytotoxic.*

In some type II reactions, antibody binding to a specific target cell receptor does not lead to cell death, but rather to a change in function. For example, in Graves disease and myasthenia gravis, autoantibodies against cell surface hormone receptors and postsynaptic neurotransmitter receptors, respectively (Fig. 3-4), may activate or inhibit cell activation (see below). In Graves disease, autoantibody against thyroid-stimulating hormone (TSH) receptors elicits thyroxin production, giving rise to thyrotoxicosis. In myasthenia gravis, autoantibodies to

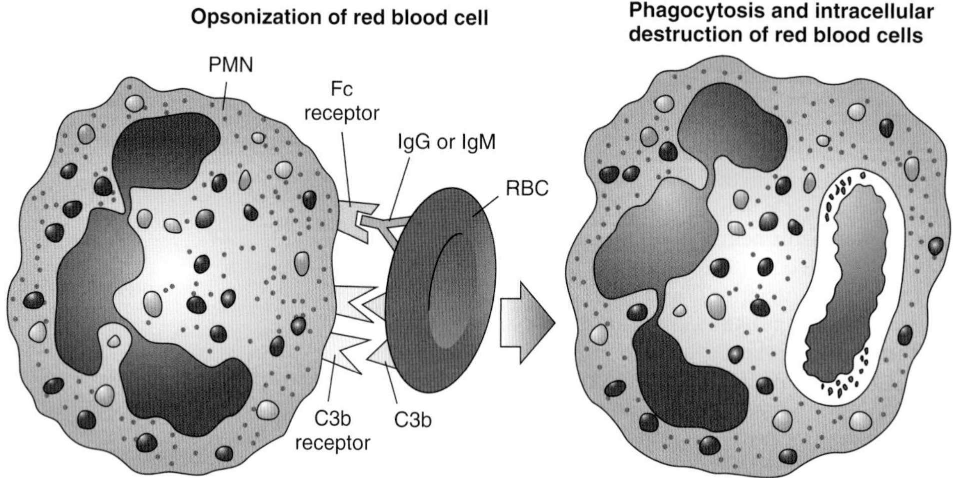

FIGURE 3-3. In a type II hypersensitivity reaction, opsonization by antibody or complement leads to phagocytosis via either Fc or C3b receptors, respectively. Ig, immunoglobulin; PMN, polymorphonuclear leukocyte; RBC, red blood cell.

acetylcholine receptors on postsynaptic membranes block acetylcholine binding and mediate internalization or destruction of receptors, thereby preventing effective synaptic transmission. Patients with myasthenia gravis suffer from muscle fatigue.

Some type II reactions result from antibody against a structural connective tissue component. Classic examples are Goodpasture syndrome and the bullous skin diseases, pemphigus, and pemphigoid. In these disorders, circulating antibodies bind intrinsic connective tissue antigens and evoke destructive local inflammatory responses. In Goodpasture syndrome, antibody binds the noncollagenous domain of type IV collagen, which is a major structural component of pulmonary and glomerular basement membranes (Fig. 3-5). Local complement activation results in neutrophil chemotaxis and activation, tissue injury, pulmonary hemorrhage, and glomerulonephritis. Direct complement-mediated damage to glomerular and alveolar basement membranes via membrane attack complexes may also be involved.

Antibodies (often termed inhibitors) may bind to infused coagulation factors used as therapy in hemophiliacs who lack tolerance to such agents. Rarely, they react with endogenous coagulation factors as part of an autoimmune response. Such antibodies inhibit the biologic activity of the coagulation factor and may result in a bleeding tendency in a previously normal person. Similar antibody-mediated inhibition of activity may also occur with infused therapeutic agents, such as monoclonal antibodies. This depression of protein activity is often classified as a type II reaction.

In summary, type II hypersensitivity reactions are directly or indirectly cytotoxic through the action of antibodies

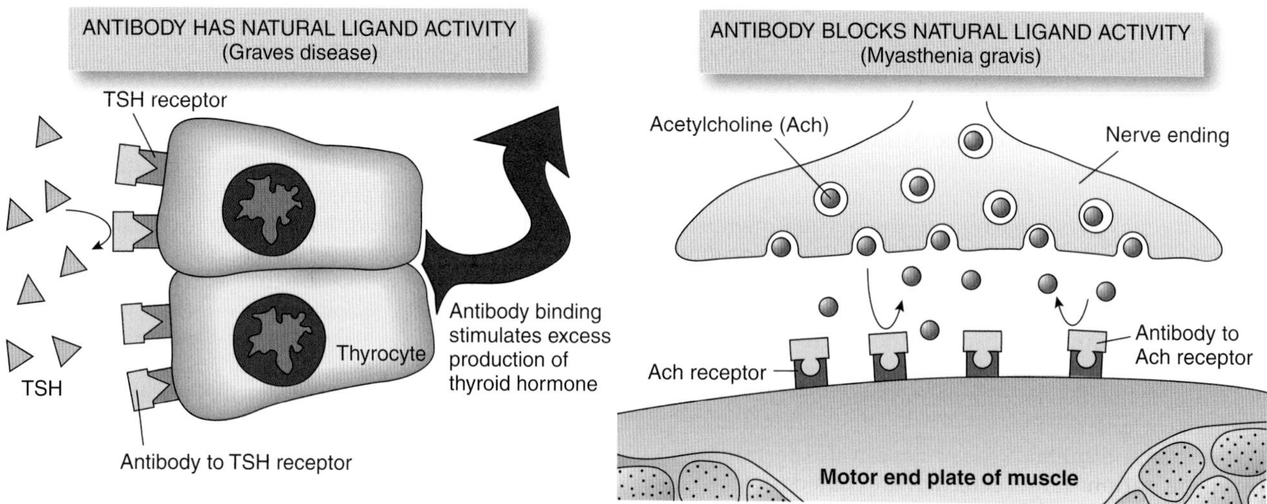

FIGURE 3-4. In a type II hypersensitivity reaction, antibodies bind to a cell surface receptor and induce activation (e.g., thyroid-stimulating hormone [TSH] receptors in Graves disease) or inhibition/destruction (e.g., acetylcholine receptors in myasthenia gravis).

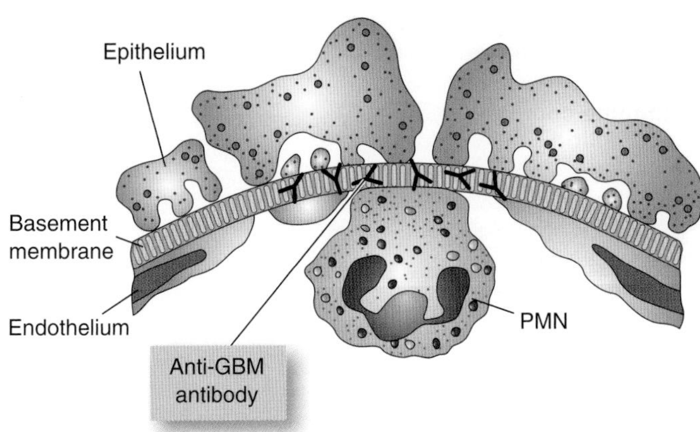

FIGURE 3-5. Goodpasture syndrome involves a type II hypersensitivity reaction in which antibody binds to a structural antigen, activates the complement system, and leads to the recruitment of tissue-damaging inflammatory cells. Several complement-derived peptides (e.g., C5a) are potent chemotactic factors. GBM, glomerular basement membrane; PMN, polymorphonuclear leukocyte.

against antigens on cell surfaces or in connective tissues. Complement participates in many of these events. It may directly mediate lysis, or it may act indirectly by opsonization and phagocytosis or chemotactic attraction of phagocytic cells, which produce a variety of tissue-damaging products. Complement-independent reactions, such as ADCC, also play a role in type II hypersensitivity.

Immune Complex Reactions (Type III)

Type III hypersensitivity reactions are mediated by immune complexes. Antigen–antibody complexes involving IgM, IgG, and, occasionally, IgA antibodies may be formed either in the circulation and then deposited in the tissues, or in situ. Immune complexes fix complement, which promotes recruitment of neutrophils and monocytes. Activation of inflammatory cells by immune complexes and complement, with consequent release of potent inflammatory mediators, is directly responsible for injury (Fig. 3-6). Immune complexes have been implicated in many human diseases. The most compelling cases are those in which demonstration of immune complexes in injured tissue correlates with development of injury. Examples include cryoglobulinemic vasculitis associated with hepatitis C infection, Henoch–Schönlein purpura (in which IgA deposits are found at sites of vasculitis), and systemic lupus erythematosus (SLE) (anti–double-stranded DNA in vasculitic lesions). Some forms of glomerulonephritis also feature the deposition of immune complexes at the glomerular basement membrane.

Physicochemical characteristics of the immune complexes, such as size, charge, and solubility, in addition to Ig isotype, determine whether immune complex deposits in tissue and fix complement. Such immune complexes elicit inflammatory responses by activating complement, thereby recruiting neutrophils and monocytes. These activated phagocytes release tissue damage mediators, such as proteases and reactive oxygen species. Several specialized forms of type III hypersensitivity disease are defined as follows:

- **Serum sickness** is an acute, self-limited disease that typically occurs 6 to 8 days after therapeutic administration of a foreign protein, such as an immune serum produced in an animal. The disease is now rare but can occur in patients given semi-purified serum preparations, such as antilymphocyte globulin. Experimental serum sickness serves as a model for type III hypersensitive reactions because the mechanism of tissue injury that occurs mimics that seen in human type III hypersensitivity. It is characterized by fever, arthralgias, vasculitis, and acute glomerulonephritis. Serum levels of exogenously injected antigen remain constant until about day 6, after which they fall rapidly (Fig. 3-6). At the same time, immune complexes (containing IgM or IgG bound to antigen) appear in the circulation. Some circulating complexes deposit in tissues, such as renal glomeruli and blood vessel walls. Immune complexes fix complement, leading to the generation of C3a and C5a, which increase vascular permeability. C5a is also a potent neutrophil chemoattractant. Other neutrophil chemotactic mediators that play a role include leukotriene B_4 and IL-8. Recruited neutrophils are activated through contact with, and ingestion of, immune complexes. Activated cells release inflammatory mediators, including proteases, reactive oxygen intermediates, and arachidonic acid products, which collectively produce tissue injury (see Chapter 2).
- The **Arthus reaction** refers to a type III hypersensitivity reaction in the vasculature (Fig. 3-7). This condition is seen in dermal blood vessels after local injection of an antigen to which an individual was previously sensitized. The circulating antibody and locally injected antigen diffuse down concentration gradients toward each other to form complex deposits in walls of small blood vessels. The walls of affected vessels contain numerous neutrophils and show evidence of damage, with edema and hemorrhage into surrounding tissue. The presence of fibrin creates the classic appearance of immune complex–induced vasculitis, namely, fibrinoid necrosis. The Arthus reaction is a prototype for many forms of vasculitis (e.g., cutaneous vasculitides that characterize certain drug reactions).

Cell-Mediated Hypersensitivity Reactions (Type IV)

Type IV reactions, although cell mediated, often occur together with antibody reactions, which can make it difficult to distinguish them. The type of tissue response is largely determined by the nature of the inciting agent. *Classically, delayed-type hypersensitivity is a tissue reaction, mainly involving lymphocytes and mononuclear phagocytes, occurring in response to a soluble protein antigen, and reaching peak intensity after 24 to 48 hours.* Hence, type IV reactions are often termed **delayed hypersensitivity**. A classic example is the contact sensitivity response to poison ivy. Although the chemical ligands in poison ivy (e.g., urushiol) are not proteins, they bind covalently to cell proteins, the products of which are recognized by antigen-specific lymphocytes.

In delayed-type hypersensitivity reactions (Fig. 3-8), foreign protein antigens or chemical ligands first interact with accessory cells that express HLA class II molecules (Fig. 3-8A). Accessory cells (macrophages and dendritic cells) secrete IL-12, which along with processed and presented antigen, activate $CD4^+$ T cells (Fig. 3-8B). Activated $CD4^+$ T cells secrete IFN-γ and IL-2, which respectively activate more macrophages and elicit T-lymphocyte proliferation (Fig. 3-8C). In turn, the cytokines recruit and activate lymphocytes, monocytes, fibroblasts, and other inflammatory cells. If

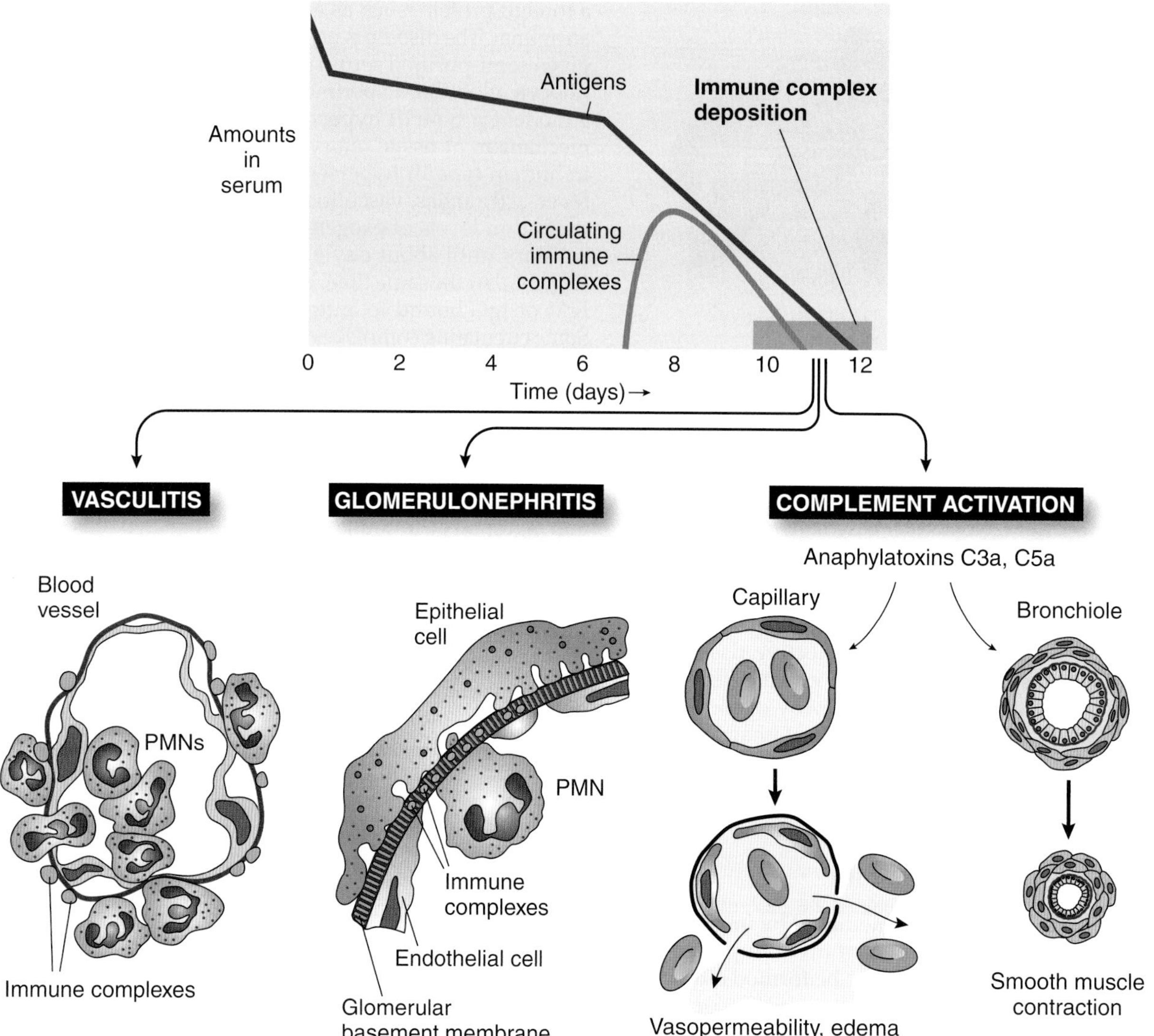

FIGURE 3-6. In type III hypersensitivity, immune complexes are deposited and can lead to complement activation and the recruitment of tissue-damaging inflammatory cells. This schematic illustrates the series of events that occur in acute serum sickness. The ability of immune complexes to mediate tissue injury depends on size, solubility, net charge, and ability to fix complement. PMN, polymorphonuclear leukocyte.

the antigenic stimulus is eliminated, the reaction spontaneously resolves after about 48 hours. Chronic inflammation associated with autoimmune diseases (e.g., type 1 diabetes, chronic thyroiditis, Sjögren syndrome, and primary biliary cirrhosis) is largely the result of type IV hypersensitivity.

Another mechanism by which T cells (especially CD8$^+$) mediate tissue damage is direct lysis of target cells (Fig. 3-9). This mechanism is important in destroying and eliminating cells infected by viruses, transplanted tissues, and even tumor cells.

In contrast to delayed-type hypersensitivity reactions, cytotoxic CD8$^+$ T cells specifically recognize target antigens in the context of MHC class I molecules. Foreign antigens are actively presented together with self-MHC antigens. In graft rejection, foreign MHC antigens are themselves potent activators of CD8$^+$ T cells. Once activated by antigen, cytotoxic cell proliferation is aided by helper cells and mediated by soluble growth factors, such as IL-2 (Fig. 3-9C); the population of antigen-specific cytotoxic cells thus expands. Cell killing occurs via several mechanisms (Fig. 3-9D; see also Chapter 1). Cytolytic T cells (CTLs) secrete perforins that form pores in target cell membranes and introduce granzymes that activate intracellular caspases, leading to apoptosis. CTLs can also kill targets by engaging Fas ligand (FasL, on the CTL) and Fas (on the target). FasL–Fas interaction triggers apoptosis of the Fas-bearing cell.

IMMUNODEFICIENCY DISEASES

Immunodeficiency diseases are classified as congenital (primary) or acquired (secondary), and by the particular defective host defense system. **Primary immunodeficiencies are classified as B cell or humoral, T cell or cellular, or combined and affecting both systems.** This scheme is

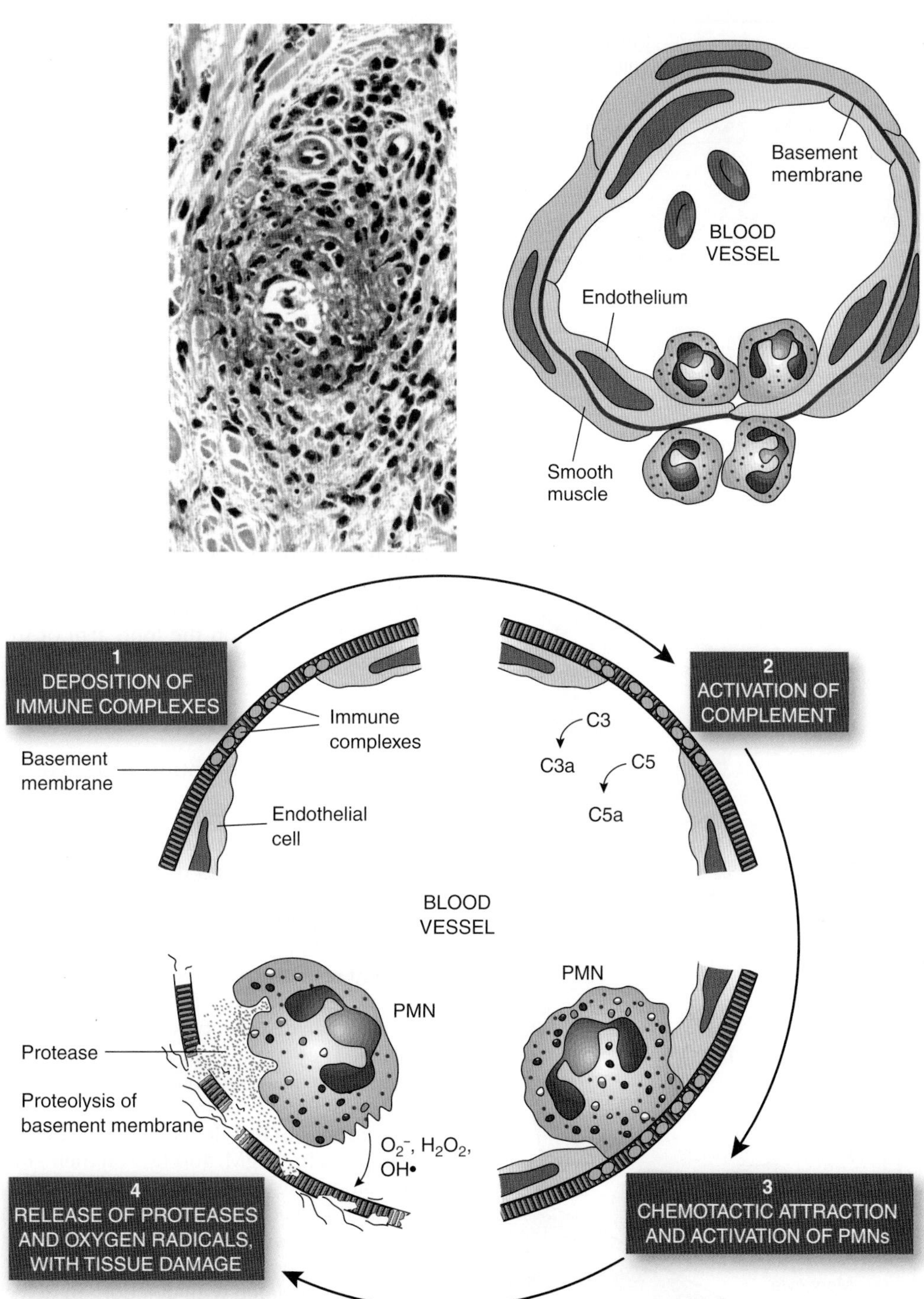

FIGURE 3-7. The Arthus reaction is a type III hypersensitivity reaction characterized by the deposition of immune complexes and the induction of an acute inflammatory response within blood vessel walls. Some vasculitic lesions exhibit fibrinoid necrosis. H_2O_2, hydrogen peroxide; O_2^-, superoxide anion; OH•, hydroxyl radical; PMN, polymorphonuclear leukocyte.

useful, but it should be recognized that a primary defect within one aspect of the immune system may have farther-reaching effects. In contrast to the low prevalence of congenital immunodeficiencies, acquired immune deficits, such as AIDS, are common.

Functional defects in lymphocytes can be localized to particular stages in the ontogeny of the immune system, or the interruption of discrete immune activation events (Fig. 3-10).

Antibody Deficiency Diseases

There are a variety of immunoglobulin isotype and subclass deficiencies, including selective deletions of immunoglobulin heavy chains and selective loss of light-chain expression (Table 3-2). Some patients have normal immunoglobulin levels but fail to make antibodies against specific antigens, usually polysaccharides. The clinical manifestations of these

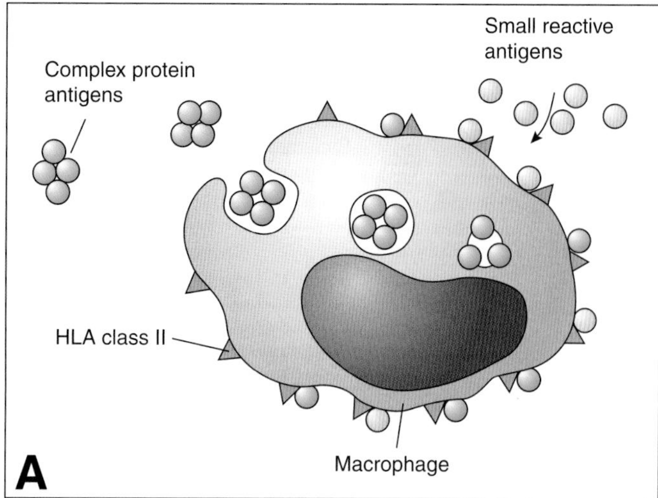

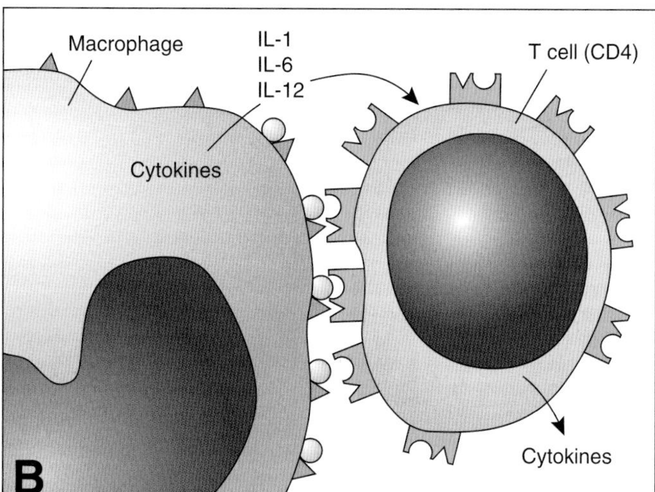

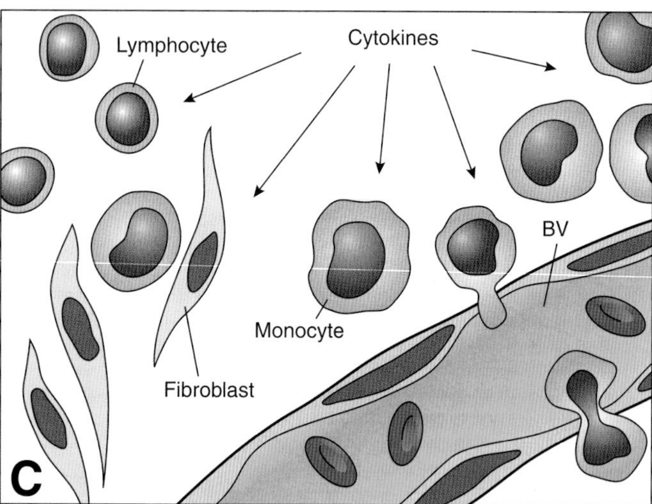

FIGURE 3-8. In a type IV (delayed-type) hypersensitivity reaction, complex antigens are phagocytized, processed, and presented on macrophage cell membranes in conjunction with major histocompatibility complex class II antigens. Antigens are, in turn, recognized via T-cell receptors expressed on histocompatible T lymphocytes. **A.** Antigen-specific, histocompatible, cytotoxic T lymphocytes bind presented antigens and are activated. **B, C.** Activated cytotoxic T cells secrete cytokines that amplify the response. BV, blood vessel; CD, cluster of differentiation; HLA, human leukocyte antigen; IL, interleukin.

entities are highly variable; some patients suffer from life-threatening bacterial infections, varying from meningitis to mucosal infections, whereas others are asymptomatic.

Bruton X-Linked Agammaglobulinemia

Bruton X-linked agammaglobulinemia (XLA) typically presents in boys younger than 1 year, when protective maternal antibody levels have declined. Up to 10% of XLA patients do not present until they are teenagers, and recent studies suggest that perhaps 10% of adults diagnosed with "common variable immunodeficiency (CVID)" (see below) actually have XLA. Patients develop recurrent infections of mucosal surfaces (e.g., sinusitis and bronchitis), pyoderma, meningitis, and septicemia. Severe hypogammaglobulinemia involves all Ig isotypes. Some persons develop viral hepatitis or chronic enterovirus infections of the CNS or large joints. Immunization with live attenuated poliovirus can lead to paralytic poliomyelitis. About one third of XLA patients suffer from a poorly understood form of arthritis, possibly caused by enteroviruses or *Ureaplasma.*

There are no mature B cells in peripheral blood or plasma cells in lymphoid tissues. Pre-B cells, however, can be detected. The genetic defect, on the long arm of the X chromosome, inactivates the gene for B-cell tyrosine kinase (Bruton tyrosine kinase), an enzyme critical to B-lymphocyte maturation (Table 3-2).

Selective Immunoglobulin A Deficiency

This is the most common primary immunodeficiency syndrome, characterized by normal serum levels of IgM and IgG and low serum (<7 mg/dL) and secretory concentrations of IgA. The incidence ranges from 1 in 18,000 in Japan to 1 in 400 among northern Europeans. Some 90% of patients are asymptomatic; the remainder may present with chronic or recurrent respiratory or gastrointestinal infections. They have a 10-fold greater risk of developing autoimmune diseases, such as celiac disease, type 1 diabetes, SLE, and rheumatoid arthritis. They are also at increased risk for allergic disease and occasionally anaphylactic, reactions to IgA-containing transfused blood products.

Patients with IgA deficiency have peripheral blood B cells that express IgA, IgM, and IgD on their surface (although the expression of IgA is often reduced). The varied and poorly understood defects result in an inability of such cells to mature and effectively synthesize and secrete IgA (Table 3-2). There may be a common origin with CVID (see below). Some cases have been associated with deletions or defects in chromosome 18. Patients with concomitant IgG subclass deficiencies are more likely to be clinically affected.

Common Variable Immunodeficiency

CVID is a heterogeneous group of disorders with severe hypogammaglobulinemia and attendant infections (Table 3-2), apparently owing to a variety of defects in B-lymphocyte maturation or T cells that regulate this maturation. Some relatives of patients with CVID have selective IgA deficiency. Affected patients present with recurrent severe pyogenic infections, especially pneumonia and diarrhea, the latter often due to infection with *Giardia lamblia.* Recurrent attacks of herpes simplex virus are common; herpes zoster develops in one fifth of patients. CVID appears years to decades after birth,

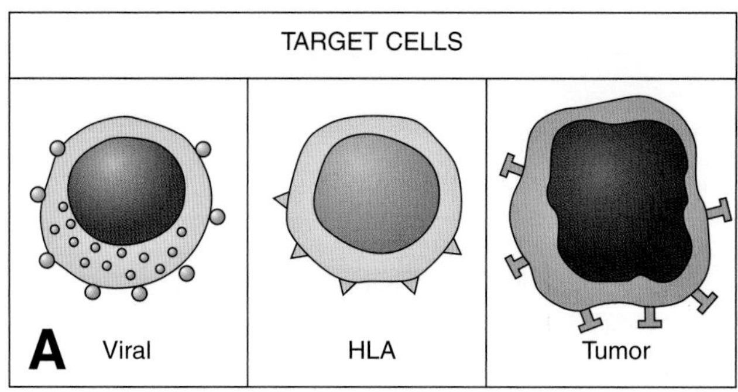

TARGET ANTIGENS
- Virally coded membrane antigen
- Foreign or modified histocompatibility antigen
- Tumor-specific membrane antigens

B
T-helper (CD4)
T-Cytotoxic (CD8)

RECOGNITION OF ANTIGEN BY T CELLS
- T-helper cells recognize antigen plus class II molecules
- T-cytotoxic/killer cells recognize antigen plus class I molecules

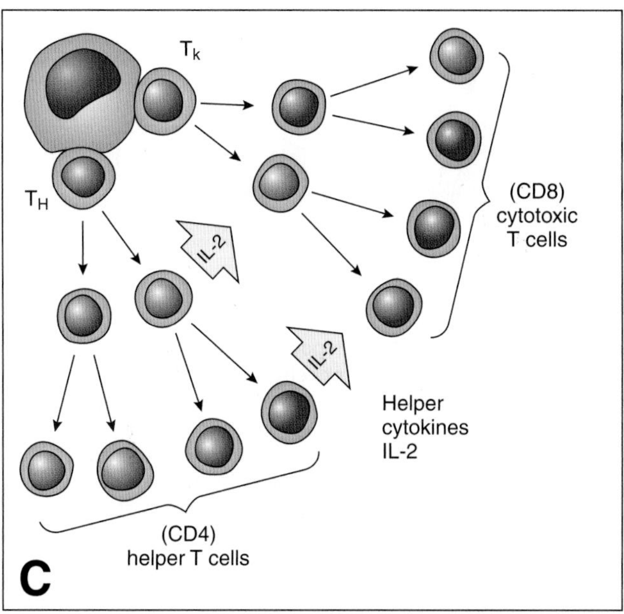

ACTIVATION AND AMPLIFICATION
- T-helper cells activate and proliferate, releasing helper molecules (e.g., IL-2)
- T-cytotoxic/killer cells proliferate in response to helper molecules

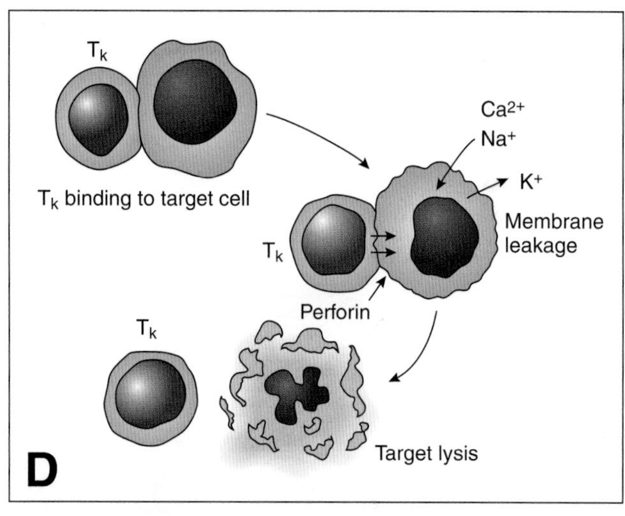

TARGET CELL KILLING
- T-cytotoxic/killer cells bind to target cell
- Killing signals perforin release and target cell loses membrane integrity
- Target cell undergoes lysis

FIGURE 3-9. In T-cell–mediated cytotoxicity, potential target cells include (A) virus-infected host cells, malignant host cells, and foreign (histoincompatible transplanted) cells. B. Cytotoxic T lymphocytes recognize foreign antigens in the context of human leukocyte antigen (HLA) class I molecules. **C.** Activated T cells secrete lytic compounds (e.g., perforin and other mediators) and cytokines that amplify the response. **D.** Apoptosis (target cell killing) is mediated by perforin and involves influx of Ca^{2+} and Na^+ and efflux of K^+. Ca^{2+}, calcium ion; CD, cluster of differentiation; IL, interleukin; K^+, potassium ion; Na^+, sodium ion; T_H, T helper; T_K, T killer.

with a mean age at onset of 25 years. It occurs in between 1 in 50,000 and 1 in 200,000 people. Inheritance patterns vary. CVID features several maturational and regulatory defects of the immune system. Cancers are increased in CVID, including a 50-fold greater incidence of gastric cancer. Interestingly, lymphoma is 300 times more common in women with this disease than in affected men. Malabsorption secondary to lymphoid hyperplasia and inflammatory bowel diseases occurs more frequently in the general population. Patients are also more susceptible to other autoimmune disorders, including hemolytic anemia, neutropenia, thrombocytopenia, and pernicious anemia.

Hyper-Immunoglobulin M Syndrome

Hyper-IgM (HIM) syndrome is often classified as a humoral immunodeficiency because Ig production is disordered. Patients have subnormal IgG, IgA, and IgE levels, and elevated IgM concentrations. There is an X-linked form that results from defects in CD40 ligand (type 1 hyper-IgM) and an autosomal recessive type because of defects in CD40 (type 3 hyper-IgM). Circulating B cells bear only IgM and IgD. The "switch" to other heavy-chain isotypes from IgD/IgM is defective. An interaction of the CD40 receptor on B-cell membranes with CD40 ligand is required for isotype switching (Fig. 3-10). Infants

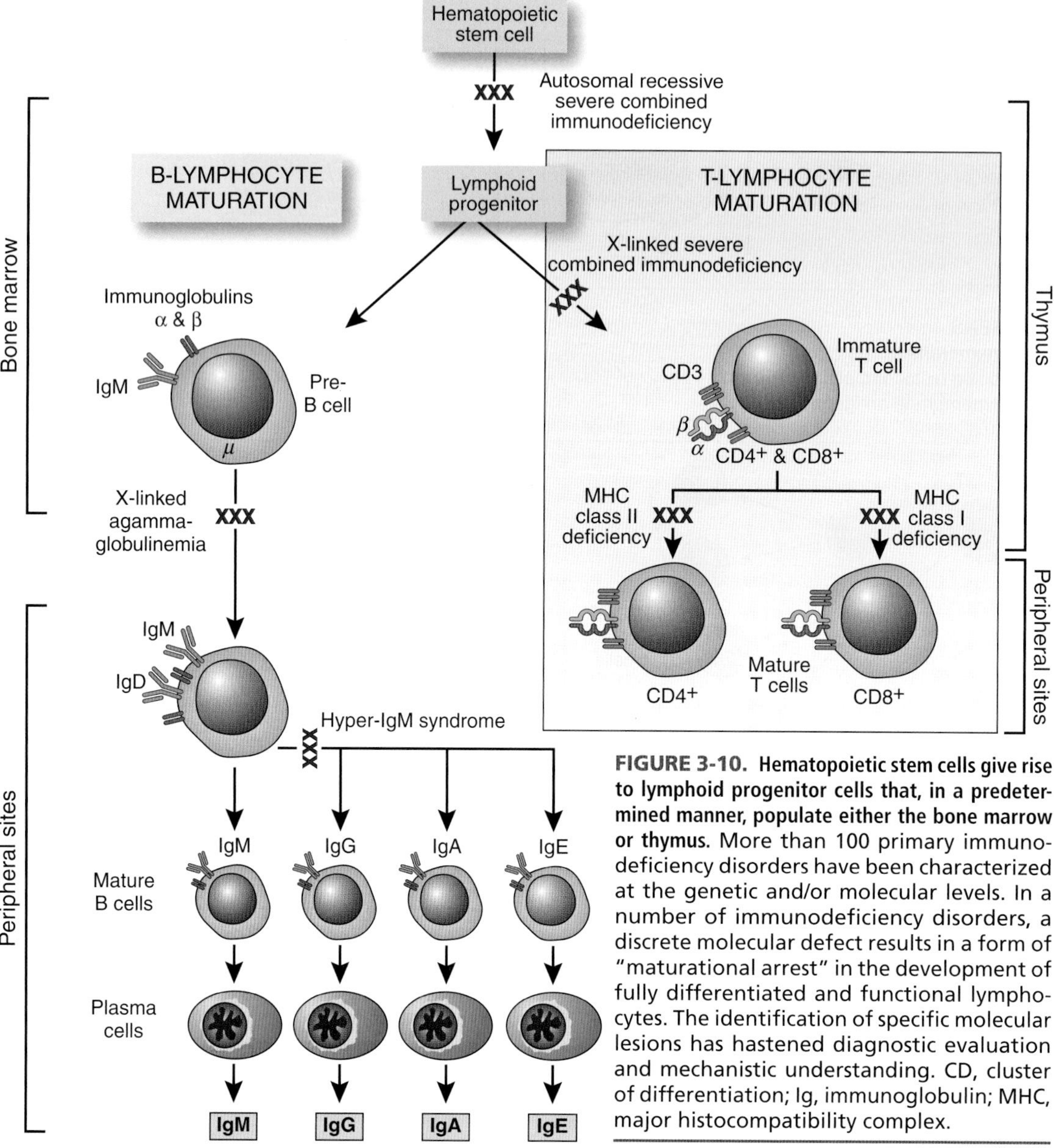

FIGURE 3-10. Hematopoietic stem cells give rise to lymphoid progenitor cells that, in a predetermined manner, populate either the bone marrow or thymus. More than 100 primary immunodeficiency disorders have been characterized at the genetic and/or molecular levels. In a number of immunodeficiency disorders, a discrete molecular defect results in a form of "maturational arrest" in the development of fully differentiated and functional lymphocytes. The identification of specific molecular lesions has hastened diagnostic evaluation and mechanistic understanding. CD, cluster of differentiation; Ig, immunoglobulin; MHC, major histocompatibility complex.

with X-linked disease suffer from pyogenic and opportunistic infections, especially with *Pneumocystis*, and also tend to develop autoimmune diseases involving the formed elements of blood. These are especially autoimmune hemolytic anemia, thrombocytopenic purpura, and recurrent severe neutropenia.

T-Cell Immunodeficiencies

T-cell immunodeficiencies are often part of a constellation of abnormalities and may effect predominantly T cells or both B and T cells (combined immunodeficiencies) (Table 3-3).

DiGeorge Syndrome

In its complete form, DiGeorge syndrome is a severe T-cell immunodeficiency disorder in which serum Igs are reduced because of lack of T-helper activity. Although variable, some infants present with conotruncal great vessel and cardiac defects and severe hypocalcemia (due to hypoparathyroidism). Others show characteristically abnormal facial features. Infants who survive the neonatal period are subject to recurrent and chronic viral, bacterial, fungal, and protozoal infections.

DiGeorge syndrome is caused by defective development of the third and fourth pharyngeal pouches, which give rise to thymic epithelium and parathyroid glands and influence conotruncal cardiac development. Most patients have a deletion on the long arm of chromosome 22; thus, DiGeorge syndrome is considered to be a form of the "22q11 deletion syndrome." In the absence of a functional thymus, T-cell maturation is interrupted at the pre–T-cell stage. The immunologic defect has been corrected by transplanting thymic tissue. Most affected patients have "partial" DiGeorge syndrome, in which a small remnant of thymus is present. With time, many individuals recover T-cell function without treatment. Some persons with 22q11 mutations suffer only from conotruncal cardiac defects.

Table 3-2

Primary Humoral Immunodeficiency Disorders

Disease	Mode of Inheritance	Locus/Gene
Agammaglobulinemia	XL	Xq21.3/*BTK*
Selective antibody class/subclass deficiencies		
γ1 isotype	AR	14q32.33
γ2 isotype	AR	14q32.33
Partial γ3 isotype	AR	14q32.33
γ4 isotype	AR	14q32.33
IgG subclass ± IgA deficiency	uncertain	
α_1 isotype	AR	14q32.33
α_2 isotype	AR	14q32.33
ε isotype	AR	14q32.33
IgA deficiency	Varied	—
Common variable immunodeficiency	Varied	—

AR, autosomal recessive; BTK, Bruton tyrosine kinase; Ig, immunoglobulin; XL, X-linked.

Chronic Mucocutaneous Candidiasis

This disease results from impaired T-cell function and is characterized by susceptibility to candidal infections and endocrinopathy (hypoparathyroidism, Addison disease, and diabetes mellitus). Most T-cell functions are intact, but the response to *Candida* antigens is deficient.

A series of defects in T-cell development underlie this syndrome. Patients with this disorder react to *Candida* antigens differently than do normal individuals. Unlike normal responses in which Th1 (IL-2/IFN-γ) cells predominate and effectively control candidal infections, affected persons mount a Th2 (IL-4/IL-6) helper-cell response, which is ineffective in resisting the organism.

Combined Immunodeficiency Diseases

Severe combined immunodeficiencies are conspicuously heterogeneous and are often life-threatening (Table 3-3).

Severe Combined Immunodeficiency

SCID encompasses over 20 disorders associated with deficiencies in T-cell and B-cell development and function. Affected infants present in the first few months of life with recurrent, often severe infections, diarrhea, and failure to thrive. Some forms of SCID have nonimmunologic developmental defects. SCID is usually fatal within the first year of life unless an immune system can be provided by stem cell transplantation.

SCID is consistently marked by defective T-cell development and function. In some types, B-cell development is also affected. Because B cells require T-cell–derived signals for optimal antibody production, most patients have defective cellular and humoral immunity. NK-cell development and function are variably affected. Current classifications of SCID include several categories (see Table 3-3).

Table 3-3

Severe Combined Immunodeficiency (SCID): Molecular Lesions

Disease	Locus/Gene
T−/−B+/−NK−/−	
IL2RG	Cytokine receptor common γ-chain
JAK3	Tyrosine kinase JAK3
T−/−B+/−NK+/−	
CD3D	CD3 complex, δ subunit
CD3E	CD3 complex, ε subunit
CD3G	CD3 complex, γ subunit
CIITA	MHC class II transactivator
RFXANK	MHC class II transactivator
FRX5	MHC class II transactivator
RXAP	MHC class II transactivator
ZAP70	TCR-associated protein of 70 kd
TAP1	Transporter-associated antigen processing 1
TAP2	Transporter-associated antigen processing 2
T−/−B−/−NK−/−	
ADA	Adenosine deaminase
PNP	Purine nucleoside phosphoacylase
T−/−B−/−NK+/−	
RAG1	Recombinase-activating gene 1
RAG2	Recombinase-activating gene 2

This is a partial list of SCID disorders.

MHC, major histocompatibility complex; TCR, T-cell receptor.

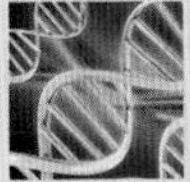

MOLECULAR PATHOGENESIS: More than a dozen molecular lesions have been described in T−/−B+/−NK+ SCID patients. For instance, mutations in genes (*CD3D*, *CD3E*, and *CD3G*) that encode each subunit (δ, ε, and γ) of the TCR-associated CD3 complex have been described. These patients all show defects in T-lymphocyte function, but clinical features have varied. Other patients lack $CD4^+$ T cells in association with various defects in expression of MHC class II molecules. Yet another group of patients is deficient in $CD8^+$ T cells.

Mutations in the genes for enzymes in the purine nucleotide salvage pathway, adenosine deaminase (*ADA*), and purine nucleoside phosphorylase (*PNP*) result in T−/−B−/−NK− SCID.

The most common form of SCID in the United States (50% of cases) is caused by mutations within *IL2RG; this gene* encodes the cytokine receptor common γ-chain, which is shared by receptors for IL-2, IL-4, IL-7, IL-9, IL-15, and IL-21. Defects result in complete absence of T cells and NK cells (90% of cases) but normal numbers of B cells. Immunoglobulin production is severely impaired because of the T-cell defect. Signaling downstream of the IL receptors with the common γ-chain requires activation of JAK3 tyrosine kinase. Not surprisingly, T−/−B−/−NK− SCID patients with mutations in *JAK3* have been identified.

The accumulation of toxic purine metabolites results in death of immature, proliferating lymphocytes (and other cell types). ADA deficiency accounts for 15% of all SCID patients in the United States. PNP deficiency is very rare.

AUTOIMMUNITY

Both the innate and adaptive immune systems have the capacity to injure host tissues. This process gives rise to a large number of human diseases, some entirely caused by self-reactivity, whereas others are mediated secondarily by autoreactivity. Broadly speaking, human autoimmune diseases are divided into those affecting primarily one organ (e.g., type 1 diabetes) and those whose effects extend to multiple body systems (e.g., SLE).

Immune Tolerance

An abnormal or injurious autoimmune response to self-antigens implies loss of **immune tolerance**. Tolerance to self-antigens is an active process and requires contact between self-antigens and immune cells. In fetal life, tolerance is readily established to antigens that trigger vigorous immune responses in adults. Several mechanisms induce and maintain tolerance, actively and continuously. Thus, in tolerance, potentially harmful immune responses are constantly blocked or aborted. Induction of tolerance to an antigen is partly related to the dose of antigen to which cells are exposed.

Central and peripheral mechanisms both participate. In **central tolerance**, self-reactive immature T and B lymphocytes are "deleted" or changed during their maturation in the "central" thymus and bone marrow, respectively. Developing T cells that recognize self-peptides, in the context of compatible MHC molecules with high binding affinity, undergo apoptosis. These T cells are said to have been "negatively selected." The AIRE protein (*a*uto*i*mmune *re*gulator) is involved in the expression of self-antigens within the thymus, and so is important in the central expression of peripheral self-antigens to which the individual becomes tolerant. Mutations in *AIRE* cause an autoimmune polyendocrinopathy (Fig. 3-11). In the bone marrow, a similar negative selection process involves B cells. In addition, engagement of self-antigens by developing marrow B cells can reset antigen receptor gene rearrangement through a process called "receptor editing." These reprogrammed B cells thus do not recognize self. CD4$^+$ regulatory T cells also develop.

Peripheral tolerance is important in regulating T cells that escape intrathymic negative selection. Mature T lymphocytes

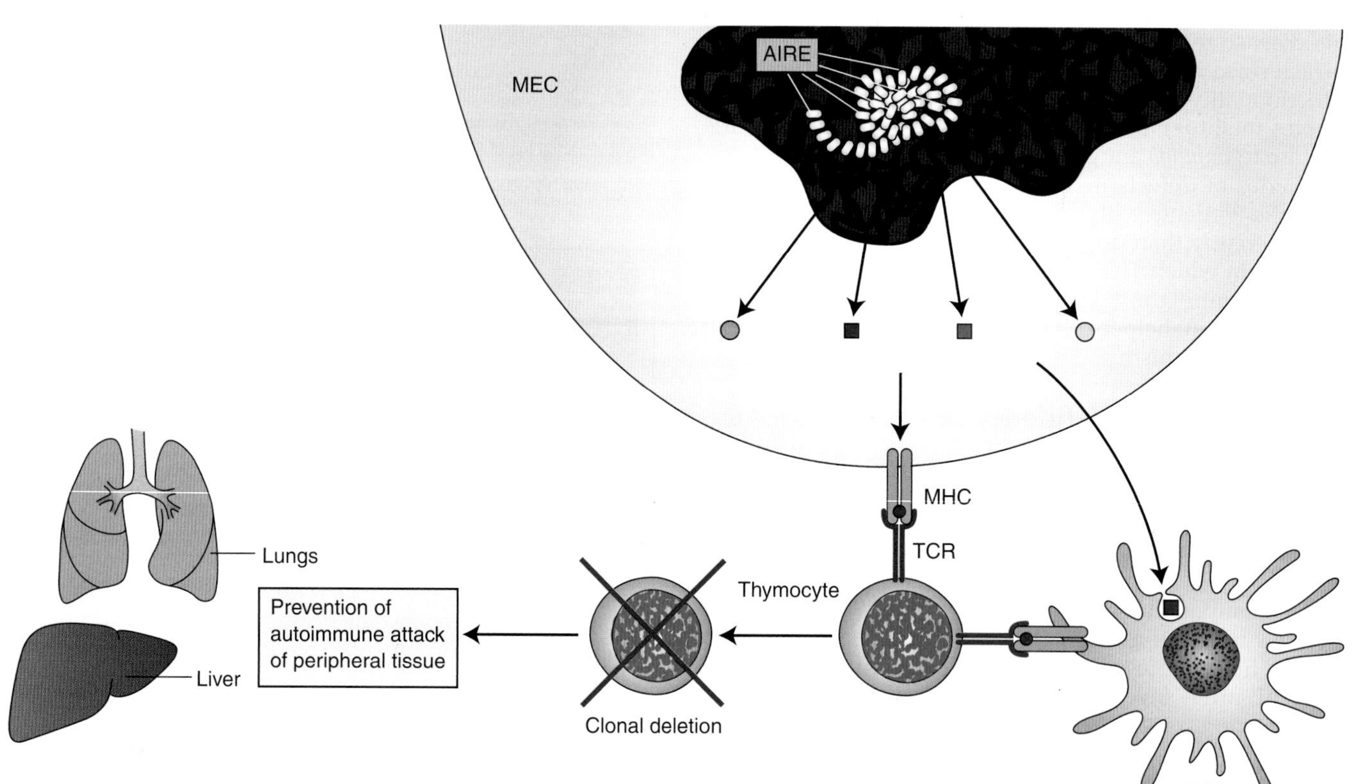

FIGURE 3-11. T-lymphocyte clonal deletion in tolerance. AIRE transcription factor activates expression of antigens normally expressed in peripheral tissues, so that they are expressed in thymic medulla epithelial cells (MEC). Antigens so regulated may include those of any tissue, the liver and lungs being shown here as representatives. Such self-antigens are presented to T lymphocytes developing in the thymus, directly by the MEC or by dendritic cells (DCs). The result is deletion of autoreactive T lymphocytes. AIRE, *a*uto*i*mmune *re*gulator; MHC, major histocompatibility complex, TCR, T-cell receptor.

are held in check in the periphery via **anergy**, suppression, or activation-induced cell death. Anergy occurs when T lymphocytes bind antigen presented by APCs in the absence of the "second signal," which is normally provided by the antigen- presenting cells (APC) and CD28 antigens on the T cell. Immune responses are suppressed by the population of regulatory T cells (T_{reg}s, noted above) generated in response to exposure to self-antigens. These T_{reg}s are $CD4^+$, constitutively express CD25 (β-chain of high-affinity IL-2 receptor), and express FOXp3 transcription factor. Mutations and polymorphisms affecting *CD25*, IL-2, or FOXp3 result in autoimmune disorders. Finally, $CD4^+$ T cells and self-reactive B cells can be deleted by several activation-initiated mechanisms (Fig. 3-12).

Theories of Autoimmunity

There are multiple explanations for the development of autoimmune diseases which are not mutually exclusive.

Breach of Immunologic Privilege

This is a rare cause of autoimmunity. Certain body areas (e.g., the anterior part of the eye) are immunologically "privileged"; the immune system has little or no contact with these areas, and tolerance is not established to tissue-specific antigens there. This allows transplantation of foreign corneas. But if "privileged" proteins should contact the immune system (through trauma, for instance), self-reactivity can occur. This accounts for **sympathetic ophthalmitis**, when trauma to one eye causes chronic autoimmune inflammation of both eyes; the immune system has become sensitized to ocular antigens it normally ignored. Post–myocardial infarction pericarditis may have a similar etiology.

Molecular Mimicry

Helper T-cell tolerance may also be overcome if foreign antigens elicit antibodies that cross-react with self-antigens, a process that is termed **molecular mimicry**. In acute rheumatic heart disease, antibodies against streptococcal bacterial antigens cross-react with tissue in joints, the nervous system, and the heart. This causes an acute febrile illness, with inflammation in and around the heart and in the joints, and sometimes in the brain (see Chapters 8 and 9). **Guillain–Barré syndrome** is a postviral autoimmune neuropathy, apparently resulting from immunity originally directed against viral products. A large number of viral diseases have been associated with autoimmune consequences—for example, postmeasles encephalomyelopathy. The extent to which this represents cross-reactivity with the host or other mechanisms is unclear (Fig. 3-13).

Polyclonal Activation and Autoimmunity

Certain environmental agents—famously, the lipopolysaccharide (LPS) that is part of the coating of Gram-negative bacteria, but also many other substances—may diffusely activate the immune system. LPS acts by binding to Toll-like receptor 4 (TLR4; see Chapter 2). Because B cells have certain TLRs, they can be powerfully activated by ligands binding these receptors, resulting in the simultaneous activation of many

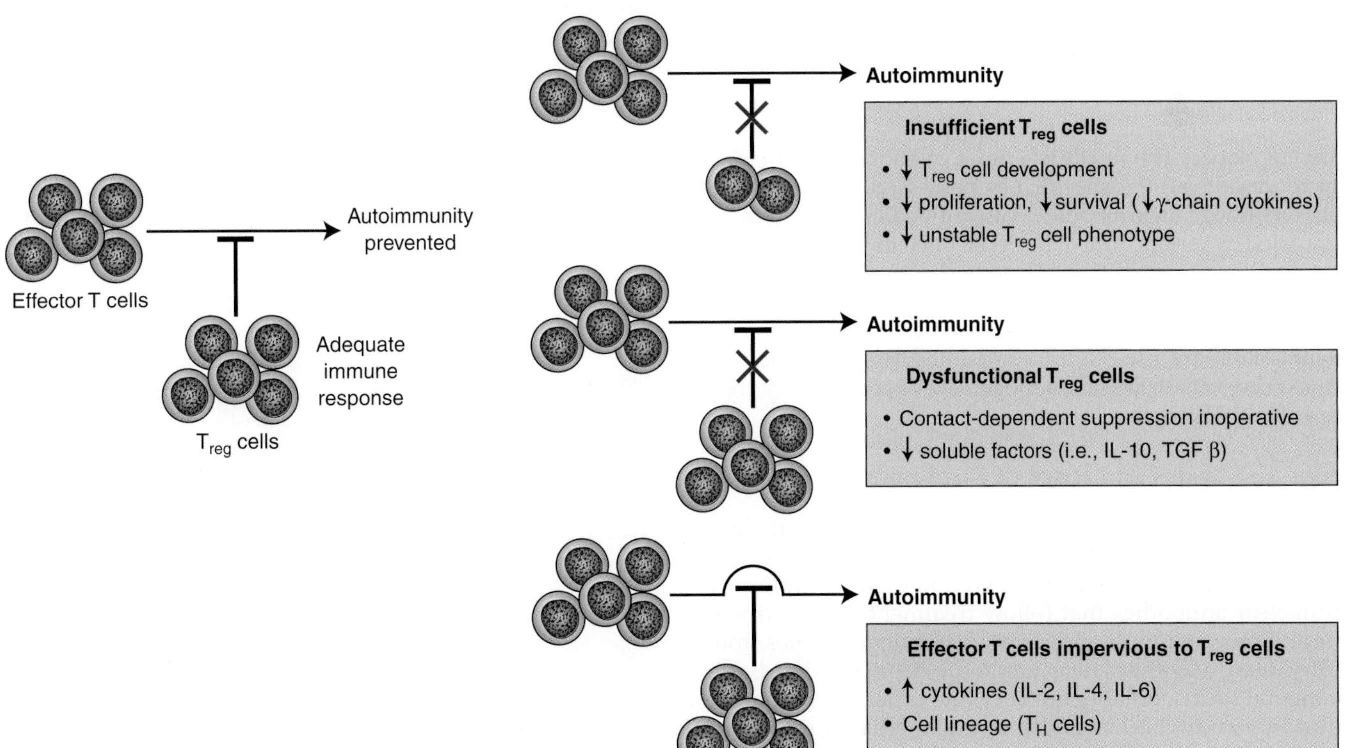

FIGURE 3-12. Regulatory T lymphocytes may inhibit autoimmunity. T_{reg}s inhibit effector T lymphocytes. Pathologic situations are shown in which T_{reg}s may be insufficient in number or impaired in functionality, or in which T effector cells may not be susceptible to the regulatory activities of T_{reg}s. IL, interleukin; TGF, transforming growth factor; T_H, T helper; T_{reg}, regulatory T cells.

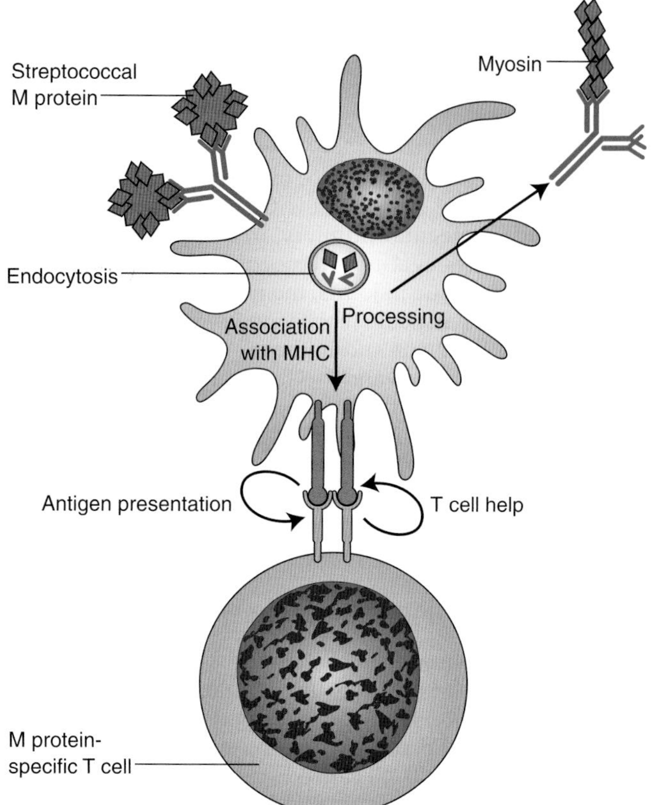

FIGURE 3-13. Molecular mimicry. In molecular mimicry, the immune system is sensitized by foreign proteins (here, *Streptococcus* M protein). M-protein–reactive T cells help B cells, which make antibody that cross-reacts with autologous cardiac myosin, to cause damage to the heart, as in rheumatic fever. MHC, major histocompatibility complex.

different clones. The result is a burst of antibody formation that represents all the specificities possessed by available B cells, including autoantibodies. Autoantibodies can thereby be stimulated by certain viral or bacterial infections. For example, Epstein–Barr virus (EBV) binds to and activates B cells, and autoantibodies are regularly present during acute EBV infection. Chronic bacterial infections, such as endocarditis and osteomyelitis, are also often accompanied by autoantibodies. In most cases, these are not pathogenic, but occasionally, they cause clinical disease.

Drugs and Toxins as Causes of Autoimmunity

Certain drugs can provoke autoantibodies and even clinical autoimmunity in ways that are still ill-defined but that involve aberrations of tolerance. Well-known examples are antinuclear antibodies that follow treatment with hydralazine and procainamide, antierythrocyte autoantibodies from methyldopa, and antiplatelet antibodies from quinine. Environmental toxins, notably mercury and other heavy metals, result in autoantibodies and immune-mediated renal and nervous system disease.

Genetics and Autoimmunity

Host genes profoundly affect susceptibility to autoimmune diseases. Concordance for certain autoimmune diseases among identical twins may reach 35%. In addition, autoimmune disease patients frequently report family members who have or had the same or similar autoimmune disorders. Except for rare inherited conditions, inheritance is complex, and multiple genes conspire together with multiple environmental factors. Among the genetic loci that influence the development of autoimmune diseases are MHC alleles (mostly class II, but class I for the spondyloarthropathies). They act together with multiple genes involving the immune system, such as IL-7 and its receptor and IL-23. As well, *TLR* genes and other genes for cytokines, cytokine receptors, and tyrosine kinases involved in immune cell activation are associated with the development of immune responses to self-antigens.

Gender and Autoimmunity

Most autoimmune diseases occur more often in females. Female to male ratios range from up to 20:1 for autoimmune thyroiditis and SLE to perhaps 3:1 for rheumatoid arthritis and multiple sclerosis. The increased susceptibility of women to autoimmunity remains incompletely understood. A large but not conclusive body of evidence supports the notion that sex hormones are involved through their influence on the immune response. However, X-chromosome gene dosage effects are also possible.

Innate Immunity as a Form of Autoimmunity

Certain inflammatory diseases are caused by improper control of the innate immune system. The periodic fever syndromes, an important cause of morbidity in many parts of the world. They are caused by genetic defects in the control of the **inflammasome** (see Chapter 2), a complex protein that regulates the conversion of pro–interleukin-1 to interleukin-1 (Fig. 3-14). The "autoinflammatory" diseases also include several inherited disorders characterized by widespread inflammation. An

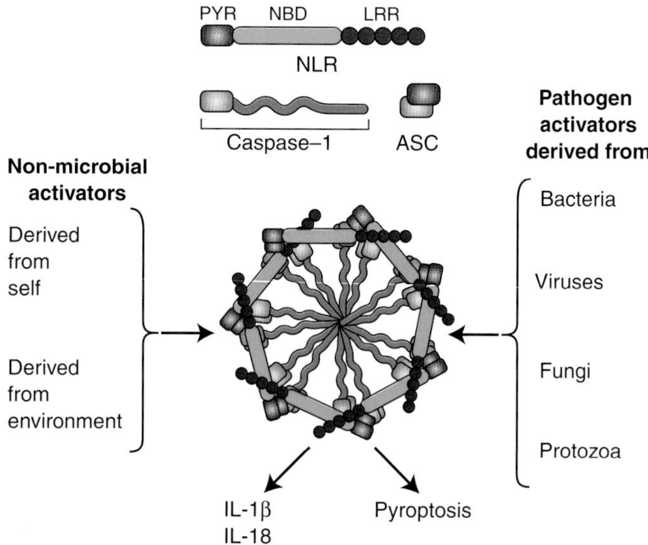

FIGURE 3-14. The inflammasome. The NLRP3 inflammasome, the best studied of these pro-inflammatory complexes, is a cluster of proteins (NLR, caspase 1, and ASC) on macrophages and other innate immune cells. Several stimuli activate it to cause production of active interleukin-1 (IL-1) and IL-18 and to elicit cell death. ASC, apoptosis-associated speck-like protein containing a caspase recruitment domain; LRR, leucine-rich repeat; NBD, nucleotide-binding domain; NLR, nod-like receptor gene; PYR, pyrin domain.

example is neonatal onset multisystem inflammatory disease (NOMID), a condition in which a mutated cryopyrin protein (a key component of the inflammasome) is constitutively activated and leads to skin inflammation and arthritis. Mutations of TRAPS, a key intracellular protein involved in TNF signaling, also results in inherited inflammatory conditions.

Inherited or acquired defects of complement control proteins (factor H and others) can result in severe microangiopathic disease (the hemolytic–uremic syndrome). Defects in red cell proteins that control complement activation can lead to paroxysmal nocturnal hemoglobinuria, a serious form of anemia and hemolysis (see Chapter 18).

EXAMPLES OF AUTOIMMUNE DISEASES

Systemic Lupus Erythematosus

SLE characteristically affects the skin, joints, serous membranes, central nervous system, and kidneys. Autoantibodies are formed against a variety of self-antigens, including (1) plasma proteins (complement components and clotting factors) and protein–phospholipid complexes, (2) cell surface antigens (lymphocytes, neutrophils, platelets, and erythrocytes), (3) ribosomes, RNA, and nuclear DNA, and (4) ribonucleoproteins and histones. The spectrum of intracellular autoantigens also includes the proteins and DNA that make up chromatin, proteins of the spliceosome complex (small nuclear RNPs [snRNPs]) and the Ro/La small cytoplasmic ribonucleoprotein particle. The most important diagnostic autoantibodies are those against nuclear antigens—in particular, antibody to double-stranded DNA (dsDNA) and to a soluble nuclear antigen complex, Sm antigen, that is part of the spliceosome. In clinical context, high titers of these two **antinuclear antibodies (ANAs)** are very suggestive of SLE. Antigen–antibody complexes form or deposit in tissues, thereby provoking a characteristic vasculitis, synovitis, and glomerulonephritis. SLE is a prototypical type III hypersensitivity reaction. Occasionally, directly cytotoxic antibodies are present, particularly antibodies against cell surface antigens of leukocytes and erythrocytes. There is also evidence that cell-mediated immune responses are involved.

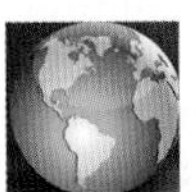

EPIDEMIOLOGY: The prevalence of SLE varies worldwide. In North America and northern Europe, it is 40 in 100,000. In the United States, it appears to be more common and severe in blacks and Hispanics. Nearly 90% of cases are in women of childbearing age, as many as 1 in 700 of whom may have this disease.

The etiology of SLE is unknown. Genetic, immunologic, and environmental factors presumably contribute (Fig. 3-15). The presence of numerous autoantibodies, particularly ANAs, suggests a loss of tolerance. Some manifestations of SLE result from tissue injury as a result of immune complex–mediated vasculitis, whereas other conditions (e.g., thrombocytopenia or the secondary antiphospholipid syndrome) are caused by autoantibodies to cell membrane molecules or serum components.

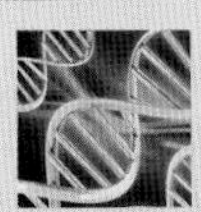

MOLECULAR PATHOGENESIS: Genetic factors clearly are important in the etiology of SLE. Although identical twins show a concordance rate of 25% for SLE, no single factor dominates the genetics of the disease. Instead, susceptibility to SLE results from the sum of small effects of multiple genes. Genome-wide association studies have identified at least 50 associations (including HLA-DR2), but each increases the risk of disease no more than twofold. An exception to this are uncommon disorders of early complement components (C2, C4, and C1q), which markedly increase the risk of SLE. About 90% of patients totally lacking C1q develop the disease. This finding suggests an important role for failure in clearance of circulating immune complexes in the etiology of the disease.

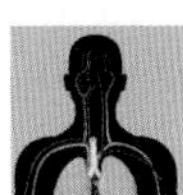

PATHOPHYSIOLOGY

ENVIRONMENT. SLE has an important genetic component, as described above. However, the observation that 75% of monozygotic twins are discordant for the disease implies an important role for nongenetic factors, be they environmental, epigenetic, or stochastic.

Ultraviolet irradiation and viral infections are two established environmental factors. For example, a typical lupus onset is a patient who presents to the clinic with malar rash and arthritis after prolonged exposure to the sun. Common viral infections also exacerbate or ignite the onset of the disorder. Both factors are thought to operate by inducing a form of pro-inflammatory cell death.

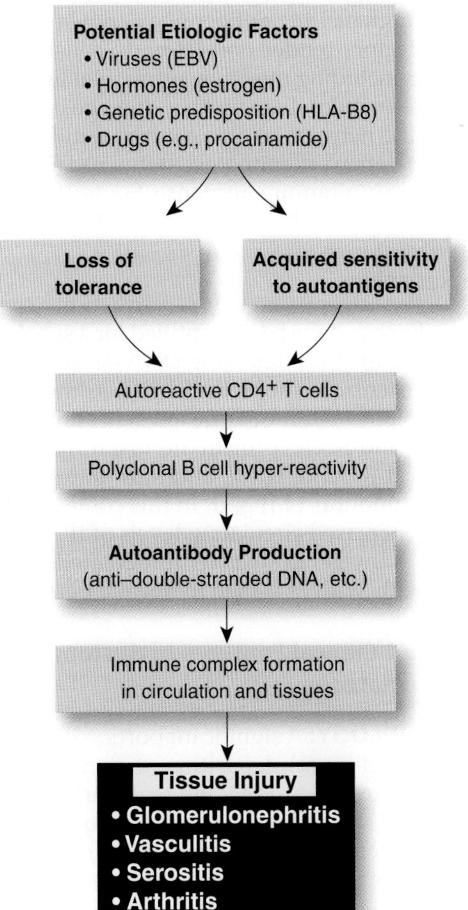

FIGURE 3-15. The pathogenesis of systemic lupus erythematosus is multifactorial. CD, cluster of differentiation; EBV, Epstein–Barr virus; HLA, human leukocyte antigen.

Other factors such as cigarette smoking, heavy metals, solvents, pesticides, and exogenous estrogens have been implicated, but definitive proof is lacking. Finally, silica exposure significantly increases the risk of developing SLE if exposure lasts more than 1 year. It has been suggested that exposure to silica, which has been demonstrated to be toxic to macrophages, may impair clearance of apoptotic cells and thus favor self-immunization and SLE.

HORMONES. SLE is predominantly a female disease. The onset of the malady before puberty and after menopause is uncommon, and the female predilection becomes less pronounced outside the reproductive age range. Finally, patients with Klinefelter syndrome, characterized by hypergonadotropic hypogonadism, are prone to the development of SLE. These observations suggest a role for endogenous sex hormones in disease predisposition.

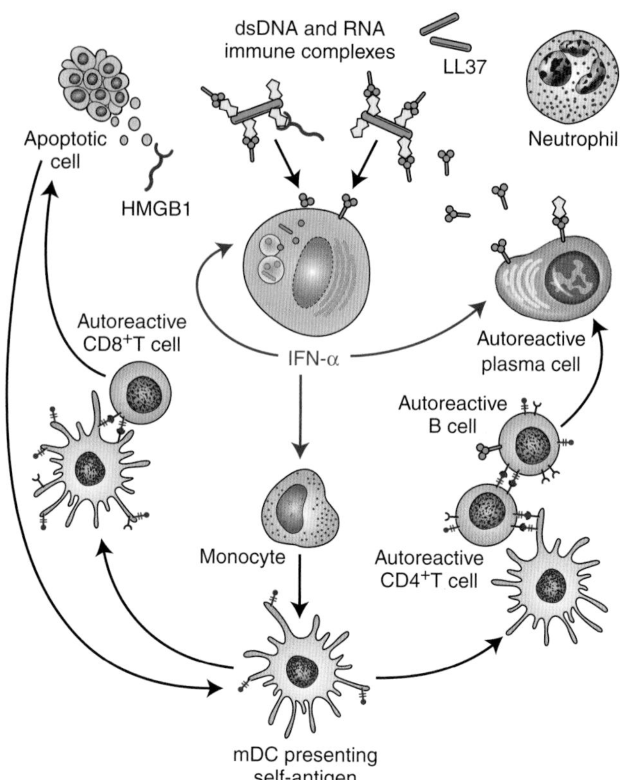

FIGURE 3-16. Immune pathogenesis of systemic lupus erythematosus. Nucleic acid complexes or Toll-like receptor agonists elicit interferon α (IFN-α) by dendritic cells (DCs). This, in turn, triggers autoantigen presentation and autoantibody production by plasma cells. CD, cluster of differentiation; dsDNA, double-stranded DNA; HMGB1, high-mobility group box 1; LL37, cathelicidin antimicrobial peptide; mDC, myeloid dendritic cell.

Immunologic Factors in the Pathogenesis of Systemic Lupus Erythematosus

Pathogenic autoantibodies produced by B cells are an important cause of tissue damage in SLE. Evidence for specific antigen-driven responses comes from the observation that, with time, the antibodies of SLE demonstrate gene rearrangements and mutations that are typical of antigen-driven, T-cell–dependent responses. Moreover, patients with SLE often have antibodies to more than one epitope on a single antigen, further suggesting a primary role for an antigen-driven process. Although inciting antigens have not been identified, a number of factors render normal body constituents more immunogenic, including infection, ultraviolet light exposure, and other environmental agents that damage cells.

The cytokine network is also abnormal in lupus and reflects (1) the systemic inflammatory status and (2) an ongoing antigen-driven autoimmune response. Some of the increased cytokines are IL-4, IL-6, IL-10, and IFN-α (Fig. 3-16).

Toll-Like Receptors

Endogenous ligands have been identified for a substantial proportion of TLRs. In SLE, circulating DNA/histone and RNA/protein complexes from apoptotic debris become endogenous ligands, especially when complexed with autoantibodies. DNA/histone and RNA/protein are taken up by dendritic cells, engage TLR9 and TLR7, and stimulate such cells to produce large amounts of IFN-α. In this context, most lupus patients have increased circulating levels of IFN-α. Levels of expression of many genes that are upregulated by IFN-α are higher in patients with SLE than in normal persons.

Pathology and Clinical Features of Systemic Lupus Erythematosus

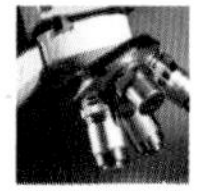

PATHOLOGY: A significant portion of injury in SLE is caused by (1) deposition of circulating immune complexes against self-antigens, particularly against DNA, (2) the occurrence of circulating immune complexes that contain nuclear antigen, (3) the presence of those immune complexes in injured tissues, as identified by immunofluorescence, and (4) the observation that immune complexes can be extracted from tissues that contain nuclear antigens. Additional evidence suggests that under certain conditions, immune complex formation also occurs in situ—that is, in tissues rather than in the circulation. Examples include antibodies against connective tissue components and perhaps the membranous form of lupus glomerulonephritis. Type II hypersensitivity reactions are also implicated in SLE because cytotoxic antibodies against red blood cell and platelet membrane proteins can cause cytopenias (see Chapter 18).

The renal lesions of SLE are largely caused by deposition of immune complexes, leading to glomerular inflammation (Fig. 3-17). IgG and complement components are demonstrated in a "lumpy-bumpy" pattern, and electron-dense complexes can be visualized by electron microscopy (see Chapter 14). T-lymphocytes infiltrate of the kidneys as well, and a variable amount of interstitial nephritis, occurs. Skin lesions are characterized by lymphocytic infiltration and by hydropic degeneration of keratinocytes.

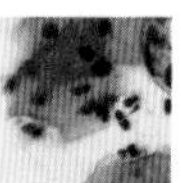

CLINICAL FEATURES: Because circulating immune complexes in SLE deposit in many tissues, virtually every organ in the body may be involved (Fig. 3-18).

- **Joint disease** is the most common manifestation of SLE; over 90% of patients have polyarthralgia. An inflammatory synovitis occurs, but unlike rheumatoid arthritis, joint destruction is unusual.
- **Skin involvement** (see Chapter 20) is common. An erythematous rash in sun-exposed sites, a malar "butterfly" rash, is characteristic. Microscopically, perivascular lymphoid infiltrates, and liquefactive degeneration of the basal cells is seen; they correlate with immunoglobulin and complement deposition along the dermal–epidermal junction ("lupus band").

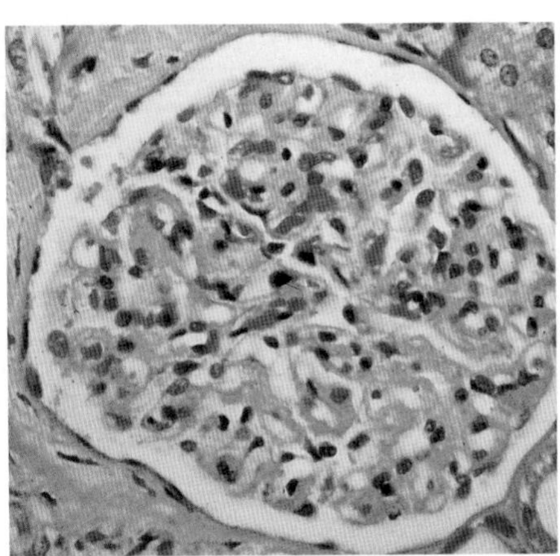
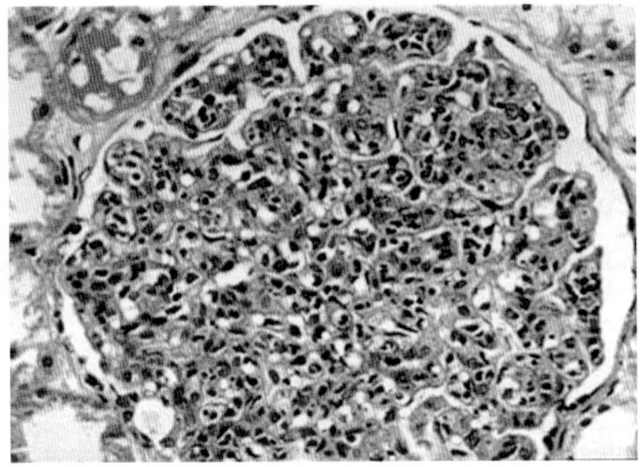

FIGURE 3-17. Glomerulonephritis in systemic lupus erythematosus. A normal glomerulus is shown at left, highlighting the inflammatory hypercellularity of the glomerulus from a patient with lupus, shown at right.

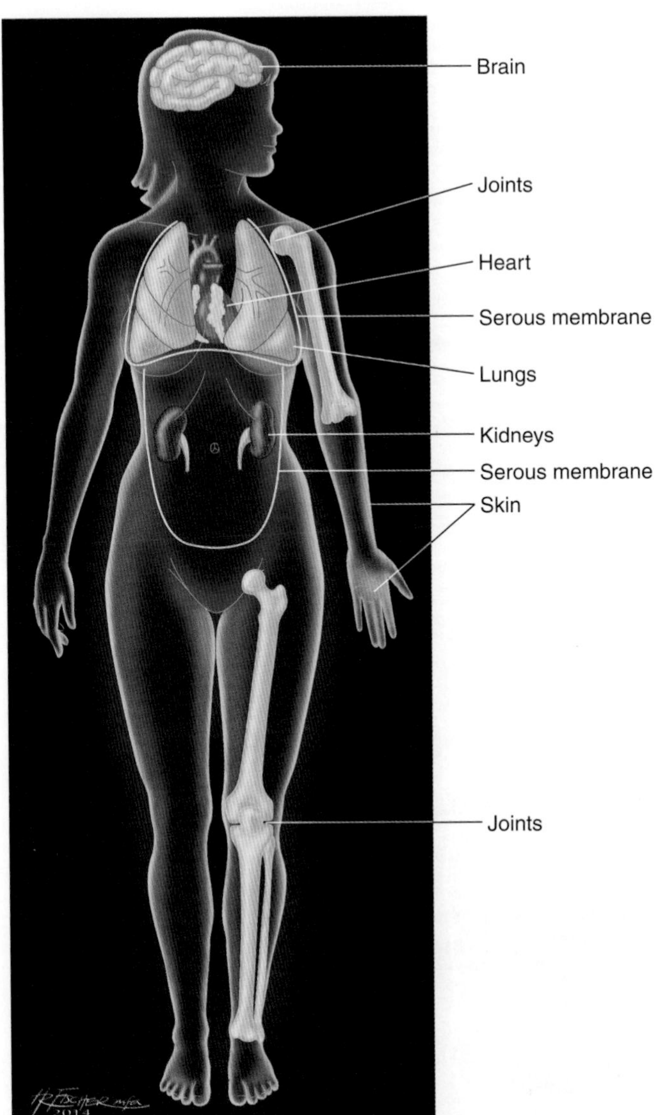

FIGURE 3-18. Organ involvement in systemic lupus erythematosus.

- **Renal disease**, especially glomerulonephritis, affects more than 50% of patients with SLE. Immune complexes that contain IgG antibodies to double-stranded DNA deposit in glomeruli and evoke various forms of glomerulonephritis. These include mesangial disease, focal proliferative nephritis, diffuse proliferative nephritis, and membranous glomerulopathy (see Chapter 14).
- **Serous membranes** are commonly involved. More than one third of patients have pleuritis and pleural effusions. Pericarditis and peritonitis occur, but less frequently.
- **Disorders of the respiratory system** occur frequently, with clinical manifestations ranging from pleural disease to upper airway and pulmonary parenchymal disease. Pneumonitis is thought to be caused by deposition of immune complexes in alveolar septa.
- **Cardiac involvement** is often seen in SLE, although congestive heart failure is rare. All layers of the heart may be involved, with pericarditis being the most common finding. **Libman–Sacks endocarditis**, which is usually not clinically significant, is characterized by small nonbacterial vegetations on valve leaflets.
- **Central nervous system disease** can manifest as psychiatric disease or vasculitis, the latter a life-threatening complication. Vasculitis can lead to hemorrhage and infarction of the brain, which may be fatal.
- **Antiphospholipid antibodies** and antibodies directed against related protein–phospholipid complexes are identified in one third of SLE patients. These antibodies, which are procoagulant, are associated with thromboembolic complications, including stroke, pulmonary embolism, deep venous thrombosis, portal vein thrombosis, and spontaneous abortions (see Chapter 18).
- Other organ involvement is less common and is often due to **vasculitis**. Lesions in the spleen are characterized by thickening and concentric fibrosis of the penicillary arteries, the so-called "onion-skin pattern."

The clinical course of SLE is extremely variable, typically with exacerbations and remissions that correlate with changes in the levels of complement and dsDNA antibodies levels. Because of immunosuppressive therapies, better recognition of mild forms of the disease, and improved antihypertensive medication, the overall 10-year survival approaches 90%. Patients with severe renal or CNS disease or with persistent systolic hypertension have the worst prognosis.

Lupus-Like Disorders

Drug-Induced Lupus

A lupus-like syndrome may be precipitated in some people by the use of certain medications, notably procainamide (for arrhythmias), hydralazine (for hypertension), and isoniazid (for tuberculosis). Drug-induced lupus ranges from asymptomatic laboratory abnormalities (positive ANA test) to a syndrome clinically similar to SLE. However, antibodies to double-stranded DNA and Sm antigen are distinctly uncommon.

Chronic Discoid Lupus

The most common variety of localized lupus erythematosus is a skin disorder, although identical lesions can occur in some cases of SLE. Erythematous, depigmented, and telangiectatic plaques occur most commonly on the face and scalp. Lesional deposition of immunoglobulins and complement at the dermal–epidermal interface is similar to that in SLE. However, unlike SLE, uninvolved skin contains no immune deposits. Although ANAs develop in about one third of the patients, antibodies to double-stranded DNA and Sm antigen are not seen. Most patients with discoid lupus are not otherwise ill, but up to 10% eventually exhibit features of systemic disease.

Rheumatoid Arthritis

RA is a systemic autoimmune disease in which many organs are affected, in addition to the joints. As an inflammatory disorder of the joints, RA has a particular predilection for involvement of the hands and wrists. Patients are usually (3:1) women, with a peak incidence in early middle age. They often complain of symmetric stiffness and pain in the joints, with swelling and warmth often noted by clinicians. Untreated, the disease can lead to destruction of cartilage and bone, loss of joint function, and considerable disability. The disease is discussed in detail in Chapter 22.

Vasculitides

Vasculitis is a term for a broad category of diseases characterized by inflammation of blood vessels of different types together with impairment of blood flow to tissues. This group of disorders is subdivided depending on the caliber of blood vessel involved and on whether there is an associated rheumatic disease. Thus, both SLE and RA can be associated with vasculitis, which is also seen in (see below), especially in children. Vasculitis is encountered in conjunction with a number of infections, particularly viral infections, and as a consequence of taking certain drugs. Vasculitides that are not associated with systemic autoimmune diseases are discussed in Chapter 8.

Sjögren Syndrome

This malady is marked by lymphocytic infiltration of exocrine glands, primarily salivary and lacrimal glands, and is clinically associated with dry mouth (**xerostomia**) and dry eyes (**xerophthalmia** or **keratoconjunctivitis sicca**). It exists as a single entity (primary SS) or occurs together with other systemic autoimmune diseases, such as SLE and RA. Primary SS is also frequently associated with involvement of other organs, including the thyroid, lungs, and kidneys (Fig. 3-19). The primary form of the disease most commonly begins in late middle age, and patients are overwhelmingly female.

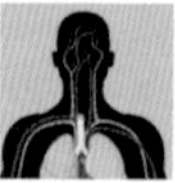

PATHOPHYSIOLOGY: The basis of lymphocyte accumulation in Sjögren syndrome is unknown. The majority of lymphocytes found in glands are $CD4^+$, with a significant $CD8^+$ minority. B cells are also present, with occasional germinal centers. It has been proposed that the primary abnormality is autoimmunity to salivary epithelial cells. Most patients with primary SS produce antibodies to the cytoplasmic RNA-associated proteins SS-A (Ro) and SS-B (La). Antinuclear antibodies are frequently present, as is rheumatoid factor. Autoantibodies to DNA or histones are rare; their presence suggests secondary SS associated with SLE.

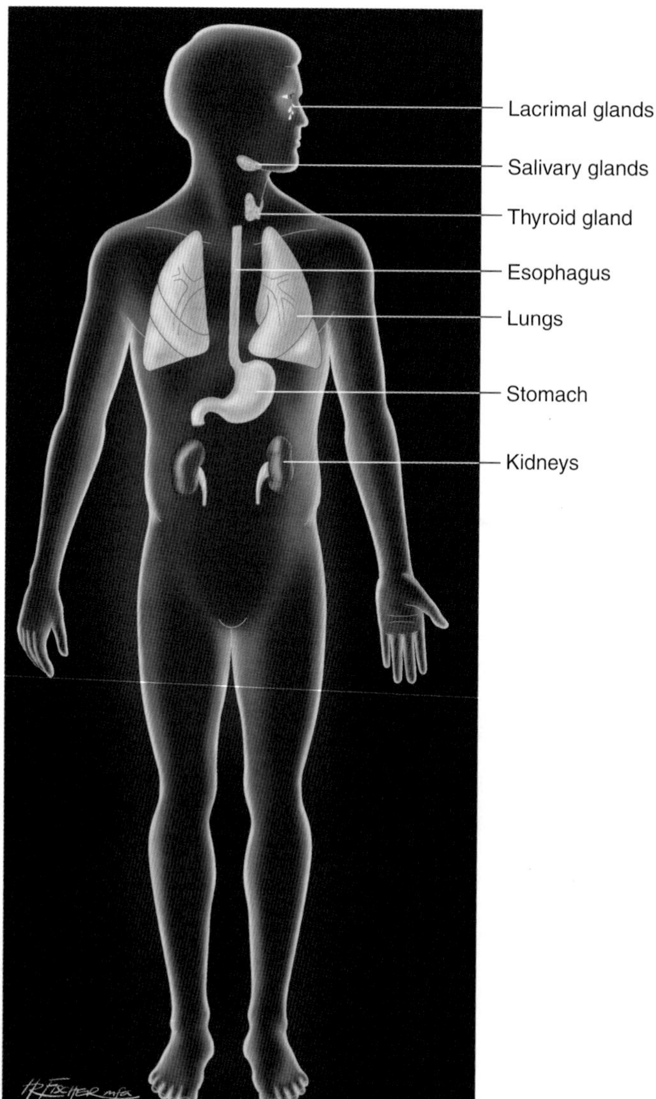

FIGURE 3-19. Organ involvement in Sjögren syndrome.

SS has become the focus for investigation of possible viral etiology for autoimmune disease. Particular attention has been paid to the possible roles of human T-cell leukemia virus 1 (HTLV-1). In Japan, seropositivity for HTLV-1 among patients with SS is 23%, compared with 3.4% among unselected blood donors. Conversely, more than three quarters of HTLV-1–seropositive people have evidence of SS.

PATHOLOGY: SS is characterized by intense lymphocytic infiltrates in salivary and lacrimal glands (see Chapter 21 and Fig. 3-20). Initially periductal, lymphocytic infiltrates eventually affect most lobules, especially the centers. Well-defined germinal centers are rare. The lymphoid infiltrates destroy acini and ducts; the latter often become dilated and filled with cellular debris. Preservation of glandular stroma helps distinguish SS from lymphoma. Late in the disease, affected glands atrophy and may be replaced by hyalinized fibrotic tissue. Owing to the absence of tears, corneas can become dry and fissured, and may ulcerate. Lack of saliva causes atrophy, inflammation, and cracking of the oral mucosa.

Involvement of extraglandular sites is also common in SS. Pulmonary disease occurs in many patients, particularly bronchial gland atrophy in association with lymphoid infiltration. SS of the lung is accompanied by thick tenacious secretions, focal atelectasis, bronchiectasis, and recurrent infections. The gastrointestinal tract can be affected, and many patients have difficulty swallowing (dysphagia). In such cases, esophageal submucosal glands are infiltrated by lymphocytes. In addition, atrophic gastritis occurs secondary to lymphoid infiltration of the gastric mucosa. Liver disease, especially primary biliary cirrhosis, is present in 5% to 10% of patients with SS and is associated with nodular lymphoid infiltrates in the liver and destruction of intrahepatic bile ducts.

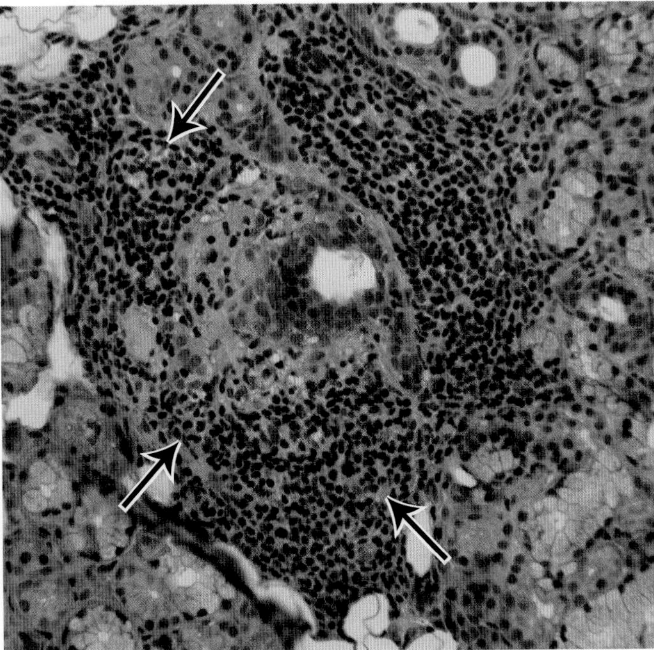

FIGURE 3-20. Histologic appearance of salivary glands in Sjögren syndrome. Note the infiltration of lymphocytes into the salivary gland tissue (*arrows*).

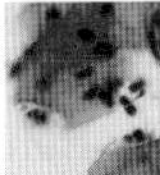

CLINICAL FEATURES: Patients with Sjögren syndrome suffer the consequences of lack of tears and saliva. They complain of eye discomfort and can develop ulcerations and infections of the cornea and conjunctivae. Dry mouth symptoms are sometimes accompanied by increased dental caries and by thrush or other mouth infections. Dryness of the skin and female genital tract also occurs. SS is associated with a 40-fold increased risk of lymphoma, probably through B-cell clonal expansion.

Systemic Sclerosis (Scleroderma)

Systemic sclerosis is an autoimmune disease of unknown origin, which is characterized by (1) excessive deposition of collagen and other connective tissue macromolecules in the skin and multiple internal organs (Fig. 3-21), (2) prominent and often severe alterations in the microvasculature, and (3) immunologic abnormalities. Systemic sclerosis is a complex and heterogeneous disease with a variety of clinical presentations, ranging from (1) limited skin involvement

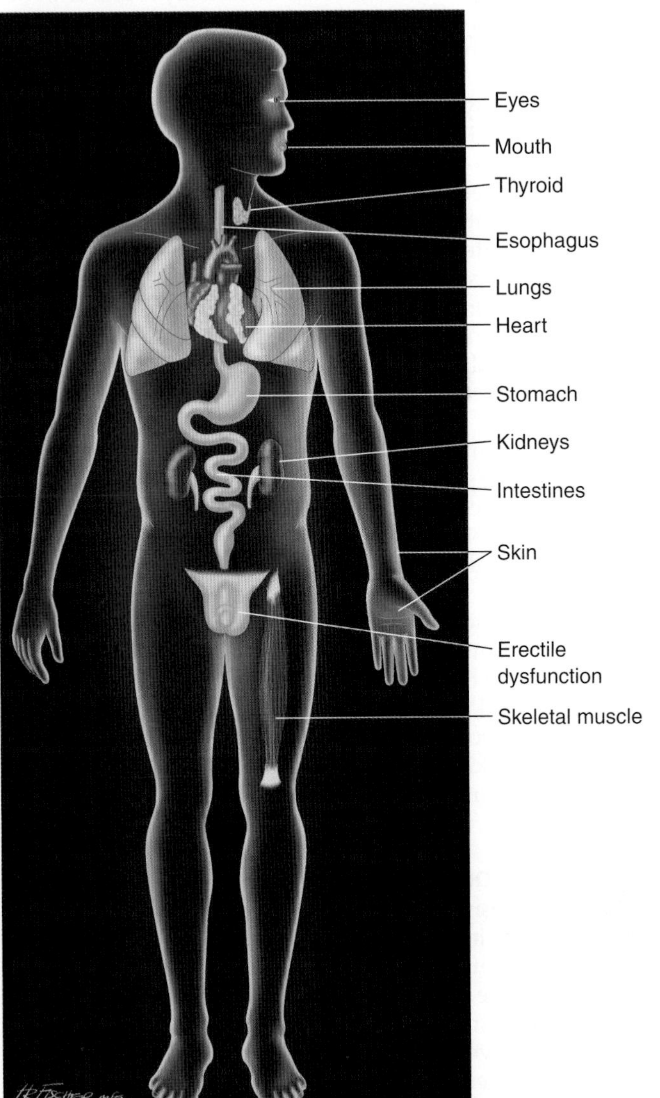

FIGURE 3-21. Organ involvement in systemic sclerosis.

and minimal systemic alterations (**limited cutaneous systemic sclerosis**, previously known as CREST syndrome; see below), (2) diffuse skin sclerosis and severe and often progressive internal organ involvement (**diffuse cutaneous systemic sclerosis**), and (3) occasionally a fulminant course (**fulminant systemic sclerosis**). Systemic sclerosis is the third most common systemic autoimmune disease (following rheumatoid arthritis and SLE) and is 3 to 8 times more frequent in women, with a peak occurrence from 40 to 50 years of age. Although systemic sclerosis is not inherited, it is accepted that genetic predisposition plays an important role in its development. Familial clusters have been reported, and there is an association between HLA-DQB1 and the characteristic autoantibodies (see below).

Abnormalities of Immunity in Systemic Sclerosis

There are normal numbers of circulating B lymphocytes, but hypergammaglobulinemia and cryoglobulinemia suggest that they may be hyperactive. The presence of specific antibodies is one of the most common manifestations of systemic sclerosis, being present in over 90% of patients. ANAs are common, but usually at lower titers than in SLE. Commonly found antibodies include nucleolar autoantibodies (primarily against RNA polymerase). Antibodies to Scl-70, a nonhistone nuclear protein topoisomerase, are found in 30% to 40% of patients with the diffuse form of systemic sclerosis. Anticentromere antibodies are associated with the CREST variant (see below). The Scl-70 autoantibody is the most common and specific for diffuse scleroderma, seen in 60% of patients. There is no correlation between ANA titer and disease severity.

Although autoantibodies are common in systemic sclerosis, they do not cause the clinical manifestations of the disease. However, owing to their high frequency and specificity for certain clinical subsets of the disease, their presence is helpful in establishing the diagnosis and predicting a likely pattern of organ involvement, severity, and progression of systemic sclerosis.

Cellular immune derangements are also seen in patients with progressive systemic sclerosis. Patients with active disease exhibit (1) reduced circulating $CD8^+$ T suppressor cells, (2) evidence of T-cell activation, alterations in functions mediated by IL-1, and (3) elevated IL-2 and soluble IL-2 receptor. Increased levels of IL-4 and IL-6 have also been described. Tissues show active mononuclear inflammation, which precedes the development of the vasculopathy and fibrosis characteristic of this disease. The infiltrates contain increased numbers of $CD4^+$ and $\gamma\delta$-T cells (which adhere to fibroblasts), as well as macrophages. Mast cells (degranulated) are also present in the skin of scleroderma patients. The incidence of other autoimmune disorders, such as thyroiditis and primary biliary cirrhosis, is increased.

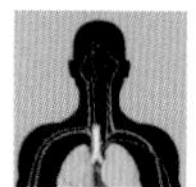

PATHOPHYSIOLOGY: The pathogenesis of systemic sclerosis is extremely complex, and the exact mechanisms involved are not well understood. The clinical and pathologic manifestations of systemic sclerosis result from three distinct processes: (1) fibroproliferative vascular lesions of small arteries and arterioles, (2) excessive and often progressive deposition of collagen and other extracellular matrix macromolecules in the skin and various internal organs, and (3) alterations of humoral and cellular immunity.

The pathogenesis of systemic sclerosis entails the following sequence of events (Fig. 3-22):

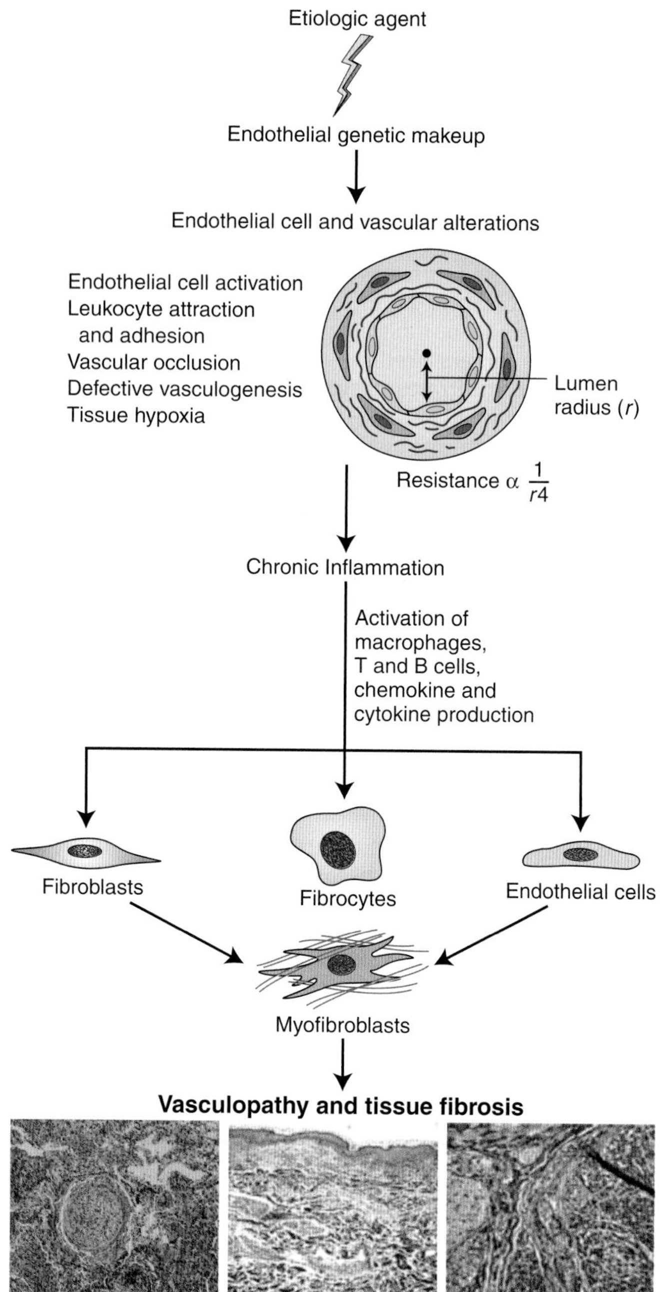

FIGURE 3-22. Involvement of endothelial cell and vascular alteration in the pathogenesis of systemic sclerosis.

1. **Microvascular injury** characterized by endothelial cell abnormalities. The endothelial cell abnormalities result from increased production of inflammatory mediators or the reduction in synthesis of protective factors, such as prostacyclin and nitric oxide.
2. **Attraction and transmigration** of inflammatory cells and fibroblast precursors into tissue.
3. **Chronic inflammation** occurs in tissue, with participation of macrophages and T and B lymphocytes, and secretion of cytokines and growth factors.
4. **Activation** of resident fibroblasts and pericytes into myofibroblasts.

5. **Fibroproliferative vasculopathy** progresses to vessel rarefaction and exaggerated and widespread accumulation of fibrotic tissue, ***the hallmark of the fibrotic process characteristic of the disease.***

Pathology of Systemic Sclerosis

The fibrotic process is the most notable characteristic of systemic sclerosis and causes most of its clinical manifestations (Fig. 3-21). The increased population of myofibroblasts produces more fibrillar type I and type III collagens and expresses α-smooth muscle actin. They also produce less extracellular matrix (ECM) degradative enzymes. The accumulation of myofibroblasts in affected tissues and the uncontrolled persistence of their elevated biosynthetic functions are crucial determinants of the extent and rate of progression of the fibrotic process in systemic sclerosis and of its clinical course, response to therapy, prognosis, and mortality. The growth factor that plays a crucial role in the fibrosis that accompanies systemic sclerosis is TGF-β. This molecule decreases the production of collagen-degrading metalloproteinases, while simultaneously upregulating the production of protease inhibitors, which prevent ECM breakdown.

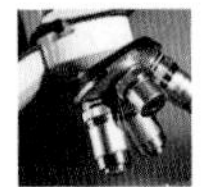

PATHOLOGY: Skin in scleroderma initially demonstrates edema, then induration. The thickened skin exhibits (1) a striking increase in collagen fibers in the reticular dermis, (2) thinning of the epidermis with loss of rete pegs and atrophy of dermal appendages (Fig. 3-23A), (3) hyalinization and obliteration of arterioles, and (4) variable mononuclear infiltrates, primarily of T cells. The stage of induration may progress to atrophy or revert to normal. Increased collagen deposition can also occur in the synovia, lungs, gastrointestinal tract, heart, and kidneys.

Lesions in arteries, arterioles, and capillaries are typical, and in some cases, may be the first demonstrable pathology. Initial subintimal edema with fibrin deposition is followed by thickening and fibrosis of the vessel wall and reduplication or fraying of the internal elastic lamina. Involved vessels may become severely narrowed or occluded by thrombi.

The kidneys are involved in more than half of patients and show marked vascular changes, often with focal hemorrhage and cortical infarcts. The interlobular arteries and afferent arterioles tend to be the most severely affected vessels. Early fibromuscular thickening of the subintima causes luminal narrowing, followed by fibrosis (Fig. 3-23B). Fibrinoid necrosis is commonly seen in afferent arterioles. Heightened pulmonary vascular reactivity ("pulmonary Raynaud phenomenon") and, later, pulmonary hypertension and diffuse interstitial fibrosis are the primary lung abnormalities. Pulmonary disease can progress to end-stage fibrosis, the so-called "honeycomb lung" (see Chapter 10).

Most patients with scleroderma display patchy myocardial fibrosis. These lesions result from focal myocardial necrosis, which may reflect focal ischemia secondary to Raynaud-like reactivity of cardiac microvasculature.

Progressive systemic sclerosis can also involve any portion of the gastrointestinal tract. Esophageal dysfunction is the most common and troublesome gastrointestinal complication.

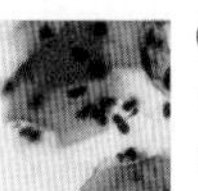

CLINICAL FEATURES: The most apparent and almost universal clinical features of systemic sclerosis are related to the progressive thickening and fibrosis of the skin. Scleroderma manifests as two distinct clinical syndromes, namely, a generalized or diffuse **(progressive systemic)** form and a **limited variant**. Progressive systemic sclerosis (diffuse scleroderma) is characterized by severe and progressive disease of the skin and early onset of all or most of the associated abnormalities of visceral organs. Symptoms usually begin with Raynaud phenomenon, namely, intermittent episodes of ischemia of the fingers, paresthesias, and pain. Raynaud phenomenon is accompanied or followed by edema of the fingers and hands; thickening and tightening of the skin; polyarthralgia; and involvement of specific internal organs. The affected skin is tight, indurated, and firmly bound

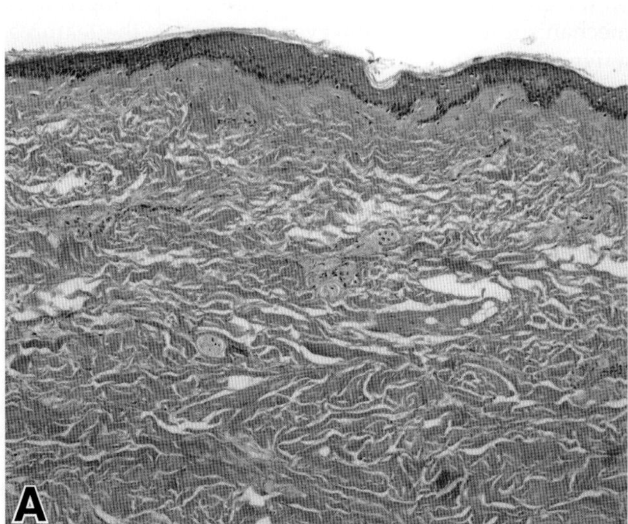

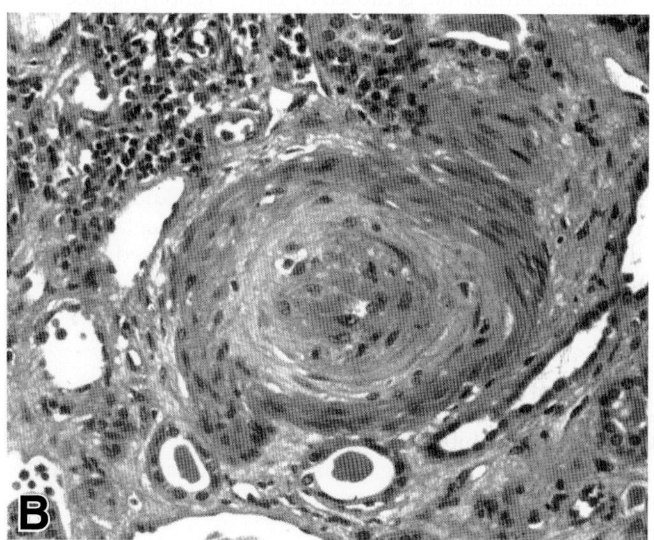

FIGURE 3-23. Histologic appearance of systemic sclerosis. A. Dermal fibrosis is characteristic of scleroderma. Dense collagen accumulation occurs beneath the epidermis. Note the absence of dermal appendages. **B.** Scleroderma that affects the kidney is manifested by vascular involvement. Here, the interlobular artery exhibits marked luminal narrowing owing to pronounced intimal thickening.

to the subcutaneous tissue. The skin over the hands and face is most frequently involved, and as the disease progresses, the sclerotic changes extend and may affect the entire body.

The typical patient with generalized scleroderma exhibits "stone facies," owing to tightening of facial skin and restricted motion of the mouth. Progression of vascular lesions in the fingers leads to ischemic ulceration of the fingertips, with subsequent shortening and atrophy of the digits. Many patients suffer from painful tendonitis and joint pain.

Other organ systems are also involved:

- **Musculoskeletal symptoms** are often the first manifestations of the disease. The severity varies from mild polyarthralgias to more severe arthralgias, but synovitis is rare. Muscle infiltration with fibrotic tissue may produce an inflammatory myopathy or a more indolent noninflammatory form.
- **Gastrointestinal symptoms** of gastroesophageal reflux and dysphagia are caused by dysfunctional esophageal sphincter motility. In severe cases, stricture may result. Impaired gastric emptying and small intestine peristalsis may cause distention, bloating, nausea, and pain. Bacterial overgrowth sometimes results in secondary malabsorption and diarrhea.
- **Pulmonary involvement** frequently results in severe respiratory disability and is the most common cause of death. Patients develop progressively worsening tachypnea and exertional dyspnea, secondary to pulmonary fibrosis and pulmonary hypertension.
- **Cardiac involvement** is not uncommon and may manifest as chest pain, arrhythmias, and conduction defects.
- **Renal disease**, known as scleroderma renal crisis, typically begins abruptly, with malignant hypertension and rapidly progressive renal insufficiency. It is often heralded by severe headache, hypertensive retinopathy, seizures, and other central nervous system symptoms. Myocardial ischemia, infarction, and left ventricular failure are occasional complications. Prompt aggressive treatment is necessary to prevent renal failure.
- **Additional symptoms** may include functional thyroid abnormalities, resulting hypothyroidism and some degree of erectile failure. The sicca syndrome (keratoconjunctivitis sicca and xerostomia) is caused by fibrosis and lymphocytic infiltration of the salivary and lacrimal glands.
- **Crest syndrome** (limited systemic sclerosis) differentiates this clinical presentation from a more severe form. The term CREST is an acronym for calcinosis, long-standing Raynaud phenomenon, esophageal dysmotility, sclerodactyly, and telangiectases. Other cutaneous manifestations include skin ulcerations, usually localized to fingertips or knuckles, and peculiar pigmentary changes, with hyperpigmentation and hypopigmentation. More severe disease, termed **diffuse systemic sclerosis,** involves more extensive cutaneous and also visceral disease.

Mixed Connective Tissue Disease

MCTD patients exhibit features of several different collagen vascular diseases, including SLE, scleroderma, and polymyositis. Almost 90% of patients are female, and most are adults (mean age, 37 years).

The pathogenesis of MCTD is poorly understood. Patients often have evidence of B-cell activation, with hypergammaglobulinemia and rheumatoid factor. ANAs are present; the most distinctive are associated with high titers of antibody to uridine-rich ribonucleoprotein (anti-U1-RNP), which is considered a sine qua non for diagnosis.

There is an association with HLA-DR4 and HLA-DR2 genotypes, suggesting a role for T cells in autoantibody production. However, there is no direct evidence that these antibodies participate in the development of any of the characteristic lesions of MCTD.

There is controversy whether the disorder is a separate disease or a heterogeneous collection of patients with nonclassical presentations of SLE, scleroderma, or polymyositis. It is unclear whether MCTD is a distinct entity or simply an overlap of findings in patients with other types of collagen vascular disease.

TRANSPLANTATION IMMUNOLOGY

Donor MHC-encoded antigens are immunogenic molecules that can stimulate rejection of transplanted tissues. Optimal graft survival occurs when recipient and donor are closely matched for histocompatibility antigens. In practice, an exact HLA match is uncommon, except between monozygotic twins. Thus, immunosuppressive therapy and vigilant monitoring of graft function are required after organ transplantation. Therapeutic advances have greatly improved transplant success rates, even when there is a degree of histoincompatibility. When host-versus-graft immune reactions (rejection) occur, a combination of immune mechanisms may injure the graft.

Both T-cell–mediated and antibody-mediated reactions participate in transplant rejection. Within the graft, antigen-presenting cells, specifically those bearing foreign MHC molecules, are recognized by host $CD8^+$ cytotoxic T lymphocytes, which mediate tissue injury. Concurrently, host $CD4^+$ T-helper cells, which augment antibody production, induce IFN-γ production and activate macrophages. In turn, IFN-γ enhances MHC expression, amplifying the immune response and resulting tissue injury. Host APCs also process foreign donor antigens, leading to $CD4^+$-mediated delayed-type hypersensitivity and $CD4^+$-mediated antibody production.

Solid organ transplant rejection reactions are usually categorized as "hyperacute," "acute," and "chronic" based on the clinical tempo of the response and pathophysiologic mechanism involved. However, in practice, the features often overlap. Categorization of transplant rejection is further complicated by the toxicity of immunosuppressive drugs, the potential for mechanical problems (e.g., vascular thrombosis), and recurrence of original disease (e.g., some types of glomerulonephritis). The next sections explain rejection in the context of renal transplantation. Similar responses occur in other transplanted tissues, although rejection as applied to each tissue type has its own unique features.

Hyperacute Rejection

Hyperacute rejection of a kidney may be so rapid as to occur intraoperatively. It manifests as a sudden cessation of urine output, darkening of the graft, and rapid development of fever and pain at the graft site. This form of rejection is mediated by preformed anti-HLA antibodies in the recipient and complement activation products, including chemotactic and other inflammatory mediators. Hyperacute rejection is catastrophic, necessitating prompt surgical removal of the grafted kidney. Histologic features include vascular congestion, fibrin–platelet thrombi within capillaries, neutrophilic vasculitis with fibrinoid necrosis, prominent interstitial edema, and neutrophil infiltrates (Fig. 3-24A). Fortunately, hyperacute rejection is distinctly uncommon when appropriate pretransplantation antibody screening has been performed.

Acute Rejection

Acute rejection is characterized by the abrupt onset of azotemia and oliguria, which may be associated with fever and graft tenderness. This complication typically involves both cell-mediated and humoral mechanisms of tissue damage. If detected early, acute rejection can be reversed with immunosuppressive therapy. Needle biopsy is often needed to differentiate acute rejection from acute tubular necrosis or toxicity associated with immunosuppressive drugs. Findings vary, depending on whether the process is mainly cellular or humoral. Acute cellular rejection is characterized by interstitial lymphocyte and macrophage infiltration, edema, lymphocytic tubulitis, and tubular necrosis (Fig. 3-24B). In the acute humoral form, which is sometimes called "rejection vasculitis," vascular damage predominates, with arteritis, fibrinoid necrosis, and thrombosis. Blood vessel involvement is an ominous sign because it usually signifies resistance to therapy.

Chronic Rejection

Patients affected with chronic rejection typically develop progressive azotemia, oliguria, hypertension, and weight gain over a period of months. Chronic rejection may be because of repeated episodes of cellular rejection, either asymptomatic or clinically apparent. Arterial and arteriolar intimal thickening cause vascular stenosis or obstruction, thickened glomerular capillary walls, tubular atrophy, and interstitial fibrosis (Fig. 3-24C). There are scattered interstitial mononuclear infiltrates. Tubules contain proteinaceous casts. Chronic rejection represents an advanced state of organ injury and does not respond to therapy. Acute and chronic rejection may overlap histologically and may vary in degree, so that unambiguous pathologic distinction is sometimes difficult.

Graft-Versus-Host Disease

The advent of transplantation of allogeneic (donor) bone marrow or hematopoietic stem cells (HSCs) harvested from peripheral blood makes possible treatment of diseases that had previously been considered terminal or untreatable. In order for the transplanted marrow/HSCs to engraft in the new host, the recipient's bone marrow and immune system must be "conditioned" (usually ablated) by cytotoxic drugs, sometimes plus radiation. If the graft includes immunocompetent lymphocytes, these donor cells may react to—"reject"—host tissues, causing graft-versus-host disease (GVHD). GVHD can also occur if a severely immunodeficient patient receives a solid organ containing many "passenger"

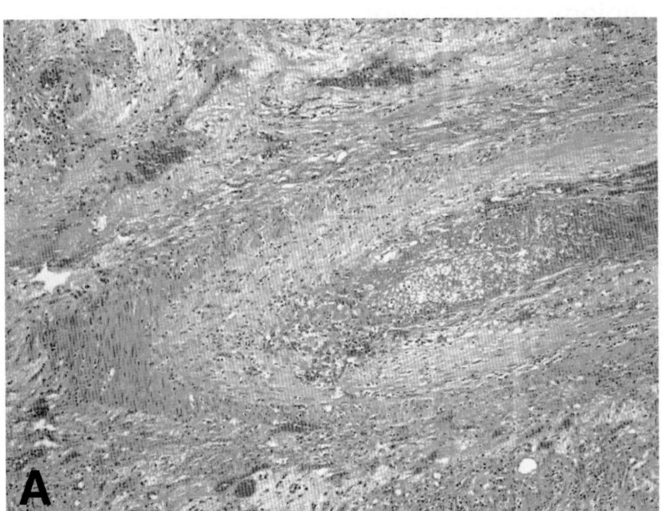

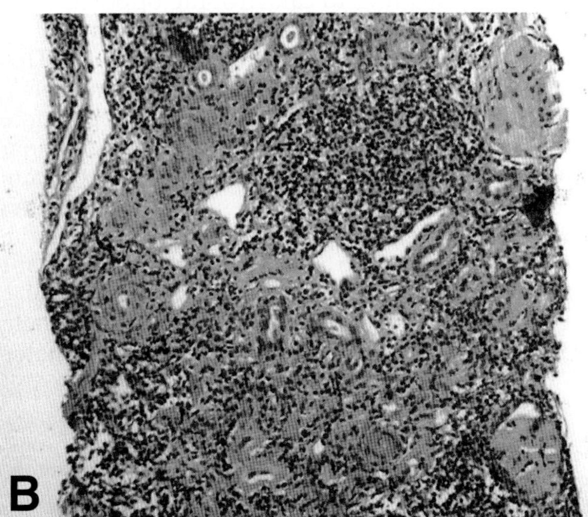

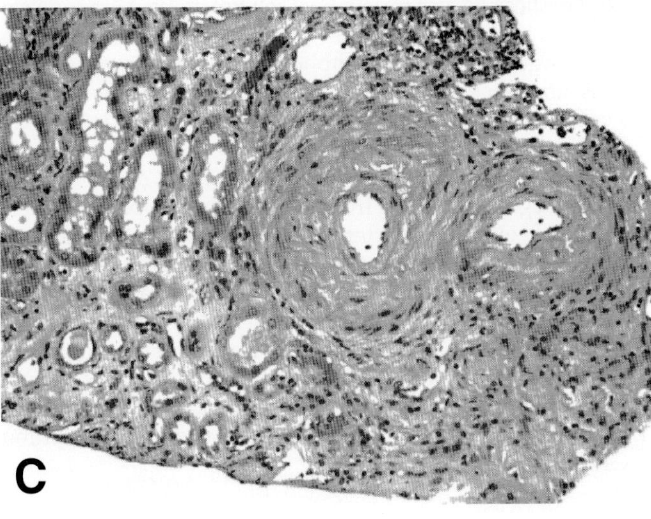

FIGURE 3-24. There are three major forms of renal transplant rejection. A. Hyperacute rejection occurs within minutes to hours after transplantation and is characterized, in part, by neutrophilic vasculitis, intravascular fibrin thrombi, and neutrophilic infiltrates. **B.** Acute cellular rejection occurs within weeks to months after transplantation and is characterized by tubular damage and mononuclear leukocyte infiltration. **C.** Chronic rejection is observed months to years after transplantation and is characterized by tubular atrophy, patchy interstitial mononuclear cell infiltrates, and fibrosis. In this example, arteries show fibrointimal thickening.

lymphocytes or is transfused with blood products containing viable HLA-incompatible lymphocytes.

The major organs affected by GVHD are the skin, gastrointestinal tract, and liver. The skin and intestine show mononuclear cell infiltrates and epithelial cell necrosis. The liver displays periportal inflammation, damaged bile ducts, and liver cell injury. Clinically, acute GVHD manifests as rash, diarrhea, abdominal cramps, anemia, and liver dysfunction. Chronic GVHD is characterized by dermal sclerosis, sicca syndrome, and immunodeficiency. Treatment of GVHD requires immunosuppression. Patients, especially those with chronic GVHD, are at a higher risk for potentially life-threatening opportunistic infections (e.g., invasive aspergillosis).

HUMAN IMMUNODEFICIENCY VIRUS AND ACQUIRED IMMUNODEFICIENCY SYNDROME

AIDS is the most common acquired immunodeficiency state worldwide. It is mainly caused by human immunodeficiency virus type 1 (HIV-1), although a small minority of patients, primarily in western Africa, are infected with HIV-2. People infected with HIV-1, if untreated, develop many immunologic defects, the most devastating of which is severely impaired cellular immunity, leading to catastrophic opportunistic infections. HIV-1 infection progresses from an initial asymptomatic state to severe immune depletion in overt AIDS. This continuum is called HIV/AIDS. Infection of CD4$^+$ (helper) T lymphocytes by HIV-1 causes depletion of this cell population, giving rise to impaired immune function and dysregulation. Because they cannot mount new immune responses, especially cell-mediated immune responses, patients with AIDS often die of opportunistic infections, principally with mycobacteria, viruses, or fungi. There is also a high incidence of malignant tumors, mainly B-cell lymphomas, and Kaposi sarcoma. Finally, HIV-1 infection in the CNS causes HIV-associated neurologic disease (HAND), which ranges from minor cognitive or motor disorders to frank dementia.

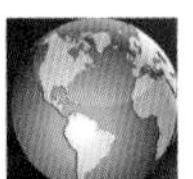

EPIDEMIOLOGY: AIDS originated in Sub-Saharan Africa, and at least three different viral strains were transmitted from chimpanzees to humans. It is now a worldwide pandemic owing to the ease of international travel and enhanced population mobility, which in many societies coincided with a rapid increase in sexually transmitted diseases. Presently, the WHO estimates that 37 million people carry HIV worldwide, with 2 million new infections and 1.2 million deaths yearly. The death rate peaked in 2005 and has declined since then. Annual new infections peaked in 1997, at 3.3 million, and have dropped subsequently. Because antiretroviral therapy (ART) reaches more people, the total number of people living with HIV infection continues to increase.

The highest prevalence is in Sub-Saharan Africa, but no country is free of HIV-1. Male homosexuals are by far the largest group of HIV-positive people in the United States and still account for most newly infected cases. In some other parts of the world, transmission may be largely by heterosexual contact or via intravenous drug users. Most AIDS patients in the United States are men, although the prevalence of HIV-1 infection in women continues to increase.

Human Immunodeficiency Virus Transmission

HIV is present in blood, semen, vaginal secretions, breast milk, and cerebrospinal fluid of infected patients. The agent is present in most of these fluids in lymphocytes and as free virus. It is transmitted via these fluids to sexual partners, drug users who share needles, and recipients of contaminated blood products. During pregnancy, infection takes place via delivery or breast milk to infants.

Virus in semen enters through tears in the rectal mucosa, particularly in anal-receptive partners. It can also infect rectal epithelial cells directly. In heterosexual contact, male-to-female transmission is more likely than the reverse, perhaps because there is more HIV in semen than in vaginal fluid. Additionally, genital lesions facilitate virus entry. The rate of HIV infection is lower in circumcised men, perhaps because the foreskin is less well keratinized than other parts of the penis and has a higher concentration of cutaneous dendritic cells (Langerhans cells).

HIV-1 is not transmitted by nonsexual, casual exposure to infected people. Furthermore, fewer than 1% of health care workers who sustained "needle sticks" or other accidental exposures to blood from HIV-positive patients became infected with HIV-1. Immediate postexposure antiretroviral prophylaxis is available (for details, see http://www.dhhr.wv.gov/oeps/std-hiv-hep/needlestick/Pages/Post-ExposureProphylaxis(PEP)FAQs.aspx).

Human Immunodeficiency Virus Type 1 Biology and Behavior

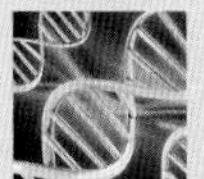

MOLECULAR PATHOGENESIS: HIV-1 is a member of the lentivirus family of retroviruses. Animal lentiviruses have been recognized for a century, but human lentiviruses have been known for less than three decades.

HIV-1 virions carry two identical 9.7-kb copies of the virus single-stranded RNA genome plus some key enzymes, such as reverse transcriptase (RNA-dependent DNA polymerase, RT) and integrase, which are needed early in the infectious cycle (see below). These are packaged in a core of viral proteins. The outermost layer, the envelope, is derived from the host cell membrane, which contain virally encoded Env glycoproteins (gp120 and gp41). In addition to the *gag*, *pol*, and *env* genes present in all replication-competent RNA viruses, HIV-1 has six other genes that code for proteins that control viral replication and certain host cell functions. Mononuclear phagocytes and CD4$^+$ helper T lymphocytes are the virus's main targets, although B lymphocytes, astrocytes, endothelial cells, and intestinal epithelium can also be infected.

The replicative cycle of HIV-1 is depicted in detail in Fig. 3-25.

Several mechanisms are responsible for the killing of infected T lymphocytes by HIV-1: (1) T-cell death prior to viral integration results from activation of caspases 1 and 3; a type of cellular death termed pyroptosis (see Chapter 1), (2) during viral integration, p-53–dependent cell-killing mechanisms are activated, and (3) postviral integration T-cell death results from the action of HIV protease. Even noninfected T cells in an infected individual undergo cell death as a result of bystander effects brought on by several mechanisms. Whatever the mechanism, there is a clear association between increasing viral burden and declining CD4$^+$ lymphocyte counts.

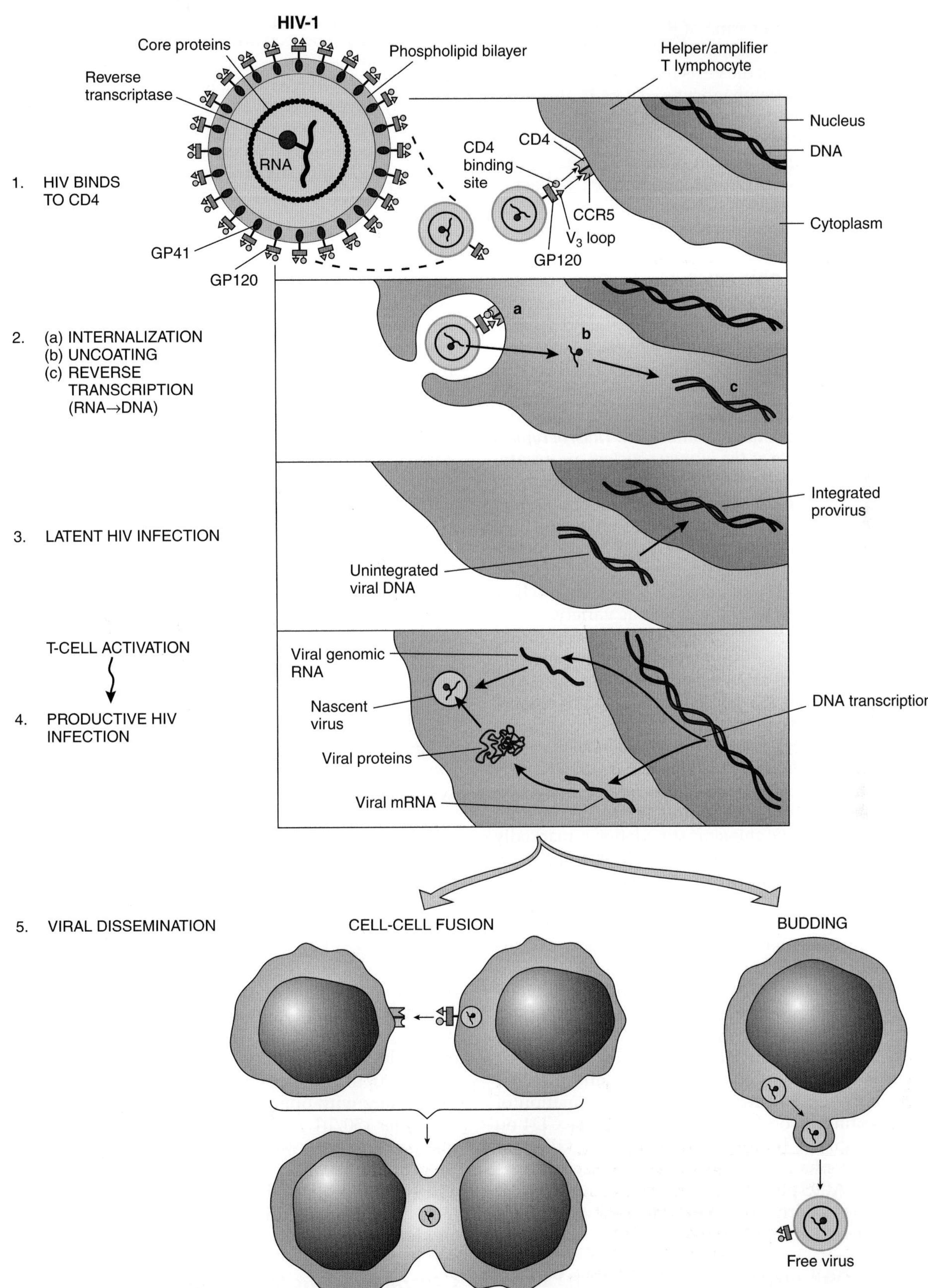

FIGURE 3-25. The life cycle of human immunodeficiency virus type 1 (HIV-1) is a multistep process that includes (1) binding CD4 receptor in conjunction with chemokine receptor (e.g., CCR5); (2) internalization, uncoating, and reverse transcription; (3) integration into host DNA as a provirus where it persists in a state of latency; (4) replication in concert with host T-cell activation; and (5) dissemination. CD, cluster of differentiation; GP, G protein; mRNA, messenger RNA; V_3, third hypervariable.

HIV-1 persists for the lifetime of the host. Even in the face of low or undetectable plasma virus levels (see below), a latent or quiescent form of the virus remains in long-lived memory T cells and tissue phagocytes. There is also evidence that the CNS, and possibly other organs, may serve as a reservoir for potential reseeding.

Initiation of viral replication in latent HIV-1 infection depends on induction of host proteins during T-cell activation. Thus, immune system activation by a variety of infectious agents may promote HIV replication.

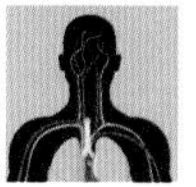

PATHOPHYSIOLOGY: HIV-1 shows an initial tropism for the subset of $CD4^+$ T cells expressing the CCR5 receptor. Such cells are predominantly found in extralymphatic sites where they have effector, host defense functions. However, the ultimate destruction of $CD4^+$ T cells by HIV-1 can disable the entire immune system because this subset of lymphocytes exerts critical regulatory and effector functions that involve both cellular and humoral immunity. ***Thus, in typical AIDS patients, all elements of the immune system are eventually crippled, including T cells, B cells, NK cells, the monocyte/macrophage lineage of cells, and immunoglobulin production.***

Eventually, total $CD4^+$ lymphocyte counts fall to less than 500 cells/µL, and helper to suppressor T-cell ratios decline from a normal of 2.0 to as little as 0.5. The numbers of $CD8^+$ (cytotoxic/suppressor) cells are variable, although in AIDS, most of these cells seem to be of the cytotoxic variety.

Defects in T-cell function are manifested by weak responses in skin testing with a variety of antigens (delayed hypersensitivity) and impaired proliferative responses to mitogens and antigens in vitro. Moreover, the deficiency of $CD4^+$ cells reduces levels of IL-2, the cytokine produced in response to antigens that stimulate cytotoxic T-cell killing. ***Thus, patients with AIDS cannot generate the antigen-specific cytotoxic T cells that are required to clear viruses and other infectious agents.***

Humoral immunity is also abnormal. Production of antibodies in response to specific antigenic stimulation is markedly decreased, often to less than 10% of normal. B cells also show poor proliferative responses in vitro to mitogens and antigens. Yet, sera of patients with AIDS usually show high levels of polyclonal immunoglobulins, autoantibodies, and immune complexes. This apparent paradox is probably explained by the concurrent infection with polyclonal B-cell–activating viruses (e.g., EBV or cytomegalovirus), which constantly stimulate B cells nonspecifically to produce immunoglobulins. A lack of $CD4^+$ lymphocytes impairs the cytotoxic T-cell proliferation that normally would eliminate B cells infected with EBV.

Lentiviruses tend to target macrophages, and infected macrophages may serve as reservoirs for dissemination of the virus. Interestingly, some macrophages express CD4 on their surfaces. Unlike T lymphocytes, which are killed by HIV, infected macrophages generally survive. Macrophages from patients with AIDS phagocytose immune complexes and opsonized particles poorly and show impaired chemotaxis and responsiveness to antigenic challenges.

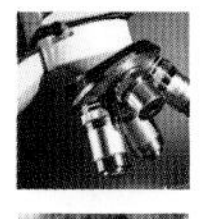

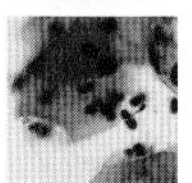

PATHOLOGY AND CLINICAL FEATURES: Patients recently infected with HIV-1 may have an acute, usually self-limited flu-like illness, termed the **acute retroviral syndrome**. It clinically resembles infectious mononucleosis. This occurs 2 to 3 weeks after exposure to HIV, before the appearance of antibodies against the virus. Less commonly, patients present with neurologic symptoms that suggest encephalitis, aseptic meningitis, or a neuropathy. Fever, myalgia, lymphadenopathy, sore throat, and a macular rash are common. Most of these symptoms resolve within 2 to 3 weeks, although lymphadenopathy, fever, and myalgia may persist for a few months. Seroconversion occurs 1 to 10 weeks after the onset of this acute illness. Thus, HIV-1 enzyme immunoassay and Western blot testing, which depend on the presence of anti–HIV-1 *gag* antibodies, are negative during the initial stage of the infection. Most patients recover from this initial illness because their immune system mounts a cytotoxic T-cell counterattack, although a small proportion progress rapidly to frank AIDS within a few months. After the initial acute syndrome, most newly infected individuals enter a period of latency and slow immune system decline, which averages approximately 10 years before they reach a state of serious immune compromise. If symptoms go unrecognized or untreated, the eventual outcome is fulminant immunodeficiency and its fatal complications (Fig. 3-26).

Persistent generalized lymphadenopathy refers to palpable lymph node enlargement at two or more extrainguinal sites, persisting for more than 3 months in a person infected with HIV. The disorder develops either as part of the acute HIV syndrome or within a few months of seroconversion. Axillary, inguinal, and posterior cervical nodes are most affected, although any group of lymph nodes can be involved. Persistent generalized lymphadenopathy does not have any prognostic significance with respect to the progression of HIV infection to AIDS.

Most patients infected with HIV express detectable viral antigens and antibodies within 6 months. Patients generally experience an initial period of intense viremia, with very high viral loads, during the acute retroviral syndrome. This is accompanied by a corresponding sharp drop in their absolute number of $CD4^+$ T cells (Fig. 3-26). As a patient's immune system begins to recognize the new infection, viral load drops, and $CD4^+$ T-cell count begins to climb. This control of HIV-1 infection occurs via a vigorous cytotoxic T-cell response. Viral replication continues but is constrained by the immune response. During this time, infected individuals are generally asymptomatic. However, the rapidity with which HIV-1 evolves within each host ensures that it represents a continually moving antigenic target for the body's immune system.

The long interval between HIV-1 entry and the appearance of clinical symptoms of AIDS is related to the small number of initially infected T lymphocytes (see above) and viral latency. At some time, $CD4^+$ T-cell counts start to decrease. Patients generally remain asymptomatic until their $CD4^+$ counts fall below 500/µL. Nonspecific constitutional symptoms may appear, along with opportunistic infections. Once $CD4^+$ levels are under 150/µL and CD4 to CD8 ratios are less than 0.8, the disease progresses rapidly. A variety of bacteria, viruses, and fungi attack immunocompromised patients. Kaposi sarcoma and lymphoproliferative disorders, especially virus-related lymphoproliferative disorders (see Chapter 18), may appear, and neurologic disease is common.

Central Nervous System Infection

Symptoms of CNS dysfunction occur in one third of AIDS patients, and postmortems have revealed CNS pathology in more than three fourths of cases. HIV is thought to enter the brain via infected blood monocytes shortly after it enters the body where it resides in microglial cells and perivascular

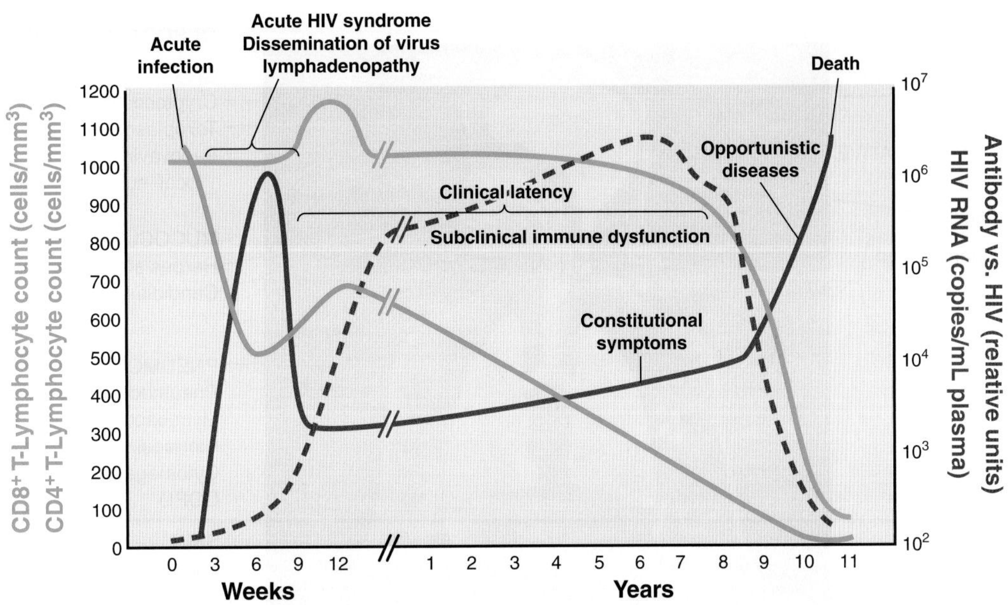

FIGURE 3-26. Human immunodeficiency virus type 1 (HIV-1)–mediated destruction of the cellular immune system results in AIDS. The infectious and neoplastic complications of AIDS can affect practically every organ system. CD, cluster of differentiation.

macrophages. HIV infection of neurons is not common, but HIV gene products produced by infected brain phagocytes are toxic for neurons and cause apoptosis via several mechanisms. Antiretroviral drugs cross the blood–brain barrier poorly, so HIV-1 infection can progress independently of HIV-1 infection outside the CNS. Longer survival among the HIV-positive population has led to greater numbers of patients with discernible neurologic deficits.

About 1% of whites are homozygous for major deletions in the *CCR5* gene (see above). ***These people may remain uninfected despite extensive exposure to the virus.*** Heterozygosity for the mutant CCR5 allele provides partial protection against HIV infection, and if infections do occur, they usually progress more slowly. Carriage of a single mutant allele is found in up to 20% of whites, but is largely absent in blacks and Asians.

Opportunistic Infections

It is important to recognize that while most immunocompetent patients will have only one infection at a time, HIV-1–infected patients often develop multiple severe infections simultaneously. A number of the many opportunistic agents that occur in HIV-1/AIDS patients is summarized in Figure 3-27.

The majority of patients with HIV-1/AIDS suffer from opportunistic pulmonary infections, although this has been greatly reduced through the use of prophylactic antibiotics. *Pneumocystis jiroveci* (formerly *Pneumocystis carinii*) pneumonia may occur in patients with advanced HIV-1 disease. Lung infections with CMV and *Mycobacterium avium-intracellulare* are less common. Patients with AIDS are also susceptible to *Legionella* infections.

Diarrhea occurs in over 75% of patients, often representing simultaneous infections with more than one organism. The most frequent pathogens are protozoans, including *Cryptosporidium, Isospora belli*, and *G. lamblia*. *M. avium-intracellulare* and *Salmonella* species are the most common bacterial causes of diarrhea in AIDS patients. CMV infection of the gastrointestinal tract can manifest as a colitis associated with watery diarrhea in patients whose CD4 counts are under 50 cells/mm^3.

Cryptococcal meningitis is a devastating complication and represents 5% to 8% of all opportunistic infections in patients with AIDS. Other CNS infectious complications include cerebral toxoplasmosis; primary CNS lymphoma; encephalitis caused by herpes simplex, varicella, or CMV; and progressive multifocal leukoencephalopathy, which is due to JC virus.

Virtually, all patients with AIDS develop some form of skin disease, infections being the most prominent. *Staphylococcus aureus* is the most common, causing bullous impetigo, deeper purulent lesions (ecthyma), and folliculitis. Chronic mucocutaneous herpes simplex infection is so characteristic of AIDS that it is considered an index infection in establishing the diagnosis. Skin lesions produced by *Molluscum contagiosum* and human papilloma virus (HPV) are also common, as are scabies and infections with *Candida* species. A varicella zoster eruption in someone under the age of 50 should raise the question of a possible occult HIV-1 infection.

Among the most common causes of death in patients with HIV/AIDS is hepatitis C virus (HCV) infection (see Chapter 12). In some studies, over one fourth of deaths among HIV-positive individuals are from hepatitis C. A very high percentage of HIV-positive intravenous drug abusers are also infected with HCV. There is evidence that coinfection with HIV and HCV accelerates the course of disease with both viruses.

Kaposi sarcoma (KS) is an otherwise rare, multicentric, malignant neoplasm (see Chapters 4 and 20). It is characterized by cutaneous and (less commonly) visceral nodules, in which endothelium-lined channels and vascular spaces are admixed with spindle-shaped cells (see Chapter 20). Patients with AIDS, especially homosexuals rather than intravenous drug users, are at very high risk for KS. In fact, KS in an otherwise healthy person under age 60 is strong evidence for AIDS. Unlike the classic indolent variety of KS, the tumor in AIDS is usually aggressive, often involving viscera, such as the gastrointestinal tract or lungs. Lung involvement frequently leads to death.

A strain of herpesvirus—human herpes virus-8 (HHV8)—is implicated in all forms of KS, including that associated with

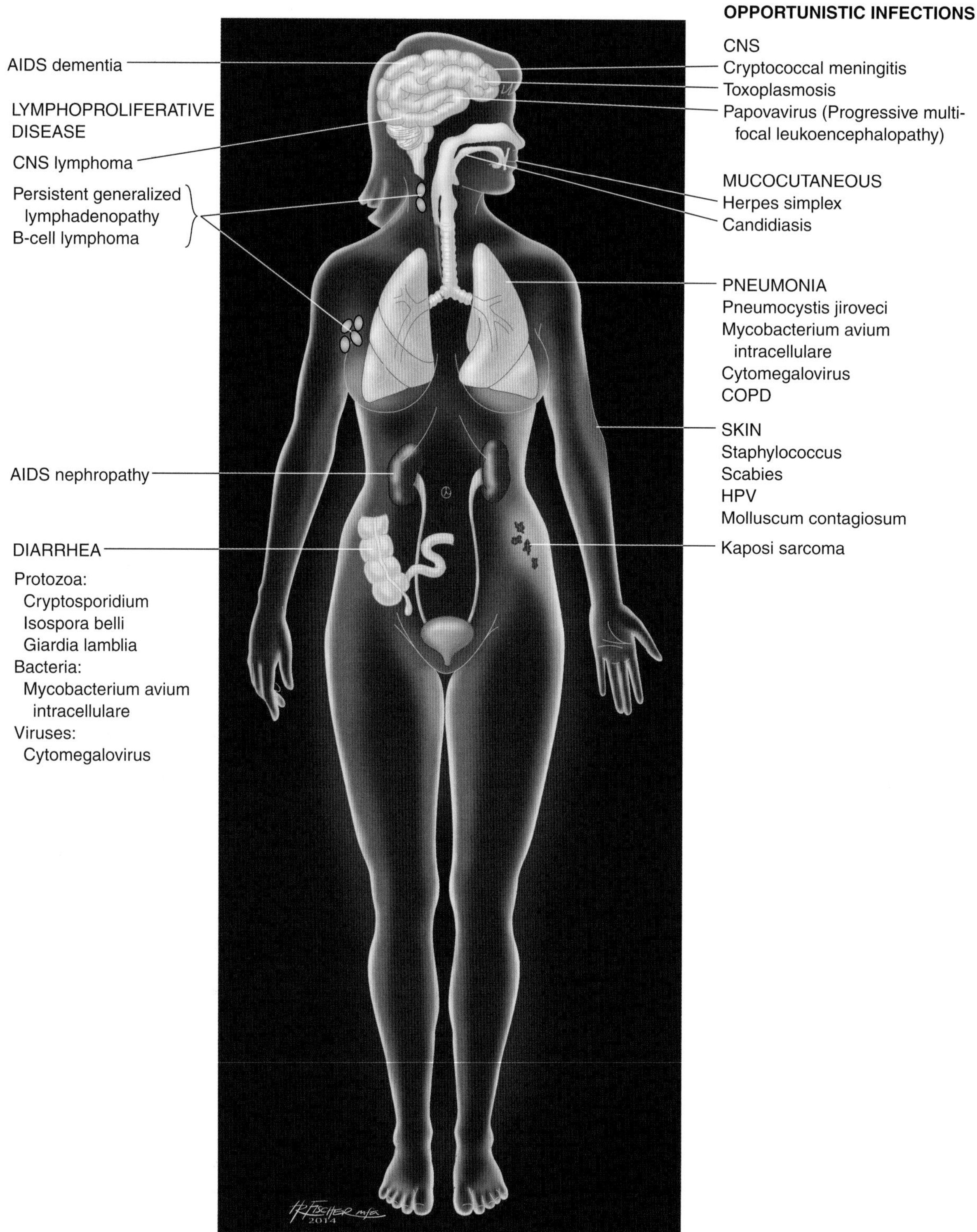

FIGURE 3-27. Generalized time course of human immunodeficiency virus type 1 (HIV-1) infection. Important events in the development of HIV-1 infection are shown, including the clinical syndrome, virus loads, and $CD4^+$ and $CD8^+$ lymphocyte population dynamics over time. CD, cluster of differentiation.

AIDS. The virus has been detected in both KS spindle cells and endothelial cells. The finding of HHV8 in the blood strongly predicts later development of KS. In fact, 75% of HIV-infected people with HHV8 in the blood developed KS within 5 years. It is thought that HHV8 is sexually transmitted because almost all homosexual HIV carriers are infected, but only one fourth of heterosexual drug users with HIV infection harbor HHV8.

B-cell lymphoproliferative diseases are common in AIDS patients. Congenital and acquired immunodeficiency states are associated with B-cell hyperplasia, usually manifested as generalized lymphadenopathy. This lymphoproliferative syndrome may be followed by the appearance of high-grade B-cell lymphomas. In fact, patients who have been subjected to immunosuppressive therapy for renal transplants are at a 35-times-greater risk of developing lymphoma, and in one third of these cases, the tumor is confined to the CNS. Lymphomas in chronically immunodeficient patients may manifest as invasive polyclonal B-cell proliferations or monoclonal B-cell lymphomas. EBV infection has been closely associated with these lesions.

B-cell hyperplasia and generalized lymphadenopathy precede malignant lymphoproliferative disease. HIV-associated lymphomas are usually of the large cell variety, as in other immunodeficiency conditions, although small cell lymphomas are sometimes seen. A conspicuous feature of AIDS-associated lymphomas is their preference for extranodal primary sites, particularly the brain, gastrointestinal tract, liver, and bone marrow. The EBV genome has also been demonstrated in many AIDS-related lymphomas, especially in the CNS.

Human Immunodeficiency Virus Type 2

In 1985, otherwise healthy prostitutes in Senegal were discovered to harbor antibodies that cross-reacted with a monkey retrovirus, now termed **simian immunodeficiency virus (SIV)**. A year later, a retrovirus similar to HIV-1 was isolated from West African patients with AIDS who were negative for antibodies against HIV-1. The infection is now endemic in West Africa and occurs in countries with social and economic ties to this part of the world.

HIV-2 is morphologically similar to HIV-1, and the immunodeficiency state associated with HIV-2 infection is indistinguishable from AIDS caused by HIV-1. The risk factors for infection in both diseases seem to be similar. People infected with HIV-2 tend to progress to AIDS more slowly than those infected with HIV-1 and may require differences in treatment.

ANTIRETROVIRAL THERAPY AND ITS CONSEQUENCES

HIV infection represents a novel challenge in treatment. Therapy focuses on HIV proteins that are obligatory for HIV replication and sufficiently different from normal cellular proteins to offer clear targets for pharmacotherapy. Initial agents were designed to inhibit the function of HIV reverse transcriptase and protease. Combining compounds that inhibit RT with drugs that inhibit PR has been the mainstay of ART. The use of ART revolutionized AIDS treatment, thereby reducing AIDS-related mortality and increasing all indices of health in HIV-1–infected patients. Newer medications that target CCR5 and HIV-1 integrase and other HIV-1–related functions have been added often in combination with an antiretroviral therapeutic armamentarium (**HAART therapy, highly active antiretroviral therapy**).

Immune Reconstitution Inflammatory Syndrome

The introduction of effective antiretroviral therapy has led to an unanticipated consequence, namely, the complications of sudden widespread suppression of HIV-1 replication, termed IRIS. This syndrome affects about one sixth of patients, usually shortly after ART begins.

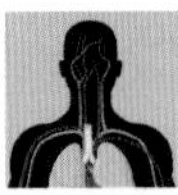

PATHOPHYSIOLOGY: The sudden increase in both CD4 and CD8 memory cells following ART can be dangerous. As memory cells, their repertoire reflects previous contact with foreign antigens. The presence of unresolved infections then magnifies these populations, leading to exaggerated immune responses.

The triggers for IRIS are largely infectious agents. The so-called paradoxical IRIS occurs when residual microbial antigens drive the T-cell responses in unresolved infections. Typically, this type of IRIS occurs 3 to 6 months after ART begins. A second type of IRIS, which is called the unmasking form, reflects the ability of a previously unsuspected infection to stimulate unrestrained inflammation. In general, IRIS due to undiagnosed pathogens occurs sooner than the paradoxical form.

Human Immunodeficiency Virus Type 1 Persistence

HIV-positive cells remain in the body so that eradication of the virus from the body is not a realistic expectation with therapies currently available. Among therapy-adherent patients in late-stage disease, about 30% did not achieve success in therapy as defined by suppression of viral load and increase in the $CD4^+$ count in the blood.

4 Neoplasia

David S. Strayer ▪ Emanuel Rubin

LEARNING OBJECTIVES

- Define and distinguish between the terms "neoplasia," "cancer," "malignant," and "benign."
- Name two cell populations that do not undergo neoplasia.
- Distinguish between the biologic behavior and morphologic characteristics of benign and malignant neoplasms.
- Discuss whether hamartomas and choristomas should be considered as neoplasms.
- Provide examples as to how the tissue of origin is used to classify benign tumors.
- Define the terms "papilloma" and "polyp."
- Distinguish between "adenocarcinoma," "squamous cell carcinoma," "sarcoma," and "lymphoma."
- List and describe five histologic characteristics distinguishing benign and malignant tumors.
- In what cases do marker studies help determine tumor origin?
- Distinguish between direct extension of a tumor and metastatic spread.
- Define "carcinoma in situ."
- List routes of metastatic spread of cancer and site examples.
- Outline the temporal sequence of events necessary for tumor metastasis.
- Distinguish between tumor staging and grading.
- Describe the TNM system of cancer staging.
- Distinguish between oncogenes and tumor suppressor genes.
- Define the term "driver mutation."
- What are the roles of HIF-1α and VEGF in tumor angiogenesis?
- Distinguish between energy production in most normal and neoplastic cells.
- Describe the term "monoclonal" as it applies to cancer.
- What are the unique properties that distinguish cancer stem cells from other stem cell populations?
- How may the term "Darwinian selection" be used to describe cancer subclones?
- Describe the origin of the term proto-oncogene.
- What are the major classes of gene function likely to be involved in oncogenes?
- How can ligands and ligand receptors drive the initial stages of oncogenesis?
- Describe two cellular receptors often involved in oncogenesis.
- What is the mechanism by which Ras family proteins are involved in oncogenesis?
- What role do kinases play in abnormalities of cell proliferation?
- Define transcription factors that are frequently activated during oncogenesis.
- What are several mechanisms likely to lead to genetic instability in neoplasia?
- Cite a common example of oncogene activation by translocation.
- Define how "loss of heterozygosity" plays a role in oncogenesis.
- Explain the two-hit hypothesis as it relates to Rb and retinoblastoma.
- By what mechanism does *Rb* function as a tumor suppressor?
- How does p53 function as "guardian of the genome?"
- Define the term "dominant negative."
- What sequence of events involving telomeres provokes the DNA damage response?
- Define the term "anoikis" and differentiate it from apoptosis.
- Describe and define epigenetic mechanisms in neoplasia.
- Describe the mechanism by which microRNAs may serve as tumor suppressors.
- Distinguish between tumor-specific and tumor-associated antigens.
- Why might immune checkpoint inhibitors be valuable as agents for cancer therapy?
- What is the source of aflatoxin B_1 and how does it interact with tumor suppressor genes?
- Give examples of radiation exposure resulting in cancer.
- Distinguish between the roles of DNA and RNA viruses in the causation of human cancer.
- What distinguishes pediatric cancers from those in adults?
- How do studies of migrant populations aid in distinguishing environmental and genetic factors in carcinogenesis?

THE PATHOLOGY OF NEOPLASIA

A **neoplasm** (Greek, *neo*, "new," + *plasma*, "thing formed") is the autonomous growth of tissues that have escaped normal restraints on cell proliferation. Tumors that remain localized are considered **benign,** whereas those that spread to distant sites are called **malignant,** or **cancer**. The neoplastic process entails not only cell proliferation but also variable modification of the differentiation of the involved cell types.

The incidence of neoplastic disease increases with age, and longer life spans in modern times enlarge the population at risk. Neoplasms are derived from cells that can multiply. Thus, mature neurons and cardiac myocytes do not give rise to tumors. The resemblance of neoplastic cells to their cells of origin usually enables conclusions about their sources and potential behavior. However, a tumor mimics its tissue of origin to a variable degree. Some closely resemble their parent structures whereas others seem to be collections of cells that are so primitive that the tumor's origin cannot be identified.

Benign Versus Malignant Tumors

Although exceptions are known, benign tumors basically do not penetrate (invade) across adjacent tissue borders, nor do they spread (metastasize) to distant sites. They remain as localized overgrowths in the area in which they arise. Benign tumors tend to be more differentiated than malignant ones—that is, they more closely resemble their tissue of origin.

In common usage, **the terms "benign" and "malignant" refer to a tumor's overall biologic behavior rather than its morphologic characteristics**. However, tumors can usually be identified as benign or malignant by virtue of their morphologic characteristics, although the biologic behavior of some types of tumors may not correlate with their histologic appearance. Some tumors that appear histologically malignant may not metastasize in a patient. Thus, basal cell carcinomas of the skin may invade subjacent structures locally but rarely metastasize and are not life-threatening. By contrast, some tumors that exhibit benign histologic characteristics may be lethal. For example, aggressive meningiomas do not metastasize, but their local invasiveness may cause death by compromising vital structures. For many endocrine tumors (e.g., islet cell tumors of the pancreas), metastatic potential is not predictable from histologic features, and a tumor's benign or malignant nature can only be determined on the basis of the clinical history and the presence or absence of metastases.

Tumor-like Conditions

Hamartomas

These lesions are focal benign overgrowths of one or more mature cellular elements of a normal tissue and are often arranged irregularly. Many hamartomas are clonal and have defined DNA rearrangements, and so may be classified as true neoplasms.

Choristomas

Also called **heterotopias,** choristomas are minute aggregates of normal tissue components in aberrant locations. They are not true tumors. Examples include pancreatic rests in the walls of gastrointestinal (GI) organs and adrenal tissue in the renal cortex.

CLASSIFICATION OF NEOPLASMS

Labeling a tumor as benign or malignant is a prediction of its eventual biologic behavior and clinical outcome. As of yet, such predictions are not based on scientific principles but rather on accumulated experience and historical correlations between histologic patterns and clinical courses.

Primary Descriptors of Tumors

The primary descriptor of any tumor, benign or malignant, is its cell or tissue of origin. The classification of benign tumors is the basis for the names of their malignant variants. *The suffix "oma" for benign tumors is preceded by reference to the cell or tissue of origin.* For example, a benign tumor that resembles chondrocytes is called a **chondroma** (Fig. 4-1). Tumors of epithelial origin are given a variety of names on the basis of what is believed to be their outstanding characteristic. Thus, a benign tumor of the squamous epithelium may be called simply **epithelioma** or, when branched and exophytic, may be termed **papilloma**. Benign tumors arising from glandular epithelium, such as in the colon or the endocrine glands, are named **adenoma**. Accordingly, we refer to a **thyroid adenoma** or a **pancreatic islet cell adenoma**.

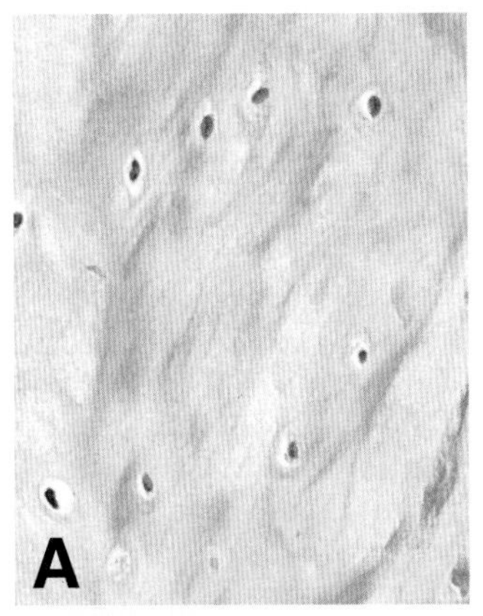

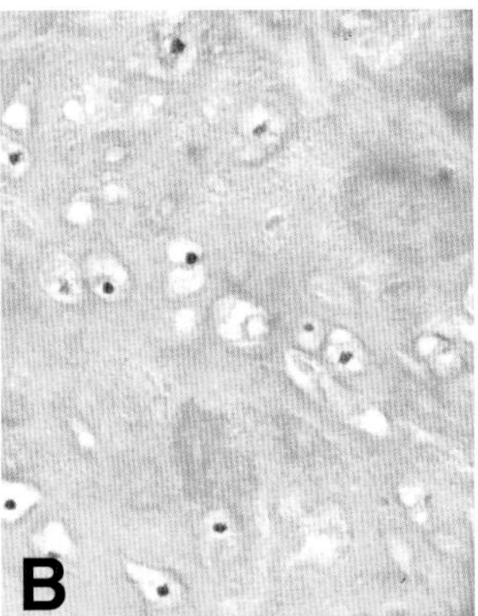

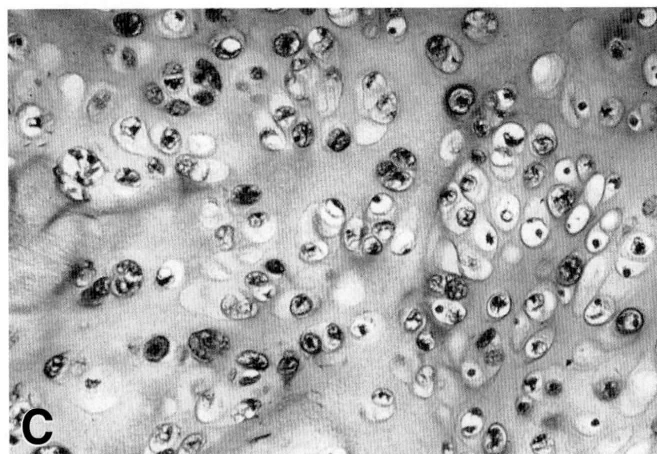

FIGURE 4-1. **Cartilaginous lesions. A.** Normal cartilage. **B.** A benign chondroma closely resembles normal cartilage. **C.** Chondrosarcoma of bone. The tumor is composed of malignant chondrocytes, which have bizarre shapes and irregular hyperchromatic nuclei, embedded in a cartilaginous matrix. Compare A and B. (Figure 4-1C: From Bullough PG, Vigorita VJ. *Atlas of Orthopaedic Pathology*. New York, NY: Gower Medical Publishing, 1984.)

Benign tumors that arise from germ cells and contain derivatives of different germ layers are labeled **teratoma**. These tumors occur principally in the gonads and occasionally in the mediastinum and may contain a variety of structures, such as skin, neurons and glial cells, thyroid, intestinal epithelium, and cartilage. Certain benign growths, recognized clinically as tumors, are not truly neoplastic but rather represent overgrowth of normal tissue elements. Examples are vocal cord polyps, skin tags, and hyperplastic polyps of the colon. ***Although historically the suffix "oma" referred to benign tumors, there are many exceptions.*** For example, tumors called melanomas, mesotheliomas, seminomas, and lymphoma are all malignant even though they carry the suffix "oma." Most hamartomas are not even true neoplasms but disorganized developmental medleys of multiple structures.

In general, the malignant counterparts of benign tumors usually carry the same name, except that the suffix **"carcinoma"** ***is applied to epithelial cancers and*** **"sarcoma"** *to those of mesenchymal origin.* For instance, a malignant tumor of the stomach, which is glandular in nature, is a **gastric adenocarcinoma** or **adenocarcinoma of the stomach** (Fig. 4-2). **Squamous cell carcinoma** is an invasive tumor of the skin or other organs lined by a squamous epithelium (e.g., the esophagus). Squamous cell carcinomas also arise in the metaplastic squamous epithelium of the bronchus or endocervix. **Urothelial cell carcinoma** is a malignant neoplasm of the bladder or ureters. By contrast, we speak of **chondrosarcoma** (see Fig. 4-1) or **fibrosarcoma**. Sometimes the name of the tumor suggests the tissue of origin, as in **osteogenic sarcoma** or **bronchogenic carcinoma**. Some tumors display neoplastic elements of different cell types but are not germ cell tumors. For example, **fibroadenoma** of the breast, composed of epithelial and stromal elements, is benign, whereas, as the name implies, **adenosquamous carcinoma** of the uterus or the lung is malignant. Tumors of the hematopoietic system are a special case in which the relationship to the blood is indicated by the suffix "emia." Thus, **leukemia** refers to a malignant proliferation of leukocytes. Tumors in which historically the histogenesis was poorly understood may be given an eponym—for example, Hodgkin disease or Ewing sarcoma.

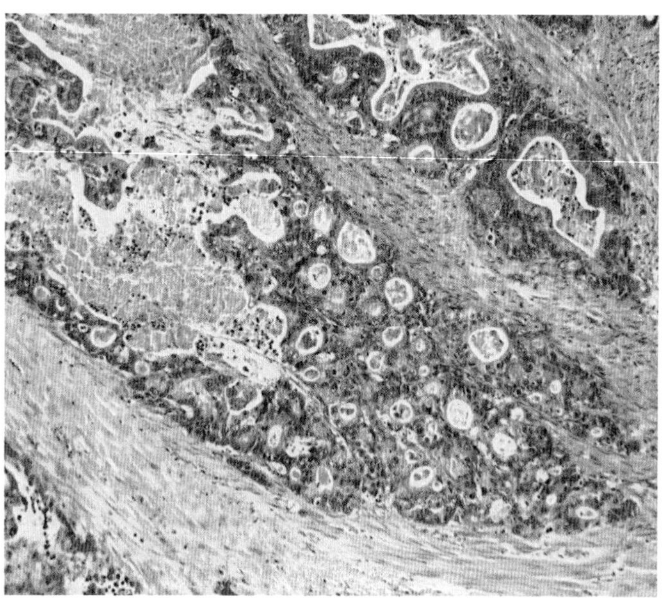

FIGURE 4-2. Adenocarcinoma of the stomach. Irregular neoplastic glands infiltrate the gastric wall.

Distinguishing Benign From Malignant Tumors Through Histology

Some of the histologic features that are considered in differentiating benign from malignant tumors include the following:

- **Degree of cellular atypia:** This term refers to the extent to which the tumor departs from the appearance of its normal tissue or cellular counterparts (see Fig. 4-1). An example is the difference between normal cartilage, a benign chondroma, and a malignant chondrosarcoma. In general, the magnitude of cellular atypia (termed **anaplasia** when severe) correlates with the aggressiveness of the tumor. Cytologic evidence of atypia includes (1) variation in size and shape of cells and cell nuclei **(pleomorphism),** (2) enlarged and hyperchromatic nuclei with coarsely clumped chromatin and prominent nucleoli, (3) atypical mitoses, and (4) bizarre cells, including tumor giant cells (Fig. 4-3).
- **Mitotic activity:** Many malignant tumors show high mitotic rates. For some tumors (e.g., smooth muscle malignancies, leiomyosarcomas), a diagnosis of malignancy is based on finding even a few mitoses. Nonetheless, high mitotic activity is not obligatory to consider a tumor as malignant.
- **Growth pattern:** Malignant neoplasms often exhibit disorganized growth, which may be expressed as sheets of cells, arrangements around blood vessels, papillary structures, whorls, rosettes, and so forth. Malignant tumors often suffer from compromised blood supply and show ischemic necrosis.
- **Invasion:** Malignancy is proved by the demonstration of invasion, particularly of blood vessels and lymphatics. In some circumstances (e.g., squamous carcinoma of the cervix or carcinoma arising in an adenomatous polyp), the diagnosis of malignant transformation is made principally on the basis of local invasion.
- **Metastases:** The presence of metastases identifies a tumor as malignant. If a metastatic tumor is not preceded by a diagnosed primary cancer, the site of origin may not be readily apparent from histologic characteristics alone. In such cases, demonstration of specific tumor markers may establish the correct origin.

Marker Studies of Tumor Origin

Some metastatic tumors may be so undifferentiated microscopically as to preclude even the distinction between epithelial and mesenchymal origin. Determination of cell lineage of undifferentiated tumors is more than an academic exercise because therapeutic decisions are often based on the appropriate identification of the cell of origin. Tumor markers are products of neoplasms that can be detected in the cells themselves or in body fluids. To identify such marker, pathologists often rely on the preservation of characteristics that identify progenitor cells or, in some cases, the synthesis of specialized substances by neoplastic cells. Such materials may be unique to the neoplastic cells such as fetal proteins or those synthesized in excess (monoclonal immunoglobulins) by some plasma cell tumors (multiple myeloma). Among these,

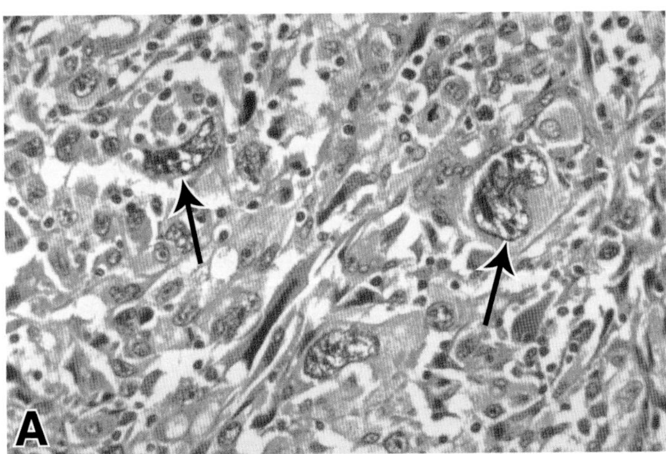

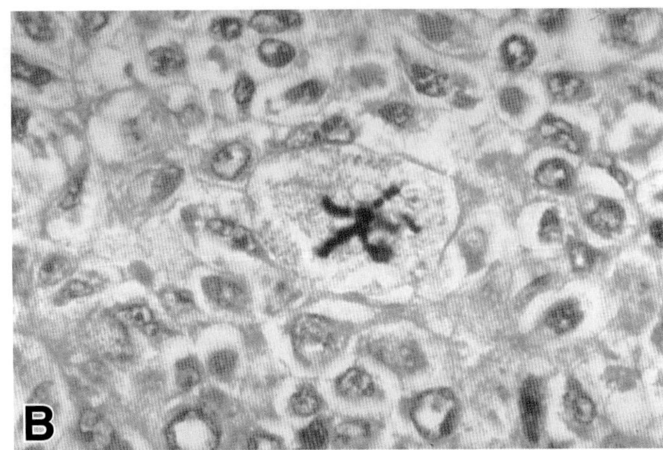

FIGURE 4-3. Anaplastic features of malignant tumors. A. The cells of this anaplastic carcinoma are highly pleomorphic (i.e., they vary in size and shape). The nuclei are hyperchromatic and are large relative to the cytoplasm. Multinucleated tumor giant cells are present (*arrows*). **B.** A malignant cell in metaphase exhibits an abnormal mitotic figure.

diagnostically useful markers are such diverse products as enzymes, hormones, and cytoskeletal and junctional proteins. Although no one tumor marker allows unequivocal distinction between benign and malignant cells, such markers are often useful in classifying their cellular origin.

Tumor markers can be detected in tissue sections by immunologic techniques (immunohistochemistry, immunofluorescence) (Fig. 4-4) and by molecular studies (in situ hybridization). Table 4-1 contains examples of marker studies that are used to identify the tissue of origin of tumors. In addition to their use in identifying the lineages of malignancies, tumor-associated antigens are also used in other ways. Blood levels of tumor antigens are helpful in following the development of metastases and progression of the tumor after the primary neoplasm has been treated. Representative examples include carcinoembryonic antigen (CEA) for GI tumors, cancer antigen (CA 125) for ovarian carcinoma, and prostate-specific antigen (PSA) for prostate cancer.

INVASION AND METASTASIS

Two properties that are unique to cancer cells are the ability to invade locally and the capacity to metastasize to distant sites. These characteristics are responsible for the vast majority of deaths from cancer; the primary tumor itself (e.g., breast or colon cancer) is usually amenable to surgical resection.

Direct Extension of Cancer

Most carcinomas begin as localized growths confined to the epithelium where they arise. As long as these early cancers do not penetrate the basement membrane on which the epithelium rests, such tumors are called ***carcinoma in situ*** (Fig. 4-5). In this stage, it is unfortunate that in situ tumors are asymptomatic because they are invariably curable. When in situ tumors acquire invasive potential, and extend through the underlying basement membrane, they can compromise neighboring tissues and metastasize. In situations in which cancer arises from cells that are not confined by a basement membrane—such as connective tissue cells, lymphoid elements, and hepatocytes—an in situ stage is not defined.

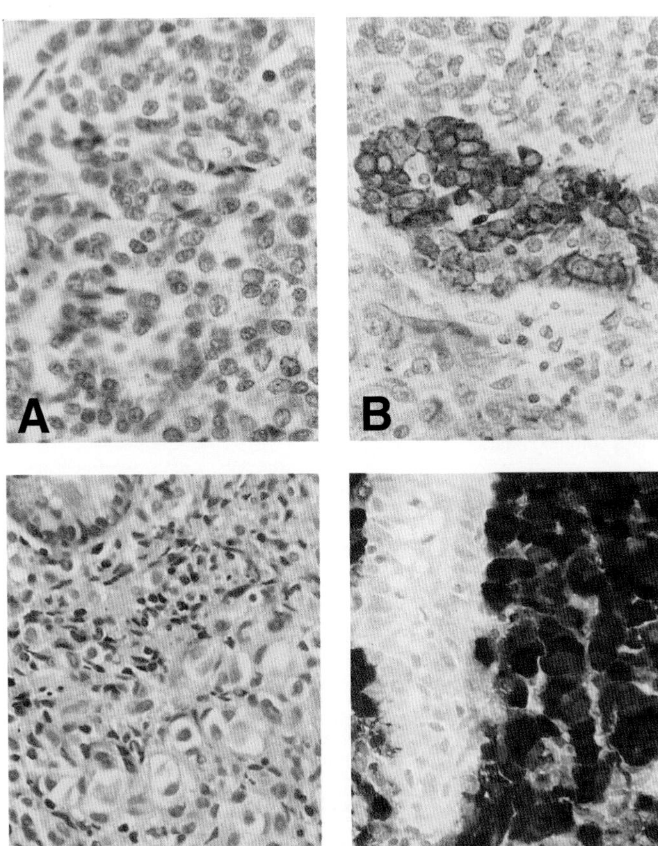

FIGURE 4-4. Tumor markers in the identification of undifferentiated neoplasms. A. A poorly differentiated metastatic bladder cancer is difficult to identify as a carcinoma with the hematoxylin and eosin stain. **B.** A section of the tumor depicted in **A** is positive for cytokeratin with an immunoperoxidase stain and is identified as carcinoma. **C.** A metastasis to the colon of an undifferentiated malignant melanoma is not pigmented, and its origin is unclear. **D.** An immunoperoxidase stain of the tumor shown in **C** reveals numerous cells positive for S-100 protein, a commonly used marker for cells of melanocytic origin.

Table 4-1

Frequently Used Markers to Identify Tumors

Marker	Target Cells
Epithelial cells	
Cytokeratins (CKs)	Carcinomas, mesothelioma
CK7	Many nongastrointestinal adenocarcinomas
CK20	Gastrointestinal and ovarian carcinomas, urothelial carcinomas, Merkel cell tumor
Epithelial membrane antigen (EMA)	Carcinomas, mesothelioma, some large cell lymphomas
Ber-Ep4	Most carcinomas, but not in mesothelioma
B72.3 (tumor associated)	Many adenocarcinomas, but not in mesothelioma
Carcinoembryonic antigen (CEA)	Many adenocarcinomas of endodermal origin but not in others (e.g., renal, mesothelioma)
Mesothelial cells	
CK5/6	Mesothelioma
Vimentin	Mesothelioma
HBME	Mesothelioma, thyroid tumors
Calretinin	Mesothelioma
Melanocytes	
HMB-45	Malignant melanoma
S-100 protein	Malignant melanoma, glial cells
Mel A	Malignant melanoma
Neuroendocrine and neural cells	
Chromogranins, particularly chromogranin A	Neuroendocrine tumors
Synaptophysin	Neuroendocrine tumors
CD57	Neuroendocrine tumors, T and NK cells, Schwann cells
Glial cells	
Glial fibrillary acidic protein (GFAP)	Astrocytoma and other glial tumors
Mesenchymal cells	
Vimentin	Most sarcomas
Desmin	All types of muscle tumors
Muscle-specific actin	Muscle tumors, myofibroblast tumors
CD99	Ewing sarcoma, peripheral neuroectodermal tumors (PNETs), acute lymphoid, and myeloid leukemias
Specific organs	
Prostate-specific antigen (PSA)	Prostatic cancer
Prostate-specific alkaline phosphatase (PSAP)	Prostate cancer
Thyroglobulin	Thyroid cancer
α-Fetoprotein (AFP)	Hepatocellular carcinoma, yolk sac tumor
HepPar1	Hepatocellular carcinoma
WT1	Wilms tumor, some mesotheliomas
Placental alkaline phosphatase (PLAP)	Seminoma, embryonal carcinoma
Human chorionic gonadotropin (hCG)	Trophoblastic tumors
CA19-9	Pancreatic and gastrointestinal carcinomas
CA125	Ovarian carcinoma, endometrial carcinoma, some other nongynecologic tumors (pancreas, mesothelioma)
Calcitonin	Medullary carcinoma of the thyroid
CD markers	
CD1	Some T-cell leukemias, Langerhans cell proliferations
CD2	T cells, T-cell malignancies
CD3	T cells, T-cell malignancies
CD4	T cells, T-cell malignancies, monocytes, monocytic malignancies
CD5	T cells, some B-cell malignancies
CD8	Suppressor T cells, some T-cell malignancies
CD10 (common ALL antigen, CALLA)	Acute lymphoblastic leukemia, some B-cell lymphomas, renal cell carcinomas
CD15	Reed-Sternberg cells, some T cells, some myeloid leukemias, many adenocarcinomas, but not in mesothelioma
CD19	B cells, B-cell malignancies
CD20	B cells, B-cell malignancies
CD30	Hodgkin disease, anaplastic large cell lymphoma
CD33	Myeloid leukemias
CD34	Acute myeloid or lymphoblastic leukemias, some spindle cell tumors
CD117 (c-Kit)	Chronic myeloid leukemia, gastrointestinal stromal tumors, seminomas, also tumors of lung, breast, endometrium, urinary bladder
Non-CD leukemia/lymphoma markers	
κ Light chain	B-cell malignancies
λ Light chain	B-cell malignancies
TdT	Acute lymphoblastic leukemia
Bcl-1 and cyclin D1	Mantle cell lymphoma
von Willebrand factor (vWF)	Vascular neoplasms
CD31	Vascular neoplasms, endothelial cells
CD34	Bone marrow stem cells, vascular neoplasms (endothelial cells)
Lectins	Vascular neoplasms
CD43	Almost all leukocytes
CD56	NK cells

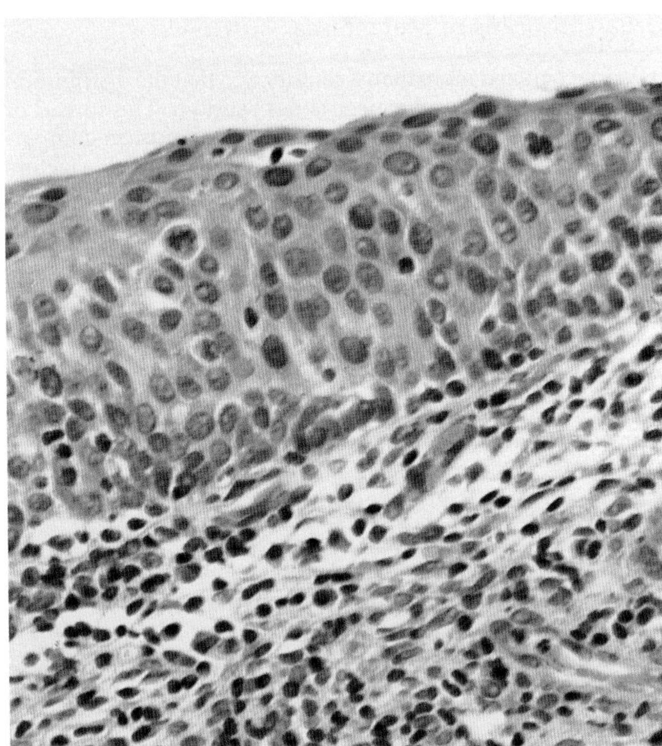

FIGURE 4-5. Carcinoma in situ. A section of the uterine cervix shows neoplastic squamous cells occupying the full thickness of the epithelium and confined to the mucosa by the underlying basement membrane.

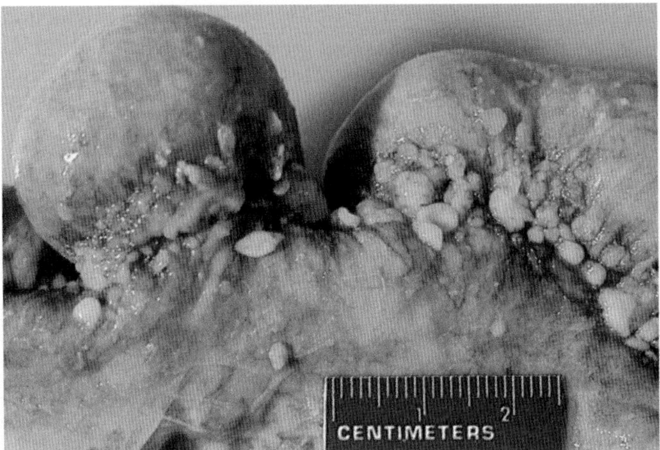

FIGURE 4-6. Peritoneal carcinomatosis. The mesentery attached to a loop of small bowel is studded with small nodules of metastatic ovarian carcinoma.

Malignant tumors growing within the tissue of origin may also extend beyond the confines of that organ to involve adjacent tissues. The growth of the cancer is occasionally so extensive that replacement of the normal tissue results in functional insufficiency of the organ. Such a situation is common in primary liver cancer. Brain tumors, such as astrocytomas, infiltrate the brain until they compromise vital regions. The direct extension of malignant tumors within an organ may also be life-threatening because of their location. A common example is intestinal obstruction produced by colon cancer.

The invasive growth pattern of cancers may secondarily impair the function of an adjacent organ. Squamous carcinoma of the cervix frequently grows beyond the genital tract to obstruct the ureters or produce vesicovaginal fistulas. Neglected cases of breast cancer are often complicated by extensive skin ulceration. Even small tumors can produce severe consequences when they invade vital structures. The agonizing pain of pancreatic carcinoma results from direct extension of the tumor to the celiac nerve plexus. Tumor cells that reach serous cavities (e.g., those of the peritoneum or pleura) spread easily by direct extension or can be carried by the fluid to new locations on the serous membranes. The most common example is the seeding of the peritoneal cavity by certain types of ovarian cancer (Fig. 4-6).

Metastatic Spread

Metastasis (Greek, "displacement") is the migration of malignant cells from one site to another noncontiguous site. The invasive properties of malignant tumors bring them into contact with blood and lymphatic vessels, which they can also penetrate, and through which they disseminate to distant sites.

Hematogenous Metastases

Cancer cells often invade capillaries and venules, but thicker-walled arterioles and arteries are relatively resistant to their attack. Before they can form viable metastases, circulating tumor cells must lodge in the vascular bed of the metastatic site (Fig. 4-7). Here they attach to, and then traverse, the walls of blood vessels and lymphatics. Often, the location of a primary tumor with regard to blood or lymph flow determines the distribution of the initial metastases from that tumor. Thus, abdominal tumors that seed the hepatic portal system often cause liver metastases; other tumors penetrate veins that eventually drain into the vena cava and hence to the lungs. Breast cancers first metastasize to regional lymph nodes because of

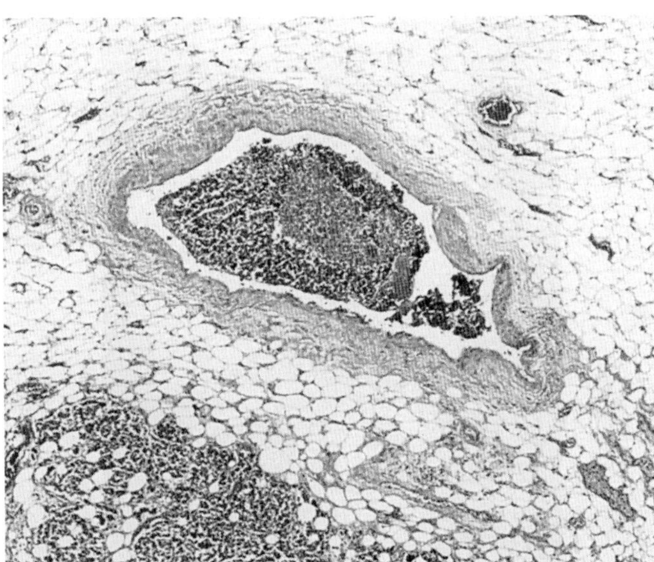

FIGURE 4-7. Hematogenous spread of cancer. A malignant tumor (*bottom*) has invaded adipose tissue and penetrated into a small vein.

the direction of lymphatic flow. More widespread metastatic disease may result from extensive early dissemination of tumor cells in the circulation or from secondary spread from early metastatic foci.

Lymphatic Metastases

Basement membranes envelop only large lymphatic channels; lymphatic capillaries lack them. Having invaded lymphatic vessels, tumor cells are carried to regional draining lymph nodes. There, they first lodge in the marginal sinus and then extend throughout the node. Lymph nodes bearing metastatic deposits may be enlarged to many times their normal size, often exceeding the diameter of the primary lesion (Fig. 4-8).

The regional lymphatic pattern of metastasis is exemplified by breast cancer. The initial metastases are almost always lymphatic and have considerable prognostic significance. Cancers that arise in the lateral aspect of the breast characteristically spread to axillary lymph nodes; those arising in the medial portion drain to the internal mammary thoracic lymph nodes.

A graphic example of the relationship of lymphatic anatomy to the spread of malignant tumors is afforded by cancers of the testis. Rather than metastasizing to inguinal nodes, as do other tumors of the male external genitalia, testicular cancers typically involve the draining abdominal periaortic nodes. The explanation lies in the descent of the testis from an intra-abdominal site to the scrotum, during which it is accompanied by its own lymphatic supply.

Seeding of Body Cavities

Malignant tumors that arise in organs adjacent to body cavities (e.g., ovaries, GI tract, lung) may shed malignant cells into these spaces. Such sites include the peritoneal and pleural cavities, although occasional seeding of the pericardial, joint, and subarachnoid spaces is observed. Tumors in these locations often produce fluid (e.g., ascites, pleural effusions), sometimes in large quantities. Mucinous adenocarcinoma may also secrete copious amounts of mucin in these areas.

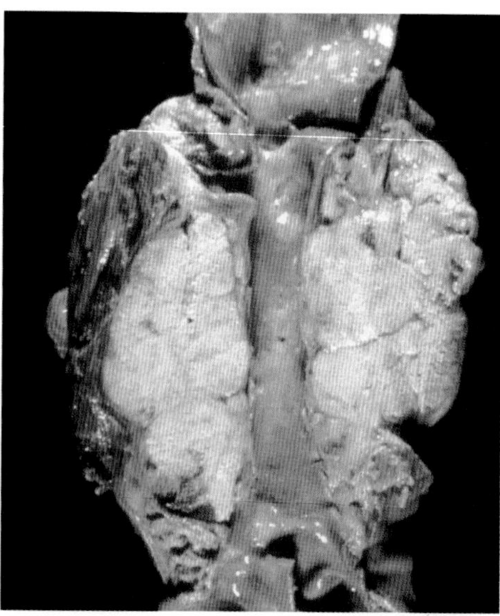

FIGURE 4-8. Metastatic carcinoma in periaortic lymph nodes. The aorta has been opened and the nodes bisected.

Organ Tropisms of Metastases

It was recognized more than a century ago that the distribution of metastases in breast cancer is not random. The spread of tumor cells to specific secondary sites depends on compatibility between the tumor cells (the seed) and favorable factors in the secondary site (the soil). For example, cancers of the breast, prostate, and thyroid metastasize to bone, a tropism that suggests a favored "soil." Conversely, despite their size and abundant blood flow, neither the spleen nor skeletal muscle is a common site of metastases.

Steps in Invasion and Metastasis

Tumor spread is a multistep process, with each step potentially representing major genetic and epigenetic modifications in tumor cells and their behavior.

Malignant cells go through several steps to establish a metastasis (Fig. 4-9):

- **Invasion of the basement membrane underlying the tumor** requires that the previously stationary cells of solid tumors become mobile. Cancer cells develop specialized structures, **invadopodia**, which express matrix metalloproteinases and other proteinases. The tumor cells degrade extracellular matrix (ECM) and promote interaction with integrins in the ECM, which serve as guides.
- **Movement through the ECM** is furthered by the epithelial-mesenchymal transition (EMT) of tumor cells. In this process, the initially polarized nonmobile tumor cells become more like mesenchymal cells, that is, nonpolarized and mobile. The EMT is triggered in large part by hypoxia, which promotes the production of HIF-1α thereby activating numerous genes. Tumors co-opt normal stromal cell functions, trigger inflammatory reactions, and recruit additional tumor cells to the area to overcome anatomic and other barriers to invasion.
- **Penetration of vascular or lymphatic channels** occurs initially by solitary tumor cells that have already undergone EMT. These cells move more rapidly than do cell clusters and **intravasate** (penetrate) into blood vessels. Tumor-associated capillaries are not completely invested by pericytes and permit further penetration. By contrast, compact cell collections preferentially transfer to the lymph nodes, where they generally remain in place. Collective cell migration to lymph nodes appears to be independent of spread through blood vessels, and each may be the preferred mode of dissemination for specific tumors. In lymph nodes, communications between lymphatics and venous tributaries allow the cells access to the systemic circulation.
- **Survival within circulating blood or lymph** requires that tumor cells must avoid anoikis (apoptosis triggered by loss of ECM anchors). **Circulating tumor cells** are unlikely to survive for long in the circulation, being filtered out in the pulmonary circulation. Nevertheless, if detected within blood as circulating tumor cells (CTC), they may serve as a useful diagnostic marker for otherwise occult tumors.
- **Homing to a new site and exiting from the circulation** requires "preparation of the soil" into premetastatic niches, which undergo repeated remodeling by cytokines and enzymes produced by the marrow-derived cells in response to tumor-produced factors. In the circulation, tumor cells bind to and activate platelets. Similar interactions serve to tether tumor cells to the endothelium and to endothelial-bound

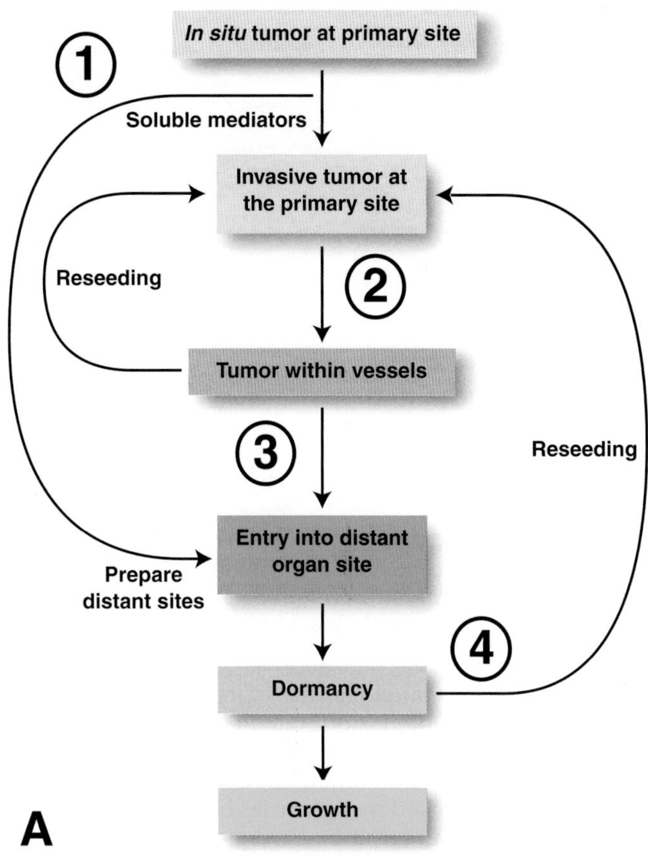

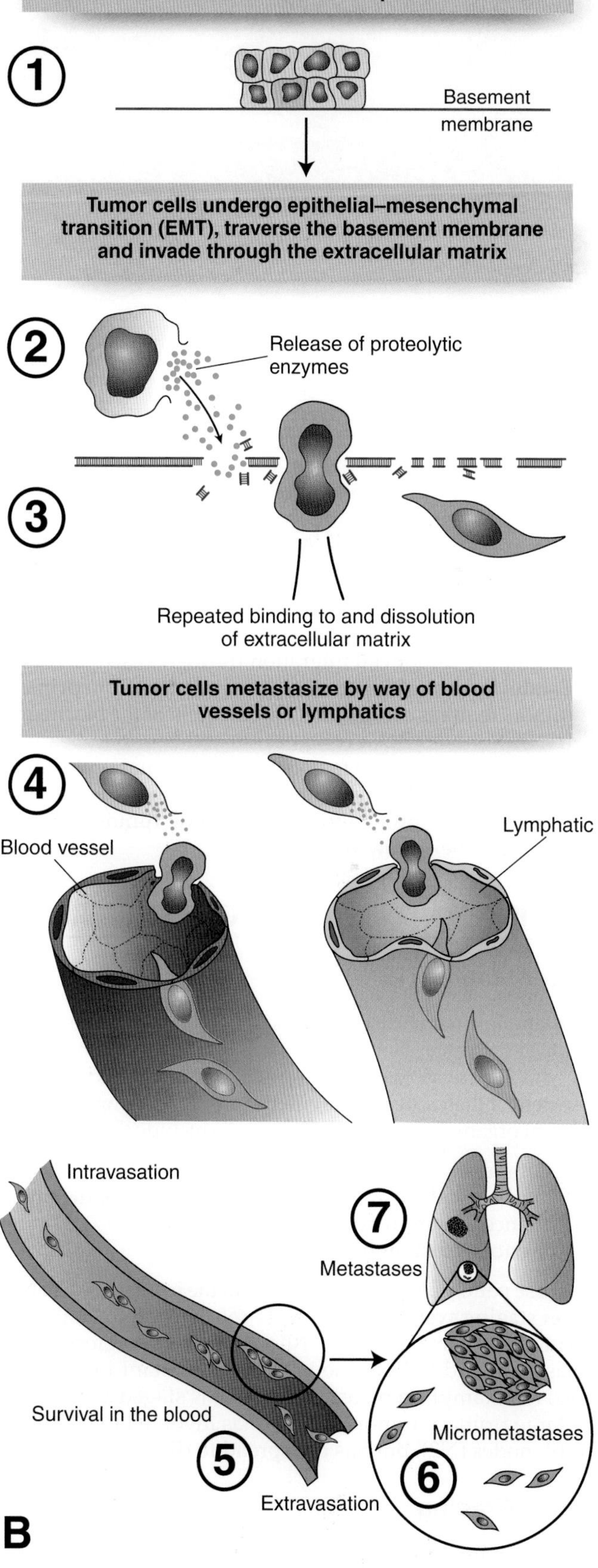

FIGURE 4-9. Mechanisms of tumor invasion and metastasis. **A.** Initial behavior of tumor at primary site. **B.** Subsequent invasive behavior of tumor. The mechanism by which a malignant tumor initially penetrates a confining basement membrane and then invades the surrounding extracellular environment involves several steps. (*1*) The tumor first acquires the ability to bind components of the extracellular matrix. These interactions are mediated by the expression of a number of adhesion molecules. (*2*) The tumor undergoes epithelial–mesenchymal transition (EMT) and traverses the basement membrane. (*3*) Proteolytic enzymes are then released from the tumor cells, and the extracellular matrix is degraded. (*4*) After moving through the extracellular environment, the invading cancer penetrates blood vessels and lymphatics by the same mechanisms. (*5*) After survival in blood vessels or lymphatics, the tumor exits the vascular system. (*6*) It establishes micrometastases at the site where it leaves the vasculature. (*7*) These micrometastases grow into gross masses of metastatic tumor.

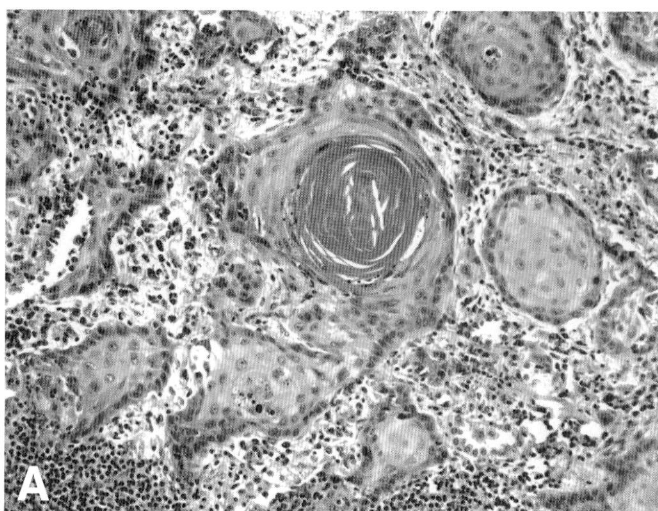

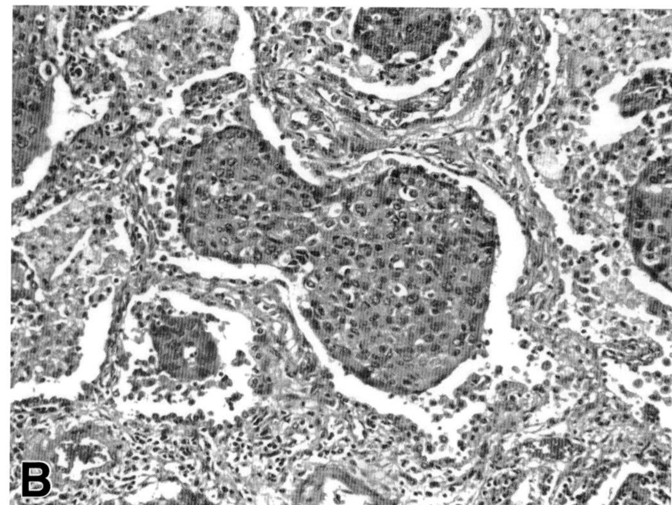

FIGURE 4-10. Cytologic grading of squamous cell carcinoma of the lung. A. Well-differentiated (grade 1) squamous cell carcinoma. The tumor cells bear a strong resemblance to normal squamous cells and synthesize keratin, as evidenced by epithelial pearls. **B.** Poorly differentiated (grade 3) squamous cell carcinoma. The malignant cells are difficult to identify as being of squamous origin.

leukocytes. Malignant cells appear to secrete proteins that dissolve tight junctions between endothelial cells, thereby facilitating tumor cell migration through vascular walls.

- **Establishment of a micrometastasis** distant from primary tumors requires complex synchronization of the biochemistry, ECM, and cellular composition of the soon-to-be metastatic site. Among the factors that enable micrometastatic foci to persist is the recruitment of bone marrow–derived hematopoietic progenitor cells to guide tumor cells and stimulate their growth.

STAGING AND GRADING OF CANCERS

Cancer Staging

In an attempt to predict the clinical behavior of a malignant tumor and to establish criteria for therapy, most cancers are staged; they are assessed using protocols that help determine the extent of their spread. The criteria used for staging vary with different organs. Commonly used criteria include the following:

- Tumor size
- Extent of local growth, whether within or out of the organ
- Presence of lymph node metastases
- Presence of distant metastases

These patterns have been codified in the international **TNM cancer staging system,** in which "T" refers to the size and local extent of the primary tumor, "N" to the level of regional node metastases, and "M" to the presence of distant metastases. Thus, for example, a breast cancer that is staged at T3N2M0 is a large primary tumor (T3) that has involved two axillary lymph nodes (N2), but has not spread to distant sites (M0).

Cancer Grading

Well-differentiated tumors are referred to as low grade, and poorly differentiated ones are regarded as high grade. Cytologic and histologic grading include the degree of anaplasia and the number of proliferating cells. Anaplasia is determined from the shape and regularity of the cells and from the presence of distinct differentiated features, such as gland-like structures in adenocarcinomas or epithelial pearls in squamous carcinomas (Fig. 4-10). The presence of such characteristics identifies a tumor as well differentiated. By contrast, the cells of poorly differentiated malignancies bear little resemblance to their normal counterparts. Evidence of rapid growth is provided by (1) large numbers of mitoses, (2) atypical mitoses, (3) nuclear pleomorphism, and (4) tumor giant cells. Most grading schemes classify tumors into three or four grades of increasing malignancy. The general correlation between the cytologic grade and the biologic behavior of a neoplasm is not invariable: there are many examples of tumors of low cytologic grades that exhibit substantial malignant properties. Thus, in most cases, staging is a more important criterion than grading in predicting a tumor's course and influencing therapeutic decisions.

TUMOR CELL EVASION OF NORMAL REGULATION

Cancer develops as a consequence of genetic changes in cells, and several critical cellular processes prevent tumor development, including cell-cycle regulation, DNA repair, and regulation of telomerase activity. Tumor cells escape from controlled proliferation as a result of mutations that have the effects of both activating and inactivating certain genes. Generally, activating mutations stimulate passage through the cell cycle. The genes affected by such mutations have traditionally been called **oncogenes**. Inactivating mutations, by contrast, usually prevent the inhibitory influences of **tumor suppressor genes**.

Most cancers develop because multiple mutations accumulate in dividing cells. Incipient tumors become malignant by undergoing serial genetic changes that lead to the acquisition of hallmarks of cancers. The order in which these changes arise vary from tumor to tumor, but eventually a neoplasm amasses most or all of them. Thus, certain attributes and genes may contribute to one tumor but not to others, or may suppress oncogenesis in one context but encourage it in another.

HALLMARKS OF CANCER

At its root, the process of neoplasia begins with the occurrence of a mutation **(driver mutation)** in a gene that gives a cell a growth advantage over its neighbors. The clonal derivatives of this initial mutated cell expand in number over the course of several years; with expansion the likelihood of a second driver mutation within the same clone increases, resulting in cells with two mutations, now better able to more effectively proliferate in the local environment. With an increasing number of cells, additional driver mutations within the clone become ever more likely, ultimately resulting in an invasive clone of cells capable of metastasis. Hence, oncogenesis may be seen as a "Darwinian" process in which a small number of random driver mutations (perhaps few as three) yielding more effective cell growth and competition with neighboring cells results in cancer.

However, this does not answer the question as to what is the source of the driver mutations. Although the somatic mutation rate is small per cell division (10^{-7} per gene per division), the large number of cells and divisions occurring in an adult result in an estimate that every gene will be mutated at least once in one cell. ***Statistical study demonstrates that the lifetime risk of cancer of a particular organ is highly correlated with the total number of stem cell divisions needed to maintain that organ.*** Estimates suggest that environmental and hereditary factors contribute 35% of the risk for cancer development. However, 65% of the risk is stochastic and related to inevitable chance errors in somatic DNA replication in cells. Hence, much of the risk of cancer is related to random chance, also known as "bad luck."

It should be stressed that **driver mutations** may affect both DNA sequences that encode proteins and noncoding sequences. In the latter case, altered sequences and levels of untranslated RNAs and of regulatory regions may drive oncogenesis. In addition, tumors accumulate large numbers of mutations not implicated in carcinogenesis, which are termed **passenger mutations**.

Other mutations may affect tumor development and progression. It is clear that there are several basic activities that distinguish cells of solid malignancies from their normal counterparts. (Hematologic cancers develop and spread differently, and so share some, though not all, of these characteristics.) The following hallmarks or attributes of malignant tumors are significant:

- **Unregulated cellular proliferation:** In normal tissues, progression through the cell cycle is carefully regulated. However, cancer cells proliferate independently of normal restraints to multiplication.
- **Cellular immortalization:** Although normal cells in tissue culture have a limited potential for replication, cancer cells can multiply indefinitely. Thus, malignant cells circumvent the process of senescence and retain the ability to reproduce (see Chapter 1).
- **Evasion of programmed cell death:** Programmed cell death (see Chapter 1) can be activated by such factors as genomic instability and inhospitable cellular microenvironments. Cancer cells often develop mutations that circumvent such suicide programs.
- **Stimulation of vascular proliferation:** Expansion of solid tumors requires increased supplies of nutrients and oxygen. This, in turn, necessitates proliferation of blood vessels. Thus, tumor cells secrete signaling molecules that stimulate **angiogenesis** (i.e., formation of new blood vessels).
- **Inactivation of tumor suppressors:** Normally many genes interact to limit cell-cycle transit, maintain genomic stability, and regulate other key functions. During tumorigenesis, these endogenous tumor suppressors are evaded or inactivated.
- **Invasion and metastasis:** Death from cancer is usually caused by tumor dissemination (metastasis). To accomplish such spread, tumor cells must be able to surmount anatomic barriers, for example, the basement membrane. They must then traverse intervening connective tissues, enter blood vessels and lymphatics, identify fertile sites for implantation, exit the vasculature, and ultimately establish colonies far from their origin.

Additional Processes that Facilitate Growth and Spread of Tumors

Some mechanisms play supporting roles in developing and maintaining many cancers but may not be obligatory for tumor development.

- **Genomic instability:** Most human cancer cells show increased susceptibility to random mutation. This allows tumor cells to evolve quickly and to achieve genotypes that favor cancer maintenance and progression.
- **Altered epigenetic regulation:** Epigenetics refers to management of gene function by mechanisms independent of DNA coding sequences. Among the modalities involved are covalent modifications of DNA and DNA-associated proteins (such as histones), noncoding RNAs, altered messenger RNA (mRNA) translation, and posttranslational modifications of gene products.
- **Altered bioenergetics:** Generally, cancer cells favor glycolysis over oxidative phosphorylation for ATP generation. This metabolic change requires increased glucose utilization, which has many consequences for the cell's metabolic needs and products.
- **Immune avoidance:** A body of clinical and experimental evidence suggests that the immune system may protect from tumor production and progression. However, the nature of the interactions between tumors and host immunity remains a subject of study.
- **Inflammation:** Inflammatory cells infiltrate most developing solid tumors and secrete diverse factors that facilitate tumor development and progression.

Tumor-Induced Angiogenesis

Angiogenesis is the formation of new blood vessels from preexisting small blood vessels. In order to grow beyond about 2 mm in diameter, tumors need more nutrient and oxygen supply than preexisting blood vessels can provide. Most tumors experience hypoxia, which induces expression of **hypoxia-induced factors (HIFs),** especially **HIF-1α**. In turn, HIF-1α elicits production of angiogenic growth factors, which stimulate formation of new tumor-associated blood vessels. This process is obligatory for a primary tumor to grow and metastasize.

Vascular Endothelial Growth Factor

The VEGF family is a major mediator of oncogenesis and is made by the cells of most tumors. As noted above, tumor cells produce HIF-1α when they sense insufficient oxygen.

HIF-1α is a transcription factor that upregulates diverse genes, including VEGFs. The family of VEGFs binds to and activates a family of receptors that stimulates several signaling pathways (Fig. 4-11). Consequences include endothelial cell proliferation, protection from apoptosis, enhanced cell migration and increased vascular permeability. The last effect leads to leakage of such blood components as fibrinogen into the area. Once outside blood vessels, fibrinogen generates a fibrin matrix that facilitates endothelial cell migration and angiogenesis.

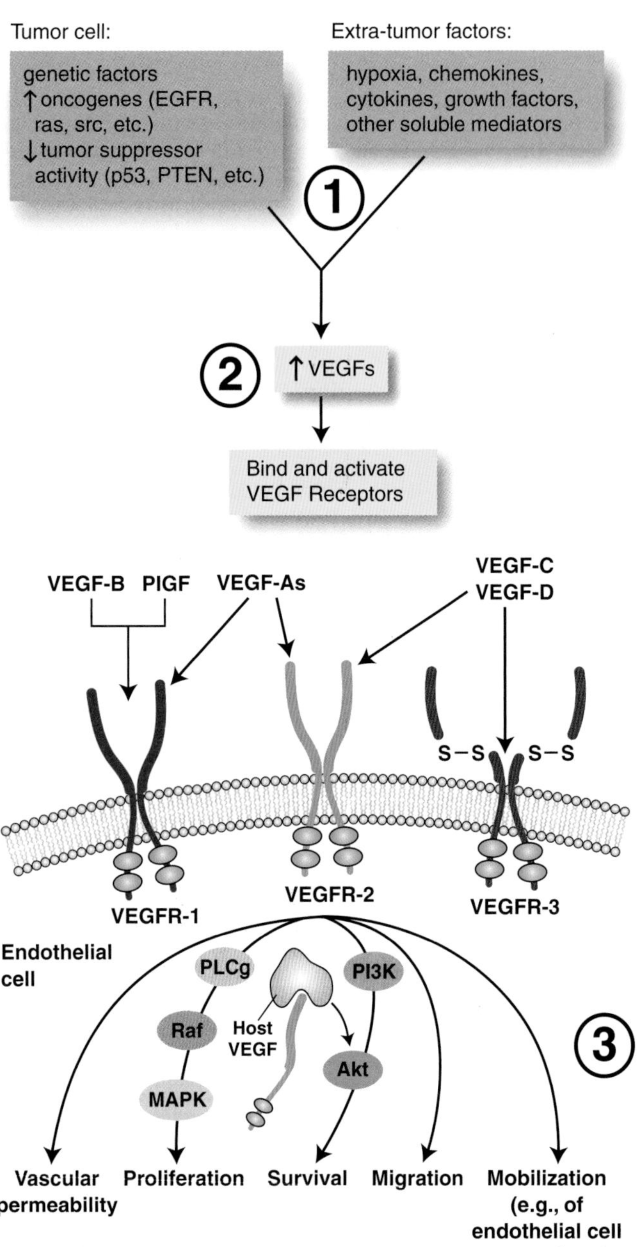

FIGURE 4-11. The vascular endothelial growth factor (VEGF) system and its effects. (*1*) Under the influence of factors generated by tumor cells (*left;* increased expression of certain oncogenes or decreased activity or tumor suppressors) or coming from other sources (tumor-related stroma, external environment, etc.), several VEGFs are produced. (*2*) These bind the several VEGF receptors (VEGFRs), the principal of which is VEGFR-2. (*3*) Downstream signaling from these receptors has diverse effects on vascular endothelium, including increasing vascular permeability, activating cell proliferation and survival mechanisms, inducing in-migration of endothelial cells, and mobilizing progenitor cells to the area, to help form new blood vessels. EGFR, epidermal growth factor receptor; PlGF, placental growth factor; PTEN, phosphatase and tensin homolog; PLC, phospholipase C; MAPK, mitogen-activated protein kinase; PI3K, phosphatidylinositol-3 kinase.

Cancer Cell Metabolism

Cancer cells have different needs from normal cells. As their proliferative rate generally far exceeds that of normal cells, they must produce the structural components of daughter cells at a rate that sustains their mitotic activity. Thus, the synthesis of proteins, lipids, and other molecules must be faster than that of normal cells.

Tumor cells generate energy mainly by aerobic glycolysis in the cytosol, producing pyruvate and two ATPs. This compares to mitochondrial oxidative phosphorylation, which generates 36 ATPs, CO_2, and H_2O. Pyruvate contributes to protein, lipid, and other macromolecular synthesis. Tumor cells can also generate energy from multiple carbon sources including lactate and glutamate. Acetate may also be taken up by tumor cells, where it can be made into acetyl-CoA, to be used mostly for lipid synthesis.

CANCER STEM CELLS AND TUMOR HETEROGENEITY

Most Cancers Are Monoclonal

Most cancers arise from a single transformed cell. This conclusion is best established for proliferative disorders of the lymphoid system, in which clonality is easiest to assess.

Monoclonality has also been demonstrated for many solid tumors. One of the best examples of this principle utilized glucose-6-phosphate dehydrogenase in women who were heterozygous for its two isozymes, A and B (Fig. 4-12).

Cancer Stem Cells

Like the pluripotent somatic stem cells found in normal tissue, which can both replenish their own numbers (self-renewal) and differentiate into mature cells (see Chapter 2), cancers also have a small population of malignant cells with such capabilities. These are called **cancer stem cells (CSCs)**. Their existence has been best demonstrated in hematologic malignancies like acute myeloid leukemia, but there is also strong evidence for their existence in an increasing number of solid tumors (Fig. 4-13).

Tumors Derive from Cancer Stem Cells

CSCs are the cells from which many human tumors arise. They divide infrequently, which allows them to evade destruction by cytotoxic chemotherapeutic agents that preferentially kill rapidly dividing cells. Thus, although chemotherapy may destroy the bulk of the rapidly dividing cells in a malignant tumor, residual CSCs may survive to regenerate the cancer. CSCs have evolved to evade apoptosis and senescence and therefore are likely to be less sensitive to cancer therapies than their normal tissue counterparts.

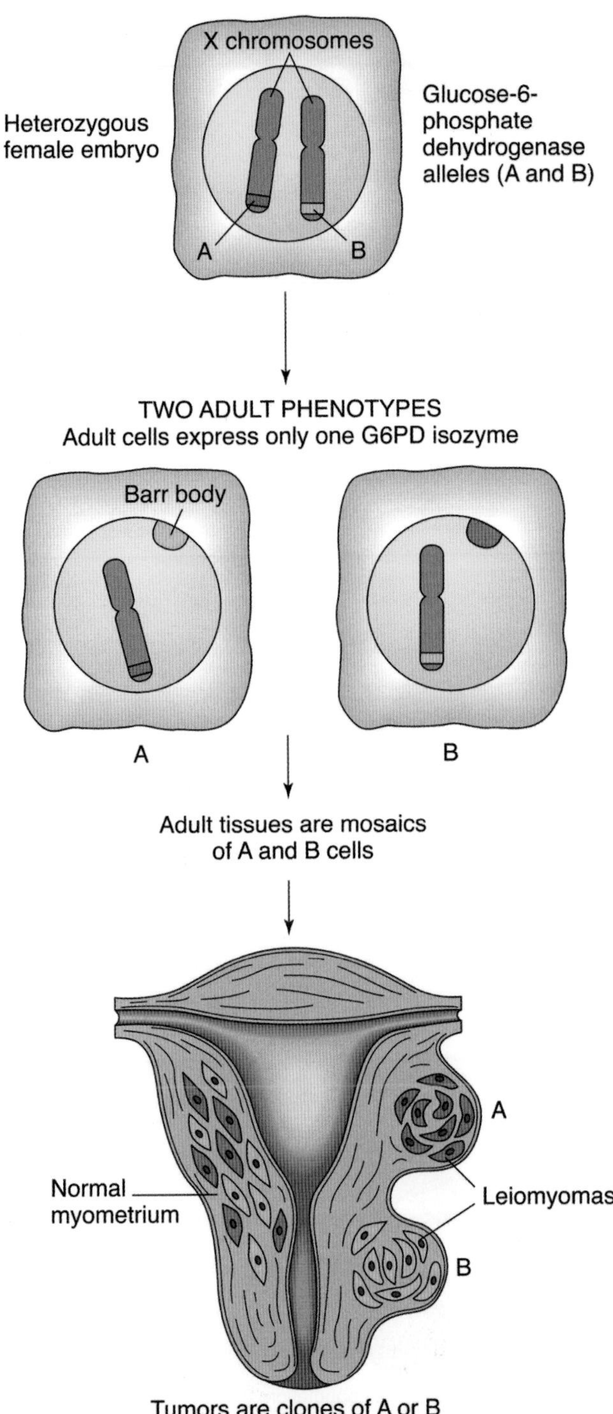

FIGURE 4-12. Monoclonal origin of human tumors. Some females are heterozygous for the two alleles of glucose-6-phosphate dehydrogenase (G6PD) on the long arm of the X chromosome. Early in embryogenesis, one of the X chromosomes is randomly inactivated in every somatic cell and appears cytologically as a Barr body attached to the nuclear membrane. As a result, the tissues are a mosaic of cells that express either the A or the B isozyme of G6PD. Leiomyomas of the uterus have been shown to contain one or the other isozyme (A or B) but not both, a finding that demonstrates the monoclonal origin of the tumors.

Clonal Evolution

The original explanation of tumor heterogeneity holds that tumor cells progressively accumulate new mutations as they proliferate. A tumor in which many cells are dividing can thus, over time, generate a diverse population of genetically different cells. Some of these cells may be destined for death, although others will become genetically distinct subclones of the original malignant cells (Fig. 4-13A). Darwinian-style selection—whether due to localized hypoxia, differences in proliferation rates, potential for invasion and metastasis, therapy, and so forth—governs which subclones will grow and which will die, and which will metastasize and which will remain localized. The implications of this phenomenon are substantial. Some malignant tumors may represent constantly shifting therapeutic targets. They exhibit incredible plasticity in adapting to a changing chemotherapeutic milieu via the ability to shift phenotypes rapidly to evade antineoplastic drugs, and then to shift back (Fig. 4-14).

THE CONCEPT OF ONCOGENES

Transfer of specific genes from human cancer cells **(oncogenes)** in vitro can impart a transformed phenotype to normal recipient cells. Such genes were initially described in viruses, which had the property of conferring a neoplastic phenotype to human cells in culture (v-oncogenes). Transforming human tumor genes were later found to be mutant versions of normal genes **(proto-oncogenes)**, which dysregulated cellular proliferation. Such genes are designated with the letter "c," referring to *cytoplasmic* (e.g., *c-myb*).

Mechanisms of Cell Proliferation

Among the key genes often altered during oncogenesis are those that stimulate cell proliferation. They are in the biochemical pathways that guide entry into and progression of the cell cycle. These include the following (Fig. 4-15):

- Growth factors
- Cell surface receptors
- Intracellular signal transduction pathways
- DNA-binding nuclear proteins (transcription factors)

Growth Factor–Related Signaling and Oncogenesis

Cell proliferation normally reflects a balance between forces driving cells to divide and the cell cycle regulators discussed above. In acquiring the ability to multiply without restraint, cancer cells must be able to circumvent dependence on outside stimulatory influences. They usually accomplish this by mimicking those influences. To understand how this occurs, one must first review how receptor–ligand interactions drive cells into mitosis. A general schematic relating the roles of ligand–receptor interactions in tumor development is shown in Figure 4-15.

Tumor-driving mutations may occur at any step of this process. The consequence of such mutations is that proteins are produced that drive cellular proliferation without the normal restraints that match cell numbers to the body's needs.

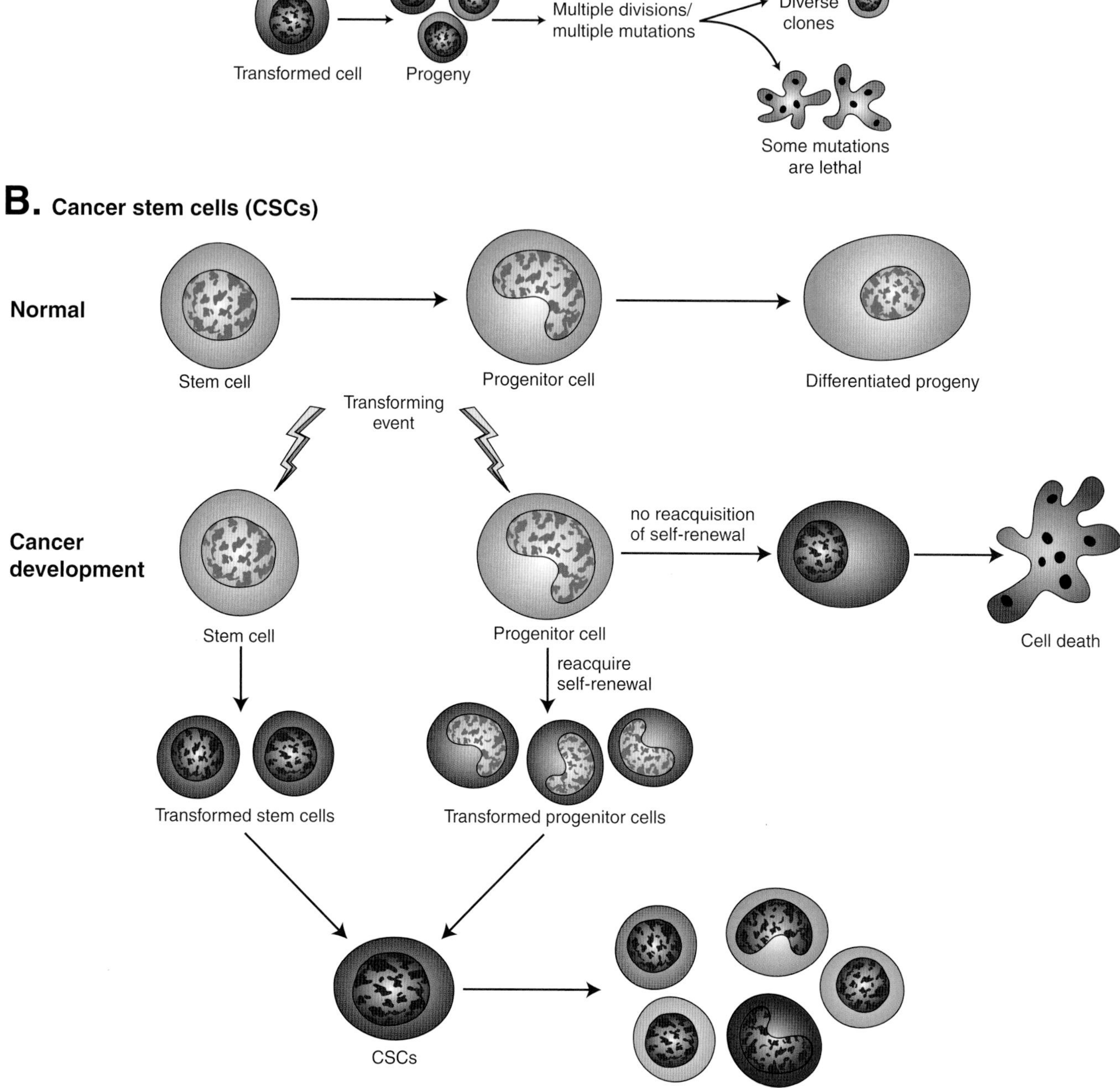

FIGURE 4-13. Tumor stem cells and tumor heterogeneity. A. Linear progression of tumor clonal evolution. Proliferating cancer progenitor cells eventually develop a variety of mutations, with different individual cells acquiring different mutations, leading to heterogeneity in the tumor cell population. Some such mutations are inconsistent with cell survival, whereas others facilitate cancer progression. This model is most consistent with critical enabling primordial mutations in a stem cell that must be retained throughout subsequent tumor evolution. **B. Cancer stem cells and progenitor cells.** Normally (*above*) stem cells give rise to committed progenitor cells. These then produce terminally differentiated cells. An oncogenic stimulus (*below*) to a stem cell may lead to an expanded pool of transformed stem cells. These become cancer stem cells (CSCs). Alternatively, the oncogenic stimulus may affect a committed progenitor cell. If the latter recapitulates a program of self-renewal, the resulting transformed progenitor may become a CSC. If it does not activate the self-renewal program, resulting differentiated progeny will be produced and eventually die. CSCs generated either via transformation of stem cells or transformation of committed progenitors may then be the antecedents of a heterogeneous malignant cell population.

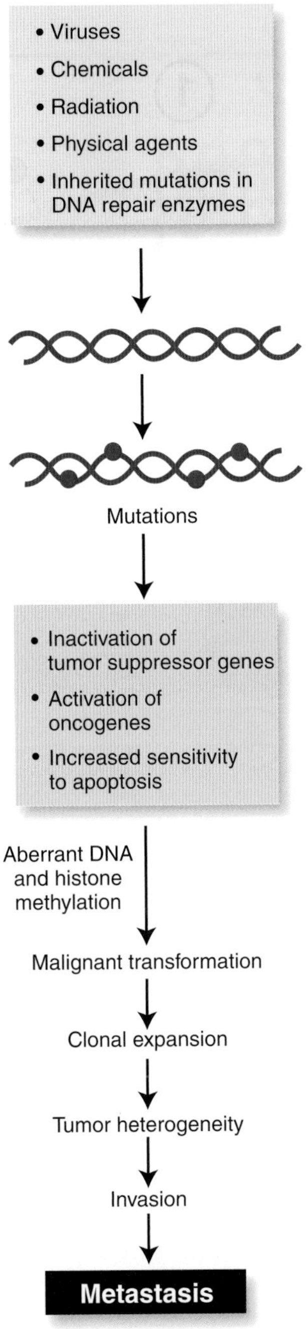

FIGURE 4-14. Summary of the general mechanisms of cancer.

Ligands, Receptors, and Cell Proliferation

Ligands

Some ligands may drive cell multiplication in early stages of oncogenesis, with tumor cells eventually becoming independent of those molecules. Sometimes, the developing (or developed) tumor cell itself produces such ligands, resulting in an autocrine trigger to cell division. Some such stimulatory molecules occasionally act as oncoproteins by virtue of being overexpressed through **gene amplification** (increase in gene copy number) (Table 4-2).

Receptors

There are several basic classes of receptors that stimulate or inhibit cell proliferation (Table 4-3). Except for the steroid hormone receptors, these are cell membrane molecules that respond to ligands produced by other cells. Receptor–ligand interactions normally cause changes in the receptors, after which they serve as docking sites for one or more intracellular signaling networks.

The changes that ligands elicit in receptors reflect the specifics of the receptor:

- **Receptor tyrosine kinases (RTKs)** possess intrinsic kinase activity that causes the receptor to undergo phosphorylation after recognizing its ligand.
- **Nonkinase receptors** include many that undergo structural rearrangements, allowing them to initiating downstream signaling. These types of receptors often associate with nonreceptor tyrosine kinases (**NRTKs**; see below), which mediate further signaling.
- **G-protein–coupled receptors (GPCRs)** are the most common type of membrane receptors. Upon binding their ligands—which include very diverse types of molecules—GPCRs change conformation. In so doing, they activate GTP-related nucleotide exchange factors. Some GPCRs transduce mitogenic signals triggered by such ligands as prostaglandins, endothelin, and thrombin. These receptors may be amplified in cancers or they may mediate stimulatory autocrine or paracrine signals.

Receptor proteins are among the most important transforming proteins and are widely implicated in oncogenesis (see Table 4-2). They *often drive tumor formation via mutations that render them constitutively active, independently of their ligands.*

Signaling Downstream After Receptor Activation

Once a receptor binds to its ligand, downstream signaling pathways are stimulated.

What follows depends on many factors including (1) the type of receptor activated, (2) whether its activation entails tyrosine kinase activity, and (3) the molecular species that are activated. Pathways that may be set in motion include the following:

- **Ras:** Members of the Ras family are small guanine nucleotide-binding proteins that may be activated by tyrosine kinases via a linker protein. To understand activated Ras and Ras-related oncogenesis, the Ras cycle should be appreciated (Fig. 4-16).
- Many malignant tumors possess a mutated form of Ras, which does not undergo deactivation and is constitutively activated.
- Activation of many GPCRs stimulates a similar type of response, but by a different group of proteins, called heterotrimeric G proteins. Unlike Ras, these G proteins tend not to be mutated in cancers. Rather, they may be overexpressed, also resulting in constitutive activation of downstream signaling.
- **Phosphatidylinositol-3 (PI3) kinase:** This family of enzymes is generally activated by RTKs and GPCRs. Family members add a phosphate group to a phosphatidylinositol lipid to create the small molecule phosphatidylinositol-3-phosphate (PI(3)P), as well as more heavily phosphorylated derivatives such as PI(3,4,5)P_3. These mediate many proliferation-related and cell survival reactions.

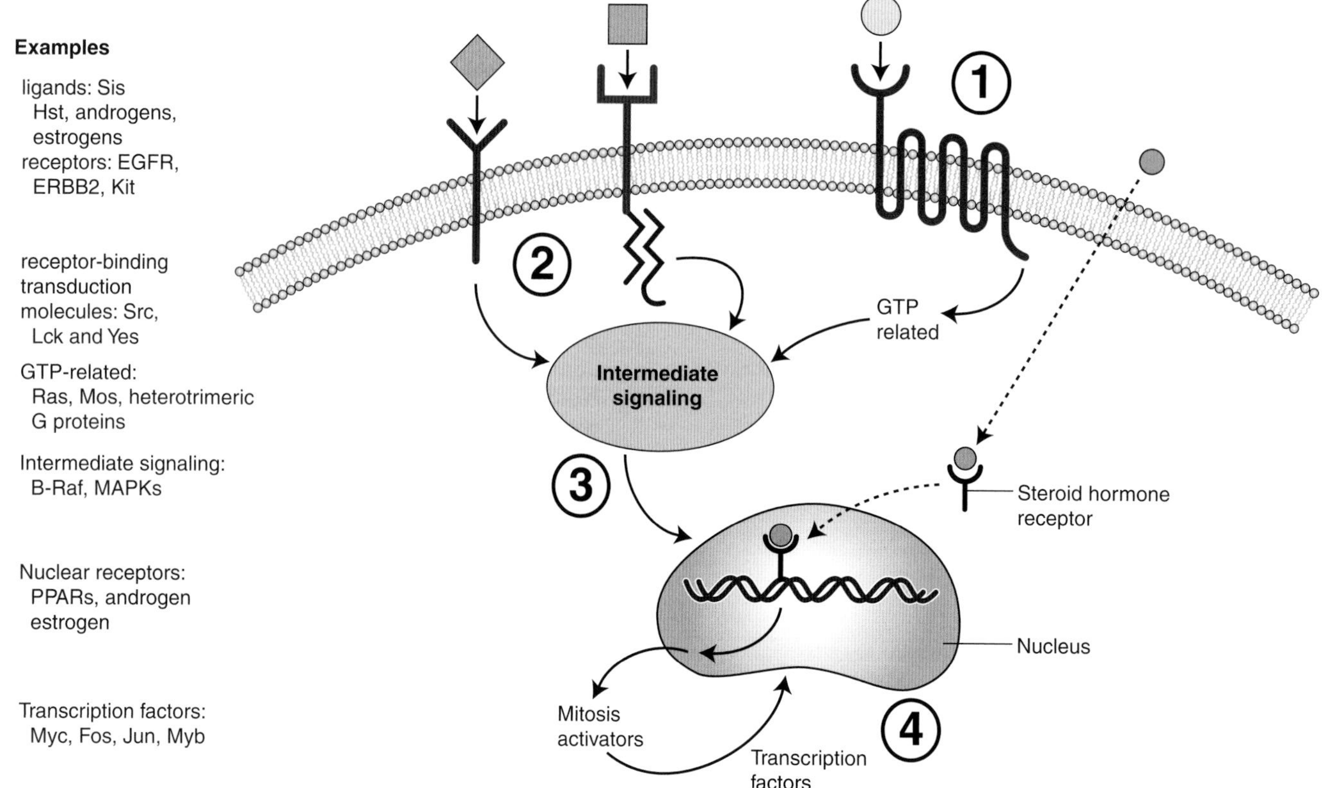

FIGURE 4-15. Signaling paradigms in cellular transformation. (*1*) Extracellular ligands bind to cell membrane receptors. (*2*) One of several pathways of signaling is then activated. The receptor itself can activate intracellular signaling (*left*). A protein that binds to the activated receptor may trigger intracellular signaling (*center*). The receptor may be a G-protein–coupled receptor, which stimulates guanine nucleotide–related signaling. Or, the ligand may traverse the cell membrane to activate receptors within the cytosol directly, without a cell membrane intermediate (*far right*). (*3*) In the first three cases, cellular intermediates of many types are activated. (*4*) The result for all pathways is activation of transcription, particularly of proteins that help take the cell through the cell cycle. Shown at the *left* are examples of proto-oncogenes and other cellular products that act in each capacity. EGFR, epidermal growth factor receptor; ERBB2, receptor tyrosine-protein kinase erbB-2; GTP, guanosine triphosphate; MAPKs, mitogen-activated protein kinases; PPARs, peroxisome proliferator-activated receptors.

- **Phospholipase C:** This family of enzymes is commonly activated by diverse types of receptors, especially GPCRs, but also others. They cleave certain phospholipids and so participate in the generation of inositol phosphate signaling intermediates and diacylglycerol. These both drive cellular multiplication via calcium signaling pathways and protein kinase C, respectively.
- **Mitogen-activated protein kinases (MAPKs):** These enzymes mediate many different types of signaling reactions involved in cell proliferation. MAPKs may be triggered by upstream proteins such as Ras (after RTK activation), GPCRs, or other mechanisms. Some very important driver mutations for malignancy (e.g., b-Raf) occur among these proteins, frequently generating constitutive activation.

Transcriptional Activation

The key element for cancer cells proliferation without restraint is the array of genes whose transcriptional activities are turned on or off. When transcription factors drive oncogenesis, the genetic changes responsible usually entail increased production of wild-type proteins. Thus, driver mutations of transcription factors may entail, for example, translocations that place them under the control of more vigorous promoters. Many transcription factors are implicated in oncogenesis. Among the best-known examples are as follows:

- **Myc:** A ubiquitous transcription factor that may control transcription of as many as 10% to 15% of all human genes.
- **Fos and Jun:** Together, these proteins form the **AP-1** (activation protein-1) transcription factor. Increased AP-1 activity promotes cellular proliferation and survival (Fig. 4-17) and is generally a result of increased signaling via several pathways, including MAPK and the protein kinase C family (PKC; see above).
- **Androgen and estrogen receptors:** These cytoplasmic receptor proteins act both as receptors and as transcription factors. They translocate to the nucleus on binding their cognate ligands. Once in the nucleus, they act as transcription factors. Depending on the cell type, steroid sex hormone receptors may stimulate cell proliferation. Thus, estrogen receptors promote mammary epithelial cell proliferation and are important in the progression of many breast cancers. Similarly, in many prostate cancers, androgens cause prostatic tumor cells to proliferate.

Table 4-2

Common Proteins That Drive Cell Proliferation, Their Activities, and Activation

Activity	Name of Protein	Nature of Mutation	Explanation
Ligand	Hst	Amplification	Growth factor in FGF family
	Sis	Derepression (autocrine stimulation)	PDGF, β subunit
	FGF3	Amplification	
RTK	Kit	Activating point mutation	Receptor for stem cell factor
	Her2/neu (ErbB2)	Amplification	Constitutively activated
	EGFR	Mutations, amplification	Constitutively activated
	Met	Translocation	HGF receptor
	Ret	Point mutation, translocation	Constitutively activated
Intracellular signaling intermediate	Ras (K-Ras, N-Ras, H-ras)	Point mutation	GTP-binding protein, three different *RAS* genes, activated in different settings
	B-Raf	Point mutation	Tyrosine kinase
	Src	Point mutation	Tyrosine kinase
	Abl	Translocation	Mutant protein, Bcr-Abl
Transcription factor	Myc (c-Myc, N-Myc, L-Myc)	Amplification, translocation	Directs transcription of up to 15% of human genes
	Fos	Amplification	Part of AP-1, with Jun
	Myb	Point mutations	Promotes hematopoietic stem cell proliferation
	Rel	Amplification, point mutations	Member of NFκB family, expressed mainly in lymphocytes
	Ets	Translocation	Large family; fusion products may drive tumorigenesis

AP-1, activation protein-1; EGFR, epidermal growth factor receptor; FGF, fibroblast growth factor; GTP, guanosine triphosphate; HGF, human growth factor; NF, nuclear factor; PDGF, platelet-derived growth factor; RTK, receptor tyrosine kinase.

As noted above, however, cell proliferation mediated by these and similar receptors need not necessarily require exogenous hormones. Autocrine stimulation may occur when the tumor cells themselves produce the requisite androgen or estrogen. The ability of the tumor to progress thus becomes independent of exogenous sources of the stimulatory hormone, and the tumor is resistant to hormone antagonist therapies.

Table 4-3

Types of Signal-Transducing Receptors Important in Tumorigenesis

Receptor Category	Prototypical Ligands
Tyrosine kinase (RTK)	EGF, IGF-I, insulin
G-protein–coupled receptor (GPCR)	Prostaglandins, RANTES, SDF-1
Nuclear receptors	Androgens, estrogens, other steroid hormones
Serine/threonine kinases	TGF-β
Kinase-associated receptors	GH, TCR, IL-2
Extracellular matrix receptors	Fibronectin, collagen, laminin

EGF, epidermal growth factor; GH, growth hormone; IGF-I, insulin-like growth factor-1; IL-2, interleukin-2; RANTES, SDF-1, TCR, T-cell receptor; TGF-β, transforming growth factor-β.

GENETIC INSTABILITY IN CANCER

Genomic instability is a key contributor to the multiple changes that lead to cancer. Although not universal in tumors, **chromosomal instability (CI)** entails additions or deletions of entire chromosomes, or portions thereof, to yield variable cellular karyotypes. Typically, about one fourth of alleles are lost in malignancies.

Mechanisms of Altered Activation of Cellular Genes

There are three general mechanisms by which proto-oncogenes become activated:

- A mutation in a proto-oncogene leads to **constitutive production of an abnormal protein**.
- Increased expression of a proto-oncogene causes **overproduction of a normal gene product**.
- Activation or expression of proto-oncogenes is regulated by numerous auto-inhibitory mechanisms that safeguard against inappropriate activity. Many mutations

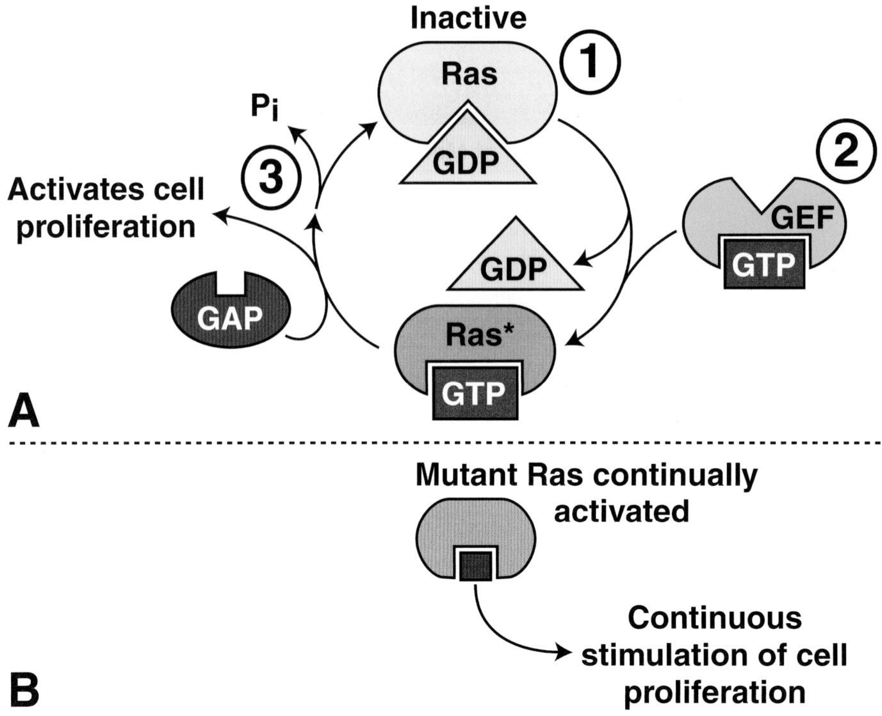

FIGURE 4-16. Mechanism of action of Ras. A (upper). Normal. The Ras protein, $p21^{Ras}$, exists in two conformational states, determined by the binding of either guanosine diphosphate (GDP) or guanosine triphosphate (GTP). (*1*) Normally, most of the $p21^{Ras}$ is in the inactive GDP-bound state. (*2*) An external stimulus, or signal, triggers the exchange of GTP for GDP, an event that converts Ras to the active state. (*3*) Activated $p21^{Ras}$, which is associated with the plasma membrane, binds GTPase-activating protein (GAP) from the cytosol. The binding of GAP has two consequences. In association with other plasma membrane constituents, it initiates the effector response. At the same time, the binding of GAP to Ras GTP stimulates by about 100-fold the intrinsic GTPase activity of Ras, promoting hydrolysis of GTP to GDP and the return of Ras to its inactive state. **B (lower).** Mutated Ras protein is locked into the active GTP-bound state because of an insensitivity of its intrinsic GTPase to GAP or because of a lack of the GTPase activity itself. As a result, the effector response is exaggerated, and the cell is transformed. GEF, guanine nucleotide exchange factor.

in proto-oncogenes render them **insensitive to normal auto-inhibitory and regulatory constraints** and provoke constitutive activation.

Tumor suppressor genes (1) may suffer mutations that increase production of an abnormal protein that either lacks or interferes with tumor suppression; (2) their effectiveness is rendered useless when a regulatory target is overexpressed, overwhelming a normally expressed suppressor; or (3) their expression is impaired, whether by an inactivating mutation or epigenetic inactivation.

Mechanisms of Genetic Instability

Several mechanisms of genetic instability contribute to tumorigenesis. These include (1) point mutations, (2) translocations, (3) amplifications and deletions, (4) loss or gain of whole chromosomes, and (5) epigenetic changes. These types of instability occur in many ways. Among the most important is the loss—whether by inheritance, mutation, or epigenetic inactivation—of proteins that protect the cell from mutations. These include cell-cycle regulatory proteins (checkpoints, mutational error correcting proofreaders, mitosis-related chromosomal sorting proteins, etc.) and proteins that mediate DNA repair functions.

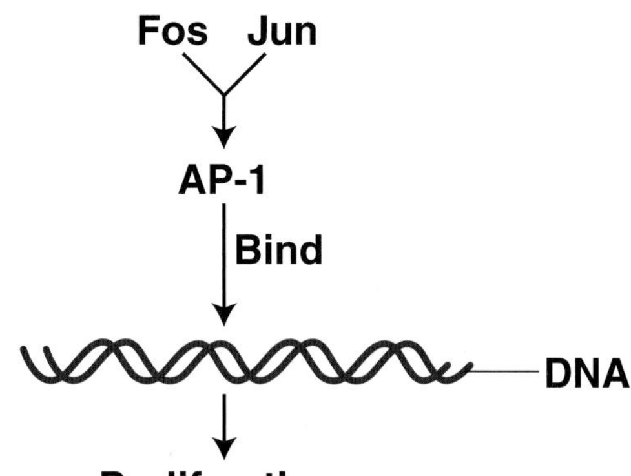

FIGURE 4-17. Activating protein-1 (AP-1) complex. The AP-1 transcription factor complex is formed by the protein products of two proto-oncogenes, Fos and Jun. When these factors form a heterodimer, they bind DNA and direct transcription of genes whose products are involved in cell proliferation, tumor cell invasion and metastasis, angiogenesis, and inhibiting apoptosis.

Defects in DNA Repair Systems

An understanding of how defects in DNA repair contribute to oncogenesis was derived in part from observations made in familial cancer syndromes. For example, a type of colon cancer syndrome, hereditary nonpolyposis colon cancer (HNPCC, Lynch syndrome), entails a 75% lifetime risk for colon cancer. The large majority of HNPCC patients have mutations in DNA mismatch repair enzymes MLH1 or MSH2.

Xeroderma pigmentosum (XP), a hereditary syndrome characterized by enhanced sensitivity to UV light and development of skin cancer, reflects defects in nucleotide excision repair (NER) enzymes. Detection of double-strand breaks (DSBs) and the initiation of repair processes involve the ATM protein. Mutations in ATM and other enzymes involved in DSBs repair are associated with a high frequency of malignant tumors.

Oncogene Activation by Point Mutation

Conversion of proto-oncogenes into oncogenes may involve (1) point mutations, (2) deletions, or (3) chromosomal translocations. The first oncogene identified in a human tumor was activated *HRAS* in a bladder cancer. This gene had only a point mutation in codon 12, which led to the substitution of valine for glycine in the H-ras protein. Subsequent studies of other cancers have revealed point mutations involving other codons of the *ras* gene, suggesting that these positions are critical for the normal function of the ras protein. Since the discovery of mutations in *HRAS*, alterations in other growth-regulatory genes have been described.

Activating, or gain-of-function, mutations in proto-oncogenes are usually somatic rather than germline because germline mutations in proto-oncogenes, which are known to be important regulators of growth during development, are lethal in utero. There are several exceptions to this rule. For example, mutated *c-ret* is incriminated in the pathogenesis of certain heritable endocrine cancers, and *c-met*, which encodes the receptor for hepatocyte growth factor, is associated with a hereditary form of renal cancer.

Oncogene Activation by Chromosomal Translocation

Chromosomal translocation may lead to production of a new, abnormal, protein. A part of one chromosome including part or all of a coding region (e.g., a proto-oncogene) may detach and move to another chromosome, where it now resides adjacent to the coding region of another gene. The result is a new protein, sharing sequence homology with the original ones, but active in driving oncogenesis in a way that the originals are not.

This process has been implicated in the pathogenesis of several human leukemias and lymphomas. The first and still the best-known example of an acquired chromosomal translocation in a human cancer is the **Philadelphia chromosome**, which is found in 95% of patients with chronic myelogenous leukemia (CML; Fig. 4-18). The *c-abl* proto-oncogene on chromosome 9 is translocated to chromosome 22, where it is placed in juxtaposition to a site known as the breakpoint cluster region (*bcr*). The *c-abl* gene and *bcr* region unites to produce a hybrid oncogene that codes for an aberrant protein with high tyrosine kinase activity, thereby generating mitogenic and antiapoptotic signals. The chromosomal translocation that produces the Philadelphia chromosome is an example of oncogene activation by formation of a chimeric (fusion) protein. Inhibition of the resulting abnormal kinase by therapy with imatinib causes long-term remissions in CML.

Amplifications and Deletions

Genetic amplifications are duplications of variably sized regions of chromosomes. These changes not infrequently affect oncogenes or drug resistance genes.

Activation by Gene Amplification

The *ERBB2* proto-oncogene is amplified in up to a third of breast and ovarian cancers. The gene (also called *HER2/neu*) encodes a receptor-type tyrosine kinase that structurally resembles the EGF receptor. Amplification of *ERBB2* in breast and ovarian cancers (Fig. 4-19) is associated with poor overall survival and decreased time to relapse. In this context, an antibody targeted against **HER2/neu** (trastuzumab) is now used as adjunctive therapy for breast cancers that overexpress this protein.

Inactivation by Deletion

Deletions, naturally, are lost chromatin. These can vary from tiny pieces to whole arms of chromosomes. Just as amplifications tend to occur at sites of oncogenes, deletions that come to our attention in cancer cells tend to affect tumor suppressor gene function.

TUMOR SUPPRESSORS

Cells possess complex mechanisms that guard against tumor development. The molecular guardians responsible for this protection are called **tumor suppressors** and the genes that encode them, **tumor suppressor genes (TSGs).** Major activities of tumor suppressors are illustrated in Figure 4-20. If an incipient tumor is to develop successfully, it must generally inactivate one or more TSGs or their products. Such a mutation creates a deficiency of a normal gene product that exerts a negative regulatory control of cell growth and thereby suppresses tumor formation (**"loss of function mutations"**). TSG encode *negative* transcriptional regulators of virtually every process in multistep carcinogenesis, from cell division through invasion and metastasis.

Because both alleles of tumor suppressor genes must be inactivated to produce a deficit that allows the development of a tumor, the normal suppressor gene is functionally dominant. In this circumstance, the heterozygous state is sufficient to protect against cancer. **Loss of heterozygosity** (see above) in a tumor suppressor gene by deletion or somatic mutation of the remaining normal allele predisposes to tumor development.

Suppressor Genes in Carcinogenesis

TSGs are incriminated in the pathogenesis of both hereditary and spontaneous cancers in humans. Two such genes have been particularly well studied. For example, the Rb and p53 gene products serve to restrain cell division in many tissues, and their absence or inactivation is linked to the development of malignant tumors. In this context, oncogenic DNA viruses encode products that interact with these suppressor proteins, thereby inactivating their function. *Thus, the mechanisms underlying the development of some tumors associated with germline and somatic mutations and carcinogenic infections with DNA viruses involve the same gene products.*

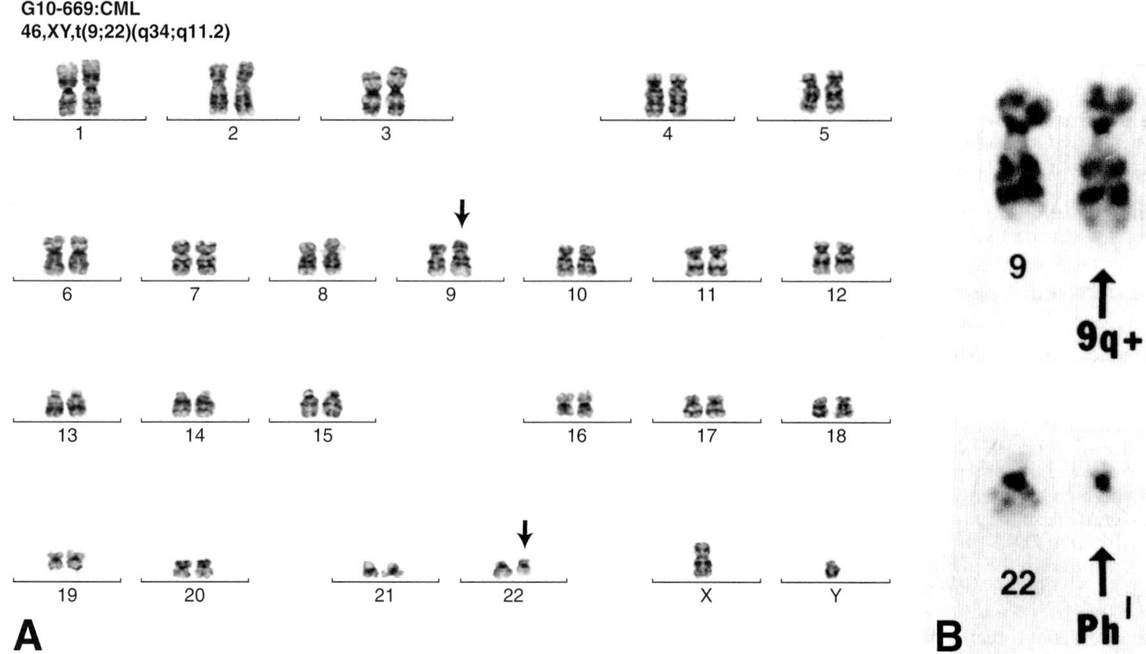

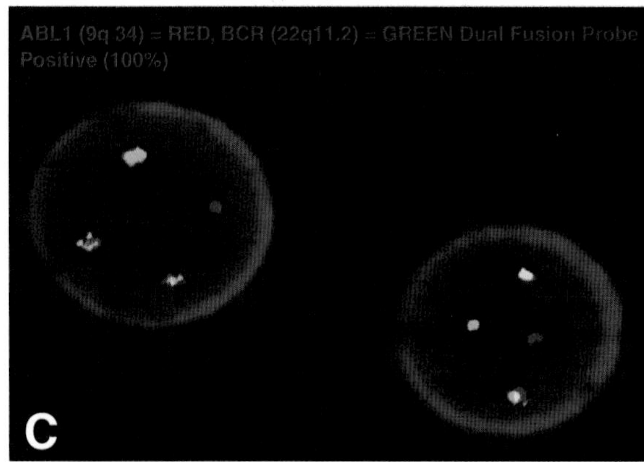

FIGURE 4-18. The t(9;22) translocation in chronic myelogenous leukemia (CML). A. Abnormal karyotype with the shortened chromosome 22 and the longer chromosome 9 highlighted. **B.** Higher magnification of the translocated chromosomes. **C.** Fluorescence in situ hybridization. This assay demonstrates the fusion chromosome using a red ABL chromosome 9 probe and a green BCR chromosome 22 probe, the joining of which yields a yellow signal. Two tumor cells are shown. Each has one normal chromosome 9 and one normal chromosome 22.

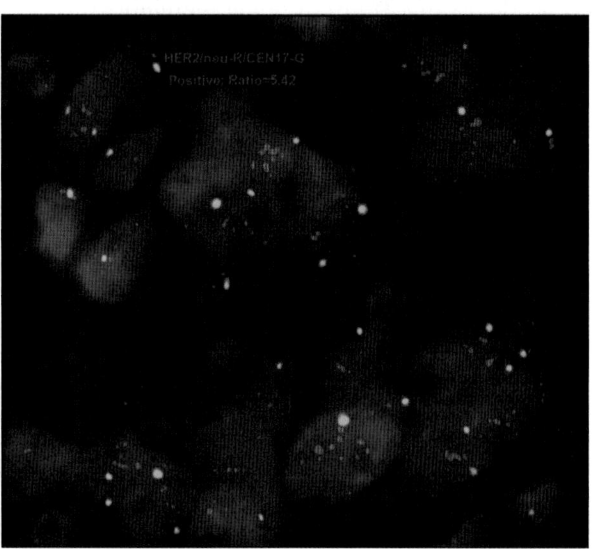

FIGURE 4-19. ***ERBB2*** **amplification in human cancers.** ERBB2 also called HER2/neu amplification in a human breast cancer (fluorescence in situ hybridization), showing the multiple copies (red fluorescence) as minute bodies. As a chromosome control, a green probe for chromosome 17 is shown.

Retinoblastoma Gene

Retinoblastoma, a rare childhood cancer, is the prototype of a human tumor in which the origin is attributed to the inactivation of a specific TSG (Rb) located on the long arm of chromosome 13. About 40% of cases are associated with a germline mutation; the remainder are sporadic. In sporadic cases of retinoblastoma, the child begins life with two normal *Rb* alleles in all somatic cells, but both are inactivated by somatic mutations in the retina. Because somatic mutations in the *Rb* gene are uncommon, the incidence of sporadic retinoblastoma is very low (1/30,000).

In patients with *hereditary* retinoblastoma, all somatic cells carry one missing or mutated allele of the *Rb* gene. This heterozygous state is not associated with any observable changes in the retina because 50% of the *Rb* gene product is sufficient to prevent the development of disease. If the remaining normal *Rb* allele is inactivated by deletion or mutation (loss of heterozygosity), the absence of the Rb gene product allows the development of retinoblastoma, in which both alleles of the *Rb* gene are inactive in **all tumor cells**. Thus, the *Rb* gene exerts a tumor suppressor function, and the development of hereditary retinoblastoma is associated with two genetic events (Knudson's "two-hit" hypothesis) (Fig. 4-21). Children who inherit a mutant *Rb* gene also suffer a 200-fold increased

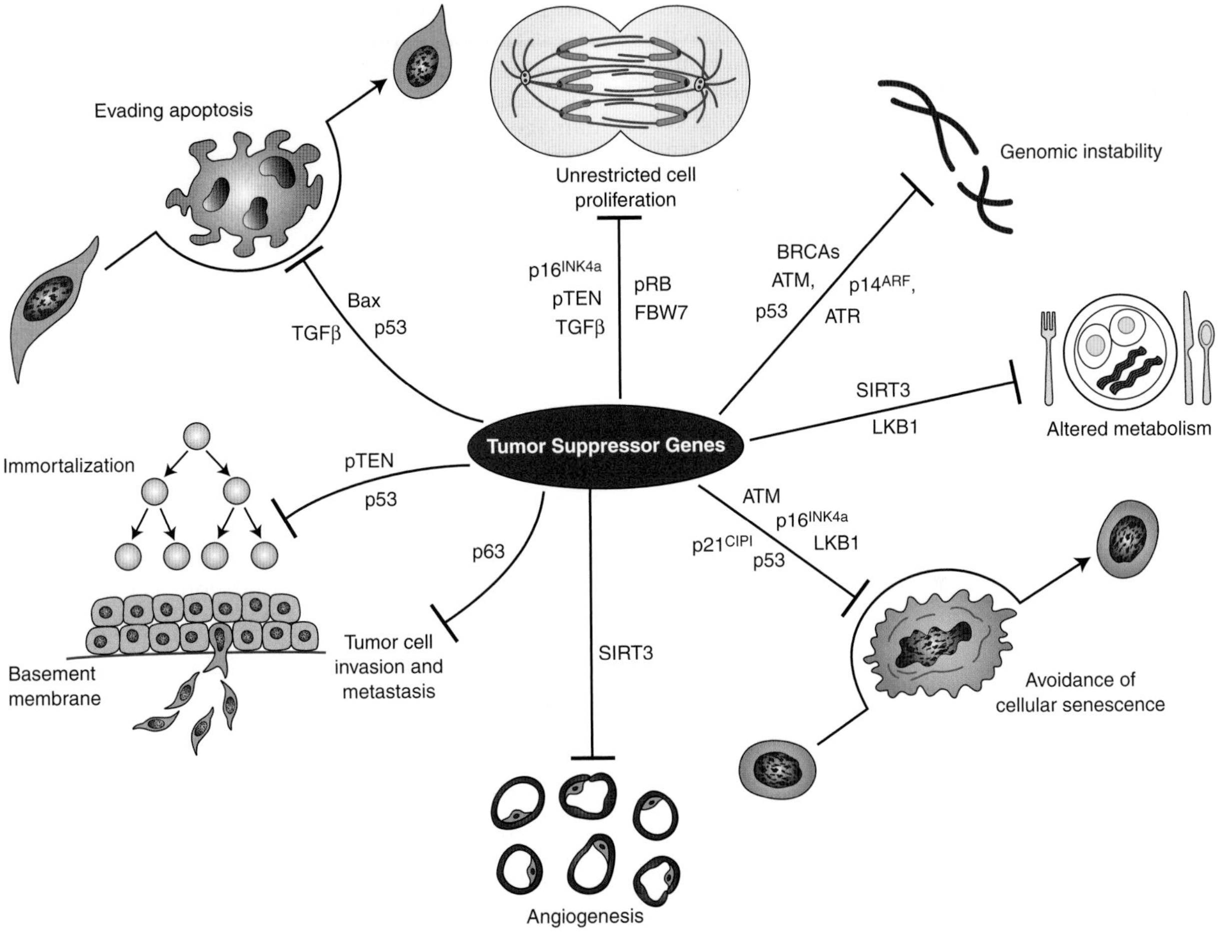

FIGURE 4-20. Tumor-related activities that are targeted by important tumor suppressor genes and representative tumor suppressors involved. The major hallmarks of malignant tumors each is antagonized by multiple tumor suppressor gene products. Those hallmarks, and the tumor suppressor activities that work against them, are illustrated here ATM, ataxia telangiectasia mutated; TGF, transforming growth factor; LKB, liver kinase B; pTEN, phosphatase and tensin homolog; ATR, ataxia telangiectasia and RAD3 related; pRB, RB gene protein.

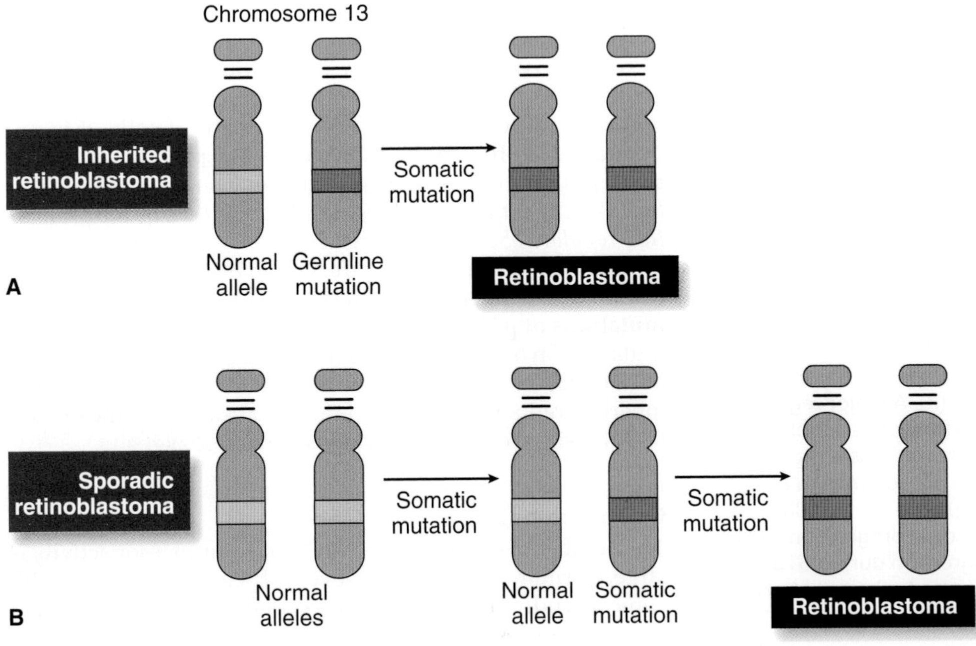

FIGURE 4-21. The "two-hit" origin of retinoblastoma. A. A child with the inherited form of retinoblastoma is born with a germline mutation in one allele of the retinoblastoma gene located on the long arm of chromosome 13. A second somatic mutation in the retina leads to the inactivation of the functioning *Rb* allele and the subsequent development of a retinoblastoma. **B.** In sporadic cases of retinoblastoma, the child is born with two normal *Rb* alleles. It requires two independent somatic mutations to inactivate *Rb* gene function and allow the appearance of a neoplastic clone.

risk of developing mesenchymal tumors in early adult life. More than 20 different cancers have been described, with osteosarcoma being by far the most common. Chromosomal analysis has demonstrated abnormalities of the *Rb* locus in 70% of cases of osteosarcoma and in many instances of small cell lung cancer, carcinomas of the breast, bladder and pancreas, and other human tumors.

Rb genes function at the most critical checkpoint in the cell cycle. **Inactivating** mutations in Rb genes permit unregulated cell proliferation by allowing cells to escape the G_1 restriction (R) checkpoint and proceed to the G_1–S phase transition (Fig. 4-22). In addition, certain products of human DNA viruses (e.g., human papillomavirus [HPV]) inactivate the Rb protein by binding to it, thereby leading to dysregulated cell growth.

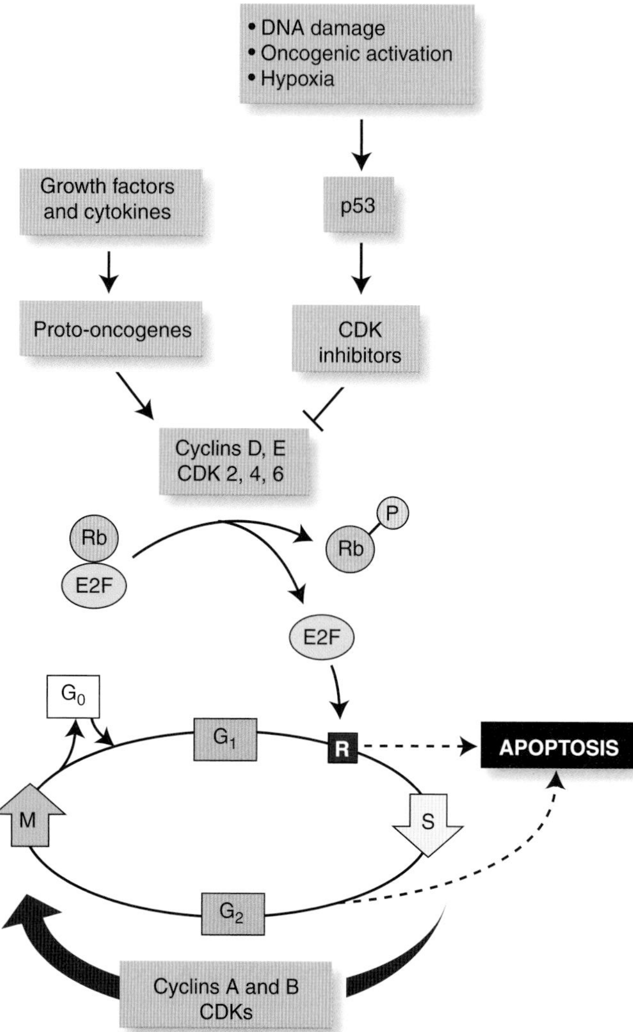

FIGURE 4-22. Regulation of the cell cycle. Cells are stimulated to enter G_1 from G_0 by growth factors and cytokines via proto-oncogene activation. A critical juncture in the transition of cells from G_1 to S phase is the restriction point (R). A major regulatory event in this process is the phosphorylation of retinoblastoma (Rb) by cyclin-dependent kinases (CDKs), which causes the release of the transcriptional activator E2F. CDKs are suppressed by CDK inhibitors (cyclin kinase inhibitors [CKIs]) that are regulated by p53. Tumor suppressor proteins block cell-cycle progression largely within G_1. Interruption of cell-cycle progression during G_1 and G_2 may lead to apoptosis as a default pathway. S, G_2, and M phases are also regulated by cyclins, CDKs and CKIs.

The *p53* Gene Family

The *p53* tumor suppressor gene is a mediator of growth arrest, senescence, and apoptosis. Therefore, loss of its function is, not unexpectedly, associated with cancer. In response to DNA damage, oncogenic activation of other proteins, and other stresses (e.g., hypoxia), p53 levels rise. Increased amounts of p53 enhance the synthesis of cyclin–dependent kinase (CDK) inhibitors resulting in the inactivation of CDK complexes and lead to cell arrest at the G_1/S checkpoint. Hence, cells are prevented from entering the S phase of the cell cycle. Such arrested cells may either repair DNA damage or undergo apoptosis. In addition, stimulation of gene transcription by p53 promotes the synthesis of proteins that enhance DNA repair. In this manner, p53 acts as a "guardian of the genome" by (1) restricting uncontrolled cellular proliferation under circumstances in which cells with abnormal DNA might propagate, (2) eliciting DNA repair (Fig 4-23), and (3) playing a key role in detecting acquired DNA mismatches. Acquired mismatches in DNA bases are detected by *ATM* if they occur in resting cells damaged by, for example, radiation or by *ATR* if they occur during DNA replication. These proteins then activate one of two kinases, Chk2 or Chk1, respectively. The latter phosphorylates p53 (Fig. 4-24), which causes it to dissociate from its inhibitor, MDM2, and thereby activating the p53 damage response.

The *p53* gene is located on the small arm of chromosome 17, and its protein product is present in virtually all normal tissues. This gene is deleted or mutated in 75% of cases of colorectal cancer and frequently in breast cancer, small cell carcinoma of the lung, hepatocellular carcinoma, astrocytoma, and numerous other tumors. *In fact, mutations of p53 seem to be the most common genetic change in human cancer.* Many tumors exhibit deletion of both *p53* alleles, in which case the cell contains no *p53* gene product. By contrast, in some cancers, the malignant cells express one normal *p53* allele and one mutant version. In these instances, the mutant p53 protein forms complexes with the normal p53 protein and that effect inactivates the function of the normal suppressor gene. When a mutant allele inactivates the normal one, the former is said be a **dominant negative** gene. Theoretically, a cell containing one mutant *p53* allele (i.e., a heterozygote) might have a growth advantage over normal cells, a situation that would increase the number of cells at risk for a second p53 mutation (loss of heterozygosity) and the consequent development of cancer. Since p53 is so important in the life and death of cells, it is understandable that both its activity and protein levels are tightly regulated. *Thus, most human cancers display either inactivating mutations of p53 or abnormalities in the proteins that regulate p53 activity* (Fig. 4-24).

***Li-Fraumeni syndrome* refers to an inherited predisposition to develop cancers in many organs owing to germline mutations of p53.** Persons with this condition carry germline mutations in one *p53* allele, but their tumors display mutations at both alleles. This situation is similar to that determining inherited retinoblastoma and is another example of the two-hit hypothesis (see Fig. 4-21) and loss of heterozygosity.

Other Tumor Suppressor Genes

The number of genes that display tumor suppressor activity is large. Germline mutations in several TSGs are associated with clinical syndromes that display a propensity for development of malignancies.

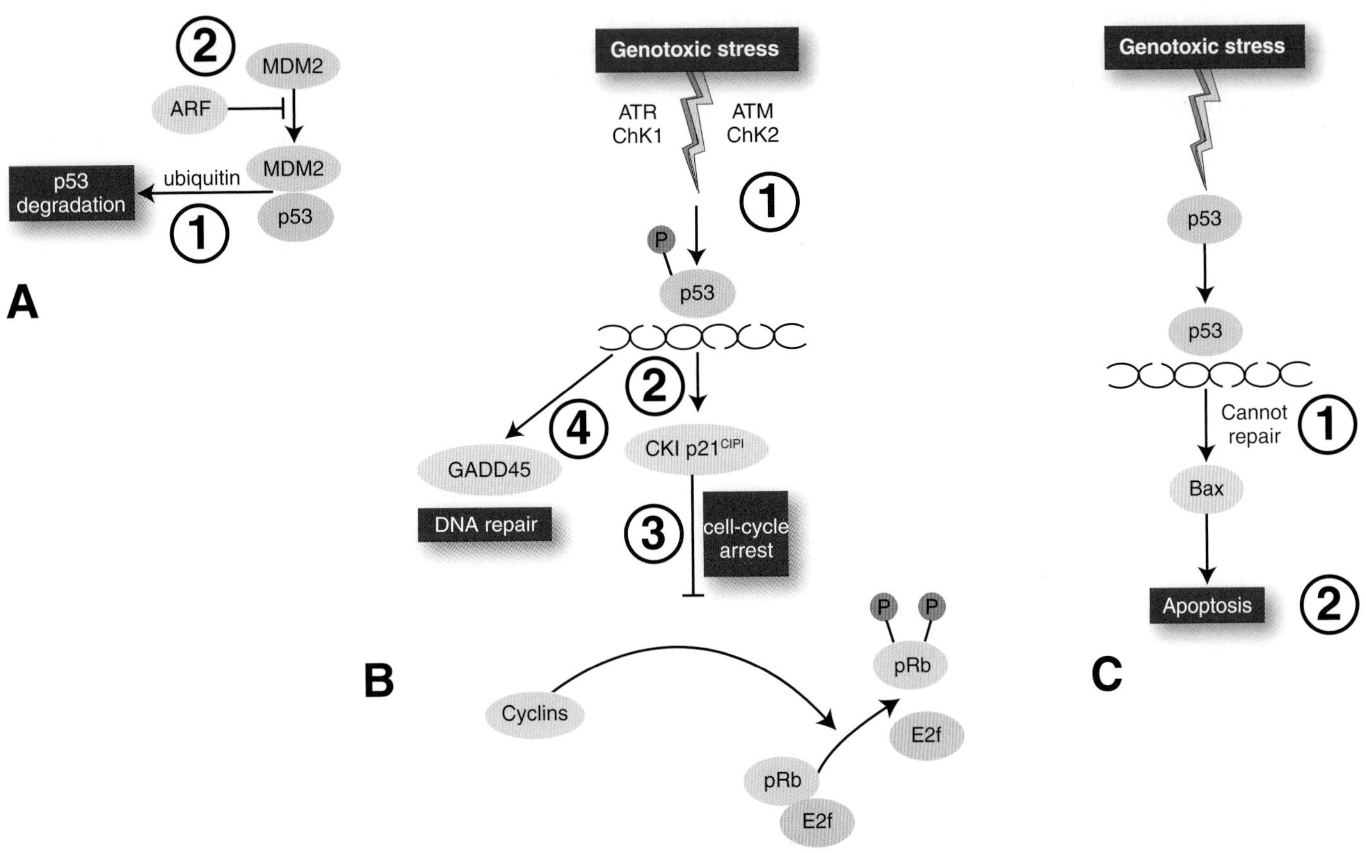

FIGURE 4-23. A. Regulation of p53 and MDM2 (murine double minute). (*1*) MDM2 is an E3 ubiquitin ligase that binds to and directs the inactivation of p53. *2* MDM2 activity is inhibited by the tumor suppress p14ARF. **B.** (*1*) In response to genotoxic stress (e.g., ionizing radiation, carcinogens, mutagens), ATR (ATM and Rad3 related) and ATM (ataxia telangiectasia mutated) increase p53, which does two things. (*2*) It binds to DNA and upregulates transcription of several genes, including cyclin kinase inhibitor (CKI) p21CIP1/WAF1. (*3*) It also induces cell-cycle arrest by preventing release of E2F from retinoblastoma protein (pRB). (*4*) GADD45 promotes DNA repair. **C.** (*1*) Should DNA repair not be possible, p53 directs increased transcription of the proapoptotic protein Bax. (*2*) Increased Bax triggers apoptosis.

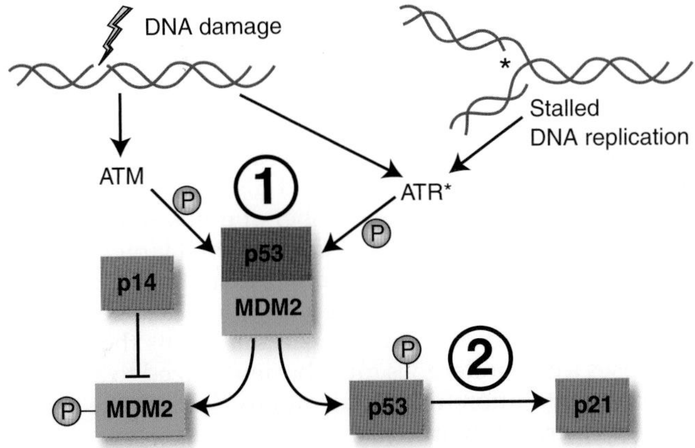

FIGURE 4-24. Linkage of DNA damage and replication stress to cell-cycle arrest, via p53. (*1*) Both DNA damage and other interference with DNA replication activate the kinases ATM (ataxia telangiectasia mutated) and ATR (ATM and Rad3 related). These kinases phosphorylate p53, releasing it from binding to its inhibitor murine double minute (MDM2). (*2*) Activated p53 stimulates p21 (also called p21CIIP1/WAF1).

- ***APC* gene:** This gene is implicated in the pathogenesis of familial adenomatous polyposis coli (APC) and most sporadic colorectal cancers (see Chapter 11). The normal *APC* gene product causes the degradation of β-catenin, an intracellular protein that transmits signals from E-cadherin, a cell surface adhesion protein. β-Catenin upregulates several genes that facilitate cell-cycle progression. Hence, a nonfunctional APC gene product allows excessive cell proliferation. Mutations in both *APC* and β-catenin genes have also been described in other malignant tumors, including malignant melanoma and ovarian cancer.
- ***BRCA1* and *BRCA2*:** *BRCA1* (breast cancer-1) and *BRCA2* are TSGs that encode proteins important in DNA repair. These include correction of DSBs, cell-cycle checkpoint control, and regulation of aspects of mitosis. Germline mutations in these genes create genomic instability in cells of both the breast and ovary. By age 70, women who inherit mutations in *BRCA1* suffer an 80% cumulative risk of breast cancer and a 35% cumulative risk of ovarian cancer. In women who have germline *BRCA2* mutations, the lifetime cumulative risk of breast cancer is 50% and that of ovarian cancer is 10% to 15% (see Chapter 17). The large

majority of women with germline mutations in *BRCA1* or *BRCA2* are heterozygous in their germline, and the breast and ovarian cancers that develop exhibit somatic mutations in the remaining normal allele; resulting in loss of heterozygosity (LOH).

- ***PTEN.*** Phosphatase and tensin homolog (*PTEN*) on chromosome 10 is a potent TSG and after p53 is the second most frequently mutated gene in human cancer. Normal PTEN is essential for the maintenance of chromosomal stability, and its loss causes conspicuous changes in chromosomes. The importance of PTEN lies in its suppression of sporadic (i.e., nonhereditary) tumor development. Monoallelic loss or mutation in *PTEN* is commonly seen in a variety of tumors, including cancers of the brain, breast, colon, lung, and prostate. Homozygous mutations of *PTEN* are also frequent in many tumors, especially endometrial carcinomas and glioblastomas.
- PTEN protein has multiple functions, including effects on response to DNA damage, apoptosis, cell-cycle progression, aging, chemotaxis, and angiogenesis. Normally PTEN dephosphorylates phosphoinositol trisphosphate (PIP3), a lipid-signaling intermediate that activates numerous targets. Inadequate PTEN activity permits PIP3 to accumulate and thereby constitutively activate a variety of signaling pathways. These include the AKT and mTOR pathways (Fig. 4-25), which are involved in cell proliferation and survival and which are key in cancer development.

The resulting activation of these signaling pathways enhances metabolic activity and triggers an increase in cell receptors for glucose and amino acids, thereby adding to their availability for the tumor cell's biosynthetic needs.

- ***NF-1.*** Neurofibromatosis (NF) type 1 is related to germline mutations of the *NF-1* gene, which encodes *neurofibromin*, a negative regulator of *ras*. Inactivation of *NF-1* permits unopposed *ras* function and thus promotes cell growth. Patients with neurofibromatosis-1 are at a substantial risk for the development of neurogenic sarcomas.

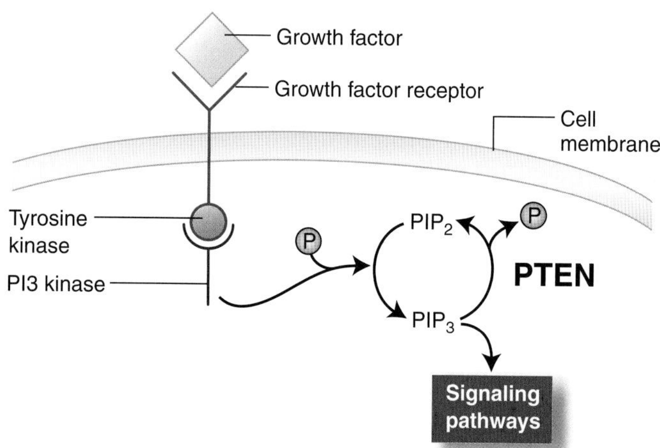

FIGURE 4-25. Signaling function of phosphatase and tensin homolog (PTEN). Normal binding of a growth factor to its receptor leads to phosphorylation of phosphatidylinositol-4,5-bisphosphate (PIP2) to produce the important signaling molecule phosphatidylinositol-3,4,5-trisphosphate (PIP3). The level of PIP3 is regulated by its dephosphorylation by PTEN.

- ***VHL.*** This protein is part of a ubiquitin ligase that targets HIF transcription factors, which are critical in tumor angiogenesis (see above) for degradation. Inactivation of the *VHL* creates a defect in ubiquitin conjugation, giving rise to increased HIF-1α, an angiogenic factor that activates transcription of genes important in cellular responses to low-oxygen environments. These include (1) increases cellular intake of glucose for anaerobic glycolysis, (2) stimulation of angiogenesis, and (3) activation of several critical growth factors.
  - Carcinogenicity associated with the inactivation of VHL is caused in large part by the action of HIF-1α in promoting tumor growth. Interestingly, similar activation of HIF-1α occurs in the oxygen-starved cores of many tumors, even in the absence of *VHL* mutation. In those settings, HIF-1α degradation is impaired by decreased activity of a cofactor for ubiquitination.
  - The normal VHL protein has additional tumor suppressor activities independent of HIF-1α. These include (1) promotion of apoptosis, (2) increased cellular immobilization by adherence to matrix proteins, and (3) repression of certain cell activation responses.

Tumor Suppressors and Senescence

No single paradigm explains all of oncogene-induced senescence. The centrality of the DNA damage response via Rb and p53 is generally accepted, but senescence entails complex signaling (Fig. 4-26) and perturbation of any member of a participating pathway could facilitate development of malignancy.

For example, ongoing telomere shortening in normal cells eventually leads to senescence. Tumor suppressor activities that elicit senescence are critical defenses against oncogenesis. They include components of the DNA damage response system, such as ATM, ATR, Chk 1 and 2, the cell-cycle regulators p53 and Rb, and many others.

ROLE OF CELLULAR SENESCENCE

Senescence is a process that maintains cell viability when a cell can no longer contribute to cell division. Senescent cells are growth arrested and viable but remain unable to proliferate. This state was reported initially in cultured normal human fibroblasts. After a certain number of mitoses (usually 40 to 45), the cells stopped dividing but remained alive. The upper limit of the number of mitoses is called the Hayflick limit, after its original discoverer. It largely reflects the effects of telomere depletion in preventing cell cycling when a cell's telomeres become very short (see below and Chapter 1). Clearly, this mechanism that limits the number of mitoses a cell undergoes must be neutralized to allow for endless proliferation (immortalization). Several effectors of senescence are known:

- **The DNA damage response (DDR):** Because DNA polymerases "fall off" as they approach the ends of chromosomes, telomere lengths decrease with each cell division. Once telomeres have shortened to a certain point, they elicit DDR. DNA damage-sensing proteins activate p53 and cdc25, after which the cell stops dividing, subsequently either the offending DNA damage is corrected or the cell is directed into senescence or apoptosis pathways (Fig. 4-27).

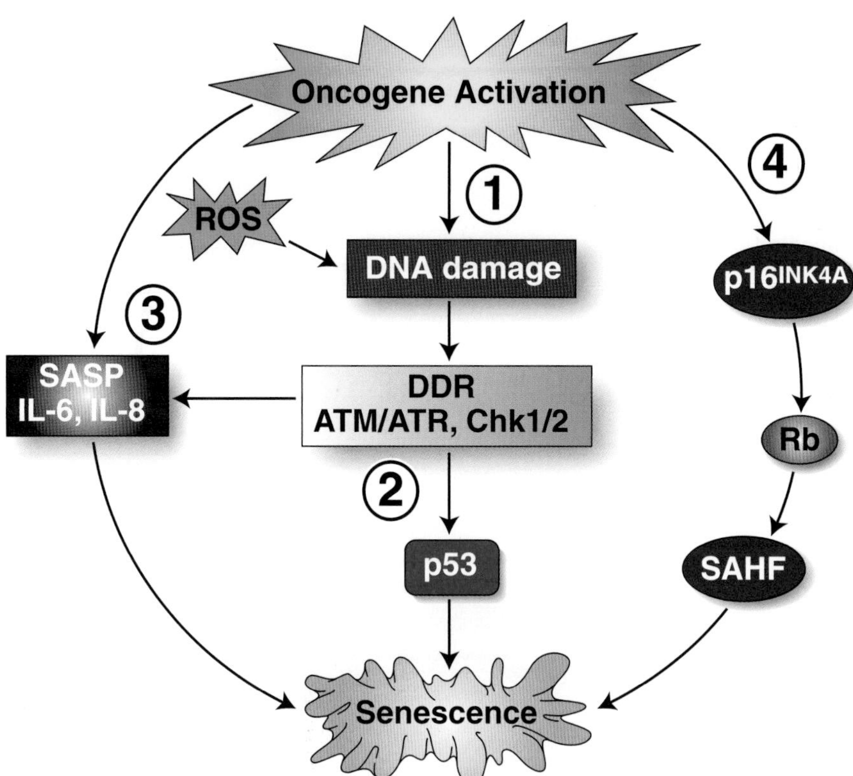

FIGURE 4-26. Oncogene-induced senescence (OIS). Oncogenic stress can elicit cellular responses that eventuate in cellular senescence. (*1*) Excessive cell division, a result of oncogene activation, for example, causes oxidative stress and DNA damage to accumulate. (*2*) As a consequence, the DNA damage response (DDR) is activated, with p53 expression blocking cell-cycle progression. (*3*) The same DDR may also activate the senescence-associated secretory phenotype (SASP), which leads affected cells to secrete cytokines that maintain the senescent state (interleukin-6 [IL-6], IL-8). SASP can also be activated directly by the excessive oncogene activity. (*4*) Oncogene activation may directly activate the tumor suppressor p16^{INK4A}, which in turn activates Rb. This leads to the formation of senescence-associated heterochromatin (SAHF), which restricts expression of cell-cycle drivers.

- **Telomerase activation:** Expression of telomerase allows repair of telomeres and maintenance of genomic stability in the face of continuing cell proliferation. *Telomerase activation permits—but does not directly cause—the emergence of cancer* (Fig. 4-28).
- **Tumor suppressors:** Key among these proteins are p16^{INK4a} and Rb, which induce certain proteins to associate with the cell's DNA. This event results in termination of cell transit through S phase.
- **Cytokines:** Cells secrete factors, including interleukin (IL)-6 and IL-8, that help trigger the senescent phenotype. Together with their receptors, they assist in maintaining the senescence. These cytokines elicit in transcriptional regulation that inhibits cellular proliferation and promotes senescence.

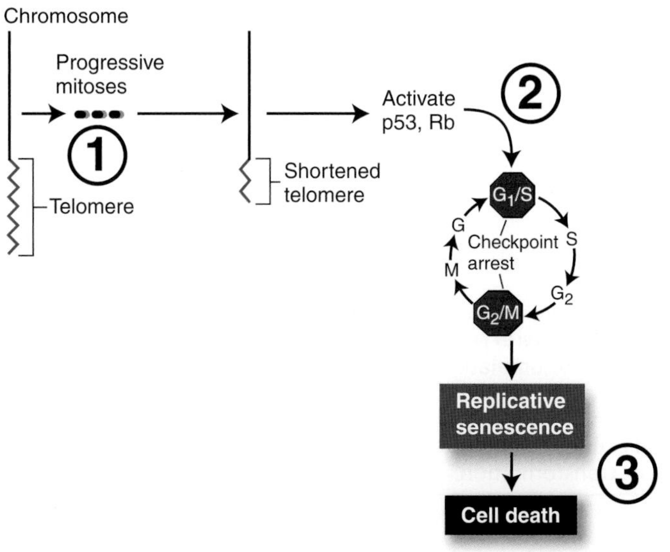

FIGURE 4-27. The sequence of events resulting from DNA instability as a result of telomere shortening and leading to cell death. This sequence occurs when the tumor suppressors p53 and Rb are intact. (*1*) Progressive telomere shortening activates p53 and Rb. (*2*) This leads to cell-cycle arrest at the G_1/S and G_2/M checkpoints. (*3*) Consequent replicative senescence triggers cell death programs.

Programmed Cell Death

The total number of cells in any organ reflects a balance between cell division and cell death. Interference with this intricate equilibrium can incite tumor development. Cell death programs encompass several different pathways (see Chapter 1), dysfunction of which is often a fundamental requirement for tumor development. The best understood of these is apoptosis and its cousin, anoikis.

Apoptosis as an Inhibitor of Cancer

Apoptosis eliminates damaged or abnormal cells. Apoptotic pathways are activated by (1) errors in DNA replication or repair, (2) detected genetic or metabolic instability, (3) loss of anchoring connections to the extracellular matrix (ECM) **(anoikis)**, and (4) other stimuli. Because many triggers for apoptosis are among the attributes of tumor cells, it is not surprising that those cells often evolve mechanisms to disable it. Cancers may avoid PCD by impairing proapoptotic activities and by augmenting prosurvival functions.

There are many known pro- and antiapoptotic proteins that interact. The best known is p53. The gene for this protein, ***TP53***, is mutated in over half of human cancers. This protein is activated when oncogenic danger is sensed, for example, if damage to cellular DNA cannot be repaired

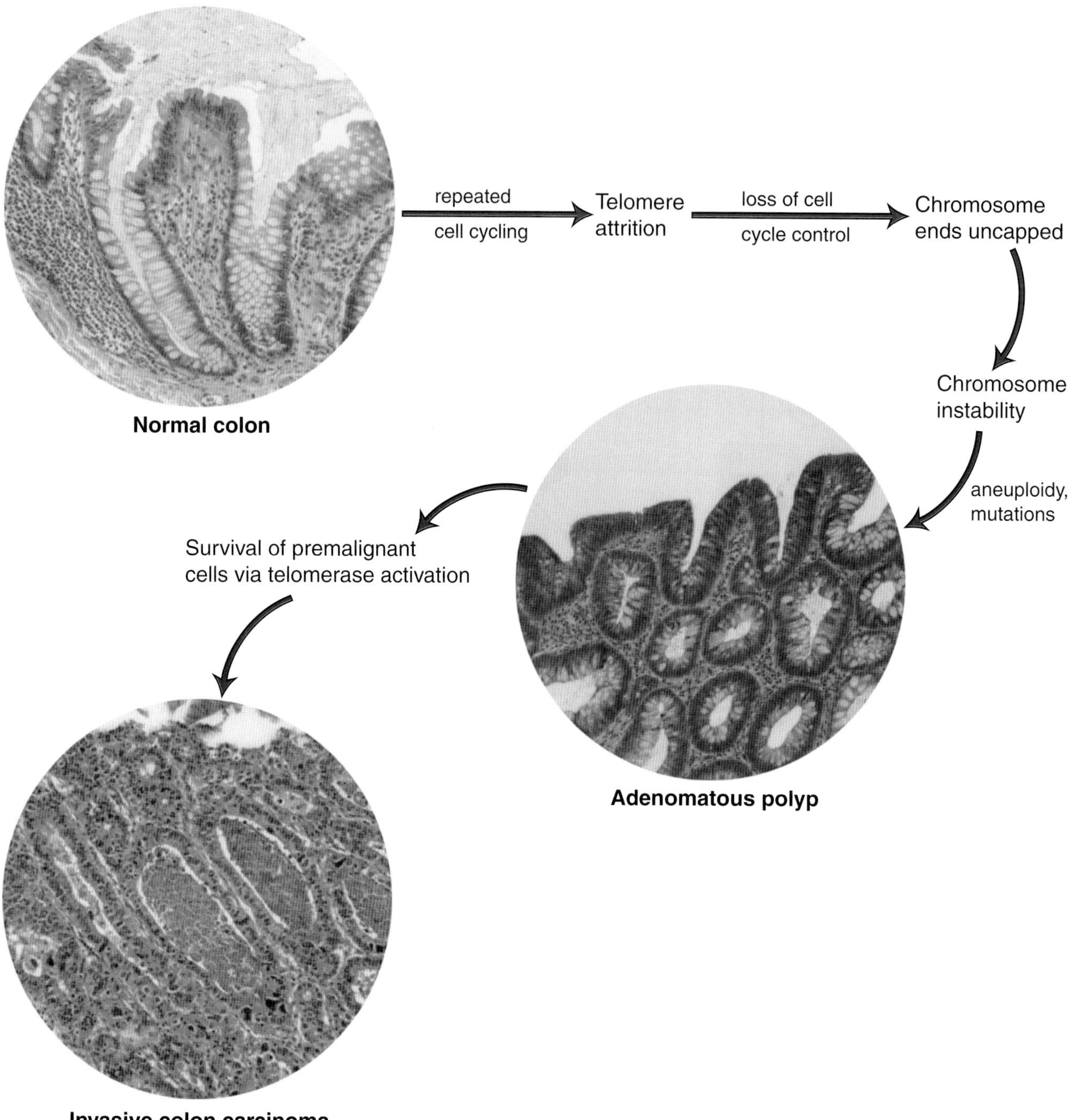

FIGURE 4-28. Role of telomere attrition and subsequent telomere activation in carcinogenesis. Normal colonic mucosa features continuous epithelial renewal, with resulting shortening of telomeres, which leads to uncapping of chromosomal ends. Accumulated DNA damage may impair cell-cycle control, allowing development of a variety of mutations. At first, a benign accumulation of colonic epithelial cells (i.e., a colonic adenomatous polyp [or tubular adenoma; see Chapter 11]) grows. The preservation of abnormal cells by telomerase activation allows further mutation to occur and eventuates in malignant transformation.

(see Chapter 1). Activated p53 upregulates transcription of proapoptotic Bcl-2–like proteins and downregulates their prosurvival cousins.

The prototypical example of the effectiveness of inhibiting apoptosis in human cancer is follicular lymphoma (see Chapter 18) in which the prosurvival (antiapoptosis) protein, Bcl-2, is constitutively activated by a translocation [t(14:8)] that places its expression under the control of the immunoglobulin heavy-chain promoter. As a result, insufficient elimination of excess neoplastic B cells occurs.

EPIGENETIC MECHANISMS AND CANCER

Tumorigenesis and tumor suppression cannot be understood solely in terms of changes in coding DNA sequence. Regulation of the amounts of proteins in cells influences cell behavior at least as profoundly as the DNA sequences that encode those proteins. **Epigenetics** is the umbrella term for the mechanisms that control gene expression, independently of DNA base sequences. The most important epigenetic mechanisms that are involved in neoplasia are listed in Table 4-4.

Environmental Stimuli and Epigenetic Regulators

The epigenome is highly dynamic and responds to modulation by nutrition, stress, pharmacologic and toxic agents, and other influences. For example, identical twins diverge increasingly over time in patterns of DNA methylation. In fact, patterns of CpG methylation of specific genes change over the course of years in any given individual. The ways in which the cellular milieu influences epigenetic regulation are largely obscure. What is known suggests that this impact may be fundamental to the processes by which tumors originate and spread.

DNA Methylation at CpG Islands

The promoters of many genes contain disproportionate concentrations of CpG dinucleotides, called "**CpG islands**." (The *p* represents the interbase phosphodiester bond.) These islands are inhomogeneously distributed in the genome. They predominate in the promoter regions of many genes and in repetitive DNA sequences, particularly transposable elements (see below).

DNA Hypermethylation

Some genes important in oncogenesis are highly susceptible to downregulation by promoter methylation. CpG methylation may also complement mutation. It may complete the inactivation of tumor suppressor gene alleles. Thus, if one allele of the DNA mismatch-repair gene *MLH1* is mutated in a colon cancer, the other is likely to be inactivated by promoter methylation.

Hypomethylation

On average, the DNA of most cancer cells is hypomethylated, compared with their normal tissue counterparts. This occurs in repetitive DNA sequences, as well as in exons and introns of protein-encoding genes. The extent of DNA hypomethylation may increase as oncogenesis advances from a benign proliferation to a malignant tumor. Undermethylation destabilizes DNA structure and favors recombination during mitosis, leading to increased deletions, translocations, chromosomal rearrangements, and aneuploidy, all of which contribute to malignant progression. Decreased methylation of genes associated with cell proliferation may increase transcription of such genes. The same principle applies to latent human tumor viruses (e.g., HPV, Epstein–Barr virus), hypomethylation of which may induce tumor development.

Table 4-4

Major Mechanisms of Epigenetic Regulation That Affect Oncogenesis

Mechanism	Example
Covalent modifications of DNA	CpG methylation
Covalent modifications of histones	Acetylation
Remodeling/repositioning of nucleosomes	Incorporation of histone variants
Small noncoding RNAs	MicroRNAs
Long noncoding RNAs	Pseudogene transcripts

MicroRNAs as Tumor Suppressors

Understanding of the role of miRNAs in oncogenesis grew out of the finding that a specific area of the genome in a B-lymphocytic leukemia (see Chapter 18) tended to be disrupted in the leukemic cells. Surprisingly the affected region did not code for a known protein but for a small RNA species that acted as a tumor suppressor. Loss of that miRNA tumor suppressor was linked to the development of that type of leukemia. *Since then, over 1000 miRNAs have been discovered and functions relating to neoplasia have been ascribed to many of these* (Table 4-5).

Actions of miRNAs

miRNAs may be encoded anywhere in the genome: intergenic DNA, introns, exons, 3′ untranslated regions (UTRs), and so forth. They are usually transcribed by RNA polymerase II (pol II), the same enzyme that transcribes protein-encoding genes. The initial transcripts that will eventually become miRNAs are often long (>1 kb). These are processed to precursor miRNAs about 70 bases long, which are exported (Fig. 4-29) to the cytosol. There, they are processed further and incorporated as single strands, about 22 bases long, into an RNA-induced silencing complex **(RISC)**. RISC includes an enzyme (Argonaute, or Ago) that can cleave target mRNAs.

If the recognition sequence (bases 2–8) of an miRNA matches an mRNA—usually the 3′ UTR—perfectly or nearly perfectly, Ago may degrade the targeted transcript. If miRNA complementarity for an mRNA is imperfect, translation of the latter is blocked without degrading the target. miRNAs are thus promiscuous, and any individual miRNA may regulate many different transcripts.

miRNAs and Cancer

miRNAs are critical controllers of many activities, such as embryogenesis and development, cell cycling, differentiation, apoptosis, and maintaining stem cell pluripotency ("stemness"). They also regulate many steps in oncogenesis.

miRNAs may inhibit tumor suppressor proteins or may themselves act as tumor suppressors. They may also upregulate cell proliferation and so act as oncogenes. In some cases, one miRNA species, or clusters of related species, may promote tumor development in some tissues but suppress it in others. Examples of cancer-related activities for few of the numerous miRNAs are shown in Table 4-5.

Epigenetic Regulators in Cancers

Tumor development, progression, and dissemination all entail extensive disequilibrium at every level of epigenetic activity.

Table 4-5

Examples of MicroRNAs (miRNAs) That Act as Oncogenes, Tumor Suppressors, or Both, and the Tumor Types for Which They Display Those Activities

Oncogenic miRNAs		Tumor Suppressor miRNAs		miRNAs That Act as Both Suppressors and Oncogenes	
miRNA	**Organ**	**miRNA**	**Organ**	**miRNA**	**Organ**
miR-21	Breast, CLL, colorectal, esophagus, glioblastoma, liver, lung, pancreas, prostate	miR-143	Breast, CLL, colorectal, lung, prostate	miR-23 group	Bladder (o), breast (o), CLL (o), prostate (s)
miR-23	Bladder, breast, CLL	let-7group[a]	ALL, breast, CLL colorectal, lung, pancreas	miR-23 group	Bladder (o), breast (o), CLL (o), prostate (s)
miR-221	AML, bladder, CLL, glioblastoma, liver, pancreas, prostate, thyroid	miR-145	Bladder, breast, colorectal, lung, ovary, prostate	miR-181 group	ALL (o), AML (s), breast (o), CLL (s), glioblastoma (s), pancreas (o), prostate (o), thyroid (o)
miR-17–92 cluster[b]	ALL, CML, colorectal, lung, ovary			miR-125 group	ALL (o, s), AML (o), breast (s), glioblastoma (s), liver (s), ovary (s), pancreas (o), prostate (s), thyroid (s)

[a]The let-7 group includes let-7-a-a1 through -a3, -b through -g, -i, and miR-98.
[b]The miR17-92 cluster includes structurally homologous miRs 17-3p, 17-5p, 18a, 19a, 19b-1, 20a, and 92a-1.
ALL, acute lymphoblastic leukemia; AML, acute myeloblastic leukemia; CLL, chronic lymphocytic leukemia; CML, chronic myeloid leukemia.

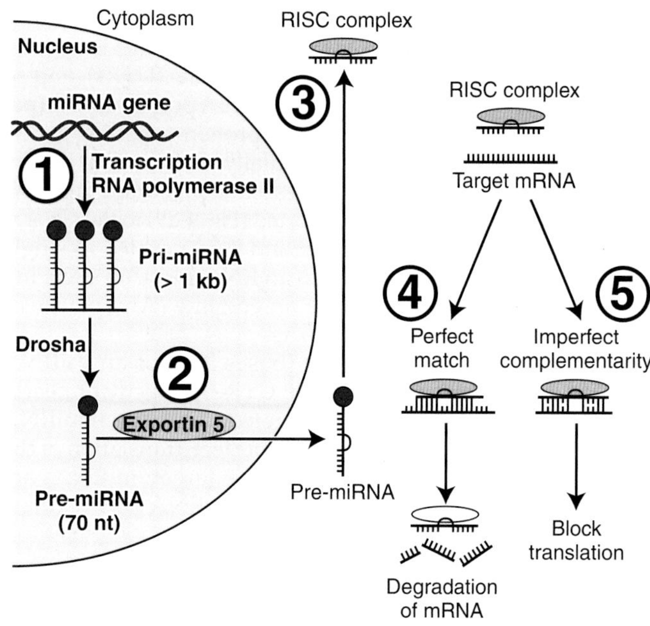

FIGURE 4-29. Production, modification, and activities of microRNAs (miRNAs). (*1*) Most miRNAs are transcribed by RNA polymerase II, the same enzyme that transcribes messenger RNAs (mRNAs) for protein production. (*2*) However, the original transcript, which is often more than 1 kb in length, is processed by an enzyme, Drosha, to a shorter form, which is called a pre-miRNA. (*3*) This form is exported from the nucleus. In the cytosol, it joins an RNA-induced silencing complex (RISC), where the pre-miRNA is tailored further to the final miRNA by an enzyme called Dicer. A member of this complex, a protein called Argonaute, or Ago, can cleave targeted mRNAs. The nature of the effect of miRNAs depends on the extent of complementarity with a particular mRNA. (*4*) If the nucleotides 2–8 of the miRNA align with the 3′-untranslated region of a target perfectly, the target is digested and degraded. (*5*) If, on the other hand, the complementarity is imperfect, the miRNA inhibits translation of the target mRNA.

For example, a transcriptional activating function may be overactive in a tumor and so upregulate an oncogene, but the same function may be blocked with respect to a tumor suppressor in the same cancer. Epigenetic processes in addition to miRNA include the following:

- **DNA methylation:** As noted above, cancer cell genomes are generally hypomethylated. This causes general genomic instability and extensive derepression of transcription of many genes, especially oncogenes. At the same time, site-specific hypermethylation (e.g., of tumor suppressor genes) also characterizes cancers.
- **Histone modifications:** Many tumors show a general loss of histone acetylation, especially associated with silencing of TSGs. Histone deacetylase (HDAC) overexpression is common in cancers, a phenomenon that has stimulated development of therapeutic HDAC inhibitors. However, histone acetylases (HACs) are also often abnormal in cancers, and it is the specific interplay of both HACs and HDACs relative to tumor suppressor genes and oncogenes that determines the result—which genes are activated and which are repressed. Other types of histone-modifying enzymes, such as the methylating enzyme EZH2, are also often involved in silencing tumor suppressor genes.
- **Nucleosome positioning:** Altered chromatin structure in cancer accompanies changes in DNA methylation and histone derivatives. Thus, nucleosome localization in tumor cells differs from that in their nonmalignant cellular counterparts.
- **Noncoding RNAs:** Levels of specific noncoding RNAs, both short and long noncoding RNA species, in cancer differ greatly from those in normal cells. About 3% of the human genome encodes proteins, but over 90% of the human genome is actively transcribed. Many DNA sequence changes associated with cancer and other diseases occur within the regions that encode these untranslated RNAs.

The Role of the Immune System in Carcinogenesis

The notion that the immune system plays a role in suppressing tumor development is rooted in the concept of tumors as non-self-entities, with unique "tumor-specific antigens" that can elicit protective immunologic responses. This principle has been extensively demonstrated in experimental animals.

People with immune deficiencies, such as patients with AIDS, are also more prone to cancers than are immunocompetent persons. However, the tumors that develop in this setting bear little resemblance to most human cancers. The tumors that occur in immunocompromised humans and animals are almost always virus induced and, again, dissimilar to the tumors that normally afflict people (e.g., lung, colon) that are not connected to infectious agents. The immune deficits in such cases can be seen as defects in viral clearance rather than as antitumor surveillance or defense mechanisms. Recent evidence based on therapeutic trials suggest that natural immune checkpoints, which are normally presumed to prevent autoimmune reactivity, prevent immune response to many cancers.

Tumor Antigens

Most human cancers reflect somatic mutations that may theoretically produce mutant proteins, which in turn can serve as targets of the immune system. In addition, normal proteins may be overexpressed, and posttranslational modifications of normal proteins may produce altered antigens. Tumor antigens that are not associated with oncogenic viruses may be categorized as follows:

- **Tumor-specific antigens (TSAs):** These represent products of somatic mutations or alterations in protein (and other) processing, unique to tumors.
- **Tumor-associated antigens (TAAs):** These reflect the production of normal proteins, either in excess or in a setting different from their normal expression.

Tumor-Specific Antigens

Most tumor-related mutations occur in intracellular proteins, which could theoretically offer immunologic targets. However, most TSAs tend to be specific for individual patients' tumors, and not for tumor types, making immunologic targeting for therapy complicated and highly personalized. Nevertheless, because TSAs are expressed only by the cancer cells and not in normal tissues, there should be no preexisting immune tolerance to them and they are theoretically candidates for tumor immunotherapy.

Tumor-Associated Antigens

TAAs are molecules that are shared between cancer cells and normal cells and include the following:

- **Differentiation antigens:** These molecules are seen on normal cells of the same derivation as the cancer cells. As an example, CD20, which is a normal B-cell differentiation antigen, is expressed by some lymphomas, and anti-CD20 antibody (rituximab) is effective treatment for such tumors.
- **Oncofetal antigens:** These antigens are made by normal embryonic and fetal structures and by several cancers (e.g., carcinoembryonic antigen, α-fetoprotein).
- **Overexpressed antigens:** These are normal proteins that are overproduced in certain malignant cells (e.g., prostate-specific antigen, HER2/neu).

Because TAAs represent a class of antigens that is principally recognized as "self" by the immune system, and so have elicited tolerance, they do not lead to effective immunologic responses.

To date, the evidence for natural control of neoplasia by immunologically mediated mechanisms (immune surveillance) in humans is scanty. The potential development of effective cancer immunotherapy is complicated by tumor mechanisms that evade immunologic destruction. Among escape routes from immune attack are production of immunosuppressive cytokines, resistance to lysis by cytotoxic lymphocytes, inhibition of apoptotic signaling, and changes in antigenic profiles.

Various homeostatic mechanisms in the immune system suppress T-cell reactivity against self-components. Such "immune checkpoints" presumably protect against inappropriate autoimmune reactivity but also prevent T-cell–mediated reactions against some neoplasms. Immune checkpoint inhibitors, which are monoclonal antibodies that interfere with such checkpoint function, have proven useful in cancer therapy.

CHEMICAL CARCINOGENS

Many compounds known to be potent carcinogens are relatively inert in terms of chemical reactivity because most, although not all, chemical carcinogens require metabolic activation before they can react with cell constituents. For this reason, tests of chemicals for mutagenicity are carried out in cellular systems. Initially, a culture of *Salmonella* bacteria was used (the Ames test). Cultured human cells are now increasingly used for assays of mutagenicity. At least 90% of known carcinogens are mutagenic in these systems. Moreover, most, but not all, mutagens are carcinogenic. This close correlation between carcinogenicity and mutagenicity presumably occurs because both reflect damage to DNA. Although not infallible, in vitro mutagenicity assays have proved to be valuable tools in screening for the carcinogenic potential of chemicals. Chemical carcinogenesis needs both the mutagen and also a proliferative stimulus in the form of a second, noncarcinogenic, irritating chemical. In experimental models of chemical carcinogenesis, the first effect is called **initiation**. The action of the second noncarcinogenic irritant chemical is termed **promotion**. *Thus, chemical carcinogenesis is a multistep process that ultimately involves numerous mutations.*

Metabolic Activation of Carcinogens

The International Agency for Research in Cancer (IARC) has listed about 75 chemicals as human carcinogens. Most of these chemicals cause cancer after metabolic activation. The direct-acting carcinogens are inherently reactive enough to bind covalently to cellular macromolecules. A number of organic compounds, such as nitrogen mustard, *bis*(chloromethyl) ether, and benzyl chloride, as well as certain metals are included in this category. Most organic carcinogens, however, require conversion to an ultimate, more reactive compound. This conversion is enzymatic and, for the most part, is effected by the cellular systems involved in drug metabolism and detoxification. Many cells in the body, particularly liver cells, possess enzyme systems that can convert procarcinogens to their active forms. Yet each carcinogen usually has its own spectrum of target tissues, sometimes limited to a single organ, as noted for several well-understood chemical carcinogens:

- **Polycyclic aromatic hydrocarbons**: Originally derived from coal tar, these are among the most extensively studied carcinogens. These compounds have a broad range of target organs. The specific type of cancer produced varies with the route of administration and includes tumors of the skin, soft tissues, and breast. Polycyclic hydrocarbons have been identified in cigarette smoke; it has been suggested, but not proved, that they are involved in the production of lung cancer. Polycyclic hydrocarbons are metabolized by cytochrome P450–dependent mixed function oxidases to electrophilic epoxides, which in turn react with proteins and nucleic acids.
- **Alkylating agents:** These agents are often used as chemotherapeutic drugs (e.g., cyclophosphamide, cisplatin, busulfan) that transfer alkyl groups (e.g., methyl, ethyl) to macromolecules, including guanines within DNA. Although such drugs destroy cancer cells by damaging DNA, they also injure normal cells. Thus, alkylating chemotherapy carries a significant risk for the appearance of solid and hematologic malignancies at a later time.
- **Aflatoxin:** Aflatoxin B_1 is a natural product of the fungus *Aspergillus flavus.* Like the polycyclic aromatic hydrocarbons, aflatoxin B_1 is metabolized to an epoxide, which can bind covalently to DNA. Aflatoxin B_1 is among the most potent liver carcinogens recognized, producing tumors in fish, birds, rodents, and primates. Since *Aspergillus* sp. are ubiquitous, contamination of vegetable foods exposed to the warm and moist conditions, particularly peanuts and grains, may result in the formation of significant amounts of aflatoxin B_1. The agent results in liver tumors, which exhibit a specific inactivating mutation in the *p53* gene (G:C→T:A transversion at codon 249).
- **Aromatic amines and azo dyes:** Aromatic amines and azo dyes commonly produce bladder and liver tumors, respectively, when fed to experimental animals. Both aromatic amines and azo dyes are primarily metabolized in the liver. Occupational exposure to aromatic amines in the form of aniline dyes has resulted in bladder cancer.
- **Nitrosamines:** These are a subject of considerable study because it is suspected that they may play a role in human GI neoplasms and possibly other cancers. The simplest nitrosamine, dimethylnitrosamine, produces kidney and liver tumors in rodents, although unambiguous evidence of cancer induction in humans is lacking. However, the extremely high incidence of esophageal carcinoma in the Hunan province of China (100 times higher than in other areas) has been correlated with the high nitrosamine content of the diet. Nitrosamines may also be implicated in other GI cancers because nitrites, commonly added to preserve processed meats and other foods, may react with other dietary components to form nitrosamines.
- **Metals:** A number of metals or metal compounds can induce cancer, often by inhalation, but the carcinogenic mechanisms are unknown. Most metal-induced cancers occur in occupational settings.

PHYSICAL CARCINOGENESIS

Ultraviolet Radiation and Skin Cancers

The popular tanned complexion has been accompanied not only by cosmetic deterioration of facial skin but also by an increased incidence of the major skin cancers.

Cancers attributed to sun exposure, namely, basal cell carcinoma, squamous carcinoma, and melanoma, occur predominantly in people of the white race. The skin of people of the darker races is protected by the increased concentration of melanin pigment, which absorbs UV radiation.

It appears that only certain portions of the UV spectrum are associated with tissue damage, and a carcinogenic effect occurs at wavelengths between 290 and 320 nm. *The effects of UV radiation on cells include enzyme inactivation, inhibition of cell division, mutagenesis, cell death, and cancer.* The most important biochemical effect of UV radiation is the formation of **pyrimidine dimers** in DNA, a type of DNA damage that is not seen with any other carcinogen. Unless efficiently eliminated by the nucleotide excision repair pathway, genomic injury produced by UV radiation is mutagenic and carcinogenic. **Xeroderma pigmentosum** is a rare autosomal recessive disease demonstrating extreme sensitivity to sunlight. It is accompanied by a high incidence of skin cancers, including basal cell carcinoma, squamous cell carcinoma, and melanoma. Both the neoplastic and nonneoplastic disorders of the skin in xeroderma pigmentosum are attributed to an impairment in the excision of UV-damaged DNA.

Relationship of Radiation and Cancer

The evidence that radiation can lead to cancer is incontrovertible and comes from many sources (Fig. 4-30). Early examples of cancer produced by radiation include the experience of early radiologists who developed squamous cell cancer of the hand and osteosarcoma occurred among workers who painted radium-containing material onto watches to create luminous dials. Another example of occupational exposure to a radioactive element is the high rate of lung cancer in uranium miners who inhaled radioactive dust and radon gas.

Iodine is concentrated by the thyroid. If radioactive iodine isotopes are inhaled or ingested, that gland will experience highly concentrated exposure to radioactivity. An explosive increase in the incidence of thyroid cancer among children in geographical areas contaminated by the nuclear catastrophe at Chernobyl in Ukraine in 1986 has been linked to the release of radioactive iodine isotopes in that incident.

The risk of **solid tumors,** especially breast cancer, is particularly high among adult women who were treated with thoracic radiation for Hodgkin disease as children. Long-term survivors of childhood Hodgkin disease, who were treated with radiation therapy, have almost a 20-fold increased risk of developing a second neoplasm. Thorium dioxide (Thorotrast), a material avidly ingested by phagocytic cells, was used a few decades ago for radionuclide imaging. The persistence in the liver of a long-lived radioisotope resulted in the development of hepatic angiosarcomas.

The survivors of the nuclear bomb explosions in Japan suffered from a number of cancers. They exhibited a more than 10-fold increase in the incidence of leukemia, which peaked 5 to 10 years after exposure and then declined to background

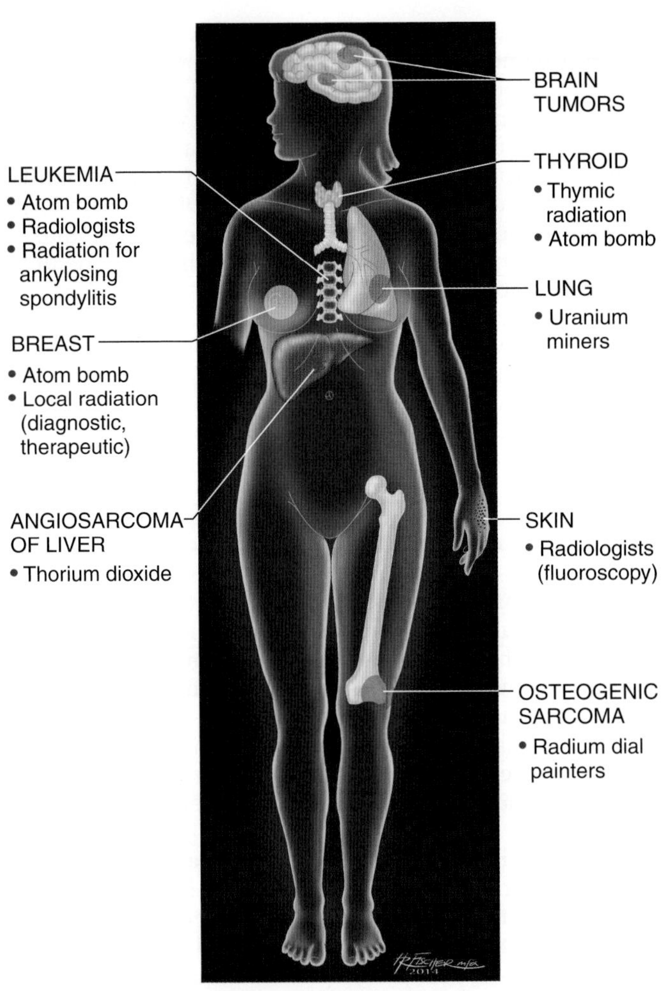

FIGURE 4-30. **Radiation-induced cancers.**

rates. Two thirds were cases of acute leukemia; the remainder were chronic myelogenous leukemia. The frequency of solid tumors, although not as great as that for leukemia, was clearly increased for the breast, lung, thyroid, GI tract, and urinary tract. The incidence of malignant tumors showed a dose–response relationship.

Low-level Radiation and Cancer

Studies demonstrate that the risk of developing cancer at low radiation doses are very low but not zero. Although DNA damage appears to occur proportionately to the dose of gamma radiation, there is considerable uncertainty as to the extent to which DNA repair mechanisms may be protective at low radiation doses or dose rates.

Radon

The finding that some homes in the United States are contaminated with radon has elicited considerable public concern. Radon is a radioactive gas derived from the decay of uranium 238 (^{238}U), which is found in soil and rock formations. Although radon is itself inert, its decay products include radioactive isotopes of bismuth, lead, and polonium, which are chemically active and which bind to particulates and lung tissues. Recent large-scale studies report that people who dwell in homes containing high concentrations of radon gas have an increased risk of developing lung cancer. The risk is by far the greatest for smokers, but it is said to be present in nonsmokers.

Asbestos Exposure and Mesothelioma

Pulmonary asbestosis and asbestosis-associated cancer are discussed in Chapter 10.

Dietary Influences on Cancer

Numerous epidemiologic studies have attempted to identify possible relationships between dietary factors and the occurrence of a variety of cancers. Such investigations have particularly emphasized the roles of dietary fats, red meat, and fiber. The results of studies comparing different ethnic groups or societies across international borders have often not been accepted as accurate and in fact have sometimes yielded misleading conclusions. Prospective cohort studies comparing like populations are usually more reliable. Some such cohort studies have indicated correlations between consumption of animal (but not vegetable) fat and an increased risk of breast cancer. This relationship was limited to premenopausal women, and there is a suggestion that nonlipid components of food containing animal fats may be involved. Despite claims that eating fruits and vegetables helps to prevent cancer, there is little evidence that these dietary constituents protect from tumor development. Although there is a popular notion that high intake and blood concentrations of vitamin D may be associated with a lower incidence of some cancers, a recent review indicates that this is not the case. Obesity itself, without identification of particular dietary constituents, has been linked to an increased risk for some cancers, including acute myeloid leukemia. In conclusion, the beneficial effects of dietary constituents on cancer risk are at best limited and are often controversial. The consequences of a specific type of diet on longevity are largely limited to reduced cardiovascular disease.

VIRUSES AND HUMAN CANCER

Only a few viruses demonstrably cause human cancers; viral infections are responsible for an estimated 15% of human cancers. The strongest associations between specific viruses and tumors in humans involve the following:

- Human T-cell leukemia virus type I (HTLV-I; RNA retrovirus) and T-cell leukemia/lymphoma
- Hepatitis B virus (HBV; DNA virus) and hepatitis C virus (HCV; RNA virus) and primary hepatocellular carcinoma
- Human papilloma virus (HPV; DNA virus) squamous carcinomas of the cervix, anus and vulva, and some oropharyngeal cancers
- Epstein–Barr virus (EBV; DNA virus) and certain forms of lymphoma and nasopharyngeal carcinoma
- Human herpes virus 8 (HHV8; DNA virus) and Kaposi sarcoma

Worldwide, infections with hepatitis B and C viruses and HPVs alone account for 80% of all virus-associated human cancers.

Human T-Cell Leukemia Virus

The one human cancer that has been firmly linked to infection with an RNA retrovirus is the rare adult T-cell leukemia, which is endemic in southern Japan and the Caribbean basin and occurs sporadically elsewhere. The etiologic agent, HTLV-I, is tropic for $CD4^+$ T lymphocytes and has also been incriminated in the pathogenesis of a number of neurologic disorders. It is estimated that leukemia develops in 3% to 5% of people infected with HTLV-I, and then only after a latency period of 30 to 50 years. A closely related virus, HTLV-II, has been associated with only a few cases of lymphoproliferative disorders.

The HTLV-I genome contains no known oncogene and does not integrate at specific sites in the host DNA. Viral oncogenicity appears to be mediated mainly by the viral transcriptional activator Tax. This protein not only drives transcription of the viral genome but also promotes the activity of other genes involved in cell proliferation, such as NFκB and IL-2 receptor. Tax also downregulates a cell-cycle control protein, $p16^{INK4a}$, and p53. Lymphocyte transformation in vitro by HTLV-I is initially polyclonal and only later monoclonal. Tax therefore probably initiates transformation, but additional genetic events are required for the complete malignant phenotype.

Hepatitis B and C Viruses

Epidemiologic studies have established a strong link between primary hepatocellular carcinoma and chronic infection with HBV, a DNA virus, and HCV, an RNA virus (see Chapter 12). Two mechanisms have been invoked to explain the mechanism of carcinogenesis in virus-related liver cancer. One theory holds that the inability of some people to clear these infections leads to continued hepatocyte proliferation, owing to ongoing liver injury, a situation that eventuates in malignant transformation. However, a small subset of patients with HBV infection develop hepatocellular carcinomas in noncirrhotic livers. A second theory implicates a virally encoded protein, HBx, in the pathogenesis of HBV-induced liver cancer. The *HBx* gene product upregulates a number of cellular genes. It also binds to and inactivates p53. The underlying mechanisms in HBV-induced carcinogenesis are still controversial and require further investigation.

It has not been shown that HCV is directly oncogenic. Tumors, when they develop in HCV-infected patients, tend to do so 20 or more years after primary infection, and then usually in the context of cirrhosis and chronic liver injury. However, some data suggest that expression of HCV core protein may contribute to the pathogenesis of hepatocellular carcinoma, and one of the HCV nonstructural proteins activates NFκB.

Proteins Encoded by DNA Viruses

Four DNA viruses (HPV, EBV, HBV, HHV8) are incriminated in human cancers. The transforming genes of oncogenic DNA viruses exhibit virtually no homology with cellular genes. However, the viruses have genes that encode protein products that bind to and inactivate the products of tumor suppressor genes (e.g., *Rb*, *p53*).

Human Papilloma Virus

HPVs induce lesions in humans that progress to squamous cell carcinoma. They manifest a pronounced tropism for epithelial tissues, and their full productive life cycle occurs only in squamous cells. More than 140 distinct HPVs have been identified, and most are associated with benign lesions of squamous epithelium, including warts, laryngeal papillomas, and condylomata acuminata (genital warts) of the vulva, penis, and perianal region. Occasionally, condylomata acuminata and laryngeal papillomas undergo malignant transformation to squamous cell carcinoma. At least 20 HPV types are associated with cancer of the uterine cervix, especially HPV types 16 and 18 (see Chapter 16). The major oncoproteins encoded by HPV are E5, E6, and E7. E6 binds to p53 and targets it for degradation. It also activates telomerase expression and promotes tumor development via other mechanisms that are independent of p53. E7 binds to Rb, thereby releasing its inhibitory effect on E2F transcriptional activity and allowing cell-cycle progression.

Epstein–Barr Virus

EBV is a human herpesvirus that is so widely disseminated that 95% of adults in the world have antibodies to it. The agent infects B lymphocytes, transforming them into lymphoblasts. In a small proportion of primary infections with EBV, this lymphoblastoid transformation is manifested as infectious mononucleosis, a short-lived benign lymphoproliferative disease. However, EBV is also intimately associated with the development of certain human cancers. A number of EBV genes are implicated in lymphocyte immortalization, including (1) Epstein–Barr nuclear antigens (EBNAs); (2) certain untranslated nuclear EBV RNAs, called EBER1 and EBER2; and (3) latency-associated membrane proteins (LMPs). About 40 miRNAs are also encoded by EBV, some of which activate or repress specific cellular genes.

Burkitt Lymphoma

EBV was the first virus to be unequivocally linked to the development of a human tumor. African Burkitt lymphoma (BL) is a B-cell tumor, in which the neoplastic lymphocytes invariably contain EBV and its related antigens (see Chapter 18). The tumor has also been recognized in non-African populations, but in those cases only about 20% carry EBV genomes. The localization of BL to equatorial Africa is not understood, but prolonged stimulation of the immune system by endemic malaria may be important. Therefore, the multistep pathogenesis of African BL may be viewed as follows:

1. Infection and polyclonal lymphoblastoid transformation of B cells by EBV
2. Proliferation of B cells and inhibition of suppressor T cells induced by malaria
3. Deregulation of *c-myc* by translocation in a single transformed B cell, with effects on other signaling pathways
4. Uncontrolled proliferation of a malignant clone of B lymphocytes

Other EBV-Associated Tumors

EBV markers have been identified in about half of cases of classical Hodgkin lymphoma, in which the virus infects Reed–Sternberg cells. A number of T-cell and NK lymphomas have also been found to harbor EBV, as well as 5% of gastric carcinomas. In addition, congenital or acquired immunodeficiency states can be complicated by the development of EBV-induced B-cell proliferative disorders. Lymphoid neoplasia occurs in immunosuppressed renal transplant recipients 30 to 50 times more often than in the general population.

Human Herpesvirus 8

Kaposi sarcoma (KS) is a vascular tumor that was originally described in elderly eastern European men and later observed in Sub-Saharan Africa. KS is today the most common neoplasm associated with AIDS. The neoplastic cells contain sequences of a novel herpesvirus, HHV8, also known as KS-associated herpesvirus (KSHV). HHV8 is present in virtually all specimens of KS, whether from HIV-positive or HIV-negative patients, and appears to be necessary—but not sufficient—for development of KS. Like other DNA viruses, the HHV8 viral genome encodes proteins that interfere with the p53 and Rb tumor suppressor pathways. Some viral proteins also inhibit apoptosis and act in multiple ways to accelerate cell-cycle transit. The virus encodes an inhibitor of the normal regulator of NFκB (i.e., IκB), resulting in unrestrained activation of NFκB.

INHERITED CANCER SYNDROMES

Cancer syndromes attributed to inherited mutations comprise only 1% of cancers. These mutations principally involve tumor suppressor and DNA repair genes. As previously discussed for *Rb,* inheritance of a single mutated allele of a tumor suppressor gene results in a heterozygous state and high risk for LOH (i.e., inactivation of the normal allele). What is inherited in this setting is a high degree of susceptibility to developing cancer. Although the germline genotype of such people is heterozygous, both tumor suppressor alleles are inactivated in the tumors that develop in these individuals.

Hereditary tumor syndromes can be arbitrarily divided into three categories:

1. Inherited malignant tumors (e.g., Rb, WT, many endocrine tumors)
2. Inherited tumors that remain benign or have a malignant potential (e.g., APC)
3. Inherited syndromes associated with a high risk of malignant tumors (e.g., Bloom syndrome, ataxia telangiectasia)

These syndromes highlight tumor suppressor activities and the genes that cause them. However, many inherited syndromes entail a different spectrum of tumors than the significance of the mutated gene(s) would suggest. For example, decreased PTEN is very common in many malignancies (see above), but germline loss of PTEN (Cowden syndrome) is mainly associated with benign hamartomas.

Most of these are discussed in chapters dealing with specific organs, and selected examples are given in Table 4-6.

Many of the inherited germline mutations cited above (e.g., *BRCA1* or *VHL* genes) lead to specific tumor syndromes. However, it remains unclear why alterations in certain genes tend to affect some organs but not others. Thus, the importance of BRCA1 in repair of DNA double-strand breaks is well established, but it is obscure why germline mutations in this gene lead mainly to breast and ovarian cancers and not to a comparable incidence of other types of cancer.

NEOPLASMS OF INFANCY AND CHILDHOOD

Pediatric Malignancies

The incidence of childhood cancer is 1.3 per 10,000 per year in children younger than 15 years of age. Mortality is determined by the intrinsic behavior of the tumor and its response to therapy, but overall, the death rate for childhood cancer is one third of the incidence. Almost half of all such malignancies are acute leukemias and lymphomas. The former, particularly acute lymphoblastic leukemia, make up one third of childhood cancers. Most of the rest are neuroblastomas, brain tumors, Wilms tumors, retinoblastomas, bone cancers, and soft tissue sarcomas.

Genetic influences in the development of childhood tumors are well studied in the case of retinoblastoma (as noted above), Wilms tumor, and osteosarcoma. Interactions of heritable factors and environmental influences in the pathogenesis of malignant tumors in both children and adults are discussed in Chapter 5.

Unlike adults, in whom most cancers are of epithelial origin (e.g., carcinomas of the lung, breast, and GI tract), most malignant tumors in children arise from hematopoietic, nervous, and soft tissues (Fig. 4-31). Many childhood cancers are part of developmental complexes (Table 4-7). Examples include short-arm deletions of chromosome 11, especially 11p13, causing Wilms tumor associated with aniridia, genitourinary malformations, and mental retardation (WAGR complex), and hemihypertrophy of the body with Wilms. Loss of the long arm of chromosome 13 is associated with retinoblastoma owing to the loss of the *Rb* tumor suppressor gene. Some tumors are evident at birth and obviously develop in utero. In addition, abnormally developed organs, persistent organ primordia, and displaced organ rests are all liable to neoplastic transformation.

SYSTEMIC EFFECTS OF CANCER

The symptoms of cancer are, for the most part, referable to local effects of the primary tumor or its metastases. However, in a minority of patients, cancer produces remote effects that are not attributable to tumor invasion or to metastasis and are collectively called **paraneoplastic syndromes**.

Fever

It is not uncommon for cancer patients to present initially with fever of unknown origin that cannot be explained by an infectious disease. Fever attributed to cancer correlates with tumor growth, disappears after treatment, and reappears on recurrence. The most common cancers in which this occurs are Hodgkin disease, renal cell carcinoma, and osteosarcoma, although many other tumors are occasionally complicated by fever. Tumor cells may themselves release pyrogens, or the inflammatory cells in the tumor stroma can produce IL-1, a cytokine that acts to promote fever.

Anorexia and Weight Loss

A paraneoplastic syndrome of anorexia, weight loss, and cachexia is common in patients with cancer, often appearing before its malignant cause becomes apparent. For example,

Table 4-6

Selected Hereditary Conditions Associated With an Increased Risk of Cancer

Syndrome	Gene	Predominant Malignancies	Gene Function	Inheritance[a]
Chromosomal instability syndromes				
Bloom syndrome	*BLM*	Many sites	DNA repair	R
Fanconi anemia	Multiple genes	Acute myelogenous leukemia	DNA repair	R
Hereditary skin cancer				
Familial melanoma	*CDKN2 (p16)*	Malignant melanoma	Cell-cycle regulation	D
Xeroderma pigmentosum	*XP group*	Squamous cell carcinoma of skin; malignant melanoma	DNA repair	R
Endocrine system				
Hereditary paraganglioma and pheochromocytoma	*SDHD*	Paraganglioma; pheochromocytoma	Oxygen sensing and signaling	D
Multiple endocrine neoplasia (MEN) type 1	*MEN1*	Pancreatic islet cell tumors	Transcriptional regulation	D
MEN type 2	*RET*	Thyroid medullary carcinoma; pheochromocytoma (MEN type 2A)	Receptor tyrosine kinase; cell-cycle regulation	D
Breast cancer				
Breast/ovary cancer syndrome	*BRCA1*	Carcinomas of ovary, breast, fallopian tube, and prostate	DNA repair	D
Site-specific breast cancer	*BRCA2*	Female and male breast carcinoma; carcinomas of prostate, pancreas, and ovary	DNA repair (Fanconi pathway)	D/R
Breast cancer	*PALB2*	Breast, pancreas	DNA repair (Fanconi pathway)	D/R
Nervous system				
Retinoblastoma	*RB*	Retinoblastoma	Cell-cycle regulation	D
Phacomatoses				
Neurofibromatosis type 1	*NF1*	Neurofibrosarcomas; astrocytomas; malignant melanomas	Regulator of ras-mediated signaling	D
Neurofibromatosis type 2	*NF2*	Meningiomas; schwannomas	Regulator of cytoskeleton	D
Tuberous sclerosis	*TSC1*	Renal cell carcinoma; astrocytoma	Regulator of cytoskeleton	D
Gastrointestinal system				
Familial adenomatous polyposis	*APC*	Colorectal carcinoma	Cell-cycle regulation; migration and adhesion	D
Hereditary nonpolyposis colorectal carcinoma (HNPCC; Lynch syndrome)	*hMSH2, hMSH6, MLH1, hPMS1, hPMS2*	Carcinomas of colon, endometrium, ovary, and bladder; malignant melanoma	DNA repair	D
Juvenile polyposis coli	*DPC4/Smad4*	Colorectal carcinoma; endometrial carcinoma	TGF-β signaling	D
Peutz–Jeghers syndrome	*LKB1/STK11*	Stomach, small bowel, and colon carcinomas	Serine threonine kinase	D
Kidney				
Hereditary papillary renal cell carcinoma	*MET*	Papillary renal cell carcinoma	Receptor tyrosine kinase; cell-cycle regulation	D
Wilms tumor	*WT*	Wilms tumor	Transcriptional regulation	D
Von Hippel-Lindau	*VHL*	Renal cell carcinoma	Regulator of adhesion	D
Multiple sites				
Carney complex	*PRKARIA*	Testicular neoplasms, thyroid carcinoma	cAMP signaling	D
Cowden syndrome	*PTEN*	Colorectal, breast, and thyroid carcinomas	Protein tyrosine phosphatase	D
Li-Fraumeni syndrome	*TP53*	Breast carcinoma, soft tissue sarcomas, brain tumors, leukemia	Transcriptional regulation	D
Werner syndrome	*WRN*	Soft tissue sarcomas	DNA repair	R
Ataxia telangiectasia	*ATM*	Lymphoma, leukemia	Cell signaling and DNA repair	R

[a]D, autosomal dominant; R, autosomal recessive.

ATM, mutated AT (gene); cAMP, cyclic adenosine 3′,5′-monophosphate; PTEN, phosphatase and tensin homolog; TGF-β, transforming growth factor-β.

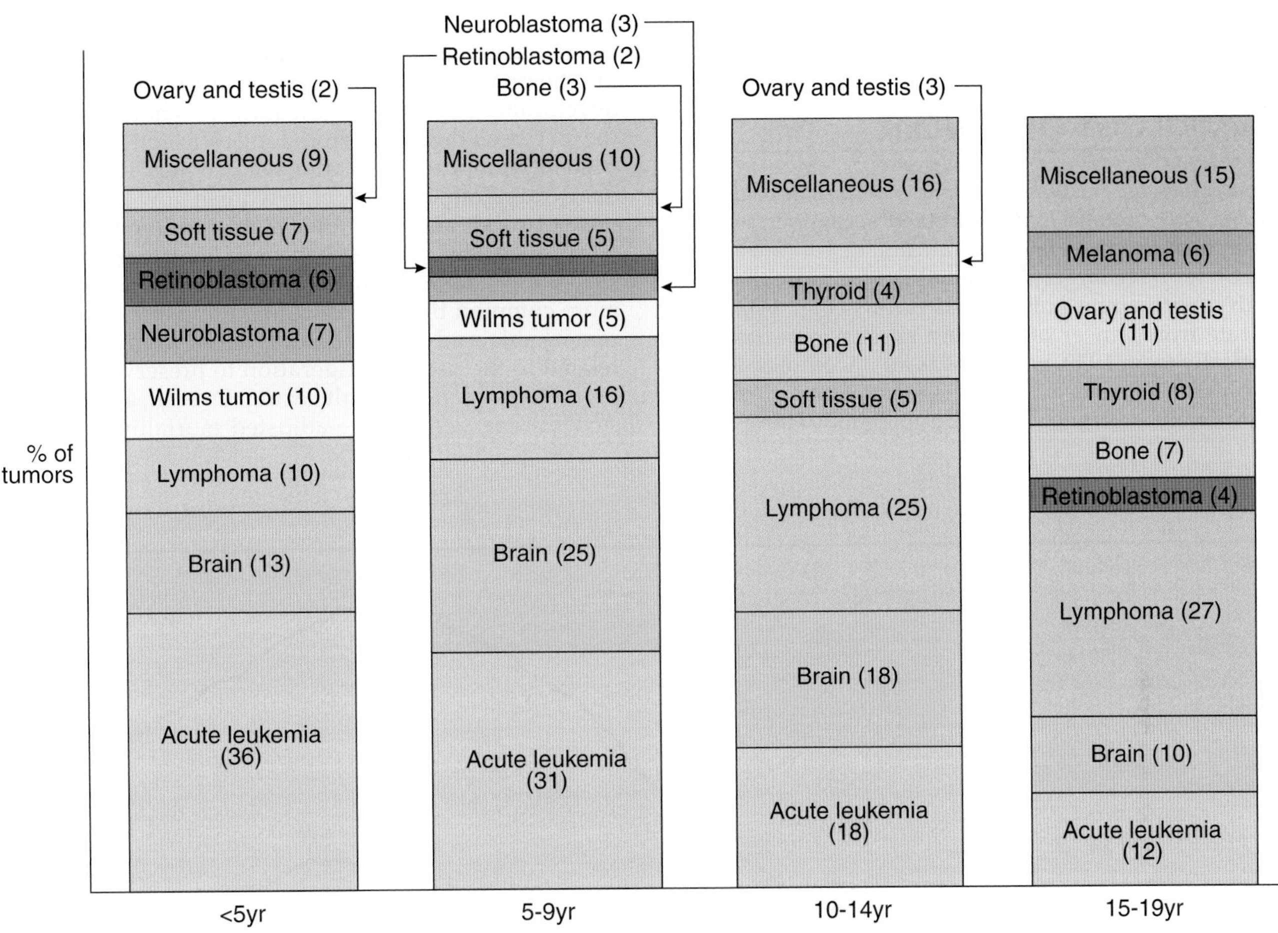

FIGURE 4-31. Distribution of childhood tumors according to age and primary site.

a small asymptomatic pancreatic cancer may be suspected only on the basis of progressive and unexplained weight loss. Although cancer patients often decrease their caloric intake because of anorexia and abnormalities of taste, restricted food intake does not explain the profound wasting so common among them. The mechanisms responsible for this phenomenon are poorly understood. It is known, however, that unlike starvation, which is associated with a lowered metabolic rate, cancer is often accompanied by an elevated metabolic rate. It has been demonstrated that TNF-α and other

Table 4-7

Clinical Features of the Autosomal Chromosomal Syndromes[a]

Syndromes	Features
Trisomic syndromes	
Chromosome 21 (Down syndrome 47,XX or XY, +21)	Epicanthic folds, speckled irides, flat nasal bridge, congenital heart disease, simian crease of palms, Hirschsprung disease, increased risk of leukemia
Chromosome 18 (47,XX or XY, +18)	Female preponderance, micrognathia, congenital heart disease, horseshoe kidney, deformed fingers
Chromosome 13 (47,XX or XY, +13)	Persistent fetal hemoglobin, microcephaly, congenital heart disease, polycystic kidneys, polydactyly, simian crease
Deletion syndromes	
5p– syndrome (cri du chat 46,XX or XY, 5p–)	Cat-like cry, low birth weight, microcephaly, epicanthic folds, congenital heart disease, short hands and feet, simian crease
11p– syndrome (46,XX or XY, 11p–)	Aniridia, Wilms tumor, gonadoblastoma, male genital ambiguity
13q– syndrome (46,XX or XY, 13q–)	Low birth weight, microcephaly, retinoblastoma, congenital heart disease

[a]All of these syndromes are associated with mental retardation.

cytokines (interferons, IL-6) can produce a wasting syndrome in experimental animals.

EPIDEMIOLOGY OF CANCER

Cancer accounts for one fifth of the total mortality in the United States and is the second leading cause of death after ischemic cardiovascular diseases. For most cancers, death rates in the United States have largely remained flat for more than half a century, with some notable exceptions (Fig. 4-32). The death rate from cancer of the lung among men has risen dramatically from 1930, when it was an uncommon tumor, to the present, when it is by far the most common cause of death from cancer in men. The entire epidemic of lung cancer deaths is attributable to smoking. Among women, smoking did not become fashionable until World War II. Considering the time lag needed between starting to smoke and the development of cancer of the lung, it is not surprising that the increased death rate from lung cancer in women did not become significant until after 1965. In the United States, the death rate from lung cancer in women now exceeds that for breast cancer, and it is now, as in men, the most common fatal cancer. By contrast cancer of the stomach, which in 1930 was by far the most common cancer in men and was more common than breast cancer in women, has shown a remarkable and sustained decline in frequency possibly related to the use of refrigeration to preserve meats as opposed to smoking and salt curing. Overall, after decades of steady increases, the age-adjusted mortality as a result of

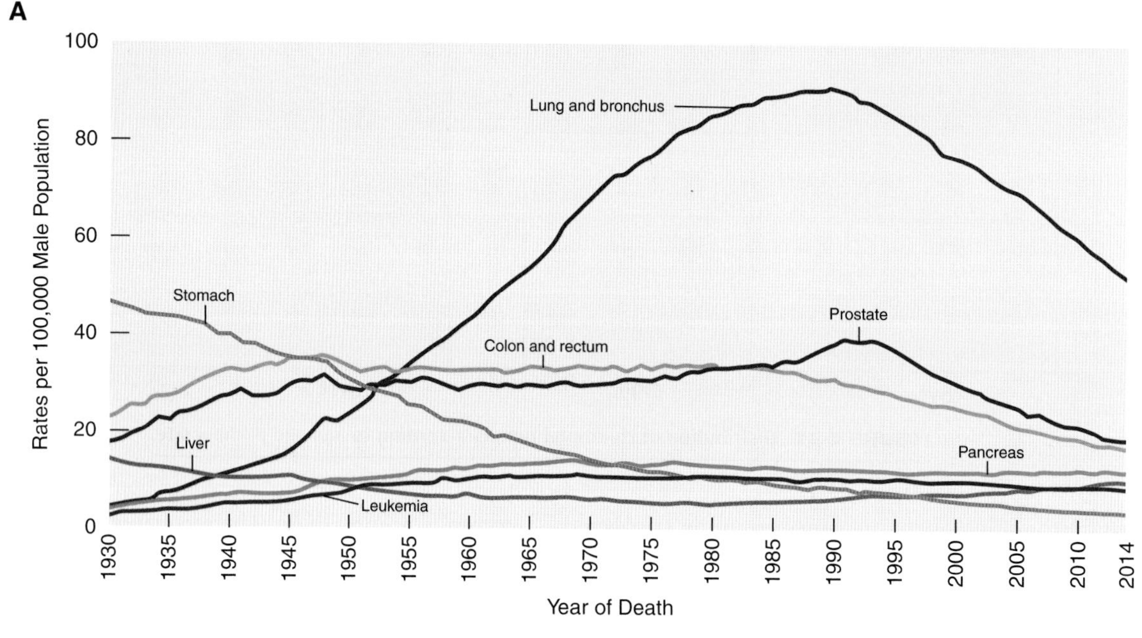

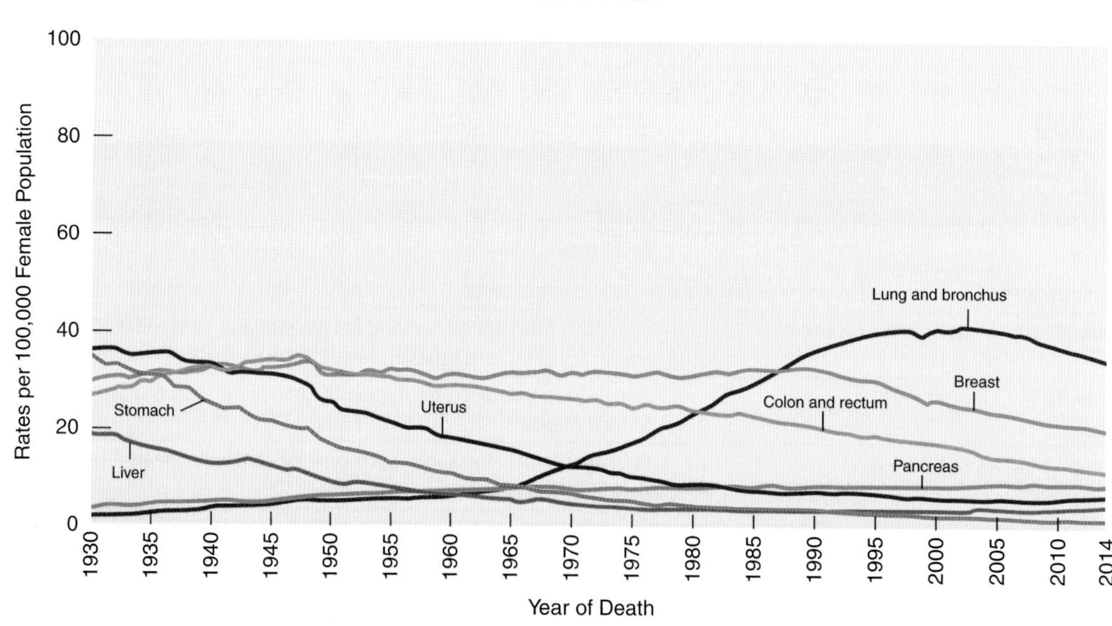

FIGURE 4-32. Cancer death rates in the United States, 1930 to 2014, among men (**A**) and women (**B**). From Cancer Facts & Figures. Atlanta, American Cancer Society, 2017.

Table 4-8

Most Common Tumor Types in Men and Women

Tumor Type: Men	% of Cases	Tumor Type: Women	% of Cases
Prostate	19	Breast	30
Lung and bronchus	14	Lung and bronchus	12
Colon and rectum	9	Colon and rectum	8
Urinary bladder	7	Uterine corpus	7
Melanoma of the skin	6	Thyroid	5
Kidney and renal pelvis	5	Melanoma of the skin	4
Non-Hodgkin lymphoma	5	Non-Hodgkin lymphoma	4
Leukemia	4	Leukemia	3
Oral cavity and pharynx	4	Pancreas	3
Liver and intrahepatic bile duct	3	Kidney and renal pelvis	3
All other sites	24	All other sites	21

Data from Cancer Facts & Figures. Atlanta, American Cancer Society, 2017

all cancers has now reached a plateau. The ranking of the incidence of tumors in men and women in the United States is shown in Table 4-8.

Individual cancers have their own age-related profiles, but for most, increased age is associated with an increased incidence. The most striking example of the dependency on age is carcinoma of the prostate, in which the incidence increases 30-fold between men ages 50 and 85 years. Certain neoplastic diseases, such as acute lymphoblastic leukemia in children and testicular cancer in young adults, show different age-related peaks of incidence.

Geographic and Ethnic Differences

The differences in cancer incidence among populations are often striking and the causes for such differences are often speculative at best. A striking example is the range in incidence of **esophageal carcinoma,** which varies from extremely low in Mormon women in Utah to a value some 300 times higher in the female population of northern Iran. Particularly high rates of esophageal cancer are noted in a so-called Asian esophageal cancer belt, which includes the great land mass stretching from Turkey to eastern China. The causes of esophageal cancer are obscure, but it is known that it disproportionately affects the poor in many areas of the world, and the combination of alcohol abuse and smoking is associated with a particularly high risk.

The rates for skin cancers vary with skin color and exposure to the sun. Thus, particularly high rates have been reported in northern Australia, where the population is principally of English origin and sun exposure is intense. Increased rates of skin cancer have also been noted among the white population of the American Southwest. The lowest rates are found among people with pigmented skin (e.g., Japanese, Chinese, Indians). The rates for African blacks, despite their heavily pigmented skin, are occasionally higher than those for Asians because of the higher incidence of melanomas of the soles and palms in the former.

Studies of Migrant Populations

Although planned experiments on the etiology of human cancer are hardly feasible, certain populations have unwittingly performed such experiments by migrating from one environment to another. Initially at least, the genetic characteristics of such people remain the same, but the new environments differ in climate, diet, infectious agents, occupations, and so on. *Consequently, epidemiologic studies of migrant populations have provided many intriguing clues to the factors that may influence the pathogenesis of cancer.* The United States, which has been the destination of one of the greatest population movements of all time, is the source of most of the important data in this field.

Colorectal, Breast, Endometrial, Ovarian, and Prostatic Cancers

Emigrants from low-risk areas in Europe and Japan to the United States exhibit an increased risk of colorectal cancer in the United States. Moreover, their offspring continue at higher risk and reach the incidence levels of the general American population. This rule for colorectal cancer also prevails for cancers of the breast, endometrium, ovary, and prostate.

Hodgkin Disease

In general, in poorly developed countries the childhood form of Hodgkin disease is the one reported most often. In developed Western countries, by contrast, the disease is most common among young adults, except in Japan. Such a pattern is characteristic of certain viral infections. Further evidence for an environmental influence is the higher incidence of Hodgkin disease in Americans of Japanese descent than Japanese dwelling in Japan.

5 Developmental and Genetic Diseases

Linda A. Cannizzaro

LEARNING OBJECTIVES

- Describe the etiology and manifestations of neonatal respiratory distress syndrome.
- Define the term "hyaline membrane" and discuss its origin in the newborn.
- Discuss Rh and ABO serology with regard to erythroblastosis fetalis.
- Discuss theories about the etiology of sudden infant death syndrome (SIDS).
- What are the etiologic categories responsible for birth defects?
- Discuss "critical stages" in human embryogenesis.
- Compare the results of embryonic injury during the first week of postconception to those occurring between weeks 2 and 8.
- Contrast the use of the term "dysplasia" in neoplasia and in developmental abnormalities.
- Discuss deformation, malformation, developmental sequence, and developmental association.
- Explain how Potter complex illustrates both malformations and deformations.
- Apply the "general principles of teratology" to a specific known teratogen, such as thalidomide.
- Describe the characteristics of fetal alcohol syndrome.
- Discuss the TORCH complex.
- Review the terminology of human chromosomal abnormalities.
- Compare X chromosome monosomy in males and females.
- Discuss the etiology and pathophysiology of Down syndrome.
- Enumerate human trisomies resulting in live births.
- Describe common syndromes associated with numeric aberrations of the sex chromosomes.
- Define the term "lyonization" and discuss its role in numeric aberrations of the sex chromosomes.
- Define "mutational hotspots."
- Distinguish between "haploinsufficiency" and "dominant-negative mutations."
- Describe the etiology and consequences of major autosomal dominant diseases of connective tissue (osteogenesis imperfecta, Ehlers–Danlos syndrome, and Marfan syndrome).
- Explain the loss of tumor suppressor function in neurofibromatosis types I and II.
- Discuss why autosomal recessive diseases are most common in inbred pedigrees.
- Explain how a defect in the *CFTR* gene results in the clinical spectrum of cystic fibrosis.
- Define and discuss the term "lysosomal storage diseases."
- Differentiate the etiology, pathogenesis, and clinical syndromes associated with Gaucher, Tay–Sachs, and Niemann–Pick diseases.
- Describe the etiology and pathogenesis common to the mucopolysaccharidoses, using Hurler disease as an example.
- Describe the etiology and pathogenesis common to the glycogenoses, using Pompe disease as an example.
- Distinguish between classic PKU (hyperphenylalaninemia) and malignant hyperphenylalaninemia.
- How does the expression and transmission of X-linked dominant and recessive disorders differ in males and females?
- Describe several common X-linked recessive diseases.
- Using fragile X syndrome as a model, describe the inheritance of trinucleotide repeat disorders. Also, define the terms "premutation" and "genetic anticipation."
- What are the unique characteristics associated with the expression and inheritance of mitochondrial diseases?
- Describe the effect of genetic imprinting on the transmission of genetic diseases.
- Describe multifactorial inheritance in terms of common diseases.

DISEASES OF PREMATURITY, INFANCY, AND CHILDHOOD

Diseases of prematurity, infancy, and childhood have a number of causes. They may (1) appear at or proximate to birth or during the perinatal period solely and may be the result of prematurity, (2) result from genomic abnormalities, or (3) reflect interactions between genetic defects and environmental influences. The period of early childhood has been traditionally subdivided into several stages, including the neonatal (the first 4 weeks) and infancy (the first year). Each of these periods has its own anatomic, physiologic, and immunologic characteristics, which determine which diseases occur and how they manifest. Causes and mechanisms of morbidity and mortality in the neonatal period differ greatly from those in infancy and childhood.

Neonatal Respiratory Distress Syndrome

RDS is the leading cause of morbidity and mortality among premature infants, accounting for half of neonatal deaths in the United States. Its incidence varies inversely with gestational age and birth weight. Over half of infants born younger than 28 weeks' gestational age develop RDS, compared with one fifth of infants born between 32 and 36 weeks. Additional risk factors for RDS include (1) neonatal asphyxia, (2) maternal diabetes, (3) cesarean delivery, (4) precipitous delivery, and (5) twin pregnancy.

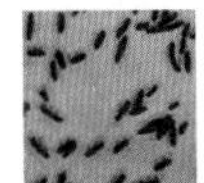

ETIOLOGIC FACTORS: *The pathogenesis of RDS of the newborn is intimately linked to surfactant deficiency* (Fig. 5-1). When a newborn starts breathing, type II cells release their surfactant stores. Surfactant reduces surface tension and decreases the affinity of alveolar surfaces for each other. This effect allows alveoli to remain open when the baby exhales and reduces resistance to reinflating the lungs. If surfactant function is inadequate, as it is in many premature infants with immature lungs, alveoli collapse when the baby exhales and resist expansion with the next breath. The energy required for the second breath must then overcome the stickiness within alveoli. Inspiration, therefore, requires considerable effort, and the alveolar lining becomes damaged when adherent alveolar walls pull apart. As a result, injured alveoli leak plasma constituents, including fibrinogen and albumin, into airspaces. These proteins bind surfactant and further impair its function, thereby exacerbating respiratory insufficiency.

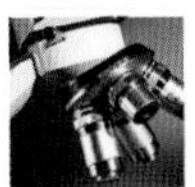

PATHOLOGY: Alveolar ducts become lined by conspicuous, eosinophilic, fibrin-rich, amorphous structures, called **hyaline membranes**, hence the original term **hyaline membrane disease** (Fig. 5-2). Collapsed alveoli have thick walls, capillaries are congested, and lymphatics are filled with proteinaceous material.

Many alveoli are perfused with blood but not ventilated by air, which leads to hypoxia and acidosis and further compromises the ability of type II pneumocytes to produce surfactant. Intra-alveolar hypoxia induces pulmonary arterial vasoconstriction, thus increasing right-to-left shunting through the ductus arteriosus, through the foramen ovale, and within the lung itself. The resulting pulmonary ischemia further aggravates alveolar epithelial damage and injures alveolar capillary endothelium. Leak of protein-rich fluid into alveolar spaces from the injured vascular bed contributes to the typical clinical and pathologic features of RDS.

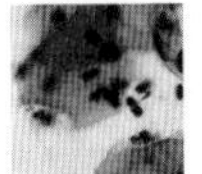

CLINICAL FEATURES: Most newborns destined to develop RDS appear normal at birth. The first symptom, appearing usually within an hour of birth, is increased respiratory effort, with forceful intercostal retraction and the use of accessory neck muscles. Respiratory rate increases to more than 100 breaths/min, and the baby becomes cyanotic.

If labor threatens a preterm pregnancy, administration of corticosteroids to mothers hastens fetal lung maturation and decreases the incidence of RDS in preterm babies. The use of animal-derived surfactants (porcine or bovine),

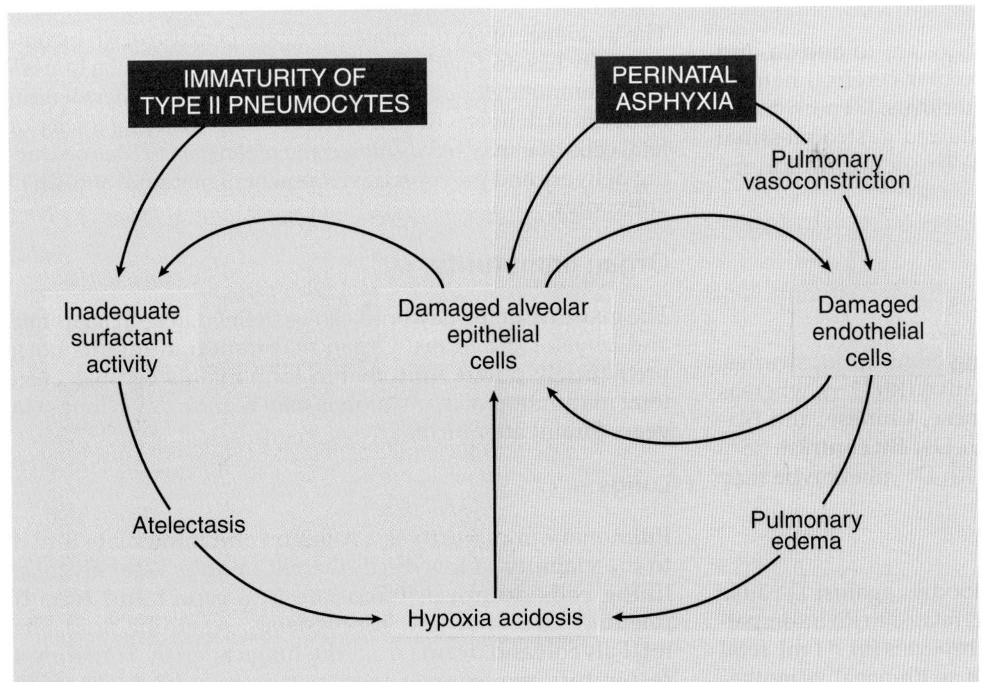

FIGURE 5-1. Pathogenesis of respiratory distress syndrome in the neonate. Immaturity of the lungs and perinatal asphyxia are the major pathogenetic factors.

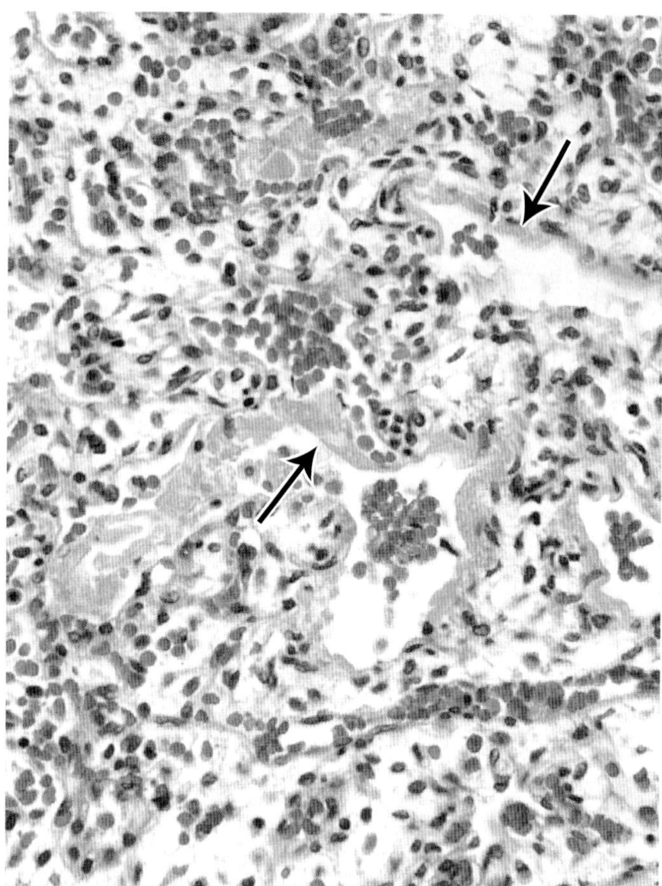

FIGURE 5-2. The lung in respiratory distress syndrome of the neonate. Alveoli are atelectatic, and dilated alveolar ducts are lined by fibrin-rich hyaline membranes (*arrows*).

combined with improved ventilatory therapy, has dramatically improved the survival of infants with RDS. Currently, even very small premature infants have an 85% to 90% chance of survival.

The major complications of RDS relate to anoxia and acidosis and include (1) intraventricular cerebral hemorrhage, (2) persistent patent ductus arteriosus, (3) necrotizing enterocolitis (the most common acquired gastrointestinal emergency in newborns), and (4) bronchopulmonary dysplasia.

Erythroblastosis Fetalis

Rh Incompatibility

The distribution of Rh antigens among ethnic groups varies. In American whites, 15% are Rh negative (Rh D−), whereas only 8% of blacks are Rh D−. Japanese, Chinese, and Native Americans are essentially all Rh D+. By contrast, 35% of Basque people, among whom the Rh D− phenotype may have arisen, are Rh D−.

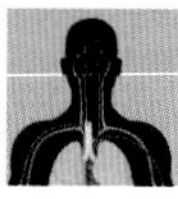

PATHOPHYSIOLOGY: Antibodies against D cause 90% of erythroblastosis fetalis related to Rh incompatibility. Rh-positive fetal erythrocytes (in >1 mL fetal blood) enter the circulation of an Rh-negative mother at the time of delivery and elicit maternal antibodies to the fetal D antigen (Fig. 5-3). ***Because the fetal blood required to sensitize a mother is introduced into her circulation only at the time of delivery, the disease does not ordinarily affect her first fetus. However, at subsequent pregnancies, when a now sensitized mother again carries an Rh-positive fetus, much smaller quantities of fetal D antigen boost antibody titer. The resulting IgG antibodies cross the placenta and thus cause hemolysis in the fetus.*** This cycle is magnified in multiparous women, the severity of erythroblastosis increasing progressively with each subsequent pregnancy. However, even after multiple pregnancies, only 5% of Rh-negative women ever deliver infants with erythroblastosis fetalis.

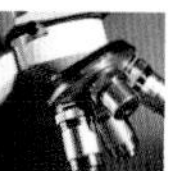

PATHOLOGY AND CLINICAL FEATURES: The severity of hemolysis in erythroblastosis fetalis varies from mild to fatal anemia.

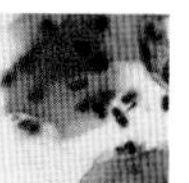

- **Death in utero** occurs in the most extreme form of the disease, and severe maceration is evident on delivery. Many erythroblasts are seen in organs that are not extensively autolyzed.
- **Hydrops fetalis** is the most serious form of erythroblastosis fetalis in liveborn infants. ***It is characterized by severe edema due to congestive heart failure caused by severe anemia.*** Affected infants generally die unless adequate exchange transfusions with Rh-negative cells correct the anemia and treat the hemolysis.

Kernicterus, or **bilirubin encephalopathy,** is a neurologic condition associated with severe jaundice and is characterized by bile staining of the brain, particularly the basal ganglia, pontine nuclei, and cerebellar dentate nuclei. Bilirubin derived from the destruction of erythrocytes and catabolism of the released heme is poorly conjugated by the immature liver, which is deficient in glucuronyl transferase. Severe kernicterus leads initially to the loss of the startle reflex and athetoid movements and progresses to lethargy and death in 75% of cases.

Prevention and Treatment

The incidence of erythroblastosis fetalis because of Rh incompatibility has declined to <1% of women at risk when human anti-D immunoglobulin (RhoGAM) is given to mothers within 72 hours of delivery. RhoGAM neutralizes the antigenicity of fetal cells that may have entered the maternal circulation during delivery and prevents development of maternal anti-Rh D antibodies.

Organ Immaturity

The maturity of the newborn can be defined in both anatomic and physiologic terms. Organ maturation in infants born prematurely differs from that in term infants because even total maturation of many organs may require days (lungs) to years (brain) after birth.

Lungs

Pulmonary immaturity is a common and immediate threat to the viability of low–birth-weight infants. Fetal alveolar lining cells do not differentiate into type I and type II pneumocytes until late in pregnancy. Amniotic fluid fills fetal alveoli and drains from the lungs at birth. Sometimes respiratory movements of immature infants are sluggish

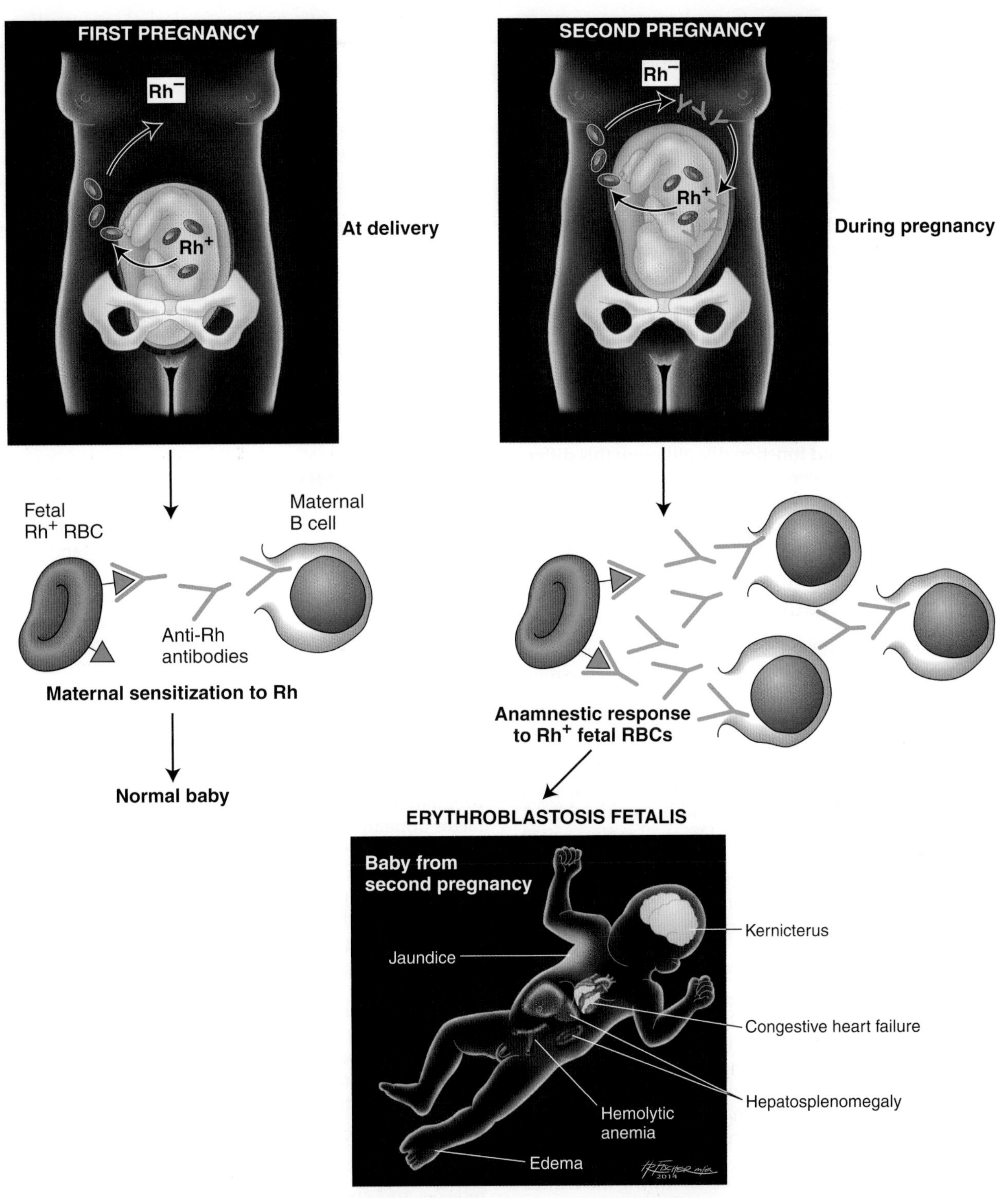

FIGURE 5-3. Pathogenesis of erythroblastosis fetalis because of maternal–fetal Rh incompatibility. Immunization of an Rh-negative mother with Rh-positive erythrocytes in the first pregnancy leads to formation of anti-Rh antibodies of the immunoglobulin (Ig) G type. These antibodies cross the placenta and damage the Rh-positive fetus in subsequent pregnancies. RBCs, red blood corpuscles.

and do not fully expel amniotic fluid from their lungs. Respiratory embarrassment may ensue, a syndrome called **amniotic fluid aspiration**, but that actually represents retained amniotic fluid. Air passages contain desquamated squamous cells **(squames)** and lanugo hair from the fetal skin and protein-rich amniotic fluid. RDS may occur in term or near-term infants. Clinically, this syndrome mimics that seen in premature infants who lack adequate surfactant (see above). A high proportion of **term infants** with RDS suffer from genetic deficiencies of one of the hydrophobic surfactant proteins (SP-B or SP-C) or have mutations in the ATP- binding cassette transporter (ABCA3), which is responsible for transporting surfactant phospholipids and proteins to the alveolar space.

Liver

The liver of premature infants is morphologically similar to that of adults, except for conspicuous extramedullary hematopoiesis. However, the hepatocytes tend to be functionally immature. Because the fetal liver is deficient in glucuronyl transferase, a lack of conjugation of bilirubin often leads to **neonatal jaundice** (see Chapter 12). This enzyme deficiency is aggravated by the rapid destruction of fetal erythrocytes, a process that increases the supply of bilirubin.

Brain

The brain of immature newborns differs from that of the adult, morphologically and functionally, although this difference is rarely fatal. Still, incomplete CNS development often contributes to poor vasomotor control, hypothermia, feeding difficulties, and recurrent apnea.

Sudden Unexpected Infant Death Syndrome and Sudden Infant Death Syndrome

Nearly 4,000 cases of SUIDS in children younger than 1 year of age occur yearly in the United States. SUIDS is classified as sudden infant death syndrome (SIDS) if no explanation for the death is apparent after thorough investigation, which optimally includes death scene examination, autopsy, and clinical history. Hence, the diagnosis of SIDS is made only after excluding other specific causes of sudden death, such as infection, hemorrhage, aspiration, and homicide. About 40% of SUID cases are classified as SIDS, the leading cause of death in infants between 1 and 12 months of age with most cases occurring before 6 months. Typically, victims of SIDS are apparently healthy young infants who went to sleep without any hint of an impending calamity but did not wake up.

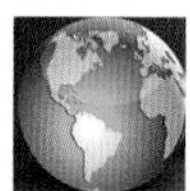

EPIDEMIOLOGY: The incidence of SIDs in the United States has decreased from 1.2 in 1,000 live births in 1992 to 0.4 in 1,000 live births in 2015. The major reduction occurred with the adoption of caregiver guidelines (Back to Sleep) emphasizing placement of babies on their back for sleep, use of firm mattresses, safe cribs, and several additional guidelines to reduce inadvertent overlaying and suffocation.

The majority of deaths from SIDS occur during the winter months, and a significantly higher percentage of infants dying of SIDS are reported to have experienced upper respiratory infections within the previous 4 weeks. However, deaths involving active infections are by definition excluded.

Maternal risk factors for SIDS are as follows:

- Low socioeconomic status (poor education, unmarried mother, and poor prenatal care)
- Black or Native American parentage in the United States independent of economic status; in other countries, indigenous populations like Maoris in New Zealand and Aborigines in Australia
- Age younger than 20 years at first pregnancy
- Maternal cigarette smoking or alcohol consumption during and after pregnancy
- Use of illicit drugs during pregnancy
- High parity

Risk factors for the infant are more controversial. The consensus includes the following:

- Low birth weight.
- Prematurity.
- An illness, often respiratory, within the last 4 weeks before death.
- Subsequent siblings of SIDS victims.
- Survivors of a life-threatening event, for example, an episode of some combination of apnea, color change, marked alteration in muscle tone, choking, or gagging. A definite cause, such as seizures or aspiration after vomiting, is known in only half the cases of an apparent life-threatening event.

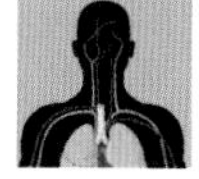
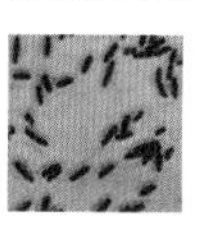

PATHOPHYSIOLOGY AND ETIOLOGIC FACTORS: Although the original definition of SIDS excludes from the diagnosis known causes, a more expansive definition helps to improve understanding of both molecular and environmental factors involved.

Channelopathies, namely, inherited abnormalities in cell membrane ion channels, are responsible for 10% to 12% of cases of SIDS, although this percentage may be higher (up to about 30%) between 6 and 12 months of age. Various inherited arrhythmia syndromes have also been implicated in sudden infant death. All involve more than one different mutation, producing clustered phenotypes.

Now that publicity about SIDS related to prone sleeping position has diminished the event, **maternal smoking during pregnancy** accounts for 80% or more of SIDS deaths. The key factor appears to be exposure to nicotine in utero. There is a dose–response effect; the likelihood of an infant developing SIDS is a function of the number of cigarettes smoked by the mother during pregnancy.

Significant abnormalities have been detected in the brains of infants dying of SIDS, including hypoplasia of the arcuate nucleus, decreased serotonin receptors, and impaired muscarinic cholinergic activity, in favor of increased nicotinic activity. Comparable abnormalities are seen in experimental animals exposed to nicotine in utero and are associated with depressed ventilatory responses to hypercarbia and hypoxia. Low levels of serotonin, a brain chemical involved in regulating breathing and other vital functions, have been found in the brainstems of SIDS victims. Furthermore, prospective studies of babies who later died of SIDS demonstrated abnormal activity of the autonomic nervous system, including depressed gasping reflexes and anomalous regulation of heart rhythm. Hence, although the exact pathophysiologic mechanisms underlying SIDS remain obscure, delayed maturation or maldevelopment of the brainstem functions appears to be involved. These relate to arousal and response to a variety of events involving stress to cardiorespiratory function.

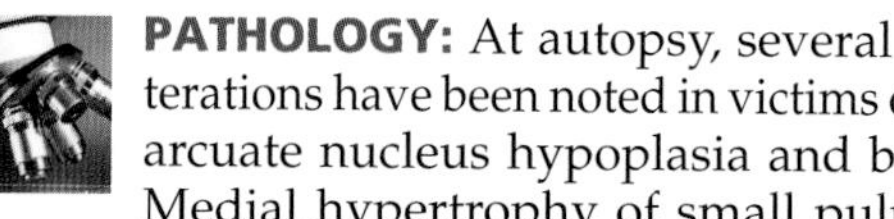

PATHOLOGY: At autopsy, several morphologic alterations have been noted in victims of SIDS, including arcuate nucleus hypoplasia and brainstem gliosis. Medial hypertrophy of small pulmonary arteries, persistence of extramedullary hematopoiesis in the liver, right ventricular hypertrophy, and increased periadrenal brown fat have also been seen and suggest a degree of chronic hypoxia. However, except for brainstem abnormalities, none of these changes occur with any regularity. Petechiae on the surfaces of the lungs, heart, pleura, and thymus are reported in most infants dying of SIDS but apparently reflect terminal events.

CONGENITAL ABNORMALITIES

Each year, about 250,000 babies in the United States are born with a birth defect. Worldwide, at least 1 in 50 newborns has a major congenital anomaly, 1 in 100 has a defect that can be attributed to a single-gene abnormality, and 1 in 200 has a major chromosomal abnormality. ***A specific cause is not apparent in more than two thirds of all birth defects*** (Fig. 5-4). No more than 6% can be attributed to uterine factors such as maternal metabolic imbalances or infections during pregnancy or environmental exposures (drugs, chemicals, and radiation). Others are caused by genomic defects and only a small number by chromosomal abnormalities. Currently, about 70% are not associated with any known genetic or other cause.

Developmental and genetic disorders are classified as follows:

- Errors of morphogenesis
- Adverse transplacental influences
- Chromosomal abnormalities
- Single-gene defects
- Polygenic inherited diseases

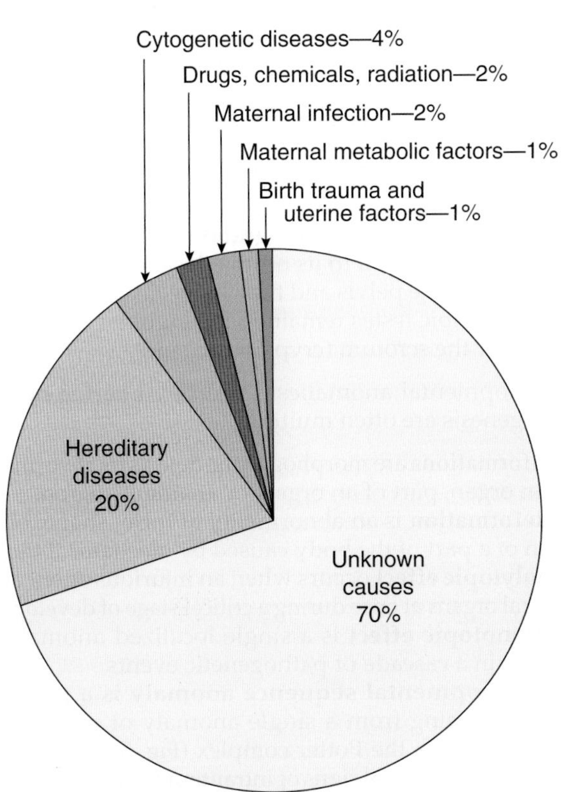

FIGURE 5-4. Causes of birth defects in humans. Most birth defects have unknown causes.

ERRORS OF MORPHOGENESIS

Normal intrauterine and postnatal development depends on sequential activation and repression of numerous genes. A fertilized ovum (zygote) has all the genes of an adult, but most of them are inactive. As zygotes enter cleavage stages of development, individual genes or sets of genes are specifically activated at different stages of embryogenesis. Thus, ***abnormal gene activation in early embryonic cells can cause death. Likewise, exogenous toxins acting on preimplantation embryos do not produce errors of morphogenesis or malformations*** (Fig. 5-5). ***The most common consequence is death of the embryo, which often goes unnoticed or is perceived as heavy, delayed, menstrual bleeding.***

Cells that comprise two- and four-cell embryos (blastomeres) are equipotent; each can give rise to an adult organism. If such cells separate at this stage, identical twins or quadruplets can result. Because blastomeres are equipotent and interchangeable, loss of a single blastomere at this stage does not have serious consequences. Injury during the first 8 to 10 days after fertilization may cause incomplete separation of blastomeres, to yield conjoined twins (Siamese twins) often linked at the head (craniopagus), thorax (thoracopagus), or rump (ischiopagus). Conjoined twins may be asymmetric; one is well developed and the other rudimentary or hypoplastic. The latter is always abnormal and may reside within the body of the better-developed sibling (fetus in fetu). Some congenital teratomas, especially in the sacrococcygeal area, are actually asymmetric twins.

Complex developmental abnormalities affecting multiple organ systems are usually due to injuries during early organogenesis. This period is characterized by the formation of the so-called **developmental fields**, in which rapidly dividing cells interact to determine their developmental fate through irreversible differentiation of groups of cells. ***The developmental stage of primordial organ system formation is most susceptible to teratogenesis, owing to faulty gene activity or effects of exogenous toxins*** (Fig. 5-5). Impaired morphogenesis may affect (1) cells and tissues, (2) organs or organ systems, and (3) anatomic regions.

Terminology for Morphogenetic Errors

- **Agenesis** is the complete absence of an organ primordium. It may manifest as (1) total lack of an organ (e.g., unilateral or bilateral renal agenesis), (2) the absence of part of an organ, such as agenesis of the corpus callosum of the brain, or (3) lack of specific cell types in an organ, such as the absence of testicular germ cells in congenital Sertoli cell–only syndrome.
- **Aplasia** is persistence of an organ anlage or rudiment, without the mature organ. In pulmonary aplasia, for example, the main bronchus ends blindly in a nondescript mass of rudimentary ducts and connective tissue.
- **Hypoplasia** refers to reduced size, owing to incomplete development of all or part of an organ, as in micrognathia (small jaw) and microcephaly (small brain and head).
- **Dysraphic anomalies** are defects caused by failure of apposed structures to fuse. In spina bifida, the spinal canal does not close completely, and overlying bone and skin do not fuse, leaving a midline defect.
- **Involution failure** refers to persistence of embryonic or fetal structures that normally involute during development.

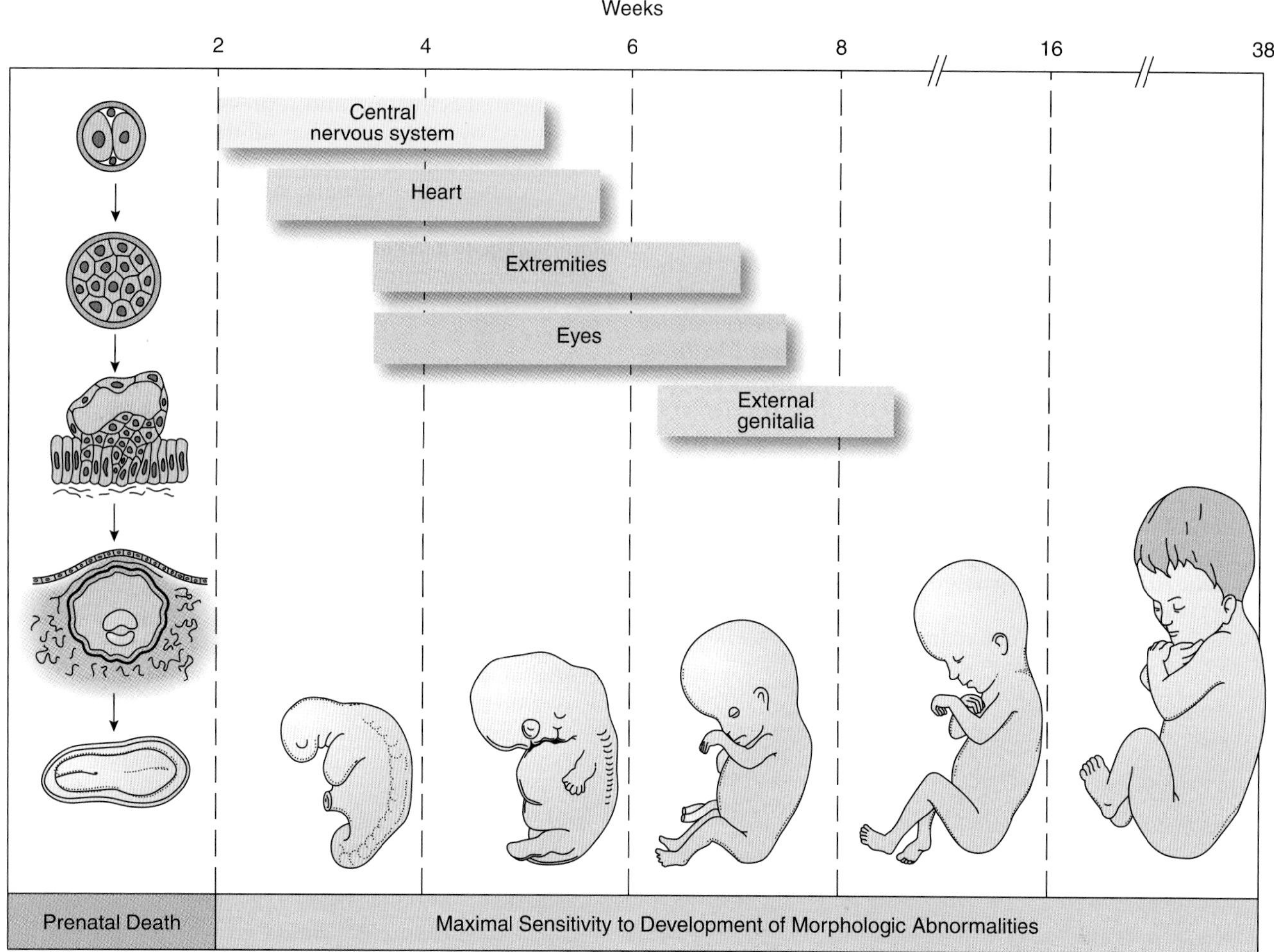

FIGURE 5-5. Sensitivity of specific organs to teratogenic agents at critical stages of human embryogenesis. Exposure to adverse influences in preimplantation and early postimplantation stages of development (*far left*) leads to prenatal death. Periods of maximal sensitivity to teratogens (*horizontal bars*) vary for different organ systems, but overall are limited to the first 8 weeks of pregnancy.

Thus, a persistent thyroglossal duct results from incomplete involution of the tract that connects the base of the tongue with the developing thyroid.

- **Division failures** are caused by incomplete programmed cell death in embryonic tissues (see Chapter 1). Fingers and toes are formed at the distal ends of limb buds by loss of cells between cartilage-containing primordia. If these cells do not undergo apoptosis, fingers are conjoined or incompletely separated (syndactyly.)
- **Atresia** refers to incomplete formation of a normal body orifice or tubular passage. Many hollow organs originate as cell strands and cords. Esophageal atresia is characterized by localized absence of the lumen, which was not fully established in embryogenesis.
- **Dysplasia** is caused by abnormal histogenesis. (This context is different from "dysplasia" in precancerous epithelial lesions; see Chapters 1 and 4). In tuberous sclerosis, for example, aggregates of normally developed cells are arranged into grossly visible "tubers."
- **Ectopia,** or **heterotopia,** refers to a normally formed organ outside its normal anatomic location. Thus, heterotopic parathyroid glands may arise within the thymus in the anterior mediastinum.
- **Dystopia** is inadequate migration of an organ from its site of development to its normal location. Thus, kidneys originate in the pelvis and then move in a cephalad direction. Dystopic testes remain in the inguinal canal and do not enter the scrotum (cryptorchidism).

Developmental anomalies caused by interference with morphogenesis are often multiple:

- **Malformations** are morphogenetic defects or abnormalities of an organ, part of an organ, or anatomic region.
- A **deformation** is an abnormality of form, shape, or position of a part of the body caused by mechanical forces.
- A **polytopic effect** occurs when an injurious agent affects several organs at once during a critical stage of development.
- A **monotopic effect** is a single localized anomaly that results in a cascade of pathogenetic events.
- A **developmental sequence anomaly** is a pattern of defects arising from a single anomaly or pathogenetic mechanism. In the Potter complex (Fig. 5-6), pulmonary hypoplasia, external signs of intrauterine fetal compression, and morphologic changes of the amnion are all related to oligohydramnios (severely reduced amount of amniotic fluid), resulting from any cause.

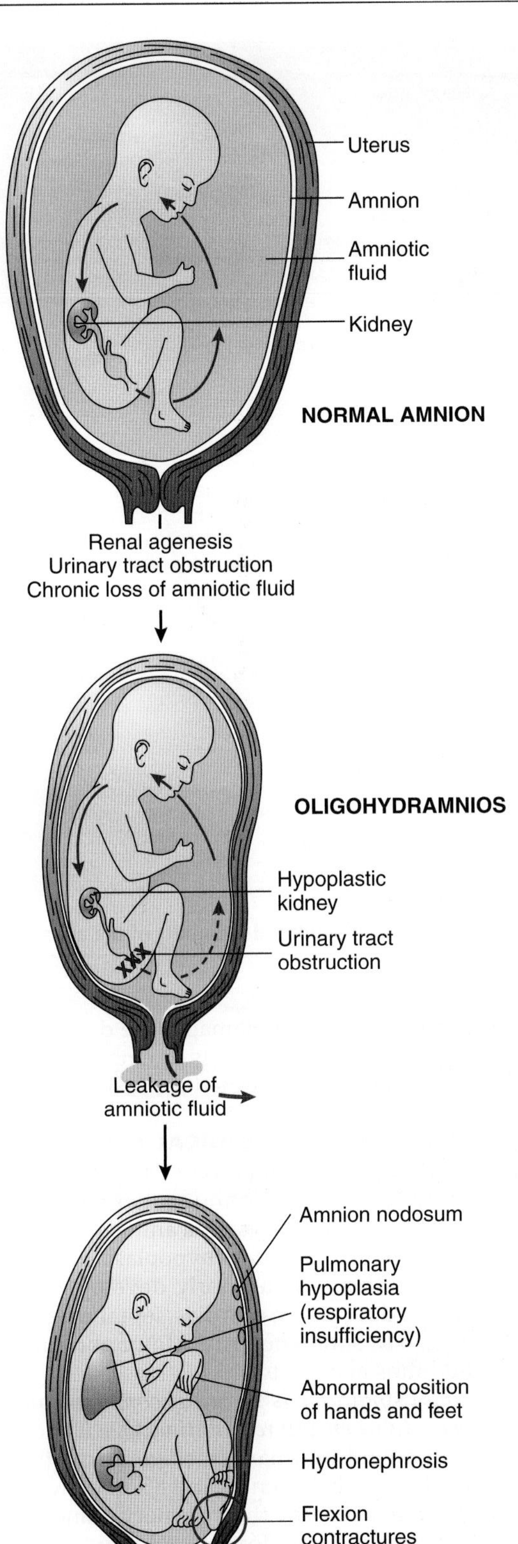

FIGURE 5-6. Potter complex. The fetus normally swallows amniotic fluid and, in turn, excretes urine, thus maintaining a normal volume of amniotic fluid. In the face of urinary tract disease (e.g., renal agenesis or urinary tract obstruction) or leakage of amniotic fluid, the volume of amniotic fluid becomes reduced, a situation called **oligohydramnios.** Oligohydramnios results in a spectrum of congenital abnormalities called **Potter sequence,** which includes pulmonary hypoplasia and contractures of the limbs. The amnion has a nodular appearance.

- A **developmental association,** or **syntropy,** describes multiple anomalies that arise concurrently but have different pathogeneses. Congenital anomalies in a child with multiple defects are not necessarily interrelated and do not automatically imply exposure to an exogenous teratogen or a common genetic defect.

PRINCIPLES OF TERATOLOGY

Teratology is the study of developmental anomalies (Greek *teraton,* "monster"). **Teratogens** are chemical, physical, or biologic agents that cause developmental anomalies. Although only a few teratogens have been *proven* in humans, many drugs and chemicals are teratogenic in animals and are thus potentially dangerous for humans. Exposure to a teratogen may result in a malformation, but not invariably. Such observations have led to the formulation of general principles of teratology:

- **Susceptibility to teratogens is variable.** Key determinants are the genotypes of the fetus and mother, although other factors play a role.
- **Susceptibility to teratogens is specific for each embryologic stage.** Most agents are teratogenic only at particular times in development (Fig. 5-5). Thus, maternal rubella infection can cause congenital rubella syndrome, but only if the mother is infected within the first 20 weeks of pregnancy.
- **Mechanisms of teratogenesis are specific for each agent.** Teratogenic drugs may inhibit crucial enzymes or receptors, interfere with formation of mitotic spindles, or impair energy production, thereby inhibiting normal morphogenesis.
- **Teratogenesis is dose dependent and may be idiosyncratic.** Thus, an absolutely safe dose cannot be predicted for every woman.
- **Teratogens may produce death, growth retardation, malformation, or functional impairment.** The outcome depends on complex interactions between a teratogen, the maternal organism, and the fetal–placental unit.

Proven teratogens include most cytotoxic drugs, alcohol, some antiepileptic drugs, heavy metals, and thalidomide. Many drugs and chemicals have been declared safe for use during pregnancy because they are not teratogenic in laboratory animals. However, the fact that a drug is not teratogenic for mice or rabbits does not necessarily mean that it is innocuous for humans, as is the case with thalidomide.

Teratogens rarely cause major errors of morphogenesis after the third month of pregnancy. Yet, functional and, to a lesser degree, structural abnormalities may occur in children exposed to exogenous teratogens during later trimesters. Although organs are formed by the end of the first trimester, most continue to restructure and mature at prescribed rates. For example, the CNS does not attain functional maturity for several years after birth and thus remains susceptible to adverse exogenous influences for this interval. ***Most anatomic defects arising in the last two trimesters of pregnancy are deformations.*** Responsible forces may be external (e.g., amniotic bands in the uterus) or intrinsic (e.g., fetal hypomobility caused by CNS injury).

Malformations

Anencephaly and Other Neural Tube Defects

Anencephaly is congenital absence of the cranial vault. In this dysraphic defect of neural tube closure, cerebral hemispheres are completely missing or reduced to small masses at the base of the skull. Normally, the neural tube closes in a craniocaudad direction, so a more distal defect in this process causes abnormalities of the vertebral column. **Spina bifida** is an incomplete closure of the spinal cord or vertebral column or both. Protrusion of the meninges through a defect in the vertebral column is called **meningocele**. In a **myelomeningocele**, a meningocele also contains herniated spinal cord. Neural tube defects are discussed in Chapter 24.

Thalidomide-Induced Malformations

Limb reduction deformities are rare congenital defects of mostly obscure origin that affect 1 in 5,000 liveborn infants. They have been known for ages. In the 1960s, a dramatic increase in the incidence of limb reduction deformities in Germany and England was linked to maternal ingestion of a sedative, thalidomide, early in pregnancy. This derivative of glutamic acid is teratogenic between the 28th and 50th days of pregnancy. Many children born to mothers exposed to thalidomide had skeletal deformities and pleomorphic defects in other organs, mostly the ears (**microtia** and **anotia**) and heart. Typically, their arms were short and malformed (Fig. 5-7), resembling the flippers of a seal **(phocomelia)**, or sometimes even completely missing **(amelia)**. The CNS was unaffected, and these children had normal intelligence. Once the link between phocomelia and thalidomide was established, the drug was banned (1962), but not before an estimated 3,000 such children had been born. Thanks to action by the U.S. FDA less than 20 of those were born in the United States. Thalidomide impairs limb growth by blocking angiogenesis and, perhaps, by inducing caspase-8–dependent apoptosis. The same properties make it useful in treating certain malignancies, for example, multiple myeloma.

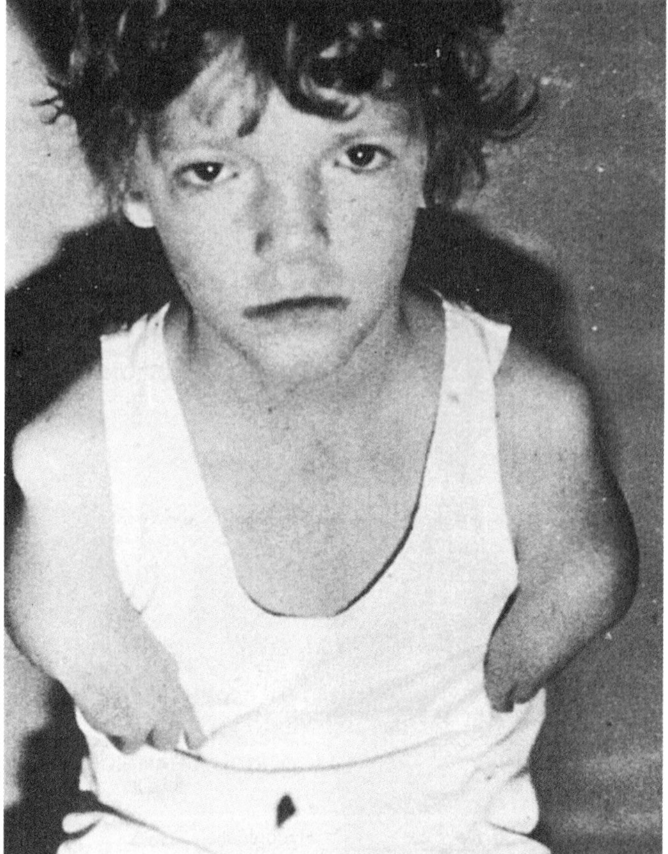

FIGURE 5-7. Thalidomide-induced deformity of the arms.

Fetal Alcohol Syndrome

Fetal alcohol syndrome is a complex of abnormalities caused by excessive maternal consumption of alcoholic beverages during pregnancy. It includes (1) growth retardation, (2) CNS abnormalities, and (3) characteristic facial dysmorphology. Not all children harmed by maternal alcohol abuse show the full spectrum of abnormalities. In such cases, the term **fetal alcohol effect** is used.

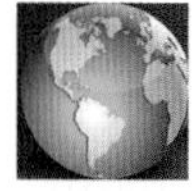

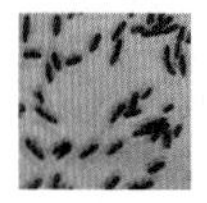

EPIDEMIOLOGY AND ETIOLOGIC FACTORS: The incidence of fetal alcohol syndrome ranges from 0.2 to 2.0 cases per 1,000 live births in the United States, but may be as high as 20 to 150 cases per 1,000 in populations with high rates of alcoholism, ***mild mental deficiency and emotional disorders related to fetal alcohol effect are far more common than full-blown fetal alcohol syndrome.*** The minimum amount of alcohol that causes fetal injury is not well established. Children with the full syndrome are usually born to mothers who are chronic alcoholics. Heavy alcohol consumption during the first trimester of pregnancy is particularly dangerous. The mechanism by which alcohol damages the developing fetus is poorly understood although effects on embryonic transcription factors have been demonstrated in vitro.

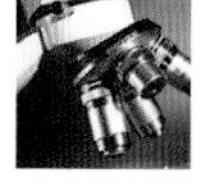

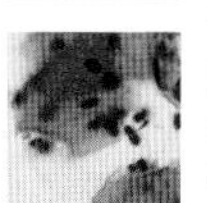

PATHOLOGY AND CLINICAL FEATURES: Infants born to alcoholic mothers often show prenatal growth retardation, which continues after birth. They may also have microcephaly, epicanthal folds, short palpebral fissures, maxillary hypoplasia, thin upper lip, micrognathia, and a poorly developed philtrum. One third may have cardiac septal defects, which often close spontaneously. Minor abnormalities of the joints and limbs may occur.

Fetal alcohol syndrome is the most common cause of acquired but preventable mental retardation. One fifth of children with fetal alcohol syndrome have intelligence quotients (IQs) below 70, and 40% are between 70 and 85. Even with normal IQ, these children tend to have short memory spans and exhibit impulsive behavior and emotional instability.

TORCH Complex

TORCH refers to a complex of signs and symptoms produced by fetal or neonatal infection with *Toxoplasma* (T), rubella (R), cytomegalovirus (C), or herpes simplex virus (H). The "O" in TORCH represents "others," including syphilis, varicella-zoster virus (chicken pox), parvovirus B19, and HIV. The term reminds pediatricians that these fetal and newborn infections may be indistinguishable from one another, and testing for all TORCH agents should be done in suspected cases (Fig. 5-8).

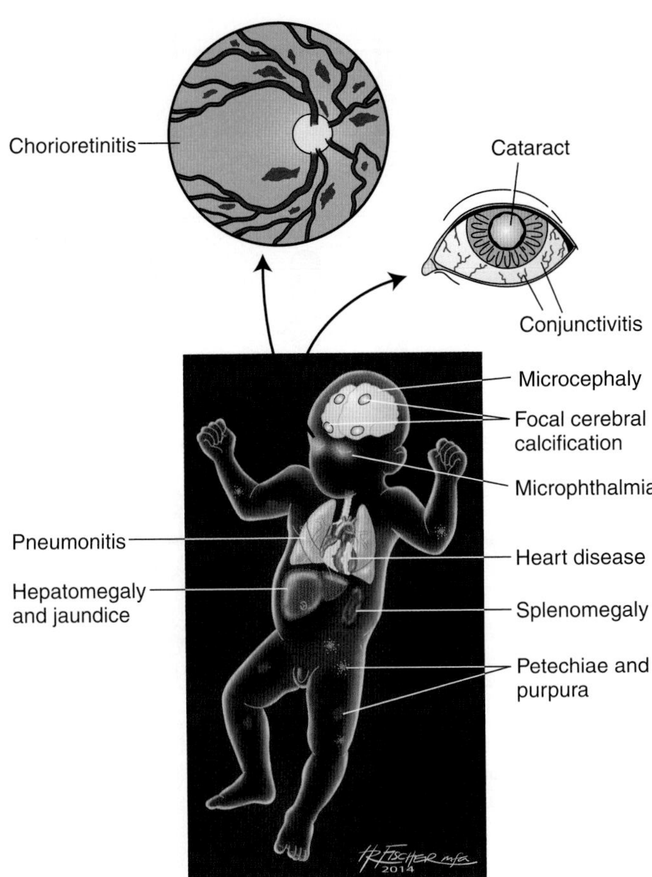

FIGURE 5-8. TORCH complex. Children infected in utero with *Toxoplasma*, rubella virus, cytomegalovirus, or herpes simplex virus show remarkably similar effects.

Table 5-1

Pathologic Findings in the Fetus and Newborn Infected With TORCH Agents

General	Prematurity
	Intrauterine growth retardation
Central nervous system	Encephalitis
	Microcephaly
	Hydrocephaly
	Intracranial calcifications
	Psychomotor retardation
Ear	Inner ear damage with hearing loss
Eye	Microphthalmia (R)
	Chorioretinitis (TCH)
	Pigmented retina (R)
	Keratoconjunctivitis (H)
	Cataracts (RH)
	Glaucoma (R)
	Visual impairment (TRCH)
Liver	Hepatomegaly
	Liver calcifications (R)
	Jaundice
Hematopoietic system	Hemolytic and other anemias
	Thrombocytopenia
	Splenomegaly
Skin and mucosae	Vesicular or ulcerative lesions (H)
	Petechiae and ecchymoses
Cardiopulmonary system	Pneumonitis
	Myocarditis
	Congenital heart disease
Skeleton	Various bone lesions

C, cytomegalovirus; H, herpesvirus; R, rubella virus; T, *Toxoplasma.*

Infections with TORCH agents affect 1% to 5% of all liveborn infants in the United States. They are major causes of neonatal morbidity and mortality. Severe damage caused by these organisms is largely irreparable, and prevention is the best approach.

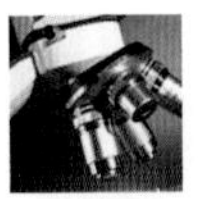

PATHOLOGY: Clinical and pathologic findings in symptomatic newborns vary. Only a minority show the entire spectrum of abnormalities (Table 5-1). Growth retardation and abnormalities of the brain, eyes, liver, hematopoietic system, and heart are common.

CNS lesions are the most serious changes in TORCH-infected children. In acute encephalitis, foci of necrosis are initially surrounded by inflammatory cells. Later, these lesions calcify, most prominently in congenital toxoplasmosis. Microcephaly, hydrocephalus, and abnormally shaped gyri and sulci (microgyria) are common. Radiologically, abnormal cerebral cavities (porencephaly), missing olfactory bulbs, and other major brain defects may occur. Severe CNS injury results in psychomotor retardation, neurologic defects, and seizures.

Ocular defects are sometimes prominent, particularly with rubella, in which over two thirds of patients have cataracts and microphthalmia. Glaucoma and retinal malformations (coloboma) occasionally occur. Chorioretinitis usually bilateral, is common with rubella, *Toxoplasma*, and cytomegalovirus (CMV). Keratoconjunctivitis is the most common eye lesion in neonatal herpes infection. Sensorineural hearing loss is common in infants with otherwise asymptomatic congenital CMV infection.

Cardiac anomalies occur in many children with the TORCH complex, in congenital rubella, patent ductus arteriosus, and septal defects are the most common. Pulmonary artery stenosis and complex cardiac anomalies are occasionally observed.

Congenital Syphilis

The organism that causes syphilis, *Treponema pallidum*, is transmitted to the fetus by a mother who had been infected during pregnancy or within 2 years before the pregnancy. About 1 in 2,000 liveborn infants in the United States have congenital syphilis. One third of pregnancies in syphilitic women end in stillbirth. *T. pallidum* may invade a fetus any time in pregnancy. Early infections mostly cause abortion, but 50% to 80% of neonates who survive early transmission of *T. pallidum* show congenital infection. Grossly visible signs of congenital syphilis appear only in fetuses infected after the

16th week of pregnancy. Because spirochetes grow in all fetal tissues, clinical presentations vary.

Children with congenital syphilis often appear normal at first or show changes characteristic of the TORCH complex. Early lesions teem with spirochetes and show perivascular infiltrates of lymphocytes and plasma cells, and granuloma-like lesions, called **gummas**. Many infants are asymptomatic and only develop stigmata of congenital syphilis in the first few years of life. Late symptoms of congenital syphilis appear many years later and reflect slowly evolving tissue destruction and repair. Symptoms appearing in the first 2 years of life (early congenital syphilis) involve neurologic disease, deafness, and bone deformities, and are similar to those seen in secondary syphilis.

If penicillin is given during pregnancy or in the first 2 years of postnatal life, most symptoms of congenital syphilis are prevented.

Structural Chromosome Alterations

Chromosomal defects result from breakage and reunion of homologous and nonhomologous autosomal and sex chromosome segments, often during meiosis. Chromosomal breakage can also occur spontaneously or result from exposure to clastogenic agents, such as viruses, radiation, or various chemicals. Structural abnormalities that occur in human chromosomes are reviewed in Figure 5-9.

Causes of Chromosomal Abnormalities

Most major chromosomal defects are incompatible with life. They are usually lethal to a developing conceptus and lead to early death and spontaneous abortion. Embryos with a significant loss of genetic material (e.g., autosomal monosomies) rarely survive pregnancy. Even though X chromosome monosomy (45,X) may be compatible with life, more than 95% of such embryos are lost during pregnancy. The absence of an X chromosome in male fetuses (45,Y) invariably leads to early abortion.

Genesis of Numerical Aberrations

The causes of chromosomal aberrations are obscure. Exogenous factors, such as radiation, viruses, and chemicals, can (1) affect mitotic spindles or DNA synthesis, (2) disturb mitosis and meiosis, and (3) cause breakage in human chromosomes, all of which increase the risk of chromosomal defects. Changes in chromosome numbers arise primarily from nondisjunction, which occurs more commonly in both maternal and paternal gametes of older parents.

Nondisjunction

Nondisjunction refers to failure of paired chromosomes or chromatids to separate and move to opposite poles of the spindle at anaphase, during mitosis or meiosis. This malfunction creates aneuploidy if only one pair of chromosomes fails to separate. It results in polyploidy if the entire set does not divide, and all the chromosomes are segregated into a single daughter cell. Aneuploidy caused by nondisjunction in somatic cells leads to one daughter cell with trisomy (2n + 1) and the other with monosomy (2n − 1). Aneuploid germ cells have two copies of the same chromosome (n + 1) or lack the affected chromosome entirely (n − 1).

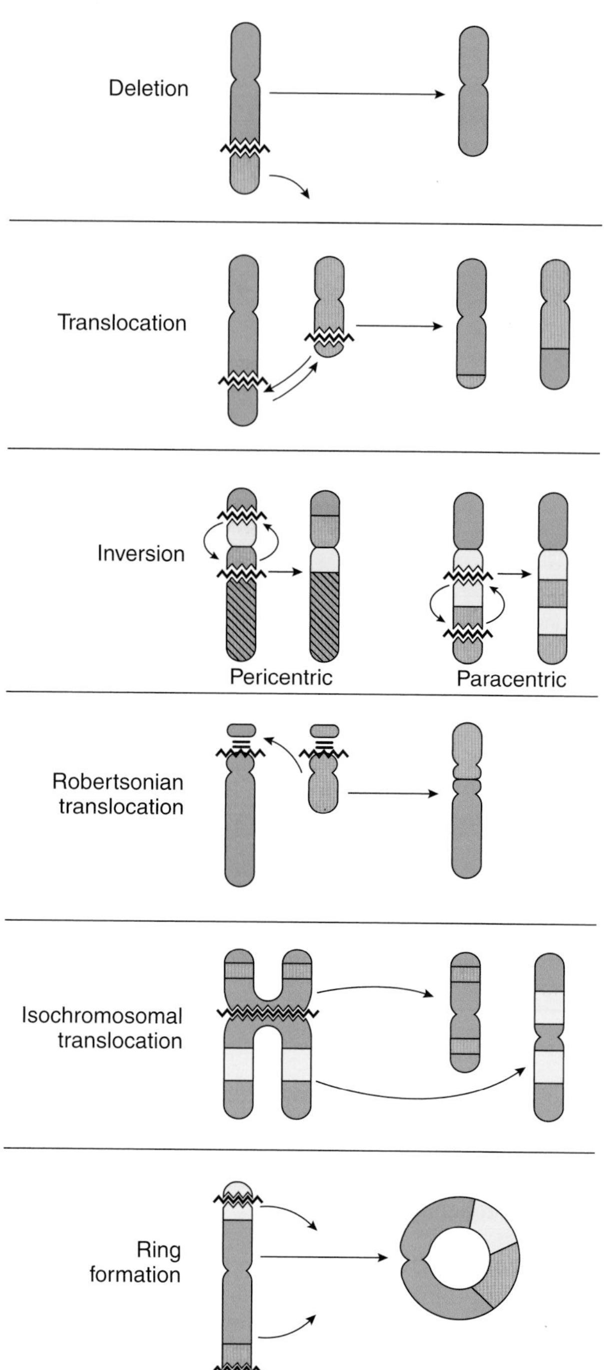

FIGURE 5-9. Structural abnormalities of human chromosomes. The **deletion** of a portion of a chromosome leads to the loss of genetic material and a shortened chromosome. A **reciprocal translocation** involves breaks on two nonhomologous chromosomes, with exchange of the acentric segments. An **inversion** requires two breaks in a single chromosome. If the breaks are on opposite sides of the centromere, the inversion is **pericentric**; it is **paracentric** if the breaks are on the same arm. A **Robertsonian translocation** occurs when two nonhomologous acrocentric chromosomes break near their centromeres, after which the long arms fuse to form one large metacentric chromosome. **Isochromosomes** arise from faulty centromere division, which leads to duplication of the long arm (iso q) and deletion of the short arm, or the reverse (iso p). **Ring chromosomes** involve breaks of both telomeric portions of a chromosome, deletion of the acentric fragments, and fusion of the remaining centric portion.

Chromosomal Aberrations During Pregnancy

Chromosomal abnormalities identified in liveborn infants at birth differ from those in early spontaneous abortions. At birth, the common chromosomal abnormalities are trisomies 21 (most frequent), 18, 13, and X or Y (47,XXX; 47,XXY; and 47,XYY). ***About 0.3% of all infants have a chromosomal abnormality, but up to 35% of spontaneous abortions have one.*** The most common chromosomal abnormalities in spontaneous abortions are, in descending order of frequency, 45,X, then trisomies 16, 21, and 22. Importantly, trisomy of almost any chromosome occurs in spontaneous abortions. The reason for these differences is presumably related to survival in utero.

Effects of Chromosomal Aberrations

Autosomal trisomies give rise to developmental abnormalities. Affected fetuses usually die during pregnancy or shortly after birth. Trisomy 21, which causes Down syndrome, is an exception, and people with this condition may survive for years. X chromosome trisomy may bring on in abnormal development but is not lethal.

Mitotic nondisjunction in embryonic cells early in development results in **mosaicism**, in which chromosomal aberrations are transmitted in some cell lineages but not others. ***The body thus has two or more karyotypically different cell lines.*** Mosaicism may involve autosomes or sex chromosomes, and the phenotype depends on the chromosome involved and the extent of mosaicism. Autosomal mosaicism was once thought to be rare but probably occurs fairly frequently, and mosaicism involving sex chromosomes is common. In fact, aneuploidy and mosaicism of sex chromosomes are the most important causes of infertility or abnormal development. Phenotypes in patients with mosaicism depend on the ratio of abnormal and normal cells and are more severe when the proportion of abnormal cells is higher.

Table 5-2

Chromosomal Nomenclature

Numerical designation of autosomes	1–22
Sex chromosomes	X, Y
Addition of a whole or part of a chromosome	+
Loss of a whole or part of a chromosome	–
Numerical mosaicism (e.g., 46/47)	/
Short arm of chromosome (petite)	p
Long arm of chromosome	q
Isochromosome	i
Ring chromosome	r
Deletion	del
Insertion	ins
Translocation	t
Derivative chromosome (carrying translocation)	der
Terminal	ter
Representative Karyotypes	
Male with trisomy 21 (Down syndrome)	47,XY, +21
Female with Robertsonian translocation between chromosomes 14 and 21	45,XX,t(14;21)(q10;q10)
Cri du chat syndrome (male) with deletion of a portion of the short arm of chromosome 5	46,XY, del(5p)
Male with ring chromosome 19	46,XY, r(19)
Turner syndrome with monosomy X	45,X
Mosaic Klinefelter syndrome	47,XXY/46,XY

CHROMOSOMAL SYNDROMES

Structural alterations that may result in clinical disorders include trisomies, translocations, deletions, and chromosomal breakage (Tables 5-2 and 5-3).

Trisomy 21: Down Syndrome

Trisomy 21 is the most common cause of mental retardation. Liveborn infants represent only a fraction of all conceptuses with this defect because two thirds abort spontaneously or die in utero. Advances in treating infections, congenital heart defects, and leukemia—the leading causes of death in Down syndrome—have increased the life expectancy of persons with trisomy 21.

EPIDEMIOLOGY: *The incidence of trisomy 21 rises dramatically with increasing maternal age; older mothers are at increased risk to have children with Down syndrome* (Fig. 5-10). Up to the mid-30s, a woman's risk of giving birth to a trisomic child is about 1 in 300 to 900 liveborn infants. By age 45, the incidence is 1 in 25. Nevertheless, 80% of children with Down syndrome are born to mothers under 35 years, perhaps because women in this age group conceive more often and have not been screened. ***The risk of a second child with Down syndrome is comparable to that of the normal population, regardless of maternal age, unless the syndrome is associated with translocation of chromosome 21.***

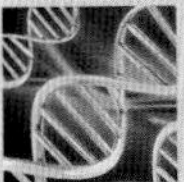

MOLECULAR PATHOGENESIS: Chromosome 21 is the smallest human autosome, containing less than 2% of all human DNA. It is an acrocentric chromosome, and all functional 200 to 250 genes are on the long arm (21q). The region responsible for the full Down syndrome phenotype is in band 21q22.2, a 4-Mb region of DNA, called the **Down syndrome critical region** (DSCR).

Mechanisms that explain how three copies of *DSCR* genes occur in somatic cells are as follows:

- **Nondisjunction** in the first meiotic division of gametogenesis (meiosis I) accounts for the majority (92% to 95%) of patients with trisomy 21. The extra chromosome 21 is maternal in about 95% of such cases.
- **Translocation** of an extra long arm of chromosome 21 to another acrocentric chromosome causes 5% of cases.
- **Mosaicism** for trisomy 21 reflects nondisjunction during mitosis of a somatic cell early in embryogenesis (2%).

The maternal age effect is related to maternal nondisjunction events, virtually all during maternal meiosis I. Down syndrome caused by translocation or mosaicism is not related to maternal age.

Down syndrome caused by translocation of an extra portion of chromosome 21 occurs in two situations. Either parent may be

Table 5-3

Clinical Features of the Autosomal Chromosomal Syndromes

Syndromes	Features
Trisomic Syndromes	
Chromosome 21 (Down syndrome 47,XX or XY, +21)	Epicanthic folds, speckled irides, flat nasal bridge, congenital heart disease, simian crease of palms, Hirschsprung disease, increased risk of leukemia
Chromosome 18 (47,XX or XY, +18)	Female preponderance, micrognathia, congenital heart disease, horseshoe kidney, deformed fingers
Chromosome 13 (47,XX or XY, +13)	Persistent fetal hemoglobin, microcephaly, congenital heart disease, polycystic kidneys, polydactyly, simian crease
Deletion Syndromes	
5p− syndrome (cri du chat 46,XX or XY, 5p−)	Cat-like cry, low birth weight, microcephaly, epicanthic folds, congenital heart disease, short hands and feet, simian crease
11p− syndrome (46,XX or XY, 11p−)	Aniridia, Wilms tumor, gonadoblastoma, male genital ambiguity
13q− syndrome (46,XX or XY, 13q−)	Low birth weight, microcephaly, retinoblastoma, congenital heart disease

All of these syndromes are associated with mental retardation.

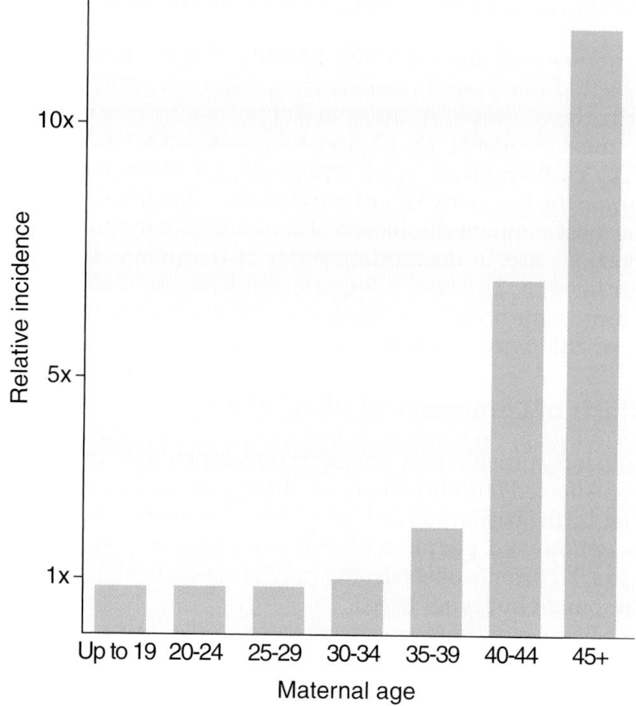

FIGURE 5-10. Incidence of Down syndrome in relation to maternal age. A conspicuous increase in the frequency of this disorder is seen beyond the age of 35 years.

a phenotypically normal carrier of a balanced translocation, or a translocation may arise de novo during gametogenesis. These translocations are typically Robertsonian, tending to involve only acrocentric chromosomes, with short arms consisting of a satellite and stalk (chromosomes 13, 14, 15, 21, and 22). Translocations between these chromosomes are particularly common because they cluster during meiosis and are liable to break and recombine more than other chromosomes. The most common translocation in Down syndrome (50%) is fusion of the long arms of chromosomes 21 and 14, followed in frequency (40%) by similar fusion involving two chromosomes 21.

If the translocation is inherited from a parent, a balanced translocation has been converted to an unbalanced one. Then, one would expect a one in three chance of Down syndrome among offspring of a carrier of a balanced Robertsonian translocation. However, early loss of most embryos with trisomy 21 means that the actual incidence is only 10% to 15% with a maternal translocation and less than 5% if the father is the carrier (Fig. 5-11).

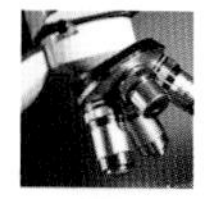
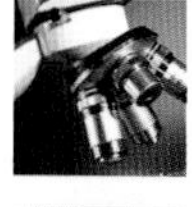
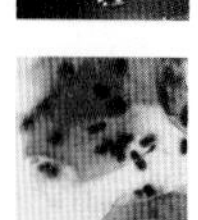

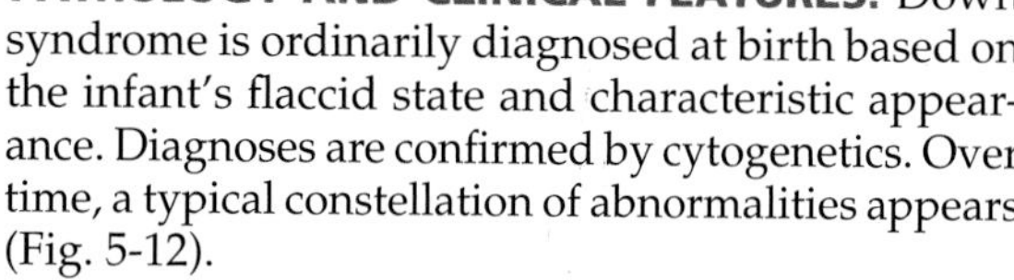

PATHOLOGY AND CLINICAL FEATURES: Down syndrome is ordinarily diagnosed at birth based on the infant's flaccid state and characteristic appearance. Diagnoses are confirmed by cytogenetics. Over time, a typical constellation of abnormalities appears (Fig. 5-12).

- **Mental status:** Children with Down syndrome are invariably mentally retarded; their average IQ is 30 to 60. Their cognitive skills decrease as they grow older, and they are at a very high risk for early-onset Alzheimer disease.
- **Craniofacial features:** Face and occiput tend to be flat, with a low-bridged nose, reduced interpupillary distance, and oblique palpebral fissures. Epicanthal folds of the eyes impart an Asian appearance, which accounts for the obsolete term **mongolism**. Irides are speckled with **Brushfield spots**. Ears are enlarged, low set, and malformed. A prominent tongue, typically lacking a central fissure, protrudes through an open mouth.
- **Heart:** One third of children with Down syndrome have cardiac malformations. The incidence is even higher in aborted fetuses. Anomalies include atrioventricular canal, ventricular and atrial septal defects, tetralogy of Fallot, and patent ductus arteriosus (see Chapter 9).
- **Skeleton:** These children tend to be small, owing to shorter than normal bones of the ribs, pelvis, and extremities. Their hands are broad and short with a "simian crease," a single transverse crease across the palm. The middle phalanx of the fifth finger is hypoplastic and curves inward.
- **Gastrointestinal tract:** Duodenal stenosis or atresia, imperforate anus, and Hirschsprung disease (megacolon) occur in 2% to 3% of these children (see Chapter 11).
- **Reproductive system:** Men are invariably sterile, owing to arrested spermatogenesis. A few women with Down syndrome have given birth to children, 40% of whom had trisomy 21.
- **Immune system:** Affected children are unusually susceptible to respiratory and other infections, although there is no clear pattern of immune defects.
- **Hematologic disorders:** Patients with Down syndrome have a particularly high risk of developing leukemia at all ages. ***The risk of leukemia in Down syndrome children***

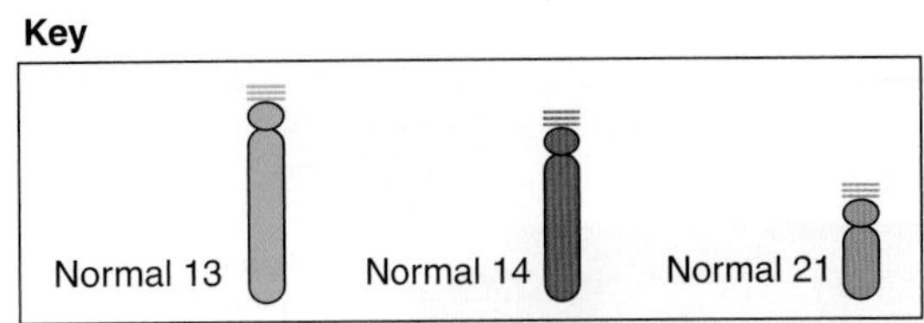

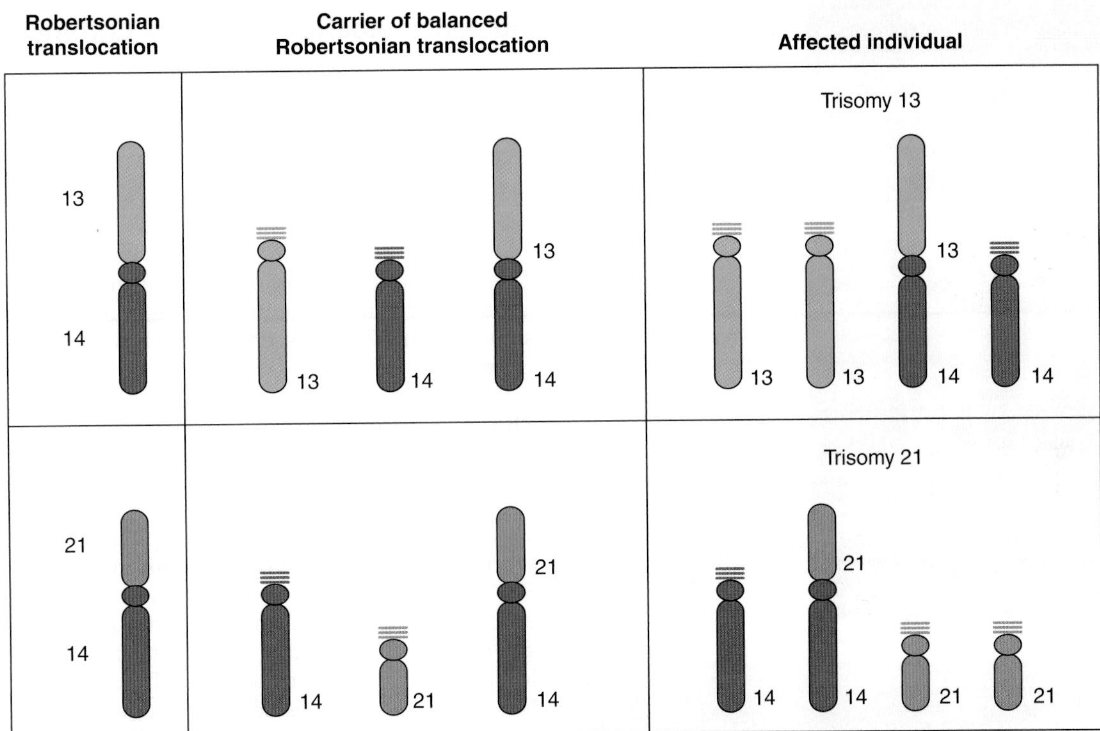

FIGURE 5-11. Robertsonian translocations and trisomy. From Genetics Home Reference. U.S. National Library of Medicine, U.S. Department of Health & Human Services, Bethesda, MD, 2017. Available at https://ghr.nlm.nih.gov/art/large/robertsonian-translocation.jpeg

under 15 years of age is 10- to 20-fold higher than normal. In children under 4 years of age, acute myeloid leukemia predominates. In older individuals, acute lymphoblastic leukemia is most common.

- **Neurologic disorders:** There is no clear pattern of neuropathology in Down syndrome, nor are there characteristic changes on the electroencephalogram. *The association of Down syndrome with Alzheimer disease is related to the presence of the gene for the amyloid precursor protein on the triplicated chromosome 21.* By age 35, characteristic Alzheimer lesions are universal in these patients (see Chapter 24). Senile plaques and cerebral blood vessels in both Alzheimer disease and Down syndrome always contain β-amyloid protein; Alzheimer disease causes the sharp decline in survival in Down syndrome subjects over 45 years of age. Only about 25% live for more than 60 years of age, in which case most have Alzheimer disease.
- **Life expectancy:** In the first decade of life, the presence or absence of congenital heart disease largely determines survival in Down syndrome. Only 5% of those with normal hearts die before age 10, but one fourth of those with heart disease die by that age. Life expectancy in patients who reach age 10 is about 55 years, which is more than 20 years lower than that of the general population. Only 10% reach age 70.

Trisomy of Chromosomes 18 and 13

Trisomy 18, or Edwards syndrome, occurs in 1 of 3,000 to 8,000 live births and is the second most common autosomal trisomy syndrome. It causes mental retardation and affects females three times more often than males. Virtually, all infants with trisomy 18 have severe cardiac malformations, and survival of more than a few months is rare. Other anomalies include clenched hands with overlap of fingers, intrauterine growth retardation, rocker bottom feet, micrognathia, prominent occiput, microphthalmia, low-set ears, and renal anomalies. Given the severe congenital defects, about 95% abort spontaneously. About 50% of liveborn trisomy 18 patients die within 1 week, and 90% die within a year. The risk of bearing a fetus with trisomy 18 is higher in women older than 35 years. This trisomy may occur as a mosaic with more moderate phenotypic expression.

Trisomy 13, or Patau syndrome, is rare. It occurs in 1 in 20,000 to 25,000 births and is associated with severe mental and growth retardation. Significant malformations include cleft lip and cleft palate, plus severe nervous system and cardiac malformations. This syndrome is also associated with increased maternal age. Trisomy 21, trisomy 18, and trisomy 13 are the only known trisomies in liveborn infants.

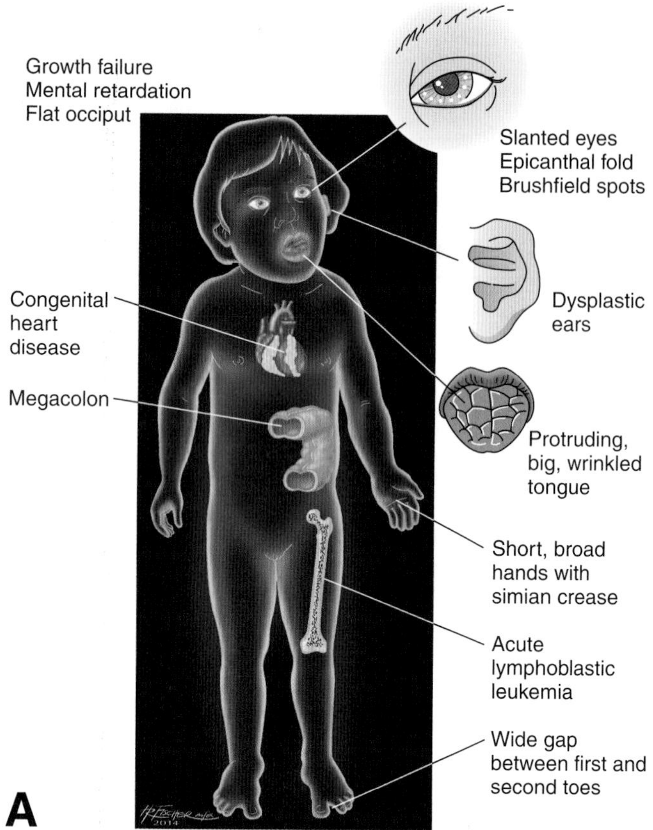

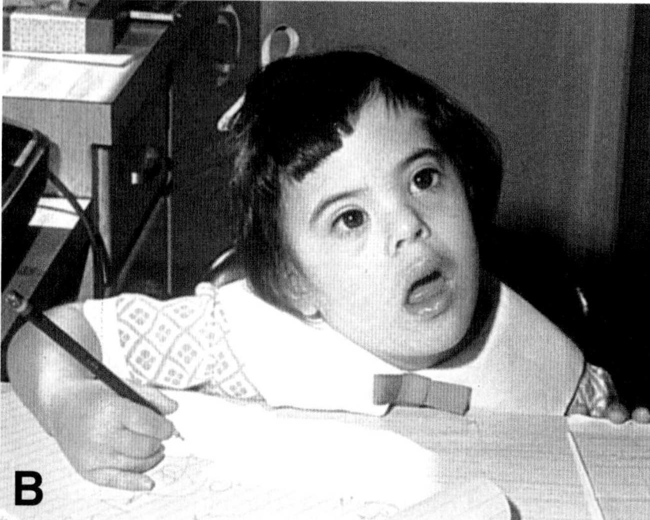

FIGURE 5-12. **A.** Clinical features of Down syndrome. **B.** A young girl with the facial features of Down syndrome.

Chromosomal Deletion Syndromes

Deletion of an entire autosomal chromosome (i.e., monosomy) is usually not compatible with life. However, several syndromes arise from deletions of parts of several chromosomes (Table 5-3). Most of these congenital syndromes are sporadic, but in a few instances, reciprocal translocations occur in the parents. Virtually, all of these deletion syndromes have phenotypes that exhibit low birth weight, mental retardation, microcephaly, and craniofacial and skeletal abnormalities. Cardiac and urogenital malformations are also common. **5p− syndrome (cri du chat)** is the best-known deletion syndrome because the high-pitched cry of the infant is like that of a kitten and calls attention to the disorder. It features intellectual disability and delayed development, microcephaly, low birth weight, and hypotonia in infancy.

Numerical Aberrations of Sex Chromosomes

Additional sex chromosomes (Fig. 5-13) cause less severe clinical manifestations than do extra autosomes and are less likely to disturb the critical stages of development. Additional X chromosomes probably cause less severe phenotypes because of **lyonization**, a normal process by which each cell only has one active X chromosome.

The contrast between the X and Y chromosomes is striking. The X chromosome is one of the larger chromosomes containing about 2,000 genes. By contrast, the much smaller Y chromosome has only 78 genes, one of which is the testis-determining gene (*SRY*).

The Y Chromosome

In humans, genes on the Y chromosome are key determinants of gender phenotype. Thus, people who are XXY (Klinefelter syndrome; see below) have a male phenotype, whereas those who are XO (Turner syndrome) are female. The intronless *SRY* gene near the end of the short arm of the Y chromosome encodes the testis-determining factor (TDF), also called the **sex-determining region Y protein** or **SRY protein**, which initiates male sex determination. Mutations in *SRY* create XY females, whereas translocations that add *SRY* to an X chromosome produce XX males. A small proportion of infertile men with azoospermia or severe oligospermia exhibit small deletions in parts of the Y chromosome.

The X Chromosome

Males carry only one X chromosome but have the same amount of products from that chromosome for almost all loci as do females. This seeming discrepancy is explained by the **Lyon effect:**

- In females, one X chromosome is irreversibly inactivated early in embryogenesis and is detectable in interphase nuclei as a clump of heterochromatin attached to the inner nuclear membrane, the **Barr body**. The inactive X chromosome is extensively methylated at gene control regions and transcriptionally repressed. Nevertheless, a significant minority of X-linked genes escapes inactivation and continues to be expressed by both X chromosomes. The probability that an X chromosome is inactive seems to correlate with levels of *XIST*, an X-linked DNA sequence that is transcribed to an RNA species expressed only by the inactive partner.
- Either the paternal or maternal X chromosome is inactivated randomly.
- X chromosome inactivation is permanent and transmitted to progeny cells, so paternally or maternally derived X chromosomes are propagated clonally. ***All females are thus mosaic for paternal and maternal X chromosomes.*** Mosaicism in females for glucose-6-phosphate dehydrogenase was a key in demonstrating the monoclonal origin of neoplasms (see Chapter 4).

Gametes: Ovum \ Sperm	X	Y	XY	O
X	46,XX Normal ♀	46,XY Normal ♂	47,XXY Klinefelter ♂	45,X Turner ♀
XX	47,XXX ♀	47,XXY Klinefelter ♂	48,XXXY Klinefelter ♂	46,XX Normal ♀
XXX	48,XXXX ♀	48,XXXY Klinefelter ♂	49,XXXXY Klinefelter ♂	47,XXX Triple X ♀
O	45,X Turner ♀	45,Y LETHAL	46,XY LETHAL	44 LETHAL

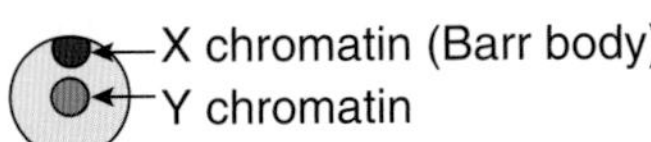

FIGURE 5-13. Numerical aberrations of sex chromosomes. Nondisjunction in either the male or female gamete is the principal cause of these abnormalities.

If one X chromosome is entirely nonfunctional, individuals with XXY (Klinefelter syndrome) or XO (Turner syndrome) karyotypes should be phenotypically normal. The fact that they are not indicates that inactivated X chromosomes still partly function. Indeed, a part of the X chromosome short arm is known to escape inactivation. This pseudoautosomal region can pair with a homologous region on the short arm of the Y chromosome and undergo meiotic recombination. Genes in this location are present in two functional copies in both males and females. Thus, patients with Turner syndrome (45,X) are haploinsufficient for these genes, and those with more than two X chromosomes (e.g., Klinefelter syndrome) have more than two functional copies. A gene in this region, *SHOX*, is associated with height, and its haploinsufficiency in Turner syndrome may explain the short stature of patients with Turner syndrome. Extra copies of *SHOX* may explain the increased stature in other sex chromosome aneuploidy conditions, such as 47,XXX; 47,XYY; 47,XXY; and 48,XXYY. Several other genes outside the pseudoautosomal region also escape X inactivation. ***Mental retardation in phenotypic boys and girls with extra X chromosomes correlates roughly with the number of X chromosomes.***

Klinefelter Syndrome (47,XXY)

In Klinefelter syndrome, males have a Y chromosome plus two more X chromosomes. This is the most important clinical condition involving trisomy of sex chromosomes (Fig. 5-14). It is a prominent cause of male hypogonadism and infertility.

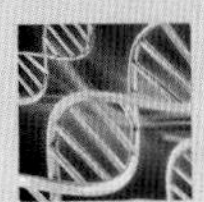

MOLECULAR PATHOGENESIS: Most men with Klinefelter syndrome (80%) have one extra X chromosome (47,XXY). A minority are mosaics (46,XY/47,XXY) or have more than two X chromosomes (48,XXXY). ***Regardless of the number of supernumerary X chromosomes (even up to 4), the Y chromosome ensures a male phenotype.*** Additional X chromosomes correlate with more abnormal phenotypes, despite inactivation of the extra X chromosomes. Presumably, the same genes that escape inactivation in normal females are functional in Klinefelter syndrome.

Klinefelter syndrome occurs in 1 per 1,000 male newborns, about the incidence of Down syndrome. Interestingly, half of all 47,XXY conceptuses are miscarried. The additional X chromosome(s) results from meiotic nondisjunction during gametogenesis. In half of cases, nondisjunction in paternal meiosis I leads to sperm with both X and Y chromosomes. Fertilization of a normal egg by such a sperm yields a 47,XXY karyotype.

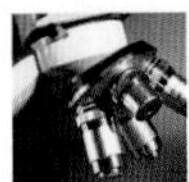

PATHOLOGY: After puberty, the intrinsically abnormal testes do not respond to gonadotropin stimulation and show later regressive changes. Seminiferous tubules display atrophy, hyalinization, and peritubular fibrosis. Germ cells and Sertoli cells are usually absent, and the tubules become dense cords of collagen. Leydig cells are increased in number and are functionally impaired, as evidenced by low testosterone levels in the face of elevated luteinizing hormone (LH) levels.

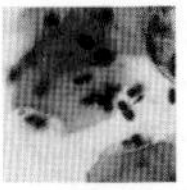

CLINICAL FEATURES: The diagnosis of Klinefelter syndrome is usually made after puberty because the main manifestations of the disorder during childhood are behavioral and psychiatric. Gross mental retardation is uncommon, but average IQ is somewhat reduced.

Children with Klinefelter syndrome tend to be tall and thin, with relatively long legs (eunuchoid body habitus). Normal testicular growth and masculinization do not occur at puberty, and the testes and penis remain small. Feminine characteristics include a high-pitched voice, gynecomastia, and a female pattern of pubic hair (female escutcheon). Azoospermia results in infertility. These changes reflect hypogonadism and a resulting lack of androgens. Serum testosterone is low to normal, but LH and FSH are high, indicating normal pituitary function. High circulating estradiol levels increase the

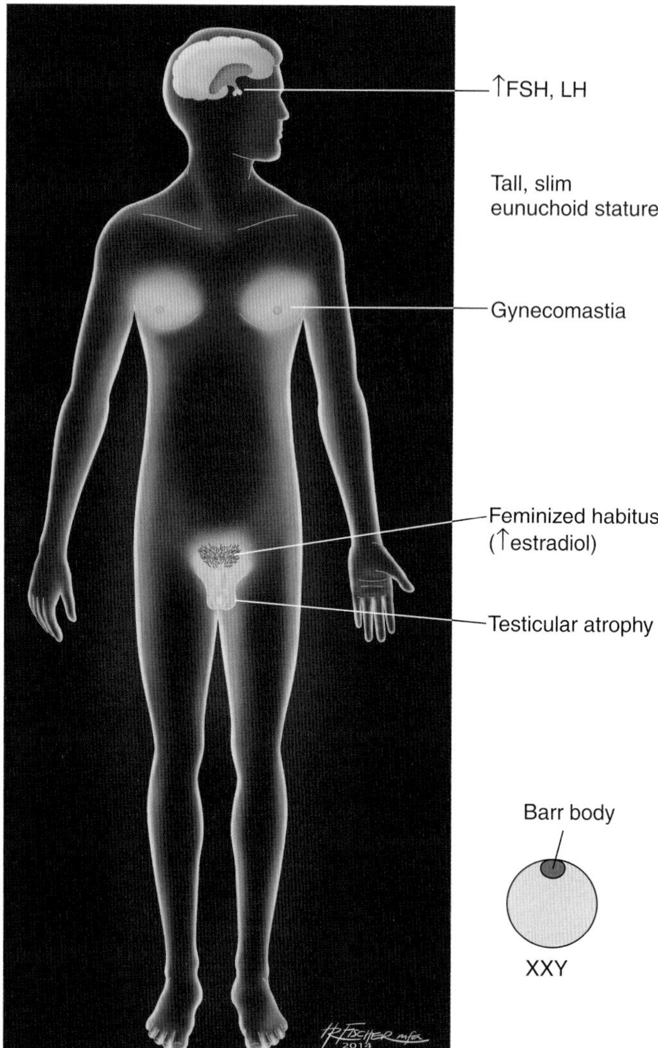

FIGURE 5-14. Clinical features of Klinefelter syndrome. FSH, follicle-stimulating hormone; LH, luteinizing hormone.

estradiol-to-testosterone ratio, which determines the degree of feminization. Treatment with testosterone will virilize these patients but does not restore fertility.

The XYY Male

Interest in the XYY phenotype (1 in 1,000 male newborns) comes from studies suggesting that this karyotype is significantly more prevalent in male prisoners than in the general population. However, the idea that XYY "supermales" show antisocial behavior because of an extra Y chromosome has not been substantiated, and the topic remains controversial. Acknowledged features of the XYY phenotype are tall stature, a tendency toward cystic acne, and some problems in motor and language development. Y chromosome aneuploidy results from meiotic nondisjunction in the father.

Turner Syndrome

Turner syndrome is the spectrum of abnormalities that derives from **complete or partial X chromosome monosomy in a phenotypic female**. It occurs in 1 in 5,000 females. In three fourths of cases, the single X chromosome is of maternal origin, suggesting that the meiotic error tends to be paternal. The incidence of Turner syndrome does not correlate with maternal age, and the risk of producing a second affected female infant is not increased.

The 45,X karyotype is one of the most common aneuploidies in human conceptuses, but almost all are aborted spontaneously. Because patients with Turner syndrome survive normally after birth, it is unclear why the lack of an X chromosome is lethal during fetal development. It is believed that homologs of Y genes in the pseudoautosomal region of the X chromosome escape inactivation and are critical for survival of female embryos.

About half of patients with Turner syndrome lack an entire X chromosome (monosomy X). The remainder are mosaics or have structural aberrations of the X chromosome, such as isochromosome of the long arm, translocations, and deletions. Mosaic patients with Turner syndrome who have a Y chromosome in some cells have a 20% risk of developing a germ cell cancer and should have prophylactic removal of the abnormal gonads.

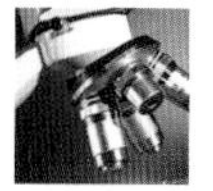

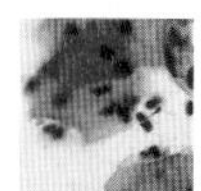

PATHOLOGY AND CLINICAL FEATURES: The clinical hallmarks of Turner syndrome are sexual infantilism with primary amenorrhea and sterility (Fig. 5-15). The disorder is usually discovered when the absence of menarche brings the child to medical attention. Virtually, all of these women are under 5 ft (152 cm) in height. Other clinical features include a short, webbed neck (pterygium colli), low posterior hairline, wide carrying angle of the arms (cubitus valgus), broad chest with widely spaced nipples, and hyperconvex fingernails. Half of patients have renal anomalies, the most common being horseshoe kidney and malrotation. Many have facial abnormalities, including a small mandible, prominent ears, and epicanthal folds. Defective hearing and vision are common, and up to 20% are mentally retarded. Pigmented nevi become

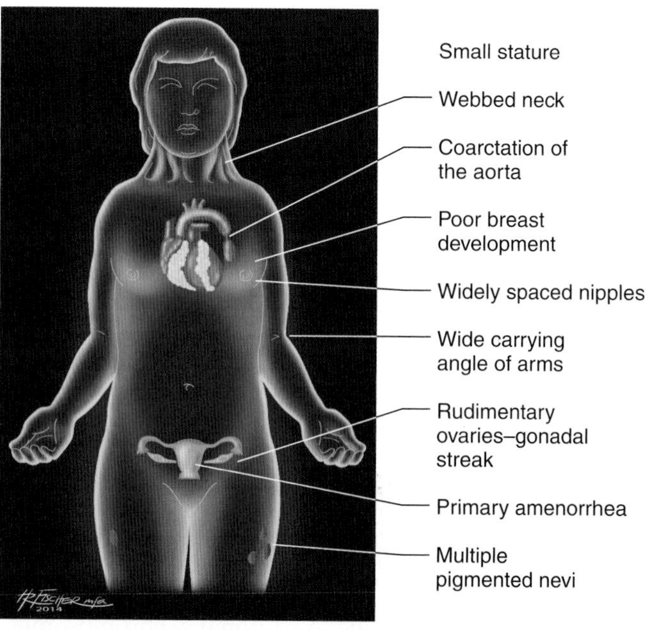

FIGURE 5-15. Clinical features of Turner syndrome.

prominent with age. For unknown reasons, women with Turner syndrome are at a significant risk for chronic autoimmune thyroiditis and goiter.

Cardiovascular anomalies occur in almost half of patients with Turner syndrome: coarctation of the aorta in 15% and a bicuspid aortic valve in up to one third. Essential hypertension occurs in some patients, and dissecting aneurysm of the aorta may occasionally be lethal.

Ovaries of women with Turner syndrome show a curious acceleration of normal aging. Normal female fetal ovaries initially contain 7 million oocytes each, less than half of which survive until birth. Relentless loss of oocytes continues, so that by menarche, only about 5% (400,000) remain. At menopause, 0.1% survive. By contrast, ovaries of fetuses with Turner syndrome contain oocytes at first but lose them rapidly. None remain by 2 years of age. The ovaries become fibrous streaks, but the uterus, fallopian tubes, and vagina develop normally. Thus, menopause in children with Turner syndrome may be considered to occur long before menarche. Children with Turner syndrome are treated with growth hormone and estrogens, and most experience for a normal, albeit infertile, life.

Syndromes in Females With Multiple X Chromosomes

One extra X chromosome in a phenotypic female (i.e., a 47,XXX karyotype) is the most frequent abnormality of sex chromosomes in women. It occurs at about the same rate as Klinefelter syndrome. Most of these women are of normal intelligence but may have some difficulty in speech, learning, and emotional responses. Minor physical anomalies are seen, such as epicanthal folds and clinodactyly (inward curvature of the fifth finger). These women are usually fertile, but their children are more susceptible to congenital defects.

FUNCTIONAL CONSEQUENCES OF MUTATIONS

A biochemical pathway represents the sequential actions of a series of enzymes, which are encoded by specific genes. A typical pathway can be represented by the conversion of a substrate (A) through intermediate metabolites (B and C) to a final product (D).

A single-gene defect can have several consequences:

- **Failure to complete a metabolic pathway:** The endproduct (D) is not formed because an enzyme needed to complete a metabolic sequence is missing.
- **Accumulation of unmetabolized substrate:** The enzyme that converts the initial substrate to the first intermediary metabolite may be missing so the initial substrate accumulates in excess.
- **Storage of an intermediary metabolite:** An intermediary metabolite, which is normally quickly processed into the final product and is present only in minute amounts, accumulates if the enzyme for its metabolism is lacking.
- **Formation of an abnormal endproduct:** A mutant gene encodes an abnormal protein.

Mutation Hotspots

Certain regions of the genome mutate at a much higher rate than average. These "hotspots" are usually DNA sequences with inherent instability. They have an increased tendency toward unequal crossing over or may be predisposed to single-nucleotide substitutions. The best-characterized hotspot is the dinucleotide CG or CpG sites.

The cytosines in CpG p-phosphate dinucleotides can be methylated to 5-methylcytosine. In mammals, CpG methylation commonly represses gene transcription. Such an ***epigenetic*** change affects gene expression by mechanisms other than changes in DNA base sequences (see Chapter 4). 5-Methylcytosines can undergo spontaneous deamination to thymine. If this occurs in a gamete, it can become a fixed mutation in the offspring. Regions of the genome that have higher concentrations of CpGs are known as **CpG islands**. Many mammalian genes have CpG islands in their promoter regions.

Autosomal Dominant Disorders

If only one mutated allele is sufficient to cause disease when its paired allele on the homologous autosome is normal, the mutant trait is considered to be dominant. The features of autosomal dominant traits are as follows (Fig. 5-16):

- Males and females are affected equally because the mutant gene is on an autosome. Thus, father-to-son transmission (which is absent in X-linked disorders) may occur.
- The trait encoded by the mutant gene can be transmitted to successive generations (unless reproductive capacity is compromised).
- Unaffected members of a family do not transmit the trait to their offspring. Unless the disease represents a new mutation, everyone with the disease has an affected parent.
- Proportions of normal and diseased offspring of patients with the disorder are about equal because most affected people are heterozygous, and their normal mates do not carry the defective gene.

Biochemical Basis of Autosomal Dominant Disorders

There are several major mechanisms by which a single mutated allele may cause disease even when the other allele is normal.

- If the gene product is rate limiting in a complex metabolic network (e.g., a receptor or an enzyme), having half of the normal amount of gene product may be insufficient for a normal phenotype. This is known as **haploinsufficiency**.
- In some diseases, an extra copy of an allele gives rise to an abnormal phenotype. An example of this is Charcot–Marie–Tooth disease type IA, which is caused by duplication of the *peripheral myelin protein-22* gene.
- A mutant protein may be insensitive to normal regulation. For example, mutations in the *RET* proto-oncogene in families with multiple endocrine neoplasia type 2 (MEN2) increase the activity of a tyrosine kinase that stimulates cell proliferation.
- In **dominant-negative mutations**, the aberrant product of the mutant allele interferes with the function of the normal allele. Mutations in genes for structural proteins (e.g., collagens and cytoskeletal constituents) cause abnormal molecular interactions and disrupt normal morphologic patterns.

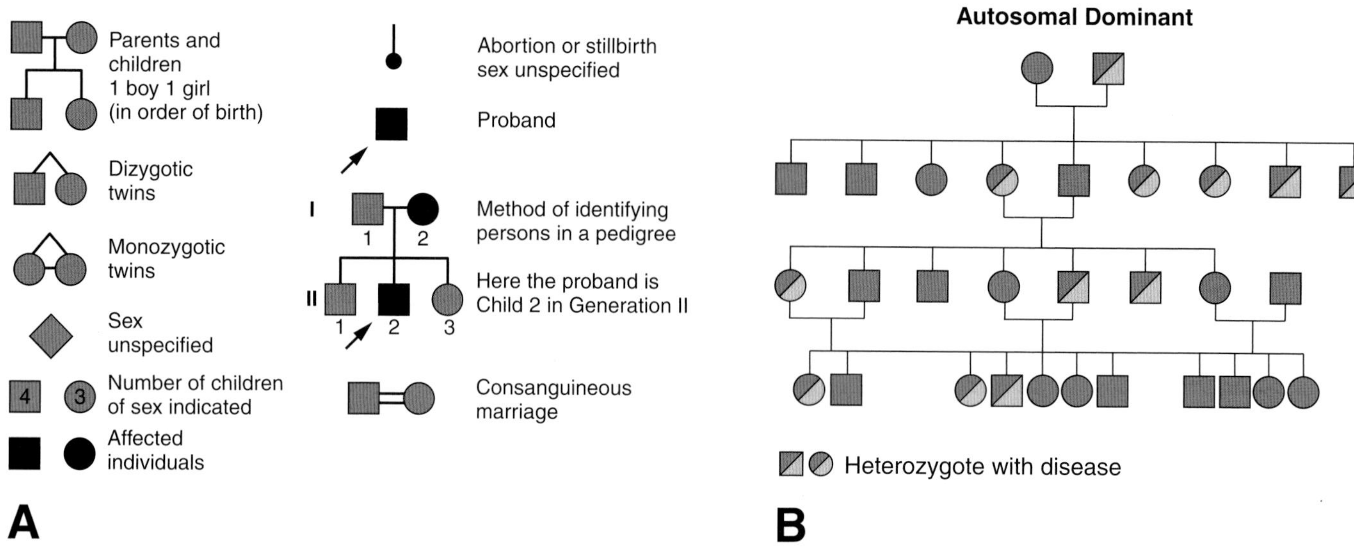

FIGURE 5-16. **A. Definition of symbols in a pedigree.** Males, squares; females, circles. A line drawn between a square and a circle represents a mating of that male and female. Two lines drawn between a square and a circle indicate a consanguineous mating in which the two individuals are related, usually as second cousins. Children of a mating are connected to a horizontal line, called the sibship line, by short vertical lines. The children of a sibship are always listed in order of birth, the oldest being on the left. Other conventions concerning twins and identification of probands and affected individuals are shown in the figure. **B. Autosomal dominant inheritance.** Only symptomatic individuals transmit the trait to the next generation, and heterozygotes are symptomatic. Both males and females are affected.

More than 1,000 human diseases are inherited as autosomal dominant traits, although most are rare. Examples of human autosomal dominant diseases are shown in Table 5-4.

Inherited Connective Tissue Diseases

This discussion is limited to three of the most common and best-studied diseases of connective tissue: Marfan syndrome, Ehlers–Danlos syndrome, and osteogenesis imperfecta. Even in these well-delineated disorders, the clinical phenotypes often overlap. Thus, some patients in a family may develop the joint dislocations typical of Ehlers–Danlos syndrome, whereas others suffer from multiple fractures more characteristic of OI. Still others with the same genetic defect may have no symptoms. The pathogenesis of all three conditions is attributed to both dominant-negative and haploinsufficiency effects, depending on the nature of the mutation. In general, "null" alleles that result in reduced levels of a normal protein result in haploinsufficiency, whereas alleles that produce a structurally altered product are often associated with dominant-negative effects.

Marfan Syndrome

Marfan syndrome is an autosomal dominant disorder of connective tissue affecting many organs, including the heart, aorta, skeleton, eyes, and skin. In all, 15% to 30% of cases are de novo mutations that occur once in 20,000 live births. Marfan syndrome affects males and females equally and shows no ethnic or geographical bias. About 1 in 3,000 to 5,000 persons have Marfan syndrome.

Table 5-4

Representative Autosomal Dominant Disorders

Disease	Frequency	Chromosome
Familial hypercholesterolemia	1/500	19p
von Willebrand disease	1/8,000	12p
Hereditary spherocytosis (major forms)	1/5,000	14, 8
Hereditary elliptocytosis (all forms)	1/2,500	1, 1p, 2q, 14
Osteogenesis imperfecta (types I–IV)	1/10,000	17q, 7q
Ehlers–Danlos syndrome (all types)	1/5,000	2q
Marfan syndrome	1/5,000	15q
Neurofibromatosis type 1	1/3,500	17q
Huntington chorea	1/15,000	4p
Retinoblastoma	1/14,000	13q
Wilms tumor	1/10,000	11p
Familial adenomatous polyposis	1/10,000	5q
Acute intermittent porphyria	1/15,000	11q
Hereditary amyloidosis	1/100,000	18q
Adult polycystic kidney disease	1/1,000	16p

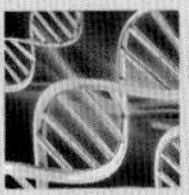

MOLECULAR PATHOGENESIS: The cause of Marfan syndrome is a missense mutation in the gene for *fibrillin-1 (FBN1)*, on the long arm of chromosome 15. **Fibrillins** belongs to a family of collagen-like connective tissue proteins. There are now about a dozen genetically distinct fibrillins, and over 100 mutations are known. They are present in many tissues, in the form of **microfibrils**, thread-like filaments that form larger fibers and are organized into rods, sheets, and interlaced networks. These fibers are scaffolds for elastin deposition during embryonic development, after which they remain as a component of elastic tissues (e.g., elastin is deposited on lamellae of microfibrillar fibers in the concentric rings of elastin in the aortic wall). Deficiencies in the amount and distribution of microfibrillar fibers occur in skin, which renders the elastic fibers incompetent to resist normal stress. Fibrillin also binds to TGF-β, a multifunctional protein that regulates cell proliferation and is upregulated in a variety of inflammatory diseases (see Chapters 2 and 4). Patients with Marfan syndrome have increased TGF-β in the aorta, cardiac valves, and lungs, possibly because of decreased fibrillin-1. There is currently dispute as to whether dominant-negative effects that produce interference with TGF-β or haploinsufficiency are responsible for the pathogenesis of Marfan syndrome.

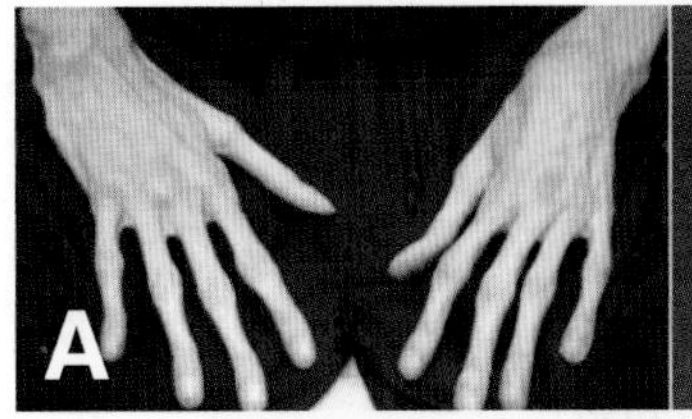

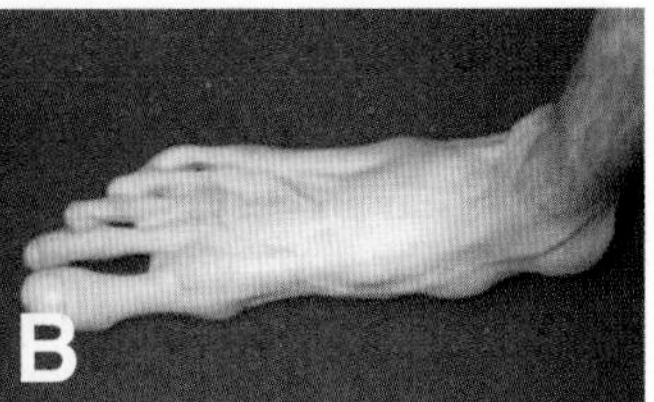

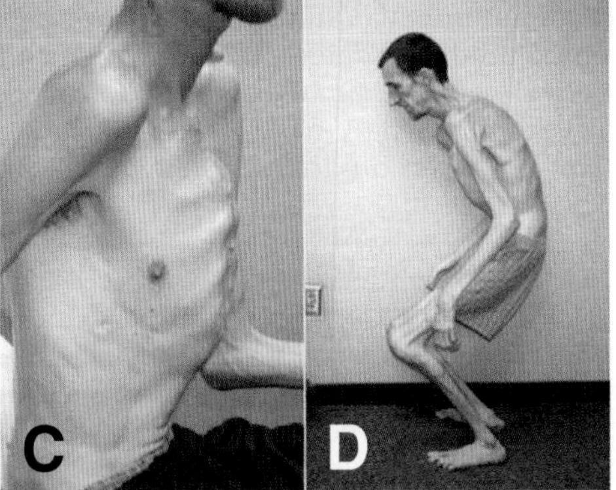

FIGURE 5-17. **Features of Marfan syndrome. A, B.** Long, slender digits (arachnodactyly). **C, D.** Tall slender build with disproportionately long arms, legs, fingers and toes, and a breastbone that protrudes outward or dips inward.

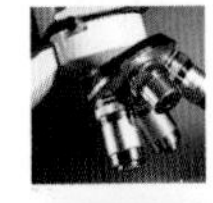

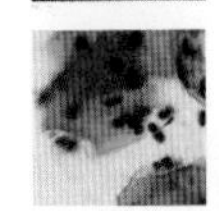

PATHOLOGY AND CLINICAL FEATURES: People with Marfan syndrome are usually (but not always) tall, with greater lower body length (pubis to sole) than upper body length. They are slender in habitus, reflecting a paucity of subcutaneous fat, and have long, thin extremities and fingers (arachnodactyly) (Fig. 5-17).

- **Skeletal system:** The skull in Marfan syndrome is usually long (dolichocephalic), with prominent frontal eminences. Disorders of the ribs cause pectus excavatum (concave sternum) and pectus carinatum (pigeon breast). Tendons, ligaments, and joint capsules are weak, leading to hyperextensibility of the joints (double-jointedness), dislocations, hernias, and often severe kyphoscoliosis.
- **Cardiovascular system:** ***The most important defect is in the aorta, where the tunica media is weak.*** This leads to variable dilation of the ascending aorta and a high incidence of dissecting aneurysms, usually of the ascending aorta. Expansion of the aortic ring results in aortic regurgitation, which may be severe enough to produce angina pectoris and congestive heart failure (see Chapter 9). Patients most often die of cardiovascular disorders.
- **Eyes:** Ocular changes are common in Marfan syndrome. These include dislocation of the lens (ectopia lentis), severe myopia as a result of elongation of the eye, and retinal detachment.

Untreated men with Marfan syndrome usually died in their 30s, and untreated women often succumbed in their 40s. However, antihypertensive therapy and replacement of the ascending aorta and aortic valve with prosthetic grafts have significantly improved longevity. Although there is no cure, life expectancy has increased significantly over the past few decades and now approaches that of the average person.

Ehlers–Danlos Syndromes

EDS are inherited disorders of connective tissue that feature remarkable hyperelasticity and fragility of the skin, joint hypermobility, and often a bleeding diathesis.

EDS is clinically and genetically heterogeneous. Different forms may be inherited as autosomal dominant, recessive, or X-linked traits. The worldwide prevalence of all types is approximately 1 in 5,000 (Table 5-4). Multiple genes on several chromosomes are associated with EDS, including the *ADAMTS2* gene at the terminal region of chromosome 5q. Procollagen cannot be processed correctly without an enzyme encoded by this gene. As a result, collagen fibrils are not assembled properly; they appear ribbon-like and disorganized. Cross-links or chemical interactions between collagen fibrils are also affected. ***Whatever the underlying biochemical defect, the result is deficient or defective collagen.*** Depending on the type of EDS, these molecular lesions are associated with conspicuous weakness of supporting structures of the skin, joints, arteries, and viscera.

Classical EDS types 1 and 2 occur in 1 in 20,000 to 50,000 people. Both are autosomal dominant and affect types I and V collagen. Type 1 EDS typically presents with severe skin involvement, but in type 2 disease, the skin is only mildly to moderately affected. More than 50% of classic EDS is caused by mutations in the *COL5A1*, *COL5A2*, and *COL1A1* genes on chromosomes 9, 2, and 17, respectively. These gene mutations cause significant changes in the structure of connective tissue, which elicits the characteristic features of the classic types of EDS.

Hypermobility EDS type 3 affects 1 in 10,000 to 15,000 and can be either autosomal dominant or autosomal recessive. Joint hypermobility and chronic musculoskeletal pain are the most prominent features of EDS type 3; skin manifestations are less severe. Mutations of *TNXB* located at 6p21.3 prevent production of tenascin-X protein, which disrupts the normal organization of collagen fibrils and elastic fibers and leads to hypermobility.

Vascular EDS type 4 affects 1 in 100,000 to 250,000 individuals. These patients exhibit characteristic facial features (small chin, thin nose and lips, and sunken cheeks), slight body habitus, and translucent skin, through which veins appear prominently. This form of EDS is more serious than other types because autosomal dominant mutations in *COL3A1* on chromosome 2 produce a defect in type III collagen, resulting in fragile blood vessels that are liable to rupture. Some 25% of patients with EDS type 4 experience significant complications by age 20, and more than 75% have life-threatening problems before age 40.

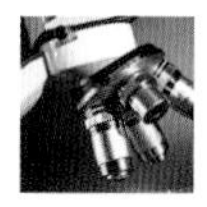

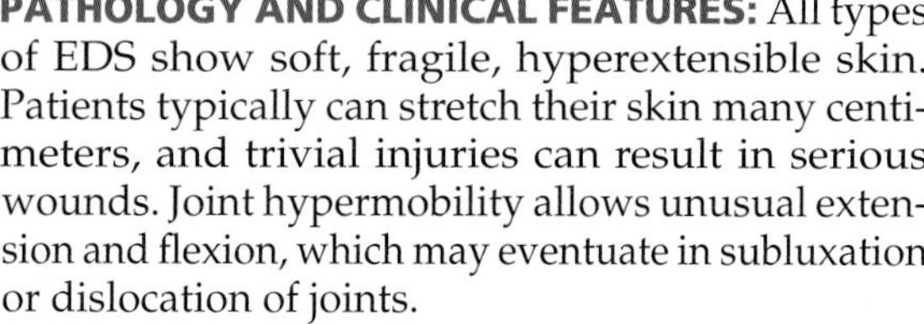

PATHOLOGY AND CLINICAL FEATURES: All types of EDS show soft, fragile, hyperextensible skin. Patients typically can stretch their skin many centimeters, and trivial injuries can result in serious wounds. Joint hypermobility allows unusual extension and flexion, which may eventuate in subluxation or dislocation of joints.

Many people with clinical abnormalities suggesting EDS do not match any of the documented types of this disorder. Further characterization of such cases is likely to expand the classification of EDS.

Osteogenesis Imperfecta

OI, or brittle bone disease, is a group of inherited disorders in which a generalized abnormality of connective tissue is expressed principally as fragility of bone. The disorder is inherited as an autosomal dominant trait, although rare cases are transmitted as autosomal recessives.

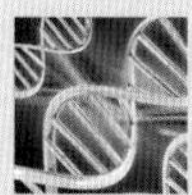

MOLECULAR PATHOGENESIS: *Genetic defects in the eight types of OI are heterogeneous, but all affect type I collagen synthesis, helical structure, or, rarely, other structural proteins in bone.* The genes most commonly involved are *COL1A1* and *COL1A2*, which are required to form mature type I collagen. The combined incidence of all forms is 1 in 20,000 live births in the United States.

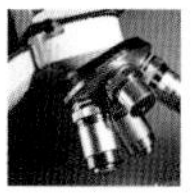

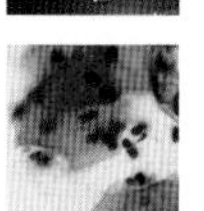

PATHOLOGY AND CLINICAL FEATURES:

- **Type I** OI is characterized by a normal appearance at birth, but fractures of many bones occur during infancy and at the time the child learns to walk. Children with type I OI typically have blue sclerae because the deficiency in collagen fibers makes sclerae translucent so that choroidal veins are visible. Fractures and fusion of the bones of the middle ear restrict their mobility and often cause hearing loss. Type I collagen is normal, but the quantity is reduced by half (haploinsufficiency).
- **Type II** OI is usually fatal in utero or shortly after birth. Abnormal forms of collagen are the result of glycine substitution.
- **Type III** OI causes progressive deformities. It is ordinarily detected at birth by the baby's short stature and misshapenness caused by fractures in utero. Dental defects and hearing loss are common. Unlike other OI types, type III is often inherited as an autosomal recessive trait.
- **Type IV** OI resembles type I, but sclerae are normal, and the phenotype is more variable.

Neurofibromatosis

The neurofibromatosis includes two distinct autosomal dominant disorders characterized by development of multiple neurofibromas, which are benign Schwann cell tumors of peripheral nerves. These disorders involve all cells derived from the neural crest, including melanocytes, Schwann cells, and endoneurial fibroblasts. Thus, type 1 includes disorders of pigmentation as well as neural tumors. In both neurofibromatosis types I and II, the responsible genetic mutations result in loss of a tumor suppressor function (see Chapter 4) and a defect in the regulation of cell growth.

Neurofibromatosis Type I (von Recklinghausen Disease)

Neurofibromatosis type I (NF1) is characterized by (1) disfiguring neurofibromas, (2) areas of dark pigmentation of the skin (café au lait spots), (3) pigmented lesions of the iris (Lisch nodules), (4) freckles in the groin or axilla, (5) optic nerve gliomas, (6) skeletal abnormalities, including thinning of the cortices of long bones, and (7) increased risk for childhood acute myeloid leukemia (Fig. 5-18). It is one of the more common autosomal dominant disorders, occurring once in 4,000 people of all races. The *NF1* gene has a very high rate of mutation, and over 500 mutations are known. Half of cases are sporadic rather than familial.

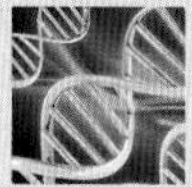

MOLECULAR PATHOGENESIS: Germline mutations in the *NF1* gene on the long arm of chromosome 17 include deletions, missense mutations, and nonsense mutations. The gene product, *neurofibromin*, belongs to a family of GTPase-activating proteins (GAPs), which inactivate the ras protein (see Chapter 4). In this sense, NF1 is a classic tumor suppressor.

Neurofibromatosis Type II (Central Neurofibromatosis)

NF2 is a syndrome defined by bilateral tumors of the eighth cranial nerve (acoustic neuromas) and, commonly, by meningiomas and gliomas. NF2 is much less common than NF1, occurring in 1 in 40,000 to 45,000 people. Most patients have bilateral acoustic neuromas, but the condition can be diagnosed if a unilateral eighth nerve tumor occurs with two or more of the following: neurofibroma, meningioma, glioma, schwannoma, or juvenile posterior lenticular opacity.

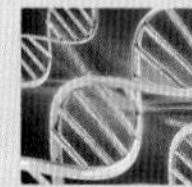

MOLECULAR PATHOGENESIS: The *NF2* gene is on the long arm of chromosome 22 (22q,11.1-13.1). Unlike NF1, tumors in NF2 often show deletions or loss of heterozygous DNA markers in the affected chromosome. *NF2* encodes a tumor suppressor, **merlin** or **schwannomin**, a member of a superfamily of proteins that links the cytoskeleton to the cell membrane.

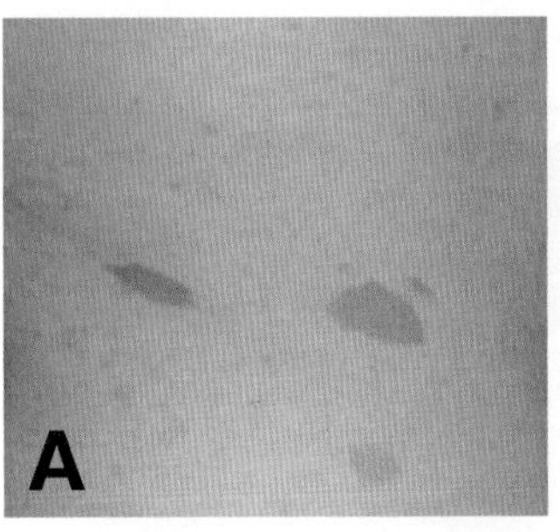

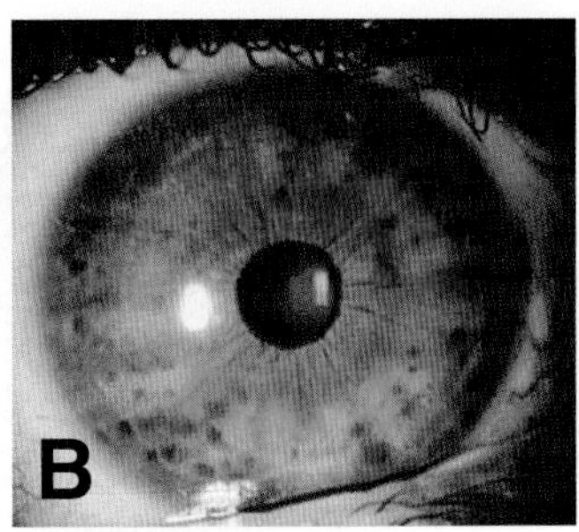

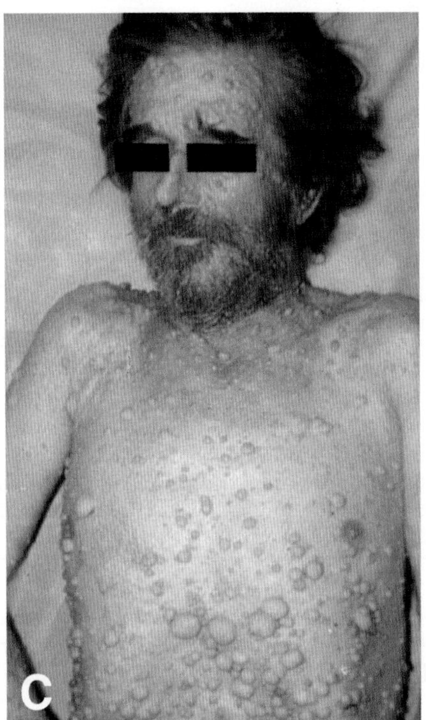

FIGURE 5-18. **Features of neurofibromatosis type 1. A.** Café au lait spots. **B.** Lisch nodules. **C.** Multiple cutaneous neurofibromas on the face and trunk.

Achondroplastic Dwarfism

This condition is an autosomal dominant, hereditary disease of epiphyseal chondroblastic development that leads to inadequate endochondral bone formation (discussed in Chapter 22).

Familial Hypercholesterolemia

Familial hypercholesterolemia is an autosomal dominant disorder characterized by high levels of LDLs in the blood and cholesterol deposition in arteries, tendons, and skin. It is one of the most common autosomal dominant disorders, affecting 1 in 500 adults in the United States in its heterozygous form. Only 1 person in 1 million is homozygous for the disease. In this condition, there is a striking acceleration of atherosclerosis and its complications.

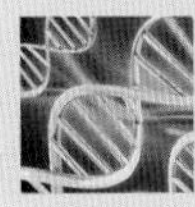

MOLECULAR PATHOGENESIS: The gene on the short arm of chromosome 19 that encodes the cell surface receptor for low-density lipoprotein (LDLR) is mutated in familial hypercholesterolemia. The LDL receptor removes LDL from the blood, a process that occurs mainly in the liver. Over 1,000 unique allelic variants are known. The LDL receptor is made in the endoplasmic reticulum, transferred to the Golgi, and transported to the cell surface, where it resides in clathrin-coated pits. Once it binds LDL, the receptor and its ligand are internalized by receptor-mediated endocytosis and processed in lysosomes. For additional details, see Chapter 8.

AUTOSOMAL RECESSIVE DISORDERS

Most genetic metabolic diseases show autosomal recessive inheritance (Table 5-5). The facts that recessive genes are uncommon and the need for two mutant alleles to cause clinical disease determines the key characteristics of autosomal recessive inheritance.

Most mutant genes responsible for autosomal recessive disorders are rare in the general population because those homozygous for the trait often die before reproductive age. However, a few autosomal recessive diseases, such as sickle cell anemia and cystic fibrosis (CF), are common. New mutations for recessive diseases are difficult to identify clinically because heterozygotes are asymptomatic. Nonconsanguineous mating of two such heterozygotes would occur by chance, and many generations later, if at all. Hence, rare autosomal recessive diseases occur most often in consanguineous matings.

Biochemical Basis of Autosomal Recessive Diseases

Autosomal recessive diseases are usually caused by deficiencies in enzymes rather than structural proteins. A mutation that

Table 5-5

Representative Autosomal Recessive Disorders

Disease	Frequency	Chromosome
Cystic fibrosis	1/2,500	7q
α-Thalassemia	High	16p
β-Thalassemia	High	11p
Sickle cell anemia	High	11p
Myeloperoxidase deficiency	1/2,000	17q
Phenylketonuria	1/10,000	12q
Gaucher disease	1/50,000	1q
Tay–Sachs disease	1/300,000	15q
Hurler syndrome	1/100,000	22p
Glycogen storage disease Ia (von Gierke disease)	1/100,000	17
Wilson disease	1/50,000	13q
Hereditary hemochromatosis	1/1,000	6p
α_1-Antitrypsin deficiency	1/7,000	14q
Oculocutaneous albinism	1/20,000	11q
Alkaptonuria	<1/100,000	3q
Metachromatic leukodystrophy	1/100,000	22q

inactivates an enzyme rarely causes an abnormal phenotype in heterozygotes; most cellular enzymes operate at substrate concentrations well below saturation, so an enzyme deficiency is easily corrected simply by increasing the amount of substrate. In autosomal recessive diseases caused by impaired catabolism of dietary substances (e.g., phenylketonuria and galactosemia) or cellular constituents (e.g., Tay–Sachs and Hurler), increased substrate concentrations in heterozygotes overcome partial lack of the enzyme. By contrast, loss of both alleles in a homozygote results in complete loss of enzyme activity, which cannot be corrected by such mechanisms.

Cystic Fibrosis

CF is characterized by (1) chronic pulmonary disease, (2) deficient exocrine pancreatic function, and (3) other complications of inspissated/thickened mucus in several organs, including the small intestine, liver, and reproductive tract. A defective chloride channel, namely, the cystic fibrosis transmembrane conductance regulator (CFTR), is responsible.

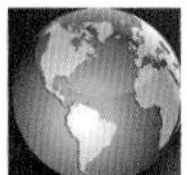

EPIDEMIOLOGY: Cystic fibrosis is most common among whites. Among white Americans, about 1 in 29 people carry a mutation of the *CF* gene. One in 46 Hispanic Americans, 1 in 65 black Americans, and 1 in 90 Asian Americans carry a *CF* gene mutation.

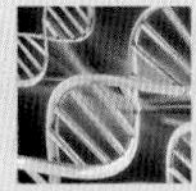

MOLECULAR PATHOGENESIS: The *CFTR* gene is on the long arm of chromosome 7 (Table 5-5). It encodes a protein that functions as a chloride ion transporter in most epithelial cells. Its two ATPase domains drive transporter function. It also has two domains that anchor the transporter as a transmembrane spanning protein. Two R domains with phosphorylation sites for cAMP-dependent protein kinase A (PKA) regulate chloride channel activity.

Secretion of chloride anions by mucus-secreting epithelial cells controls the parallel secretion of fluid and thus the viscosity of the mucus. Mutations in CFTR perturb this process (Fig. 5-19). The most common (ΔF_{508} 70%) mutation in the white population is loss of 3 bp, which deletes a phenylalanine (F) residue, producing an abnormally folded protein that is degraded.

Pathologic consequences of CF arise from abnormally thick mucus, which obstructs airway lumina, pancreatic and biliary ducts, and the fetal intestine.

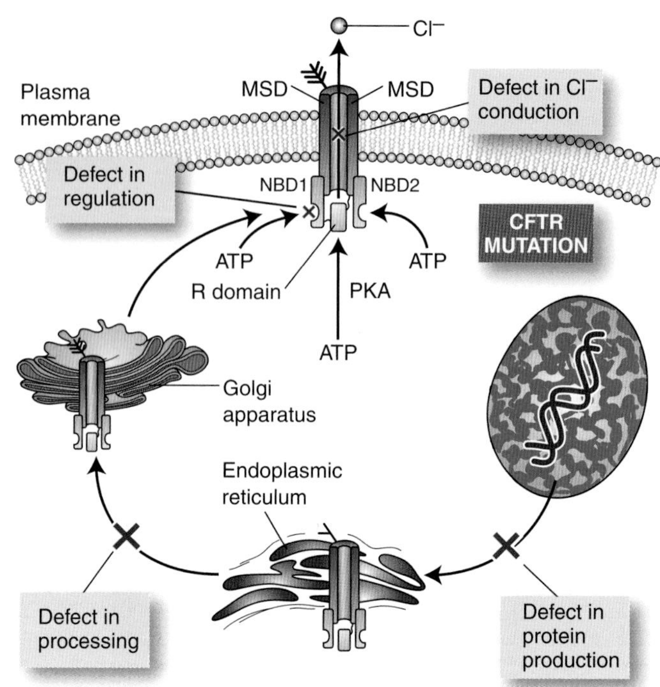

FIGURE 5-19. Cellular sites of disruption in the synthesis and function of the cystic fibrosis transmembrane conductance regulator (CFTR) in cystic fibrosis. ATP, adenosine triphosphate; Cl^-, chloride ion; MSD, membrane-spanning domain; NBD, nucleotide-binding domain; PKA, protein kinase A.

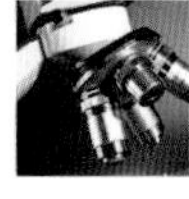

PATHOLOGY: CF affects many organs that produce exocrine secretions (Fig. 5-20).

Respiratory Tract

Lung disease causes most morbidity and mortality in CF. The earliest lesion is obstruction of bronchioles by mucus, with secondary infection and inflammation of bronchiolar walls. Recurrent cycles of obstruction and infection result in **chronic bronchiolitis** and **bronchitis**, which increase in severity as the disease progresses, and may lead to secondary pulmonary hypertension. Bronchial mucous glands undergo hypertrophy and hyperplasia, and airways are distended by thick, tenacious secretions. Widespread **bronchiectasis** is apparent by age 10 and often earlier. Late in the disease, large bronchiectatic cysts, and lung abscesses are common.

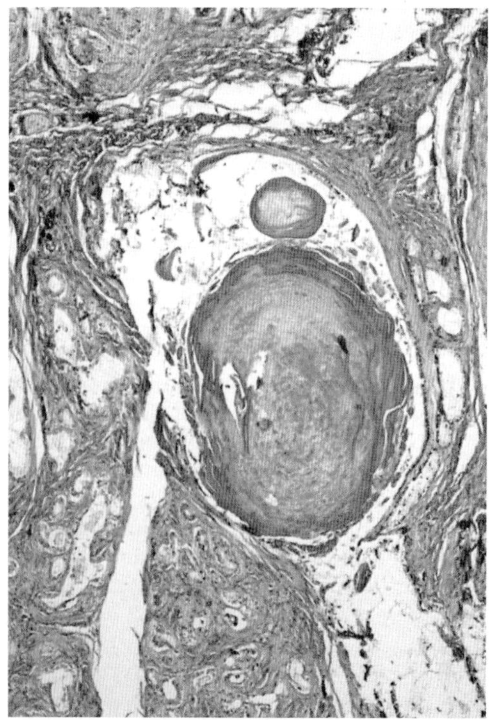

FIGURE 5-20. Intraductal concretion and acinar atrophy in the pancreas of a patient with cystic fibrosis.

Pancreas

Most patients (85%) with CF have a form of **chronic pancreatitis**, and in long-standing cases, little or no functional exocrine pancreas remains. Inspissated secretions in central pancreatic ducts produce secondary dilation and cystic change of the distal ducts. Recurrent pancreatitis leads to loss of acinar cells and extensive fibrosis so that the pancreas may become simply cystic fibroadipose tissue containing islets of Langerhans. The finding of pancreatic cysts and fibrosis led to the original name of "mucoviscidosis."

Liver

Inspissated mucous secretions in the intrahepatic biliary system obstruct bile flow in draining areas of the affected ducts and in one fourth of patients result in focal **secondary biliary cirrhosis**. Inspissated concretions clog bile ducts and ductules. Sometimes (<5%), hepatic lesions, which include chronic portal inflammation and septal fibrosis, are sufficiently widespread to appear as the clinical manifestations of biliary cirrhosis.

Gastrointestinal Tract

Shortly after birth, a normal newborn passes the intestinal contents that have accumulated in utero (meconium). The most important lesion of the gut in CF is small bowel obstruction in newborns, **meconium ileus**, which is due to failure to pass meconium in the immediate postpartum period. This occurs in 5% to 10% of newborns with CF and reflects the failure of pancreatic secretions to digest meconium, possibly augmented by the greater viscosity of small bowel secretions.

Reproductive Tract

Almost all boys with CF have atrophy or fibrosis of the vas deferens, epididymis, and seminal vesicles. These lesions are caused by luminal obstruction by inspissated secretions early in life and even in utero. Thus, only 2% to 3% of males are fertile, with spermatozoa absent from the semen in the rest. A minority of women with CF are fertile. Many suffer from anovulatory cycles as a result of poor nutrition and chronic infections. Moreover, the cervical mucous plug is abnormally thick and tenacious.

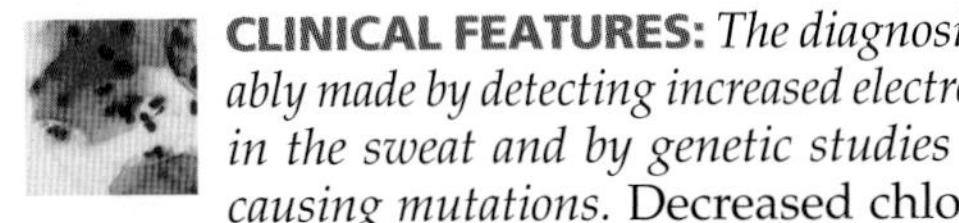

CLINICAL FEATURES: *The diagnosis of CF is most reliably made by detecting increased electrolyte concentrations in the sweat and by genetic studies that show disease-causing mutations.* Decreased chloride conductance in CF results in failure of chloride reabsorption by cells of sweat gland ducts and thus to the accumulation of sodium chloride in the sweat. The skin in children with CF is salty and may even display salt crystals after vigorous sweating.

Pulmonary symptoms of CF begin with cough, which becomes productive of large amounts of tenacious and purulent sputum. Repeated bouts of infectious bronchitis and bronchopneumonia become progressively more frequent, and eventually dyspnea develops. Respiratory failure and cardiac complications of pulmonary hypertension (cor pulmonale) occur later.

The most common organisms that infect the respiratory tract in CF are *Staphylococcus* and *Pseudomonas* spp. As the disease advances, *Pseudomonas* may be the only organism cultured from the lung. ***In fact, recovery of Pseudomonas spp., particularly the mucoid variety, from the lungs of a child with chronic pulmonary disease is virtually diagnostic of CF.*** Infection with *Burkholderia cepacia* is associated with **cepacia syndrome**, a very severe pulmonary infection that is highly resistant to antibiotics and is commonly fatal.

Failure of pancreatic exocrine secretion leads to fat and protein malabsorption, causing bulky, foul-smelling stools (steatorrhea), nutritional deficiencies, and growth retardation. Postural drainage of airways, antibiotic therapy, and pancreatic enzyme supplementation are mainstays of treatment. Molecular prenatal diagnosis of CF is now accurate in 95% of cases.

In 1959, children with CF in the United States rarely survived for 1 year. With improved therapies, life expectancy has increased to 40 years.

LYSOSOMAL STORAGE DISEASES

Lysosomes are membrane-bound collections of hydrolytic enzymes that digest macromolecules (see Chapter 1). Lysosomal digestive enzymes are called "acid hydrolases" because their optimal activities occur at an acidic pH (pH 3.5 to 5.5). This environment is maintained by an ATP-dependent proton pump in the lysosomal membrane. These enzymes degrade virtually all types of biologic macromolecules, including lipids, glycoproteins, and mucopolysaccharides. Extracellular macromolecules that are internalized by endocytosis or phagocytosis and intracellular constituents that are subjected to autophagy are digested in lysosomes to their basic components. End products may be transported across lysosomal membranes into the cytosol, where they are reused for the synthesis of new macromolecules.

Virtually, all lysosomal storage diseases result from mutations in genes for lysosomal hydrolases. Some 50 acid hydrolases are nucleases, proteases, glycosidases, lipases, phosphatases, sulfatases, and phospholipases. Deficiency in one of these acid hydrolases can prevent the catabolism of the normal macromolecular substrate of that enzyme. As a result, undigested substrates accumulate in and engorge, lysosomes, thereby expanding the lysosomal compartment of the cell. Resulting lysosomal distention impairs other critical cellular activities, particularly in the brain and heart, and lead to poor cellular function or cell death.

Lysosomal storage diseases are classified by the material retained in the lysosomes. Thus, when accumulated substrates are sphingolipids, they are termed **sphingolipidoses**. Storage of mucopolysaccharides (glycosaminoglycans) results in the **mucopolysaccharidoses**. Over 50 lysosomal storage diseases are known, but we limit our discussion to the more important ones.

Sphingolipidoses

Sphingolipidoses are lysosomal storage diseases characterized by accumulation of lipids derived from the turnover of obsolete cell membranes. Cerebrosides, gangliosides, sphingomyelin, and sulfatides are all sphingolipid components of membranes of a variety of cells. These substances are degraded within lysosomes by complex pathways that produce sphingosine and fatty acids (Fig. 5-21). Deficiencies of acid hydrolases that mediate specific steps in these pathways lead to accumulation of undigested intermediate substrates in lysosomes and hence a metabolic disorder.

Gaucher Disease

Gaucher disease is characterized by accumulation of glucosylceramide, mainly in macrophage lysosomes.

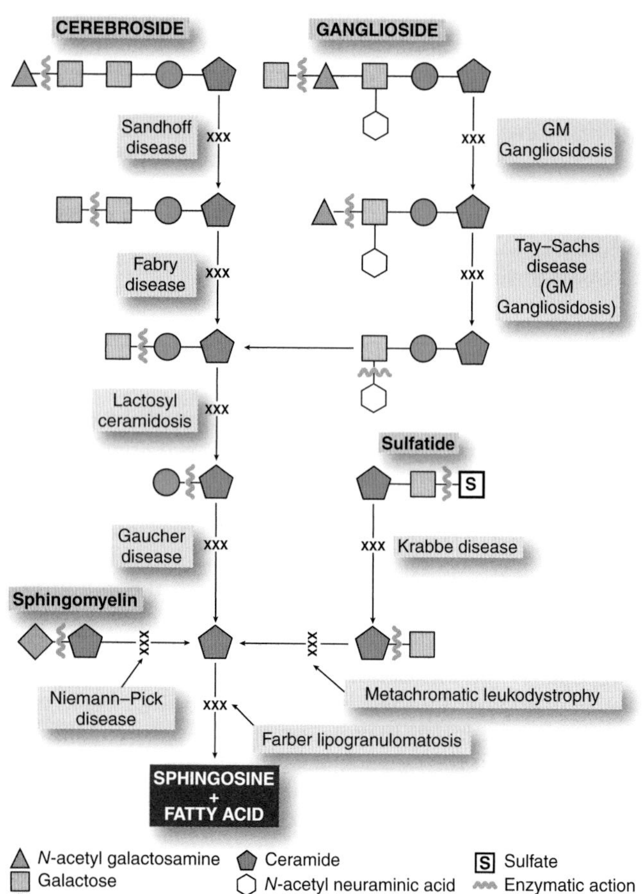

FIGURE 5-21. Disturbances of lipid metabolism in various sphingolipidoses.

MOLECULAR PATHOGENESIS: The abnormal enzyme in Gaucher disease is glucocerebrosidase, a lysosomal acid β-glucosidase. The enzyme deficiency can be traced to a variety of single base mutations in the *β-glucosidase* gene, on the long arm of chromosome 1. Each of the clinical types of the disease (see below) exhibits heterogeneous mutations in this gene, although the molecular basis for the phenotypic differences remains unclear.

The glucosylceramide that accumulates in Gaucher cells of the spleen, liver, bone marrow, and lymph nodes derives principally from catabolism of membranes of senescent leukocytes, which are rich in cerebrosides. When membrane degradation is blocked by a lack of glucocerebrosidase, the intermediate metabolite, glucosylceramide, accumulates. In the brain, this material originates from turnover of plasma membrane gangliosides in the CNS.

PATHOLOGY: The hallmark of this disorder is the presence of **Gaucher cells**, lipid-laden macrophages characteristically seen in the red pulp of the spleen, liver sinusoids, lymph nodes, lungs, and bone marrow, although they may appear in virtually any organ. These cells are derived from resident macrophages in the respective organs (e.g., Kupffer cells in the liver and alveolar macrophages in the lung).

Gaucher cells are large (20 to 100 μm), with eccentric nuclei and clear cytoplasm (Fig. 5-22). They have a characteristic fibrillar appearance, which has been likened to "wrinkled tissue paper" and are intensely positive with the PAS stain. The material is stored in enlarged lysosomes and appears as parallel layers of tubular structures.

Splenomegaly is virtually universal in Gaucher disease. In the adult form of the disorder, spleens may weigh up to 10 kg. The cut surface of the enlarged spleen is firm and pale and often contains sharply demarcated infarcts. The red pulp shows nodular and diffuse infiltrates of Gaucher cells and moderate fibrosis.

The liver is usually enlarged by Gaucher cells within sinusoids, but hepatocytes are not affected. However, in severe cases, hepatic fibrosis and even cirrhosis may ensue. Bone marrow involvement varies, but appears as radiologic abnormalities in 50% to 75% of cases.

Gaucher cells may also be found in many other organs, including lymph nodes, lungs, endocrine glands, skin, GI tract, and kidneys, but symptoms referable to involvement of these organs are uncommon.

In the infantile (neuronopathic) form of the disease, Gaucher cells are also seen in the brain parenchyma, where they may stimulate gliosis and microglial nodules.

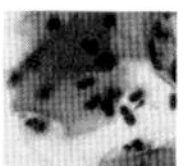

CLINICAL FEATURES: Gaucher disease is classified into three distinct forms, based on the age at onset and degree of neurologic involvement:

- **Type 1 (chronic non-neuronopathic):** This variant is the most common of the lysosomal storage diseases. It occurs in 1 in 40,000 to 60,000 in the general population, but in 1 in 500 to 800 of those with Ashkenazi Jewish ancestry. Thus, the carrier rate is 1 in 12 Ashkenazi Jews. The age at onset is variable; some cases are diagnosed in infants and others at age 70. The severity of clinical manifestations also varies widely. Most cases are diagnosed as adults and present initially as painless splenomegaly and complications of hypersplenism, including anemia, leukopenia, and thrombocytopenia. Hepatomegaly is common, but clinical liver disease is infrequent. Bone involvement manifests as pain and pathologic fractures and can cause disability severe enough to confine a patient to a wheelchair. The life expectancy of

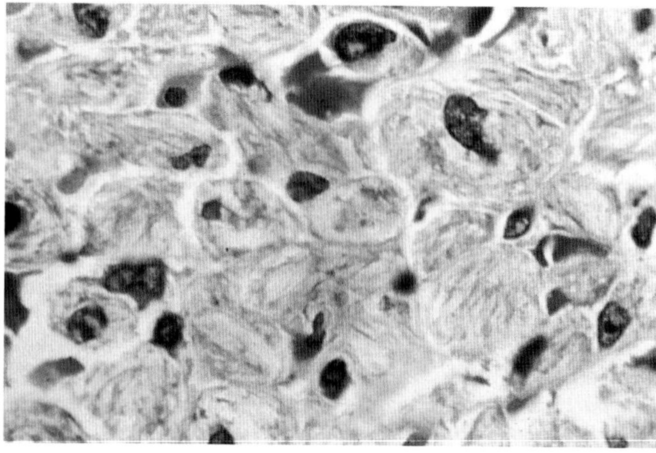

FIGURE 5-22. The spleen in Gaucher disease. Typical Gaucher cells have foamy cytoplasm and eccentrically located nuclei.

most patients with type 1 Gaucher disease is normal. The disease is now treated by administering modified acid glucose cerebrosidase, although its high cost limits its use. Marrow transplantation is also effective but is little used because of the attendant risks. Prenatal diagnosis is based on β-glucosidase activity in amniotic fluid or chorionic villi. Prenatal DNA testing is now routinely available. Because there are numerous mutations, sequencing of the affected gene is sometimes necessary to confirm the diagnosis.

- **Type 2 (acute neuronopathic):** Type 2 Gaucher disease is rare and quite different from type 1 in age at onset and clinical presentation. It usually presents by age 3 months with hepatosplenomegaly and has no ethnic predilection. Within a few months, infants show neurologic signs, with a classic triad of trismus, strabismus, and backward flexion of the neck. Further neurologic deterioration rapidly ensues. Most patients die by age 3 years.
- **Type 3 (subacute neuronopathic):** This form is also rare and combines features of types 1 and 2. Neurologic deterioration starts later than in type 2 and progresses more slowly, with most living until about age 30.

Tay–Sachs Disease (GM_2 Gangliosidosis Type 1)

Tay–Sachs disease is a catastrophic infantile form GM_2 gangliosidoses, in which this material is deposited in CNS neurons, owing to a failure of lysosomal degradation. Tay–Sachs disease is inherited as an autosomal recessive trait and is mainly seen in Ashkenazi Jews, among whom the carrier rate is about 1 in 30, with homozygotes seen in 1 in 4,000 live newborns. By contrast, the incidence in non–Jewish American populations is less than 1 in 100,000. Tay–Sachs disease is caused by a genetic mutation in the *hexosaminidase A* gene on chromosome 15. Numerous mutations in the gene have been reported with significant frequencies in specific populations. The carrier frequency in French Canadians is similar to that in Ashkenazi Jews, but with different mutations. Screening programs for heterozygous Ashkenazi Jews have reduced disease incidence by 90%. The other GM_2 gangliosidoses are very rare.

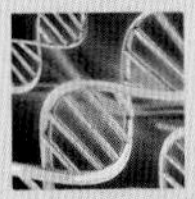

MOLECULAR PATHOGENESIS: Gangliosides are glycosphingolipids, with a ceramide and an oligosaccharide chain that contains *N*-acetylneuraminic acid (Fig. 5-21). They are located in the outer leaflet of the plasma membrane of animal cells, particularly in brain neurons.

Lysosomal catabolism of ganglioside GM_2 (1 of 12 gangliosides in the brain) requires β-hexosaminidases (A and B), which have α and β subunits and need GM_2-activator protein. Deficiency in any of these components results in clinical disease.

Tay–Sachs mutations in the gene that codes for the α subunit of hexosaminidase A result in defective synthesis of this enzyme. An insertion of four nucleotides in exon 11 accounts for over two thirds of the carriers among Ashkenazi Jews.

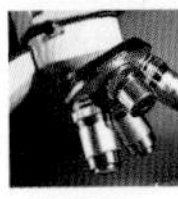

PATHOLOGY: GM_2 ganglioside accumulates in lysosomes of all organs in Tay–Sachs disease, but it is most prominent in brain neurons and cells of the retina. The size of the brain varies with the length of survival of affected infants. Early cases are marked by brain atrophy, but the organ weight may be as much as doubled in those who survive beyond a year. Neurons are markedly distended with stored lipids. By electron microscopy, neurons are stuffed with "membranous cytoplasmic bodies," which are concentric whorls of membranous material. As disease progresses, neurons are lost, and many lipid-laden macrophages are conspicuous in the cortical gray matter. Eventually, gliosis becomes prominent, and myelin and axons in the white matter die.

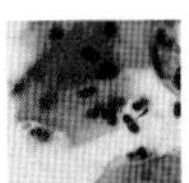

CLINICAL FEATURES: Tay–Sachs disease presents between 6 and 10 months of age with progressive weakness, hypotonia, and decreased attentiveness. Motor and mental deterioration, often with generalized seizures, follows rapidly. Vision is seriously impaired. Retinal ganglion cell involvement is detected by ophthalmoscopy as a **cherry-red spot** in the macula. This feature reflects the pallor of the affected cells, which enhances the prominence of blood vessels underlying the central fovea. Most children with Tay–Sachs disease die before 4 years of age.

Niemann–Pick Disease

NPD is a form of sphingolipidosis involving dysfunctional catabolism of cell membrane sphingolipids. Macrophage lysosomes in many cells, especially in the liver and the brain, store **sphingomyelin**. There are several variants of this disorder; types A and B are caused by mutations in the *SMPD1* gene, which encodes the enzyme acid sphingomyelinase; type C is caused by mutations in the *NPC1* and *NPC2* genes, which encode lipid transport proteins.

Type A NPD appears in infancy, with hepatosplenomegaly and progressive neurodegeneration. Death occurs by 3 years of age. Type B NPD is more variable, with hepatosplenomegaly, minimal neurologic symptomatology, and survival to adulthood. Type C NPD is biochemically, genetically, and clinically distinct from types A and B.

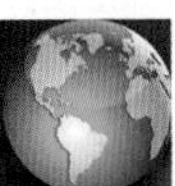

EPIDEMIOLOGY: The incidence of type A NPD is 1 in 40,000 among Ashkenazi Jews. In all other populations, both types A and B NPD occur in 1 in 250,000. For type C, the incidence is 1 in 100,000. The total incidence for all types in the general population is thus 1 in 100,000.

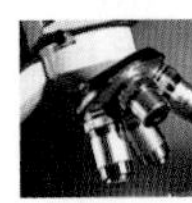

PATHOLOGY: The characteristic storage cell in NPD is a foam cell, that is, an enlarged (20 to 90 μm) macrophage whose cytoplasm is distended by uniform vacuoles containing sphingomyelin and cholesterol. Foam cells are particularly abundant in the spleen, lymph nodes, and bone marrow but also occur in the liver, lungs, and GI tract. The spleen is enlarged, often massively, with foam cells distributed diffusely throughout the red pulp. Lymph nodes enlarged by foam cells are seen in many locations. Hematopoietic tissues in bone marrow may be displaced by aggregates of foam cells. The liver is enlarged by stored sphingomyelin and cholesterol in lysosomes of both Kupffer cells and hepatocytes.

The brain is the most important organ involved in type A NPD, and neurologic damage is the usual cause of death. Half of children with type A disease have cherry-red retinal spots, as in Tay–Sachs disease.

Table 5-6

Mucopolysaccharidoses

Type	Eponym	Location of Gene	Clinical Features
I H	Hurler	4p16.3	Organomegaly, cardiac lesions, dysostosis multiplex, corneal clouding, death in childhood
I S	Scheie	4p16.3	Stiff joints, corneal clouding, normal intelligence, longevity
II	Hunter	X	Organomegaly, dysostosis multiplex, mental retardation, death earlier than 15 years of age
III	Sanfilippo	12q14	Mental retardation
IV	Morquio	16q24	Skeletal deformities, corneal clouding
V	Obsolete	—	—
VI	Maroteaux–Lamy	5q13–14	Dysostosis multiplex, corneal clouding, death in second decade
VII	Sly	7q21.1–22	Hepatosplenomegaly, dysostosis multiplex

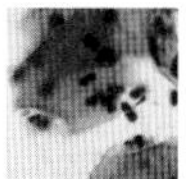

CLINICAL FEATURES: Type A NPD manifests in early infancy with conspicuous spleen and liver enlargement and psychomotor retardation. Motor and intellectual function is lost over time. Children usually die before 3 years of age. Most type B NPD patients present in childhood with marked hepatosplenomegaly. Pulmonary infiltration with sphingomyelin-laden macrophages eventually impairs respiratory function. However, these patients have few neurologic symptoms and may survive for years. Progressive neurologic disease is the hallmark of type C Niemann–Pick disease and causes disability and early death in all cases beyond early childhood.

Mucopolysaccharidoses

MPSs are lysosomal diseases in which **glycosaminoglycans (mucopolysaccharides)** accumulate in many organs. All are inherited as autosomal recessive traits, except for Hunter syndrome, which is X-linked recessive. These rare diseases are caused by deficiencies in any of the 12 lysosomal enzymes that catabolize glycosaminoglycans (Fig. 5-23). Six abnormal phenotypes are described, each varying with the specific enzyme deficiency (Table 5-6).

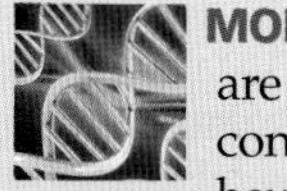

MOLECULAR PATHOGENESIS: Glycosaminoglycans are large polymers of repeating disaccharide units containing *N*-acetylhexosamine and a hexose or hexuronic acid. Either disaccharide may be sulfated. The accumulated GAGs (dermatan sulfate, heparan sulfate, keratan sulfate, and chondroitin sulfate) in MPSs all derive from cleavage of proteoglycans, which are important extracellular matrix constituents. GAGs are degraded stepwise by removing sulfates or sugar residues. Thus, a deficiency in any one of the glycosidases or sulfatases causes undegraded GAGs to accumulate. A special case is deficiency of an *N*-acetyltransferase, which leads to deposition of heparan sulfate in Sanfilippo C disease.

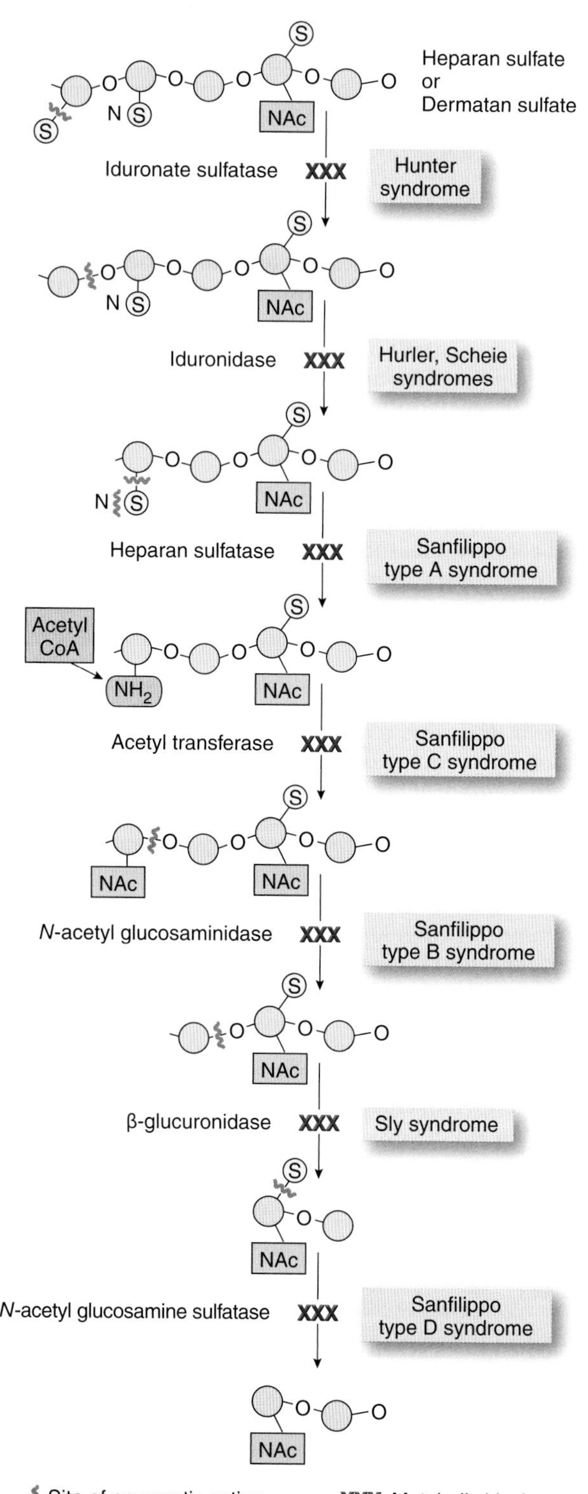

FIGURE 5-23. Metabolic blocks in various mucopolysaccharidoses that affect the degradation of heparan sulfate and dermatan sulfate with resulting syndromes. Acetyl CoA, acetyl coenzyme A; NAc, *N*-acetyl moiety.

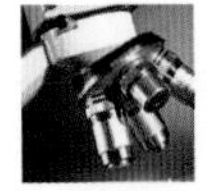

PATHOLOGY: Although the severity and location of lesions in MPSs vary with the specific enzyme deficiency, most of these syndromes share common features. Underprocessed Pompe GAGs tend to accumulate in connective tissue cells, mononuclear phagocytes (including Kupffer cells), endothelial cells, neurons, and hepatocytes. Affected cells are swollen with clear cytoplasm. Stains for metachromasia confirm the presence of GAGs. The most critical lesions involve the CNS, skeleton, and heart, although hepatosplenomegaly and corneal clouding are common.

- Initially, the **CNS** only accumulates GAGs, but as the disease advances, extensive neurons die and gliosis occurs, terminating in cortical atrophy. Communicating hydrocephalus, owing to meningeal involvement, is common.
- **Skeletal deformities** result from GAG accumulation in chondrocytes, a process that eventually interferes with normal endochondral ossification. Abnormal foci of osteoid and woven bone are common in the deformed skeleton.
- **Cardiac** involvement is often severe, with thickening and distortion of valve leaflets, chordae tendineae, and endocardium. Coronary arteries are frequently narrowed owing to proliferation of intimal smooth muscle cells containing GAG deposits.
- **Hepatosplenomegaly** is secondary to distention of Kupffer cells and hepatocytes and accumulation of GAG-filled macrophages in the spleen.

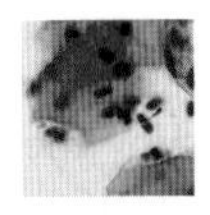

CLINICAL FEATURES: Hurler syndrome (MPS I) is the most severe clinical form of MPS and is the prototype for these syndromes. Deficiency of α-L-iduronidase located on chromosome 4 results in buildup of heparin sulfate and dermatan sulfate in various tissues (Fig. 5-23). The clinical features of other varieties of MPS are summarized in Table 5-6. The symptoms of Hurler syndrome appear at 6 months to 2 years of age. Children typically show skeletal deformities, enlarged livers and spleens, characteristic facies, and joint stiffness. The combination of coarse facial features and dwarfism reminiscent of gargoyles on Gothic cathedrals accounts for the old term, **gargoylism**, for this syndrome.

Children with Hurler syndrome suffer developmental delay, hearing loss, corneal clouding, and progressive mental deterioration, as well as increased intracranial pressure, as a result of communicating hydrocephalus. Most patients die from recurrent pulmonary infections and cardiac complications before they reach 10 years of age.

Prenatal diagnosis is possible for MPS and is routine in families with a history of Hurler syndrome or Hunter syndrome. Enzyme replacement therapy and bone marrow transplantation may reduce non-neurologic symptoms and pain.

Glycogenoses (Glycogen Storage Diseases)

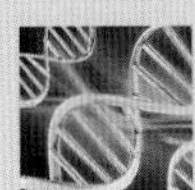

MOLECULAR PATHOGENESIS: The glycogenoses are a group of at least 14 inherited disorders characterized by glycogen accumulation, mainly in the liver, skeletal muscle, and heart. Each entity reflects a deficiency of one of the enzymes involved in glycogen metabolism (Fig. 5-24). Save for X-linked phosphorylase kinase deficiency, all glycogen storage diseases are autosomal recessive traits. In the United States, they occur once in 20,000 to 25,000 births.

Glycogen is a large glucose polymer (20,000 to 30,000 glucose units per molecule) that is stored in most cells as a ready source of energy during fasting, although its function is different in each organ. Liver and muscle are particularly rich in glycogen. The liver stores glycogen not for its own use but rather to supply glucose to the blood quickly, particularly to benefit the brain. By contrast, glycogen in skeletal muscle is used as a local fuel when oxygen or glucose supplies fall. Glycogen is degraded by several enzymes, deficiency in any of which leads to accumulation of glycogen. Significant organ involvement varies with the specific enzyme defect. Some mainly affect the liver, whereas others principally cause cardiac or skeletal muscle dysfunction. Symptoms of glycogenosis may reflect accumulation of glycogen itself (Pompe disease and Andersen disease) or lack of the glucose normally derived from glycogen degradation (von Gierke disease and McArdle disease). We discuss only several representative examples of the known glycogenoses.

- **von Gierke Disease (Type IA Glycogenosis):** In von Gierke disease, glucose-6-phosphatase is lacking. Glycogen accumulates in the liver, and symptoms include the inability of the liver to convert glycogen to glucose, leading to hepatomegaly and hypoglycemia. The disorder usually presents in infancy or early childhood. Growth is commonly stunted, but with treatment, the prognosis for normal mental development and longevity are generally good.
- **Pompe Disease (Type II Glycogenosis):** Pompe disease is a lysosomal storage disease that involves virtually all organs and results in death from heart failure before the age of 2. Juvenile and adult variants are less common and have a better prognosis. The incidence of the disease is 1 in 140,000 for the infantile type and 1 in 60,000 for adult disease. Type II glycogenosis is caused by a mutation in the gene for the lysosomal enzyme acid maltase/acid α-glucosidase (GAA) located on the long arm of chromosome 17. It leads to inexorable accumulation of undegraded glycogen in lysosomes of many different cells. Patients do not develop hypoglycemia because cytoplasmic metabolic pathways of glycogen synthesis and degradation are intact. Without enzyme replacement therapy, the hearts of babies with infantile-onset Pompe disease progressively thicken and enlarge. These babies die before 1 year of age from cardiorespiratory failure or respiratory infection. For persons with late-onset Pompe disease, the prognosis depends on the age of onset. In general, the later the age of onset, the slower the disease progresses. Ultimately, survival depends on the extent of respiratory muscle involvement.
- **McArdle Disease (Type V Glycogenosis):** In McArdle disease, glycogen accumulates in skeletal muscles, owing to a lack of muscle phosphorylase, the enzyme that releases glucose-1-phosphate from glycogen. There are two autosomal recessive forms of this disease: childhood onset and adult onset. The gene for myophosphorylase, *PYGM* (the muscle type of the glycogen phosphorylase gene), is on chromosome 11. Symptoms usually appear in adolescence or early adulthood and consist of muscle cramps and spasms during exercise, which may lead to myocytolysis and myoglobinuria. Aerobic exercise and high-protein diets have been effective therapies in some patients.

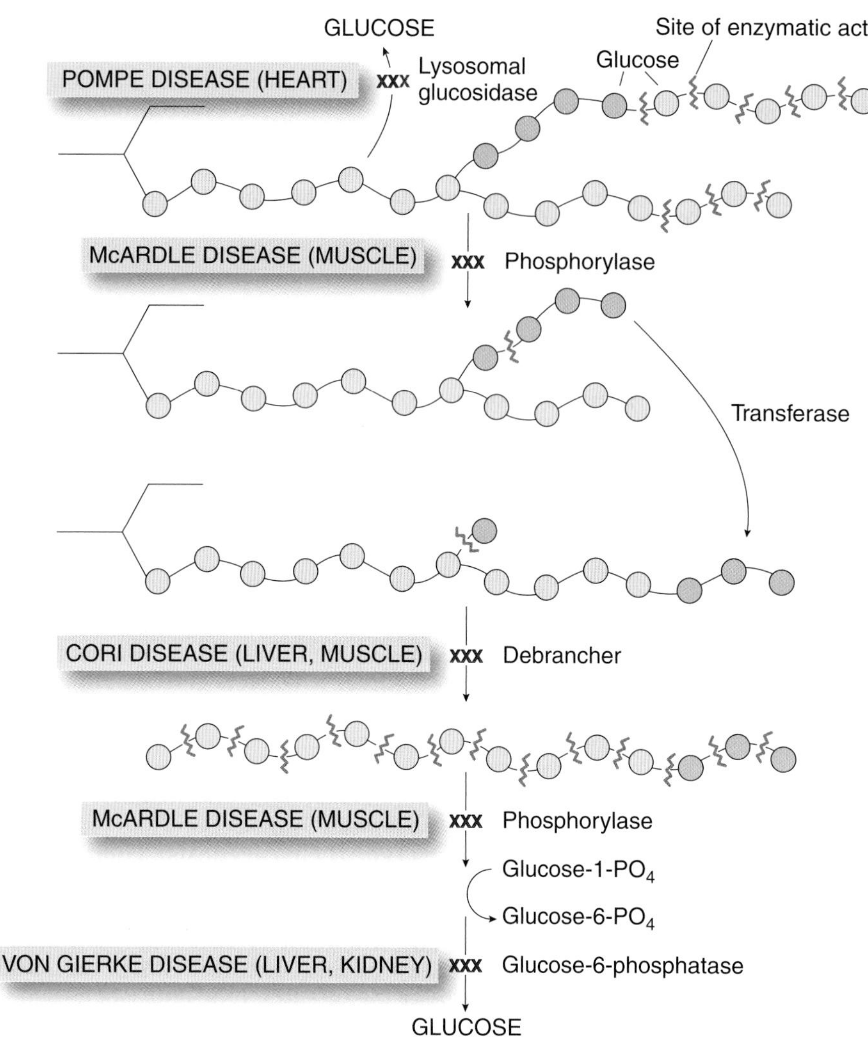

FIGURE 5-24. Sequential catabolism of glycogen and enzymes that are deficient in various glycogenoses. Glycogen is a long-chain branched polymer of glucose residues connected by α-1,4 linkages, except at branch points, where an α-1,6 linkage is present. Phosphorylase hydrolyzes α-1,4 linkages to a point three glucose residues distal to an α-1,6–linked sugar. These three glucose residues are transferred to the chain linked by α-1,4 bonds, by the bifunctional debrancher enzyme amylo-1,6-glucosidase. Subsequently, the same enzyme removes the α-1,6–linked sugar at the original branch point. This creates a linear α-1,4 chain, which is degraded by phosphorylase to glucose-1-phosphate. Following the conversion to glucose-6-phosphate, glucose is released by the action of glucose-6-phosphatase. A small proportion of glycogen is totally degraded within lysosomes by acid α-glucosidase. A *red X* indicates a metabolic block and its associated glycogen storage disease.

Inborn Errors of Amino Acid Metabolism

Heritable disorders of the metabolism of many amino acids have been described (Table 5-7). Some are lethal in early childhood; others are clinically insignificant. Some of these are addressed in chapters on specific organs. This discussion focuses on examples provided by defects in the metabolism of phenylalanine and tyrosine (Fig. 5-25).

Phenylketonuria

PKU **(hyperphenylalaninemia)** is an autosomal recessive deficiency of the hepatic enzyme phenylalanine hydroxylase. A high circulating levels of phenylalanine leads to progressive mental deterioration in the first few years of life. The incidence of PKU is 1 per 10,000 in white and Asian populations, but it varies widely across different geographic areas. It is most frequent (1 in 5,000) in Ireland and Western Scotland and among Yemenite Jews.

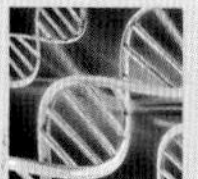

MOLECULAR PATHOGENESIS: Phenylalanine is an essential amino acid derived exclusively from the diet. It is oxidized in the liver to tyrosine by phenylalanine hydroxylase (PAH). Deficiency in PAH causes hyperphenylalaninemia and formation of phenylketones by the transamination of phenylalanine. Phenylpyruvic acid and its derivatives are excreted in the urine, but phenylalanine itself, rather than its metabolites, causes the neurologic damage central to this disease. Thus, hyperphenylalaninemia is actually a more appropriate name than PKU.

Classic PKU is caused by mutations in the *PAH* gene on the long arm of chromosome 12. Up to 400 mutations are known, most causing a deficiency in PAH.

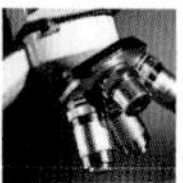

PATHOLOGY: The mechanism of neurotoxicity in hyperphenylalaninemia in infancy is not clear. Several processes have been implicated: competitive interference with amino acid transport systems in the brain, inhibition of neurotransmitter synthesis, and disturbance of

Table 5-7

Representative Inherited Disorders of Amino Acid Metabolism

Phenylketonuria (hyperphenylalaninemia)
Tyrosinemia
Histidinemia
Ornithine transcarbamylase deficiency (ammonia intoxication)
Carbamoyl phosphate synthetase deficiency (ammonia intoxication)
Maple syrup urine disease (branched-chain ketoacidemia)
Arginase deficiency
Arginosuccinic acid synthetase deficiency (citrulline accumulation)

other metabolic processes. These effects presumably impair neuronal development and myelin synthesis. PAH is not always totally lacking; those with more than 5% activity exhibit (1) non-PKU hyperphenylalaninemia, (2) do not suffer neurologic damage, and (3) develop normally.

Malignant hyperphenylalaninemia occurs in fewer than 5% of infants with the disease. In this case, dietary restriction of phenylalanine does not arrest neurologic deterioration. These patients have a deficiency in tetrahydrobiopterin (BH_4), a cofactor required for hydroxylation of phenylalanine by PAH. At first, infants with malignant hyperphenylalaninemia are phenotypically indistinguishable from those with classic PKU, but BH_4 deficiency also interferes with the synthesis of the neurotransmitters dopamine (tyrosine hydroxylase dependent) and serotonin (tryptophan hydroxylase dependent). Thus, brain damage in malignant hyperphenylalaninemia most likely involves more than a simple elevation in phenylalanine levels.

CLINICAL FEATURES: Affected infants appear normal at birth, but mental retardation is evident within a few months. By 12 months, untreated infants have lost about 50 IQ points, which means that a child who would otherwise have normal intelligence has become severely retarded. Infants with PKU tend to have fair skin, blond hair, and blue eyes because the inability to convert phenylalanine to tyrosine results in reduced melanin synthesis. They exude a "mousy" or "musty" odor, owing to the production of phenylacetic acid.

The main treatment for classic PKU patients is a strict phenylalanine-restricted diet supplemented by a medical formula containing amino acids and other nutrients. In the United States, the current recommendation is that the PKU diet should be maintained for life. Patients who are diagnosed early and maintain a strict diet can have a normal life span with normal mental development. However, recent studies suggest that neurocognitive and psychosocial development and growth are slightly suboptimal if the diet is not supplemented with amino acids.

In developed countries, the clinical phenotype of classic PKU is now more of historic interest than a significant concern. About 10 million newborns worldwide are screened annually for hyperphenylalaninemia by a simple blood test (Guthrie test), and new cases are promptly treated.

Tyrosinemia

There are three types of tyrosinemia. The most severe is type I, a rare (1 in 100,000) autosomal recessive inborn error of tyrosine catabolism caused by a shortage of the enzyme fumarylacetoacetate hydrolase (FAH) coded for by a gene on chromosome 15. It manifests as acute liver disease in early infancy or as a more chronic disease of the liver, kidneys, and brain in children.

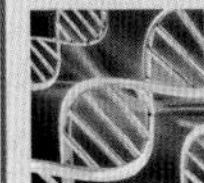

MOLECULAR PATHOGENESIS: Blood levels of tyrosine and its metabolites are elevated. Fumarylacetoacetate hydrolase, the last enzyme in the catabolic pathway that converts tyrosine to fumarate and acetoacetate, is deficient in both acute and chronic forms of type I tyrosinemia. In the acute form, there is no enzyme activity, although children with chronic disease have variable residual activity. Cell injury in hereditary tyrosinemia is attributed to abnormal toxic metabolites, namely, succinylacetone and succinylacetoacetate.

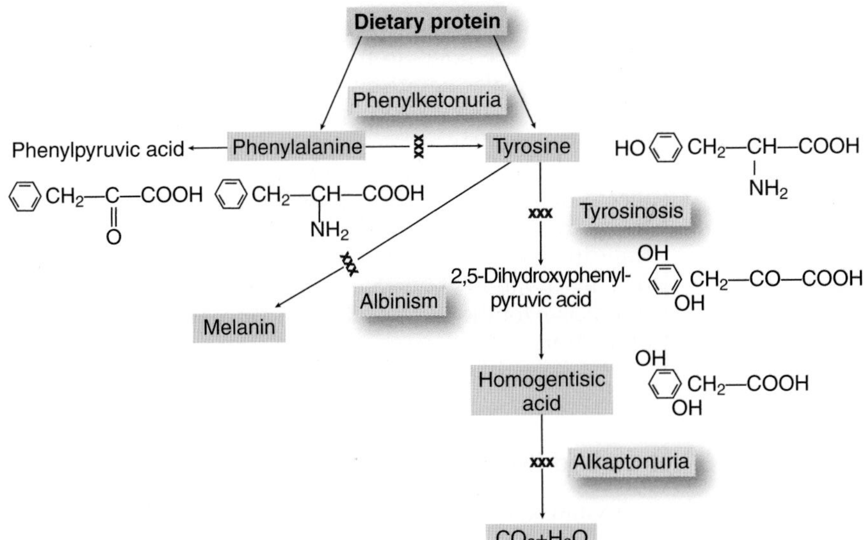

FIGURE 5-25. Diseases caused by disturbances of phenylalanine and tyrosine metabolism.

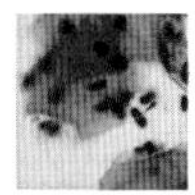

CLINICAL FEATURES: **Acute tyrosinemia** manifests in the first few months of life as hepatomegaly, edema, failure to thrive, and a cabbage-like odor. Within a few months, infants die of hepatic failure.

Chronic tyrosinemia is characterized by cirrhosis of the liver, renal tubular dysfunction (Fanconi syndrome), and neurologic abnormalities. Hepatocellular carcinoma occurs in more than one third of these patients. Most children die before the age of 10. Liver transplantation corrects hepatic metabolic abnormalities and prevents the neurologic crises. Combined liver–kidney transplants have also been performed. Analysis of amniotic fluid for succinylacetone or of fetal cells for FAH establishes the diagnosis prenatally.

Albinism

Albinism is a heterogeneous group of at least 10 inherited disorders in which absent or reduced biosynthesis of melanin causes hypopigmentation. Type 1 albinism is caused by defects in the production of melanin pigment. Type 2 albinism is caused by a defect in the *OCA2* gene, which interferes with the metabolism of tyrosine, a precursor of melanin. People with this type have slight coloring at birth.

The most common type is oculocutaneous albinism (OCA), a family of closely related diseases that (with one rare exception) are autosomal recessive traits. In OCA, melanin pigment is absent or reduced in the skin, hair follicles, and eyes. The frequency of OCA in whites is 1 per 18,000 in the United States and 1 in 10,000 in Ireland. Blacks have the same high frequency of OCA as the Irish.

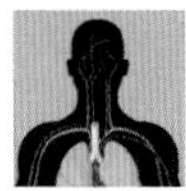

PATHOPHYSIOLOGY: Two major forms of OCA are distinguished by the presence or absence of tyrosinase, the first enzyme in the biosynthetic pathway that converts tyrosine to melanin (Fig. 5-25).

Tyrosinase-positive OCA is the most common type of albinism in whites and blacks. Patients typically begin life with complete albinism, but with age, a small amount of clinically detectable pigment accumulates. A defect in the *OCA2* (15q), which may encode a tyrosine transport protein, prevents melanin synthesis.

Tyrosinase-negative OCA is the second most common type of albinism and is characterized by complete absence of tyrosinase (11q) and melanin: melanocytes are present but contain unpigmented melanosomes. Affected people have snow-white hair, pale pink skin, blue irides, and prominent red pupils, owing to an absence of retinal pigment. They typically have severe ophthalmic problems, including photophobia, strabismus, nystagmus, and poor visual acuity.

The skin of all types of albinos is strikingly sensitive to sunlight. Exposed skin areas require strong sunscreens. These patients have an increased risk for squamous cell carcinomas of sun-exposed skin. Interestingly, albinos seem to have a below-normal frequency of malignant melanoma.

X-LINKED DISORDERS

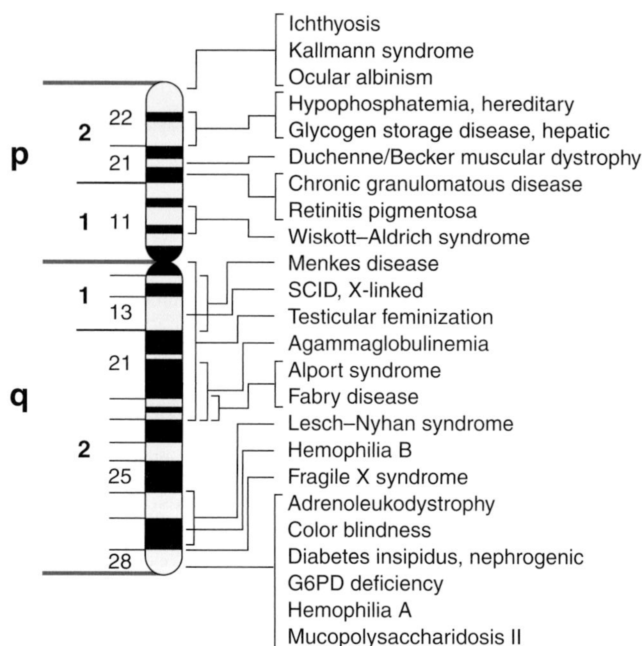

FIGURE 5-26. Localization of representative inherited diseases on the X chromosome. G6PD, glucose-6-phosphate dehydrogenase; SCID, severe combined immunodeficiency (syndrome).

The expression of X-linked disorders (Fig. 5-26) is different in males and females. Females, with two X chromosomes, may be homozygous or heterozygous for a given trait. It follows that clinical expression of a trait in a female is variable, depending on whether it is dominant or recessive. Males, having only one X chromosome, are hemizygous for that trait and express it, regardless of whether it is dominant or recessive.

X-linked traits are not transmitted from father to son: a symptomatic father donates only a normal Y chromosome to his male offspring. By contrast, he always donates his abnormal X chromosome to his daughters, who are thus obligate carriers of the trait. The disease thus skips a generation in males because female carriers transmit it to grandsons of a symptomatic male.

X-Linked Dominant Traits

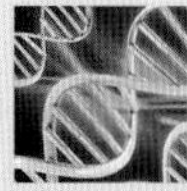

MOLECULAR PATHOGENESIS: X-linked dominance refers to the expression of a trait only in females because the hemizygous state in males precludes distinction between dominant and recessive inheritance.

Only a few X-linked dominant disorders are known, including familial hypophosphatemic rickets and ornithine transcarbamylase deficiency. Phenotypic variation in these traits in females may reflect, at least in part, the Lyon effect (i.e., inactivation of one X chromosome), which produces mosaicism for the mutant allele, and inconstant expression of the trait.

X-Linked Recessive Traits

Most X-linked traits are recessive; that is, heterozygous females do not manifest clinical disease. Table 5-8 lists representative X-linked recessive disorders.

Table 5-8

Representative X-Linked Recessive Diseases

Disease	Frequency in Males
Fragile X syndrome	1/4,000
Hemophilia A (factor VIII deficiency)	1/10,000
Hemophilia B (factor IX deficiency)	1/70,000
Duchenne–Becker muscular dystrophy	1/3,500
Glucose-6-phosphate dehydrogenase deficiency	Up to 30%
Lesch–Nyhan syndrome (HPRT deficiency)	1/10,000
Chronic granulomatous disease	Not rare
X-linked agammaglobulinemia	Not rare
X-linked severe combined immunodeficiency	Rare
Fabry disease	1/40,000
Hunter syndrome	1/70,000
Adrenoleukodystrophy	1/100,000
Menkes disease	1/100,000

HPRT, hypoxanthine-guanine phosphoribosyltransferase.

X-Linked (Duchenne and Becker) Muscular Dystrophies

The muscular dystrophies are devastating muscle diseases. Most are X linked, although a few are autosomal recessive. The X-linked muscular dystrophies are among the most common human genetic diseases, occurring in 1 per 3,500 boys, an incidence approaching that of CF. The most common X-linked recessive disorders include ***Duchenne muscular dystrophy (DMD)*** and ***Becker muscular dystrophy (BMD)***. DMD, the most common variant, is a fatal progressive degeneration of muscle that appears before the age of 4 years. It is associated with mutations in the *dystrophin* gene, the largest gene on the X chromosome. Dystrophin connects the cytoskeleton to the extracellular matrix and is thus crucial for function and survival of myocytes. DMD is characterized by rapid progression of muscle degeneration, with eventual loss of skeletal muscle control, respiratory failure, and death. BMD is allelic with DMD but is milder and causes slowly progressive muscle weakness of the legs and pelvis (see Chapter 23).

Hemophilia A (Factor VIII Deficiency)

Hemophilia A (see Chapter 18) is an X-linked recessive disorder of blood clotting, resulting in spontaneous bleeding, mainly into joints, muscles, and internal organs. It is caused by a deficiency of coagulation factor VIII secondary to a mutation in the *factor VIII* gene.

Red-Green Color Blindness

Red-green color blindness is a very common trait in humans. Between 7% of men and 0.5% of women are affected. It is most commonly inherited as an X-linked recessive condition, but mutations involving as many as 19 chromosomes and 56 genes have been implicated in rare forms of this disorder.

Fabry Disease

Fabry disease is an X-linked lysosomal storage disease. Recessive mutations cause deficiency of **α-galactosidase A**, resulting in accumulation of globotriaosylceramide and other glycosphingolipids in endothelial and smooth muscle cells throughout the vasculature. Deposition is greatest in coronary arteries, renal glomeruli, cardiac myocytes, and components of the cardiac conduction system. A particular type of tumor, angiokeratoma, is a characteristic cutaneous manifestation of Fabry disease. The microvasculature becomes increasingly compromised, causing progressive vascular insufficiency, with cerebral, renal, and cardiac infarcts. Patients die in early adulthood from complications of their vascular disease. Therapy with recombinant α-D-galactosidase A shows promise in arresting the disease.

TRINUCLEOTIDE REPEAT DISEASES

Fragile X Syndrome

Fully 20% of heritable mental retardation is as a result of X-linked disorders, and one fifth of these reflect an inducible fragile site on the X chromosome. A **fragile site** represents a specific locus, or band, on a chromosome that breaks easily. Fragile sites are detected in cytogenetic preparations as a nonstaining gap or constriction.

FXS is second only to Down syndrome as a genetic cause of mental retardation. The prevalence of FXS in males is 1 in 3,600 to 4,000 and 1 in 4,000 to 6,000 in females.

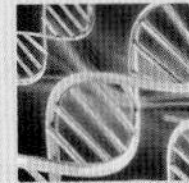

MOLECULAR PATHOGENESIS: Mutations in the *FMR1* gene cause FXS. This gene encodes a protein called fragile X mental retardation 1 protein (FMRP), which helps regulate production of other proteins and plays a role in synapse development. Nearly all cases of fragile X syndrome are caused by a mutation in which DNA in the 5′-untranslated region, known as the CGG triplet repeat, which is expanded within *FMR1*. In normal persons, this DNA segment is repeated from 5 to 45 times. In people with FXS, however, it is repeated over 200 times. The abnormally expanded CGG silences the gene through a mechanism involving methylation of selected nucleotides. The resultant loss or deficiency of the protein disrupts CNS functions and causes the symptoms of fragile X syndrome (Fig 5-27).

Males and females with 50 to 200 repeats of the CGG segment are said to have *FMR1* gene **premutation**. About 1 in 260 females and 1 in 800 males are carriers of fragile X premutation. Most people with premutation are intellectually normal, although sometimes they have lower-than-normal amounts of FMRP. As a result, premutation may cause mild versions of the physical features of fragile X syndrome and present as emotional problems, such as anxiety or depression. Some children with a premutation may have learning disabilities or autistic-like behavior.

Within fragile X families, the probability of being affected is related to position in the pedigree; later generations are more likely than earlier ones to be affected **(genetic anticipation)**.

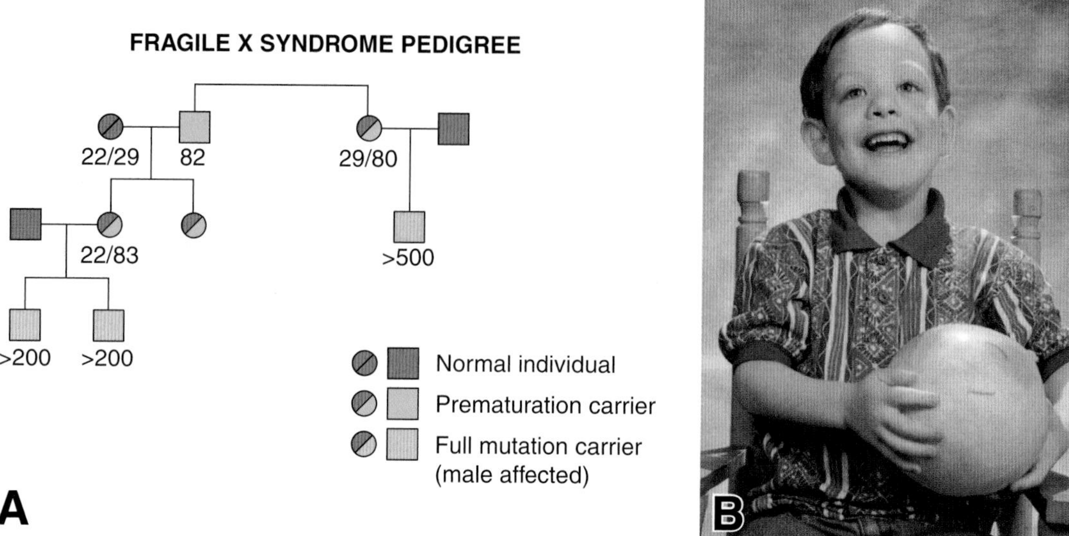

FIGURE 5-27. **A. Inheritance pattern of fragile X syndrome.** The number of copies of the trinucleotide repeat (CGG) in each X chromosome is shown below selected members in this pedigree. Expansion occurs primarily during meiosis in females. When the number of repeats exceeds ~200, the clinical syndrome is manifested. Individuals shaded orange carry a premutation and are asymptomatic. **B. Male diagnosed with fragile X syndrome.**

This is due to progressive triplet repeat expansion (Fig. 5-27). Although small expansions tend to be asymptomatic, they can enlarge, particularly during meiosis in females, leading to larger expansions in successive generations. As noted, expansions with over 200 repeats are associated with mental retardation and are considered full mutations of the *FMR1* gene locus. Expansion of a premutation to a full mutation during gametogenesis occurs only in females (Fig. 5-27). Thus, daughters of men with premutations (carriers) are never clinically symptomatic but always harbor the premutation. However, sisters of transmitting males occasionally produce affected daughters. *The frequency of conversion of a premutation to a full mutation in female carriers (i.e., the probability that their sons will have fragile X syndrome) varies with the length of the expanded tract.* Premutations with more than 90 repeats are almost always converted to full mutations. Hence, the risk of the disorder increases in succeeding generations of fragile X families. Because the syndrome is recessive, most daughters of carrier males transmit mental retardation to 50% of their sons.

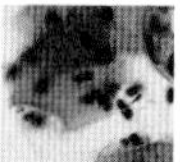

CLINICAL FEATURES: A male newborn with FXS appears normal, but during childhood, typical features appear, including increased head circumference and elongated face, large protruding ears (Fig. 5-27B), joint hyperextensibility, enlarged testes, and hypotonia. Mental retardation is profound, and IQ scores vary from 20 to 60.

Molecular DNA diagnostic testing is now available to identify fragile X premutation carriers and those with the full fragile X syndrome mutation.

Huntington Disease

HD is the most common genetic cause of chorea and leads to premature death. It is associated with abnormalities of muscle coordination and psychomotor and cognitive functions. The disease is transmitted as an autosomal dominant trait and reflects an expansion of a CAG repeat within the *HTT/IT15* gene, which encodes the protein **Huntingtin**. Expanded CAG repeats determine several other neurodegenerative disorders in addition to HD and are discussed in detail in Chapter 24 (Table 5-9).

Table 5-9

Representative Diseases Associated With Trinucleotide Repeats

Disease	Location	Sequence	Normal Length	Premutation	Full Mutation
Huntington disease	4p16.3	CAG	10–30	—	40–100
Kennedy disease	Xq21	CAG	15–25	—	40–55
Spinocerebellar ataxia	6p23	CAG	20–35	—	45–80
Fragile X syndrome	Xq27.3	CGG	5–44	50–200	200–1,000
Myotonic dystrophy	19q13	CTG	5–35	37–50	50–2,000
Friedreich ataxia	9q13	GAA	7–30	—	120–1,700

Myotonic Dystrophy

DM, the most common form of autosomal muscular dystrophy, is caused by expansion of a CTG repeat in the 3′-untranslated region of the *DM* gene on chromosome 19q. The disease is discussed in detail in Chapter 23.

Friedreich Ataxia

FA is an autosomal recessive degenerative disease associated with expansion of a GAA repeat. It affects the CNS and is also characterized by cardiomyopathy and type 2 diabetes. FA is the most common inherited ataxia, affecting 1 in 50,000 people in the United States, with males and females affected equally. The estimated carrier prevalence is 1 in 110. The affected gene codes for frataxin, a protein involved in iron transport into mitochondria. Because the defect is in an intron (which is removed from the mRNA transcript between transcription and translation), abnormal frataxin (FXN) protein is not produced. Instead, it causes gene silencing and loss of *frataxin* gene protein (see Chapter 24). Affected individuals have 200 to 1,700 repeats in the first intron of the *FXN* gene.

MITOCHONDRIAL DISEASES

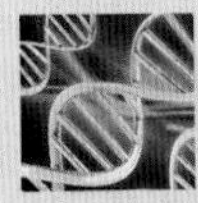

MOLECULAR PATHOGENESIS: Proteins in mitochondria are encoded by both nuclear and mitochondrial genes. Most mitochondrial respiratory chain proteins are encoded by nuclear genes, but 13 such proteins are products of the mitochondrial genome. The remaining 1,500 or so proteins in mitochondria are nuclear encoded. A few rare, autosomal recessive (Mendelian) disorders are caused by defects in nuclear-encoded mitochondrial proteins. However, most inherited defects in mitochondrial function result from mutations in the mitochondrial genome itself.

To understand these conditions, an explanation of the unique genetics of the mitochondria is needed. These features include the following:

- **Maternal inheritance:** All vertebrate mitochondria are inherited from the mother via the ovum, which has up to 300,000 copies of mitochondrial DNA (mtDNA).
- **Variability of mtDNA copies:** The number of mitochondria and the number of copies of mtDNA per mitochondrion vary in different tissues. Each mitochondrion has 2 to 10 mtDNA copies, and varying tissue needs for ATP correlate with the DNA content per mitochondrion.
- **Threshold effect:** Because any given cell has many mitochondria, and thus hundreds or thousands of mtDNA copies, mutations in mtDNA lead to mixed populations of mutant and normal mitochondrial genomes, a situation called **heteroplasmy**. The phenotype of mtDNA mutations reflects the severity of the mutation, the proportion of mutant genomes, and the tissue's demand for ATP. Different tissues need different amounts of ATP to sustain their metabolism; the brain, heart, and skeletal muscle have particularly high-energy demands.
- **High mutation rate:** The rate of mtDNA mutation is much higher than that of nuclear DNA, owing (at least in part) to less DNA repair capacity.

Diseases caused by mutations in the mitochondrial genome mainly affect the nervous system, heart, and skeletal muscle. Functional deficits in all of these disorders are traced to impaired oxidative phosphorylation (OXPHOS). **OXPHOS diseases** are divided into several classes: nuclear mutations, mtDNA point mutations, mtDNA deletions, and undefined defects.

All inherited mitochondrial diseases are rare and have variable clinical presentations for the reasons discussed above. The first human mtDNA disease described was **Leber hereditary optic neuropathy**, which is characterized by progressive loss of vision. Various mitochondrial myopathies (skeletal and cardiac) and encephalomyopathies are known (see Chapter 23).

GENETIC IMPRINTING

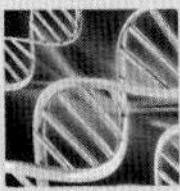

MOLECULAR PATHOGENESIS: Phenotypes associated with some genes differ, depending on whether the allele is inherited from the mother or father. This phenomenon is called **genetic imprinting**. For imprinted genes, either the maternal or paternal allele is maintained in an inactive state. This normal physiologic process results from CpG methylation (see above) in regulatory regions of imprinted allele, such that the nonimprinted allele provides the sole biologic function for that locus. If the nonimprinted allele is disrupted via mutation, the imprinted allele remains inactive and cannot compensate for the missing function. *Imprinting occurs in meiosis during gametogenesis, and the pattern of imprinting is maintained to variable degrees in different tissues. It is reset during meiosis in the next generation, so the selection of a given allele for imprinting can vary from one generation to the next.*

Genetic imprinting is illustrated by certain hereditary diseases, whose phenotype is determined by the parental source of the mutant allele. Prader–Willi syndrome (PWS) and **Angelman syndrome (AS)** provide examples of the effect of imprinting on genetic diseases. Both disorders are associated with (heterozygous) deletion in the region of 15(q11-13).

The phenotypes of these disorders are remarkably different. PWS features hypotonia, hyperphagia with obesity, hypogonadism, mental retardation, and characteristic facies. By contrast, AS patients are hyperactive, display inappropriate laughter, have different facies from that in PWS, and suffer from seizures.

PWS develops because critical genes in the maternal locus are normally silenced by imprinting, and the same region on the paternal chromosome is deleted, resulting in lack of expression. The opposite applies in Angelman syndrome. The paternal gene is normally imprinted and silenced, and the maternal locus is inactivated by mutation or deletion. Critical genes silenced by methylation in the maternal 15q11-13 region include *SNRPN* (encoding small nuclear ribonucleoprotein polypeptide), *NDN* (encoding necdin), and a cluster of small nucleolar RNAs (snoRNAs) In AS, *UBE3A*, which encodes a ubiquitin ligase, is mutated or deleted in the maternal chromosome and epigenetically silenced (in the paternal chromosome).

Each of these disorders is now routinely diagnosed by FISH or DNA analysis to detect the microdeletion of genes in 15q11-13 and by DNA methylation studies to detect uniparental disomy of maternal/paternal genes. This pattern is similar to loss of heterozygosity in tumor suppressor genes by aberrant methylation in some cases of cancer (see Chapter 4).

MULTIFACTORIAL INHERITANCE

Most normal human traits are not inherited as simple dominant or recessive Mendelian attributes. Many result from interplay between multiple genes and environmental, epigenetic, and other factors. These reflect multifactorial inheritance. Thus, such inheritance determines height, skin color, and body habitus. Similarly, most chronic disorders of adults—diabetes, atherosclerosis, many forms of cancer, arthritis, and hypertension—are diseases that are understood to "run in families," but in which inheritance does not follow simple patterns. Many birth defects (e.g., cleft lip and palate, pyloric stenosis, and congenital heart disease) are also transmitted via such complex mechanisms (Table 5-10).

Multifactorial inheritance entails multiple genes interacting with each other and with environmental factors to produce disease in an individual. Such inheritance leads to familial aggregation that does not obey simple Mendelian rules. Thus, inheritance of polygenic diseases is studied by population genetics, rather than by analysis of individual families.

The number of involved genes for any such disease is not known. Thus, in an individual case, the risk of a particular disorder cannot be quantified. The probability of disease can only be suggested from the numbers of relatives affected, the severity of their disease, and statistical projections based on population analyses. Although monogenic inheritance implies a specific risk of disease (e.g., 25%, 50%), the probability of symptoms in first-degree relatives of someone with a polygenic disease is usually only about 5% to 10%.

Over one fourth of all genes in normal humans demonstrate polymorphic alleles. Such heterogeneity creates wide variability in susceptibility to many diseases, made yet more complex by interactions with the environment.

- **Expression of symptoms is proportional to the number of mutant genes.** Close relatives of an affected person have more mutant genes than the population at large and more chance of expressing the disease. The probability of disease is highest in identical twins.
- **Environmental factors influence expression of the trait.** Thus, concordance for the disease may occur in only one third of monozygotic twins.
- **Risk in first-degree relatives (parents, siblings, and children) is the same (5% to 10%).** The probability of disease is much lower in second-degree relatives.
- **The likelihood of a trait's expression in later offspring is influenced by its expression in earlier siblings.** If one or more children are born with a multifactorial defect, the chance it will recur in later offspring is doubled. For simple Mendelian traits, by contrast, the probability is independent of the number of affected siblings.
- **The more severe the defect, the greater the risk of transmitting it to offspring.** Patients with more severe polygenic defects probably have more mutant genes. Their children thus will more likely inherit more abnormal genes than offspring of less severely affected parents.
- **Some diseases with multifactorial inheritance also show gender predilection.** Thus, pyloric stenosis is more common in males, whereas congenital hip dislocation is more common in females. Such differential susceptibility is thought to reflect different thresholds for expression of mutant genes in the two sexes. ***As a rule, if there is an altered sex ratio in the incidence of a polygenic defect, a member of the less commonly affected sex who expresses the defect has a much greater probability of transmitting the abnormality.***

Table 5-10

Representative Diseases Associated With Multifactorial Inheritance

Adults	Children
Hypertension	Pyloric stenosis
Atherosclerosis	Cleft lip and palate
Diabetes, type 2	Congenital heart disease
Allergic diathesis	Meningomyelocele
Psoriasis	Anencephaly
Schizophrenia	Hypospadias
Ankylosing spondylitis	Congenital hip dislocation
Gout	Hirschsprung disease

Cleft Lip and Cleft Palate

At the 35th day of gestation, the frontal prominence fuses with the maxillary process to form the upper lip. This process is under the control of many genes, and disturbances in gene expression (hereditary or environmental) at this time interfere with proper fusion, resulting in cleft lip, with or without cleft palate (Fig. 5-28). This anomaly may also be part of a systemic malformation syndrome caused by teratogens (e.g., rubella and anticonvulsants) and often occurs in children with chromosomal abnormalities.

The incidence of cleft lip, with or without cleft palate, is 10 per 10,000 live births. The incidence of cleft palate alone is 6 per 10,000 live births. If one child is born with a cleft lip, the chances are 4% that a second child will have the same defect. If the first two children are affected, the risk of cleft lip in the third child increases to 9%. The more severe the defect, the greater the probability of transmitting cleft lip. Although 75% of cases of cleft lip occur in boys, the sons of women with cleft lip have a fourfold higher risk for the defect than do sons of affected fathers.

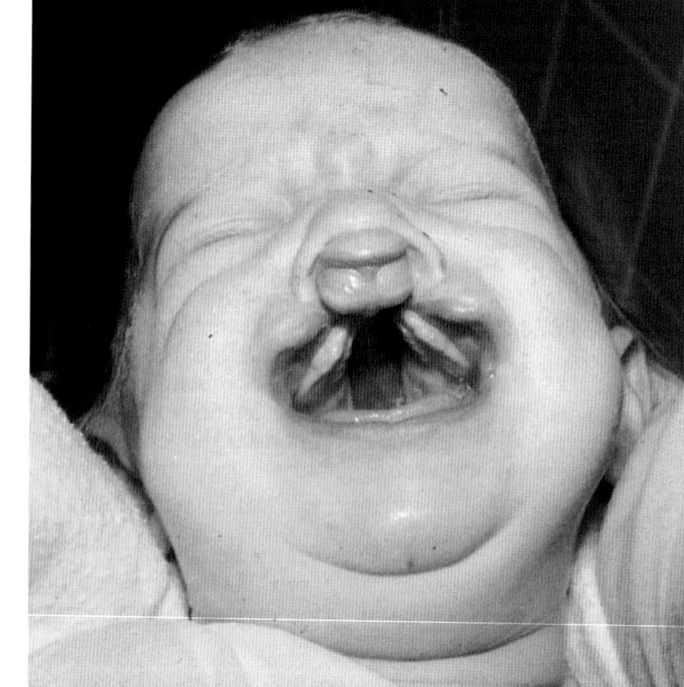

FIGURE 5-28. Cleft lip and palate in an infant.

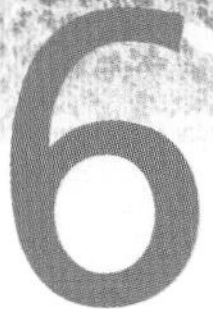

6 Infectious and Parasitic Diseases

David A. Schwartz

LEARNING OBJECTIVES

- Distinguish between the modes of replication of prions, bacteria, viruses, protozoa, and parasitic worms.
- Define the properties that contribute to the virulence of organisms.
- List several age-specific factors important in infection.
- Describe the pathogenetic mechanisms by which viral infections cause disease.
- Define the key difference between infection with RNA and DNA viruses.
- What agent and host factors are responsible for the symptoms resulting from infection by respiratory viruses?
- What are the routes of infection and pathogenetic mechanisms responsible for the common viral exanthems?
- What factors in the pathogenesis of mumps are responsible for the symptoms of the disease?
- List common infections resulting from DNA viruses.
- What are the distinguishing characteristics of herpes virus diseases?
- What is the characteristic histopathology of varicella-zoster infection?
- Describe the pathogenesis of Epstein–Barr virus infections.
- Define and provide examples of the following terms: endotoxin, exotoxin, cytotoxin, neurotoxin, and enterotoxin.
- List the common gram-positive pyogenic cocci and describe the pathogenetic mechanisms and tissue pathology associated with each organism.
- What is the role of the capsule in pneumococcal virulence?
- List important bacterial infections of childhood and describe the pathogenetic mechanisms and tissue pathology associated with each disease.
- Describe the pathogenesis of disease resulting from infection by different strains of *Escherichia coli*.
- Describe the pathogenesis and tissue pathology produced by infections with *Salmonella*, *Shigella*, and *Vibrio* bacteria.
- List gram-negative bacteria associated with pulmonary infections and describe the pathogenetic mechanisms and tissue pathology associated with each organism.
- List diseases associated with clostridial infection and describe the pathogenesis and tissue pathology associated with each.
- List the animal reservoir and insect vector (if present) associated with brucellosis, bubonic plague, and anthrax.
- Describe the pathogenesis of bubonic plague.
- List diseases associated with nonvenereal treponematoses infections and describe the pathogenesis and tissue pathology associated with each.
- Describe the target cell associated with the pathogenesis of rickettsial infections.
- Describe the pathogenesis and tissue pathology associated with leprosy.
- What factors predispose to superficial candidiasis at different body sites?
- Describe the pathogenesis and tissue pathology associated with malaria.
- What factors distinguish malignant malarial disease from milder infection?
- Describe the pathogenesis and tissue pathology associated with enteric protozoal diseases, including amebiasis, cryptosporidiosis, and giardiasis.
- Distinguish between the various types of leishmaniasis infections in terms of pathogenesis and organ/tissue pathology.
- Distinguish between acute and chronic Chagas disease in terms of pathogenesis and tissue pathology, including myocarditis, megaesophagus, and megacolon.
- Describe the pathogenesis and tissue pathology associated with African trypanosomiasis.
- Describe the pathogenesis and tissue pathology associated with filarial nematode infections.
- Explain why eating sushi containing raw freshwater fish may lead to parasitic disease.
- Describe a foodborne disease associated with the ingestion of a tissue nematode in terms of pathogenesis and organ/tissue pathology.
- Describe the pathogenesis and tissue pathology associated with schistosomiasis.

TISSUE DAMAGE AND INFECTIOUS DISEASE

Infectious diseases represent many of the familiar taxa: bacteria, fungi, protozoa, and various parasitic worms. Yet, some infectious agents do not qualify as completely independent organisms. Viruses cannot replicate by themselves and are obligate intracellular parasites that hijack the replicative machinery of susceptible cells.

There is great diversity in how various infectious diseases are acquired. Many of these maladies, such as influenza, syphilis, and tuberculosis, are contagious (i.e., transmissible from person to person). Yet, many others, such as legionellosis, histoplasmosis, and toxoplasmosis, are not contagious but are acquired from the environment. *Legionella* bacteria normally replicate in aquatic amebas but can infect humans via aerosolized water or through microaspiration of contaminated water. Other infectious agents come from many diverse sources, such as animals, insects, soil, air, inanimate objects, and the endogenous microbial flora of the human body.

Perhaps, the greatest paradox is that certain retroviruses have actually been incorporated into the human genome and are passed from generation to generation. Their function is unclear, but their possible activation during placentation has led to speculation that such endogenous retroviruses may have allowed placental mammals to evolve.

Just as there is diversity in how pathogens are acquired, the mechanisms by which they produce disease vary. Some cause mechanical injury (e.g., filarial worms blocking lymphatics), some synthesize toxic proteins released into the tissue environment, others are toxic in and of themselves, and still others are intracellular parasites that hijack the cells metabolic machinery. Often, the injury is more the result of misdirected or excessive host defense, rather than a direct effect of the pathogen.

INFECTIVITY AND VIRULENCE

Virulence is the complex of properties that allow an organism to establish infection and to cause disease or death. The organism must (1) gain access to the body, (2) avoid multiple host defenses, (3) accommodate to growth in the human milieu, and (4) parasitize human resources. Virulence reflects both the structures inherent in the offending microbe and the interplay of those factors with host defense mechanisms.

HOST DEFENSE MECHANISMS

The means by which the body prevents or contains infections are known as defense mechanisms (Table 6-1). There are major anatomic barriers to infection—the skin and the aerodynamic filtration system of the upper airway—that prevent most organisms from ever penetrating the body. The mucociliary blanket of the airways is also an essential defense, expelling organisms that gain access to the respiratory system. Microbial flora normally resident in the gastrointestinal tract and in various body orifices compete with outside organisms, preventing them from gaining sufficient nutrients or binding sites in the host. The body's orifices are also protected by secretions that possess antimicrobial properties, both nonspecific (e.g., lysozyme and interferon) and specific (secretory immunoglobulin A [IgA]). In addition, gastric acid and bile chemically destroy many ingested organisms.

Table 6-1

Host Defenses Against Infection
Skin
Tears
Normal bacterial flora
Gastric acid
Bile
Salivary and pancreatic secretions
Filtration system of nasopharynx
Mucociliary blanket
Bronchial, cervical, urethral, and prostatic secretions
Neutrophils
Monocytes
Complement
Stationary mononuclear phagocyte system
Immunoglobulins
Cell-mediated immunity

Effect of Differences in Host Membrane Receptors

The first step in infection is often a highly specific interaction of a binding molecule on an infecting organism with a receptor molecule on the host. If the host lacks a suitable receptor, the organism cannot attach to the target. Thus, *Plasmodium vivax*, one of the organisms that causes human malaria, infects human erythrocytes by using Duffy blood group determinants on the cell surface as receptors. Many people, particularly blacks, lack these determinants and are not susceptible to infection with *P. vivax*. As a result, *P. vivax* malaria is absent from much of Africa. Similar racial or geographic differences in susceptibility are apparent for many infectious agents, including *Coccidioides immitis* and *Coccidioides posadasii*, which are 14 times more common in blacks and 175 times more frequent in Filipinos than in whites.

Effect of Age

The effect of age on the outcome of exposure to many infectious agents is well illustrated by infections of the fetus. Some organisms produce more severe disease in utero than in children or adults. Infections of the fetus with cytomegalovirus (CMV), rubella virus, parvovirus B19, and *Toxoplasma gondii* interfere with fetal development. Normally, the fetus is protected by maternal IgG (generated by a specific previous infection) that passively crosses the placenta. In acute infection of a pregnant woman who lacks neutralizing antibody, certain pathogens may cross the placenta. These infections are usually subclinical or produce minimal disease in the mother. Depending on the organism and timing of exposure, fetal infection can produce minimal damage, major congenital abnormalities, or death.

Age also affects the course of common illnesses, such as the diverse viral and bacterial diarrheas. In older children and adults, these infections cause discomfort and inconvenience, but rarely severe disease. The outcome can be different in children under 3 years of age, who cannot compensate for rapid volume loss resulting from profuse diarrhea. The World Health Organization (WHO) estimates that acute diarrheal diseases remain the second leading cause of death in children under 5 years of age and kill 1.5 million children yearly.

Other examples include infection with *Mycobacterium tuberculosis*, which produces severe, disseminated tuberculosis in children under the age of 3 years. By contrast, older people tend to fare much better.

Maturity, however, is not always an advantage in infections. Epstein–Barr virus (EBV) is more likely to cause symptomatic infections in adolescents and adults than in younger children. Varicella-zoster virus causes chickenpox in children but produces more severe disease in adults, who are more likely to develop viral pneumonia.

The elderly fare more poorly with almost all infections than do younger persons. Common respiratory illnesses, such as influenza and pneumococcal pneumonia, are more often fatal in those older than 65 years. An example of the susceptibility of the aged to infectious disease occurred during the 2002 to 2003 outbreak of the newly emergent severe acute respiratory syndrome (SARS) coronavirus. The case fatality rate was less than 1% for people younger than 24 years, but was greater than 50% for those over 65 years.

Effect of Human Behavior

The link between behavior and infection is probably most obvious for sexually transmitted diseases. Syphilis, gonorrhea, urogenital chlamydial infections, AIDS, and a number of other infectious diseases are transmitted primarily by sexual contact.

Other aspects of behavior also influence the risk of acquiring infections. Humans contract brucellosis and Q fever, which are primarily bacterial diseases of domesticated farm animals, by close contact with infected animals or their secretions. These infections occur in farmers, herders, meat processors, and, in the case of brucellosis, people who drink unpasteurized milk. Transmission of a number of parasitic diseases is strongly affected by behavior. Schistosomiasis is acquired when waterborne parasite larvae penetrate the skin of a susceptible host. It is primarily a disease of farmers who work in fields irrigated by infected water. The larvae of hookworm and *Strongyloides stercoralis* live in humid soil and penetrate the skin of the feet in people who walk barefoot. Shoes are probably the single most important factor in limiting infection with soil-transmitted nematodes. Anisakiasis and diphyllobothriasis are helminthic diseases acquired by eating incompletely cooked fish. Toxoplasmosis is a protozoan infection transmitted from animals to humans by ingestion of incompletely cooked, infected meat, or by exposure to infected cat feces. Botulism, a food poisoning caused by a bacterial toxin, is contracted by ingestion of improperly canned food that contains the toxin.

As humans change their behavior, they open up new possibilities for infectious diseases. Although the agent of Legionnaires disease is common in the environment, aerosols generated by cooling plants, faucets, and humidifiers provide the means for causing human infections.

Effect of Compromised Host Defenses

Disruption or absence of any of the complex host defenses results in increased numbers and severity of infections. Damage to epithelial surfaces by trauma or burns can lead to invasive bacterial or fungal infections. Injury to the airway mucociliary apparatus, as in smoking or influenza, impairs clearance of inhaled microorganisms and gives rise to an increased incidence of bacterial pneumonia. Congenital absence of certain complement components prevents formation of a fully functional membrane attack complex and permits disseminated, and often recurrent, *Neisseria* infections (see Chapter 2). Diseases such as diabetes mellitus and the use of chemotherapeutic drugs and corticosteroids may interfere with neutrophil production or function and increase the likelihood and severity of infections with bacteria or fungi.

Compromised hosts are often attacked by organisms that are innocuous to normal people. For example, patients deficient in neutrophils frequently develop life-threatening bloodstream infections with commensal microorganisms that normally populate the skin and gastrointestinal tract. Such organisms that mainly cause disease in hosts with impaired defenses are called **opportunistic pathogens**.

VIRUSES

Viruses range in size from 20 to 300 nm and consist of RNA or DNA surrounded by a protein shell. Some are also enveloped in lipid membranes. ***Viruses do not metabolize or reproduce independently. They are obligate intracellular parasites and require living cells in order to replicate.*** After invading cells, they divert intracellular biosynthetic and metabolic pathways to synthesizing virus-encoded nucleic acids and proteins.

Viruses often cause disease by killing infected cells. By contrast, rotavirus, a common cause of diarrhea, interferes with the function of infected enterocytes without immediately killing them. The agent prevents enterocytes from synthesizing proteins that transport molecules from the intestinal lumen, thereby causing diarrhea.

Viruses may also promote the release of chemical mediators that elicit inflammatory or immunologic responses. The symptoms of the common cold are caused by the release of bradykinin from infected cells. Other viruses cause cells to proliferate and form tumors. Human papillomaviruses (HPVs), for instance, cause squamous cell proliferative lesions, which include benign warts and squamous cell carcinoma (see Chapter 4).

Some viruses infect and persist in cells without interfering with cellular functions, a process known as **latency**. Latent viruses often emerge to produce disease years after a primary infection. Opportunistic infections may reflect reactivation of latent virus infections. CMV and herpes simplex viruses are commonly present as latent agents and emerge in people with impaired cell-mediated immunity.

Finally, some viruses may reside within cells, either by integrating into their genomes or by remaining episomal. Such viruses can cause those cells to generate tumors. Epstein-Barr virus (EBV) causes endemic Burkitt lymphoma in Africa and other tumors in different settings. Infection with human T-cell leukemia virus-1 (HTLV-1) gives rise to a form of T-cell leukemia/lymphoma.

RNA Viruses

RNA viruses generally follow different paths to causing disease than do most DNA viruses. They need different enzymes for their infectious cycles, and many aspects of their biology do not have correlates among DNA viruses. One of the key differences between some RNA viruses and many DNA viruses is that the polymerases of some important pathogenic RNA viruses (e.g., HIV-1 and hepatitis C virus [HCV]) do not proofread the strand being synthesized. This has two important consequences. First, the mutation rate—and thus the plasticity of these viruses in circumventing therapies—is very high. Second, a greater proportion of daughter virions is inactive.

PATHOGENETIC MECHANISMS OF RNA VIRUSES

Respiratory Viruses

The Common Cold (Coryza)

The common cold (coryza) is an acute, self-limited upper respiratory tract disorder caused by infection with a variety of RNA viruses, including over 110 distinct rhinoviruses and several coronaviruses.

Rhinoviruses and coronaviruses have a tropism for respiratory epithelium and optimally reproduce at temperatures well below 37°C (98.6°F). Thus, infection remains confined to the cooler passages of the upper airway; they do not destroy respiratory epithelium and produce no visible alterations. Infected cells release chemical mediators, such as bradykinin, which produce most of the symptoms associated with colds, namely, increased mucus production, nasal congestion, and Eustachian tube obstruction.

Influenza

Influenza is an acute, usually self-limited, infection of the upper and lower airways, caused by influenza virus. The virus is enveloped, and contains single-stranded RNA. Influenza spreads from person to person by virus-containing respiratory droplets and secretions. When it reaches the respiratory epithelial cell surface, a viral glycoprotein (hemagglutinin) binds to sialic acid residues on human respiratory epithelium, after which the agent enters the cell. Once inside, the virus directs the cell to produce progeny viruses, which results in necrosis and desquamation of ciliated respiratory tract epithelium and a predominantly lymphocytic inflammatory infiltrate. Extension of infection to the lungs leads to necrosis, sloughing of alveolar lining cells, and the histologic appearance of viral pneumonitis. Destruction of ciliated epithelium cripples mucociliary clearance and predisposes to bacterial pneumonia.

Parainfluenza and Respiratory Syncytial Virus

The parainfluenza viruses cause acute upper and lower respiratory tract infections, particularly in young children. They are the most common cause of croup (laryngotracheobronchitis), which is characterized by stridor on inspiration and a "barking" cough. RSV is the most common cause of bronchiolitis and pneumonia in children younger than 1 year. Parainfluenza viruses infect and kill ciliated respiratory epithelial cells and elicit an inflammatory response. In very young children, this process frequently extends into the lower respiratory tract, causing bronchiolitis and pneumonitis. Local edema of laryngotracheitis may compress the upper airway enough to obstruct breathing and cause croup.

RSV produces necrosis and sloughing of bronchial, bronchiolar, and alveolar epithelium, and is associated with a predominantly lymphocytic inflammatory infiltrate. Multinucleated syncytial cells are sometimes seen in infected tissues.

Viral Exanthems

Measles (Rubeola)

Measles virus is an enveloped, single-stranded RNA paramyxovirus that causes an acute illness, characterized by upper respiratory tract symptoms, fever, and rash. The virus is transmitted to humans by respiratory aerosols and secretions.

The initial site of infection is the mucous membranes of the nasopharynx and bronchi. Two surface glycoproteins, "H" and "F," mediate viral attachment and fusion with respiratory epithelium. The virus then spreads to regional lymph nodes and the bloodstream, resulting in widespread dissemination and prominent involvement of the skin and lymphoid tissues. ***The rash results from the action of T lymphocytes on virally infected vascular endothelium.*** Measles virus produces necrosis of infected respiratory epithelium, with a predominantly lymphocytic inflammatory infiltrate, and a vasculitis of small blood vessels in the skin. Lymphoid hyperplasia is often prominent in cervical and mesenteric lymph nodes, spleen, and appendix. In lymphoid tissues, the virus sometimes causes fusion of infected cells, producing multinucleated giant cells containing up to 100 nuclei, with both intracytoplasmic and intranuclear inclusions. These cells, termed **Warthin–Finkeldey giant cells** (Fig. 6-1), are pathognomonic for measles.

Rubella (German Measles)

Rubella virus is an enveloped, single-stranded RNA virus that causes a mild, self-limited systemic disease, usually associated with a rash (also known as "German measles"). Many infections are so mild that they go unnoticed. However, in pregnant women, rubella is a destructive fetal pathogen. The virus infects respiratory epithelium and then disseminates through the bloodstream and lymphatics. The rubella rash is believed to result from an immune response to the disseminated virus. In most patients, rubella is a mild, acute febrile illness, with rhinorrhea, conjunctivitis, postauricular

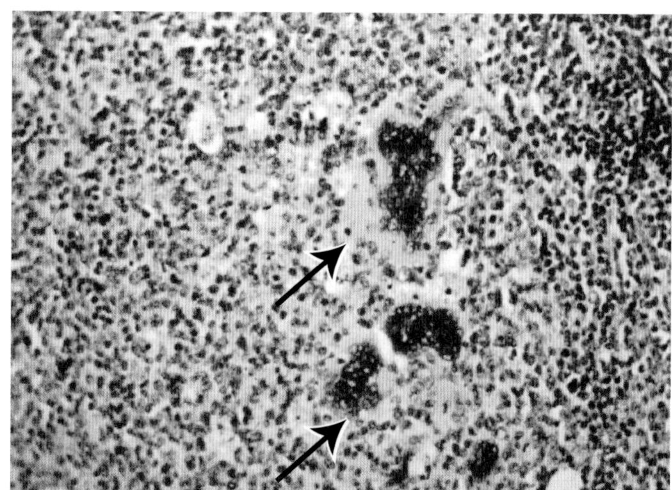

FIGURE 6-1. Warthin–Finkeldey giant cells in measles. A hyperplastic lymph node from a patient with measles showing several multinucleated giant cells (*arrows*).

lymphadenopathy and a rash that spreads from face to trunk and extremities. However, in the fetus, the heart, eye, and brain are the organs most often affected. Severe brain involvement can produce microcephaly and mental retardation, and sensorineural deafness is common (see Chapter 5).

Mumps

Mumps virus is a paramyxovirus, an enveloped, single-stranded RNA virus. It causes an acute, self-limited systemic illness, characterized by parotid gland swelling and meningoencephalitis, which spreads from person to person via the respiratory route. Mumps begins as a viral infection of respiratory tract epithelium. The virus then disseminates through the blood and lymphatic systems to other sites, most commonly the salivary glands (especially parotids), central nervous system (CNS), pancreas, and testes. Over half of infections involve the CNS, with symptomatic disease in 10%. Epididymo-orchitis occurs in 20% of males infected after puberty. Mumps virus causes necrosis of infected cells, eliciting a predominantly lymphocytic inflammatory infiltrate. Affected salivary glands are swollen, their ducts lined by necrotic epithelium, and their interstitium infiltrated with lymphocytes. In mumps, epididymo-orchitis, the swelling of testicular parenchyma, confined within the tunica albuginea, produces focal infarcts. Mumps orchitis is usually unilateral and, thus, rarely causes sterility.

Intestinal Infections

Rotavirus and Norwalk Virus

Rotavirus is a double-stranded RNA virus, which produces profuse watery diarrhea that can lead to dehydration and death if untreated. Rotavirus infection spreads from person to person by the oral–fecal route. Infection is most common among children, who shed huge amounts of virus in the stool. Rotavirus infects enterocytes of the upper small intestine, disrupting absorption of sugars, fats, and various ions. The resulting osmotic load causes a net loss of fluid into the bowel lumen and produces diarrhea and dehydration. Infected cells are shed from intestinal villi, after which the regenerating epithelium initially lacks full absorptive capabilities.

Pathologic changes in rotavirus infection are largely confined to the duodenum and jejunum. The intestinal villi are shortened, and there is a mild infiltrate of neutrophils and lymphocytes.

Norwalk virus is a member of a group of caliciviruses, which are responsible for one third of all outbreaks of diarrheal disease. The pathophysiology of the disease is similar to that of rotavirus infection.

Viral Hemorrhagic Fevers

Viral hemorrhagic fevers are a group of at least 20 distinct viral infections that cause varying degrees of hemorrhage, shock, and often death. There are many similar viral hemorrhagic fevers in different parts of the world, usually named for the area where they were first described. Four viral families are involved—the Bunyaviridae, Flaviviridae, Arenaviridae, and Filoviridae. On the basis of differences in routes of transmission, vectors, and other epidemiologic characteristics, viral hemorrhagic fevers have been divided into four epidemiologic groups (Table 6-2): mosquito-borne; tick-borne; zoonotic; and

Table 6-2

Viral Hemorrhagic Fevers

Vector	Viral Fever
Mosquitoes	Yellow fever
	Rift valley fever
	Dengue hemorrhagic fever
	Chikungunya hemorrhagic fever
Ticks	Omsk hemorrhagic fever
	Crimean hemorrhagic fever
	Kyasanur forest disease
Rodents	Lassa fever
	Bolivian hemorrhagic fever
	Argentine hemorrhagic fever
	Korean hemorrhagic fever
Fruit bats	Ebola virus disease

the filoviruses, Marburg, and Ebola virus, in which the route of transmission is uncertain but likely to involve bats as a natural reservoir.

Yellow Fever

Yellow fever is an acute hemorrhagic fever, sometimes associated with extensive hepatic necrosis and jaundice, which is caused by an insect-borne flavivirus, an enveloped, single-stranded RNA virus. The virus is restricted to both jungle and urban areas in Africa and South America. The natural viral reservoir is tree-dwelling monkeys, which are unaffected by the virus. Humans acquire jungle yellow fever by being bitten by *Aedes* mosquitoes that have fed on infected monkeys or humans.

On inoculation by the mosquito, the virus multiplies within tissue and vascular endothelium and then disseminates through the bloodstream. It has a tropism for liver cells, where it sometimes produces extensive acute hepatocellular destruction. Extensive damage to the endothelium of small blood vessels may lead to the loss of vascular integrity, hemorrhages, and shock. The disease causes coagulative necrosis of hepatocytes, beginning in the middle of hepatic lobules and spreading toward the central veins and portal tracts, sometimes producing confluent necrosis in the middle of the hepatic lobules (i.e., midzonal necrosis). Necrotic hepatocytes lose their nuclei and become intensely eosinophilic apoptotic bodies (**Councilman bodies**).

Ebola Hemorrhagic Fever

Ebola virus is an RNA virus belonging to the Filoviridae family; it causes a hemorrhagic disease with a high mortality rate in humans in several regions of Africa. The only other filovirus pathogenic to humans is Marburg virus, which produces Marburg hemorrhagic fever. In the wild, the virus infects humans, gorillas, chimpanzees, and monkeys, with fruit bats serving as a possible natural reservoir. The virus can also be transmitted via bodily secretions and blood. *Ebola virus results in the most widespread destructive tissue lesions of all viral hemorrhagic fever agents.* The virus replicates massively in endothelial cells, mononuclear phagocytes, and hepatocytes.

Necrosis is most severe in the liver, kidneys, gonads, spleen, and lymph nodes. The liver characteristically shows hepatocellular necrosis, Kupffer cell hyperplasia, Councilman bodies, and microsteatosis. The lungs are usually hemorrhagic. Petechial hemorrhages are seen in the skin, mucous membranes, and internal organs. Injury to the microvasculature and increased endothelial permeability are important causes of shock.

DNA Viruses

DNA viruses may be (1) enveloped or nonenveloped, (2) either single-stranded or double-stranded, and (3) have either a linear or circular genome. Many, for example, herpesvirus, are able to survive in the human body in a latent stage without causing symptoms. Because DNA viruses replicate within the cell nucleus, the infectious process requires that the viral DNA be delivered to that site. Different viruses use different mechanisms to achieve this effect.

Adenovirus

Adenoviruses are nonenveloped DNA viruses that are isolated from the respiratory and intestinal tracts of humans and animals. Certain serotypes are common causes of acute respiratory disease and adenovirus pneumonia. In addition, some adenoviruses are important causes of chronic pulmonary disease in infants and young children. Adenoviruses spread via direct contact, fecal–oral transmission, and, occasionally, waterborne transmission. Pathologic changes feature necrotizing bronchitis and bronchiolitis, in which sloughed epithelial cells and inflammatory infiltrate fill damaged bronchioles. Interstitial pneumonitis is characterized by areas of consolidation, with extensive necrosis, hemorrhage, and a mononuclear inflammatory infiltrate. Adenovirus infection is associated with two distinctive types of intranuclear inclusions—Cowdry type A inclusions and smudge cells (Fig. 6-2), which appear in bronchiolar epithelial cells and alveolar lining cells. Cytopathic effects appear as granular, slightly enlarged nuclei containing eosinophilic bodies intermixed with clumped basophilic chromatin. The eosinophilic bodies coalesce, forming larges masses that end as a central, granular, ill-defined mass surrounded by a halo (Cowdry A inclusions). The second type of inclusion, which is more common and probably corresponds to a late-stage infected cell, is the "smudge cell." The nucleus is rounded or ovoid, large and completely occupied by a granular amphophilic to deeply basophilic mass. There is no halo, and the nuclear membrane and nucleus are indistinct.

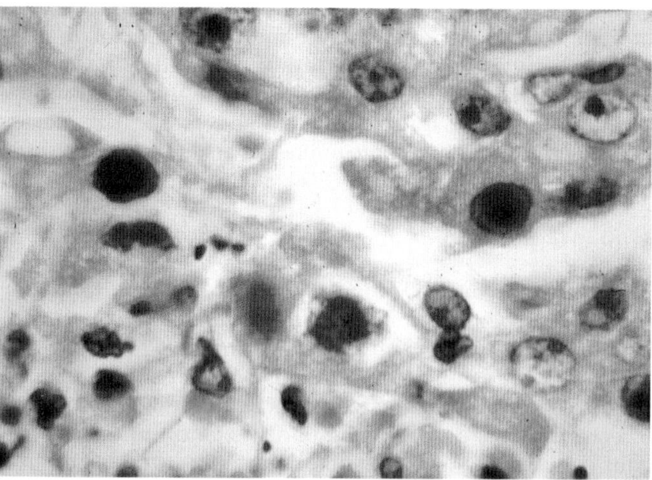

FIGURE 6-2. Adenovirus infection of the liver from a child. The two forms of viral inclusions are present: smudge cells and Cowdry A inclusions.

Human Parvovirus (Erythrovirus) B19

Human parvovirus B19, now called erythrovirus, is a single-stranded DNA virus that causes **erythema infectiosum (fifth disease)**, a benign self-limited febrile illness in children. It also produces systemic infections, characterized by rash, arthralgias, and transient interruption in erythrocyte production in nonimmune adults. The virus spreads from person to person by the respiratory route. It is not known which cells, other than erythroid precursors, support viral replication, but the agent probably multiplies in the respiratory tract before it spreads to erythropoietic cells. Human parvovirus B19 gains entry to erythroid precursor cells via the P-erythrocyte antigen and produces characteristic cytopathic effects in those cells. Nuclei of affected cells are enlarged, and chromatin is displaced peripherally by central, glassy, eosinophilic inclusion bodies (giant pronormoblasts).

Herpesviruses

The virus family Herpesviridae includes a large number of enveloped DNA viruses, many of which infect humans. Almost all herpesviruses express some common antigenic determinants, and many produce type A nuclear inclusions (see above). The most important pathogenic human herpesviruses (HHVs) are varicella-zoster virus (VZV, or HHV-3); herpes simplex virus 1 and 2 (HSV-1 and -2); EBV (HHV-4); HHV6, the cause of roseola; CMV (HHV-5); and Kaposi sarcoma–associated herpesvirus (HHV-8), a human oncovirus that causes Kaposi sarcoma, primary effusion lymphoma, and some types of Castleman disease. ***These viruses are distinguished by their capacity to remain latent for long periods of time.***

Varicella-Zoster Infection (Chicken Pox and Herpes Zoster)

First, exposure to VZV produces chickenpox, an acute systemic illness characterized by a generalized vesicular skin eruption (Fig. 6-3). The virus then becomes latent, and its reactivation many years later causes herpes zoster ("shingles"), a localized vesicular skin eruption. VZV is restricted to human hosts and spreads from person to person primarily by the respiratory route. It can also be spread by contact with secretions from skin lesions. The virus is present worldwide and is highly contagious.

VZV initially infects the respiratory tract or conjunctival epithelium. There it reproduces and spreads through the blood and lymphatic systems. Many organs are infected during this viremic stage, but skin involvement usually dominates the clinical picture. The virus spreads from the capillary endothelium to the epidermis, where its replication destroys the basal cells. As a result, the upper layers of the epidermis separate from the basal layer to form vesicles. During primary infection, VZV establishes latent infection in perineuronal satellite cells of the dorsal nerve root ganglia. Transcription of viral genes continues during latency, and viral DNA can be demonstrated years after the initial infection.

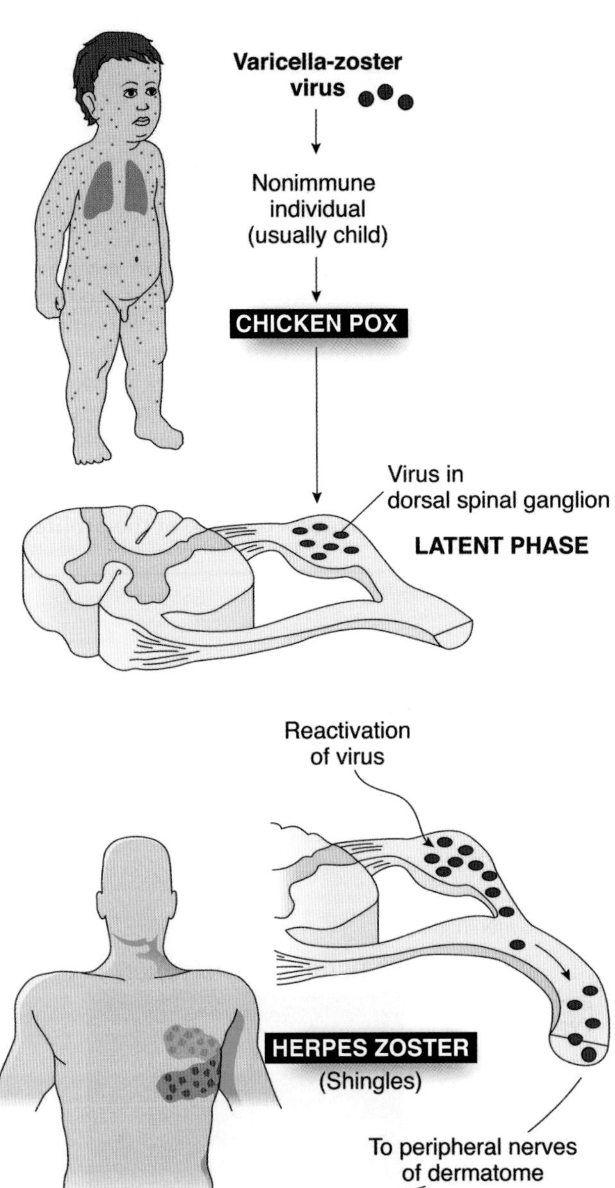

FIGURE 6-3. Varicella (chickenpox) and herpes zoster (shingles). Varicella-zoster virus (VZV) in droplets is inhaled by a nonimmune person (usually a child) and initially causes a "silent" infection of the nasopharynx. This progresses to viremia, seeding of fixed macrophages, and dissemination of VZV to skin (chickenpox) and viscera. VZV resides in a dorsal spinal ganglion, where it remains dormant for many years. Latent VZV is reactivated and spreads from ganglia along the sensory nerves to the peripheral nerves of sensory dermatomes, causing shingles.

Shingles occurs when viral replication takes place in ganglion cells and the agent travels down the sensory nerve from a single dermatome. It then infects the corresponding epidermis, producing a localized, painful vesicular eruption. The risk of shingles in an infected person increases with age, and most cases occur among the elderly. Impaired cell-mediated immunity also increases the risk of VZV reactivation. The skin lesions of chickenpox and shingles are identical and also resemble lesions caused by HSV (see below). Vesicles fill with neutrophils, soon erode, and become shallow ulcers. In infected cells, VZV produces a characteristic cytopathic effect, with nuclear homogenization and intranuclear (Cowdry type A) inclusions. Multinucleated cells are common (Fig. 6-4). Over several days, vesicles become pustules, which then rupture and heal.

Herpes Simplex Viruses

HSVs are common human viral pathogens (Table 6-3) with two different forms (Fig. 6-5):

- **HSV-1** is transmitted in oral secretions and typically causes disease "above the waist," including oral, facial, and ocular lesions.
- **HSV-2** is transmitted in genital secretions and typically causes genital ulcers and neonatal herpes infection.

Primary HSV disease occurs at a site of initial viral inoculation, such as the oropharynx, genital mucosa, or skin. The virus infects epithelial cells, producing progeny viruses and destroying basal cells in the squamous epithelium, with resulting formation of vesicles. Cell necrosis also elicits an inflammatory response, initially dominated by neutrophils and then followed by lymphocytes. Primary infection resolves when humoral and cell-mediated immunity to the virus develop.

Latent infection is established in a manner analogous to that of VZV. The virus invades sensory nerve endings in the oral or genital mucosa, ascends within axons, and establishes a latent infection in sensory neurons within corresponding ganglia. Various factors, such as intense sunlight, emotional stress, febrile illness and, in women, menstruation, can induce reactivation of latent HSV infection. Both HSV-1 and HSV-2 can cause severe protracted and disseminated disease in immunocompromised persons.

Epstein–Barr Virus

EBV causes infectious mononucleosis, a disorder characterized by fever, pharyngitis, lymphadenopathy, and increased circulating lymphocytes. The virus is also associated with several cancers, including **African Burkitt lymphoma, B-cell lymphoma** in immunosuppressed patients, and **nasopharyngeal carcinoma** (see Chapters 4 and 18).

In areas of the world where children live in crowded conditions, EBV infection usually occurs before 3 years of

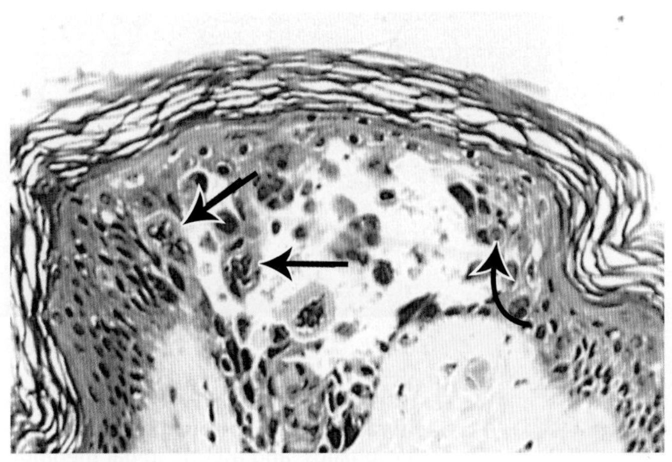

FIGURE 6-4. Varicella. Photomicrograph of the skin from a patient with chickenpox showing an intraepidermal vesicle. Multinucleated giant cells (*straight arrows*) and nuclear inclusions (*curved arrow*) are present.

Table 6-3

Herpes Simplex Virus (HSV) Diseases

Viral Type	Common Presentations	Infrequent Presentations
HSV-1	Oral–labial herpes	Conjunctivitis, keratitis
		Encephalitis
		Herpetic whitlow
		Esophagitis[a]
		Pneumonia[a]
		Disseminated infection[a]
HSV-2	Genital herpes	Perinatal infection
		Disseminated infection[a]

[a]These conditions usually occur in immunocompromised hosts.

age, and infectious mononucleosis is rare. In developed countries, infection occurs in adolescence, and two thirds of those newly infected develop clinically evident infectious mononucleosis.

EBV spreads from person to person primarily through contact with infected oral secretions (Fig. 6-6). Once it enters the body, EBV remains for life, analogous to latent infections with other herpesviruses. A few people (10% to 20%) shed the virus intermittently. Transmission requires close contact with infected individuals. The virus first binds to and infects nasopharyngeal cells and then B lymphocytes, which carry the virus throughout the body. The result is a generalized infection of lymphoid tissues predominantly involving the lymph nodes and spleen. In most patients, lymphadenopathy is symmetric and most striking in the neck. The nodes are movable, discrete, and tender. General nodal architecture is preserved. Germinal centers are enlarged and display indistinct margins because of the proliferation of immunoblasts.

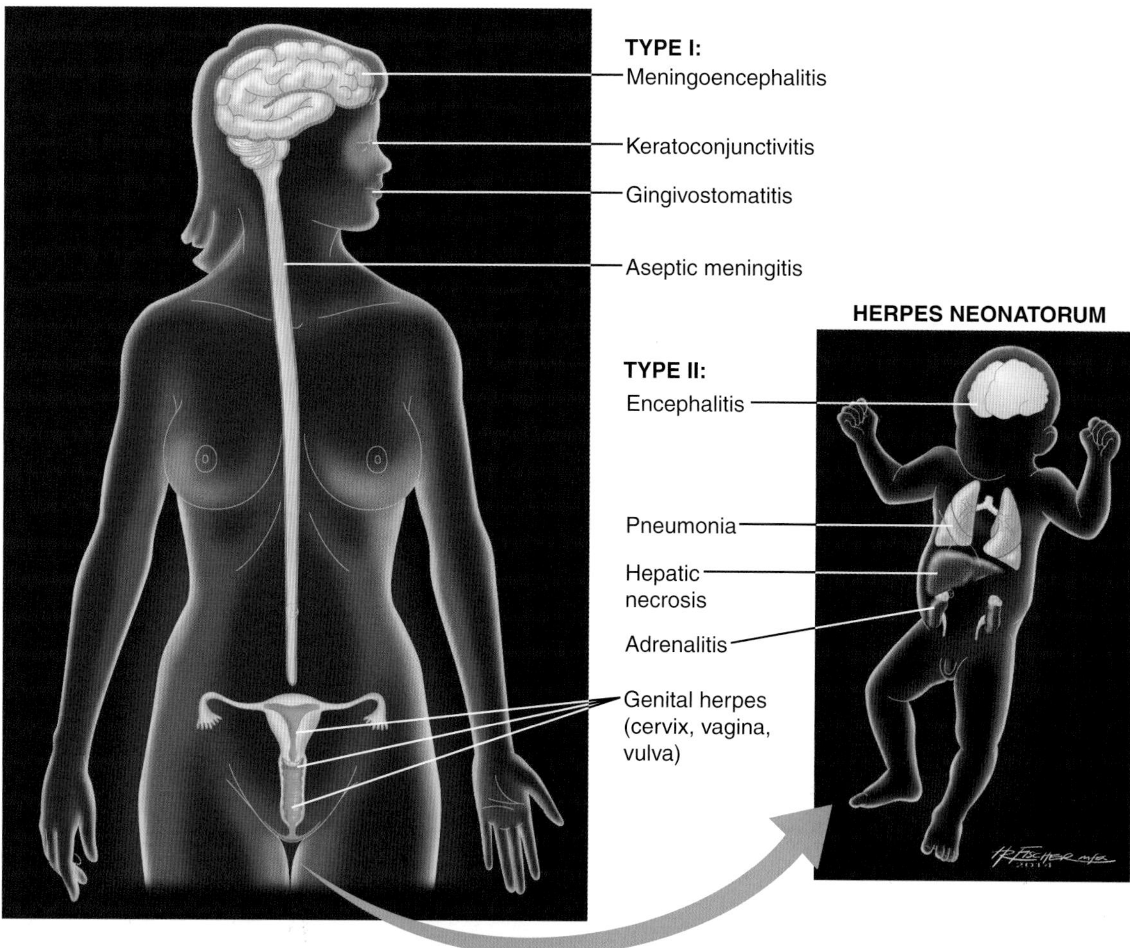

FIGURE 6-5. Herpesvirus infections. Herpes simplex virus type 1 (HSV-1) infects a nonimmune adult, causing gingivostomatitis ("fever blister" or "cold sore"), keratoconjunctivitis, meningoencephalitis, and aseptic spinal meningitis. HSV-2 infects the genitalia of a nonimmune adult, involving the cervix, vagina, and vulva. HSV-2 infects the fetus as it passes through the birth canal of an infected mother. The infant's lack of a mature immune system results in disseminated infection with HSV-1. The infection is often fatal, involving lung, liver, adrenal glands, and central nervous system.

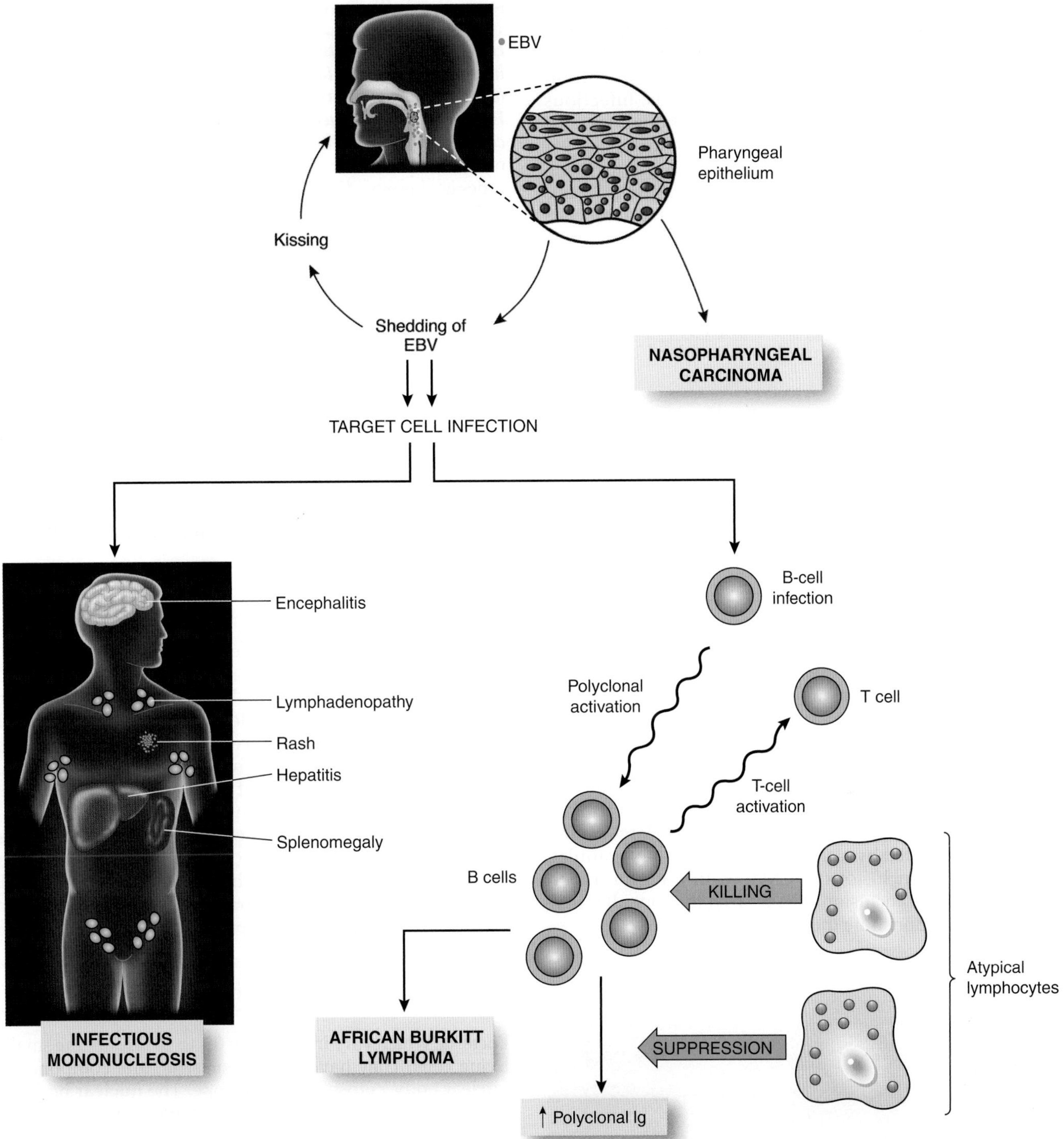

FIGURE 6-6. Role of Epstein–Barr virus (EBV) in infectious mononucleosis, nasopharyngeal carcinoma, and Burkitt lymphoma. EBV invades and replicates within the salivary glands or pharyngeal epithelium and is shed into the saliva and respiratory secretions. In some people, the virus transforms pharyngeal epithelial cells, leading to nasopharyngeal carcinoma. In persons who are not immune from childhood exposure, EBV causes infectious mononucleosis. EBV infects B lymphocytes, which undergo polyclonal activation. These B cells stimulate the production of atypical lymphocytes, which kill virally infected B cells and suppress the production of immunoglobulins. Some infected B cells are transformed into immature malignant lymphocytes of Burkitt lymphoma. Ig, immunoglobulin.

EBV is a polyclonal activator of B cells. In turn, activated B cells stimulate the proliferation of specific killer T lymphocytes and suppressor T cells. The former destroy virally infected B cells, whereas suppressor cells inhibit the production of immunoglobulins by B cells. Infectious mononucleosis is characterized by lymphocytosis and **atypical lymphocytes**, which are activated T cells that exhibit lobulated, eccentric nuclei and vacuolated cytoplasm. Lymph nodes contain occasional large hyperchromatic cells with polylobular nuclei that resemble Reed–Sternberg cells of Hodgkin disease. In fact, lymph node histology may be difficult to distinguish from that of Hodgkin disease or other lymphomas (see Chapter 18). Patients with infectious mononucleosis develop a specific **heterophile antibody**—an immunoglobulin detected by its affinity for sheep erythrocytes, whose presence is used as a standard diagnostic test for the disease.

Cytomegalovirus

CMV is a congenital and opportunistic pathogen that usually produces asymptomatic infection. However, the fetus (see Chapter 5) and immunocompromised patients are particularly vulnerable to its destructive effects. CMV infects various human cells, including epithelial cells, lymphocytes, and monocytes, and establishes latency in white blood cells. Normal immune responses rapidly control the infection. However, virus is shed periodically in body secretions. Like other herpesviruses, CMV may remain latent for life. Fetal CMV disease most commonly involves the brain, inner ears, eyes, liver, and bone marrow. Severely affected fetuses may have microcephaly, hydrocephalus, cerebral calcifications, hepatosplenomegaly, and jaundice. Microscopically lesions of fetal CMV disease show cellular necrosis and a characteristic cytopathic effect, consisting of marked cellular and nuclear enlargement, with nuclear and cytoplasmic inclusions. The giant nucleus, which is usually solitary, contains a large central inclusion surrounded by a clear zone. The smaller, granular, intracytoplasmic inclusions of CMV occur after formation of the intranuclear inclusion (Fig. 6-7), so that not all CMV-infected cells demonstrate them.

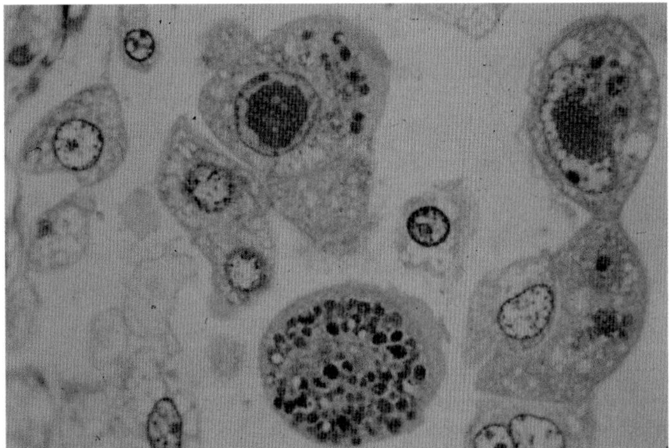

FIGURE 6-7. Cytomegalovirus (CMV) pneumonitis. Two type II pneumocytes display enlarged nuclei containing solitary CMV inclusions surrounded by a clear zone. The cell at the *bottom* shows numerous intracytoplasmic CMV inclusions.

Human Papillomaviruses

HPVs elicit proliferative lesions of squamous epithelium, including common warts, flat warts, plantar warts, anogenital warts (condyloma acuminatum), and laryngeal papillomatosis. Some HPV serotypes produce squamous cell dysplasias and squamous cell carcinomas of the genital tract and oropharynx. HPVs are nonenveloped, double-stranded DNA viruses. Over 100 HPV types are known, different ones causing different lesions. Thus, HPV types 1, 2, and 4 produce common warts and plantar warts. Types 6, 10, 11, and 40 through 45 lead to anogenital warts. Types 16, 18, and 31 are associated with squamous carcinomas of the female genital tract (see Chapters 4 and 16).

HPV infection begins with viral inoculation into a stratified squamous epithelium, where the virus enters the nuclei of basal cells. Infection stimulates proliferation of the squamous epithelium, producing the various HPV-associated lesions. The rapidly growing squamous epithelium replicates innumerable progeny viruses, which are shed in the degenerating superficial cells. HPV infections produce lesions, which vary in appearance and biologic behavior. Most show thickening of affected epithelium. Some HPV-infected cells display characteristic **koilocytosis**, with large squamous cells that contain shrunken nuclei enveloped in large cytoplasmic vacuoles (koilocytes).

PRIONS

Prions are essentially misfolded proteins that aggregate in the CNS and cause progressive neurodegeneration. The prion protein (PrP) exists in a normal isoform and in a pathogenic form. The latter is transmissible and can be considered as infectious in limited circumstances. Of particular importance is the uncommon persistence of these infectious agents. Normal methods of sterilization do not inactivate them, so they may be transmitted via surgical instruments or electrodes. All prion diseases feature spongiform encephalopathy. Diseases associated with prions include Kuru, sporadic, familial, and new variant Creutzfeldt—Jackob disease (nvCJD), fatal familial insomnia, and Gerstmann–Sträussler–Scheinker syndrome (for additional detail, see Chapter 24).

BACTERIAL INFECTIONS

Bacteria, which vary in size from 0.1 to 10 µm, are the smallest living cells. They have three basic structural components: a nuclear body, cytosol, and envelope. The **nuclear body** consists of a single, coiled, circular molecule of double-stranded DNA, with associated RNA and proteins. It is not separated from the cytoplasm by a special membrane, a feature that distinguishes bacteria, as prokaryotes, from eukaryotes. The **cytosol** is densely packed with ribosomes, proteins, and carbohydrates and lacks the structured organelles, such as mitochondria and Golgi apparatus, of eukaryotic cells. The **bacterial envelope** is a permeability barrier and is also actively involved in transport, protein synthesis, energy generation, DNA synthesis, and cell division.

Many bacterial diseases are caused by organisms that normally inhabit the human body. The gastrointestinal tract, upper respiratory tract, skin, and vagina are all home to diverse bacteria. These microorganisms are normally commensal and cause no harm. However, if they gain access to usually sterile sites, or if host defenses are impaired, they can produce extensive destruction. *Staphylococcus aureus, Streptococcus pneumoniae*, and *Escherichia coli* are normal flora that are also major human pathogens.

Bacteria are classified by the structural features of their envelope. The simplest envelope, which is possessed by mycoplasmas, consists of only a phospholipid–protein bilayer membrane. Most bacteria, however, have a rigid cell wall that surrounds the cell membrane. Two types of bacterial cell walls are identified by their Gram-stain properties. **Gram-positive bacteria** have a cell wall that contains teichoic acids and a thick peptidoglycan layer. **Gram-negative bacteria** have outer membranes that enclose a lipopolysaccharide component, known as endotoxin, which is a potent mediator of the shock that complicates infections with these organisms.

The lipopolysaccharide (LPS), or endotoxin, in the outer membranes of gram-negative bacteria activates complement, coagulation, fibrinolysis, and bradykinin systems (see Chapter 2). It also induces release of primary inflammatory mediators, including TNF, IL-1, and various colony-stimulating factors. Endotoxin may cause shock, complement depletion, and disseminated intravascular coagulation.

In contrast to endotoxins, which are part of the bacterial structure, many bacteria secrete toxins (exotoxins) that damage human cells, either at the site of bacterial growth or at distant sites. Exotoxins are often named for the site or mechanism of their activity. Thus, those that act on the nervous system are neurotoxins; those that affect intestinal cells are enterotoxins. Those that kill target cells, such as diphtheria toxin or some of the *Clostridium perfringens* toxins, are known as cytotoxins. Others may disturb normal functions of their target cells and damage or kill them. Examples include the diarrheogenic toxin of *Vibrio cholerae* or the neurotoxin of *Clostridium botulinum*. *C. perfringens* produces over 20 highly diverse toxins.

Many bacteria damage tissues by eliciting inflammatory or immune responses. The capsule of *S. pneumoniae* protects it from phagocytosis, while activating the host's inflammatory response. Within the lung, the encapsulated organism causes exudation of fluid and cells that fill alveoli. This inflammation impairs breathing but does not, at least initially, limit the organism's proliferation. *Treponema pallidum*, the spirochete that causes syphilis, persists in the body for years and evokes inflammatory and immune responses that continuously damage host tissues.

Many common bacterial infections (e.g., *S. aureus* skin infections) are characterized by purulent exudates, but tissue responses to bacteria are highly variable. In some cases, such as cholera, botulism, and tetanus, there is no inflammatory response at critical sites of cellular injury. Other bacterial infections, including syphilis and Lyme disease, lead to a predominantly lymphocytic and plasma cellular response. Still others (e.g., brucellosis) are characterized by granuloma formation.

Pyogenic Gram-Positive Cocci

Staphylococcus aureus

S. aureus is a gram-positive coccus that normally resides on the skin and is readily inoculated into deeper tissues. ***It is the most common cause of suppurative infections of the skin, joints, and bones and is a leading cause of infective endocarditis.*** *S. aureus* spreads by direct contact with colonized surfaces or persons. Many *S. aureus* infections begin as localized infections of skin and skin appendages, causing cellulitis and abscesses. The organism, equipped with destructive enzymes and toxins, sometimes invades beyond the initial site, spreading by blood or lymphatics to almost any location in the body. ***Bones, joints, and heart valves are the most common sites of metastatic S. aureus infections.*** *The organism* also causes several distinct diseases by elaborating toxins that are carried to distant sites.

For example, Staphylococcal food poisoning is caused by preformed toxin present in the food at the time it is eaten. **Toxic shock syndrome toxin-1,** an exotoxin released by some Staphylococcal strains, impairs the ability of mononuclear phagocytes to clear other potentially toxic substances, such as endotoxin (for details, see Chapter 16). When *S. aureus* is introduced into a previously sterile site, infection usually produces suppuration and abscesses. These range from microscopic foci to lesions several centimeters in diameter, which are filled with pus and bacteria.

Coagulase-Negative Staphylococci

Coagulase-negative staphylococci, which are usually derived from normal flora, are the major cause of infections involving medical devices, including intravenous catheters, prosthetic heart valves, heart pacemakers, orthopedic prostheses, cerebrospinal fluid shunts, and peritoneal catheters. Coagulase-negative staphylococci readily contaminate foreign bodies, on which they proliferate slowly, inducing inflammatory responses that damage adjacent tissue. Bacteria present on an intravascular surface can spread through the bloodstream to cause metastatic infections. However, they lack the enzymes and toxins that permit *S. aureus* to cause extensive local tissue destruction. Some strains of coagulase-negative staphylococci produce a polysaccharide gel biofilm, which enhances their adherence to foreign objects and protects them from host antimicrobial defenses and from many antibiotics.

Streptococcus pyogenes (Group A Streptococcus)

Streptococcus pyogenes, also known as Group A streptococcus, is one of the most common human pathogens, causing diseases of diverse organ systems, from acute self-limited pharyngitis to major illnesses such as rheumatic fever (Fig. 6-8). Suppurative diseases caused by *S. pyogenes* occur at sites of bacterial invasion and consequent tissue necrosis and usually involve acute inflammatory responses. Such diseases include pharyngitis, impetigo, cellulitis, myositis, pneumonia, and puerperal sepsis. Nonsuppurative diseases caused by *S. pyogenes* are remote from the site of bacterial invasion and include rheumatic fever (discussed in Chapter 9) and acute poststreptococcal glomerulonephritis (see Chapter 14). These two diseases are characterized by (1) affected organs far from the sites of streptococcal invasion, (2) a time delay after the acute infection, and (3) immune reactions. *S. pyogenes* also produces several exotoxins, including erythrogenic toxins and cytolytic toxins **(streptolysins S and O)**. Erythrogenic toxins cause the rash of scarlet fever. Streptolysin S lyses bacterial protoplasts (L forms) and probably destroys neutrophils after they ingest *S. pyogenes*.

The pathogenesis of specific forms of streptococcal disease is as follows:

- **Streptococcal Pharyngitis:** The bacterium attaches to epithelial cells by binding to fibronectin on their surfaces. It produces hemolysins, DNAase, hyaluronidase, and streptokinase, which allow it to damage and invade human tissues.

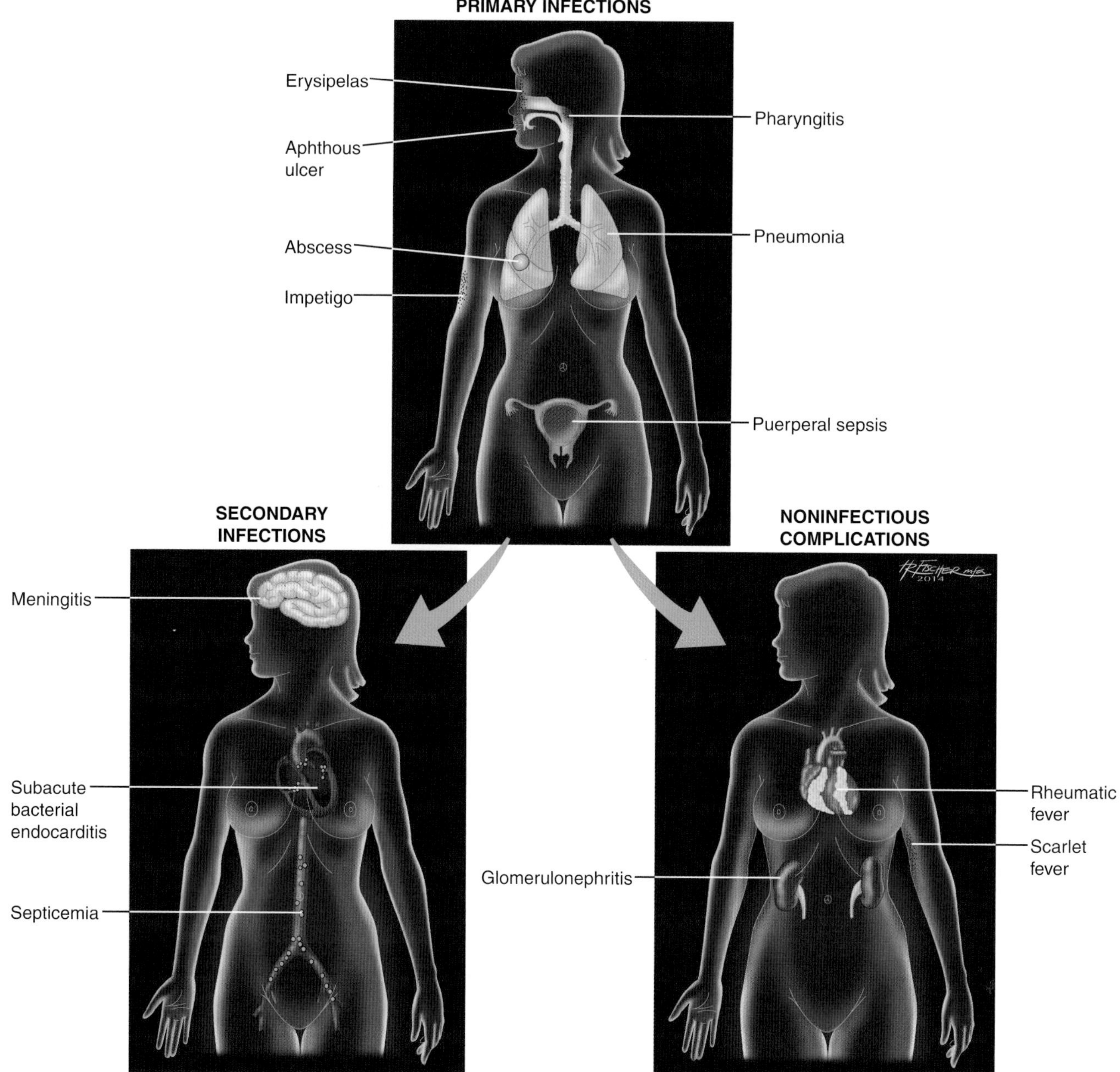

FIGURE 6-8. **Streptococcal diseases.**

A bacterial cell wall component, **M protein**, protrudes from cell walls of virulent strains and prevents complement deposition, thereby protecting bacteria from phagocytosis. The invading organism elicits acute inflammation, often producing an exudate of neutrophils in the tonsillar fossae. Scarlet fever **(scarlatina)** describes a punctate red rash on the skin and mucous membranes, which is seen with some infections.

- **Erysipelas:** *S. pyogenes* infection may result in a diffuse, edematous, acute inflammatory reaction in the epidermis and dermis, which extends into subcutaneous tissues. It usually begins on the face and spreads rapidly. The inflammatory infiltrate is principally composed of neutrophils and is most intense around vessels and adnexae of the skin. Cutaneous microabscesses and small foci of necrosis are common.
- **Impetigo (pyoderma):** Distinct strains of *S. pyogenes* (or sometimes *S. aureus*) result in a localized, intraepidermal infection. The disease spreads from person to person by direct contact and most commonly affects children aged 2 to 5 years. Infection begins with skin colonization with the causative organism, which is inoculated into the skin by trauma or an insect bite. An intraepidermal pustule, forms, ruptures, and leaks a purulent exudate (Fig. 6-9). **Streptococcal cellulitis** results when infection spreads to loose connective tissue, frequently on the extremities in the context of impaired lymphatic drainage.

Streptococcus pneumoniae (Pneumococcus)

S. pneumoniae, also called **pneumococcus**, causes pyogenic infections, primarily of the lungs **(pneumonia)**, middle ear

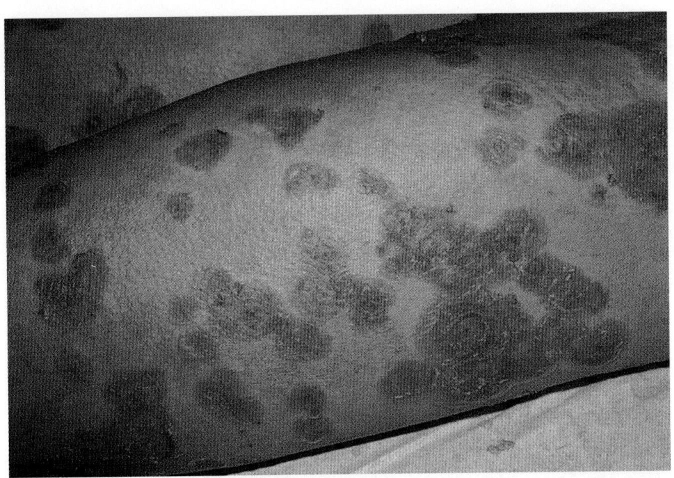

FIGURE 6-9. **Streptococcal impetigo.** The lower extremities exhibit numerous erythematous papules, with central ulceration and the formation of crusts.

(otitis media), sinuses (**sinusitis**), and meninges **(meningitis). It is *one of the most common human bacterial pathogens.*** The organism is an aerobic, gram-positive diplococcus. Most strains that cause clinical disease have a capsule. The organisms are commensal in the oropharynx, and virtually everyone has been colonized at some time.

Pneumococcal disease begins when the bacterium gains access to sterile sites, usually in the oropharynx. Pneumococcal sinusitis and otitis media are usually preceded by a viral illness, which injures the protective ciliated epithelium and fills affected air spaces with nutrient-rich fluid, where pneumococci thrive. These localized infections can spread to the adjacent meninges. Likewise, damage to the defense mechanisms of the lower respiratory tract (i.e., the mucociliary blanket and cough response) by viral respiratory illnesses, smoking, and alcoholism allows *S. pneumoniae* to reach the alveoli and results in pneumococcal pneumonia.

In the alveoli, the bacteria elicit an acute inflammatory response, multiply to fill alveoli, and spread to other alveoli. Their polysaccharide capsule prevents the formation of the opsonin C3b, thereby allowing the organisms to spread unimpeded by phagocytes. As a result, alveoli fill with proteinaceous fluid, neutrophils, and bacteria. *S. pneumoniae* then spreads rapidly to involve an entire lobe or several lobes of the lung (lobar pneumonia).

Group B Streptococci

Group B streptococci are gram-positive bacteria that cause several thousand neonatal infections in the United States each year, although they are part of the normal vaginal flora in 10% to 30% of women. Most babies born to colonized women acquire the organisms as they pass through the birth canal. Particular risk factors associated with infection include premature delivery and low levels of maternally derived IgG antibodies against the organism. The infant's lack of a functional reserve for granulocyte production also plays a role. Group B streptococcal infection may be limited to the lungs or CNS or be widely disseminated. The involved tissues show a pyogenic response, often with large numbers of gram-positive cocci.

Bacterial Infections of Childhood

Diphtheria

Infection with Corynebacterium diphtheriae—an aerobic, gram-positive rod—may lead to cardiac and neurologic disturbances because of exotoxin production.

Humans are the only known reservoir for *C. diphtheriae*, and most people are asymptomatic carriers. The organism spreads from person to person in respiratory droplets or oral secretions, which than enter the pharynx and proliferate, often on the tonsils. Diphtheria exotoxin is a protein composed of two peptide chains held together by a disulfide bond, which is encoded by a lysogenic β-bacteriophage. The B subunit binds glycolipid receptors on target cells, and the A subunit acts within the cytoplasm on elongation factor 2 to interrupt protein synthesis. The heart, nerves, and kidneys are most susceptible to damage. The toxin is one of the most potent known: one molecule can kill a cell.

The characteristic lesions of diphtheria are thick, gray, leathery pseudomembranes composed of sloughed epithelium, necrotic debris, neutrophils, fibrin, and bacteria. The material lines affected respiratory passages (Fig. 6-10). The epithelial surface beneath the membranes is denuded, and the submucosa is acutely inflamed and hemorrhagic. The inflammation often causes swelling in surrounding soft tissues, which can be severe enough to cause respiratory compromise. When the heart is affected, the myocardium displays fat droplets in the myocytes and focal necrosis. Diphtheria is now distinctly uncommon because of early immunization.

Pertussis (Whooping Cough)

Bordetella pertussis, a small gram-negative coccobacillus, is highly contagious, spreading from person to person by

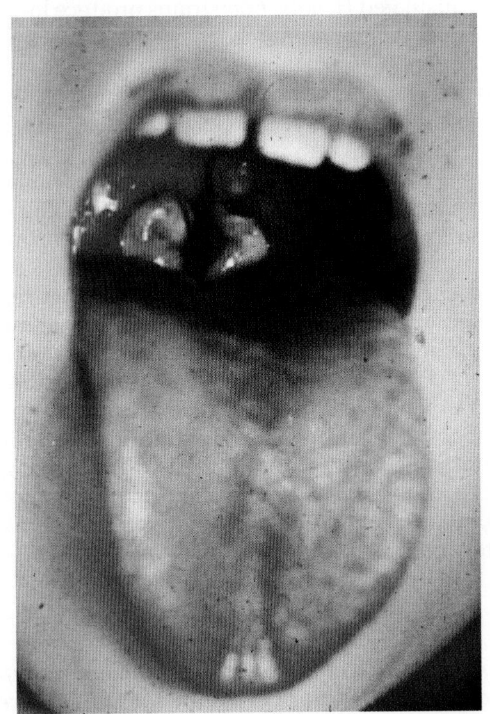

FIGURE 6-10. **Child with characteristic diphtheric membrane in the oropharynx.**

respiratory aerosols. Humans are the only reservoir of infection. In susceptible populations, pertussis is primarily a disease of children under 5 years although it is rare in developed countries owing to infantile immunization. *B. pertussis* initiates infection by attaching to the cilia of respiratory epithelial cells. The organism then elaborates a cytotoxin that kills ciliated cells. Progressive destruction of ciliated respiratory epithelium and the ensuing inflammatory response cause local respiratory symptoms. Several other toxins include a "pertussis toxin," which causes a characteristic lymphocytosis, and a toxin that blocks bacterial phagocytosis.

B. pertussis causes an extensive tracheobronchitis, with necrosis of ciliated respiratory epithelium and an acute inflammatory response. With the loss of the protective mucociliary blanket, there is increased risk of pneumonia from aspirated oral bacteria. Coughing paroxysms followed by a long, high-pitched inspiration (the "whoop," which gives the disease its name) and vomiting make aspiration likely. Secondary bacterial pneumonia is the most common cause of death.

Haemophilus influenzae

Haemophilus influenzae is a major pediatric pathogen, causing infections involving the middle ear, sinuses, facial skin, epiglottis, lungs, and joints. It is a leading cause of bacterial meningitis worldwide. The bacteria is an aerobic, gram-negative coccobacillus whose encapsulated strains cause over 95% of the invasive infections. *H. influenzae* only infects humans and spreads from person to person, mainly in respiratory droplets and secretions. It resides in the human nasopharynx of 20% to 50% of healthy adults. However, only 3% to 5% are encapsulated and elaborate an IgA protease, which facilitates local survival in the respiratory tract.

The incidence of serious disease peaks at 6 to 18 months of age, when maternally acquired immunity wanes prior to the acquisition of native immunity.

Unencapsulated *H. influenzae* strains produce local disease by spreading to sterile locations, such as the sinuses or middle ear, most often in association with a viral upper respiratory tract illness. The unencapsulated organisms proliferate and elicit a transient acute inflammatory response, which injures only local tissue. By contrast, the capsular polysaccharide of *H. influenzae* type B allows the bacteria to evade phagocytosis and invade tissue, promoting bacteremic infections, which may result in epiglottitis, facial cellulitis, septic arthritis, and meningitis.

H. influenzae elicits strong acute inflammatory responses. *H. influenzae* meningitis like other acute bacterial meningitides, has a predominantly acute inflammatory leptomeningeal infiltrate, sometimes involving the subarachnoid space. In pneumonia, alveoli become filled with neutrophils and macrophages, containing bacilli and fibrin. The bronchiolar epithelium is necrotic and infiltrated by macrophages. Epiglottitis, characterized by swelling and acute inflammation of the epiglottis, aryepiglottic fold, and pyriform sinuses, may completely obstruct the upper airway.

Neisseria meningitides (Meningococcus)

Meningococcus produces disseminated blood-borne infections, often accompanied by shock and profound disturbances in coagulation (Fig. 6-11). The aerobic organism appears as paired, bean-shaped, gram-negative cocci and spreads from person to person, primarily via respiratory droplets. Some 5% to 15% of the population carries meningococcus as commensals in the nasopharynx and develop protective antibodies specific to their colonizing strain. Meningococcal diseases appear as sporadic cases, clusters of cases, and epidemics. Most infections in industrialized countries are sporadic and affect children under the age of 5 years. Epidemic disease occurs mostly in crowded quarters, such as among military recruits in barracks.

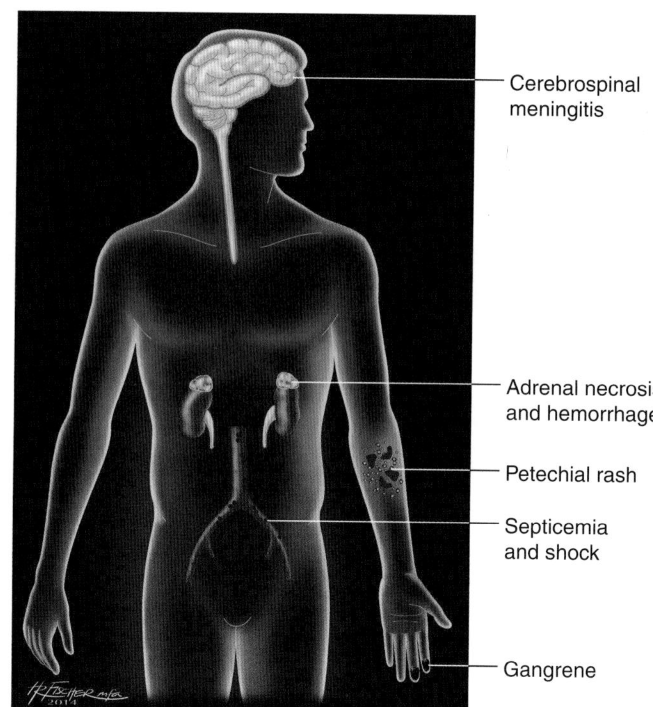

FIGURE 6-11. Meningococcemia. Meningococcal infections have a variety of clinical manifestations, including meningitis, septicemia, shock, and associated complications.

Upon colonizing the upper respiratory tract, *Neisseria meningitidis* attaches to nonciliated respiratory epithelium by means of its pili. Most exposed people then develop protective bactericidal antibodies and may become carriers. If the organism spreads to the bloodstream before protective immunity develops, it can proliferate rapidly and cause fulminant meningococcal disease. Many of the systemic effects of meningococcal disease are caused by the lipopolysaccharide endotoxin, which promotes an increase in TNF production and activation of complement and coagulation cascades. Disseminated intravascular coagulation, fibrinolysis, and shock follow.

If disease is confined to the CNS, the leptomeninges and subarachnoid space are infiltrated with neutrophils, and the underlying brain parenchyma is swollen and congested. When disseminated, meningococcal septicemia is characterized by diffuse damage to the endothelium of small blood vessels, with widespread petechiae and purpura in the skin and viscera. Rarely (4% of cases), vasculitis and thrombosis produce hemorrhagic necrosis of both adrenals, termed **Waterhouse–Friderichsen syndrome**.

Sexually Transmitted Bacterial Diseases

Details of important sexually transmitted bacterial diseases, including gonorrhea, granuloma inguinale, and chancroid, may be found in Chapter 16.

Enteropathogenic Bacterial Infections

Escherichia coli

***E. coli* is among the most frequent and important human bacterial pathogens, causing over 90% of all urinary tract infections and many cases of diarrheal illness worldwide.** It is also a major opportunistic pathogen, frequently causing pneumonia and sepsis in immunocompromised hosts, and meningitis and sepsis in newborns.

E. coli comprises a group of antigenically and biologically diverse, aerobic (facultatively anaerobic), gram-negative bacteria. Most strains are intestinal commensals. However, the bacteria may be aggressive when they gain access to usually sterile body sites, such as the urinary tract, meninges, or peritoneum. Strains of *E. coli* that produce diarrhea possess specialized virulence properties, usually plasmid borne, that cause intestinal disease.

E. coli is also the most common cause of enteric gram-negative sepsis. The topic of sepsis is discussed in Chapter 2.

Escherichia coli Diarrhea

There are four distinct strains of *E. coli* that cause diarrhea:

- **ENTEROTOXIGENIC *E. coli*** gives rise to diarrhea in poor tropical areas and probably causes most "traveler's diarrhea." It is acquired from contaminated water and food. Enterotoxigenic strains produce diarrhea by adhering to the intestinal mucosa and elaborating one of several enterotoxins that cause secretory dysfunction of the small bowel. One of the enterotoxins is similar to cholera toxin, and another acts on guanylyl cyclase. Enterotoxigenic *E. coli* produces no distinctive macroscopic or light-microscopic alterations in the intestine.
- **ENTEROPATHOGENIC *E. coli*** is responsible for diarrheal illness in poor tropical areas, especially in infants and young children. The organism is not invasive and causes disease by adhering to and deforming the microvilli of the intestinal epithelial cells Enteropathogenic *E. coli* produces diarrhea, vomiting, fever, and malaise and remains a problem in underdeveloped areas.
- **ENTEROHEMORRHAGIC *E. coli*** (serotype 0157:H7) causes a bloody diarrhea, which may be followed by the **hemolytic–uremic syndrome** (see Chapter 8). The source of infection is usually ingestion of contaminated meat or milk. Bacteria adhere to colonic mucosa and elaborate an enterotoxin (verotoxin), virtually identical to Shiga toxin (see below) that destroys the epithelial cells.
- **ENTEROINVASIVE *E. coli*** causes foodborne dysentery, which is clinically and pathologically indistinguishable from that caused by *Shigella*, with which it shares extensive DNA and biochemical similarity. It invades and destroys mucosal cells of the distal ileum and colon. As in shigellosis, the mucosa of the distal ileum and colon is acutely inflamed and focally eroded, and is sometimes covered by an inflammatory pseudomembrane.

Urinary Tract Infections

These infections occur in more than 10% of the human population, often repeatedly and are most common in sexually active women and in people of both sexes who have abnormalities of the urinary tract. The bacteria are usually flora derived from fecal contamination of the perineum and periurethral areas, which gain access to the sterile urinary tract by ascending from the distal urethra. Women are more prone to urinary tract infections because their shorter urethra is a less effective mechanical barrier. Abnormalities of the urinary tract and catheterization account for most urinary tract infections in men. Uropathogenic *E. coli* organisms have specialized adherence factors (Gal-Gal) on the pili, which enable them to bind sugar residues on the uroepithelium.

Infections initially produce an acute inflammatory infiltrate, usually in the bladder mucosa, which spills into the urine. The blood vessels of the submucosa are dilated and congested. Chronic infections exhibit an inflammatory infiltrate of neutrophils and mononuclear cells. Infection may ascend to involve the kidney and result in chronic pyelonephritis and renal failure (see Chapter 14).

Salmonella Enterocolitis and Typhoid Fever

The bacterial genus *Salmonella* contains over 1,500 biochemically and genetically related gram-negative rods, which cause *Salmonella* enterocolitis and typhoid fever.

Salmonella Enterocolitis (*Salmonella* Food Poisoning)

Salmonella enterocolitis is an acute, self-limited (1 to 3 days) gastrointestinal illness acquired by eating food containing nontyphoidal *Salmonella* strains. These bacteria infect diverse animal species and contaminate foodstuffs derived from infected animals. The organism can spread from person to person by the fecal–oral route, particularly among small children. *Salmonella* proliferates in the small intestine and invades enterocytes in the distal small bowel and colon. The nontyphoidal *Salmonella* species elaborate several toxins that injure intestinal cells. The mucosa of the ileum and colon is acutely inflamed and sometimes superficially ulcerated.

Typhoid Fever

Typhoid fever is an acute systemic illness caused by infection with *Salmonella typhi*. **Paratyphoid fever** is a similar but milder disease that results from infection with *Salmonella paratyphi*. Humans are the only natural reservoir, and disease is acquired from infected patients or chronic carriers. The disease is spread primarily by ingestion of contaminated water and food, especially dairy products, and shellfish.

S. typhi attaches to and invades the small bowel mucosa without causing clinical enterocolitis. Invasion tends to be most prominent in the ileum in areas overlying Peyer patches. The organisms are engulfed by macrophages, after which they block the respiratory burst of the phagocytes and multiply within these cells. Infected cells spread first to regional lymph nodes, then throughout the body via the lymphatics and bloodstream, affecting mononuclear macrophages in lymph nodes, bone marrow, liver, and spleen (Fig. 6-12). Infection of macrophages stimulates IL-1 and TNF production, thereby causing the prolonged fever, malaise, and wasting characteristic of typhoid fever.

The earliest pathologic change in typhoid fever is degeneration of the intestinal epithelium brush border. As bacteria invade, Peyer patches become hypertrophic, which can progress to capillary thrombosis and necrosis of overlying mucosa with the characteristic ulcers oriented along the long axis of the bowel (Fig. 6-13). These ulcers frequently bleed and occasionally perforate, causing infectious peritonitis. Systemic dissemination of the organisms leads to focal granulomas in

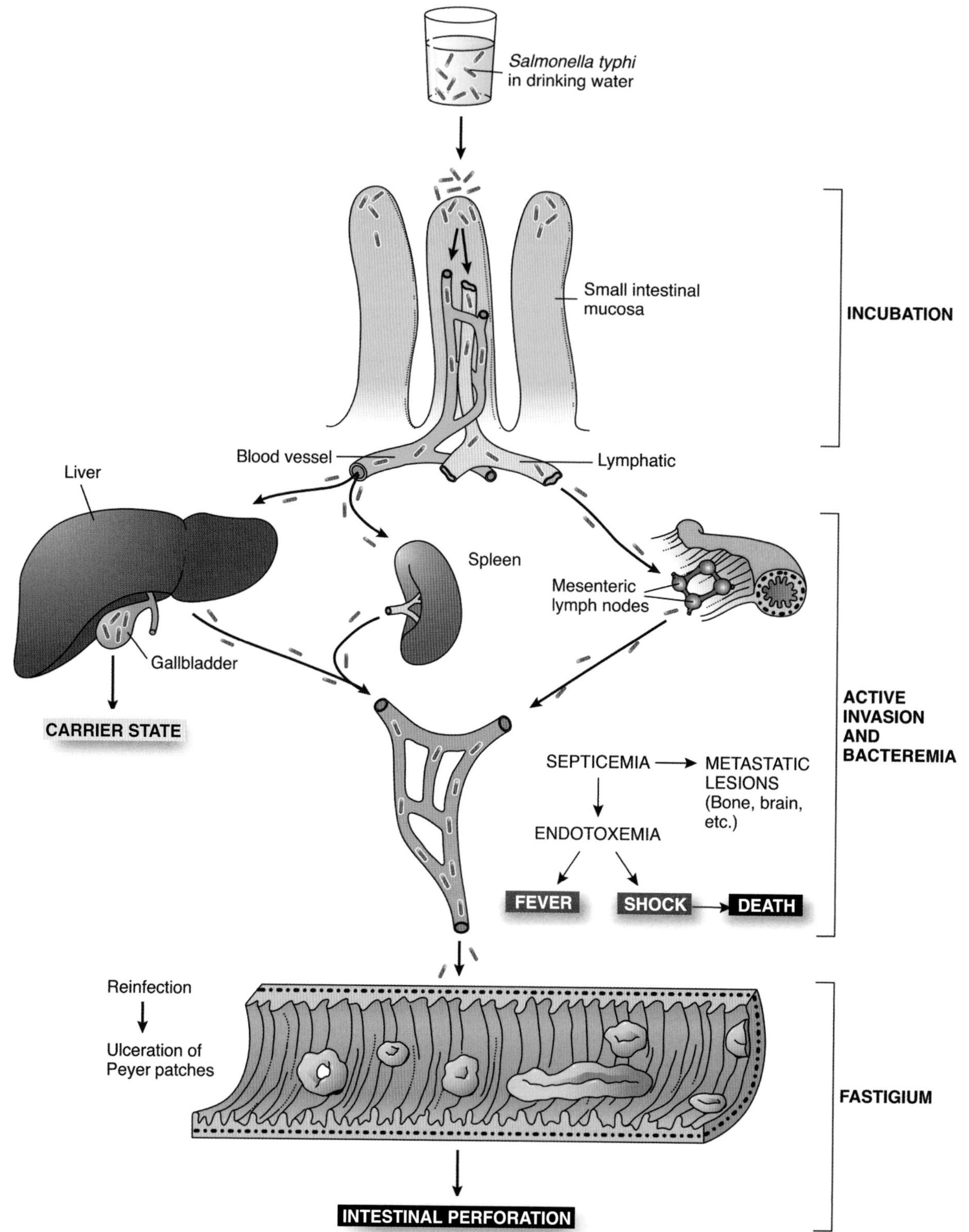

FIGURE 6-12. Stages of typhoid fever. Incubation (10 to 14 days). Water or food contaminated with *Salmonella typhi* is ingested. Bacilli attach to the villi in the small intestine, invade the mucosa, and pass to the intestinal lymphoid follicles and draining mesenteric lymph nodes. The organisms proliferate further within mononuclear phagocytic cells of the lymphoid follicles, lymph nodes, liver, and spleen. Bacilli are sequestered intracellularly in the intestinal and mesenteric lymphatic system. **Active invasion/bacteremia** (1 week). Organisms are released and produce a transient bacteremia. The intestinal mucosa becomes enlarged and necrotic, forming characteristic mucosal lesions. The intestinal lymphoid tissues become hyperplastic and contain "typhoid nodules"—aggregates of macrophages ("typhoid cells") that phagocytose bacteria, erythrocytes, and degenerated lymphocytes. Bacilli proliferate in several organs, reappear in the intestine, are excreted in stool, and may invade through the intestinal wall. **Fastigium** (1 week). Dying bacilli release endotoxins that cause systemic toxemia. **Lysis** (1 week). Necrotic intestinal mucosa sloughs, producing ulcers, which hemorrhage or perforate into the peritoneal cavity.

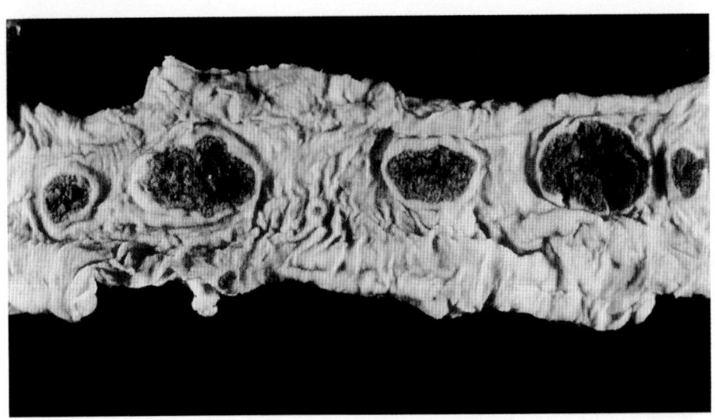

FIGURE 6-13. Ulcers of the terminal ileum in fatal typhoid fever. The ulcers have a longitudinal orientation because they are located over hyperplastic and necrotic Peyer patches.

the liver, spleen, and other organs. These are termed **typhoid nodules** and are composed of aggregates of macrophages ("typhoid cells") containing ingested bacteria, erythrocytes, and degenerated lymphocytes.

Shigellosis

This disease is caused by species of *Shigella* with *Shigella dysenteriae* being the most virulent. Shigellosis is a self-limited disease that typically presents with abdominal pain and bloody, mucoid stools. The organisms are spread from person to person by the fecal–oral route. Because they have no animal reservoir and do not survive well outside the stool, ingestion of fecally contaminated food or water or contact with a contaminated surface is the usual route of infection.

Shigellae are among the most virulent enteropathogens, with as few as 10 to 100 ingested organisms producing disease. The agent proliferates rapidly in the small bowel and attaches to enterocytes, where it is endocytosed and replicated within the cytoplasm. Replicating shigellae kill infected cells and then spread to adjacent cells. Shigellae also produce **Shiga toxin**, similar to the verotoxin of *E. coli* O157:H7. This toxin interferes with 60S ribosomal subunits and inhibits protein synthesis, thereby causing watery diarrhea by interfering with fluid absorption in the colon. Although shigellae extensively damage the epithelium of the ileum and colon, they rarely invade beyond the intestinal lamina propria, so bacteremia is uncommon. The distal colon is almost always affected, with the mucosa becoming edematous, acutely inflamed, and focally eroded. Ulcers appear first on the edges of mucosal folds, perpendicular to the long axis of the colon. A patchy inflammatory pseudomembrane, composed of neutrophils, fibrin, and necrotic epithelium, is commonly found on the most severely affected areas. Regeneration of infected colonic epithelium occurs rapidly, and healing is usually complete within 10 to 14 days.

Cholera

Cholera is a severe diarrheal illness caused by the enterotoxin of V. cholerae, an aerobic, curved gram-negative rod. The organism proliferates in the lumen of the small intestine and causes profuse watery diarrhea, rapid dehydration, and (if fluids are not restored) shock and death within 24 hours of the onset of symptoms.

Cholera is acquired by ingesting *V. cholerae*, mainly in contaminated food or water. Epidemics spread readily in areas where human feces pollute the water supply. Shellfish and plankton may serve as a natural reservoir for the organism.

Bacteria that survive passage through the stomach thrive and multiply in the mucous layer of the small bowel. They do not invade the mucosa but cause diarrhea by elaborating a potent exotoxin, **cholera toxin**, which is composed of A and B subunits. The latter binds to GM_1 ganglioside in the enterocyte cell membrane. The A subunit then enters the cell, where it activates adenylyl cyclase to produce a rise in cell cyclic adenosine 3′,5′-monophosphate (cAMP) content. The consequence is massive secretion of sodium and water by the enterocyte into the intestinal lumen (Fig. 6-14). Most fluid secretion occurs in the small bowel, where there is a net loss of water and electrolytes. *V. cholerae* causes little visible alteration in the affected intestine, which appears grossly normal or only slightly hyperemic. The intestinal epithelium remains intact but depleted of mucus.

Campylobacter jejuni

Campylobacter jejuni is a curved gram-negative rod, morphologically similar to the vibrios, which causes an acute, self-limited, inflammatory diarrheal illness.

Infection is acquired through contaminated food or water. The bacteria inhabit the gastrointestinal tracts of many animal species, forming a significant reservoir for infection that is often acquired from consumption of raw milk and inadequately cooked poultry and meat. *C. jejuni* can also spread from person to person by the fecal–oral route.

Ingested *C. jejuni* that survives gastric acidity multiplies in the alkaline environment of the upper small intestine. The agent elaborates several toxic proteins, and infection results in a superficial enterocolitis, primarily involving the terminal ileum and colon, with focal necrosis of intestinal epithelium and acute inflammation. In severe cases, infection progresses to small ulcers and patchy inflammatory exudates (pseudomembranes) composed of necrotic cells, neutrophils, fibrin, and debris. Epithelial crypts in the colon often fill with neutrophils, forming the so-called crypt abscesses. These changes resolve in 7 to 14 days. Gastrointestinal infections with *C. jejuni* have been associated with Guillain–Barré syndrome.

Yersinia Infections

Yersinia enterocolitica and *Yersinia pseudotuberculosis* are gram-negative, coccoid or rod-shaped bacteria found in the feces of wild and domestic animals. *Y. pseudotuberculosis* is also often seen in domestic birds, including turkeys, ducks, geese, and canaries. *Y. enterocolitica* is more likely to be acquired from contaminated meat, and *Y. pseudotuberculosis* from contact with infected animals. *Y. enterocolitica* proliferates in the ileum and invades the mucosa, causing ulceration and necrosis of Peyer patches. It migrates by way of lymphatics to mesenteric lymph nodes. Fever, diarrhea (sometimes bloody), and abdominal pain begin 4 to 10 days after mucosal penetration. Abdominal pain in the right lower quadrant has led to an incorrect diagnosis of appendicitis. Arthralgia, arthritis, and erythema nodosum are complications. *Y. pseudotuberculosis* penetrates ileal mucosa, localizes in ileal–cecal lymph nodes, and produces abscesses and granulomas in the lymph nodes, spleen, and liver. Fever, diarrhea, and abdominal pain may also suggest appendicitis.

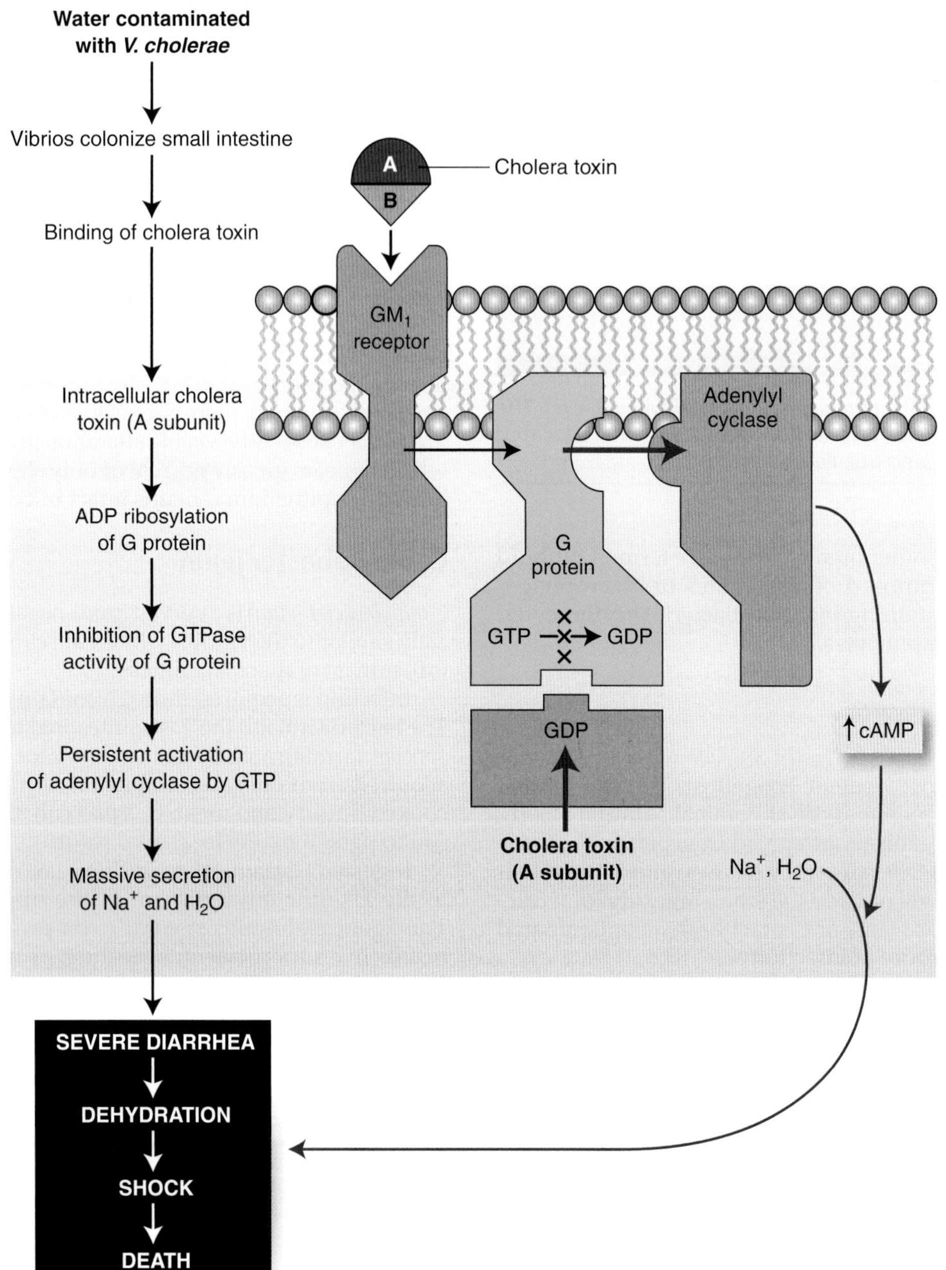

FIGURE 6-14. Cholera. Infection comes from water contaminated with *Vibrio cholerae* or food prepared with contaminated water. *Vibrios* traverse the stomach, enter the small intestine, and propagate. Although they do not invade the intestinal mucosa, *Vibrios* elaborate a potent toxin that induces a massive outpouring of water and electrolytes. Severe diarrhea ("rice water stool") leads to dehydration and hypovolemic shock. ADP, adenosine diphosphate; cAMP, cyclic adenosine 3′,5′-monophosphate; GDP, guanosine diphosphate; GM_1 ganglioside; GTP, guanosine triphosphate; Na^+, sodium ion.

Pulmonary Infections With Gram-Negative Bacteria

Klebsiella and Enterobacter

Klebsiella and *Enterobacter* species are short, encapsulated, gram-negative bacilli, which cause 10% of all hospital-acquired (nosocomial) infections, involving the lungs, urinary tract, biliary tract, and surgical wounds. Person-to-person transmission by hospital personnel is a special hazard.

Klebsiella and *Enterobacter* are inhaled and multiply in the alveolar spaces. The pulmonary parenchyma becomes consolidated, and a mucoid exudate of macrophages, fibrin, and edema fluid fills the alveoli. As the exudate accumulates, alveolar walls become compressed and then necrotic. Numerous small abscesses may coalesce and lead to cavitation. *Klebsiella* and *Enterobacter* infections are sometimes complicated by fulminating, often fatal, septicemia.

Legionella

Legionella pneumophila is a minute aerobic bacillus that has the cell wall structure of a gram-negative organism but reacts poorly with Gram stains. The bacteria are present in small numbers in natural bodies of fresh water. They survive chlorination and proliferate in devices, such as cooling towers, water heaters, humidifiers, and evaporative condensers. Infection occurs when people inhale aerosols from contaminated sources. The disease is not contagious, and the organism is not part of normal human flora.

Legionella cause two distinct diseases, namely, pneumonia and **Pontiac fever**. *Legionella* pneumonia begins when the organisms arrive in the terminal bronchioles or alveoli, where they are phagocytosed by alveolar macrophages. The bacteria replicate within phagosomes and protect themselves by blocking fusion of lysosomes with the phagosomes. The multiplying *Legionella* are released and infect freshly arriving macrophages. When immunity develops, macrophages are activated and cease to support such intracellular growth. Conditions that interfere with native respiratory defenses, such as smoking, alcoholism, and chronic lung diseases, increase the risk of developing *Legionella* pneumonia.

The disease is an acute and usually patchy bronchopneumonia but may show a lobar pattern of infiltration. Affected alveoli and bronchioles are filled with an exudate composed of proteinaceous fluid, fibrin, macrophages and neutrophils, and microabscesses. Alveolar walls become necrotic and are destroyed. Many macrophages show eccentric nuclei, pushed aside by cytoplasmic vacuoles containing *L. pneumophila*. As the pneumonia resolves, the lungs heal with little permanent damage.

Pontiac fever is a self-limited, flu-like illness associated with fever, malaise, myalgias, and headache. It differs from Legionnaires disease in that it lacks pulmonary consolidation and resolves spontaneously in 3 to 5 days.

Pseudomonas aeruginosa

This organism only infrequently infects humans, but in hospital environments, it colonizes moist environmental surfaces and is associated with pneumonia, wound infections, urinary tract disease, and sepsis in debilitated or immunosuppressed persons. The bacterium is an aerobic, gram-negative rod that requires moisture and only minimal nutrients. *Pseudomonas aeruginosa* produces a proteoglycan that surrounds and protects the bacteria from mucociliary action, complement, and phagocytes. It also elaborates an array of proteins that allow it to attach to, and invade injured epithelial cells, which have exposed surface molecules that serve as binding sites for the pili of the bacteria. The organism releases extracellular enzymes—including an elastase, an alkaline protease, and a cytotoxin—which facilitate tissue invasion and necrosis and the distinctive ability to invade blood vessel walls. The agent also causes systemic pathologic effects through endotoxin and several systemically active exotoxins.

Pseudomonas infection produces an acute inflammatory response. The bacterium often invades small arteries and veins, causing thrombosis and hemorrhagic necrosis, particularly in the lungs and skin. Blood vessel invasion predisposes to dissemination and sepsis and causes multiple nodular lesions in the lungs. Gram stains of necrotic tissue infected with *Pseudomonas* commonly show blood vessel walls densely infiltrated with organisms.

CLOSTRIDIAL DISEASES

Clostridia are gram-positive, spore-forming, anaerobic bacilli. The vegetative bacilli are found in the gastrointestinal tract of herbivorous animals and humans. Anaerobic conditions promote vegetative division. Aerobic environments lead to sporulation. Spores pass in animal feces and contaminate soil and plants and survive well in unfavorable environments. Under anaerobic conditions, spores revert to vegetative cells, thereby completing the cycle. ***During sporulation, vegetative cells degenerate, and their plasmids produce a variety of specific toxins that cause widely differing diseases, depending on the species*** (Fig. 6-15).

- **Food poisoning and necrotizing enteritis** are caused by enterotoxins of *C. perfringens*. The disease is an acute, generally benign, diarrheal disease, usually lasting less than 24 hours. The bacteria are omnipresent in the environment, contaminating soil, water, air samples, clothing, dust, and meat. Spores survive cooking and germinate to yield vegetative forms, which proliferate when food is allowed to stand without refrigeration. The vegetative bacteria sporulate in the small bowel, where they produce several exotoxins, which are cytotoxic to enterocytes and cause loss of intracellular ions and fluid. Certain types of food, including meats, gravies, and sauces, are ideal substrates for *C. perfringens*.
- **Gas gangrene** is produced by myotoxins of *C. perfringens* and, occasionally, *C. novyi*, *C. septicum*, and other species. The disease is a necrotizing, gas-forming infection that begins in contaminated wounds and spreads rapidly to adjacent tissues. It can be fatal within hours of onset and follows anaerobic deposition of *C. perfringens* into extensive devitalized tissue, as in severe penetrating trauma. Tissue necrosis is the result of phospholipase myotoxins that destroy the membranes of muscle cells, leukocytes, and erythrocytes. Affected tissues rapidly become mottled and then frankly necrotic. Muscle may even liquefy. The overlying skin becomes tense, as edema and gas expand underlying soft tissues. A striking feature is the paucity of neutrophils, which are destroyed by the myotoxin.
- **Tetanus** (lockjaw) is due to *C. tetani* neurotoxin. The organism is present in the soil and lower intestine of many animals. Disease occurs when the *C. tetani* contaminates wounds and proliferates in tissue, releasing its exotoxin (**tetanospasmin**), which is transported retrograde through the ventral roots of peripheral nerves to the anterior horn cells of the spinal cord. The toxin then crosses the synapse and binds to ganglioside receptors on presynaptic terminals of motor neurons in the ventral horns. In that location, it is internalized and selectively cleaves a protein that mediates exocytosis of synaptic vesicles, thereby blocking the release of inhibitory neurotransmitters. This blockade permits unopposed neural stimulation and sustained contraction of skeletal muscles (**tetany**). Spastic rigidity often begins in the muscles of the face (hence the term **lockjaw**), which causes a fixed grin (**risus sardonicus**). Rigidity of the muscles of the back produces a backward arching (**opisthotonos**). Abrupt stimuli, including noise, light, or touch, can precipitate painful generalized muscle spasms. If they occur in the respiratory and laryngeal musculature, they may be fatal.
- **Botulism** is a paralyzing disease resulting from neurotoxins of *C. botulinum*. The spores are widely distributed in

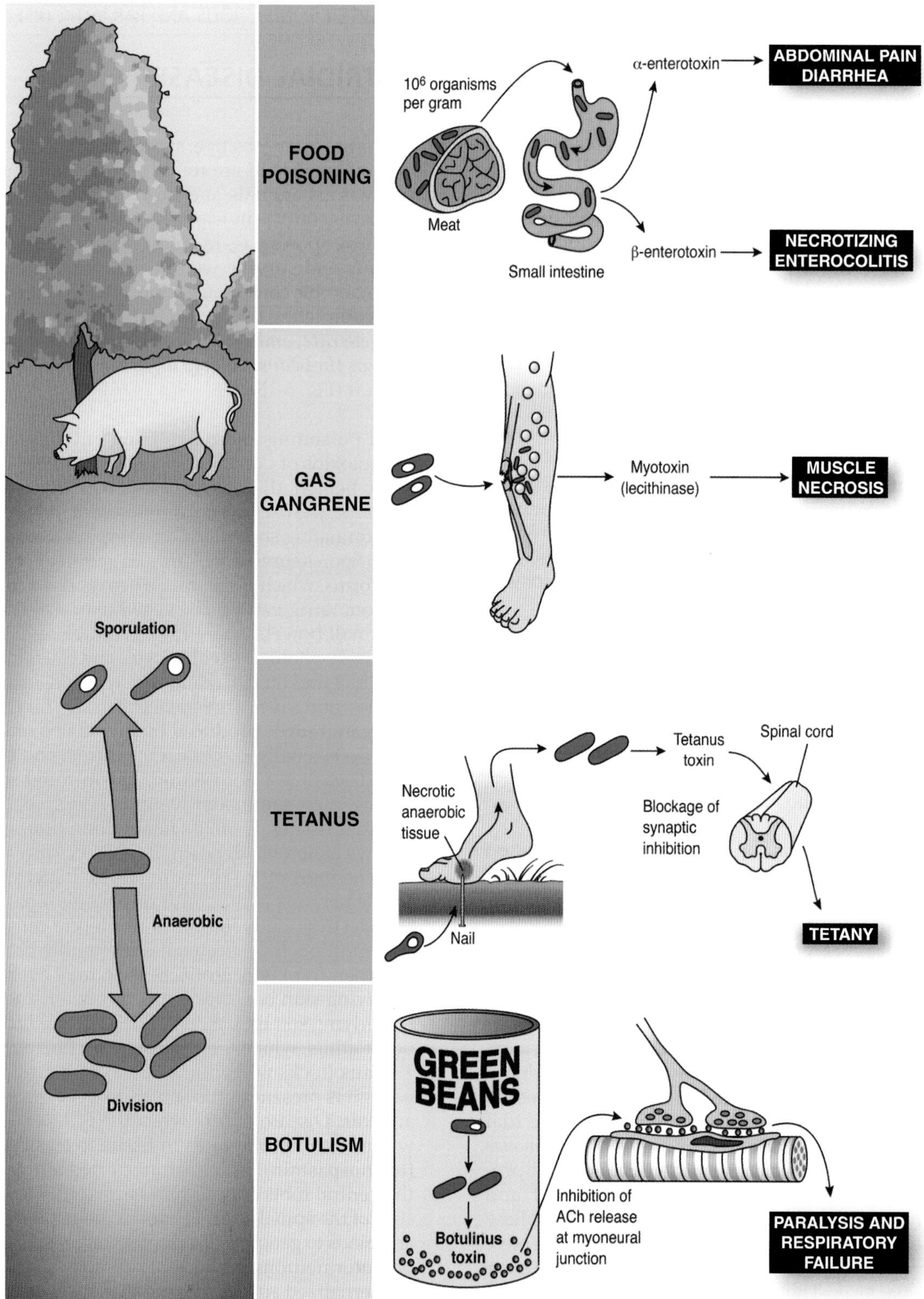

FIGURE 6-15. **Clostridial diseases.** Clostridia in the vegetative form (bacilli) inhabit the gastrointestinal tract of humans and animals. Spores pass in the feces, contaminate soil and plant materials, and are ingested or enter sites of penetrating wounds. Under anaerobic conditions, they revert to vegetative forms. Plasmids in the vegetative forms elaborate toxins that cause several clostridial diseases. **Food poisoning and necrotizing enteritis.** Meat dishes left to cool at room temperature grow large numbers of clostridia ($>10^6$ organisms per gram). When contaminated meat is ingested, *Clostridium perfringens* types A and C produce α enterotoxin in the small intestine during sporulation, causing abdominal pain and diarrhea. Type C also produces β enterotoxin. **Gas gangrene.** Clostridia are widespread and may contaminate a traumatic wound or surgical operation. *C. perfringens* type A elaborates a myotoxin (α toxin), an α lecithinase that destroys cell membranes, alters capillary permeability, and causes severe hemolysis following intravenous injection. The toxin causes necrosis of previously healthy skeletal muscle. **Tetanus.** Spores of *Clostridium tetani* are present in soil and enter the site of an accidental wound. Necrotic tissue at the wound site causes spores to revert to the vegetative form (bacilli). Autolysis of vegetative forms releases tetanus toxin. The toxin is transported in peripheral nerves and (retrograde) through axons to the anterior horn cells of the spinal cord. The toxin blocks synaptic inhibition, and the accumulation of acetylcholine in damaged synapses leads to rigidity and spasms of the skeletal musculature (tetany). **Botulism.** Improperly canned food is contaminated by the vegetative form of *Clostridium botulinum*, which proliferates under aerobic conditions and elaborates a neurotoxin. After the food is ingested, the neurotoxin is absorbed from the small intestine and eventually reaches the myoneural junction, where it inhibits the release of acetylcholine (ACh). The result is a symmetric descending paralysis of cranial nerves, trunk, and limbs, with eventual respiratory paralysis and death.

nature and are resistant to drying and boiling. The toxin is most often present in foods that have been improperly home canned, resulting in suitable anaerobic conditions for the growth of the vegetative cells that produce the neurotoxin. **Infantile botulism** is caused by absorption of toxin from organisms proliferating in infants' intestines. Ingested botulinum neurotoxin resists gastric digestion and is readily absorbed into the blood from the proximal small intestine, reaching the cholinergic nerve endings at the myoneural junction. The most common neurotoxin, serotype A, binds gangliosides at presynaptic nerve terminals and inhibits acetylcholine release. This effect results in a descending paralysis, first affecting cranial nerves and causing blurred vision, photophobia, dry mouth, and dysarthria. Weakness progresses to involve the neck muscles, extremities, diaphragm, and accessory muscles of breathing and can progress rapidly to complete respiratory arrest and death. Injections of small amounts of botulinum toxin are used cosmetically to paralyze facial muscles and alleviate wrinkles.

- **Pseudomembranous enterocolitis** is caused by exotoxins made by *C. difficile.* The bacteria produce an acute necrotizing infection of the terminal small bowel and colon, which can be lethal. *C. difficile* resides in the colon in some healthy individuals. A change in intestinal flora, often because of antibiotic administration (e.g., clindamycin) or other insults such as bowel surgery, allows the organism to flourish. Although noninvasive, toxins produced by the bacteria cause fluid secretion and destroy mucosal cells, resulting in an acute inflammatory response. Lesions range from focal colitis limited to a few crypts and only detectable on biopsy, to massive confluent mucosal ulceration. Inflammation initially involves only the mucosa, but it can extend into the submucosa and muscularis propria. An inflammatory exudate, "pseudomembrane" of cellular debris, neutrophils, and fibrin, often forms over affected areas of the colon.

Bacterial Infections With Animal Reservoirs or Insect Vectors

A group of uncommon bacterial diseases require contact with a particular animal species either directly or via a specific insect vector for infection. Such infections are often localized to areas where host animals and required vectors are present. Thus, the disease may be limited to persons engaged in particular occupations associated with animal or to geographic regions where host and vector co-occur.

Examples of these diseases are as follows:

- **Brucellosis** is a chronic febrile disease acquired from domestic animals, including sheep, goats, cattle, swine, and dogs. Each animal reservoir is associated with a particular *Brucella* species. Humans acquire the bacteria by contact with infected blood or tissue, ingesting contaminated meat or milk, or inhaling contaminated aerosols. Brucellosis is an occupational hazard among ranchers, herders, veterinarians, and slaughterhouse workers. Bacteria enter the circulation through skin abrasions, lungs, conjunctiva, or oropharynx and spread in the bloodstream to the liver, spleen, lymph nodes, and bone marrow. They multiply in macrophages, causing lymphadenopathy and hepatosplenomegaly. In those infected with *Brucella abortus* from cattle, noncaseating granulomas of the liver occur. The organisms usually cannot be demonstrated histologically. Periodic release of bacteria from infected phagocytic cells may be responsible for the episodic febrile illness named **undulant fever**. Brucellosis is a systemic infection that can involve any organ or organ system, with an insidious onset in half of cases. It is characterized by a multitude of somatic complaints, such as fever, sweats, anorexia, fatigue, weight loss, and depression and complications involving the bones and joints and including spondylitis of the lumbar spine and suppuration in large joints.
- **Bubonic plague** is a bacteremic, often fatal disease that results from infection with *Yersinia pestis*, a short gram-negative rod. It characteristically features enlarged, painful regional lymph nodes **(buboes)**. In the United States, up to 30 to 40 cases of plague occur annually, mostly in the desert Southwest. Between 2,000 and 3,000 cases of plague are reported worldwide each year, although, historically, the disease has been associated with major pandemics (e.g., the *Black Death*). *Y. pestis* infection is an endemic zoonosis in many parts of the world, where the organisms are found in wild rodents, such as rats, squirrels, and prairie dogs. Fleas transmit it from animal to animal, with most human infections resulting from bites of infected fleas. Some infected humans develop **pneumonic plague** and shed large numbers of organisms in aerosolized respiratory secretions, allowing person-to-person transmission. After inoculation into the skin by the vector, the organism is phagocytosed by neutrophils and macrophages. Those bacteria engulfed by macrophages survive and replicate intracellularly. They are then carried to regional lymph nodes, where they continue to multiply, producing extensive hemorrhagic necrosis. The organisms disseminated via the bloodstream and lymphatics produce a necrotizing pneumonitis, enabling pneumonic spread of the disease. Affected lymph nodes (buboes) are frequently enlarged and fluctuant as a result of extensive hemorrhagic necrosis. Infected patients often develop necrotic, hemorrhagic skin lesions, hence the name "Black Death" for this disease. **Septicemic plague** occurs when bacteria do not produce buboes but enter directly into the blood. Patients rapidly die of overwhelming bacterial growth in the bloodstream. All blood vessels contain bacilli, and fibrin casts surround the organisms in renal glomeruli and dermal vessels.
- **Anthrax** is a necrotizing disease caused by *Bacillus anthracis*, which is a large, spore-forming, gram-positive rod. The major reservoirs are goats, sheep, cattle, horses, pigs, and dogs. Spores form in the soil, often from dead animals and resist heat, desiccation, and chemical disinfection for years. Humans can be infected when spores enter the body through breaks in the skin, by inhalation, or by ingestion. Human disease may also result from exposure to contaminated animal by-products or via deliberate spore dissemination (bioterrorism). The spores of *B. anthracis* germinate in the human body to yield vegetative bacteria that multiply and release a potent necrotizing toxin. In most of cases of **cutaneous anthrax**, infection remains localized and is eventually eliminated by host immune responses. If the infection disseminates, as occurs when the organisms are inhaled or ingested, the resulting widespread tissue destruction is usually fatal. *B. anthracis* produces extensive tissue necrosis at the sites of infection, with only a mild infiltrate of neutrophils. Cutaneous lesions are ulcerated, contain numerous organisms, and are covered by a black scab. Pulmonary infection produces a necrotizing, hemorrhagic pneumonia, associated with hemorrhagic necrosis

of mediastinal lymph nodes and widespread septicemic dissemination of the organism.

- **Listeriosis** is a systemic multiorgan infection caused by *Listeria monocytogenes*, a small, motile, gram-positive coccobacillus. It is particularly important as a cause of perinatal disease in newborn babies. The organism is widespread in surface water, soil, vegetation, feces of healthy persons, many species of wild and domestic mammals, and several species of birds. However, spread of infection from animals to humans is rare. Because *L. monocytogenes* grows at refrigerator temperatures, outbreaks have been traced to unpasteurized milk, cheese, and dairy products. After phagocytosis by host cells, the organisms enter phagolysosomes, where acidic pH activates *Listeriolysin O*, an exotoxin that disrupts the vesicular membrane and allows bacteria to escape into the cytoplasm. After replicating, bacteria usurp host cytoskeleton contractile elements to form elongated protrusions that are engulfed by adjacent cells. Thus, *Listeria* spread from one cell to another without exposure to the extracellular environment, thereby evading host defenses. Listeriosis of adults is characterized by meningoencephalitis and septicemia, but may be localized to the skin, eyes, lymph nodes, endocardium, or bone. Maternal infection early in pregnancy may lead to abortion or premature delivery. Infected infants rapidly develop respiratory distress, hepatosplenomegaly, cutaneous and mucosal papules, leukopenia, and thrombocytopenia. Neurologic sequelae of neonatal listeriosis are common, and the mortality is high.

Infection Caused by Branching Filamentous Organisms

Actinomycosis

Actinomyces are branching, filamentous, gram-positive rods that normally reside in the oropharynx, gastrointestinal tract, and vagina. Actinomycosis is a slowly progressive, suppurative, fibrosing infection, which involves the jaw (termed "lumpy jaw"), thorax, or abdomen. It is caused by a number of anaerobic and microaerophilic bacteria, the most common being *Actinomyces israelii*. The bacterium is not ordinarily virulent and resides in the body as a saprophyte. To cause disease, it must be inoculated into deeper tissues and have an anaerobic atmosphere necessary for bacterial proliferation. Infection is associated with trauma and tissue necrosis, beginning as a nidus of proliferating organisms that attract an acute inflammatory infiltrate. A series of abscesses forms and is connected by sinus tracts, which burrow across normal tissue boundaries and into adjacent organs. The lesion may eventually reach an external surface or mucosal membrane to produce a draining sinus. The walls of abscesses and tracts consist of granulation tissue, often thick, densely fibrotic, and chronically inflamed. Within abscesses and sinuses are pus and colonies of organisms, which can grow to several millimeters and be visible to the naked eye as hard, yellow **sulfur granules**. Histologically, colonies are rounded, basophilic grains with scalloped eosinophilic borders (Fig. 6-16A). Individual filaments of *Actinomyces* are readily visible on Gram staining or silver impregnation (Fig. 6-16B).

Spirochetal Infections

Spirochetes are long, slender, helical bacteria with specialized cell envelopes that permit them to move by flexion and rotation. The thin organisms are below the resolving power of routine light microscopy so darkfield microscopy or silver impregnation is needed to visualize them. They have the basic cell wall structure of gram-negative bacteria, but stain poorly with the Gram stain.

Three genera of spirochetes, *Treponema*, *Borrelia*, and *Leptospira*, cause human disease (Table 6-4). Because they are adept at evading host inflammatory and immunologic defenses, all diseases caused by these organisms are chronic or relapsing.

Syphilis

The disease is discussed in Chapter 16.

Nonvenereal Treponematoses

Tropical and subtropical areas are home to nonvenereal, chronic diseases caused by treponemes indistinguishable from *T. pallidum*, the causative agent of syphilis. Like syphilis, they result from inoculation of the organism into mucocutaneous surfaces. The disorders also pass through clearly defined clinical and pathologic stages, including a primary lesion at the site of inoculation, secondary skin eruptions, a latent period, and a tertiary late stage.

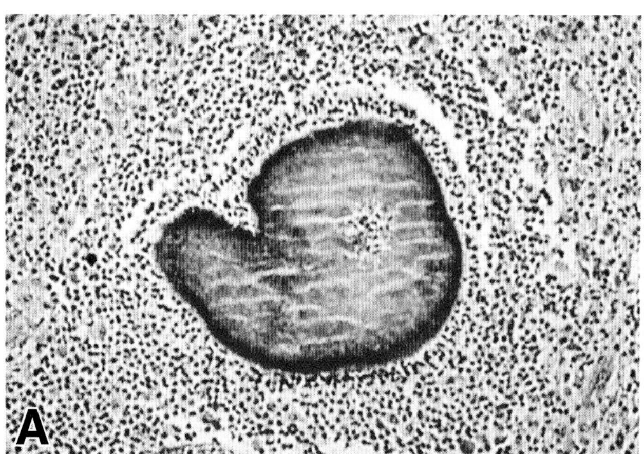

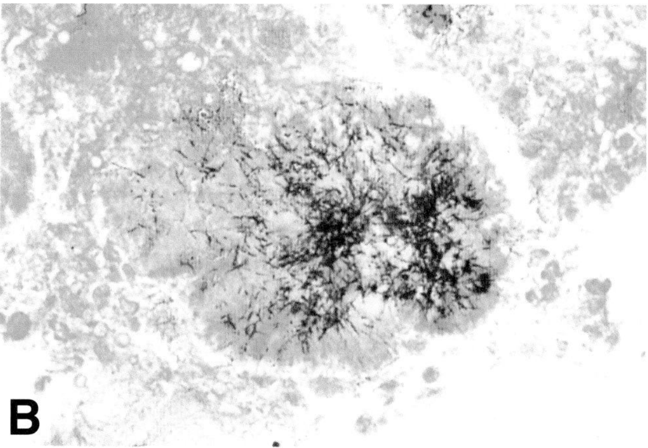

FIGURE 6-16. Actinomycosis. A. A typical sulfur granule lies within an abscess. **B.** The individual filaments of *Actinomyces israelii* are readily visible with the silver impregnation technique.

Table 6-4

Spirochete Infections

Disease	Organism	Clinical Manifestation	Distribution	Mode of Transmission
Treponemes				
Syphilis	*Treponema pallidum*	See text	Common worldwide	Sexual contact, congenital
Bejel	*Treponema endemicum* (*T. pallidum*, subspecies *endemicum*)	Mucosal, skin. and bone lesions	Middle East	Mouth-to-mouth contact
Yaws	*Treponema pertenue* (*T. pallidum* subspecies *pertenue*)	Skin and bone	Tropics	Skin-to-skin contact
Pinta	*Treponema carateum*	Skin lesions	Latin America	Skin-to-skin contact
Borrelia				
Lyme disease	*Borrelia burgdorferi*	See text	North America, Europe, Russia, Asia, Africa, Australia	Tick bite
Relapsing fever	*Borrelia recurrentis*	Relapsing flu-like illness	Worldwide	Tick bite, louse bite, and related species
Leptospira				
Leptospirosis	*Leptospira interrogans*	Flu-like illness, meningitis	Worldwide	Contact with animal urine

- **Yaws** is predominantly a disease of children and adolescents spread by skin-to-skin contact. Primary and disseminated (or secondary) yaws involve dermal lesions, which show hyperkeratosis, papillary acanthosis, and an intense neutrophilic infiltrate of the epidermis. The epidermis at the apex of the papilloma lyses to form a shallow ulcer, and plasma cells invade the upper dermis. Spirochetes are numerous in the dermal papillae. During a latent period or 5 years or more, treponemes are borne by the blood to bones, lymph nodes, and skin. The lesions in the late stage include cutaneous gummas, which are destructive to the face and upper airway, and periostitis, characteristically of the tibia.
- **Bejel** (also known as "endemic syphilis") is transmitted from an infected infant to the breast of the mother. The causative agent, *Treponema pallidum endemicum*, is morphologically and serologically indistinguishable from the agent of syphilis and may produce primary disease on the nursing breast. Later stage disease progresses much as syphilis.

Lyme Disease

Lyme disease is a chronic systemic infection that begins with a characteristic skin lesion and later manifests as cardiac, neurologic, or joint disturbances. The causative agent is a large, microaerophilic spirochete belonging to the genus *Borrelia*, most commonly *Borrelia burgdorferi*. The spirochete is transmitted from its animal reservoir to humans by the bite of the minute *Ixodes* tick found in wooded areas, where it usually feeds on mice and deer.

Lyme disease, the most common tick-borne illness in the United States, is predominantly found along the eastern seaboard from Maryland to Massachusetts and in the Midwest in Minnesota and Wisconsin. *B. burgdorferi* reproduces locally at the site of inoculation, spreads to regional lymph nodes, and disseminates throughout the body via the bloodstream. Like other spirochetal diseases, Lyme disease is chronic, with remissions and exacerbations.

Three clinical stages are described as follows:

- **Stage 1:** The characteristic skin lesion, **erythema chronicum migrans**, appears at the site of the tick bite, beginning 3 to 35 days after the bite as an erythematous macule or papule and growing into an erythematous patch 3 to 7 cm in diameter. The patch is often intensely red at its periphery, with some central clearing, imparting an annular appearance. The organism elicits a chronic inflammatory infiltrate, composed of lymphocytes and plasma cells, which is accompanied by fever, fatigue, headache, arthralgias, and regional lymphadenopathy.
- **Stage 2:** The second stage begins weeks to months after the skin lesion and is characterized by exacerbation of migratory musculoskeletal pains and cardiac and neurologic abnormalities.
- **Post-treatment Lyme disease syndrome** may occur in a small percentage of treated cases. It begins months to years after initial infection, with joint, skin, and neurologic abnormalities. Over half of these patients have arthralgia and severe arthritis of the large joints, especially the knee. The histopathology of affected joints is virtually indistinguishable from that of rheumatoid arthritis, including villous hypertrophy and a conspicuous mononuclear infiltrate in the subsynovial lining area. In patients who die of the disease, organisms are seen at autopsy in virtually every organ affected, including the skin, myocardium, liver, CNS, and musculoskeletal systems.

Leptospirosis

Leptospirosis is a worldwide zoonosis that features infection with spirochetes of the genus *Leptospira*. Although usually mild and self-limited, severe infections may entail hepatic and renal failure, which may prove fatal. *Leptospires* penetrate abraded skin or mucous membranes following contact with infected rats, contaminated water, or mud. The disease is uncommon in the United States, but is occasionally found in slaughterhouse workers and trappers, and among destitute people in urban areas. In severe cases, *Leptospires* are initially present in the blood and cerebrospinal fluid, but soon disappear. After IgM antibodies appear, recurrent symptoms are now associated with signs of meningeal irritation and the presence of white cells in the CSF. Jaundice may be followed by hepatic and renal failure and the appearance of widespread hemorrhages and shock (**Weil disease**).

At autopsy, tissues are bile stained, and hemorrhages are seen in many organs. The principal lesion is a diffuse vasculitis with capillary injury. Liver shows dissociation of liver cell plates, erythrophagocytosis by Kupffer cells, minimal necrosis of hepatocytes, neutrophils in the sinusoids, and a mixed inflammatory cell infiltrate in portal tracts. Renal tubules are swollen and necrotic. Spirochetes are numerous in tubular lumina, and particularly in bile-stained casts (Fig. 6-17).

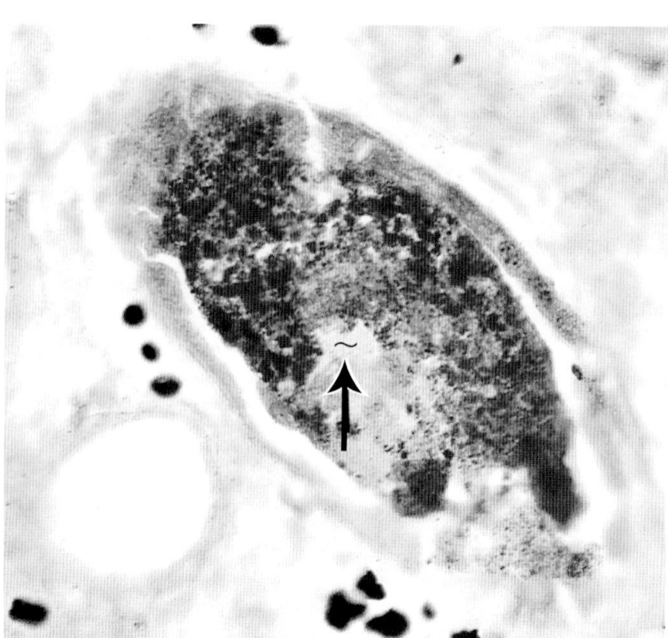

FIGURE 6-17. **Leptospirosis.** A distal renal tubule is obstructed by a bile-stained mass of hemoglobin and cellular debris. A leptospire (*arrow*) is in the center of this mass.

Chlamydial Infections

Chlamydiae are obligate intracellular parasites that are smaller than most other bacteria. Because they cannot make ATP, they must parasitize the metabolic machinery of a host cell to reproduce. The life cycle involves two morphologic forms. The **elementary body** is the smaller, metabolically inactive form, which survives extracellularly and attaches to the appropriate host cell, induces endocytosis, and forms a vacuole. After transforming into the larger, metabolically active form, namely, the **reticulate body**, it commandeers host cell metabolism to fuel chlamydial replication. The reticulate body divides repeatedly, forming daughter elementary bodies and destroying the host cell. Necrotic debris elicits inflammatory and immunologic responses that further damage infected tissue. Chlamydial infections are widespread among birds and mammals. Three species of chlamydiae (*Chlamydia trachomatis*, *Chlamydia psittaci*, and *Chlamydia pneumoniae*) cause human infection.

Chlamydia trachomatis

C. trachomatis contains a number of strains (serovars), which cause three distinct types of disease. Genital and neonatal disease and lymphogranuloma venereum are both discussed in Chapter 16.

Trachoma is a chronic infection of the eye with *C. trachomatis* that causes progressive scars of the conjunctiva and cornea. Only humans are naturally infected, and poor personal hygiene and inadequate public sanitation are common factors. The disease is spread mostly by direct contact, but may also be transmitted by fomites, contaminated water, and, probably, flies. Subclinical infections are an important reservoir. In endemic areas, infection is acquired early in childhood, becomes chronic, and eventually progresses to blindness.

When *C. trachomatis* is inoculated into the eye, it reproduces in the conjunctival epithelium, inciting a mixed acute and chronic inflammatory infiltrate. Histologic examination of early lesions shows chronic inflammation, lymphoid aggregates, focal degeneration, and chlamydial inclusions in the conjunctiva. As trachoma progresses, lymphoid aggregates enlarge, and the conjunctiva becomes scarred and focally hypertrophic. The cornea is invaded by blood vessels and fibroblasts, forming a scar that is eventually opacified.

Psittacosis (Ornithosis)

Psittacosis is a self-limited pneumonia transmitted to humans by the inhalation of the excreta or feather dust of birds infected with *C. psittaci*. The organism first infects pulmonary macrophages, which carry the organism to the phagocytes of the liver and spleen, where it reproduces. It then spreads via the bloodstream, causing systemic infection, with particularly diffuse involvement of the lungs. *C. psittaci* reproduces in alveolar lining cells, whose destruction elicits an inflammatory response. The pneumonia is a predominantly interstitial, lymphocytic infiltrate. Dissemination of the infection is characterized by foci of necrosis in the liver and spleen and diffuse mononuclear cell infiltrates in the heart, kidneys, and brain.

Rickettsial Infections

The rickettsiae are small, gram-negative, coccobacillary bacteria that are intracellular pathogens, which cannot replicate outside a host. Human infections result from insect bites. Unlike chlamydiae, rickettsiae replicate by binary fission. They synthesize their own ATP and can also obtain ATP from the host. The organisms induce endocytosis by target cells and replicate in their cytoplasm. Rickettsiae have cell wall structures like gram-negative bacteria, but do not stain well with the Gram stain.

Humans are accidental hosts for most species of *Rickettsia*. The organisms reside in animals and insects and do not require humans for perpetuation. Several species of *Rickettsia* cause different human diseases (Table 6-5) that share many common

Table 6-5

Rickettsial Infections

Disease	Organism	Distribution	Transmission
Spotted-fever group (genus Rickettsia)			
Rocky mountain spotted fever	*Rickettsia rickettsii*	Americas	Ticks
Queensland tick fever	*Rickettsia australis*	Australia	Ticks
Boutonneuse fever, Kenya tick fever	*Rickettsia conorii*	Mediterranean, Africa, India	Ticks
Siberian tick fever	*Rickettsia sibirica*	Siberia, Mongolia	Ticks
Rickettsialpox	*Rickettsia akari*	United States, Russia, Central Asia, Korea, Africa	Mites
Flea-borne spotted fever	*Rickettsia felis*	North and South America, Europe, Australia	Ticks
Typhus group			
Louse-borne typhus (epidemic typhus)	*Rickettsia prowazekii*	Latin America, Africa, Asia	Lice
Murine typhus (endemic typhus)	*Rickettsia typhi*	Worldwide	Fleas
Scrub typhus	*Orientia tsutsugamushi*	South Pacific, Asia	Mites
Q fever	*Coxiella burnetti*	Worldwide	Inhalation

features. ***In humans, the target cells for all rickettsiae are capillary and small vessel endothelial cells.*** The organisms reproduce within these cells, killing them in the process and producing a necrotizing vasculitis. Human rickettsial infections are traditionally divided into the "**spotted-fever group**" and the "**typhus group**."

Rocky Mountain Spotted Fever

RMSF is an acute, potentially fatal, systemic vasculitis that is usually accompanied by headache, fever, and rash, and is acquired through bites of infected ticks, the vectors for *Rickettsia rickettsii.* The organism is transmitted from mother to progeny ticks, thereby maintaining a natural reservoir for human infection. Such disease occurs when the organism in tick salivary glands is introduced into the skin during feeding. Rickettsiae spread via lymphatics and small blood vessels to the systemic and pulmonary circulation where they enter vascular endothelial cells. In these sites, they reproduce in the cytoplasm and are then shed from the damaged endothelium into the vascular and lymphatic systems, resulting in a systemic vasculitis. The rash is produced by inflammatory damage to cutaneous vessels and is the most visible manifestation of the generalized vascular injury. However, *R. rickettsii* can also spread to vascular smooth muscle and endothelium of larger vessels. Extensive damage to blood vessel walls causes loss of vascular integrity throughout the body, fluid exudation and disseminated intravascular coagulation, and shock. Damage to pulmonary capillaries can produce pulmonary edema and acute alveolar injury. Necrosis and reactive hyperplasia of vascular endothelium are often associated with thrombosis of small-caliber vessels. Vessel walls are infiltrated initially with neutrophils and macrophages and later by lymphocytes and plasma cells. Microscopic infarcts and extravasation of blood into surrounding tissues are common.

Typhus Group Rickettsial Infections

- **Epidemic (Louse-Borne) typhus** is a now an uncommon systemic vasculitis transmitted by the bites of infected lice. It is caused by *Rickettsia prowazekii*, an organism that has a human–louse–human life cycle (Fig. 6-18). Unlike other rickettsial diseases, it can establish latent infection and produce recrudescent disease (Brill–Zinsser disease) many years after the primary infection. The pathologic findings produced by *R. prowazekii* are similar to those in RMSF and other rickettsial diseases. Collections of mononuclear cells are found in various organs (e.g., skin, brain, and heart). The infiltrate includes mast cells, lymphocytes, plasma cells, and macrophages, frequently arranged as **typhus nodules** around arterioles and capillaries. Throughout the body, the endothelium of small blood vessels is focally necrotic and hyperplastic, and the walls contain inflammatory cells. Historically, epidemic typhus has been responsible for innumerable deaths in malnourished and abused populations.
- **Endemic typhus** is similar to epidemic typhus but tends to be milder. Humans are infected with *Rickettsia typhi*, interrupting the rat–flea–rat cycle of transmission. The organism may become airborne and, if inhaled, causes pulmonary infection.
- **Scrub typhus (Tsutsugamushi fever)** is an acute, febrile illness of humans caused by *Orientia tsutsugamushi* (previously *Rickettsia tsutsugamushi*). Rodents are the natural mammalian reservoir, from which the organism is passed to trombiculid mites known as chiggers. While feeding, mites inoculate the organisms into the skin. Rickettsemia and lymphadenopathy follow shortly thereafter. Severe infections are complicated by myocarditis, meningoencephalitis, and shock.

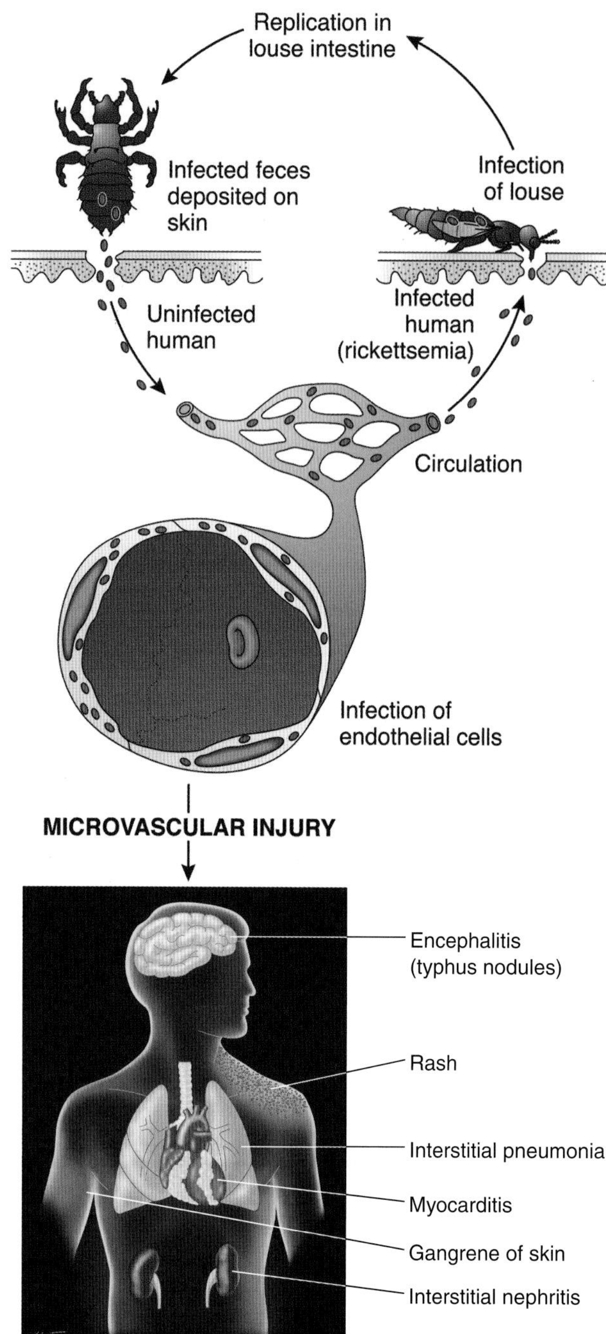

FIGURE 6-18. Epidemic typhus (louse-borne typhus). *Rickettsia prowazekii* has a man–louse–man life cycle. The organism multiplies in endothelial cells, which detach, rupture, and release organisms into the circulation (rickettsemia). A louse taking a blood meal becomes infected with rickettsiae, which enter the epithelial cells of its midgut, multiply, and rupture the cells, thereby releasing rickettsiae into the lumen of the louse intestine. Contaminated feces are deposited on the skin or clothing of a second host, penetrate an abrasion, or are inhaled. The rickettsiae then enter endothelial cells, multiply, and rupture the cells, thus completing the cycle.

Mycoplasmal Infections

At less than 0.3 μm in greatest dimension, mycoplasmas are the smallest free-living **prokaryotes**. They lack the rigid cell walls of more complex bacteria. Mycoplasmas are widespread, geographically, and ecologically, as saprophytes and parasites of many animals and plants. Many *Mycoplasma* species inhabit the human body, but only three are pathogenic: *Mycoplasma pneumoniae, Mycoplasma hominis* (discussed in Chapter 10), and *Ureaplasma urealyticum* (discussed in Chapter 16). The diseases associated with these organisms are shown in Table 6-6.

MYCOBACTERIAL INFECTIONS

Mycobacteria are distinctive organisms, 2 to 10 μm in length, with cell wall architecture similar to that of gram-positive bacteria. However, they also contain large amounts of lipid that renders the organism difficult to demonstrate by Gram stain. ***The waxy lipids of the cell wall make the mycobacteria "acid fast" (i.e., they retain carbolfuchsin staining after rinsing with acid alcohol).***

Mycobacteria grow more slowly than other pathogenic bacteria, and their diseases are chronic and slowly progressive. They produce no known toxins, but damage human tissues by inducing inflammatory and immune responses. Most mycobacterial pathogens replicate within cells of the monocyte/macrophage lineage and elicit granulomatous inflammation. The outcome of mycobacterial infection is largely determined by the host's capacity to contain the organism through cell-mediated immune responses.

The two main mycobacterial pathogens, *M. tuberculosis* and *Mycobacterium leprae*, only infect humans and have no environmental reservoir. Other pathogenic mycobacteria are environmental organisms that only occasionally cause human disease.

Tuberculosis

The disease is discussed in Chapter 10.

Leprosy

Leprosy (Hansen disease), caused by *M. leprae*, is a chronic, slowly progressive, destructive process that involves peripheral nerves, skin, and mucous membranes.

Leprosy is transmitted from person to person, after years of intimate contact with the nasal secretions or ulcerated lesions of infected persons. The mode of infection is unclear, but probably involves inoculation of bacilli into the respiratory tract or open wounds.

Table 6-6

Mycoplasmal Infections

Organism	Disease
Mycoplasma pneumoniae	Tracheobronchitis
	Pneumonia
	Pharyngitis
	Otitis media
Ureaplasma urealyticum	Urethritis
	Chorioamnionitis
	Postpartum fever
Mycoplasma hominis	Postpartum fever

M. leprae multiplies best at low temperatures, and lesions tend to occur in cooler parts of the body (e.g., hands and face). Leprosy exhibits a bewildering variety of clinical and pathologic features. Lesions vary from the small, insignificant, and self-healing macules of tuberculoid leprosy to the diffuse, disfiguring, and sometimes fatal ones of lepromatous leprosy (Fig. 6-19). This extreme variation in disease presentation probably reflects differences in immune reactivity.

Most (95%) persons have a natural protective immunity to *M. leprae* and are not infected, despite intimate and prolonged exposure. Susceptible individuals (5%) range from anergic patients who have little or no resistance and develop **lepromatous leprosy**, to patients with high resistance, who manifest **tuberculoid leprosy**. Most patients, in between these extremes, have **borderline leprosy**.

Lepromatous leprosy: This form of leprosy exhibits multiple, tumor-like lesions of the skin, eyes, testes, nerves, lymph nodes, and spleen. Nodular or diffuse infiltrates of foamy macrophages contain myriad bacilli (Fig. 6-20). The epidermis is stretched thinly over the nodules, and beneath it is a narrow, uninvolved "clear zone" of the dermis. Rather than destroying the bacilli, macrophages seem to act as microincubators that contain numerous organisms, which appear as aggregates of acid-fast material, called "globi." The dermal infiltrates expand slowly to distort and disfigure the face, ears, and upper airway, and to destroy the eyes, eyebrows and eyelashes, nerves, and testes. The nodular skin lesions of lepromatous leprosy may ulcerate and coalesce to produce a lion-like appearance ("leonine facies"). Involvement of the upper airways leads to chronic nasal discharge and voice change. Infection of the eyes may cause blindness.

Tuberculoid leprosy is characterized by a single lesion or very few lesions of the skin, usually on the face, extremities, or trunk. Microscopically, lesions show well-formed, circumscribed dermal granulomas, with epithelioid macrophages, Langhans giant cells, and lymphocytes. Nerve fibers are almost invariably swollen and infiltrated with lymphocytes, and their destruction accounts for the sensory deficit associated with tuberculoid leprosy. The term "tuberculoid leprosy" is used because the granulomas vaguely resemble those of tuberculosis but lack caseation. The lesions of tuberculoid leprosy cause minimal disfigurement and are not infectious.

Mycobacterium avium–Intracellulare Complex

Mycobacterium avium and *Mycobacterium intracellulare* are similar species, which cause identical diseases, and are grouped as *M. avium–intracellulare* (MAI) complex, or simply MAI. The agents cause two types of disease: (1) a rare, slowly progressive granulomatous pulmonary disease in immunocompetent persons and (2) a progressive systemic disease in patients with AIDS. ***MAI infection is the third most common opportunistic infection in AIDS patients in the United States.*** The disease is discussed in Chapter 10.

Atypical Mycobacteria

Several other species of environmental mycobacteria present in surface water, dust, and dirt occasionally produce human disease, which is acquired by inhalation, inoculation, or ingestion of environmental material. These bacteria, including MAI, are often lumped together as the "atypical mycobacteria" (in contrast to *M. tuberculosis*, regarded as the "typical" *Mycobacterium*). The atypical mycobacteria are biologically diverse, and the uncommon diseases that they produce in humans differ in circumstances of acquisition, pathology, clinical presentations, and therapies.

FUNGAL INFECTIONS

The few fungi that cause human disease act, for the most part, as "opportunists" that infect people with impaired defenses. Corticosteroid administration, antineoplastic therapy, and congenital or acquired T-cell deficiencies all predispose to mycotic infections. Fungi, larger and more complex than bacteria, vary in size from 2 to 100 μm and possess nuclear membranes and cytoplasmic organelles, such as mitochondria and endoplasmic reticulum.

There are two morphologic types of fungi: yeasts and molds.

- **Yeasts** are unicellular forms of fungi. They are round or oval cells that reproduce by budding, a process by which daughter organisms pinch off from a parent. Some yeasts produce buds that do not detach but instead create **pseudohyphae** (i.e., chains of elongated yeast cells that resemble hyphae).
- **Molds** are multicellular filamentous fungal colonies, with branching tubules, or **hyphae**, 2 to 10 μm in diameter. The mass of tangled hyphae in the mold form is called a **mycelium**. Some hyphae are separated by septa that are located at regular intervals; others are nonseptate.
- **Dimorphic fungi** may grow as yeasts or molds, depending on their environment.

Fungal Agents Associated with Pulmonary Disease

Several of the more commonly encountered fungal pathogens produce pulmonary disease and are associated with granulomatous inflammation, often accompanied by necrosis (e.g., *Histoplasma*, *Coccidioides*, *Cryptococcus*, and *Blastomyces*). *Aspergillus* may also produce invasive disease. *Pneumocystis* infections are invariably associated with immunodeficiency states, such as HIV/AIDS, drug therapy for neoplastic disease, or transplantation. Details of infection with these agents are presented in Chapter 10.

Candida

Yeasts of the genus *Candida* include the most common opportunistic pathogens. Many are endogenous human flora. However, when host defenses are compromised, they can cause disease, which is most often mucosal and superficial. Commonly affected sites include oral infections (thrush), esophagitis, and vulvovaginitis (Table 6-7).

Candidal infections of deep tissues, much less common than superficial infections, can be life-threatening. The most common deep sites affected are the brain, eye, kidney, and heart. Deep infections, with candidal sepsis and disseminated candidiasis, occur only in immunologically compromised people and are often fatal.

Candida is relegated to superficial, nonsterile sites via mechanical barriers, inflammatory cells, humoral immunity, cell-mediated immunity, and resident bacterial flora. In turn, the normal resident florae limit the number of fungal organisms. Antibiotic therapy is the most common precipitating factor for candidiasis because its use suppresses competing bacterial florae. Under conditions of unopposed growth, the

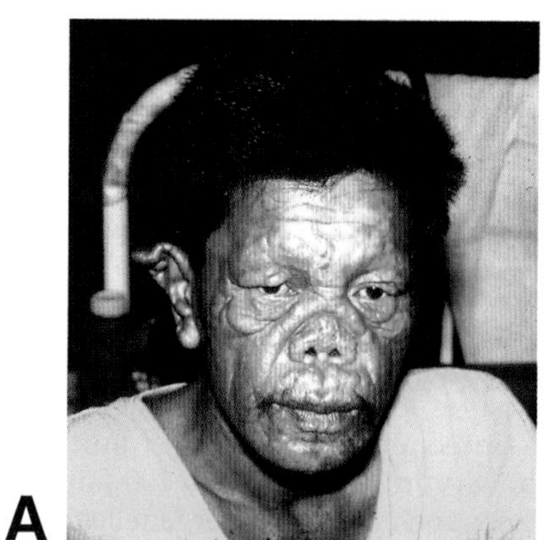

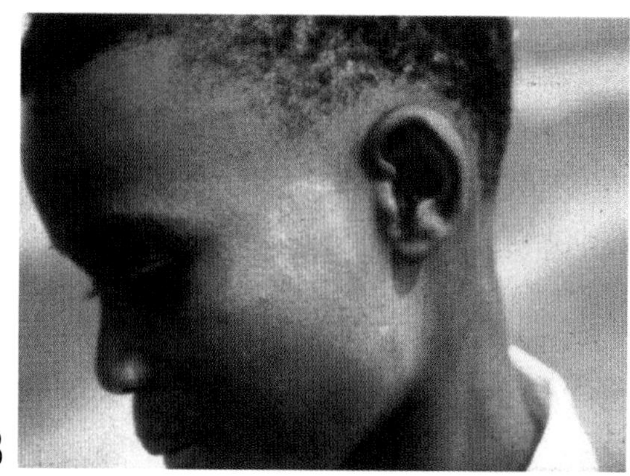

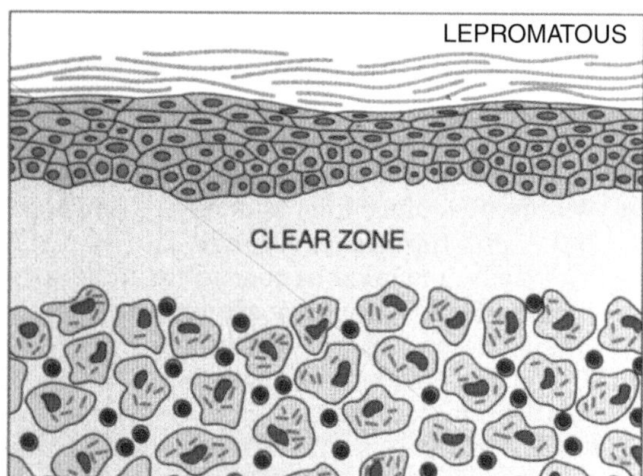

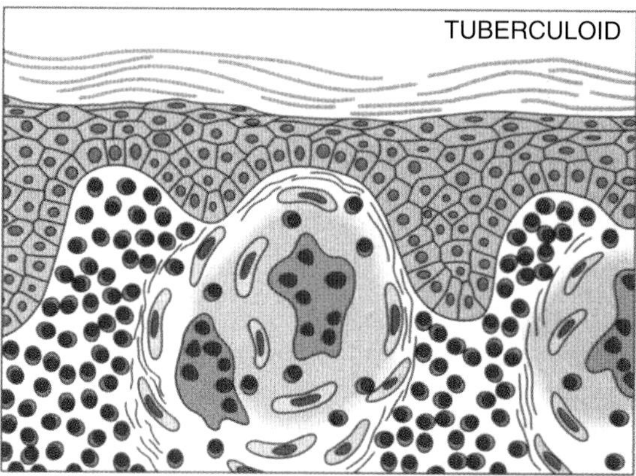

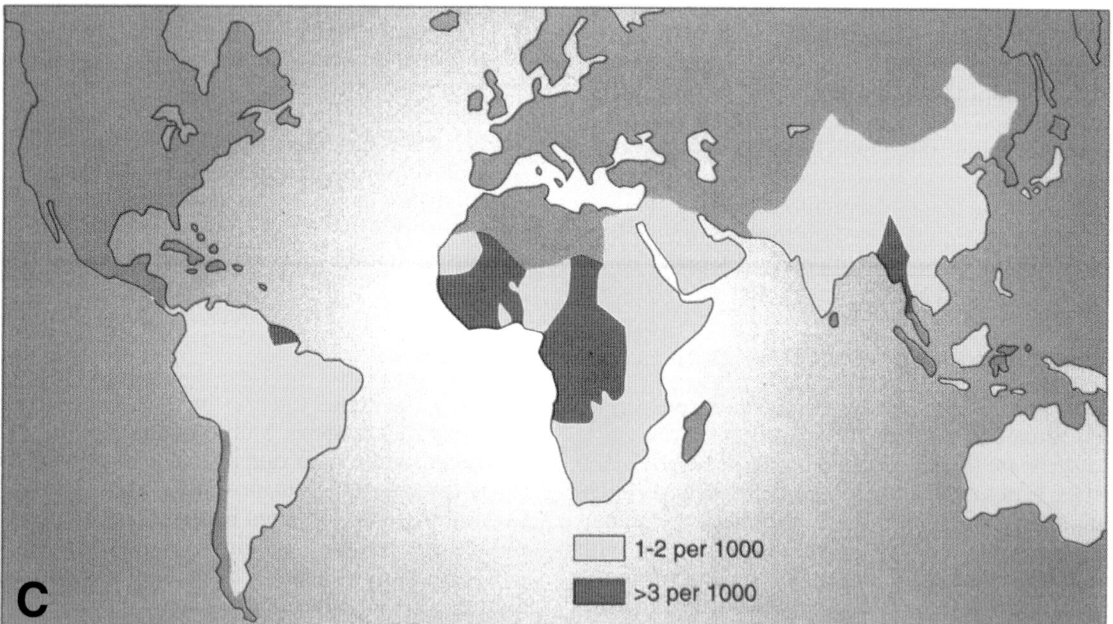

FIGURE 6-19. **A.** (*Top*) **Leonine facies of lepromatous leprosy.** There is diffuse involvement, including a loss of eyebrows and eyelashes and nodular distortions of the face and ears, the exposed (cool) parts of the body. The septum and bone of the nose are damaged, producing "saddle nose" deformity. This Filipino patient also had deformities of the hands and feet. (*Bottom*) The nodular skin lesions of advanced lepromatous leprosy. Swelling has flattened the epidermis (loss of rete ridges). A characteristic "clear zone" of uninvolved dermis separates the epidermis from tumor-like accumulations of macrophages, each containing numerous lepra bacilli (*Mycobacterium leprae*). **B.** (*Top*) **Tuberculoid leprosy** on the cheek showing a hypopigmented macule with a raised, infiltrated border. The central portion may be hypesthetic or anesthetic. (*Bottom*) Macular skin lesion of tuberculoid leprosy. Skin from the raised "infiltrated" margin of the plaque contains discrete granulomas that extend to the basal layer of the epidermis (without a clear zone). The granulomas are composed of epithelioid cells and Langhans giant cells and are associated with lymphocytes and plasma cells. Lepra bacilli are rare. **C. Distribution of leprosy.** Prevalence is greatest in tropical regions of Africa, Asia, and Latin America.

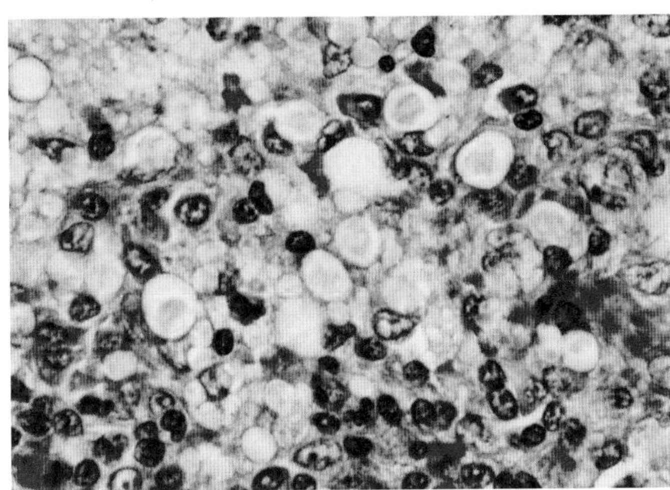

FIGURE 6-20. Lepromatous leprosy. A section of skin shows a tumor-like mass of foamy macrophages. The faint masses within the vacuolated macrophages are enormous numbers of lepra bacilli.

Table 6-7

Candidal Infections

Disease	Predisposing Conditions
Superficial infections	
Intertrigo (opposed skin surfaces)	Maceration
Paronychia (nail beds)	Maceration
Diaper rash	Maceration
Vulvovaginitis	Alteration in normal flora
Thrush (oral)	Decreased cell-mediated immunity
Esophagitis	Decreased cell-mediated immunity
Deep infections	
Urinary tract infections	Indwelling urinary catheters
Sepsis and disseminated infection	Neutropenia, indwelling vascular catheters, and change in normal flora

yeast converts to its invasive form (hyphae or pseudohyphae), invades superficially, and elicits an inflammatory or immunologic response.

Superficial infections of the skin, oropharynx (Fig. 6-21A), and esophagus feature organisms in the most superficial epithelial layers, which lead to acute inflammatory infiltrates (Fig. 6-21B). The yeasts are round, 3 to 4 μm in diameter, and display septate hyphae. Deep infections consist of multiple microscopic abscesses, which contain yeast, hyphae, necrotic debris, and neutrophils.

Dermatophyte Infections

Dermatophytes are fungi that cause localized superficial infections of keratinized tissues, including the skin, hair, and nails. Dermatophyte infections are minor illnesses, but are among the most common skin diseases for which medical help is sought. They are resident in soil, on animals, and on humans. Most dermatophyte infections in temperate countries are acquired by direct contact with people who have infected hairs or skin scales. The agent proliferates within the superficial keratinized tissues and spreads centrifugally from the initial site, producing round, expanding lesions with sharp margins. The appearance once suggested that a worm was responsible for the disease, hence the names **ringworm** and **tinea** (from the Latin *tinea*, meaning "worm").

Dermatophyte infections produce thickening of the squamous epithelium, with increased numbers of keratinized cells and a mild lymphocytic inflammatory infiltrate in the dermis.

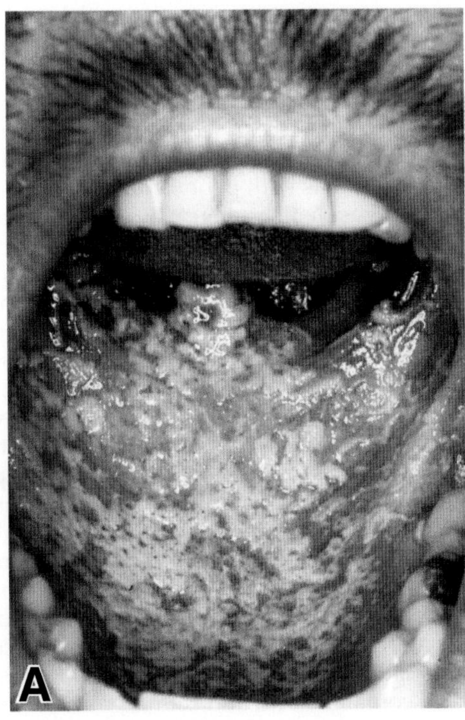

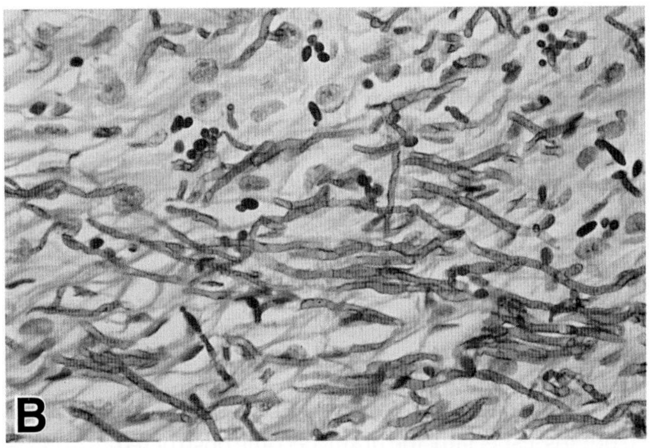

FIGURE 6-21. Candidiasis. A. The oral cavity of a patient with acquired immunodeficiency syndrome is covered by a white, curd-like exudate containing numerous fungal organisms. **B.** A periodic acid–Schiff stain showing numerous septate hyphae and yeast forms. *A*, From Farrar WE, Wood MJ, Innes JA, Tubbs H. *Infectious Diseases Text and Color Atlas*. 2nd ed. New York, NY: Gower Medical Publishing, 1992.

Hyphae and spores of the infecting dermatophytes are confined to the nonviable portions of the skin, hair, and nails.

PROTOZOAL INFECTIONS

Protozoa are single-celled eukaryotes that fall into three general classes: **amebae, flagellates,** and **sporozoites**. Amebae move by projection of cytoplasmic extensions termed **pseudopodia**. Flagellates move through thread-like structures, flagella, which extend out from the cell membrane. Sporozoites do not have organelles of locomotion and also differ from amebae and flagellates in their mode of replication.

Protozoa cause human disease by diverse mechanisms. Some, such as *Entamoeba histolytica*, are extracellular parasites that digest and invade human tissues. Others, such as plasmodia, are obligate intracellular parasites that replicate in, and kill, human cells. Still others, such as trypanosomes, damage human tissue largely by inflammatory and immunologic responses. Some protozoa (e.g., *T. gondii*) can establish latent infections and cause reactivation disease in immunocompromised hosts.

Malaria

Malaria is a mosquito-borne, hemolytic, febrile illness which affects over 200 million people worldwide and kills more than 1 million yearly. Four *Plasmodium* species cause malaria: *Plasmodium falciparum*, *P. vivax*, *Plasmodium ovale*, and *Plasmodium malariae*. *P. falciparum* causes the most severe disease and accounts for most deaths. All infect and destroy human erythrocytes, causing recurrent paroxysms of chills, high fever, anemia, and splenomegaly.

Malaria is transmitted by the bite of the female *Anopheles* mosquito. *P. falciparum* and *P. vivax* are the most common pathogens, although *P. vivax* is rare in Africa, where much of the black population lacks the erythrocyte cell surface receptors required for infection.

The life cycle of the *Plasmodium* is complex, requiring both human and mosquito hosts. The rupture of infected erythrocytes containing the merozoite stage (see Fig. 6-22) releases pyrogens and causes the chills and fever of malaria. Anemia results from (1) loss of circulating infected erythrocytes and (2) sequestration of cells in the enlarging spleen and liver by the fixed mononuclear phagocytes, which results in hepatosplenomegaly. The liver, spleen, and lymph nodes are darkened ("slate gray") by macrophages filled with hemosiderin and malarial pigment, the endproduct of parasitic digestion of hemoglobin.

P. falciparum infestation produces **malignant malaria**, a particularly aggressive disease. Its activity is related, in large part, to the altered flow characteristics and adhesive properties of infected erythrocytes, which results in adherence of erythrocytes to endothelial cells of small blood vessels. Capillaries of deep organs, especially the brain, become obstructed, leading to ischemia of the brain, kidneys, and lungs. Brains of patients who die of cerebral malaria show congestion and thrombosis of small blood vessels in the white matter, which are rimmed with edema and hemorrhage ("ring hemorrhages") (Fig. 6-23). Obstruction of renal blood flow produces acute renal failure, whereas intravascular hemolysis results in hemoglobinuric nephrosis (**blackwater fever**). In the lung, damage to alveolar capillaries generates pulmonary edema and acute alveolar damage.

Toxoplasmosis

Toxoplasmosis is a worldwide infectious disease caused by a protozoan, *T. gondii*. Most infections are asymptomatic, but if they occur in a fetus or immunocompromised host, devastating necrotizing disease may result. *T. gondii* infects many mammals and birds as intermediate hosts. The domestic cat serves as final host when it becomes infected by ingesting *Toxoplasma* cysts. Therefore, cat feces may cause infection when oocysts contaminate the hands and food of people who live in close proximity to cats.

Toxoplasmosis may also be acquired by eating infectious forms of the organism, often by ingesting incompletely cooked meat (lamb and pork) that carries *Toxoplasma* tissue cysts. **Congenital infection** is acquired by transplacental transmission of infectious forms from an acutely infected (usually asymptomatic) mother to the fetus. Serious consequences are discussed in Chapter 5.

In most *T. gondii* infections, little tissue destruction occurs before the immune response brings the active phase of the infection under control. *T. gondii* establishes latent infection, however, by forming dormant tissue cysts in some infected cells, which survive for decades in host cells. If an infected person loses cell-mediated immunity, such as in AIDS, the organism can emerge from its encysted form and re-establish a destructive infection.

The brain is most commonly affected and exhibits a multifocal necrotizing encephalitis accompanied by paresis, seizures, alterations in visual acuity, and changes in mentation. *Toxoplasma* encephalitis in immunocompromised patients is fatal if not treated with antiprotozoal agents.

Enteric Protozoal Infections

Amebiasis

Amebiasis refers to infection with *E. histolytica*, which principally involves the colon. The parasite is named for its lytic actions on tissue. Intestinal infection ranges from asymptomatic colonization to severe invasive infection with bloody diarrhea. On occasion, the organisms spread beyond the colon to involve other organs, most commonly the liver. Humans are the only known reservoir for the organism, which reproduces in the colon and passes in the feces. Hence, amebiasis is acquired by ingestion of materials contaminated with human feces and is most common in areas with poor sanitation.

E. histolytica has distinct stages: the cyst, the precyst, and the trophozoite (see Fig. 6-24). **Cysts** are the infecting stage and are found only in stools because they do not invade tissue. Upon ingestion, cysts traverse the stomach and excyst in the lower ileum, where they form immature trophozoites, which then grow to full size. These organisms thrive in the colon with the cecum most often being affected, and feed on bacteria and human cells. The trophozoites develop into cysts through an intermediate form, the precyst. Patients with symptomatic disease pass both cysts and trophozoites, but only the former are infectious. Invasion begins with the attachment of a trophozoite to a colonic epithelial cell. The parasite kills target cells by elaborating a lytic protein that breaches the cell membrane. Lesions begin as small foci of necrosis, which progress to ulcers (Fig. 6-25A). Undermining of the ulcer margin and confluence of expanding ulcers lead to irregular sloughing of the mucosa. The ulcer bed is gray and necrotic and contains fibrin and cellular debris. The exudate

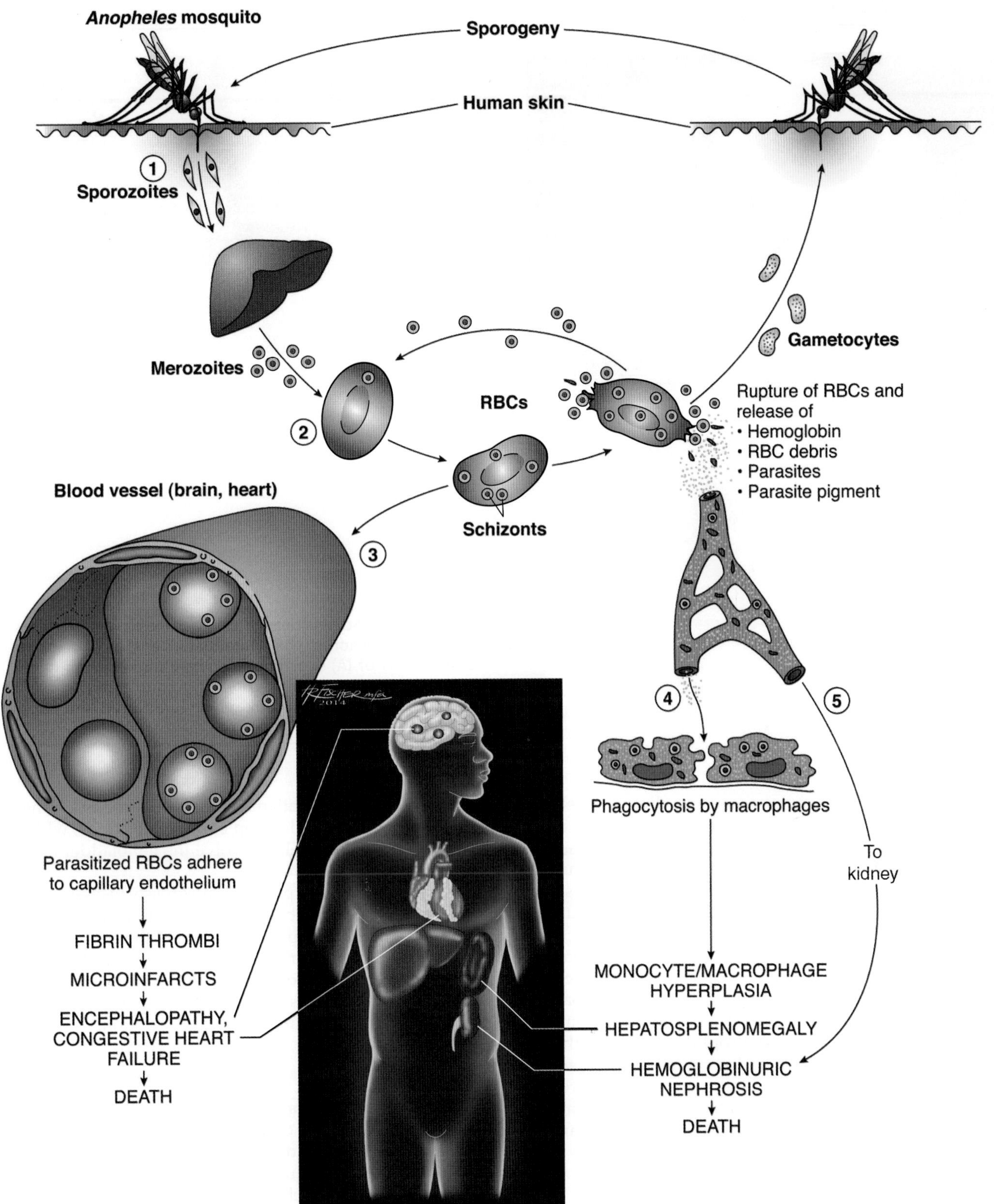

FIGURE 6-22. Life cycle of malaria. An *Anopheles* mosquito bites an infected person, taking blood that contains microgametocytes and macrogametocytes (sexual forms). In the mosquito, sexual multiplication (sporogony) produces infective sporozoites in the salivary glands. (*1*) During the mosquito bite, sporozoites are inoculated into the bloodstream of the vertebrate host. Some sporozoites leave the blood and enter the hepatocytes, where they multiply asexually (exoerythrocytic schizogony) and form thousands of uninucleated merozoites. (*2*) Rupture of hepatocytes releases merozoites, which penetrate erythrocytes and become trophozoites, which then divide to form numerous schizonts (intraerythrocytic schizogony). Schizonts divide to form more merozoites, which are released on the rupture of erythrocytes and re-enter other erythrocytes to begin a new cycle. After several cycles, subpopulations of merozoites develop into microgametocytes and macrogametocytes, which are taken up by another mosquito to complete the cycle. (*3*) Parasitized erythrocytes obstruct capillaries of the brain, heart, kidney, and other deep organs. Adherence of parasitized erythrocytes to capillary endothelial cells causes fibrin thrombi, which produce microinfarcts. These result in encephalopathy, congestive heart failure, pulmonary edema, and frequently death. Ruptured erythrocytes release hemoglobin, erythrocyte debris, and malarial pigment. (*4*) Phagocytosis leads to monocyte/macrophage hyperplasia and hepatosplenomegaly. (*5*) Released hemoglobin produces hemoglobinuric nephrosis, which may be fatal. RBCs, red blood cells.

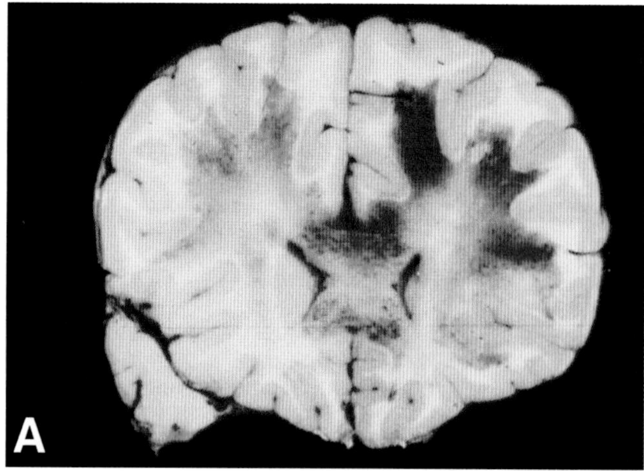

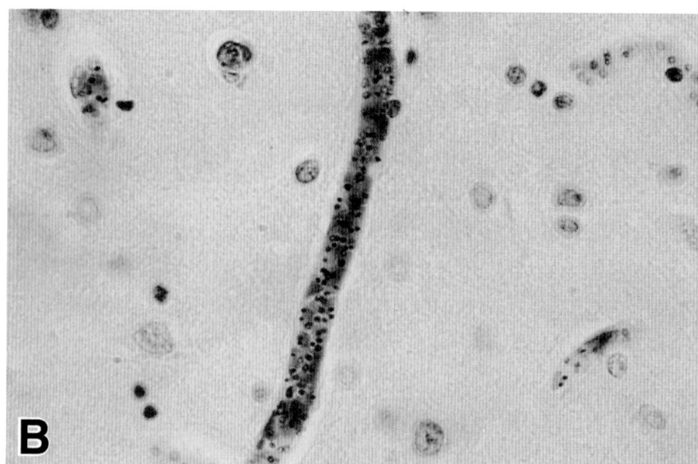

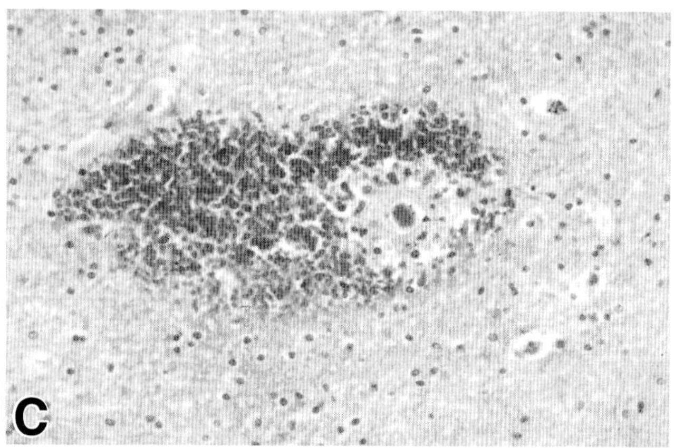

FIGURE 6-23. **Acute falciparum malaria of the brain. A.** There is severe diffuse congestion of the white matter and focal hemorrhages. **B.** A section of **(A)** showing a capillary packed with parasitized erythrocytes. **C.** Another section of **(A)** displaying a ring hemorrhage around a thrombosed capillary, which contains parasitized erythrocytes in a fibrin thrombus.

raises the undermined mucosa, causing chronic amebic ulcers, whose shape has been described as resembling a flask or a bottle neck. Trophozoites are found on the ulcer surface, in the exudate, and in the crater (Fig. 6-25B). They are also frequent in the submucosa, muscularis propria, serosa, and small veins of the submucosa. As ulcers enlarge, acute and chronic inflammatory cells accumulate.

Amebic liver abscesses form when trophozoites that have invaded submucosal veins of the colon enter the portal circulation, reach the liver, and kill hepatocytes. A slowly expanding necrotic cavity filled with a dark brown, odorless, semisolid material results (Fig. 6-26). Neutrophils are rare within the cavity, but trophozoites are found along the edges adjacent to hepatocytes. Amebic liver abscesses may expand or rupture through the capsule, resulting in infection extending into the peritoneum, diaphragm, pleural cavity, lungs, or pericardium.

Cryptosporidiosis

Cryptosporidiosis, an enteric infection with protozoa of the genus *Cryptosporidium*, can cause diarrhea, predominantly in persons with compromised immunity; it is a potentially life-threatening illness. The disease is acquired by ingesting *Cryptosporidium* oocysts, which are shed in the feces of infected humans and animals. The oocysts survive passage through the stomach and release forms that attach to the microvillus surface of the small bowel, while remaining extracellular. They reproduce on the luminal surface of the gut, from stomach to rectum, forming progeny that also attach to the epithelium. In immunocompetent people, infection is terminated by immune responses. Patients with AIDS and some congenital immunodeficiencies develop chronic infections, which may spread from the bowel to involve the gallbladder and intrahepatic bile ducts.

Cryptosporidiosis produces no grossly visible alterations. The organisms are visible microscopically as round, 2- to 4-µm blebs attached to the luminal surface of the epithelium. In the small intestine, moderate or severe chronic inflammation in the lamina propria and villous atrophy are directly related to the density of the parasites. The colon displays a chronic active colitis, with minimal architectural disruption.

Giardiasis

Giardiasis, an infection of the small intestine caused by the flagellated protozoan *Giardia lamblia*, is characterized by abdominal cramping and diarrhea.

The disorder is acquired by ingesting infectious cyst forms of the organism, which are shed in the feces of infected humans and animals. Infection spreads directly from person to person and also through contaminated water or food. *Giardia* is often acquired from wilderness water sources, where infected animals, such as beavers and bears, serve as the reservoir. Infection may be epidemic, and outbreaks have occurred in orphanages and institutions.

G. lamblia has two stages: trophozoites and cysts; the latter survive gastric acidity and rupture in the duodenum and jejunum to release trophozoites. These trophozoites attach to small bowel epithelial microvilli and reproduce. Giardiasis produces no grossly visible alterations. Microscopic examination

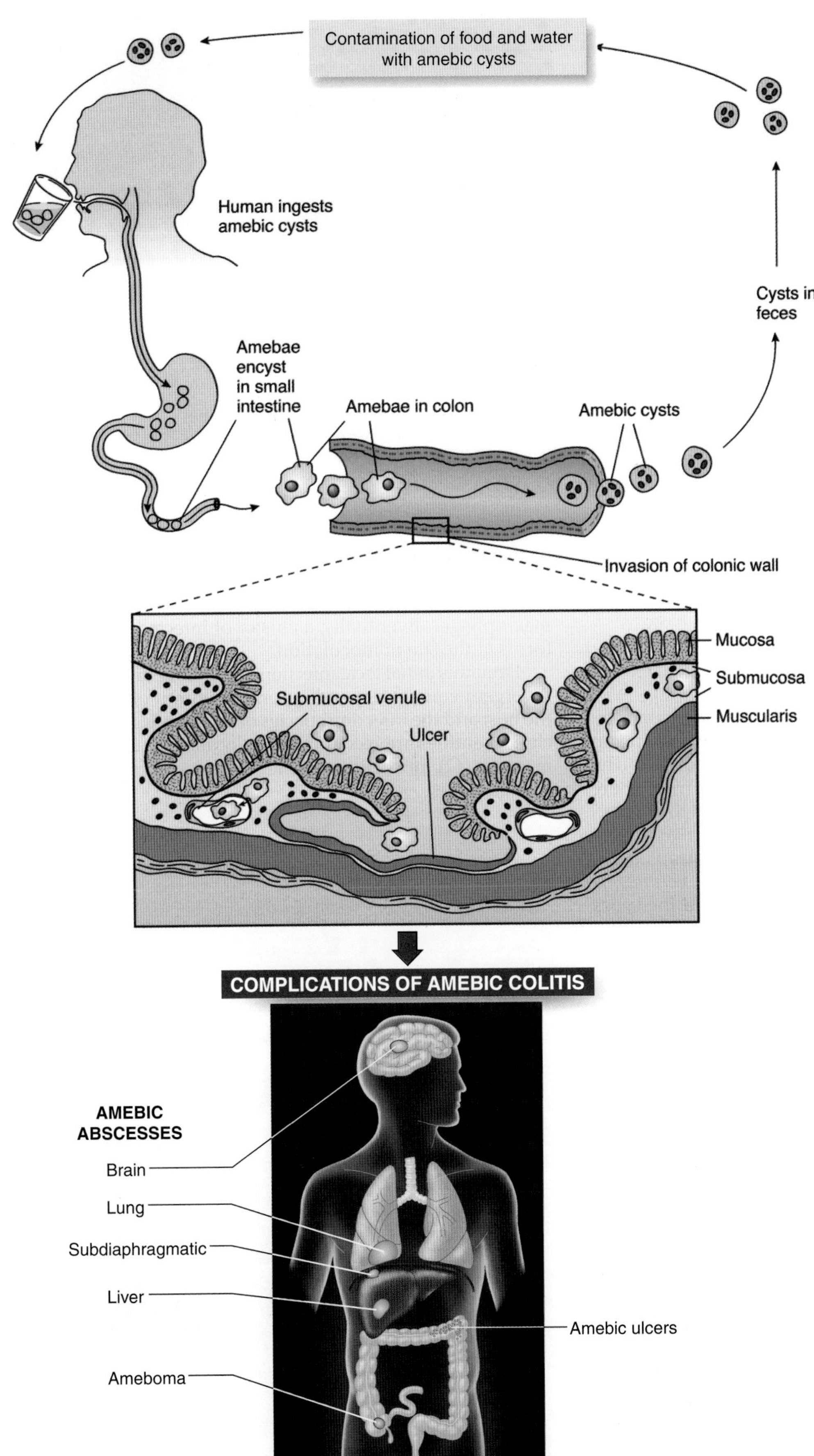

FIGURE 6-24. Amebic colitis and its complications. Amebiasis results from the ingestion of food or water contaminated with amebic cysts. In the colon, the amebae penetrate the mucosa and produce flask-shaped ulcers of the mucosa and submucosa. The organisms may invade submucosal venules, thereby disseminating the infection to the liver and other organs. The liver abscess can expand to involve adjacent structures.

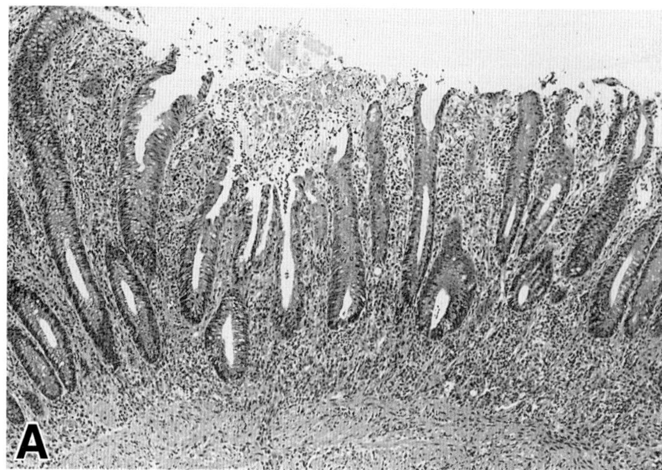

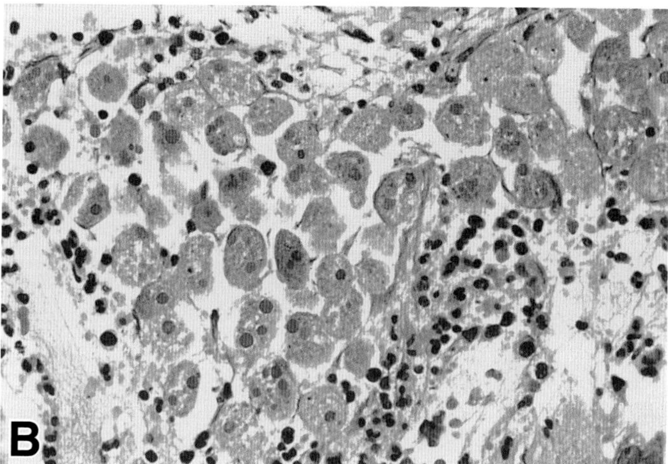

FIGURE 6-25. Intestinal amebiasis. A. The colonic mucosa showing superficial ulceration beneath a cluster of trophozoites of *Entamoeba histolytica.* The lamina propria contains excess acute and chronic inflammatory cells, including eosinophils. **B.** Higher power view showing numerous trophozoites in the luminal exudate.

shows minimal associated mucosal changes, with crescentic or semilunar-shaped *Giardia* trophozoites on villous surfaces and within crypts (Fig. 6-27). They are most numerous in the duodenum and proximal small intestine.

Leishmaniasis

Leishmanias are protozoans that are transmitted to humans by *Phlebotomus* sandflies, which acquire the agent by feeding on infected animals, including dogs and ground squirrels. The disease occurs most often in less developed countries where humans live in close proximity to animal hosts and the fly vector (Fig. 6-28). Leishmaniasis comprises a spectrum of clinical syndromes, from indolent, self-resolving cutaneous ulcers to fatal disseminated disease. There are numerous *Leishmania* species, which differ in their natural habitats and the types of disease that they produce.

Infection begins when the organisms are inoculated into human skin by a sandfly bite. The *Leishmanias* are phagocytosed by mononuclear phagocytes and transformed into amastigotes, which reproduce within the macrophage. Daughter amastigotes eventually rupture from the cell and spread to other macrophages. Eventually, a cluster of infected macrophages forms at the site of inoculation.

From this initial local infection, the disease may take widely divergent courses depending on the immunologic status of the host and the infecting species of *Leishmania.* Three distinct clinical entities are recognized: (1) localized cutaneous leishmaniasis, (2) mucocutaneous leishmaniasis, and (3) visceral leishmaniasis.

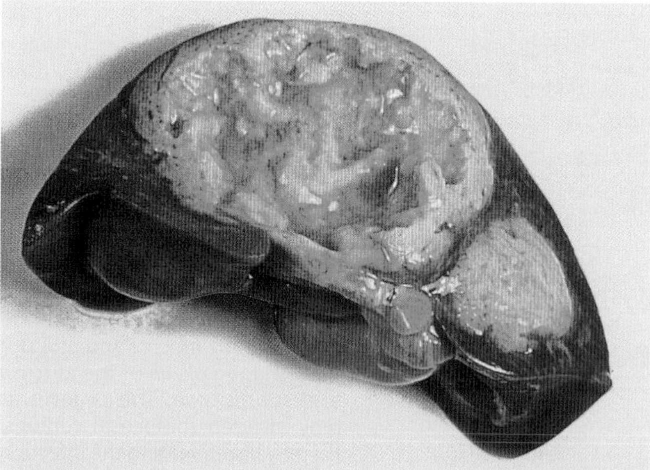

FIGURE 6-26. Amebic abscesses of the liver. The cut surface of the liver showing multiple abscesses containing "anchovy paste" material.

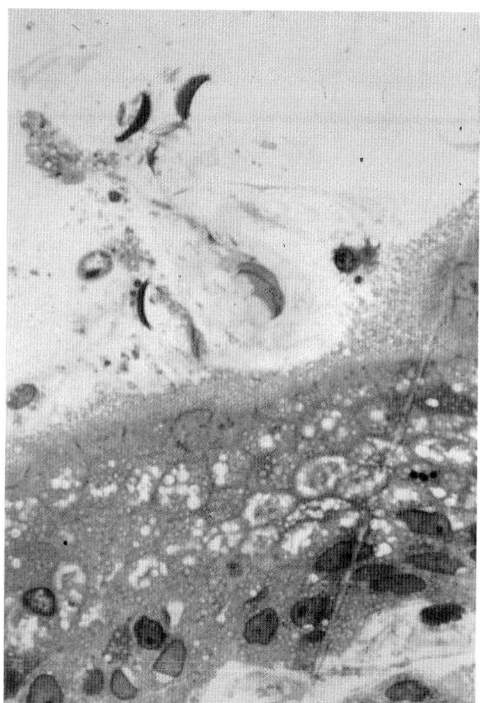

FIGURE 6-27. Giardiasis. Crescent-shaped trophozoites of *Giardia lamblia* are present overlying the small intestinal mucosa.

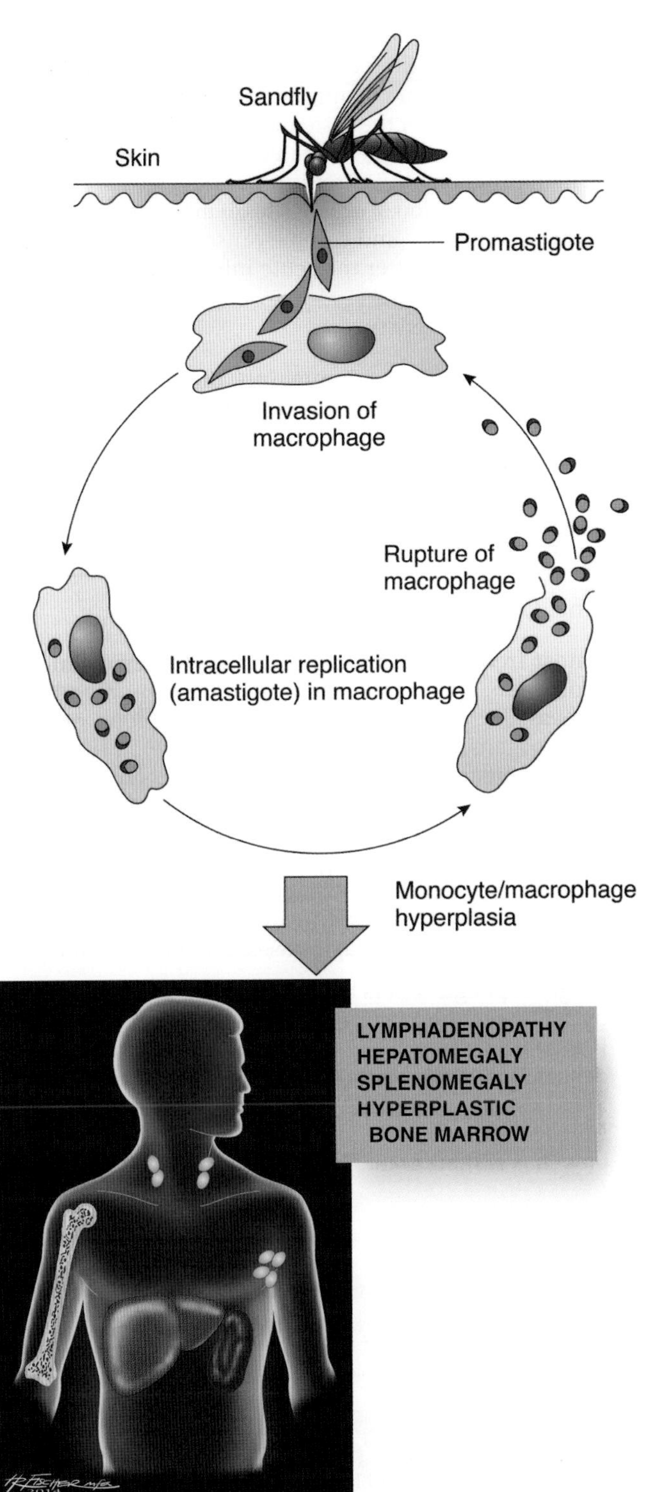

FIGURE 6-28. Leishmaniasis. Blood-sucking sandflies ingest amastigotes from an infected host. These are transformed in the sandfly gut into promastigotes, which multiply and are injected into the next vertebrate host. There they invade macrophages, revert to the amastigote form, and multiply, eventually rupturing the cell. They then invade other macrophages, thus completing the cycle.

Localized Cutaneous Leishmaniasis

Several *Leishmania* species in Central and South America, Northern Africa, the Middle East, India, and China cause a localized skin disease, also known as "oriental sore" or "tropical sore." The disease begins as a collection of amastigote-filled macrophages that ulcerate the overlying epidermis. In tissue sections, amastigotes in macrophages appear as multiple regular cytoplasmic dots, termed **Leishman–Donovan bodies**. With progressive development of cell-mediated immunity, macrophages are activated and kill the intracellular parasites. The lesion slowly becomes a more mature granuloma, with epithelioid macrophages, Langhans giant cells, plasma cells, and lymphocytes. Over the course of months, the cutaneous ulcer heals spontaneously.

Mucocutaneous Leishmaniasis

Mucocutaneous leishmaniasis is caused by infection with *Leishmania braziliensis*. Most cases occur in Central and South America, where rodents and sloths are reservoirs.

The early course and pathologic changes are similar to those of localized cutaneous leishmaniasis. A solitary ulcer appears, expands, and resolves. Years afterward, an ulcer develops at a mucocutaneous junction, such as the larynx, nasal septum, anus, or vulva. Although the mucosal lesion progresses slowly, it is highly destructive and disfiguring and erodes mucosal surfaces and cartilage (Fig. 6-29). Destruction of the nasal septum sometimes produces a "tapir nose" deformity. The patient may die if the ulcers obstruct the airways.

Visceral Leishmaniasis (Kala Azar)

Kala azar is produced by several subspecies of *Leishmania donovani*. Reservoirs of the agent and susceptible age groups vary in different parts of the world, including India and parts of Europe. Infection begins with localized collections of infected macrophages at the site of a sandfly bite (Fig. 6-28); the macrophages spread the organisms throughout the mononuclear phagocyte system. *L. donovani* are mostly destroyed by cell-mediated immune responses, but 5% of patients develop visceral leishmaniasis. Children and malnourished people are especially susceptible. The liver (Fig. 6-30A), spleen, and lymph nodes become massively enlarged because macrophages in these organs are filled with proliferating leishmanial amastigotes (Fig. 6-30B). Normal organ architecture is gradually replaced by sheets of parasitized macrophages. Eventually, these cells accumulate in other organs, including the heart and kidney. Light-skinned people develop a characteristic darkening of the skin; *kala azar* means "black sickness" in Hindi.

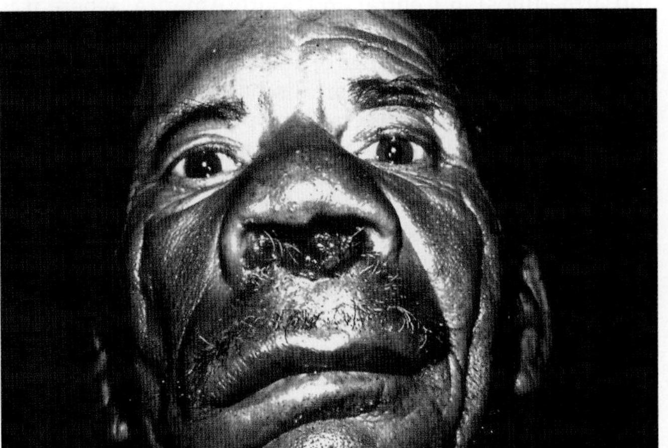

FIGURE 6-29. Mucocutaneous leishmaniasis. There is a complete destruction of the basal septum and mucocutaneous ulceration.

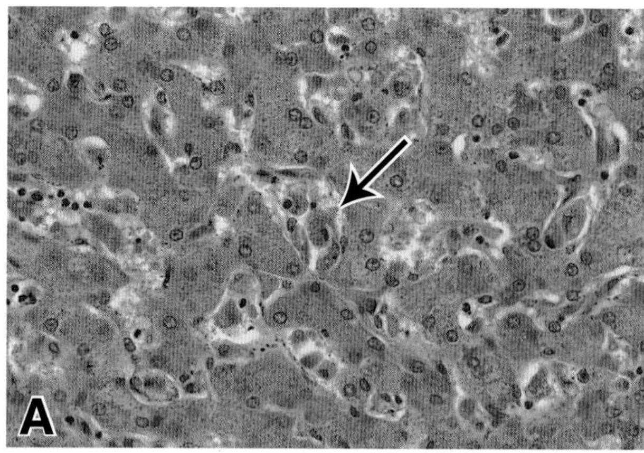

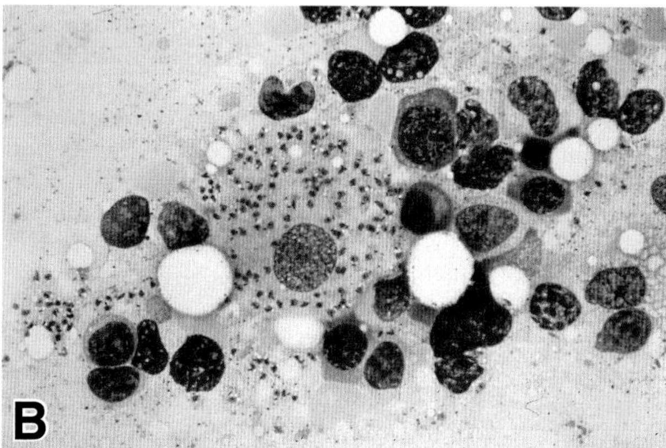

FIGURE 6-30. **Visceral leishmaniasis. A.** A photomicrograph of an enlarged liver showing prominent Kupffer cells distended by leishmanial amastigotes (*arrows*). **B.** A bone marrow aspirate from a patient with visceral leishmaniasis. Numerous leishmanial amastigotes are present, some of which are intracytoplasmic.

Chagas Disease (American Trypanosomiasis)

Chagas disease is an insect-borne, zoonotic infection by the protozoan *Trypanosoma cruzi*, which causes a systemic infection of humans. Acute manifestations and long-term sequelae occur in the heart and gastrointestinal tract. Infection is endemic in wild and domesticated animals (e.g., rats, dogs, goats, cats, and armadillos) in Central and South America, where it is transmitted to humans by the reduviid ("kissing") bug found in mud or thatched dwellings of the rural and suburban poor.

Infective forms of *T. cruzi* are discharged in the feces of the reduviid bug; itching and scratching promote contamination of the wound. The trypomastigotes penetrate at the site of the bite or at other abrasions, or may enter the mucosa of the eyes or lips. Once inside the body, they lose their flagella and undulating membranes, round up to become amastigotes, and enter macrophages, where they undergo repeated divisions. Amastigotes also invade other sites, including cardiac myocytes and brain. Within host cells, amastigotes differentiate into trypomastigotes, which break out and enter the bloodstream. There they are then ingested in a subsequent bite of a reduviid bug where they renew the cycle of infection.

T. cruzi infects and reproduces in cells at sites of inoculation, forming localized nodular inflammatory lesions, termed **chagomas**. The organism then disseminates throughout the body via the bloodstream. Strains of *T. cruzi* differ in their predominant target cells; infections of cardiac myocytes, gastrointestinal ganglion cells, and meninges cause the most significant disease. Parasitemia and widespread cellular infection are responsible for the systemic symptoms of acute Chagas disease. The onset of cell-mediated immunity eliminates the acute manifestations, but chronic tissue damage may continue. Progressive destruction of cells at sites of infection—particularly the heart, esophagus, and colon—causes organ dysfunction, manifested decades after the acute infection.

Acute Chagas Disease

Acute Chagas disease predominantly affects the heart, which is enlarged and dilated, with a pale, focally hemorrhagic myocardium. Many parasites are seen in the heart, and amastigotes are evident within pseudocysts in myofibers (Fig. 6-31) with results that may be lethal. Extensive chronic inflammation and phagocytosis of parasites are conspicuous. Lethal meningeal involvement may also occur.

Chronic Chagas Disease

The most frequent and serious consequences of infection develop years after acute infection. In the chronic phase of the illness, *T. cruzi* is no longer present in blood or tissue. Infected organs have been damaged, however, by chronic, progressive inflammation. Chronic myocarditis is characterized by a dilated heart, which demonstrates extensive interstitial fibrosis, hypertrophied myofibers, and focal lymphocytic inflammation, often involving the cardiac conduction system. In endemic regions, chronic Chagas disease is a leading cause of dysrhythmia and heart failure in young adults. Conditions associated with chronic Chagas disease include the following:

- **Megaesophagus** refers to dilation of the esophagus caused by failure of the lower esophageal sphincter (achalasia). It is common in chronic Chagas disease and results from destruction of parasympathetic ganglia in the wall of the lower esophagus, leading to difficulty in swallowing.
- **Megacolon,** which refers to massive dilation of the large bowel, is similar to megaesophagus in that the myenteric

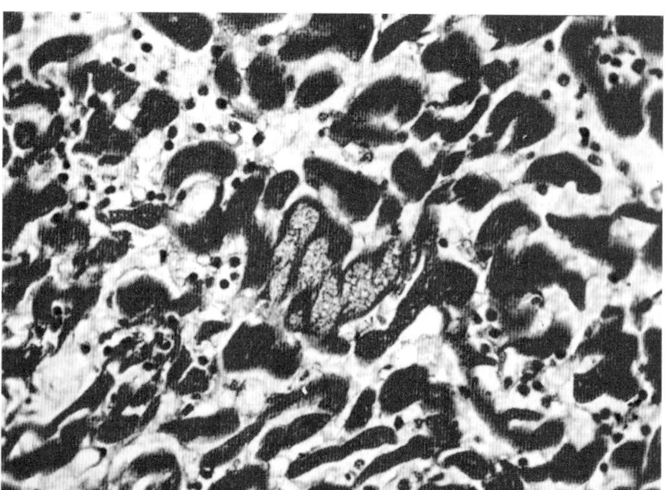

FIGURE 6-31. **Acute Chagas myocarditis.** The myofibers in the center contain numerous amastigotes of *Trypanosoma cruzi* and are surrounded by edema and chronic inflammation.

plexus of the colon is destroyed. The progressive aganglionosis of the colon causes severe constipation.

- **Congenital Chagas disease** occurs in some pregnant women with parasitemia. Infection of the placenta and fetus leads to spontaneous abortion. In the infrequent live births, the infants die of encephalitis within a few days or weeks.

African Trypanosomiasis

African trypanosomiasis, popularly termed **sleeping sickness**, is an infection with *Trypanosoma brucei gambiense* or *Trypanosoma brucei rhodesiense*, which gives rise to life-threatening meningoencephalitis. The protozoa are transmitted by several species of blood-sucking tsetse flies of the genus *Glossina*. Humans are the only important reservoir for this trypanosome.

Gambian trypanosomiasis is a chronic infection often lasting more than a year. By contrast, East African (Rhodesian) trypanosomiasis is a rapidly progressive infection that kills the patient in 3 to 6 months. The organisms are curved flagellates, 15 to 30 μm in length. Although they can be demonstrated in blood or cerebrospinal fluid, they are difficult to find in infected tissues.

Trypanosomes have a complex life cycle that commences with the fly biting an infected animal or human after which it ingests trypomastigotes with the donor blood (Fig. 6-32). The organisms multiply in the fly's saliva as infective metacyclic trypomastigotes, which are then injected into the lymphatics and blood vessels of a new host. After disseminating in the bone marrow and tissue fluids, some eventually invade the CNS. After replicating by binary fission in the blood, lymph, and spinal fluid, trypomastigotes are ingested by another fly to complete the cycle.

African trypanosomiasis involves immune complex formation by trypanosomal antigens and antibodies. Autoantibodies to antigens of the erythrocytes, brain, and heart may participate in the pathogenesis of this disease. The trypanosome evades immune attack in mammals by periodically altering its glycoprotein antigen coat. Thus, each wave of circulating trypomastigotes features different antigenic variants which keep a step ahead of the immune response.

T. brucei multiplies at sites of inoculation, occasionally producing localized nodular lesions, termed "primary chancres." Generalized involvement of the lymph nodes and spleen is prominent early in the disease. Affected nodes and spleen show foci of lymphocyte and macrophage hyperplasia. Infection eventually localizes to small blood vessels of the CNS, where replicating organisms elicit a destructive vasculitis with endothelial cell hyperplasia and dense perivascular infiltrates of lymphocytes, macrophages, and plasma cells, which causes destruction of neurons, demyelination, and gliosis. The result is a progressive decrease in mentation characteristic of sleeping sickness (Fig. 6-33). In *T. brucei rhodesiense* infection, the organisms also localize to blood vessels in the heart, sometimes causing a fulminant myocarditis.

Primary Amebic Meningoencephalitis

Amebic meningoencephalitis is a fatal illness caused by *Naegleria fowleri*, a free-living, ameba that inhabits ponds and lakes. Although rare, several recent outbreaks have been reported in the United States. These affected people who swam or bathed in water containing high concentrations of the organism. *N. fowleri* is inoculated into the nasal mucosa when a person swims or dives. Amebae invade the olfactory nerves, migrate into

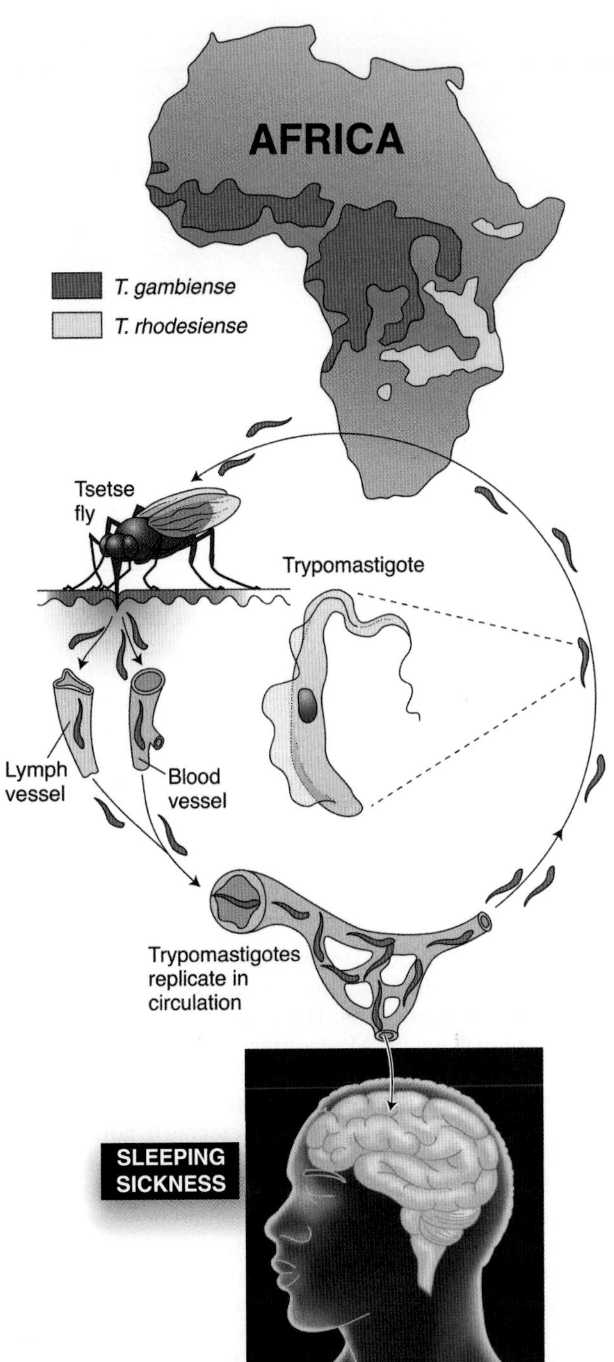

FIGURE 6-32. African trypanosomiasis (sleeping sickness). The distribution of Gambian and Rhodesian trypanosomiasis is related to the habitats of the vector tsetse flies (*Glossina* spp.). A tsetse fly bites an infected animal or human and ingests trypomastigotes, which multiply into infective, metacyclic trypomastigotes. During another fly bite, these are injected into lymphatic and blood vessels of a new host. A primary chancre develops at the site of the bite (stage 1a). Trypomastigotes replicate further in the blood and lymph, causing a systemic infection (stage 1b). Another fly ingests hypomastigotes to complete the cycle. In stage 2, invasion of the central nervous system by trypomastigotes leads to meningoencephalomyelitis and associated symptoms, including lethargy and daytime somnolence. Patients with Rhodesian trypanosomiasis may die within a few months. *T. gambiense*, *Trypanosoma brucei gambiense*; *T. rhodesiense*, *Trypanosoma brucei rhodesiense*.

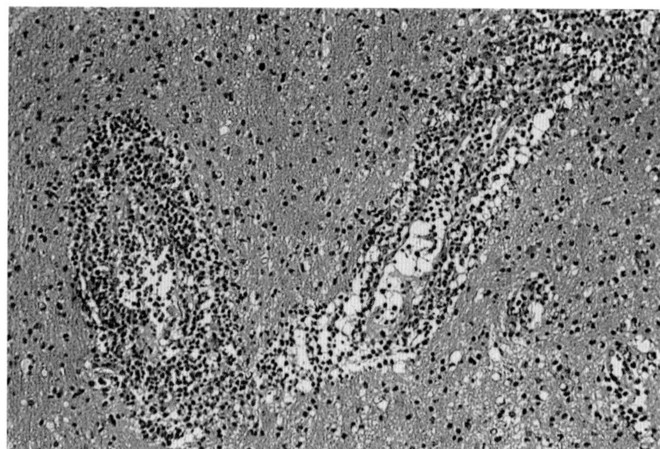

FIGURE 6-33. African trypanosomiasis. A section of brain from a patient who died from infection with *Trypanosoma brucei rhodesiense* showing a perivascular mononuclear cell infiltrate.

the olfactory bulbs, and then proliferate in the meninges and brain. The brain is swollen and soft, with vascular congestion and a purulent meningeal exudate. The amebae invade the brain along the Virchow-Robin spaces and cause massive tissue damage. The olfactory tract and bulbs are enveloped and destroyed, and there is an exudate between the bulb and the inferior surface of the temporal lobe. Meningitis can extend the full length of the spinal cord. The disease is rapidly fatal.

HELMINTHIC INFECTION

Helminths, or worms, the largest and most complex organisms capable of living within the human body, are among the most common human pathogens. Their adult forms range from 0.5 mm to over 1 m in length. Most are visible to the naked eye. They are multicellular animals with differentiated tissues, including specialized nervous tissues, digestive tissues, and reproductive systems. Their maturation from eggs or larvae to adult worms is complex, often involving multiple morphologic transformations (molts). Some undergo these metamorphoses in different hosts before attaining adulthood, and the human host may be only one in a series that supports this maturation process. Within the human body, the helminths frequently migrate from the port of entry through several organs to a site of final infection. Most helminths that infect humans are well adapted to human parasitism, causing limited or no host tissue damage. With few exceptions, they do not multiply in the human body.

Helminths cause disease in various ways. A few compete with their human host for certain nutrients. Some grow to block vital structures, producing disease by mass effect. Most, however, cause dysfunction by eliciting destructive inflammatory and immunologic responses. For example, morbidity in schistosomiasis, the most destructive helminthic infection, results from granulomatous responses to schistosome eggs deposited in tissue. Helminths include both roundworms and flatworms. Eosinophils contain basic proteins toxic to some helminths and are a major component of inflammatory responses to these organisms. Parasitic helminths are categorized based on overall morphology and the structure their digestive tissues.

- **Roundworms (nematodes)** are elongate cylindrical organisms with tubular digestive tracts.
- **Flatworms (trematodes)** are dorsoventrally flattened organisms with digestive tracts that end in blind loops.
- **Tapeworms (cestodes)** are segmented organisms with separate head and body parts; they lack a digestive tract and absorb nutrients through their outer walls.

Filarial Nematodes

Lymphatic Filariasis

Lymphatic filariasis (Bancroftian and Malayan filariasis) is an inflammatory parasitic infection of lymphatic vessels caused by the roundworms *Wuchereria bancrofti* and *Brugia malayi*. Infection with the former is widespread in southern Asia, the Pacific, Africa, and parts of South America. The latter infection is localized to coastal southern Asia and western Pacific islands. These and similar organisms are known as filarial worms because of their thread-like appearance.

Humans, the only definitive host of these filarial nematodes, acquire infection from the bites of several genera of mosquitoes. The insects transmit infectious larvae, which then migrate to lymphatics and lymph nodes. After maturing into adult forms over several months, worms mate, and the female releases microfilariae into lymphatics and the bloodstream. Adult worms inhabit the lymphatics, most frequently in inguinal, epitrochlear, and axillary lymph nodes, testis, and epididymis. There they cause acute lymphangitis and, in a minority of infected subjects, lymphatic obstruction, which leads to severe lymphedema. In its most severe form, the condition is known as elephantiasis. The manifestations of filariasis result from inflammatory responses to degenerating adult worms in the lymphatics, which appear dilated, with a thickened endothelial lining. In adjacent tissues, worms are surrounded by chronic inflammation, including eosinophils and, at times, a granulomatous reaction. After repeated bouts of lymphangitis, lymph nodes and lymphatics become densely fibrotic, often containing calcified remnants of the worms.

Other Filarial Diseases

Onchocerciasis

Onchocerciasis ("river blindness") is a chronic inflammatory disease of the skin, eyes, and lymphatics caused by the filarial nematode *Onchocerca volvulus*, transmitted by bites of blackflies. Adult worms live as coiled tangled masses, termed onchocercal nodules, in the deep dermis and subcutis over bony prominences of the skull, scapula, ribs, iliac crest, trochanter, sacrum, and knee. They do not cause tissue damage or elicit inflammatory responses. However, gravid females release millions of microfilariae, which migrate into the skin, eyes, lymph nodes, and deep organs, producing corresponding onchocercal lesions. Ocular onchocerciasis results from migration of microfilariae into all regions of the eye, from the cornea to the optic nerve head. When microfilariae die, they incite vigorous inflammatory and immune responses. Inflammatory damage to the cornea, choroid, or retina causes partial or total loss of vision.

Loiasis

Loiasis is an infection by the filarial nematode *Loa loa*, the African "eyeworm," which is prevalent in the rain forests of Central and West Africa. Humans and baboons are the definitive hosts, and infection is transmitted by mango flies. Adult worms (4 cm long) migrate in the skin and, occasionally, cross the eye beneath the conjunctiva, making the patient acutely aware of this infection (Fig. 6-34). Gravid worms discharge microfilariae, which circulate in the blood during the day but reside in capillaries of the skin, lungs, and other organs at night. Migrating worms cause no inflammation, but static ones are surrounded by eosinophils, other inflammatory cells, and a foreign-body giant cell reaction. Rarely, those infected may develop acute generalized loiasis, characterized by obstructive fibrin thrombi, containing degenerating microfilariae in small vessels of most organs. Brain involvement, with obstruction of vessels by filarial thrombi, may cause lethal and sudden diffuse cerebral ischemia.

Intestinal Nematodes

The adult forms of several nematode species (Table 6-8) reside in the human bowel, but rarely cause symptomatic disease. Clinical symptoms occur almost exclusively in patients with very large numbers of worms or who are immunocompromised. Heavy infections may be complicated by vomiting, malnutrition, and sometimes intestinal obstruction; in the case of hookworm infection, blood loss and anemia are common (Fig. 6-35). Humans are the exclusive or primary hosts for all of intestinal nematodes. Infection spreads from person to person via eggs or larvae passed in the stool or deposited in the perianal region. Infection is most prevalent in settings where handwashing and hygienic disposal of feces are lacking (e.g., less developed countries). Warm, moist climates are required for the infectious forms of many intestinal nematodes to survive outside the body. These worms are, thus, endemic in tropical and subtropical climates.

Table 6-8

Intestinal Nematodes

Species	Common Name	Site of Adult Worm	Clinical Manifestations
Ascaris lumbricoides	Roundworm	Small bowel	Allergic reactions to lung migration; intestinal obstruction
Ancylostoma duodenale	Hookworm	Small bowel	Allergic reactions to cutaneous inoculation and lung migration; intestinal blood loss
Necator americanus	Hookworm	Small bowel	Allergic reactions to cutaneous inoculation and lung migration; intestinal blood loss
Trichuris trichiura	Whipworm	Large bowel	Abdominal pain and diarrhea; rectal prolapse (rare)
Strongyloides stercoralis	Threadworm	Small bowel	Abdominal pain and diarrhea; dissemination to extraintestinal sites in immunocompromised persons
Enterobius vermicularis	Pinworm	Cecum, appendix	Perianal and perineal itching

Tissue Nematodes

Trichinosis

Humans acquire trichinosis by eating inadequately cooked meat that contains encysted *Trichinella spiralis* larvae. The larvae are found in the skeletal muscles of various carnivorous or omnivorous wild and domesticated animals, including pigs, rats, bears, and walruses. Pork and improperly processed game are the most common sources of human trichinosis (Fig. 6-36).

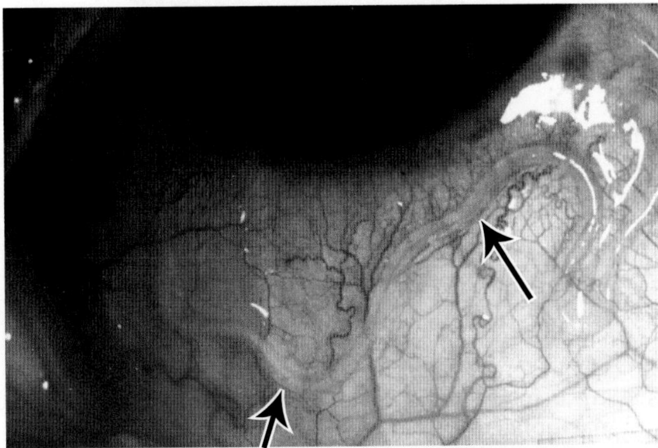

FIGURE 6-34. Loiasis. A thread-like *Loa loa* (*arrows*) is migrating in the subconjunctival tissues. From Farrar WE, Wood MJ, Innes JA, Tubbs H. *Infectious Diseases Text and Color Atlas*. 2nd ed. New York, NY: Gower Medical Publishing, 1992.

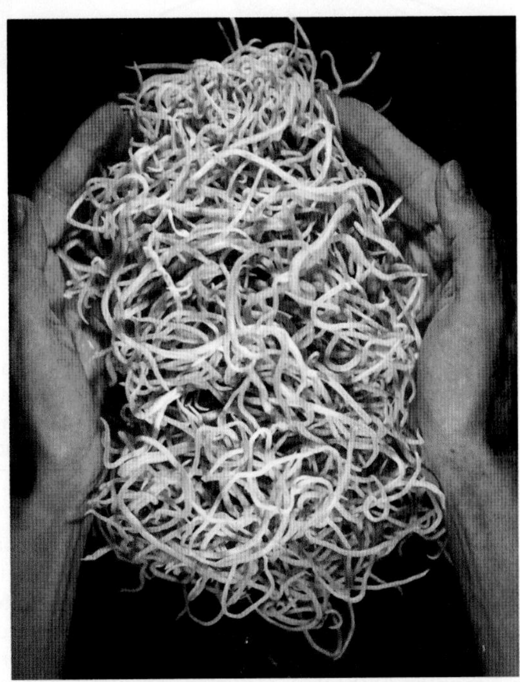

FIGURE 6-35. Ascariasis. This mass of over 800 worms of *Ascaris lumbricoides* obstructed and infarcted the ileum of a 2-year-old girl in South Africa.

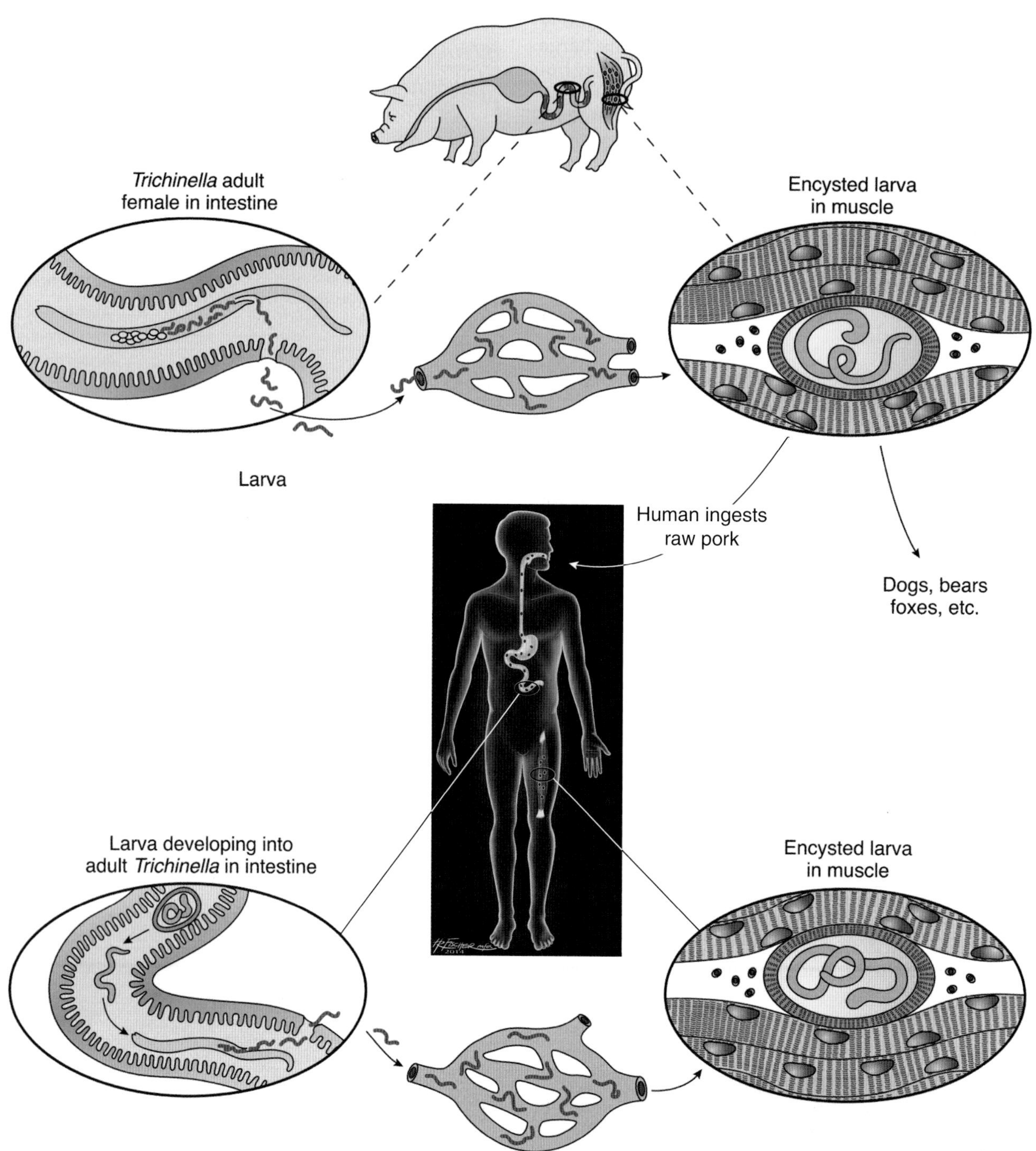

FIGURE 6-36. Trichinosis. After being ingested by the pig, cysts of *Trichinella* are digested in the gastrointestinal tract, liberating larvae that mature to adult worms. Female worms release larvae that penetrate the intestinal wall, enter the circulation, and lodge in striated muscle, where they encyst. When humans ingest inadequately cooked pork, the cycle is repeated, resulting in the muscle disease characteristic of trichinosis.

In the small bowel, *T. spiralis* larvae emerge from the ingested tissue cysts and burrow into the intestinal mucosa, where they develop into adult worms. The adults mate, and the female liberates larvae that invade the intestinal wall and enter the circulation. Production of larvae may continue for 1 to 4 months, until the worms are finally expelled from the intestine. The larvae can invade nearly any tissue but survive only in striated skeletal muscle, where they encyst and remain viable for years. When a larva infects a myocyte, the cell undergoes basophilic degeneration and swelling, eliciting an intense inflammatory infiltrate rich in eosinophils and macrophages. Eosinophilia may be extreme (over 50% of all leukocytes).

Larvae grow to 10 times their initial size, fold on themselves, and develop a capsule. Inflammation then subsides, and after years, the larvae die, and the cysts calcify. The resulting

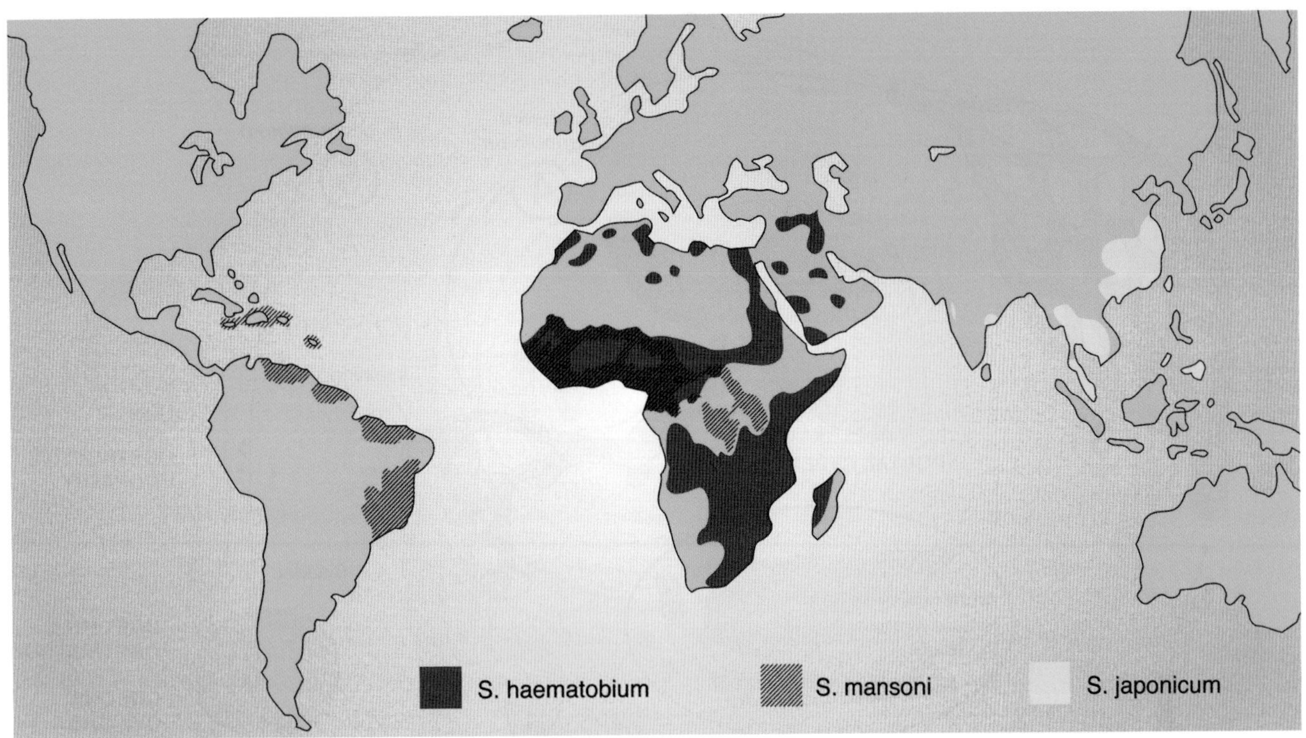

FIGURE 6-37. Distribution of schistosomiasis caused by ***Schistosoma mansoni, Schistosoma haematobium,*** and ***Schistosoma japonicum***.

myositis is especially prominent in the diaphragm, extrinsic ocular muscles, tongue, intercostal muscles, gastrocnemius, and deltoids. Sometimes the CNS or heart is also inflamed, causing meningoencephalitis or myocarditis. Several years later, the larvae die, and the cysts calcify.

Trematodes (Flukes)

Schistosomiasis

Schistosomiasis (bilharziasis) is the most important human helminthic disease, causing greater morbidity and mortality than all other worm infections. Intense inflammatory and immune responses damage the liver, intestine, or urinary bladder. Three species of schistosomes, namely, *Schistosoma mansoni*, *Schistosoma haematobium*, and *Schistosoma japonicum*, are the causative agents, which are found in distinct geographic regions, as dictated by the distribution of their specific host snail species (Fig. 6-37).

Schistosomes have complicated life cycles, alternating between asexual generations in their invertebrate host (snail) and sexual generations in the vertebrate host (for details, see Fig. 6-38). Female *S. mansoni* and *S. japonicum* deposit eggs in intestinal venules, whereas *S. haematobium* lays eggs in those of the urinary bladder. Embryos develop as the eggs pass through these tissues. When larvae are mature, eggs pass through the wall of the intestine or the bladder and are discharged in feces or urine.

The tissue lesions are circumscribed granulomas or a cellular infiltrate of eosinophils and neutrophils around an egg, which obstruct microvascular blood flow and produce ischemic damage to adjacent tissue. The result is progressive scarring and dysfunction in affected organs.

The site of involvement is determined by the tropism of the particular schistosome species.

- *S. mansoni* inhabits the branches of the inferior mesenteric vein, thereby affecting the distal colon and liver.
- *S. haematobium* winds its way to the veins serving the rectum, bladder, and pelvic organs.
- *S. japonicum* deposits eggs predominantly in the branches of the superior mesenteric vein, thereby damaging the small bowel, ascending colon, and liver.

Liver disease caused by *S. mansoni* or *S. japonicum* begins as periportal granulomatous inflammation (Fig. 6-39) and progresses to dense periportal fibrosis (pipestem fibrosis). In severe hepatic schistosomiasis, obstruction of portal blood flow and portal hypertension are prominent. *S. mansoni* and *S. japonicum* also damage the intestine, where granulomatous responses produce inflammatory polyps and foci of mucosal and submucosal fibrosis.

In urogenital schistosomiasis, caused by *S. haematobium*, eggs are most numerous in the bladder, ureter, and seminal vesicles, although they may also reach the lungs, colon, and appendix. Eggs in the bladder and ureters provoke a granulomatous reaction, inflammatory protuberances, and patches of mucosal and mural fibrosis, which may obstruct urine flow and cause secondary inflammatory damage. Bladder disease produced by *S. haematobium* is a cause of squamous cell carcinoma of the bladder. In areas where *S. haematobium* is prevalent, this is the most common form of cancer.

Clonorchiasis

Clonorchiasis is an infection of the hepatic biliary system by the Chinese liver fluke, *Clonorchis sinensis*. Although the

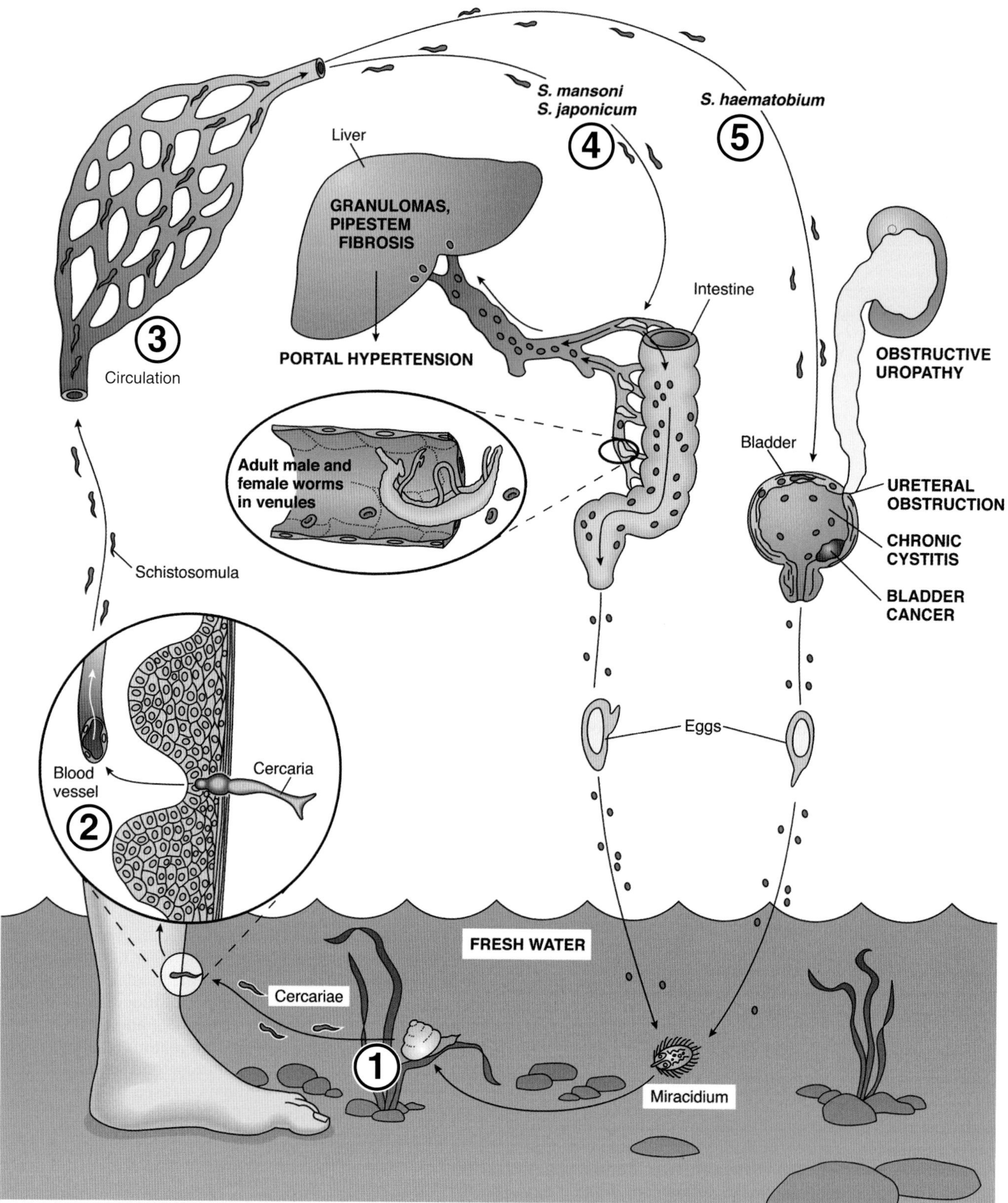

FIGURE 6-38. Life cycle of *Schistosoma* and clinical features of schistosomiasis. The schistosome egg hatches in water, liberates a miracidium that penetrates a snail, and develops through two stages to a sporocyst to form the final larval stage, the cercaria. (*1*) The cercaria escapes from the snail into water, "swims," and penetrates the skin of a human host. (*2*) The cercaria loses its forked tail to become a schistosomulum, which migrates through tissues, penetrates a blood vessel, and (*3*) is carried to the lung and later to the liver. In hepatic portal venules, the schistosomula become sexually mature and form pairs, each with a male and a female worm, the female worm lying in the gynecophoral canal of the male worm. The organism causes lesions in the liver, including granulomas, portal ("pipestem") fibrosis, and portal hypertension. (*4*) The female worm deposits immature eggs in small venules of the intestine and rectum (*Schistosoma mansoni* and *Schistosoma japonicum*) or (*5*) of the urinary bladder (*Schistosoma haematobium*). The bladder infestation leads to obstructive uropathy, ureteral obstruction, chronic cystitis, and bladder cancer. Embryos develop during passage of the eggs through tissues, and larvae are mature when eggs pass through the wall of the intestine or urinary bladder. Eggs hatch in water and liberate miracidia to complete the cycle.

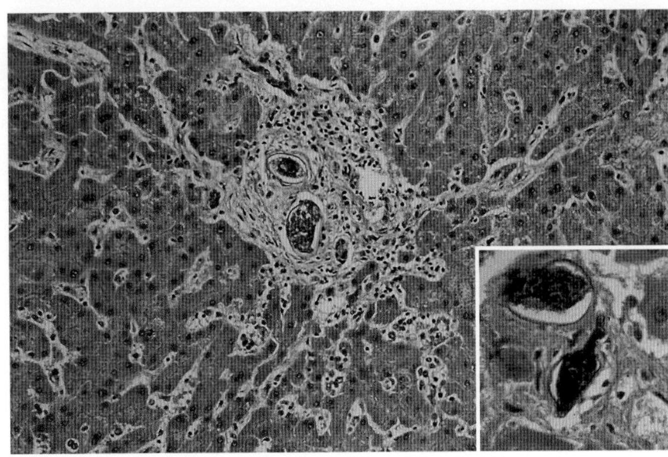

FIGURE 6-39. Hepatic schistosomiasis. A hepatic granuloma surrounds a degenerating egg of *Schistosoma mansoni*. A higher power of the organism is shown in the inset.

fluke usually causes only mild symptoms, it is sometimes associated with bile duct stones, cholangitis, and bile duct cancer.

The disease is endemic in East Asia, where it is acquired by ingesting inadequately cooked freshwater fish containing *C. sinensis* larvae. The larvae emerge in the duodenum, enter the common bile duct through the ampulla of Vater, eliciting an inflammatory response that does not eliminate the worm, but causes dilation and fibrosis of the ducts. Sometimes the worms cause calculus formation in the hepatic bile ducts, leading to ductal obstruction. The adult *Clonorchis* persists in the ducts for decades, and long-standing infection is associated with an increased incidence of bile duct cancer (cholangiocarcinoma).

In heavy infections, the liver may be greater than three times its normal size. In such cases, the liver is punctuated with thick-walled dilated bile ducts. Microscopically, the epithelial duct lining is initially hyperplastic and then metaplastic with surrounding stroma becoming fibrotic.

Table 6-9

Tapeworm Infections

Species	Human Disease	Source of Human Infection
Taenia saginata	Adult tapeworm in intestine	Beef
Taenia solium	Adult tapeworm in intestine; cysticercosis	Pork, human feces
Diphyllobothrium latum	Adult tapeworm in intestine	Fish
Echinococcus granulosus	Hydatid cyst disease	Dog feces

Cestodes: Intestinal Tapeworms

Taenia saginata, *Taenia solium*, and *Diphyllobothrium latum* are tapeworms that infect humans, growing to their adult forms within the intestine (Table 6-9). The presence of these adult worms rarely damages the human host.

Infections are acquired by eating inadequately cooked beef (*T. saginata*), pork (*T. solium*), or fish (*D. latum*) containing larvae. Tapeworm life cycles involve cystic larval stages in animals and worm stages in the human. The life cycles of beef and pork tapeworms require that the animals ingest material tainted with infected human feces. The cystic larval forms develop in the animals' muscles. Modern cattle and pig farming practices, plus meat inspection, have largely eliminated beef and pork tapeworms in industrialized countries, but infection remains common in the underdeveloped world. Fish tapeworm infection is prevalent in areas where raw, pickled, or partly cooked freshwater fish is common fare. Tapeworm infections are usually asymptomatic. The fish tapeworm (*D. latum*) takes up vitamin B_{12}, and a small number ($<2\%$) of infected persons develop pernicious anemia.

7 The Amyloidoses

Philip Hawkins

LEARNING OBJECTIVES

- List the common biochemical properties of amyloidogenic proteins.
- What physiologic circumstances further the deposition of amyloid?
- How is amyloid deposition in tissue detected?
- Define and characterize AA amyloidosis, AL amyloidosis, and ATTR amyloidosis. What is the nature of the amyloid protein deposited in each case, and what organ systems are most often affected?

CONSTITUENTS OF AMYLOID

Amyloid refers to a group of diverse extracellular protein deposits that have (1) common morphologic properties, (2) affinities for specific dyes, and (3) a characteristic appearance under polarized light. All proteins that form amyloid are folded, so as to share common ultrastructural and physical properties, despite different amino acid sequences. **Amyloidosis** encompasses the clinical disorders caused by localized or systemic amyloid deposition. Protein misfolding and aggregation are increasingly being recognized in various other diseases. However, amyloidosis—the disease directly caused by extracellular amyloid deposition—is a precise term with critical implications for patients with a specific group of life-threatening disorders.

More than 25 different unrelated proteins can form amyloid in vivo, and clinical amyloidosis is classified by the identity of the fibril protein. Amyloid deposition is remarkably diverse; it can be systemic or localized, acquired or hereditary, life-threatening or merely incidental. Clinical consequences occur when amyloid accumulates sufficiently to disrupt the structure of tissues or organs and to impair function. Patterns of organ involvement vary among the amyloidoses, but clinical phenotypes overlap greatly. In **systemic amyloidosis**, virtually any tissue may be involved. This form of the disease is often fatal, although prognosis has improved owing to better treatments for many of the underlying conditions. **Localized amyloid deposits** are confined to a particular organ or tissue and range from being clinically silent to life-threatening (e.g., cardiac amyloidosis). In addition to clinical disorders classified as amyloidoses, localized amyloid deposits are seen in other important disorders, including Alzheimer disease (see Chapter 24), prion disorders, and pancreatic islets in type 2 diabetes mellitus (see Chapter 19).

MOLECULAR PATHOGENESIS: Amyloid-forming proteins can exist in two different stable structures: (1) **a native form** and (2) massive refolding of the native form into predominantly **β-sheets** that can autoaggregate in a highly ordered manner to produce characteristic fibrils. Such amyloid fibrils are rigid, nonbranching, 10 to 15 nm in diameter, and indeterminate in length. Acquired biophysical properties that are common to all amyloid fibrils include (1) insolubility in physiologic solutions, (2) relative resistance to proteolysis, and (3) the ability to bind **Congo red dye** in a spatially ordered manner to produce the diagnostic green birefringence under cross-polarized light (Fig. 7-1).

There are several circumstances in which amyloid deposition occurs (Fig. 7-2):

- ***Sustained, abnormally high abundance of certain proteins that are normally present at low levels.*** Examples are serum amyloid A (SAA) protein in chronic inflammation and β_2-microglobulin in renal failure, which underlie susceptibility to AA and Aβ_2M amyloidosis, respectively (see below).
- ***Normal concentrations of a normal, but to some extent inherently amyloidogenic, protein over a prolonged period.*** Transthyretin in senile amyloidosis (ATTR) and β-protein in Alzheimer disease are prototypes.
- ***Presence of an acquired or inherited variant protein with an abnormal, markedly amyloidogenic structure.*** There are certain monoclonal immunoglobulin light chains in AL amyloidosis and genetic amyloidogenic variants of transthyretin, lysozyme, apolipoprotein AI, and fibrinogen A α-chain in hereditary amyloidosis.

Although it is not clear why only the 20 or so known amyloidogenic proteins adopt amyloid folding and persist as fibrils in vivo, a unifying theme is that amyloid precursors are relatively unstable. Even under normal physiologic conditions, these proteins can exist in partly unfolded states. They lose tertiary structure but retain β-sheet secondary structure, and can autoaggregate into protofilaments and thence mature amyloid fibrils.

Amyloid deposits not only consist mainly of these protein fibrils but also contain some common minor constituents, including certain **glycosaminoglycans (GAGs)**, the normal plasma protein **serum amyloid P component (SAP)**, and various other trace proteins, such as **apolipoprotein E (apoE)**, **laminin**, and **collagen IV**.

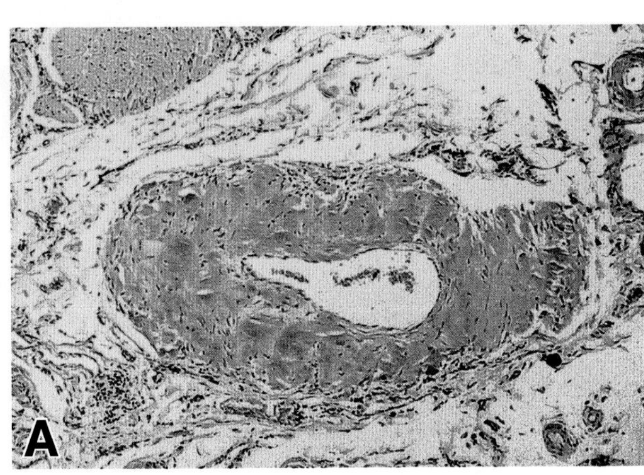

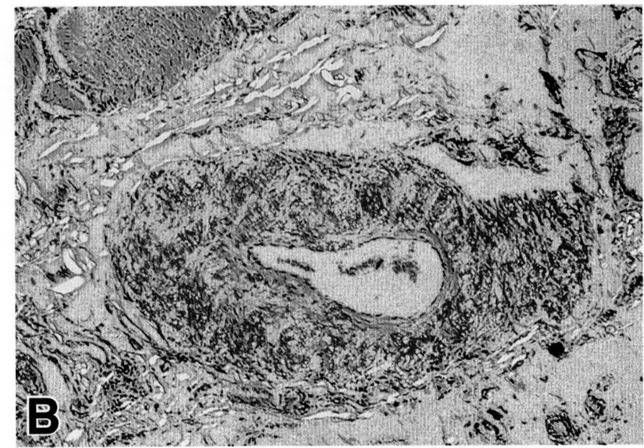

FIGURE 7-1. AL amyloid involving the wall of an artery stained with Congo red showing under (A) ordinary light and (B) polarized light. Note the red-green birefringence of the amyloid and a silvery appearance of collagen.

The genetic and/or environmental factors that determine individual susceptibility and timing of amyloid deposition are unclear, although several factors may be at play:

- Once the process has begun, further accumulation of amyloid is unremitting as long as there is a continuous supply of the respective precursor protein. Initiation of amyloid accumulation may involve a "seeding" process, consistent with observations that amyloid deposition can be remarkably rapid following its initiation.
- Both increasing age and male sex appear to be potent susceptibility factors in wild-type transthyretin (TTR) amyloid deposition. Clinical sequelae of this kind of amyloid are almost unheard of before age 60 years, and more than 90% of patients are male.
- The factors that influence the anatomic distribution of amyloid deposits are also unclear, but there is reasonable consistency related to the organ involvement associated with AA and most hereditary types of amyloidosis. In the latter, the fibril protein has the same structure in all individuals. By contrast, the organ distribution in AL amyloidosis is extremely heterogeneous, probably reflecting the unique sequence of the respective monoclonal Ig light chain in each patient.

Amyloid precursor proteins

Increased synthesis (e.g., SAA or L-chains) | Constitutive synthesis (e.g., TTR) | Mutant forms (e.g., TTR in FAP)

Protein precursor pool

Native protein conformation

Fibrillogenic microenvironment → Amyloidogenic conformation

Tissue amyloid deposits → Fibril formation

Proteolysis and turnover of amyloid → Pruning of amyloid proteins

FIGURE 7-2. General scheme for amyloidogenesis. FAP, familial amyloidotic polyneuropathy; SAA, serum amyloid A; TTR, transthyretin.

The pathologic effects of amyloid are because of its physical presence. Extensive deposits may total kilograms and are structurally disruptive. They impair normal function, as do strategically located smaller deposits (e.g., in glomeruli or nerves). It is possible that amyloid fibrils or prefibrillar aggregates may sometimes be directly cytotoxic, although amyloid deposits evoke little or no local inflammatory reaction.

STAINING PROPERTIES OF AMYLOID

The staining properties and general appearance of amyloid are governed primarily by its compact and proteinaceous nature. Because of this, amyloid has few morphologic features visible on light microscopy. With routine stains (hematoxylin and eosin), amyloid is amorphous, glassy, and almost cartilage-like, appearing much like many other proteins. However, the nature and organization of amyloid deposits allow it to be stained in specific ways.

CONGO RED: All types of amyloid stain red with the Congo red dye and exhibit red-green birefringence when viewed under cross-polarized light (Fig. 7-1). The fibrillar deposits organized in one plane exhibit one color, and those opposite to that plane appear the other color. Congo red is the stain most commonly used for the diagnosis of amyloidosis, although published techniques vary in their sensitivity and specificity.

THIOFLAVIN T: Although not entirely specific for amyloid, staining with thioflavin T allows amyloid to fluoresce when viewed in ultraviolet light.

SPECIFIC ANTIBODIES: Immunohistochemistry is the best way to characterize amyloid, although its success varies with the fibril protein type.

ELECTRON MICROSCOPY: By electron microscopy, amyloid features straight, rigid, nonbranching fibrils of indeterminate length, 10 to 15 nm in diameter (Fig. 7-3).

CLINICAL CLASSIFICATION OF THE AMYLOIDOSES

Amyloidoses are classified according to the identity of the amyloid proteins (Table 7-1).

Acquired Amyloidosis

Acquired systemic amyloidosis is thought to be the cause of death in about 1 in 1,000 individuals in Western countries, and it is probably underdiagnosed among the elderly, who are likely to be at greatest risk of developing it. Systemic AL amyloidosis is the most common and serious type, accounting for over 60% of cases. Although less serious, dialysis-related β_2-microglobulin amyloidosis affects about 1 million patients on long-term renal replacement therapy worldwide. Senile transthyretin amyloidosis, which predominantly involves the heart, occurs in about one quarter of persons older than 80 years.

Reactive Systemic Amyloidosis (AA Amyloidosis)

AA amyloidosis is a complication of chronic infections and inflammatory diseases, or any condition that leads to long-term overproduction of the acute-phase reactant serum amyloid A (SAA). The amyloid fibrils are composed of cleavage fragments of SAA (i.e., AA protein). AA amyloidosis occurs in 1% to 5% of patients with rheumatoid arthritis, juvenile idiopathic arthritis, and Crohn disease, and it is more common in those with untreated lifelong autoinflammatory diseases, such as familial Mediterranean fever. Most patients present with proteinuria, and although liver and gastrointestinal involvement may occur later, clinically significant cardiac or neuropathic involvement is very rare.

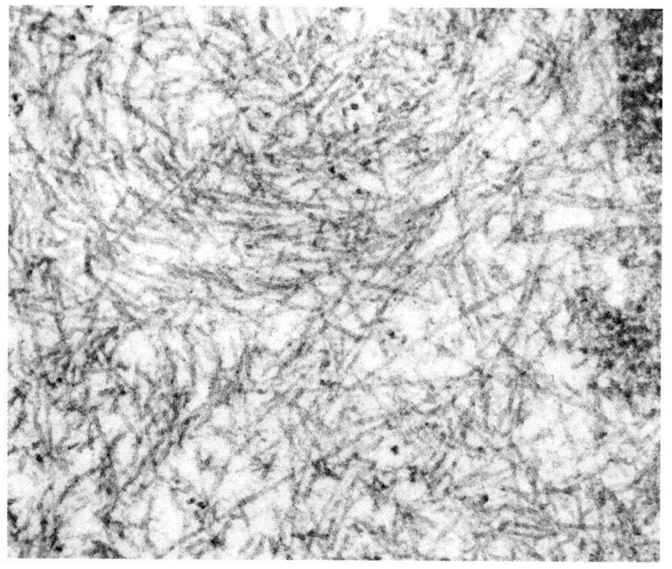

FIGURE 7-3. Amyloid deposits in tissue. Parallel and interlacing arrays of fibrils are evident in this electron micrograph.

Table 7-1

Classification of Human Amyloids

Amyloid Protein	Protein Precursor	Clinical Setting
AL	κ or λ immunoglobulin light chain	Multiple myeloma, plasma cell dyscrasias, and primary amyloid
AH	γ Immunoglobulin chain	Waldenström macroglobulinemia
Aβ_2M	β_2-Microglobulin	Hemodialysis related
ATTR	Transthyretin	Familial amyloidotic polyneuropathy (FAP), normal TTR in senile systemic amyloid
AA	Apo serum AA	Persistent acute inflammation, familial Mediterranean fever, certain malignancies
AApoAI	Apolipoprotein AI	FAP Iowa
AApoAII	Apolipoprotein AII	Familial
AApoAIV	Apolipoprotein AIV	Sporadic, age associated
Aβ	β-Protein precursor	Alzheimer disease, Down syndrome, HCHWA, Dutch
ABri	ABriPP	Familial dementia, British
ADan	ADanPP	Familial dementia, Danish
APrP	Prion protein	CJD, scrapie, BSE, GSS, Kuru
ACys	Cystatin C	HCHWA, Icelandic
ALys	Lysozyme	Hereditary systemic amyloidosis, Ostertag type
AFib	Fibrinogen	Hereditary renal amyloidosis
AGel	Gelsolin	Familial amyloidosis, Finnish
ACal	(Pro)calcitonin	Medullary carcinoma of the thyroid
AANF	Atrial natriuretic factor	Isolated atrial amyloid
AIAPP	Islet amyloid polypeptide	Type 2 diabetes, insulinomas
AIns	Insulin	Iatrogenic
APro	Prolactin	Pituitary, age associated
AMed	Lactadherin	Senile aortic, media
AKer	Keratoepithelin	Cornea, familial
ALac	Lactoferrin	Cornea

Apo, apolipoprotein; BSE, bovine spongiform encephalopathy; CJD, Creutzfeldt–Jakob disease; GSS, Gerstmann–Sträussler–Scheinker syndrome; HCHWA, hereditary cerebral hemorrhage with amyloid TTR, transthyretin.

MOLECULAR PATHOGENESIS: ***AA protein is a single polypeptide chain consisting of the 76-residue N-terminal portion of the 104-residue SAA.*** SAA is an apolipoprotein particle and is the product of a set of genes located on chromosome 11. It is highly conserved in evolution and is a major acute-phase reactant. Most SAA in plasma is produced by hepatocytes under transcriptional regulation by cytokines, IL-1, IL-6, and TNF-α. Circulating SAA can rise from normal levels (≤3 mg/L) to over 2,000 mg/L within 24 to 48 hours of an acute stimulus and remains elevated indefinitely in the presence of chronic inflammation.

Long-term overproduction of SAA is a prerequisite for the deposition of AA amyloid, but it is not known why the latter occurs in only some individuals. SAA isoforms are complex, but homozygosity for particular types seems to favor amyloidogenesis, as may ethnic differences in susceptibility.

The function of SAA is not known, but it serves as a sensitive acute-phase protein with enormous dynamic range, making it an empirical clinical marker. It can be used to monitor the extent and activity of many infective, inflammatory, necrotic, and neoplastic diseases. Frequent long-term monitoring of SAA is vital in managing all patients with AA amyloidosis because the primary inflammatory process must be controlled to reduce SAA production.

In the Western world, the most common predisposing conditions are chronic inflammatory diseases, particularly rheumatoid arthritis. Tuberculosis and leprosy are important causes of AA amyloidosis in some parts of the world. Chronic osteomyelitis, bronchiectasis, chronically infected burns and decubitus ulcers, and chronic pyelonephritis of paraplegia are other well-recognized associations. Hodgkin disease and renal carcinoma often cause a major acute-phase response and are the malignancies most commonly associated with systemic AA amyloid.

Because AA amyloid deposits are widely distributed, random biopsies are often used to make the diagnosis. However, clinically AA amyloidosis is dominated by progressive proteinuria. Treatment entails measures to suppress the underlying inflammatory disorder. Prognosis is now often excellent among patients in whom the causative acute-phase response can be substantially suppressed, but half of patients with persistent inflammation die within 10 years of diagnosis.

Amyloidosis Associated With Monoclonal B-Cell Dyscrasias (AL Amyloidosis)

Systemic AL occurs in 2% of people with monoclonal B-cell dyscrasias. AL fibrils are derived from monoclonal Ig light chains. These are unique in each patient so that AL amyloidosis is highly heterogeneous in terms of organ involvement and overall clinical course. Virtually any organ other than the brain may be directly affected, but the kidneys, heart, liver, and peripheral nerves are the most significant.

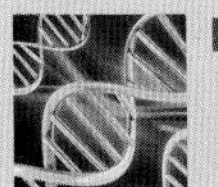

MOLECULAR PATHOGENESIS: ***AL amyloid fibrils are usually derived from the N-terminal region of monoclonal Ig light chains and consist of the whole or part of the variable (V_L) domain.*** AL fibrils develop more commonly from λ than from κ light chains, despite the fact that κ-chains are more common among normal immunoglobulins and monoclonal gammopathies.

B-cell dyscrasias underlying systemic AL amyloidosis are heterogeneous and include almost any clonal proliferation of differentiated B cells: multiple myeloma, Waldenström macroglobulinemia, and, occasionally, other malignant lymphomas or leukemias. However, over 80% of cases are associated with low-grade and otherwise "benign" monoclonal gammopathies that may be difficult to detect (see Chapter 18).

Dialysis-Related Amyloidosis (β_2-Microglobulin Amyloidosis)

β_2-Microglobulin amyloid deposition occurs in patients with dialysis-dependent chronic renal failure. It mainly affects articular and periarticular structures, and typically causes arthralgia of the shoulders, knees, wrists and small joints of the hand, joint swelling, and carpal tunnel syndrome. The precursor protein is β_2-microglobulin, which is the invariant chain of the MHC class I molecule, and is expressed by all nucleated cells. It is synthesized at an average rate of 150 to 200 mg/day and is normally filtered freely at the glomerulus, reabsorbed, and catabolized by proximal tubular cells. Decreasing renal function causes a proportionate rise in concentration. β_2-Microglobulin amyloidosis occurs in patients who have been on hemodialysis for several years and peritoneal dialysis for 5 to 10 years. The disorder is present in 20% to 30% of patients within 3 years of starting dialysis for end-stage renal failure. Although it is a systemic disease, manifestations outside the musculoskeletal system are unusual.

Senile Transthyretin Amyloidosis (ATTR Amyloidosis)

In the elderly, clinically silent systemic deposits of wild-type "senile" TTR amyloid are common, involving the heart and blood vessel walls, smooth and striated muscle, fat tissue, renal papillae, and alveolar walls. Unlike most other forms of systemic amyloidosis, including hereditary TTR amyloid caused by point mutations in the *transthyretin* gene, the spleen and renal glomeruli are rarely affected. The brain is not involved, although symptomatic leptomeningeal deposits can occasionally occur in familial TTR amyloidosis. ATTR amyloidosis almost always presents with restrictive cardiomyopathy, and other than carpal tunnel syndrome, deposits elsewhere rarely attain clinical significance. Most patients are over 70 years old, and there is a very strong male preponderance. Cardiac failure progresses, and death usually occurs within about 5 years.

Endocrine Amyloidosis

Hormone-producing tumors may have amyloid deposits in their stroma (see Chapter 19). These are probably composed of hormone peptides; in the case of medullary carcinoma of the thyroid, fibril subunits are derived from procalcitonin.

In insulinomas, the amyloid fibril protein is called islet amyloid polypeptide (or **amylin**) and shows homology with calcitonin gene–related peptide. It has subsequently been shown to be the same protein as in the amyloid of the islets of Langerhans in type 2 diabetes.

Amyloid and the Brain

The brain is a common and important site of amyloid deposition, although there are no deposits in the cerebral parenchyma itself in any acquired systemic amyloidosis. However, cerebrovascular and oculoleptomeningeal amyloid deposits, which can be clinically significant, do occasionally occur in hereditary TTR amyloidosis.

The common forms of brain amyloid are associated with Alzheimer disease, the most common type of dementia. Intracerebral amyloid plaques derived from the normal cellular prion protein, PrP^C, are sometimes seen in acquired and hereditary spongiform encephalopathy (see Chapter 24).

Hereditary Amyloidosis

In hereditary systemic amyloidosis, mutations in the genes for transthyretin, cystatin C, gelsolin, lysozyme, fibrinogen A α-chain, apolipoprotein AI, and, rarely, apolipoprotein AII lead to the deposition of mutant proteins as amyloid (see Table 7-1). These diseases are all inherited dominantly with variable penetrance, and present clinically from teenage to old age, though usually in mid-adult life. Hereditary transthyretin amyloidosis is by far the most common, usually presenting as a syndrome of familial amyloid polyneuropathy with peripheral and autonomic neuropathy or cardiomyopathy. ***Of patients presenting with non-AA systemic amyloidosis, 5% to 10% have hereditary forms of the disease.***

Familial Amyloidotic Polyneuropathy (Variant Transthyretin [ATTR] Amyloidosis)

Familial amyloidotic polyneuropathy (FAP) is associated with heterozygous point mutations in the *TTR* gene. It is an autosomal dominant syndrome, with onset between the third and seventh decades. The disease is characterized by progressive and disabling peripheral and autonomic neuropathy and varying degrees of visceral amyloid involvement. The latter includes cardiac amyloidosis, which can be the sole clinical feature in some cases. Typically, the disease progresses inexorably, causing death within 5 to 15 years.

MORPHOLOGIC FEATURES OF AMYLOIDOSIS

Amyloid fibrils are usually first deposited near subendothelial basement membranes. Because amyloid accumulates along stromal networks, deposits take on the configurations of the organs involved. Morphologic differences in amyloid deposition among organs simply reflect differences in stromal organization. For example, in the renal medulla, amyloid is laid down longitudinally, parallel to tubules and vasa recta, whereas in glomeruli, amyloid (Fig. 7-4) follows lobular glomerular architecture. Deposits in the liver accompany the arteries of the portal triads or are placed along central veins and radiate into the parenchyma along liver cell plates (Fig. 7-5).

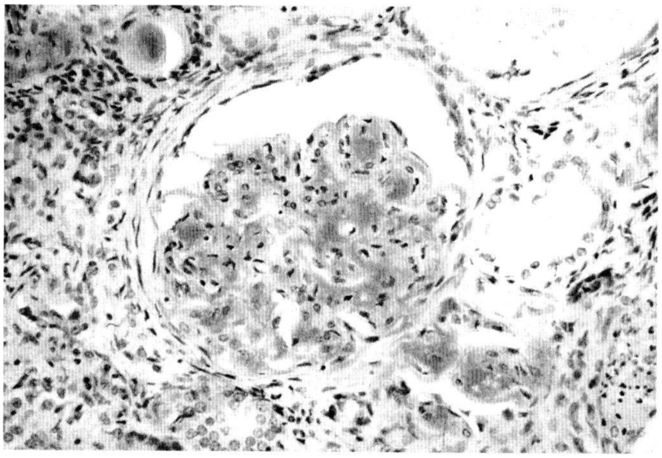

FIGURE 7-4. Microscopic appearance of AA amyloid in a glomerulus. Note the lobular pattern of the amyloid deposit and the involvement of the afferent arteriole.

Amyloid adds interstitial material at the sites of deposition, thereby increasing the size of affected organs. This increase may be counterbalanced by the deposition of amyloid in blood vessels (Fig. 7-6), which can impair circulation and lead to organ atrophy. Affected organs may thus increase or decrease in size. Amyloid deposits are essentially avascular, so the involved organs are commonly pale and firm.

Regardless of whether amyloid is laid down in a systemic or localized manner, deposits tend to occur between parenchymal cells and their blood supply, thus interfering with normal nutrition and gas exchange. Amyloid may eventually entrap parenchymal cells and produce cell strangulation, atrophy, and death.

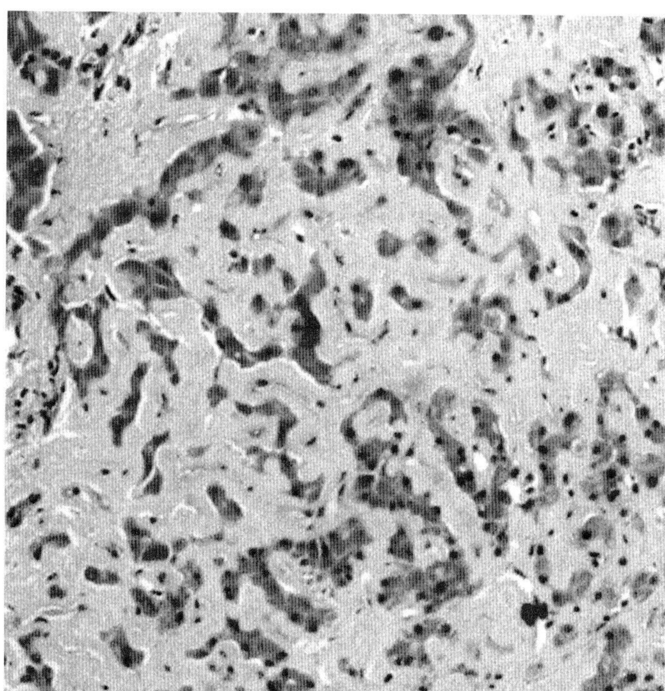

FIGURE 7-5. Hepatic amyloidosis. Amyloid is deposited along the sinusoids. Note the atrophic hepatocytes.

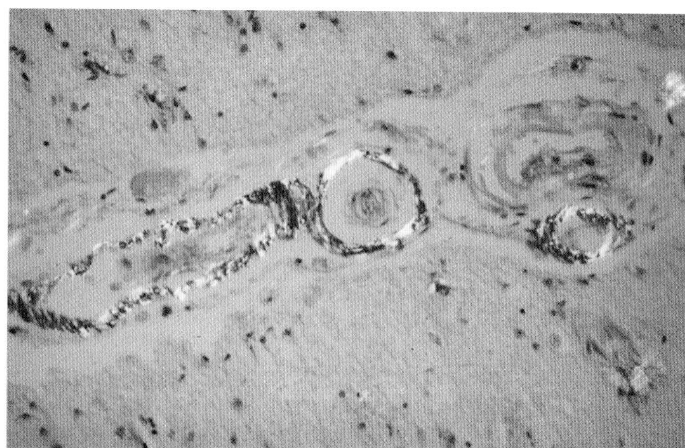

FIGURE 7-6. Cerebrovascular amyloid in a case of Alzheimer disease. The section was stained with Congo red and examined under polarized light.

CLINICAL FEATURES AND ORGAN INVOLVEMENT

No single set of symptoms points unequivocally to amyloidosis as a diagnosis. The symptoms depend on the underlying disease and the type and organ locations of the amyloid deposits. Amyloidosis may also be diagnosed unexpectedly in the course of evaluation for something unrelated, with no clinical manifestations referable to the amyloidosis itself. In other cases, for example, unexplained renal and cardiac dysfunction may be the presenting conditions (for relevant details, see Chapters 9 and 14).

TREATMENT OF AMYLOIDOSIS

Systemic amyloidosis is a progressive disease that, without effective treatment, is ultimately fatal in most cases. The long-held belief that amyloid deposition is irreversible and inexorably progressive is evidently incorrect and simply reflects the usually persistent nature of the conditions that underlie it. Many case reports have described improvement in organ function when the underlying conditions have been controlled, suggesting that amyloid deposits may regress.

8 Blood Vessels and Hemodynamic Disorders

Avrum I. Gotlieb[1] ▪ Amber Chang Liu[1] ▪ Bruce M. McManus[2] ▪ Michael F. Allard[2] ▪ Robert Yanagawa[2]

LEARNING OBJECTIVES

- Correlate the anatomic structure and function of the various blood vessels.
- Discuss the structural specializations of the microcirculation allowing for fluid and solute exchange.
- Correlate the structural features of the lymphatic system with their role in fluid homeostasis.
- Compare and contrast active and passive hyperemia, and list possible factors contributing to each.
- List three major causes of edema.
- Define the term "effusion," and provide several examples of anatomic locations where it occurs.
- Differentiate between shock and hypotension.
- Discuss the pathogenesis and etiology of the major classifications of shock.
- Define the term "distributive shock," and provide examples of its subcategories.
- List and define examples of the specialized terminology used in describing the hemorrhagic process (such as "hematoma").
- Differentiate between a thrombus and an embolus.
- List three major factors that may provoke arterial thrombosis.
- Define one factor important in arterial but not venous thrombosis.
- List the potential fates of arterial thrombi.
- Define atherosclerosis and provide an overview of its natural history.
- Differentiate the factors important in differentiating preclinical and clinically apparent atherosclerosis.
- List the major components of an atheroma and their location within the artery.
- Differentiate between a "simple," "fibrofatty," and "complicated" plaque.
- Provide a histologic description of two precursor lesions of atherosclerosis.
- Provide a brief overview of plaque initiation and formation concentrating on the pathogenesis of the lesions.
- Define the factors that lead to the generation of clinically significant plaques, concentrating on structural changes within the lesion associated with plaque destabilization.
- What are the causes and consequences of plaque rupture?
- List the major complications of atherosclerosis and their anatomic sites.
- List major risk factors for atherosclerosis, and provide a brief explanation for the pathophysiologic role of each.
- Provide a brief description of the role of high- and low-density lipoprotein in lipid metabolism and atherosclerosis.
- Contrast and compare forms of heritable dyslipoproteinemia.
- Define the terms "xanthoma" and "arcus lipoides," and discuss their significance.
- Distinguish between primary and secondary hypertension, and provide several clinical examples of the latter.
- Describe the characteristic vascular changes associated with "benign" and "malignant" hypertension.
- Define the term "aneurysm," and list the characteristics used to classify it.
- Discuss the pathogenesis and pathology of abdominal aortic aneurysms.
- What is a major causative factor in the pathogenesis of subarachnoid hemorrhage?
- Differentiate between aneurysms, dissecting aneurysms, and false aneurysms.
- List several congenital and acquired risk factors for venous thrombosis.
- What are the potential fates of thrombi of the deep veins?
- List the risk factors for varicose veins.
- Provide examples of venous varicosities at sites other than the legs.
- Define the term "embolism," and provide a common example associated with significant morbidity and mortality.
- Describe the pathogenesis of a pulmonary arterial embolism and how it may result in death.
- Describe the evolution of a paradoxical embolism.
- What are the sources of embolism other than thrombi?

[1]Blood Vessels
[2]Hemodynamic Disorders

- Differentiate between pale and red infarctions, and provide examples of each.
- Differentiate between fibromuscular dysplasia, Mönckeberg medial sclerosis, and atherosclerosis in terms of pathogenesis, clinical effects, and anatomic location.
- Describe the major mechanisms of vessel injury that result in vasculitis.
- Differentiate between ANCA and immune complex–mediated vasculitis.
- Distinguish between polyarteritis nodosa and giant cell arteritis in terms of pathogenesis and clinical findings.
- Distinguish between granulomatosis with polyangiitis (GPA) and allergic granulomatosis and angiitis (AGA) in terms of pathogenesis and clinical findings.
- Distinguish between Takayasu arteritis and Kawasaki disease in terms of pathogenesis and clinical findings.
- List several common benign tumors of capillaries.
- Describe the etiology and pathology of Kaposi sarcoma.

ANATOMY OF BLOOD VESSELS

Arteries

The vascular portion of the circulatory system is composed of a variety of blood vessel compartments that are categorized by size, structure, and function. These include arteries, which are conducting and resistance vessels; capillaries; and veins (Fig. 8-1). Because blood vessels are ubiquitous in the body, diseases of the blood vessels are expressed in all organ systems. In a notable example, ischemic heart disease, expressed as damage to cardiac myocytes leading to failure of cardiac function, is almost always the result of disease of the arteries supplying the heart. Such cardiac disease is discussed in Chapter 9, but the provoking lesion, the disease of arteries termed atherosclerosis, is discussed here.

Elastic Arteries

The largest blood vessels in the body, the aorta and the elastic arteries, are conduits for blood flow to smaller arterial branches and are composed of three layers (Fig. 8-1).

- **Tunica intima:** This structure consists of a single layer of endothelial cells, a subendothelial compartment containing a few smooth muscle cells, and an extracellular matrix that extends to the luminal side of the internal elastic lamina. The aortic intima is thicker than that of the other elastic arteries and contains matrix proteins, including collagen, proteoglycans, and small amounts of elastin. Occasional resident lymphocytes, macrophages, dendritic cells, and other blood-derived inflammatory cells are also present.
- **Tunica media:** The next (and thickest) layer outward is the tunica media. It is bounded by internal and external elastic laminae and displays numerous elastic laminae and smooth muscle cells within an extracellular connective tissue matrix. In the aorta, the media is organized into lamellar units, each consisting of two concentric elastic laminae, with smooth muscle cells and their associated matrix in between the laminae. In elastic arteries, elastic fibers are interposed between smooth muscle cells and serve to minimize energy loss during the pressure changes between systole and diastole; in doing so, they dampen pulsations within the system. Nutrition of the small elastic arteries is provided by diffusion from the lumen. However, larger vessels are nourished by the **vasa vasorum**, small vessels that penetrate into the outer two thirds of the media. The tunica media also contains autonomic nerve fibers that influence vascular contractility.
- **Tunica adventitia:** The most external vessel wall layer contains fibroblasts, connective tissue, nerves, and small vessels that give rise to the vasa vasorum. Occasional inflammatory cells, including collections of lymphocytes, may also be present in the adventitia.

Muscular Arteries

Blood conducted by the elastic arteries is distributed to individual organs through large muscular arteries (Figs. 8-1 and 8-2). The tunica media of a muscular artery lacks prominent bands of elastin, but a conspicuous internal elastic lamina and usually an external elastic lamina are present. Owing to the lack of heavy elastin layers, muscular arteries contract more efficiently. The intima of muscular arteries, similarly to that of the aorta, also contains small numbers of smooth muscle cells, connective tissue, and occasional inflammatory cells. Vasa vasorum are present in the outer wall of thicker muscular arteries but not in smaller ones. As the vascular tree branches further, the tunica media becomes thinner, and except for the endothelium, the tunica intima disappears.

The small muscular arteries are important regulators of blood flow. Their narrow lumens increase resistance (**resistance vessels**), thereby reducing blood pressure to levels appropriate for the exchange of water and plasma constituents across downstream thin-walled capillaries. These vessels help maintain systemic pressure by regulating total peripheral resistance.

Arterioles

Arterioles are the smallest parts of the arterial system. They have an endothelial lining surrounded by one or two layers of smooth muscle cells. No elastic layers are evident. The smallest arterioles regulate blood flow by vasomotion (change in an artery's caliber), thereby controlling blood distribution through the capillary tree.

The Microcirculation

The blood vessels of the microcirculation are less than 100 μm in diameter. Blood from an arteriole enters capillaries, which freely anastomose with each other. The large aggregate surface area of capillaries determines that velocity is low, which along with capillary length further enhances microvascular exchange (Fig. 8-2). The density of capillaries in a tissue also influences microvascular exchange by affecting the diffusion distance. For example, in tissues with high oxygen demands, such as the heart, capillary density is very high. Entry into the capillary system is guarded by precapillary sphincters, except for **thoroughfare channels**, which bypass capillaries and are always open. Because not all capillaries are always open, blood flow to a structure can be increased by recruiting additional capillaries. **The sum of blood flow through the capillary bed, the thoroughfare channels, and the arteriovenous anastomoses determines the regional blood flow**.

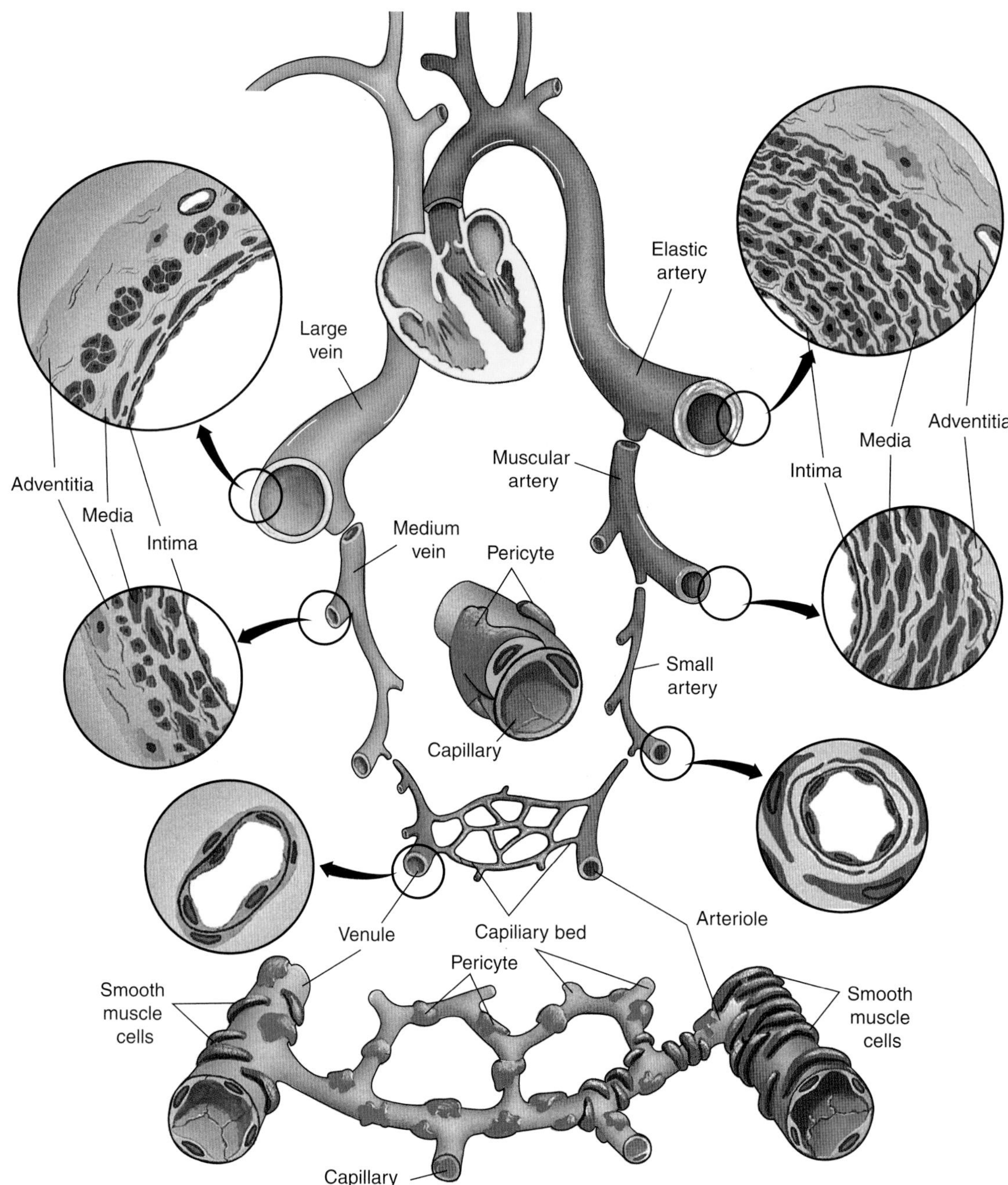

FIGURE 8-1. Subdivisions and histologic structure of the vascular system. Each subdivision is subject to a set of pathologic changes conditioned by the structure–function relationship of that part of the system. For example, the aorta, an elastic artery subject to great pressure, frequently shows a pathologic dilation (aneurysm) if the supporting elastic media is damaged. Muscular arteries are the most significant sites of atherosclerosis. Small arteries, particularly arterioles, are sites of hypertensive changes. Capillary beds, venules, and veins each display their own types of pathologic changes.

Capillaries

In the capillaries, the endothelium is supported only by sparse smooth muscle cells. The capillary endothelium provides for exchange of solutes and cells between blood and extracellular fluid. A necessary feature of this exchange is the aforementioned marked lowering of pressure, which prevents intravascular fluid from being shifted into the extracellular space.

The capillary endothelium is a semipermeable membrane, in which exchange of plasma solutes with extracellular fluid is controlled by molecular size and charge. The permeability of capillaries depends on their endothelial cells and their junctions. Brain capillaries are highly impermeable because junctions between endothelial cells are tightly sealed. Transport in other capillary beds is mediated either by passage of molecules through incomplete cell junctions or by pinocytosis, that is, traverse of substances through the cytoplasm by vesicular transport. In some locations such as the renal glomeruli, the capillary endothelium itself may have permanent channels through discontinuous gaps (**fenestrae**).

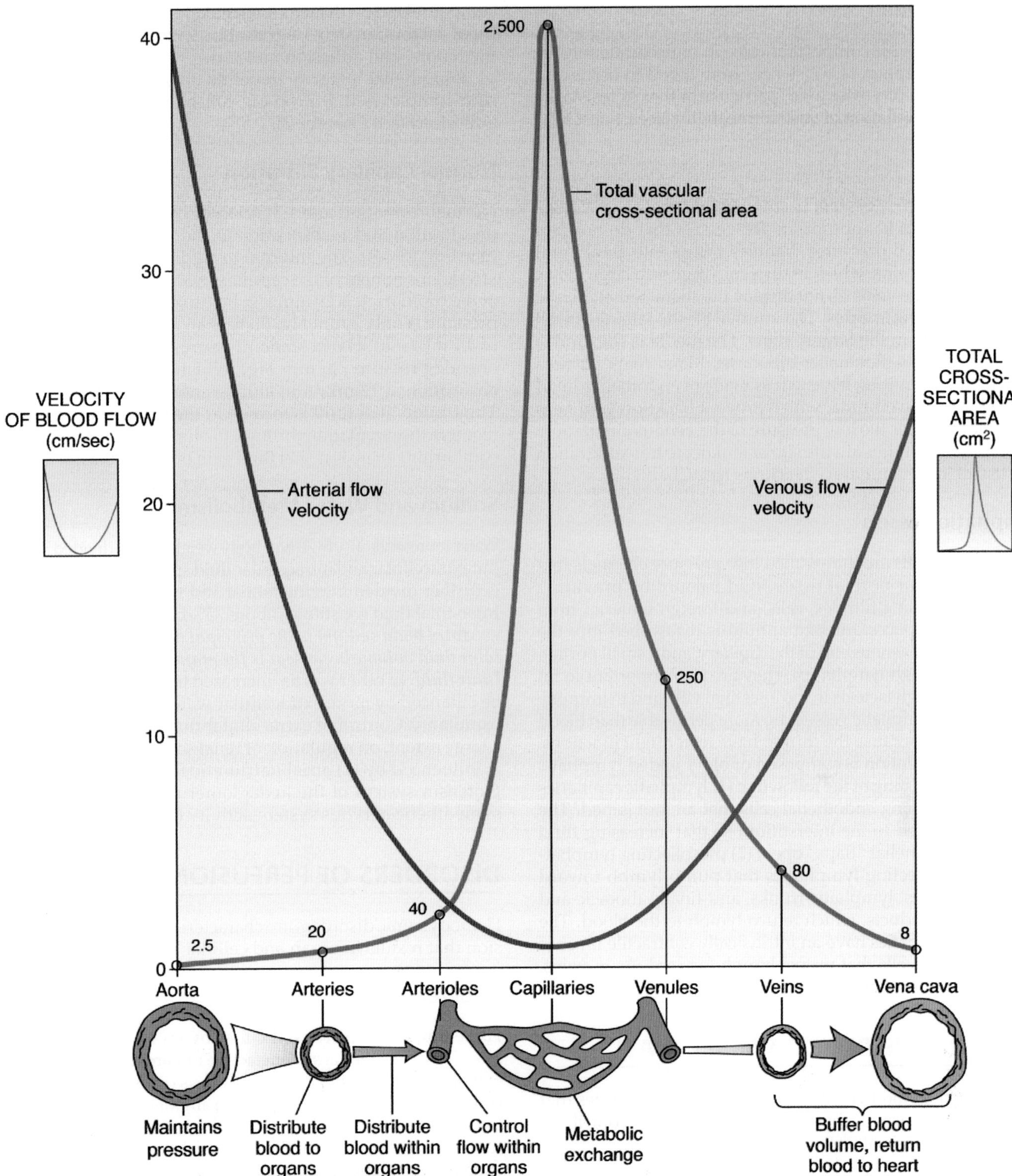

FIGURE 8-2. Relationship between velocity of blood flow and cross-sectional area in the vasculature. The vascular tree is a circuit that conducts blood from the heart through large-diameter, low-resistance conducting vessels to small arteries and arterioles, which lower blood pressure and protect the capillaries. The capillaries are thin walled and allow the exchange of nutrients and waste products between tissue and blood, a process that requires a very large surface area. The circuit back to the heart is completed by the veins, which are distensible and provide a volume buffer that acts as a capacitance for the vascular circuit.

The Endothelium

Endothelial cells play important roles in anticoagulation, facilitation of migration of substances from blood to tissue and back, regulation of vessel tone (particularly that of resistance arteries), and regulation of vasopermeability (see Chapter 2).

Veins

Venules are the first vessels to collect blood from capillaries. Their thin media is appropriate for vessels that do not face high intraluminal pressures. Venules merge into small- and medium-sized veins, which in turn converge into large veins. The walls of large veins do not display the characteristic elastic lamellae of elastic arteries. The internal elastic lamina is well developed only in the largest veins. The media is thin and is virtually absent in the smaller tributaries. Many veins, particularly in the extremities, have valves made of endothelial-lined folds of the tunica intima, which prevent backflow and help move blood under the low pressure of the venous circulation. Postcapillary venules are the site of leukocyte transmigration into tissue in inflammatory reactions (see Chapter 2).

Lymphatic Vessels

Lymphatic vessels are thin-walled low-pressure channels that are important for normal tissue fluid balance by providing drainage of plasma filtrates, cells, and foreign material from the interstitial spaces. Interstitial fluid is reabsorbed into the circulation at the venous end of the capillary, and a small portion is drained through lymphatics. They are also important in fat digestion, through lacteals in the intestinal villi, and in immune surveillance. Lymphatic vessels are more permeable than blood vessels, in part because the former have fewer tight junctions. Lymphatic circulation is composed of blind-ended lymphatic capillaries, consisting of the following: (1) lymphatic capillaries having overlapping endothelial cells that are not joined. The cells are anchored to the interstitium so that increasing fluid forces the endothelial "flaps" open; (2) precollecting lymphatics; and (3) collecting lymphatics that pump lymph toward the lymph nodes, lymphatic trunks, and finally thoracic and right lymphatic ducts, which return lymph to the blood. The collecting lymphatics have an intrinsically contractile layer of smooth muscle cells that propel lymph forward. As in veins, intraluminal valves prevent backflow.

CELLS OF THE BLOOD VESSEL WALL

The cells of the blood vessel wall have unique properties that are critical for normal physiologic functions and contribute to the pathogenesis of vascular diseases.

Endothelial Cells

Endothelial cells are metabolically active and are intimately involved in a number of biologic functions, including vascular permeability, coagulation, platelet regulation, fibrinolysis, inflammation, immunoregulation, and repair. They also modulate vascular smooth muscle cell function through paracrine pathways. Endothelial cells form unique mechanotransduction structures that modulate the effects of luminal hemodynamic shear stress on the vessel wall. By virtue of mechanical sensing, endothelial cell membranes may deform. This effect activates biochemical signaling and leads to the expression of vasoactive compounds, growth factors, coagulation/fibrinolytic/complement factors, matrix degradation enzymes, inflammatory mediators, and adhesion molecules.

Endothelial integrity depends on several types of adhesion complexes that promote cell–substratum and cell–cell adhesions (see Chapter 2).

Normal Capillary Filtration

Normal formation and retention of interstitial fluid depend on filtration and reabsorption at the level of the capillaries (Starling forces). The internal or hydrostatic pressure in the arteriolar segment of the capillary is 32 mm Hg. At the middle of the capillary, it is 20 mm Hg. Because interstitial hydrostatic pressure is only 3 mm Hg, there is an outward fluid filtration of 14 mL/min. Hydrostatic pressure is opposed by plasma oncotic pressure (26 mm Hg), which results in osmotic reabsorption at 12 mL/min at the venous end of the capillary. Thus, interstitial fluid is formed at the rate of 2 mL/min and reenters the circulation through the lymphatics. As a result, in equilibrium, there is no net fluid gain or loss in the interstitium.

Sodium and Water Metabolism

Water represents 50% to 70% of body weight and is divided between the extracellular and intracellular fluid spaces. Extracellular fluid is further divided into interstitial and vascular compartments. Interstitial fluid constitutes about 75% of the extracellular fluid.

Total body sodium is the principal determinant of extracellular fluid volume because it is the major cation in the extracellular fluid. In other words, increased total body sodium must be balanced by more extracellular water to maintain constant osmolality. Control of extracellular fluid volume depends, to a large extent, on regulation of renal sodium excretion, which is influenced by (1) atrial natriuretic factor, (2) the renin–angiotensin system of the juxtaglomerular apparatus, and (3) sympathetic nervous system activity (see Chapter 14).

DISORDERS OF PERFUSION

Hemodynamic disorders are characterized by disturbed perfusion that results in organ and cellular injury.

Hyperemia

Hyperemia may be caused either by an increased supply of blood from the arterial system (**active hyperemia**) or by impaired exit of blood through venous pathways (**passive hyperemia** or **congestion**). Active hyperemia is an augmented supply of blood to an organ. It is usually a physiologic response to increased functional demand, as in the heart and skeletal muscle during exercise or notably during inflammation. Passive hyperemia, or congestion, is engorgement of an organ with venous blood. Clinically acute passive congestion is a consequence of acute left or right ventricular failure. Generalized increases in venous pressure, usually from chronic heart failure, lead to slower blood flow and a consequent increase in blood volume in many organs, including the lung, liver, spleen, and kidneys.

Lung

In the lung, the result of passive hyperemia is the accumulation of transudate in the alveolus, which is called **pulmonary edema** (Fig. 8-3). This is often accompanied by the release of

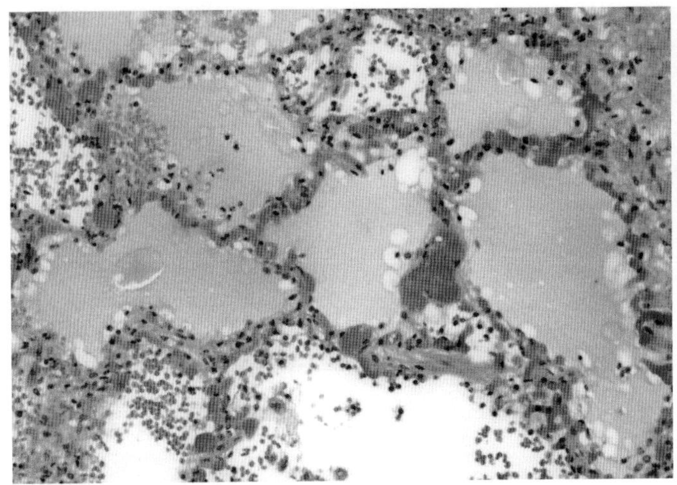

FIGURE 8-3. Pulmonary edema. A patient with congestive heart failure showing pink-staining fluid in the alveoli. Centre for Heart Lung Innovation James Hogg Lung Registry, St. Paul's Hospital, University of British Columbia.

erythrocytes into the alveolus and the phagocytosis of such cells by alveolar macrophages, resulting in characteristic **heart failure cells** marked by accumulated hemosiderin (Fig. 8-4). **Pulmonary hypertension** occurs when the pressure is transmitted to the pulmonary arterial system. This may lead to right-sided heart failure and consequent generalized systemic venous congestion. The morphologic changes associated with pulmonary hypertension are discussed in Chapter 10.

Liver

The hepatic veins empty into the vena cava inferior to the heart, so the liver is particularly vulnerable to acute or chronic passive congestion (see Chapter 12). The central veins of hepatic lobules become dilated. During passive liver congestion, the sinusoids dilate, and centrilobular hepatocytes undergo pressure atrophy (Fig. 8-5A). Grossly, the cut surface of a chronically congested liver exhibits dark foci of centrilobular congestion surrounded by paler zones of unaffected peripheral portions of the lobules. The result is a reticulated appearance that resembles a cross section of a nutmeg ("nutmeg liver") (Fig. 8-5B).

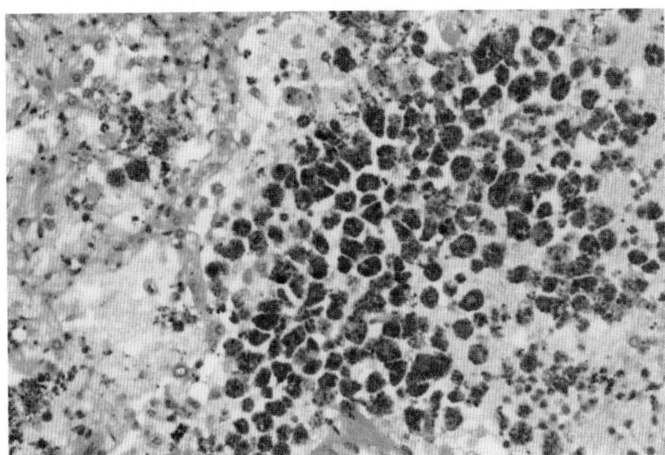

FIGURE 8-4. Passive congestion of lung. Hemosiderin-laden macrophages in the lung of a patient with congestive heart failure.

Spleen

Increased intravascular pressure in the liver, from cardiac failure or an intrahepatic obstruction to blood flow (e.g., cirrhosis), generates higher pressure in the splenic vein and congestion of the spleen. The organ becomes enlarged and tense, and the cut section oozes dark blood. If congestion is long-standing, the spleen displays enlargement, fibrosis, and the formation of calcified foci of old hemorrhage (Gamna–Gandy bodies). The enlarged spleen sometimes displays excessive functional activity (**hypersplenism**), which causes hematologic abnormalities (e.g., thrombocytopenia).

Venous congestion impedes blood flow through the capillaries, thereby increasing hydrostatic pressure, promoting edema formation (see below).

EDEMA

Edema refers to excess fluid in interstitial tissue spaces. **Local edema**, in most instances, occurs with inflammation. Local edema of a limb, usually the leg, results from venous or lymphatic obstruction.

Generalized edema describes swelling of visceral organs and the skin of the trunk and lower extremities. It refers to a global disorder of fluid and electrolyte metabolism, most often due to heart failure. **Anasarca** is extreme generalized edema, a condition evidenced by conspicuous fluid accumulation in subcutaneous tissues, visceral organs, and body cavities. Edema fluid may accumulate in body spaces, such as the pleural cavity (**hydrothorax**), peritoneal cavity (**ascites**), or pericardial space (**hydropericardium**).

Causes of Edema

- **Increased hydrostatic pressure** results in greater filtration of fluid into the interstitial space and its retention as edema. Decompensated heart disease and left ventricular failure cause acute pulmonary edema. Venous obstruction in the lower extremity causes edema of the leg. Obstruction to portal blood flow in cirrhosis of the liver contributes to the formation of abdominal fluid (ascites).
- **Decreased plasma oncotic pressure** as a result of decreased plasma protein (predominantly albumin) levels tends to promote generalized edema. This may result from a failure of synthesis as a result of malnutrition or liver disease or as a result of protein loss, which may occur in renal disease.
- **Lymphatic obstruction** results in localized edema when the normal excess of fluid filtered into the interstitial space cannot be removed by the lymphatic circulation. Such lymphatic obstruction may result from (1) neoplasia, (2) fibrosis as a result of irradiation or inflammation, for example, **elephantiasis**, massive lymphedema of the legs and scrotum resulting from the response to filarial worm infestation, or (3) as a side effect of ablative surgery, such as nodal dissection in the case of mastectomies.

The Role of Sodium Retention

Generalized edema and ascites invariably reflect increased total body sodium, as a consequence of renal sodium retention. When peripheral edema is first detectable clinically, extracellular fluid volume has already expanded by at least 5 L. The most common conditions in which generalized edema is found include congestive heart failure, cirrhosis of the liver, nephrotic

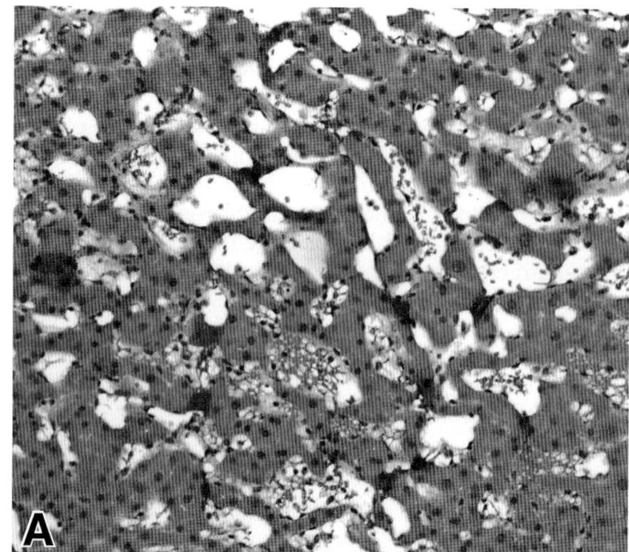

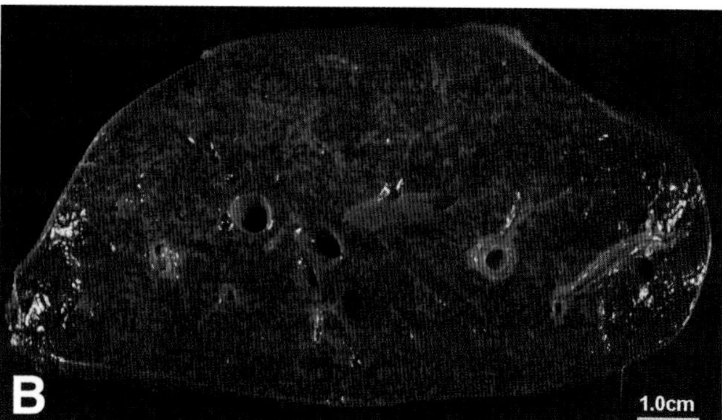

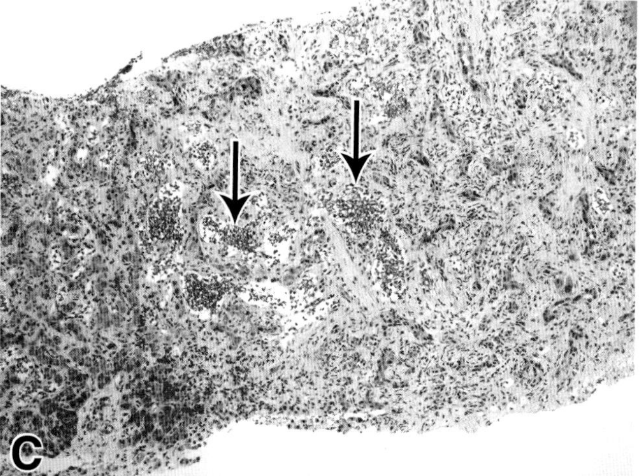

FIGURE 8-5. **Passive congestion of liver. A.** A photomicrograph of liver showing dilated centrilobular sinusoids. The intervening plates of hepatocytes exhibit pressure atrophy. **B.** A gross photograph of liver showing nutmeg appearance, reflecting congestive failure of the right ventricle. **C.** Late changes in chronic passive congestion characterized by dilated sinusoids (*arrows*) and fibrosis. (Note the blue staining of collagen in this trichrome stain.) Proliferated bile ducts are on the right.

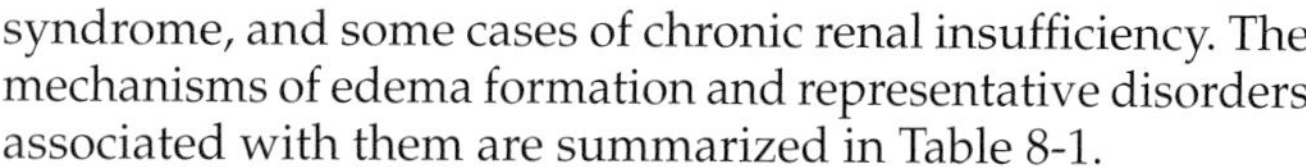

syndrome, and some cases of chronic renal insufficiency. The mechanisms of edema formation and representative disorders associated with them are summarized in Table 8-1.

Fluid Accumulates in Body Cavities

The accumulation of fluid within a body space or cavity is termed an **effusion**.

- **Pleural effusion** (fluid in the pleural space) may result from any generalized tendency to form edema (as discussed above), but is also a frequent response to an inflammatory process or tumor in the lung or on the pleural surface.
- **Pericardial effusion** occurs with pericardial infections, metastatic neoplasms to the pericardium, uremia, and systemic lupus erythematosus. It is also occasionally encountered after cardiac operations (**postpericardiotomy syndrome**) or radiation therapy for cancer. Hemorrhage into the pericardial sack (**hemopericardium**) may occur with trauma or following postischemic cardiac rupture. Such hemorrhage, particularly if rapid, may result in **cardiac tamponade**. This condition is accompanied by a precipitous fall in cardiac output, which is often fatal, because pericardial cavity pressure exceeds the cardiac filling pressure.
- **Peritoneal effusion**, also called **ascites**, is usually the result of cirrhosis of the liver, abdominal neoplasms, pancreatitis, cardiac failure, the nephrotic syndrome, or hepatic venous obstruction (Budd–Chiari syndrome). Patients with severe ascites accumulate many liters of fluid and have hugely distended abdomens. The resultant increase in abdominal pressure is associated with anorexia and vomiting, reflux esophagitis, dyspnea, ventral hernia, and leakage of fluid into the pleural space.

Table 8-1

Disorders Associated With Edema

Increased hydrostatic pressure	
Arteriolar dilation	Inflammation
	Heat
Increased venous pressure	Venous thrombosis
	Congestive heart failure
	Cirrhosis (ascites)
	Postural inactivity (e.g., prolonged standing)
Hypervolemia	Sodium retention (e.g., decreased renal function)
Decreased oncotic pressure	
Hypoproteinemia	Nephrotic syndrome
	Cirrhosis
	Protein-losing gastroenteropathy
	Malnutrition
Increased capillary permeability	
	Inflammation
	Burns
	Adult respiratory distress syndrome
Lymphatic obstruction	
	Cancer
	Postsurgical lymphedema
	Inflammation

SHOCK

Shock is a condition of profound hemodynamic and metabolic disturbance characterized by failure of the circulatory system to maintain an appropriate blood supply to the microcirculation, with consequent inadequate perfusion of vital organs and failure to remove metabolites. Absent compensatory mechanisms, shock becomes irreversible and leads to organ system failure and death.

Shock is not synonymous with low blood pressure. Hypotension is a late sign in shock and indicates failure of compensatory mechanisms by which extreme vasoconstriction maintains arterial blood pressure in the case of critical failure of peripheral blood flow.

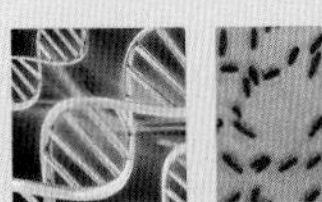

MOLECULAR PATHOGENESIS AND ETIOLOGIC FACTORS: Decreased perfusion in shock most commonly results from decreased cardiac output, owing either to the inability of the heart to pump normal venous return (**cardiogenic shock**) or to decreased effective blood volume. The latter results in decreased venous return (**hypovolemic shock**). Systemic vasodilation, with or without increased vascular permeability, is referred to as a **distributive** shock. This condition has several key subcategories, namely, **septic, anaphylactic, and neurogenic** shock (Fig. 8-6).

- **Cardiogenic shock** is caused by myocardial pump failure. It usually arises after massive myocardial infarction, although myocarditis may also be responsible. Disorders that prevent left or right heart filling reduce cardiac output, resulting in "obstructive" shock. Such conditions include pulmonary embolism, cardiac tamponade, and (rarely) atrial myxoma.
- **Hypovolemic shock** is a consequence of pronounced decreases in blood or plasma volume, caused by loss of fluid from the vascular compartment. Hemorrhage, fluid loss from severe burns, diarrhea, excessive urine formation, perspiration, and trauma all can trigger hypovolemic shock.
- **Septic shock** is an aftermath of severe systemic microbial infections. The pathogenesis of septic shock is complex (see Fig. 8-6) and is discussed in detail in Chapter 2.
- **Anaphylactic shock** stems from a systemic type I hypersensitivity reaction, which generates widespread vasodilation and increased vascular permeability.
- **Neurogenic shock** can follow acute injury to the brain or spinal cord, which impairs neural control of vasomotor tone and causes generalized vasodilation.

In hypovolemic and cardiogenic shock, lower cardiac output and resultant decreased tissue perfusion are the key steps in the progression from reversible to irreversible shock. In the case of both anaphylactic and neurogenic shock, the subsequent redistribution of blood to the periphery, with or without increased vascular permeability, reduces the effective circulating blood and plasma volume and leads to the same consequences as in hypovolemic shock.

Cellular hypoxia commonly follows an initial decrease in tissue perfusion. This does not initially result in irreversible injury; a vicious circle of decreasing tissue perfusion and further cell injury is perpetuated by injury to endothelial cells. The ensuing loss of fluid from the vasculature reduces blood volume and cardiac output. Ultimately, metabolic acidosis supervenes, with damage to multiple organ systems.

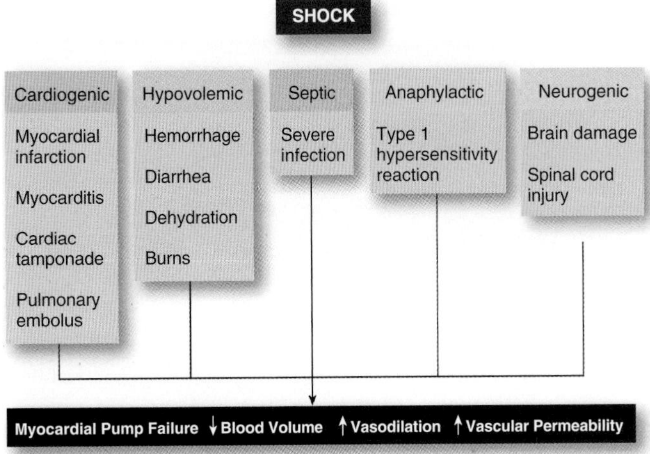

FIGURE 8-6. Classification of shock. Shock results from (1) an inability of the heart to pump adequately (cardiogenic shock), (2) decreased effective blood volume as a consequence of severely reduced blood or plasma volume (hypovolemic shock), or (3) widespread vasodilation (septic, anaphylactic, or neurogenic shock). Increased vascular permeability may complicate vasodilation by contributing to reduced effective blood volume.

HEMOSTASIS AND THROMBOSIS

Normal hemostasis requires that a resting nonthrombotic state be maintained within the vascular system, but that the hemostatic system responds instantly to vascular damage and forms a clot.

Hemorrhage is a discharge of blood outside the vascular compartment into a nonvascular space or outside the body. The most common and obvious cause is trauma. Severe atherosclerosis may so weaken the wall of the abdominal aorta that it balloons to form an aneurysm, which may then rupture and bleed into the retroperitoneal space (as discussed below). A severe decrease in the number of platelets (**thrombocytopenia**) or deficiency of a coagulation factor is often associated with spontaneous hemorrhage without apparent trauma.

Specialized terminology that describes hemorrhagic processes includes the following:

- **Hematoma:** Hemorrhage into soft tissue. Such collections of blood can be merely painful, as in a muscle bruise, or fatal, if located in the brain.
- **Hemothorax:** Hemorrhage into the pleural cavity.
- **Hemopericardium:** Hemorrhage into the pericardial space.
- **Hemoperitoneum:** Bleeding into the peritoneal cavity.
- **Hemarthrosis:** Bleeding into a joint space.
- **Purpura:** Diffuse superficial hemorrhages in the skin, up to 1 cm in diameter.
- **Ecchymosis:** A large superficial hemorrhage in the skin (Fig. 8-7). It is purple at first, then turns green, and finally yellow before resolving. This sequence of events reflects progressive oxidation of bilirubin released from the hemoglobin of degraded erythrocytes. A good example of an ecchymosis is a "black eye."
- **Petechiae:** Pinpoint hemorrhages, usually in the skin or conjunctiva (Fig. 8-8). This lesion represents the rupture of a capillary or arteriole and occurs in conjunction with coagulopathies or vasculitis. Petechiae may also be caused by microemboli from infected heart valves (bacterial endocarditis) (Fig. 8-8).

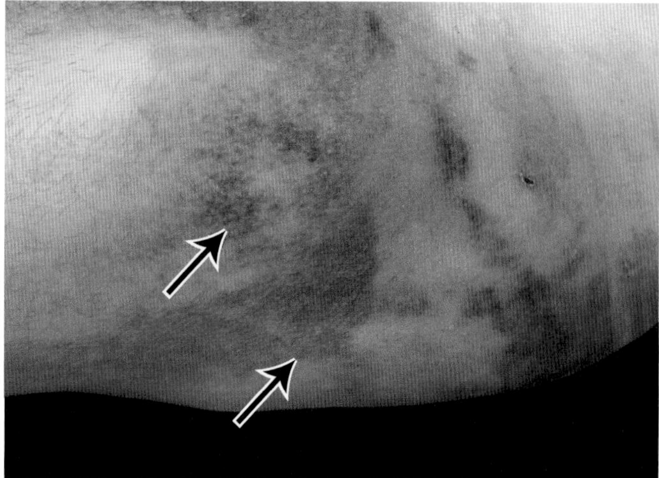

FIGURE 8-7. Ecchymosis. Superficial diffuse hemorrhage (*arrows*) on the thigh caused by blunt force trauma. Courtesy of Dr. Charles Lee, Department of Pathology and Laboratory Medicine, University of British Columbia.

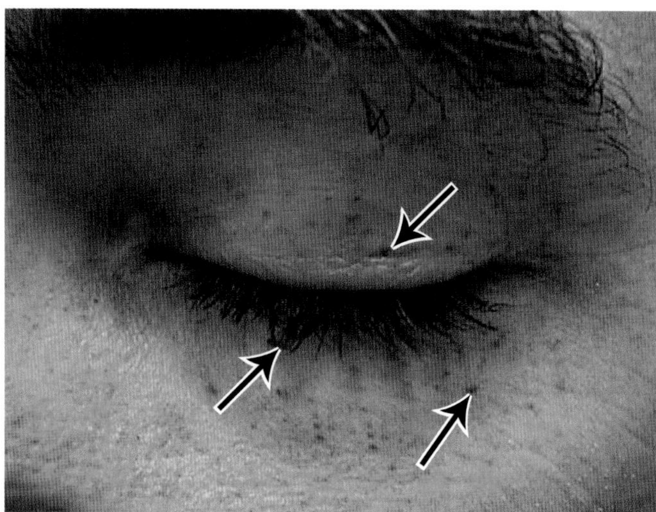

FIGURE 8-8. Petechiae. Periorbital microhemorrhages (*arrows*) appear as punctate red foci. Courtesy of Dr. Greg J. Davis, Department of Pathology, University of Kentucky College of Medicine.

THROMBOSIS

Thrombosis refers to the pathologic formation of a **thrombus**, defined as an aggregate of coagulated blood containing platelets, fibrin, and entrapped cellular elements, all within a vascular lumen. By definition, a thrombus adheres to vascular endothelium and should be distinguished from a simple blood clot, which depends only on activation of the coagulation cascade and can form in vitro or even postmortem. Similarly, a thrombus differs from a hematoma, which follows hemorrhage and subsequent clotting outside the vascular system. Thrombi may form when (1) endothelial function is altered, (2) endothelial continuity is lost, or (3) when blood flow in a vessel becomes abnormal, such as turbulent or static.

Details of the complex processes that maintain normal hemostasis are found in Chapter 18.

Arterial Thrombosis

The pathogenesis of arterial thrombosis involves principally the following three factors:

- **Damage to endothelium**, usually by **atherosclerosis**, disturbs the anticoagulant properties of the vessel wall and serves as a nidus for platelet aggregation and fibrin formation. Atherosclerosis is discussed in detail below.
- **Alterations in blood flow**, whether from turbulence in an aneurysm or at sites of arterial bifurcation, are conducive to thrombosis. Slowing of blood flow in narrowed arteries favors thrombosis.
- **Increased coagulability of the blood**, for example, polycythemia vera or in association with some cancers, entails an increased risk of thrombosis.

The vessels most commonly involved in arterial thrombosis are coronary, cerebral, mesenteric and renal arteries, and arteries of the lower extremities. Less commonly, arterial thrombosis occurs in other disorders, including inflammation of arteries (arteritis), trauma, and blood diseases. Thrombi are common in **aneurysms** (localized dilations of the lumen) of the aorta and its major branches, in which the distortion of blood flow, combined with intrinsic vascular disease and, in particular, atherosclerosis, promotes thrombosis.

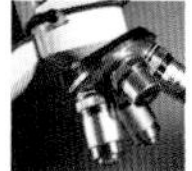

PATHOLOGY: Arterial thrombi attached to vessel walls are soft, friable, and dark red at first, with fine alternating bands of yellowish platelets and fibrin, termed lines of Zahn (Fig. 8-9). Arterial thrombi have several possible fates:

- **Lysis**, owing to the potent thrombolytic activity of the blood.
- **Propagation** (i.e., increase in size), because the thrombus acts as a focus for further thrombosis.
- **Organization**, the eventual invasion of connective tissue elements, which causes a thrombus to become firm and grayish white.
- **Canalization**, by which new lumens lined by endothelial cells form in an organized thrombus (Fig. 8-10). Its functional significance tends to be uncertain.
- **Embolization**, in which part or all of the thrombus becomes dislodged, travels through the circulation, and lodges in

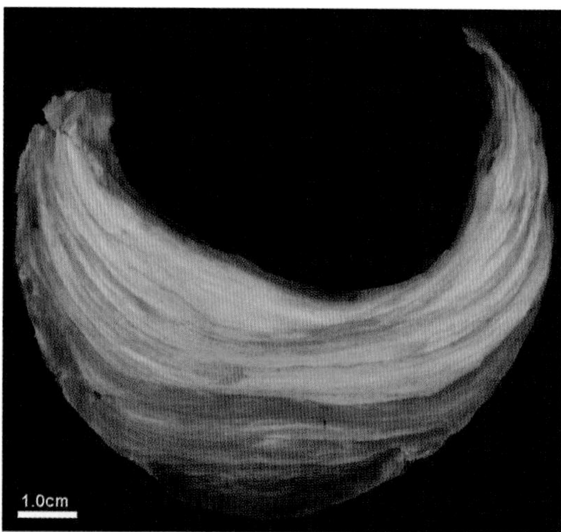

FIGURE 8-9. Arterial thrombus. Gross photograph of a thrombus from an aortic aneurysm showing the laminations of fibrin and platelets known as the lines of Zahn.

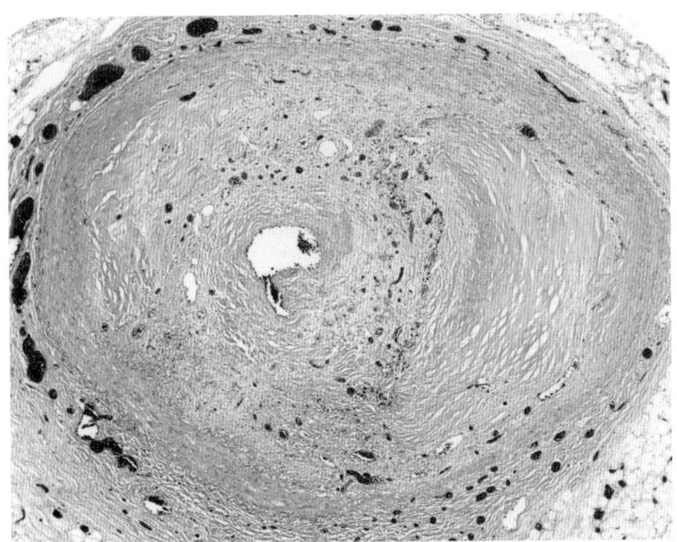

FIGURE 8-10. Canalization of thrombus. Photomicrograph of the left anterior descending coronary artery showing severe atherosclerosis and canalization.

a blood vessel some distance from the site of thrombus formation (see below for further discussion).

The organized structure of a thrombus reflects a tight interaction between platelets and fibrin and differs in appearance from a postmortem clot or one formed in a test tube. Determination of whether a clot formed during life (antemortem clot) or after death (postmortem clot) is often important in a medical autopsy and in forensic pathology. Lines of Zahn characterize a thrombus formed during life, whereas a postmortem clot has a more gelatinous structure. Postmortem clots settle into a lower region containing many red blood cells, resulting in a reddish, gelatinous appearance ("currant jelly"). An upper overlying clot is firmer and yellow white, representing coagulated plasma without red blood cells ("chicken fat").

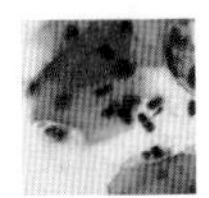

CLINICAL FEATURES: *Arterial thrombosis due to atherosclerosis is the most common cause of death in industrialized countries.* Because most arterial thrombi occlude the vessel, they often lead to ischemic necrosis of tissue supplied by that artery (i.e., an **infarct**). Thus, thrombosis of a coronary or cerebral atherosclerotic plaque (Fig. 8-11) results in a **myocardial infarct** (heart attack) or **cerebral infarct** (stroke), respectively. Other end arteries that are often affected by atherosclerosis and suffer thrombosis include mesenteric arteries (intestinal infarction), renal arteries (kidney infarcts), and arteries of the leg (ischemic leg gangrene).

ATHEROSCLEROSIS

Atherosclerosis is characterized by the progressive accumulation of (1) inflammatory, immune, and smooth muscle cells, (2) lipids, and (3) connective tissue in the intima of large- and medium-sized elastic and muscular arteries. The classic atherosclerotic lesion is best described as a fibroinflammatory lipid plaque termed an **atheroma**. These plaques develop over several decades (Tables 8-2 and 8-3). Their continued growth encroaches on the media of the arterial wall and into the lumen of the vessel, thereby narrowing its caliber. Atherosclerotic lesions are also called atherosclerotic plaques, atheromas, fibrous plaques, or fibrofatty lesions. A comprehensive description of the pathogenesis of atherosclerosis is now possible, with the caveat that the formation, growth, and clinical presentation of the plaques vary from patient to patient.

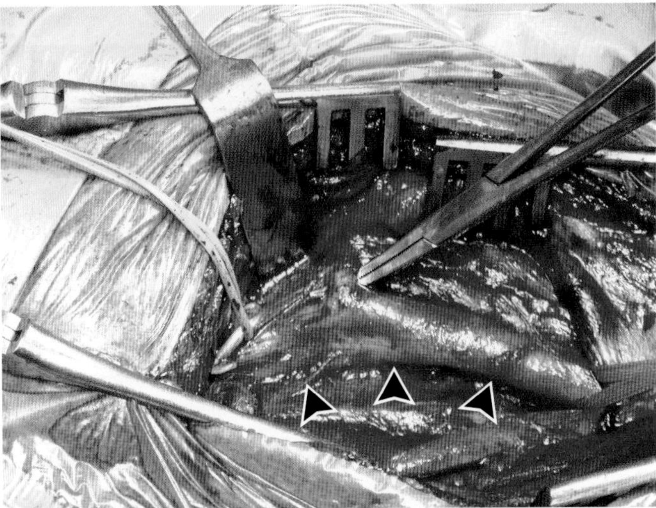

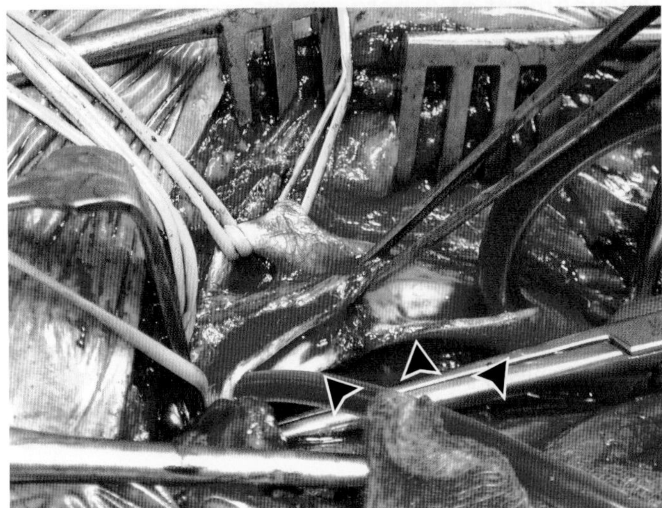

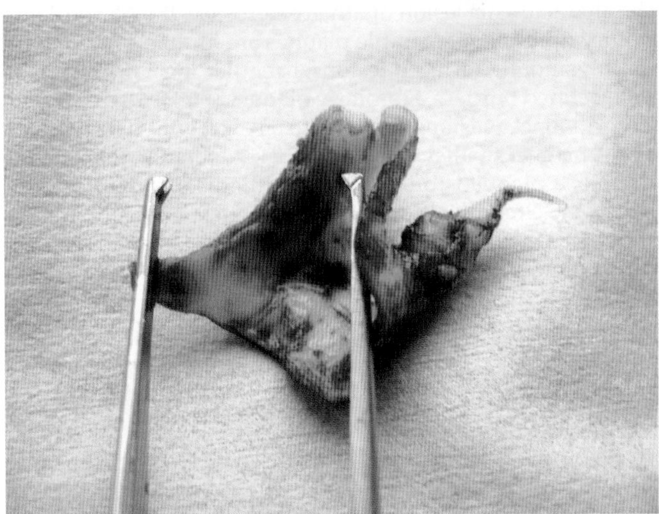

FIGURE 8-11. Endarterectomy. Intraoperative image of a carotid artery (*above, arrowheads*) postarteriotomy displaying a near-occlusive atherosclerotic plaque in situ (*middle, arrowheads*) and the atherosclerotic plaque itself after carotid endarterectomy (*below*).

Table 8-2

Atherogenesis

- Initiation and growth of fibroinflammatory lipid atheroma is a slowly evolving dynamic process with superimposed acute events.
- Risk factors accelerate progression.
- The pathogenesis is multifactorial, and thus the relative-importance of specific genetic and environmental factors may vary in individuals.
- Interactions between cellular and matrix components of the vessel wall and serum constituents, leukocytes, platelets, and physical forces regulate the formation of the fibroinflammatory lipid atheroma.

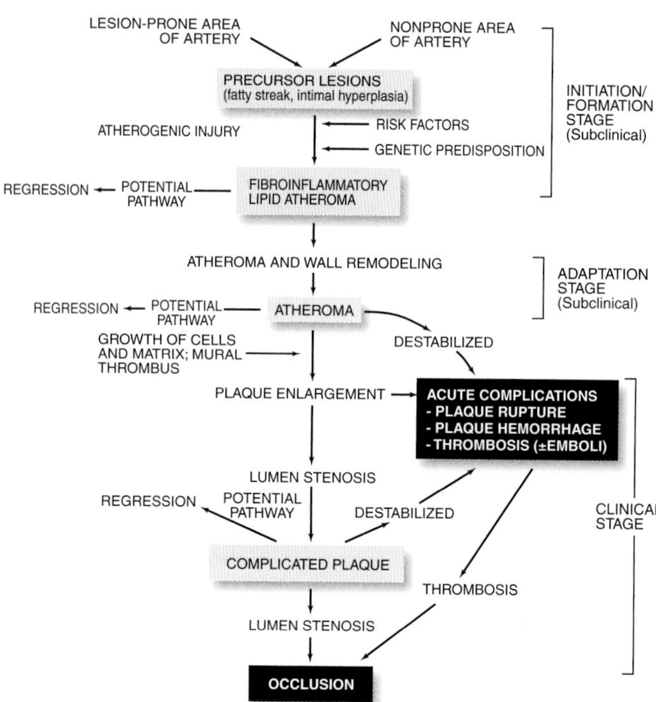

FIGURE 8-12. A unifying hypothesis for the pathogenesis of atherosclerosis.

Development of Atherogenesis

The typical atherosclerotic lesion, which is initially clinically insignificant, forms over 20 to 30 years. An exception is the case of homozygous familial hypercholesterolemia, in which lesions develop in the first decade of life. Identification of a single "master" atherogenic gene responsible for most atherosclerosis is unlikely. Rather, it seems that multiple gene polymorphisms interact with the environment and with each other.

The pathogenesis of atherosclerosis is progressive, proceeding through an initiation or formation stage and an adaptation stage, both of which are subclinical. However, as lesions enlarge and encroach into the vessel lumen, a clinical stage becomes apparent. Central to this prolonged process is the development of the **fibroinflammatory lipid plaque or atheroma** (Fig. 8-12).

The Characteristic Lesion of Atherosclerosis

The characteristic lesion of atherosclerosis is the fibroinflammatory lipid plaque. Simple plaques are focal, elevated, pale yellow, smooth-surfaced lesions, irregular in shape but with well-defined borders. Fibrofatty plaques (Fig. 8-13) represent more advanced lesions and tend to be oval, with diameters of up to 12 cm. In smaller vessels, such as the coronary or cerebral arteries, a plaque is often eccentric, that is, it occupies only part of the circumference of the lumen. In later stages, fusion of plaques in muscular arteries can give rise to larger lesions, which occupy several square centimeters.

Table 8-3

Important Components of Fibroinflammatory Lipid Atheroma

Cells	• Endothelial cells	• Lipids and lipoproteins
	• Foam cells	• Serum proteins
	• Giant cells	• Platelet and leukocyte products
	• Lymphocytes	• Necrotic debris
	• Mast cells	• New microvessels
	• Macrophages	• Hydroxyapatite crystals
Matrix	• Collagen	• Growth factors
	• Elastin	• Oxidants/antioxidants
	• Glycoproteins	• Proteolytic enzymes
	• Proteoglycans	• Procoagulant factors

Atherosclerotic plaques are initially covered by endothelium and tend to involve the intima and very little of the upper media (Fig. 8-13B). The area between the lumen and the necrotic core—the **fibrous cap**—contains smooth muscle cells, macrophages, lymphocytes, lipid-laden cells (**foam cells**), and connective tissue components. The central core features necrotic debris. Foam cells are both macrophages and smooth muscle cells that have taken up lipids. Cholesterol crystals and foreign-body giant cells may be present within the fibrous tissue and necrotic areas. Numerous inflammatory and immune cells, especially T cells, are present within a plaque.

Neovascularization is an important contributor to plaque growth and its subsequent complications. It is postulated that vessels grow inward from the vasa vasorum. They are rare in healthy coronary arteries but plentiful in atherosclerotic plaques.

A **complicated** plaque reflects erosion, ulceration, or fissuring of the plaque surface, plaque hemorrhage, mural thrombosis, calcification, and aneurysm formation (Figs. 8-13C and D, 8-14, and 8-15). Progression from a simple fibrofatty atherosclerotic plaque to a complicated lesion may occur as early as the third decade of life, but most affected persons are 50 or 60 years of age. The process heralds the advent of potential clinical disease.

The Precursor Lesion of Atherosclerosis

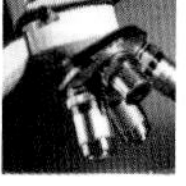

PATHOLOGY: Two distinct lesions precede atherosclerotic plaques, fatty streak, and intimal cell mass.

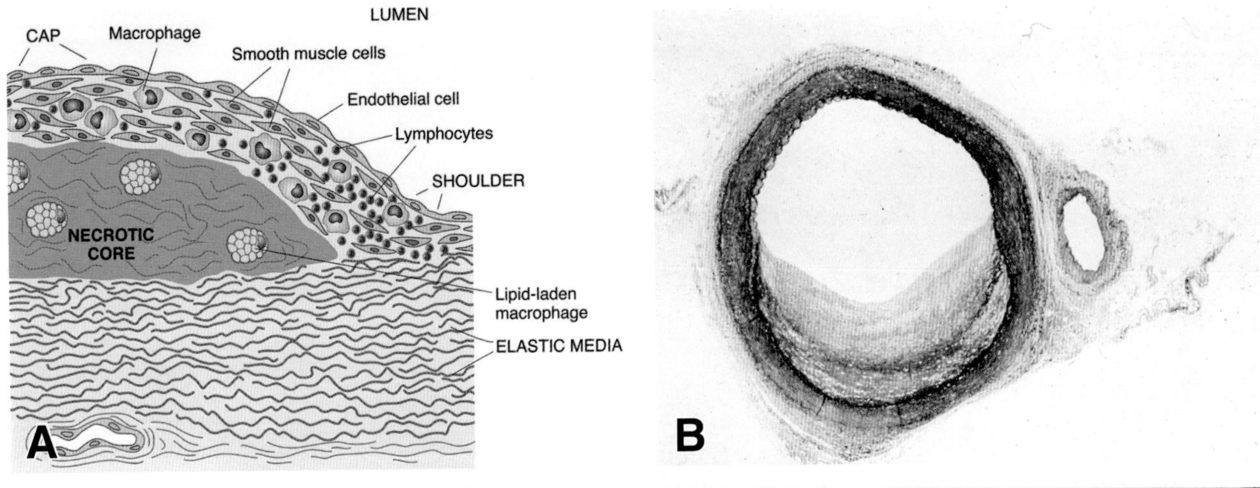

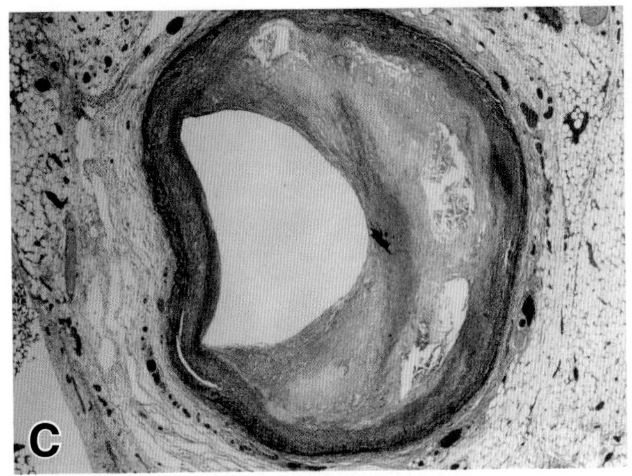

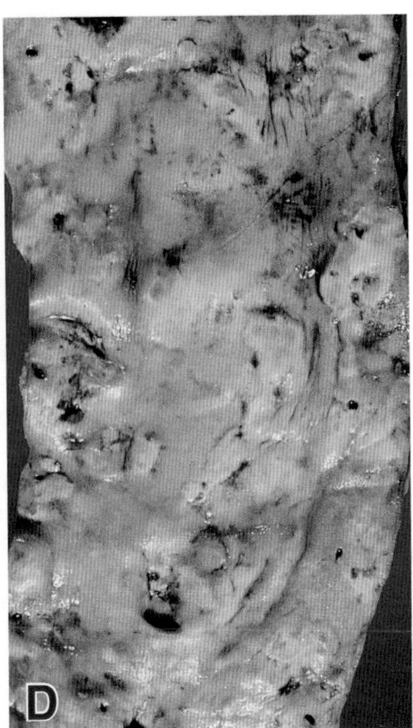

FIGURE 8-13. Fibrofatty plaque of atherosclerosis. A. In this fully developed fibrous plaque, the core contains lipid-filled macrophages and necrotic smooth muscle cell debris. The "fibrous" cap is composed largely of smooth muscle cells, which produce collagen, small amounts of elastin, and glycosaminoglycans. Also shown are infiltrating macrophages and lymphocytes. Note that the endothelium over the surface of the fibrous cap frequently appears intact. **B.** Adaptive stage with atherosclerotic plaque and vessel wall dilatation to maintain the normal size of the lumen. Normal artery wall is at the top. **C.** Stenotic coronary artery with atherosclerotic plaque. **D.** The aorta showing discrete, raised, tan plaques. Focal plaque ulcerations are also evident.

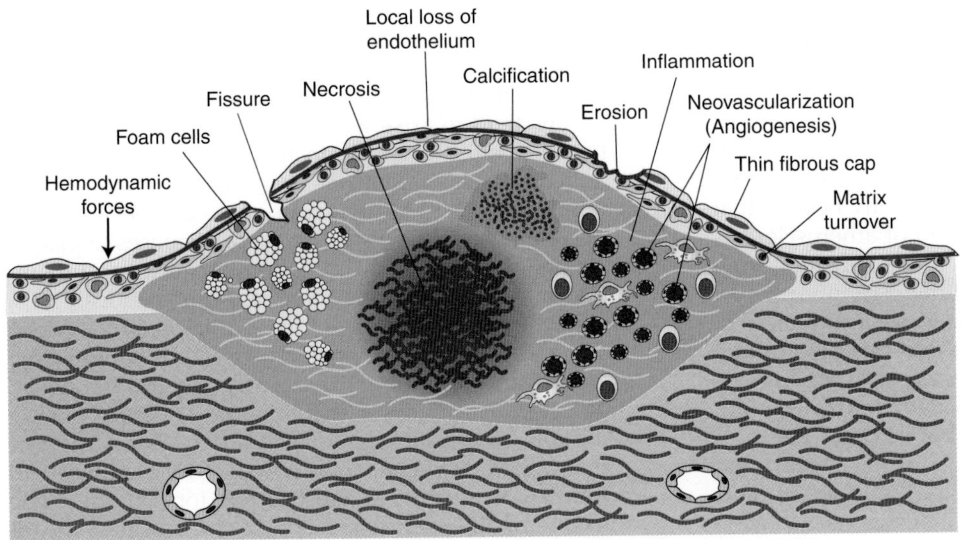

FIGURE 8-14. Complicated atherosclerotic plaque. The surface shows endothelial denudation, erosion, and fissure formation. The plaque shows a thin fibrous cap, a central necrotic core, inflammation, lipids, calcification, and neovascularization.

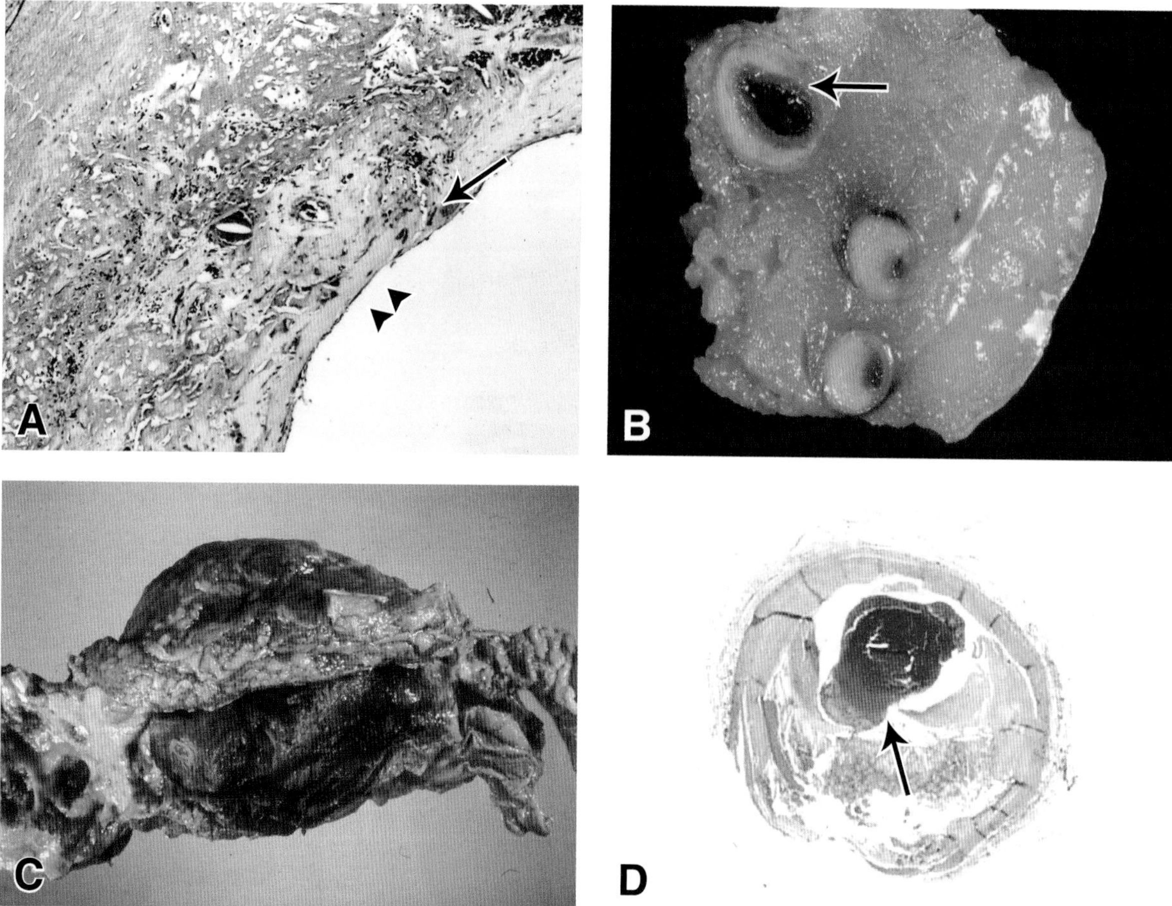

FIGURE 8-15. Complications of atherosclerosis. A. Fibroinflammatory lipid plaque. Microscopic features of plaque erosion (*arrowheads*) and fissure formation (*arrow*). **B.** Fibroinflammatory lipid plaque with occlusive luminal thrombosis (*arrow*). **C.** Abdominal aortic aneurysm with thrombus. **D.** Rupture of fibrous cap and occlusive luminal thrombosis (*arrow*) in atherosclerotic coronary artery.

- **Fatty streak:** Fatty streaks are flat or slightly elevated lesions in the intima in which intracellular and extracellular lipids accumulate. They may be seen in young children as well as in adults. Foam cells are present (Fig. 8-16). Macrophages contain the most lipid, but smooth muscle cells contain fat as well. In children, significant fatty streaks may be evident in many parts of the arterial tree, but they do not reflect the distribution of atherosclerotic lesions in adults. Fatty streaks are common in the thoracic aorta in children, but atherosclerosis in adults is far more prominent in the abdominal aorta. However, with time, fatty streaks occur in coronary arteries at locations similar to those in which atheromas occur in adulthood. Thus, many believe that fatty infiltration is a precursor lesion of atherosclerosis and that other factors are involved in the transition from fatty streak to clinically significant atherosclerotic plaque.
- **Intimal cell mass:** The intimal cell mass is another candidate for a precursor lesion of atherosclerosis. Intimal cell masses are white, thickened areas at branch points in the arterial tree. Microscopically, they contain smooth muscle cells and connective tissue but no lipid. The location of these lesions, also known as "cushions," at arterial branch sites correlates well with the locations of later atherosclerotic lesions.

Plaque Initiation and Formation Stage

1. Intimal lesions initially occur at sites that appear to be predisposed to lesion formation because of structural features, including intimal cell mass, bifurcations, branch points, and curvatures in the artery. Endothelial dysfunction and ensuing lipid accumulation may also be secondary to hemodynamic shear stress or constitutive in association with vessel wall structure. Atherosclerotic lesions tend to arise where shear stresses are low but fluctuate rapidly (e.g., branch points and bifurcations). Subendothelial smooth muscle cells accumulate in an intimal cell mass at branch points and other locations in certain vessels. This cell mass predisposes to plaque formation, particularly in the coronary arteries. Inflammatory cells, including macrophages and dendritic cells, are present in the intima of these atherosclerotic-prone areas. The distribution of atherosclerotic lesions in large vessels and differences in the location and frequency of lesions in different vascular beds support a belief in the role of hemodynamic factors (Fig. 8-18). The fact that hypertension enhances the severity of atherosclerotic lesions further suggests a role for hemodynamic factors in atherogenesis. In people at increased risk of

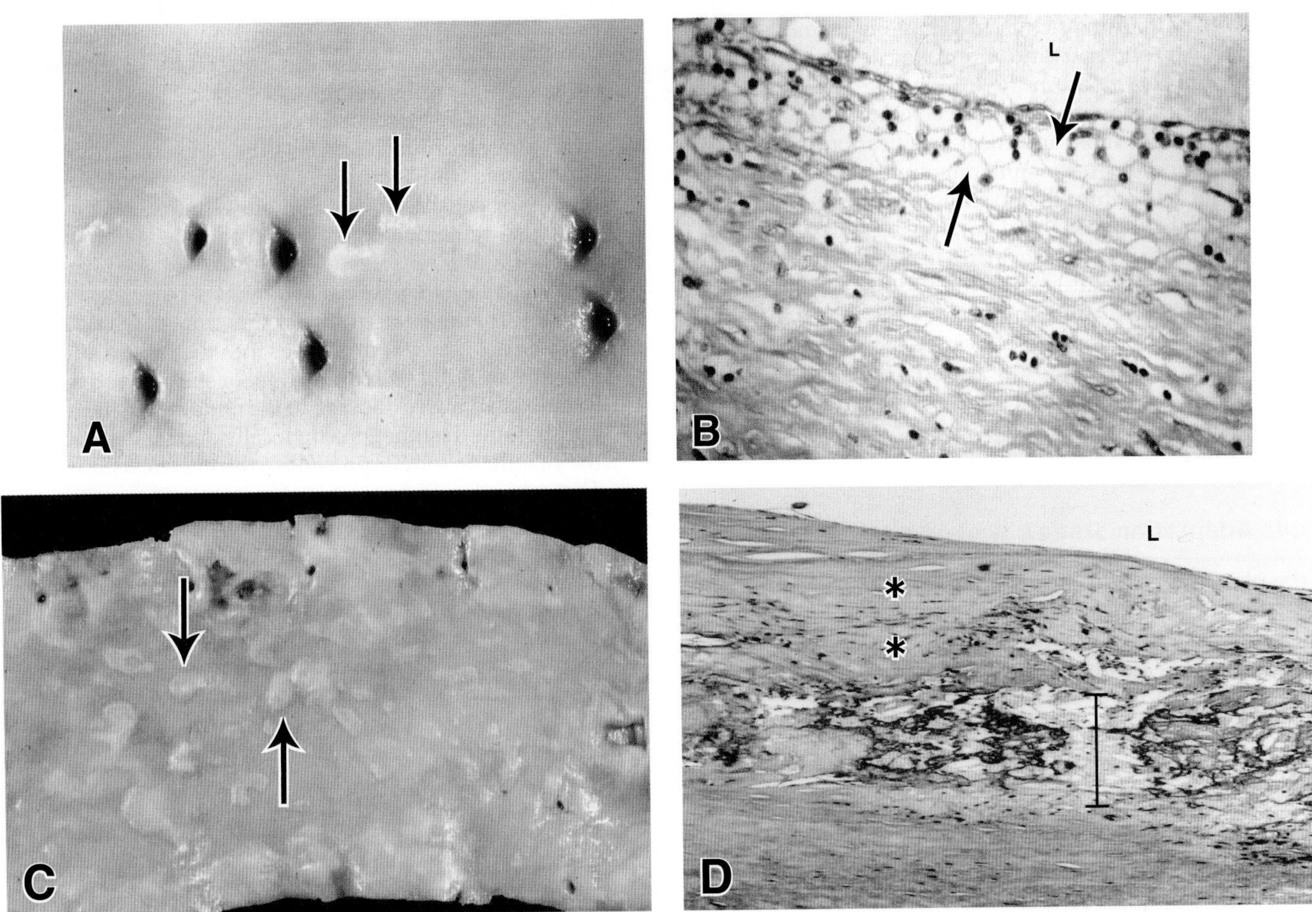

FIGURE 8-16. Fatty streak and atherosclerosis. A. Fatty streak. Gross photo of yellow fatty streaks (*arrows*) in the thoracic aorta. **B.** Fatty streak. Microscopic features of fatty streak in artery wall with intimal foam cells (*arrows*). **C.** Fibroinflammatory lipid plaques (*arrows*). Focal elevated plaques in thoracic aorta. **D.** Fibroinflammatory lipid plaques. Fibrous cap (*asterisks*) separating lumen (L) from central necrotic core (*bracket*).

atherosclerosis, lesions also occur in areas that are not necessarily predisposed to the disease.

2. Lipid accumulation depends on disruption of the integrity of the endothelial barrier through gaps between cells, cell loss, or endothelial cell dysfunction. This injury may result from hypercholesterolemia, abnormal laminar flow, reactive oxygen species, cytokine-induced inflammation, advanced glycation end products produced in diabetes, and hyperhomocysteinemia. Hypertension also promotes endothelial dysfunction. Oxidative stress in endothelial cells and macrophages induces cellular dysfunction and damage. Low-density lipoproteins (LDLs) carry lipids into the intima. Because oxidized LDL activates cell adhesion molecules, macrophages can adhere to activated endothelial cells and transmigrate between endothelial cells into the intima, bringing lipids with them. Some of these "foamy" macrophages undergo necrosis and release lipids. Alterations in types of matrix proteoglycans synthesized by the smooth muscle cells in the intima also render these sites prone to lipid accumulation by binding lipids and trapping them in the intima. Reduced egress of lipids out of the artery wall also promotes lipid accumulation.
3. Mononuclear macrophages, in addition to being central to atherogenesis by participating in lipid accumulation, also release growth factors that stimulate further accumulation of smooth muscle cells. **Oxidized LDL** induces tissue damage and recruits macrophages. It also promotes endothelial and smooth muscle cell release of chemokines, which regulate immune cell recruitment in the plaque. The combination of macrophages and endothelial cells may transform the normal anticoagulant vascular surface to a procoagulant one.
4. As a lesion progresses, mural thrombi often form on the damaged intimal surface. This effect stimulates PDGF release, thereby accelerating smooth muscle proliferation and secretion of matrix components. The thrombus may grow, lyse, or become organized and incorporated into the plaque.
5. The deeper parts of the thickened intima are poorly nourished because of a distance limitation for the diffusion of nutrients. This tissue undergoes ischemic necrosis, which is augmented by proteolytic enzymes released by macrophages (i.e., cathepsins) and tissue damage caused by oxidized LDL, reactive oxygen species, and other agents. Thus, the central necrotic core is formed. Together with specific platelet- and macrophage-derived angiogenic factors, the necrotic core initiates angiogenesis, with new vasa vasorum forming in the plaque.

6. The fibroinflammatory lipid plaque is formed, with a central necrotic core and a fibrous cap, separating the core from the blood in the lumen (Fig. 8-15). The core contains tissue debris, apoptotic cells, necrotic foam cells, cholesterol crystals, and focal calcification. Cholesterol crystals promote further inflammation. Inflammatory and immune cells infiltrate and mingle with smooth muscle cells, deposited lipids, and variably organized matrix.
7. The immune system participates in atherogenesis. Expression of HLA-DR antigens on the endothelial and smooth muscle cells of plaques implies that these cells may have undergone immunologic activation, perhaps in response to interferon released by activated T cells in the plaque. Hence, the presence of T cells reflects an autoimmune response (e.g., against oxidized LDL). Dendritic cells are also present in early lesions.

Plaque Adaptation Stage

As the plaque protrudes into the lumen (e.g., in coronary arteries), the wall of the artery remodels to maintain lumen size (Fig. 8-18). When a plaque occupies about half of the lumen, such remodeling can no longer compensate, and the arterial lumen becomes narrowed (**stenosis**). Hemodynamic shear stress, an important regulator of vessel wall remodeling, acts through the mechanotransduction properties of endothelial cells. These include the cell cytoskeleton, ion channels in the cell membrane, and the cell coat. Apoptosis and proliferation of smooth muscle cells and matrix synthesis and degradation modulate remodeling of the vessel and the atherosclerotic plaque. Even a small plaque at this stage can rupture, with catastrophic results.

Plaque Clinical Stage

1. As a plaque encroaches on the lumen, hemorrhage into the plaque may increase its size without overall plaque rupture. This hemorrhage may occur when fragile new vessels in the plaque rupture locally. Macrophages clean up the hemorrhagic material. Circulating blood may undermine the plaque, in which case the raised plaque, hemorrhage, and thrombosis combine to obstruct the vessel.
2. Complications develop in the plaque, including surface ulceration, fissure formation, calcification, and aneurysm formation. Activated mast cells at sites of erosion may release pro-inflammatory mediators and cytokines. Continued plaque growth results in severe stenosis or occlusion of the lumen. Plaque rupture and ensuing thrombosis and occlusion may precipitate catastrophic events in these advanced plaques (e.g., acute myocardial infarction). However, recent angiographic studies suggest that even plaques causing less than 50% stenosis may suddenly rupture. There are several conditions that appear to favor rupture, as noted in Figure 8-13. These include hemodynamic shear stress, fissure formation, a thin fibrous cap, reduced number of smooth muscle cells, increased matrix metalloproteinase activity, inflammation, foam cell accumulation, and focal nodular calcification.

Mechanisms in Plaque Development

- **Calcification**, sometimes involving differentiation of osteocytes and chondrocytes, occurs in areas of necrosis and elsewhere in the plaque. Oxidized lipids and inflammatory cytokines promote vascular calcification. Calcification in the artery is thought to depend on mineral deposition and resorption, which are regulated by osteoblast- and osteoclast-like cells in the vessel wall. These cells are considered to be rare precursor cells in the artery wall, derived from smooth muscle–type cells that have undergone a phenotypic transformation or possibly circulating stem/precursor cells derived from bone marrow. Calcification may also reflect changes in the physical–chemical properties of a diseased vessel wall that provoke formation of hydroxyapatite crystals.
- **Mural thrombosis** results from abnormal blood flow around the plaque, where it protrudes into the lumen and creates turbulence, reduced luminal flow or stasis. The disturbance in flow also causes damage to the endothelial lining, which may become dysfunctional or locally denuded, in which case the plaque no longer presents a thromboresistant surface. Thrombi often form at sites of erosion and fissuring on the surface of the fibrous cap. Mural thrombi in the proximal region of a coronary artery may embolize to more distal sites in the vessel.
- **Atheroma destabilization** often results in acute coronary syndromes. It may occur whenever the dynamic balance of opposing biologic and physical processes is disrupted, leading to mural thrombosis, fibrous cap rupture, or intraplaque hemorrhage, as noted above. Some ruptures are clinically silent and can heal. In a ruptured plaque, the necrotic material that comes in contact with the blood contains tissue factor (**TF**) and is highly thrombogenic. The adjacent endothelium has reduced tissue factor pathway inhibitor (TFPI) levels and lower antiplatelet and fibrinolytic activities, all favoring coagulation. The presence of circulating markers of inflammation suggests that procoagulant inflammatory mediators also participate.

Plaque Rupture

Once a plaque **ruptures**, the exposed thrombogenic material promotes clot formation in the lumen, generating an occlusive thrombus. Plaque hemorrhage may occur within a plaque, with or without a subsequent rupture of the fibrous cap. In the latter case, hemorrhage may expand the plaque, narrowing the lumen further. The hemorrhage will be resorbed over time within the plaque, leaving telltale residual hemosiderin-laden macrophages.

Most plaques that rupture show less than 50% luminal stenosis, and over 95% are less than 70% stenosed. Plaque rupture often occurs at the shoulder of the plaque, suggesting that hemodynamic shear stress weakens and tears the fibrous cap. If not repaired, endothelial loss furthers plaque erosion, weakens the fibrous cap, and exposes the plaque to blood constituents. Plaque rupture has been associated with (1) areas of inflammation, (2) large lipid core size, (3) thin fibrous cap, (4) decreased smooth muscle cells owing to apoptosis, (5) imbalance of proteolytic enzymes and their inhibitors in the fibrous cap, (6) calcification in the plaque, and (7) intraplaque hemorrhage, resulting in inside-out rupture of the fibrous cap.

Complications of Atherosclerosis

The complications of atherosclerosis depend on the location and size of the affected vessel (Fig. 8-17) and the chronicity of the process. The major complications of atherosclerosis, including ischemic heart disease (coronary artery disease), myocardial infarction, stroke, and gangrene of the extremities, account for

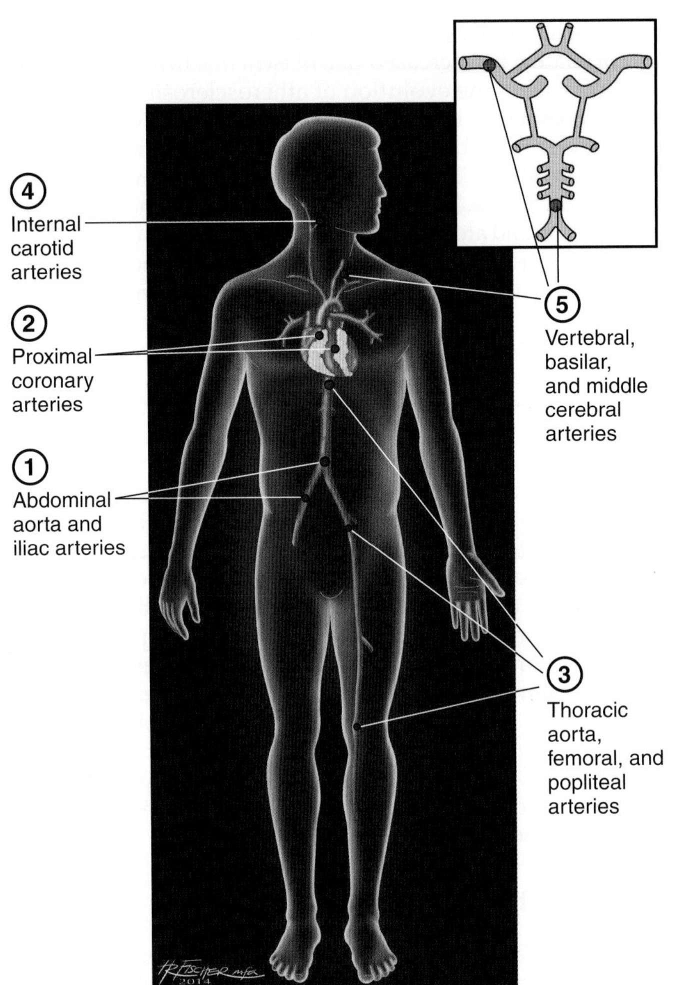

FIGURE 8-17. Sites of severe atherosclerosis in order of frequency.

more than half of the annual mortality in the United States, with ischemic heart disease being the leading cause of death. The incidence of death from ischemic heart disease in Western countries peaked in the late 1960s, then declined by more than 30%. There are wide geographic and racial variations in the frequency of the disorder.

- **Acute occlusion:** Thrombosis on an atherosclerotic plaque may abruptly occlude a muscular artery (Fig. 8-18). The consequence is ischemic necrosis (infarction) of the tissue supplied by that vessel, manifested clinically as myocardial infarction, stroke, or gangrene of the intestine or lower extremities. Some occlusive thrombi can be dissolved therapeutically by enzymes that activate plasma fibrinolytic activity, including streptokinase and tissue plasminogen activator.
- **Chronic narrowing of the vessel lumen:** As an atherosclerotic plaque grows, it may narrow the lumen, progressively reducing blood flow to tissue served by that artery. Chronic ischemia of the affected tissue causes atrophy of the organ, for example, (1) unilateral renal artery stenosis giving rise to renal atrophy, (2) mesenteric artery atherosclerosis causing intestinal stricture, or (3) ischemic atrophy of the skin in a diabetic with severe peripheral vascular disease. Such reduced blood flow to target organs may also result in muscle pain on exertion, such as angina pectoris of the heart and vascular claudication of the lower limbs.

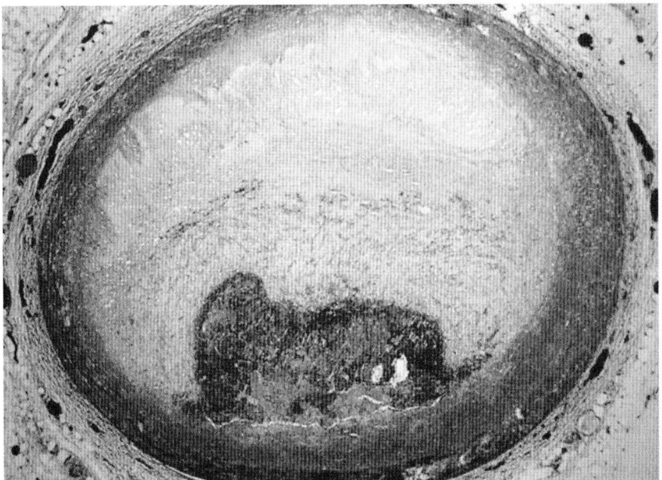

FIGURE 8-18. Coronary artery thrombosis. A microscopic section of a coronary artery showing severe atherosclerosis and a recent thrombus in the narrowed lumen.

- **Aneurysm formation:** The complicated lesions of atherosclerosis may extend into the media of elastic arteries and weaken their walls, so as to allow aneurysm formation, typically in the abdominal aorta. The reduced elastin promotes thinning and ballooning of the wall, whereas matrix metalloproteinases secreted by smooth muscle cells and macrophages break down collagen. Such aneurysms often contain thrombi, which may embolize. Sudden rupture of these aneurysms, especially in the aorta and cerebrum, precipitates a vascular catastrophe.
- **Embolism:** A thrombus formed over an atherosclerotic plaque may detach and lodge in a distal vessel. Thus, embolization from a thrombus in an abdominal aortic aneurysm may acutely occlude the popliteal artery, causing gangrene of the leg. Ulceration of an atherosclerotic plaque or disturbance of plaque by medical procedures may also dislodge atheromatous debris and produce so-called cholesterol crystal emboli, which appear as needle-shaped spaces in affected tissues (Fig. 8-19), most often the kidney, a major complication of atherosclerosis.

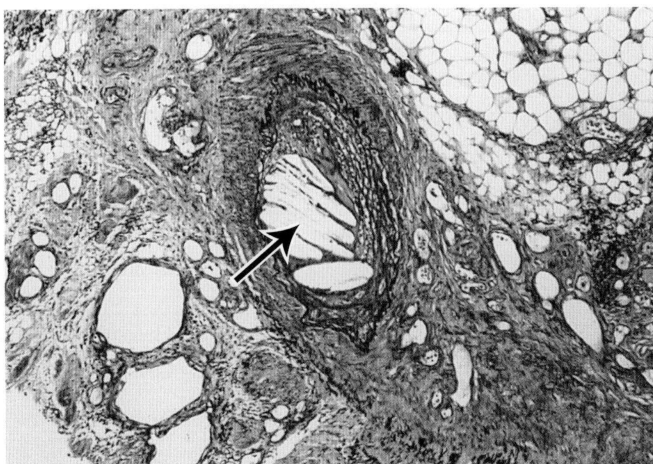

FIGURE 8-19. Cholesterol crystal embolus. Needle-shaped clefts (*arrow*) are seen in an atherosclerotic embolus that has occluded a small artery.

Risk Factors for Atherosclerosis

Factors associated with a twofold or greater risk of ischemic heart disease include the following:

- **Hypertension:** High blood pressure increases the risk of myocardial infarction. Recent evidence indicates that both diastolic and systolic hypertension contribute equally to this increased risk. Men with systolic blood pressures over 160 mm Hg have almost triple the incidence of myocardial infarction compared to those with systolic pressures under 120 mm Hg. The use of antihypertensive drugs has significantly reduced myocardial infarction and stroke.
- **Blood cholesterol level:** Serum cholesterol levels correlate with the development of ischemic heart disease and account for much of the geographic variation in the incidence of this condition. Absent genetic disorders of lipid metabolism (see below), blood cholesterol level correlates with the dietary intake of saturated fat. The use of cholesterol-lowering drugs lowers the risk of myocardial infarction. Total serum cholesterol does not necessarily predict the risk of ischemic heart disease because cholesterol is transported by atherogenic and antiatherogenic lipoproteins. Thus, therapeutic decisions are based mainly on LDL cholesterol levels.
- **Cigarette smoking:** Coronary and aortic atherosclerosis are more severe and extensive in cigarette smokers than in nonsmokers, and the effect is dose related. Thus, smoking markedly increases the risk of myocardial infarction, ischemic stroke, and abdominal aortic aneurysms.
- **Diabetes:** Diabetics are at increased risk for occlusive atherosclerotic vascular disease in many organs. However, the relative contribution of carbohydrate intolerance alone, as opposed to the hypertension and hyperlipidemias common in diabetics, is not well defined (see Chapter 19).
- **Increasing age and male sex:** Both correlate strongly with the risk of myocardial infarction, probably as reflections of accumulated effects of other risk factors.
- **Physical inactivity and stressful life patterns:** These factors correlate with increased risk of ischemic heart disease, but their role in the evolution of atherosclerosis is not clear.
- **Homocysteine:** Homocystinuria is a rare autosomal recessive disease caused by mutations in the gene encoding cystathionine synthase. The disorder causes premature and severe atherosclerosis. Mild elevations of plasma homocysteine are common and are an independent risk factor for coronary atherosclerosis and that of other large vessels. The increased risk is similar in magnitude to those of smoking and hyperlipidemia. Homocysteine is toxic to endothelial cells and impairs several anticoagulant mechanisms in endothelial cells. In addition, oxidative interactions between homocysteine, lipoproteins, and cholesterol further complicate the situation. Low dietary folate intake may aggravate genetic predispositions to hyperhomocysteinemia, but it is not known whether folic acid treatment protects from atherosclerotic vascular disease.
- **C-reactive protein:** CRP is an acute-phase reactant produced mainly by hepatocytes. It is a serum marker for systemic inflammation and has been linked to an increased risk of myocardial infarction and ischemic stroke. This observation, together with the presence of CRP in atherosclerotic plaques, suggests that systemic inflammation may contribute to atherogenesis.
- **Infection:** Seroepidemiologic studies suggest that some infectious agents may contribute to atherosclerosis. *Chlamydia pneumoniae* and cytomegalovirus have been the most studied. DNA from these and other infectious agents has been found in human atherosclerotic lesions, but the nature of this association is obscure.

Lipid Metabolism

Lipoproteins and their roles in lipid transport and metabolism play a major role in the development of atherosclerosis. Cholesterol and other lipids (mainly triglycerides) are insoluble, and lipoprotein particles function as special transporters (Table 8-4; Fig. 8-20). These particles differ in protein and lipid

Table 8-4

The Apolipoproteins

Apolipoprotein	Approximate Molecular Weight	Major Density Class	Major Sites of Synthesis in Humans	Major Function in Lipoprotein Metabolism
AI	28,000	HDL	Liver, intestine	Activates lecithin:cholesterol acyltransferase
AII	18,000	HDL	Liver, intestine	
AIV	45,000	Chylomicrons	Intestine	
B-100	250,000	VLDL, IDL, LDL	Liver	Binds to LDL receptor
B-48	125,000	Chylomicrons, VLDL, IDL	Intestine	
CI	6,500	Chylomicrons, VLDL, HDL	Liver	Activates lecithin:cholesterol acyltransferase
CII	10,000	Chylomicrons, VLDL, HDL	Liver	Activates lipoprotein lipase
CIII	10,000	Chylomicrons	Liver	Inhibits lipoprotein uptake by the liver
D	20,000	HDL		Cholesteryl ester exchange protein
E	40,000	Chylomicrons, VLDL, HDL	Liver, macrophage	Binds to E receptor system

HDL, high-density lipoprotein; IDL, intermediate-density lipoprotein; LDL, low-density lipoprotein; VLDL, very–low-density lipoprotein.

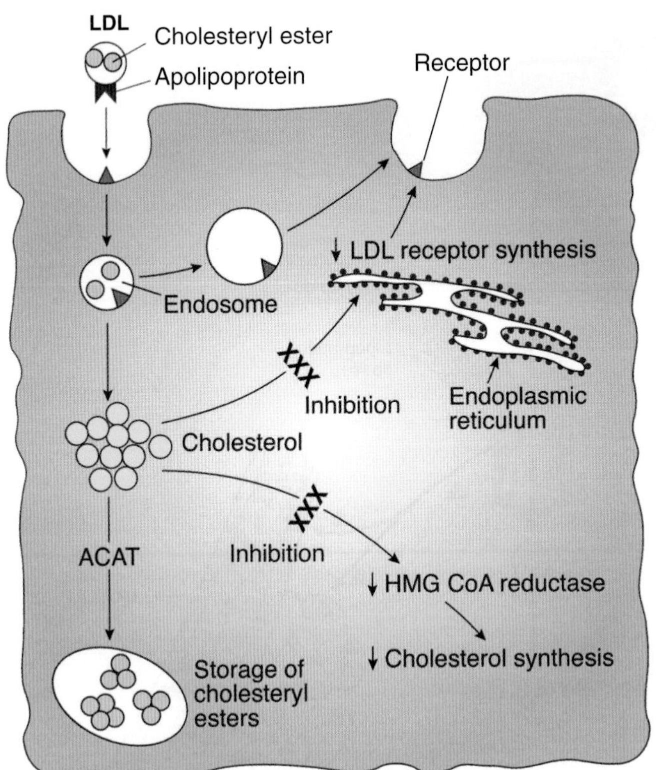

FIGURE 8-20. The relationship between circulating low-density lipoprotein (LDL) cholesterol, LDL receptors, and the synthesis of cholesterol. LDL, which contains cholesteryl esters, is taken up by cells into vesicles by a receptor-mediated pathway to form an endosome. The receptor and lipids are dissociated, and the receptor is returned to the cell surface. The exogenous cholesterol, now in the cytoplasm, causes a reduction in receptor synthesis in the endoplasmic reticulum and inhibits the activity of hydroxymethylglutaryl–coenzyme A (HMG–CoA) reductase in the cholesterol-synthesizing pathway. Excess cholesterol in the cell is esterified to cholesteryl esters and stored in vacuoles. ACAT, acyl-CoA:cholesterol acyltransferase.

composition, size, and density. They are categorized according to density as follows:

- Chylomicrons
- Very low-density lipoproteins (VLDLs)
- Low-density lioproteins (LDLs)
- High-density lipoproteins (HDLs)

Each of these has a lipid core with associated proteins (apolipoproteins) (Table 8-4). The metabolic pathways for lipoproteins containing apolipoprotein B (apoB) are two major cascades, one from the intestine (**exogenous pathway**) and the other from the liver (**endogenous pathway**) (Fig. 8-21).

High-density Lipoprotein

HDL is referred to as "good" cholesterol. ***An inverse correlation between ischemic heart disease and HDL cholesterol levels has been established.*** Factors that increase HDL levels include female gender, estrogens, vigorous exercise, and moderate alcohol consumption. Decreased HDL occurs with diets high in polyunsaturated fats, truncal obesity, diabetes, smoking, and androgen administration. ***HDL interacts with cells in the transport system to carry extrahepatic cholesterol, including that in the arterial wall, to the liver for elimination.*** The latter function has been called **reverse cholesterol transport**. The cholesterol removed from cells is principally free cholesterol, which is rapidly esterified to cholesteryl esters; transferred to LDL; and transported to smooth muscle cells, adrenal cells, and fibroblasts. In these cells, LDL is endocytosed via specific LDL receptors and catabolized. Defects in this process of cholesteryl ester transfer and exchange induce dyslipoproteinemia, increased intracellular cholesteryl ester concentrations, and premature atherosclerosis.

Low-density Lipoprotein

LDL contains apoB-100 and cholesterol esters as its main lipid entity. LDLs are heterogeneous in particle density, a characteristic that correlates with differences in atherogenicity. Macrophages, endothelial cells, and smooth muscle cells in atherosclerotic lesions can oxidize LDL, thereby increasing LDL atherogenicity, facilitating LDL recognition by the macrophage scavenger receptor, and generating massive cholesterol uptake by macrophages. Autoantibodies to oxidized LDL are detected in both plasma and plaques in patients with atherosclerosis and may be important in plaque development. Oxidized LDLs are toxic to vascular wall cells, may disrupt endothelial integrity, and promote the accumulation of cell debris within atheromas. They are also chemotactic for macrophages, thereby increasing their accumulation in atheromas.

Heritable Dyslipoproteinemia

Familial clustering of ischemic heart diseases is well documented (Table 8-5).

Familial Hypercholesterolemia

The 1985 Nobel Prize was awarded to Brown and Goldstein for discovering the LDL receptor. They identified the pathways regulating cholesterol homeostasis (Fig. 8-20) and facilitated our understanding of receptor-mediated endocytosis and regulation of cell membrane receptors. The LDL receptor is a cell surface glycoprotein that regulates plasma cholesterol by mediating endocytosis and recycling of apoE, a major plasma cholesterol transport protein. Mutations in the *LDL receptor* gene, on the short arm of chromosome 19, give rise to familial hypercholesterolemia (FH), an autosomal dominant disease for which about 1 in 500 people are heterozygotes and 1 in a million are homozygotes.

Most untreated homozygotes die from coronary artery disease before the age of 20 years. Among people under 60 years of age who have suffered a myocardial infarction, 5% are heterozygous for familial hypercholesterolemia. Such heterozygotes have plasma LDL levels that are twice the normal, whereas homozygotes exhibit a 6- to 10-fold increase in plasma LDL. Heterozygote patients also suffer from premature myocardial infarction (40 to 45 years of age in men) but at a later age than do homozygotes. In addition to accelerated accumulation of cholesterol in arteries (premature atherosclerosis), LDL cholesterol deposits in skin and tendons to form xanthomas (Fig. 8-22). In some cases (before age 10 in homozygotes), an *arcus lipoides* is present in the cornea.

More than 400 mutant alleles for familial hypercholesterolemia are known, including point mutations, insertions, and

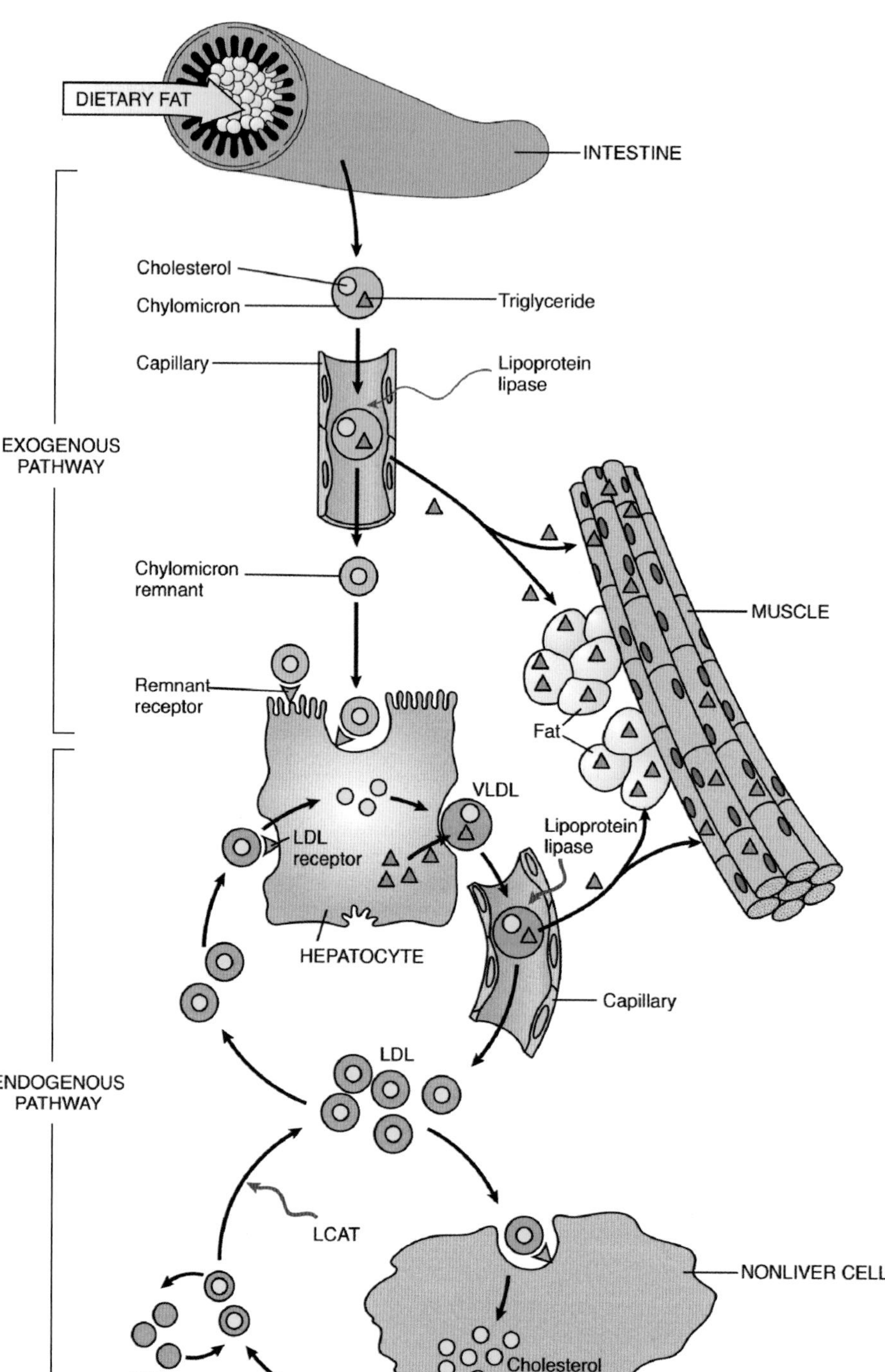

FIGURE 8-21. Exogenous and endogenous cholesterol transport pathway. In the exogenous pathway, cholesterol and fatty acids from food are absorbed through the intestinal mucosa. Fatty acid chains are linked to glycerol to form triglycerides. Triglycerides and cholesterol are packaged into chylomicrons that are returned via the lymph to the blood. The lipids are coupled to proteins by enzymes such as the microsomal transfer protein complex. In the capillaries (mainly of fat tissue and muscle, but also other tissues), the ester bonds holding the fatty acids in triglycerides are split by lipoprotein lipase. Fatty acids are removed, leaving cholesterol-rich lipoprotein remnants. These bind to special remnant receptors and are taken up by liver cells. The cholesterol of the remnant is either secreted into the intestine, largely as bile acids, or packaged as very–low-density lipoprotein (VLDL) particles, which are then secreted into the circulation. This is the first step in the endogenous cycle. In fat or muscle tissue, the triglyceride is removed from the VLDLs with the aid of lipoprotein lipase. The intermediate-density lipoprotein (IDL) particles (not shown) remain in the circulation. Some IDLs are immediately taken up by the liver via the mediation of LDL receptors for apoB/apoE. The remaining IDLs in the circulation are either taken up by nonliver cells or converted into LDLs. Most of the LDLs in the circulation bind to hepatocytes or other cells and are removed from the circulation. High-density lipoproteins take up cholesterol from cells. This cholesterol is esterified by the enzyme lecithin:cholesterol acyltransferase, after which the esters are transferred to LDLs and taken up by cells.

deletions. These mutations fall into five main classes, based on their effects on receptor protein function (Fig. 8-23).

Apolipoprotein E

Genetic variations in various apolipoproteins are also accompanied by alterations in LDL levels. Polymorphisms in apoE and variants of apolipoprotein AI and AII have been observed. Apolipoprotein E is one of the main protein constituents of VLDL and of a subclass of HDL. The gene locus that codes for apoE is polymorphic; three common alleles, E2, E3, and E4, code for three major apoE isoforms, which are responsible for 20% of the variability in serum cholesterol. In men, the apoE 3/2 phenotype is associated with a 20% lower LDL level than the most common phenotype, apoE 3/3. By contrast, the E4 allele is associated with elevated serum cholesterol. Interestingly, the E2 allele is increased and E4 decreased among male octogenarians. The E4 allele is also a major risk factor for late-onset alzheimer disease.

Lipoprotein (a)

Lp(a) is an LDL-like particle to which the glycoprotein apo(a) is attached through a disulfide bridge with apoB-100. High circulating levels of Lp(a) are associated with an increased risk

Table 8-5

Molecular Defects in Dyslipoproteinemias

Disease	Genetic Defect	Clinical Features
Apolipoprotein defects		
ApoAI deficiency	ApoA1 truncations or rearrangements (11q23)	Absent HDL, severe atherosclerosis
ApoAI variants	ApoA1 point mutations (11q23)	Reduced HDL, variable atherosclerosis
Abetalipoproteinemia (absence of both apoB-100 defects, absence of atherosclerosis and apoB-48)	Microsomal triglyceride protein mutations (4q22–24)	Ataxia, malabsorption, hemolytic anemia, visual
ApoB-100 absence	Unknown (2p24)	Mild ataxia, malabsorption, absence of atherosclerosis
ApoCII deficiency	ApoCII mutations (19q13.2)	Type I hyperlipidemia: severe hypertriglyceridemia, variable atherosclerosis
ApoE variants	ApoE mutations (19q13.2)	Type III hyperlipidemia: elevated triglycerides, premature atherosclerosis
Enzyme defects		
Lipoprotein lipase deficiency	Lipoprotein lipase mutations (8p22)	Type I hyperlipidemia: hypertriglyceridemia; minimal atherosclerosis
Hepatic lipase deficiency	Hepatic lipase mutations (15q21–23)	Elevations of IDL and HDL; severe atherosclerosis
Lecithin:cholesterol acyltransferase (LCAT) deficiency	LCAT mutations (16q22.1)	Mild hypertriglyceridemia; reduced HDL; corneal opacities; variable atherosclerosis
Receptor defect		
Familial hypercholesterolemia	LDL receptor mutations (19p13.2)	Type II hyperlipidemia: severe elevation of LDL; premature atherosclerosis

Apo, apolipoprotein; HDL, high-density lipoprotein; IDL, intermediate-density lipoprotein; LDL, low-density lipoprotein.

of atherosclerosis of the coronary arteries and larger cerebral vessels in both sexes. Plasma levels of this cholesterol-rich lipoprotein vary greatly (<1 to >140 mg/dL) and appear to be independent of LDL levels. Lp(a) plasma levels are heritable and not altered by most cholesterol-lowering drugs, although they are reduced by nicotinic acid. Taken together, this information distinguishes a risk factor that appears superficially to be related to serum cholesterol but the effect of which may actually be linked to an alteration in clot lysis. Apo(a) and plasminogen are highly homologous and contain similar domains that mediate interactions with fibrin and cell surface receptors. Thus, Lp(a) may be an important link between atherosclerosis and thrombosis.

HYPERTENSIVE VASCULAR DISEASE

Hypertension affects over 30% of the population of the United States. It is present in more than half of cases of myocardial infarction, stroke, and chronic renal disease. It is a component of "metabolic syndrome" (see Chapter 19), along with hyperglycemia, insulin resistance, dyslipidemia, and obesity. Hypertension is present in 95% or greater cases of ascending aortic dissections or rupture. At least three fourths of patients with dissecting aortic aneurysm, intracerebral hemorrhage, or myocardial wall rupture also have elevated blood pressure. Blacks are particularly plagued by hypertension and are more likely than whites to experience severe complications. In 95% of patients, hypertension occurs without an identifiable cause, a condition referred to as **primary** hypertension. Much less frequently, **secondary** hypertension may be associated with a number of defined disease states (see below). Whatever the etiology, effective treatment of hypertension prolongs life.

Data from twin and family studies indicate that genetics accounts for some 30% of blood pressure regulation. This finding may also account for the tremendous variation in patient response to blood pressure-lowering medication. Human genetic linkage and whole genome association studies have identified a host of mutations in key blood pressure-regulatory processes.

The definition of hypertension depends on a statistical estimate of the distribution of systolic and diastolic blood pressures in the general population. Both systolic and diastolic pressures are important in determining the risk of cardiovascular disease, especially that due to atherosclerosis. The mean systolic blood pressure in 20-year-old men is about 130 mm Hg, but 95% confidence limits range from 105 to 150 mm Hg. Average systolic blood pressure increases with age, so that in 80-year-olds, it reaches a mean of 170 mm Hg. The American Heart Association defines hypertension as systolic pressure above 140 mm Hg until age 80 and greater than 150 mm Hg thereafter.

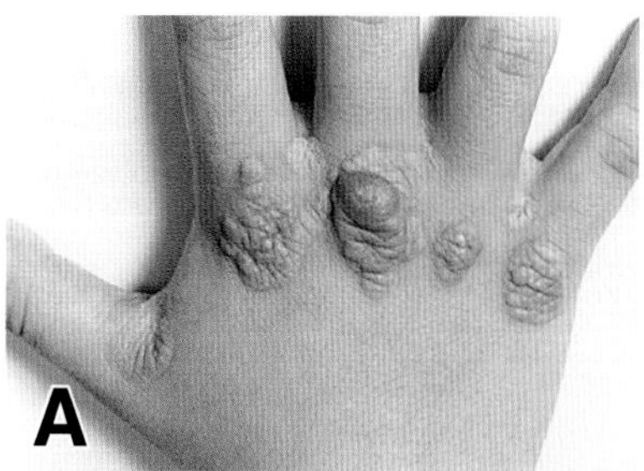

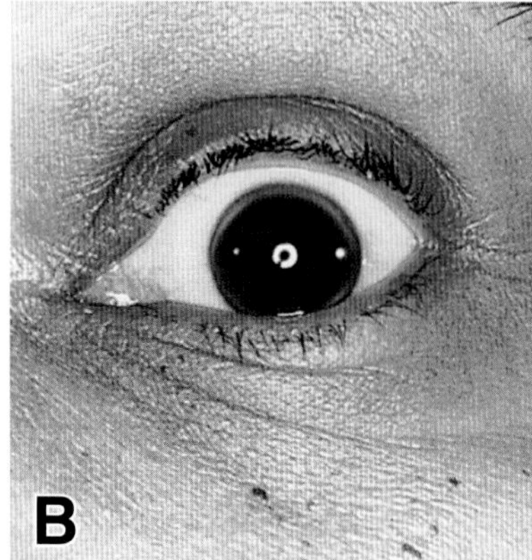

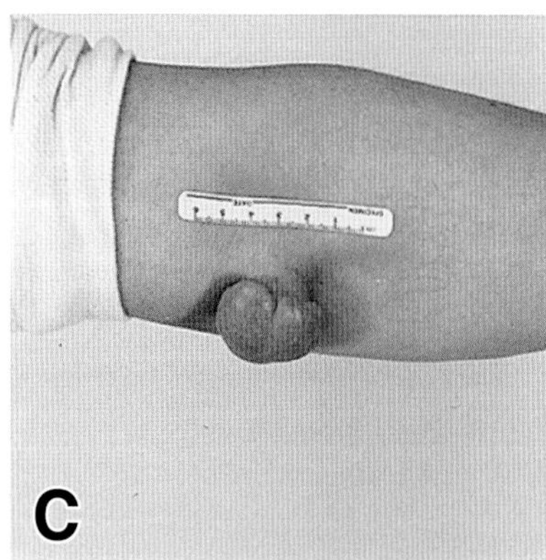

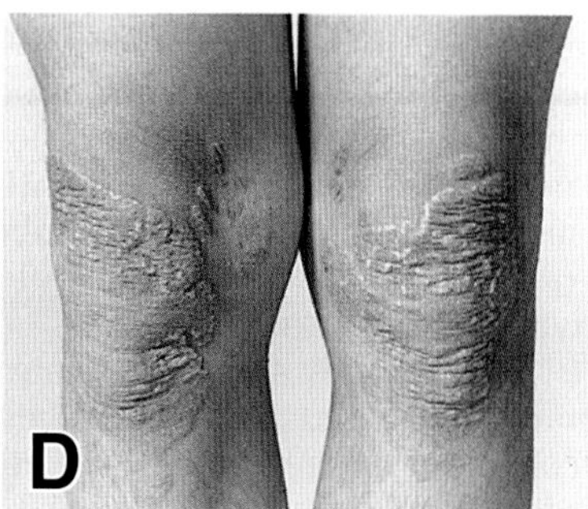

FIGURE 8-22. Xanthomas in familial hypercholesterolemia. A. Dorsum of the hand. **B.** Arcus lipoides representing the deposition of lipids in the peripheral cornea. **C.** Extensor surface of the elbow. **D.** Knees.

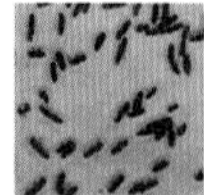

ETIOLOGIC FACTORS: Blood pressure is the product of cardiac output and systemic vascular resistance to blood flow. The most widespread hypothesis holds that primary hypertension results from an imbalance in the interactions between these mechanisms (Fig. 8-24). However, both of these functions are critically influenced by renal function and sodium homeostasis. The frequency of hypertension increases as the glomerular filtration rate (GFR) falls, even with mild renal dysfunction. Reduced GFR causes

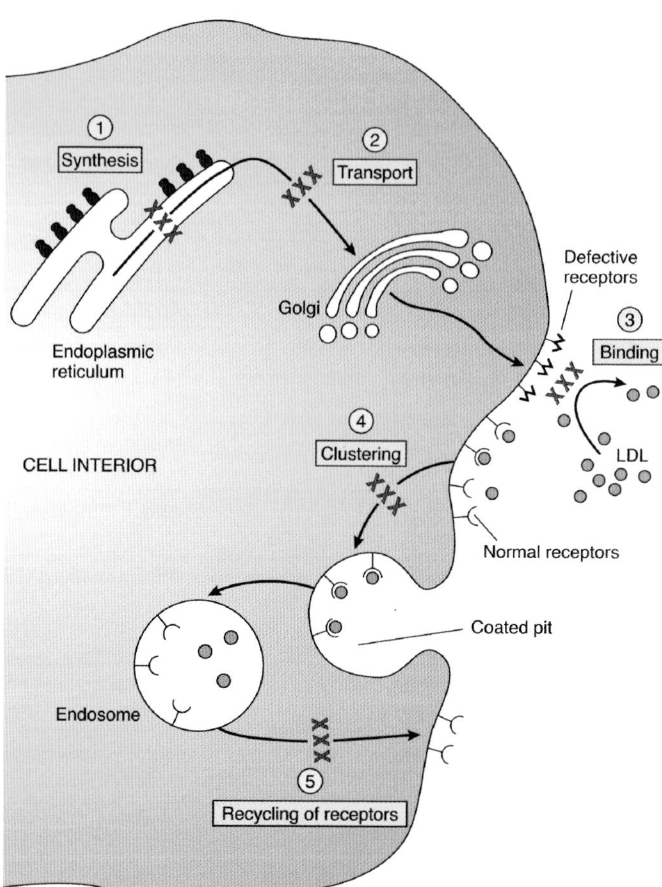

FIGURE 8-23. Mutations of the low-density lipoprotein receptor in familial hypercholesterolemia.

sodium retention and volume expansion, which should be compensated by a decrease in tubular sodium reabsorption. Impaired renal tubular sodium handling and reduced GFR are likely to be important in hypertension that afflicts patients with chronic kidney disease caused by diabetes or aging.

A complex endocrine axis centers on the renin-angiotensin system (RAS), which is both hormonal and tissue based, the latter present in many organs, including the brain. The RAS is important in the regulation of normal blood pressure, and dysregulation of RAS is implicated in over two thirds of the cases of hypertension. The **renin–angiotensin system** elevates blood pressure through the following three mechanisms:

- Increased sympathetic output
- Increased mineralocorticoid secretion
- Direct vasoconstriction

The importance of the hormonal axis in regulating blood pressure in hypertension is demonstrated by the therapeutic success of sympathetic antagonists (β-adrenergic blockers), diuretics, and inhibitors of angiotensin-converting enzyme (ACE). Nonetheless, no central defect in the renin–angiotensin axis has been identified, in part because the vasculature responds quickly to hemodynamic changes in the tissues by autoregulation.

Acquired Causes of Hypertension

Causes of hypertension are identifiable only in a small proportion of cases. These include renal artery stenosis, most forms

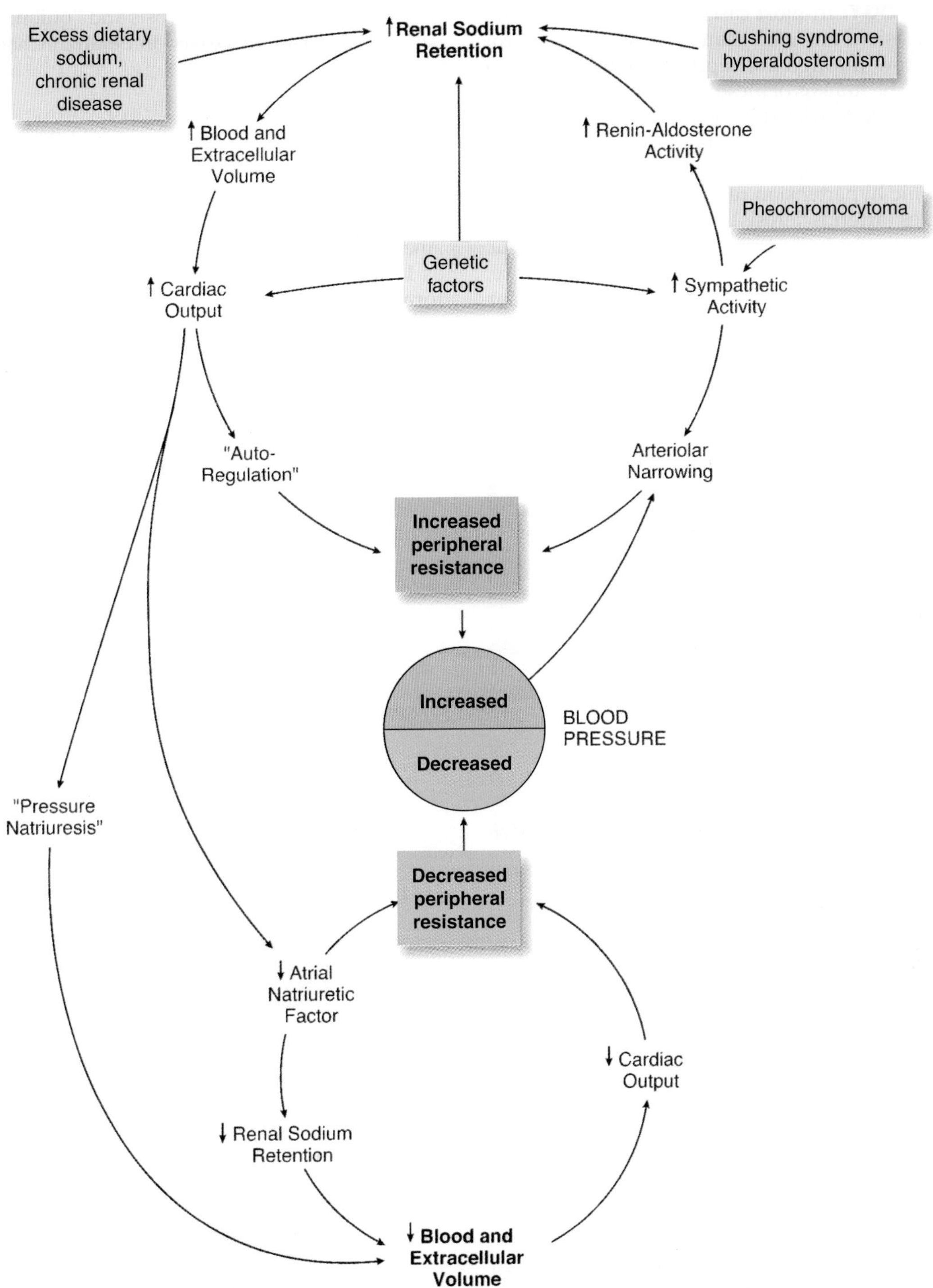

FIGURE 8-24. Factors contributing to hypertension and the counterregulatory factors that lower blood pressure. An imbalance in these factors results in the increased peripheral resistance that is responsible for most cases of essential (primary) hypertension. Note the central role of peripheral resistance.

of chronic renal disease, diabetes mellitus, primary elevation of aldosterone levels (Conn syndrome), Cushing syndrome, pheochromocytoma, hyperthyroidism, coarctation of the aorta, and renin-secreting tumors. In addition, people with severe atherosclerosis may have high systolic pressure because a sclerotic aorta cannot properly absorb the kinetic energy of pulse waves, and because they often have renovascular hypertension.

All mutations that cause hereditary hypertension constitutively increase renal sodium reabsorption. Conversely, diseases that result in sodium-losing syndromes (e.g., pseudohypoaldosteronism type I and Gitelman syndrome) are associated with profound hypotension. ***Thus, these Mendelian disorders illustrate a central role of sodium homeostasis in determining blood pressure.***

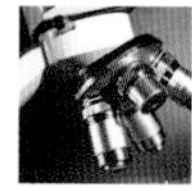

PATHOLOGY: In most cases of hypertension, the critical lesions are in resistance vessels that control blood flow through the capillary beds and in the kidney. The lumens of these small muscular arteries and arterioles may be restricted by active contraction of the vessel wall or increased vessel wall mass. Thicker vessel walls narrow vascular lumens more than do normal, thinner walls. Over time, chronic hypertension results in reactive changes in smaller arteries (arteriosclerosis) and arterioles (arteriolosclerosis) throughout the body. Kidneys affected with chronic hypertension have a contracted and granular gross appearance, and microscopically often show tubular and glomerular changes, a pattern termed nephrosclerosis. The characteristic vascular changes of mild chronic hypertension (benign or hyaline arteriosclerosis, Fig. 8-25) and of malignant hypertension (fibrinoid necrosis and "onion skinning" of vessels, Fig. 8-26) are discussed in detail in Chapter 14.

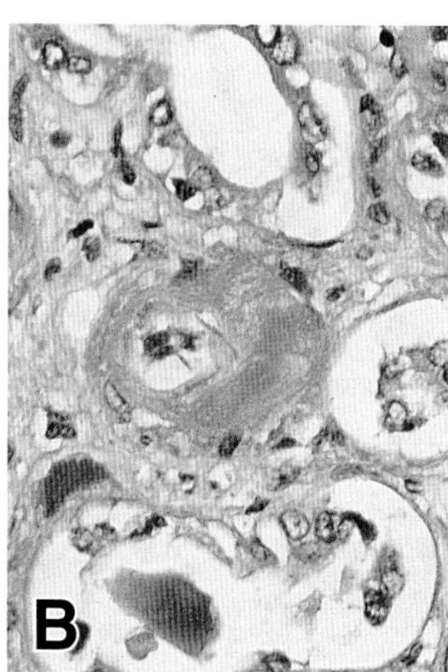

FIGURE 8-25. Benign arteriosclerosis. A. A cross section of a renal intralobular artery showing irregular thickening of the intima (*arrows*). **B.** A renal arteriole exhibits hyaline arteriolosclerosis (*center*).

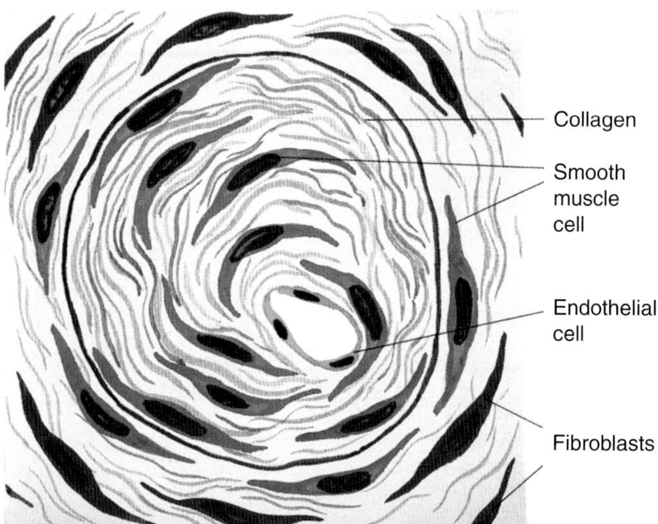

FIGURE 8-26. Arteriolosclerosis. In cases of hypertension, the arterioles exhibit smooth muscle cell proliferation and increased amounts of intercellular collagen and glycosaminoglycans, resulting in an "onion-skin" appearance. The mass of smooth muscle and associated elements tends to fix the size of the lumen and restrict the arteriole's capacity to dilate.

ANEURYSMS

Arterial aneurysms are localized dilations of blood vessels caused by a congenital or acquired weakness of the media. They are not rare, and their incidence tends to rise with age. Aneurysms of the aorta and other arteries are found in as many as 10% of unselected autopsies. The wall of an aneurysm is formed by stretched remnants of the arterial wall.

Aneurysms are classified by location, configuration, and etiology (Fig. 8-27). The location refers to the type of vessel involved—artery or vein—and the specific vessel affected, such

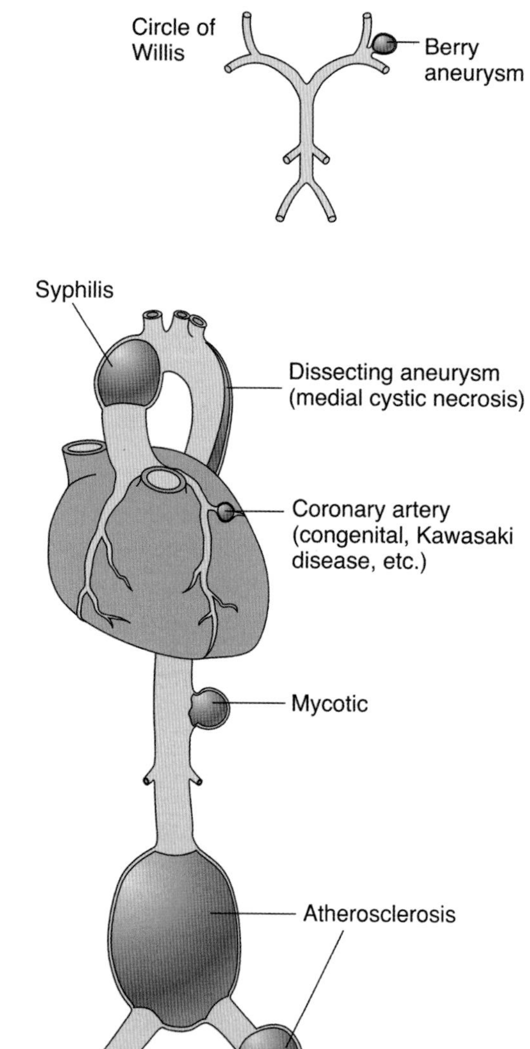

FIGURE 8-27. The locations of aneurysms. Syphilitic aneurysms are the common variety in the ascending aorta, which is usually spared by the atherosclerotic process. Atherosclerotic aneurysms can occur in the abdominal aorta or muscular arteries, including the coronary and popliteal arteries and other vessels. Berry aneurysms are seen in the circle of Willis, mainly at branch points; their rupture leads to subarachnoid hemorrhage. Mycotic aneurysms occur almost anywhere that bacteria can deposit on vessel walls.

as the aorta or popliteal artery. There are several categories of aneurysms:

- **Fusiform aneurysms** are ovoid swellings parallel to the long axis of the vessel.
- **Saccular aneurysms** are bubble-like arterial wall outpouchings at a site of weakened media.
- **Dissecting aneurysms** are actually dissecting hematomas in which blood from hemorrhage into the media separates the layers of the vascular wall.
- **Arteriovenous aneurysms** are direct conduits between an artery and a vein.
- **False (pseudo) aneurysms** are not "true aneurysms" but rather localized collections of blood between the layers of the vessels.

Abdominal Aortic Aneurysms

Abdominal aortic aneurysms are dilations that increase vessel wall diameter by at least 50%. They are the most frequent aneurysms, usually developing after the age of 50 years and invariably associated with severe atherosclerosis of the artery. The prevalence rises to 6% after age 80. They occur much more often in men than in women, and half of patients are hypertensive. Occasionally, aneurysms may be found in all parts of the thoracic aorta and in iliac and popliteal arteries.

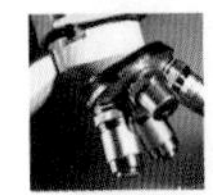

PATHOLOGY: Most abdominal aortic aneurysms occur distal to the renal arteries and proximal to the aortic bifurcation (Fig. 8-28). They are usually fusiform, but saccular varieties are occasionally seen. Although most of the symptomatic lesions are over 5 to 6 cm in diameter, they may be of almost any size. Some extend into the iliac arteries, which occasionally exhibit distinct aneurysms distal to the one in the aorta. Aneurysms that extend above the renal arteries may occlude the origin of the superior mesenteric artery and the celiac axis.

Most abdominal aortic aneurysms are lined by raised, ulcerated, and calcified (complicated) atherosclerotic lesions. The majority contain mural thrombi of varying degrees of organization, portions of which may embolize to peripheral arteries.

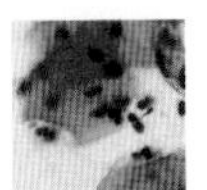

CLINICAL FEATURES: Many abdominal aortic aneurysms are asymptomatic and are discovered only after palpation of a mass in the abdomen or incidentally on radiologic examination. In some cases, the condition is brought to medical attention by the onset of abdominal pain resulting from expansion of the aneurysm. The most dreaded complication of aortic aneurysms is rupture and exsanguination into the retroperitoneum (or chest), in which case the patient presents with pain, shock, and a pulsatile mass in the abdomen. This is an acute emergency, and half of patients die, even with prompt surgical intervention. Therefore, even asymptomatic large aneurysms are often replaced by or bypassed with prosthetic grafts. ***The risk of rupture of an abdominal aortic aneurysm is a function of its size.*** Aneurysms under 4 cm in diameter rarely rupture (2%), and 25% to 40% of those larger than 5 cm rupture within 5 years of their discovery.

Aneurysms of Cerebral Arteries

The most common type of cerebral aneurysm is a saccular structure known as **berry aneurysm,** because it resembles a berry attached to a twig of the arterial tree. Berry aneurysms reflect congenital defects in arterial walls and tend to arise at branches in the circle of Willis or one of the arterial junctions. The most common sites are between the anterior cerebral and anterior communicating arteries, between the internal carotid and posterior communicating arteries, and between the first main divisions of the middle cerebral artery and the bifurcation of the internal carotid artery. These aneurysms are also discussed in Chapter 24.

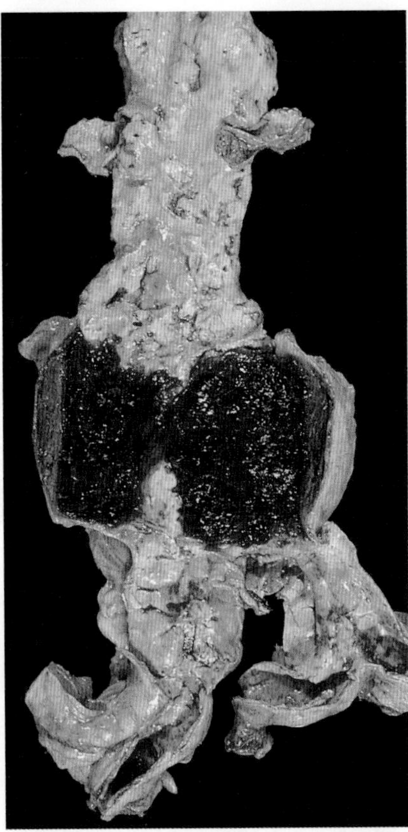

FIGURE 8-28. Atherosclerotic aneurysm of the abdominal aorta. The aneurysm has been opened longitudinally to reveal a large mural thrombus in the lumen. The aorta and common iliac arteries display complicated lesions of atherosclerosis.

Dissecting Aneurysm

The dissection occurs on a path along the length of the vessel (Fig. 8-29) and essentially represents a false lumen within the wall of the artery. Although the lesion is usually designated an aneurysm, it is actually a form of hematoma. Dissecting aneurysms most often affect the aorta, especially the ascending portion, and its major branches. Thoracic dissections may involve the ascending aorta alone (type A) or only the distal aorta (type B). Their frequency has been estimated to be as high as 1 in 400 autopsies, with men affected three times as frequently as women. They may occur at almost any age but are most common in the sixth and seventh decades. Almost all patients have a history of hypertension, and associated conditions include atherosclerosis, bicuspid aortic valve, and idiopathic aortic root dilation. The basis of dissecting aneurysms is usually weakening of the aortic media, often associated with hereditary conditions that affect connective tissue structure.

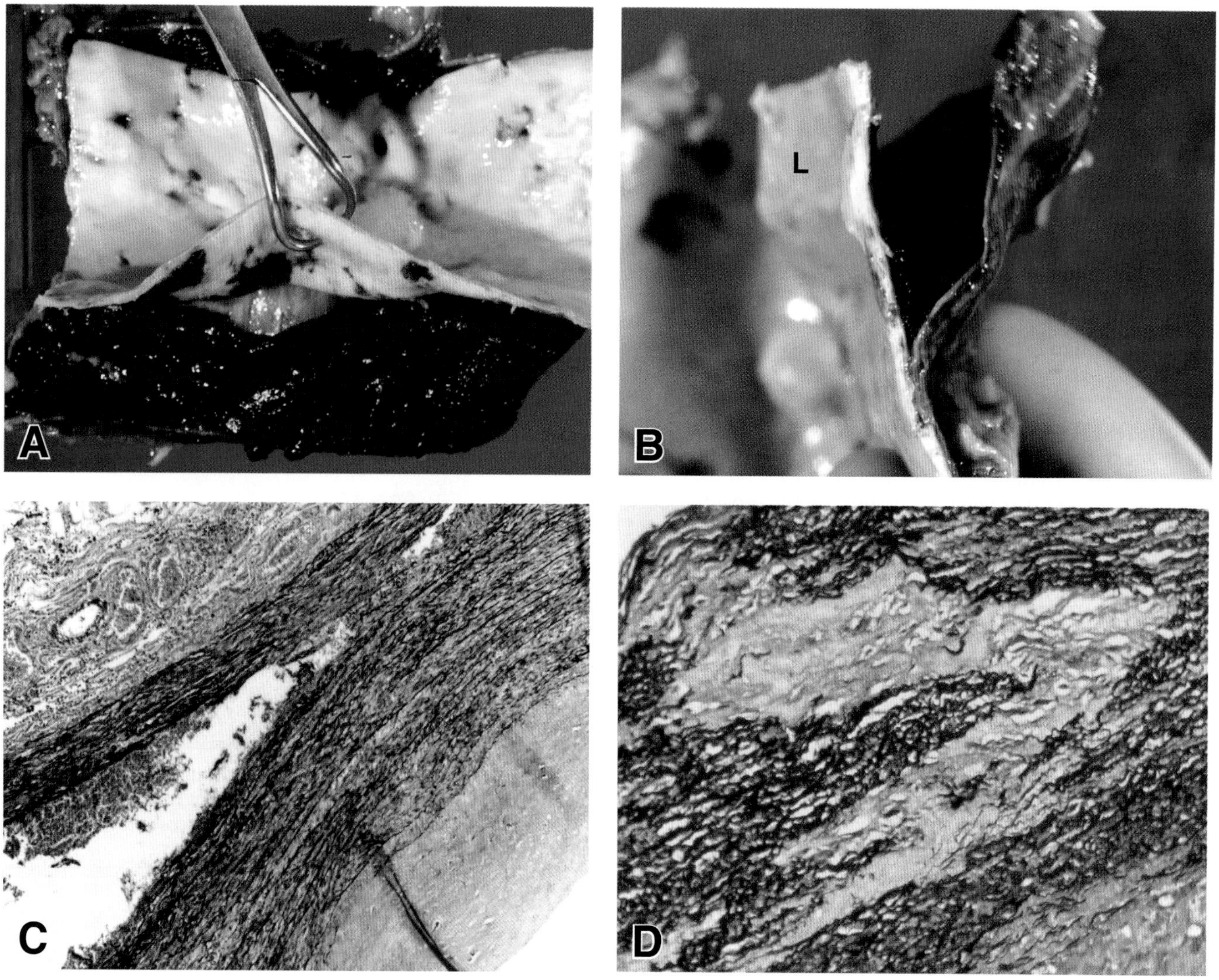

FIGURE 8-29. Dissecting aortic aneurysm. A. Thoracic aorta with metal clamps revealing the dissection and hematoma in the wall with old blood clot. **B.** The thoracic aorta has been opened longitudinally and reveals clotted blood dissecting the media of the vessel. **C.** Atherosclerotic aorta with dissection along the outer third of the media (elastic stain). **D.** A section of the aortic wall stained with aldehyde fuchsin showing pools of metachromatic material characteristic of the degenerative process known as cystic medial necrosis. L, lumen.

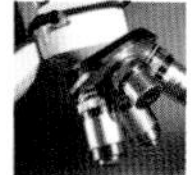

PATHOLOGY: The initial event that triggers medial dissection is controversial. Over 95% of cases have a transverse tear in the intima and internal media; hence, spontaneous laceration of the intima allows blood from the lumen to enter and dissect the media. Alternatively, hemorrhage from vasa vasorum into a media weakened by cystic medial necrosis initiates stress on the intima, which in turn creates the ubiquitous intimal tear.

Most intimal tears are in the ascending aorta, 1 or 2 cm above the aortic ring. Dissection in the media occurs within seconds and separates the inner two thirds of the aorta from the outer third. It can also involve coronary arteries; great vessels of the neck; and renal, mesenteric, or iliac arteries. Because the outer wall of the false channel of the dissecting aneurysm is thin, hemorrhage into the extravascular space—including the pericardium, mediastinum, pleural space, and retroperitoneum—frequently causes death. In 5% to 10% of cases, the blood within the dissection reenters the lumen via a second distal tear to form a "double-barreled aorta." In a comparable proportion, a reentry site produces communication of the aorta with a major artery, most often the iliac artery.

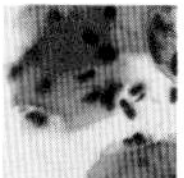

CLINICAL FEATURES: Patients typically present with acute onset of severe, "tearing" pain in the anterior chest, which is sometimes misdiagnosed as myocardial infarction. Loss of one or more arterial pulses is common, as is a murmur of aortic regurgitation. Whereas hypertension is a frequent finding in patients with dissecting aneurysms, hypotension is an ominous sign and suggests aortic rupture. Cardiac tamponade or congestive heart failure is diagnosed by the usual criteria. Prompt surgical intervention and control of hypertension have reduced overall mortality to less than 20%.

Venous Thrombosis

Venous thrombosis is often referred to as **deep venous thrombosis.** *This term is appropriate because the most common manifestation of the disorder is thrombosis of the deep venous system of the legs.*

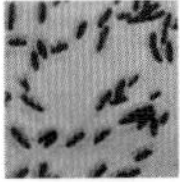

ETIOLOGIC FACTORS: Deep venous thrombosis is (with the exception of atherosclerosis) caused by the same factors that favor arterial thrombosis, endothelial injury, stasis, and a hypercoagulable state. Conditions that favor the development of deep venous thrombosis include the following:

- **Stasis** (heart failure, chronic venous insufficiency, postoperative immobilization, prolonged bed rest, hospitalization, and travel)
- **Injury and inflammation** (trauma, surgery, childbirth, and infection)
- **Hypercoagulability** (oral contraceptives, late pregnancy, and cancer)
- **Inherited thrombophilic disorders** (including factor V Leiden and prothrombin G20210A; see Chapter 18)
- **Advanced age** (venous varicosities)
- **Sickle cell disease** (see Chapter 18)

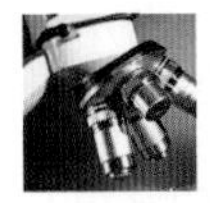

PATHOLOGY: Most (>90%) venous thromboses occur in deep veins of the legs; the rest usually involve pelvic veins. Most begin in the calf veins, often in the sinuses above venous valves. There, venous thrombi have several potential fates:

- **Lysis:** They may stay small, are eventually lysed, and pose no further danger.
- **Organization:** Many undergo organization similar to those of arterial origin. Small, organized venous thrombi may be incorporated into the vessel wall; larger ones may undergo canalization, with partial restoration of venous drainage.
- **Propagation:** Venous thrombi often serve to elicit further thrombosis and so propagate proximally to involve the larger iliofemoral veins (Fig. 8-30).
- **Embolization:** Large venous thrombi or those that have propagated proximally represent a significant hazard to life: they may dislodge and be carried to the lungs as pulmonary emboli (Fig. 8-31).

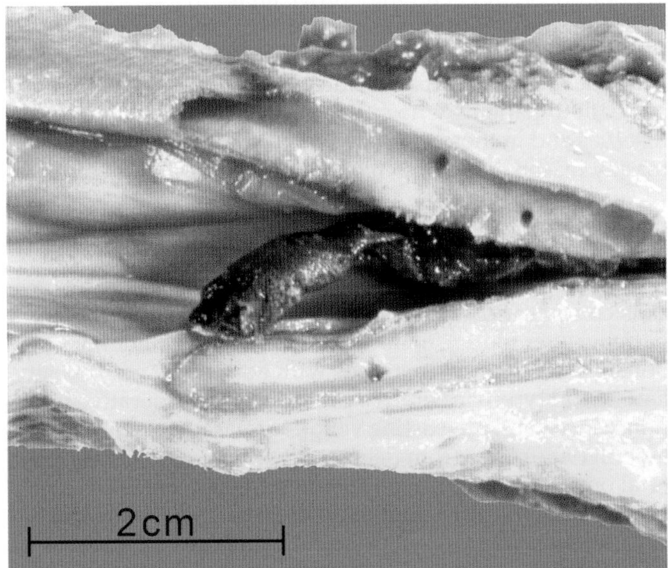

FIGURE 8-30. Venous thrombus. The femoral vein has been opened to reveal a large thrombus within the lumen.

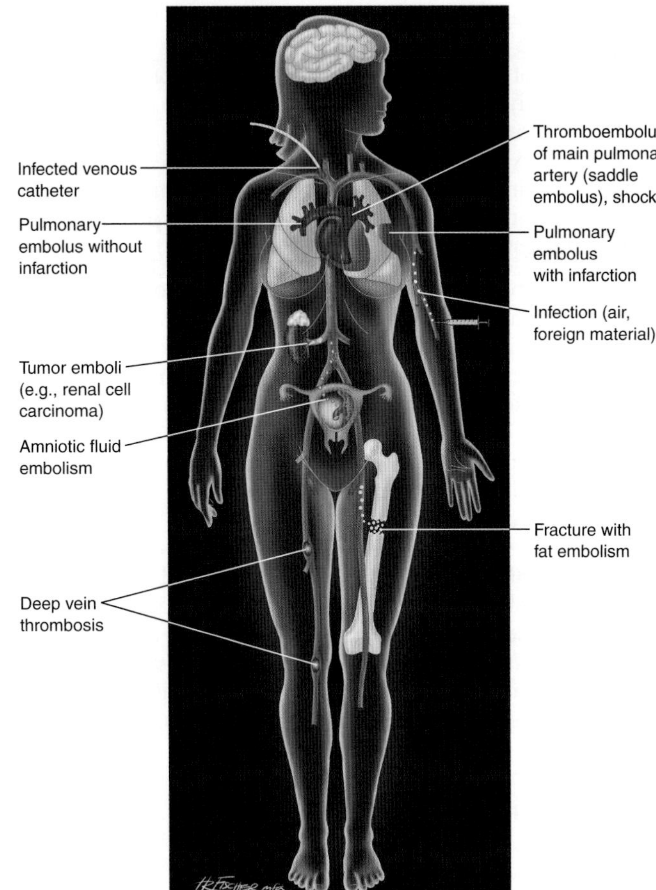

FIGURE 8-31. Sources and effects of venous emboli.

VARICOSITIES OF VEINS

Varicose Veins

Superficial varicosities of leg veins, usually in the saphenous system, are very common. They vary from a trivial knot of dilated veins to painful and disabling distension of the whole venous system of the leg, with secondary trophic disturbances. It is estimated that as much as 10% to 20% of the population has some varicosities in the leg veins, but only a fraction of these develop symptoms.

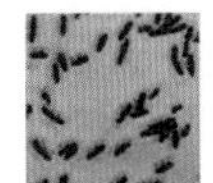

ETIOLOGIC FACTORS: There are several risk factors for varicose veins:

- **Age:** Varicose veins increase in frequency with age and may reach 50% in people over 50 years. This increased incidence may reflect age-related degenerative changes in connective tissues of venous walls, loss of supporting fat and connective tissues, and more flaccid muscle tone and inactivity.
- **Sex:** Among 30- to 50-year-olds, women are more often affected by varicose veins than men, particularly those who have experienced increased venous pressure on the iliac veins from a pregnant uterus.
- **Heredity:** There is a strong familial predisposition to varicose veins, possibly owing to inherited configurations or structural weaknesses of the walls or valves of these vessels.

- **Posture:** Leg vein pressure is 5 to 10 times higher when a person is erect rather than recumbent. As a result, the incidence of varicose veins and its complications are greater in those whose occupations require them to stand in one place for long periods.
- **Obesity:** Excessive body weight increases the incidence of varicose veins, perhaps because of increased intra-abdominal pressure or poor support to vessel walls provided by subcutaneous fat.

Incompetence of venous valves and dilation of the vein reinforce each other to produce varicosities. As the vein increases in length and diameter, tortuosities develop. Once the process begins, the varicosity extends progressively throughout the length of the affected vein. As each valve becomes incompetent, increasing strain is put on the vessel and valve below. The role of inflammation is not well studied, although elevated expression of leukocyte–endothelial adhesion molecules is reported in affected veins.

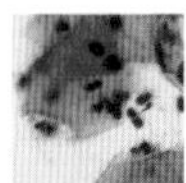

CLINICAL FEATURES: Most affected vessels and veins have little clinical effect and are mainly cosmetic problems. The principal symptoms are aching in the legs, aggravated by standing and relieved by elevation. Severe varicosities (Fig. 8-32) may give rise to trophic changes in the skin drained by the affected veins, called **stasis dermatitis**.

Varicose Veins at Other Sites

Hemorrhoids

These are dilations of the veins of the rectum and anal canal and may occur inside or outside the anal sphincter (see Chapter 11). Although there may be a hereditary predisposition, the condition is aggravated by factors that increase intra-abdominal pressure. These include constipation, pregnancy, and venous obstruction by rectal tumors. Hemorrhoids often bleed, and this may be confused with bleeding rectal cancers. Thrombosed hemorrhoids are exquisitely painful.

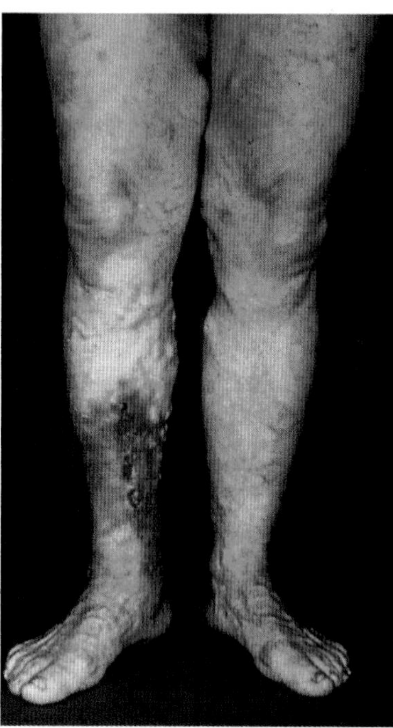

FIGURE 8-32. Varicose veins of the legs. Severe varicosities of the superficial leg veins have led to stasis dermatitis and secondary ulcerations.

Esophageal Varices

This complication of portal hypertension is caused mainly by cirrhosis of the liver (see Chapter 12). Hemorrhage from esophageal varices is a common cause of death in patients with cirrhosis.

Varicocele

This palpable scrotal mass represents varicosities of the pampiniform plexus (see Chapter 15).

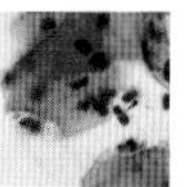

CLINICAL FEATURES: Occlusive thrombosis of femoral or iliac veins leads to severe congestion, edema, and cyanosis of the lower extremity. Symptomatic deep venous thrombosis is treated with systemic anticoagulants, and thrombolytic therapy may be useful in selected cases. In some cases, a filter is inserted into the vena cava to prevent pulmonary embolization. Venous thrombi elsewhere may also be dangerous. Thrombosis of mesenteric veins can cause hemorrhagic small bowel infarction; thrombosis of cerebral veins may be fatal; hepatic vein thrombosis (Budd–Chiari syndrome) tends to result in end-stage liver disease.

EMBOLISM

Embolism is passage through venous or arterial circulations of any material that can lodge in a blood vessel and obstruct its lumen. The most common embolus is a thromboembolus—that is, a thrombus formed in one location that detaches from a vessel wall at its point of origin and travels to a distant site. Pulmonary thromboemboli, which often originate in the deep veins of the legs, are of great clinical significance because they are not uncommon and may prove fatal.

Pulmonary embolism is the most common cause of death after major orthopedic surgery and is the most frequent nonobstetric cause of postpartum death. It is also a common cause of death in patients who suffer from chronic heart and lung diseases and in those subjected to prolonged immobilization for any reason, including inactivity associated with air travel.

Pulmonary Arterial Embolism

Pulmonary thromboemboli occur in over half of autopsies. This complication also occurs in 1% to 2% of postoperative patients over the age of 40 years. The risk of pulmonary embolism after surgery increases with advancing age, obesity, length and type of operative procedure, postoperative infection, cancer, and preexisting venous disease. Most pulmonary emboli (90%) arise from deep veins of the lower extremities; fatal ones usually form in iliofemoral veins (Fig. 8-34). Only half of patients with such emboli have signs of deep vein thrombosis. The upper extremities are rarely sources of thromboemboli.

The clinical features of pulmonary embolism are determined by the size of the embolus, the health of the patient, and whether embolization occurs acutely or chronically. Acute pulmonary

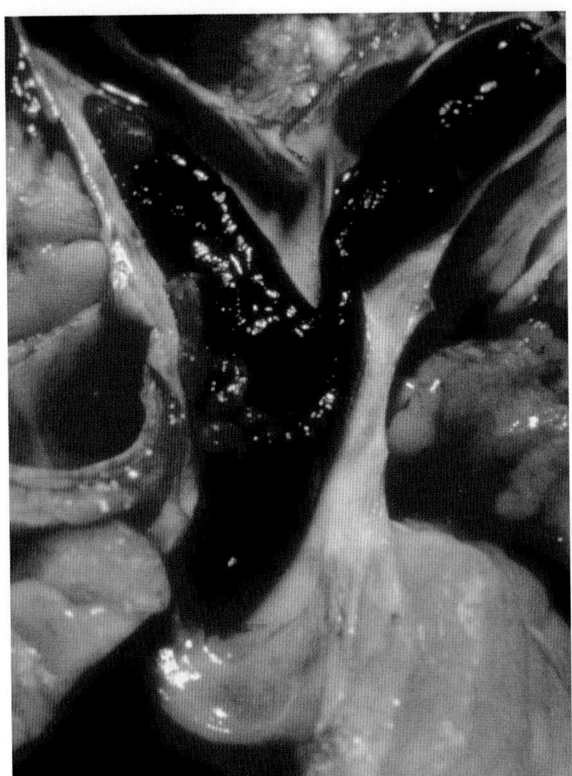

FIGURE 8-33. **Pulmonary embolism.** The main pulmonary artery and its bifurcation have been opened to reveal a large saddle embolus. Courtesy of Dr. Greg J. Davis, Department of Pathology, University of Kentucky College of Medicine.

embolism may be asymptomatic, produce pulmonary symptoms of varying severity, or result in sudden death.

Massive Pulmonary Embolism

One of the most dramatic calamities complicating hospitalization is a postoperative patient succumbing upon getting out of bed for the first time. The muscular activity dislodges a thrombus that formed as a result of the stasis from prolonged bed rest. A large pulmonary embolus may lodge at the bifurcation of the main pulmonary artery (**saddle embolus**) and obstruct blood flow to both lungs (Fig. 8-33). Large lethal emboli may also block the right or left main pulmonary arteries or their first branches. Multiple smaller emboli may lodge in secondary branches and prove fatal. With acute obstruction of more than half of the pulmonary arterial tree, the patient often experiences immediate severe hypotension (or shock) and may die within minutes.

The hemodynamic consequences of such massive pulmonary embolism are acute right ventricular failure from sudden obstruction of outflow and pronounced reduction in left ventricular cardiac output, secondary to the loss of right ventricular function. The low cardiac output is responsible for the sudden appearance of severe hypotension.

Pulmonary Infarction

Small pulmonary emboli are not ordinarily lethal. They tend to lodge in peripheral pulmonary arteries and sometimes (15% to 20% of all pulmonary emboli) produce lung infarcts. Because the bronchial artery supplies blood to the necrotic area, pulmonary infarcts are typically hemorrhagic. They tend to be pyramidal, with the base of the pyramid on the pleural surface. Patients experience cough, stabbing pleuritic pain, shortness of breath, and occasional hemoptysis. Pleural effusion is common and often bloody. With time, the blood in the infarct is resorbed, and the center of the infarct becomes pale. Granulation tissue forms on the edge of the infarct, after which it is organized to form a fibrous scar.

Paradoxical Embolism

Paradoxical embolism refers to emboli that arise in the venous circulation and bypass the lungs by traveling through an incompletely closed foramen ovale, subsequently entering the left side of the heart and blocking flow to systemic arteries. Because left atrial pressure usually exceeds that in the right, most of these cases occur in the context of a right-to-left shunt (see Chapter 9).

Arterial Thromboembolism

The heart is the most common source of arterial thromboemboli (Fig. 8-34)***, which usually arise from mural thrombi*** (Fig. 8-35) ***or diseased valves.*** These emboli tend to lodge at points where vessel lumens narrow abruptly (e.g., at bifurcations or near atherosclerotic plaques). The viability of tissue supplied by the vessel depends on the available collateral circulation and the fate of the embolus itself. The thromboembolus may propagate locally and lead to a more severe obstruction, or it may fragment and lyse. The more common sites of infarction from arterial emboli are shown in Figure 8-36.

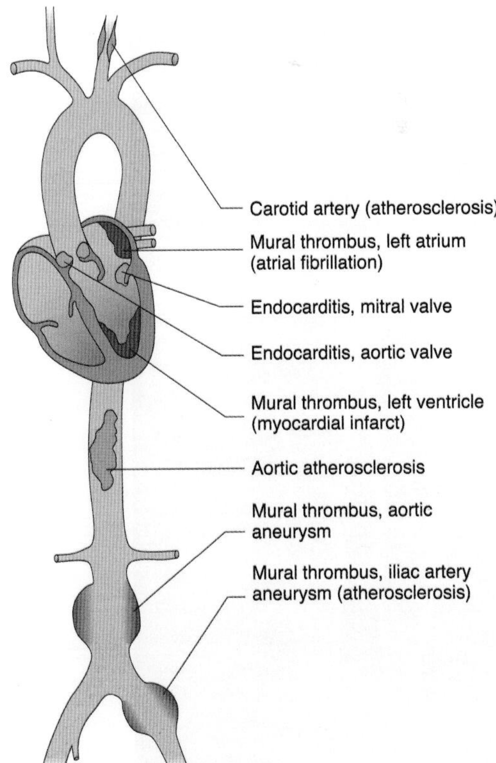

FIGURE 8-34. **Sources of arterial emboli.** Courtesy of Dr. Greg J. Davis, Department of Pathology, University of Kentucky College of Medicine.

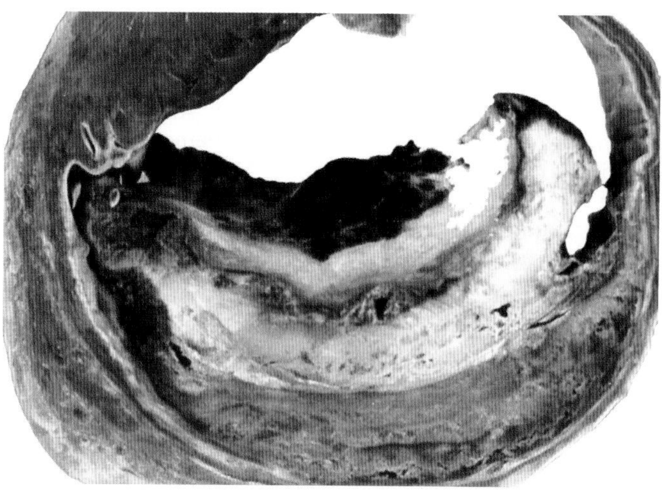

FIGURE 8-35. Mural thrombus of the left ventricle. laminated thrombus adheres to the endocardium overlying a healed aneurysmal myocardial infarct.

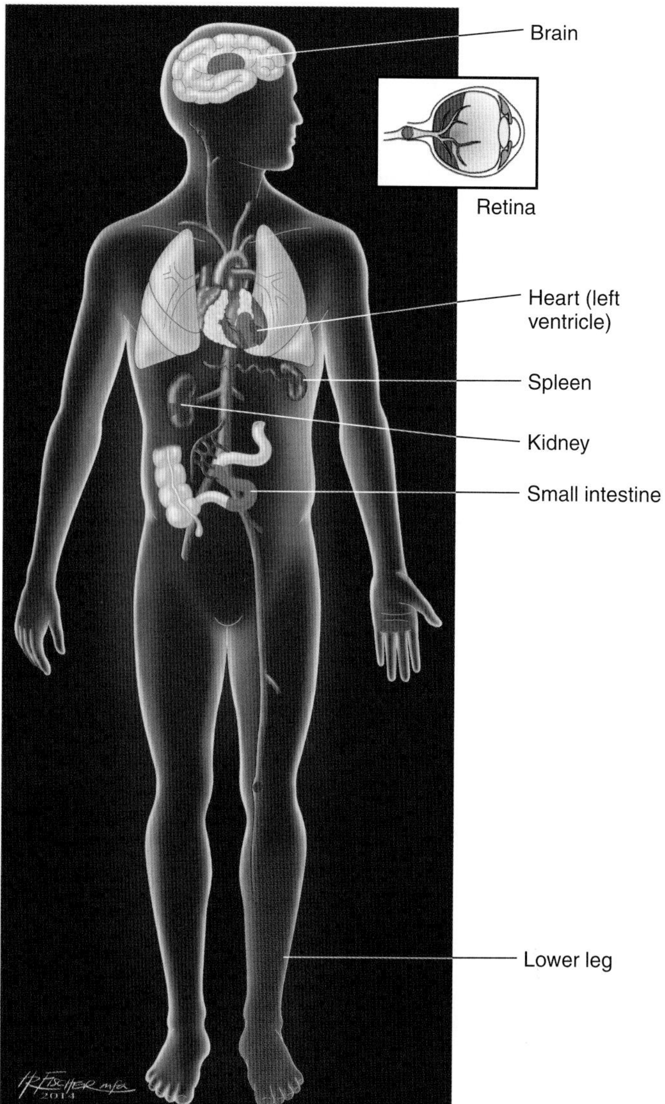

FIGURE 8-36. Common sites of infarction from arterial emboli.

Uncommon Sources of Embolism

Air Embolism

Air may enter the venous circulation through neck wounds, thoracentesis, or punctures of the great veins during invasive procedures or intraoperatively. Small amounts of circulating air are of little consequence, but quantities of 100 mL or more can result in sudden death by physically obstructing blood flow in the right side of the heart, the pulmonary circulation, and the brain.

Decompression sickness is a risk for people exposed to increased atmospheric pressure, such as scuba divers and workers in underwater occupations (e.g., tunnels and drilling platform construction). Under pressure, large amounts of nitrogen are dissolved in bodily fluids. When pressure is rapidly reduced, this gas is released from solution and gas bubbles form in the circulation and within tissues, obstructing blood flow and directly injuring cells. When acute, decompression sickness is characterized by temporary muscular and joint pain, owing to small-vessel obstruction in these tissues. However, severe involvement of cerebral blood vessels may cause coma or even death, a condition termed "the bends."

Amniotic Fluid Embolism

Amniotic fluid containing fetal cells and debris can enter the maternal circulation through open uterine and cervical veins. It is a rare maternal complication of childbirth but can be catastrophic when it occurs. This disorder usually occurs at the end of labor when the pulmonary emboli are composed of the solid epithelial constituents (squames) contained in the amniotic fluid. Of greater importance is the initiation of a potentially fatal consumptive coagulopathy caused by the high thromboplastin activity of the amniotic fluid. Such embolic disease results in sudden onset of cyanosis and shock, followed by coma and death. If the mother survives this acute episode, she may die of disseminated intravascular coagulation. Alternatively, she is at substantial risk for developing **acute respiratory distress syndrome** and ongoing neurologic complications (see Chapter 10).

Fat and Bone Marrow Embolism

Fat and marrow embolism reflect the release of emboli of fatty marrow into damaged blood vessels following severe trauma, particularly accompanying bone fractures (Fig. 8-37). In most instances, such emboli are clinically inapparent. However, in its most severe form, which may be fatal, this syndrome is characterized by respiratory failure, mental changes, thrombocytopenia, and widespread petechiae. At autopsy, innumerable fat globules are seen in the microvasculature of the lungs (Fig. 8-37B) and brain and sometimes other organs.

INFARCTION

Infarction is the process by which coagulative necrosis develops in an area distal to occlusion of an end-artery. The necrotic zone is an **infarct**. Infarcts of vital organs such as the heart, brain, and intestine are major causes of morbidity and mortality. If the victim survives, the infarct heals with a scar. The consequences of infarcts in specific organs are discussed in subsequent chapters.

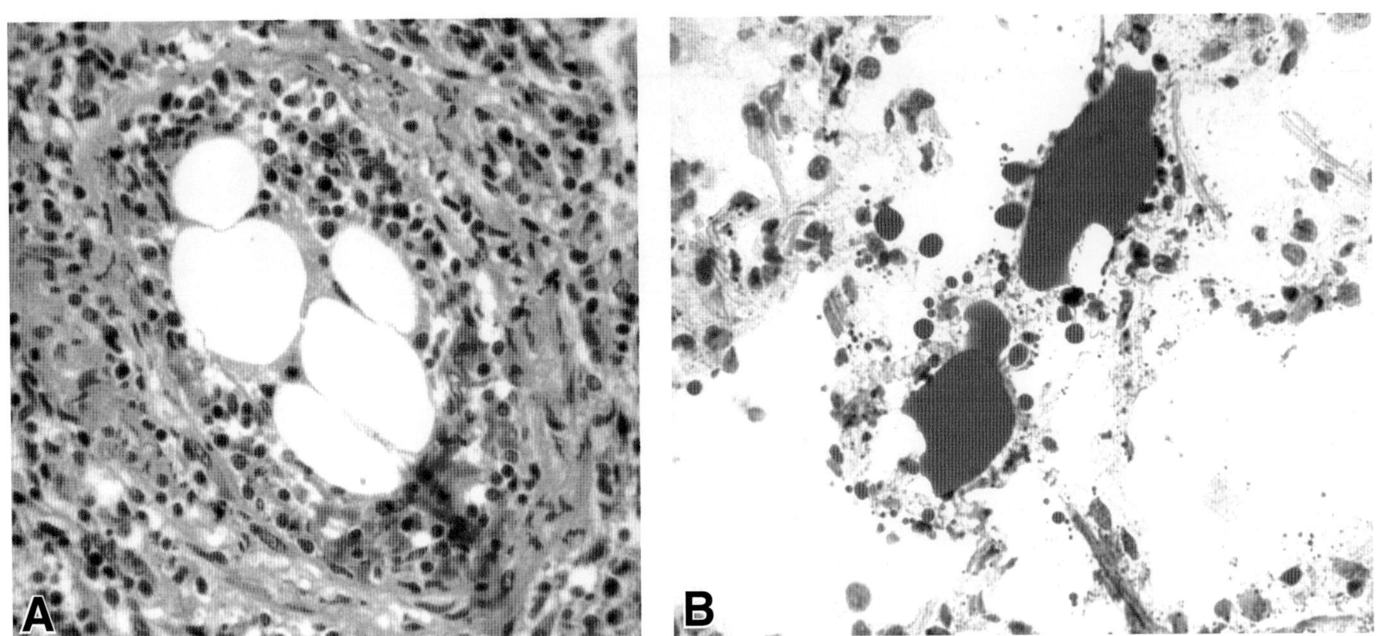

FIGURE 8-37. Fat embolism. A. The lumen of a small pulmonary artery is occluded by a fragment of bone marrow consisting of fat cells and hematopoietic elements. **B.** A frozen section of lung stained with Sudan red showing capillaries occluded by red-staining fat emboli.

Pale infarcts are typical in the heart, kidneys, and spleen (Fig. 8-38), although certain renal infarcts may be cystic. **Dry gangrene** of the leg secondary to arterial occlusion (often noted in diabetes) is actually a large pale infarct. Within 1 or 2 days after the initial hyperemia, an infarct becomes soft, sharply delineated, and light yellow (Fig. 8-39). The border tends to be dark red, reflecting hemorrhage into surrounding viable tissue. Microscopically, a pale infarct exhibits uniform coagulative necrosis.

Red infarcts may result from either arterial or venous occlusion and are also characterized by coagulative necrosis. However, they are distinguished by bleeding into the affected area from adjacent vessels. ***Red infarcts occur mainly in organs with a dual blood supply,*** such as the lung, or those with extensive collateral circulation (e.g., the small intestine and brain) (Fig. 8-40). In the brain, an infarct typically undergoes liquefactive necrosis and may become a fluid-filled cyst, which is referred to as a **cystic infarct** (Fig. 8-41).

Septic infarction results when the necrotic tissue of an infarct is seeded by pyogenic bacteria and becomes infected. Pulmonary infarcts are not uncommonly infected, presumably because necrotic tissue offers little resistance to inhaled bacteria. In the case of bacterial endocarditis, the emboli themselves are infected, and resulting infarcts are often septic.

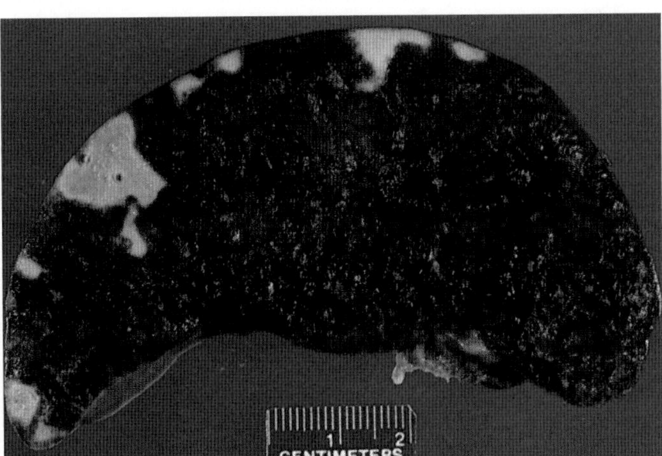

FIGURE 8-38. Spleen infarcts. A cut section of the spleen displaying multiple pale, wedge-shaped infarcts beneath the capsule.

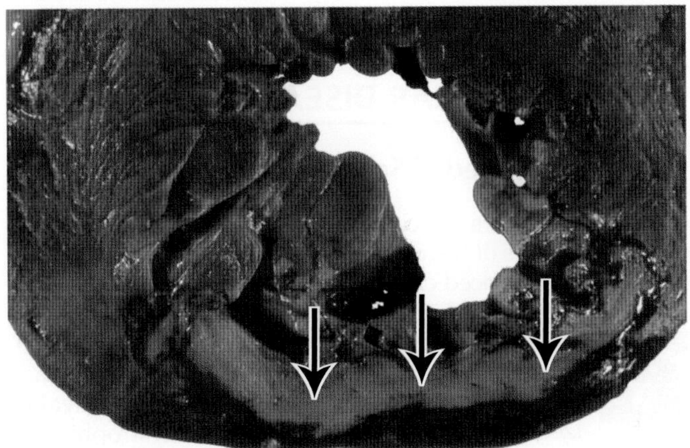

FIGURE 8-39. Acute myocardial infarct. A cross section of the left ventricle revealing a sharply circumscribed, soft, yellow area of necrosis in the posterior free wall (*arrows*).

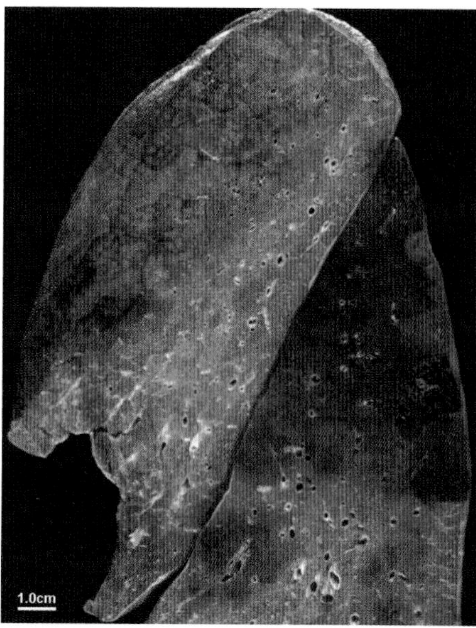

FIGURE 8-40. Red infarct. A sagittal slice of the lung showing a hemorrhagic infarct in the upper segments of the lower lobe.

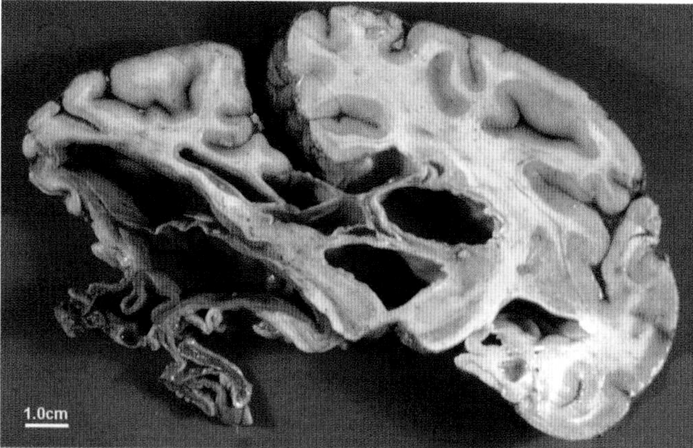

FIGURE 8-41. Cystic infarct. A cross section of the brain in the frontal plane showing a healed cystic infarct. Courtesy of Dr. Ken Berry, Department of Pathology, St. Paul's Hospital.

OTHER VASCULAR DISEASE

Mönckeberg Medial Sclerosis

The disorder occurs principally in older people and most often involves arteries of the upper and lower extremities. It is also common in advanced chronic renal disease.

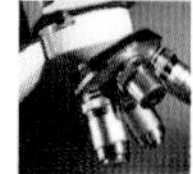

PATHOLOGY: Involved arteries are hard and dilated. Microscopically, the smooth muscle of the media is focally replaced by pale-staining, acellular, hyalinized fibrous tissue, with concentric dystrophic calcification. In most cases, the internal elastic lamina shows focal calcification. Osseous metaplasia in calcified areas is occasionally observed. Mönckeberg medial sclerosis is distinct from atherosclerosis and ordinarily does not entail any clinically significant impairment.

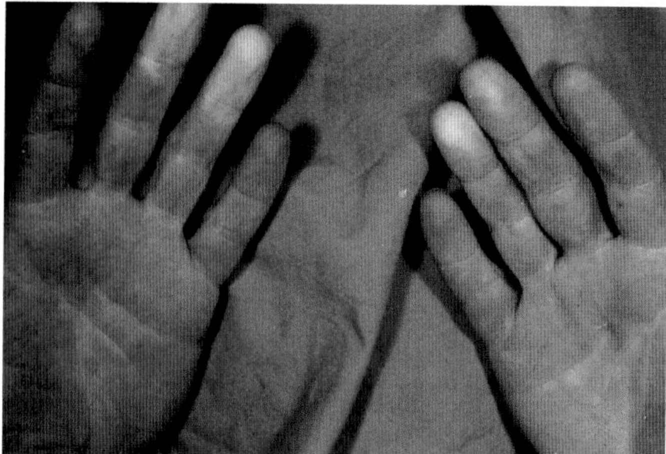

FIGURE 8-42. Raynaud phenomenon. The tips of the fingers showing marked pallor.

Raynaud Phenomenon

Raynaud phenomenon is characterized by intermittent bilateral attacks of ischemia of the fingers or toes, and sometimes the ears or nose. It is associated with severe pallor (Fig. 8-42) and is often accompanied by paresthesias and pain. Symptoms are precipitated by cold or emotional stimuli and relieved by heat. Primary cold sensitivity of the Raynaud type is more common in women and often starts in the late teens. It is bilateral and symmetric and, on rare occasions, may lead to ulcers or gangrene of the tips of digits. The hands are more commonly affected than the feet.

Raynaud phenomenon may occur as an isolated disorder or as part of systemic diseases of connective tissue (collagen vascular disorders), particularly scleroderma and systemic lupus erythematosus. Whatever its cause, the condition reflects vasospasm of the arteries and arterioles in the skin. Dysregulation of vascular tone by sympathetic nerve activity and by neurohumoral factors may play a role in its pathogenesis.

Fibromuscular Dysplasia

Fibromuscular dysplasia is a rare noninflammatory thickening of large- and medium-sized muscular arteries, which is distinct from atherosclerosis and arteriosclerosis. The cause is unknown; however, it may represent a developmental abnormality. Renal artery stenosis caused by this condition is an important cause of renovascular hypertension, although fibromuscular dysplasia may affect almost any other vessel, including carotid, vertebral, and splanchnic arteries. It is typically a disease of women during their reproductive years but may appear at any age, even in childhood.

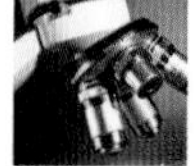

PATHOLOGY: In most cases, the distal two thirds of the renal artery and its primary branches display several areas of segmental stenoses, which represent fibrous and muscular ridges that project into the lumen. Microscopically, these segments show disorderly arrangement and proliferation of the cellular elements of the vessel wall, without necrosis or inflammation. Smooth muscle is replaced by fibrous tissue and myofibroblasts, and the media may be thinned. Other than renal hypertension, the major

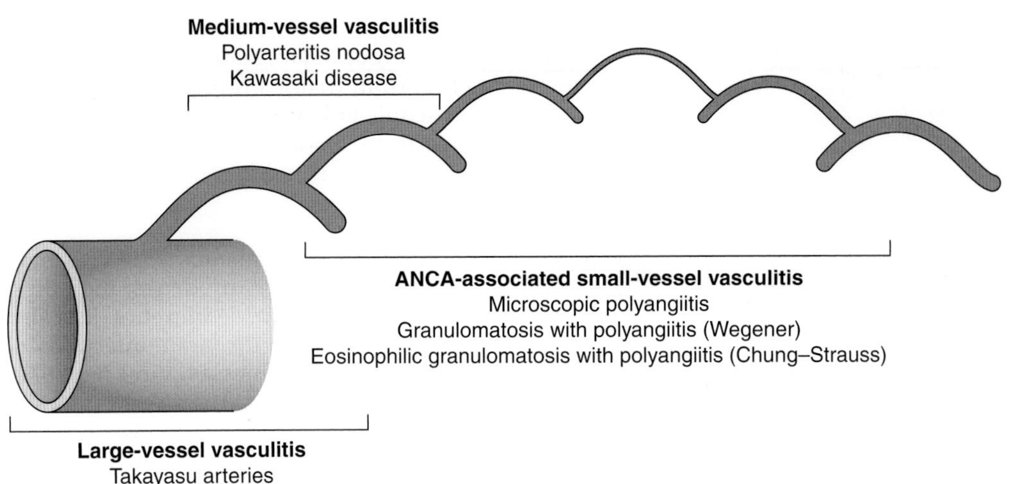

FIGURE 8-43. Inflammatory disorders of blood vessels. ANCA, antineutrophil cytoplasmic antibody. Modified from Jennette JC, Falk RJ. Pathogenesis of antineutrophil cytoplasmic autoantibody-mediated disease. *Nature Rev Rheumatol.* 2014;10(8):463-473.

complication of fibromuscular dysplasia is dissecting aneurysm, owing to thinning of the media of affected arteries.

VASCULITIS

Vasculitis, inflammation, and necrosis of blood vessels may affect arteries, veins, and capillaries (Fig. 8-43). Vessels may be damaged by immune mechanisms (see Chapter 3), infectious agents, mechanical trauma, radiation, or toxins. However, in many cases, no specific cause is determined.

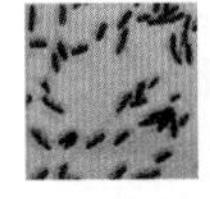

ETIOLOGIC FACTORS: Vasculitic syndromes are thought to involve immune mechanisms, including **(1) deposition of immune complexes, (2) direct attack on vessels by circulating antibodies, (3) neutrophil activation as a result of circulating antineutrophil cytoplasmic antibodies (ANCAs), and (4) various forms of cell-mediated immunity.** Agents that incite these reactions are largely unknown, although, in some instances, vasculitis is associated with viral infection.

Viral antigens may cause vasculitis. Thus, chronic infection with hepatitis B virus is associated with some cases of polyarteritis nodosa (see below). In this case, viral antigen–antibody complexes circulate and are deposited in the vascular lesions. Human vasculitis has also been associated with other viral infections, including herpes simplex, cytomegalovirus, and parvovirus, as well as with several bacterial antigens.

Small-vessel vasculitides (e.g., granulomatosis with polyangiitis; see below) are associated with circulating **antineutrophil cytoplasmic antibodies (ANCAs)**. Why these autoantibodies appear is not known, but infection may play a role in their development. ANCAs cause endothelial damage by activating neutrophils, and antibody titers correlate with disease activity in some cases. ANCAs are detected by indirect immunofluorescence assays, using patients' sera and ethanol-fixed neutrophils. Common patterns include **P-ANCA**, mostly against myeloperoxidase, and **C-ANCA**, principally against proteinase 3. (The **"P"** —perinuclear— and **"C"**—cytoplasmic—refer to the location of immunofluorescence in the commonly used diagnostic test.) When neutrophils are exposed to TNF, the cells degranulate and express myeloperoxidase and proteinase 3 at their surfaces. ANCA, which may present as a response to infection, can then bind to the surface expressed protein and activate the neutrophils, resulting in endothelial damage (Fig. 8-44).

Polyarteritis Nodosa

Polyarteritis nodosa affects medium-sized and smaller muscular arteries and, occasionally, larger arteries. Polyarteritis nodosa–like lesions may also occur in viral infections, including hepatitis B and C and HIV infection.

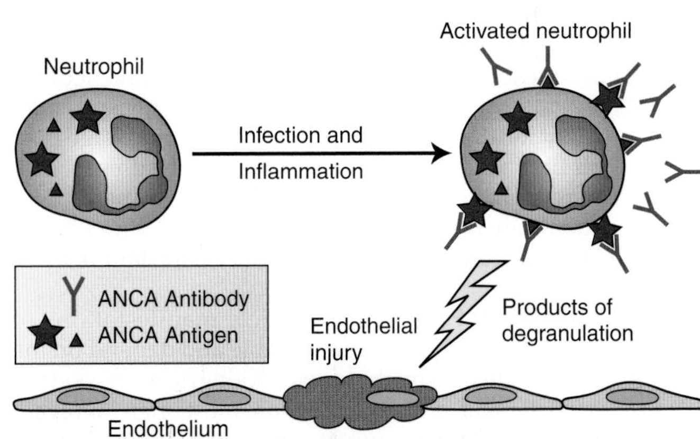

FIGURE 8-44. Model of the pathogenesis of antineutrophil cytoplasmic antibody (ANCA) vasculitis. ANCA antigens are normally found in the neutrophil cytoplasm with very little surface expression. In inflammation and infection, increased cell surface expression of ANCA antigens is induced in the neutrophils. ANCA present in the circulation owing to previous formation through unknown mechanisms binds to these ANCA antigens on the surface, leading to neutrophil activation and interaction with endothelial cells. Neutrophil degranulation releases toxic factors, including reactive oxygen species, proteinase-3, and myeloperoxidase, and other granule enzymes cause endothelial cell apoptosis and necrosis, leading to endothelial injury.

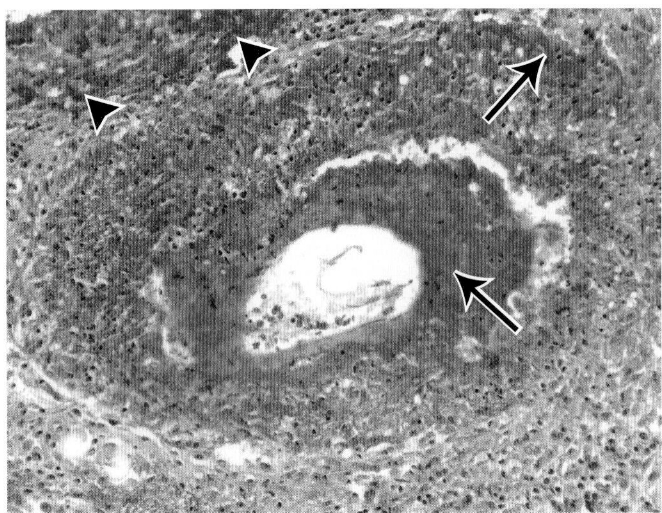

FIGURE 8-45. Polyarteritis nodosa. The intense inflammatory cell infiltrate in the arterial wall and surrounding connective tissue is associated with fibrinoid necrosis (*arrows*) and disruption of the vessel wall with hemorrhage into surrounding tissues (*arrowheads*).

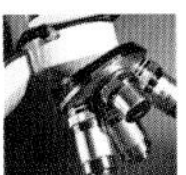

PATHOLOGY: The characteristic lesions of polyarteritis nodosa occur patchily in small- to medium-sized muscular arteries. However, on occasion, they extend into larger arteries, such as renal, splenic, or coronary arteries. Each lesion is usually less than 1 mm long and may involve part or all of the circumference of the vessel. Fibrinoid necrosis is the most prominent morphologic feature. Thrombosis and small aneurysms may occur in affected segments. The medial muscle and adjacent tissues are fused into a structureless eosinophilic mass that stains for fibrin. A vigorous acute inflammatory response envelops the area of necrosis, usually involving the entire adventitia (periarteritis), and extends through the other coats of the vessel (Fig. 8-45). Neutrophils, lymphocytes, plasma cells, and macrophages are present in varying proportions, and eosinophils are often conspicuous. Infarcts are common in involved organs. Aneurysms may rupture and, if located in a critical area, fatal hemorrhage may ensue. Over time, many vascular lesions start to heal, especially if corticosteroids have been given. Necrotic tissue and inflammatory exudate are resorbed, and the vessel is left with fibrosis of the media and conspicuous gaps in the elastic laminae.

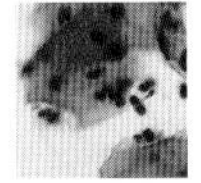

CLINICAL FEATURES: Clinical manifestations of polyarteritis nodosa are variable and depend on the organs affected by the lesions. Kidneys, heart, skeletal muscle, skin, and mesentery are most often involved, but lesions may occur in almost any organ, including the bowel, pancreas, lungs, liver, and brain. Constitutional symptoms such as fever and weight loss are common.

Without treatment, polyarteritis nodosa is usually fatal, but anti-inflammatory and immunosuppressive therapy, in the form of corticosteroids and cyclophosphamide, eventuates in remissions or cures in most patients.

Microscopic Polyangiitis

Microscopic polyangiitis refers to a broad category of inflammatory vascular lesions that are thought to represent a reaction to foreign materials (e.g., bacterial products or drugs). In the case of vascular lesions confined predominantly to skin, the term **leukocytoclastic vasculitis** (referring to nuclear debris from disintegrating neutrophils) is often applied. **Microscopic polyangiitis** affects many of the same organs as polyarteritis nodosa but is restricted to the smallest arteries and arterioles and is ***strongly associated with P-ANCA***.

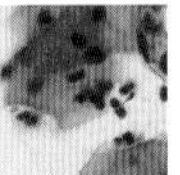

CLINICAL FEATURES: Cutaneous vasculitis may follow administration of many drugs, including aspirin, penicillin, and thiazide diuretics. It is also commonly related to such disparate infections as streptococcal and staphylococcal illnesses, viral hepatitis, tuberculosis, and bacterial endocarditis. The disease typically presents as palpable purpura, principally on the lower extremities. Microscopically, superficial cutaneous venules show fibrinoid necrosis with acute inflammation. Cutaneous vasculitis is generally self-limited (see Chapter 20).

Microscopic polyangiitis may be an isolated entity or a feature of other conditions, including collagen vascular diseases (lupus erythematosus, rheumatoid arthritis, and Sjögren syndrome), dysproteinemias, and several malignancies. Renal involvement is characterized by rapidly progressive glomerulonephritis and renal failure (see Chapter 14).

Giant Cell Arteritis

Although it most often affects the temporal artery, giant cell arteritis (temporal arteritis) may also involve other cranial arteries, the aorta (giant cell aortitis) and its branches, and occasionally other arteries. Aortic aneurysms and dissection occur. The average age at onset is 70 years, and it is rare before age 50. Giant cell arteritis is the most common vasculitis; its incidence rises with age and may reach 1% by 80 years of age. Women are slightly more often affected than men. The age at onset helps differentiate it from other vasculitides that may involve the same vessels in younger people, such as Takayasu disease.

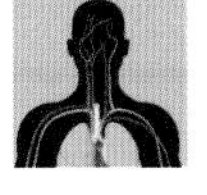

PATHOPHYSIOLOGY: The etiology of giant cell arteritis is obscure. Its association with HLA-DR4 and its occurrence in first-degree relatives support a genetic component. The lesions contain activated $CD4^+$ T-helper cells and macrophages, but B lymphocytes are lacking. Macrophages at the border of the intima and media produce matrix metalloproteinases that digest extracellular matrix. ANCA is absent in giant cell arteritis. Generalized muscle aching and widespread distribution of its manifestations are consistent with a relationship to rheumatoid diseases.

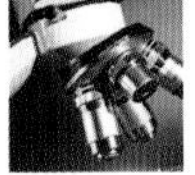

PATHOLOGY: Affected vessels are cord like and exhibit nodular thickening. Lumens are reduced to slits or may be obliterated by a thrombus (Fig. 8-46A). Microscopically, the media and intima show granulomatous inflammation; aggregates of macrophages, lymphocytes, and plasma cells are admixed with variable numbers of eosinophils and neutrophils. Giant cells tend to be distributed at the internal elastic lamina (Fig. 8-46B) but vary widely in number. Foreign-body giant cells and Langhans giant cells are both seen. Foci of necrosis are characterized by changes in the internal elastica, which becomes swollen, irregular, and fragmented, and in advanced lesions may completely disappear. Fragments of the elastica occasionally appear in

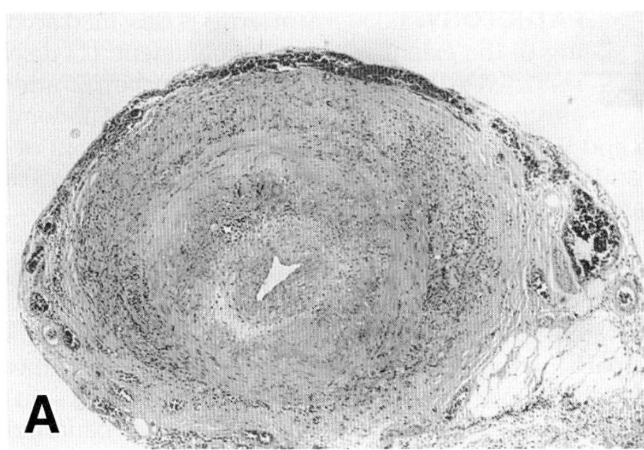

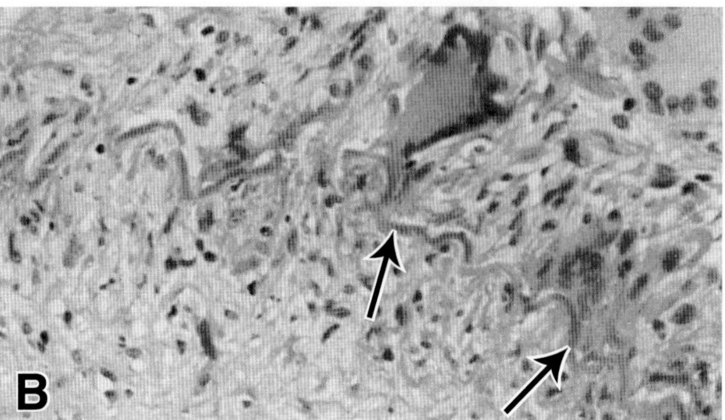

FIGURE 8-46. Temporal arteritis. A. A photomicrograph of a temporal artery showing chronic inflammation throughout the wall and a lumen severely narrowed by intimal thickening. **B.** A high-power view showing giant cells adjacent to the fragmented internal elastic lamina (*arrows*).

the giant cells. In the late stages, the intima is conspicuously thickened, and the media is fibrotic. Thrombi may obliterate the lumen, after which organization and canalization occur.

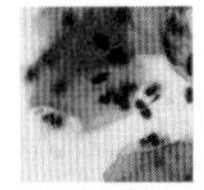

CLINICAL FEATURES: Giant cell arteritis tends to be benign and self-limited, and symptoms subside in 6 to 12 months. Patients present with headache and throbbing temporal pain. In some instances, there are early constitutional symptoms, including malaise, fever, and weight loss, plus generalized muscular aching or stiffness in the shoulders and hips. Throbbing and pain over the temporal artery are accompanied by swelling, tenderness, and redness in overlying skin. Almost half of patients have visual symptoms, which may proceed from transient to permanent blindness in one or both eyes, sometimes rapidly. Because the inflammatory process is patchy, biopsy of the temporal artery may not be diagnostic in as many as 40% of patients with otherwise classic manifestations. Response to corticosteroids is usually dramatic, and symptoms subside within days.

Granulomatosis With Polyangiitis

Granulomatosis with polyangiitis (GPA, formerly Wegener granulomatosis) is a systemic necrotizing vasculitis of unknown etiology, with granulomatous lesions of the nose, sinuses, and lungs and renal glomerular disease. Men are affected more than women, usually in their fifth and sixth decades. Over 90% of patients with GPA are positive for ANCA, 75% of whom have C-ANCA. The response to immunosuppressive therapy supports an immunologic basis for the disease.

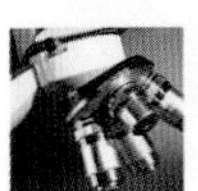

PATHOLOGY: Lesions of GPA feature parenchymal necrosis, vasculitis, and granulomatous inflammation composed of neutrophils, lymphocytes, plasma cells, macrophages, and eosinophils. Individual lesions in the lung may be as large as 5 cm across and must be distinguished from tuberculosis. Vasculitis involving small arteries and veins may be seen anywhere but occurs most frequently in the respiratory tract (Fig. 8-47), kidney, and spleen. Arteritis is characterized principally by chronic inflammation, although acute inflammation, necrotizing and non-necrotizing granulomas and fibrinoid necrosis are often present. Medial thickening and intimal proliferation are common and often cause narrowing or obliteration of the lumen.

The most prominent pulmonary feature is persistent bilateral pneumonitis, with nodular infiltrates that undergo cavitation. Chronic sinusitis and nasopharyngeal mucosal ulcers are frequent. The kidney at first shows focal necrotizing

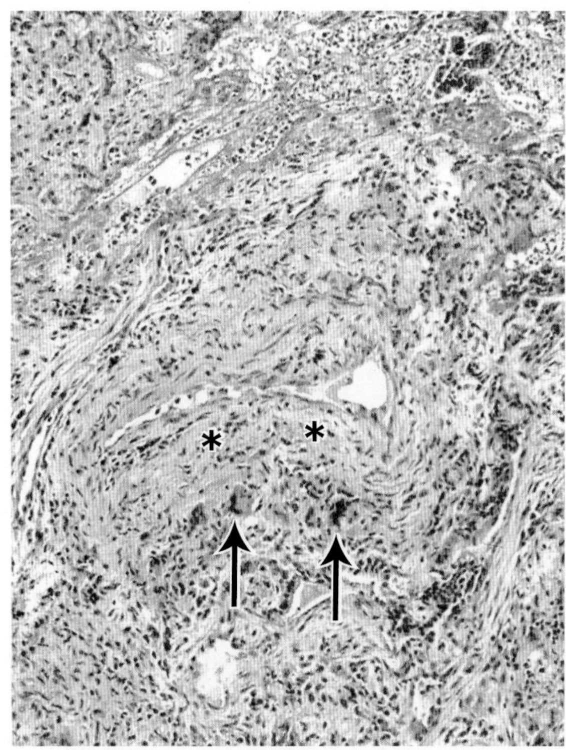

FIGURE 8-47. Granulomatosis with polyangiitis. A photomicrograph of the lung showing vasculitis of a pulmonary artery. There are chronic inflammatory cells and Langhans giant cells (*arrows*) in the wall, together with thickening of the intima (*asterisks*).

glomerulonephritis, which progresses to crescentic glomerulonephritis (see Chapter 14).

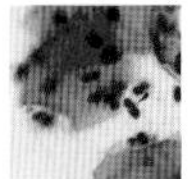

CLINICAL FEATURES: Most patients present with symptoms referable to the respiratory tract, particularly pneumonitis and sinusitis, the lung being involved in over 90% of patients. Hematuria and proteinuria are common, and glomerular disease can progress to renal failure. Rash, muscular pains, joint involvement, and neurologic symptoms occur. Most patients (80%) die within a year if untreated, with a mean survival of 5 to 6 months. Treatment with cyclophosphamide produces complete remissions or substantial disease-free intervals in most patients.

Allergic Granulomatosis and Angiitis (Churg–Strauss Syndrome)

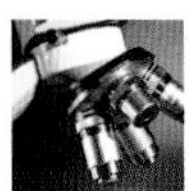

PATHOLOGY: Two thirds of patients with Churg–Strauss syndrome have P-ANCA. Widespread necrotizing lesions of small- and medium-sized arteries, arterioles, and veins are found in the lungs, spleen, kidney, heart, liver, CNS, and other organs. These lesions are granulomas and show characteristic intense eosinophilic infiltrates in and around blood vessels. The resulting fibrinoid necrosis, thrombosis, and aneurysm formation may simulate polyarteritis nodosa, although Churg–Strauss syndrome seems to be a distinct entity. Untreated, these patients have a poor prognosis, but corticosteroid therapy is almost always effective.

Takayasu Arteritis

This form of arteritis is seen worldwide. It mainly affects women (90%), most of whom are under 30 years of age. The cause of Takayasu arteritis is unknown, but an autoimmune basis has been proposed.

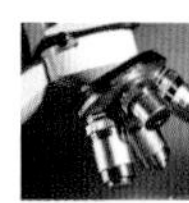

PATHOLOGY: Takayasu arteritis is classified according to the extent of aortic involvement: (1) disease restricted to the aortic arch and its branches, (2) arteritis affecting only the descending thoracic and abdominal aorta and its branches, and (3) combined involvement of the arch and descending aorta. The pulmonary artery is occasionally and the retinal vasculature is frequently affected.

The aortic wall is thickened, and the intima shows focal, raised plaques. Branches of the aorta often have localized stenosis or occlusion, which interferes with blood flow. If the subclavian arteries are affected, the synonym **pulseless disease** is used. The aorta, particularly the distal thoracic and abdominal segments, commonly shows variably sized aneurysms. Early lesions of the aorta and its main branches consist of an acute panarteritis, with infiltrates of neutrophils, mononuclear cells, and occasional Langhans giant cells. Inflammation of vasa vasorum in Takayasu arteritis resembles that observed in syphilitic aortitis. Late lesions display fibrosis and severe intimal proliferation. Secondary atherosclerotic changes may obscure the basic disease.

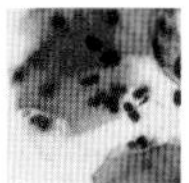

CLINICAL FEATURES: Patients with early Takayasu arteritis complain of constitutional symptoms, dizziness, visual disturbances, dyspnea and, occasionally, syncope. As the disease progresses, cardiac symptoms become more severe, with intermittent claudication of the arms or legs. Asymmetric differences in blood pressure may develop, and pulses in one extremity may sometimes actually disappear. Hypertension may reflect coarctation of the aorta or renal artery stenosis. Most patients eventually develop congestive heart failure. Loss of visual acuity ranges from field defects to total blindness. Early Takayasu arteritis responds to corticosteroids, but the later lesions require surgical reconstruction.

Kawasaki Disease

Kawasaki disease (mucocutaneous lymph node syndrome) is an acute necrotizing vasculitis of infancy and early childhood, with high fever, rash, conjunctival and oral lesions, and

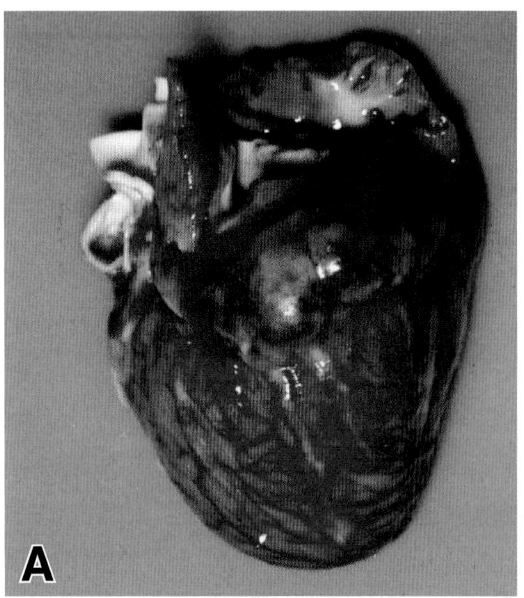

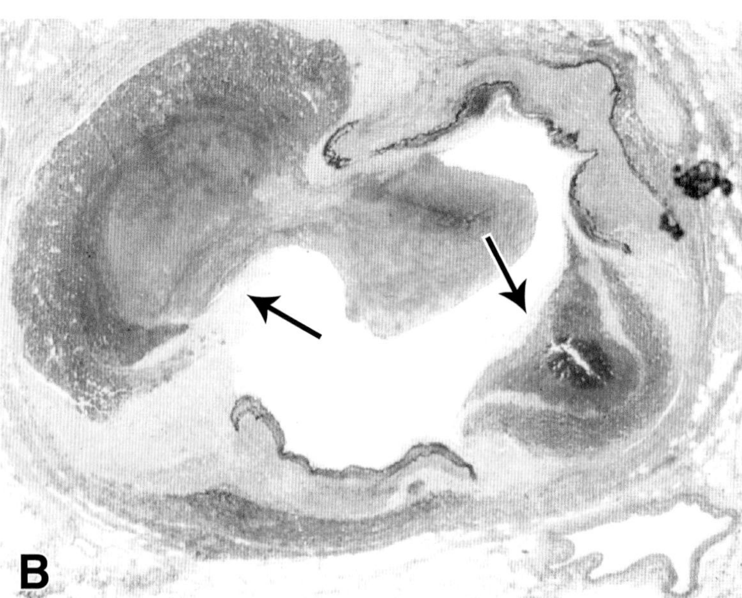

FIGURE 8-48. Kawasaki disease. A. The heart of a child who died from Kawasaki disease showing conspicuous coronary artery aneurysms. **B.** A microscopic section of a coronary artery from the same patient showing two large defects (*arrows*) in the internal elastic lamina, with two small aneurysms filled with thrombus.

lymphadenitis. In 70% of patients, vasculitis of the coronary arteries leads to coronary artery aneurysms (Fig. 8-48), 1% to 2% of which are lethal.

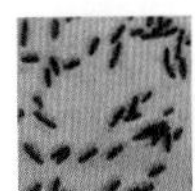

ETIOLOGIC FACTORS: Kawasaki disease is usually self-limited. An infectious etiology is strongly suspected based on epidemiologic data, but no etiologic agent has been firmly established. The disease has a high frequency in Japanese and Korean populations and individuals of Asiatic descent.

Buerger Disease

Buerger disease (thromboangiitis obliterans) is an occlusive inflammatory disease of medium- and small-sized arteries in the distal arms and legs. It once occurred almost only in young and middle-aged men who smoked heavily, but it is now also described in women. It is more common in the Mediterranean area, Middle East, and Asia.

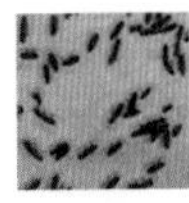

ETIOLOGIC FACTORS: The etiologic role of smoking in Buerger disease is underscored by the fact that cessation of smoking may lead to remission, and resumption of smoking to exacerbation. Yet how tobacco smoke produces the malady is obscure.

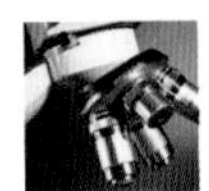

PATHOLOGY: The earliest change in Buerger disease is acute inflammation of medium- and small-sized arteries. Neutrophilic infiltrates extend to involve neighboring veins and nerves. Injury to the endothelium in inflamed areas gives rise to thrombosis and obliteration of the lumen. Small microabscesses of the vessel wall, with a central area of neutrophils surrounded by fibroblasts and Langhans giant cells, distinguish this process from thrombosis associated with atherosclerosis. Early lesions often become severe enough to cause gangrene of the extremity, leading to amputation. Late in the course of the disease, thrombi are completely organized and partly canalized.

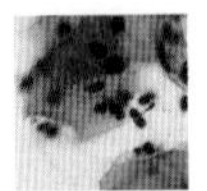

CLINICAL FEATURES: Symptoms of Buerger disease usually start between the ages of 25 and 40 years as intermittent claudication (cramping pains in muscles after exercise, quickly relieved by rest). Patients often present with painful ulceration of a digit, which progresses to destruction of the tips of the involved digits. Those who continue to smoke may slowly lose both hands and feet.

Behçet Disease

Behçet disease is a systemic vasculitis characterized by oral aphthous ulcers, genital ulcers, and ocular inflammation. Occasionally, there are lesions in the CNS, gastrointestinal tract, and cardiovascular system. Both large and small vessels show vasculitis. The mucocutaneous lesions exhibit nonspecific vasculitis of arterioles, capillaries, and venules, with infiltration of vessel walls and perivascular tissue by lymphocytes and plasma cells. Occasional endothelial cells are proliferated and swollen. Medium and large arteries show destructive arteritis, characterized by fibrinoid necrosis, mononuclear infiltration, thrombosis, aneurysms, and hemorrhage. The cause is unknown, but the effectiveness of corticosteroid treatment and an association with specific HLA subtypes suggest an immune basis.

BENIGN TUMORS OF BLOOD VESSELS

Tumors of the vascular system are common. Many are hamartomas rather than true neoplasms.

Hemangiomas

Hemangiomas usually occur in the skin but are also found in internal organs.

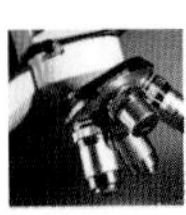

PATHOLOGY: Capillary Hemangioma. ***This lesion is composed of vascular channels with the size and structure of normal capillaries.*** Capillary hemangiomas may occur in any tissue. The most common sites are skin, subcutaneous tissues, mucous membranes of the lips and mouth, and internal viscera, including the spleen, kidneys, and liver. Capillary hemangiomas vary from a few millimeters to several centimeters in diameter. They are bright red to blue, depending on the degree of oxygenation of the blood. In the skin, capillary hemangiomas are known as **birthmarks** or **ruby spots**. The only disability is cosmetic disfiguration.

- **Juvenile Hemangioma.** Also called **strawberry hemangiomas**, these lesions are found on the skin of newborns. They grow rapidly in the first months of life, begin to fade at 1 to 3 years of age, and completely regress in most (80%) cases by 5 years of age. Juvenile hemangiomas contain packed masses of capillaries separated by connective tissue stroma (Fig. 8-49). The endothelial-lined channels are usually filled with blood. Thromboses, sometimes organized, are common. Although finger-like projections of the vascular tissue may give the impression of invasion, these growths are benign; they do not invade or metastasize.
- **Cavernous Hemangioma.** ***This term is reserved for lesions made of large vascular channels, often interspersed with small, capillary-type vessels.*** When cavernous hemangiomas occur in the skin, they are called **port wine stains**. They also appear on mucosal surfaces and visceral organs, including the spleen, liver, and pancreas. If they occur in the brain, they may enlarge slowly and cause neurologic symptoms after long quiescent periods.

A cavernous hemangioma is a red-blue, soft, spongy mass, with a diameter of up to several centimeters. Unlike capillary hemangiomas, cavernous hemangiomas do not regress spontaneously. Although the lesion is demarcated by a sharp border, it is not encapsulated. Large endothelial-lined, blood-containing spaces are separated by sparse connective tissue. Cavernous hemangiomas can undergo a variety of changes, including thrombosis, fibrosis, cystic cavitation, and intracystic hemorrhage.

Although hemangiomas are clearly benign, their origin is uncertain; they are likely to be hamartomas.

MALIGNANT TUMORS OF BLOOD VESSELS

Malignant vascular neoplasms are rare.

Angiosarcoma

These tumors occur in either sex and at any age. They begin as small, painless, sharply demarcated, red nodules. The most common locations are skin, soft tissue, breast, bone, liver, and

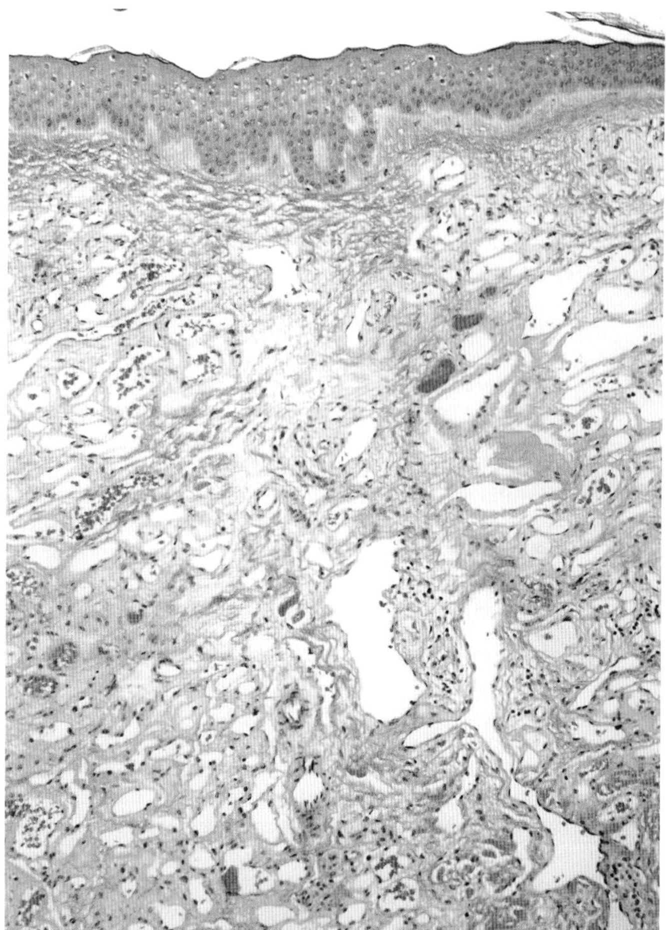

FIGURE 8-49. Juvenile hemangioma. A network of delicate, anastomosing vessels is present subcutaneously.

spleen. Eventually, most enlarge to become pale gray, fleshy masses without a capsule. These tumors often undergo central necrosis, with softening and hemorrhage.

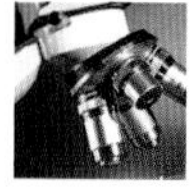

PATHOLOGY: Angiosarcomas exhibit varying degrees of differentiation, ranging from those composed mainly of distinct vascular elements to undifferentiated tumors with few recognizable blood channels (Fig. 8-50). The latter display frequent mitoses, pleomorphism, and giant cells and tend to be more malignant. Almost half of patients with angiosarcoma die of the disease.

Angiosarcoma of the liver is of special interest; it is associated with environmental carcinogens, particularly arsenic (a component of pesticides) and vinyl chloride (used in production of plastics). There is a long latent period between exposure to the chemicals and development of hepatic angiosarcoma. The earliest detectable changes are atypia and diffuse hyperplasia of the cells lining the hepatic sinusoids. The tumors are frequently multicentric and may arise in the spleen as well. Hepatic angiosarcomas are highly malignant and spread by both local invasion and metastasis.

Kaposi Sarcoma

Kaposi sarcoma is a malignant angioproliferative tumor derived from endothelial cells.

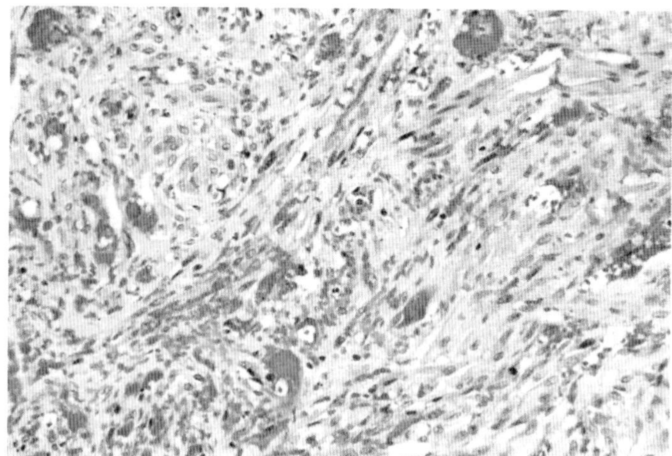

FIGURE 8-50. Angiosarcoma. Malignant spindly cells line vague channels. (*Inset*) Immunostain for CD31, an endothelial marker.

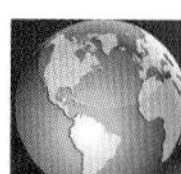

EPIDEMIOLOGY: Kaposi sarcoma was originally a sporadic tumor endemic in parts of central Africa, but was otherwise an oddity that afflicted mainly older men. Kaposi sarcoma is now seen in immunosuppressed patients, especially those with AIDS. Human herpesvirus 8 (HHV8), also called Kaposi sarcoma–associated herpes virus (KSHV), is responsible for this tumor, which arises in endothelial cells. Cofactors that determine the occurrence of Kaposi sarcoma in individuals who are at risk are not well understood.

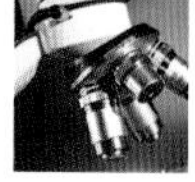

PATHOLOGY: Kaposi sarcoma begins as painful purple or brown 1-mm to 1-cm cutaneous nodules. They appear most often on the hands or feet but may occur anywhere. Their microscopic appearance is highly variable. One form resembles a simple hemangioma, with tightly packed clusters of capillaries and scattered hemosiderin-laden macrophages. Other types are highly cellular with less prominent vascular spaces (Fig. 8-51). Although Kaposi sarcoma is considered a malignant lesion and may be widely disseminated in the body, it rarely causes death.

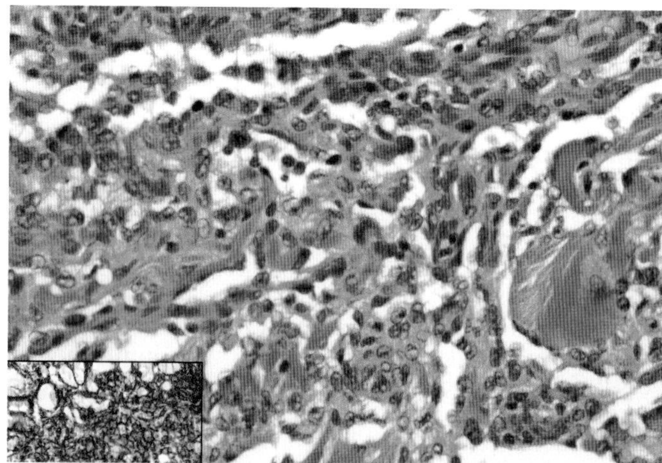

FIGURE 8-51. Kaposi sarcoma. A photomicrograph of a vascular lesion from a patient with acquired immune deficiency syndrome showing numerous poorly differentiated, spindle-shaped neoplastic cells and a vascular lesion filled with red blood cells.

9 Heart

Jeffrey E. Saffitz

LEARNING OBJECTIVES

- Identify the location of myocardial infarcts produced by the occlusion of each coronary artery.
- Classify congenital heart disease (CHD) based on the anatomic and functional findings.
- Discuss the sequelae associated with aortic stenosis.
- Differentiate between physiologic, pathologic, molecular, and cellular events associated with cardiac hypertrophy.
- Review cardiac hypertrophy, heart failure, and myocardial regeneration.
- Differentiate between left- and right-sided cardiac failure.
- Outline the mechanisms by which atherosclerosis may result in cardiac ischemia.
- List the conditions other than atherosclerosis that can limit coronary blood flow.
- What are the clinical, laboratory, and histopathologic effects associated with the forms of angina and myocardial infarcts?
- Differentiate between subendocardial and transmural infarcts.
- Provide a time course for the histopathologic changes associated with the progression of a myocardial infarct.
- Describe the causation and cellular effects of reperfusion injury.
- Describe the complications of myocardial infarction.
- Distinguish between true and false cardiac aneurysms.
- Describe the clinical and pathologic effects of hypertensive heart disease, pulmonary hypertension, and cor pulmonale.
- Define stenosis, regurgitation and insufficiency in cardiac valves and describe their effects on blood flow in the vascular circuit.
- What are the etiologic agents and conditions associated with infectious endocarditis?
- Describe the etiology, progression, and cardiac abnormalities associated with acute and chronic rheumatic fever.
- What transmissible agents are associated with myocarditis?
- List the etiologies of cardiomyopathy and describe their pathophysiologic effects.
- Define sudden cardiac death and discuss common etiologies.
- List the primary tumors of the heart.
- Define the term "pericardial effusion" and give several examples.
- List the causes of constrictive pericarditis.
- Describe the forms of tissue rejection associated with heart transplantation.

ANATOMY OF THE HEART

The heart of a normal adult man weighs 280 to 340 g (woman, 230 to 280 g) and is a two-sided pump. Blood enters each side through a thin-walled **atrium**, from which it is propelled forward by thicker muscular **ventricles**. The right ventricle is considerably thinner (<0.5 cm) than the left ventricle (1.3 to 1.5 cm) because of the low venous pressure and relatively low afterload on the right side. Blood enters the ventricles across atrioventricular valves, the mitral valve on the left and the tricuspid valve on the right. These valve leaflets are held in place by chordae tendineae, strong fibrous cords attached to the inner surface of the ventricular wall via papillary muscles. The entrances to the aorta and pulmonary arteries are guarded by the aortic and pulmonary valves, each with three semilunar cusps. The heart wall has three layers: outer epicardium, middle myocardium, and inner endocardium. The heart is surrounded and enclosed by visceral and parietal pericardia, which are separated by the pericardial cavity.

Cardiac Myocytes

The myocardium is a network of individual myocytes separated from each other by intercalated disks that contain cell–cell adhesion and electrical junctions. The contractile elements of the myocyte, the **myofilaments**, are arranged in bundles called **myofibrils**. These are separated by mitochondria and sarcoplasmic reticulum (**SR**).

Myofibrils are organized into repeating units termed **sarcomeres** (Fig. 9-1A). ***The sarcomere is the basic functional unit of the contractile apparatus.*** The sarcomere consists of a Z disk at each end and interdigitated thick and thin filaments oriented perpendicular to the Z disk. The thick filaments contain myosin heavy chains, myosin-binding protein C, and myosin light chains. The thick filaments are limited to the A band and interact with the giant sarcomeric protein, titin (27,000 amino acids), which spans from the Z disk to the M line to form a third sarcomere filament system. The thin filaments contain actin and regulatory proteins, including **α-tropomyosin-1** and the **troponin complex** (cardiac troponins I, C, and T). They extend from the Z disk through the I band and into the A band. Interaction of these myofilaments generates the force for contraction.

Contraction of cardiac muscle is initiated by increases in cytosolic free calcium. In a normal myocyte, an action potential triggers entry of calcium ions into the myocyte through voltage-gated, L-type Ca^{2+} channels in T tubules. These invaginations of the sarcolemma bring depolarizing current and resultant voltage-gated Ca^{2+} entry into intimate proximity to intracellular organelles that regulate calcium homeostasis (lateral cisterns of the SR) and the contractile apparatus itself (Fig. 9-1B). The entering calcium stimulates release of Ca^{2+} sequestered in the SR (Ca^{2+} induced Ca^{2+} release) via cardiac ryanodine receptors (RyR2). Increased cytosolic Ca^{2+} produces a conformational change in the regulatory myofilament proteins, in particular troponin, allowing cross-bridges between actin and myosin to break and reform repeatedly. As a result, the filaments slide over one another, causing myocardial contraction. ***The number of contractile sites activated and the resulting force generated are directly proportional to the concentration of Ca^{2+} near the myofibrils.***

The myocardium relaxes when cytosolic Ca^{2+} returns to its low concentration of 10^{-7} M in diastole. This process depends on calcium ATPase of the SR, which pumps Ca^{2+} from the cytosol back into the SR (Fig. 9-1B). ***Thus, myocardial relaxation is an active, energy-requiring event.***

The Conduction System

Specialized myocytes of the conducting system have two major functions: (1) they initiate heartbeats by generating electrical current through their automatic rhythmicity, which is more rapid in the sinoatrial (SA) node than more distally

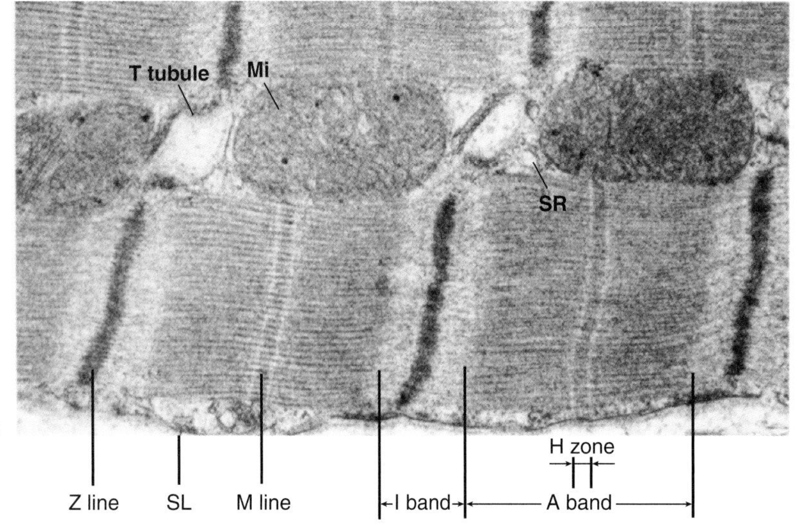

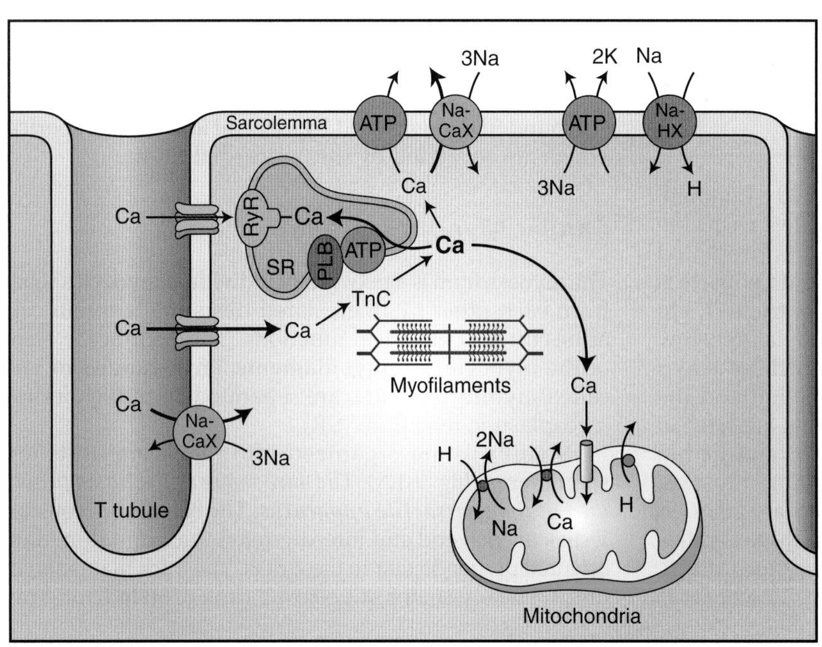

FIGURE 9-1. Ultrastructure of the myocardium. A. Electron micrograph of the left ventricle in the longitudinal plane showing the sarcolemma (SL); the sarcomeres of the myofibrils, delimited by Z lines; A bands; I bands; H zones; and M lines. Also present are mitochondria (Mi), sarcoplasmic reticulum (SR), and T tubules. The I bands and H zones are absent when the myofibrils are shortened. The structural basis for the banding is shown in the electron micrograph. The fine threads that extend at right angles to the thick (myosin) filaments are the cross-bridges that form the force-generating cross-links with actin. The amount of force that can be generated is proportional to the length of the adjoining myofilaments and is at a maximum when the sarcomeres are between 2 and 2.2 μm in length. When the sarcomeres are less than 2 μm in length, the thin filaments slide across each other and overlap, decreasing the potential for force-generating cross-links; similarly, when the sarcomeres are stretched beyond 2.2 μm, there is a decrease in force that is proportional to the widening of the H zone. This mechanism can be invoked as the basis for Starling law of the heart. **B.** Pathways regulating Ca^{2+} homeostasis and excitation–contraction coupling in cardiac myocytes. The cardiac action potential brings depolarizing current into T tubules where voltage-gated L-type Ca^{2+} channels reside in high concentrations (*green channel structures*). Influx of Ca^{2+} through these channels (ICa) stimulates release of Ca^{2+} from the SR (located in immediate proximity to the T tubule) via RyR2. The transient increase in cytosolic Ca^{2+} promotes contraction through interactions with cardiac troponin T (TnC). Resting diastolic Ca^{2+} levels are restored by reuptake into the SR and extrusion via sodium-calcium exchange (Na-CaX) and an adenosine triphosphate (ATP) pump. RyR2, ryanodine receptor-2.

in the system; and (2) they distribute this current to activate atrial and ventricular myocardium in an appropriate temporal–spatial pattern. Fibers of the atrioventricular conduction system generally conduct impulses faster (1 to 2 m/sec) than do working (contractile) atrial and ventricular fibers (0.5 to 1 m/sec). By contrast, conduction through the atrioventricular node is exceptionally slow (0.1 m/sec). Slow conduction at the atrioventricular junction delays ventricular activation and facilitates ventricular filling.

Heartbeats normally originate in the SA node, which is near the junction of the superior vena cava and the roof of the right atrium. If the node is diseased or otherwise prevented from functioning as the pacemaker, more distal components of the conduction system or even ventricular muscle itself assume the role of pacemaker. ***As a rule, the more distal the pacemaker site, the slower the heart rate.*** On leaving the SA node, an electrical impulse activates the atria. Atrial wave fronts converge on the atrioventricular (AV) node, which conducts the impulse through the common bundle (bundle of His) to the left and right bundle branches of the Purkinje system. Purkinje fibers run within the endocardium on both sides of the interventricular septum and distribute current to overlying ventricular muscles. In each cycle, ventricular contraction begins along the interventricular septum and at the apex. It progresses from apex to base, resulting in smooth and efficient ejection of blood into the great vessels.

The His bundle in normal adult heart is the only electrical connection between atria and ventricles. Additional abnormal connections may occasionally arise as small bundles or tracts of cardiac myocytes. Such "bypass tracts" can activate ventricular muscle before the normal impulse arrives via the conduction system. They are found in patients with the **Wolff–Parkinson–White syndrome** and can establish circuits that promote **supraventricular tachycardia**. Acquired defects may arise secondary to infarction, inflammatory or infiltrative disease, cardiac surgery, or cardiac catheterization.

The Heart As a Pump

In this circuit, the amount of blood handled by the right ventricle, which pumps blood to the lungs (pulmonary circulation), must, over time, exactly equal the amount of blood going through the left ventricle, which distributes blood to the body (systemic circulation). The hemodynamically important parameters are cardiac output, perfusion pressure, and peripheral vascular resistance.

- **Cardiac output** is the volume of blood pumped by each ventricle per minute and represents the total blood flow in pulmonary and systemic circuits. Cardiac output is the product of heart rate and stroke volume and, as the **cardiac index**, is often adjusted for body surface area (in m^2) as an indicator of ventricular function.
- **Perfusion pressure** (also called **driving pressure**) is the difference in dynamic pressure between two points along a blood vessel. Blood flow to any segment of the circulation ultimately depends on arterial driving pressure. However, each organ can autoregulate flow and so determine the amount of blood it receives from the circulation. Such local control of perfusion depends on continuous modulation of microvascular beds by hormonal, neural, metabolic, and hemodynamic factors.
- **Peripheral vascular resistance** is the sum of the factors that determine regional blood flow in each organ. Two thirds of the resistance in the systemic vasculature is determined by the arterioles.

The sum of all regional flows equals the **venous return**, which, in turn, determines the cardiac output. Assessment of the heart's response to inflow (preload) and outflow (afterload) relies on cardiac reflexes, as well as cardiac muscle integrity and neurohormonal regulation.

Coronary Arteries

The right and left main coronary arteries originate in, or immediately above, the sinuses of Valsalva of the aortic valve. The left main coronary artery bifurcates within 1 cm of its origin into the left anterior descending (LAD) and left circumflex coronary arteries. The latter rests in the left atrioventricular groove and supplies the lateral wall of the left ventricle (Fig. 9-2). The LAD coronary artery lies in the anterior interventricular groove and provides blood to the (1) anterior left ventricle, (2) adjacent anterior right ventricle, and (3) anterior half to one third of the interventricular septum. In the apical region, the LAD artery supplies the ventricles circumferentially (Fig. 9-2).

The right coronary artery travels along the right atrioventricular groove and feeds most of the right ventricle and posteroseptal left ventricle (Fig. 9-2), including the posterior one third to half of the interventricular septum at the base of the heart (also referred to as the "inferior" or "diaphragmatic" wall). Thus, one can predict locations of infarcts that result from occlusion of any of these major epicardial coronary arteries.

The epicardial coronary arteries are usually arranged in a so-called right coronary–dominant distribution. The pattern of dominance is defined by the coronary artery that contributes the most blood to the posterior heart. In 5% to 10% of human hearts, the left circumflex coronary artery supplies the posterior descending coronary artery (left dominant).

Blood flows in the myocardium inward from the epicardium to the endocardium. Thus, as a general rule, the endocardium is most vulnerable to ischemia when flow through a major epicardial coronary artery is compromised. Some of the small intramyocardial coronary arteries branch as they traverse the ventricular wall; others maintain a large diameter and pass to the endocardial surface without branching. Because capillary networks arising from penetrating arteries do not interconnect, the borders between viable and infarcted myocardium after coronary artery occlusion are distinct.

The epicardial portion of each coronary artery fills and expands during systole and empties and narrows during diastole. Intramyocardial arteries do the opposite and are compressed by systolic muscular pressure. Thus, blood flow in the myocardium, especially in subendocardial ventricular regions, is lower or absent in systole. Autoregulation of blood flow roughly equalizes the myocardial supply.

CONGENITAL HEART DISEASE

CHD results from faulty embryonic development, expressed as either misplaced structures (e.g., transposition of the great vessels) or arrested progression of a normal structure from an early stage to a more advanced one

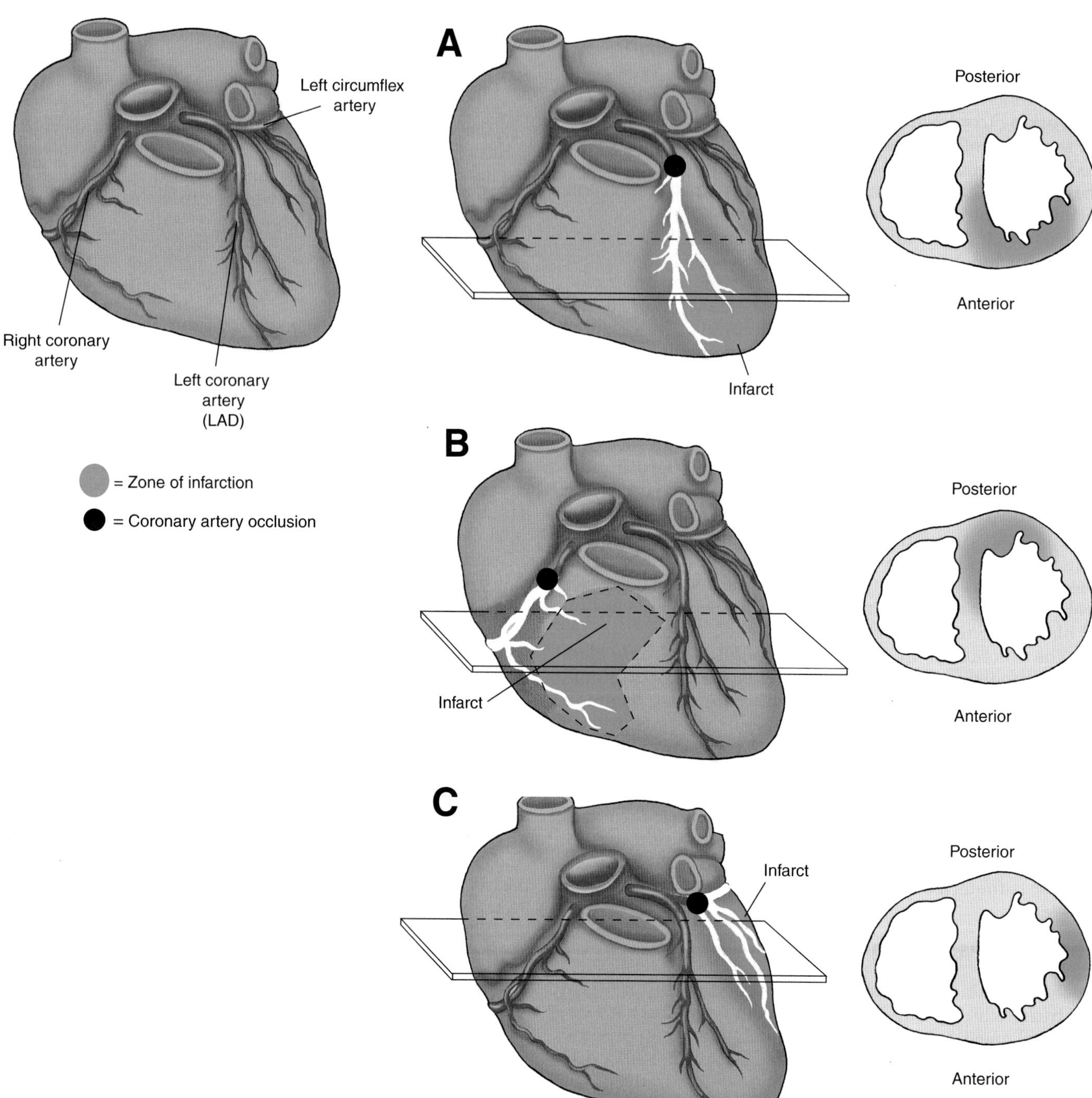

FIGURE 9-2. Position of left ventricular infarcts resulting from occlusion of each of the three main coronary arteries. A. Anterior infarct, which follows occlusion of the anterior descending branch (left anterior descending, LAD) of the left coronary artery. The infarct is located in the anterior wall and adjacent two thirds of the septum. It involves the entire circumference of the wall near the apex. **B.** A posterior ("inferior" or "diaphragmatic") infarct results from occlusion of the right coronary artery and involves the posterior wall, including the posterior one third of the interventricular septum and the posterior papillary muscle in the basal half of the ventricle. **C.** Posterolateral infarct, which follows occlusion of the left circumflex artery and is present in the posterolateral wall.

(e.g., atrial septal defect). Symptomatic CHD occurs in 1% of live births.

Causes of Congenital Heart Disease

The causes of CHD are not usually clear. Most congenital heart defects reflect multifactorial genetic, epigenetic, and environmental influences. As in other diseases with complex inheritance, risk of recurrence is greater among siblings of an affected child. Whereas CHD occurs in 1% of the general population, its incidence increases from 2% to 15% for pregnancies after the birth of a child with a heart defect. The risk of a third affected child may reach 30%. Also, infants born to mothers with CHD have an increased risk for CHD. Chromosomal abnormalities may cause CHD, most prominently Down syndrome (trisomy 21), other trisomies, Turner syndrome, and DiGeorge syndrome (22q11.2 deletion syndrome). However, chromosomal defects account for no more than 5% of cases of CHD.

Intrauterine infection can also play a role in congenital cardiac defects, for example, maternal rubella infection during the first trimester, especially during the first 4 weeks of gestation. Associations with other viral infections are suspected but are not as well documented. Maternal use of certain drugs in early pregnancy is also associated with increased cardiac defects in offspring. For example, 10% of babies with thalidomide syndrome (phocomelia) had CHD. Other drugs implicated in CHD include alcohol, amphetamines, phenytoin, lithium, and estrogens. Maternal diabetes is also associated with an increased incidence of CHD.

Types of Congenital Heart Disease

CHD can be divided into groups based on the presence or absence of shunting and the direction of the shunting.

Left-to-Right Shunt

These defects include ventricular and atrial septal defects, patent ductus arteriosus, aortopulmonary window, persistent truncus arteriosus, and hypoplastic left heart syndrome. Early left-to-right shunt reflects higher pressure on the left side of the heart.

Ventricular Septal Defect

Ventricular septal defects (VSDs) are among the most common congenital heart lesions (Table 9-1). They occur as isolated lesions or in combination with other malformations.

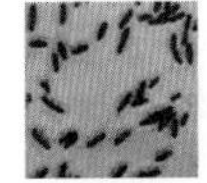

ETIOLOGIC FACTORS: The fetal heart consists of a single chamber until the fifth week of gestation, after which development of interatrial and interventricular septa and formation of atrioventricular valves from endocardial cushions divide it. A muscular interventricular septum grows upward from the apex toward the base of the heart (Fig. 9-3). It is joined by the downward-growing membranous septum, separating right and left ventricles. ***The most common VSD is related to partial or incomplete formation of the membranous portion of the septum.***

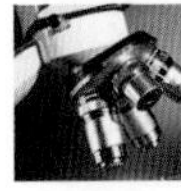

PATHOLOGY: VSDs occur as (1) a small hole in the membranous septum; (2) a large defect involving more than the membranous region (perimembranous defects); (3) defects in the muscular portion, which are more common anteriorly but can occur anywhere in the muscular septum and are often multiple; or (4) complete absence of the muscular septum (leaving a single ventricle).

Table 9-1

Relative Incidence of Specific Anomalies in Patients With Congenital Heart Disease

Ventricular septal defects: 25%–30%
Atrial septal defects: 10%–15%
Patent ductus arteriosus: 10%–20%
Tetralogy of Fallot: 4%–9%
Pulmonary stenosis: 5%–7%
Coarctation of the aorta: 5%–7%
Aortic stenosis: 4%–6%
Complete transposition of the great arteries: 4%–10%
Truncus arteriosus: 2%
Tricuspid atresia: 1%

VSDs are most common in the superior portion of the septum below the pulmonary artery outflow tract (below the crista supraventricularis, i.e., infracristal) and behind the septal leaflet of the tricuspid valve. The common bundle (bundle of His) is located immediately below the defect (inlet type). Less commonly, the defect is above the crista supraventricularis (supracristal) and just below the pulmonary valve (infra-arterial). The supracristal variety of septal defect is often associated with other defects, such as an overriding pulmonary artery (the **Taussig–Bing** type of double-outlet right ventricle), transposition of the great vessels, or persistent truncus arteriosus.

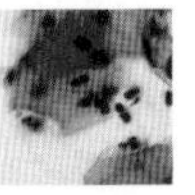

CLINICAL FEATURES: *A small septal defect may have little functional significance and may close spontaneously as the child matures.* Either hypertrophy of adjacent muscle or adherence of tricuspid valve leaflets to the margins of the hole may close the defect. In infants with large septal defects, higher left ventricular pressure creates initially a left-to-right shunt. Left ventricular dilation and congestive heart failure are common complications of such shunts. If a defect is small enough to permit prolonged survival, augmented pulmonary blood flow caused by shunting of blood into the right ventricle eventually results in thickening of pulmonary arteries and increased pulmonary vascular resistance. This increased vascular resistance may be so great that the direction of the shunt reverses and goes from right to left **(Eisenmenger complex)**. A patient with this condition displays late onset of cyanosis (i.e., tardive cyanosis), right ventricular hypertrophy, and right-sided heart failure.

Additional complications of ventricular septal defects include (1) infective endocarditis at the lesional site, (2) paradoxical (right-to-left) emboli, and (3) prolapse of an aortic valve cusp (with resulting aortic insufficiency). Large ventricular septal defects are repaired surgically, usually in infancy.

Atrial Septal Defects

Atrial septal defects (ASDs) range in severity from clinically insignificant and asymptomatic to life-threatening conditions. They arise embryologically by defects in atrial septum formation. Embryologic development of the atrial septum occurs

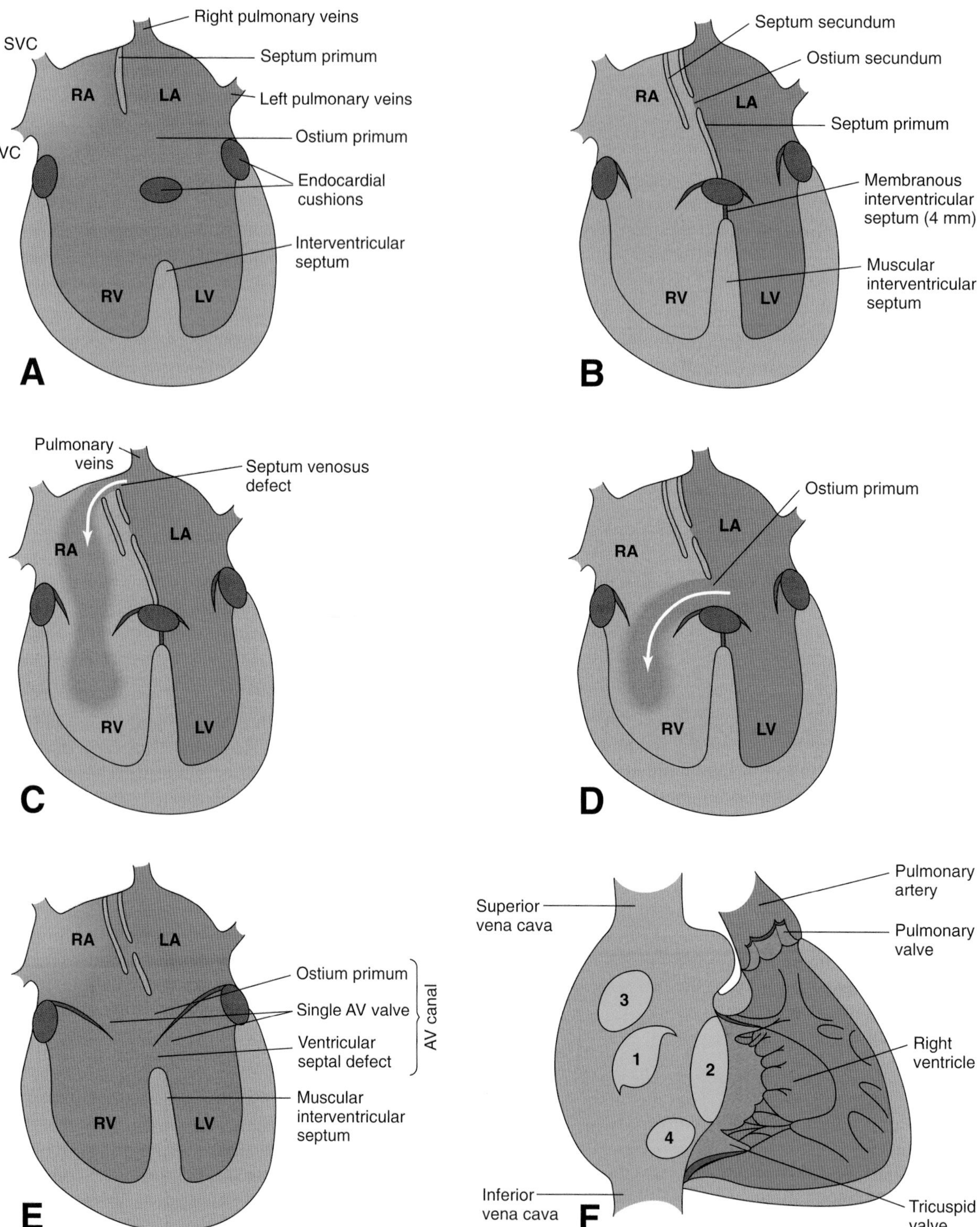

FIGURE 9-3. Pathogenesis of ventricular and atrial septal defects. A. The common atrial chamber is being separated into the right atrium (RA) and left atrium (LA) by the septum primum. Because the septum primum has not yet joined the endocardial cushions, there is an open ostium primum. The ventricular cavity is being divided by a muscular interventricular septum into right and left chambers (right ventricle [RV] and left ventricle [LV]). **B.** The septum primum has joined the endocardial cushions but, at the same time, has developed an opening in its midportion (the ostium secundum). This opening is partly overlaid by the septum secundum, which has grown down to cover, in part, the foramen ovale. Simultaneously, the membranous septum joins the muscular interventricular septum to the base of the heart, completely separating the ventricles. **C.** The sinus venosus type of atrial septal defect is located in the most cephalad region and is adjacent to the inflow of the right pulmonary veins, which thus tend to open into the RA. **D.** The ostium primum defect occurs just above the atrioventricular (AV) valve ring, sometimes in the presence of an intact valve ring. It may also, in conjunction with a defect of the valve ring and ventricular septum, form an AV canal, as shown in panel **E**. This common opening allows free communication between the atria and the ventricles. **F.** Location of atrial septal defects. In decreasing order of frequency: 1. Ostium secundum. 2. Ostium primum. 3. Sinus venosus. 4. Coronary sinus type. IVC, inferior vena cava; SVC, superior vena cava.

in a sequence that permits continued passage of oxygenated placental blood from the right atrium to the left atrium through the patent foramen, which continues until birth. Beginning at the fifth week of intrauterine life, the septum primum extends downward from the roof of the common atrium to join with the endocardial cushions, thereby closing the incomplete segment, or "ostium primum" (Fig. 9-3A). Before this closure is complete, the midportion of the septum primum develops a defect, or "ostium secundum," so that right-to-left flow continues. During the sixth week, a second septum (septum secundum) develops to the right of the septum primum, passing from the roof of the atrium toward the endocardial cushions (Fig. 9-3B). This process leaves a patent foramen, the **foramen ovale**, in the position of the original ostium secundum. The defect persists until it is sealed off after birth by fusion of the septum primum and septum secundum, whereupon it is termed the **fossa ovalis**.

PATHOLOGY: ASDs occur at a number of sites (Fig. 9-3).

- **Patent foramen ovale:** Tissue derived from the septum primum situated on the left side of the foramen ovale functions as a flap valve that normally fuses with the margins of the foramen ovale, thereby sealing the opening. An incomplete seal of the foramen ovale, which can be traversed with a probe **(probe patent foramen ovale),** occurs in 25% of normal adults. It may become a significant right-to-left shunt if right atrial pressure increases (e.g., with recurrent pulmonary thromboemboli). In this case, a right-to-left shunt develops, and emboli from the right-sided circulation pass directly into the systemic circuit. Such **paradoxical emboli** may cause infarcts in many parts of the arterial circulation, most commonly in the brain, heart, spleen, intestines, kidneys, and lower extremities.
- **Atrial septal defect, ostium secundum type:** This defect accounts for 90% of ASDs. It is a true deficiency of the atrial septum and should not be confused with a patent foramen ovale. Small defects are usually not problematic, but larger ones may allow sufficient blood to shunt from left to right to cause dilation and hypertrophy of the right atrium and ventricle. In this setting, pulmonary artery diameter may exceed that of the aorta.
- **Sinus venosus defect:** This anomaly, accounting for 5% of ASDs, occurs in the upper portion of the atrial septum, above the fossa ovalis, and near the entry of the superior vena cava (Fig. 9-3C). It is usually accompanied by drainage of right pulmonary veins into the right atrium or superior vena cava.
- **Atrial septal defect, ostium primum type:** This condition involves the region adjacent to the endocardial cushions (Fig. 9-3D) and comprises 7% of atrial septal defects. There are usually clefts in the anterior mitral valve leaflet and the septal leaflet of the tricuspid valve, which may be accompanied by a defect in the adjacent interventricular septum.
- **Atrioventricular canal:** A persistent common atrioventricular canal results from fully developed combined atrial and ventricular septal defects (Fig. 9-3E). Although quite uncommon, this defect occurs often in patients with Down syndrome. Additional defects include both complete and partial atrioventricular canals that result in ostium primum septal defects combined with ventricular septal, mitral, and tricuspid valve defects in varying degrees.
- **Coronary sinus atrial septal defect:** This is the rarest of atrial septal defects and is associated with a persistent left superior vena cava, which drains into the roof of the left atrium.

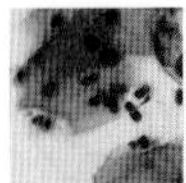

CLINICAL FEATURES: Young children with ASDs are usually asymptomatic, although they may complain of easy fatigability and dyspnea on exertion. Later in life, generally in adulthood, changes in the pulmonary vasculature may reverse blood flow through the defect and create a right-to-left shunt. Then, cyanosis and clubbing of the fingers ensue. Complications of atrial septal defects include atrial arrhythmias, pulmonary hypertension, right ventricular hypertrophy, heart failure, paradoxical emboli, and bacterial endocarditis. Symptomatic cases are treated surgically or with closure devices, which can be delivered and placed percutaneously.

Patent Ductus Arteriosus

In the early embryo, the six aortic arches connect the ventral and dorsal aortas as part of the branchial cleft system (Fig. 9-4A). The left sixth aortic arch is partly preserved as the pulmonary arteries and the **ductus arteriosus,** which convey most of the pulmonary outflow into the aorta. It constricts after birth in response to increased arterial oxygen content and becomes occluded by fibrosis **(ligamentum arteriosus)** (Fig. 9-4B).

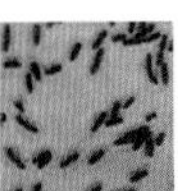

ETIOLOGIC FACTORS: Persistent PDA is one of the most common congenital cardiac defects, especially in infants whose mothers were infected with rubella virus early in pregnancy. It is also common in premature infants. In these patients, the ductus usually closes spontaneously. In full-term infants with PDA, however, the ductus has an abnormal endothelium and media, and only rarely closes spontaneously. PDAs occur in some patients with Down and DiGeorge syndromes.

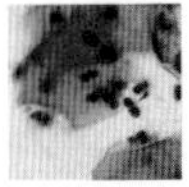

CLINICAL FEATURES: Luminal diameters of PDAs vary greatly. A small shunt has little effect on the heart, but a large one may divert blood from the aorta to the low-pressure pulmonary artery. In severe cases, left ventricular hypertrophy and heart failure ensue because of increased demand for cardiac output. The increased volume and pressure of blood in the pulmonary circulation eventually leads to pulmonary hypertension and its cardiac complications. Infective endarteritis involving the pulmonary artery side of the ductus is a frequent complication of untreated PDA.

PDA can be caused to contract and then close by instilling prostaglandin synthesis inhibitors (e.g., indomethacin) and, if necessary, can be corrected surgically or by interventional cardiac catheterization. Conversely, PDAs can be kept open after birth by administering prostaglandins (PGE_2) if survival of patients born with a cardiac defect requires a left-to-right or right-to-left shunt. Examples include patients with isolated pulmonary stenosis, complete transposition of the great vessels, or hypoplastic left heart syndrome.

Persistent Truncus Arteriosus

The truncus arteriosus is the embryonic arterial trunk that initially opens from both ventricles and is later separated into the aorta and pulmonary trunk by the spiral septum. ***Persistent truncus arteriosus is a common trunk of origin for the aorta, pulmonary arteries, and coronary arteries, resulting from absent or incomplete partitioning of the truncus arteriosus by the spiral septum. Truncus arteriosus almost always overrides (i.e., straddles) a VSD and receives blood from both ventricles.*** The valve of the truncus usually has three or four semilunar cusps but may have as few as two or as many as six. The coronary arteries arise from the base of the valve.

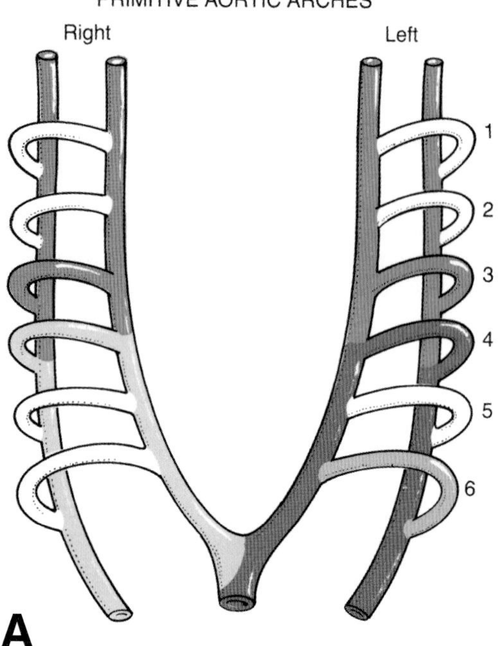

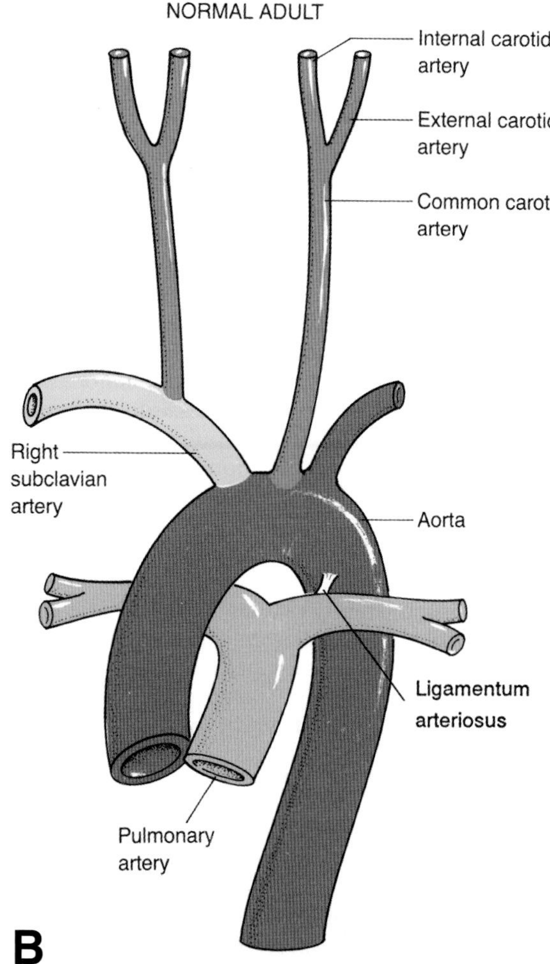

FIGURE 9-4. Derivatives of the aortic arches. A. Complete primitive aortic arch system. **B.** In the normal adult, the left fourth aortic arch is preserved as the arch of the adult aorta, and the left sixth arch gives rise to the pulmonary artery and ligamentum arteriosus (closed ductus arteriosus).

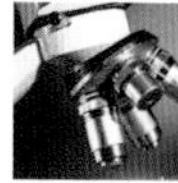

PATHOLOGY: There are several variants of truncus arteriosus that depend on the anatomic details of the defect. **Type 1** is most common and consists of a single trunk that gives rise to a common pulmonary artery and ascending aorta.

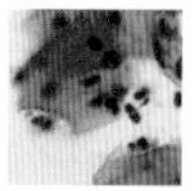

CLINICAL FEATURES: Most infants with truncus arteriosus have torrential pulmonary blood flow, causing heart failure, recurrent respiratory infections, and often early death. Pulmonary vascular disease develops if children survive, in which case cyanosis, polycythemia, and clubbing of the fingers appear. Open-heart surgery before significant pulmonary vascular changes develop is an effective treatment.

Hypoplastic Left Heart Syndrome

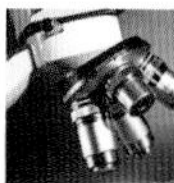

PATHOLOGY: This usually profound malformation features hypoplasia of the left ventricle and ascending aorta and hypoplasia or atresia of the left-sided valves. Severe aortic valvular stenosis or aortic atresia is often the main defect.

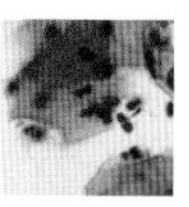

CLINICAL FEATURES: Aortic valve atresia precludes the left ventricular outflow into the aorta. As a consequence, there is an obligate left-to-right shunt through a patent foramen ovale. Cardiac output is entirely via the right ventricle and pulmonary artery. Systemic blood flow depends on flow from the pulmonary trunk to the aorta through a PDA. Because pulmonary vascular resistance is high at birth, and both the foramen ovale and ductus arteriosus are patent, newborns with hypoplastic left heart syndrome may appear well initially. As pulmonary vascular resistance falls and systemic (and especially coronary) blood flow decreases, infants become symptomatic. Without surgical correction or transplantation, over 95% die within their first month.

Right-to-Left Shunt

These defects include tetralogy of Fallot and tricuspid atresia.

Tetralogy of Fallot

Tetralogy of Fallot represents 10% of CHD. It has a familial recurrence rate of 2% to 3%, but little is known of its potential genetic and epigenetic causes.

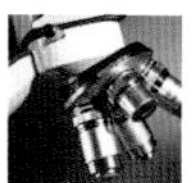

PATHOLOGY: The following four changes define tetralogy of Fallot (Fig. 9-5):

- Pulmonary stenosis
- Ventricular septal defect
- Dextroposition of the aorta so that it overrides the ventricular septal defect
- Right ventricular hypertrophy

The VSD, which may be as large as the aortic orifice, results from incomplete closure of the membranous septum and affects both the muscular septum and the endocardial cushions. In addition, development of the spiral septum, which normally divides the common truncus region into an aorta and a pulmonary artery, is abnormal. As a result, the aorta is displaced to the right and overlies the septal defect, which is immediately below the overriding aorta. Pulmonary stenosis is often as a result of subpulmonary muscular hypertrophy or an abnormal valve, which is usually funnel shaped, with the narrow part more distal.

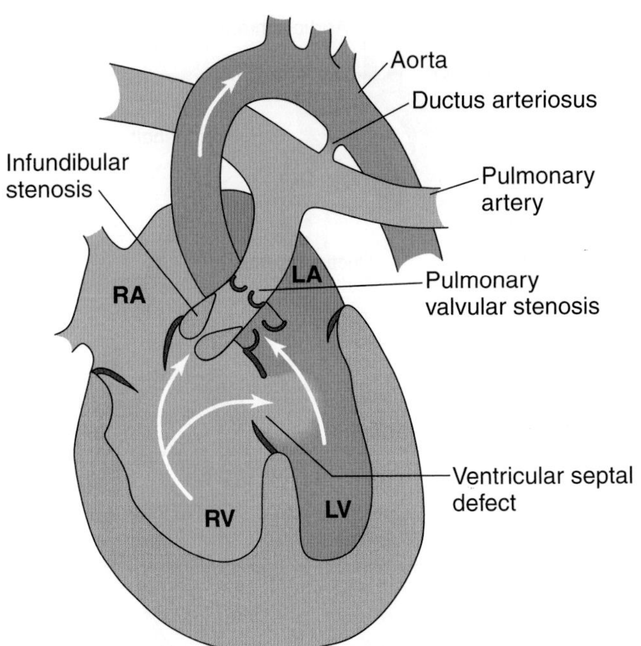

FIGURE 9-5. Tetralogy of Fallot. Note the pulmonary stenosis, which is due to infundibular hypertrophy as well as pulmonary valvular stenosis. The ventricular septal defect involves the membranous septum region. Dextroposition of the aorta and right ventricular hypertrophy are shown. Because of the pulmonary obstruction, the shunt is from right to left, and the patient is cyanotic. LA, left atrium; LV, left ventricle; RA, right atrium; RV, right ventricle.

The heart is hypertrophied and has a characteristic boot shape. Almost half of patients with tetralogy of Fallot have other cardiac anomalies, including ostium secundum atrial septal defects, PDA, left superior vena cava, and endocardial cushion defects. The aortic arch is on the right side in about 25% of cases of tetralogy of Fallot. Patency of the ductus arteriosus is actually protective because it provides a source of blood to the otherwise deprived pulmonary vascular bed.

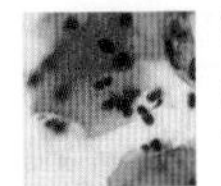

CLINICAL FEATURES: In the face of severe pulmonary stenosis, right ventricular blood is shunted through the ventricular septal defect into the aorta, causing arterial desaturation and cyanosis. Surgical correction is typically done in the first 2 years of life. Otherwise, the affected child complains of dyspnea on exertion and often assumes a squatting position to relieve the shortness of breath. Physical development is characteristically slow. Cerebral thromboses as a result of marked polycythemia may occur. Patients are also at risk for bacterial endocarditis and brain abscesses. Increasing cyanosis and shortness of breath may indicate that a beneficial PDA has closed spontaneously. Left-sided heart failure is not common. Without treatment, the prognosis of tetralogy of Fallot is dismal. However, total correction is possible with surgery, which has less than 10% mortality. After successful surgery, patients become asymptomatic and have excellent long-term prognoses.

Tricuspid Atresia

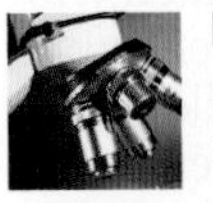

PATHOLOGY: *Tricuspid atresia, a congenital absence of the tricuspid valve, causes obligate right-to-left shunting through the patent foramen ovale.* This defect usually occurs with a VSD through which blood gains access to the pulmonary artery. In the most common type of tricuspid atresia (75% of patients), the great arteries are normal. The condition may also be associated with transpositions of the great arteries.

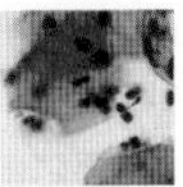

CLINICAL FEATURES: Infants with tricuspid atresia present with cyanosis because of atrial right-to-left shunt. If the VSD is small, the limitation of pulmonary blood flow can result in even worse cyanosis. In that case, a cardiac murmur is prominent. Surgical intervention tries to bypass the atretic tricuspid valve and small right ventricle. Staged surgical palliation is the goal of current therapy.

Congenital Heart Diseases Without Shunting

These defects include transposition of the great arteries, coarctation of the aorta, pulmonary stenosis, and congenital aortic stenosis as well as other uncommon malformations.

Transposition of the Great Arteries

In TGA, the aorta arises from the right ventricle and the pulmonary artery from the left ventricle. TGA has a male predominance and is more common if mothers are diabetic. It causes over half of deaths from cyanotic heart disease in the first year of life.

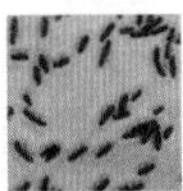

ETIOLOGIC FACTORS: Abnormal development of the spiral septum can produce aberrant positioning of the great arteries, such that the aorta is anterior to the pulmonary artery and connects to the right ventricle. Then, the pulmonary artery receives the left ventricular outflow (Fig. 9-6). Because the venous blood from the right side

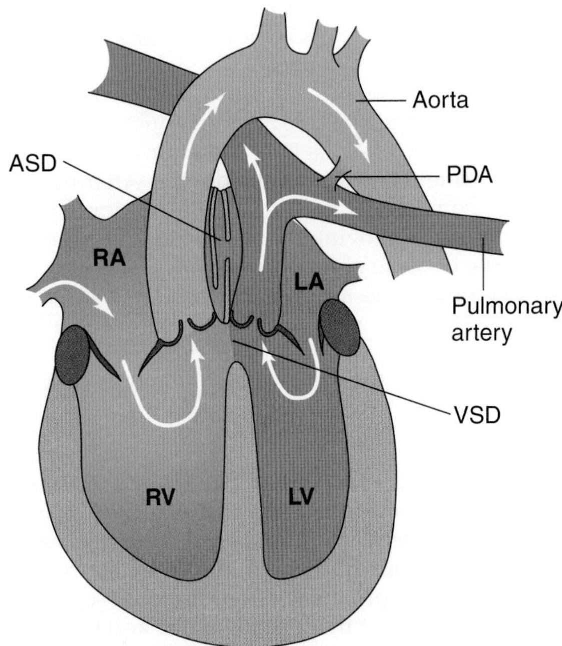

FIGURE 9-6. Complete transposition of great arteries, regular type. The aorta is anterior to, and to the right of, the pulmonary artery ("D-transposition") and arises from the right ventricle. In the absence of interatrial or interventricular connections or patent ductus arteriosus, this anomaly is incompatible with life. The volume and direction of blood flow through intracardiac communications and patent ductus arteriosus, if present, depend on pressure gradients across the communications, which can vary during early stages of extrauterine life. ASD, atrial septal defect; LA, left atrium; LV, left ventricle; PDA, patent ductus arteriosus; RA, right atrium; RV, right ventricle; VSD, ventricular septal defect.

of the heart flows to the aorta and the oxygenated blood from the lungs returns to the pulmonary artery, there are in effect two independent and parallel blood circuits for systemic and pulmonary circulations. Survival requires a communication between the circuits. Virtually, all such infants have an ASD, half have a VSD, and two thirds have a PDA.

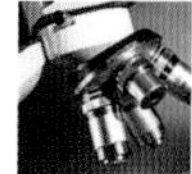

PATHOLOGY: The aorta normally arises posterior to and left of the pulmonary artery and ascends behind and right of it. In TGA, the aorta is anterior and right of the pulmonary artery **("D-transposition" or dextrotransposition)** all the way from its origin.

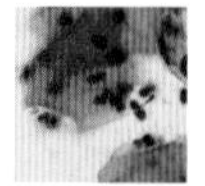

CLINICAL FEATURES: It is possible to correct the malformation within the first 2 weeks of life using an arterial-switch operation, with overall survival of 90%.

Coarctation of the Aorta

Coarctation of the aorta is a local constriction that almost always occurs immediately distal to the origin of the left subclavian artery at the site of the ductus arteriosus. The condition is two to five times more common in males than females and is associated with a bicuspid aortic valve in two thirds of cases. Mitral valve malformations, VSDs and subaortic stenosis, and berry aneurysms in the brain may also be present. Turner syndrome, in particular, is associated with coarctation.

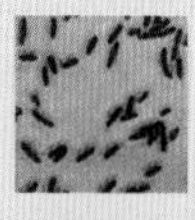

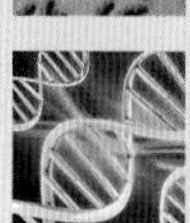

ETIOLOGIC FACTORS AND PATHOGENESIS: The pathogenesis of coarctation of the aorta reflects the pattern of flow in the ductus arteriosus in fetal life (Fig. 9-7). In utero, considerably, more blood flows through the ductus than across the aortic valve. The blood leaving the ductus is diverted into two streams by a posterior aortic shelf opposite the orifice of the ductus. After birth, the ductal orifice is obliterated, and the posterior shelf normally involutes, removing the obstruction. The shelf may not involute because of inadequate antegrade flow in the aortic arch in utero as a result of anomalies that limit left ventricular output (e.g., bicuspid aortic valve) or failure of the obstructing shelf to involute for unknown reasons. In any event, the result is the most common type of coarctation of the aorta, a **juxtaductal constriction.**

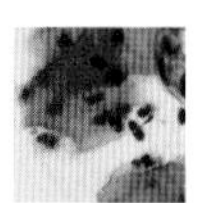

CLINICAL FEATURES: ***The clinical hallmark of coarctation of the aorta is a discrepancy in blood pressure between the upper and lower extremities.*** The pressure gradient produced by the coarctation causes hypertension proximal to the narrowed segment and, occasionally, dilation of that portion of the aorta.

Hypertension in the upper part of the body results in left ventricular hypertrophy and may cause dizziness, headaches, and nosebleeds. Hypotension below the coarctation leads to weakness, pallor, and coldness of the lower extremities. In an attempt to bridge the obstruction between the upper and lower aortic segments, collateral vessels enlarge. Chest radiography shows notching of the inner surfaces of the ribs, caused by increased pressure in markedly dilated intercostal arteries.

Most patients with coarctation of the aorta die by age 40 unless they are treated. Complications include (1) heart failure, (2) rupture of a dissecting aneurysm (secondary to cystic medial necrosis of the aorta), (3) infective endarteritis at the point of narrowing or at the site of jet-stream impingement on the wall immediately distal to the coarctation, (4) cerebral hemorrhage, and (5) stenosis or infective endocarditis of a bicuspid aortic valve. Surgical excision of the narrowed segment, preferably between 1 and 2 years of age for asymptomatic patients, is an effective treatment. Balloon dilation of the narrowed area by cardiac catheterization has also been performed.

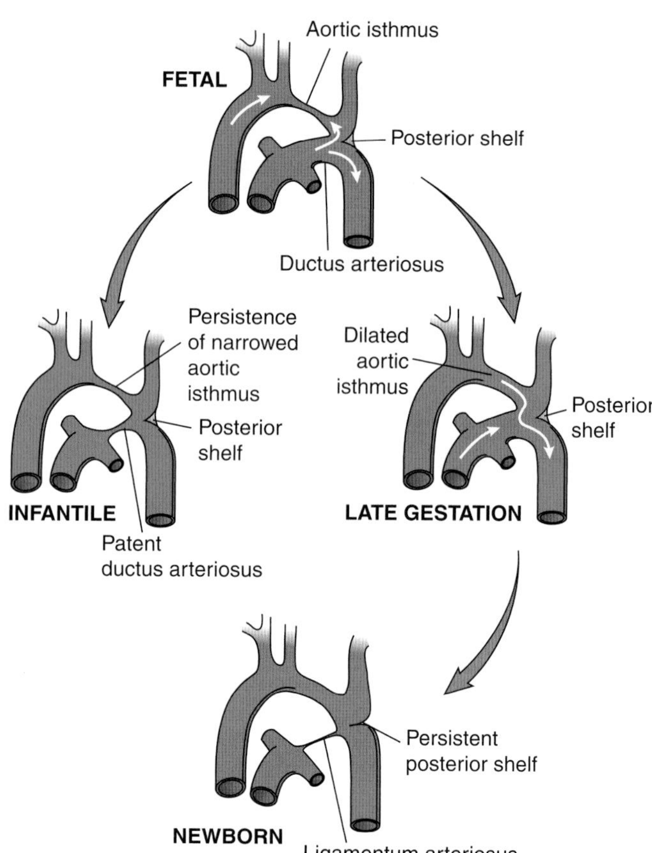

FIGURE 9-7. Pathogenesis of coarctation of the aorta. In the fetus, ductal blood is diverted into cephalad and descending streams by the posterior aortic shelf. In late fetal life, the isthmus dilates, and the increased descending blood flow is accommodated by the ductal orifice. After birth, if the shelf does not undergo the normal involution, obliteration of the ductal orifice does not permit free flow around the persistent posterior shelf, thereby creating a juxtaductal obstruction of blood flow to the distal aorta. If the aortic isthmus does not dilate during late fetal life, it remains narrow, resulting in an infantile or preductal coarctation. In this circumstance, the ductus arteriosus usually remains patent.

Pulmonary Stenosis

Pulmonary stenosis results from (1) developmental deformities from the endocardial cushion region (with involvement of the pulmonary valves), (2) an abnormality of the right ventricular infundibular muscle (subvalvular or infundibular stenosis, especially as part of tetralogy of Fallot), or (3) abnormal development of the more distal parts of the pulmonary artery tree (peripheral pulmonary stenosis). The last is more common in newborns with **Williams syndrome** and is associated with chromosomal microdeletions that include the gene encoding elastin. The syndrome is also associated with infantile hypercalcemia, mental retardation, multiple system disorders, and a distinctive facies, depending on the extent of the microdeletion.

Isolated pulmonary stenosis ordinarily involves the valve cusps, which are fused to form an inverted cone or funnel type of constriction. The artery distal to the valve may develop post-stenotic dilation after several years. In severe cases, infants have right ventricular and atrial hypertrophy. If the foramen ovale is patent, there is a right-to-left shunt, with cyanosis, secondary polycythemia, and clubbing of the fingers. Balloon dilation of the stenotic valve by cardiac catheterization can be effective.

Congenital Aortic Stenosis

Valvular Aortic Stenosis

The most common congenital aortic stenosis, bicuspid valve, arises through abnormal development of the endocardial cushions. A congenitally bicuspid aortic valve is much more frequent (4:1) in males than in females and is associated with other cardiac anomalies (e.g., coarctation of the aorta) in 20% of cases. Typically, two of the three semilunar cusps (the right coronary cusp with one of the adjacent two cusps) are fused.

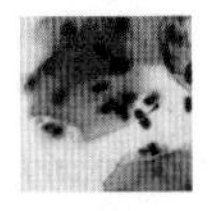

CLINICAL FEATURES: Many children with bicuspid aortic stenosis are asymptomatic. Over the years, the resulting bicuspid valve tends to become thickened and calcified, generally causing symptoms in adulthood. More severe forms of congenital aortic stenosis result in a unicommissural valve or one without any commissures. These malformations cause symptoms in early life, for example, exertional dyspnea and angina pectoris. Sudden death, principally caused by ventricular arrhythmias, is a distinct threat for patients with severe obstruction. Bacterial endocarditis sometimes complicates the condition. Valve replacement may be indicated.

Subvalvular Aortic Stenosis

This defect accounts for 10% of cases of congenital aortic stenosis and is caused by abnormal development of a band of subvalvular fibroelastic tissue or a muscular ridge. Many people with subvalvular aortic stenosis develop thickening and immobility of the aortic cusps, with mild aortic regurgitation. Bacterial endocarditis may also aggravate the regurgitation. Surgical treatment of subvalvular aortic stenosis involves excising the membrane or fibrous ridge.

Supravalvular Aortic Stenosis

This type of stenosis is much less common than the other two, and is often associated with Williams syndrome, as discussed above.

MYOCARDIAL HYPERTROPHY AND HEART FAILURE

Response of the Heart to Injury

In a normal heart, diastolic filling occurs at low atrial pressures. During systole, the ventricles contract vigorously and eject about 60% of the blood (**ejection fraction**). If the heart is injured, the clinical consequences are similar, regardless of the cause of cardiac dysfunction. The heart's ability to adapt to injury is based on the same mechanisms that cause cardiac output to rise in response to stress. ***Compensation reflects the Frank–Starling law: cardiac stroke volume is a function of diastolic fiber length; within certain limits, a normal heart will pump whatever volume the venous circulation brings to it*** (Fig. 9-8). Stroke volume is a measure of ventricular function and increases with greater ventricular end-diastolic volume, because of increased atrial filling pressure. Thus, ventricular output is augmented because the stretch on myocardial fibers increases prior to contraction (as the **preload** increases).

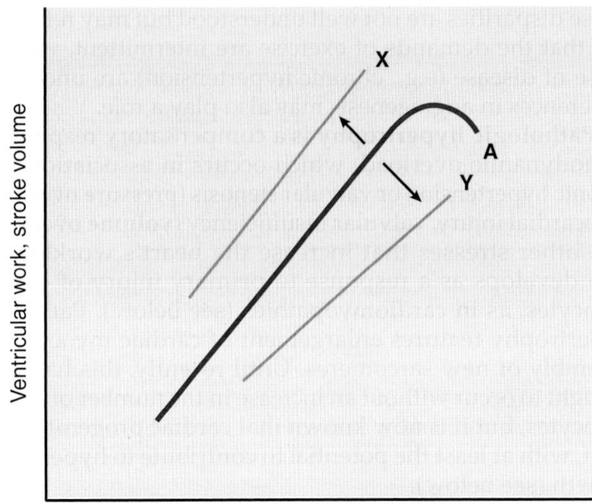

FIGURE 9-8. Relation between the work of the heart (or stroke volume) and the level of venous inflow, as measured by atrial pressure, ventricular end-diastolic volume (EDV), or end-diastolic pressure (EDP). *Curve A* indicates that as ventricular EDV, EDP, or left atrial pressure increases, the amount of work done by the heart increases linearly up to a point. Beyond this point, the work done decreases, and the heart fails. However, the downslope of this curve is reached only at very high left atrial pressures. The curve may shift upward to position *X* or downward to position *Y*, depending on whether contractility has increased (e.g., because of the action of norepinephrine) or decreased (i.e., in failure), respectively. The failing heart usually functions on the ascending limb of a depressed curve.

When there is a sudden need to increase cardiac output in a normal heart, as during exercise, catecholamine stimulation increases both heart rate and contractility. The latter is mainly mediated by modulating the activities of key proteins that regulate Ca^{2+} transients during excitation–contraction coupling. Thus, the normal relationship between end-diastolic volume and stroke volume is shifted upward (from curve A to curve X in Fig. 9-8). End-diastolic volume may also increase, thereby resulting in a large increase in cardiac output.

If a heart is injured, overall cardiac function tends to be depressed in the basal state. Higher-than-normal filling pressures are then required to maintain cardiac output (curve Y in Fig. 9-8). Moreover, in cardiac failure, catecholamine stimulation is often present in the basal state. Comparable increases in cardiac output thus require greater increases in atrial pressure in failing hearts than in normal ones. ***The most prominent feature of heart failure is an abnormally high atrial filling pressure relative to stroke volume.*** However, the absolute values of stroke volume and cardiac output are generally well maintained.

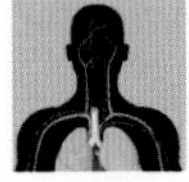

PATHOPHYSIOLOGY: Myocardial hypertrophy is an adaptive response that augments myocyte contractile strength. There is a distinction between **physiologic hypertrophy,** which develops in highly trained athletes, and **pathologic hypertrophy**, which occurs because of disease. While there is considerable overlap in the molecular mechanisms leading to these different forms of hypertrophy, there must also be important differences. The athlete's enlarged heart is highly efficient, whereas a diseased heart of similar mass is structurally and functionally deficient.

These disparities are not well understood but may reflect the fact that the demands of exercise are intermittent, whereas those of disease (e.g., chronic hypertension) are unceasing. Differences in angiogenesis may also play a role.

Pathologic hypertrophy is a compensatory response to hemodynamic overload, which occurs in association with chronic hypertension or valvular stenosis (**pressure overload**), myocardial injury, valvular insufficiency (**volume overload**), and other stresses that increase the heart's workload. It also develops as a response to primary injury of cardiac myocytes, as in cardiomyopathies (see below). Pathologic hypertrophy features enlargement of cardiac myocytes by assembly of new sarcomeres. Until recently, this had been thought to occur without an increase in the number of cardiac myocytes, but it is now known that cardiac progenitor cells exist, with at least the potential to contribute to hyperplastic growth (see below).

Pathologic hypertrophy at first entails compensatory and, possibly, reversible mechanisms, but with persistent stress, the myocardium becomes irreversibly enlarged and dilated.

***When initial impairment is severe, cardiac output is not maintained despite compensatory changes, and the result is acute, life-threatening,* cardiogenic shock.** For a lesser impairment, compensatory mechanisms (see below) maintain cardiac output by increasing diastolic ventricular filling pressure and end-diastolic volume. This effect results in congestive heart failure, which is often tolerated for years.

Pathogenesis of Hypertrophy

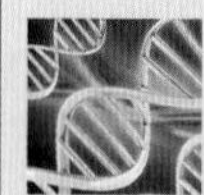

MOLECULAR PATHOGENESIS: *Receptor-mediated myocardial events that are triggered by a stimulus promote the hypertrophic response by autocrine and paracrine mechanisms.* Contractile cells respond to mechanical stimuli, such as stretching or pressure overload, by releasing ligands that activate receptor-mediated signaling pathways to produce hypertrophy (Fig. 9-9). Among the most important ligands are (1) angiotensin II (AngII), (2) endothelin-1 (ET-1), (3) norepinephrine (NE), and (4) various growth factors, including insulin-like growth factor-I (IGF-I) and transforming growth factor-I (TGF-I). Some of these mediators may also act on interstitial fibroblasts in the heart to promote synthesis and deposition of extracellular matrix. Events mediated by β-adrenergic receptors are implicated in the transition from compensatory hypertrophy to heart failure.

Apoptosis of cardiac myocytes may be important in heart failure. Pathologic hypertrophy is generally associated with an increase in cardiac myocyte apoptosis, which may accelerate transition from compensated hypertrophy to heart failure. Diverse signaling pathways in cardiac hypertrophy may exert both proapoptotic and antiapoptotic influences, the final outcome depending on the balance between them.

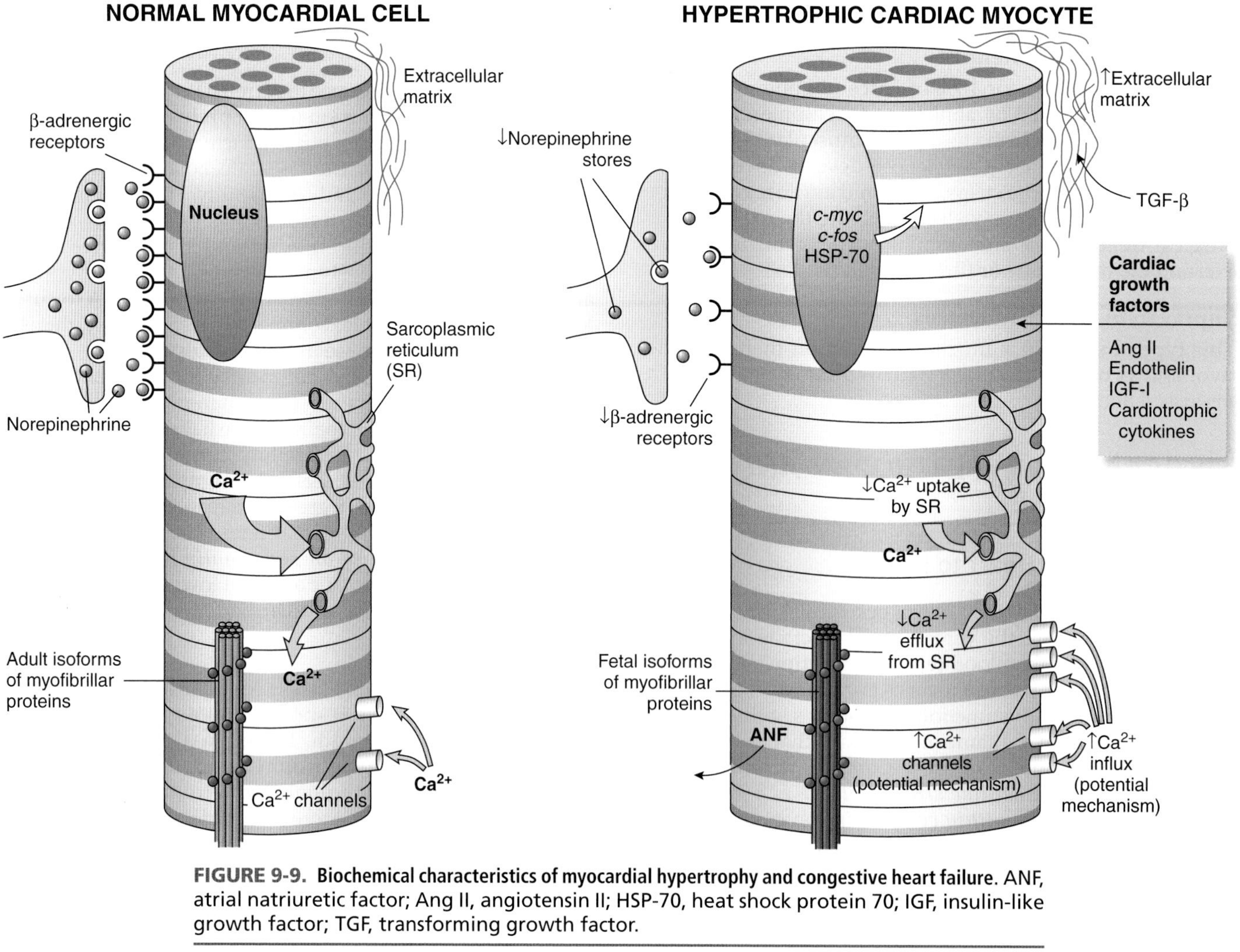

FIGURE 9-9. Biochemical characteristics of myocardial hypertrophy and congestive heart failure. ANF, atrial natriuretic factor; Ang II, angiotensin II; HSP-70, heat shock protein 70; IGF, insulin-like growth factor; TGF, transforming growth factor.

Myocardial Regeneration

The heart has traditionally been thought of as a static organ incapable of growing new myocytes to regenerate or repair damage. However, it is clear that populations of cardiac stem or progenitor cells (CPC) are distributed through the adult heart. Such cells have the ability to self-renew and are multipotent, capable of differentiating into cardiac myocytes, as well as smooth muscle and endothelial cells. Adult human myocytes show an annual rate of turnover of about 1%. Evidence indicates that new cardiac myocytes can arise directly from existing myocytes or in the case of cardiac injury, from activated CPCs. Nevertheless, the heart's regenerative capacity is quite limited and remains controversial. Current research focuses on strategies to exploit and expand this capacity in order to replace damaged or necrotic muscle.

Morphology of Heart Failure

Other than changes characteristic of specific diseases (e.g., ischemic heart disease or cardiac amyloidosis), **the morphology of failing hearts is nonspecific**. *Ventricular hypertrophy is seen in virtually all conditions associated with chronic heart failure.* Initially, only the left ventricle may be hypertrophied, as in compensated hypertensive heart disease. But when the left ventricle fails, some right ventricular hypertrophy usually follows because the increased workload is imposed on the right ventricle by the failing left ventricle. Systolic heart failure is related to abnormal ventricular emptying caused by reduced left ventricular contractility or increased afterload (i.e., hypertension or aortic stenosis). ***In most cases of systolic heart failure, the ventricles are conspicuously dilated.*** The distribution of end-organ involvement depends on whether the heart failure is predominantly left sided or right sided. Diastolic failure associated with defects in diastolic relaxation or ventricular filling is also possible.

Left-sided heart failure is most common because the most frequent causes of cardiac injury (e.g., ischemic heart disease and hypertension) primarily affect the left ventricle. To compensate for left ventricular failure, left atrial and pulmonary venous pressures rise, resulting in passive pulmonary congestion. Pulmonary alveolar capillaries fill with blood, and small ruptures allow erythrocytes to escape. As a result, alveoli contain many hemosiderin-laden macrophages (the so-called heart failure cells). If capillary hydrostatic pressure exceeds plasma osmotic pressure, fluid leaks from capillaries into alveoli. The resultant **pulmonary edema** (see Chapters 8 and 10) may be massive, with alveoli being "drowned" in a transudate. Interstitial pulmonary fibrosis results when congestion is present over an extended period.

Right-sided heart failure most commonly complicates left-sided failure, but it can develop independently as a result of intrinsic lung disease or pulmonary hypertension. The latter creates resistance to blood flow through the lung, causing right atrial pressure and systemic venous pressure to increase. Jugular veins become distended, edema accumulates in the legs, and the liver and spleen become congested. Hepatic congestion in heart failure is characterized by distended central veins, which stand out on the cut surface of the liver as dark red foci against the yellow of the cells in the lobular periphery. This gives the liver a gross appearance that has been compared to the cut surface of a nutmeg (hence "nutmeg liver"; see Chapters 8 and 12).

Diastolic heart failure, often seen in elderly patients, has become an important clinical problem because life expectancy has increased. Ventricles become progressively stiffer with advancing age and require greater filling (diastolic) pressures. Some patients exhibit signs and symptoms of heart failure even though their hearts are normal in size and have normal systolic contractile function. These patients do not tolerate increases in blood volume well and are susceptible to developing pulmonary edema in response to a fluid challenge. Their hearts typically show interstitial fibrosis, which may contribute to the decreased compliance of ventricular myocardium.

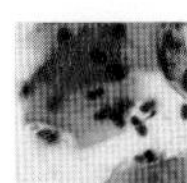

CLINICAL FEATURES: Symptoms of left-sided failure include **dyspnea on exertion** (respiratory distress with exercise), **orthopnea** (dyspnea when lying down), and **paroxysmal nocturnal dyspnea** (dyspnea that awakens patients from sleep). Dyspnea on exertion reflects the increasing pulmonary congestion that accompanies a higher end-diastolic pressure in the left atrium and ventricle. Orthopnea and paroxysmal nocturnal dyspnea result when lung blood volume increases, because of reduced blood volume in the legs during recumbency.

Although much of the clinical presentation of heart failure can be explained by venous congestion **(backward failure),** important aspects involve inadequate perfusion of vital organs **(forward failure)**. Most patients with left-sided heart failure retain sodium and water (edema) because of poor renal perfusion, decreased glomerular filtration rate, and renin-angiotensin–aldosterone system activation. Inadequate cerebral perfusion reflects confusion, memory loss, and disorientation. Reduced perfusion of skeletal muscle reflects fatigue and weakness.

ISCHEMIC HEART DISEASE

Ischemic heart disease is caused by an imbalance between myocardial oxygen requirements and the supply of oxygenated blood (Table 9-2). The heart is an aerobic organ, using oxidative phosphorylation to generate energy for contraction. Anaerobic glycolysis used by skeletal muscle under conditions of extreme physical exertion is insufficient to sustain the heart. Conditions that decrease the supply of blood (notably, atherosclerosis and thrombosis), the level of oxygen in the blood, or conditions that increase oxygen demand and hence cardiac workload all may result in ischemic heart disease.

There is great redundancy built into the supply of oxygen to the heart. Maximal blood flow to the myocardium is not impaired until about 75% of the cross-sectional area of an epicardial coronary artery (~50% of the diameter as assessed during coronary angiography) is compromised by atherosclerosis. Resting blood flow is not reduced until over 90% of the lumen is occluded. In patients with long-standing angina pectoris (transient substernal pain resulting from cardiac ischemia), the extent and distribution of collateral circulation exerts an important influence on the risk of acute myocardial infarction. In some settings (e.g., hypotension or tachycardia), the demand for oxygen and perfusion pressure may be so out of balance that myocardial infarction ensues even when a coronary artery is not sufficiently narrowed to produce ischemia alone.

Conditions Limiting Blood Supply to the Heart

Atherosclerosis and Thrombosis

Coronary arteries are conductance vessels—small muscular arteries with a prominent internal elastic lamina. Their main role is to deliver blood to the cardiac regulatory vasculature (small intramural arteries and arterioles), which controls

Table 9-2

Causes of Ischemic Heart Disease

Decreased Supply of Oxygen
Conditions that influence the supply of blood
Atherosclerosis and thrombosis
Thromboemboli
Coronary artery spasm
Collateral blood vessels
Blood pressure, cardiac output, and heart rate
Miscellaneous: arteritis (e.g., periarteritis nodosa), dissecting aneurysm, luetic aortitis, anomalous origin of coronary artery, muscular bridging of coronary artery
Conditions that influence the availability of oxygen in the blood
Anemia
Shift in the hemoglobin–oxygen dissociation curve
Carbon monoxide
Cyanide
Increased oxygen demand (i.e., increased cardiac work)
Hypertension
Valvular stenosis or insufficiency
Hyperthyroidism
Fever
Thiamine deficiency
Catecholamines

nutritive myocardial blood flow. A healthy person has substantial coronary flow reserve, and myocardial perfusion can increase it to four to eight times above the resting blood flow. In a normal heart, the large coronary arteries provide almost no resistance to blood flow, and myocardial circulation is mainly controlled by constriction and dilation of small, intramyocardial branches less than 400 μm in diameter. In advanced atherosclerosis of the main epicardial coronary arteries, luminal stenosis decreases blood pressure distal to the narrowed zone. To compensate for reduced perfusion pressure, microvessels dilate, thereby maintaining normal resting blood flow. As a result, most patients with coronary atherosclerosis do not have ischemia or angina at rest. However, the capacity of the microcirculation to dilate further is limited, so if myocardial oxygen demand with exercise exceeds the supply, the result is ischemia and angina.

Although myocardial infarction often occurs during physically demanding activities, such as running or shoveling snow, many infarcts occur at rest or even while asleep. Thus, for most people, conversion of clinically silent coronary atherosclerosis to a catastrophic myocardial infarction involves a sudden, marked decrease in myocardial blood flow, with or without increased myocardial oxygen demand. ***Coronary artery thrombosis is the event that usually precipitates acute myocardial infarction. Thrombosis typically results from spontaneous rupture of an atherosclerotic plaque, usually in a region with numerous inflammatory cells and a thin fibrous cap*** (see **Chapter 8**). The initiating event may be hemorrhage into or beneath the plaque.

Thromboemboli

Thromboembolism is a rare cause of myocardial infarction. A coronary embolus often comes from the heart itself, usually valvular vegetations from infective or nonbacterial endocarditis. Coronary emboli sometimes complicate atrial fibrillation and mitral valve disease because mural thrombi in the left atrial appendage detach. Thromboembolic occlusion of a coronary artery is also seen in patients with left ventricular mural thrombi, secondary to infarction, aneurysm, or dilated cardiomyopathy.

Coronary Collateral Circulation

Normal coronary arteries act as end arteries. Most normal hearts have anastomoses that measure 20 to 200 μm in diameter between coronary vessels. Collateral vessels do not function under normal circumstances because there is no pressure gradient between the arteries that they connect. However, a pressure differential resulting from abrupt occlusion of a coronary artery allows blood to flow from the patent artery to the ischemic area via coronary collaterals. As a result, extensive collateral connections develop in the hearts with severe coronary atherosclerosis. These collaterals may actually provide enough arterial flow to prevent infarction or to limit infarct size when a major epicardial coronary artery is suddenly occluded.

Other Conditions That Limit Coronary Blood Flow

- **Coronary arteritis** occurs in various vasculitides, such as polyarteritis nodosa or Kawasaki disease. It may cause luminal narrowing from vessel wall thickening. Local aneurysms may become occluded by thrombus.
- **Dissecting aortic aneurysms** may involve and obstruct coronary arteries. Rarely, medial necrosis and dissecting aneurysms are limited to a coronary artery.
- **Syphilitic aortitis** characteristically affects the ascending aorta, where it may obliterate a coronary artery orifice.
- **Congenital anomalous origin of a coronary artery** refers to the origin of a coronary artery from the pulmonary trunk or passage of an anomalous coronary artery between the aorta and pulmonary artery. It may cause sudden death in young, otherwise healthy individuals.
- **An intramural course of the LAD coronary artery** may result in myocardial ischemia and sudden death. The artery normally runs in the epicardial fat, but in some hearts, it dips into the myocardium for a short distance. The muscular bridge may compress the artery during systole or predisposes to coronary spasm.

Anemia or Carbon Monoxide Poisoning Also Decreases Oxygen Delivery

Anemia is a common cause of decreased myocardial oxygen delivery. Although a heart with normal circulation can survive severe anemia, narrowing of vessels as a result of coronary atherosclerosis may limit the effectiveness of compensatory increases in coronary blood flow and result in cardiac necrosis. Anemia also increases cardiac workload because increased output is required to oxygenate vital organs adequately.

Carbon monoxide (CO) poisoning decreases oxygen delivery to tissues. The high affinity of hemoglobin for CO displaces oxygen, thereby depriving tissues of oxygen. It should be noted that cigarette smoking generates significant levels of carboxyhemoglobin (a measure of CO) in the blood.

Increased Oxygen Demand May Cause Cardiac Ischemia

Any increase in cardiac workload increases the heart's need for oxygen. Conditions that raise blood pressure or cardiac output, such as exercise or pregnancy, increase myocardial oxygen demand, which may lead to angina pectoris or infarction. Disorders in this category include valvular disease (mitral or aortic insufficiency, aortic stenosis), infection, and conditions such as hypertension, coarctation of the aorta, and hypertrophic cardiomyopathy (HCM) (Table 9-2). Hyperthyroid patients have increased metabolic rates and tachycardia, leading to increased oxygen demand and greater cardiac workload. Fever also increases the basal metabolic rate, cardiac output, and heart rate.

Effects of Ischemic Heart Disease

Ischemic heart disease develops when blood flow is inadequate to meet the heart's oxygen needs. It is by far the most common type of cardiac malady in the United States and other industrialized nations, where it is the leading overall cause of death and is responsible for at least 80% of all deaths from heart disease. The principal effects of ischemic heart disease are angina pectoris, myocardial infarction, chronic congestive heart failure, and sudden death.

Angina Pectoris

Angina pectoris refers to the pain of myocardial ischemia. It typically feels like severe crushing or burning in the substernal portion of the chest, which may radiate to the left arm, jaw, or epigastrium. It is the most common symptom of ischemic heart disease. Coronary atherosclerosis tends to become symptomatic only when the luminal cross-sectional area of the affected vessel is reduced by more than 75%. A patient with angina pectoris typically has recurrent episodes of chest pain, usually brought on by physical or emotional stress. The pain is of limited duration (1 to 15 minutes) and is relieved by rest or by treatment with sublingual nitroglycerin (a potent vasodilator).

Although the most common cause of angina pectoris is severe coronary atherosclerosis, decreased coronary blood flow can result from other conditions, including coronary vasospasm (Prinzmetal angina), aortic stenosis, or aortic insufficiency.

Prinzmetal angina (variant angina) ***is an atypical form of angina that occurs at rest and is caused by coronary artery spasm.*** The mechanisms responsible are not fully understood, but endothelial dysfunction plays a major role. Spasm in structurally normal coronary arteries may be part of a systemic syndrome of abnormal arterial vasomotor reactivity, which includes migraine headache and Raynaud phenomenon. Usually, though, it develops in atherosclerotic coronary arteries, often in a portion of a vessel near an atherosclerotic plaque. In this case, coronary artery spasm may contribute to acute myocardial infarction or affect the size of an infarct, although it is generally not the principal cause of infarction.

In **unstable angina,** ***chest pain has a less predictable relationship to exercise than does stable angina; it may occur during rest or sleep and is often associated with nonocclusive thrombi over atherosclerotic plaques.*** In some cases of unstable angina, episodes of chest pain become progressively more frequent and longer over a 3- to 4-day period. Electrocardiographic changes are not characteristic of infarction, and serum levels of cardiac-specific intracellular proteins, such as the MB isoform of CK (MB-CK) or cardiac troponin T or troponin I (evidence of myocardial necrosis), remain normal. Unstable angina is also called **preinfarction angina, accelerated angina,** or **"crescendo" angina.** ***Without pharmacologic or mechanical intervention to treat the coronary narrowing, many such patients progress to myocardial infarction.***

Myocardial Infarction

A myocardial infarct is a discrete focus of ischemic necrosis of muscle in the heart. This definition excludes patchy foci of necrosis caused by drugs, toxins, or viruses. Development of an infarct is related to the duration of ischemia and the metabolic demands of the ischemic tissue. In experimental coronary artery ligation, foci of necrosis form after 20 minutes of ischemia and become more extensive as the period of total ischemia lengthens.

Chronic Congestive Heart Failure

Early mortality following acute myocardial infarction is now less than 5%. Many patients with ischemic heart disease survive longer, in which case over 75% develop chronic congestive heart failure. Contractile impairment in these people is caused by irreversible loss of myocardium (previous infarcts) and hypoperfusion of surviving muscle, which leads to chronic ventricular dysfunction ("hibernating" myocardium). Whereas some of these patients die suddenly, others develop progressive pump failure and succumb to multiorgan failure. Because their coronary artery disease is often so extensive and many have already had coronary artery bypass surgery, the only treatments available for end-stage disease in these patients are heart transplantation or the use of artificial pumps (ventricular assist devices).

Sudden Cardiac Death

In some patients, the first and only clinical manifestation of ischemic heart disease is sudden death caused by spontaneous ventricular tachycardia that degenerates into ventricular fibrillation. Some authorities only consider death to be sudden if it occurs within 1 hour of the onset of symptoms. Others regard death within 24 hours after the onset of symptoms to be sudden or require that sudden death be diagnosed only if it is unexpected. ***In any event, coronary atherosclerosis underlies most cases of cardiac death that occur during the first hour after the onset of symptoms.***

Major Risk Factors for Coronary Artery Disease

The major risk factors predisposing to coronary artery disease are (1) systemic hypertension, (2) elevated blood cholesterol, (3) cigarette smoking, and (4) diabetes mellitus. Any one of these factors significantly increases the risk of myocardial infarction, but a combination of multiple factors augments that risk by over sevenfold (risk factors are discussed in detail in Chapter 8.

Myocardial Infarcts Are Mainly Subendocardial or Transmural

There are important differences between these two types of infarction (Table 9-3).

Table 9-3

Differences Between Subendocardial and Transmural Infarcts

Subendocardial Infarcts	Transmural Infarcts
Multifocal	Unifocal
Patchy	Solid
May be circumferential	In distribution of a specific coronary artery
Coronary thrombosis rare	Coronary thrombosis common
Often result from hypotension or shock	Often cause shock
No epicarditis	Epicarditis common
Do not form aneurysms or lead to ventricular rupture	May result in aneurysm or ventricular rupture

A **subendocardial infarct** affects the inner one third to half of the left ventricle. It may arise within the territory of one of the major epicardial coronary arteries or it may be circumferential, involving subendocardial distributions of multiple coronary arteries. ***Subendocardial infarction generally results from hypoperfusion.*** It may be due to atherosclerosis in one coronary artery or due to diseases that limit myocardial blood flow globally, such as aortic stenosis, hemorrhagic shock, or hypoperfusion during cardiopulmonary bypass. Most subendocardial infarcts are not the consequences of occlusive coronary thrombi, although small particles of platelet–fibrin thrombus may be seen in the epicardial coronary artery that supplies the affected region. Circumferential subendocardial infarction caused by global hypoperfusion of the myocardium does not require that coronary artery stenosis to be present. Because necrosis is limited to the inner layers of the heart, complications that characterize transmural infarcts (e.g., pericarditis and ventricular rupture) do not follow subendocardial infarction.

A **transmural infarct** involves the full left ventricular wall thickness, usually after occlusion of a coronary artery. As a result, transmural infarcts typically conform to the distribution of one of the three major coronary arteries (Fig. 9-2).

- **Right coronary artery:** Occlusion of this vessel's proximal portion results in an infarct of the posterior basal region of the left ventricle and the posterior one third to half of the interventricular septum ("inferior" infarct).
- **LAD coronary artery:** Blockage of the LAD produces an infarct of the apical, anterior, and anteroseptal walls of the left ventricle.
- **Left circumflex coronary artery:** Obstruction of this vessel is the least common cause of myocardial infarction, and leads to infarcts of the lateral left ventricle wall.

Myocardial infarction does not occur instantaneously. Rather, it first develops in the subendocardium and progresses as a wave front of necrosis from subendocardium to subepicardium over several hours. Transient coronary occlusion may precipitate only subendocardial necrosis, but persistent occlusion eventually results in transmural necrosis. The goal of acute coronary interventions (pharmacologic or mechanical thrombolysis) is interruption and limitation of myocardial necrosis. ***The volume of arterial collateral flow is the chief determinant of transmural progression of an infarct.*** In chronic cardiac hypoperfusion, extensive collaterals, which preferentially supply the outer or subepicardial layer, often restrict infarction to the subendocardial myocardium. However, in fatal cases, acute transmural infarcts are more common than those confined to the subendocardium.

Infarcts involve the left ventricle much more often and extensively than the right ventricle. This difference may be partly explained by the greater workload imposed on the left ventricle by systemic vascular resistance and the greater thickness of the left ventricular wall. Right ventricular hypertrophy (e.g., in pulmonary hypertension) increases the incidence of right ventricular infarction. Infarction of the posterior right ventricle occurs in about one third of left ventricular posteroseptal infarcts (right coronary artery territory), but infarcts limited to the right ventricle are rare.

Development of Myocardial Infarcts

The early stages of myocardial infarction have been characterized most thoroughly in experimental animals. Within 10 seconds after ligation of a coronary artery, the affected myocardium becomes cyanotic and, rather than contracting, bulges outward during systole. If the obstruction is promptly relieved, myocardial contractions resume and there is no anatomic damage, although contractility may be depressed in the affected area for many hours **(stunned myocardium)**. This effect reflects the deleterious effects produced by oxygen radicals formed by reperfusion of acutely ischemic myocardium (see below). This reversible stage lasts for 20 to 30 minutes of total ischemia, after which damaged myocytes progressively die.

Acute myocardial infarcts are not grossly identifiable within the first 12 hours. By 24 hours, they are recognized by pallor on cut surfaces of the involved ventricle. After 3 to 5 days, they become mottled and more sharply outlined, with a central pale, yellowish, necrotic region bordered by a hyperemic zone (Fig. 9-10). By 2 to 3 weeks, the infarcted region is depressed and soft, with a refractile, gelatinous appearance. Older, healed infarcts are firm and contracted, comprising pale gray scar tissue (Fig. 9-11).

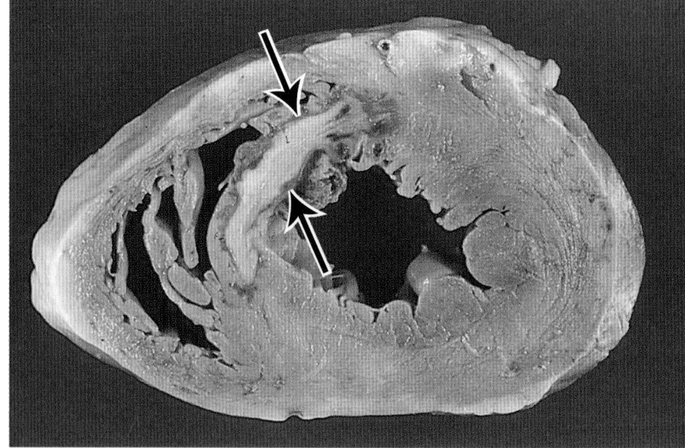

FIGURE 9-10. Acute myocardial infarct. A transverse section of the heart of a patient who died a few days after the onset of severe chest pain shows a transmural **infarct** in the anteroseptal region of the left ventricle (left anterior descending coronary artery territory). The necrotic myocardium is soft, yellowish, and sharply demarcated (*arrows*).

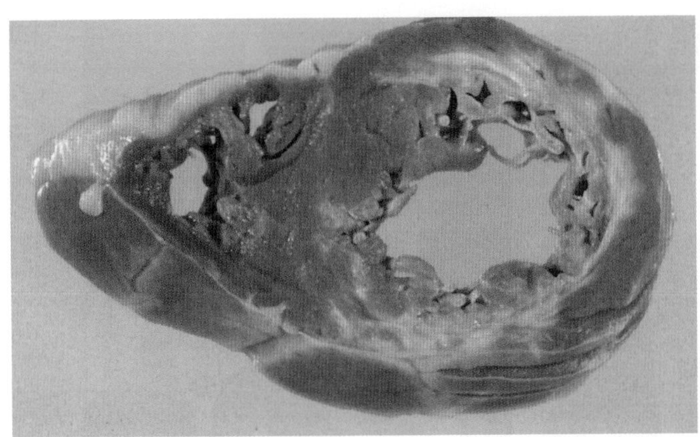

FIGURE 9-11. **Healed myocardial infarct.** A cross section of the heart from a man who died after a long history of angina pectoris and several myocardial infarctions shows near-circumferential scarring of the left ventricle.

Microscopic Characteristics of Myocardial Infarcts

THE FIRST 24 HOURS: Electron microscopy is required to discern the earliest morphologic features of ischemic injury. Reversibly injured myocytes show subtle changes of sarcoplasmic edema, mild mitochondrial swelling, and loss of glycogen (the ultrastructural correlates of stunned myocardium). After 30 to 60 minutes of ischemia, when myocyte injury has become irreversible, mitochondria are greatly swollen with disorganized cristae and amorphous matrix densities made of calcium phosphate salts. The latter are formed by massive Ca^{2+} overload in severely injured cells. Nuclei show clumping and margination of chromatin, and the sarcolemma is focally disrupted.

Loss of sarcolemmal integrity promotes release of intracellular proteins, such as myoglobin, LDH, CK, and troponins I and T. Ion gradients are also dissipated, and tissue potassium decreases as sodium, chloride, and calcium increase.

The noncontractile ischemic myocytes are stretched with each systole and become **"wavy fibers."** By 24 hours, they are deeply eosinophilic by light microscopy (Fig. 9-12) with the characteristic changes of coagulative necrosis (see Chapter 1). However, it takes several days for myocyte nuclei to disappear totally.

2 TO 3 DAYS: Polymorphonuclear leukocytes are attracted to necrotic myocytes, but they gain access only at the edge of the infarct, where blood flow is intact. They accumulate at infarct borders and reach peak concentrations at 2 to 3 days (Figs. 9-12 and 9-13). Interstitial edema and microscopic areas of hemorrhage may also appear. By 2 to 3 days, muscle cells are more clearly necrotic, nuclei disappear, and striations become less prominent. Some of the neutrophils begin to undergo karyorrhexis.

5 TO 7 DAYS: By this time, few, if any, neutrophils remain. The periphery of the infarcted region shows phagocytosis of dead muscle by macrophages. Fibroblasts begin to proliferate, and new collagen is deposited. Lymphocytes and pigment-laden macrophages are prominent. The process of replacing necrotic muscle with scar tissue starts at about 5 days, first at the edge of the infarct, gradually moving inward.

1 TO 3 WEEKS: Collagen deposition proceeds, inflammation gradually recedes, and the newly sprouted capillaries are progressively obliterated.

MORE THAN 4 WEEKS: Considerable dense fibrous tissue is present. The debris is slowly removed, and the scar is more solid and less cellular as it matures (Fig. 9-14).

This sequence of inflammatory and reparative events can be altered by local or systemic factors. For example, immediate extension of an infarct into a region that previously had patchy necrosis may not show expected changes. A large infarct tends not to mature at its center as rapidly as a smaller one. In estimating the age of a large infarct, it is more accurate to base interpretation on the outer border where repair begins, rather than on the central region. In fact, in some large infarcts, dead myocytes are not removed but rather remain indefinitely "mummified."

Reperfusion and Ischemic Myocardium

The above descriptions pertain to healing of infarcts caused by acute coronary occlusion, such as those arising from thrombotic occlusion of an epicardial coronary artery. However, blood flow may be restored to regions of evolving infarcts either because of spontaneous thrombolysis or in response to therapeutic opening of occluded coronary arteries. When that happens, the infarcts gross, and microscopic appearances change. Reperfused infarcts are typically hemorrhagic, from escape of blood through damaged microvasculature. Thus, infarcts after persistent occlusion are only grossly apparent after about 12 hours and are pale, but hemorrhage immediately highlights reperfused infarcts. Reperfusion also accelerates acute inflammation; neutrophils gain access throughout the infarct, rather than only at the periphery. They accumulate more rapidly and then disappear more rapidly. Replacement of necrotic muscle by fibrous scar also occurs more quickly, at least in areas of the infarct in which perfusion persists.

One of the most characteristic features of reperfused infarcts is **contraction band necrosis** featuring thick irregular, transverse eosinophilic bands in necrotic myocytes (Fig. 9-15). They occur whenever there is a massive influx of Ca^{2+} into cardiac myocytes. Reperfusion of ischemic myocardium causes extensive sarcolemmal damage, mediated largely by reactive oxygen species (ROS), which damage the sarcolemma and permit unrestrained entry of extracellular Ca^{2+} into myocytes. Massive Ca^{2+} influx gives rise to hypercontraction in those cells still able to contract. Contraction band necrosis is most prominent when ischemic myocardium is reperfused (e.g., after thrombolytic therapy or with prolonged cardiopulmonary bypass, during which the myocardium has sustained irreversible injury). In infarcts arising from coronary occlusion, microscopic foci of contraction band necrosis are often seen at the margins, where dynamic ebb and flow of blood create conditions that favor Ca^{2+} influx.

Complications of Myocardial Infarction

Early mortality in acute myocardial infarction (within 30 days) has dropped from 30% in the 1950s to less than 5% today. Nevertheless, the clinical course after acute infarction may be dominated by functional or mechanical complications of the infarct. These include arrhythmias, the possibility of left ventricular failure and cardiogenic shock, extension of the infarct, and rupture of the myocardium.

ARRHYTHMIAS: Virtually, all patients who have a myocardial infarct have abnormal cardiac rhythm at some time during their illness. Arrhythmias still account for half of deaths caused by ischemic heart disease, but the advent of coronary

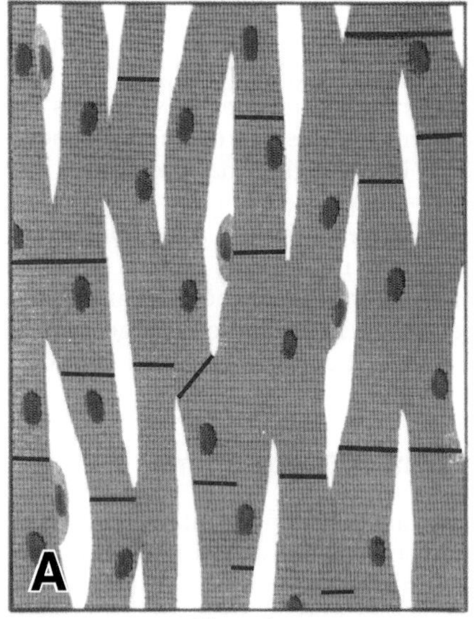

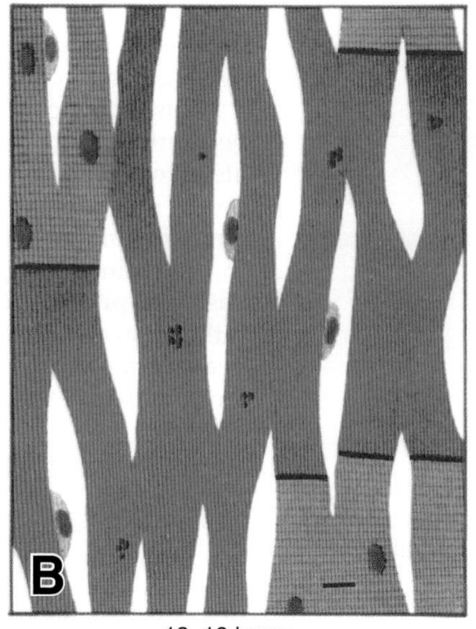

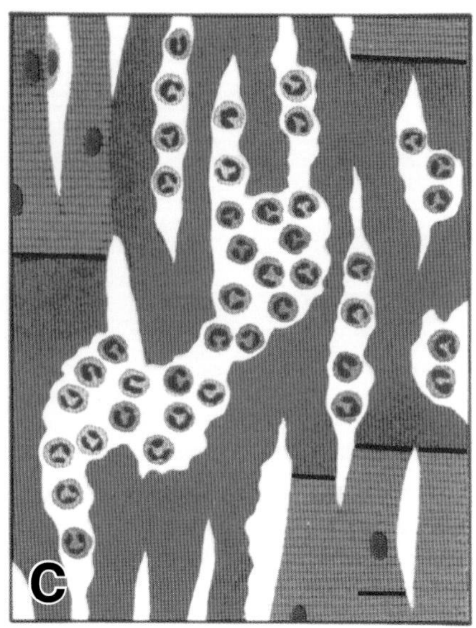

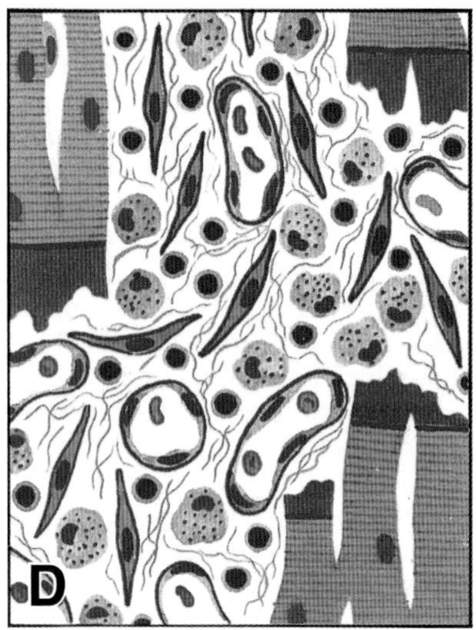

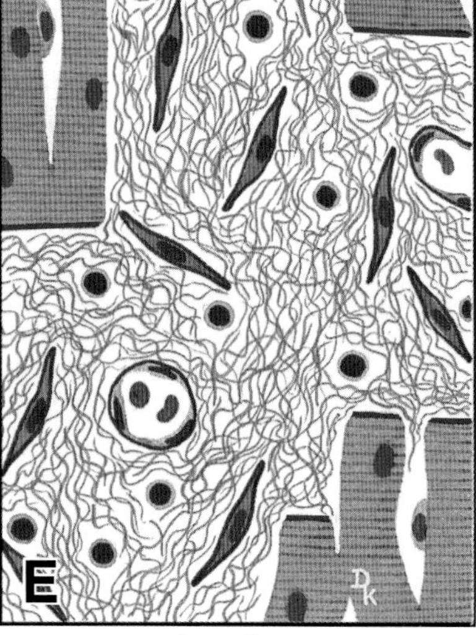

FIGURE 9-12. Development of a myocardial infarct. A. Normal myocardium. **B.** After about 12 to 18 hours, the infarcted myocardium shows eosinophilia (*red staining*) in sections of the heart stained with hematoxylin and eosin. **C.** About 24 hours after the onset of infarction, polymorphonuclear neutrophils infiltrate necrotic myocytes at the periphery of the infarct. **D.** After about 3 weeks, peripheral portions of the infarct are composed of granulation tissue with prominent capillaries, fibroblasts, lymphoid cells, and macrophages. The necrotic debris has been largely removed from this area, and a small amount of collagen has been laid down. **E.** After 3 months or more, the infarcted region has been replaced by scar tissue.

care units and defibrillators has greatly reduced early mortality. Acute infarction is often associated with paroxysmal atrial tachycardia, premature ventricular beats, sinus bradycardia, ventricular tachycardia, and sometimes ventricular fibrillation. Partial or complete heart block can also occur. The causes of these arrhythmias are often multifactorial. Acute ischemia alters conduction, increases automaticity, and promotes triggered activity related to after-depolarizations. Enhanced sympathetic activity, mediated by increased levels of local or circulating catecholamine, plays an important role.

LEFT VENTRICULAR FAILURE AND CARDIOGENIC SHOCK: Development of left ventricular failure soon after myocardial infarction is an ominous sign that generally indicates massive loss of muscle. Fortunately, cardiogenic shock occurs in fewer than 5% of cases because of the development of techniques that limit the extent of infarction (thrombolytic therapy and angioplasty) or assist damaged myocardium (intra-aortic balloon pump). Cardiogenic shock tends to develop early after infarction when 40% or more of the left ventricle has been lost; mortality is as high as 90%.

EXTENSION OF THE INFARCT: Clinically recognizable extension of an acute infarct occurs in the first 1 to 2 weeks in up to 10% of patients. In careful echocardiographic studies, half of all patients with anterior myocardial infarction showed some infarct extension during the first 2 weeks, indicating that many episodes of infarct extension are not recognized. Clinically significant infarct extension is associated with a doubling of mortality.

RUPTURE OF THE FREE WALL OF THE MYOCARDIUM: Myocardial rupture (Fig. 9-16) may occur at almost any time in the 3 weeks after acute infarction but is most common between days 1 and 4, when the infarcted wall is weakest. During this vulnerable period, the infarct is composed of soft, necrotic tissue in which the extracellular matrix has been degraded by proteases released by inflammatory cells, but new matrix deposition has not yet occurred. Once scars begin to form, rupture is less likely. Rupture of the free wall is a complication of transmural infarcts; surviving muscle overlying subendocardial infarcts prevents rupture. Interestingly, rupture usually occurs in relatively small transmural infarcts. The remaining

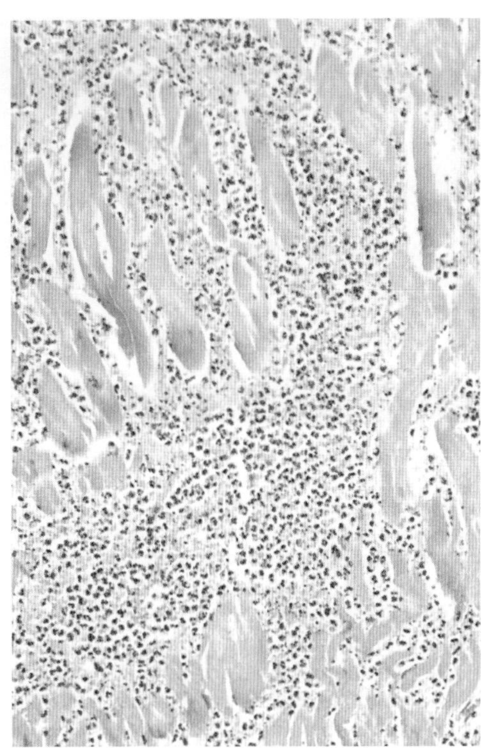

FIGURE 9-13. **Acute myocardial infarct.** The necrotic myocardial fibers, which are eosinophilic and devoid of cross-striations and nuclei, are immersed in a sea of acute inflammatory cells.

viable, contractile myocardium produces mechanical forces that may initiate and propagate tearing along the infarct's edge, where neutrophils accumulate.

Rupture of the left ventricular free wall usually results in hemopericardium and death from pericardial tamponade. Myocardial rupture accounts for 10% of deaths after acute myocardial infarction among hospitalized patients. It is more common in elderly people having a first infarct (most often women). Rarely, a ruptured ventricle may become walled off, and the patient survives with a false aneurysm.

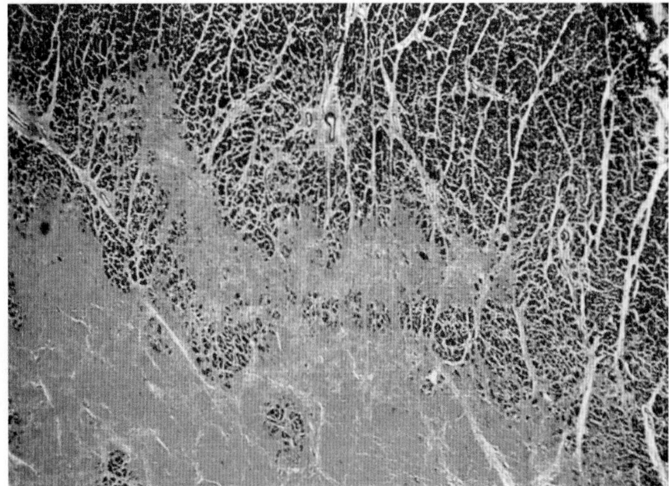

FIGURE 9-14. **Healed myocardial infarct.** A section at the edge of a healed infarct stained for collagen, which appears blue-green here, shows dense, acellular regions of collagenous matrix sharply demarcated from the adjacent viable myocardium.

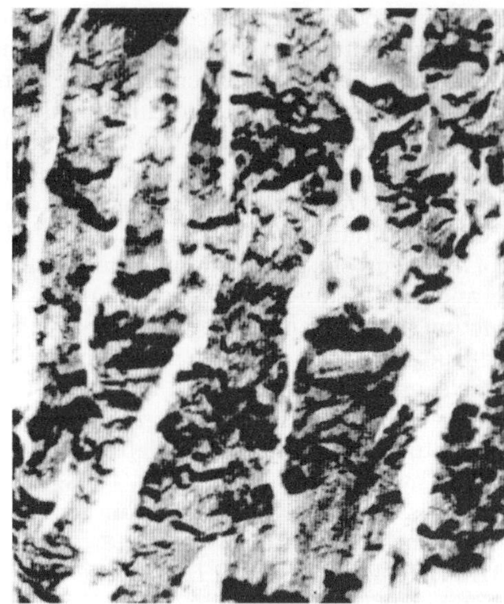

FIGURE 9-15. **Contraction band necrosis.** A section of infarcted myocardium shows prominent, thick, wavy, transverse bands in myofibers.

OTHER FORMS OF MYOCARDIAL RUPTURE: In a few patients, myocardial infarct involves the interventricular septum, which gives rise to **septal perforations**. The magnitude of the resulting left-to-right shunt and, therefore, the prognosis depend on the size of the rupture.

Rupture of a portion of a papillary muscle creates mitral regurgitation. In some cases, an entire papillary muscle is transected, in which case massive mitral valve incompetence may be fatal.

ANEURYSMS: Left ventricular aneurysms complicate 10% to 15% of transmural myocardial infarcts. The affected ventricular wall tends to bulge outward during systole in one third of such patients. As the infarct heals, the newly deposited collagenous matrix is susceptible to further stretching, although eventually, the scar tissue becomes nondistensible. Localized thinning and stretching of the ventricular wall in the region of a healing infarct is called "infarct expansion," but is actually an early aneurysm. Such an aneurysm is composed of a thin

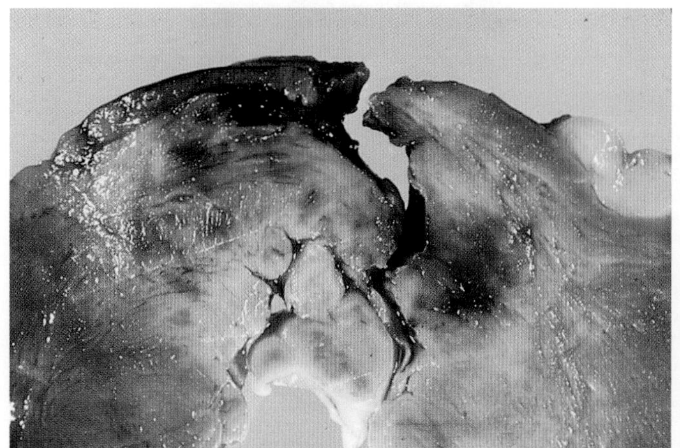

FIGURE 9-16. **Rupture of an acute myocardial infarct.** An elderly woman with a recent myocardial infarct died of cardiac tamponade. The pericardium was filled with blood, and the cut surface of the left ventricle shows a linear rupture of the necrotic myocardium.

layer of necrotic myocardium and collagenous tissue, which expands with each contraction of the heart. As evolving aneurysms become more fibrotic, their tensile strength increases. However, the aneurysms continue to dilate with each beat, thereby "stealing" some left ventricular output and increasing the workload of the heart. Patients with left ventricular aneurysms are at increased risk for ventricular tachycardia because of increased opportunities for electrical current reentry at the periphery of the aneurysm. Mural thrombi often develop within aneurysms and can be sources of systemic emboli.

A distinction should be made between "**true**" and "**false**" **aneurysms**. True aneurysms are much more common than false ones, and are caused by bulging of an intact, but weakened, left ventricular wall (Fig. 9-17). By contrast, false aneurysms result from rupture of a portion of the left ventricle that has been walled off by pericardial scar tissue. Thus, the wall of a false aneurysm is composed of pericardium and scar tissue, not left ventricular myocardium.

MURAL THROMBOSIS AND EMBOLISM: At autopsy, one third to one half of patients who die after myocardial infarction have mural thrombi overlying the infarct (Fig. 9-18). This occurs particularly often when the infarct involves the apex of the heart. In turn, half of these patients have some evidence of systemic embolization. Inflammation of the endocardium lining an infarct promotes platelet adhesion and fibrin deposition. Also, poor contractile function of the underlying myocardium allows fibrin–platelet mural thrombi to grow. Pieces of thrombus can detach and be swept away with the arterial blood, potentially causing strokes or myocardial or visceral infarcts. Documented mural thrombosis justifies anticoagulant and antiplatelet therapy.

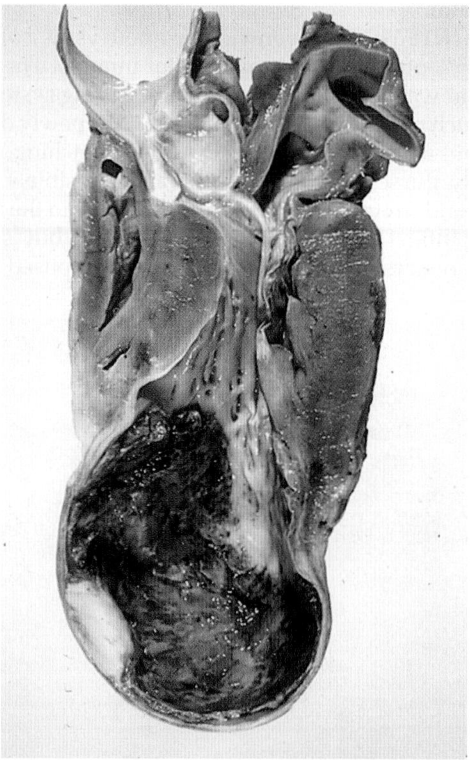

FIGURE 9-17. Ventricular aneurysm. The heart of a patient with a history of an anteroapical myocardial infarct who developed a massive ventricular aneurysm. The apex of the heart shows marked thinning and aneurysmal dilation.

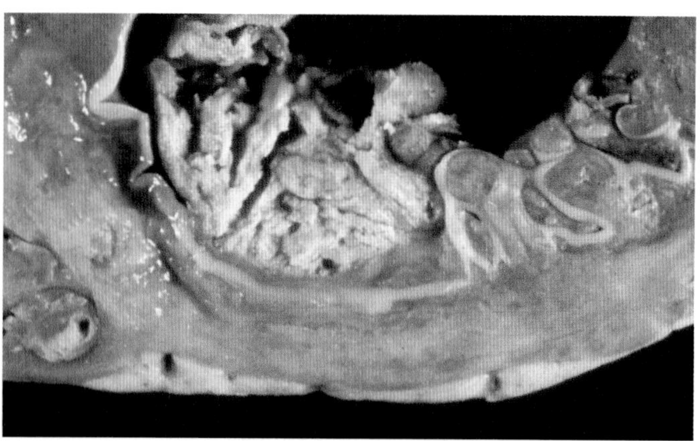

FIGURE 9-18. Mural thrombus overlying a healed myocardial infarct. In this cross section of a fixed heart, an organized, friable, grayish-white mural thrombus overlies a thickened endocardium situated over scarred myocardium.

PERICARDITIS: A transmural myocardial infarct involves the epicardium and leads to inflammation of the pericardium in 10% to 20% of patients. Pericarditis manifests clinically as chest pain and may produce a pericardial friction rub. One quarter of patients with acute myocardial infarction, particularly those with larger infarcts and congestive heart failure, develop pericardial effusions, with or without pericarditis. Less often, anticoagulant therapy may bring on hemorrhagic pericardial effusions and even cardiac tamponade.

Postmyocardial infarction syndrome (Dressler syndrome) is a delayed form of pericarditis that develops 2 to 10 weeks after infarction. A similar disorder may occur after cardiac surgery. Patients develop antibodies to heart muscle and improve with corticosteroid therapy, suggesting that the syndrome has an immunologic basis.

Therapeutic Interventions

Because the amount of myocardium that undergoes necrosis is an important predictor of morbidity and mortality, any therapy that limits infarct size should be beneficial. By definition, such treatment is directed at preventing reversibly injured, ischemic myocytes from dying and limiting infarct extension. Damaged myocytes can be salvaged for some time after the onset of ischemia if arterial blood flow resumes.

- **Restoration of arterial blood flow** is the only way to salvage ischemic myocytes permanently, although other interventions can slow ischemic injury. The most notable is hypothermia, which is used to minimize myocardial damage during cardiopulmonary bypass. Several methods have been developed to restore blood flow to myocardium damaged by an obstructed coronary artery.
- **Thrombolytic enzymes**, such as tissue plasminogen activator or streptokinase, can be infused intravenously to dissolve a clot causing vascular obstruction.
- **Percutaneous coronary intervention (PCI)** is dilation of a narrowed coronary artery by inflation with a balloon catheter. PCI can be applied as a primary procedure immediately after the onset of ischemia or as a rescue procedure if thrombolytic agents fail to restore arterial blood flow. It nearly always includes placement of a drug-eluting stent in the coronary artery to maintain its patency. Such stents provide for the slow release of drugs such as everolimus,

an inhibitor of the mTOR (mammalian target of rapamycin) pathway (see Chapters 1 and 4). This drug limits subsequent restenosis by blocking smooth muscle cell proliferative responses to local injury caused by inflation of the balloon catheter and deployment of the stent.

- **Coronary artery bypass grafting** can restore blood flow to the coronary artery segment beyond a proximal occlusion.

Procedures that restore blood flow must be performed as quickly as possible, preferably within the first few hours after symptoms begin. Beyond 12 hours, it is unlikely that much salvageable ischemic myocardium remains, although reperfusion at this point may aid infarct healing and limit maladaptive postinfarct remodeling.

Chronic Ischemic Heart Disease Can Lead to Cardiomyopathy

In a minority of patients with severe coronary atherosclerosis, myocardial contractility is impaired globally without discrete infarcts, similar to dilated cardiomyopathy (see below). This situation usually reflects a combination of ischemic myocardial dysfunction, diffuse fibrosis, and multiple small healed infarcts. However, there is a group of patients with left ventricular failure in whom cardiac dysfunction occurs without obvious infarction. These patients are said to have **ischemic cardiomyopathy**. In some, the dysfunctional myocardium has experienced repetitive episodes of ischemic injury, which causes degenerative changes in myocytes, including loss of myofibrils (hibernating myocardium). Contractile function of hibernating myocardium is restored when affected tissue is revascularized. Thus, to the extent that hibernation plays a role in ischemic cardiomyopathy, surgical revascularization may be beneficial.

HYPERTENSIVE HEART DISEASE

The World Health Organization defines hypertension as a persistent increase in systemic blood pressure above 140 mm Hg systolic or 90 mm Hg diastolic or both and is associated with damage to multiple body systems (discussed in Chapter 8). ***Chronic hypertension is one of the most prevalent and serious causes of coronary artery and myocardial disease in the United States.*** Pressure overload results first in compensatory left ventricular hypertrophy and, eventually, cardiac failure. The term **hypertensive heart disease** is used when the heart is enlarged in the absence of a cause other than hypertension.

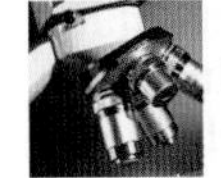

PATHOLOGY: The increased workload caused by hypertension gives rise to compensatory left ventricular hypertrophy. The left ventricular free walls and interventricular septum become thickened uniformly and concentrically (Fig. 9-19); heart weight increases, exceeding 375 g in men and 350 g in women. Hypertrophic myocardial cells are thicker, with enlarged, hyperchromatic, and rectangular ("boxcar") nuclei (Fig. 9-20).

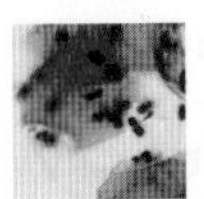

CLINICAL FEATURES: Myocardial hypertrophy clearly stimulates the heart to handle increased workload. However, there is a limit beyond which additional hypertrophy no longer compensates. This upper limit to useful hypertrophy may reflect increasing diffusion distance between the interstitial microvasculature and the center of each myofiber; if that distance is too great, oxygen supply to the myofiber will be impaired.

Diastolic dysfunction is the most common functional abnormality caused by hypertension and by itself can lead to congestive heart failure. Hypertrophy gives rise to some interstitial fibrosis, which makes the left ventricle stiffer. Hypertension is also associated with more severe coronary artery atherosclerosis. ***The combination of greater cardiac workload (systolic dysfunction), diastolic dysfunction, and narrowed coronary arteries leads to greater risk of myocardial ischemia, infarction, and heart failure.***

Congestive heart failure is the major cause of death in patients with untreated hypertension. Fatal intracerebral hemorrhage is also common. Death may occasionally result from coronary atherosclerosis and myocardial infarction, dissecting aortic aneurysm, or ruptured cerebral berry aneurysm. Renal failure supervenes when nephrosclerosis induced by hypertension becomes severe.

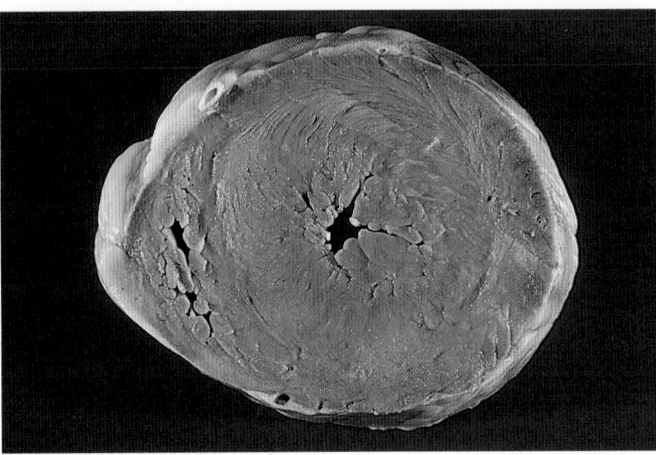

FIGURE 9-19. Hypertensive heart disease. A transverse section of the heart shows marked hypertrophy of the left ventricular myocardium without dilation of the chamber. The right ventricle is of normal dimensions.

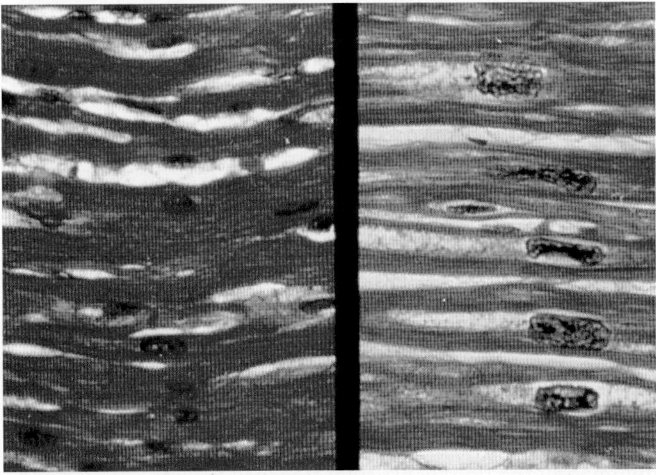

FIGURE 9-20. Hypertensive heart disease with myocardial hypertrophy. *Left.* Normal myocardium. *Right.* Hypertrophic myocardium (same magnification) showing thicker fibers and enlarged, hyperchromatic, rectangular nuclei.

COR PULMONALE

Cor pulmonale refers to right ventricular hypertrophy and dilation as a result of pulmonary hypertension. Increased pulmonary arterial pressure may reflect a disorder of lung parenchyma or, more rarely, a primary vascular disease (e.g., primary pulmonary hypertension and recurrent small pulmonary emboli). **Acute cor pulmonale** is most commonly caused by sudden, massive pulmonary embolization most commonly from deep venous thrombosis of the lower extremities. This condition precipitates acute right-sided heart failure and is a medical emergency. At autopsy, the only cardiac findings are severe right ventricular, and sometimes right atrial, dilation.

Chronic cor pulmonale is a common heart disease, accounting for 10% to 30% of heart failure in the United States, particularly right-sided failure. ***The most common causes of chronic cor pulmonale are chronic obstructive pulmonary disease and pulmonary fibrosis.*** Severe kyphoscoliosis may deform the chest wall and impede its function as a bellows, leading to hypoxemia and pulmonary vasoconstriction. Some congenital heart diseases associated with increased pulmonary blood flow (see above) are complicated by pulmonary hypertension and cor pulmonale.

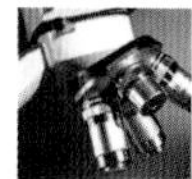

PATHOLOGY: Chronic cor pulmonale is characterized by conspicuous right ventricular hypertrophy (Fig. 9-21), which may exceed 1.0 cm in thickness (normal, 0.3 to 0.5 cm). Right ventricular and right atrial dilatations are often present. Normally, the interventricular septum is concave to the left (i.e., it is part of the left ventricle). When right ventricular hypertrophy is severe, the interventricular septum remodels by straightening or even becoming concave to the right.

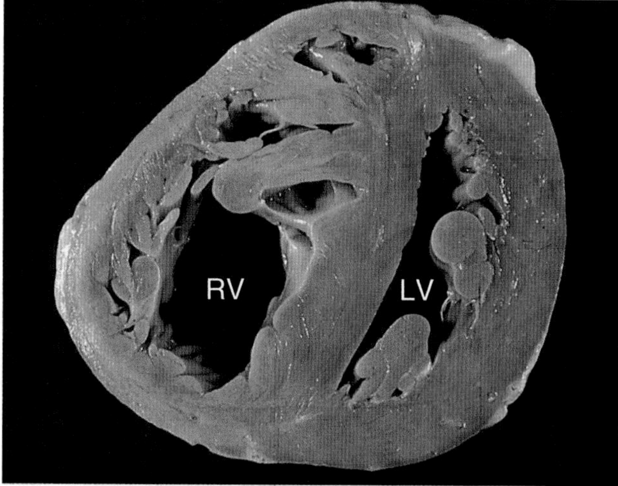

FIGURE 9-21. Cor pulmonale. A transverse section of the heart from a patient with primary (idiopathic) pulmonary hypertension shows a markedly hypertrophied right ventricle (on the left in this image). The right ventricular free wall has a thickness nearly equal to the left ventricular wall. The right ventricle is dilated. The straightened interventricular septum has lost its normal curvature toward the left ventricle as part of the remodeling process in cor pulmonale.

ACQUIRED VALVULAR AND ENDOCARDIAL DISEASES

Genetic, inflammatory, infectious, and degenerative diseases damage heart valves and impair their function. These disorders include rheumatic fever, systemic lupus erythematosus, scleroderma, polyarteritis nodosa, and bacterial endocarditis. Valvular conditions may also be the result of calcium deposits on the valves themselves.

Valve Description

Blood enters the ventricles across atrioventricular valves, the mitral valve on the left and the tricuspid valve on the right. These valve leaflets are held in place by chordae tendineae, strong fibrous cords attached to the inner surface of the ventricular wall via papillary muscles. The entrances to the aorta and pulmonary arteries through which blood leaves the heart, are guarded from regurgitation, respectively, by the aortic and pulmonary valves, each with three semilunar cusps.

The semilunar valves are structurally and functionally simple compared to atrioventricular valves. The latter consist of the valve leaflets, muscular valve annuli, and subvalvular apparatus (chordae tendineae and papillary muscles). In general, valvular stenosis involves pathologic changes of leaflets themselves, whereas regurgitation can be caused not only by abnormalities of valve leaflets but also by those of the annulus or subvalvular apparatus.

Effect of Valve Defects on the Heart

Stenosis (narrowing) of a cardiac valve features thickened or fused valve leaflets that obstruct flow and lead to **pressure overload** hypertrophy of the myocardium proximal (i.e., upstream, in terms of blood flow) to the obstruction. **Regurgitation or insufficiency** of the atrioventricular valves allows retrograde blood flow into the atria during systole, and aortic valve insufficiency permits return of blood from the aorta into the left ventricle.

Once compensatory mechanisms are exhausted, dilation and failure of the chamber proximal to the valve eventually occur. Thus, mitral stenosis results in left atrial hypertrophy and dilation. Because the left atrium decompensates and can no longer propel the pulmonary venous return through the stenotic mitral valve, blood backs up into the pulmonary venous circuit, and signs of pulmonary congestion develop. These effects are followed by right ventricular hypertrophy and even to cor pulmonale. Similarly, aortic stenosis provokes left ventricular hypertrophy and, eventually, left heart failure.

Valvular regurgitation or insufficiency also results in hypertrophy and dilation of the chamber proximal to the valve because of **volume overload**. In aortic insufficiency, the left ventricle first hypertrophies; when it can no longer accommodate the regurgitant volume and maintain adequate cardiac output, it dilates. An incompetent mitral valve elicits hypertrophy and dilation of both the left atrium and left ventricle because both experience volume overload.

Pronounced left ventricular dilation from any cause that limits cardiac contractility (e.g., congestive failure after a large myocardial infarct) may also widen the mitral valve ring and splay the left ventricular papillary muscles. These effects may be so severe that the valve leaflets do not close properly, leading to mitral regurgitation.

Mitral Valve Prolapse

MVP refers to enlargement and redundance of mitral valve leaflets. Chordae tendineae are thinned and elongated so that the leaflets billow and prolapse into the left atrium during systole (Fig. 9-22A). Also called "floppy mitral valve syndrome," MVP is the most common cause of mitral regurgitation that requires surgical valve repair or replacement. Up to 5% of adults may show echocardiographic evidence of MVP, although most will not have severe enough regurgitation to require surgery.

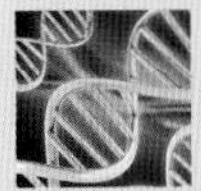

MOLECULAR PATHOGENESIS: Cases of MVP may be sporadic or appear in familial clusters. It may be transmitted as an autosomal dominant trait, with no specific gene mutations having been identified. MVP may also appear as a component of a syndrome and is particularly prevalent in patients with Marfan syndrome, Ehlers–Danlos syndrome, osteogenesis imperfecta, and other collagen-related disorders.

Prolapsed mitral valves accumulate striking amounts of myxomatous connective tissue in the center of the valve leaflet (Fig. 9-22B). Proteoglycans in the valve are increased, and electron microscopy shows fragmentation of collagen fibrils. Presumably, these changes reflect a molecular defect in the extracellular matrix that allows leaflets and chordae to enlarge and stretch under the high-pressure conditions they experience during the cardiac cycle.

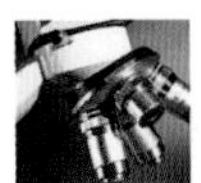

PATHOLOGY: Mitral valve leaflets are redundant and deformed (Fig. 9-22A). On cross section, they have a gelatinous appearance and slippery texture because of the accumulation of acid mucopolysaccharides (proteoglycans). Myxomatous degeneration also affects the annulus and chordae tendineae, increasing the frequency of prolapse and regurgitation. Damage to chordae may be so severe that they rupture and yield a flail mitral valve that is totally incompetent. Although the mitral valve is usually the only valve affected, myxomatous degeneration can occur in other valves, especially in patients with Marfan syndrome, 90% of whom have clinical evidence of MVP.

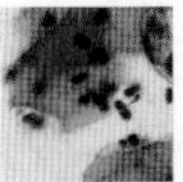

CLINICAL FEATURES: The risk of sudden death in patients with MVP, presumably as a result of ventricular tachyarrhythmias, is twice that in the general population. However, most patients with MVP are asymptomatic. Clinical recognition of MVP is based on classic auscultatory findings: a mid-to-late systolic click, caused by the snap of the redundant leaflets as they prolapse into the left atrium. Endocarditis, both infective and nonbacterial, may develop as a serious complication, and cerebral emboli are common. Significant mitral regurgitation develops in 15% of patients after 10 to 15 years of MVP, after which mitral valve repair or replacement is indicated.

Calcific Aortic Stenosis

Calcific aortic stenosis is narrowing of the aortic valve orifice caused by calcium deposition in the valve cusps and ring.

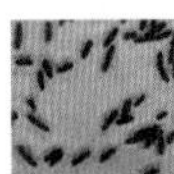

ETIOLOGIC FACTORS AND PATHOLOGY: Calcific aortic stenosis has three main causes.

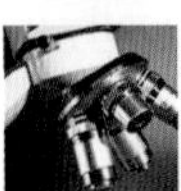

- **Rheumatic aortic valve disease** has become uncommon in the United States with the decline in acute rheumatic fever. Hence, calcific aortic stenosis is usually attributed to other causes. Details of the effects of acute and chronic rheumatic fever on the heart are discussed in detail below.
- **Degenerative (senile) calcific stenosis** develops in the elderly as a degenerative process in a tricuspid aortic valve. Valve cusps become rigidly calcified, but commissural fusion (Fig. 9-23), which is a hallmark of rheumatic aortic valves, is not seen. The mitral valve is usually normal in patients with senile calcific aortic stenosis, although the mitral annulus may also be calcified.
- **Calcific aortic stenosis** in both congenitally malformed bicuspid valves and normal ones is probably related to cumulative effects of years of turbulent blood flow around the valve. Thus, although a bicuspid valve is not inherently

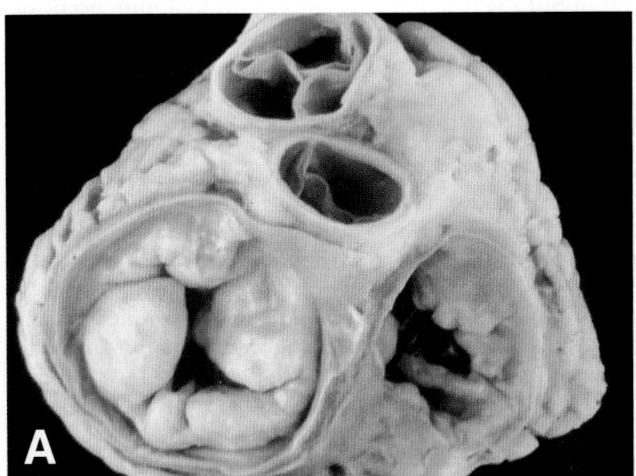

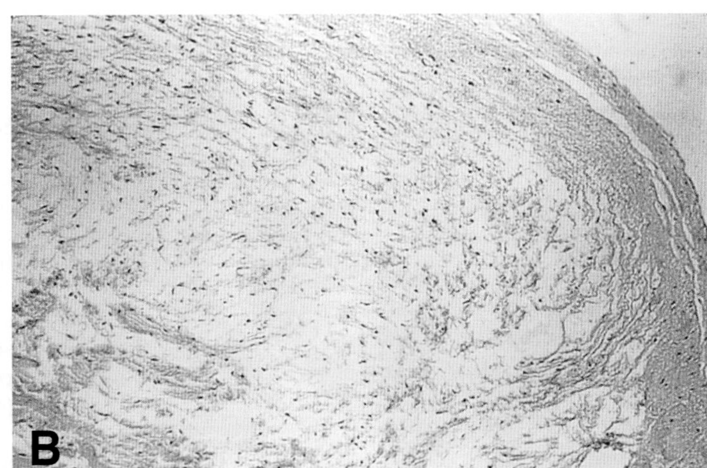

FIGURE 9-22. Mitral valve prolapse. A. A view of the mitral valve (*left*) from the left atrium showing redundant and deformed leaflets, which billow into the left atrial cavity. **B.** A microscopic section of one of the mitral valve leaflets revealing conspicuous myxomatous connective tissue in the center of the leaflet.

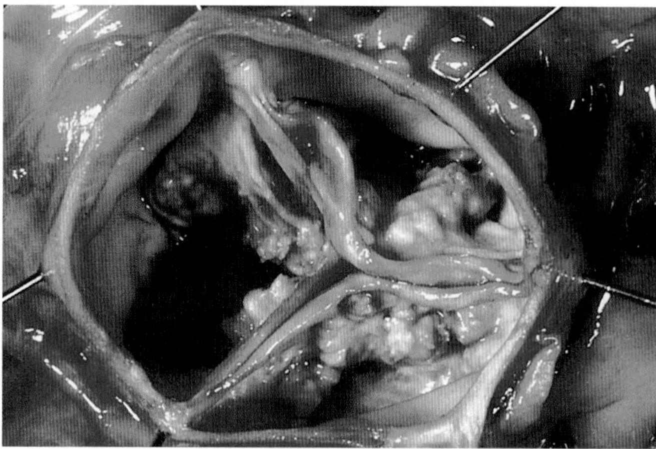

FIGURE 9-23. Calcific aortic stenosis in a three-cuspid aortic valve in an elderly person. The leaflets are heavily calcified, but there is no commissural fusion.

stenotic, its orifice is elliptical rather than round, and flow across the valve is more turbulent than with a normal tricuspid aortic valve (Fig. 9-24). Increasing cusp rigidity eventually produces functional derangements, typically in patients over age 60.

In any form of calcific aortic stenosis, calcification produces nodules restricted to the base and lower half of the cusps, and rarely involves the free margins. Without rheumatic scarring (see below), commissures are not fused, and three distinct cusps are evident.

Aortic valve calcification is not a purely passive process in which devitalized tissue becomes mineralized as the term "dystrophic calcification" seems to imply. In fact, valvular calcification is an active process involving modulation of valvular interstitial cells to an osteoblastic phenotype; new gene expression results in cell-mediated mineralization of the extracellular matrix. Many of the mechanisms and risk factors associated with valvular calcification are similar to those for atherosclerosis, but the process is resistant to drug (statin) therapy.

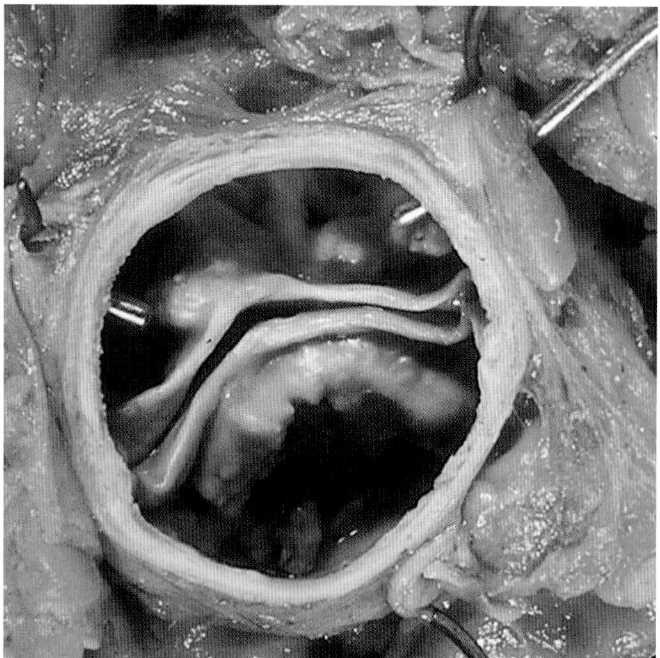

FIGURE 9-24. Calcific aortic stenosis of a congenitally bicuspid aortic valve. The two leaflets are heavily calcified, but there is no commissural fusion. Probes show the openings of the coronary ostia.

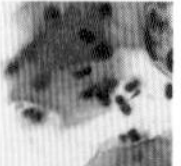

CLINICAL FEATURES: Severe aortic stenosis causes striking concentric left ventricular hypertrophy. Eventually, the ventricle dilates and fails. Valve replacement is highly successful (5-year survival rate of 85%), if done before ventricular dysfunction is irreversible. The hypertrophic left ventricle then returns to normal size.

Mitral Valve Annulus Calcification

Calcification of the mitral valve annulus occurs commonly in the elderly. It is more frequent in women and is usually without functional significance, although it often produces a murmur. However, if it is severe enough to interfere with posterior mitral leaflet excursion during systole, mitral regurgitation occurs. Unlike calcification in rheumatic valves, the leaflets are not deformed in mitral valve annulus calcification in the elderly. Calcific deposits transform the mitral ring into a rigid curved bar up to 2 cm in diameter, which may be evident radiologically.

Autoimmune Diseases Affecting Cardiac Valves and Myocardium

Rheumatic Fever

Although associated with an infectious agent (Group A β-hemolytic *Streptococcus*), the pathogenesis of the acute myocarditis and chronic valvular disease associated with infection in some persons has a strong autoimmune component, which is likely under genetic control. The disease is discussed in detail below.

Systemic Lupus Erythematosus

The heart is often involved in SLE, but cardiac symptoms are usually less prominent than other manifestations of the disease. **Libman–Sacks endocarditis** is the most striking cardiac lesion of SLE. Verrucous vegetations, up to 4 mm, occur on endocardial surfaces, most often on the mitral valve. Fibrinous pericarditis and myocarditis also occur.

Scleroderma (Progressive Systemic Sclerosis)

Cardiac involvement is second only to renal disease as a cause of death in scleroderma. The myocardium shows intimal sclerosis of small arteries, which leads to small infarcts and patchy fibrosis. As a result, congestive heart failure and arrhythmias are common. In fact, electrocardiograms show ventricular ectopy in up to two thirds of patients with scleroderma, and serious arrhythmias in one quarter. Cor pulmonale (caused by pulmonary interstitial fibrosis) and hypertensive heart disease (caused by renal involvement) are also seen.

Polyarteritis Nodosa

The heart is affected in 75% of patients with polyarteritis nodosa. Necrotizing lesions in branches of the coronary arteries cause myocardial infarction, arrhythmias, or heart block. Cardiac hypertrophy and failure as a result of renal vascular hypertension are common.

Bacterial Endocarditis

Bacteria may infect the cardiac valves. Fungi, chlamydia, and rickettsiae may also cause infective endocarditis, but do so uncommonly. ***Antimicrobial therapy changed clinical patterns of bacterial endocarditis.*** (Table 9-4).

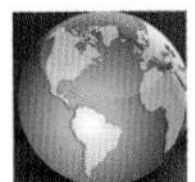

EPIDEMIOLOGY: *The most common predisposing condition for bacterial endocarditis in children currently is a congenital cardiac malformation. Mitral valve prolapse and congenital heart disease are now the most frequent bases for bacterial endocarditis in adults.*

Other Sources of Infection

- **Intravenous drug abusers** inject pathogenic organisms along with illicit drugs, and bacterial endocarditis is a notorious complication. In such patients, 80% have no underlying cardiac lesion, and the tricuspid valve is involved in half of cases. The most common source of bacteria in intravenous drug abusers is the skin, with *Staphylococcus aureus* causing more than half of the infections.
- **Prosthetic valves** are sites of infection in 15% of cases of endocarditis in adults, and 4% of patients with prosthetic valves have this complication. Staphylococci are again responsible for half of these infections. Most of the rest are caused by Gram-negative aerobic organisms, streptococci, enterococci, and fungi. Indwelling vascular catheters are another source of iatrogenic endocarditis.
- **Transient bacteremia** from any procedure may lead to infective endocarditis. Examples include dental procedures, urinary catheterization, gastrointestinal endoscopy, and obstetric procedures. Antibiotic prophylaxis is recommended during such maneuvers for patients at increased risk for bacterial endocarditis (e.g., those with a history of rheumatic fever or a cardiac murmur).
- **The elderly** are increasingly prone to developing endocarditis. Degenerative changes in heart valves, including calcific aortic stenosis and calcification of mitral annuli, predispose to endocarditis.
- **Diabetes** and **pregnancy** may also increase the incidence of bacterial endocarditis.

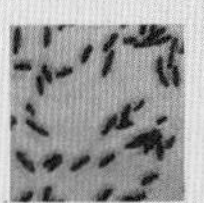
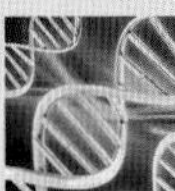

ETIOLOGIC FACTORS AND MOLECULAR PATHOGENESIS: Virulent organisms, such as *S. aureus*, can infect apparently normal valves, but the mechanism of such bacterial colonization is poorly understood. By contrast, infection of previously damaged valves by less virulent organisms has been tied to (1) hemodynamic factors, (2) formation of an initially sterile platelet–fibrin thrombus, and (3) adherence properties of the microorganisms. A key feature is abnormal blood flow across a damaged valve. Lesions form on the inflow portions of valves, where high pulsatile shear stresses occur. The pressure gradient across a narrow orifice (valve or congenital defect) produces turbulent flow at the periphery and a high-velocity jet at the center, both of which tend to denude valve endothelial surfaces. This effect leads to focal deposition of platelets and fibrin, creating small sterile vegetations that are hospitable sites for bacterial colonization and growth. Microorganisms that gain access to the circulation, as a result of dental manipulation for example, can be deposited within the vegetations. In this protected environment, there may be 10^{10} organisms per gram of tissue. Matrix metalloproteinases made by bacteria begin to destroy valves, facilitating formation of adjacent vegetations.

Table 9-4

Etiologic Factors in Bacterial Endocarditis

	Children (%)		Adults (%)	
	Newborns	<15 y	15–60 y	>60 y
Underlying disease				
Congenital heart disease	30	80	10	2
Rheumatic heart disease	—	5	25	8
Mitral valve prolapse	—	10	10	10
Valvular calcification	—	—	5	30
Intravenous drug abuse	—	—	15	10
Other	—	—	10	10
None	70	5	25	30
Microorganisms[a]				
Staphylococcus aureus	45	25	35	30
Coagulase-negative staphylococci	10	5	5	10
Streptococci	15	45	45	35
Enterococci	—	5	5	15
Gram-negative bacteria	10	5	5	5
Fungi	10	Rare	Rare	Rare
Negative culture	5	10	5	5

[a]Five perc+ent of neonatal infections are polymicrobial.

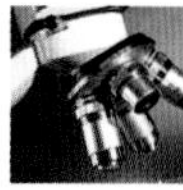

PATHOLOGY: Bacterial endocarditis most commonly involves the left-sided heart valves (mitral or aortic or both). The most common congenital heart lesions that underlie bacterial endocarditis are patent ductus arteiosus, tetralogy of Fallot, ventricular septal defect, and bicuspid aortic valve, which is an increasingly recognized risk factor, especially in men over 60 years. ***As a rule, the vegetations form on the upstream sides of the valves (i.e., the atrial side of atrioventricular valves and the ventricular side of semilunar valves), often at points where leaflets or cusps close*** (Fig. 9-25). Vegetations consist of platelets, fibrin, cell debris, and masses of organisms. The underlying valve tissue is edematous and inflamed, and may eventually become so damaged that a leaflet perforates, causing regurgitation. Lesions vary from small, superficial deposits to bulky, exuberant vegetations. The infective process may spread locally to involve valve rings or adjacent mural endocardium and chordae tendineae. ***A major complication is the detachment of infected thromboemboli and their travel to multiple systemic sites, causing infarcts or abscesses in many organs, including the brain, kidneys, intestine, and spleen.***

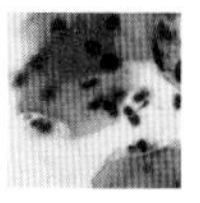

CLINICAL FEATURES: Many patients show early symptoms of bacterial endocarditis within a week of the bacteremic episode, and almost all are symptomatic within 2 weeks. Nonspecific symptoms—low-grade fever, fatigue, anorexia, and weight loss—predominate at first. Heart murmurs almost invariably develop and often change during the course of the disease. In cases lasting more than 6 weeks, splenomegaly, petechiae, and clubbing of the fingers are frequent. In one third of patients, systemic emboli are recognized at some time during the illness. One third of patients show some neurologic dysfunction because of the frequency of cerebral emboli. Mycotic aneurysms of cerebral vessels, brain abscesses, and intracerebral bleeding are observed. Pulmonary emboli typify tricuspid valve endocarditis in drug addicts.

Antibacterial therapy is effective in limiting the morbidity and mortality of bacterial endocarditis. Most patients defervesce within a week of instituting such therapy. However, prognosis depends to some extent on the offending organism and the stage at which infection is treated. ***One third of cases of S. aureus endocarditis are still fatal. The most common serious complication of bacterial endocarditis is congestive heart failure, usually caused by valvular destruction, and portending a grim prognosis.*** Myocardial abscesses and infarction secondary to coronary artery emboli may contribute to heart failure.

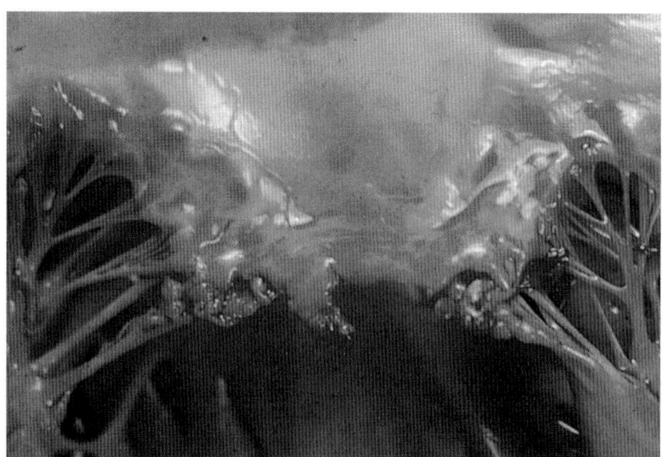

FIGURE 9-25. Bacterial endocarditis. The mitral valve shows destructive vegetations, which have eroded through the free margins of the valve leaflets.

Nonbacterial Thrombotic Endocarditis

Nonbacterial thrombotic endocarditis (NBTE), also known as marantic endocarditis, entails sterile vegetations on apparently normal cardiac valves, almost always in association with cancer or some other wasting disease. It affects mitral and aortic valves equally often. NBTE resembles infective endocarditis grossly, but it does not destroy affected valves and lacks both inflammation and microorganisms. The cause of NBTE is poorly understood. It is seen commonly as a paraneoplastic condition, usually complicating adenocarcinomas (particularly of the pancreas and lung) and hematologic malignancies.

RHEUMATIC HEART DISEASE

Rheumatic fever (RH) is a multisystem childhood disease that follows streptococcal infection. It entails an inflammatory reaction involving the myocardium and valves of the heart, joints, and central nervous system.

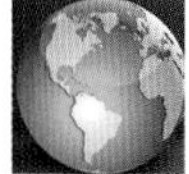

EPIDEMIOLOGY: RF is a complication of acute streptococcal infection, almost always pharyngitis (i.e., "strep" throat; see Chapter 6). The cause is *Streptococcus pyogenes*, also known as Group A β-hemolytic *Streptococcus*. In some epidemics of streptococcal pharyngitis, the incidence of RF may be as high as 3%. RF is mainly a disease of children, the median age being 9 to 11 years, although it can occur in adults. The death rate from RF has fallen drastically over the past 60 years in the United States. ***RF, though less common in developed countries, is still a leading cause of cardiac deaths in young people in less developed areas.***

MOLECULAR PATHOGENESIS: The pathogenesis of acute RF involves the triad of (1) a genetically susceptible host, (2) infection with a rheumatogenic strain of group A *Streptococcus*, and (3) an abnormal host immune response to the infection. It remains unknown why only a small number of people infected with the offending *Streptococcus* develop RF. Human leukocyte antigen (HLA) class II molecules appear to play a role in disease susceptibility; exactly how is unclear. There are similarities between some HLA class II alleles and streptococcal antigens, which may result in antibodies being directed against proteins on valves and other host tissues. Alternatively, bacterial antigens may mimic HLA molecules and so initiate an aberrant immune response. In either case, an autoimmune etiology is likely (Fig. 9-26).

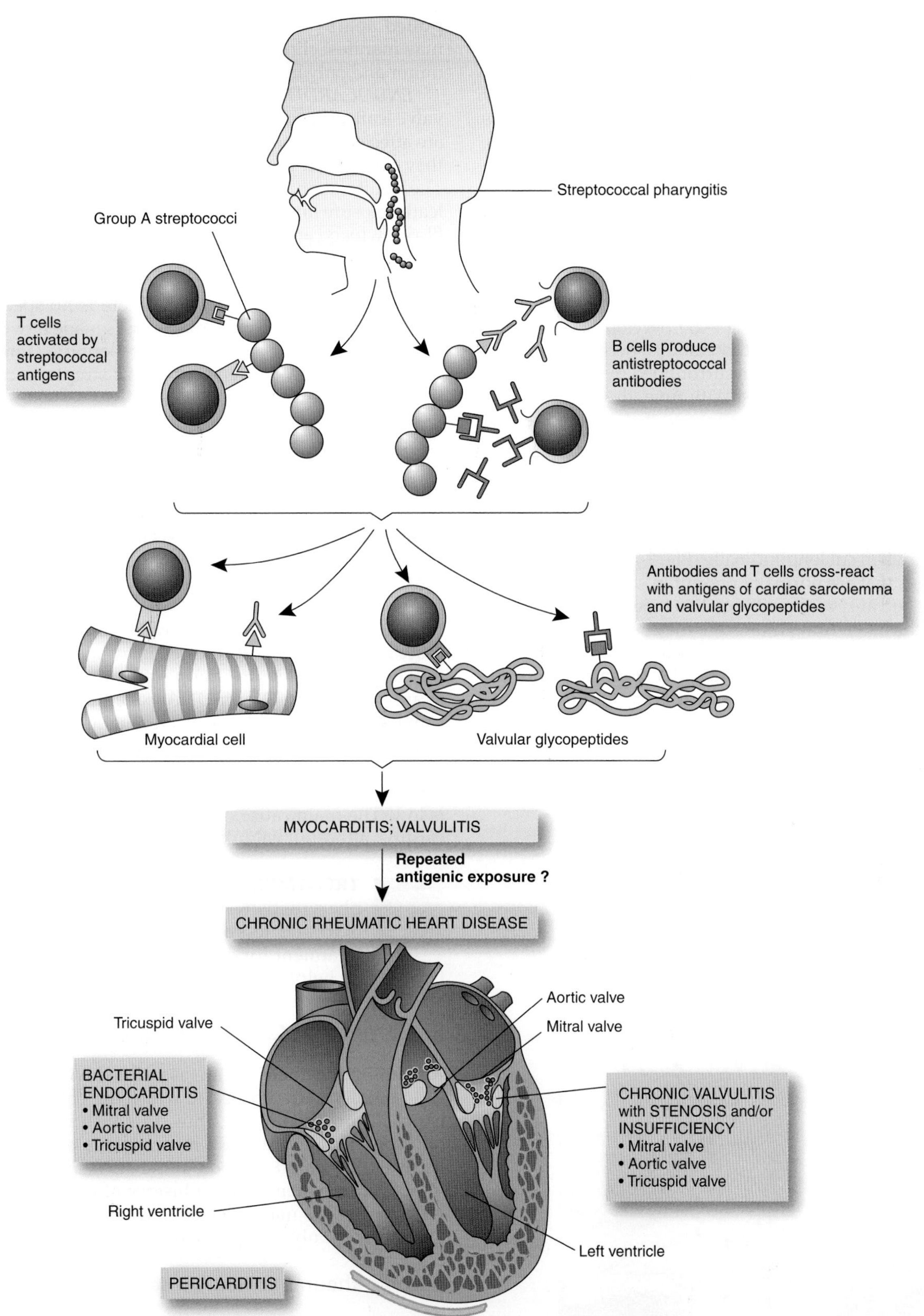

FIGURE 9-26. Biologic factors in rheumatic heart disease. The upper portion illustrates the initiating β-hemolytic streptococcal infection of the throat, which introduces the streptococcal antigens into the body and may also activate cytotoxic T cells. These antigens lead to the production of antibodies against various antigenic components of the *Streptococcus*, which can cross-react with certain cardiac antigens, including those from the myocyte sarcolemma and glycoproteins of the valves. This may be the mechanism for inflammation of the heart in acute rheumatic fever, which involves all cardiac layers (endocarditis, myocarditis, and pericarditis). This inflammation becomes apparent after a latent period of 2 to 3 weeks. Active inflammation of the valves may eventually lead to chronic valvular stenosis or insufficiency. These lesions involve the mitral, aortic, and tricuspid valves, in that order of frequency.

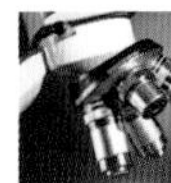

PATHOLOGY: Acute rheumatic heart disease is a pancarditis; that is, it affects all three layers of the heart as myocarditis, pericarditis, and endocarditis.

MYOCARDITIS: In severe cases of RF, a few patients may die during the earliest acute phase of the illness before the granulomatous inflammation typical of RF develops. At this early stage, the heart tends to be dilated and shows a nonspecific myocarditis, with lymphocytes and macrophages predominating, although a few neutrophils and eosinophils may be present. Fibrinoid degeneration of collagen, in which fibers become swollen, fragmented, and eosinophilic, is characteristic of this early phase.

The **Aschoff body**, which is the characteristic granulomatous lesion of rheumatic myocarditis (Fig. 9-27), develops several weeks after symptoms begin. At first, it consists of a perivascular focus of swollen eosinophilic collagen surrounded by lymphocytes, plasma cells, and macrophages. With time, the Aschoff body assumes a granulomatous appearance, with a fibrinoid central and a perimeter of lymphocytes, plasma cells, macrophages, and giant cells. In time, it is replaced by a scarred nodule.

Anitschkow cells are unusual cells within Aschoff bodies, whose nuclei contain a central band of chromatin. These nuclei have an "owl-eye" appearance in cross section, and they resemble a caterpillar when cut longitudinally (Fig. 9-27). These cells are macrophages that are normally present in small numbers but accumulate and are prominent in certain types of inflammatory diseases of the heart. Anitschkow cells may become multinucleated, in which case they are termed **Aschoff giant cells**.

PERICARDITIS: Tenacious irregular fibrin deposits are found on visceral and parietal pericardial surfaces during the acute inflammatory phase of RF. These exudates resemble the shaggy surfaces of two slices of buttered bread that have been pulled apart ("bread-and-butter pericarditis"). Pericarditis may manifest clinically as a friction rub, but it is functionally minor and only infrequently leads to constrictive pericarditis.

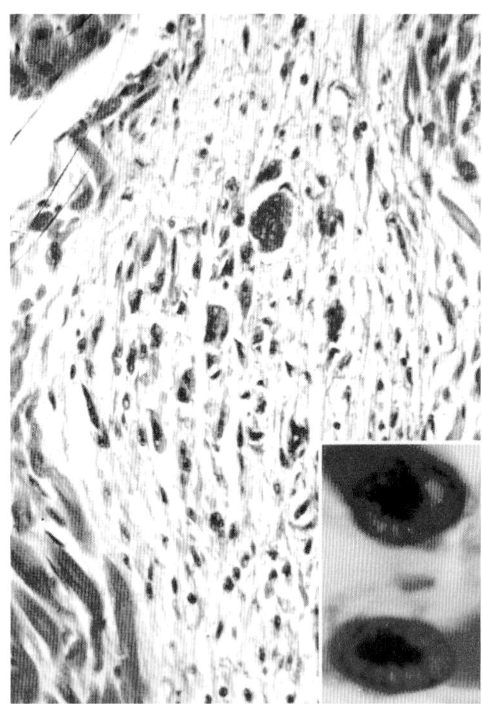

FIGURE 9-27. Acute rheumatic heart disease. An Aschoff body in the myocardial interstitium. Note collagen degeneration, lymphocytes, and a multinucleated Aschoff giant cell. *Inset.* Nuclei of Anitschkow myocytes showing "owl-eye" appearance in cross section and "caterpillar" shape longitudinally.

ENDOCARDITIS: During the acute stage of rheumatic carditis, valve leaflets become inflamed and edematous. All four valves are affected, but the left-sided valves are most injured because they close under greater pressures than the right-sided valves. The result is damage and focal loss of endothelium along valve leaflet closure lines. This leads to deposition of tiny nodules of fibrin, which can be recognized grossly as "verrucae" along the leaflets (the so-called verrucous endocarditis of acute RF).

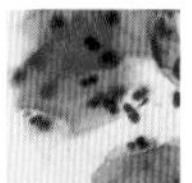

CLINICAL FEATURES: There is no specific test for RF. Clinically, the diagnosis is made if two major—or one major and two minor—criteria (**Jones criteria**) are met. Evidence of recent streptococcal infection increases the probability of RF.

The **major criteria** of acute RF include carditis (murmurs, cardiomegaly, pericarditis, and congestive heart failure), polyarthritis, chorea, erythema marginatum, and subcutaneous nodules.

The **minor criteria** are previous history of RF, arthralgia, fever, and certain laboratory tests indicating an inflammatory process (e.g., increased sedimentation rate, positive test result for C-reactive protein, and leukocytosis) and electrocardiographic changes.

Symptoms of RF begin 2 to 3 weeks after an infection with *S. pyogenes*. By then, throat cultures are usually negative. Increasing serum antibodies to Group A streptococcal antigens, such as antistreptolysin O, anti-DNAase B, and antihyaluronidase, provides concrete evidence of a recent infection with Group A *Streptococcus*. Acute symptoms of RF usually subside within 3 months, but with severe carditis, clinical activity may continue for 6 months or more. Mortality in acute rheumatic carditis is low. The main cause of death is heart failure due to myocarditis, although valvular dysfunction may also play a role.

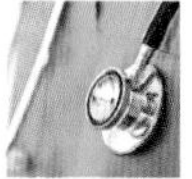

TREATMENT: Prompt treatment of streptococcal pharyngitis with antibiotics prevents a first attack of RF and, less often, recurrences. There is no specific treatment for acute RF, but corticosteroids and salicylates are helpful in managing the symptoms.

Recurrent and Chronic Rheumatic Heart Diseases

Recurrent attacks of RF are associated with types of Group A β-hemolytic streptococci to which the patient has not been exposed previously and, thus, to which immunity has not developed. The rate of RF recurrence is related to the time between the initial episode and a subsequent streptococcal infection. In patients with a history of a recent attack of RF, recurrence rates may reach 65%, whereas recurrence after 10 years affects only 5% of patients.

Chronic Rheumatic Heart Disease

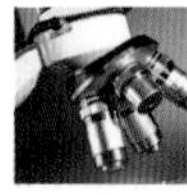

PATHOLOGY: *The myocardial and pericardial components of rheumatic pancarditis typically resolve without permanent sequelae. By contrast, valvulitis due to RF often leads to long-term structural and functional changes.* During the healing phase, valve leaflets develop diffuse fibrosis and become thickened, shrunken, and less pliable. At the same time, healing of the verrucous lesions along the lines of closure often generates fibrous "adhesions"

between leaflets, especially at the commissures (commissural fusion). The result is a stenotic valve that does not open freely because its leaflets are rigid and partially fused. Blood flow across such a valve is turbulent, which can cause even more scarring and deformation of leaflets because of chronic "wear and tear" on the valve. Severe valvular scarring may develop months or years after a single bout of acute RF.

Valves Affected

The mitral valve is the most commonly and severely affected valve in chronic rheumatic disease. It snaps shut under systolic pressure and thus bears the greatest mechanical burden of all the valves. In chronic mitral valvulitis, valve leaflets become conspicuous, irregularly thickened, and calcified, often with fusion of commissures and chordae tendineae (Fig. 9-28). In severe chronic rheumatic mitral valvular disease, valve orifices become reduced to fixed narrow slits, resembling "fish mouths" when viewed from the ventricular aspect (Fig. 9-29).

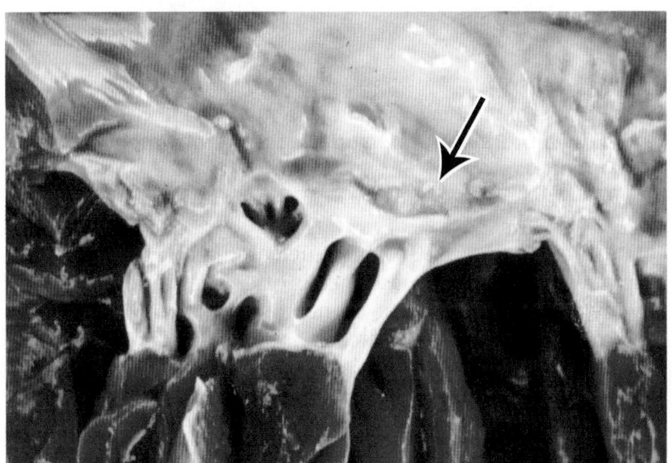

FIGURE 9-28. Chronic rheumatic valvulitis. The mitral valve leaflets are thickened and focally calcified (*arrow*), and the commissures are partially fused. The chordae tendineae are also short, thick, and fused.

Stenosis is dominant functionally, but mitral valves are also regurgitant. Chronic regurgitation produces a "jet" of blood directed at the posterior aspect of the left atrium, damaging atrial endocardium and producing focal rough, wrinkled endocardium, called "MacCallum patches."

The aortic valve, which snaps shut under diastolic pressure, is the second most commonly involved valve in rheumatic heart disease. Diffuse fibrous thickening of the cusps and fusion of the commissures cause aortic stenosis, which may be mild initially but which progresses because of the chronic effects of turbulent blood flow across the valve. Often, cusps become rigidly calcified as the patient ages, resulting in stenosis and insufficiency, although either lesion may predominate. The lower pressures experienced by the right-sided valves are usually protective. However, in recurrent RF, however, tricuspid valves may become deformed, virtually always in association with mitral and aortic lesions. Pulmonic valves are rarely affected.

Complications of Chronic Rheumatic Heart Disease

- **Bacterial endocarditis** follows episodes of bacteremia (e.g., during dental procedures). The scarred valves of rheumatic heart disease provide an attractive environment for bacteria that would bypass a normal valve.
- **Mural thrombi** form in atrial or ventricular chambers in 40% of patients with rheumatic valvular disease. They give rise to thromboemboli, which can produce infarcts in various organs. Rarely, a large thrombus in the left atrial appendage develops a stalk and acts as a ball valve to obstruct the mitral valve orifice.
- **Congestive heart failure** complicates rheumatic disease of both mitral and aortic valves.
- **Adhesive pericarditis** often follows the fibrinous pericarditis of acute attacks, but rarely causes constrictive pericarditis.

MYOCARDITIS

Myocarditis is an inflammation of the myocardium associated with myocyte necrosis and degeneration. This definition specifically excludes ischemic heart disease. The true incidence of myocarditis is difficult to establish because many cases are

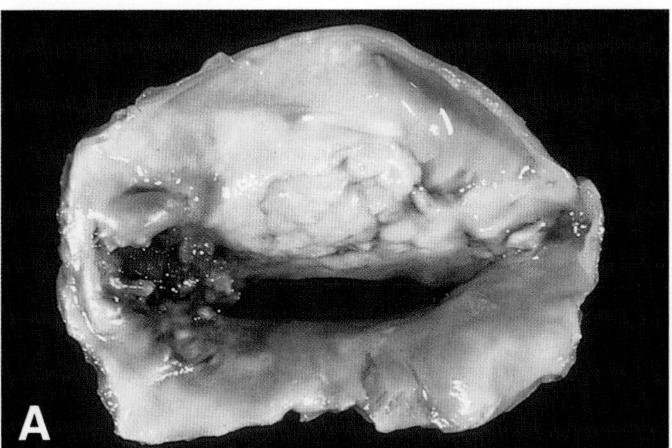

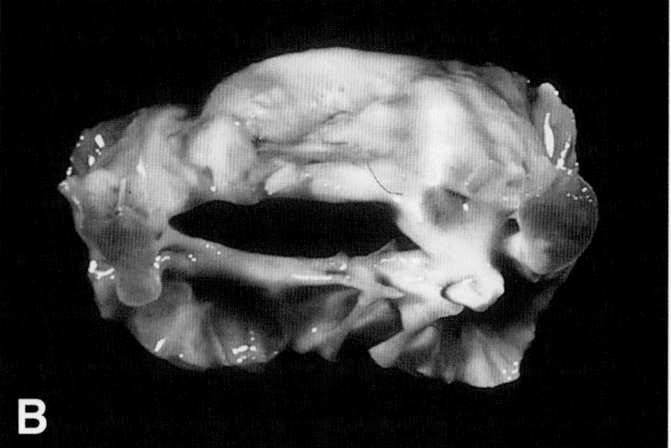

FIGURE 9-29. Chronic rheumatic valvulitis. A view of a surgically excised rheumatic mitral valve from the left atrium (**A**) and left ventricle (**B**) showing rigid, thickened, and fused leaflets with a narrow orifice, creating the characteristic "fish mouth" appearance of rheumatic mitral stenosis. Note that the tips of the papillary muscles (shown in **B**) are directly attached to the underside of the valve leaflets, reflecting marked shortening and fusion of the chordae tendineae.

Table 9-5

Causes of Myocarditis

Causes of Myocarditis
Idiopathic
Infectious
• Viral: Coxsackievirus, adenovirus, echovirus, influenza virus, human immunodeficiency virus, and many others
• Rickettsial: Typhus, Rocky Mountain spotted fever
• Bacterial: Diphtheria, staphylococcal, streptococcal, meningococcal, *Borrelia* (Lyme disease), and leptospiral infection
• Fungi and protozoan parasites: Chagas disease, toxoplasmosis, aspergillosis, cryptococcal, and candidal infection
• Metazoan parasites: *Echinococcus, Trichina*
Noninfectious
• Hypersensitivity and immunologically related diseases: Rheumatic fever, systemic lupus erythematosus, scleroderma, drug reaction (e.g., to penicillin or sulfonamide), and rheumatoid arthritis
• Radiation
• Miscellaneous: Sarcoidosis, uremia

asymptomatic. It can occur at any age but is most common in children aged 1 to 10 years. It is one of the few heart diseases that can cause acute heart failure in previously healthy children, adolescents, or young adults. Severe myocarditis precipitates arrhythmias and even sudden cardiac death. Causes of myocarditis include sequelae of rheumatic fever, as noted above, viral or nonviral infections, granulomatous disease, hypersensitivity to drugs, or giant cell myocarditis. Many cases of viral myocarditis have no demonstrable cause. In such cases, viral etiology is generally suspected, but the evidence is usually circumstantial unless polymerase chain reaction (PCR) studies identify viral genomes in heart biopsies. The most common viral causes of myocarditis are listed in Table 9-5.

MOLECULAR PATHOGENESIS: The pathogenesis of viral myocarditis involves direct viral cytotoxicity and cell-mediated immune reactions against infected myocytes. The most common viruses that infect the heart are coxsackievirus and adenovirus, both of which enter myocytes using the same cellular receptor. Once inside a myocyte, coxsackieviruses produce proteases that play a role in viral replication. These proteases may impede myocardial function and may cleave myocyte proteins, such as dystrophin.

PATHOLOGY: The hearts of patients with myocarditis who develop clinical heart failure during the active inflammatory phase show biventricular dilation and generalized myocardial hypokinesis. At autopsy, such hearts are flabby and dilated. Histologic features of viral myocarditis vary with the clinical disease severity, but with few exceptions, microscopic features are nonspecific and indistinguishable from toxic myocarditis. Most cases show patchy or diffuse interstitial, predominantly mononuclear, inflammatory infiltrates, mainly of T lymphocytes and

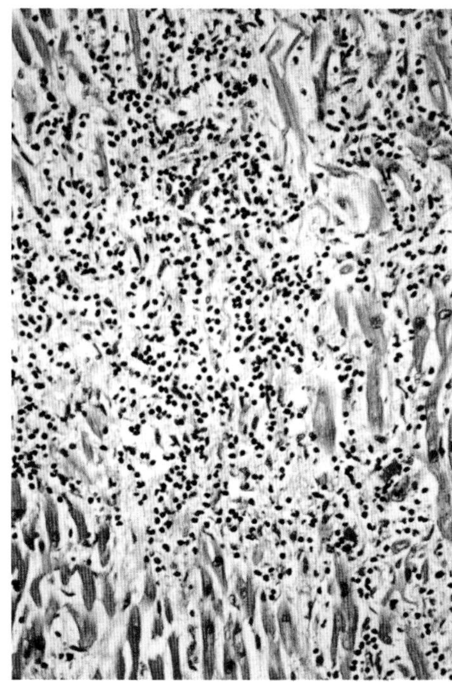

FIGURE 9-30. Viral myocarditis. The myocardial fibers are disrupted by a prominent interstitial infiltrate of lymphocytes and macrophages.

macrophages (Fig. 9-30). Multinucleated giant cells may also be present. The inflammatory cells often surround individual myocytes, and focal myocyte necrosis is seen. Most viruses that cause myocarditis also cause pericarditis.

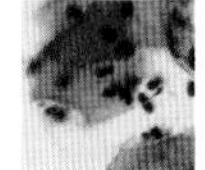

CLINICAL FEATURES: Many people with viral myocarditis have no symptoms. When symptoms do occur, they usually start a few weeks after infection. Most patients recover from acute myocarditis, although a few die of congestive heart failure or arrhythmias. There is no specific treatment for viral myocarditis; supportive measures are the rule.

Nonviral Transmissible Causing Myocarditis

Other microorganisms that gain access to the bloodstream can infect the heart. Among these, brucellosis, meningococcemia, and psittacosis often lead to infectious myocarditis. Some bacteria (e.g., diphtheria) produce cardiotoxins, which may cause fatal myocarditis. The most common cause of myocarditis in South America is a protozoan, *Trypanosoma cruzi*, the agent of Chagas disease (discussed in Chapter 6).

METABOLIC DISEASES OF THE HEART

Similar metabolic diseases of the heart are secondary to hyperthyroidism or hypothyroidism and thiamine deficiency. Thyroid hormone increases the heart rate and force of contraction. Hyperthyroidism, therefore, is characterized by tachycardia and increases cardiac workload, because of decreased peripheral resistance and increased cardiac output. It may eventually lead to angina pectoris, high-output failure, or arrhythmias (atrial fibrillation, most commonly). Contrawise patients with severe hypothyroidism (**myxedema**) experience low cardiac output, reduced heart rate, and poor myocardial contractility. The hearts of patients with myxedema are flabby and dilated, but the condition alone does not result in congestive failure. Thiamine deficiency heart disease (Beriberi) results in decreased peripheral vascular resistance and increased cardiac output, thus resembling hyperthyroidism with high-output failure.

CARDIOMYOPATHY

Cardiomyopathies are primary diseases of the myocardium exclusive of damage caused by extrinsic factors. Usually, primary cardiomyopathies are divided into the major clinicopathologic groups of **dilated cardiomyopathy (DCM)**, **hypertrophic cardiomyopathy (HCM)**, **arrhythmogenic cardiomyopathy** (ACM), and **restrictive cardiomyopathy (RCM)**. Most can be traced to genetic factors.

Dilated cardiomyopathy, the most common type and a leading indication for heart transplantation, is characterized by biventricular dilation, impaired contractility, and, eventually, congestive heart failure. DCM can develop after a large number of known insults that injure cardiac myocytes In this context, alcohol abuse, hypertension, pregnancy, and viral myocarditis predispose to secondary DCM. Diabetes mellitus and cigarette smoking are also associated with an increased incidence of **secondary DCM.** Genetic factors play a major role in idiopathic **primary DCM.**

Idiopathic Dilated Cardiomyopathy

MOLECULAR PATHOGENESIS: Many etiologies have been implicated in idiopathic DCM. Most cases probably represent an interplay between genetic, epigenetic, and environmental factors.

Genetic factors are important in the pathogenesis of DCM. At least one third of DCM patients inherited the disease as a single-gene disorder in a Mendelian pattern. The proportion may be even greater because incomplete penetrance often makes it difficult to identify early or latent disease in family members. Most familial cases seem to be transmitted as autosomal dominant traits, but autosomal recessive, X-linked recessive, and mitochondrial inheritance patterns have all been described.

Mutations in more than 50 genes have been linked to DCM. Several occur in genes encoding cytoskeletal proteins, such as lamin A/C, desmin, and metavinculin. Others affect genes such as *δ-sarcoglycan* and *dystrophin*, which are involved in anchoring the cytoskeleton and the sarcolemma to the extracellular matrix. ***These data suggest that defects in force transmission bring about the development of a dilated, poorly contracting heart.*** However, 35% to 45% of genetic causes of DCM may be related to mutations in genes encoding sarcomeric proteins, such as actin, titin, troponin T, and β- or α-myosin heavy chains. Mutations (mainly truncations) in the giant sarcomeric protein titin may alone account for up to 25% of genetic causes. Interestingly, some sarcomeric protein mutations may produce either DCM or HCM phenotypes, perhaps depending on whether they produce a defect in force generation (HCM) or force transmission. However, the link between the particular protein mutated, the location of the mutation within the functional domains of the protein, and the nature of the cardiac defect remains uncertain.

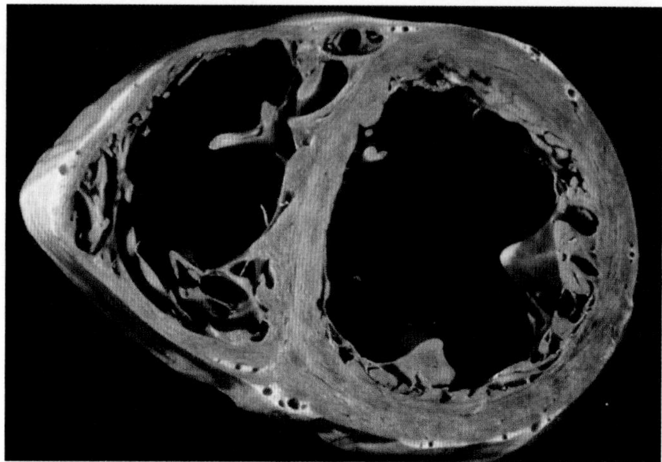

FIGURE 9-31. Idiopathic dilated cardiomyopathy. A transverse section of the enlarged heart revealing conspicuous dilation of both ventricles. Although the ventricular wall appears thinned, the increased mass of the heart indicates considerable hypertrophy.

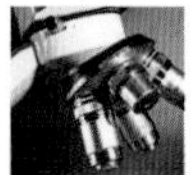

PATHOLOGY: The pathology of DCM is generally nonspecific and is similar whatever its genesis. At autopsy, the heart is invariably enlarged, with conspicuous left and right ventricular hypertrophy. Heart weight may be tripled (>900 g). As a rule, all chambers of the heart are dilated, though the ventricles are more severely affected than the atria (Fig. 9-31). At end stage, left ventricular dilation is usually so severe that the left ventricular wall appears to be of normal thickness or even thinned. The myocardium is flabby and pale, sometimes with small subendocardial scars. The left ventricle endocardium tends to be thickened, especially at the apex. Adherent mural thrombi are often present in this area.

Microscopically, DCM is characterized by atrophic and hypertrophic myocardial fibers. Cardiac myocytes, especially in the subendocardium, often show advanced degenerative changes characterized by myofibrillar loss (myocytolysis), an effect that gives cells a vacant, vacuolated appearance. Interstitial and perivascular fibrosis of myocardium is evident, especially in the subendocardial zone.

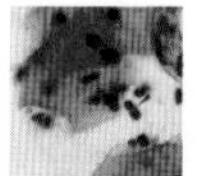

CLINICAL FEATURES: The clinical courses of idiopathic and secondary DCM are comparable. Both begin insidiously with compensatory ventricular hypertrophy and asymptomatic left ventricular dilation. Exercise intolerance usually progresses relentlessly to frank congestive heart failure, and 75% of patients die within 5 years of the onset of symptoms. Half of all deaths in DCM patients are sudden and are attributed to ventricular arrhythmias. Supportive treatment is useful, but cardiac transplantation or a ventricular assist device is eventually necessary.

Toxic Cardiomyopathy

Many chemicals and drugs cause myocardial injury, but only a few of the more important chemicals are discussed as follows:

- *ETHANOL:* Alcohol abuse is the single most common identifiable cause of DCM in the United States and Europe. The typical patient is between ages 30 and 55 years and has been drinking heavily for at least 10 years.

- *CATECHOLAMINES:* In high concentrations, catecholamines can cause focal myocyte necrosis (contraction band necrosis). Toxic myocarditis may occur in patients with pheochromocytomas, those who require high doses of inotropic drugs to maintain blood pressure, and accident victims who sustain massive head trauma.
- *ANTHRACYCLINES:* Doxorubicin (Adriamycin) and other anthracycline drugs are potent chemotherapeutic agents whose usefulness is limited by cumulative, dose-dependent, cardiac toxicity. The major clinical effect is poor myocyte contractility caused by irreversible degeneration of cardiac myocytes.
- *CYCLOPHOSPHAMIDE:* This alkylating agent is often used in high doses before bone marrow transplantation. It does not cause classic DCM but can result in pericarditis and, occasionally, massive hemorrhagic myocarditis. The latter is thought to be secondary to endothelial injury and thrombocytopenia.
- *COCAINE:* Cocaine use is often associated with chest pain and palpitations. True DCM is an unusual complication of cocaine abuse, but myocarditis, focal necrosis, and thickening of intramyocardial coronary arteries have been reported.

Hypertrophic Cardiomyopathy

Although HCM can develop for no apparent physiologic reason, it seems to be genetically determined in most patients and is an autosomal dominant trait in half of affected persons. Many people with no family history probably have spontaneous mutations or a mild form of disease not previously detected. The prevalence of HCM in the United States is about 1 in 500.

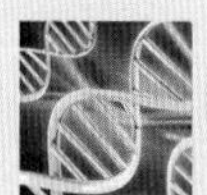

MOLECULAR PATHOGENESIS: The clinical picture of HCM is typically caused by dominant mutations in genes encoding proteins of the sarcomere. Some 80% of HCM cases for which a genetic basis is identified involve mutations in one of two genes: those encoding β-myosin heavy chain and myosin-binding protein C. Mutations in genes for cardiac troponin T, cardiac troponin I, and α-tropomyosin-1 (components of the troponin complex) account for most remaining cases. However, like DCM, there is marked allelic heterogeneity in HCM such that most mutations occur "privately" or at frequencies of less than 1%. Thus, hundreds of different mutations, mostly missense, have been identified, but their functional significance is often unknown. As noted in the discussion of DCM, different mutations in the same gene can give rise to diverse clinical phenotypes of DCM or HCM.

The mechanistic link between the mutations and the resultant clinical and pathologic phenotypes of HCM is poorly understood. In general, it is thought that the mutant protein is incorporated into the sarcomere, where it acts in a dominant-negative manner to cause a loss of sarcomeric function. ***This proposed mechanism has led to the hypothesis that HCM is related to defects in force generation as a consequence of altered sarcomeric function.*** Cardiac hypertrophy may then be a compensatory response. Other mutations may actually enhance contractility and thus lead to hypertrophy or hypertrophy may arise because a functional protein is missing, rather than by a dominant-negative effect.

Because of the risk of sudden death in HCM, there have been many attempts to use genetics to help stratify risk. Overall, the results have so far been disappointing, although some correlations have been recognized and may be useful in assessing risk in some pedigrees.

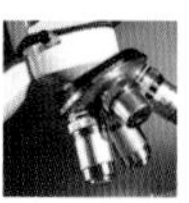

PATHOLOGY: The heart in HCM is always enlarged, but the extent of hypertrophy varies in different genetic forms. The left ventricular wall is thick, and its cavity is small, sometimes only a slit. Papillary muscles and trabeculae carneae are prominent and encroach on the lumen. More than half of cases exhibit asymmetric hypertrophy of the interventricular septum, with a ratio of septum and left ventricular free wall thickness greater than 1.5 (Fig. 9-32A). Often, the thickened, hypertrophied interventricular septum bulges into the left ventricular outflow tract early in ventricular systole, obstructing the aortic outflow tract. Both atria are commonly dilated.

***The most notable histologic feature of HCM is* myofiber disarray**, which is most extensive in the interventricular septum. Instead of the usual parallel arrangement of myocytes into muscle bundles, myofiber disarray is characterized by oblique and often perpendicular orientations of adjacent hypertrophic myocytes (Fig. 9-32B). Interstitial cells are usually hyperplastic, and intramural coronary arteries may be thick and cellular (Fig. 9-32C).

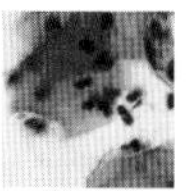

CLINICAL FEATURES: Many patients with HCM have few, if any, symptoms, and the diagnosis is commonly made during screening of the family with an affected member. Despite a lack of symptoms, such people may be at risk of sudden death, particularly during severe exertion. In fact, unsuspected HCM is often found at autopsy in young athletes who die suddenly. The clinical course tends to remain stable for many years, although, eventually, the disease can progress to congestive heart failure.

HCM responds paradoxically to pharmacologic interventions. Cardiac glycosides aggravate symptoms of HCM. Rather, HCM is treated with β-adrenergic blockers and Ca^{2+} channel blockers, which reduce contractility, decrease outflow tract obstruction, and improve left ventricular relaxation during diastole. Although surgical removal of part of the hypertrophic septum or injection of ethanol into a septal artery to cause localized infarction may relieve symptoms of obstruction, the risk of sudden death remains.

Arrhythmogenic Cardiomyopathy

ACM is a highly arrhythmogenic form of human heart disease. First described as a right ventricular disease (arrhythmogenic right ventricular cardiomyopathy), ACM is now recognized to include biventricular and left dominant forms, which may be misdiagnosed as dilated cardiomyopathy or myocarditis. It affects roughly 1 in 5,000 individuals and occurs most commonly in Mediterranean countries, where it is a leading cause of sudden death in young people.

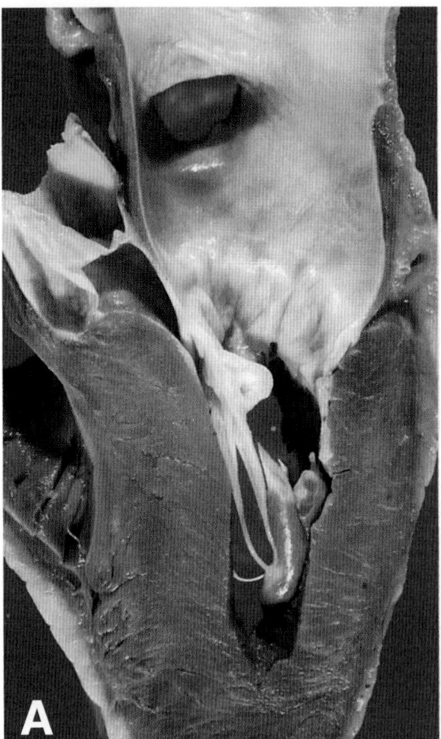

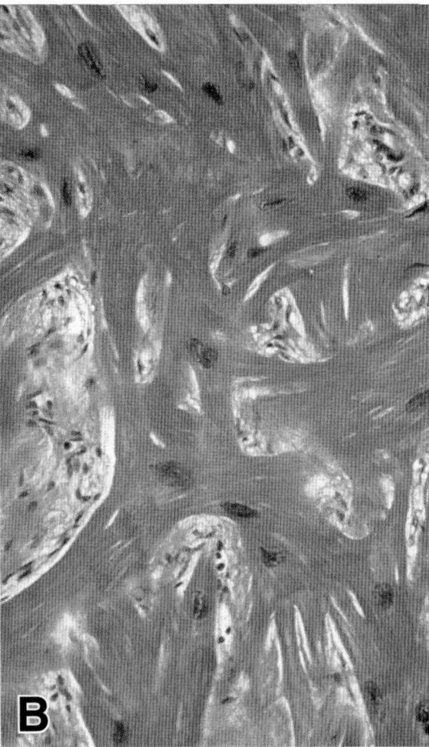

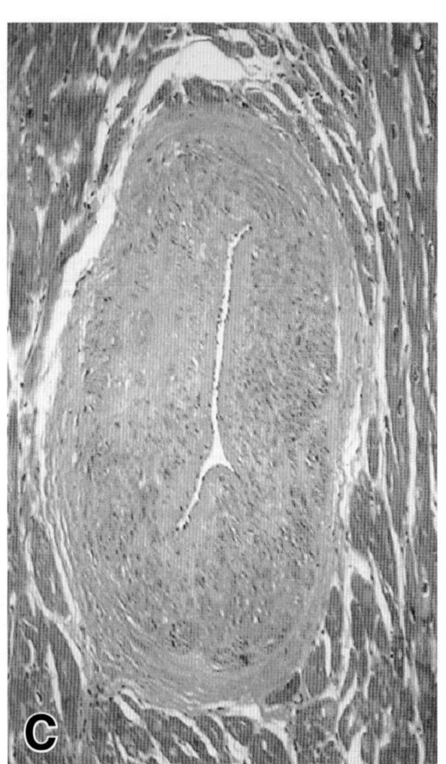

FIGURE 9-32. Hypertrophic cardiomyopathy (HCM). A. The heart has been opened to show striking asymmetric left ventricular hypertrophy. The interventricular septum is thicker than the free wall of the left ventricle and impinges on the outflow tract such that it contacts the underside of the anterior mitral valve leaflet. The left atrium is markedly enlarged. **B.** A section of the myocardium showing the characteristic myofiber disarray and hyperplasia of interstitial cells. **C.** A small intramural coronary artery showing a thickened, hypercellular media. This type of remodeling of coronary vessels could contribute to the development of angina-like symptoms in some patients with HCM.

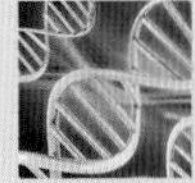

MOLECULAR PATHOGENESIS AND PATHOLOGY: ACM is associated with serious arrhythmias and sudden death, which may occur early in the disease before significant structural remodeling and contractile dysfunction develop. The classic form (ARVC) affects the right ventricular free wall. The characteristic pathologic features are degeneration of cardiac myocytes and replacement by fat and fibrous tissue, but the extent of this change can be quite variable, and it is not necessarily conspicuous in patients who die suddenly.

ACM is a familial disease, usually inherited in an autosomal dominant pattern. Its true incidence is probably underestimated because of variable penetrance, age-related progression, and large phenotypic variation. Mutations in genes encoding proteins of the desmosomes, cell–cell adhesion organelles, can be identified in more than half of individuals who fulfill these criteria.

Restrictive Cardiomyopathy

Restrictive cardiomyopathy describes a group of diseases in which myocardial or endocardial abnormalities limit diastolic filling while contractile function is normal. It is the least common category of cardiomyopathy in Western countries, but in some less developed areas (e.g., equatorial Africa, South America, and Asia), endomyocardial diseases due to parasitic infections lead to many cases of restrictive cardiomyopathy.

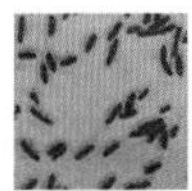
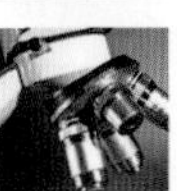

ETIOLOGIC FACTORS AND PATHOLOGY: Restrictive cardiomyopathy is caused by (1) interstitial infiltration of amyloid, metastatic carcinoma, or sarcoid granulomas; (2) endomyocardial disease that is characterized by marked fibrotic thickening of the endocardium; (3) genetic and storage diseases, including hemochromatosis and desmin-related cardiomyopathies; and (4) markedly increased interstitial fibrous tissue. The pathophysiologic consequence is a preload-dependent state, distinguished by (1) defective diastolic compliance, (2) restricted ventricular filling, (3) increased end-diastolic pressure, (4) atrial dilation, and (5) venous congestion. In many respects, these hemodynamic changes are similar to constrictive pericarditis. Many cases of restrictive cardiomyopathy are classified as idiopathic, with interstitial fibrosis as the only histologic abnormality. The disease almost invariably progresses to congestive heart failure, and only 10% of the patients survive for 10 years.

Amyloidosis

The heart is affected in most forms of **generalized amyloidosis** (see Chapter 7). In fact, restrictive cardiomyopathy is the most common cause of death in the AL amyloidosis of plasma cell dyscrasias. In **senile cardiac amyloidosis**, a protein related to prealbumin (transthyretin) is deposited in the hearts of elderly people. The disorder may be present to some extent in up to 25% of patients aged 80 years or older. It involves not only the heart (atria and ventricles) but, in many cases, the lungs as well. Senile cardiac amyloidosis is usually an incidental finding at autopsy, and rarely is functionally significant.

SUDDEN CARDIAC DEATH

Most of the 300,000 heart-related deaths in the United States are caused by spontaneous lethal ventricular tachyarrhythmias—ventricular tachycardia and ventricular fibrillation—in patients with some type of heart disease. However, some sudden deaths occur in apparently healthy persons who show coronary artery disease at autopsy but may have displayed little clinical evidence during life.

Common causes of sudden cardiac death differ in the young and old individuals. At ages younger than 35 years, HCM (idiopathic left ventricular hypertrophy) and congenital coronary anomalies account for over 75% of sudden deaths. ***In middle-aged and older adults, coronary artery disease is responsible for most sudden deaths*** (Fig. 9-33).

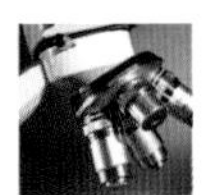

PATHOLOGY: ***Lethal arrhythmias usually arise from pathologic changes affecting conduction in the working ventricular myocardium.*** Spontaneous development of a lethal cardiac arrhythmia may be regarded as a stochastic event that arises from complex interactions between fixed anatomic substrates and acute, transient triggering events. The latter include acute ischemia, neurohormonal activation, changes in electrolytes, or other stresses. Arrhythmias are most likely when acute electrophysiologic changes (triggers) are superimposed on an existing substrate of remodeled myocardium and conduction abnormalities. Indeed, most often, sudden death involves acute ischemia (a transient triggering event) in an area of the heart containing a healed infarct (a common anatomic substrate).

Sudden Cardiac Death in Persons With Structurally Normal Hearts

Some (perhaps many) have "channelopathies," which are genetic diseases that feature mutations in genes for Na^+, K^+, and Ca^{2+} channel proteins. Although sudden death syndromes are rare, they have provided valuable insights into molecular mechanisms of lethal arrhythmias.

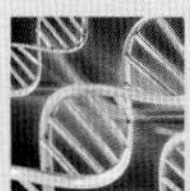

MOLECULAR PATHOGENESIS: *LONG QT SYNDROME:* This condition is defined by electrocardiographic prolonged QT intervals and T-wave abnormalities. Such persons often have a history of syncope, ventricular arrhythmias, or sudden, unexpected death. More than 10 different types of congenital long QT syndrome have been defined. Most are caused by loss-of-function mutations in genes encoding proteins that form various K^+ channels. The loss of function prolongs repolarization of the cardiac action potential (thus increasing QT intervals) and promotes arrhythmias by increasing the likelihood of after-depolarizations. Gain-of-function mutations in *SCN5A,* the gene encoding the cardiac Na^+ channel protein, can also be responsible.

BRUGADA SYNDROME: This autosomal dominant disease in a structurally normal heart displays a characteristic ST-segment elevation in right precordial leads, right bundle branch block, and susceptibility to life-threatening arrhythmias. Loss-of-function mutations in *SCN5A* are identified in 25% of cases. The disease is particularly common in some Asian populations and accounts for an appreciable proportion of sudden death in young men.

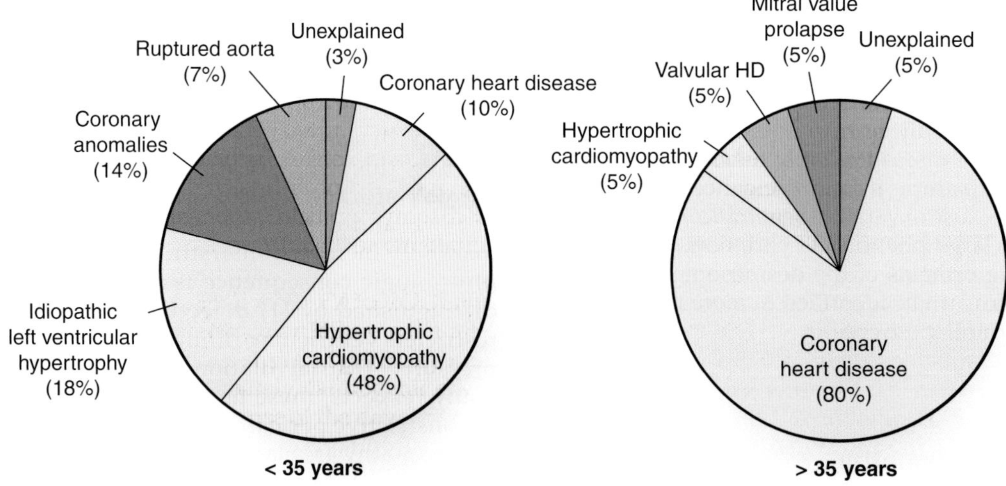

FIGURE 9-33. Different causes of sudden cardiac death in young and older adult competitive athletes. HD, heart disease.

CATECHOLAMINERGIC POLYMORPHIC VENTRICULAR TACHYCARDIA: In this condition, arrhythmias and sudden death occur in response to catecholamine surges associated with exercise or emotional stress. Mutations in genes encoding proteins that regulate intracellular Ca^{2+} homeostasis and excitation–contraction coupling, such as RyR2 and calsequestrin, are typical. These mutations promote leakage of Ca^{2+} from the SR, with resultant arrhythmias triggered by after-depolarizations.

CARDIAC TUMORS

Primary cardiac tumors are rare but can cause serious problems when they occur. The most common primary tumors include myxomas and rhabdomyomas. Less common primary tumors of the heart include angiomas, fibromas, lymphangiomas, neurofibromas, and their sarcomatous counterparts.

Myxomas

These tumors account for 30% to 50% of all primary cardiac tumors.

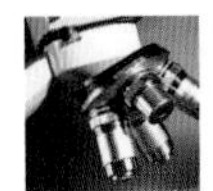

PATHOLOGY: Myxomas can occur in any cardiac chamber or on a valve, but 75% arise in the left atrium. The tumors appear as glistening, gelatinous, polypoid masses, usually 5 to 6 cm, with a short stalk (Fig. 9-34). They may be sufficiently mobile to obstruct the mitral valve orifice. Myxomas show a loose myxoid stroma containing abundant proteoglycans. Polygonal stellate cells are found within the matrix, singly or in small clusters.

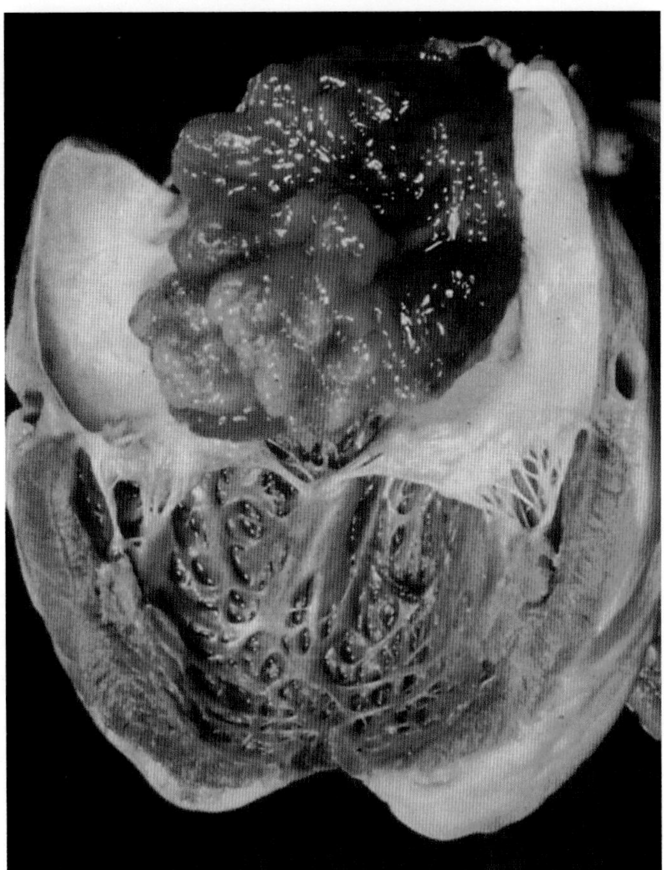

FIGURE 9-34. Cardiac myxoma. The left atrium contains a large, polypoid tumor that protrudes into the mitral valve orifice.

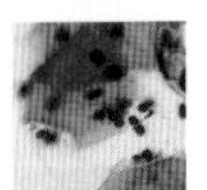

CLINICAL FEATURES: More than half of patients with left atrial myxomas have clinical evidence of mitral valve dysfunction. The tumor does not metastasize in the usual sense, but it often embolizes. Some patients with myxomas of the left heart die from tumor emboli to the brain. Surgical tumor removal is usually curative.

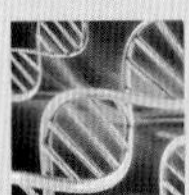

MOLECULAR PATHOGENESIS: Most cardiac myxomas are sporadic, but about 7% are part of a familial autosomal dominant syndrome that also includes pigmented lesions of the skin and adrenocortical hyperplasia. These cases have been linked to mutations in the gene encoding a regulatory subunit of cAMP-dependent protein kinase (protein kinase A), which, among other actions, appears to be a tumor suppressor gene that influences cell proliferation.

Rhabdomyomas

These tumors form nodular myocardial masses. Almost all are multiple and involve both ventricles and, in one third of cases, the atria as well. In half of the cases, the tumors project into a cardiac chamber and obstruct the lumen or a valve orifice.

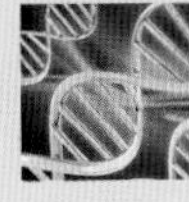

MOLECULAR PATHOGENESIS: Rhabdomyomas occur in one third of patients with tuberous sclerosis, the familial form of which is caused by mutations in *TSC1* and *TSC2*, genes that encode hamartin and tuberin, respectively. Both genes are tumor suppressors (see Chapter 4) and regulate embryonic and neonatal growth and differentiation of cardiac myocytes.

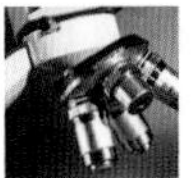

PATHOLOGY: Cardiac rhabdomyomas are pale masses, 1 mm to several centimeters. Tumor cells show small central nuclei and abundant glycogen-rich clear cytoplasm, in which fibrillar processes containing sarcomeres radiate to the margin of the cell ("spider cell"). A few cardiac rhabdomyomas have been successfully excised.

Metastatic Tumors in the Heart Are Associated With Many Common Malignancies

Of all tumors, the one most likely to metastasize to the heart is malignant melanoma. Metastatic tumors to the heart also occur in patients with common carcinomas—that is, the lung, breast, and gastrointestinal tract. Still, only a minority of patients with these tumors develop cardiac metastases. Lymphomas and leukemia may also involve the heart. Metastatic cancer involving the myocardium can result in clinical manifestations of restrictive cardiomyopathy, particularly if the cardiac tumors are associated with extensive fibrosis. Occasionally, metastatic tumors may disrupt components of the atrioventricular conduction system, giving rise to heart block or bundle branch block.

DISEASES OF THE PERICARDIUM

Pericardial Effusions

Pericardial effusions are accumulations of excess fluid within the pericardial cavity, as either a transudate or an exudate. The pericardial sac normally contains no more than 50 mL of lubricating fluid. If the pericardium is slowly distended, it can accommodate up to 2 L of fluid without notable hemodynamic consequences. However, rapid accumulation of as little as 150 to 200 mL of pericardial fluid or blood may significantly increase intrapericardial pressure and restrict diastolic filling, especially of the right atrium and ventricle resulting in cardiac tamponade.

- **Serous pericardial effusion** often complicates an increase in extracellular fluid volume, as occurs in congestive heart failure or nephrotic syndrome. The fluid has a low-protein content and few cellular elements.
- **Chylous effusion** (fluid-containing chylomicrons) results from a communication of the thoracic duct with the pericardial space, as a result of lymphatic obstruction by tumor or infection.
- **Serosanguinous pericardial effusion** may develop after chest trauma, either accidentally or after cardiopulmonary resuscitation.
- **Hemopericardium** refers to bleeding directly into the pericardial cavity. The most common cause is rupture of the ventricular free wall after a myocardial infarct. Less frequent causes are penetrating cardiac trauma, rupture of a dissecting aneurysm of the aorta, infiltration of a vessel by tumor, or a bleeding diathesis.

Cardiac tamponade *refers to a rapid accumulation of pericardial fluid, thereby restricting the filling of the heart.* Hemodynamic consequences range from a minimally symptomatic condition to abrupt cardiovascular collapse and death. As pericardial pressure increases, it eventually exceeds central venous pressure, thus limiting blood return to the heart. Cardiac output and blood pressure decrease, and **pulsus paradoxus** (an abnormal decrease in systolic pressure with inspiration) occurs in almost all patients. Acute cardiac tamponade is almost always fatal unless the pressure is relieved by removing pericardial fluid, by needle pericardiocentesis, or surgery.

Acute Pericarditis

Pericarditis is an inflammation of the visceral or parietal pericardium.

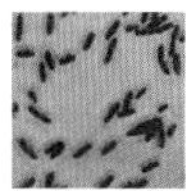

ETIOLOGIC FACTORS: The causes of pericarditis are similar to those of myocarditis (Table 9-5). In most cases, the cause of acute pericarditis is obscure and (as in myocarditis) is attributed to undiagnosed viral infection. Bacterial pericarditis is unusual in the antibiotic era. Metastatic tumors may induce serofibrinous or hemorrhagic exudative and inflammatory reactions when they involve the pericardium. Pericarditis associated with myocardial infarction and rheumatic fever is discussed above.

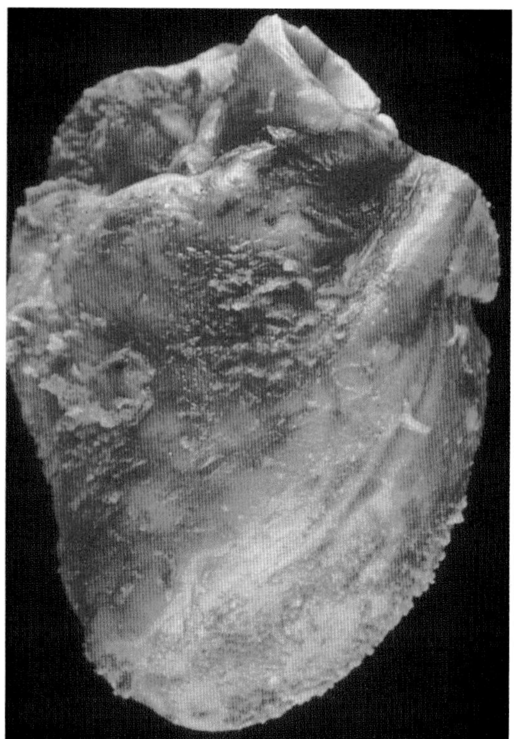

FIGURE 9-35. **Fibrinous pericarditis.** The heart of a patient who died in uremia displaying a shaggy, fibrinous exudate covering the visceral pericardium.

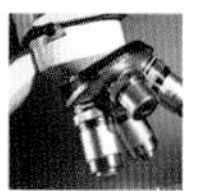

PATHOLOGY: Acute pericarditis can be **fibrinous, purulent,** or **hemorrhagic,** depending on gross and microscopic characteristics of the pericardial surfaces and fluid. The most common form is fibrinous pericarditis, in which the normal smooth, glistening pericardial surfaces are replaced by a dull, granular, fibrin-rich exudate. The rough texture of inflamed pericardial surfaces produces a characteristic friction rub on auscultation. Effusion fluid in fibrinous pericarditis is usually rich in protein, and the pericardium contains mainly mononuclear inflammatory cells. Uremia can cause fibrinous pericarditis (Fig. 9-35), but with the widespread availability of renal dialysis, uremic pericarditis is now unusual in the United States. The most common causes are viral infection and pericarditis after myocardial infarcts.

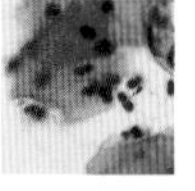

CLINICAL FEATURES: Initial manifestations of acute pericarditis are sudden, severe, substernal chest pain, sometimes referred to the back, shoulder, or neck. These symptoms differ from the pain of angina pectoris or myocardial infarction by their failure to radiate down the left arm. A characteristic pericardial friction rub is easily heard. Idiopathic or viral pericarditis is a self-limited disorder, but it may infrequently lead to constrictive pericarditis. Corticosteroids are the treatment of choice. Therapy for other specific forms of acute pericarditis varies with the cause.

Constrictive Pericarditis May Mimic Right Heart Failure

Constrictive pericarditis is a chronic fibrosing disease of the pericardium that compresses the heart and restricts inflow.

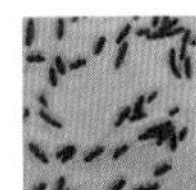
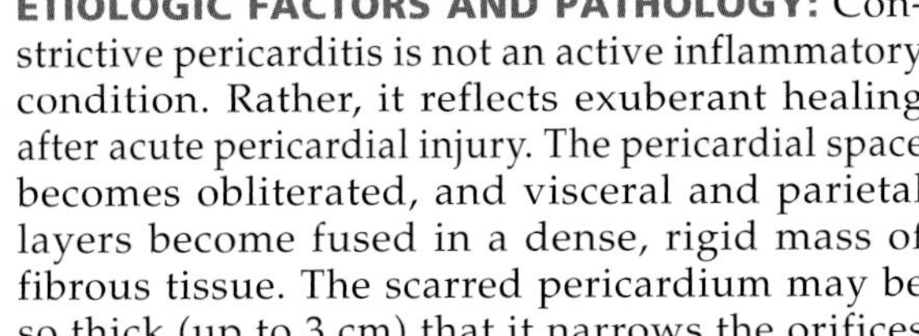

ETIOLOGIC FACTORS AND PATHOLOGY: Constrictive pericarditis is not an active inflammatory condition. Rather, it reflects exuberant healing after acute pericardial injury. The pericardial space becomes obliterated, and visceral and parietal layers become fused in a dense, rigid mass of fibrous tissue. The scarred pericardium may be so thick (up to 3 cm) that it narrows the orifices of the venae cavae. The fibrous envelope may be calcified. Tuberculosis today accounts for fewer than 15% of cases of constrictive pericarditis in industrialized countries, but it is still the major cause in underdeveloped regions. The condition is uncommon today and, in developed countries, is predominantly idiopathic.

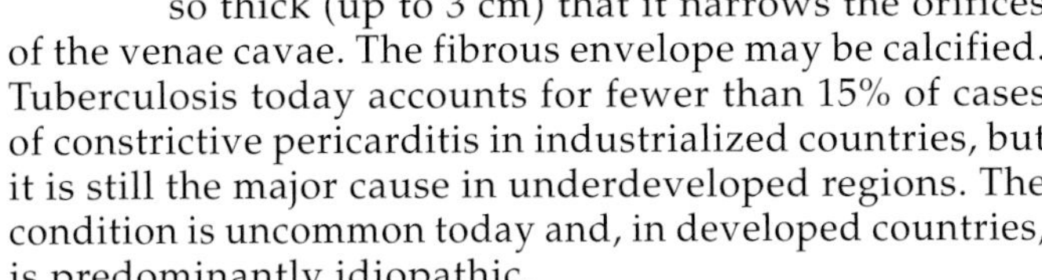

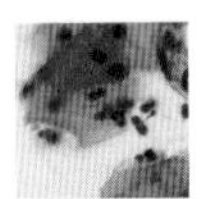

CLINICAL FEATURES: Patients with constrictive pericarditis have small, quiet hearts in which venous inflow is restricted because the rigid pericardium limits the diastolic volume of the heart. These patients have high venous pressure, low cardiac output, small pulse pressure, and fluid retention with ascites and peripheral edema. Total pericardiectomy is the treatment of choice.

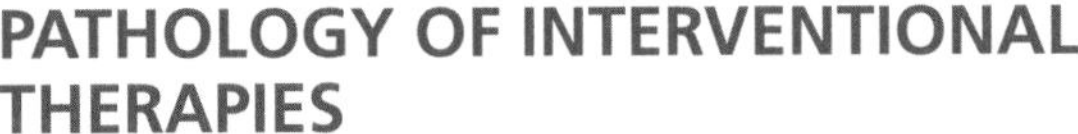

PATHOLOGY OF INTERVENTIONAL THERAPIES

Interventional percutaneous interventions (PCI) include coronary bypass grafts and valve replacement.

Prosthetic Valves

In most patients with severe valve dysfunction, valve replacement is the best prospect for long-term symptomatic improvement. Operative mortality is low, especially for patients with good preoperative myocardial function. Half of all patients with prosthetic valves are free of complications after 10 years.

TISSUE VALVES: The most commonly used tissue valve prostheses employ a mechanical frame to which glutaraldehyde fixed, porcine, aortic valve cusps, or pieces of bovine pericardium are attached. These valves have good hemodynamic characteristics, cause little obstruction, and resist thromboembolic complications. The most common cause of failure of tissue valve prostheses is tissue degeneration, with calcification and fragmentation of prosthetic valve cusps. Improved understanding of prosthetic tissue valve calcification has led to the development of treatments that improve valve longevity and performance.

MECHANICAL VALVES: The most widely used mechanical prostheses involve single or bileaflet tilting disk designs that do not obstruct blood flow across the valve and have excellent durability. However, the risk of thromboembolism makes long-term anticoagulant therapy imperative.

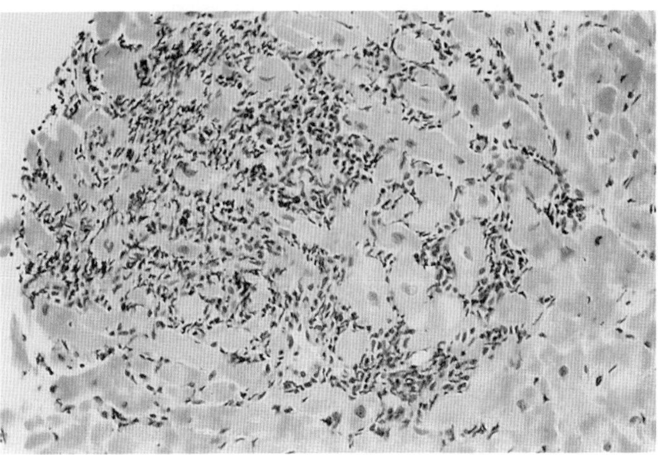

FIGURE 9-36. Cardiac transplant rejection. An endomyocardial biopsy showing lymphocytes surrounding individual myocytes and expanding the interstitium.

Heart Transplantation

The development of effective immunosuppressive regimens and surveillance endomyocardial biopsy protocols has made cardiac transplantation an effective treatment for end-stage heart disease. Allograft rejection (see Chapter 3), however, remains a major complication of cardiac transplantation.

Hyperacute rejection occurs in the presence of blood group incompatibility or major histocompatibility differences. In these situations, preformed antibodies cause immediate vascular injury to the donor heart, with diffuse hemorrhage, edema, intracapillary platelet–fibrin thrombi, vascular necrosis, and infiltration of neutrophils. Screening for blood group incompatibility has rendered this complication rare.

Acute humoral rejection is characterized by vascular deposition of antibody and complement, endothelial cell swelling, and edema. This unusual form of rejection has a worse prognosis than acute cellular rejection.

Acute cellular rejection, the most common form of allograft rejection, usually occurs in the first few months after transplantation. It begins as perivascular T-cell infiltration, which is focal and is not associated with acute myocyte necrosis. This reaction often resolves spontaneously and, therefore, does not necessitate a change in the immunosuppressive regimen. Moderate cellular rejection is characterized by T-cell infiltration into adjacent interstitial spaces, where lymphocytes surround individual myocytes and expand the interstitium (Fig. 9-36). In this instance, focal acute myocyte necrosis is also present. Moderate cellular rejection usually does not produce detectable functional impairment and tends to resolve within a few days to a week after treatment. However, additional immunosuppressive therapy is instituted because moderate cellular rejection can progress to severe rejection. The latter is characterized by vascular damage, widespread myocyte necrosis, neutrophil infiltration, interstitial hemorrhage, and functional impairment.

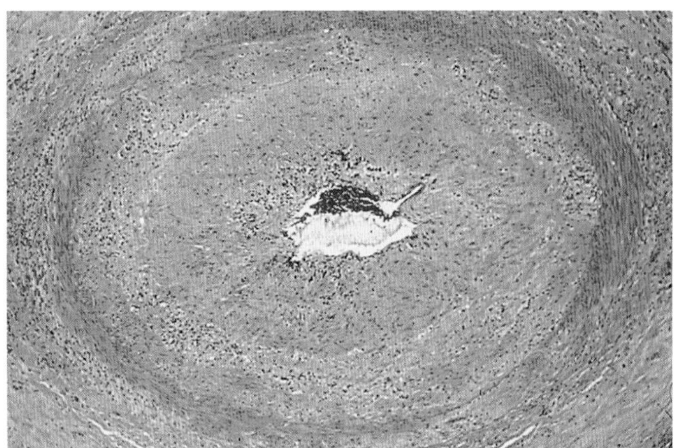

FIGURE 9-37. Chronic cardiac transplant rejection. An intramyocardial branch of a coronary artery showing prominent intimal proliferation and inflammation with concentric narrowing of the lumen.

The early stage of cellular allograft rejection is often asymptomatic. Once symptoms develop, rejection is usually advanced and has caused irrecoverable loss of cardiac myocytes. The most reliable screening procedure is endomyocardial biopsy of the right side of the interventricular septum, via cardiac catheterization.

Chronic vascular rejection, also referred to as **accelerated coronary artery disease**, is the most common cause of death in heart transplant patients beyond the first year after transplantation. Rejection affects proximal and distal epicardial coronary arteries, the penetrating coronary artery branches, and even arterioles. Accelerated coronary artery disease is characterized by concentric intimal proliferation (Fig. 9-37), which can lead to coronary occlusion and myocardial infarction. This complication is silent because the transplanted heart is denervated. Thus, extensive myocardial damage can develop before a transplant patient is aware that ischemic injury has occurred.

10 The Respiratory System

Mary Beth Beasley ▪ William D. Travis

LEARNING OBJECTIVES

- Distinguish between the components of the upper and lower respiratory system.
- List common opportunistic infectious agents associated with the tracheobronchial tree, the alveoli, and the lung interstitium.
- Describe the components of the pulmonary vasculature.
- Describe the conditions that lead to pulmonary hypoplasia.
- Distinguish between extralobar and intralobar sequestration.
- List the most significant irritant gases commonly found in the atmosphere.
- Distinguish between infectious agents most often associated with the airways and those associated with pneumonia.
- Compare *pneumococcal* and *staphylococcal* pneumonia in terms of epidemiology and tissue pathology.
- Define red and gray hepatization.
- List common opportunistic agents associated with pneumonia.
- Discuss common sources and outcomes of pulmonary infections by anaerobes.
- Describe the etiology and pathogenesis of tuberculosis.
- Describe pathogens likely to be associated with granulomatous lung inflammation.
- Compare the pathogenesis of viral versus bacterial pneumonias.
- Distinguish between three common presentations of *Aspergillus* infection of the lung.
- Define two histopathologic patterns of the acute response of bronchi and bronchioles to infectious agents.
- Distinguish between obstructive and nonobstructive bronchiectasis.
- Describe the etiology and pathogenesis of diffuse alveolar damage.
- Describe the relationship of neonatal respiratory distress syndrome and diffuse alveolar damage.
- List several clinical settings in which diffuse pulmonary hemorrhagic syndrome may occur.
- Distinguish between idiopathic and secondary eosinophilic pneumonia in terms of presentation and potential etiologies.
- List common causes of lipid pneumonias.
- Compare and contrast chronic bronchitis and emphysema in terms of etiology and histopathology.
- Distinguish between centrilobular and panacinar emphysema.
- What is the most prominent pathophysiologic response in asthma?
- List several common trigger events that may result in asthma.
- List two broad classes of pulmonary disease defined as restrictive.
- Compare and contrast common agents resulting in pneumoconiosis.
- Distinguish between hypersensitivity pneumonitis and pneumoconiosis.
- Describe the pathogenesis and pathology of sarcoidosis.
- Discuss the tissue presentation of usual interstitial pneumonia.
- Compare and contrast usual interstitial pneumonia and organizing pneumonia pattern.
- Distinguish between granulomatosis with polyangiitis, microscopic polyangiitis, and eosinophilic granulomatosis with polyangiitis.
- Discuss the pathophysiologic mechanisms that result in pulmonary hypertension and the consequent pulmonary pathology.
- Describe a common benign pulmonary neoplasm.
- Distinguish between the major forms of pulmonary carcinoma.
- Describe the association between smoking and the various major forms of pulmonary carcinoma.
- Compare the major classifications of pulmonary adenocarcinoma.
- Describe aspects of the molecular pathogenesis of pulmonary carcinoma of therapeutic significance.
- Define the terms Pancoast tumor, Pancoast syndrome, and Horner syndrome.
- Distinguish between typical and atypical carcinoid tumors of the lung.
- Describe the most common paraneoplastic syndromes associated with lung tumors.
- List common causes of pneumothorax and pleural effusions.
- Describe the etiology and pathology associated with malignant mesothelioma.

THE NORMAL RESPIRATORY SYSTEM

Anatomy

The respiratory system is divided into upper and lower zones. The upper respiratory system consists of the nose, its associated passages, and the paranasal sinuses; the pharynx; and the upper larynx. These are discussed in Chapter 21. The lower respiratory system encompasses the trachea, bronchi, and the lung and its associated components; the lobar bronchi; bronchioles alveoli; vasculature; and supporting interstitium.

TRACHEA AND BRONCHI: The trachea is a hollow tube up to 25 cm in length and 2.5 cm in diameter. The right bronchus diverges at a lesser angle from the trachea than does the left, which is why foreign material is more frequently aspirated on the right side. On entering the lung, the main bronchi divide into lobar bronchi, then into individual units, the segmental bronchi, which supply the 19 lung segments units each with its own bronchovascular supply.

The tracheobronchial tree contains cartilage and submucosal mucous glands in the wall (Fig. 10-1). The latter are compound tubular glands, which contain **mucous cells** (pale) and **serous cells** (granular, more basophilic). Although the pseudostratified epithelium appears as layers, all cells reach the basement membrane. Most cells are ciliated, but there are also mucus-secreting **(goblet)** cells and basal cells. The **basal cells,** which do not reach the surface, are precursors that differentiate into more specialized tracheobronchial epithelial cells. There are also nonciliated columnar cells, or **club cells** (formerly known as **Clara cells**), which accumulate and detoxify many inhaled toxic agents (e.g., nitrogen dioxide [NO_2]). **Neuroendocrine cells** are scattered in the tracheobronchial mucosa and contain a variety of hormonally active polypeptides and vasoactive amines.

BRONCHIOLES: Distal to the bronchi are the bronchioles, which differ from bronchi in that they lack cartilage and mucus-secreting glands in their terminal region (Fig. 10-1). Bronchiolar epithelium becomes thinner with progressive branching, until only one cell layer is present. The last purely conducting structure free of alveoli is the **terminal bronchiole**, which exhibits pseudostratified ciliated respiratory epithelium and a smooth muscle wall. Mucous cells gradually disappear from the lining of the bronchioles until they are entirely replaced in the small bronchioles by nonciliated, columnar club cells. Terminal bronchioles divide into **respiratory bronchioles**, which merge into **alveolar ducts** and **alveoli**. The gas exchange units of the lung are called **acini** and consist of respiratory bronchioles, alveolar ducts, and alveoli.

ALVEOLI: Alveoli are lined by two types of epithelium (Fig. 10-1). **Type I cells** cover 95% of the alveolar surface but comprise only 40% of alveolar epithelial cells. They are thin and have a large surface area, a combination that facilitates gas exchange. **Type II cells** produce surfactant and make up 60% of the alveolar lining cells. They are more cuboidal than type I cells and cover only 5% of the alveolar surface. Type I cells are highly vulnerable to injury. When they are lost, type II pneumocytes multiply and differentiate to form new type I cells, restoring the integrity of the alveolar surface.

Alveolar epithelial and endothelial cells are ideally arranged for gas exchange. The cytoplasm of epithelial and endothelial cells is spread very thinly on either side of a fused basement membrane, allowing efficient exchange of oxygen and carbon dioxide. An extensive capillary network supplies 85% to 95% of the alveolar surface. Away from the site of gas exchange, interstitial connective tissue is more abundant, consisting of collagen, elastin, and proteoglycans. Fibroblasts and myofibroblasts may also be present. This expanded region forms the interstitial space of the alveolar wall, where significant fluid and molecular exchange occurs.

PULMONARY VASCULATURE: The lung has a **dual blood supply** from the pulmonary and the bronchial systems. Pulmonary arteries accompany airways in a sheath of connective tissue, the **bronchovascular bundle**. The more proximal arteries are elastic and are succeeded by muscular arteries, pulmonary arterioles, and, eventually, pulmonary capillaries.

The smallest veins, which resemble the smallest arteries, join other veins and drain into the lobular septa, which are connective tissue partitions that subdivide the lung into small respiratory units. In these septa, the veins form a network separate from the bronchovascular bundles.

Bronchial arteries arise from the thoracic aorta and nourish the bronchial tree as far as the respiratory bronchioles. These arteries are accompanied by their respective veins, which drain into the azygos or hemiazygos veins.

There are no lymphatics in most alveolar walls. However, alveoli located in periphery of acini adjacent to the lobular septa, bronchovascular bundles, or pleura have lymphatics, which follow those structures. Pleural lymphatics drain toward the hilus through the bronchovascular lymphatics.

CONGENITAL ANOMALIES

BRONCHIAL ATRESIA: This abnormality most often involves the bronchus to the apical posterior segment of the left upper lobe. In infants, the lesion may result in an overexpanded part of the lung. In later life, the overexpanded lobe may also be emphysematous. Bronchial mucus accumulating distal to the atretic region may appear on radiologic examination as a mass.

PULMONARY HYPOPLASIA: This condition reflects incomplete or defective lung development. The lung is smaller than normal, with fewer and smaller acini. This is the most common congenital lesion of the lung, found in 10% of neonatal autopsies. In most cases (90%), it occurs in association with other congenital anomalies, most of which involve the thorax. The lesion may be accompanied by hypoplasia of bronchi and pulmonary vessels if the insult occurs early in gestation, as in congenital diaphragmatic hernia. Pulmonary hypoplasia is also seen in trisomies 13, 18, and 21.

ETIOLOGIC FACTORS: Two major factors may lead to pulmonary hypoplasia:

- **Congenital diaphragmatic hernia** typically occurs on the left side because the pleuroperitoneal canal fails to close. Abdominal viscera are variably present in the affected hemithorax and result in compression of the lung. The degree of hypoplasia is thus variable ranging from so severe as to be incompatible with life, to so slight as to be symptom free. Other causes of hypoplasia include abnormalities of the chest wall, pleural effusions, and ascites, as in hydrops fetalis.
- **Oligohydramnios** (low amniotic fluid volume) is usually as a result of genitourinary anomalies and is an important cause of pulmonary hypoplasia (see Chapter 5).

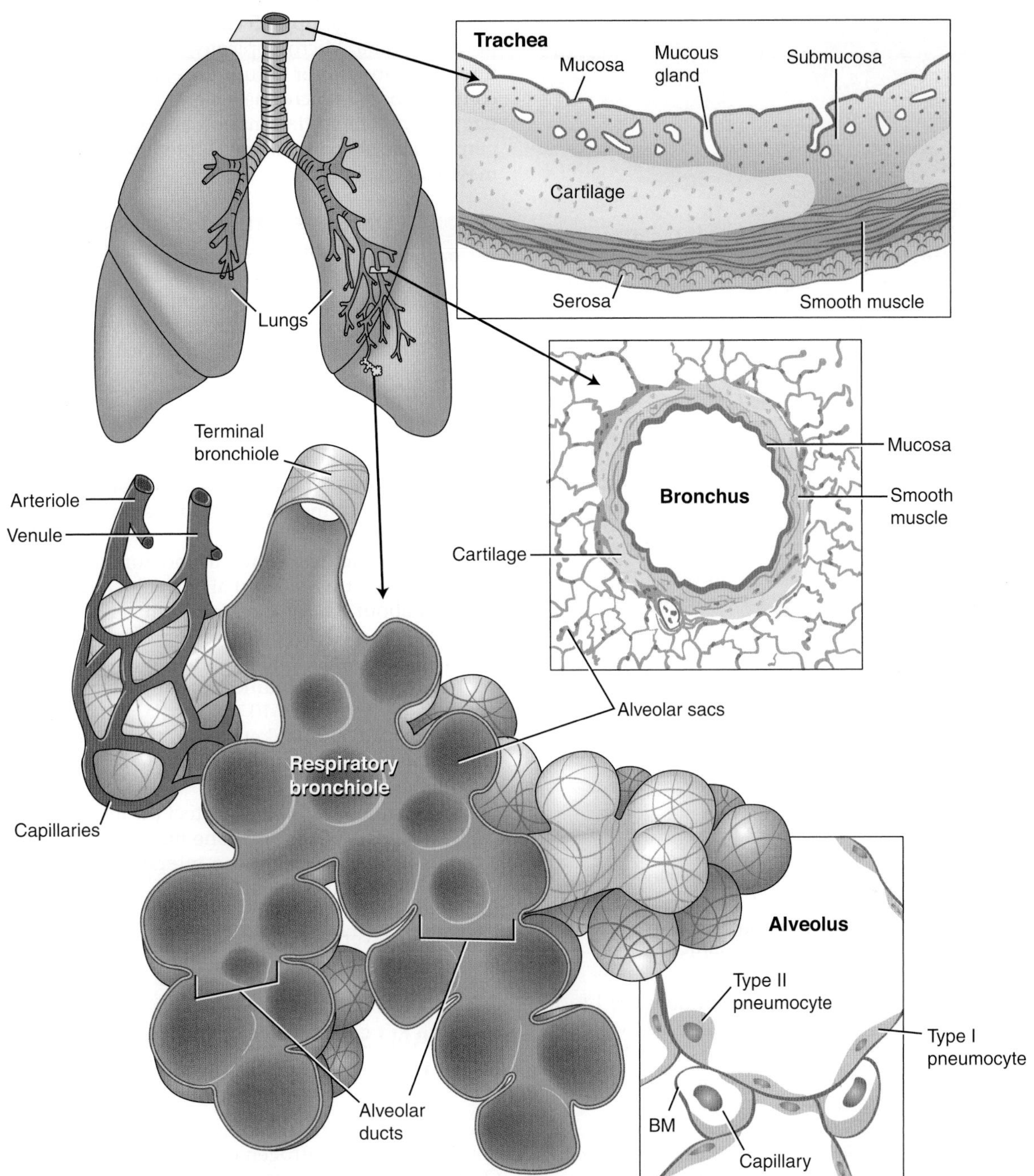

FIGURE 10-1. Anatomy of the lung. The conducting structures of the lung include (1) the trachea, which has horseshoe-shaped cartilages; (2) the bronchi, which have plates of cartilage in their walls (both the trachea and bronchi have mucus-secreting glands in their walls); and (3) the bronchioles, which do not have cartilage in their walls and terminate in the terminal bronchioles. The gas-exchanging components compose the unit distal to the terminal bronchiole, namely, the acinus. Alveoli are lined by type I cells, which are large, flat cells that cover most of the alveolar wall, and by type II cells, which secrete surfactant and are the progenitor cells of the alveolar epithelium. Gas exchange occurs at the level of the alveolar wall. BM, basement membrane.

CONGENITAL CYSTIC ADENOMATOID MALFORMATION: This common anomaly consists of abnormal bronchiolar structures of varying sizes or distribution. Most cases are seen in the first 2 years of life. The lesion usually affects one lobe of the lung and consists of multiple cyst-like spaces lined by bronchiolar epithelium and separated by loose fibrous tissue (Fig. 10-2). Some patients have other congenital anomalies. The most common presenting symptoms are respiratory distress and cyanosis. Surgical resection is the treatment of choice.

BRONCHOGENIC CYSTS: These are discrete, extrapulmonary, fluid-filled masses lined by respiratory epithelium and limited by walls that contain muscle and cartilage. They

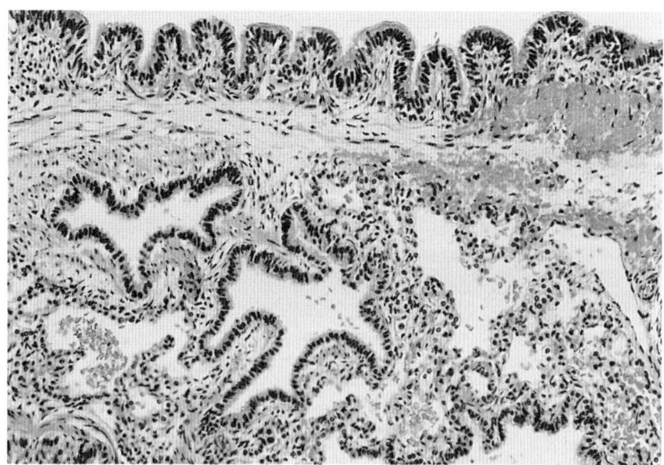

FIGURE 10-2. Congenital cystic adenomatoid malformation. Multiple gland-like spaces are lined by bronchiolar epithelium.

are most commonly found in the middle mediastinum. In newborns, a bronchogenic cyst may compress a major airway and cause respiratory distress. Later in life, secondary infections of cysts may lead to hemorrhage and perforation. Many bronchogenic cysts are asymptomatic and are found on routine chest radiographs.

EXTRALOBAR SEQUESTRATION: Extralobar sequestration is a mass of lung tissue that is not connected to the bronchial tree and is located outside the visceral pleura. An abnormal artery, usually arising from the aorta, supplies the sequestered tissue.

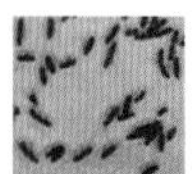

ETIOLOGIC FACTORS: This lesion is thought to originate from an outpouching of the foregut, distinct from the pulmonary anlage, but later loses its connection to the original foregut. It occurs three to four times more often in males than in females and is associated with other anomalies in two thirds of patients.

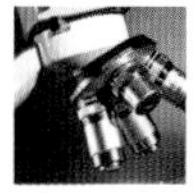

PATHOLOGY: Extralobar sequestrations are 1 to 15 cm pyramidal or round masses, covered by pleura. Microscopically, dilated bronchioles, alveolar ducts, and alveoli are noted. Infection or infarction may alter the histologic appearance.

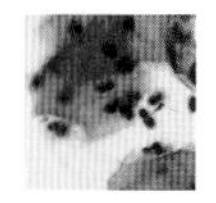

CLINICAL FEATURES: In half of cases, extralobar sequestration is detected before 1 month of age and is recognized by 2 years of age in 75% of patients. The condition is often associated with congenital cystic adenomatoid malformation. In the neonatal period, extralobar sequestration may cause dyspnea and cyanosis, often in the first day of life. In older children, recurrent bronchopulmonary infections often bring it to medical attention. Surgical excision is curative.

INTRALOBAR SEQUESTRATION: Intralobar sequestrations are masses of lung tissue in the visceral pleura, isolated from the tracheobronchial tree and supplied by a systemic artery. These are felt to be acquired abnormalities.

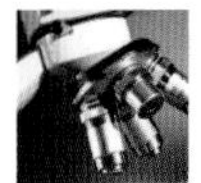

PATHOLOGY: Intralobar sequestrations are almost always found in a lower lobe and are generally unilateral. On gross examination, the sequestered tissue shows the result of chronic recurrent pneumonia, with end-stage fibrosis and honeycomb cystic changes. These cysts range up to 5 cm in diameter and lie in a dense fibrous stroma. Microscopically, the cystic spaces are mostly lined by cuboidal or columnar epithelium, and the lumen contains foamy macrophages and eosinophilic material. Interstitial chronic inflammation and follicular lymphoid hyperplasia are often prominent. Acute and organizing pneumonia may be seen.

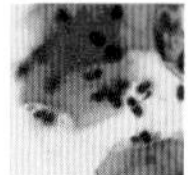

CLINICAL FEATURES: Most cases are discovered in adolescents or young adults. Only one fourth of patients are in the first decade of life, and the lesion is rarely identified in infants. Cough, sputum production, and recurrent pneumonia are seen in almost all patients. Surgical resection is often indicated.

PULMONARY DEFENSE MECHANISMS

The respiratory system has effective defense mechanisms to cope with the numerous particulates and infectious agents inhaled on inspiration.

The **nose and trachea** warm and humidify air entering the lung. The nose traps almost all particles over 10 μm in diameter and about half of those of 3 μm aerodynamic diameter (Fig. 10-3). (Aerodynamic diameter refers to the way particles behave in air rather than to their actual size.)

The **mucociliary blanket** of the airway epithelium disposes of particles 2 to 10 μm in diameter. The ciliary beat drives the mucous blanket toward the trachea. Particles that land on it are thus removed from the lungs and swallowed or coughed up.

Alveolar macrophages protect the alveolar space. These cells are derived from the bone marrow, probably undergo a maturation division in the interstitium of the lung and then enter the alveolar space. They are particularly effective in dealing with particles with aerodynamic diameters under 2 μm. Very small particles are not phagocytosed and are exhaled.

IRRITANTS DERIVED FROM AIR POLLUTION AND INDUSTRIAL ACCIDENTS

The most important irritant gases in the atmosphere are oxidants (ozone and nitrogen oxides) and sulfur dioxide (SO_2). Oxidants derive from the action of sunlight on automobile exhaust and are important in major urban areas. SO_2 is produced mainly by burning fossil fuels. These gases, plus particulate carbon carrying toxins from diesel exhaust, may also compound adverse effects of tobacco smoke. Indeed, inhabitants of urban and more polluted areas have worse pulmonary function (e.g., reduced expiratory flow rates) than do those who reside in cleaner environments. Respiratory infections are also more common in young children who live in regions of high pollution. However, these effects are small in the healthy population.

In people with chronic pulmonary disease, the situation is different: experimentally, ozone makes airways more reactive, an effect related to airway inflammation. ***Thus, air pollution may exacerbate symptoms in asthmatic people and in those with established respiratory disease. In high concentrations, irritant gases produce serious morphologic and functional effects.***

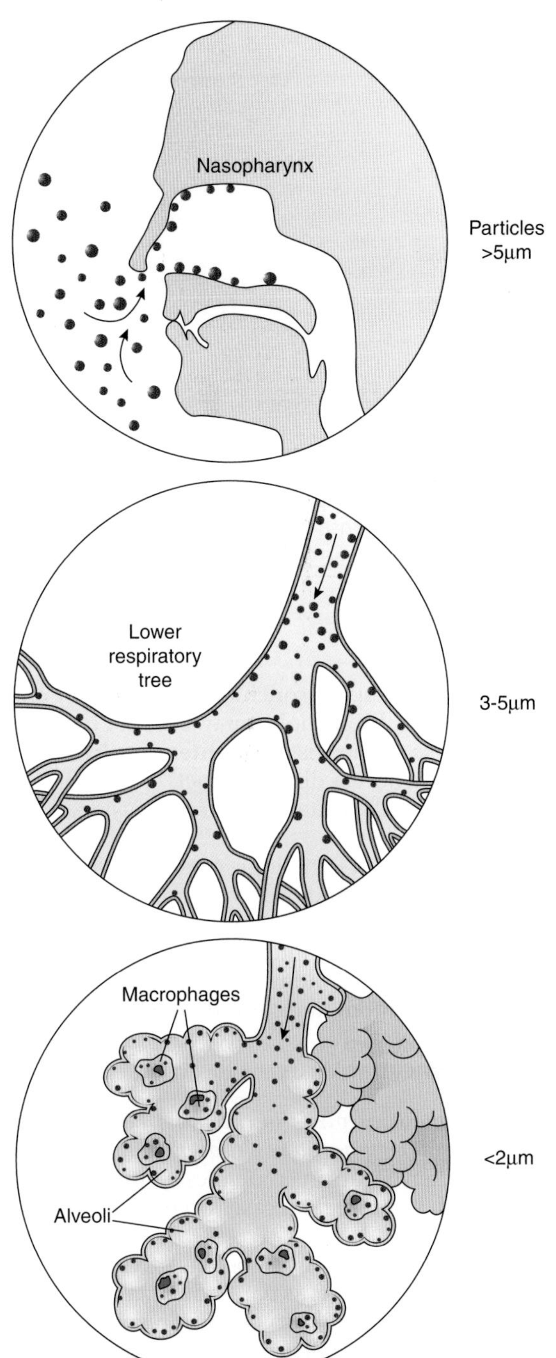

FIGURE 10-3. Deposition of particles in the respiratory tract. Large particles are trapped in the nose. Intermediate-sized particles deposit on the bronchi and bronchioles and are removed by the mucociliary blanket. Smaller particles terminate in the airspaces and are removed by macrophages. Very small particles behave as a gas and are breathed out.

INFECTIONS OF THE LUNG

Airway Infections

Infectious agents that cause disease in the respiratory system predominantly affect the airways, the alveoli, or parenchyma although there is considerable overlap.

Many viral infectious agents that involve the intrapulmonary airways tend to affect the more peripheral airways (producing bronchiolitis). Examples include influenza virus, respiratory syncytial virus (RSV), adenovirus, and measles. Both the bacteria *Bordetella pertussis* and *Mycoplasma pneumoniae* also predominantly affect the airways and are also discussed below. Severe symptomatic infections occur more often in infants and children, and recovery is the rule. Symptoms include cough, a feeling of tightness in the chest, and, in extreme cases, shortness of breath and even cyanosis.

Influenza

Influenza is an acute, usually self-limited, infection of the upper and lower airways, caused by influenza virus that results in tracheobronchitis. These viruses are enveloped and contain single-stranded RNA.

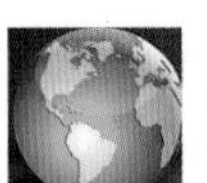

EPIDEMIOLOGY: There are three distinct types of influenza virus that cause human disease, namely, influenza A, influenza B, and influenza C. Influenza A is by far the most common and causes the most severe disease. Influenza is highly contagious, and epidemics frequently spread around the world. New strains emerge regularly, often from animal hosts in parts of the world, largely the Far East, where humans and animals, especially fowl, live in close contact. Influenza strains are identified by their type (A, B, and C), serotype of their hemagglutinin (H) and neuraminidase (virus subtype), geographic site of origin, strain number, and year of isolation (Fig. 10-4).

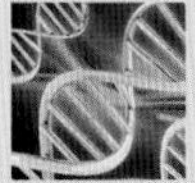

PATHOGENESIS: Influenza spreads from person to person by virus-containing respiratory droplets and secretions. When the virus reaches the respiratory epithelial cell surface, a viral glycoprotein (hemagglutinin) that binds to sialic acid residues on human respiratory epithelium, after which the virus enters the cell. Infection usually involves both the upper and lower airways. Influenza virus causes necrosis and desquamation of ciliated respiratory tract epithelium and a predominantly lymphocytic inflammatory infiltrate. In severe cases of infection, the appearance of the bronchi is dramatic. The surface of the airway is fiery red, reflecting acute inflammation and congestion of the mucosa. Extension of infection to the lungs leads to necrosis, sloughing of alveolar lining cells, and the histologic appearance of viral pneumonitis. Destruction of ciliated epithelium cripples mucociliary clearance, predisposing to bacterial pneumonia, especially with *Staphylococcus aureus* and *Streptococcus pneumoniae*.

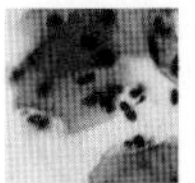

CLINICAL FEATURES: Rapid onset of fever, chills, myalgia, headaches, weakness, and nonproductive cough are characteristic. Symptoms may be primarily those of an upper respiratory infection or those of tracheitis, bronchitis, and pneumonia. Prevention by killed viral vaccines specific to epidemic strains variably effective. Such pneumonia has been the leading cause of death in some previous epidemics.

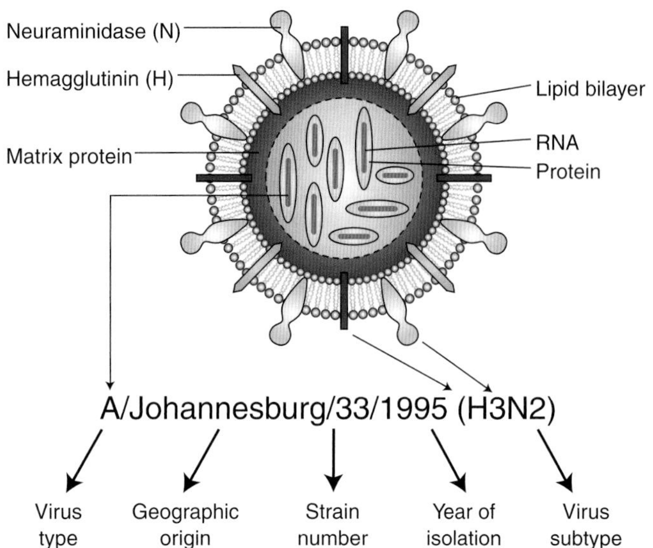

FIGURE 10-4. Nomenclature of influenza virus strains. The virus type (A, B, or C) is based on nucleoprotein characteristics encoded by the *NP* gene of the virus. The H classification is based on the hemagglutinin (most commonly H1, H2, or H3, also H5) encoded by the *HA* gene. The N classification is based on the type of neuraminidase (N1 or N2) encoded by the *NA* gene.

Parainfluenza Virus

The parainfluenza viruses cause acute upper and lower respiratory tract infections, particularly in young children. The four serotypes of these enveloped, single-stranded RNA viruses belong to the paramyxovirus family. They are the most common cause of croup (laryngotracheobronchitis), which is characterized by stridor on inspiration and a "barking" cough.

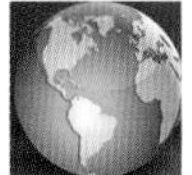

EPIDEMIOLOGY: Croup is common in children under the age of 3 years. The virus spreads from person to person via infectious respiratory aerosols and secretions. Infection is highly contagious; disease is present worldwide.

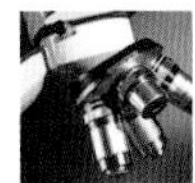

PATHOLOGY: Parainfluenza viruses infect and kill ciliated respiratory epithelial cells and elicit an inflammatory response. ***In very young children, this process frequently extends into the lower respiratory tract, causing bronchiolitis and pneumonitis.*** In young children, in whom the trachea is narrow and the larynx is small, the local edema of laryngotracheitis compresses the upper airway enough to obstruct breathing and cause croup. Parainfluenza infection is associated with fever, hoarseness, and cough. A barking cough is characteristic, as is inspiratory stridor. In older children and adults, symptoms are usually mild.

Adenovirus

Adenoviruses are nonenveloped DNA viruses that are isolated from the respiratory and intestinal tracts of humans and animals. Certain serotypes are common causes of acute respiratory disease and pneumonia in military recruits. Some adenoviruses are important causes of chronic pulmonary disease in infants and young children, resulting in serious sequelae, with extensive bronchiolitis (Fig. 10-5) and then healing by fibrosis. Bronchioles may become obliterated or occluded by loose fibrous tissue **(obliterative bronchiolitis).** Adenoviruses spread via direct contact, fecal–oral transmission, and, occasionally, waterborne transmission.

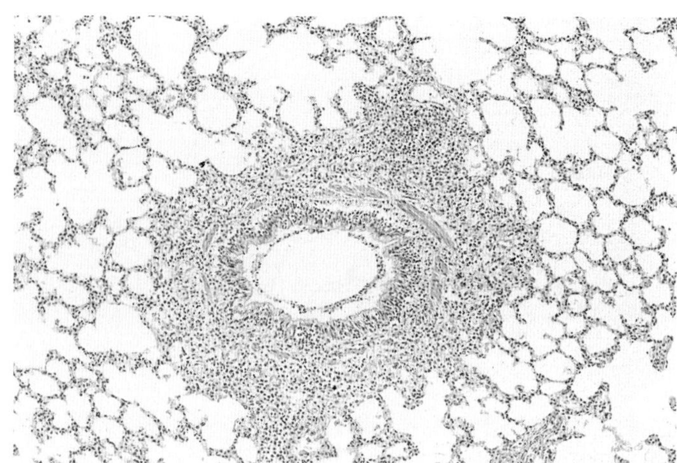

FIGURE 10-5. Bronchiolitis caused by adenovirus. The wall of this bronchiole shows an intense chronic inflammatory infiltrate with local extension into the surrounding peribronchial tissue.

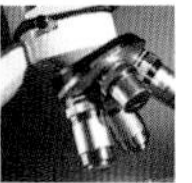

PATHOLOGY: Pathologic changes include necrotizing bronchitis and bronchiolitis, in which sloughed epithelial cells and inflammatory infiltrate fill damaged bronchioles. Interstitial pneumonitis is characterized by areas of consolidation, with extensive necrosis, hemorrhage, and a mononuclear inflammatory infiltrate.

Respiratory Syncytial Virus

Respiratory syncytial virus is the most common cause of bronchiolitis and pneumonia in children younger than 1 year. The infection often occurs in epidemics in nurseries. It is usually self-limited, but rare fatal cases occur.

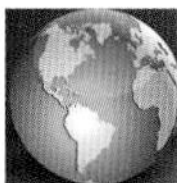

EPIDEMIOLOGY: RSV belongs to the same family, Paramyxoviridae, as parainfluenza virus. It spreads rapidly from child to child in respiratory aerosols and secretions, particularly in daycare centers, hospitals, and other settings, where small children are confined.

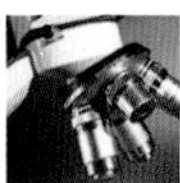

PATHOLOGY: RSV produces necrosis and sloughing of bronchial, bronchiolar, and alveolar epithelium, associated with a predominantly lymphocytic inflammatory infiltrate. Peribronchiolar inflammation and disorganization of the epithelium are evident. Severe overdistention may be found without obvious bronchiolar obstruction, possibly owing to displacement of surfactant from the bronchiolar surface.

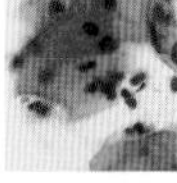

CLINICAL FEATURES: Infants and young children with RSV bronchiolitis or pneumonitis present with wheezing, cough, and respiratory distress, sometimes accompanied by fever. The illness is usually self-limited, resolving in 1 to 2 weeks. In older children and adults, RSV produces much milder disease.

Measles

Measles virus is an RNA paramyxovirus that causes an acute illness, characterized by upper respiratory tract symptoms, fever, and rash. At one time a major cause of bronchiolitis in children, the disease is rarely a problem in developed countries where immunization is widespread. Imported disease has produced a number of cases in the United States among children whose parents have shunned childhood vaccines.

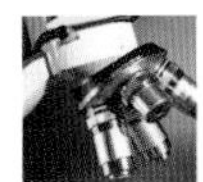

PATHOLOGY: The initial site of measles infection is the mucous membranes of the nasopharynx and bronchi. Two surface glycoproteins, "H" and "F," mediate viral attachment and fusion with respiratory epithelium. The virus then spreads to regional lymph nodes and the bloodstream, leading to widespread dissemination and characteristic involvement of the skin and lymphoid tissues. Infection is characterized by very large (100 μm) multinucleated giant cells with nuclear inclusions and large eosinophilic cytoplasmic inclusions (Fig. 10-6). Measles virus produces necrosis of infected respiratory epithelium, with a predominantly lymphocytic inflammatory infiltrate, and a vasculitis of small blood vessels in the skin.

Bordetella Pertussis (Whooping Cough)

This bacterium commonly infects the airways and is the cause of whooping cough. Prior to now common vaccination, the disease commonly led to the development of bronchiectasis. However, the disease has seen a modest increase in frequency related to parental resistance to childhood immunization. Clinically, whooping cough is typified by fever and severe prolonged bouts of coughing, followed by a characteristic deep whooping inspiration.

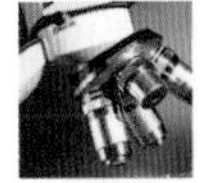

PATHOLOGY: *B. pertussis* initiates infection by attaching to the cilia of respiratory epithelial cells. The organism then elaborates a cytotoxin that kills ciliated cells. Progressive destruction of ciliated respiratory epithelium and the ensuing inflammatory response cause local respiratory symptoms. The infection results in an extensive tracheobronchitis and an acute inflammatory response. Severe bronchial and bronchiolar inflammation is found in fatal cases.

Mycoplasma Pneumoniae (Atypical Pneumonia)

Somewhat misleadingly named, most cases of mycoplasma pneumonia predominantly affect airway and produce tracheobronchitis. Alveolar or interstitial pneumonia occurs only in severe cases. Unlike lobar pneumonia, atypical pneumonia begins insidiously and is often referred to as "walking pneumonia." Leukocytosis is absent or slight, and the course is prolonged. Respiratory symptoms may be minimal or severe, and chest radiography may show patchy intra-alveolar pneumonia or interstitial infiltrates. Infection more characteristically causes a bronchiolitis, with a neutrophilic intraluminal exudate and intense lymphoplasmacytic infiltration in bronchiolar walls (Fig. 10-7). *Mycoplasma* lack rigid cell walls that most bacteria possess. They grow slowly and are difficult to culture by traditional methods. Diagnosis is, therefore, usually established by serologic detection of *M. pneumoniae* antibodies or cold agglutinins. Erythromycin is effective, and the infection is only rarely fatal.

Causative Agents of Pneumonia

Pneumonia is defined as an inflammation predominantly of the alveoli although the lung interstitium is often also affected. This is in distinction to infectious airway disease discussed above. Bacteria are the predominant agent responsible for pneumonia although viruses and fungi may be implicated.

Bacterial pneumonia was once divided into lobar pneumonia or bronchopneumonia, but these terms, although still used, have little clinical relevance today. In **lobar pneumonia,** an entire lobe is consolidated (Fig. 10-8), whereas **bronchopneumonia** refers to scattered solid foci in the same or several lobes (Fig. 10-9). In contrast to airway disease, agents responsible for pneumonia are most often bacterial with *S pneumoniae* (pneumococcus), *Klebsiella pneumoniae*, and *Staphylococcus* being of particular concern.

FIGURE 10-6. Measles pneumonitis. This multinucleated giant cell shows single, eosinophilic, refractile inclusions within each of the nuclei, as well as multiple, irregular, eosinophilic, cytoplasmic inclusions.

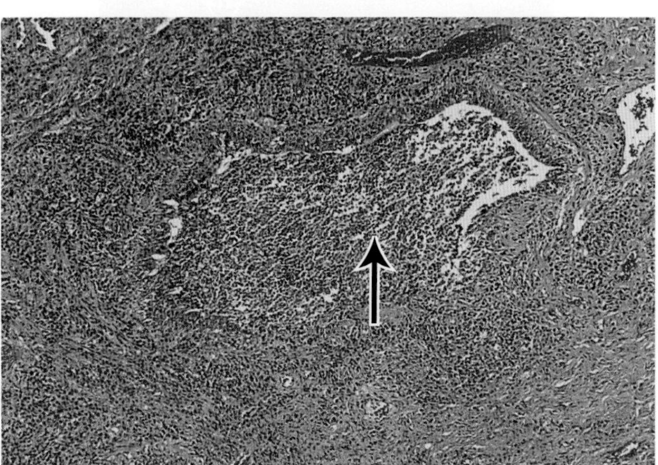

FIGURE 10-7. Mycoplasma pneumonia. Chronic bronchiolitis with a neutrophilic luminal exudate (*arrow*).

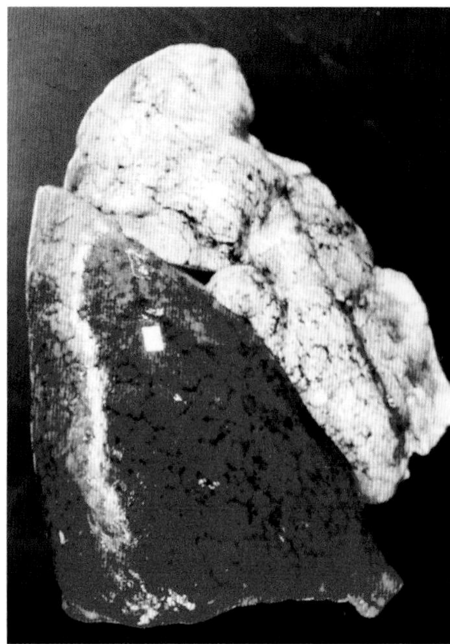

FIGURE 10-8. Lobar pneumonia. The entire left lower lobe is consolidated and in the stage of red hepatization. The upper lobe is normally expanded.

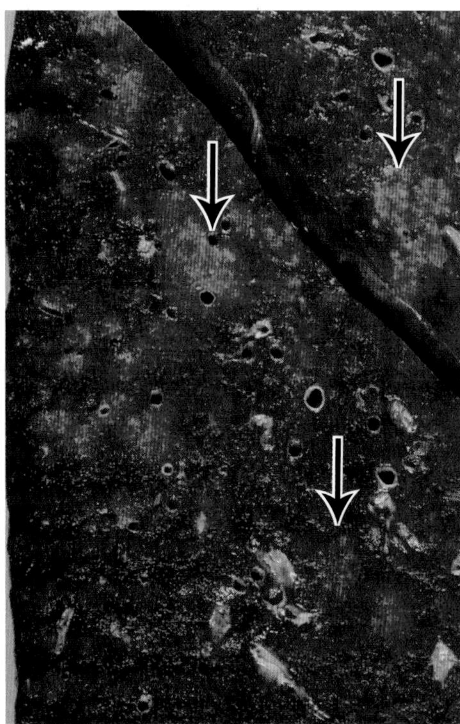

FIGURE 10-9. Bronchopneumonia. Scattered foci of consolidation (*arrows*) are centered on bronchi and bronchioles.

ETIOLOGIC FACTORS: *S. pneumoniae* (pneumococcus) was the classic cause of lobar pneumonia, but with antibiotic therapy, involvement of a lobe tends to be incomplete, and more than one lobe is usually affected. By contrast, bronchopneumonia is still a common cause of death. It typically develops in terminally ill patients, usually in dependent and posterior portions of the lung. Scattered irregular foci of pneumonia are centered on terminal bronchioles and respiratory bronchioles. Bronchiolitis is seen, with polymorphonuclear exudates in adjacent alveoli. Large contiguous areas of alveolar involvement do not occur in bronchopneumonia.

Bacterial pneumonias occur in three settings:

- **Community-acquired pneumonia** arises outside the hospital in people with no primary disorder of the immune system. The term is also used loosely to denote lobar pneumonia.
- **Nosocomial pneumonia** is an infection that develops in hospital environments and tends to affect compromised patients.
- **Opportunistic pneumonia** afflicts people whose immune status is defective.

Bacterial pneumonias are best classified by etiologic agent, as clinical and morphologic features, and thus therapies, often vary with the causative organism.

Most bacteria that cause pneumonia are normal inhabitants of the oropharynx and nasopharynx that reach alveoli by aspiration of secretions. Other routes of infection include inhalation from the environment, hematogenous dissemination from an infectious focus elsewhere, and (rarely) spread of bacteria from an adjacent site. Emergence of a virulent organism in the oropharyngeal flora often precedes the development of pneumonia. Predisposing conditions usually entail depressed host defenses related to cigarette smoking, chronic bronchitis, alcoholism, severe malnutrition, wasting diseases, and poorly controlled diabetes. Debilitated or immunosuppressed patients in the hospital often have altered oropharyngeal flora, and as many as 25% develop nosocomial pneumonia.

Pneumococcal Pneumonia

Antibiotic therapy notwithstanding, *S. pneumoniae* (pneumococcus) pneumonia remains a significant problem. It is mainly a disease of young to middle-aged adults. It is rare in infants, less common in the elderly, and much more frequent in men than women.

The organism is an aerobic, Gram-positive diplococcus. Most strains that cause clinical disease have a capsule. There are over 80 antigenically distinct serotypes of pneumococcus; antibody to one does not protect from infection with another. These are commensal organisms in the oropharynx, and virtually, everyone has been colonized at some time.

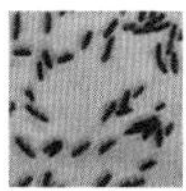

ETIOLOGIC FACTORS: Pneumococcal pneumonia is mostly a result of altered respiratory tract defenses and predisposing infections. For example, a viral upper respiratory infection (e.g., influenza) stimulates bronchial secretions. These provide a hospitable environment for *S. pneumoniae*, which are normal flora of the nasopharynx, to proliferate. The thin, watery secretions carry the organisms into the alveoli, thereby initiating an inflammatory response. The remarkably severe acute inflammation suggests that immunologic mechanisms may be involved. Aspiration of pneumococci may also follow impaired epiglottic reflexes, as occurs with exposure to cold, anesthesia, and alcohol intoxication. Lung injury caused, for example, by congestive heart failure or irritant gases also increases susceptibility to pneumococcal pneumonia.

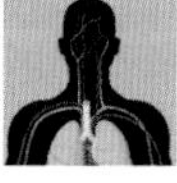

PATHOPHYSIOLOGY: The lower respiratory tract is protected by the mucociliary blanket and cough response, which normally expel organisms that reach the lower airways. Insults that interfere with respiratory defenses, including influenza, other viral respiratory illnesses, smoking, and alcoholism, allow *S. pneumoniae* to reach the alveoli. Once there, the organisms proliferate and elicit an acute inflammatory response. As the bacteria multiply and fill alveoli, they spread to other alveoli. In an immunocompetent person, antipneumococcal antibodies act as opsonins, but a host not previously exposed to the specific infecting strain of *S. pneumoniae* must use the alternative complement pathway to opsonize the bacteria. The pneumococcal capsule protects the bacteria against phagocytosis by alveolar macrophages mediated via the opsonin C3b. Consequently, the organism can proliferate and spread unimpeded by phagocytes until antibody is produced. In the lungs, *S. pneumoniae* spreads rapidly to involve an entire lobe or several lobes (lobar pneumonia).

PATHOLOGY: In the earliest stage of pneumococcal pneumonia, protein-rich edema fluid with abundant organisms fills the alveoli (Fig. 10-10). Marked capillary congestion leads to massive outpouring of polymorphonuclear leukocytes and intra-alveolar hemorrhage (Fig. 10-11). Because the color and firm consistency of the affected lung are reminiscent of the liver, this stage has been aptly named **"red hepatization"** (Fig. 10-10).

The next phase, two or more days later (depending on the success of treatment), involves lysis of neutrophils and appearance of macrophages, which phagocytose the fragmented leukocytes and other inflammatory debris. At this stage, the congestion has diminished, but the lung is still firm (**gray hepatization**) (Fig. 10-10). The alveolar exudate is then removed, and the lung gradually returns to normal.

A number of complications may follow pneumococcal pneumonia:

- **Pleuritis (inflammation of the pleura)**, often painful, is common, because the pneumonia readily extends to the pleura.
- **Pleural effusion** (fluid in the pleural space) is common but usually resolves.
- Empyema/**pyothorax (pus in the pleural space)** results from infection of a pleural effusion and may heal with extensive fibrosis.
- **Bacteremia** occurs during the early stages of pneumococcal pneumonia in more than 25% of patients and may lead to endocarditis or meningitis. Patients whose spleens have been removed often die of this bacteremia.
- **Pulmonary fibrosis** is a rare complication of pneumococcal pneumonia. The intra-alveolar exudate organizes to form intra-alveolar plugs of granulation tissue, known as **organizing pneumonia**. Gradually, increasing alveolar fibrosis gives rise to a shrunken and firm lobe, a rare complication known as **carnification**.
- **Lung abscess (localized collection of pus)** is an unusual complication of pneumococcal pneumonia.

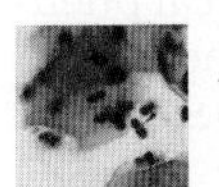

CLINICAL FEATURES: Pneumococcal pneumonia begins abruptly, with fever and chills. Chest pain due to pleural involvement is common. Sputum is characteristically "rusty," because it is derived from altered blood in alveolar spaces. Radiologic studies show alveolar filling in large areas of lung, producing a solid appearance that extends to entire lobes or segments. Before antibiotic therapy, about one third of patients died. Current antibiotic treatment for pneumococcal pneumonia is effective, and although symptoms resolve rapidly, radiographic lesions still take several days to clear. Patients with prior splenectomies

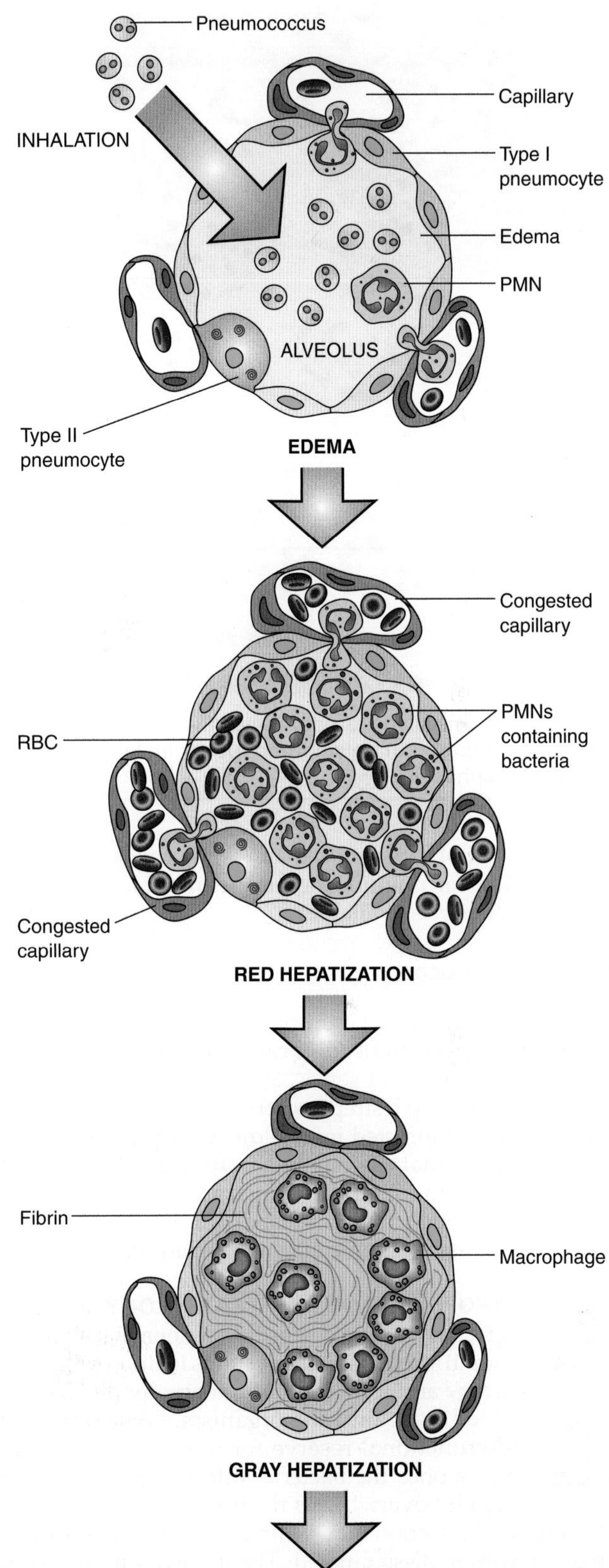

FIGURE 10-10. Pathogenesis of pneumococcal lobar pneumonia. Pneumococci, characteristically in pairs (diplococci), multiply rapidly in alveolar spaces and produce extensive edema. They incite an acute inflammatory response in which polymorphonuclear leukocytes and congestion are prominent (red hepatization). As the inflammatory process progresses, macrophages replace the polymorphonuclear leukocytes and ingest debris (gray hepatization). The process usually resolves, but complications may ensue. PMN, polymorphonuclear neutrophil; RBC, red blood cell.

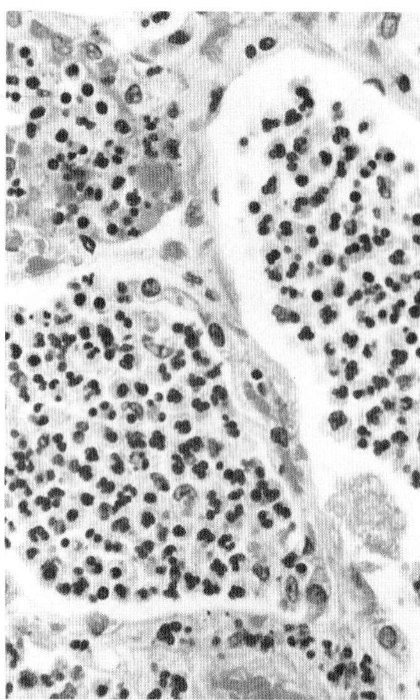

FIGURE 10-11. Pneumococcal pneumonia. Alveoli are packed with an exudate composed of polymorphonuclear leukocytes and occasional macrophages.

are at high risk of rapid, fulminant septic shock and death. Immunization for pneumococcal pneumonia, particularly among the elderly, is available.

Group B Streptococci

Group B streptococci are Gram-positive bacteria that grow in short chains. They are the leading cause of neonatal pneumonia and also meningitis and sepsis. Several thousand neonatal infections with Group B streptococci occur in the United States each year; 30% of infected infants die. Group B streptococci are part of the normal vaginal flora in 10% to 30% of women. Most babies born to colonized women acquire the organisms as they pass through the birth canal. Group B streptococci infrequently cause pyogenic infections in adults.

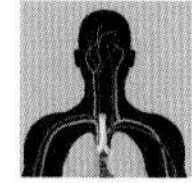

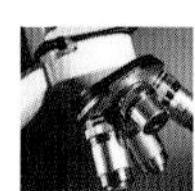

PATHOPHYSIOLOGY AND PATHOLOGY: Particular risk factors associated with the development of neonatal Group B streptococcal infections include premature delivery and low levels of maternally derived IgG antibodies against the organism. Newborns have little functional reserve for granulocyte production, so once the bacterial infection is established, it rapidly overwhelms the body's defenses. Group B streptococcal infection may be limited to the lungs or CNS or may be widely disseminated. The involved tissues show a pyogenic response, often with overwhelming numbers of Gram-positive cocci.

Other Streptococcal Pneumonias

Pulmonary infections with Group A *Streptococcus pyogenes* typically follow viral respiratory tract infections. Such an infection is distinctly unusual in a community setting but is occasionally encountered in debilitated patients.

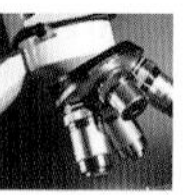

PATHOLOGY: On gross examination, the lungs of patients who die of streptococcal pneumonia are heavy, with bloody edema. Dry consolidation (hepatization) is not a feature of this disease. Microscopically, alveoli are filled with fibrin-containing fluid, but neutrophils are few. Alveolar necrosis may follow prolonged pneumonia. Empyema is a common complication.

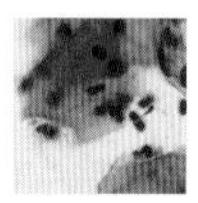

CLINICAL FEATURES: Patients with streptococcal pneumonia have abrupt fever, dyspnea, cough, chest pain, hemoptysis, and often cyanosis. Radiographically, a bronchopneumonia pattern is observed; lobar consolidation is not seen. Intensive antibiotic therapy is indicated.

Streptococcal pneumonia in the newborn is usually caused by Group B streptococci (*Streptococcus agalactiae*), a normal resident of the female genital tract. Symptoms are similar to those of the infantile respiratory distress syndrome. The infants, however, are often full term, have severe toxemia, and may die within a few hours.

Staphylococcal Pneumonia

Although staphylococci account for only 1% of community-acquired bacterial pneumonias, *S. aureus*, a Gram-positive coccus, is a common pulmonary superinfection after influenza and other viral respiratory tract infections. Repeated episodes of staphylococcal pneumonia are seen in patients with cystic fibrosis, owing to colonization of bronchiectatic airways. Nosocomial staphylococcal pneumonia typically occurs in chronically ill people, who are prone to aspiration, and in intubated patients. As noted above, it is a common causative agent of pneumonia in intensive care units. The organism may also be responsible for respiratory tract infections, including pneumonia in young infants, especially those under 2 months of age.

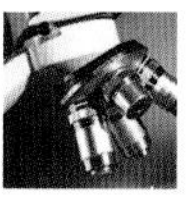

PATHOLOGY: Like staphylococcal infections elsewhere, staphylococcal pneumonia is characterized by abscess development. The multiple foci of staphylococcal pneumonia produce many small abscesses. In infants and, less often, in adults, these may lead to **pneumatoceles**, thin-walled cystic spaces lined primarily by respiratory tissue. Pneumatoceles may enlarge rapidly and compress surrounding lung or rupture into the pleural cavity and cause a tension pneumothorax. A pneumatocele develops when an abscess breaks into an airway, allowing drainage of purulent material and expansion of the former abscess by the pressure of inspired air. Cavitation and pleural effusions are common complications of staphylococcal pneumonia, but empyema is infrequent. Staphylococcal pneumonia requires aggressive therapy, particularly because *S. aureus* is often antibiotic resistant.

Legionella Pneumonia

In 1976, a mysterious respiratory disease with high mortality broke out at an American Legion convention in Philadelphia.

The responsible organism, *Legionella pneumophila*, is a fastidious bacterium that is difficult to grow in culture. Serologic and histologic studies showed that several previously unrecognized epidemics of the same disease had occurred. *Legionella* organisms thrive in aquatic environments, and outbreaks of pneumonia have been traced to contaminated water in air-conditioning cooling towers, evaporative condensers, and construction sites. Person-to-person spread does not occur, and there is no animal or human reservoir.

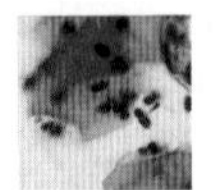

PATHOLOGY: *Legionella* organisms are Gram-negative but are difficult to visualize without silver impregnation or immunofluorescent stains. In fatal *Legionella* pneumonia, multiple lobes show bronchopneumonia, with large confluent areas. Alveoli contain fibrin and inflammatory cells, with either neutrophils or macrophages predominating. Necrosis of inflammatory cells (leukocytoclasis) may be extensive. If the patient survives for several weeks, the exudate may show fibrous organization. Empyema occurs in one third of cases. *Legionella* organisms are usually abundant within and outside the phagocytic cells.

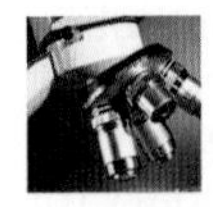

CLINICAL FEATURES: *Legionella* pneumonia tends to begin abruptly, with malaise, fever, muscle aches and pains and, curiously, abdominal pain. A productive cough is usual, and chest pain due to pleuritis occasionally occurs. Mortality is 10% to 20%, especially in immunocompromised patients.

Klebsiella and Enterobacter Pneumonia

K. pneumoniae are short, encapsulated, Gram-negative bacilli. Other than *S. pneumoniae*, *Klebsiella* is the only organism that causes lobar pneumonia with any frequency. However, it accounts for only about 1% of community-acquired pneumonias although it is a common organism in nosocomial (hospital-acquired) infections. *Klebsiella* pneumonia occurs mostly in middle-aged, often alcoholic, men. Diabetes and chronic lung disease also increase the risk. Secondary pneumonia caused by these bacteria may complicate influenza or other respiratory viral infections. *Enterobacter* are related organisms with a similar profile of pathogenicity and are responsible for 10% of pneumonia cases in intensive care units, ranking third after *S. aureus* and *Pseudomonas aeruginosa*.

PATHOLOGY: The pathologic stages of *Klebsiella* pneumonia are not as distinctly defined as those in pneumococcal pneumonia, but acute-phase congestion and hemorrhage are less pronounced. The organism has a thick, gelatinous capsule, giving the cut lung surface a characteristic mucoid appearance. Another distinctive feature of *Klebsiella* pneumonia is increased size of the affected lobe, causing the fissure to "bulge" toward the unaffected region. There is a tendency toward tissue necrosis and abscess formation. A serious complication is **bronchopleural fistula** (i.e., a communication between the bronchial airway and the pleural space).

The onset of *Klebsiella* pneumonia is less dramatic than that of pneumococcal pneumonia, but the disease may be more dangerous. Before antibiotics, mortality from *Klebsiella* pneumonia was 50% to 80%. Even with prompt antibiotic treatment, mortality remains considerable.

Opportunistic Pneumonias Caused by Gram-Negative Bacteria

Pneumonias caused by Gram-negative organisms, most commonly *Escherichia coli* and *P. aeruginosa*, have become more common with the advent of immunosuppressive and cytotoxic therapies, treatment with broad-spectrum antibiotics, and AIDS.

ESCHERICHIA COLI: *E. coli* pneumonia may follow bacteremia after abdominal and urogenital surgery, even in patients who are not immunosuppressed. It is also seen in cancer patients given chemotherapy and in people with chronic lung or heart disease. It occurs as a bronchopneumonia and responds poorly to treatment.

PSEUDOMONAS AERUGINOSA: *Pseudomonas* pneumonia is most common in patients who are immunocompromised or who have burns or cystic fibrosis. A history of antibiotic treatment for another infection is common. Often, an infectious vasculitis, with large numbers of organisms in blood vessel walls, results in pulmonary infarction. Antibiotic treatment of *Pseudomonas* pneumonia is often unsatisfactory.

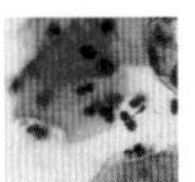

CLINICAL FEATURES: Because pneumonia caused by opportunistic Gram-negative organisms afflicts patients who are often already severely ill, symptoms of pneumonia may be less obvious than in healthy persons. Increased malaise, fever, and labored breathing are often the first signs of pneumonia. If pneumonia remains untreated, the organisms may invade the blood to produce fatal septicemia. Treatment requires parenteral antibiotics, but, unfortunately, pseudomonas is resistant to most in current use.

Pneumonias Caused by Anaerobic Organisms

Many anaerobic organisms are normal commensals of the oral cavity, especially in people with poor dental hygiene. These include certain streptococci, fusobacteria, and *Bacteroides* sp. Swallowing disorders, as in stuporous alcoholics, anesthetized patients, and people subject to seizures, predisposes to aspirating anaerobic bacteria. Resulting pulmonary infections cause necrotizing pneumonias, which often give rise to lung abscesses.

Lung abscesses are localized accumulations of pus, with destruction of pulmonary parenchyma, including alveoli, airways, and blood vessels; anaerobic bacteria are responsible in over 90% of cases. Infections are typically polymicrobial, often with fusiform bacteria and *Bacteroides* spp. Not surprisingly, alcoholism is the most common condition predisposing to lung abscess. Drug overdoses, epilepsy, and neurologic impairment also increase the risk. Other causes of lung abscess include necrotizing pneumonias, bronchial obstruction, infected pulmonary emboli, penetrating trauma, and extension of infection from adjacent tissues.

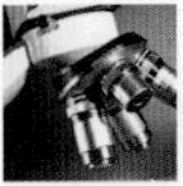

PATHOLOGY: Lung abscesses typically range from 2 to 6 cm; 10% to 20% have multiple cavities, usually arising after a necrotizing pneumonia or a shower of septic pulmonary emboli. The right side of the lung is more often involved than the left because the right main bronchus follows the direction of the trachea more closely at its bifurcation. Acute lung abscesses are not distinctly separated from the surrounding lung parenchyma. They contain abundant polymorphonuclear leukocytes and, depending on the age of the lesion, variable numbers of macrophages and necrotic tissue debris. Initially, they are surrounded by hemorrhage, fibrin, and inflammation, but as they age, a fibrous wall forms around the margin. Lung abscesses differ from abscesses elsewhere in that they may drain spontaneously into an airway. The cavity thus formed contains air, necrotic debris, and inflammatory exudate (Fig. 10-12), creating an air–fluid level that is easily seen radiographically. The cavity lining eventually becomes covered with regenerating squamous epithelium. Walls of old abscesses may be lined by ciliated respiratory epithelium, making them difficult to distinguish from bronchiectasis.

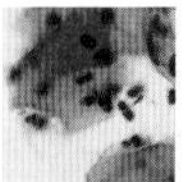

CLINICAL FEATURES: Almost all patients with lung abscess present with fever and cough, characteristically producing large amounts of foul-smelling sputum. Many patients complain of pleuritic chest pain, and 20% develop hemoptysis.

Complications of lung abscess include rupture into the pleural space, which causes empyema, and severe hemoptysis. Abscess drainage into a bronchus may spread infection to other parts of the lung. Despite vigorous antimicrobial therapy, principally directed against anaerobic bacteria, the mortality of lung abscess remains 5% to 10%.

Psittacosis

Psittacosis is a zoonotic lung infection caused by inhalation of *Chlamydia psittaci* in dust contaminated with excreta from birds, among which the disease is endemic. Human disease generally derives from pets and often parrots. The disease is uncommon with 10 cases per year reported in the United States although the true incidence of human disease may be higher. Psittacosis is characterized by severe systemic symptoms, with fever, malaise, and muscle aches, but surprisingly few respiratory symptoms other than cough. Chest radiographs may be negative, and when abnormal, they show irregular consolidation and an interstitial pattern. The pathologic patterns in most cases are unknown, but the disease is likely to be an interstitial pneumonia. In fatal cases, varying degrees of diffuse alveolar damage are present, together with edema, intra-alveolar pneumonia, and necrosis.

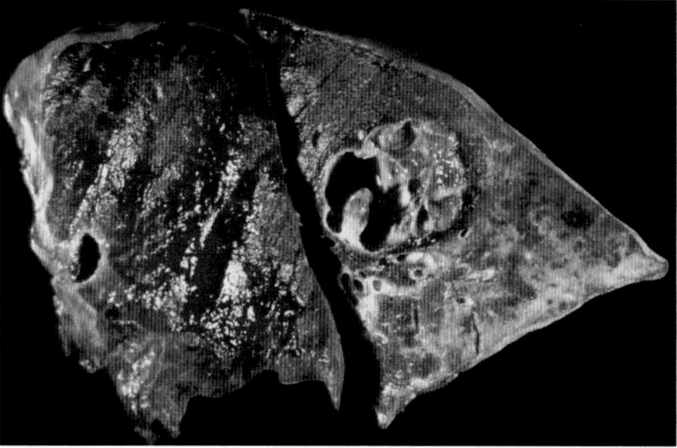

FIGURE 10-12. Pulmonary abscess. A large cystic abscess contains a purulent exudate and is lined by a fibrous wall. Pneumonia is present in the surrounding pulmonary parenchyma.

Anthrax Pneumonia and Pneumonic Plague

Recent world events have focused attention on infectious agents that could be used as weapons of bioterrorism. Chief among these are ***Bacillus anthracis*** and ***Yersinia pestis***.

B. anthracis, a Gram-positive, spore-forming bacillus, is the causative agent of anthrax. Anthrax occurs in many species of domestic animals, but human infection is rare. Transmission is via direct contact with the spores; person-to-person transmission is uncommon. Cutaneous anthrax is rarely fatal, but inhalational anthrax has a high mortality. Anthrax spores are extremely resistant to drying. When inhaled, they are transported to mediastinal lymph nodes, where bacilli emerge and disseminate rapidly through the bloodstream to other organs, including the lungs. Hemorrhagic necrosis of infected organs ensues, along with severe hemorrhagic mediastinitis related to local lymphadenopathy. In the lungs, the disease is manifested by hemorrhagic bronchitis and confluent areas of hemorrhagic pneumonia.

Y. pestis, the causative agent of **plague**, produces two main forms of infection, a bubonic form and a pneumonic form. The disease is a zoonosis of many small rodents and is transmitted to humans by an arthropod vector. In pneumonic plague, the organisms are inhaled directly, and disease may be spread from person to person. The lungs typically show extensive hemorrhagic bronchopneumonia, pleuritis, and mediastinal lymph node enlargement. Untreated disease progresses rapidly and is highly fatal.

Granulomatous Bacterial Pulmonary Infections

Granulomatous pulmonary infections are defined by the formation of the characteristic tissue lesion, the granuloma. The classic and most common causative agent is *Mycobacterium tuberculosis*, which is associated with **caseating granulomas** having a distinctive necrotic (caseous) center. Several other bacterial and fungal pathogens (see below) are also associated with some degree of granuloma formation, but they are not as distinctive and "well formed" as those found in tuberculosis.

Tuberculosis

Although tuberculosis was the scourge of the industrialized world in the 19th and early 20th centuries, its prevalence declined quickly as living and working conditions improved during the 20th century and with the introduction of antituberculosis drugs. However, the infection has recently reemerged, particularly drug-resistant strains and among patients with AIDS. The malady is divided into primary and secondary (or reactivation) tuberculosis.

PRIMARY TUBERCULOSIS: The disease is acquired after initial exposure to *M. tuberculosis*, most commonly from inhaling infected aerosols generated when a person with cavitary secondary tuberculosis coughs. Inhaled organisms multiply in the alveoli because alveolar macrophages cannot readily kill them.

PATHOLOGY: The **Ghon lesion** is the first lesion of primary tuberculosis and features a peripheral parenchymal granuloma, often in the upper lobes. When this lesion is associated with an enlarged mediastinal lymph node, a **Ghon complex** is formed (Fig. 10-13). On gross examination, the healed, subpleural

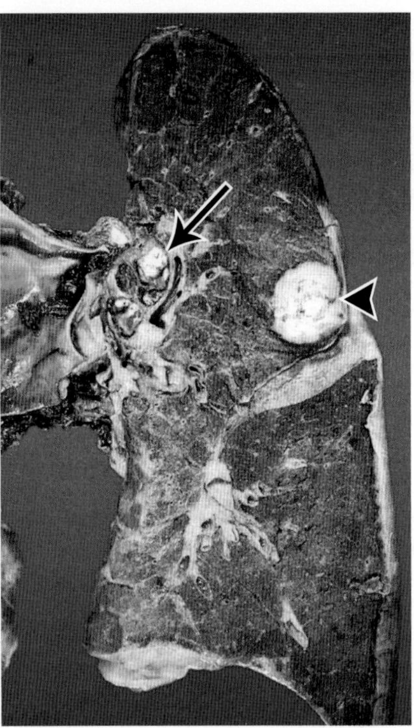

FIGURE 10-13. **Primary tuberculosis.** A healed Ghon complex is represented by a subpleural nodule (*arrowhead*) and involved hilar lymph nodes (*arrow*).

Ghon nodule is 1 to 2 cm in diameter, well circumscribed, and centrally necrotic. In later stages, it is fibrotic and calcified. Microscopically, a tuberculous granuloma is characterized by central caseous necrosis (Fig. 10-14) and varying degrees of fibrosis. The microscopic features of draining hilar lymph nodes are similar to those of the peripheral parenchymal lesion.

Most (>90%) primary tuberculous infections are asymptomatic; lesions remain localized and heal. Sometimes, there is self-limited extension to the pleura, with a secondary pleural effusion. Less often, primary tuberculosis is not limited but spreads to other parts of the lung (**progressive primary tuberculosis**). This usually occurs in young children or immunosuppressed adults. In this situation, the initial lesion enlarges, producing necrotic areas up to 6 cm. Central liquefaction results in cavities, which may expand to occupy most of the lower lobe. At the same time, draining lymph nodes display similar histologic changes. Erosion of a bronchus by the necrotizing process leads to further pulmonary dissemination of the disease.

SECONDARY TUBERCULOSIS: This stage represents reactivation of primary pulmonary tuberculosis or new infection in someone previously sensitized by primary tuberculosis.

PATHOLOGY: The initial reaction to *M. tuberculosis* is different in secondary tuberculosis. A cellular immune response occurs after a latent interval and gives rise to the formation of many granulomas and extensive tissue necrosis. Apical and posterior segments of the upper lobes are most commonly involved, but the superior segment of the lower lobe is also often affected; no part of the lung is excluded. A diffuse, fibrotic, poorly defined lesion develops, with focal areas of caseous necrosis. Often, these foci heal and calcify, but some may erode into bronchi, after which drainage of infectious material creates a tuberculous cavity.

Tuberculous cavities range from under 1 cm to large, cystic areas occupying almost the entire lung. Most measure 3 to 10 cm. They prefer the apices of the upper lobes (Fig. 10-15) but may occur anywhere in the lung. The cavity wall is composed of (1) an inner, thin, gray membrane encompassing soft necrotic nodules; (2) a middle zone of granulation tissue; and (3) an outer collagenous border. The lumen is filled with caseous material containing acid-fast bacilli. Cavities often communicate with a bronchus, and the release of infectious material into airways spreads infection within the lung. The walls of healed tuberculous cavities eventually become fibrotic and calcified.

Secondary tuberculosis is associated with a number of complications:

- **Miliary tuberculosis** refers to the presence of multiple, small (size of millet seeds), tuberculous granulomas (Fig. 10-16) in many organs. The organisms disseminate from the lung or other sites via the blood, usually during secondary tuberculosis, but occasionally in primary disease.
- **Hemoptysis** (bloody cough) is caused by erosion of a tuberculous lesion into small pulmonary arteries adjacent to the cavity wall. It may be severe enough to drown patients in their own blood.
- **Bronchopleural fistula** occurs when a subpleural cavity ruptures into the pleural space. In turn, tuberculous empyema and pneumothorax result.
- **Tuberculous laryngitis** is a consequence of coughing up infectious material.

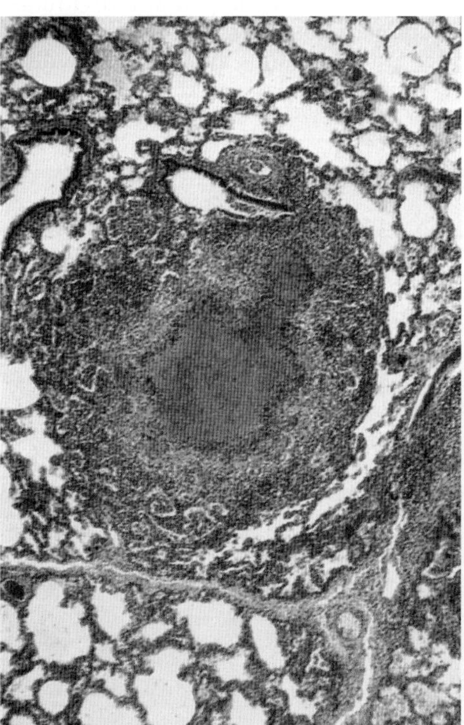

FIGURE 10-14. **Necrotizing granuloma caused by *Mycobacterium tuberculosis*.** A small tuberculous granuloma with conspicuous central caseation is present in the pulmonary parenchyma. The necrotic center is surrounded by histiocytes, giant cells, and fibrous tissue.

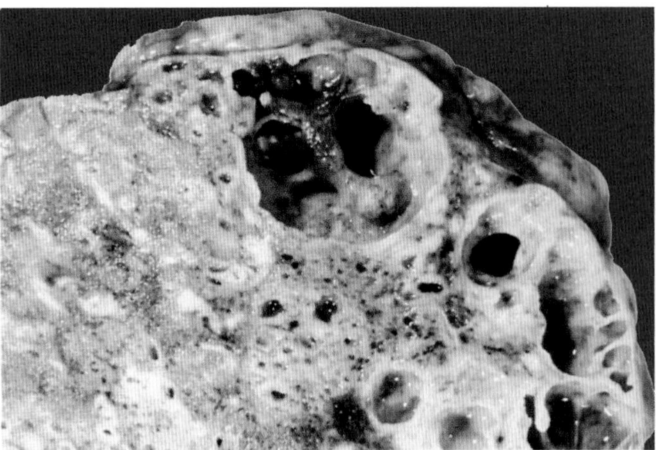

FIGURE 10-15. Cavitary tuberculosis. The apex of the left upper lobe shows tuberculous cavities surrounded by consolidated and fibrotic pulmonary parenchyma that contains small tubercles.

- **Intestinal tuberculosis** follows swallowing of the same tuberculous material.
- **Aspergilloma** is a fungal mass arising by superinfection of a persistent open cavity with *Aspergillus*; the fungi may fill the entire cavity.

MYCOBACTERIUM AVIUM-INTRACELLULARE (MAI): In immunodeficient patients, whose ability to mount a granulomatous reaction may be impaired, MAI pneumonia is characterized by an extensive infiltrate of macrophages and innumerable acid-fast organisms. MAI may colonize airways of older, immunocompetent individuals with underlying pulmonary disorders, such as bronchiectasis, or it may produce granulomatous inflammation with or without cavitation.

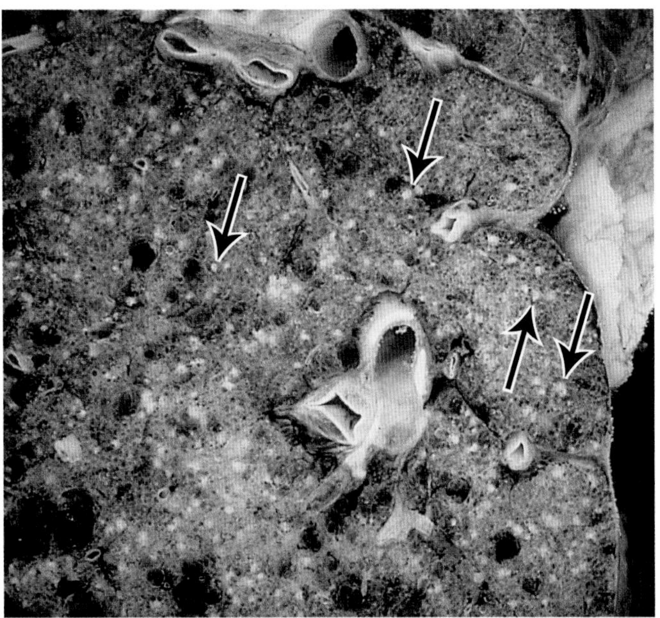

FIGURE 10-16. Miliary tuberculosis. Multiple millimeter-sized nodules (*arrows*) are scattered throughout the lung parenchyma.

Actinomycosis

Actinomycosis is caused by infection with actinomycetes; the usual pulmonary organism is *Actinomyces israeli*. Although actinomycetes resemble fungi in appearance, they are anaerobic, Gram-positive, filamentous bacteria. They normally inhabit the mouth and nose and infect the lung by aspiration of oropharyngeal contents or by extension from an actinomycotic subdiaphragmatic abscess or liver abscess.

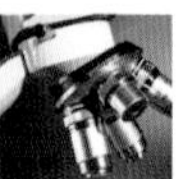

PATHOLOGY: Lung lesions of actinomycosis consist of multiple, interconnecting, small lung abscesses. The abscess margins are granulomatous, but central necrotic areas are purulent and contain colonies of thin, branching, filamentous, Gram-positive bacteria. Clubbed basophilic filaments, noted at the colony margins, are visible to the naked eye as small yellow particles (**sulfur granules**). The abscesses may extend to the pleura and produce bronchopulmonary fistulas and empyema. They may also invade the chest wall.

Nocardia

Nocardia is a Gram-positive filamentous bacterium that causes an acute progressive or chronic bacterial pneumonia. *Nocardia asteroides* is the most common *Nocardia* sp. to cause pneumonia. Infection is mostly seen in immunocompromised patients, particularly those with lymphoma, neutropenia, chronic granulomatous disease of childhood, and pulmonary alveolar proteinosis.

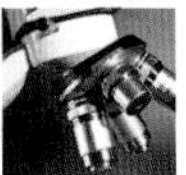

PATHOLOGY: Histologically, lungs show abscesses (Fig. 10-17A), which may have granulomatous features in chronic infections. The organisms are delicate, beaded, thin filaments, which branch mostly at right angles (Fig. 10-17B). They are best seen with Gram or Gomori methenamine silver stains (Fig. 10-17B) and are also weakly acid fast.

Viral Pneumonias

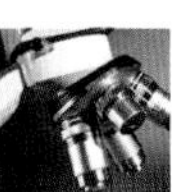

PATHOLOGY: In addition to producing bronchiolitis in the more peripheral airways, viral infections may initially affect the alveolar epithelium and elicit interstitial mononuclear infiltrates (Fig. 10-18). Hyaline membranes and necrosis of type I epithelial cells create an appearance indistinguishable from diffuse alveolar damage from other causes discussed below. Sometimes, alveolar damage is indolent, and the disease is characterized by type II pneumocyte hyperplasia and chronic interstitial inflammation. Unlike most bacterial infections, in which intra-alveolar neutrophilic exudates predominate and the interstitium is only incidentally involved (Fig. 10-19), interstitial pneumonia predominates.

Cytomegalovirus (CMV) pneumonia entails intense interstitial lymphocytic infiltration. Alveoli are lined by type II cells that have regenerated to cover the epithelial defect left by necrosis of type I cells. The infected alveolar cells are very large (cytomegaly) with a single, basophilic nuclear inclusion, a peripheral halo and multiple, indistinct cytoplasmic, basophilic inclusions (Fig. 10-20).

Measles infection involves both the airways and the parenchyma. Interstitial pneumonia, a well-characterized

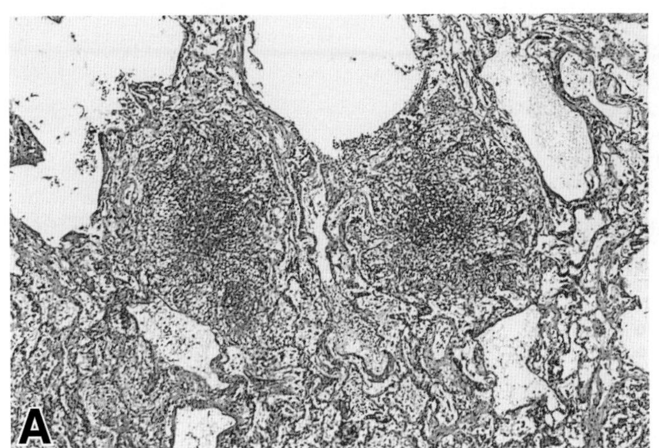
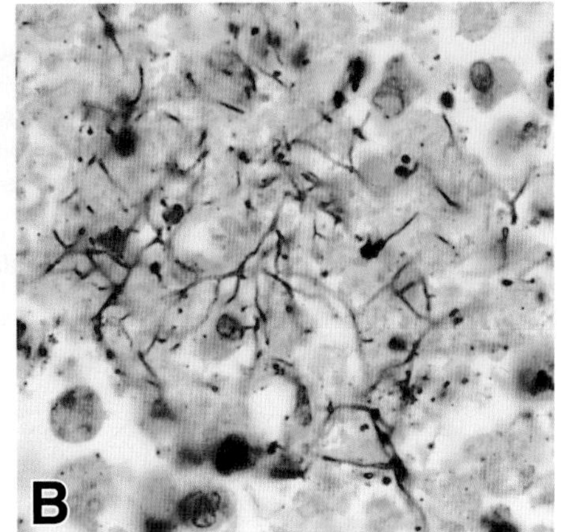

FIGURE 10-17. **Nocardiosis. A.** The lung showing abscesses consisting of focal collections of acute inflammation. **B.** The organisms are thin, filamentous, branching bacteria (Gomori methenamine silver stain).

complication of measles, is rarely fatal, except in immunocompromised, previously unexposed individuals.

Varicella infection (chickenpox and herpes zoster) produces disseminated, focally necrotic lung lesions, and interstitial pneumonia. Pulmonary involvement is usually asymptomatic, except in immunocompromised hosts, in whom it may be fatal. The viral inclusions are nuclear, eosinophilic, and refractile and are surrounded by a clear halo. Multinucleation can occur.

Herpes simplex can cause a necrotizing tracheobronchitis as well as diffuse alveolar damage. Viral inclusions are identical to those seen in varicella infection.

Adenovirus causes necrotizing bronchiolitis and bronchopneumonia. Two types of nuclear inclusions are seen: eosinophilic nuclear inclusions surrounded by a clear halo and "smudge cells," which demonstrate indistinct, basophilic, nuclear inclusions that fill the entire nucleus and are surrounded by only a thin rim of chromatin (Fig. 10-21).

Influenza virus typically produces interstitial pneumonitis and bronchiolitis similar to those seen in other viral pneumonias. It does not produce characteristic viral cytopathic changes. Morphologic features vary from interstitial pneumonia and bronchiolitis to diffuse alveolar damage. In some cases, extensive hemorrhage is present. With most strains of influenza, bacterial superinfection may be a dangerous complication.

Severe Acute Respiratory Syndrome and Middle East Respiratory Syndrome

In early 2002, an epidemic of severe pneumonia was traced to Guangdong Province of China. Because outbreaks occurred in Hong Kong, Vietnam, and Singapore, the disease swept around the globe via international air travel. This emerging clinical disease, SARS, eventually spread to the United States, Canada, and Europe. The causative agent is a novel coronavirus, termed the SARS-associated coronavirus (SARS-CoV). This agent is derived from a nonhuman host, probably bats, with civets and other animals as likely intermediate hosts. SARS is a potentially fatal viral respiratory illness, with an incubation period of 2 to 7 days and symptoms lasting up to 10 days. While this initial pandemic was spreading globally in 2003, there were over 8,000 known cases and 775 deaths, a case fatality rate of almost 10%. Although the last infected human case occurred in mid-2003, SARS-CoV has not been eradicated and has the potential to reemerge.

More recently, a similar coronavirus agent has been responsible for MERS, which has occurred predominately in the Arabian Peninsula, with a secondary focus in Korea. The disease was first described in 2012 and showed peak activity in 2014 and 2015, with occasional cases still occurring. The disease reservoir is likely to be camels and is spread by personal contact. Lungs of patients who died from SARS show diffuse alveolar damage, as discussed below. Multinucleated syncytial cells without viral inclusions have also been observed.

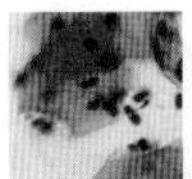

CLINICAL FEATURES: Clinically, SARS begins with fever and headache, followed shortly by cough and dyspnea. Coryza is often absent, and diarrhea is common. The presentation of MERS is similar, featuring fever, cough, sore throat, and gastrointestinal symptoms. Patients with either disease can develop adult respiratory distress syndrome (ARDS; see Chapter 10) and are at high risk of complications and death. Many patients recover, but the case fatality rate for SARS is 10% and as high as 30% in MERS. Age is a significant risk factor for severe disease for both. No specific treatments are available.

Fungal Infections

Many fungal pathogens such as *Histoplasma*, *Coccidioides*, *Cryptococcus*, and *Blastomyces* produce a granulomatous pattern of infection in the lung, often associated with necrosis. The first two agents produce disease closely resembling tuberculosis. *Aspergillus* may form granulomas or produce an invasive pattern of disease.

Histoplasmosis

Histoplasmosis, a disease of the midwestern and southeastern United States, particularly the Mississippi and Ohio River Valleys, is caused by inhalation of *Histoplasma capsulatum* in infected dust, commonly from bird droppings.

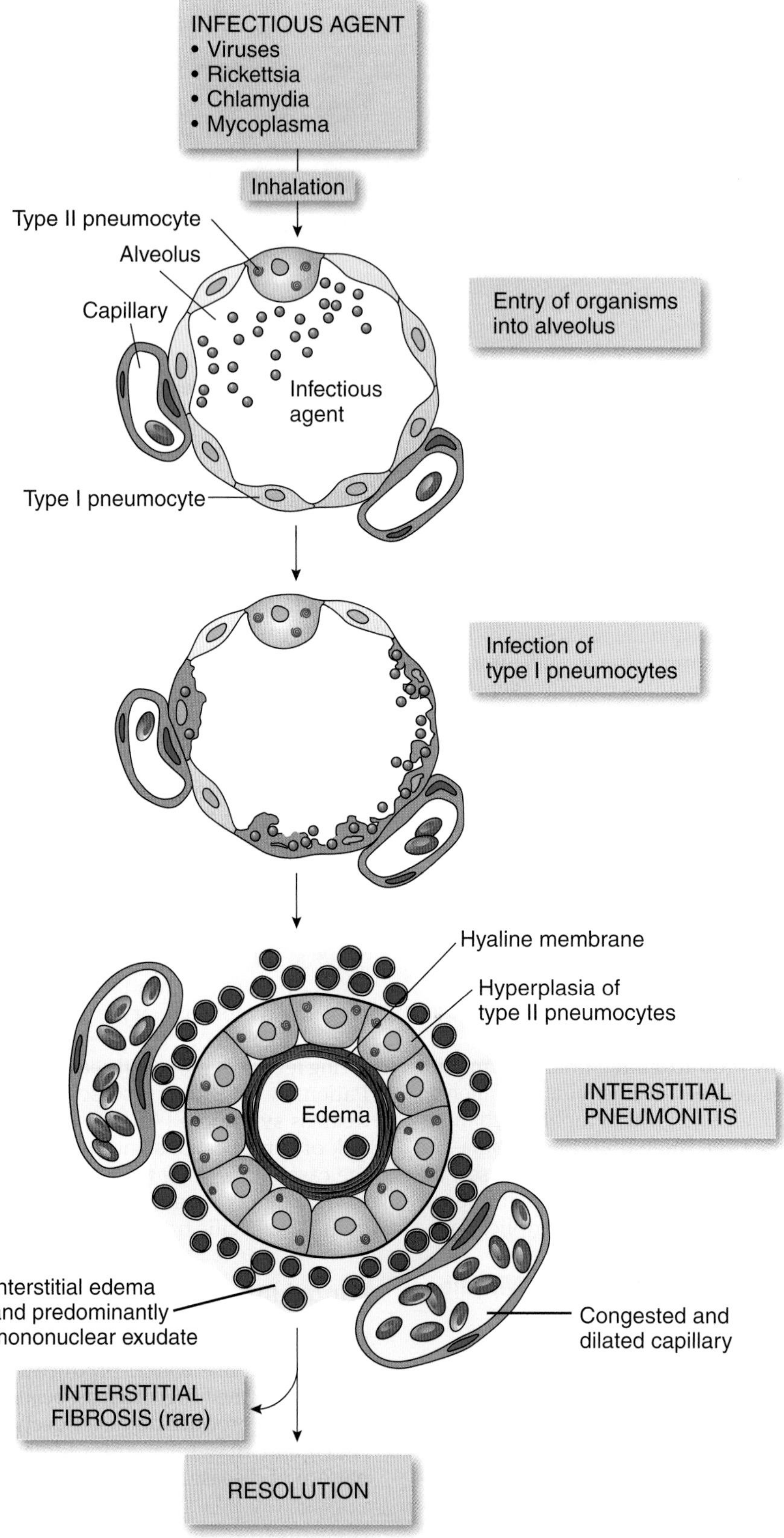

FIGURE 10-18. Pathogenesis of interstitial pneumonia. Although interstitial pneumonia is most commonly caused by viruses, other organisms may also cause significant interstitial inflammation. Type I cells are the most sensitive to damage, and loss of their integrity leads to intra-alveolar edema. The proteinaceous exudate and cell debris form hyaline membranes, and type II cells multiply to line the alveoli. Interstitial inflammation is characterized mainly by mononuclear cells. The disease usually resolves completely but occasionally progresses to interstitial fibrosis.

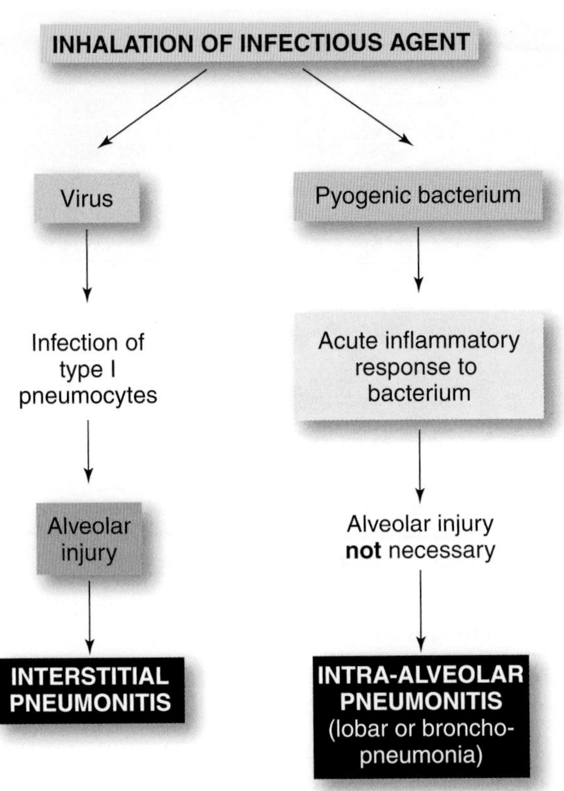

FIGURE 10-19. **Pathogenesis of interstitial and intra-alveolar pneumonitis.**

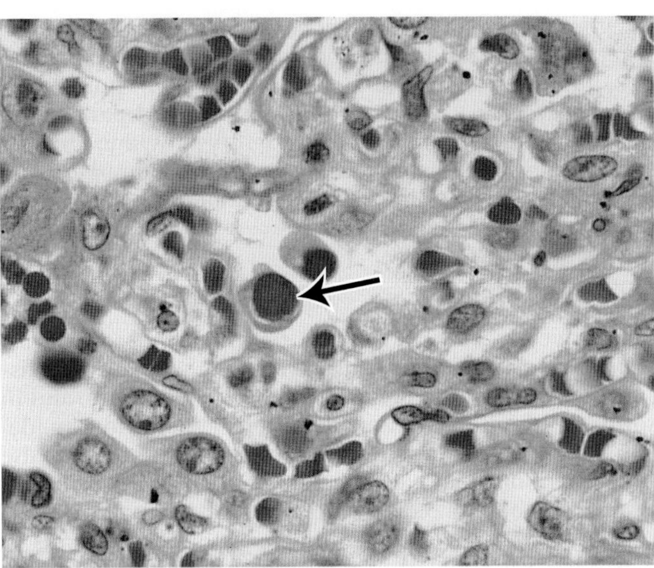

FIGURE 10-21. **Adenovirus pneumonia.** The "smudge" cell in the center (*arrow*) contains a smudgy basophilic nuclear inclusion.

PATHOLOGY: Histoplasmosis resembles tuberculosis clinically and pathologically. Most infections are asymptomatic and result in lesions like Ghon complexes, including a parenchymal granuloma and similar changes in the draining lymph nodes. The granulomas are particularly prone to calcify, often with a concentric laminar pattern. In the acute phase, numerous organisms are seen within macrophages. Granulomatous inflammation follows, often with central areas of necrosis. The granulomas heal by fibrosis and calcification, but central necrotic areas may persist. The spherical organisms are best seen with a silver stain as 2 to 4 μm in diameter with narrow-based budding.

In a few cases, pulmonary lesions progress or reactivate, giving rise to a progressive fibrotic and necrotic lesion that closely resembles reactivation tuberculosis. However, histoplasmosis lesions are more fibrotic than those of tuberculosis, and cavitation is less common. The reason for progression is not known, although large infective doses and poor host responses are usually considered to be responsible. Immunocompromised patients are at particular risk for the dissemination of *Histoplasma* within the lungs and spread to other organs.

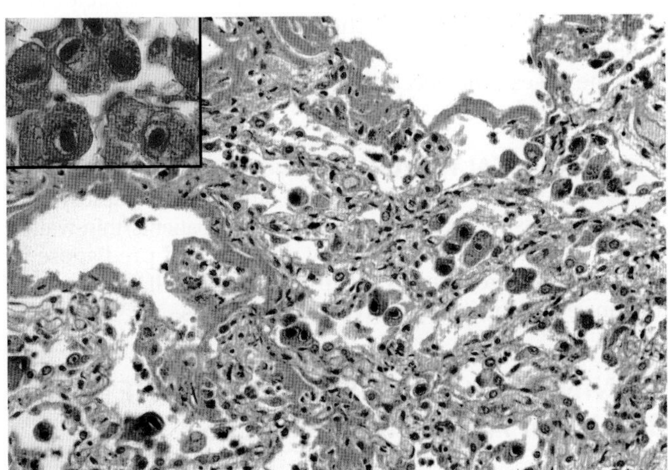

FIGURE 10-20. **Cytomegalovirus pneumonitis.** Infected alveolar cells are enlarged and display the typical dark blue nuclear inclusions. *Inset.* A higher power view showing infected alveolar cells that display a single basophilic nuclear inclusion with a perinuclear halo and multiple, indistinct, basophilic, cytoplasmic inclusions.

Coccidioidomycosis

Coccidioidomycosis is caused by inhalation of spores of *Coccidioides immitis* and was originally known as San Joaquin Valley fever, after the location where the disease has been endemic for many years. However, the infection is widespread throughout the southwestern part of the United States and shares many of the clinical and pathologic features of histoplasmosis and tuberculosis. In histologic sections, the organism is a spherule, 30 to 100 μm, with a thick refractile wall. Spherules contain innumerable 2- to 5-μm endospores. Empty spherules or endospores that have been released into the tissue may also be visible.

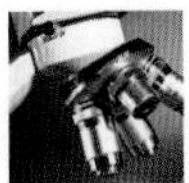

PATHOLOGY: In most instances, lesions of coccidioidomycosis are limited to a peripheral parenchymal granuloma, with or without lymph node granulomas. Sometimes, the lesion is slowly progressive. In immunocompromised hosts, the disease may progress rapidly, with release of endospores into the lung, in which case the tissue reaction is often purulent as well as granulomatous.

Cryptococcosis

Cryptococcosis results from the inhalation of spores of *Cryptococcus neoformans*, which are often found in pigeon droppings.

Lung lesions range from small parenchymal granulomas to several large granulomatous nodules, pneumonic consolidation, and even cavitation. Most serious cases of pulmonary cryptococcosis occur in immunocompromised patients, in whom the organisms proliferate extensively within alveolar spaces, with little tissue reaction. The organisms are 4 to 6 μm, but may be larger, with narrow-based budding and a thick mucoid capsule.

Blastomycosis

Blastomycosis is an uncommon condition caused by *Blastomyces dermatitidis.* It is concentrated in the Missouri, Mississippi, and Ohio river basins in the United States, and in southern Manitoba and northwestern Ontario in Canada. Clinical and pathologic features resemble those of the fungi mentioned above. Initial infection produces a lesion resembling a Ghon complex or progressive pneumonitis. Unlike tuberculous Ghon complexes, the focal lesions of blastomycosis show central necrosis and a purulent reaction, surrounded by granulomatous inflammation. The organisms are 8 to 15 μm, have a thick refractile wall, and exhibit broad-based budding.

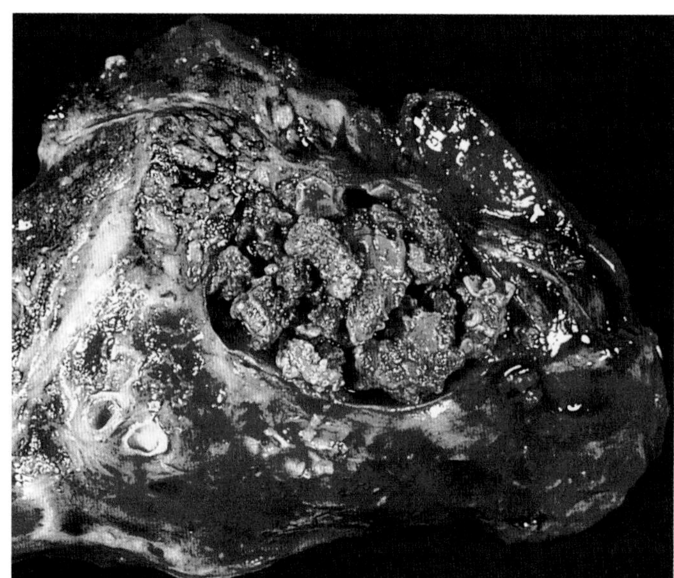

FIGURE 10-22. ***Aspergillus* fungus ball.** The lung contains a cavity filled with a fungus ball.

Aspergillosis

Lung infections by *Aspergillus* spp., usually *Aspergillus niger* or *Aspergillus fumigatus,* occur as follows:

- **Invasive aspergillosis:** This is the most serious form of *Aspergillus* infection, occurring almost exclusively as an opportunistic infection in people with compromised immunity. The lungs show patchy, multifocal consolidation, and, occasionally, cavities. Extensive blood vessel invasion, most often arterial, results in occlusion, thrombosis, and infarction of lung tissue. Invasive aspergillosis is a fulminant pulmonary infection that is not amenable to therapy.
- **Aspergilloma ("fungus ball" or mycetoma):** *Aspergillus* spp. may grow in preexisting cavities, such as those caused by tuberculosis or bronchiectasis, where they proliferate to form fungus balls (Fig. 10-22). They most often present with hemoptysis, arising either from the underlying condition or, less commonly, fungal infection of the cavity wall.
- **Allergic bronchopulmonary aspergillosis (ABPA):** Certain asthmatics have an unusual immunologic reaction to *Aspergillus* that is characterized by (1) transient pulmonary infiltrates on chest radiographs, (2) eosinophilia of blood and sputum, (3) skin sensitivity and serum precipitins to *A. fumigatus* antigens, and (4) increased serum IgE.

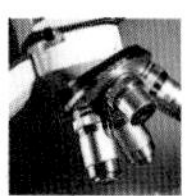

PATHOLOGY: ABPA is invariably associated with proximal (central) bronchiectasis, involving segmental bronchi and the next two to four orders of subsegmental bronchi. There are bronchial and bronchiolar mucous plugs, eosinophilic infiltrates, and Charcot–Leyden crystals (Fig. 10-23A and B). Bronchocentric granulomatosis and eosinophilic pneumonia may be present. The bronchial mucus may contain septate, fungal hyphae, with 45-degree branching. Interestingly, the peripheral bronchial tree is spared.

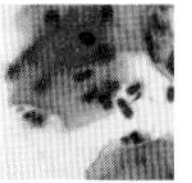

CLINICAL FEATURES: Patients with ABPA have wheezing, chest pain, and cough, and often have thick mucous plugs. Systemic corticosteroids usually control acute episodes.

Pneumocystis

Pulmonary infections with *Pneumocystis jiroveci* (formerly known as *Pneumocystis carinii*) most often cause pneumonia in immunosuppressed patients or those with immunodeficiencies such as HIV/AIDS. Patients receiving immunosuppressive drugs after organ transplantation or chemotherapy for malignant disease are particularly at risk.

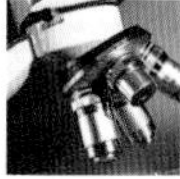

PATHOLOGY: The classic lesions of *Pneumocystis* pneumonia are interstitial infiltrates of plasma cells and lymphocytes and hyperplasia of type II pneumocytes. Alveoli are filled with a characteristic foamy exudate, in which the organisms appear as small bubbles in a background of proteinaceous exudate(Fig. 10-24). In some cases, *Pneumocystis* also produces diffuse alveolar damage (see below).

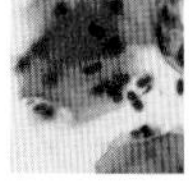

CLINICAL FEATURES: At one extreme, symptoms may be minimal, whereas at the other, there is rapidly progressive respiratory failure. In AIDS patients, thin-walled parenchymal cysts may develop and predispose to pneumothorax. Treatment is with trimethoprim–sulfamethoxazole and, in severe cases, adjunctive corticosteroids.

NONINFECTIOUS DISEASES OF THE BRONCHI AND BRONCHIOLES

Most bronchial and bronchiolar diseases are acute conditions. Chronic bronchitis is discussed later. Although the diseases discussed below are not, in themselves, infectious in origin,

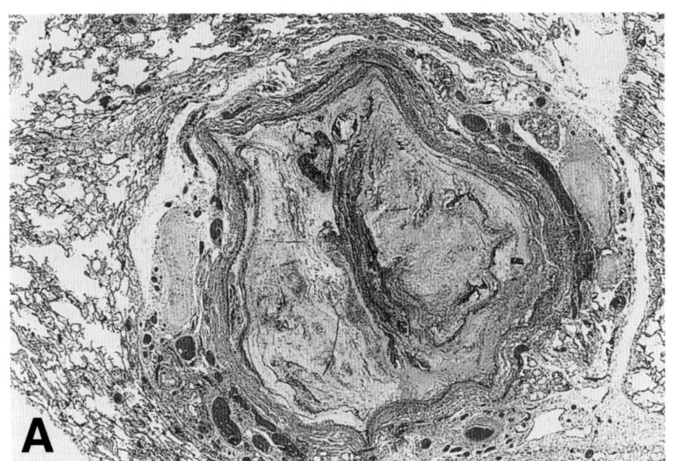

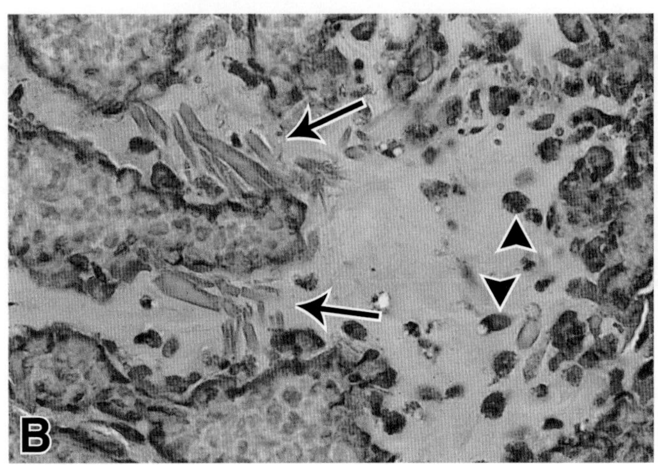

FIGURE 10-23. Allergic bronchopulmonary aspergillosis. A. A dilated bronchus is filled with a mucous plug that has dense layers of eosinophilic infiltrates. **B.** Higher magnification showing numerous eosinophils (*arrowheads*) and Charcot–Leyden crystals (*arrows*).

they can represent the response of the airway to either an infectious or noninfectious insult.

Bronchocentric Granulomatosis

Bronchocentric granulomatosis is a nonspecific granulomatous inflammation centered on bronchi or bronchioles (Fig. 10-25). ***This histologic pattern occurs in a number of clinical settings and is not a distinct clinical entity.***

Asthmatic patients, for the most part, have allergic bronchopulmonary aspergillosis (see above).

Nonasthmatic patients with bronchocentric granulomatosis are likely to have an infection, especially tuberculosis or fungi such as *H. capsulatum*. The disorder can also be a manifestation of immune problems, including rheumatoid arthritis, ankylosing spondylitis, and granulomatosis with polyangiitis (formerly known as Wegener granulomatosis). Patients with bronchocentric granulomatosis of either allergic or nonallergic type generally respond well to corticosteroid therapy.

Constrictive Bronchiolitis

In constrictive bronchiolitis, an initial inflammatory bronchiolitis is followed by bronchiolar scarring and fibrosis, with progressive narrowing and, eventually, complete destruction of the airway lumen. **Obliterative bronchiolitis** is a synonym.

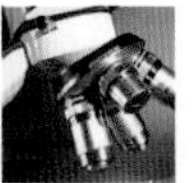

PATHOLOGY: Bronchioles show chronic mural inflammation and varying amounts of fibrosis between the epithelium and smooth muscle, with resultant narrowing of the lumen. These lesions are often focal and may be difficult to identify. The surrounding lung is usually normal. This pattern of fibrosis is seen in several situations, including (1) bone marrow transplantation (graft-versus-host disease), (2) lung transplantation (chronic rejection), (3) collagen vascular diseases (especially rheumatoid arthritis), (4) postinfectious disorders (especially viral infections), (5) after inhalation of toxins (SO_2, ammonia, and phosgene), and (6) ingestion of certain drugs (penicillamine). It may also be

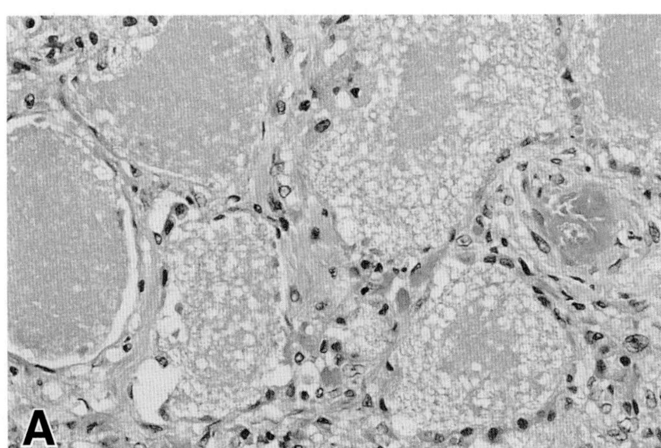

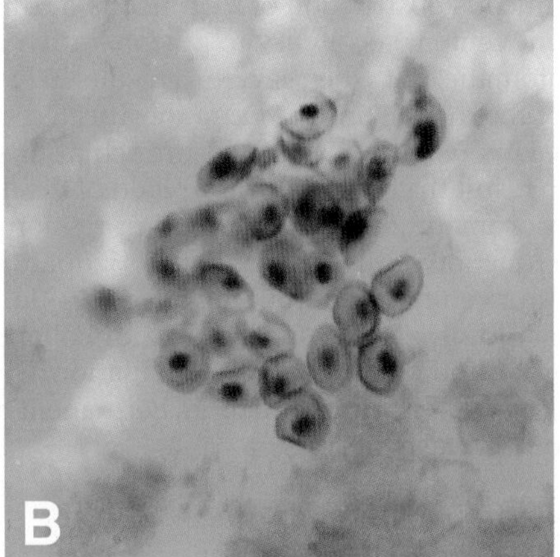

FIGURE 10-24. *Pneumocystis jiroveci* pneumonia. A. The alveoli are filled with a foamy exudate, and the interstitium is thickened and contains a chronic inflammatory infiltrate. **B.** A centrifuged bronchoalveolar lavage specimen impregnated with silver showing a cluster of *Pneumocystis* cysts.

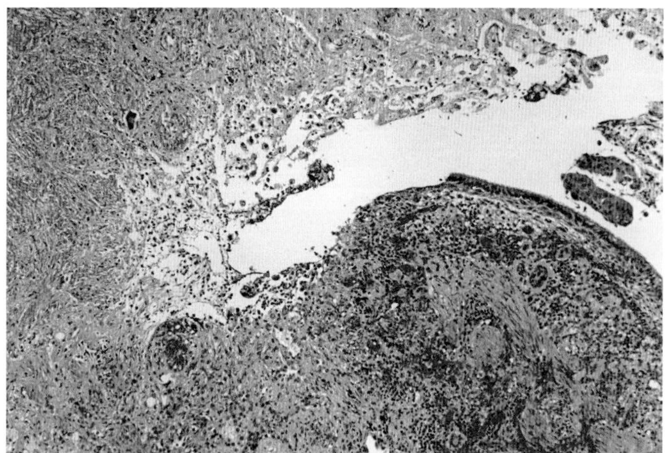

FIGURE 10-25. **Bronchocentric granulomatosis.** This bronchiole shows ulceration and necrosis of the mucosa and submucosa with granulomatous inflammation. The patient had granulomatosis polyangiitis (formerly known as Wegener granulomatosis) with lung involvement in the pattern of bronchocentric granulomatosis.

idiopathic. Most patients have a relentless progressive clinical course. Although many patients are treated with steroids, no therapy is effective for this disease.

Bronchial Obstruction

Bronchial obstruction in adults occurs mostly because of endobronchial extension of primary lung tumors, although mucous plugs, aspirated gastric contents or foreign bodies may also be responsible, especially in children. If obstruction is partial, trapped air may cause overdistention of the distal affected segment; complete obstruction results in atelectasis. Areas distal to the obstruction may also develop pneumonia, abscesses, and bronchiectasis (see later).

Atelectasis is the collapse of expanded lung tissue. If the air supply is obstructed, gas transfers from the alveoli to the blood, causing the affected region to collapse. Atelectasis occurs as an important postoperative complication of abdominal surgery, because of mucous obstruction of a bronchus or diminished respiratory movement secondary to postoperative pain. It is often asymptomatic, but when severe, it results in hypoxemia and a shift of the mediastinum *toward* the affected side.

Atelectasis is usually caused by bronchial obstruction but may also result from direct compression of the lung (e.g., hydrothorax or pneumothorax). If the compression is severe enough, the function of the affected lung is jeopardized, and the mediastinum shifts *away* from the affected side.

In long-standing atelectasis, the area of collapsed lung becomes fibrotic and displays bronchial dilation, in part owing to infection distal to the obstruction. Permanent bronchial dilation (bronchiectasis) results.

Bronchiectasis

Bronchiectasis may be obstructive or nonobstructive. **Obstructive bronchiectasis** is localized and occurs distal to a mechanical obstruction of a central bronchus. Examples include tumors, inhaled foreign bodies, mucous plugs in asthma, or lymph node enlargement. **Nonobstructive bronchiectasis** usually follows respiratory infections or defects in airway defenses from infection. It may be localized or generalized.

Localized nonobstructive bronchiectasis was once common, usually after childhood bronchopulmonary infections with measles, pertussis, or other bacteria. Cases still occur following bronchopulmonary infection, usually with adenovirus or RSV.

Generalized bronchiectasis is, for the most part, secondary to inherited impairment in host defense mechanisms or acquired conditions that permit introduction of infectious organisms into the airways. Acquired disorders that predispose to bronchiectasis include (1) neurologic diseases that impair consciousness, swallowing, respiratory excursions, and the cough reflex; (2) incompetence of the lower esophageal sphincter; (3) nasogastric intubation; and (4) chronic bronchitis. The main **inherited conditions** associated with generalized bronchiectasis are cystic fibrosis, dyskinetic ciliary syndromes, hypogammaglobulinemias, and deficiencies of specific immunoglobulin (Ig) G subclasses.

Kartagener syndrome is one of the immotile cilia syndromes (ciliary dyskinesia) and consists of the triad of dextrocardia (with or without situs inversus), bronchiectasis, and sinusitis. It is caused by defects in the outer or inner dynein arms of cilia, which generate or regulate cilia beats, respectively. Other dyskinetic ciliary syndromes include **radial spoke deficiency** ("Sturgess syndrome") and absence of the central doublet of cilia. In these diseases, cilia are deficient throughout the body. Both men and women are sterile, because of impaired ciliary mobility in the vas deferens and the fallopian tube. In the respiratory tract, ciliary defects are associated with repeated upper and lower respiratory tract infections and thus bronchiectasis.

Generalized bronchiectasis is usually bilateral and is most common in the lower lobes, the left more than the right. Localized bronchiectasis may occur wherever there was obstruction or infection. Bronchi are dilated, with thick, white, or yellow walls. Bronchial lumens often contain dense, mucopurulent secretions. Severe inflammation of bronchi and bronchioles results in destruction of all components of the bronchial wall. Collapse of distal lung parenchyma causes damaged bronchi to dilate. Inflammation of central airways leads to mucus hypersecretion and abnormalities of the surface epithelium, including squamous metaplasia and increased goblet cells. Lymphoid follicles are often seen in bronchial walls, and distal bronchi and bronchioles are scarred and often obliterated. Bronchial arteries enlarge to supply the inflamed bronchial wall and fibrous tissue. A vicious circle may be established in which pools of mucus become infected, which further promotes destruction of the bronchial walls.

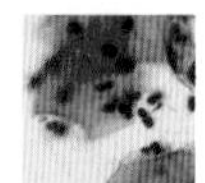

CLINICAL FEATURES: Patients with bronchiectasis have chronic cough, often producing several hundred milliliters of mucopurulent sputum a day. Hemoptysis is common because bronchial inflammation erodes the walls of adjacent bronchial arteries. Dyspnea and wheezing are variable, depending on the extent of the disease. Pneumonia is common, and patients with long-standing cases are at risk of chronic hypoxia and pulmonary hypertension. Acute, reversible bronchial dilation may follow bacterial or viral respiratory infections; it may take months before the bronchi return to normal size.

DISEASES OF THE ALVEOLI

Diffuse alveolar damage (DAD) is a pattern of reaction of alveolar epithelial and endothelial cells to a variety of acute insults (Table 10-1). The clinical expression of severe DAD is **acute respiratory distress syndrome (ARDS)**. In ARDS, apparently normal lungs sustain damage that progresses rapidly to respiratory failure. Lung compliance is impaired (usually requiring mechanical ventilation), with hypoxemia and extensive bilateral radiologic opacities ("white-out"). ARDS mortality exceeds 50%, and in patients over 60 years of age, it is as high as 90%.

ETIOLOGIC FACTORS: DAD is a final common pathologic pathway triggered by a large variety of insults (Table 10-1), including infections, sepsis, shock, aspiration of gastric contents, inhalation of toxic gases, near-drowning, radiation pneumonitis, and many drugs and other chemicals. The common pathogenic link is acute alveolar epithelial and endothelial cell injury. ***Unless a specific infectious agent is identified, the trigger for DAD is not evident from the lung histology alone.*** In some patients, no cause is found. Such idiopathic DAD is referred to clinically as **acute interstitial pneumonia** (AIP).

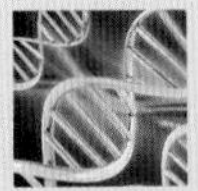

MOLECULAR PATHOGENESIS: Endothelial cell injury allows protein-rich fluid to leak from alveolar capillaries into the interstitial space (Fig. 10-26). Loss of type I pneumocytes permits fluid to enter alveolar spaces, where plasma proteins form fibrin-containing precipitates (hyaline membranes) on the injured alveolar walls (Fig. 10-27). In response to cell injury in DAD, inflammatory cells accumulate in the interstitium. Although lacking type I pneumocytes, alveolar basement membranes remain intact and act as scaffolds for type II pneumocytes, which proliferate to replace the normal alveolar epithelial lining.

Table 10-1

Important Causes of Acute Respiratory Distress Syndrome

Nonthoracic Trauma	Infection	Aspiration	Drugs and Therapeutic Agents
Shock due to any cause	Gram-negative septicemia	Near-drowning	Heroin
Fat embolism	Other bacterial infections	Aspiration of gastric contents	Oxygen
	Viral infections		Radiation
			Paraquat
			Cytotoxic drugs

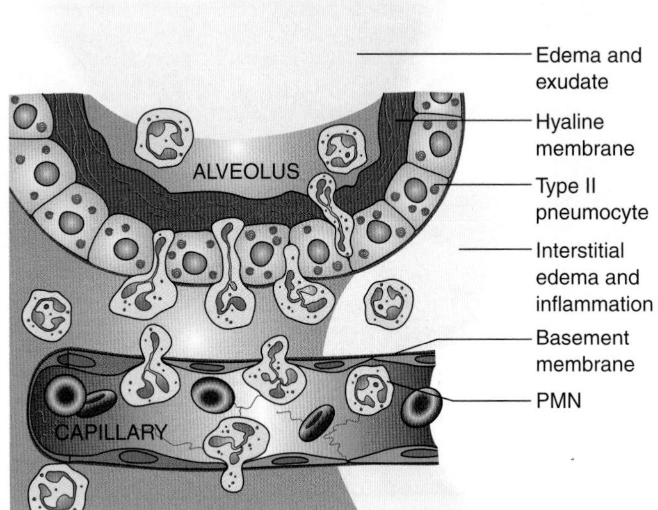

FIGURE 10-26. Diffuse alveolar damage (acute respiratory distress syndrome [ARDS]). In ARDS, type I cells die as a result of diffuse alveolar damage. Intra-alveolar edema follows, after which there is formation of hyaline membranes composed of proteinaceous exudate and cell debris. In the acute phase, the lungs are markedly congested and heavy. Type II cells multiply to line the alveolar surface. Interstitial inflammation is characteristic. The lesion may heal completely or progress to interstitial fibrosis. PMN, polymorphonuclear neutrophil.

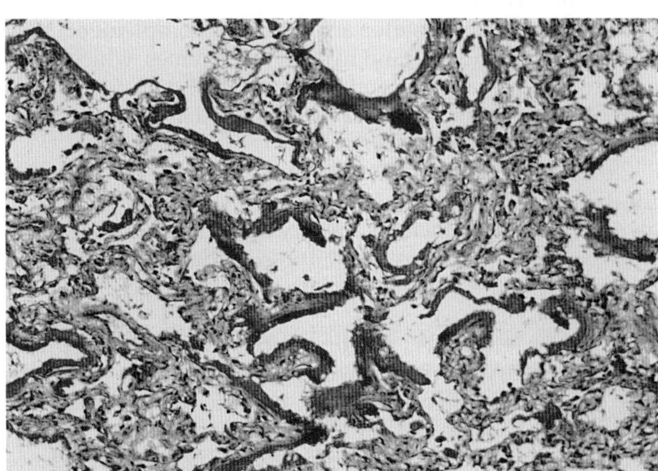

FIGURE 10-27. Diffuse alveolar damage, acute (exudative) phase. Alveolar septa are thickened by edema and a sparse inflammatory infiltrate. Alveoli are lined by eosinophilic hyaline membranes.

If the patient survives the acute phase of ARDS, fibroblasts proliferate in the interstitial space and deposit collagen in the alveolar walls (Fig. 10-28). With complete recovery, the alveolar exudate and hyaline membranes are resorbed, and normal alveolar epithelium is restored. Fibroblast proliferation ceases, the extra collagen is metabolized, and patients regain normal lung function. In patients who do not recover, DAD can progress to end-stage fibrosis, in which remodeling of lung architecture produces many cyst-like spaces throughout the lung **(honeycomb lung)**. These spaces are separated by thick fibrous walls lined by type II pneumocytes, bronchiolar epithelium, or squamous cells.

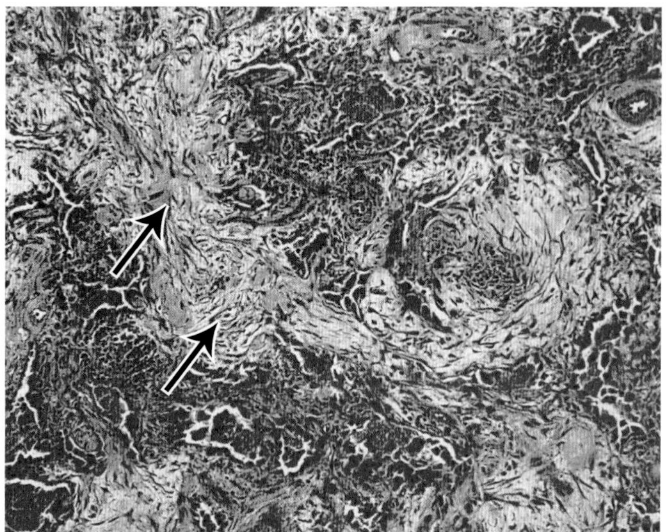

FIGURE 10-28. Diffuse alveolar damage, acute and organizing phase. The alveolar walls are thickened by fibroblasts and loose connective tissue (*arrows*).

Mechanisms of acute injury in DAD are not entirely clear. It is thought that activation of complement (e.g., by endotoxin in the case of Gram-negative septicemia) leads to sequestration of neutrophils in the marginating pool. Only a small proportion, perhaps one third, of neutrophils actively circulates in the blood; most of the rest are in the lung. Normally, they cause no damage there, but after activation by complement, they release oxygen radicals and hydrolytic enzymes, which damage pulmonary capillary endothelium. However, neutrophils cannot be obligatory for DAD because ARDS can develop in severely neutropenic patients.

In DAD following toxic gas inhalation or near-drowning, the damage is mostly at the alveolar epithelial surface. Normal alveolar epithelial junctions are very tight, but epithelial injury disrupts these junctions, permitting exudation of fluid and proteins from the interstitium into alveolar spaces.

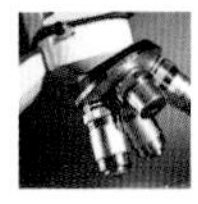

PATHOLOGY: The first step is the **exudative phase of DAD**, which develops within a week after pulmonary insult. Edema, hyaline membranes, and leakage of plasma proteins are evident, as is accumulation of inflammatory cells (Fig. 10-27). The earliest evidence of alveolar injury is seen by electron microscopy as degenerative changes in endothelial cells and type I pneumocytes. This is followed by sloughing of type I cells, thereby denuding basement membranes. Interstitial and alveolar edema is prominent by the first day but soon recedes. **Hyaline membranes** appear by the second day and are the most conspicuous morphologic feature of the exudative phase after 4 to 5 days. They are eosinophilic and glassy, consisting of precipitated plasma proteins and debris from sloughed epithelial cells. Interstitial inflammation, with lymphocytes, plasma cells, and macrophages, develops early and peaks in about a week. Toward the end of the first week and persisting during the subsequent **organizing stage**, regularly spaced, cuboidal type II pneumocytes become arrayed along the denuded alveolar septa. Alveolar capillaries and pulmonary arterioles may contain fibrin thrombi. If DAD is fatal, the lungs are heavy, edematous, and, virtually, airless.

The organizing phase of DAD starts about a week after the initial injury and is marked by fibroblast proliferation within the alveolar walls (Fig. 10-28). Interstitial inflammation and proliferated type II pneumocytes persist, but hyaline membranes are no longer formed. Alveolar macrophages digest the remnants of hyaline membranes and other debris. Loose fibrosis expands alveolar septa but resolves in mild cases. In severe DAD, fibrosis progresses to restructuring of the pulmonary parenchyma.

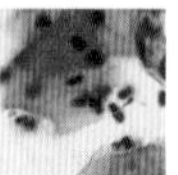

CLINICAL FEATURES: Patients destined to develop ARDS have a symptom-free interval for a few hours after the initial insult. Tachypnea and dyspnea mark the onset of ARDS. Blood gas analyses show arterial hypoxemia and decreased pCO_2. As ARDS progresses, dyspnea worsens, and the patient becomes cyanotic. Diffuse, bilateral, interstitial, and alveolar infiltrates are noted radiologically. Increasing inspired oxygen concentrations does not restore adequate blood oxygenation, necessitating mechanical ventilation.

Patients who survive ARDS may recover normal pulmonary function, but in severe cases, they are left with scarred lungs, respiratory dysfunction, and, in some instances, pulmonary hypertension.

Common Causes of Diffuse Alveolar Damage

Shock

ARDS often follows shock from any cause, including sepsis, trauma, or blood loss, the pulmonary consequences of which are often called "shock lung." The pathogenesis of DAD associated with shock is poorly understood but is likely multifactorial. Tissue necrosis in organs damaged by trauma or ischemia may lead to release of vasoactive peptides into the circulation. These enhance vascular permeability in the lung. Disseminated intravascular coagulation may damage alveolar capillaries, and fat emboli from bone fractures may obstruct the distal capillary bed of the lung. The pathogenesis of endothelial cell injury in endotoxic shock is discussed in Chapter 2.

Aspiration

Aspiration of gastric contents introduces acid with a pH less than 3.0 into the alveoli. The severe chemical injury to the alveolar lining cells leads to DAD. In near-drowning, aspiration of water produces pulmonary injury and ARDS.

Drug-Induced Diffuse Alveolar Damage

Many drugs cause DAD, especially cytotoxic chemotherapeutic agents. Of which best known is bleomycin. Bizarre, atypical, hyperchromatic nuclei in type II cells are particularly common in drug-induced disease. Damage progresses even when the offending agent is discontinued, but corticosteroid treatment may be helpful. Drugs other than chemotherapeutic agents that may cause DAD include nitrofurantoin, amiodarone, and penicillamine.

Acute Interstitial Pneumonia

AIP is a clinical term for diffuse alveolar damage of unknown cause.

Neonatal Respiratory Distress Syndrome

Neonatal respiratory distress syndrome (NRDS) results from immaturity of the surfactant system at birth, usually because of severe prematurity. The advent of surfactant replacement therapy and better ventilatory techniques have increased survival and decreased the frequency of complications of NRDS in older premature infants. However, very premature infants may still develop **bronchopulmonary dysplasia (BPD)**. Previously, BPD reflected damage to lung acini and subsequent repair, which led to atelectasis, fibrosis, and destruction of clusters of acini. With the advent of surfactant replacement therapy, the necrotizing bronchiolitis and alveolar septal fibrosis of BPD have largely disappeared, and decreased alveolarization is the main finding now. NRDS and BPD are discussed in further detail in Chapter 5.

Uncommon Alveolar Diseases

Although the following diseases are uncommon, they may be associated with serious morbidity. Several of the conditions (e.g., diffuse hemorrhagic syndromes and some forms of eosinophilic pneumonia) have an autoimmune or allergic etiology. Others, such as the lipid pneumonias, relate to either exogenous or endogenous lipids that accumulate within the airways alveoli or interstitium.

Diffuse Pulmonary Hemorrhage Syndromes

Diffuse alveolar hemorrhage can occur in diverse clinical settings (Table 10-2). These diseases are characterized by acute hemorrhage (intra-alveolar red blood cells) or chronic hemorrhage (hemosiderosis). In virtually all of these disorders, neutrophils infiltrate the alveolar capillary walls (**neutrophilic capillaritis**), reminiscent of leukocytoclastic vasculitis seen in other organs, such as the skin. This finding tends to be most prominent in hemorrhagic syndromes associated with polyangiitis with granulomatosis (formerly known as Wegener granulomatosis) or systemic lupus erythematosus.

Some diffuse pulmonary hemorrhage syndromes are associated with characteristic immunofluorescence patterns. ***Linear fluorescence along alveolar walls*** is seen in antibasement membrane antibody disease, or Goodpasture syndrome. **Goodpasture syndrome** entails a triad: (1) diffuse alveolar hemorrhage, (2) glomerulonephritis, and (3) circulating cytotoxic autoantibody to a component of basement membranes. Cross-reactivity between alveolar and glomerular basement membranes accounts for the simultaneous attack on the lung and kidney (for details, see Chapters 8 and 14). A ***granular pattern*** occurs in immune complex–associated diseases, such as systemic lupus erythematosus. ***Pauci-immune disorders*** show no significant deposition of immunoglobulin in tissue. They include antineutrophil cytoplasm antibody (ANCA)-associated diseases, such as polyangiitis with granulomatosis, microscopic polyangiitis, or idiopathic pulmonary hemorrhage syndromes. In these disorders, no etiology or immunologic mechanism can be determined. Idiopathic disease is characterized by diffuse alveolar bleeding similar to that of Goodpasture syndrome but without renal involvement or antibasement membrane antibodies. It is microscopically indistinguishable from the lung of Goodpasture syndrome (Table 10-2).

Table 10-2

Conditions of Pulmonary Hemorrhage

Disease	Immunologic Mechanism	Immunofluorescence Pattern
Goodpasture syndrome	Antibasement membrane antibody	Linear
Microscopic polyangiitis	Antineutrophilic cytoplasmic antibody (ANCA)	Negative/pauci-immune
Systemic lupus erythematosus	Immune complexes	Granular
Mixed cryoglobulinemia		
Henoch–Schönlein purpura		
Immunoglobulin A disease		
Granulomatosis with polyangiitis (formerly known as Wegener granulomatosis)	ANCA	Negative or pauci-immune
Idiopathic glomerulonephritis		
Idiopathic pulmonary hemorrhage	No immunologic marker	

Eosinophilic Pneumonia

Eosinophilic pneumonia entails accumulation of eosinophils in alveolar spaces. The disease is classified as **idiopathic** or **secondary** to an underlying illness (Table 10-3).

Idiopathic Eosinophilic Pneumonia

IEP occurs with varying degrees of clinical severity and lung involvement:

- **Simple eosinophilic pneumonia** (Löffler syndrome) is a mild condition characterized by fleeting pulmonary infiltrates, which usually resolve within a month and are accompanied by peripheral blood eosinophilia. Patients are often asymptomatic.
- **Acute eosinophilic pneumonia** is characterized by acute (<7 days) symptoms, including fever, hypoxemia, and diffuse interstitial and alveolar infiltrates on chest radiographs. The etiology is likely to be a hypersensitivity reaction. Peripheral blood eosinophilia is often absent, but bronchoalveolar lavage consistently contains increased eosinophils. Histologically, the lung shows eosinophilic pneumonia, accompanied by features of diffuse alveolar damage (e.g., hyaline membranes). Patients respond dramatically to corticosteroids.
- **Chronic eosinophilic pneumonia** is of unknown etiology, but an allergic diathesis is noted in some patients. Patients

Table 10-3

Types of Eosinophilic Pneumonia

Types of Eosinophilic Pneumonia
Idiopathic
Chronic eosinophilic pneumonia
Acute eosinophilic pneumonia
Simple eosinophilic pneumonia (Löffler syndrome)
Secondary Eosinophilic Pneumonia
Infection
Parasitic
Tropical eosinophilic pneumonia
Ascaris lumbricoides, *Toxocara canis*, filaria
Dirofilaria
Fungal
Aspergillus
Drug induced
Antibiotics
Cytotoxic drugs
Anti-inflammatory agents
Antihypertensive drugs
L-Tryptophan (eosinophilic fasciitis)
Immunologic or systemic diseases
Allergic bronchopulmonary aspergillosis
Eosinophilic granulomatosis with polyangiitis (formerly known as Churg–Strauss syndrome)
Hypereosinophilic syndrome

have fever, night sweats, weight loss, cough productive of eosinophils, and dyspnea. Alveolar spaces are flooded with eosinophils, alveolar macrophages, and a proteinaceous exudate (Fig. 10-29). Some cases may also show an eosinophilic interstitial pneumonia. Hyperplasia of type II pneumocytes may be prominent. Eosinophilic abscesses, with central masses of necrotic eosinophils surrounded by palisaded macrophages, are sometimes found. The chest radiograph is diagnostic and has been described as "the photographic negative of pulmonary edema"; it is characterized by peripheral alveolar infiltrates with sparing of the hilum. The response to corticosteroids is dramatic and helps confirm the diagnosis. However, the disease may recur.

Secondary Eosinophilic Pneumonia

Eosinophilic pneumonia can occur in a variety of clinical settings, including parasitic or fungal infection, drug toxicity, and systemic disorders, such as eosinophilic granulomatosis with polyangiitis (formerly known as Churg–Strauss syndrome) (Table 10-3). In industrialized countries, the most frequent cause of eosinophilic pneumonia is drug hypersensitivity, including reactions to antibiotics, anti-inflammatory agents, cytotoxic drugs, and antihypertensive agents. The pulmonary disease resolves without long-term sequelae. The clinical presentations and histologic findings are the same, as described above.

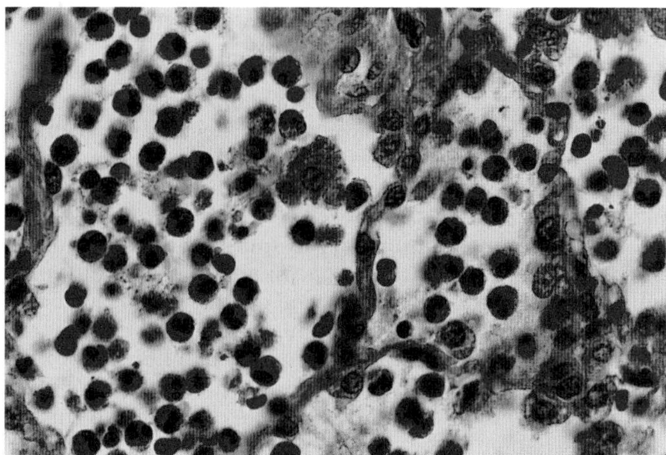

FIGURE 10-29. **Eosinophilic pneumonia.** Alveolar spaces are filled with an inflammatory exudate composed of eosinophils and macrophages. Alveolar septa are thickened by the presence of numerous eosinophils.

Infectious eosinophilic pneumonia is most commonly associated with parasitic disease (**tropical eosinophilic pneumonia**). Migration of parasites through the lung elicits an acute, self-limited, respiratory illness, characterized clinically by fever, a cough productive of sputum containing eosinophils, and transient pulmonary infiltrates.

Lipid Pneumonias

Pneumonias characterized by the presence of lipid may be either endogenous or exogenous in origin. **Endogenous lipid pneumonia** is also called "golden pneumonia," as a result of the characteristic golden yellow color, resulting from lipid accumulation within alveolar macrophages. The disease is a localized condition distal to an obstructed airway and is often related to neoplastic disease. Bronchial obstruction leads to retention of secretions and breakdown products of inflammatory and epithelial cells. Although the protein component is readily digested, lipids are phagocytosed by macrophages, which fill alveoli distal to the obstruction. **Exogenous lipid pneumonia** is caused by the inhalation of oil-containing substances and is most common in older individuals, who take nose drops or laxatives at bedtime and aspirate during sleep. The pneumonia is gray, greasy, and poorly demarcated. Foamy macrophages are seen in alveolar and interstitial spaces (Fig. 10-30). Large oil droplets in both locations are surrounded by foreign-body granulomas. Patients with exogenous disease are usually asymptomatic; the condition comes to medical attention when a mass simulating an infection or a tumor is seen on a chest radiograph.

OBSTRUCTIVE PULMONARY DISEASES

Several diseases, including chronic bronchitis, emphysema, asthma, and, in some classifications, cystic fibrosis (discussed

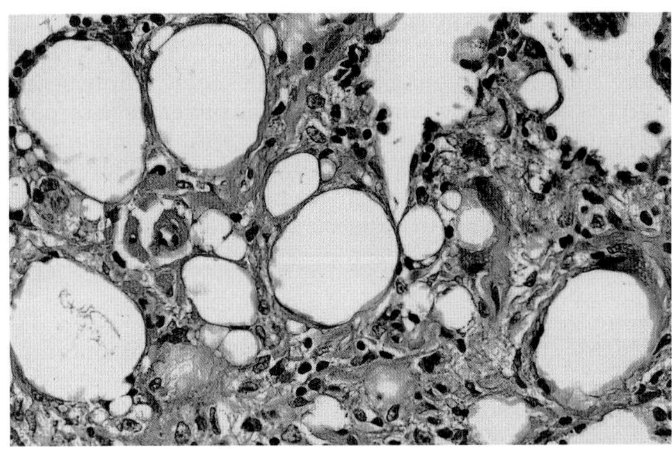

FIGURE 10-30. Exogenous lipoid pneumonia (mineral oil aspiration). The cystic spaces are empty because the lipid was washed out during tissue processing. A giant cell reaction is also present.

in detail in Chapter 5), are grouped because they all entail obstruction to airflow in the lungs.

Chronic obstructive pulmonary disease (COPD) includes chronic bronchitis and emphysema, in which forced expiratory volume, measured by spirometry, is decreased.

Airflow can be reduced by increasing resistance to airflow or by reducing outflow pressure. In the lung, narrowed airways produce increased resistance, whereas loss of elastic recoil results in diminished pressure. Airway narrowing occurs in chronic bronchitis or asthma, and emphysema causes loss of recoil.

Chronic Bronchitis

Chronic bronchitis is clinically defined as productive cough without a discernable cause for 50% or more days during a two-year or more period. The pathologic definition of the disease is less satisfactory because its morphologic alterations are a continuum; mild chronic bronchitis may show normal histology.

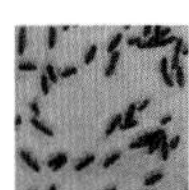

ETIOLOGIC FACTORS: ***Because 90% of chronic bronchitis cases are smokers, the disease mainly reflects the consequences of cigarette smoke.*** Chronic bronchitis occurs in less than 5% of nonsmokers and over 25% of heavy smokers. The frequency and severity of acute respiratory tract infections are increased in patients with chronic bronchitis; conversely, infections have been incriminated in its etiology and progression. Chronic bronchitis occurs more often in people in areas of substantial air pollution and in workers exposed to toxic industrial inhalants, but the effects of cigarette smoking far outweigh other contributing factors.

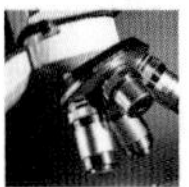

PATHOLOGY: The main pathology in chronic bronchitis is increased bronchial mucus-secreting tissue. Two types of cells line bronchial mucous glands: the more abundant pale mucous cells and basophilic, granular serous cells. ***In chronic bronchitis, mucous cells undergo hyperplasia and hypertrophy, and both individual acini and glands enlarge*** (Fig. 10-31).

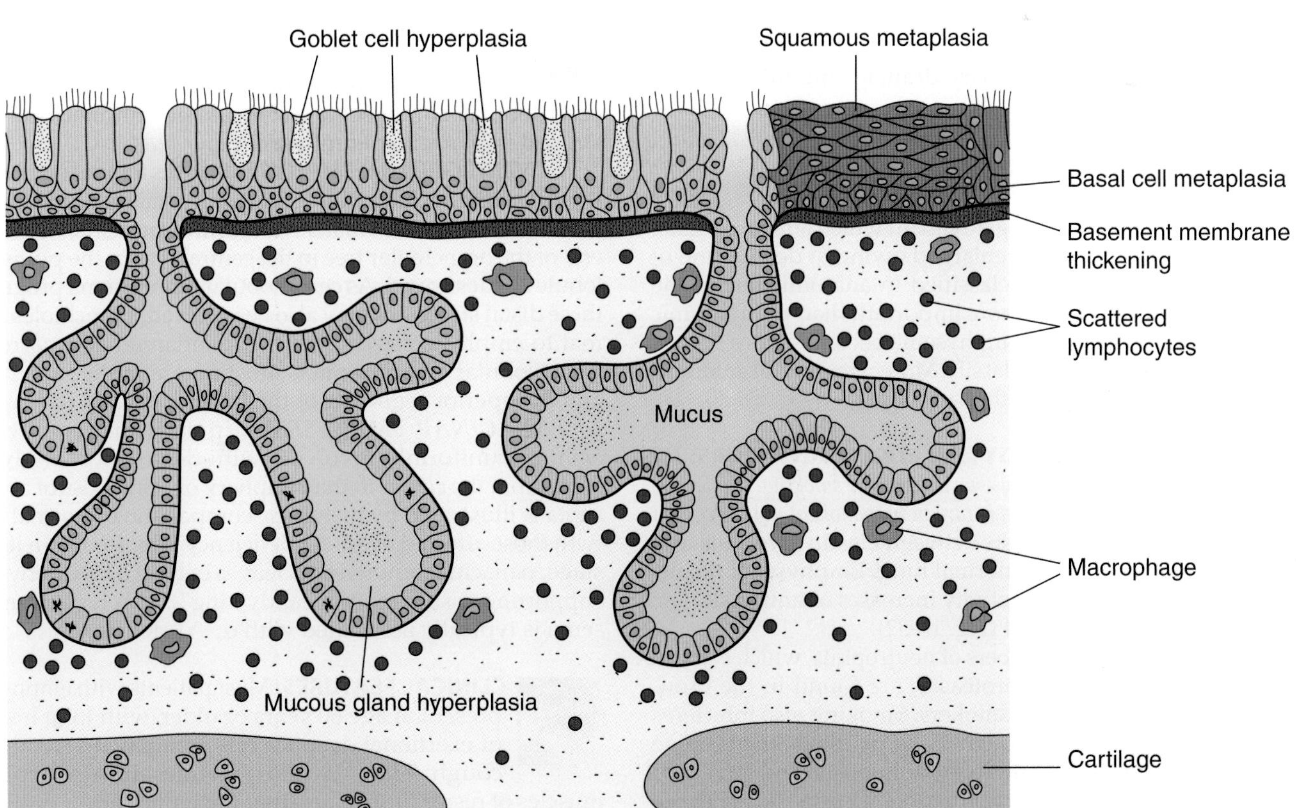

FIGURE 10-31. Chronic bronchitis. Morphologic changes in chronic bronchitis.

Other morphologic changes in chronic bronchitis are variable and include the following:

- Excess mucus in central and peripheral airways
- "Pits" on the surface of the bronchial epithelium, which represent dilated ducts into which several bronchial glands open
- Thickening of the bronchial wall by mucous gland enlargement and edema, encroaching on the bronchial lumen
- Increased numbers of goblet cells (hyperplasia) in the bronchial epithelium
- Increased smooth muscle, which may indicate bronchial hyperreactivity
- Squamous metaplasia of the bronchial epithelium, reflecting epithelial damage from tobacco smoke, an effect that is probably independent of the other changes seen in chronic bronchitis

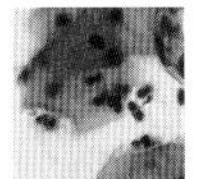

CLINICAL FEATURES: Chronic bronchitis is often accompanied by emphysema (see below), and separating the contributions of each in an individual patient may be difficult. In general, patients with mainly chronic bronchitis have had a productive cough for many years. Exertional dyspnea and cyanosis supervene, and cor pulmonale may ensue. The combination of cyanosis and edema as a result of cor pulmonale has led to the label "blue bloater" for such patients.

In patients with advanced chronic bronchitis, multiple factors such as pulmonary infections (particularly with *Haemophilus influenzae* and *S. pneumoniae*), thromboembolism, left ventricular failure, and major episodes of air pollution may precipitate acute respiratory failure, with progressive hypoxemia and hypercapnia. People with chronic bronchitis must be warned to stop smoking. Prompt antibiotic treatment of pulmonary infections, use of bronchodilator drugs, and, occasionally, bronchopulmonary drainage are mainstays of treatment.

Emphysema

Emphysema is a chronic lung disease in which airspaces distal to terminal bronchioles are enlarged owing to destruction of their walls. Although it is classified in anatomic terms, the severity of emphysema is more important than the anatomic type. In practical terms, as emphysema becomes more severe, it becomes more difficult to classify. Moreover, several anatomic patterns may be present in the same lung.

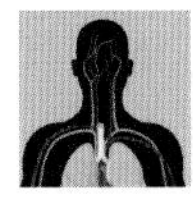

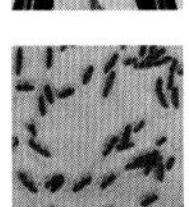

PATHOPHYSIOLOGY AND ETIOLOGIC FACTORS: *The major cause of emphysema is cigarette smoking. Moderate-to-severe emphysema is rare in nonsmokers.* It is thought that a balance exists between elastin synthesis and catabolism in the normal lung. Emphysema results when elastolytic activity increases or antielastolytic activity is reduced (Fig. 10-32).

Increased numbers of neutrophils, which contain serine elastase and other proteases, are found in the bronchoalveolar lavage fluid of smokers. Smoking also interferes with α_1-antitrypsin (α_1-AT) activity by oxidizing methionine residues in the protein. In this way, unopposed and increased elastolytic activity leads to destruction of elastic tissue in the walls of distal airspaces, impairing elastic recoil. At the same time, other cellular proteases may be involved in injury to the airspace walls.

α_1-ANTITRYPSIN DEFICIENCY: Hereditary lack of α_1-AT accounts for about 1% of patients with COPD and is much more common in young people with severe emphysema. α_1-AT is a circulating inhibitor of serine proteases (a serpin), including elastase, trypsin, chymotrypsin, thrombin, and bacterial proteases. Made in the liver, it accounts for 90% of blood antiproteinase activity. In the lung, it inhibits neutrophil elastase, an enzyme that digests elastin and other alveolar wall components.

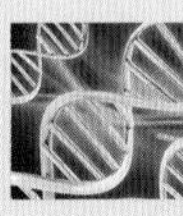

MOLECULAR PATHOGENESIS: The amount and type of α_1-AT is determined by a pair of codominant protease inhibitor (*Pi*) alleles at the *serpinA1 locus*. The most common allele is *PiM, and the most common genotype is PiMM.* Some mutant forms fail to fold properly and are thus targeted for proteasomal degradation in liver cells. Other mutant forms may polymerize and accumulate within hepatocytes. The most serious abnormality involves the *PiZ* allele. Because the abnormal protein is poorly secreted by the liver, plasma α_1-AT in *PiZZ* homozygotes is only 15% to 20% of normal. These people are at risk for cirrhosis of the liver and emphysema. **Most patients with clinically diagnosed emphysema under age 40 have α_1-AT deficiency (*PiZZ*).** In *PiZZ* homozygotes who do not smoke, emphysema begins between ages 45 and 50; those who smoke develop it 5 to 10 years earlier. Heterozygotes for the PiZ mutation show little, if any, increased risk for lung disease.

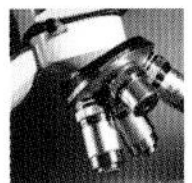

PATHOLOGY: Emphysema is morphologically classified according to the location of the lesions within the pulmonary acinus (Fig. 10-33). Only the proximal acinus (the respiratory bronchiole) is affected in centrilobular emphysema, whereas the entire acinus is destroyed in panacinar emphysema.

CENTRILOBULAR EMPHYSEMA: This form of emphysema is most common. It usually accompanies cigarette smoking and is symptomatic. The clusters of terminal bronchioles near the end of the bronchiolar tree in the central part of the pulmonary lobule are destroyed. As centrilobular emphysema progresses, these distal structures may also be involved. Bronchioles proximal to emphysematous spaces are inflamed and narrowed. Centrilobular emphysema is most severe in the upper lobes and in superior segments of the lower lobes.

PANACINAR EMPHYSEMA: In panacinar emphysema, acini are uniformly involved, with destruction of alveolar septa from the center to the periphery of acini. Loss of alveolar septa is illustrated by histologic comparison of normal lungs with those affected by α_1-AT deficiency (Fig. 10-34). In its final stage, panacinar emphysema leaves behind a lacy network of supporting tissue ("cotton-candy lung"). This type of emphysema is typically associated with α_1-AT deficiency.

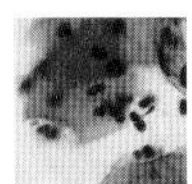

CLINICAL FEATURES: Most patients with emphysema present at age 60 years or older, with long histories of exertional dyspnea but minimal, nonproductive cough. They have lost weight and use accessory muscles of respiration to breathe. Tachypnea and a prolonged expiratory phase are typical. Radiologically, the lungs are overinflated: diaphragms are depressed, and the posteroanterior diameter is increased (barrel chest). Bronchovascular

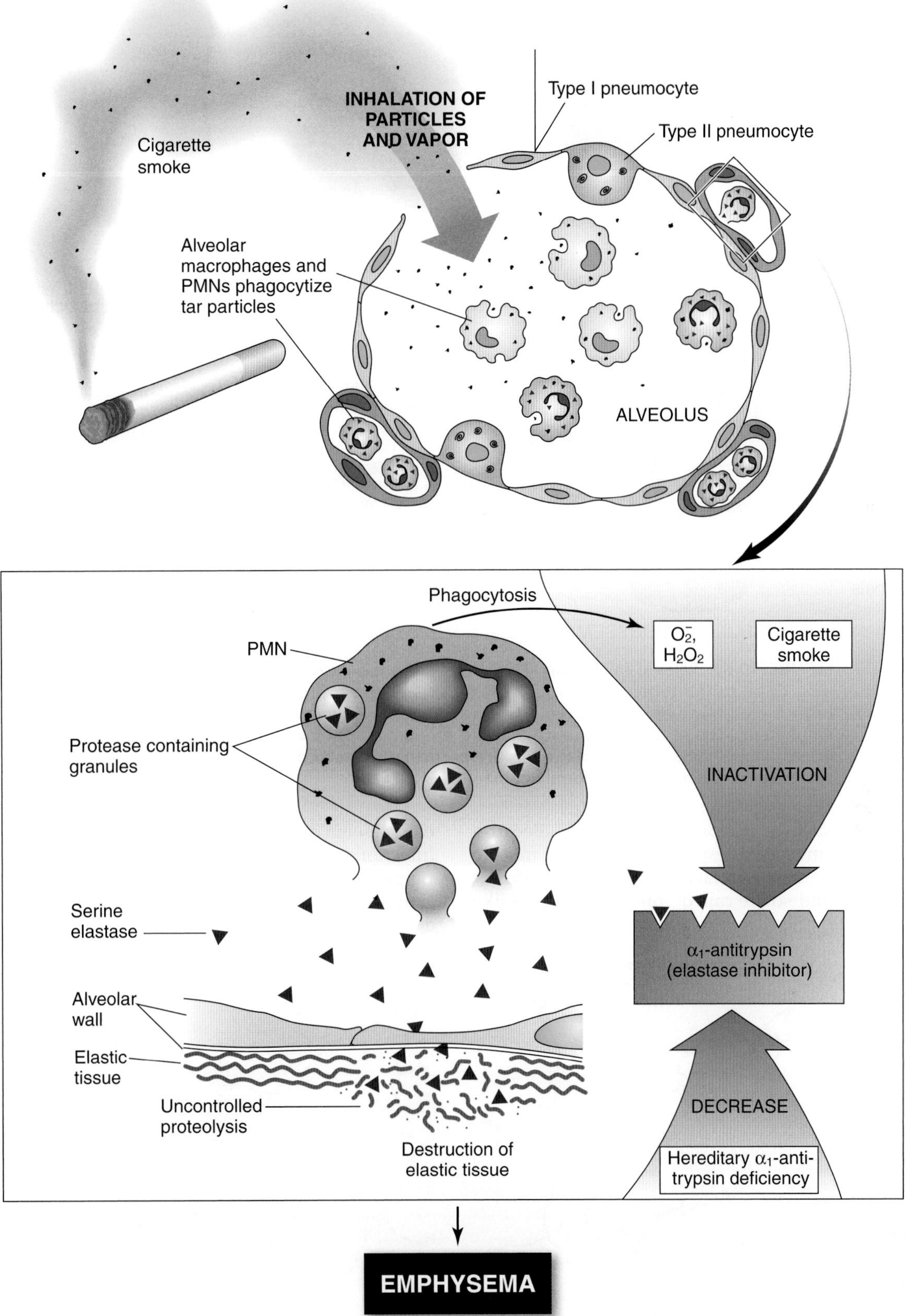

FIGURE 10-32. **The proteolysis–antiproteolysis theory of the pathogenesis of emphysema.** Cigarette (tobacco) smoking is closely related to the development of emphysema. Some products in tobacco smoke induce an inflammatory reaction. The serine elastase in polymorphonuclear leukocytes, a particularly potent elastolytic agent, injures the elastic tissue of the lung. Normally, this enzyme activity is inhibited by α_1-antitrypsin, but tobacco smoke, directly or through the generation of free radicals, inactivates α_1-antitrypsin (protease inhibitor). H_2O_2, hydrogen peroxide; O_2^-, superoxide ion; PMN, polymorphonuclear neutrophil.

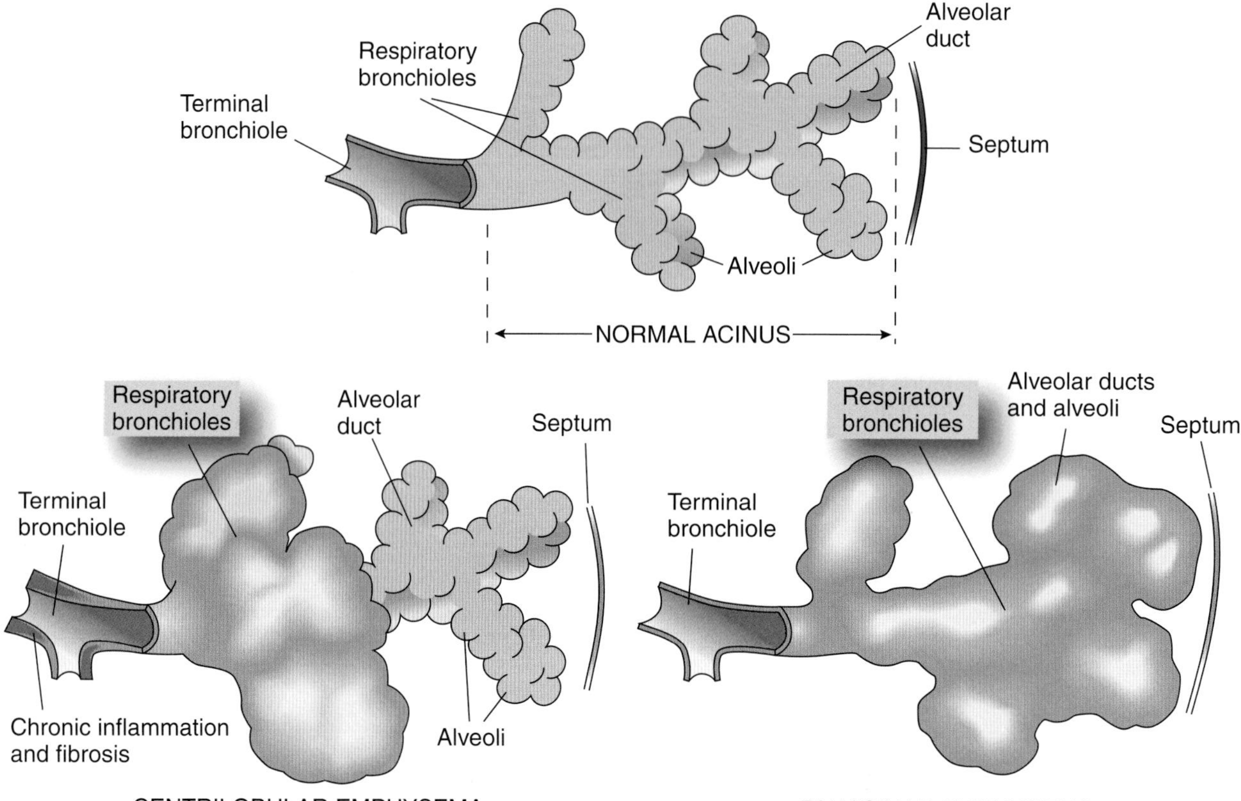

FIGURE 10-33. Types of emphysema. The acinus is the gas-exchanging structural unit of the lung distal to the terminal bronchiole. It consists of (from proximal to distal) respiratory bronchioles, alveolar ducts, alveolar sacs, and alveoli. In centrilobular (proximal acinar) emphysema, the respiratory bronchioles are predominantly involved. In paraseptal (distal acinar) emphysema, the alveolar ducts are particularly affected. In panacinar (panlobular) emphysema, the acinus is uniformly damaged.

markings do not reach the peripheral lung fields. Because these patients have increased respiratory rates and minute volumes, they can maintain arterial hemoglobin saturation at near-normal levels and so are called "pink puffers." Unlike patients with predominantly chronic bronchitis, those with emphysema are not at higher risk for recurrent pulmonary infections and are not so prone to develop cor pulmonale. Emphysema entails an inexorable decline in respiratory function and progressive dyspnea, for which no treatment is adequate.

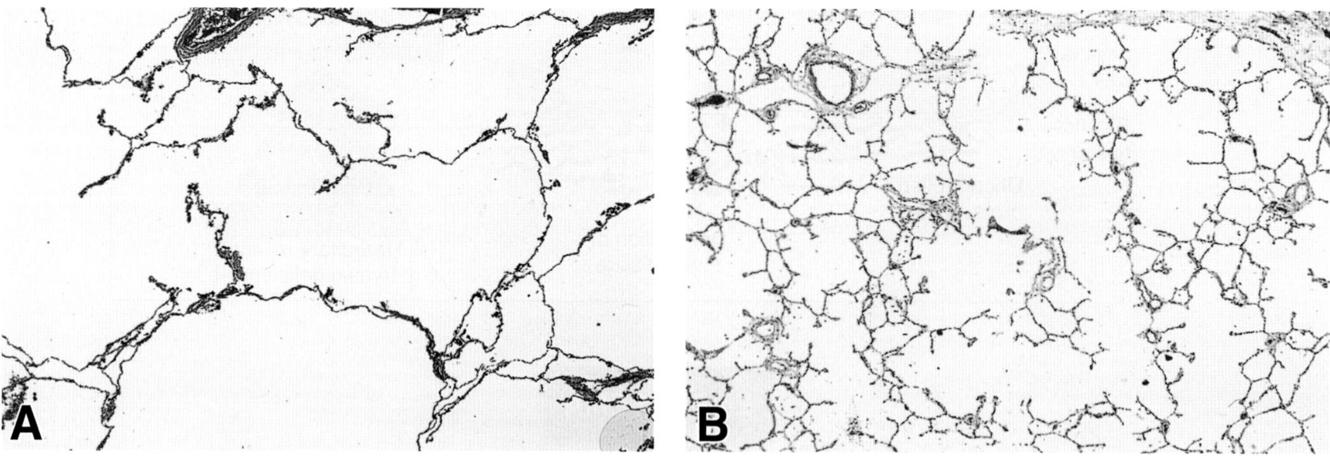

FIGURE 10-34. Panacinar emphysema. A. The lung, from a patient with α_1-antitrypsin deficiency, showing large, irregular airspaces and a markedly reduced number of alveolar walls. **B.** Extensive loss of alveolar walls in **A** is emphasized by comparison with this section of normal lung at the same magnification.

Asthma

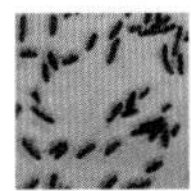

ETIOLOGIC FACTORS: Asthma was once divided into **extrinsic (allergic)** and **intrinsic (idiosyncratic)** forms, depending on inciting factors. It is now described in terms of the different inciting factors and the common effector pathways.

Bronchial hyperresponsiveness in asthma generally reflects inflammatory reactions to diverse stimuli. After exposure to an inciting factor (e.g., allergens, drugs, cold, and exercise), inflammatory mediators released by activated macrophages, mast cells, eosinophils, and basophils trigger bronchoconstriction, increased vascular permeability, and mucous secretion. Resident inflammatory cells release chemotactic factors, which, in turn, recruit more effector cells and amplify the response of the airways. Inflammation of bronchial walls may also injure the epithelium, stimulating nerve endings and initiating neural reflexes that further aggravate and propagate the bronchospasm.

In a sensitized person, an inhaled allergen interacts with T_H2 cells and IgE antibody bound to the surface of mast cells, which are interspersed among the bronchial epithelial cells (Fig. 10-35). T_H2 cells and mast cells release mediators of type I (immediate) hypersensitivity, including histamine, bradykinin, leukotrienes, prostaglandins, thromboxane A_2, and platelet-activating factor (PAF), as well as cytokines such as interleukin (IL)-4 and IL-5. These inflammatory mediators lead to (1) **smooth muscle contraction,** (2) **mucous secretion,** and (3) **increased vascular permeability and edema**. Each of these effects is a potent, albeit reversible, cause of airway obstruction.

ALLERGIC ASTHMA: This is the most common form of asthma and is usually seen in children. One third to one half of all patients with asthma have known or suspected reactions to allergens, such as pollens, animal hair or fur, and house dust contaminated with mites. Allergic asthma correlates strongly with skin-test reactivity. Half of children with asthma have substantial or complete remission of symptoms by age 20, but in many, asthma may recur after age 30.

INFECTIOUS ASTHMA: A common precipitating factor in childhood asthma is a viral respiratory tract infection rather than an allergic stimulus. In children under 2 years of age, RSV is the usual agent; in older children, rhinovirus, influenza, and parainfluenza are common inciting organisms. Inflammatory responses to viral infection in susceptible people may trigger an episode of bronchoconstriction.

EXERCISE-INDUCED ASTHMA: Exercise can precipitate bronchospasm in more than half of all asthmatics. In some patients, it may be the only inciting factor. Exercise-induced asthma is related to the magnitude of heat or water loss from airway epithelium. The more rapid the ventilation (severity of exercise) and the colder and drier the air breathed, the more likely is an attack of asthma. The mechanisms underlying exercise-induced asthma are unclear.

OCCUPATIONAL ASTHMA: More than 80 different occupational exposures have been linked to asthma. Some substances may provoke allergic asthma via IgE-related hypersensitivity. Examples include animal handlers, bakers, and workers exposed to wood and vegetable dusts, metal salts, pharmaceutical agents, and industrial chemicals. Direct release of mediators of smooth muscle contraction after contact with an offending agent occurs in byssinosis ("brown lung") in cotton workers.

DRUG-INDUCED ASTHMA: Drug-induced bronchospasm occurs mostly in patients with known asthma. The best-known offender is aspirin, but other nonsteroidal anti-inflammatory agents have also been implicated.

AIR POLLUTION: Massive air pollution, usually occurring during temperature inversions, may cause bronchospasm in patients with asthma and other preexisting lung diseases. Gases such as SO_2, nitrogen oxides, and ozone are commonly implicated, but particulate carbon, carrying toxic chemicals in diesel exhaust, may also participate.

EMOTIONAL FACTORS: Psychological stress can aggravate or precipitate attacks of bronchospasm in as many as half of asthmatics. Vagal efferent stimulation is thought to be the underlying mechanism.

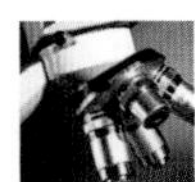

PATHOLOGY: The pathology of asthma has been studied in autopsies of patients who died in **status asthmaticus** (severe acute asthma that is unresponsive to therapy). Grossly, the lungs are highly distended with air, and airways are filled with thick, tenacious, adherent mucous plugs. Microscopically, these plugs (Fig. 10-36A) contain strips of epithelium and many eosinophils. Charcot–Leyden crystals, derived from phospholipids of the eosinophil cell membrane, may also be seen. In some cases, mucoid casts of the airways (Curschmann spirals) are expelled with coughing as are are compact clusters of epithelial cells (Creola bodies).

One of the most characteristic features of status asthmaticus is hyperplasia of bronchial smooth muscle. Bronchial submucosal mucous glands are also hyperplastic (Fig. 10-36A). The submucosa is edematous, with a mixed inflammatory infiltrate containing variable numbers of eosinophils. The epithelium does not show the normal pseudostratified appearance and may be denuded, with only basal cells remaining (Fig. 10-36B). The basal cells are hyperplastic, and squamous metaplasia and goblet cell hyperplasia are seen. Bronchial epithelial basement membranes are thickened, owing to an increase in collagen deep to the true basal lamina.

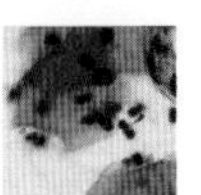

CLINICAL FEATURES: Asthmatic patients typically have paroxysms of wheezing, dyspnea, and cough. Attacks may alternate with asymptomatic periods or be superimposed on a background of chronic airway obstruction. Most asthmatic patients, even when apparently well, have some persistent airflow obstruction. A typical attack of asthma begins with tightness in the chest and nonproductive cough. Inspiratory and expiratory wheezes appear, respiratory rate increases, and the patient becomes dyspneic. The expiratory phase is particularly prolonged. The attack often ends with fits of severe coughing and expectoration of thick, mucus-containing Curschmann spirals, eosinophils, and Charcot–Leyden crystals.

Status asthmaticus is accompanied by severe bronchoconstriction that does not respond to drugs that usually abort the acute attack. It is a serious condition and requires hospitalization. Patients in status asthmaticus have hypoxemia and often hypercapnia. Severe episodes may be fatal. The cornerstone of asthma treatment includes administration of β-adrenergic agonists, inhaled corticosteroids, cromolyn sodium, methylxanthines, and anticholinergic agents. The inhalation of bronchodilators often provides dramatic relief.

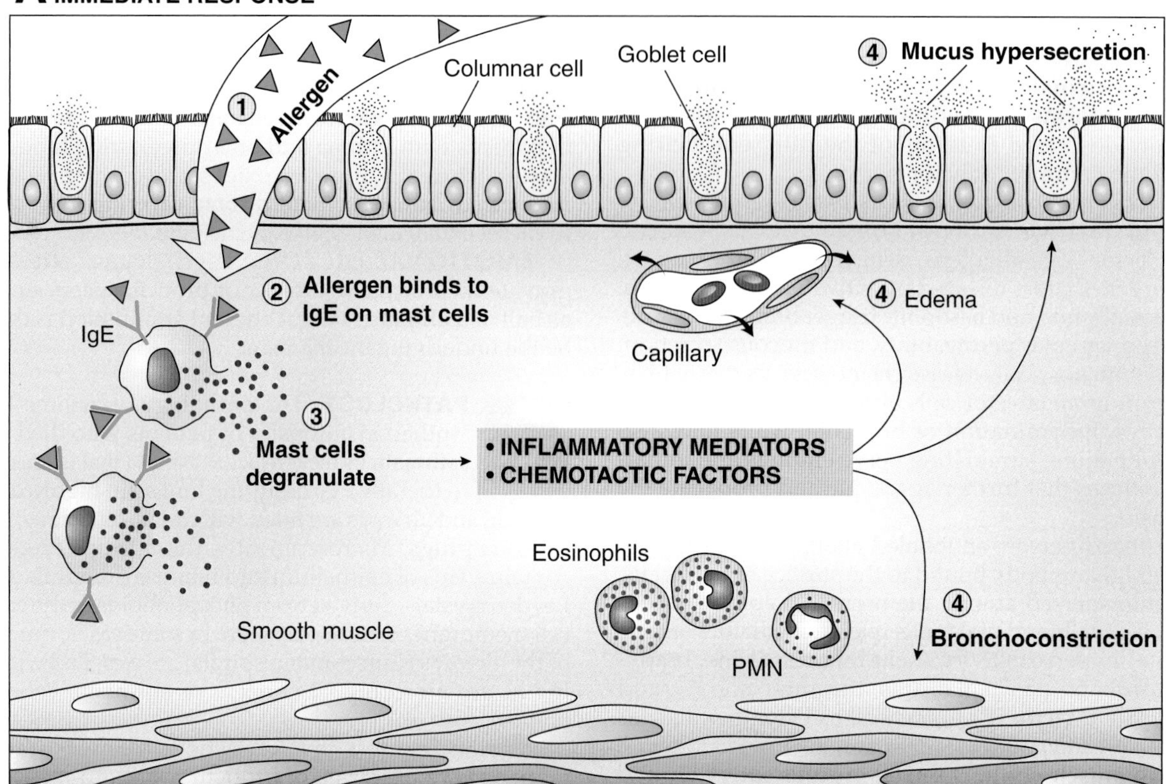

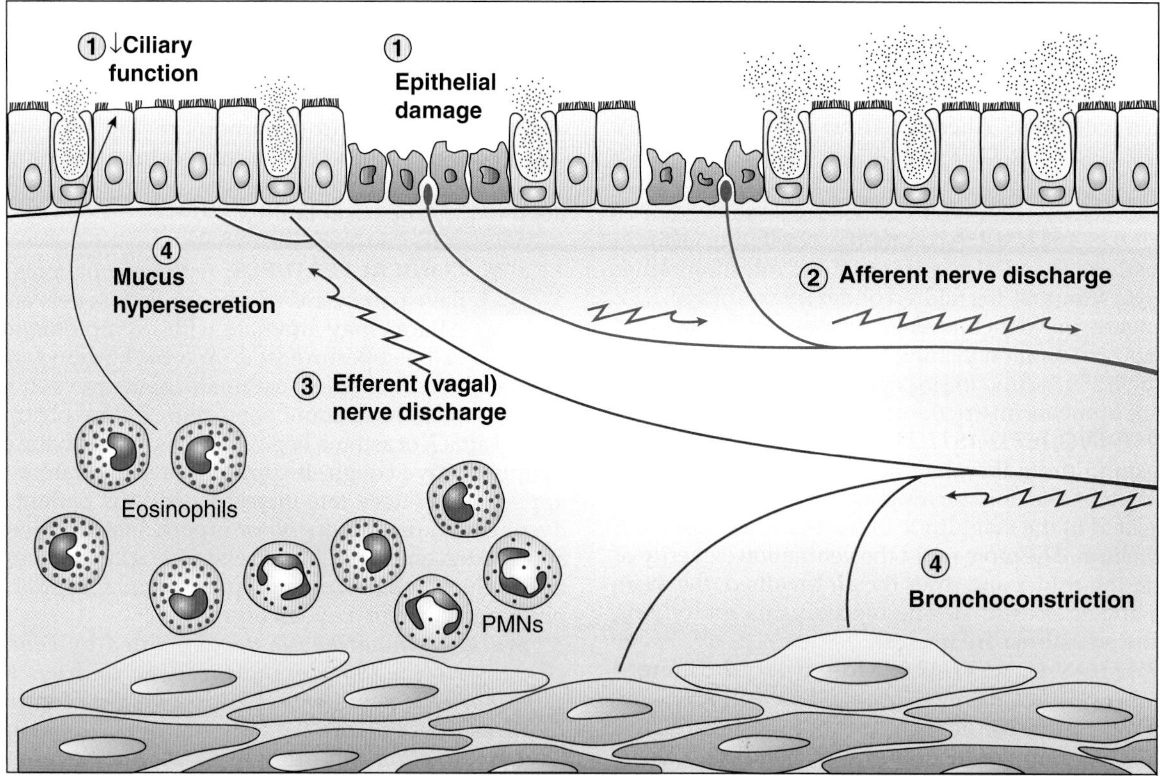

FIGURE 10-35. Pathogenesis of asthma. A. Immunologically mediated asthma. Allergens interact with immunoglobulin E (IgE) on mast cells, either on the surface of the epithelium or, when there is abnormal permeability of the epithelium, in the submucosa. Released mediators may react locally or by vagal reflexes. **B.** Discharge of eosinophilic granules further impairs mucociliary function and damages epithelial cells. Epithelial cell injury stimulates nerve endings (*in red*) in the mucosa, initiating an autonomic discharge that contributes to airway narrowing and mucus secretion. PMNs, polymorphonuclear neutrophils.

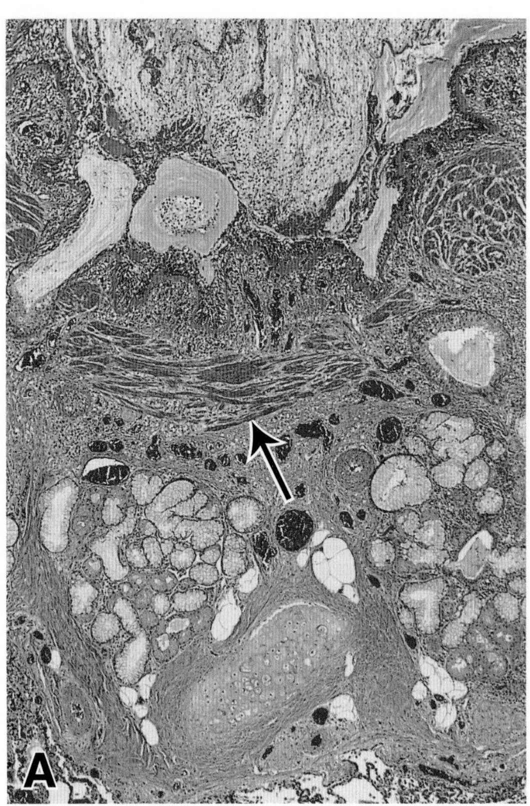

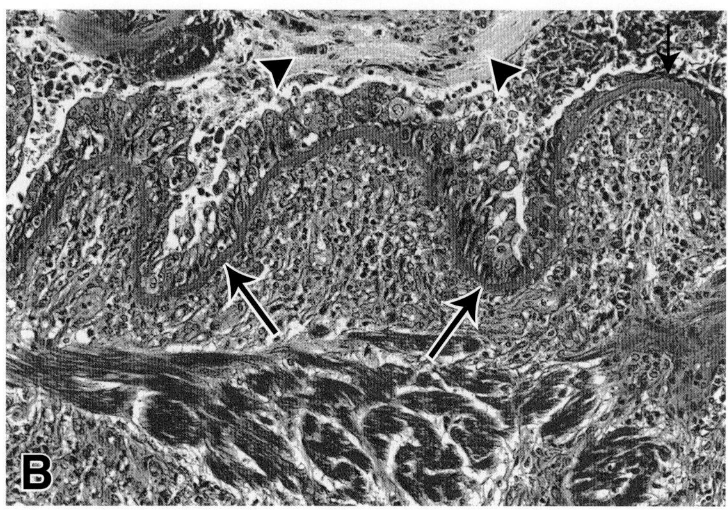

FIGURE 10-36. Asthma. A. A section of lung from a patient who died in status asthmaticus revealing a bronchus containing a luminal mucous plug, submucosal gland hyperplasia, and smooth muscle hyperplasia (*arrow*). **B.** Higher magnification showing hyaline thickening of the subepithelial basement membrane (*long arrows*) and marked inflammation of the bronchiolar wall, with numerous eosinophils. The mucosa exhibits an inflamed and metaplastic epithelium (*arrowheads*). The epithelium is focally denuded (*short arrow*).

RESTRICTIVE PULMONARY DISEASES

Restrictive lung diseases result from either a decrease in the functional lung volume or a reduction in the compliance (elasticity) of the lung. The pneumoconioses are occupational diseases that are associated with pulmonary fibrosis, resulting in loss of both functional volume and elasticity. The interstitial lung diseases are complex although primarily restrictive may also demonstrate some degree of obstructive disease.

Pneumoconioses Are Occupational in Nature

Pneumoconioses are pulmonary diseases caused by mineral dust inhalation. Over 40 inhaled minerals cause lung lesions and radiographic abnormalities. Most, like tin, barium, and iron, are innocuous and simply accumulate in the lung. However, some lead to crippling lung diseases, which are related to destruction of functional parenchymal tissue as a result of fibrosis. The specific types of pneumoconioses are named by the substance inhaled (e.g., silicosis, asbestosis, and talcosis).

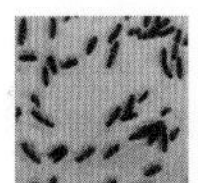

ETIOLOGIC FACTORS: ***The key factor in the genesis of symptomatic pneumoconioses is the capacity of inhaled dusts to stimulate fibrosis*** (Fig. 10-37). Thus, small amounts of silica produce extensive fibrosis, whereas coal and iron are only weakly fibrogenic.

The most dangerous particles are those that reach the farthest periphery (i.e., the smallest bronchioles and acini). Particles 2.5 to 10 μm in diameter deposit on bronchi and bronchioles and are removed by mucociliary action. Smaller particles (<2.5 μm) reach acini, and the tiniest ones (<100 nm) may penetrate alveolar walls and enter the bloodstream. Alveolar macrophages ingest inhaled particles and are the main defenders of the alveolar space. Most phagocytosed particles ascend to the mucociliary carpet, to be coughed up or swallowed. Others migrate into the lung interstitium and thence into lymphatics. Many ingested particles accumulate in and about respiratory bronchioles and terminal bronchioles. Others are not phagocytosed but migrate through epithelial cells into the interstitium.

Silicosis

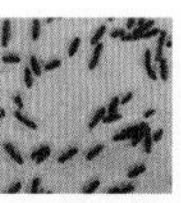

ETIOLOGIC FACTORS: The biologic effects of silica particles depend on a number of factors, some involving the particle itself and others related to the host response.

After their inhalation, silica particles are ingested by alveolar macrophages. Silicon hydroxide groups on the particle's surface form hydrogen bonds with phospholipids and proteins. This interaction damages cellular membranes and so kills the macrophages. The dead cells release free silica particles and fibrogenic factors. The released silica is then reingested by macrophages, and the process is amplified.

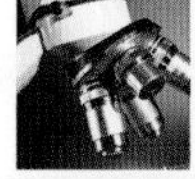

PATHOLOGY: Simple nodular silicosis is the most common form of silicosis and is almost inevitable in any worker with long-term exposure to silica. By 10 to 40 years after initial exposure to silica, the lungs contain silicotic nodules less than 1 cm in diameter (usually 2 to 4 mm). Histologically, they have a characteristic whorled appearance, with concentrically arranged collagen forming the largest part of the nodule (Fig.10-38). At the periphery are aggregates of mononuclear cells, mostly lymphocytes and fibroblasts. Polarized light reveals doubly refractile needle-shaped silicates within the nodule. Hilar nodes may be enlarged and calcified, often at their edges ("eggshell calcification").

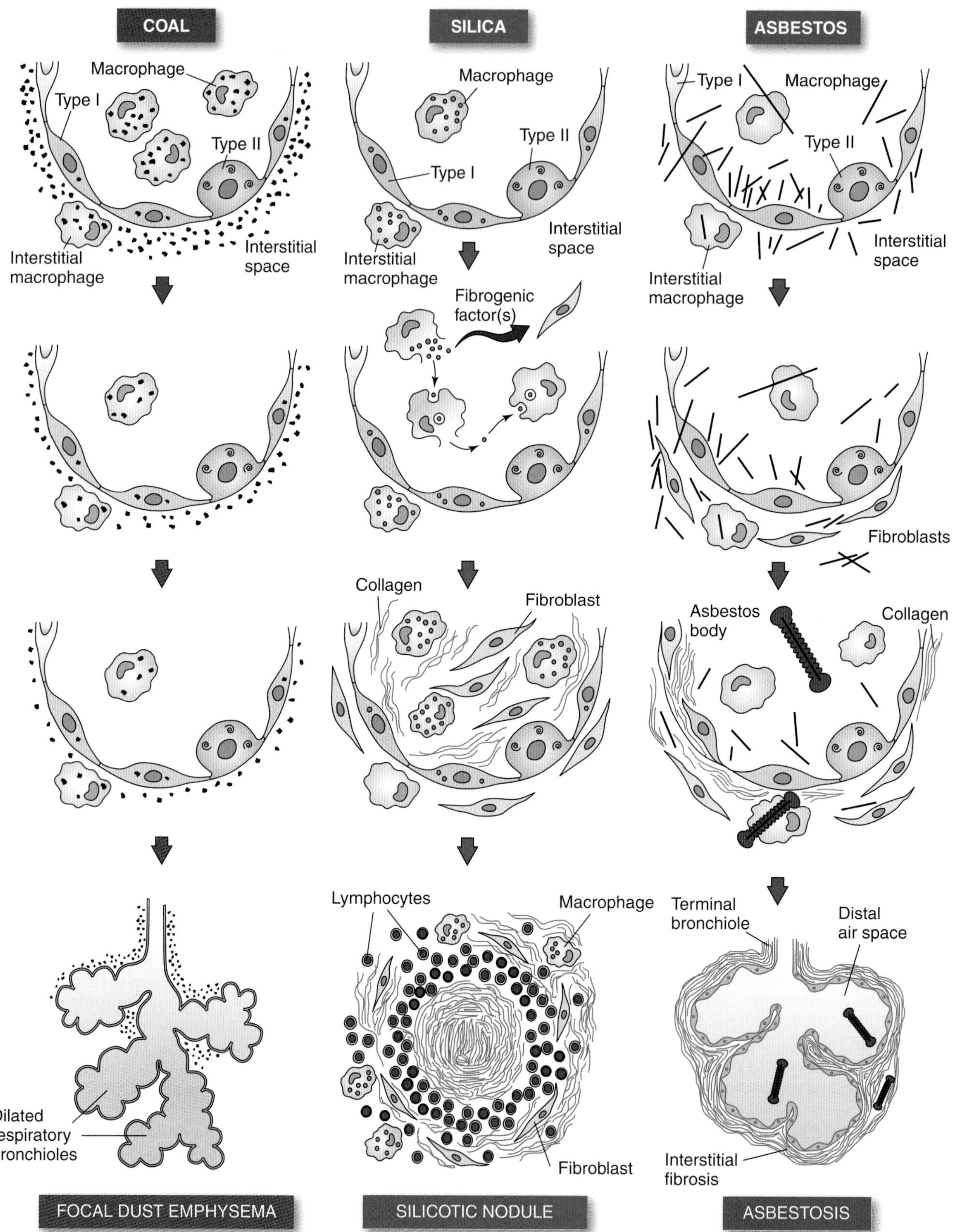

FIGURE 10-37. Pathogenesis of pneumoconioses. The three most important pneumoconioses are illustrated. In simple coal workers' pneumoconiosis, massive amounts of dust are inhaled and engulfed by macrophages. The macrophages pass into the interstitium of the lung and aggregate around respiratory bronchioles, which subsequently dilate. In silicosis, silica particles are toxic to macrophages, causing them to die and release a fibrogenic factor. In turn, the released silica is again phagocytosed by other macrophages. The result is a dense fibrotic nodule, the silicotic nodule. Asbestosis is characterized by considerable interstitial fibrosis. Asbestos bodies are the classic features.

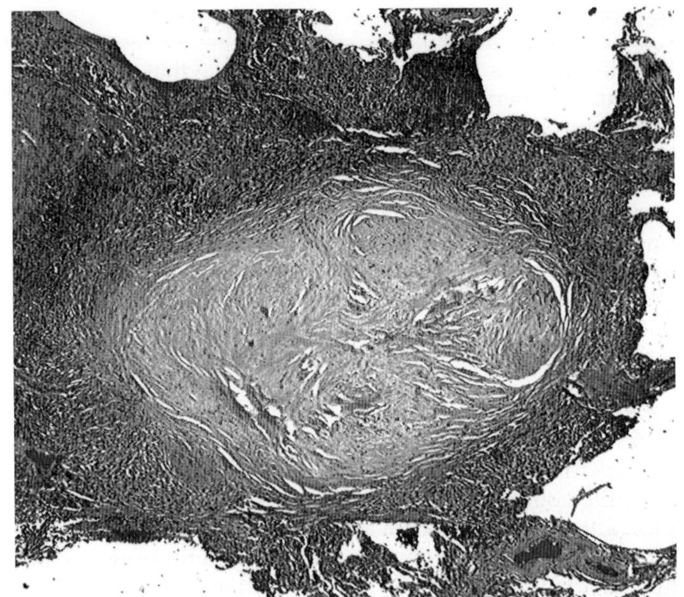

FIGURE 10-38. **Silicosis.** A silicotic nodule is composed of concentric whorls of dense, sparsely cellular collagen.

Simple silicosis does not usually impair respiration significantly. If silicosis may continue, it results in **progressive massive fibrosis,** which relates to the amount of silica in the lung. Nodular masses greater than 2 cm in diameter occur in a background of simple silicosis. Disability is caused by destruction of lung tissue that was incorporated into the nodules. Simple silicosis is usually a radiologic diagnosis without significant symptoms. Dyspnea on exertion and later at rest suggests progressive massive fibrosis or other complications of silicosis.

Coal Workers' Pneumoconiosis

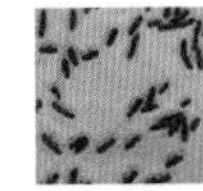

ETIOLOGIC FACTORS: Coal dust is composed of amorphous carbon and other constituents of the earth's surface, including variable amounts of silica. Anthracite (hard) coal contains significantly more quartz than does bituminous (soft) coal. Workers who inhale large amounts of quartz particles, such as those who work within mines, are at greater risk than those working above ground or loading coal for transport. In this context, amorphous carbon by itself is not fibrogenic. It does not kill alveolar macrophages, but is simply a nuisance dust that causes innocuous anthracosis. By contrast, silica is highly fibrogenic, and inhaled anthracotic particles may thus give rise to **anthracosilicosis**.

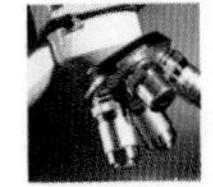

PATHOLOGY: Focal dust emphysema, a disease of coal miners, resembles centrilobular emphysema but differs in that affected spaces are smaller and more regular and lack inflammation of the bronchioles. The lesions mainly distend, rather than destroy, alveolar walls. Coal workers' pneumoconiosis (CWP) is typically divided into **simple CWP** or **complicated CWP** (a.k.a., progressive massive fibrosis). In the latter, destructive **coal-dust macules** form at multiple sites scattered throughout the lung as 1- to 4-mm black foci. Microscopically, coal-dust macules contain many carbon-laden macrophages, which surround distal respiratory bronchioles, extend to fill adjacent alveolar spaces and infiltrate peribronchiolar interstitial spaces. Nodules consist of dust-laden macrophages associated with a fibrotic stroma. **Complicated CWP** is associated with lesions 2.0 cm or greater in size and may cause significant respiratory impairment.

Asbestos-Related Diseases

Asbestos includes a group of fibrous silicate minerals that occur as thin fibers. Because of its heat resistance, it has been used in insulation, construction materials, and automotive parts and products. There are a number of natural types of asbestos that can be divided into two mineralogic groups, namely, amphiboles and chrysotile. Amphiboles are associated with lung diseases, whereas the effects of chrysotile fibers are controversial. Exposure to asbestos can cause asbestosis, benign pleural effusion, pleural plaques, diffuse pleural fibrosis, rounded atelectasis, and mesothelioma (Table 10-4).

ASBESTOSIS: Asbestosis refers to diffuse interstitial fibrosis resulting from inhalation of asbestos fibers. Development of asbestosis requires heavy exposure to asbestos of the type historically seen in certain asbestos miners, millers, and insulators. The first lesion to occur is an alveolitis that is directly related to asbestos exposure. Release of inflammatory mediators by activated macrophages and the fibrogenic character of the free asbestos fibers in the interstitium promote interstitial pulmonary fibrosis.

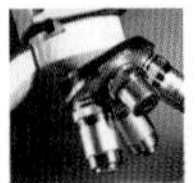

PATHOLOGY: Asbestosis is characterized by bilateral, diffuse interstitial fibrosis, and asbestos bodies in the lung (Figs. 10-39 and 10-40). In early stages, fibrosis occurs in and around alveolar ducts and respiratory bronchioles, and in the periphery of the acinus. When the fibers deposit in bronchioles and respiratory bronchioles, they incite a fibrogenic response, leading to mild chronic airflow obstruction. Thus, asbestos may produce obstructive as well as restrictive defects. As the disease progresses, fibrosis spreads beyond the peribronchiolar location and, eventually, results in an end-stage or "honeycomb" lung. Asbestosis is usually more severe in the lower zones of the lung.

Asbestos bodies are found in the walls of bronchioles or within alveolar spaces, often engulfed by alveolar macrophages. The particles have a distinctive morphology, consisting of a

Table 10-4

Asbestos-Related Lung Disease
Pleural Lesions
Benign pleural effusion
Parietal pleural plaques
Diffuse pleural fibrosis
Rounded atelectasis
Interstitial Lung Disease
Asbestosis
Malignant Mesothelioma
Carcinoma of the lung (in smokers)

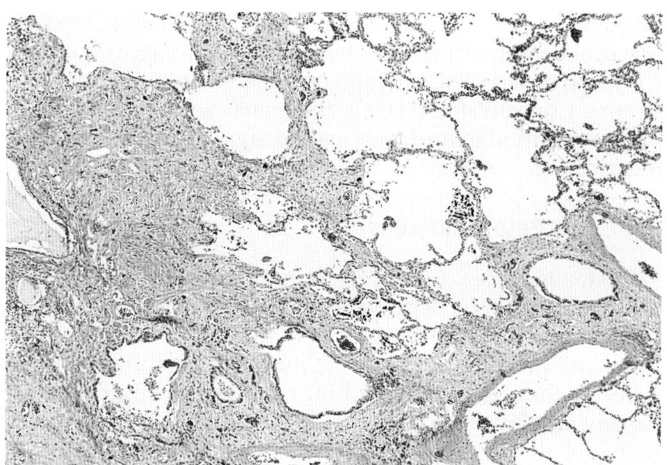

FIGURE 10-39. Asbestosis. The lung shows patchy, dense, interstitial fibrosis. Courtesy of the Joint Pathology Center.

clear, thin asbestos fiber (10 to 50 µm long) surrounded by a beaded iron-protein coat. By light microscopy, they are golden brown (Fig. 10-40) and react strongly with the Prussian blue stain for iron. Finding asbestos bodies incidentally at autopsy does not warrant a diagnosis of asbestosis; the lungs must also show diffuse interstitial fibrosis. **Pleural plaques**, mainly on parietal and diaphragmatic pleura, develop 10 to 20 years after exposure to asbestos but also occur in individuals with no known history of exposure. Grossly, pleural plaques are pearly white and have a smooth or nodular surface. Histologically, they consist of acellular, dense, hyalinized fibrous tissue, with numerous slit-like spaces in a parallel manner ("basket-weave pattern"). Pleural plaques are not predictors of asbestosis, nor do they evolve into mesotheliomas.

MESOTHELIOMA: ***The relation between asbestos exposure and malignant mesothelioma is firmly established.*** Sometimes, exposure has been reported to be indirect and slight (e.g., wives of asbestos workers who wash their husbands' clothes). Most cases of mesothelioma are seen in workers with heavy occupational exposure to asbestos. This malignancy is discussed below with diseases of the pleura.

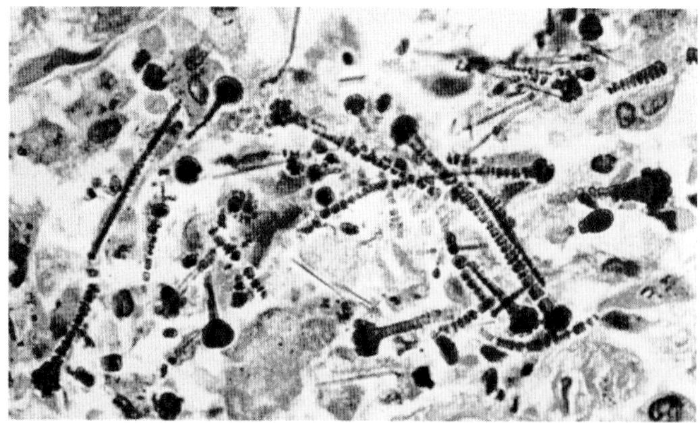

FIGURE 10-40. Asbestos bodies. These ferruginous bodies are golden brown and beaded, with a central, colorless, nonbirefringent core fiber. Asbestos bodies are encrusted with protein and iron.

Berylliosis

Berylliosis refers to the pulmonary disease that follows the inhalation of beryllium. Today, this metal is used principally in structural materials in aerospace, industrial ceramics, and nuclear industries. Exposure to beryllium may also develop in those who mine and extract beryllium ores. Berylliosis occurs as either an acute chemical pneumonitis or chronic pneumoconiosis. In the acute form, symptoms begin within hours or days after inhalation of metal particles and manifest pathologically as diffuse alveolar damage. Some 10% of such patients progress to chronic disease, although chronic berylliosis is often observed in workers without any history of an acute illness. Chronic berylliosis differs from other pneumoconioses in that exposure may be brief and minimal. It may be the result of a hypersensitivity reaction. Pulmonary lesions are indistinguishable from those of sarcoidosis (see below). Multiple noncaseating granulomas are distributed along the pleura, septa, and bronchovascular bundles. The disease may progress to end-stage fibrosis and **honeycomb lung** (see below). Patients with chronic berylliosis often have an insidious onset of dyspnea 15 years or more after the initial exposure.

Talcosis

Talc consists of magnesium silicates that are used in several industries as lubricants and in cosmetics and pharmaceuticals. Cosmetic talc is more than 90% pure and, rarely, causes lung disease. Talcosis lesions vary from tiny nodules to severe fibrosis. People who inject illicit drugs that include talc as a carrier may develop vascular and interstitial granulomas in the lung and variable fibrosis. Arterial changes of pulmonary hypertension are common and are associated with cor pulmonale. Although there have been claims of an association between use of talc products in the female genital area and ovarian cancer, current studies indicate that such risk, if it occurs at all, is extremely small.

Interstitial Lung Diseases Associated With Inflammatory Infiltrates

Many pulmonary disorders that are characterized by interstitial inflammatory infiltrates have similar clinical and radiologic presentations and are grouped as interstitial, infiltrative, or restrictive diseases. These may be acute or chronic and of known or unknown etiology, varying from minimally symptomatic to severely incapacitating and lethal interstitial fibrosis. Resultant restrictive lung diseases are characterized by decreased lung volume and impaired oxygen-diffusing capacity on pulmonary function studies.

Hypersensitivity Pneumonitis

Inhalation of many antigens leads to hypersensitivity pneumonitis (also called extrinsic allergic alveolitis), with acute or chronic interstitial inflammation in the lung. Such antigens are legion and are often encountered in occupational settings. Resulting diseases are labeled accordingly (e.g., **farmer's lung** occurs in people exposed to *Micropolyspora faeni* from moldy hay). Hypersensitivity pneumonitis may also be caused by fungi that grow in stagnant water in air conditioners, swimming pools, hot tubs, and central heating units. Skin tests and serum precipitating antibodies are often used to confirm the diagnosis. However, in chronic hypersensitivity pneumonitis, an inciting antigen is often not identified.

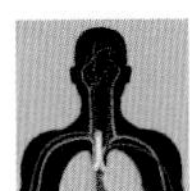

PATHOPHYSIOLOGY: Acute hypersensitivity pneumonitis is characterized by neutrophilic infiltrates in alveoli and respiratory bronchioles; chronic lesions show mononuclear cells and granulomas, typical of delayed hypersensitivity. Most cases have serum IgG precipitating antibodies against the offending agent. Hypersensitivity pneumonitis represents a combination of immune complex–mediated (type III) and cell-mediated (type IV) hypersensitivity reactions, although the precise contribution of each is still debated (Fig. 10-41). Importantly, most people who have serum precipitins to inhaled antigens do not develop hypersensitivity pneumonitis, suggesting a genetic component in host susceptibility.

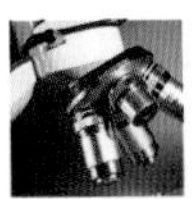

PATHOLOGY: The histologic appearance in florid cases of chronic hypersensitivity pneumonitis is virtually diagnostic. Microscopic features are bronchiolocentric cellular interstitial pneumonia, noncaseating granulomas, and organizing pneumonia (Fig. 10-42A and B). The interstitial infiltrate consists of lymphocytes, plasma cells, and macrophages and varies from severe to subtle; eosinophils are uncommon. Poorly formed noncaseating granulomas are seen in two thirds of cases (Fig. 10-42B), as is organizing pneumonia (see below) (Fig. 10-42A). In the end stage, interstitial inflammation recedes, leaving pulmonary fibrosis, which may resemble usual interstitial pneumonia.

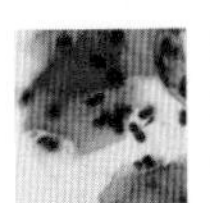

CLINICAL FEATURES: Hypersensitivity pneumonitis may present as acute, subacute, or chronic pulmonary disease, depending on the frequency and intensity of exposure to the offending antigen. Farmer's lung is the prototype of hypersensitivity pneumonitis. After a lag period of 4 to 6 hours following exposure, the worker rapidly develops dyspnea, cough, and mild fever. Symptoms remit within 24 to 48 hours but return on re-exposure; with time, the disorder becomes chronic. Patients with chronic hypersensitivity pneumonitis demonstrate a gradual onset of dyspnea and cor pulmonale. Pulmonary function studies show a restrictive pattern, with decreased compliance, reduced diffusion capacity, and hypoxemia. In the chronic stage, airway obstruction may be troublesome. Removing the offending antigen is the only adequate treatment for hypersensitivity pneumonitis. Steroid therapy may be effective in acute forms and for some chronically affected patients.

Sarcoidosis

Sarcoidosis is a granulomatous disease of unknown etiology. In this disorder, the lung is the organ most often involved, but lymph nodes, skin, eye, and other organs are also common targets.

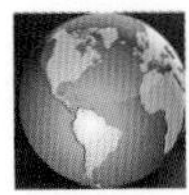

EPIDEMIOLOGY: Sarcoidosis occurs worldwide and affects all races and both sexes, but with strong racial and ethnic predilections. In North America, it is much more common among blacks than whites (15:1), but it is uncommon in tropical Africa.

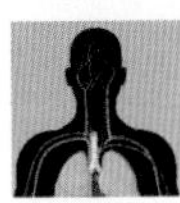

PATHOPHYSIOLOGY: The pathogenesis of sarcoidosis remains obscure, but there is a consensus that helper/inducer T-lymphocyte responses to exogenous or autologous antigens are exaggerated. These cells accumulate in affected organs, where they secrete lymphokines and recruit macrophages, which help form noncaseating granulomas. $CD4^+$ to $CD8^+$ T cell ratios are 10:1 in organs with sarcoid granulomas, but are 2:1 in uninvolved tissues. Nonspecific polyclonal activation of B cells by T-helper cells leads to hyperglobulinemia, a characteristic feature of active sarcoidosis.

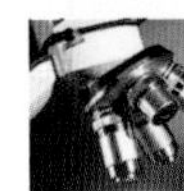

PATHOLOGY: Pulmonary sarcoidosis most often affects the lungs and hilar lymph nodes. Histologically, multiple sarcoid granulomas are scattered in the interstitium of the lung (Fig. 10-43). The distribution is distinctive—along the pleura and interlobular septa and around bronchovascular bundles (Fig. 10-43A). Frequent bronchial or bronchiolar submucosal infiltration by sarcoid granulomas accounts for the high diagnostic yield (≅90%) on bronchoscopic biopsy. Granulomas in airways may occasionally be so prominent as to lead to airway obstruction (endobronchial sarcoid).

Granulomatous vasculitis is seen in two thirds of open lung biopsies from patients with sarcoidosis. Although **asteroid bodies** (star-shaped crystals) (Fig. 10-43B) and **Schaumann bodies** (small lamellar calcifications) are commonly encountered, they are not specific for sarcoidosis and may be seen in many granulomatous processes.

Interstitial fibrosis is not prominent in pulmonary sarcoidosis. However, progressive pulmonary fibrosis may give rise to honeycomb lung, respiratory insufficiency, and cor pulmonale.

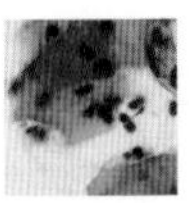

CLINICAL FEATURES: Sarcoidosis is most common in young adults of both sexes. **Acute sarcoidosis** has an abrupt onset, usually followed by spontaneous remission within 2 years and an excellent response to steroids. **Chronic sarcoidosis** begins insidiously, and patients are more likely to have persistent or progressive disease. Sarcoidosis causes several chest radiographic patterns, the most classic of which is bilateral hilar adenopathy, with or without interstitial pulmonary infiltrates. It may also affect the skin (erythema nodosum), mostly in women. Black patients tend to have more severe uveitis, skin disease, and lacrimal gland involvement. Cough and dyspnea are the major respiratory complaints. However, the disease can be mild and may be discovered as an incidental finding on a chest radiograph.

No laboratory test is specific for the diagnosis of sarcoidosis. Transbronchial lung biopsy via a fiberoptic bronchoscope often reveals granulomas. Serum angiotensin-converting enzyme (ACE) levels are elevated in two thirds of patients with active sarcoidosis, and a 24-hour urine calcium is frequently increased. These laboratory data, together with supportive clinical and radiologic findings, allow the diagnosis of sarcoidosis to be made with high probability.

The prognosis in pulmonary sarcoidosis is favorable; most patients do not develop clinically significant sequelae. In 60% of patients, pulmonary sarcoidosis resolves, but this is less likely in older patients and those with extrathoracic disease, particularly in the bone and skin. Corticosteroid therapy is effective for active sarcoidosis.

Usual Interstitial Pneumonia

Usual interstitial pneumonia (UIP) is one of the most common types of interstitial pneumonia, with an annual incidence of 6 to 14 cases per 100,000 people. It has a slight male predominance

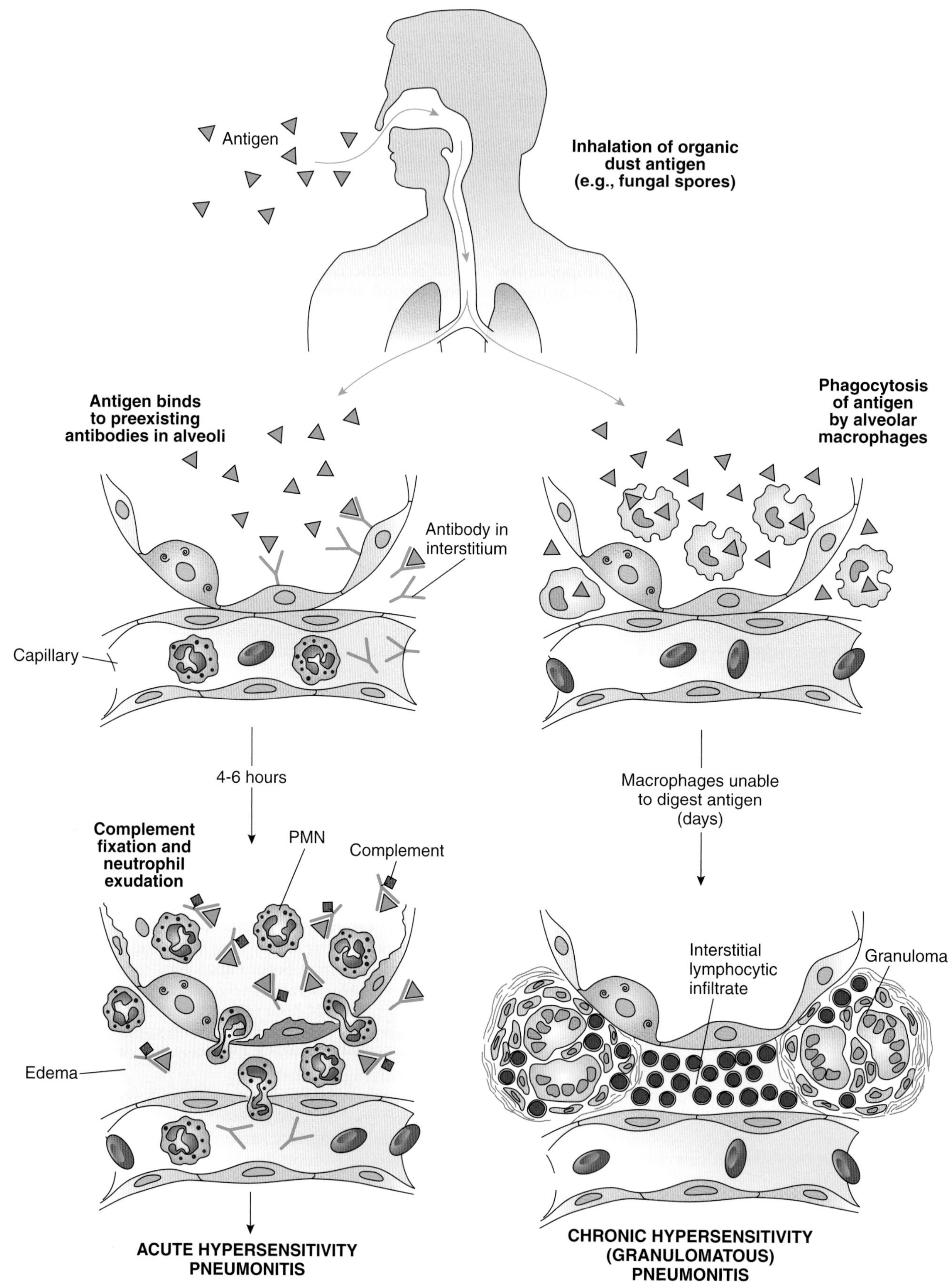

FIGURE 10-41. **Hypersensitivity pneumonitis.** An antigen–antibody reaction occurs in the acute phase and leads to acute hypersensitivity pneumonitis. If exposure is continued, this is followed by a cellular or subacute phase, with formation of granulomas and chronic interstitial pneumonitis. PMN, polymorphonuclear neutrophil.

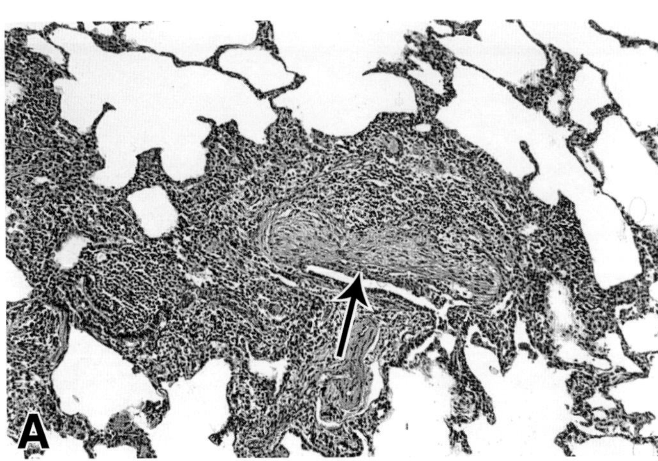

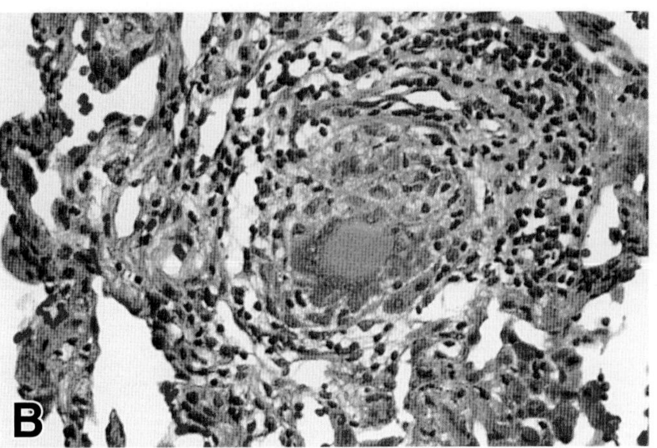

FIGURE 10-42. Hypersensitivity pneumonitis. A. A lung biopsy specimen showing a mild peribronchiolar chronic inflammatory interstitial infiltrate, with a focus of intraluminal organizing fibrosis (*arrow*). **B.** Focal poorly formed granulomas were scattered in the lung biopsy specimen.

and a mean age at onset of 50 to 60 years. UIP is the histologic pattern present on biopsy, and the clinical term **idiopathic pulmonary fibrosis** (IPF) is applied when the disease is determined to be of unknown origin.

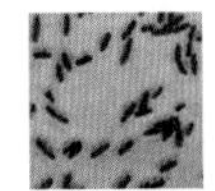

ETIOLOGIC FACTORS: The etiology of IPF is unknown, but immunologic, viral, and genetic factors probably contribute. Some patients have histories of flu-like illnesses, suggesting viral involvement. Mutations in telomerase genes, particularly telomerase reverse transcriptase (TERT), surfactant protein C, and *MUC5B*, are common in familial IPF, but involve less than one third of cases; the genetic abnormality, if any, is unknown in most patients.

In 20% of cases, histologic characteristics of UIP accompany autoimmune diseases, including rheumatoid arthritis, systemic lupus erythematosus, scleroderma, and many others, suggesting impaired immunity. Autoantibodies (e.g., antinuclear antibodies) occur but antigen has yet been identified. Activated alveolar macrophages may release cytokines, which recruit neutrophils. These, in turn, damage alveolar walls, stimulating a series of events that culminates in interstitial fibrosis.

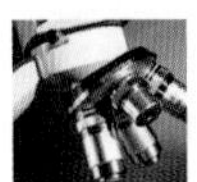

PATHOLOGY: UIP is a histologic pattern that occurs in several clinical settings (e.g., autoimmune disease, chronic hypersensitivity pneumonitis, drug toxicity, and asbestosis). Many cases have no identifiable etiology and are so considered idiopathic (IPF). The lungs are small in UIP, and fibrosis tends to be worse in the lower lobes, in the subpleural regions, and along the interlobular septa. Retraction of the scars, especially of the lobular septa, gives the pleural surface of the lung a hobnail appearance, reminiscent of cirrhosis of the liver. Fibrosis is often patchy, with areas of dense scarring and honeycomb cystic change (Fig. 10-44A).

The histologic hallmark of UIP is patchy interstitial fibrosis, with areas of normal lung adjacent to fibrotic areas (Fig. 10-44B). The fibrosis is of different ages, which has been called "**temporal heterogeneity.**" Areas of loose fibroblastic tissue **(fibroblast foci)** may be adjacent to dense collagen (Fig. 10-44C). The fibrosis is most pronounced beneath the pleura and adjacent to the interlobular septa (Fig. 10-44B).

Bronchiolar epithelium grows into the dilated airspaces, which may be damaged but unrecognizable proximal respiratory

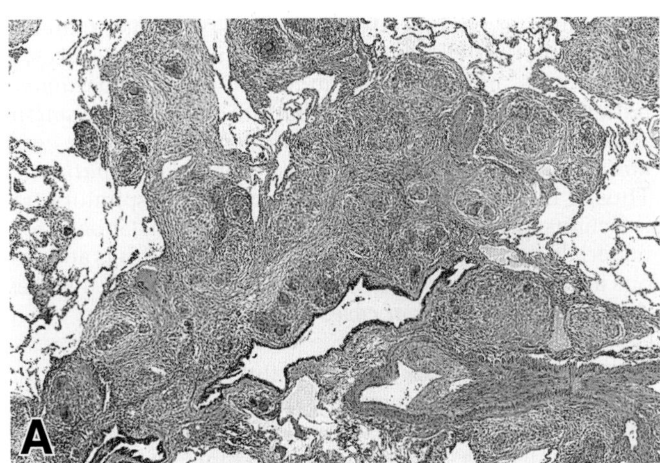

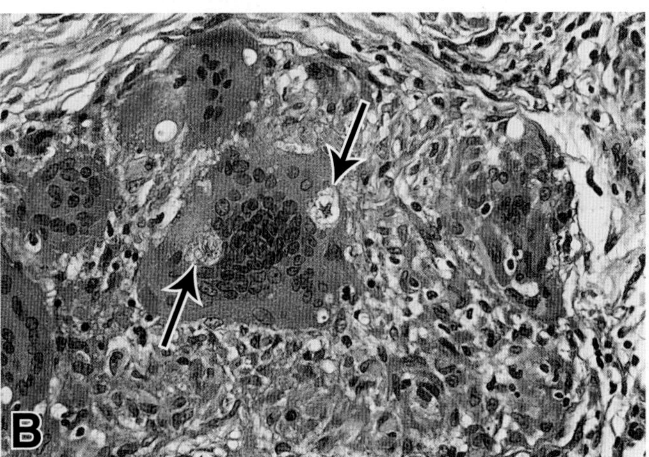

FIGURE 10-43. Sarcoidosis. A. Multiple noncaseating granulomas are present along the bronchovascular interstitium. **B.** Noncaseating granulomas consist of tight clusters of epithelioid macrophages and multinucleated giant cells. Several asteroid bodies are present (*arrows*).

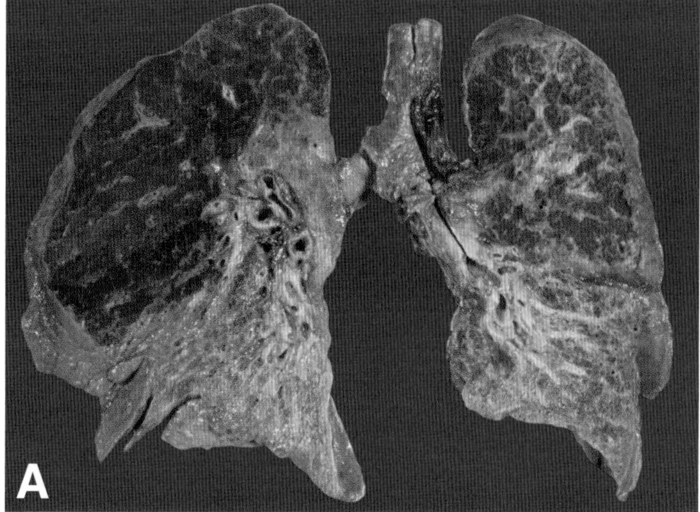

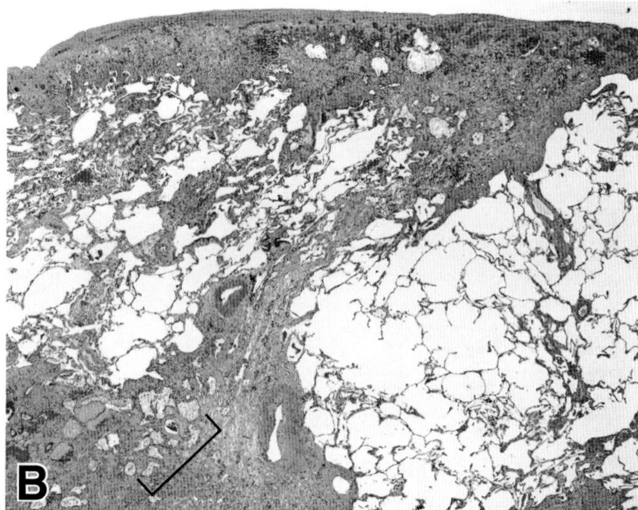

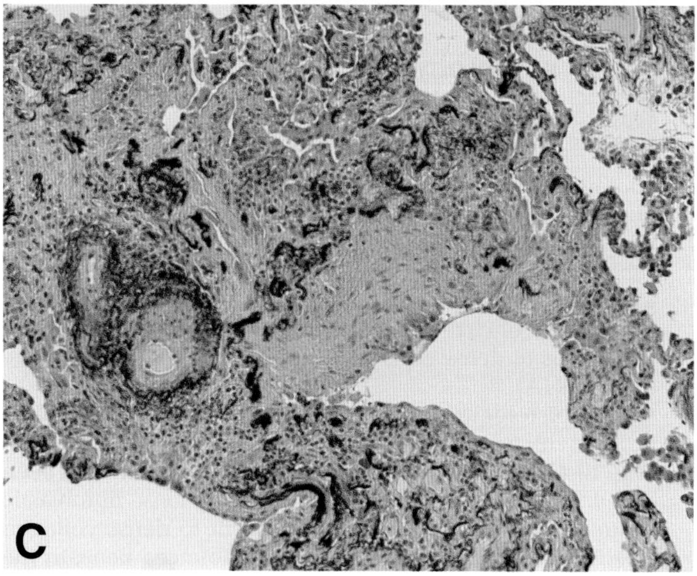

FIGURE 10-44. **Usual interstitial pneumonitis. A.** A gross specimen of the lung showing patchy dense scarring with extensive areas of honeycomb cystic change, predominantly affecting the lower lobes. This patient also had polymyositis. **B.** A microscopic view showing patchy subpleural fibrosis with microscopic honeycomb fibrosis (*bracket*). The areas of dense fibrosis display remodeling, with loss of the normal lung architecture. **C.** Elastin stain highlighting the fibroblastic focus in green, which contrasts with the adjacent area of yellow staining of dense collagen and black staining of collapsed elastic fibers.

bronchioles (Fig. 10-45). The areas of dense scarring fibrosis cause remodeling of the lung architecture, leading to alveolar wall collapse and formation of cystic spaces. These tend to be lined by bronchiolar or cuboidal epithelium and contain mucus, macrophages, or neutrophils (Fig. 10-44A), changes often described as **"honeycomb lung."** Extensive vascular changes of intimal fibrosis and medial thickening may be associated with pulmonary hypertension.

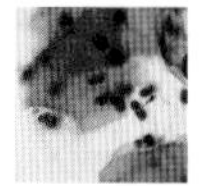

CLINICAL FEATURES: UIP begins insidiously, with gradual onset of dyspnea on exertion and dry cough, usually for 1 to 3 years. Patients have restrictive lung disease by pulmonary function testing. Finger clubbing is common, especially late in the disease. The classic auscultatory finding is late inspiratory crackles and fine ("Velcro") rales at the lung bases. Tachypnea at rest, cyanosis, and cor pulmonale eventually follow. The prognosis is bleak, with a mean survival of 4 to 6 years. Patients are treated with corticosteroids and sometimes cyclophosphamide, but lung transplantation generally offers the only hope of survival.

Organizing Pneumonia Pattern (Cryptogenic Organizing Pneumonia)

In organizing pneumonia pattern (cryptogenic organizing pneumonia), polypoid plugs of tissue fill alveolar spaces, alveolar ducts, and bronchiolar lumens. ***Organizing pneumonia pattern, previously called bronchiolitis obliterans-organizing pneumonia (BOOP) is not specific for any etiologic agent, and its cause cannot be determined from the histopathology.*** Thus, it is seen in many settings, including respiratory tract infections (particularly viral bronchiolitis), inhalation of toxic materials, after administration of a number of drugs and various inflammatory processes (e.g., collagen vascular diseases). ***A substantial number of cases are idiopathic.***

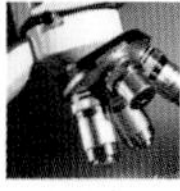

PATHOLOGY: Organizing pneumonia pattern demonstrates patchy areas of loose organizing fibrosis and chronic inflammatory cells in distal airways, adjacent to normal lung. Plugs of organizing fibroblastic tissue occlude bronchioles (bronchiolitis obliterans), alveolar ducts, and surrounding alveoli

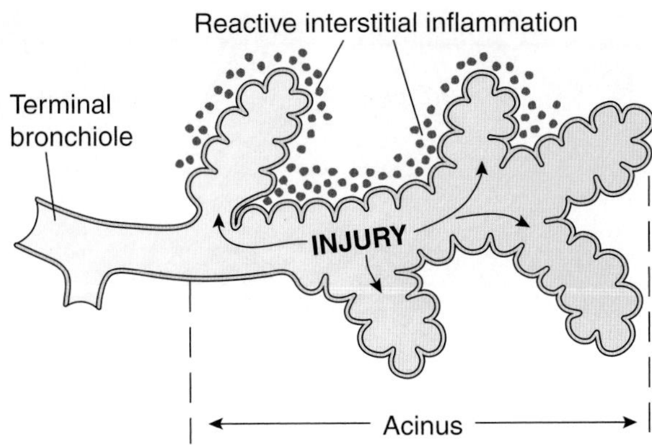

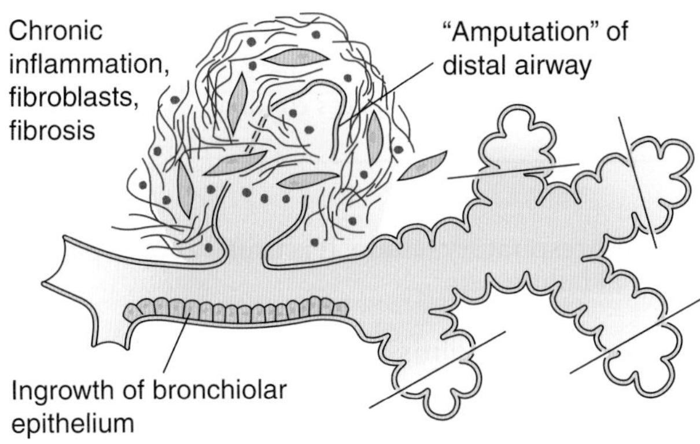

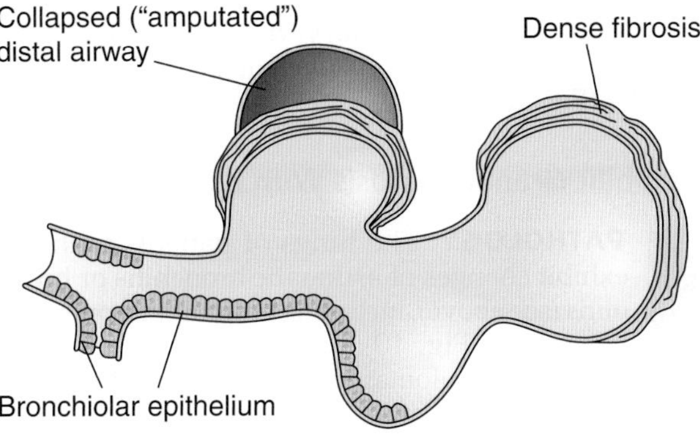

FIGURE 10-45. Pathogenesis of honeycomb lung. Honeycomb lung is the result of a variety of injuries. Interstitial and alveolar inflammation destroys ("amputates") the distal part of the acinus. The proximal parts dilate and become lined by bronchiolar epithelium.

(organizing pneumonia; Fig. 10-46). Alveolar-organizing pneumonia tends to predominate, and lung architecture is preserved.

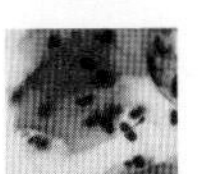

CLINICAL FEATURES: The average age at presentation is 55. The onset is acute, with fever, cough, and dyspnea, often with a history of a flu-like illness 4 to 6 weeks previously. Some patients may have predisposing conditions. Pulmonary function studies demonstrate a restrictive ventilatory pattern. Corticosteroid therapy is effective, and some patients recover within weeks to months, even without therapy.

Langerhans Cell Histiocytosis

Langerhans cell histiocytosis entails diverse histiocyte proliferations. Different presentations of Langerhans cell histiocytosis (LCH) have been called **eosinophilic granuloma, Hand–Schüller–Christian disease,** and **Letterer–Siwe disease** (for details, see Chapters 18 and 22). LCH can affect the lung as a distinctive form of interstitial lung disease. In adults, LCH is ***primarily seen in cigarette smokers*** and may occur as an isolated lesion (previously **pulmonary eosinophilic granuloma**) or as diffuse cystic lung disease. Extrapulmonary manifestations, such as bone lesions or diabetes insipidus, occur in 10% to 15% of cases. In children, lung involvement may occur in association with the multisystemic Letterer–Siwe disease or Hand–Schüller–Christian disease.

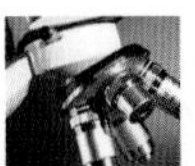

PATHOLOGY: Histologically, pulmonary LCH appears as scattered nodular infiltrates, with a stellate border extending into the surrounding interstitium (Fig. 10-47A). These lesions are frequently subpleural or centered on bronchioles. They contain varying proportions of Langerhans cells admixed with lymphocytes, eosinophils, and macrophages. Langerhans cells are round to oval, with a moderate amount of eosinophilic cytoplasm and prominently grooved nuclei, and small inconspicuous nucleoli (Fig. 10-47B). As the disease progresses, lesions cavitate and become fibrotic, sometimes ending as honeycomb lung. Parenchyma adjacent to the nodular lesions often shows marked accumulation of intra-alveolar macrophages, as a result of respiratory bronchiolitis caused by smoking. Whether pulmonary LCH is a neoplastic proliferation or an abnormal immunologic response to antigens within cigarette smoke is unclear.

VASCULAR DISEASES OF THE LUNG

Vascular pulmonary disease may result from an intrinsic inflammatory vasculitis or much more commonly be as evidence of pulmonary hypertension.

Vasculitis and Granulomatosis

Many pulmonary conditions result in vasculitis, most of which are secondary to other inflammatory processes, such as necrotizing granulomatous infections. Only a few primary idiopathic vasculitis syndromes affect the lung, the most important of which are granulomatosis with polyangiitis (GPA formerly known as Wegener granulomatosis), microscopic polyangiitis, and eosinophilic granulomatosis with polyangiitis (EGPA formerly known as Churg–Strauss granulomatosis). Details of the systemic effects of the vasculidities may be found in Chapter 8. Pulmonary manifestations of primary idiopathic vasculitis are briefly reviewed.

Granulomatosis With Polyangiitis

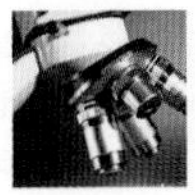

PATHOLOGY: GPA in the lung is characterized by necrotizing granulomatous inflammation, parenchymal necrosis, and vasculitis. Most cases show multiple

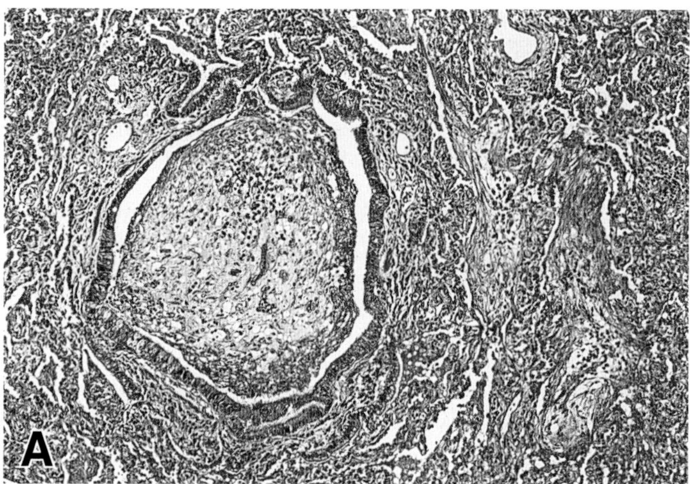

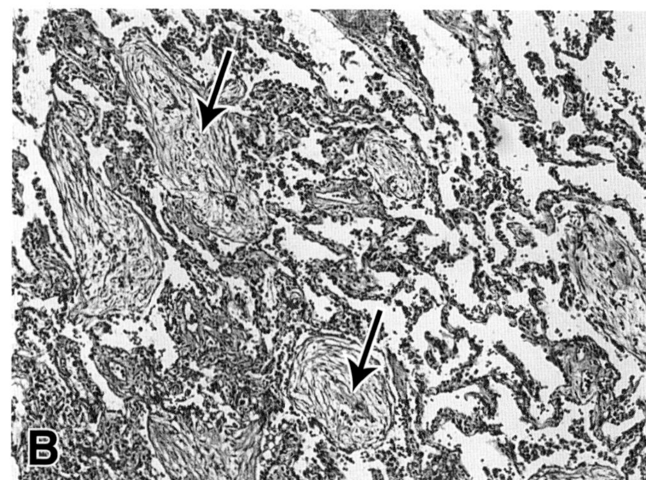

FIGURE 10-46. Organizing pneumonia pattern. A. Polypoid plugs of loose fibrous tissue are present in a bronchiole and adjacent alveolar ducts and alveoli. **B.** Alveolar spaces contain similar plugs of loose organizing connective tissue (*arrows*).

bilateral nodules, averaging 2 to 3 cm, with irregular edges and tan-brown or hemorrhagic cut surfaces, and frequent central cavitation.

Nodules of parenchymal consolidation show (1) tissue necrosis; (2) granulomatous inflammation with a mixture of lymphocytes, plasma cells, neutrophils, eosinophils, macrophages, and giant cells; and (3) fibrosis. Necrosis is accompanied by neutrophilic microabscesses or large basophilic zones of "geographical" necrosis with irregular serpiginous borders (Fig. 10-48A). Patterns of GPA granulomas include palisading macrophages along the border of the large necrotic zones, loosely clustered multinucleated giant cells, and scattered giant cells. Vasculitis may affect arteries (Fig. 10-48B), veins, or capillaries and may show acute, chronic, or granulomatous inflammation. Organizing pneumonia is common at the edges of the nodules of inflammatory consolidation. The lungs often display acute or chronic alveolar hemorrhage. "Neutrophilic capillaritis," with neutrophils in alveolar walls, is common. Diffuse pulmonary hemorrhage, an important complication of GPA, is a fulminant life-threatening crisis with severe respiratory failure. It is usually accompanied by acute renal failure.

Microscopic Polyangiitis

Microscopic polyangiitis is a pauci-immune vasculitis involving arterioles, venules, and capillaries. Almost all patients also show evidence of glomerulonephritis, and microscopic polyangiitis has emerged as one of the more common causes of "pulmonary–renal syndrome." Lung biopsies demonstrate alveolar hemorrhage with neutrophilic capillaritis (Fig. 10-49).

Eosinophilic Granulomatosis With Polyangiitis

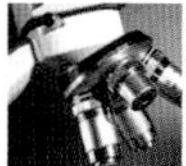

PATHOLOGY: The lungs of patients with EGPA exhibit changes of asthmatic bronchitis or bronchiolitis (see above), including eosinophilic pneumonia, vasculitis (Fig. 10-50A), parenchymal necrosis (Fig. 10-50B), and granulomatous inflammation. Infiltrates of

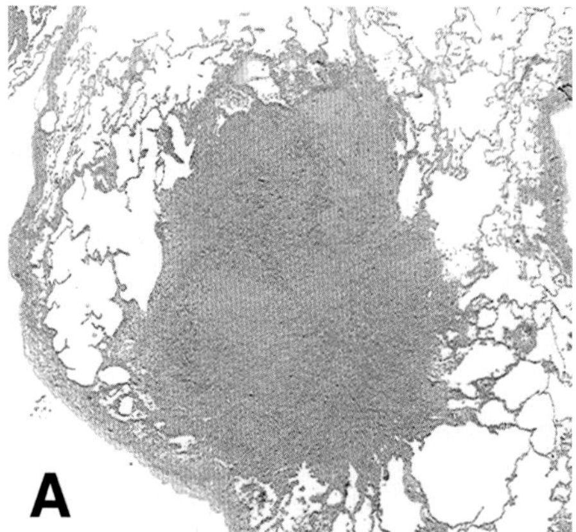

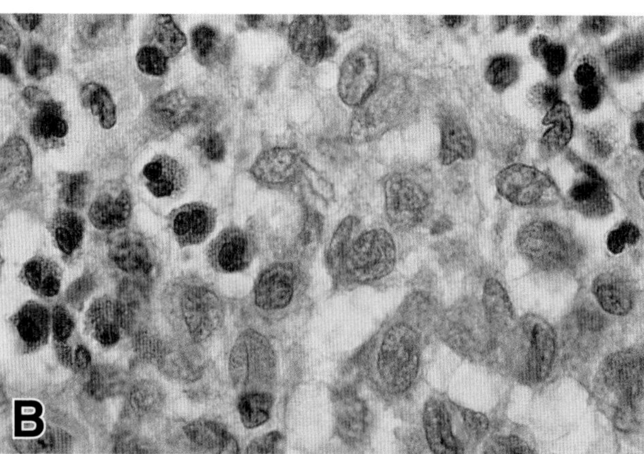

FIGURE 10-47. Langerhans cell histiocytosis. A. The nodular interstitial infiltrate has a stellate shape, with extension of cells into adjacent alveolar septa. **B.** Higher power view showing Langerhans cells with moderate amount of eosinophilic cytoplasm and prominently grooved nuclei. Eosinophils are present.

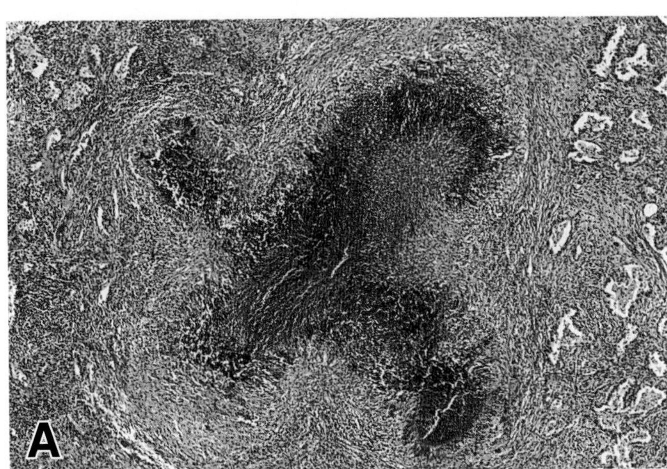

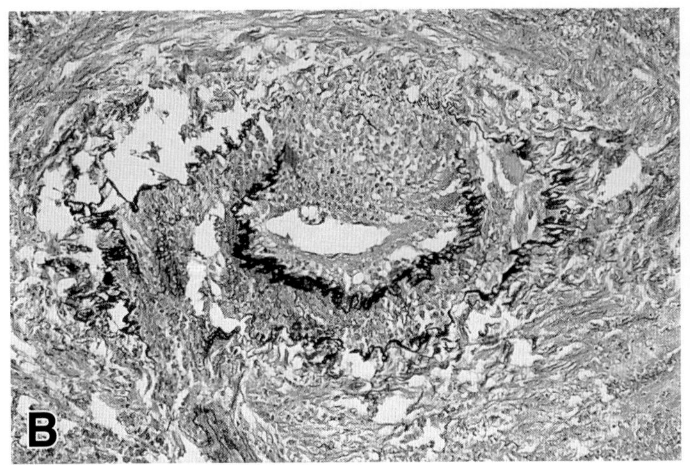

FIGURE 10-48. Granulomatosis with polyangiitis (formerly known as Wegener granulomatosis). **A.** This large area of necrosis has a "geographical" pattern with serpiginous borders and a basophilic center. **B.** Vasculitis in this artery is characterized by a focal, eccentric, transmural chronic inflammatory infiltrate that destroys the inner and outer elastic laminae (elastic stain).

eosinophils may be seen in any anatomic compartment of the lung. Involvement of blood vessel walls causes vasculitis and damage to airway walls and results in bronchitis or bronchiolitis. The vasculitis includes eosinophils, lymphocytes, plasma cells, macrophages, giant cells, and neutrophils (Fig. 10-50A). Necrotic foci have eosinophilic centers, owing to accumulation of dead eosinophils (Fig. 10-50B). Patients present with one or more of the following pulmonary symptoms: allergic rhinitis, asthma, peripheral eosinophilia, and eosinophilic infiltrative disease (eosinophilic pneumonia or eosinophilic enteritis).

Pulmonary Hypertension

Elevated pulmonary arterial pressure is defined as a mean pressure over 25 mm Hg at rest. Increased pulmonary blood flow or vascular resistance may produce higher pulmonary arterial pressure. Whatever the cause, increased pulmonary artery pressure alters pulmonary artery histology (Fig. 10-51). The Heath and Edwards grading system was devised to determine whether the arterial changes of pulmonary hypertension could be reversed with corrective cardiac surgery. Grades 1, 2, and 3 are generally reversible; grade 4 and above are not.

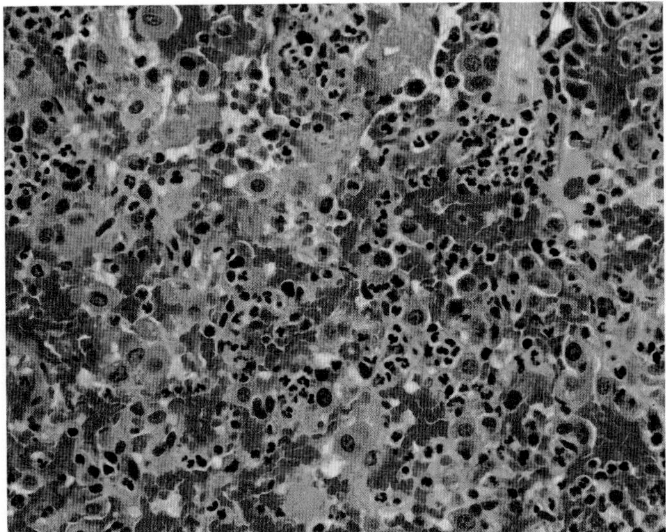

FIGURE 10-49. Microscopic polyangiitis. Alveolar walls are thickened owing to prominent infiltration by neutrophils.

- **Grade 1:** Medial hypertrophy of muscular pulmonary arteries and appearance of smooth muscle in pulmonary arterioles.
- **Grade 2:** Intimal proliferation with increasing medial hypertrophy.
- **Grade 3:** Intimal fibrosis of muscular pulmonary arteries and arterioles, which may be occlusive (Fig. 10-52A).
- **Grade 4:** Plexiform lesions, dilation, and thinning of pulmonary arteries. These nodular lesions are composed of irregular interlacing blood channels and further obstruct pulmonary blood flow (Fig. 10-52B).
- **Grade 5:** Plexiform lesions in combination with dilation or angiomatoid lesions. Rupture of dilated thin-walled vessel, with parenchymal hemorrhage and hemosiderosis, is also present.
- **Grade 6:** Fibrinoid necrosis of arteries and arterioles.

Even mild pulmonary atherosclerosis is uncommon if pulmonary arterial pressure is normal. However, atherosclerosis is seen in the largest pulmonary arteries with all grades of pulmonary hypertension. Increased pressure in the lesser circulation results in hypertrophy of the right ventricle **(cor pulmonale)**.

Pulmonary hypertension may be precapillary or postcapillary in origin. Precapillary hypertension is caused by left-to-right cardiac shunts, primary pulmonary hypertension, thromboembolism, pulmonary fibrosis, and hypoxia. Postcapillary hypertension includes pulmonary veno-occlusive disease and hypertension secondary to left-sided cardiac disorders, such as mitral stenosis and aortic coarctation. Pulmonary hypertension resulting from diseases of the lung is discussed below. Cardiac diseases resulting in pulmonary hypertension are detailed in Chapter 9.

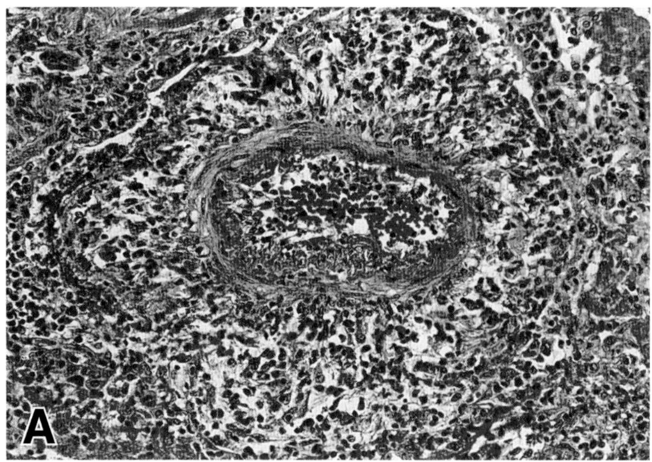

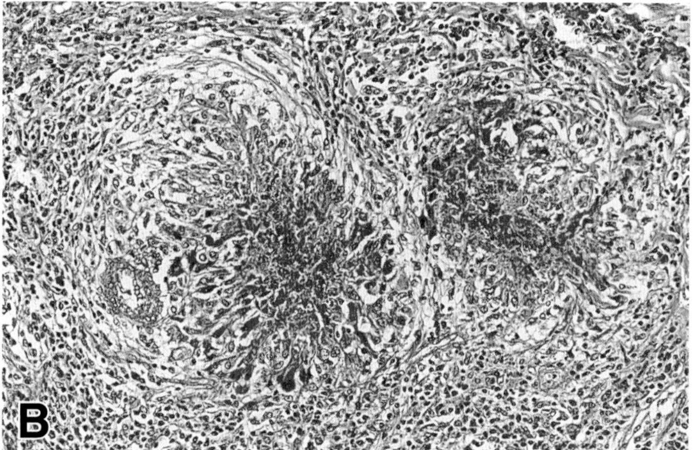

FIGURE 10-50. Allergic granulomatosis with polyangiitis (formerly known as Churg–Strauss syndrome). **A.** An artery showing severe vasculitis consisting of a dense infiltrate of chronic inflammatory cells and eosinophils. **B.** A necrotic ("allergic") granuloma has a central eosinophilic area of necrosis surrounded by palisading macrophages and giant cells.

Primary Pulmonary Hypertension

Primary pulmonary hypertension is a rare precapillary disorder caused by increased pulmonary arterial tone. The condition is often idiopathic, but some cases are hereditary and have been associated with mutations of bone morphogenetic protein receptor type 2 (*BMPR2*), activin receptor-like kinase 1 (*ALK1*), and endoglein (*ENG*). Pulmonary arterial hypertension may also be encountered in association with underlying collagen vascular diseases or may be induced by drugs or toxins (an example being the diet drug "phen-phen"). This disorder occurs at all ages but is most common in young women in their 20s and 30s. It presents with insidious onset of dyspnea. With time, severe pulmonary hypertension, typically associated with plexiform lesions histologically, eventually ensues, and patients die of cor pulmonale. Although medical treatment is mostly ineffective, recent use of prostacyclin analogs, endothelin receptor antagonists, and phosphodiesterase-5 inhibitors has led to a 5-year survival of about 30%. Heart–lung transplantation is often indicated.

Recurrent Pulmonary Emboli

Multiple thromboemboli in smaller pulmonary vessels often result from asymptomatic, episodic showers of small emboli from the periphery. They gradually limit pulmonary circulation and lead to pulmonary hypertension. In addition to the vascular lesions of pulmonary hypertension, organized thromboemboli are evidenced by fibrous bands ("webs") that extend across the lumina of small pulmonary arteries. If the condition is diagnosed during life, placement of a filter in the inferior vena cava usually prevents further embolization.

Hypoxemia and Pulmonary Hypertension

Any disorder that produces hypoxemia can constrict small pulmonary arteries and causes pulmonary hypertension. Predisposing conditions include chronic airflow obstruction (chronic bronchitis), interstitial lung disease, and living at high altitude. Severe kyphoscoliosis or extreme obesity (**Pickwickian syndrome**) may impede ventilation and produce hypoxemia and pulmonary hypertension.

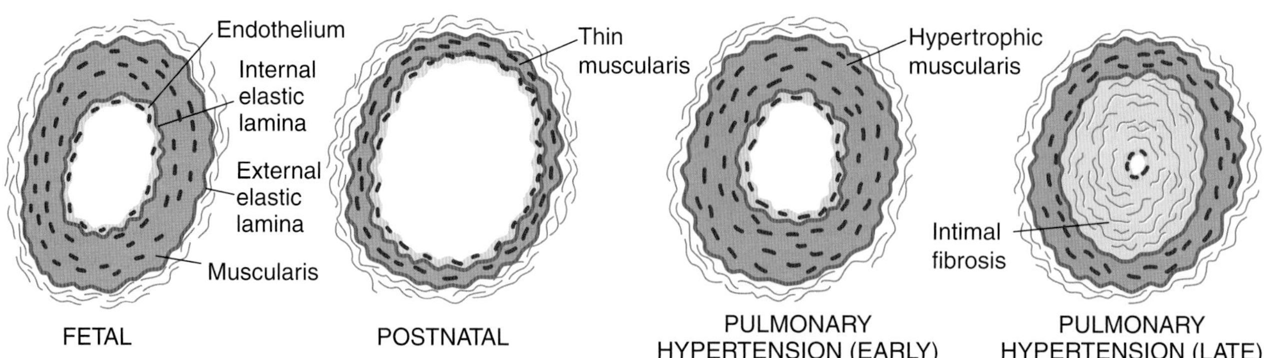

FIGURE 10-51. Histopathology of pulmonary hypertension. In late gestation, the pulmonary arteries have thick walls. After birth, the vessels dilate, and the walls become thin. Mild pulmonary hypertension is characterized by thickening of the media. As pulmonary hypertension becomes more severe, there is extensive intimal fibrosis and muscle thickening.

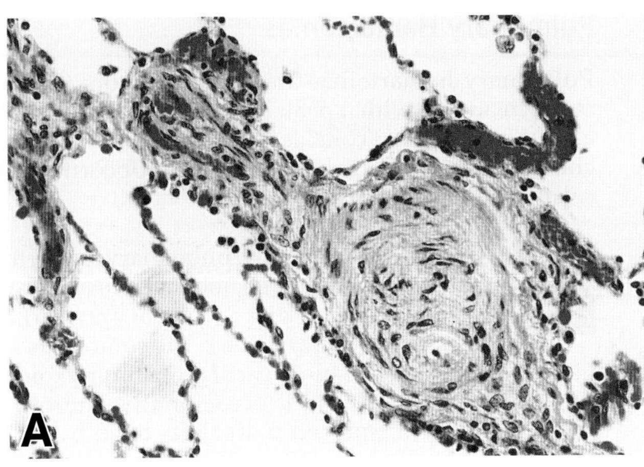

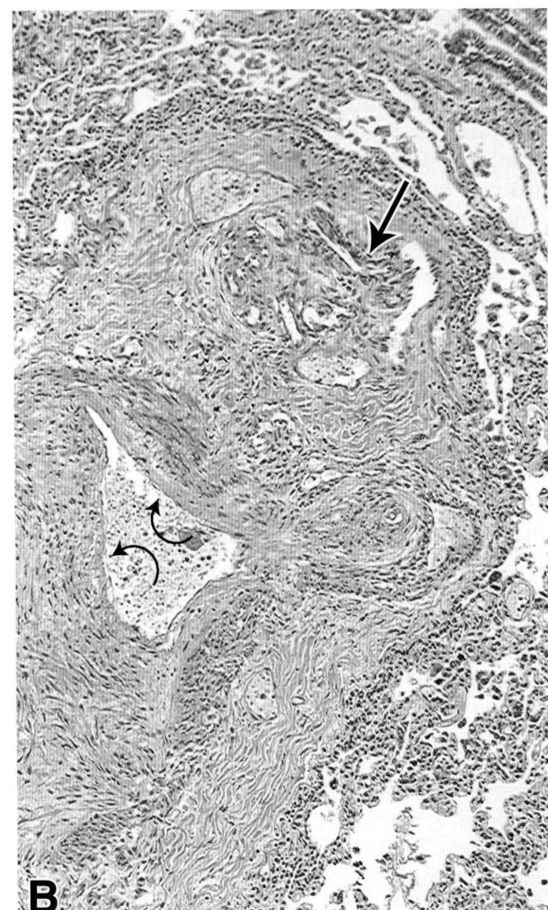

FIGURE 10-52. Pulmonary arterial hypertension. A. A small pulmonary artery is virtually occluded by concentric intimal fibrosis and thickening of the media. **B.** A plexiform lesion (*arrow*) is characterized by a glomeruloid proliferation of thin-walled vessels adjacent to a parent artery, which shows marked hypertensive changes of intimal fibrosis and medial thickening (*curved arrows*).

Pulmonary Veno-Occlusive Disease

PVOD is a rare condition of uncertain etiology in which small pulmonary veins and venules, and at times large veins and arteries, are occluded by loose, sparsely cellular, intimal fibrosis (Fig. 10-53). PVOD may follow viral infections, exposure to toxic agents, and chemotherapy.

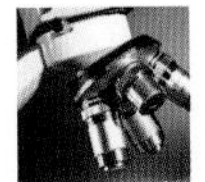

PATHOLOGY: Pulmonary veno-occlusive disease produces severe pulmonary hypertension. Grossly, the lung shows brown induration and atherosclerosis of large pulmonary arteries. Microscopically, small veins and venules are partly or totally occluded, and larger veins show eccentric intimal thickening. Moderate alveolar wall fibrosis and foci of hemosiderosis are common. Pulmonary arteries show recent thrombi and lesions of severe pulmonary hypertension.

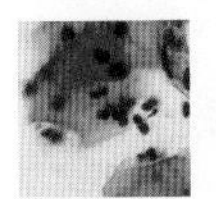

CLINICAL FEATURES: The clinical presentation of progressive dyspnea is similar to that of primary pulmonary hypertension, but pulmonary veno-occlusive disease has a more fulminant course. There is no effective therapy, and heart–lung transplantation may be undertaken.

Pulmonary Edema

Pulmonary edema leads to decreased gas exchange in the lung, causing hypoxia and retention of carbon dioxide (**hypercapnia**) and is also discussed in Chapters 8 and 9.

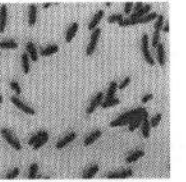

ETIOLOGIC FACTORS AND PATHOLOGY: The most common causes of pulmonary edema relate to hemodynamic alterations in the heart that increase perfusion pressure in pulmonary capillaries and block effective lymphatic drainage. These conditions include left ventricular failure (the most common cause), mitral stenosis, and mitral insufficiency. Disruption of capillary permeability is the cause of pulmonary edema in acute lung injury associated with adult respiratory distress syndrome.

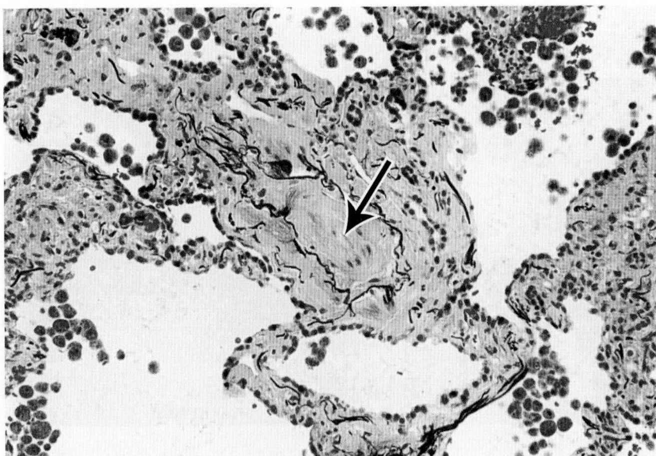

FIGURE 10-53. Veno-occlusive disease of the lung. This pulmonary vein is occluded by intimal fibrosis (*arrow*; Movat stain).

Pulmonary edema may be interstitial or alveolar. Interstitial edema is the earliest phase and is an exaggeration of normal fluid filtration. Lymphatics become distended, and fluid accumulates in the interstitium of lobular septa and around veins and bronchovascular bundles. Edema results in shunting of blood flow from the lung bases to the upper lobes, and increased airflow resistance occurs because of edema of the bronchovascular tree. Patients are often asymptomatic in this early stage.

When the fluid can no longer be accommodated in the interstitial space, it spills into the alveoli, which is called **alveolar edema**. The patient becomes acutely short of breath, and bubbly rales are heard. In extreme cases, frothy fluid is coughed up or wells up out of the trachea.

Microscopically, the edematous lung shows severely congested alveolar capillaries and alveoli filled with a homogeneous, pink-staining fluid permeated by air bubbles. If pulmonary edema is caused by alveolar damage, cell debris, fibrin, and proteins form **hyaline membranes, as seen in diffuse alveolar damage**.

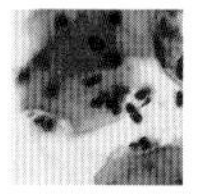

CLINICAL FEATURES: Fluid accumulation may go unnoticed initially, but eventually, dyspnea and coughing become prominent. If edema is severe, large amounts of frothy pink sputum are expectorated. Hypoxemia is manifested as cyanosis. Pulmonary function is restricted in interstitial pulmonary edema because fluid accumulation in the interstitial space causes reduced pulmonary compliance (e.g., stiffening of the lung tissue). Thus, increased respiratory work is required to maintain ventilation. Because alveolar walls are thickened, there is a greater barrier to exchange of oxygen and carbon dioxide. The latter is less affected than the former, resulting in hypoxia with near-normal carbon dioxide levels. Mismatch between ventilation (which is reduced) and perfusion (which persists) contributes to development of hypoxemia in patients with pulmonary edema.

PULMONARY NEOPLASMS

Lung cancers are by far the most common and clinically important of the lung malignancies. Histologic subtyping of carcinomas is of increasing clinical importance.

Pulmonary Hamartomas

Pulmonary hamartomas are benign tumors that typically occur in adults, with a peak in the sixth decade of life. They account for 10% of "coin" lesions discovered incidentally on chest radiographs. A characteristic ("popcorn") pattern of calcification is often seen by x-ray.

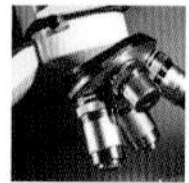

PATHOLOGY: Grossly, pulmonary hamartomas are solitary, circumscribed, lobulated masses, averaging 2 cm in diameter, with a white or gray, cartilaginous cut surface (Fig. 10-54A). The tumor has elements usually present in the lung: cartilage, fibromyxoid connective tissue, fat, bone, and, occasionally, smooth muscle (Fig. 10-54B), interspersed with clefts lined by respiratory epithelium. Hamartomas are well circumscribed and shell out from the surrounding lung parenchyma. Most are seen in the periphery, but 10% occur in a central endobronchial location. The latter may cause symptoms due to bronchial obstruction.

Carcinoma of the Lung

Squamous cell carcinoma, adenocarcinoma, large cell carcinoma, and small cell carcinoma are the major forms of lung cancer. The first three types have traditionally been lumped together from a clinical standpoint as "non–small cell lung carcinoma" (NSCLC). However, this usage is discouraged because the molecular pathology and therapeutic modalities differ between the types. Regarded as a rare tumor as recently as 1945, lung cancer is the most common cause of cancer mortality worldwide. In the United States, where it is the leading cause of cancer death in both men and women, 85% to 90% of lung cancers occur in cigarette smokers. Cigarette smoking is associated with all forms of lung cancer. Most never-smokers who develop lung cancer have an adenocarcinoma. The lifetime risk of developing lung cancer in smokers is 12% to 17%. In nonsmokers, the risk is 1%. The peak age for lung cancer is between 60 and 70 years, with most patients between 50 and 80 years. The former male predominance has decreased somewhat as smoking increased among women.

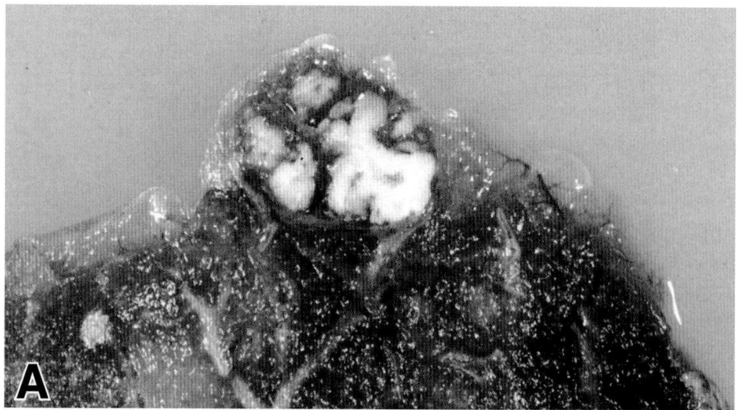

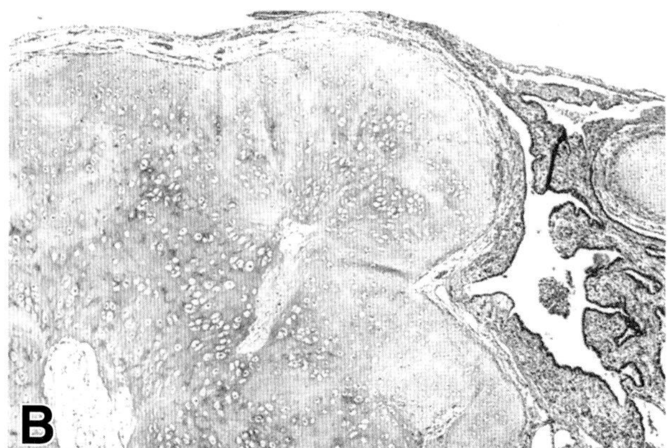

FIGURE 10-54. Pulmonary hamartoma. A. The cut surface of a sharply circumscribed, peripheral pulmonary nodule showing a lobulated structure. **B.** A photomicrograph revealing nodules of hyaline cartilage separated by connective tissue lined by respiratory epithelium.

Cigarette smoking is also an important factor in the induction of **lung cancer** that is associated with certain occupational exposures. For instance, uranium miners have an increased rate of lung cancer, presumably because of inhalation of radon daughters. The rate of lung cancer among miners who smoke is considerably higher than that in nonminers with similar smoking habits. Another example is the case of asbestos workers. Whereas heavy smokers in the general population have a risk of lung cancer some 10 to 20 times greater than nonsmokers, asbestos workers who have interstitial pulmonary fibrosis and smoke heavily have a risk about 50 times that of nonsmokers.

Lung cancer presents in early stages in 30% of patients. The primary treatment is surgical resection, but the remaining 70% of lung cancers present as advanced, unresectable disease. Treatment for the latter is mostly chemotherapy or radiation. In selected cases, tyrosine kinase inhibitors and other targeted therapies have utility.

Histologic Subtypes of Lung Carcinoma

Squamous Cell Carcinoma

Squamous cell carcinoma is the second most common histologic type of lung cancer, accounting for 20% of all lung cancers in the United States; it is more common in men than in women (Table 10-5). After injury to the bronchial epithelium, such as occurs with cigarette smoking, regeneration from the pluripotent basal layer commonly entails squamous metaplasia. The metaplastic epithelium follows the same sequence of dysplasia, carcinoma in situ, and invasive tumor seen at other sites normally lined by squamous epithelium, such as the cervix or skin.

Most squamous cell carcinomas arise centrally in the lung, from major or segmental bronchi, although 10% originate in the periphery. They tend to be firm, gray white, 3 to 5 cm, ulcerated lesions that extend through the bronchial wall into the adjacent lung parenchyma (Fig. 10-55A). Central cavitation is frequent. On occasion, a central squamous carcinoma occurs as an endobronchial tumor.

Table 10-5

Frequency of Lung Carcinoma Histologic Types by Gender

Subtype	Males	Females	Males and Females
Adenocarcinoma	32.9	40.5	36.4
Squamous cell carcinoma	23.8	15.6	20
Small cell carcinoma	13.0	14.7	13.8
Large cell carcinoma	3.6	2.9	3.3
Other carcinomas	23.7	21.8	22.8
Carcinoid	2.0	3.5	2.7
Adenosquamous carcinoma	1.0	1.0	1.0

NCI SEER Data, Histologically Confirmed, 2006–2010. Data is from Surveillance, Epidemiology, and End Results (SEER) Program of the National Cancer Institute.

These tumors vary widely in degrees of squamous differentiation. Many show overt keratinization or intercellular bridges. Well-differentiated tumors have keratin "pearls," which are small round nests of brightly eosinophilic aggregates of keratin surrounded by concentric ("onion skin") layers of squamous cells (Fig. 10-55B). Individual cell keratinization also occurs, in which the cytoplasm becomes glassy and intensely eosinophilic. Intercellular bridges in some well-differentiated squamous cancers are slender gaps between adjacent cells, traversed by fine strands of cytoplasm. By contrast, some squamous tumors are very poorly differentiated; they lack keratinization and are difficult to distinguish from large cell, small cell, or spindle cell carcinomas.

Adenocarcinoma

Worldwide, adenocarcinoma has overtaken squamous cell carcinoma as the most common subtype of lung cancer in most countries, and it is the most common type in nonsmokers. In the United States, it accounts for 36% of all invasive lung malignancies (Table 10-5). It tends to arise in the periphery and is often associated with pleural fibrosis and subpleural scars, which can lead to pleural puckering (Fig. 10-56). Adenocarcinoma classification has recently been revised.

Atypical Adenomatous Hyperplasia

AAH is recognized as a putative precursor lesion for adenocarcinomas. AAH is a well-demarcated lesion, usually less than 5 mm, with atypical proliferation of epithelial cells along the alveolar septa. It remains unclear whether all foci of AAH progress to carcinoma or if all adenocarcinomas arise via this sequence of events.

Adenocarcinoma In Situ

Adenocarcinoma in situ (AIS), once called bronchioloalveolar carcinoma, is a localized (<3 cm) preinvasive form of adenocarcinoma, in which tumor cells grow only along preexisting alveolar walls (lepidic growth) (Fig. 10-57). It accounts for 1% to 5% of lung adenocarcinomas. Patients with AIS are usually cured by surgical resection.

Minimally Invasive Adenocarcinoma

Minimally invasive adenocarcinoma (MIA) shows a limited invasive component (<0.5 cm) and lacks pleural or lymphovascular invasion. MIA has the same favorable prognosis as adenocarcinoma in situ.

AIS and MIA typically appear as ill-defined tan lesions, which may be difficult to distinguish from surrounding normal tissue. Most lesions are nonmucinous, with club cells (formerly known as Clara cells) or type II pneumocytes. Only rarely are they mucinous (Fig. 10-58). In nonmucinous tumors, cuboidal cells grow along the alveolar walls. Mucinous tumors contain columnar cells with abundant apical cytoplasm filled with mucus, sometimes with a goblet cell appearance. Particularly for mucinous tumors, the possibility that the tumor is metastatic from another site must be excluded.

Invasive Adenocarcinomas

Most lung adenocarcinomas are invasive. They typically consist of a mixture of growth patterns. Invasive tumors are classified based on the predominant growth pattern.

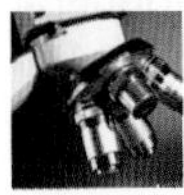

PATHOLOGY: Invasive lung adenocarcinomas appear mostly as irregular 2 to 5 cm masses but may be so large as to replace an entire lobe. On cut section,

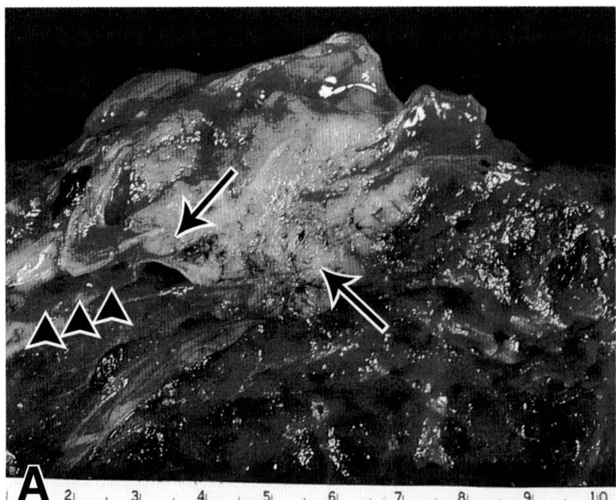

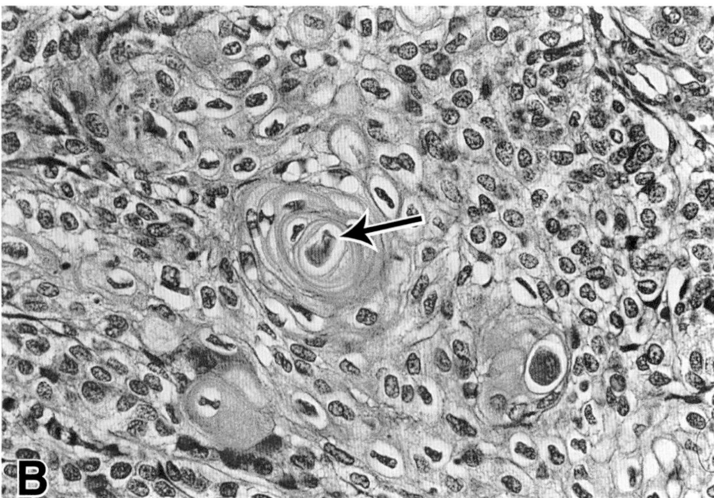

FIGURE 10-55. Squamous cell carcinoma of the lung. A. The tumor (*large arrow*) grows within the lumen of a bronchus (*arrowheads* highlight the course of the bronchus) and invades the adjacent intrapulmonary lymph node (*small arrow*). **B.** A photomicrograph showing well-differentiated squamous cell carcinoma with a keratin pearl (*arrow*) composed of cells with brightly eosinophilic cytoplasm.

nonmucinous tumors are grayish white. Mucinous tumors may be glistening or gelatinous, depending on the amount of mucin production. Central adenocarcinomas may grow endobronchially and invade bronchial cartilage.

Most invasive adenocarcinomas contain mixtures of lepidic, acinar, papillary, micropapillary, and solid patterns (Figs. 10-59 and 10-60). Solid adenocarcinomas with mucus formation are poorly differentiated tumors. They are different from large cell carcinomas by having mucin detected with mucicarmine or periodic acid–Schiff (with diastase digestion) stains (Fig. 10-60D). Invasive mucinous adenocarcinomas show solid mucoid cut surfaces and have tall columnar cells with apical cytoplasmic mucin.

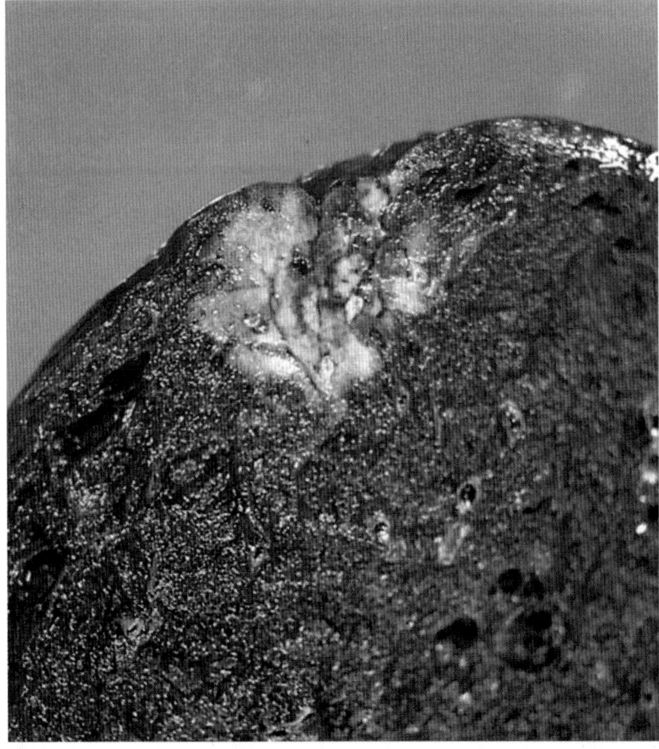

FIGURE 10-56. Invasive adenocarcinoma of the lung. A peripheral tumor of the right upper lobe has an irregular border and a tan or gray cut surface and causes puckering of the overlying pleura.

Large Cell Carcinoma

Large cell carcinoma is a diagnosis of exclusion: a poorly differentiated tumor lacking squamous or glandular differentiation. It is not a small cell carcinoma. This tumor type accounts for 30% of invasive lung tumors in the United States (Table 10-5). The cells are large and exhibit ample cytoplasm. Nuclei frequently show prominent nucleoli and vesicular chromatin. Some large cell carcinomas, called **large cell neuroendocrine carcinoma**, grow like carcinoid tumors (see below), with an organoid pattern, trabecular growth, peripheral palisading of cells, and rosette formation. By immunohistochemistry or ultrastructure, they show evidence of neuroendocrine differentiation.

Small Cell Lung Carcinoma

Small cell carcinoma (formerly known as "oat-cell" carcinoma) is a highly malignant epithelial tumor of the lung that exhibits neuroendocrine features. It accounts for 14% of all lung cancers in the United States (Table 10-5) and is strongly associated with cigarette smoking. SCLCs grow and metastasize rapidly: 70% of patients are first seen at advanced stages. These tumors often cause paraneoplastic syndromes, including **diabetes insipidus, ectopic adrenocorticotropic hormone (ACTH; corticotropin) syndrome,** and **Eaton–Lambert syndrome** (see below).

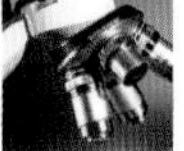

PATHOLOGY: SCLCs are usually perihilar masses, with extensive lymph node metastases. They are soft and white, often with extensive hemorrhage and necrosis. The tumor typically spreads along bronchi in a submucosal and circumferential manner.

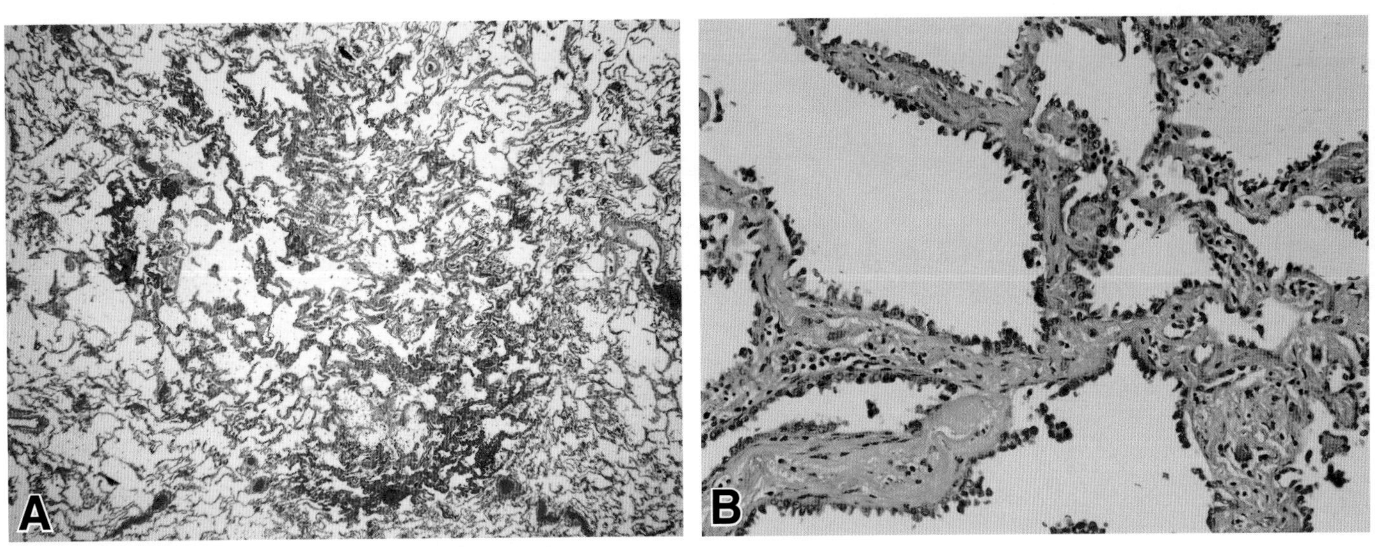

FIGURE 10-57. Adenocarcinoma in situ. A. This circumscribed nonmucinous tumor grows purely with a lepidic pattern. No foci of invasion or scarring are seen. **B.** A layer of atypical pneumocytes lines the alveolar walls.

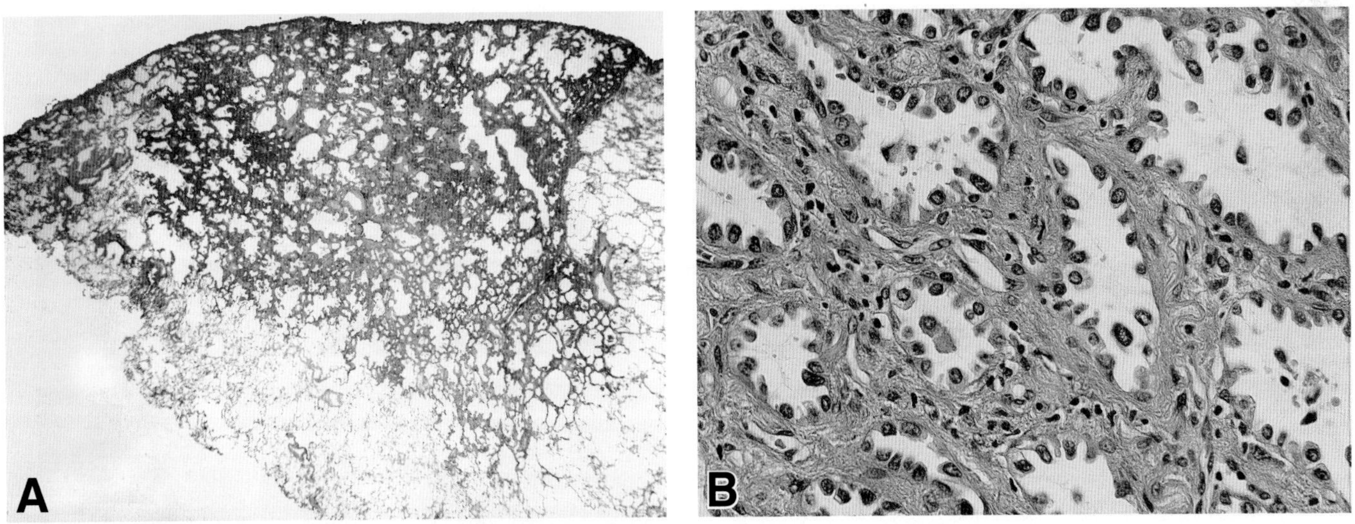

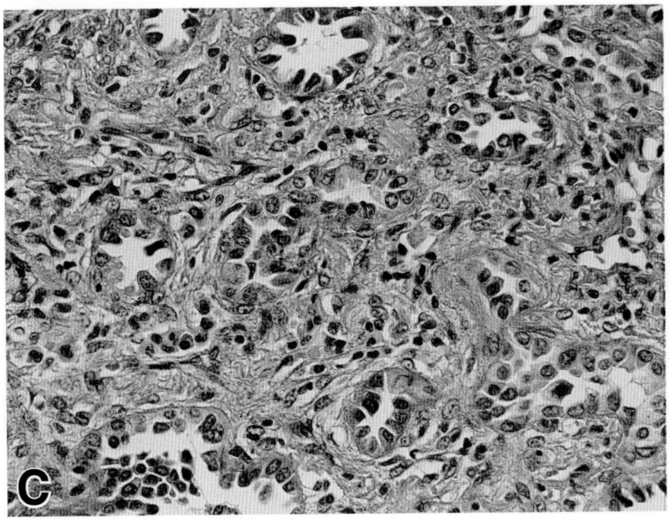

FIGURE 10-58. Minimally invasive adenocarcinoma. A. This nonmucinous adenocarcinoma consists primarily of lepidic growth with a small (<0.5 cm) area of invasion. **B.** The lepidic component showing alveolar walls lined by atypical pneumocytes. **C.** From the area of invasion, these acinar glands are invading in the fibrous stroma.

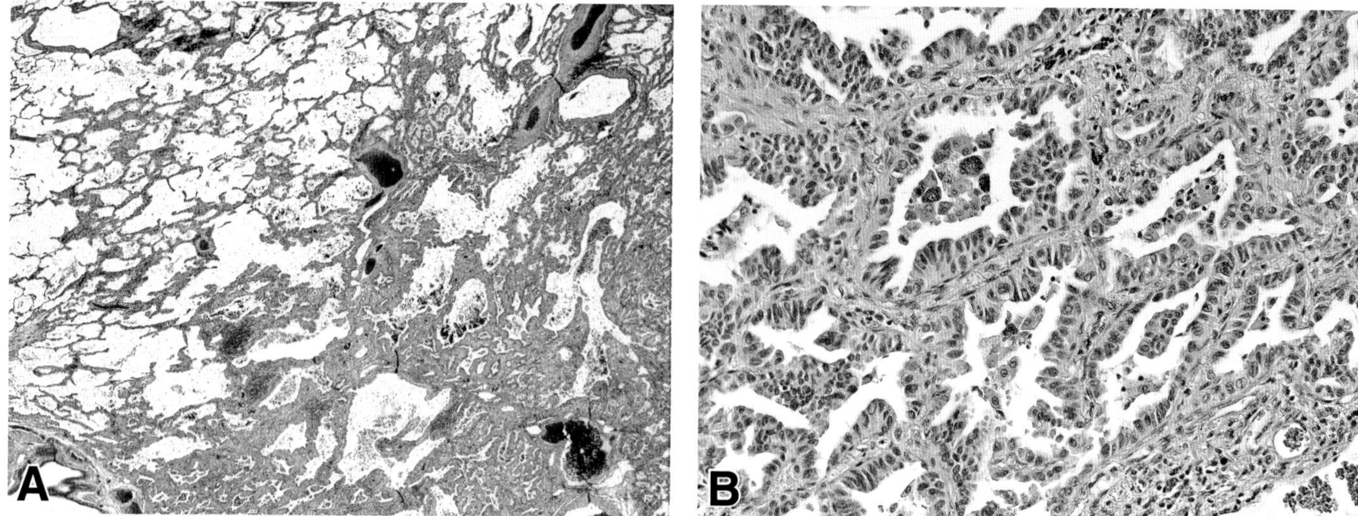

FIGURE 10-59. Adenocarcinoma with lepidic-predominant pattern. A. The tumor showing mostly lepidic growth and an area of invasive acinar adenocarcinoma. **B.** Lepidic pattern consists of a proliferation of type II pneumocytes and Clara cells along the surface alveolar walls.

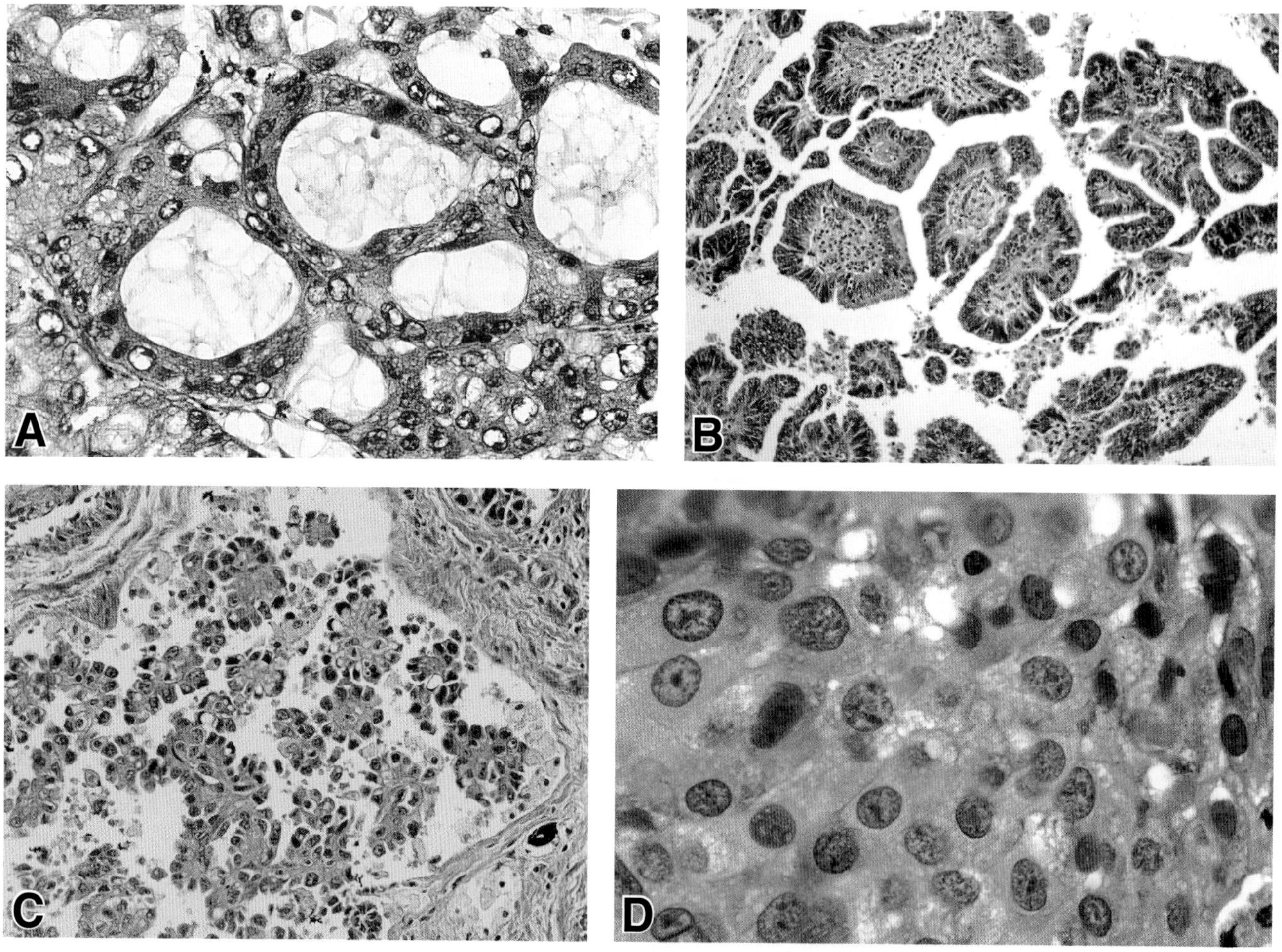

FIGURE 10-60. Invasive adenocarcinoma of the lung. A. Acinar adenocarcinoma composed of round to oval-shaped malignant glands. **B. Papillary adenocarcinoma** consists of malignant cuboidal to columnar tumor cells growing on the surface of fibrovascular cores. **C. Micropapillary adenocarcinoma** consists of small papillary clusters of glandular cells growing within this airspace, most of which do not show fibrovascular cores. **D.** Solid adenocarcinoma with mucin formation consists of solid sheets of tumor cells with several red intracytoplasmic mucin droplets that stain positively with the mucicarmine stain.

Small cell carcinomas have sheets of small, round, oval, or spindle-shaped cells with scant cytoplasm. Their nuclei are distinctive, showing finely granular nuclear chromatin and absent or inconspicuous nucleoli (Fig. 10-61). Most tumors express detectable neuroendocrine markers, such as CD56, chromogranin, or synaptophysin. Mitotic rates are very high, and necrosis is frequent and extensive. Although termed "small cell," the diameter of the neoplastic cells is usually that of three small resting lymphocytes. Unlike other lung cancers, small cell tumors, at least initially, are very sensitive to chemotherapy, which is the mainstay of treatment for this tumor type. However, the long-term prognosis is grim.

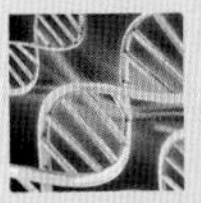

MOLECULAR PATHOGENESIS: No single mutation determines the development of lung cancer, but some are common and allow for targeted chemotherapy.

Although tumors commonly have multiple mutations, great interest lies in defining "driver" mutations. These are causative agents rather than late occurring passengers in the stepwise process of oncogenesis. Such drivers, particularly when they result in gain of function in tyrosine kinases, are potential targets for targeted drug therapy and are in use for selected cases of adenocarcinoma.

- **Epidermal growth factor receptor *(EGFR)*:** Activating mutations in the tyrosine kinase domain of this gene (*epidermal growth factor receptor*) are of particular interest in lung adenocarcinomas, owing to the responsiveness of mutated tumors to tyrosine kinase inhibitors targeted against this receptor, such as erlotinib and gefitinib. These mutations occur in 10% to 15% of lung adenocarcinomas in the United States, with higher percentages in nonsmokers and women. Some 40% to 60% of East Asians have *EGFR* mutations.
- **Echinoderm microtubule-associated protein-like 4 and anaplastic lymphoma kinase *(EML4-ALK)* translocations:** Fusion between echinoderm microtubule-associated protein-like 4 (EML4) and anaplastic lymphoma kinase (ALK) is encountered in 5% of advanced pulmonary adenocarcinomas, most frequently in nonsmokers. Tumors harboring this translocation are responsive to targeted therapy with crizotinib.
- ***K-ras:*** Mutations in this oncogene occur in 25% of adenocarcinomas, 20% of large cell carcinomas, and 5% of squamous carcinomas, but rarely in small cell cancers. These mutations correlate with cigarette smoking and with a poor prognosis. No effective targeted molecular therapy is available for *K-ras* mutations.
- ***Myc:*** Overexpression of this oncogene occurs in 10% to 40% of small cell carcinomas but is rare in other types.
- ***p53:*** Mutations of *p53* are identified in more than 80% of small cell carcinomas and 50% of non–small cell tumors.
- **Retinoblastoma *(Rb)*:** Mutations in the *retinoblastoma (Rb)* gene occur in over 80% of small cell cancers and 25% of non–small cell carcinomas.
- **Chromosome 3 (3p):** Deletions on the short arm of this chromosome are frequently found in all types of lung cancers.
- ***bcl-2:*** This proto-oncogene encodes a protein that inhibits apoptosis (see Chapter 1). It is expressed in 25% of squamous cell carcinomas and 10% of adenocarcinomas.
- ***PTEN:*** This tumor suppressor gene regulates cell survival signaling and is deficient by one of a number of mechanisms (loss of heterozygosity, mutation, promoter methylation, etc.) in many non–small cell lung cancers. Loss of PTEN is associated with poor prognosis and drug resistance.
- **Fibroblast growth factor receptor-1 (*FGFR1*):** Amplification of FGFR1 has been reported in 20% of squamous cell carcinomas, and FGFR inhibitors are currently the subject of clinical testing.

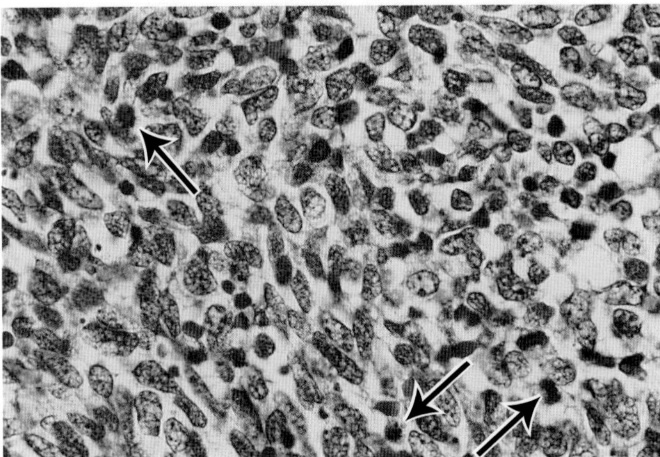

FIGURE 10-61. Small cell carcinoma of the lung. This tumor consists of small oval to spindle-shaped cells with scant cytoplasm, finely granular nuclear chromatin and conspicuous mitoses (*arrows*).

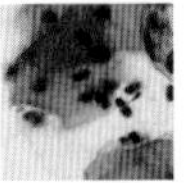

CLINICAL FEATURES: Lung cancer can produce cough, dyspnea, hemoptysis, chest pain, obstructive pneumonia, and pleural effusion. Lymphangitic spread of the tumor within the lung may interfere with oxygenation. A lung cancer (usually squamous) in the apex of the lung (Pancoast tumor) may extend to involve the eighth cervical and first and second thoracic nerves, leading to shoulder pain that radiates down the arm in an ulnar distribution (Pancoast syndrome). A Pancoast tumor may also paralyze cervical sympathetic nerves and cause Horner syndrome on the affected side, with (1) depression of the eyeball (enophthalmos), (2) ptosis of the upper eyelid, (3) constriction of the pupil (miosis), and (4) absence of sweating (anhidrosis). Tumor growth within the mediastinum can cause superior vena cava syndrome (owing to tumorous obstruction of this vein) and nerve entrapment syndromes.

PARANEOPLASTIC SYNDROMES: Disorders associated with lung cancer include acanthosis nigricans, dermatomyositis/polymyositis, clubbing of the fingers, and myasthenic syndromes, such as Eaton–Lambert syndrome and progressive multifocal encephalopathy. Endocrine syndromes are also seen. Examples are Cushing syndrome and syndrome of inappropriate release of antidiuretic hormone (SIADH) in small cell carcinomas, and hypercalcemia (secretion of a parathormone-like substance) in squamous cell cancers. Small cell carcinomas may also be associated with a paraneoplastic syndrome of encephalomyelitis and sensory impairment.

METASTASES: Lung cancers metastasize most often to regional lymph nodes, particularly hilar and mediastinal nodes, and to the brain, bone, and liver. Extranodal metastases often involve the adrenal gland, but adrenal insufficiency is uncommon.

Tumor stage is the single most important predictor of prognosis. The staging system for lung cancer is based primarily on tumor size, extent of spread in the lung and chest, lymph node involvement, distant metastases, and malignancy involving the pleural fluid. Some NSCLCs can be treated with chemotherapy. As noted above, patients whose tumors express certain *EGFR* mutations or *ALK* gene rearrangements show better progression-free survival if treated with tyrosine kinase inhibitors. Patients with advanced-stage adenocarcinoma, but not squamous cell carcinoma, may respond to a folate antimetabolite, pemetrexed. Overall survival for all patients with NSCLC was 15% for the past few decades. However, advanced lung cancer patients with *EGFR* mutations or *ALK* gene rearrangements show improved 2-year progression-free survival, from 20% to 60%, with tyrosine kinase inhibitors. Although the molecular landscape of lung cancer is evolving rapidly, small cell carcinomas still have 5-year survival of only 5% or less.

Carcinoid Tumors

There are two subtypes of carcinoid tumors of the lung, namely, **typical carcinoid** and a more aggressive **atypical carcinoid** variant. These tumors are thought to arise from the resident neuroendocrine cells normally present in the bronchial epithelium. Carcinoid tumors account for 2% to 3% of all primary lung cancers in the United States (Table 10-5), show little sex predilection, and are not related to cigarette smoking. Although neuropeptides are readily demonstrated in the tumor cells, most are endocrinologically silent. However, a small subset of cases is associated with an endocrinopathy (see Chapter 11).

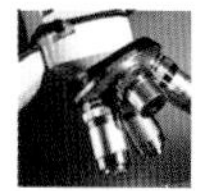

PATHOLOGY: Carcinoid tumors are found throughout the lung. Central carcinoid tumors tend to have a large endobronchial component, with fleshy, smooth, polypoid masses protruding into bronchial lumens (Fig. 10-62A).

These neoplasms are characterized by organoid growth patterns and uniform cytologic features: eosinophilic, finely granular cytoplasm and nuclei with finely granular chromatin (Fig. 10-62B). **Atypical carcinoid tumors** differ from typical carcinoids by (1) increased mitoses, with 2 to 10 mitoses per mm^2 of tumor; (2) tumor necrosis; (3) areas of increased cellularity and architectural disorganization; and (4) nuclear pleomorphism and hyperchromatism with a high nuclear to cytoplasmic ratio. Regional lymph node metastases occur in 15% of patients with typical carcinoids and 50% of those with atypical carcinoids.

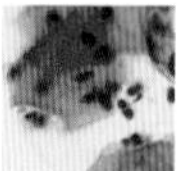

CLINICAL FEATURES: Carcinoid tumors grow slowly, so half of patients are asymptomatic at presentation. They are often discovered incidentally as a mass in a chest radiograph. If a patient is symptomatic, the most common pulmonary manifestations are hemoptysis, postobstructive pneumonitis, and dyspnea. Carcinoid tumors can occur at any age, bronchial carcinoids are the most common lung tumor in childhood.

Pulmonary Lymphomas

All lymphomas, both Hodgkin and non-Hodgkin types, may involve the lung, and most are metastatic (see Chapter 18). Primary pulmonary lymphomas are rare, the most common being **extranodal marginal zone B-cell lymphoma**. These tumors are thought to arise from *m*ucosa-*a*ssociated *l*ymphoid *t*issue of the lung and are sometimes designated "MALT" lymphomas. They are low-grade tumors, generally with a favorable prognosis.

Tumors Metastatic to the Lung

Lung metastases are encountered at autopsy in one third of all fatal cancers. In fact, metastatic tumors are the most common malignancies in the lung. They are typically multiple and circumscribed. On x-rays, large metastatic nodules in the lungs are called "cannonball" metastases (Fig. 10-63).

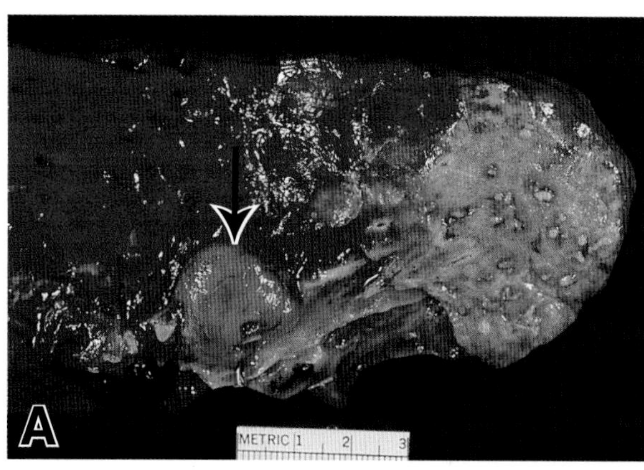

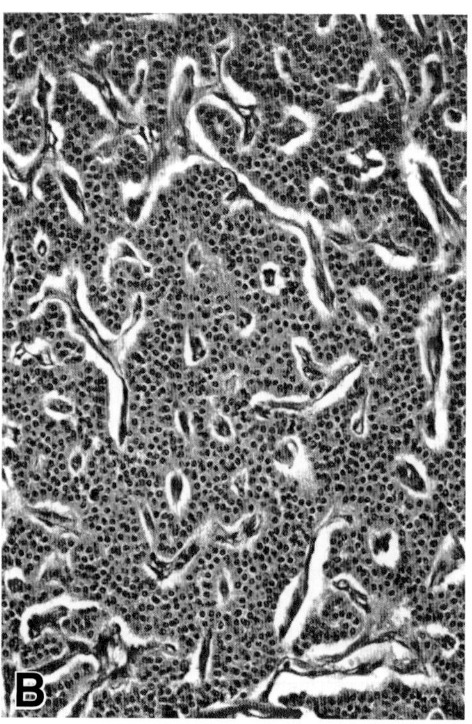

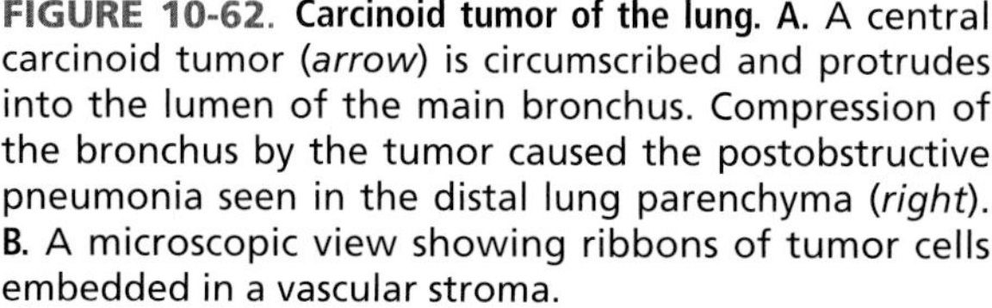

FIGURE 10-62. Carcinoid tumor of the lung. A. A central carcinoid tumor (*arrow*) is circumscribed and protrudes into the lumen of the main bronchus. Compression of the bronchus by the tumor caused the postobstructive pneumonia seen in the distal lung parenchyma (*right*). **B.** A microscopic view showing ribbons of tumor cells embedded in a vascular stroma.

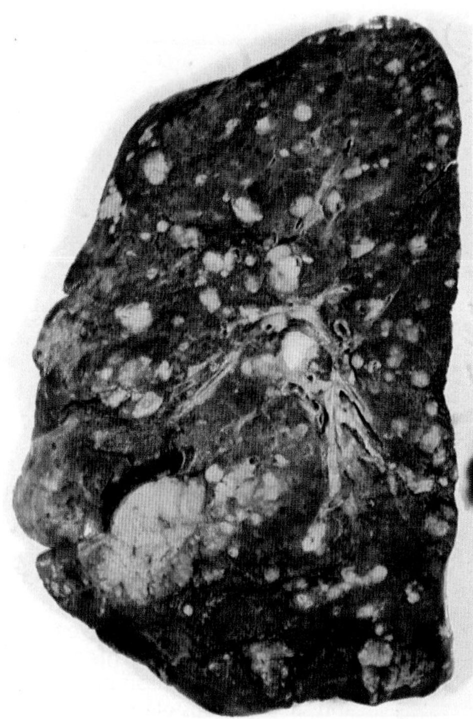

FIGURE 10-63. **Metastatic carcinoma of the lung.** A section through the lung shows numerous nodules of metastatic carcinoma corresponding to "cannonball" metastases seen radiologically.

Histologically, most metastases resemble their primary tumors. Rarely, metastatic tumors show lepidic growth, particularly mucinous types, in which cases the usual primary site is the pancreas or stomach.

THE PLEURA

Pneumothorax

Pneumothorax refers to the presence of air in the pleural cavity; it may occur with traumatic perforation of the pleura or may be "spontaneous." Traumatic causes include penetrating wounds of the chest wall (e.g., a stab wound or a rib fracture), after therapeutic aspiration of fluid from the pleura (thoracentesis), pleural or lung biopsies, transbronchial biopsies, and positive pressure–assisted ventilation.

Spontaneous pneumothorax is typically seen in young adults. For example, a young man may develop acute chest pain and shortness of breath during vigorous exercise. A chest radiograph shows collapse of the lung on the side of the pain and a large collection of air in the pleural space. The cause is rupture, usually of a subpleural emphysematous bleb. In most cases, spontaneous pneumothorax resolves by itself, but some patients require withdrawal of the air.

Tension pneumothorax refers to unilateral pneumothorax extensive enough to shift the mediastinum to the opposite side, with compression of the opposite lung. The condition may be life-threatening and must be relieved by immediate drainage.

Bronchopleural fistula is a serious condition in which there is free communication between an airway and the pleura. It is usually iatrogenic, caused by the interruption of bronchial continuity by biopsy or surgery. It may also be due to extensive infection and necrosis of lung tissue, in which case the infection is more important than the air.

Pleural Effusion

Normally, only a small amount of fluid in the pleural cavity lubricates the space between the lungs and chest wall. Fluid is secreted into the pleural space by the parietal pleura and absorbed by the visceral pleura. Effusions vary from a few milliliters, detectable only radiologically, to massive accumulations that shift the mediastinum and the trachea to the opposite side.

HYDROTHORAX: Hydrothorax is an effusion that resembles water (is edematous). It may be due to increased capillary hydrostatic pressure or decreased serum osmotic pressure. Important causes of hydrothorax are collagen vascular diseases (notably systemic lupus erythematosus and rheumatoid arthritis) and asbestos exposure.

PYOTHORAX: A turbid effusion full of polymorphonuclear leukocytes (pyothorax) results from infections of the pleura. It may be caused by a penetrating wound that introduces pyogenic organisms into the pleural space, but more commonly is a complication of bacterial pneumonia that extends to the pleural surface.

EMPYEMA: This disorder is a variant of pyothorax in which thick pus accumulates within the pleural cavity, often with loculation and fibrosis.

HEMOTHORAX: Blood in the pleural cavity as a result of trauma or rupture of a vessel (e.g., dissecting aneurysm of the aorta) is hemothorax. A pleural effusion may be blood stained in tuberculosis, cancers involving the pleura, and pulmonary infarction.

CHYLOTHORAX: Chylothorax is the accumulation of milky, lipid-rich fluid (chyle) in the pleural cavity owing to lymphatic obstruction. It is a rare complication of mediastinal tumors, such as lymphoma.

Pleuritis

Pleuritis, or inflammation of the pleura, results from extension of any pulmonary infection to the visceral pleura, bacterial infections within the pleural cavity, viral infections, collagen vascular disease or, pulmonary infarction that involves the lung surface. The most striking symptom is sharp, stabbing chest pain on inspiration. It is often associated with pleural effusions.

TUMORS OF THE PLEURA

Malignant Mesothelioma

Malignant mesothelioma is a neoplasm of mesothelial cells. It is most common in the pleura, but also occurs in the peritoneum, pericardium, and tunica vaginalis of the testis.

Some 3,000 new cases of malignant mesothelioma develop yearly in the United States. About 60% to 80% of male patients report exposure to asbestos, but in women, the tumor is more often idiopathic. Mesothelioma typically develops after a long latency period, which averages 30 or 40 years.

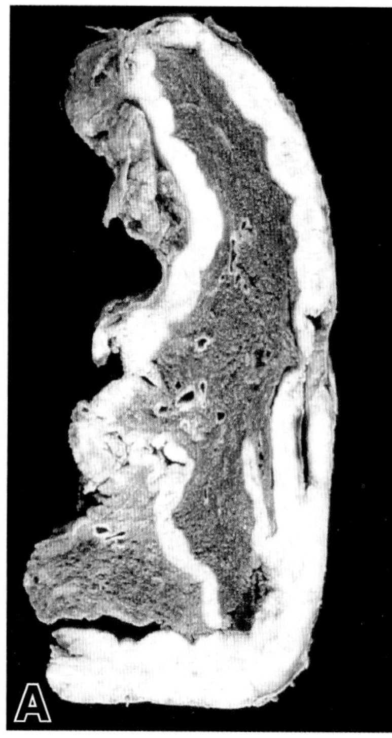

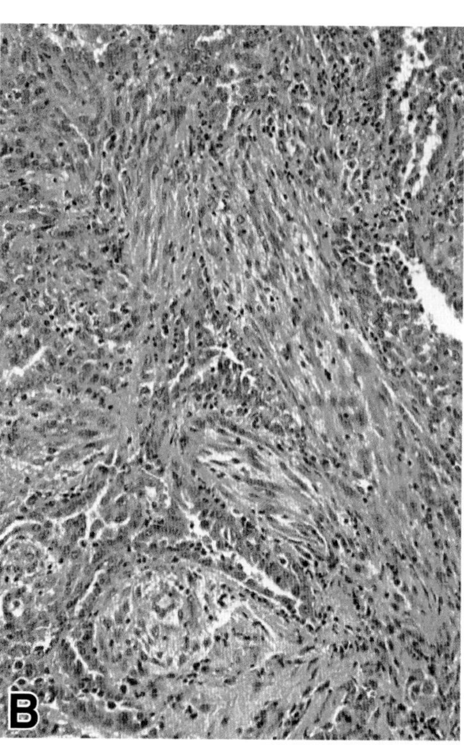

FIGURE 10-64. **Pleural malignant mesothelioma.** **A.** The lung is encased by a dense pleural tumor that extends along the interlobar fissures but does not involve the underlying lung parenchyma. **B.** This mesothelioma is composed of a biphasic pattern of epithelial and sarcomatous elements.

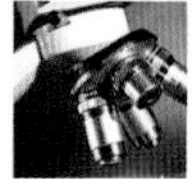

PATHOLOGY: Grossly, pleural mesotheliomas often encase and compress the lung, extending into fissures and interlobar septa, a distribution often referred to as a "pleural rind" (Fig. 10-64A). Invasion of pulmonary parenchyma is generally limited to the periphery adjacent to the tumor. Lymph nodes tend to be spared. Microscopically, classic mesotheliomas show both epithelial and sarcomatous patterns (Fig. 10-64B). Glands and tubules that resemble adenocarcinoma are admixed with sheets of spindle cells similar in appearance to a fibrosarcoma. In some instances, only one or the other component is present; if it is epithelial, the tumor may be difficult to distinguish from adenocarcinoma.

Immunohistochemistry is essential for differentiating mesothelioma from pulmonary adenocarcinoma. Both are positive for cytokeratins; but primary lung adenocarcinomas often, but not always, express thyroid transcription factor 1 (TTF-1), but epithelial mesotheliomas tend to be negative for markers of metastatic adenocarcinomas such as CEA, Leu-M1, B72.3, and BER-EP4. By contrast, mesotheliomas are typically positive for calretinin, WT-1, and D2-40 (podoplanin), for which adenocarcinomas are typically negative.

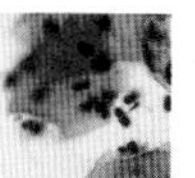

CLINICAL FEATURES: The average age of patients with mesothelioma is 60 years. Patients first present with a pleural effusion or a pleural mass, chest pain, and nonspecific symptoms such as weight loss and malaise. Pleural mesotheliomas tend to spread locally within the chest cavity, invading and compressing major structures. Metastases can occur to the lung parenchyma and mediastinal lymph nodes as well as to extrathoracic sites such as the liver, bones, peritoneum, and adrenals. Treatment is largely ineffective, and the prognosis is poor; few patients survive longer than 18 months after diagnosis.

11 The Gastrointestinal Tract

Leana Guerin ▪ Frank Mitros

LEARNING OBJECTIVES

- Distinguish between esophageal webs, Schatzki rings, Zenker diverticula, and Plummer–Vinson syndrome.
- Define achalasia. What infectious agent is often associated with secondary achalasia?
- What are the pathologic and clinical features of systemic sclerosis as related to the esophagus?
- Define and distinguish between "sliding" and paraesophageal hiatal hernias in terms of anatomic abnormality and clinical features.
- List etiologic, pathologic, and clinical features of gastroesophageal reflux disease.
- Define Barrett esophagus. What pathology and clinical features are associated with the condition?
- Distinguish between Barrett esophagus and eosinophilic esophagitis in terms of pathology and clinical presentation.
- List common etiologic agents causing infective esophagitis and discuss the histopathology associated with each.
- Describe the etiology and anatomic abnormality associated with Mallory–Weiss and Boerhaave syndromes.
- Compare and contrast esophageal squamous cell carcinoma and esophageal adenocarcinoma in terms of epidemiology, etiologic factors, histopathology, and clinical presentation.
- Describe the role of *Helicobacter pylori* infection in chronic gastritis in terms of histopathology and clinical significance.
- Describe the etiology and histopathology of autoimmune gastritis.
- List important etiologic factors in the development of peptic ulcer disease.
- What pathophysiologic factors distinguish duodenal and gastric ulcers? How does the histopathology and clinical presentation of the two conditions differ?
- What diseases are associated with risk and increased severity of peptic ulcer disease?
- Distinguish between intestinal and diffuse gastric adenocarcinoma. Which of these is associated with linitis plastica?
- List three clinical scenarios associated with the occurrence of gastric neuroendocrine tumors.
- Define Meckel diverticulum, intussusception, pneumatosis cystoides intestinalis.
- Distinguish between the etiology and pathophysiology of specific (isolated) and generalized malabsorption.
- What pathophysiologic processes, intestinal histopathology, and clinical features are associated with celiac disease?
- Compare and contrast the etiology, histopathology, and clinical presentation of Whipple disease and giardiasis.
- What clinical conditions may be associated with intestinal ischemia? What are the histopathologic and clinical features of the disease?
- Compare and contrast the anatomic location, histopathology, and clinical presentation of Crohn disease and ulcerative colitis.
- What organisms are common etiologic agents of toxigenic diarrhea?
- What organisms are common etiologic agents of enteroinvasive intestinal disease?
- Compare and contrast the pathophysiology and histopathology resulting from toxigenic and enteroinvasive bacterial diseases of the intestine.
- What are the two common viral agents of infectious diarrhea?
- Describe the pathology and clinical features of intestinal neuroendocrine tumors (carcinoid tumors).
- Describe the etiology and histopathology of appendicitis. Define the term mucocele.
- Describe the etiology, pathogenesis, pathology, and clinical features of Hirschsprung disease.
- Define the term pseudomembranous colitis and describe the histopathology associated with the disease. What are the most common causes and associated clinical features?
- Differentiate between diverticulosis and diverticulitis in terms of etiology, pathology, and clinical presentation.
- Differentiate between hyperplastic colonic and rectal polyps and sessile serrated adenomas in terms of histopathology and malignant potential.
- Discuss the etiology and molecular pathology of "traditional" (tubular and villous) adenomas of the colon.
- Differentiate the pathology of tubular and villous adenomas of the colon in terms of structure, degree of dysplasia, and frequency of occurrence.
- Discuss the molecular and histopathology of familial adenomatous polyposis.

- List risk factors for and the molecular pathogenesis of colorectal adenocarcinoma.
- Describe the pathology of colorectal cancers correlating such with TNM staging. What are common clinical presentations of the disease?
- Discuss the molecular pathogenesis and pathology of Lynch syndrome.
- Define the term hemorrhoid and discuss the histopathology and clinical presentation of the disease.

The Esophagus

ANATOMY

The adult esophagus, a 23- to 25-cm conduit for food and liquid into the stomach, contains striated and smooth muscle in its upper portion and smooth muscle alone in its lower portion, which exits the thorax through the diaphragm. Muscle sphincters at both ends control flow; microscopically, the esophagus has a mucosa, muscularis mucosae, submucosa, muscularis propria, and adventitia. The mucosa is lined by a nonkeratinizing, stratified squamous epithelium. The esophageal submucosa contains mucous glands, a rich lymphatic plexus, and nerve fibers. A transition to gastric mucosa at the **gastroesophageal (GE) junction** occurs abruptly at the level of the diaphragm. Lymphatics of the upper third of the esophagus drain to cervical lymph nodes, those of the middle third to mediastinal nodes, and those of the lower third to celiac and gastric lymph nodes. These anatomic features are significant in the spread of esophageal cancer.

CONGENITAL DISORDERS

Tracheoesophageal Fistula

Esophageal atresia occurs in 1 in 3,500 births and stenosis in 1 in 50,000 births. Atresia may be present alone or, more often, is associated with tracheoesophageal fistula. Congenital stenoses are usually in the distal esophagus and reflect abnormal wall architecture.

Esophageal atresia, with or without tracheoesophageal fistula, is the most common esophageal congenital anomaly (Fig. 11-1). Atresia without a fistula appears in only about 8% of cases. Half of patients have other congenital anomalies, 25% being other gastrointestinal malformations. One fifth have VACTERL syndrome (vertebral defects, anal atresia, cardiac defects, tracheoesophageal fistula, renal dysplasia, and limb abnormalities).

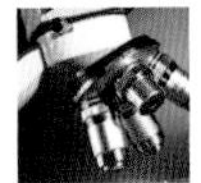

PATHOLOGY: In about 85% of tracheoesophageal fistulas, the upper portion of the esophagus ends in a blind pouch, and the superior end of the lower segment communicates with the trachea (Fig. 11-1). ***In this type of atresia, the upper blind sac soon fills with mucus, which the infant then aspirates.*** Surgical correction is feasible but difficult.

Another type of fistula is a communication between the proximal esophagus and the trachea; the lower esophageal pouch communicates with the stomach. ***Infants with this condition aspirate shortly after birth.*** In an **H-type fistula,** there is a communication between an intact esophagus and an intact trachea. In some cases, this lesion is first symptomatic in adulthood, presenting with repeated pulmonary infections.

Rings and Webs

ESOPHAGEAL WEBS: Occasionally, a thin mucosal membrane projects into the esophageal lumen. Webs are usually single and thin (2 mm) and occur anywhere in the esophagus. They have a core of fibrovascular tissue lined by normal mucosa and submucosa. Middle-aged women are most affected and present with difficulty swallowing (dysphagia). They are often successfully treated by dilation; if needed, webs can be excised.

PLUMMER–VINSON (ALSO CALLED PATERSON–KELLY) SYNDROME: This rare disorder is characterized by (1) a cervical esophageal web, (2) mucosal lesions of the mouth and pharynx, and (3) iron-deficiency anemia. Dysphagia, often associated with aspiration of swallowed food, is the most common clinical manifestation. Ninety percent of cases occur in women. ***Carcinoma of the oropharynx and upper esophagus is a possible complication.***

SCHATZKI RING: This lower esophageal narrowing is usually seen at the gastroesophageal junction. The upper surface of the mucosal ring has stratified squamous epithelium, whereas the lower surface exhibits columnar epithelium. Although they are seen in up to 14% of barium examinations, Schatzki rings are

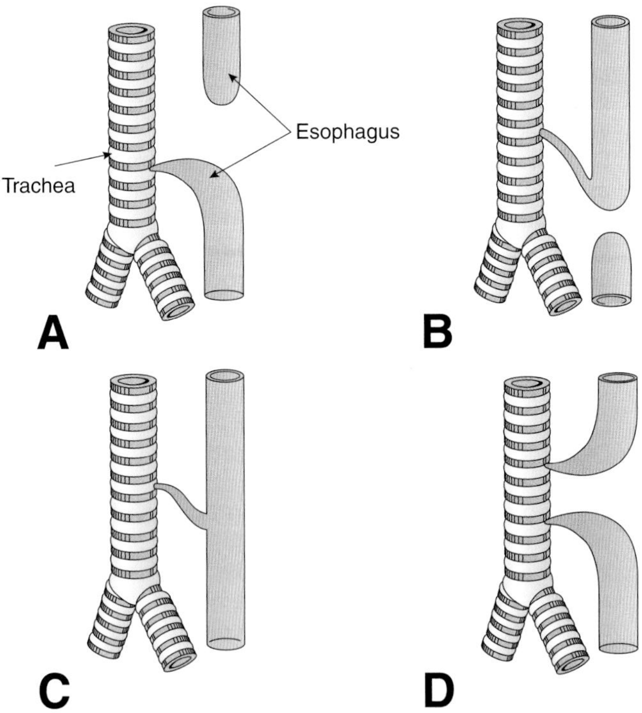

FIGURE 11-1. Congenital tracheoesophageal fistulas. A. The most common type (85% of cases) is a communication between the trachea and the lower portion of the esophagus. The upper segment of the esophagus ends in a blind sac. **B.** In a few cases, the proximal esophagus communicates with the trachea. **C.** H-type fistula without esophageal atresia. **D.** Tracheal fistulas to both a proximal esophageal pouch and distal esophagus.

usually asymptomatic. Patients with narrow Schatzki rings, however, may complain of intermittent dysphagia. Dilation can be done if necessary.

Esophageal Diverticula

A **true diverticulum** is an outpouching of the esophageal wall that contains all layers. If a sac has no muscular layer, it is a **false diverticulum** (or pseudodiverticulum). Esophageal diverticula occur in the hypopharyngeal area above the upper esophageal sphincter, in the middle esophagus, and immediately proximal to the lower esophageal sphincter.

ZENKER DIVERTICULUM: Zenker diverticula are uncommon lesions that appear high in the esophagus and affect men more than women. These false diverticula probably reflect disordered function of cricopharyngeal musculature. Most affected people who come to medical attention are older than 60 years, suggesting that Zenker diverticula are acquired.

Zenker diverticula can enlarge conspicuously and accumulate a large amount of food. The typical symptom is regurgitation of food eaten some time previously (occasionally days), without dysphagia. Patients may develop recurrent aspiration pneumonia. When symptomatic, these lesions are surgically removed or treated endoscopically.

MOTOR DISORDERS

Automatic coordination of muscular movement during swallowing is a **motor function** and results in free passage of food through the esophagus. The hallmark of motor disorders is difficulty in swallowing, or **dysphagia**. Dysphagia is often an awareness that food is not moving downward and in itself is not painful. Pain on swallowing is referred to as **odynophagia**. Motor disorders can be caused by the following:

- **Systemic diseases of skeletal muscle** (in the upper esophagus), such as myasthenia gravis, dermatomyositis, amyloidosis, hypothyroidism, and myxedema
- **Neurologic diseases** affecting nerves to skeletal or smooth muscle (e.g., cerebrovascular accidents and amyotrophic lateral sclerosis)
- **Peripheral neuropathy** associated with diabetes or alcoholism

Achalasia

Achalasia, once called cardiospasm, involves failure of the lower esophageal sphincter to relax with swallowing and poor peristalsis in the body of the esophagus. As a result of these defects in both the outflow tract and esophageal pumping mechanisms, food is retained in the esophagus, and the organ hypertrophies and dilates.

Achalasia is an inflammatory disease that causes loss of inhibitory neurons in the esophageal myenteric plexus. Chronic inflammation (mainly T cells) in the myenteric plexus leads to neuritis and ganglionitis and, eventually, to ganglion cell loss and fibrosis. The cause of the inflammation is unknown, but genetic, viral, and autoimmune factors have been suggested. Degenerative changes in the dorsal motor nucleus of the vagus and extraesophageal vagus nerves may also contribute. In Latin America, secondary achalasia is a common complication of **Chagas disease**, in which ganglion cells are destroyed by the protozoan *Trypanosoma cruzi.* Amyloidosis, sarcoidosis, and infiltrative malignancies may also cause achalasia.

Dysphagia (to both solids and liquids), occasionally odynophagia and regurgitation of material retained in the esophagus, are common symptoms of achalasia. Squamous cell carcinoma may develop in long-standing cases. Treatment may include endoscopic balloon dilation, botulinum toxin injection of the lower esophageal sphincter, endoscopic myotomy, or surgical myotomy of the lower esophageal sphincter. Patients may develop gastroesophgeal reflux after treatment.

Systemic Sclerosis

Systemic sclerosis (scleroderma) causes fibrosis in many organs and involves the GI tract 80% of the time (see Chapter 3). Any segment of the tubal gut may be affected. The esophagus is most frequently impacted, often with severely abnormal esophageal muscle function. The lower esophageal sphincter may be so impaired that the lower esophagus and upper stomach are no longer distinct functional entities and are visualized as a common cavity. Peristalsis may be impaired throughout the esophagus.

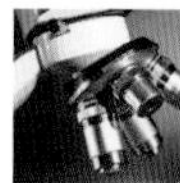

PATHOLOGY: Fibrosis is present in the esophageal smooth muscle (especially the inner muscularis propria). Nonspecific inflammation is also evident. Small arteries and arterioles show intimal fibrosis, which may contribute to fibrosis of the wall.

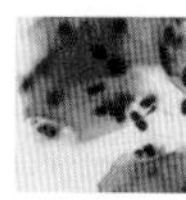

CLINICAL FEATURES: Patients have dysphagia, regurgitation, and heartburn caused by peptic esophagitis, owing to reflux of acid from the stomach. Severe reflux changes may occur (see below).

HIATAL HERNIA

Hiatal hernia is a protrusion of the stomach into the chest through an enlarged diaphragmatic opening. There are two basic types of hiatal hernia (Fig. 11-2).

Sliding Hernia

Enlargement of the diaphragmatic hiatus and laxity of the circumferential connective tissue allow a cap of gastric mucosa to move upward, above the diaphragm. This common condition accounts for 85% of hiatal hernias and is usually asymptomatic. The most commonly associated symptom is gastroesophageal reflux, although it is unclear whether hernias are the causes or results of reflux.

Paraesophageal Hernia

In this uncommon form of hiatal hernia, a portion of gastric fundus herniates through a defect in the diaphragmatic connective tissue that defines the esophageal hiatus and lies beside the esophagus. The hernia progressively enlarges, and the hiatus grows increasingly wide. These events can compress the esophagus, leading to decrease in reflux of gastric contents. In extreme cases, the entire stomach and other abdominal organs can herniate into the thorax.

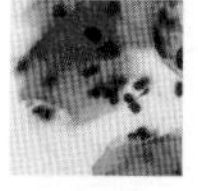

CLINICAL FEATURES: Symptoms of sliding hiatal hernia, mostly heartburn and regurgitation, reflect reflux of gastric contents into the esophagus, primarily owing to incompetence of the lower esophageal sphincter. Classically, symptoms are worse when subjects recline because this position facilitates acid reflux. Dysphagia,

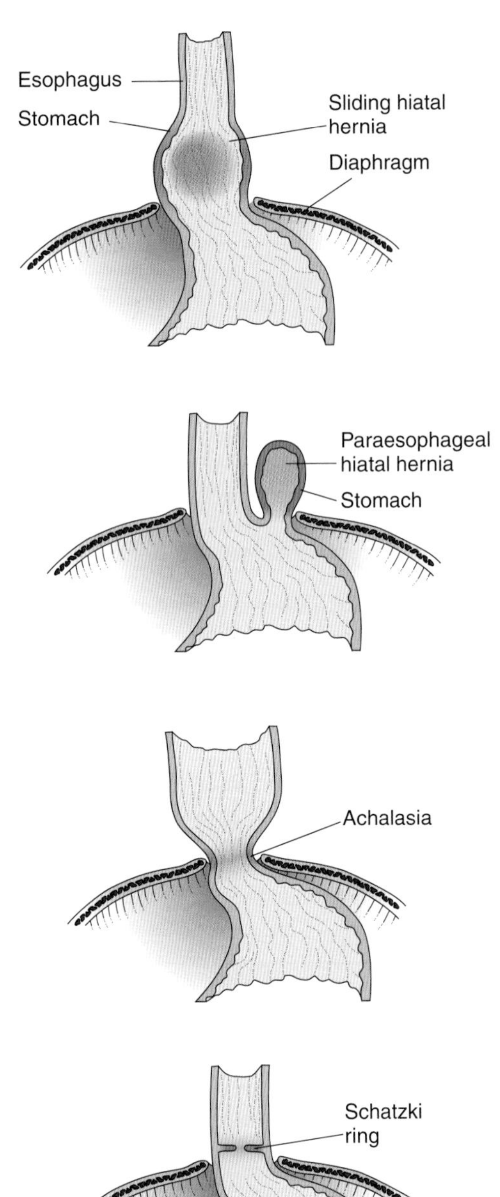

FIGURE 11-2. **Disorders of the esophageal outlet.**

fullness after meals, shortness of breath, painful swallowing, and, occasionally, bleeding peptic ulcers may be seen in paraesophageal hernias. Large hernias carry a risk of gastric volvulus or intrathoracic gastric dilation.

Sliding hiatal hernias generally do not require surgery, and symptoms are treated medically. An enlarging paraesophageal hernia should be corrected surgically, even if it is asymptomatic.

ESOPHAGITIS

Gastroesophageal Reflux Disease

This is by far the most common type of esophagitis. It often occurs together with sliding hiatal hernias but may develop as the result of an incompetent lower esophageal sphincter in the absence of any anatomic lesion.

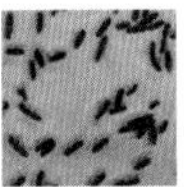

ETIOLOGIC FACTORS: The main barrier to reflux of gastric contents into the esophagus is the lower esophageal sphincter. Episodic reflux is normal, particularly after a meal. The mucosa is partially protected by the alkaline secretions of submucosal glands. Esophagitis results when episodes are frequent and prolonged. Agents that decrease lower esophageal sphincter pressure (e.g., alcohol, chocolate, fatty foods, and cigarette smoking) also cause reflux, as may certain central nervous system (CNS) depressants (e.g., morphine and diazepam), abdominal obesity, pregnancy, estrogen therapy, and the presence of a nasogastric tube. Acid damages the esophageal mucosa, but the combination of acid plus pepsin is particularly injurious. Moreover, gastric fluid often contains refluxed bile from the duodenum, which magnifies injury to the esophageal mucosa. Alcohol, hot beverages, and spicy foods may also injure the mucosa directly.

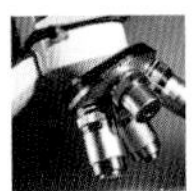

PATHOLOGY: The first grossly evident effect of gastroesophageal reflux is hyperemia. Affected areas are susceptible to superficial mucosal erosions and ulcers, which often appear as vertical linear streaks. Mild injury to the squamous epithelium is manifested as cell swelling (hydropic change; see Chapter 1). With continued injury, hyperplasia develops: the basal epithelium is thickened, and the papillae of the lamina propria are elongated and approach the surface (Fig. 11-3). Capillary vessels in the papillae are often dilated. Lymphocytes, neutrophils, and eosinophils infiltrate the epithelium. Mucosal ulceration develops in severe cases. Esophageal stricture may occur if the ulcer persists and damages the esophageal wall deep to the lamina propria. In this circumstance, reactive fibrosis can narrow the esophageal lumen.

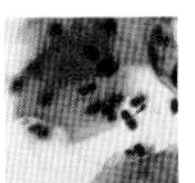

CLINICAL FEATURES: Gastroesophageal reflux disease (GERD) can occur at any age and can be nonerosive, erosive, or involved by Barrett esophagus (see below). Heartburn and dysphagia are the usual presenting symptoms and generally respond to agents that reduce gastric acidity, for example, proton pump inhibitors. In cases of erosive GERD, ulceration, hematemesis, and stricture may occur.

Barrett Esophagus

Barrett esophagus is a result of chronic GERD. For unknown reasons, its incidence has been increasing in recent years, particularly among white men. This disorder usually occurs in the lower third of the esophagus but may extend higher.

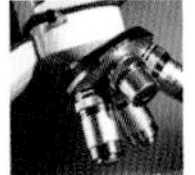

PATHOLOGY: Metaplastic Barrett epithelium partially involves the circumference of short esophageal segments or may line the entire lower esophagus (Fig. 11-4A). The diagnostic feature of Barrett esophagus is a distinctive "specialized epithelium." By endoscopy, it has a typical salmon-pink color and is an admixture of intestine-like epithelium with well-formed goblet cells, mixed with gastric foveolar cells (Fig. 11-4B). Complete intestinal metaplasia, with Paneth cells and absorptive cells, occurs occasionally. Inflammatory changes are often superimposed on these alterations. Dysplasia develops in this epithelium in a minority of patients (Fig. 11-4C). ***The risk of Barrett esophagus***

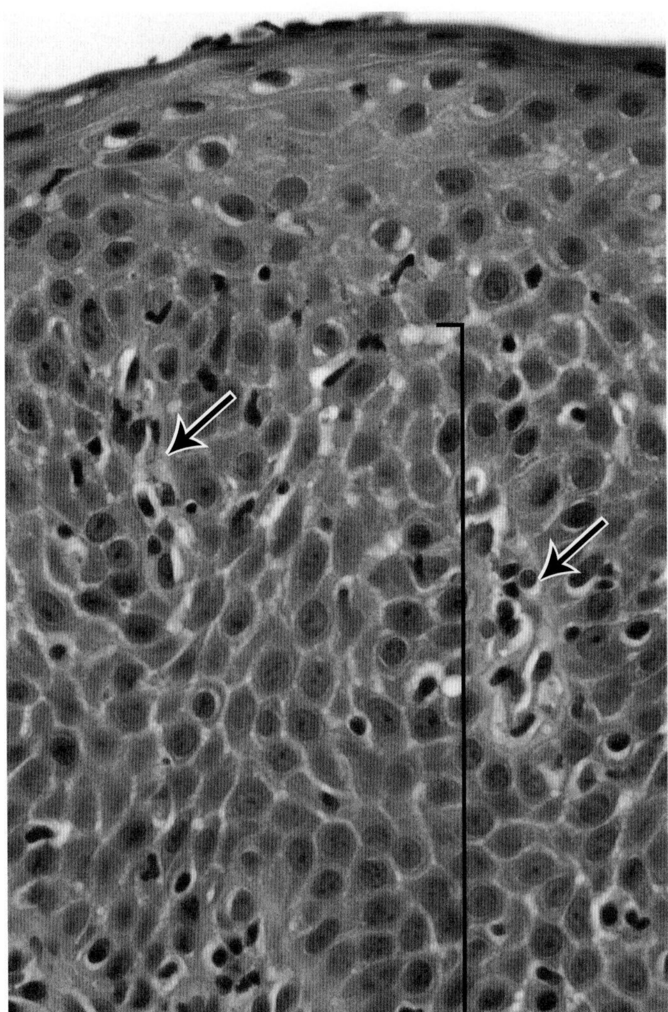

FIGURE 11-3. Reflux esophagitis. Biopsy from a patient with long-standing heartburn. Note the basal hyperplasia (*bracket*) and papillae (*arrows*), squamous hyperplasia, and inflammation.

transforming into adenocarcinoma correlates with the length of esophagus involved and the degree of dysplasia. Dysplasia in Barrett esophagus is currently classified as negative, indefinite, low grade, or high grade. The cytology and architecture of high-grade dysplasia overlap intramucosal adenocarcinoma, the latter definitively identified by invasion into the lamina propria (Fig. 11-4D).

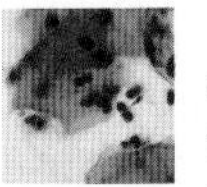

CLINICAL FEATURES: The diagnosis of Barrett esophagus is established by endoscopy with biopsy, usually after complaints of GERD, although many do not report reflux symptoms. Men predominate (3:1). The prevalence of the lesion increases with age, and most patients are diagnosed after age 60. Smokers have twice the risk of Barrett esophagus as nonsmokers. Obesity and white race are other risk factors.

Patients with Barrett esophagus are followed closely to detect early microscopic evidence of dysplastic mucosa. Many cases, particularly low-grade dysplasia (or even microscopic foci of high-grade dysplasia), regress after pharmacologic reduction in gastric acidity. However, high-grade dysplasia and intramucosal carcinoma require intervention. Techniques used to ablate these lesions (short of esophagectomy) include endoscopic mucosectomy, laser treatment, and photodynamic therapy.

Eosinophilic Esophagitis

A diagnosis of eosinophilic esophagitis requires clinical–pathologic correlation. Although the pathogenesis is not completely understood, allergies to ingested food and inhaled allergens likely play a prominent role. Patients often complain of dysphagia or feeling food "sticking" upon swallowing, which they may relate to specific foodstuffs. Affected individuals are often first identified after they fail to improve on standard antireflux therapy. The incidence of eosinophilic esophagitis is increasing, likely from a combination of greater disease prevalence and enhanced awareness of the entity.

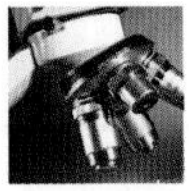

PATHOLOGY: On endoscopy, eosinophilic esophagitis shows concentric mucosal rings (called trachealization or "felinization" because it resembles the trachea or cat esophagus), vertical linear furrows, narrow esophagus, strictures, and small white plaques or exudates (Fig. 11-5A). Some patients have a normal-appearing esophagus at endoscopy. Because the disease can be quite patchy, multiple biopsies from various levels of esophagus should be assessed. The epithelium shows hyperplasia (papillary and basal layer hyperplasia), intercellular edema, increased intraepithelial eosinophils (≥15 per high-power field), superficial layering of eosinophils, eosinophilic microabscesses, and prominent degranulation of eosinophils (Fig. 11-5B). Deeper samples may display subepithelial fibrosis and eosinophils in the lamina propria.

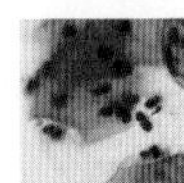

CLINICAL FEATURES: Eosinophilic esophagitis can present at any age and is more common in males. Adults typically complain of dysphagia to solids or food impaction, whereas children may suffer food intolerance, vomiting, feeding difficulties, or failure to thrive. Many patients have a personal or family history of atopy (asthma, allergic rhinitis, eczema, and atopic dermatitis), and some may have a mild increase in blood eosinophils. Eliminating inciting food from the diet leads to remission in many patients. Swallowed corticosteroids, leukotriene inhibitors, and other immunomodulators are also used to treat eosinophilic esophagitis.

Infective Esophagitis

Candida Esophagitis

This fungal infection became common as the numbers of immunocompromised patients increased owing to chemotherapy for malignant disease, immunosuppression after organ transplantation, or AIDS. Esophageal candidiasis also occurs in patients with diabetes, in those receiving antibiotics or acid-suppressive therapy, or in people using inhaled or swallowed corticosteroids. It is uncommon in the absence of known predisposing factors. Dysphagia and severe pain on swallowing are the usual symptoms.

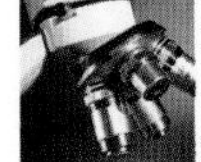

PATHOLOGY: In mild cases, a few, small elevated, white mucosal plaques are surrounded by a hyperemic zone in the middle or lower third of the esophagus. In severe cases, confluent pseudomembranes lie on a hyperemic and edematous mucosa. Candidal pseudomembranes

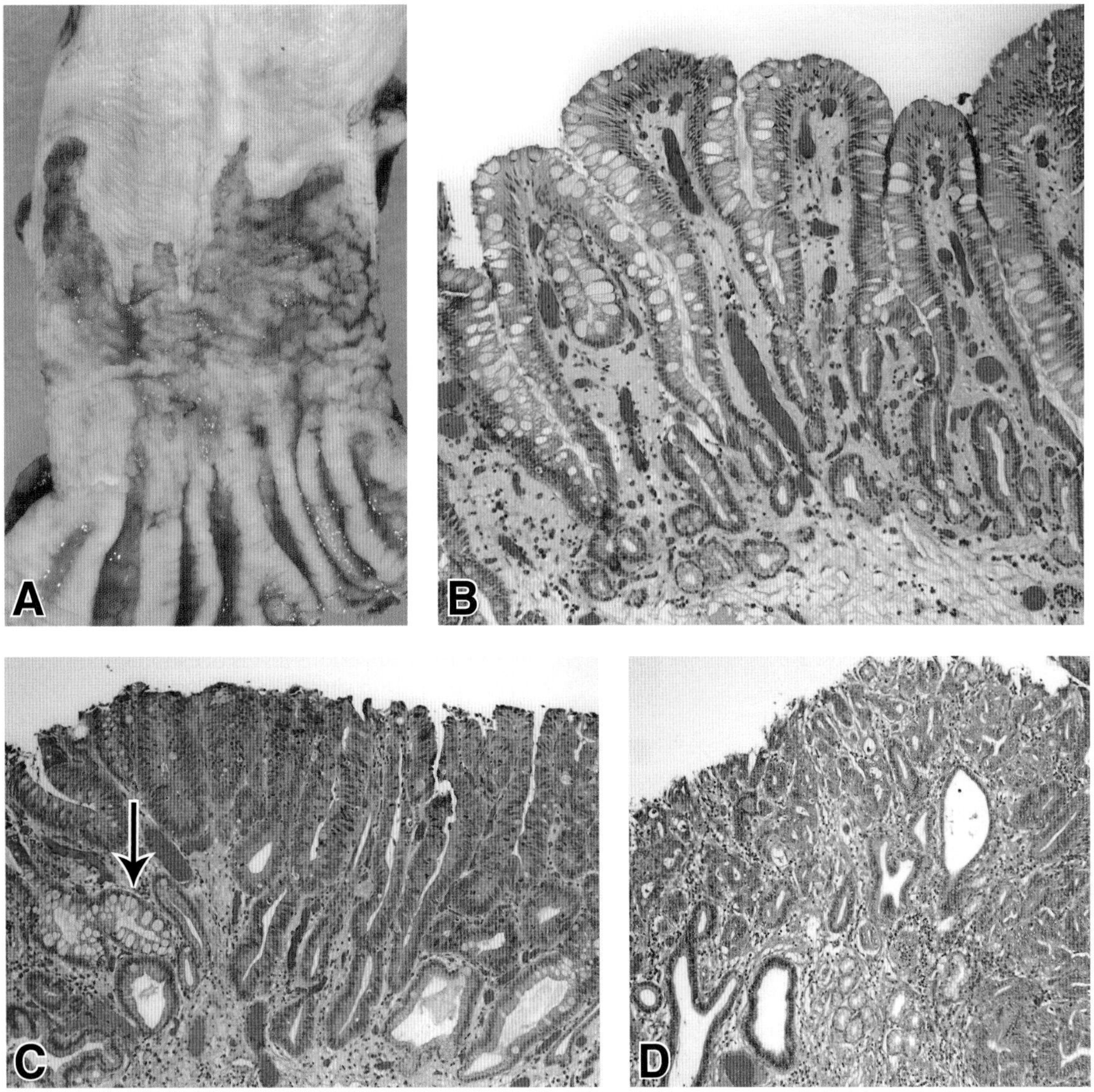

FIGURE 11-4. Barrett esophagus. A. The presence of the tan tongues of epithelium interdigitating with the more proximal squamous epithelium is typical of Barrett esophagus. **B.** The specialized epithelium has a villiform architecture and is lined by cells that are foveolar gastric-type cells and intestinal goblet-type cells. **C. High-grade dysplasia.** Markedly, dysplastic glands predominate with hyperchromatic nuclei and early architectural distortion. Intestinalized, nondysplastic glands persist (*arrow*). **D. Intramucosal adenocarcinoma.** Malignant glands are restricted to the mucosa.

contain fungal forms, necrotic debris, and fibrin. *Candida* may involve only the superficial epithelium, but invasion deeper into the esophageal wall can give rise to disseminated candidiasis or fibrosis, sometimes severe enough to create a stricture.

Herpetic Esophagitis

Esophageal infection with herpesvirus type I most commonly follows transplantation of solid organs or bone marrow. Patients complain of odynophagia. On occasion, herpetic esophagitis may occur in otherwise healthy people.

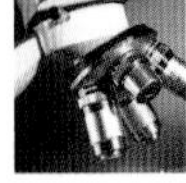

PATHOLOGY: Well-developed lesions of herpetic esophagitis grossly resemble those of candidiasis. Early cases show vesicles, small erosions, or plaques; as infection progresses, these coalesce into larger lesions. Epithelial cells exhibit typical nuclear herpetic inclusions and occasional multinucleation. Necrosis of infected cells incites ulceration. Candidal or bacterial superinfection may cause pseudomembranes.

Cytomegalovirus Esophagitis

Involvement of the esophagus or other segments of the GI tract with CMV usually reflects systemic viral disease in severely immunosuppressed patients (e.g., those with AIDS and transplant recipients). Mucosal ulceration, as in herpetic esophagitis, is common. Characteristic CMV inclusion bodies are seen in endothelial cells and fibroblasts of granulation tissue.

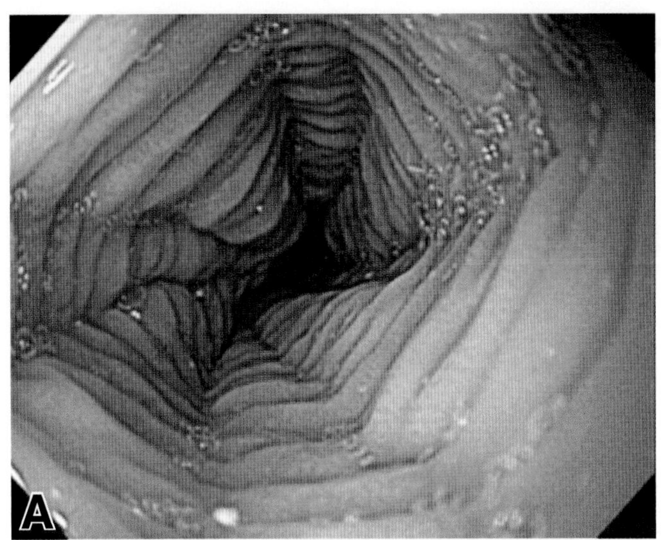

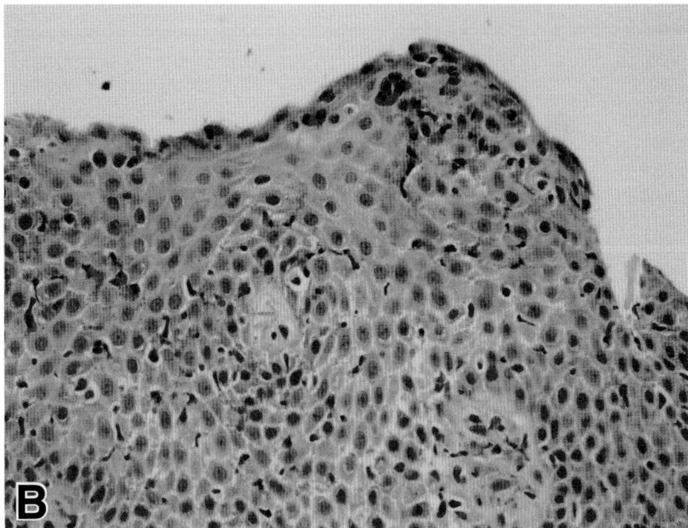

FIGURE 11-5. Eosinophilic esophagitis. A. Endoscopic view of an esophagus from a patient with eosinophilic esophagitis showing concentric mucosal rings (called trachealization or felinization because of its resemblance to the trachea or cat esophagus), vertical linear furrows, and small white plaques/exudates. **B.** Microscopic image showing epithelial hyperplasia (papillary and basal layer hyperplasia), intercellular edema, increased intraepithelial eosinophils (≥15 per high-power field), superficial layering of eosinophils, eosinophilic microabscesses, and prominent degranulation of eosinophils.

Chemical Esophagitis

Chemical injury to the esophagus usually reflects accidental poisoning in children, attempted suicide in adults, or contact with medication ("pill esophagitis"). Strong alkaline agents (e.g., lye) or potent acids (e.g., sulfuric or hydrochloric acids), which are used in various cleaning solutions, can produce chemical esophagitis. Alkaline chemicals are particularly insidious because they are generally odorless and tasteless and so easily swallowed before protective reflexes come into play.

ESOPHAGEAL VARICES

Esophageal varices are dilated veins beneath the mucosa that are prone to rupture and hemorrhage (also see Chapter 12). They arise in the lower third of the esophagus, almost always in patients with hepatic cirrhosis and portal hypertension. Gastroesophageal anastomoses link lower esophageal veins to the portal system. If portal pressure exceeds a critical level, these anastomoses dilate in the upper stomach and lower esophagus. Without treatment, varices rupture in approximately one third of patients, eliciting life-threatening hemorrhage. Reflux injury or infective esophagitis can contribute to variceal bleeding. Esophageal banding and a variety of medications are used to prevent esophageal varices from rupturing.

LACERATIONS AND PERFORATIONS

Lacerations of the esophagus result from external trauma, such as automobile accidents or medical instrumentation, or from severe vomiting, during which intraesophageal pressure may reach 300 mm Hg. Forceful retching may cause mucosal tears, first in the gastric epithelium and then extending into the esophagus.

Mallory–Weiss syndrome refers to severe retching, often associated with alcoholism. Such retching creates mucosal lacerations of the upper stomach and lower esophagus. These tears cause patients to vomit bright red blood. Bleeding may be so severe as to require transfusion of many units of blood. Perforation into the mediastinum, called **Boerhaave syndrome**, may result.

Esophageal perforation, whether from trauma, vomiting, or iatrogenic incidents, can be catastrophic. It is a well-known occurrence in newborns, occasioned by suctioning or feeding with a nasogastric tube. However, it may also occur spontaneously.

The major nonneoplastic esophageal disorders are summarized in Figure 11-6.

NEOPLASMS OF THE ESOPHAGUS

Esophageal Squamous Carcinoma

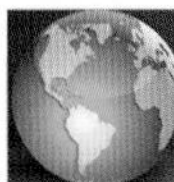

EPIDEMIOLOGY: Worldwide, most esophageal cancers are squamous cell carcinomas. Esophageal cancer is the eighth most common cancer, but in the United States, adenocarcinoma is now more common (see below).

Global geographic variations in the incidence of esophageal squamous carcinoma are striking: areas of high incidence often abut areas of low incidence. The greatest frequency is in China, Iran, South America, and South Africa. In the United States, black men have a much higher incidence than whites, and American urban dwellers are at greater risk than those in rural areas. Esophageal squamous cell carcinoma is more common in older men.

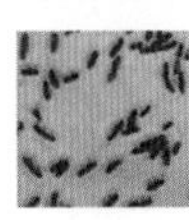

ETIOLOGIC FACTORS: The variable distribution of esophageal squamous carcinomas, even among relatively

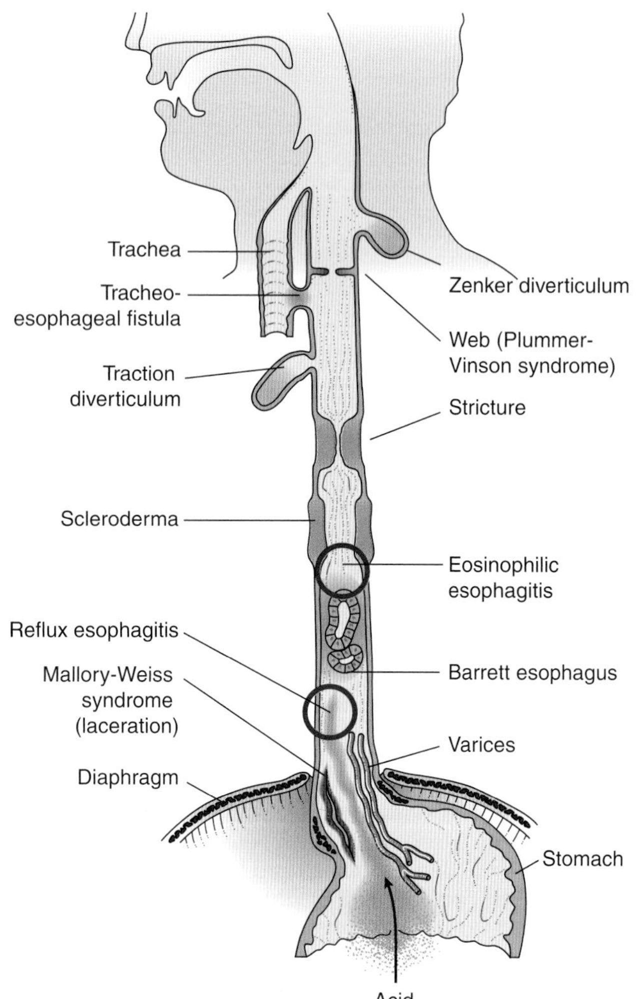

FIGURE 11-6. Nonneoplastic disorders of the esophagus.

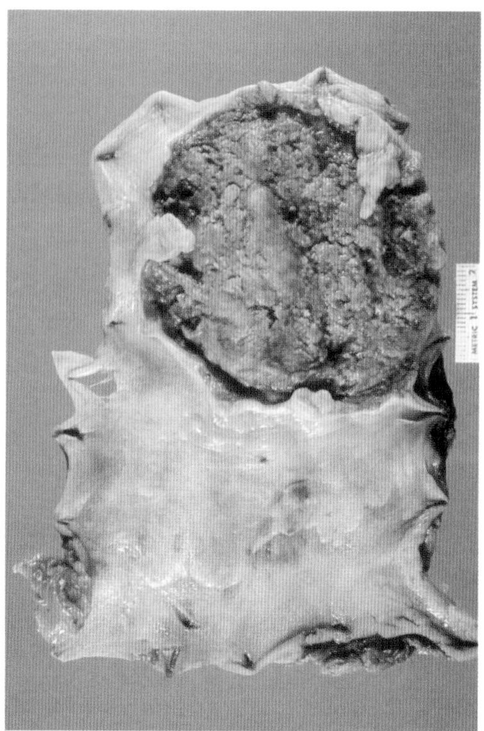

FIGURE 11-7. Esophageal squamous cell carcinoma. There is a large ulcerated mass present in the squamous mucosa with normal squamous mucosa intervening between the carcinoma and the stomach.

homogeneous populations, suggests that environmental factors strongly affect its development. The most common factors are smoking and alcohol, which have a synergistic rather than additive effect. Other putative contributors include diet, consumption of large amounts of hot beverages, HPV infection, radiation exposure, dietary nitrates and nitrosamines, vitamin deficiencies, genetic factors, Plummer–Vinson syndrome, achalasia, and prior caustic injury.

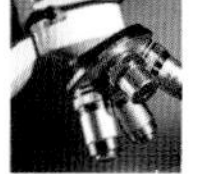

PATHOLOGY: About half of cases of esophageal squamous cell carcinoma involve the middle and upper thirds of the esophagus. Tumors may be endophytic or exophytic (Fig. 11-7). They can also be infiltrating, growing mainly in the wall. Bulky polypoid tumors tend to obstruct early, but ulcerated ones are more likely to bleed. Infiltrating tumors gradually narrow the lumen by circumferential compression. Extension of tumor into mediastinal structures is often a major problem.

Neoplastic squamous cells range from well differentiated, with squamous "pearls," to poorly differentiated, without evident squamous differentiation. Some tumors have a predominant spindle cell population of tumor cells.

The rich lymphatic drainage of the esophagus provides a route for most metastases. Tumors of the upper third spread to cervical, internal jugular, and supraclavicular nodes. Those of the middle third metastasize to paratracheal and hilar lymph nodes and to nodes in the aortic, cardiac, and paraesophageal regions. Because the lower third of the esophagus is supplied by the left gastric artery, lower esophageal tumors spread via accompanying lymphatics to retroperitoneal, celiac, and left gastric nodes. Metastases to liver and lung are common, although almost any organ may be affected.

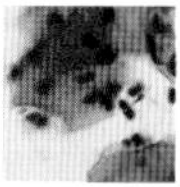

CLINICAL FEATURES: Dysphagia is the most common presenting complaint, but by the time this occurs, most tumors are inoperable. Patients may become cachectic from anorexia, difficulty in swallowing, and the remote effects of a cancer. Odynophagia occurs in half of patients. Persistent pain suggests extension to the mediastinum or to spinal nerves. Compression of the recurrent laryngeal nerve causes hoarseness, and tracheoesophageal fistula presents clinically as a chronic cough. Treatment is similar to esophageal adenocarcinoma (see below).

Adenocarcinoma of the Esophagus

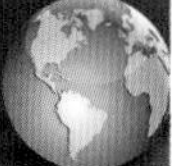

EPIDEMIOLOGY: In North America, Western Europe, and Australia, esophageal adenocarcinoma is far more common than squamous cancer. The incidence of esophageal adenocarcinoma is increasing faster than that of any solid tumor: it has increased sevenfold in the United States in the past 30 years. Men are affected more often than women.

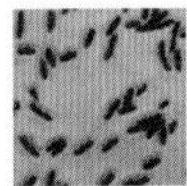

ETIOLOGIC FACTORS: Most esophageal adenocarcinomas arise from Barrett esophagus and so have similar underlying risk factors. These include white race, male sex, obesity, GERD, diet, tobacco use, and genetic factors. Other risk factors that result in increased gastric acid production or reflux include lower esophageal sphincter dilation or myotomy, scleroderma, Zollinger–Ellison syndrome, and medications that relax the lower esophageal sphincter.

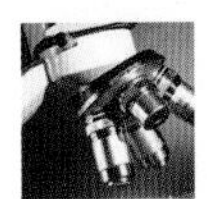

PATHOLOGY: The majority of esophageal adenocarcinomas involve the distal esophagus or GE junction and can extend into the proximal stomach. Tumors may be flat, ulcerated, polypoid, or fungating. Often, there is surrounding nonneoplastic Barrett mucosa that can be seen grossly or microscopically.

These tumors range from well differentiated to poorly differentiated tumors, with essentially no glandular differentiation. Some poorly differentiated adenocarcinomas have signet ring morphology.

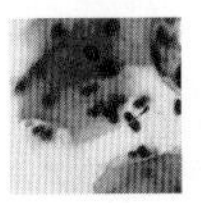

CLINICAL FEATURES: The symptoms and clinical course of esophageal adenocarcinoma are similar to those of squamous carcinoma. Symptoms generally appear in white, obese men with histories of GERD. Diagnosis and staging are typically done using endoscopy with ultrasound. Advanced disease requires neoadjuvant chemotherapy and radiation treatment, which can then be followed by surgical resection in patients who have a good clinical response.

Endoscopic surveillance is commonly done in the United States for people with Barrett esophagus. The goal is to identify and treat precursor lesions and early adenocarcinoma.

The Stomach

ANATOMY

The stomach is commonly divided into four regions: the cardia, fundus, body (corpus), and antrum (Fig. 11-8A and B). The **cardia** separates the esophagus from the rest of the stomach. The **fundus** and **body** are identical except that the fundus is the curve of the stomach that bulges above the gastroesophageal junction. Acid and intrinsic factor are produced in these regions. The **antrum** is the distal stomach, ending in the duodenum, and the pyloric sphincter.

The histology of the stomach is quite distinct in the cardia, fundus/body, and antrum. The mucosal layer of the entire stomach is a characteristic foveolar epithelium (Fig. 11-9A) and is characterized by the shallow pits covering the entire gastric surface.

The glands underlying the foveolae are characteristic features of the regions of the stomach. The glands of the cardia (Fig. 11-9B) are loosely packed and lined by cells containing neutral mucus. The glands of the gastric fundus and body (Fig. 11-9C) are where the acid-producing parietal cells (Fig. 11-9D) are located. These cells also produce intrinsic factor. They are large and polygonal, with slightly granular pink cytoplasm. Deeply in these glands, chief cells predominate; they have a granular blue cytoplasm marking production of pepsinogen. The deepest aspect of the glands is also home to neuroendocrine cells, namely, the enterochromaffin-like (ECL) cells.

The antral (or pyloric) mucosa (Fig. 11-9E) also contains loosely packed glands lined by cells that make neutral mucus. However, it is by the presence of neuroendocrine cells that the antrum differs from the cardia. Gastrin-producing G cells (Fig. 11-9F) are numerous here. There are also enterochromaffin (EC) cells, which produce serotonin and somatostatin, producing D cells.

ACUTE GASTRITIS

Acute usually occurs in specific clinical situations, including severe physiologic stress such as trauma, widespread burns, increased intracranial pressure, or sepsis. At times, acute gastritis may be related to back diffusion of hydrogen ions related to the ingestion of alcohol, aspirin, or other nonsteroidal anti-inflammatory drugs (NSAIDs). Superficial ulcers related to burns are called Curling ulcers; ulcers related to

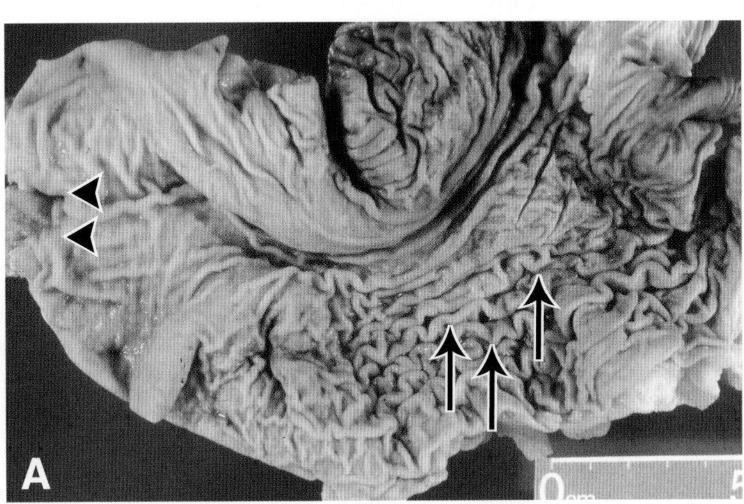

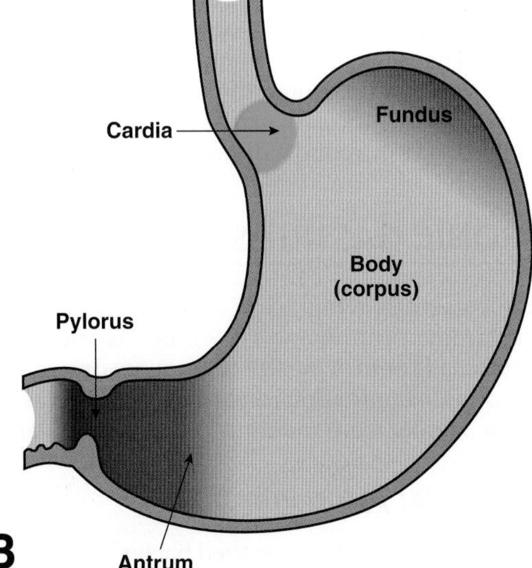

FIGURE 11-8. Anatomy of the stomach. A. A **normal stomach** from an autopsy. The rugal folds are readily seen in the body (*arrows*). The sweep of the lesser curvature leads into the V-shaped antrum (*arrowheads*). **B.** Anatomic regions of the stomach.

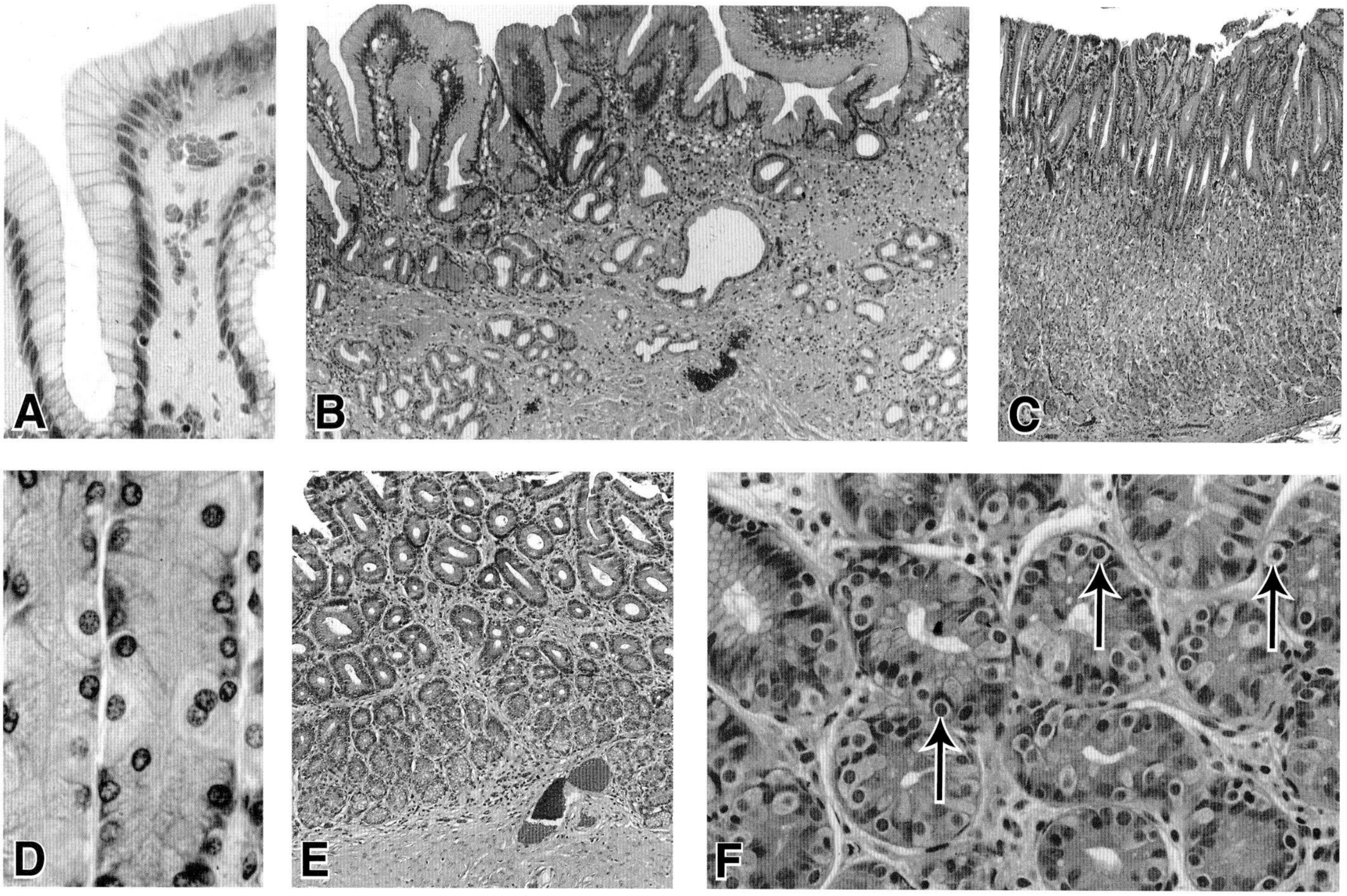

FIGURE 11-9. Histology of the stomach. A. The **foveolar epithelium. B.** The gastric **cardia. C.** The gastric **body. D. Parietal** cells (pink) and **chief cells** (granular blue). **E.** The gastric **antrum. F. Gastrin**-producing cells in antrum; they resemble fried eggs (*arrows*) (see text for further description).

increased intracranial pressure are Cushing ulcers. Unlike chronic peptic ulcers, which are usually in the antrum or the junction of the body and antrum, ulcers of acute gastritis are usually shallow and multiple and found in the acid-producing mucosa of the body (Fig. 11-10A and B). Acute gastritis itself is usually hemorrhagic (acute hemorrhagic gastritis) but can show a significant fibroinflammatory reaction (acute erosive gastritis). These processes can be life-threatening, and patients with predisposing conditions are treated prophylactically.

CHRONIC GASTRITIS

Chronic gastritis refers to an increase in inflammatory cells in the lamina propria and is common worldwide. It may be asymptomatic or may present with vague dyspeptic symptoms. Endoscopic examination is less accurate in assessing gastritis than are similar examinations for esophagitis and colitis.

Helicobacter pylori Infection

Helicobacter are short rod-shaped bacteria with a unique habitat on the surface of foveolar cells. In some countries, over 80% of people are infected, whereas in the United States, the prevalence varies from 4% to 30%. Over the past 30 years, recognition and subsequent treatment of *H. pylori* gastritis have led to a continuing reduction in its prevalence.

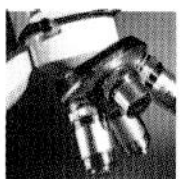

PATHOLOGY: *Helicobacter* (Fig. 11-11D) are small curvilinear bacilli found in the mucin-covered surface of foveolar cells. *Helicobacter* gastritis tends to be localized. In most cases, the antrum is mostly affected, but with advancing time, or after therapy with proton pump inhibitors, the more proximal stomach may become involved. Inflammation starts in the lamina propria (Fig. 11-11A) because the organisms reside only in a superficial layer of mucus. The bacteria are not found in the absence of foveolar cells or in association with intestinal-type epithelium. Thus, areas of intestinal metaplasia are devoid of organisms. Lymphoid aggregates, which are often present in *Helicobacter* gastritis (Fig. 11-11B), feature a mixture of lymphocytes and plasma cells, although neutrophils are often present. They can accumulate in foveolae to form "pit abscesses" (Fig. 11-11C). The presence of such neutrophils does not denote acute gastritis, which is an entirely different process (see above). Rather, they indicate an active chronic gastritis, with ongoing flares of inflammation in an underlying chronic gastritis.

Significance of *Helicobacter* Infection

The most common problem related to chronic *Helicobacter* gastritis is ***peptic ulcer disease***. Duodenal ulcers occur in 10% to 20% of patients with antral-predominant gastritis. This is the main pattern in Western countries, where for years, duodenal ulcer disease had been epidemic. Recognition of the role of

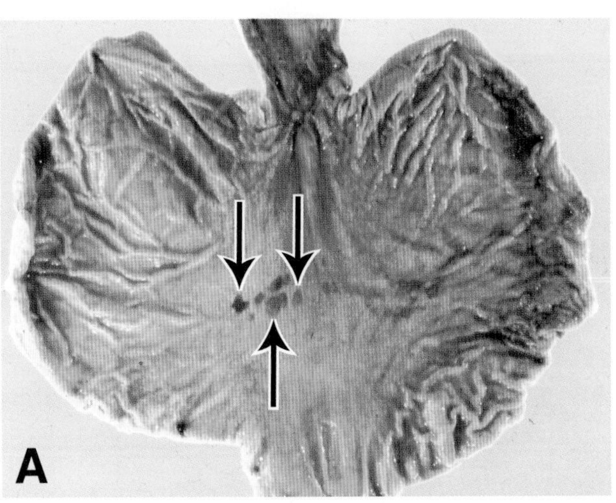

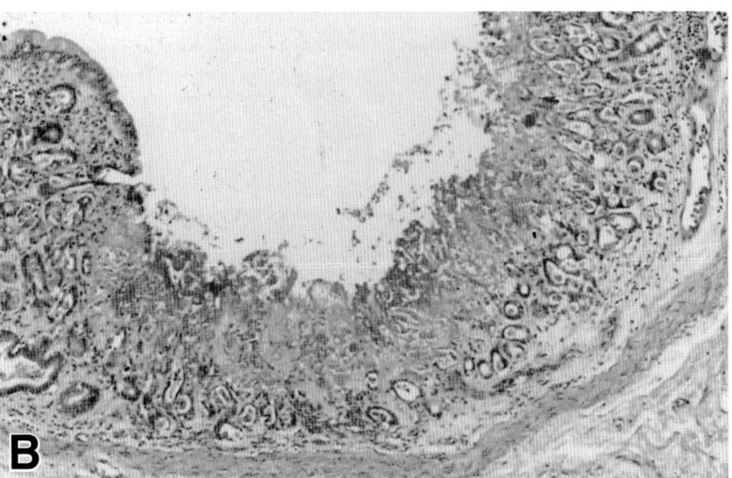

FIGURE 11-10. Acute gastritis. A. Several shallow erosions/ulcers are scattered in the gastric body (*arrows*). **B.** There is an area of erosion with hemorrhage.

Helicobacter has greatly lessened the incidence of duodenal ulcers and their complications. The disease is now largely treated medically, and surgical intervention is rarely necessary.

H. pylori infection involving the gastric body increases the risk for ***gastric cancer***. The magnitude of this risk is difficult to ascertain because the involved stomach often shows intestinal metaplasia, and *H. pylori* may no longer be readily identifiable. Still, it is widely held that *H. pylori* infection is the most common known cause of gastric cancer.

Active Chronic Gastritis Without Identified *Helicobacter*

In many cases, this condition likely represents prior therapy with antibiotics and ant acid drugs, which eradicated the organisms. Other infections (e.g., CMV), or adverse drug effects, may also be responsible. Similar gastric inflammation occurs in patients with idiopathic inflammatory bowel disease, particularly Crohn disease.

Autoimmune Gastritis

The target of the autoimmune reaction in autoimmune gastritis is gastric parietal cells, hence its limitation to the gastric fundus and body. Without parietal cells, the stomach does not produce acid, and clinical achlorhydria results. Also, lost is the other product of the parietal cells, namely, intrinsic factor, which mediates absorption of vitamin B_{12} in the distal small intestine.

Immunologically mediated destruction of parietal cells is associated with production of antiparietal cell and anti-intrinsic factor antibodies. With careful sampling from the proximal (body) and distal (antrum) stomach, the diagnosis can be established long before loss of vitamin B_{12} results in clinical anemia, known as ***pernicious anemia*** (see Chapter 18). Unlike other forms of chronic gastritis, the antrum is spared from inflammation and metaplasia. Hyperplasia of antral G cells occurs because there is no feedback inhibition, because there is no acid production. These G cells consequently produce large amounts of gastrin, which exerts a trophic effect on neuroendocrine cells of the proximal stomach. Hyperplasia of these cells predisposes to the development neuroendocrine tumors (see below).

The histologic appearance of autoimmune gastritis (Fig. 11-12A and B) is well defined. Parietal cells are absent, and there is significant mononuclear inflammation and intestinal and pseudopyloric metaplasia. In time, neuroendocrine hyperplasia may become prominent. Autoimmune gastritis indicates a significant predisposition to other autoimmune diseases (e.g., type 1 diabetes, hypothyroidism, and Addison disease) (see Chapter 3) in both the patient and family members.

Reactive (Chemical) Gastropathy

While it is clear that exposure to NSAIDs can alter the gastric mucosa, it is not clear when these changes represent a clinically significant condition. These agents lead to hyperplasia of foveolar cells, resulting in loss of the normal nearly flat surface.

The most common drug effect is caused by proton pump inhibitors. In the gastric body, glands lined by parietal cells show luminal dilation and some protrusion into these lumens by parietal cell cytoplasm. Many patients develop fundic gland polyps (see below). Because acid production is blocked, antral G cells visibly multiply and produce excess gastrin. This causes proliferation of neuroendocrine cells of the gastric body.

PEPTIC ULCER DISEASE

"Peptic ulcer disease" refers to focal destruction of the mucosa of the stomach and small intestine, mainly the proximal duodenum. Duodenal ulcers have declined greatly in frequency over the past 30 years.

Although the disease mostly affects the distal stomach and duodenum, peptic ulceration may occur as far proximally as the esophagus and as far distally as the Meckel diverticulum with gastric heterotopia. Many clinical and epidemiologic features distinguish gastric from duodenal ulcers; the common factors that unite them are gastric hydrochloric acid secretion and *H. pylori* infection.

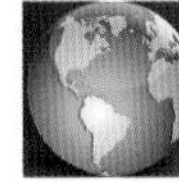

EPIDEMIOLOGY: Peptic ulcers may occur at any age (including infancy), but the peak incidence has progressively changed, so that it is now between age 30 and 60. Gastric ulcers usually afflict the

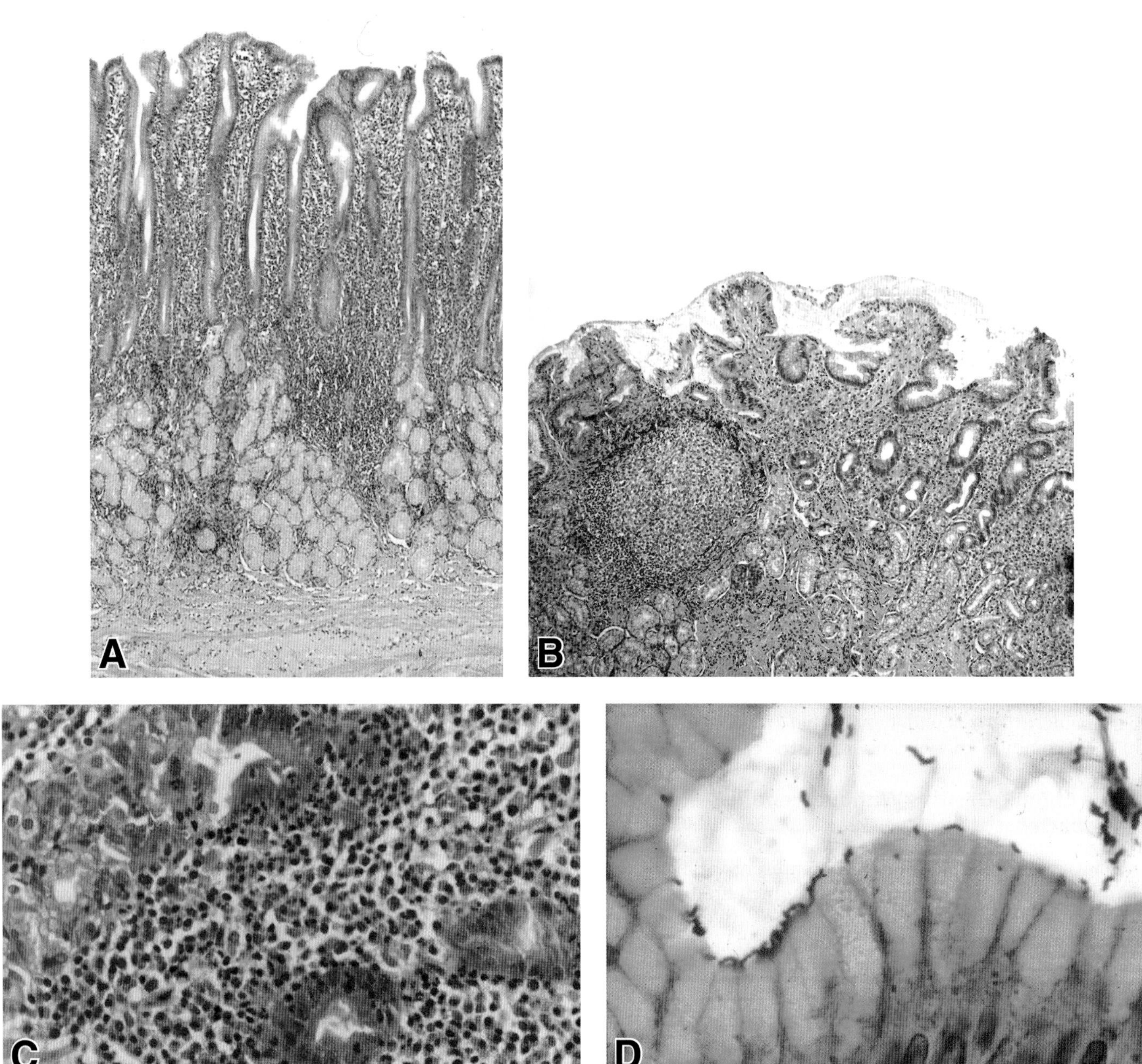

FIGURE 11-11. ***Helicobacter*** **gastritis. A.** There is a superficial dense lymphoplasmacytic infiltrate in the lamina propria. **B.** A lymphoid aggregate; when present, these are highly suggestive of *Helicobacter.* **C.** Neutrophils are scattered in the lamina propria infiltrate and can penetrate the glandular epithelium. **D.** The Warthin–Starry stain highlighting the small curvilinear organisms at the foveolar surface.

middle-aged and elderly and affect both sexes equally. Duodenal ulcers are more common in males.

ETIOLOGIC FACTORS: No single agent seems to be responsible, although many etiologies have been proffered.

***H. PYLORI*:** *H. pylori* is isolated from the gastric antrum of virtually all patients with duodenal ulcers. However, only a small minority of those carrying the bacterium have duodenal ulcer disease. Thus, *H. pylori* infection seems to be necessary but not sufficient for peptic duodenal ulcers to develop. Such ulcers heal more quickly after treatment for *H. pylori* infection and recur less often.

Just how *H. pylori* infection predisposes to duodenal ulcers is not completely clear, but several mechanisms have been proposed. Cytokines produced by inflammatory cells in response to the infection stimulate gastrin release and suppress somatostatin secretion. Interleukin 1β (IL-1β), an acid inhibitor, is a key mediator of inflammation in *H. pylori*–infected gastric mucosa. These effects, plus release of histamine metabolites from the organism itself, may stimulate basal gastric acid secretion. In addition, luminal cytokines from the stomach may enter and injure duodenal epithelium.

H. pylori infection may also block inhibitory signals from the antrum to G cells and the parietal cell region, thereby

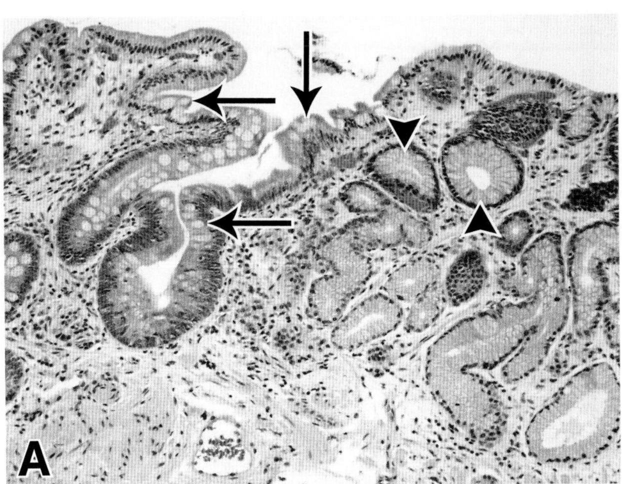

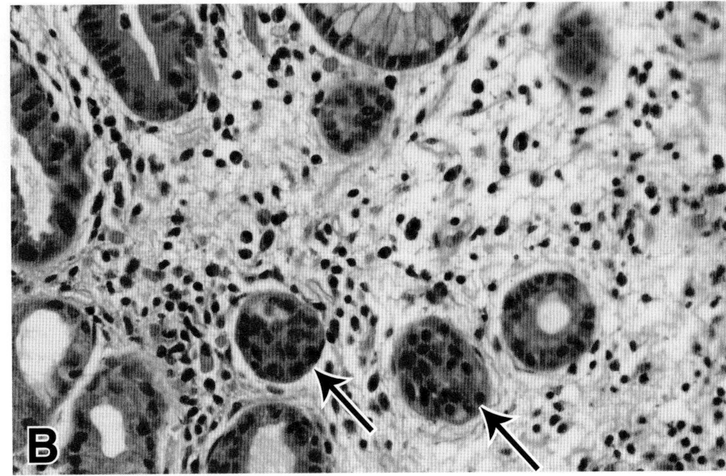

FIGURE 11-12. Autoimmune gastritis. A. The gastric body is atrophic and devoid of parietal cells. There is intestinal metaplasia (goblet cells; *arrows*) and pseudopyloric metaplasia (*arrowhead*). **B.** Elsewhere in the body, there are micronodules composed of enterochromaffin-like cells (*arrows*). Note: These biopsies were from the stomach of one of the authors (FAM).

increasing gastrin release and impairing inhibition of gastric acid secretion. Such an effect might increase acid load in the duodenum and contribute to duodenal ulceration. Acidification of the duodenal bulb leads to islands of metaplastic gastric mucosa in the duodenum in many patients with peptic ulcers. Such gastric epithelium in the duodenum is sometimes colonized with *H. pylori*, similar to the gastric mucosa, and infection of the metaplastic epithelium by *H. pylori* may render the mucosa more susceptible to peptic injury (Fig. 11-13).

H. pylori infection is also important in the pathogenesis of gastric ulcers because the organism causes most of the chronic gastritis that underlies this disease. About 75% of patients with gastric ulcers harbor *H. pylori.* The other 25% of cases may reflect the influences of other types of chronic gastritis. The gastric and duodenal factors that have been implicated as possible mechanisms in the pathogenesis of duodenal ulcers are summarized in Figure 11-14.

HCl SECRETION: Hyperacidity caused by increased hydrochloric acid secretion is necessary for peptic ulcers to form and persist in the stomach and duodenum. This is evidenced principally by the following: (1) all patients with duodenal ulcers and almost all with gastric ulcers are gastric acid secretors; (2) experimental ulcer production in animals requires acid; (3) hypersecretion of acid is present in many, but not all, patients with duodenal ulcers; and (4) surgical and medical treatment that reduces acid production results in the healing of peptic ulcers. Gastric secretion of pepsin, which may also play a role in peptic ulceration, parallels that of hydrochloric acid.

DIET: Despite the folk wisdom that spicy food and caffeine are ulcerogenic, there is little evidence that any food or beverage, including coffee and alcohol, leads to the development or persistence of peptic ulcers.

DRUGS: Aspirin is an important contributor to duodenal, and especially gastric, ulcers. Other nonsteroidal anti-inflammatory agents and analgesics have been incriminated in peptic ulcerogenesis. Prolonged treatment with high doses of corticosteroids may also increase the risk of peptic ulceration.

CIGARETTE SMOKING: Smoking is a definite risk factor for duodenal and gastric ulcers, particularly gastric ulcers.

GENETIC FACTORS: First-degree relatives of people with duodenal or gastric ulcers have a threefold higher risk of developing an ulcer—but only at the same site. Monozygotic twins show much higher (50%) concordance for these ulcers than do dizygotic twins, indicating that environmental factors are also involved.

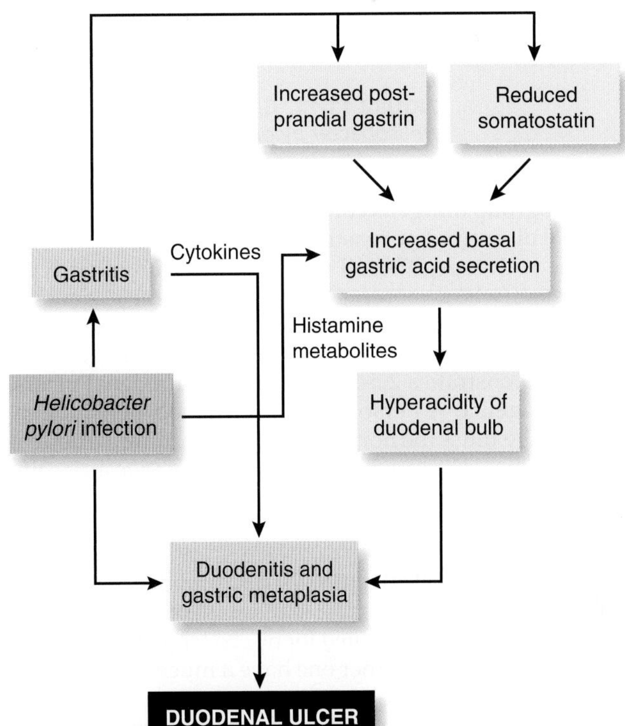

FIGURE 11-13. Possible mechanisms in the pathogenesis of duodenal ulcer disease associated with *Helicobacter pylori* infection.

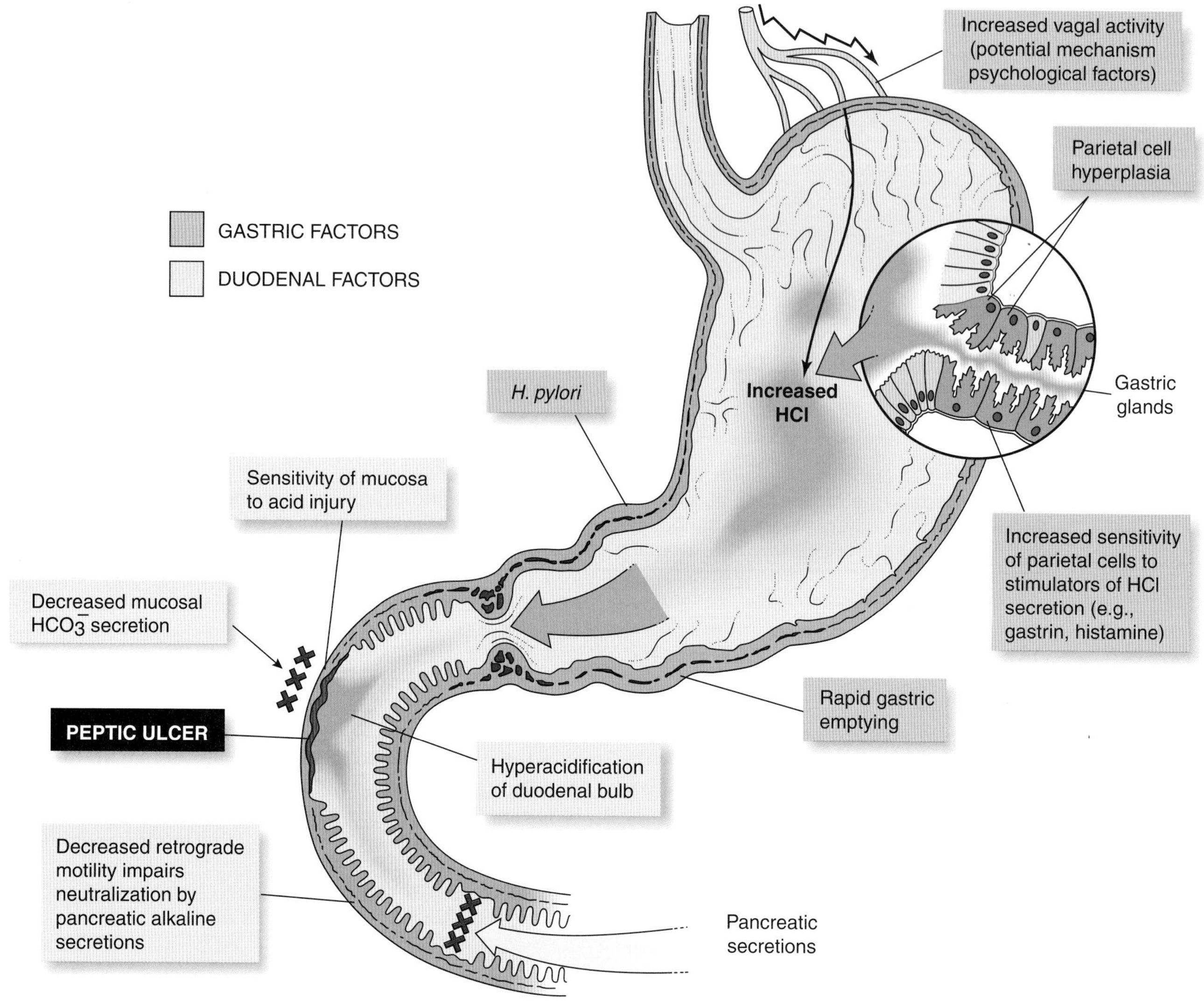

FIGURE 11-14. Gastric and duodenal factors in the pathogenesis of duodenal peptic ulcers. *H. pylori, Helicobacter pylori*; HCl, hydrochloric acid; HCO_3^-, bicarbonate.

Blood-group antigens correlate with peptic ulcer disease. Duodenal ulcers (but not gastric ulcers) occur 30% more often in people with type O blood than in those with other types. Nonsecretors (who do not secrete blood-group antigens in saliva or gastric juice) have a 50% higher risk of duodenal ulcers. Those who are both type O and nonsecretors (10% of white people) demonstrate a 2.5-fold increase in duodenal ulcers.

Pepsinogen I: A person with high blood pepsinogen I levels has five times the normal risk of developing a duodenal ulcer. Hyperpepsinogenemia has been attributed to autosomal dominant inheritance and may reflect an inherited tendency to increased parietal cell mass.

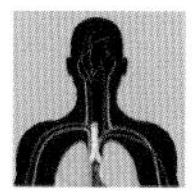

PATHOPHYSIOLOGY: Gastric and duodenal ulcers occur together in the same patient far more often than can be accounted for by chance alone. Moreover, patients with either one have a much greater risk of developing the other later.

Duodenal Ulcers: A number of other factors have been related to duodenal ulcer formation:

- Excess acid formation as a result of (1) increased parietal cell mass, (2) excess gastric acid secretion resulting from altered G-cell responses, (3) accelerated gastric emptying, (4) increased sensitivity to gastric secretagogues, and (5) reduced postprandial duodenal pH.
- Impaired mucosal defenses.

Gastric Ulcers: Gastric ulcers almost invariably arise in the setting of epithelial injury by *H. pylori* or chemical gastritis. Most patients with gastric ulcers secrete less acid than do those with duodenal ulcers and even less than normal people. Intense gastric hypersecretion, such as occurs in the Zollinger—Ellison syndrome (see below), is associated with severe ulceration of the duodenum but rarely of the stomach. The concurrence of gastric ulcers and gastric hyposecretion suggests the following:

- The gastric mucosa may in some way be particularly sensitive to low concentrations of acid.
- Something other than acid (e.g., NSAIDs) may damage the mucosa (or be present for a prolonged period).
- Reflux of bile (particularly deoxycholic acid and lysolecithin) and pancreatic secretions may contribute to the development of gastric ulcers.

Diseases Associated with Peptic Ulcers

The risk for and severity of peptic ulcer disease are increased in patients with (1) cirrhosis, (2) end-stage renal disease with hemodialysis, (3) kidney transplants, and (4) multiple endocrine neoplasia type 1 (see Chapter 19).

As noted above, Zollinger—Ellison syndrome causes severe peptic ulceration. It is characterized by gastric hypersecretion, caused by a gastric-producing islet cell adenoma of the pancreas. Peptic ulcers are also increased in people heterozygous for mutant α_1-antitrypsin with long-standing pulmonary dysfunction.

PATHOLOGY: Most peptic ulcers arise in the (1) lesser gastric curvature, (2) antral and prepyloric regions, and (3) first part of the duodenum.

Gastric ulcers are usually single and smaller than 2 cm. Ulcers on the lesser curvature are often associated with chronic gastritis; those on the greater curvature are commonly related to NSAID usage. Edges tend to be sharply punched out, with overhanging margins. Deeply penetrating ulcers produce a serosal exudate that may cause the stomach to adhere to nearby structures. Scarring of ulcers in the prepyloric region may be severe enough to cause pyloric stenosis. Grossly, chronic peptic ulcers sometimes resemble ulcerated gastric carcinomas. They differ from cancer by their tendency to produce radiating folds in the surrounding mucosa, their lack of a raised border, and a "clean" (fibrin-covered)-appearing base (Fig. 11-15).

Duodenal ulcers are ordinarily on the anterior or posterior wall of the first part of the duodenum, near the pylorus. They are usually solitary, but it is not uncommon to find paired ulcers on both walls, the so-called "kissing ulcers."

Gastric and duodenal ulcers are histologically similar (Fig. 11-16A and B). From the lumen inward, there are several layers: (1) a superficial zone of fibrinopurulent exudate, (2) necrotic tissue, (3) granulation tissue, and (4) fibrotic tissue with variable degrees of chronic inflammation at the depth of the ulcer's base. Ulceration may penetrate muscle layers, interrupting them with scar tissue after healing. Blood vessels at the margins of the ulcer are often thrombosed. Mucosal margins tend to be slightly hyperplastic. With healing, mucosa grows over ulcerated areas as a single epithelial layer. Duodenal ulcers are usually accompanied by peptic duodenitis, with Brunner gland hyperplasia and gastric mucin cell metaplasia.

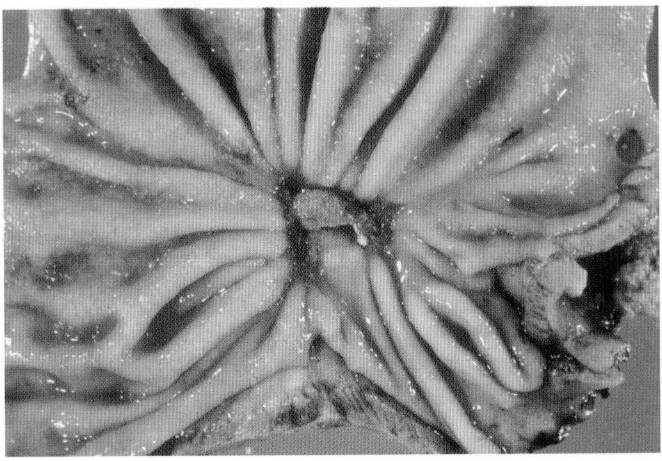

FIGURE 11-15. Gastric ulcer. There is a characteristic sharp demarcation from the surrounding mucosa, which has prominent radiating folds. The base of the ulcer is covered with fibrin, giving it a gray color.

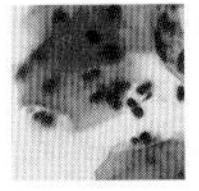

CLINICAL FEATURES: The symptoms of gastric and duodenal ulcers tend to not be distinguishable by history or physical examination. Classic duodenal ulcers are characterized by epigastric pain 1 to 3 hours after a meal or that awakens a patient at night. Alkali and food relieve these symptoms. Dyspeptic symptoms often associated with gallbladder disease, such as fatty food intolerance, distention, and belching, occur in half of patients with peptic ulcers.

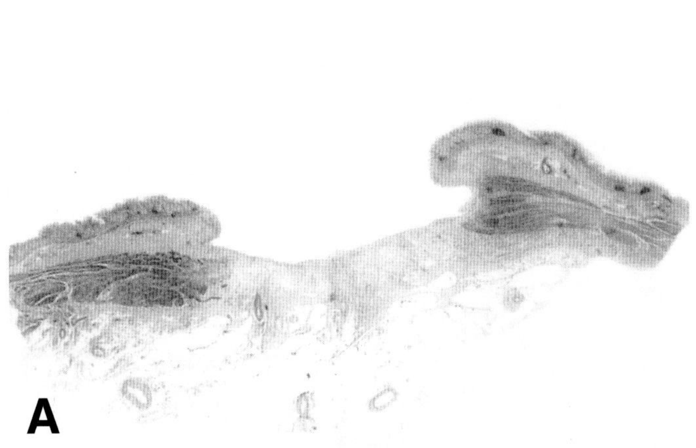

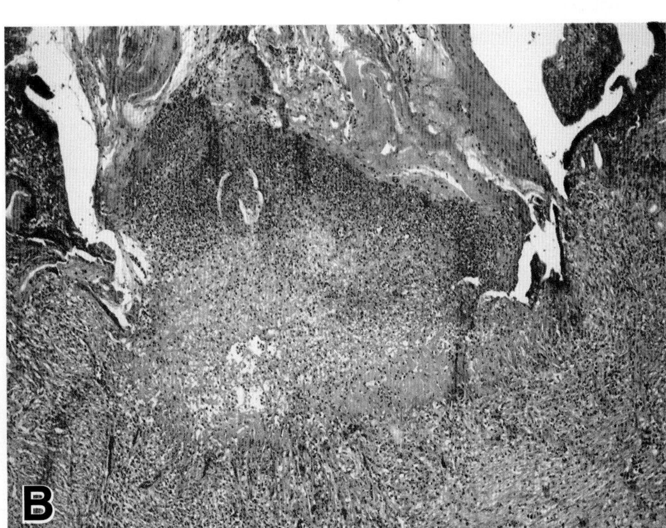

FIGURE 11-16. Gastric ulcer. A. The destructive nature of this lesion is shown by the loss of the underlying muscle in the muscularis propria with replacement by fibrous tissue. **B.** Classic appearance of peptic ulcer with superficial fibrin exudate over necrosis, followed by granulation tissue and fibrosis in the deep aspect.

The major complications of peptic ulcer disease are (1) hemorrhage, (2) obstruction, and (3) perforation with peritonitis. Of these, the most common is bleeding, which occurs in up to 20% of patients. It is often occult and may manifest as iron-deficiency anemia or occult blood in stools. Massive life-threatening bleeding is a well-known complication of active peptic ulcers.

Perforation is a serious complication that occurs in 5% of patients. In one third of these, there are no antecedent symptoms of a peptic ulcer. Duodenal ulcers perforate more often than do gastric ulcers, mostly on the anterior wall of the duodenum. Because the anterior gastric and duodenal walls are undefended by contiguous tissue, perforations there are more likely to lead to generalized peritonitis and to air in the abdominal cavity (**pneumoperitoneum**). Perforation carries a high mortality rate, which is 10% to 40% for gastric ulcers, 2 to 4 times more than for duodenal ulcers (10%).

ENLARGED RUGAL FOLDS

Enlarged rugal folds may be caused by a proliferation of parietal cells (Zollinger—Ellison [Z-E] syndrome). The cause is gastrin production by a neuroendocrine tumor (NET, gastrinoma). Most cases are sporadic, in which case the gastrinomas are more commonly duodenal than pancreatic. A minority of cases are related to multiple endocrine neoplasia syndrome type 1 (MEN1). Gastrinomas in Z-E patients may occur in the duodenum, pancreas, or gastric antrum, and they may be multiple and exceedingly small. Rugal folds are enlarged owing to increased numbers of hypertrophied parietal cells; the rugae consequently have a characteristic bumpy appearance. Patients with Z-E syndrome have intractable peptic ulcer disease, with the ulcers often being multiple and in unusual locations.

BENIGN NEOPLASMS

Polyps are endoscopically or grossly identifiable elevations of the mucosa. In the stomach, unlike the colon, the vast majority are not true neoplasms.

Fundic Gland Polyps

They are mucosal elevations composed of cystically dilated glands, which are lined by a mixture of parietal cells, chief cells, and neutral mucous cells (Fig. 11-17A and B). They were first described in patients with familial adenomatous polyposis (FAP; see below); in affected patients, myriad such polyps carpet the proximal gastric mucosa. Rarely, fundic gland polyps in these patients show focal dysplasia. Far more common are isolated or small numbers of fundic polyps in the ever-increasing number of patients taking proton pump inhibitors. The mechanism for their formation is unknown, but they appear to be innocuous.

Hyperplastic Polyps

This term is something of a misnomer because these polyps have nothing but the name in common with polyps of the colon (see below). They occur in the setting of chronic gastritis or reactive gastropathy, may be single or multiple, and are exaggerated focal responses to mucosal injury. Gastric hyperplastic polyps consist of hyperplastic foveolar cells, sometimes forming small cysts, and an inflamed lamina propria. Reactive atypia may be present, particularly if there are surface erosions. They are sometimes called "hyperplastic/inflammatory" polyps, reflecting the manner in which they arose. These lesions are not inherently precancerous. However, their malignant potential is that of the background mucosa from which they arose.

Gastric Adenomas

True adenomas of the stomach occur far less often than adenomas of the colon. Although gastric adenomas can be related to gastric carcinoma, the very close relationship of adenoma to carcinoma seen in the colon is not present. Gastric adenomas are usually single except in FAP and several other uncommon syndromes, and can be of foveolar- or intestinal-type mucosa. By definition, dysplastic changes are present (Fig. 11-18). Intestinal-type adenomas are far more common and usually arise in stomachs with intestinal metaplasia. Nuclei tend to be

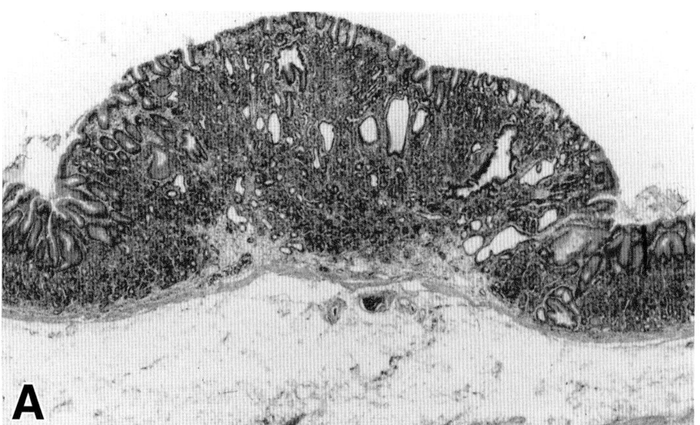

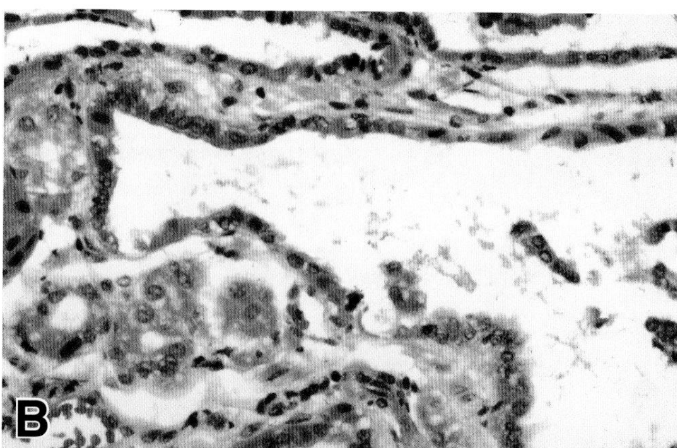

FIGURE 11-17. Fundic gland polyp. A. Low-power view showing the polyp as a slight elevation above the surrounding body-type mucosa. **B.** The cystically dilated glands contain parietal and chief cells.

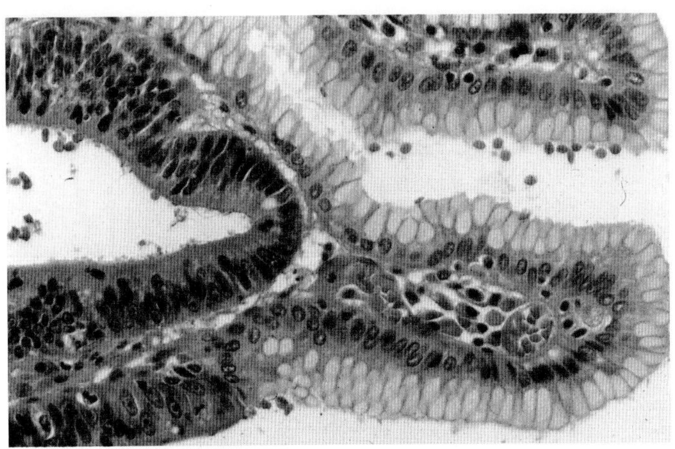

FIGURE 11-18. Gastric adenoma. There is sharp demarcation between the glandular epithelium with enlarged, hyperchromatic pencil-shaped nuclei (*left*) and adjacent normal foveolar epithelium (*right*).

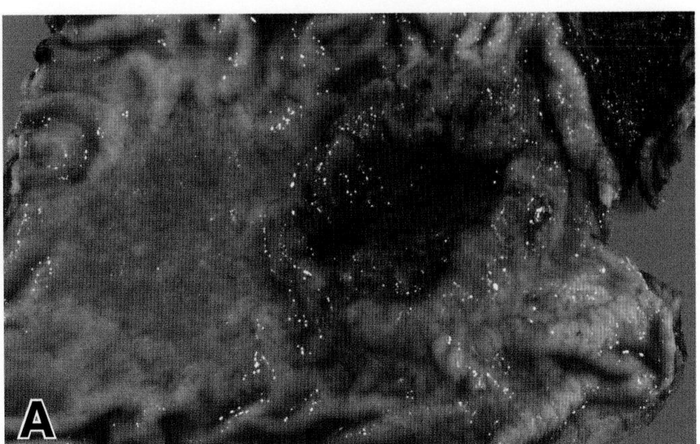

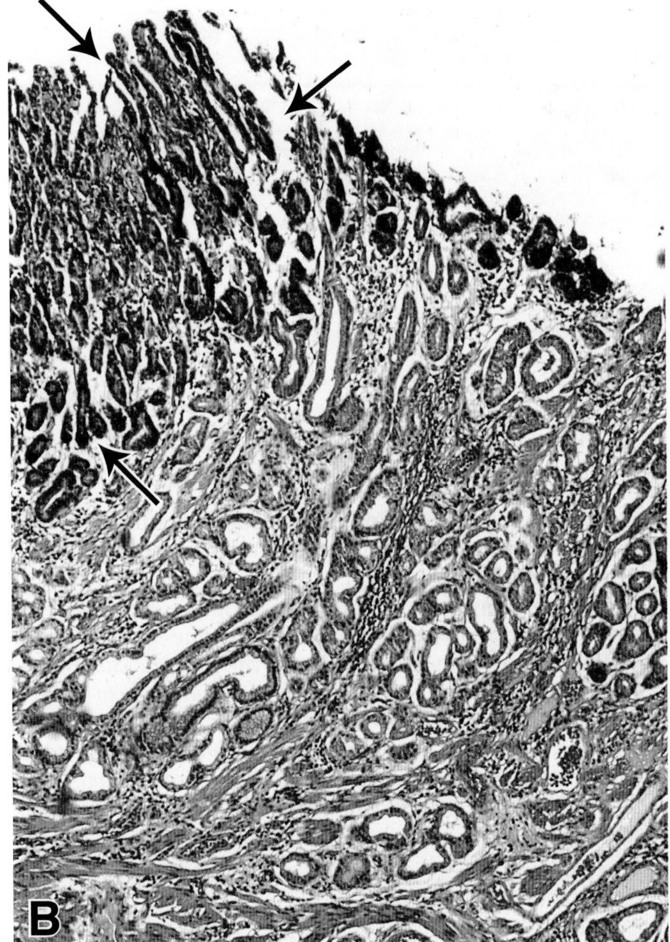

FIGURE 11-19. Gastric carcinoma. A. This large antral lesion is clearly distinguished from a benign ulcer by its raised firm edges and necrotic base. **B.** Microscopically, there are innumerable poorly formed glands (*arrows*) replacing mucosa in this intestinal-type carcinoma.

enlarged, elongated, and hyperchromatic, like their intestinal counterparts. By contrast, foveolar-type adenomas have no relationship to intestinal metaplasia; there does appear to be a relationship to FAP.

MALIGNANT NEOPLASMS

Adenocarcinoma

EPIDEMIOLOGY: Although gastric adenocarcinoma has declined markedly in incidence in Western countries over the past century, many Eastern countries have a far higher incidence. The most important factor appears to be differences in the prevalence of *Helicobacter* and chronic gastritis. With improved recognition and treatment of *Helicobacter* infections, gaps between the West and East are narrowing. Diets high in smoked or pickled foods are associated with a higher cancer rate, whereas consumption of fresh vegetables and leafy greens has the opposite effect. Genetic factors also play a significant role, particularly with some types of gastric cancer.

PATHOLOGY: The gross appearance of gastric cancer is variable. Most carcinomas form large polypoid masses or growths with significant ulceration (Fig. 11-19A and B). The tumors differ from benign peptic ulcers by their large size, raised firm irregular borders, and ragged ulcer surfaces. A minority of cancers infiltrate the gastric wall deeply, beneath a surface that may seem deceptively intact. The infiltrating cells elicit a prominent desmoplastic response. This results in a rigid thick-walled stomach, an appearance that has been classically described as **linitis plastica** (Fig. 11-20A to C).

Gastric carcinoma has traditionally been separated into two categories, intestinal and diffuse, with some cases showing overlap. The term "intestinal" in this context mainly describes the architecture, rather than the cell type. These tumors form glands or papillae, as well as some solid areas; mucin production may occur. This is the more common pattern and is the one associated with chronic gastritis. It is declining in incidence because of its relationship to *Helicobacter.*

Diffuse gastric carcinoma contains poorly cohesive cells that infiltrate the gastric wall, often with striking desmoplasia. Although the diffusely infiltrating cells may have a signet ring appearance, other cells may more mimic histiocytes or even lymphocytes. The incidence of this tumor has been more stable in all countries. It has a clearer genetic component and

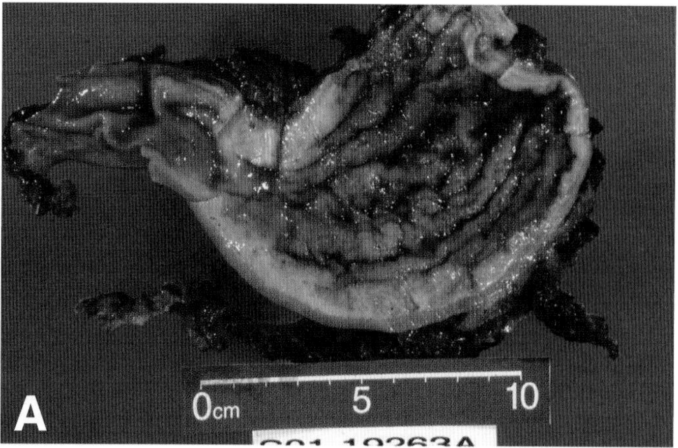

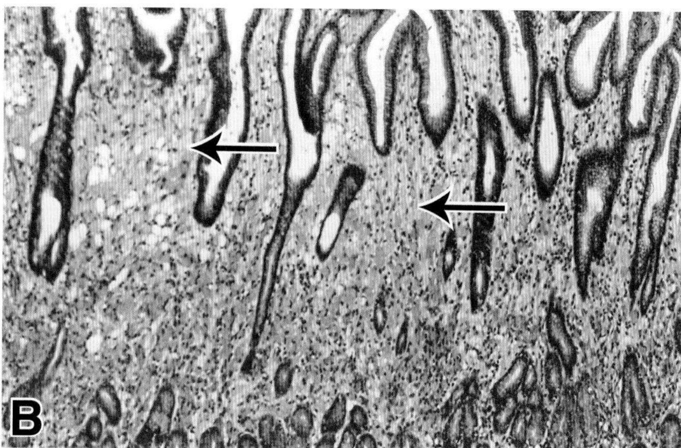

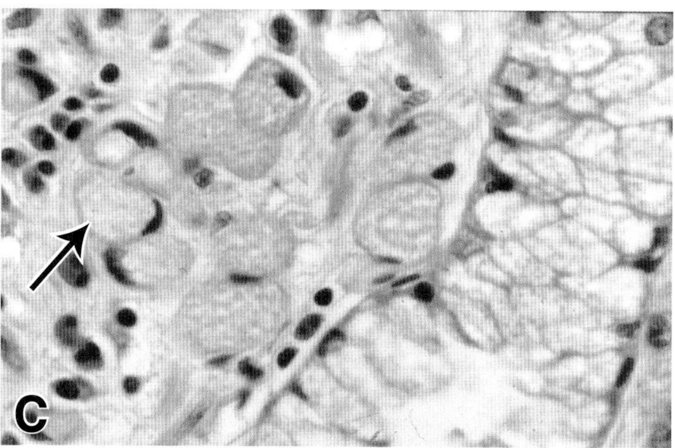

FIGURE 11-20. Gastric carcinoma. A. The wall is white and thickened owing to the diffuse infiltrate of tumor cells. The mucosal surface is deceptively free of mass lesions. **B.** The infiltrate fills and expands the lamina propria (*arrows*) but leaves glands and surface epithelium intact. **C.** The tumor cells in this diffuse-type cancer are present next to an intact gland. Note the signet ring appearance (*arrow*).

is associated with an uncommon autosomal dominant condition caused by inactivating germline mutations in *CDH1*, the gene that encodes E-cadherin.

There are complex systems describing the character and depth of gastric carcinomas, but there is one simple fact of paramount importance: *patients with early gastric cancer (i.e., tumors confined to the mucosa and submucosa) are likely to survive. The prognosis for patients with late cancers (i.e., lesions that extend beyond the submucosa into the muscularis propria or beyond) is dismal. In this context, the distinction between "early" and "late" refers to the anatomic location of the tumor rather than temporal considerations.*

Extranodal Lymphomas

The gastrointestinal tract is the most common location for extranodal lymphomas, and the stomach is the most common portion of the GI tract affected. Most gastric lymphomas are either extranodal marginal zone lymphomas of mucosa-associated lymphoid tissue (MALT lymphoma; see Chapter 18) or diffuse large B-cell lymphomas. Both are associated with *Helicobacter* infection; eradication of the organisms leads to remission in the striking majority of cases.

Gastrointestinal Stromal Tumors

GISTs occur throughout the GI tract but are particularly common in the stomach. Such tumors do not derive from smooth muscle but rather from the interstitial cells of Cajal, which normally reside in the muscularis propria and are pacemakers.

The tumors are usually large and bulky, arising in the muscularis propria (Fig. 11-21A and B). They may show central ulceration in the overlying mucosa and so present with bleeding.

It is not possible to distinguish clearly between benign and malignant GISTs, the site of origin being the most important indicator. Fortunately, most gastric GISTs are less likely to show aggressive behavior. Imatinib, a drug that inhibits the tyrosine kinase activity of c-kit (CD 117), shows impressive antitumor effects in cases of gastric GIST.

Neuroendocrine Tumors

These tumors were once called "carcinoids," but that term is being replaced by the term NETs. Similar to GISTs, the site of origin is the major determinant of likely behavior. The best predictive features within a given site are the size and mitotic rate (proliferative activity may be assessed immunohistochemically by Ki67).

This is especially so for gastric NETs. There are three major clinical scenarios in which gastric NETs are found:

- Autoimmune gastritis results in a proliferation of ECL cells in the body and fundus. Propelled by prominent and continuing hypergastrinemia, a clinically evident neoplasm is formed. Patients with NETs arising in autoimmune gastritis often have multiple visible tumors (Fig. 11-22).
- Gastric NETs may arise in the hypergastrinemic state associated with Z-E syndrome (see above).
- Gastric NETs sometimes arise spontaneously and are often aggressive.

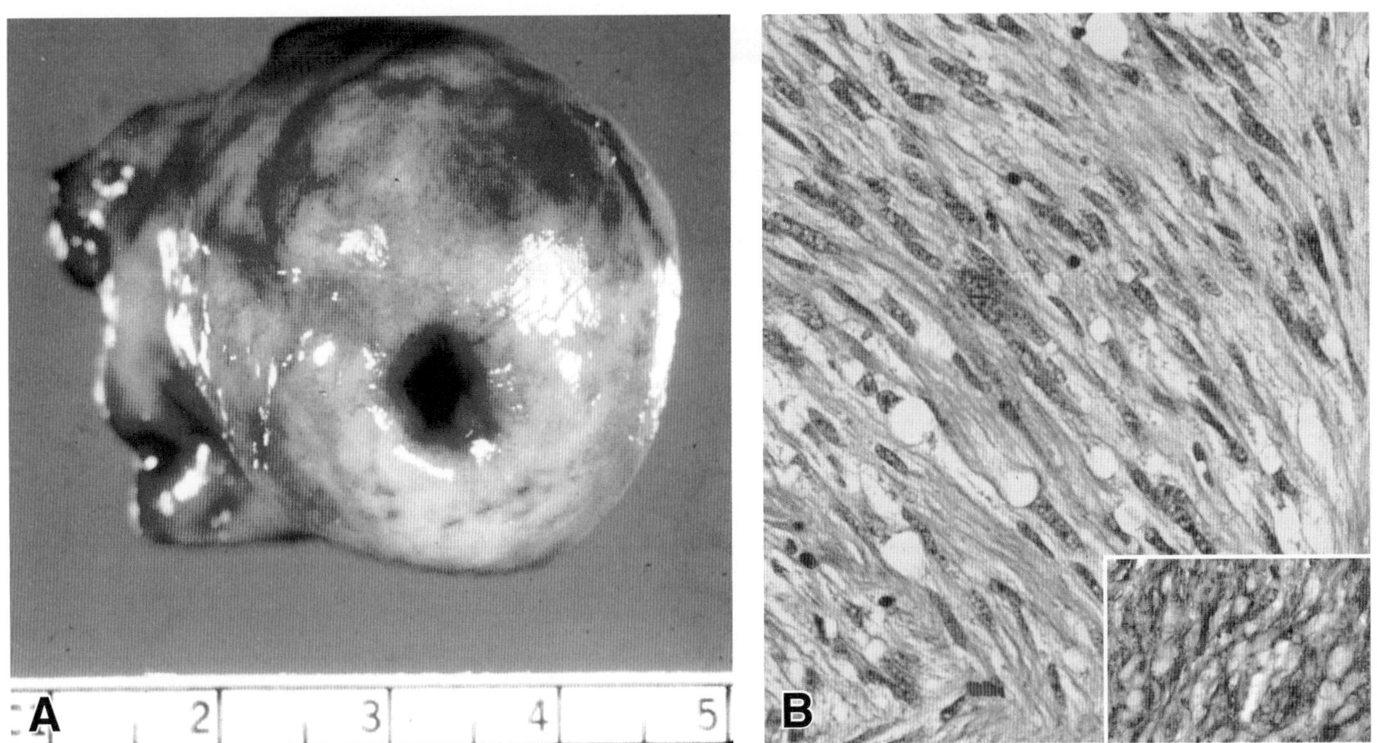

FIGURE 11-21. Gastrointestinal stromal tumor. A. The resected tumor is submucosal and covered by mucosa with a deep central ulcer. **B.** Microscopic appearance of tumor cells that are spindled and have cytoplasmic vacuoles. (*Inset*) Immunohistochemical stain positive for c-kit.

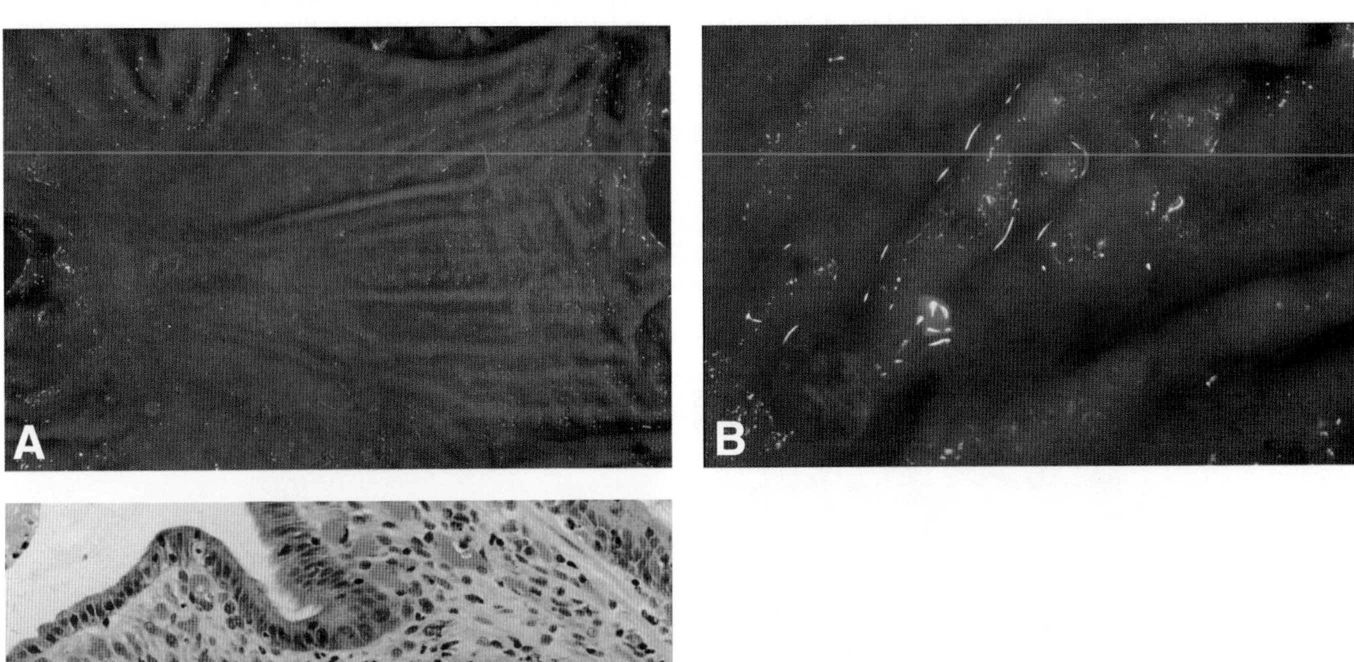

FIGURE 11-22. Neuroendocrine tumor (NET) of stomach. **A, B.** Multiple small elevated mucosal nodules dot the severely atrophic mucosa in this patient with autoimmune gastritis and pernicious anemia. **C.** Microscopically, the bland-appearing NET cells push aside the atrophic mucosa.

The Small Intestine

ANATOMY

The small intestine extends from the pylorus to the ileocecal valve and, depending on its muscle tone, is from 3.5 to 6.5 m long. It is divided into three regions as follows:

1. **The duodenum** extends to the ligament of Treitz.
2. **The jejunum** is the proximal 40% of the remainder of the small intestine.
3. **The ileum** is the distal 60%.

The duodenum is almost entirely retroperitoneal and thus fixed. The remainder of the small intestine, which is disposed in redundant loops, is movable. The C-shaped duodenum surrounds the head of the pancreas. It receives biliary drainage from the liver and pancreatic secretions through the common bile duct.

The small intestinal wall has four layers: mucosa, submucosa, muscularis, and serosa. In the retroperitoneal duodenum, however, only the anterior wall is covered by a serosa. The duodenal submucosa consists of vascularized connective tissue and scattered lymphocytes, plasma cells and macrophages, and occasional mast cells and eosinophils. In the proximal duodenum, the submucosa is occupied by Brunner glands, branched structures with mucous and serous cells. These secrete mucus and bicarbonate, which protect the duodenal mucosa from peptic ulceration. Mucosal lymphatics and venous capillaries drain into a highly developed system of lymphatic and venous plexuses in the submucosa.

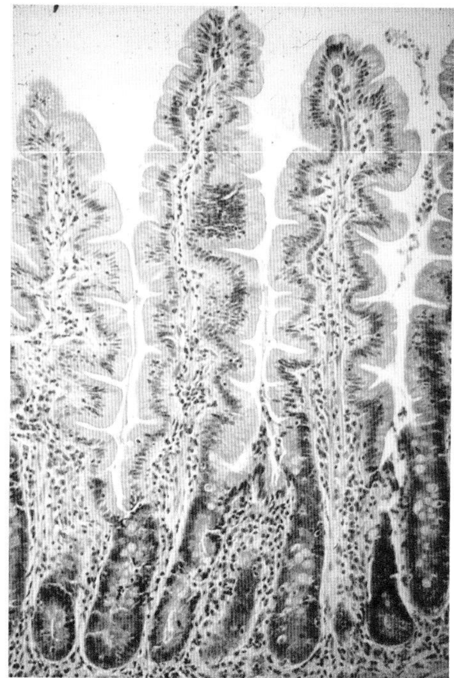

FIGURE 11-23. Intestinal villi from the proximal jejunum. The villi are several times longer than the crypts that gave rise to them. The lamina propria normally contains a mixture of lymphocytes and plasma cells with some scattered eosinophils.

The distinctive feature of intestinal mucosa is its unique villi (Fig. 11-23), 0.5- to 1-mm-long and finger-like. Villi in the proximal duodenum tend to be broad and blunted, but in the distal duodenum and proximal jejunum, they are more slender. Shorter, finger-shaped villi are the rule in the distal jejunum and ileum. The villous columnar epithelium sits on a basement membrane. A lamina propria and muscularis mucosae separate the mucosa from the submucosa. The connective tissue of the lamina propria forms the core of the villus and surrounds the crypts of Lieberkühn at the base of the villi. The normal lamina propria contains lymphocytes, plasma cells, and macrophages. Plasma cells here mainly secrete immunoglobulin A (IgA) into the intestinal lumen or the lamina propria itself. Scattered eosinophils and mast cells and a few smooth muscle cells and fibroblasts are present. This cellular composition reflects the roles of the lamina propria in preventing bacteria from penetrating the mucosa and segregating foreign material that breaches the mucosa. Lymphoid nodules are scattered throughout the mucosa and aggregate into visible Peyer patches (Fig. 11-24A and B). The villous columnar epithelial cells are mainly absorptive, whereas those lining the crypts are the source of cell renewal and secretion. There are normally a moderate number of intraepithelial T lymphocytes.

Absorptive cells, or enterocytes (Fig. 11-25), are the main lining cells of intestinal villi, which also contain a few goblet and endocrine cells. Enterocytes are tall, with basal nuclei and microvilli extending from their surfaces into the lumen, thereby hugely increasing the absorptive area.

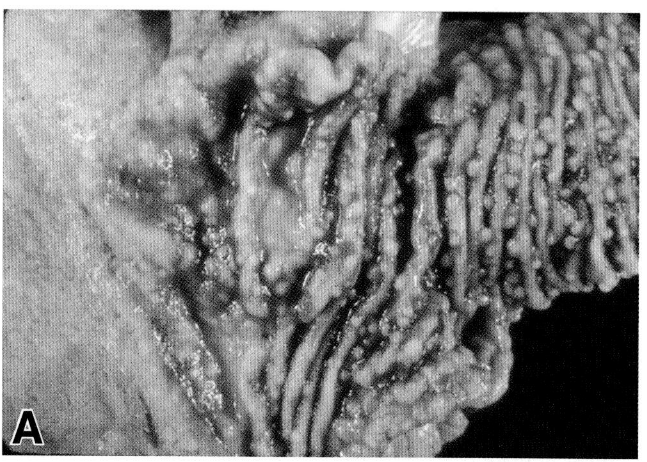

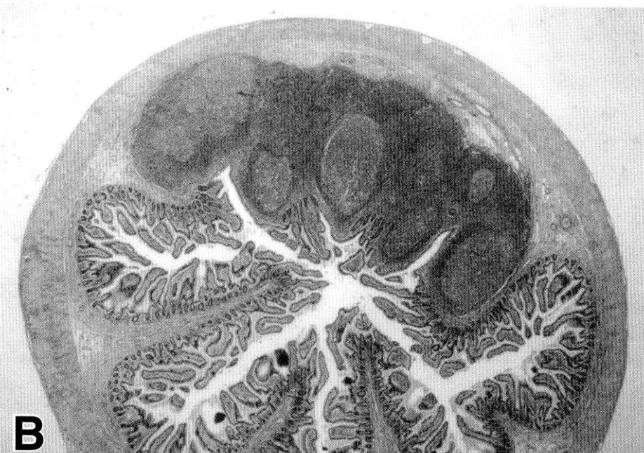

FIGURE 11-24. A. Peyer patches are particularly prominent in the terminal ileum; they are small dome-shaped mucosal mounds. **B.** The Peyer patch is composed of lymphoid tissue, often with prominent germinal centers, displacing the epithelial structures.

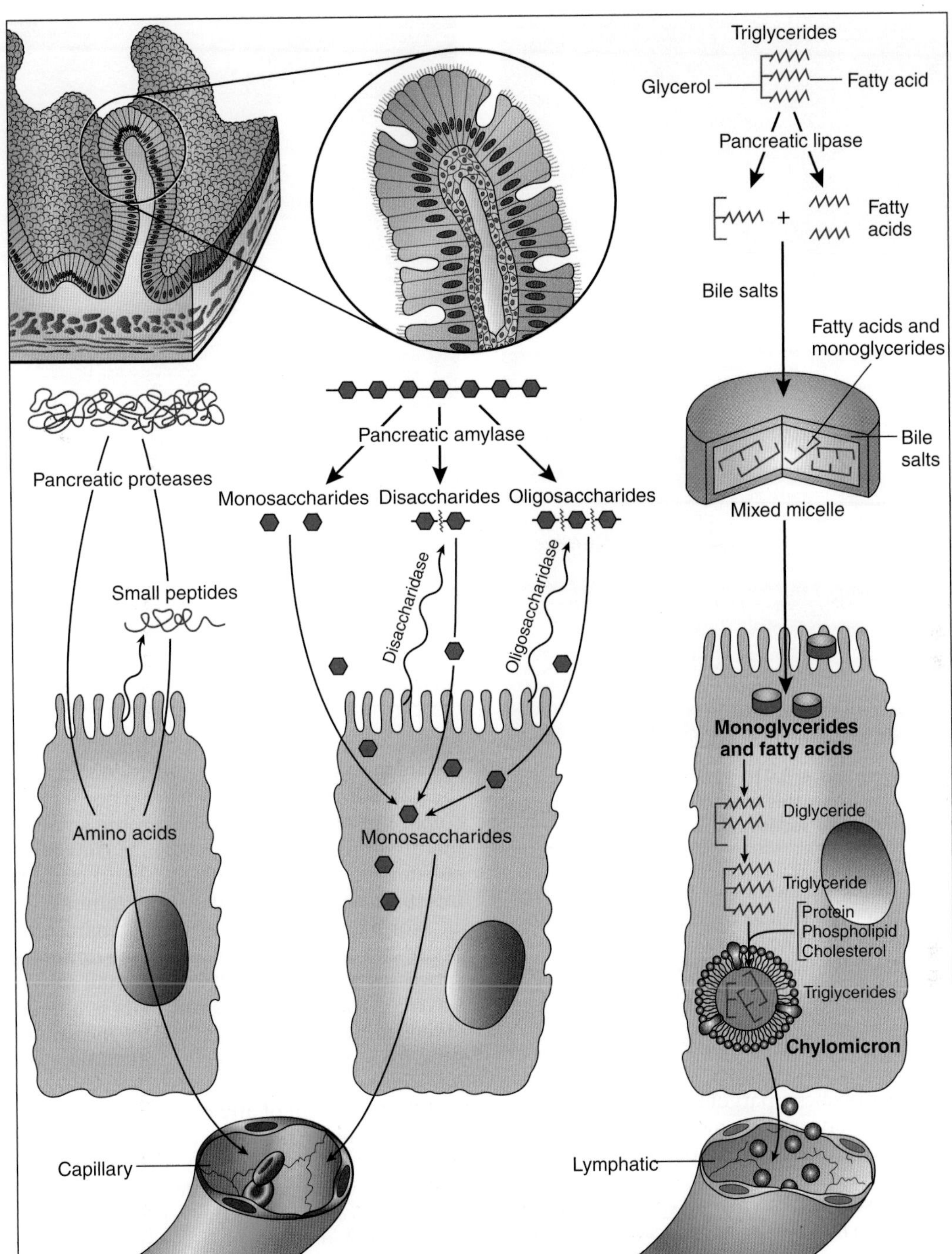

FIGURE 11-25. Mechanisms of nutrient absorption in the small intestine.

CONGENITAL AND NEONATAL DISORDERS

Meckel Diverticulum

This anomaly is the most commonly encountered clinically significant congenital disorder affecting the small intestine. It is solitary and is a true diverticulum, containing all layers of the intestinal wall. It is a remnant of the vitelline duct and so extends from the antimesenteric side of the distal ileum. Males are more affected than females. Most Meckel diverticula are asymptomatic, but bleeding, perforation, or obstruction as a result of intussusception may occur. The bleeding and perforation result from peptic ulceration, owing to the presence of heterotopic gastric tissue with parietal cells. Heterotopic pancreatic tissue may also be present. Rarely, neoplasms develop, usually neuroendocrine tumors.

Necrotizing Enterocolitis

NEC is unfortunately not uncommon and is more frequent and severe in premature and low–birth-weight infants. Signs of obstruction and perforation may occur. The ileocecal region is most commonly affected; in fatal cases, the area of involvement may be much more extensive. The onset of NEC usually follows the start of enteral feeding. Its pathogenesis is poorly understood, but it appears

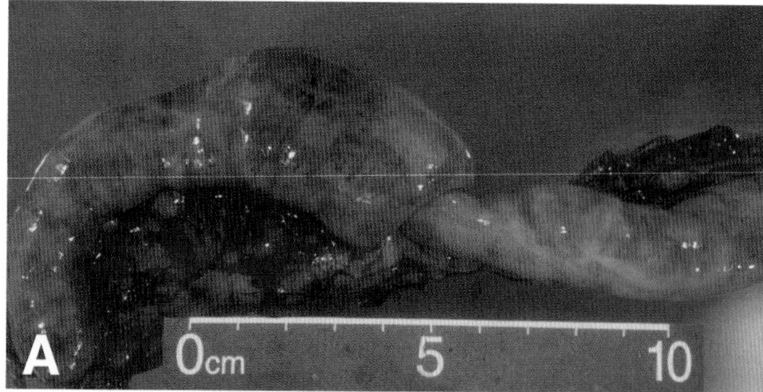

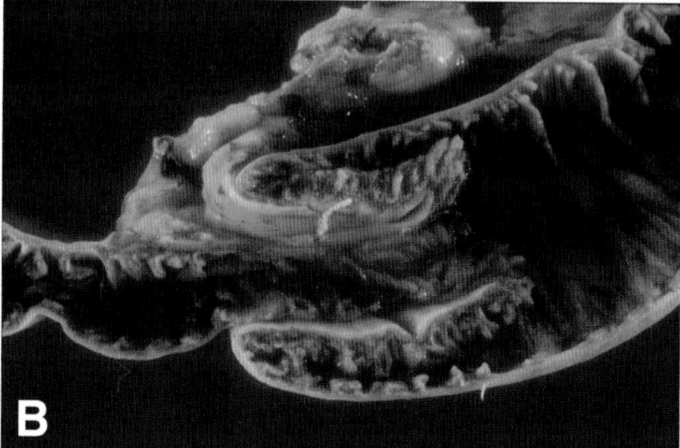

FIGURE 11-26. **Intussusception. A, B.** The proximal ileum has telescoped into the distal ileum in this case of **intussusception**; the anatomy is well seen in the cut section.

to be multifactorial, involving factors such as solute loading and bacterial proliferation, as well as diversion of blood flow away from abdominal organs. The bowel resembles that seen in ischemic damage. Pneumatosis cystoides intestinales (see below) is frequent. Healing may result in stenosis.

Intussusception

In this setting, peristalsis pushes a part of bowel distally, causing it to telescope into the adjacent segment (Fig. 11-26A and B). The mesentery and blood vessels accompany the bowel and can become compressed, resulting in edema, ischemic damage, and entrapment. Intussusception can reverse spontaneously or sometimes a barium enema may reduce it. Surgical removal may be necessary. In children, there is usually no causative anatomic defect, other than lymphoid hyperplasia. This may be physiologic for age, but in some, rotavirus or adenovirus may be implicated in causing the hyperplasia. In adults, there is often a neoplastic luminal process, with the mass serving as a point of traction.

Pneumatosis Cystoides Intestinales

The small intestine and colon are most commonly affected (Fig. 11-27). Pneumatosis almost always complicates another condition, such as NEC. In adults, it may be seen in pulmonary disease such as emphysema or complicating processes such as endoscopic polypectomy, ischemia, *Clostridium difficile* colitis, or AIDS. Entrapped gas may cause a mass effect that can be mistaken for a neoplastic process.

Gas may enter the bowel by several routes. In pulmonary disease, air from ruptured blebs may track through the retroperitoneum and follow the vascular adventitia into the bowel

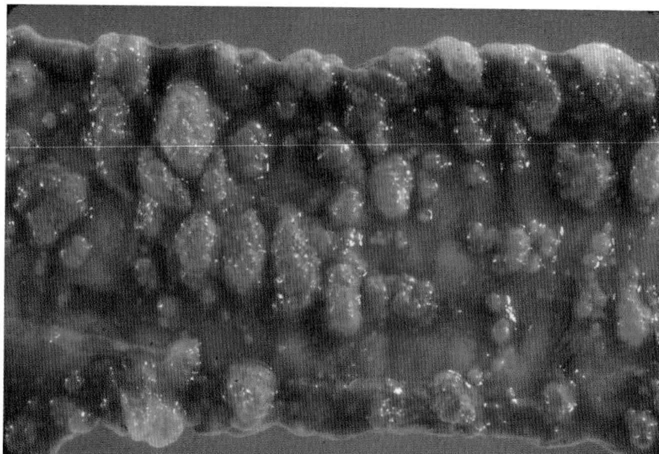

FIGURE 11-27. **Multiple gas-filled blebs protrude into the lumen in case of pneumatosis cystoides intestinales.**

wall. Increased intra-abdominal pressure may force gas through minute mucosal defects. Finally, some cases result from gas formed by luminal anaerobic organisms. The prognosis is related to the underlying condition.

MALABSORPTION

Malabsorption is a term that covers diverse clinical conditions in which important nutrients are inadequately absorbed by the gut. Some nutrient absorption occurs in the stomach and colon, but only absorption from the small intestinal lumen, mainly in the proximal portion, is clinically important. Two substances are preferentially absorbed by the distal small intestine, namely, bile salts and vitamin B_{12}.

Normal intestinal absorption is characterized by a luminal phase and an intestinal phase. In the luminal phase (i.e., those processes that occur within the small intestinal lumen), the physicochemical state of nutrients is altered so they can be taken up by absorptive cells. **The intestinal phase** includes processes occurring in cells and transport channels of the intestinal wall. Each phase has several critical components, and derangement of any one or more can impair absorption.

In the luminal phase, adequate amounts of pancreatic enzymes and bile acids are secreted into the duodenum in normal physicochemical conditions. Also, a regulated flow of gastric contents into the duodenum and a high duodenal pH are needed. Normal pancreatic enzyme excretion into the duodenum requires adequate pancreatic exocrine function and unobstructed flow of pancreatic juice.

Supplying bile in normal quantity and quality to the duodenum requires (1) adequate liver function, (2) unobstructed bile flow, and (3) intact enterohepatic bile salt circulation. Enterohepatic circulation of bile begins with absorption of most intestinal bile salts from the distal ileum and ends with their excretion into the duodenum through the bile ducts. Normally, 95% of intestinal bile salts are recycled via this circuit; 5% are excreted in the stool. Normal functioning of the enterohepatic circulation requires (1) normal intestinal microflora, (2) normal ileal absorptive function, and (3) an unobstructed biliary system.

Intestinal-Phase Malabsorption

Abnormalities in any of the four parts of the intestinal phase may cause malabsorption, although some diseases affect more than one of these components.

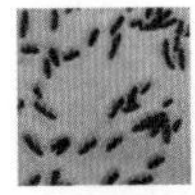

ETIOLOGIC FACTORS: ***Microvilli:*** Intestinal disaccharidases and oligopeptidases are integrally bound to microvillous membranes. Disaccharidases are essential for sugar absorption because only monosaccharides can be absorbed by intestinal epithelial cells. Oligopeptides and dipeptides may be absorbed by alternate routes that do not require peptidases. Abnormal microvillous function may be primary—as in primary disaccharidase deficiencies—or secondary, if there is damage to villi, as in celiac disease (see below). Enzyme deficiencies (e.g., of lactase) entail intolerance to the respective disaccharides.

Absorptive Area: The considerable length of the small bowel and the amplification of its surface by the intestinal folds (valves of Kerckring) provide a large absorptive surface. Severe diminution in this area may cause malabsorption. Surface area may be decreased by (1) small bowel resection (short-bowel syndrome), (2) gastrocolic fistula (bypassing the small intestine), or (3) mucosal damage due to various small intestinal diseases (celiac disease, tropical sprue, and Whipple disease).

Metabolic Function of Absorptive Cells: For their subsequent transport to the circulation, nutrients in absorptive cells are metabolized within these cells. Monoglycerides and free fatty acids are reassembled into triglycerides and coated with proteins (apoproteins) to make chylomicrons and lipoprotein particles. Specific metabolic dysfunction occurs in abetalipoproteinemia associated with erythrocyte acanthocytosis (see Chapter 18), in which absorptive cells cannot synthesize the apoprotein required for assembling lipoproteins and chylomicrons. Nonspecific damage to small intestinal epithelial cells occurs in celiac disease, tropical sprue, Whipple disease, and hyperacidity due to gastrinoma (Z-E syndrome).

Transport: Nutrients are moved from the intestinal epithelium through the intestinal wall via blood capillaries and lymphatic vessels. Impaired transport of nutrients through these conduits is probably important in malabsorption due to Whipple disease, intestinal lymphoma, and congenital lymphangiectasia.

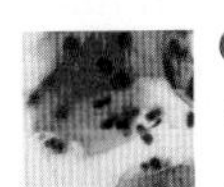

CLINICAL FEATURES: Malabsorption may be specific or generalized:

- **Specific or isolated malabsorption** refers to an identifiable molecular defect that brings on malabsorption of one nutrient. Examples are disaccharidase deficiencies (e.g., lactase deficiency) and vitamin B_{12} insufficiency (pernicious anemia) from lack of intrinsic factor. Anemias may be caused by deficiencies of iron, folic acid, vitamin B_{12}, or a combination of these. A bleeding diathesis may be caused by vitamin K deficiency; malabsorption of vitamin D and calcium may result in tetany, osteomalacia (in adults), or rickets (in children).
- **Generalized malabsorption,** which occurs when absorption of several or all major nutrient classes is impaired, gives rise to generalized malnutrition. In adults, this appears as weight loss and sometimes cachexia; in children, it is "failure to thrive" with poor growth and weight gain. **Steatorrhea** (fat in the stools) is a hallmark of generalized malabsorption.

Lactase Deficiency

The intestinal brush border contains disaccharidases that are important for absorption of carbohydrates. Lactose is present in milk and other dairy products and is one of the most common disaccharides in the diet. The availability of nonhuman milk historically favored lactase production, perhaps inducing cattle-herding societies (e.g., Europeans) to acquire lactose tolerance, whereas non–cattle herders (e.g., Native Americans and Asians) remained lactose intolerant.

Acquired lactase deficiency is widespread. Symptoms typically begin in adolescence, with abdominal distention, flatulence, and diarrhea after consuming dairy products. Removing milk and dairy products from the diet provides relief. Diseases that injure the intestinal mucosa (e.g., celiac disease) may also cause acquired lactase deficiency. Congenital lactase deficiency is rare but may be lethal if not recognized.

Celiac Disease (Gluten-Sensitive Enteropathy)

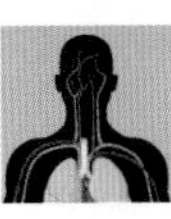

PATHOPHYSIOLOGY: Gluten is found in wheat, rye, and barley; the main culprit appears to be a peptide fraction of gluten, namely, **gliadin**. Other environmental factors may also be operative. Many patients have evidence of previous infection with adenovirus 12; a protein component of this virus shows homology with α-gliadin. GSE is an immunologic disorder that occurs in genetically susceptible individuals. The fact that a significant percentage of people with type 1 diabetes, another immunologic disorder (see Chapter 19), have GSE is further confirmation of autoimmunity. Separate genes involved in the major histocompatibility complex, namely, class I *HLA-B8*, class II *HLA-DR3*, and *DQW2*, are present in almost all patients (Fig. 11-28). Although many patients with these genes do not have GSE, it is thought that the absence of these genes virtually excludes the diagnosis.

Both cellular immunity and antibodies are involved in the pathogenesis of GSE. Activated mucosal T lymphocytes cause mucosal injury via release of cytokines; antigen–antibody complex deposition with complement activation may also lead to injury. A number of serologic tests are useful in diagnosing GSE, the most important of these being **tissue transglutaminase (tTG)**.

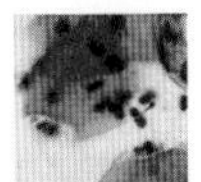

CLINICAL FEATURES: The classic symptoms of GSE are abdominal discomfort and diarrhea. With more advanced disease and consequent increased difficulty in absorbing fat, steatorrhea develops. Eventually, severe malnutrition can ensue with weight loss, muscle wasting, and hypoalbuminemia with edema. Osteoporosis and short stature compared with siblings are also reported.

The past several decades have seen a particularly wide swing of the pendulum. Early on GSE was very much underdiagnosed because the process was not considered unless the patient had several classic findings. With the current realization that GSE can manifest much more subtly than previously believed, many symptoms or conditions are attributed to GSE without unequivocal evidence. Care must be taken because the diagnosis requires strong clinical, serologic, or histologic evidence.

Treatment of GSE is exclusion of gluten from the diet and is usually quite effective. However, gluten is ubiquitous and adhering to the diet can be difficult. As well, diet change has been known to lead to a placebo effect, underscoring the need for concrete evidence before diagnosing GSE.

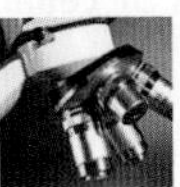

PATHOLOGY: The histologic hallmark of GSE is both increased inflammation and architectural derangement in the small intestinal villi. The previously accepted classic histology of the disease included total or near-total loss of villi, resulting in a flat mucosa, plus an increase in lamina propria inflammation, including lymphocytes, plasma cells, and some eosinophils.

In recent years, there has been an increased emphasis on the character of the inflammation, in particular, the increase in intraepithelial lymphocytes. T lymphocytes are normally

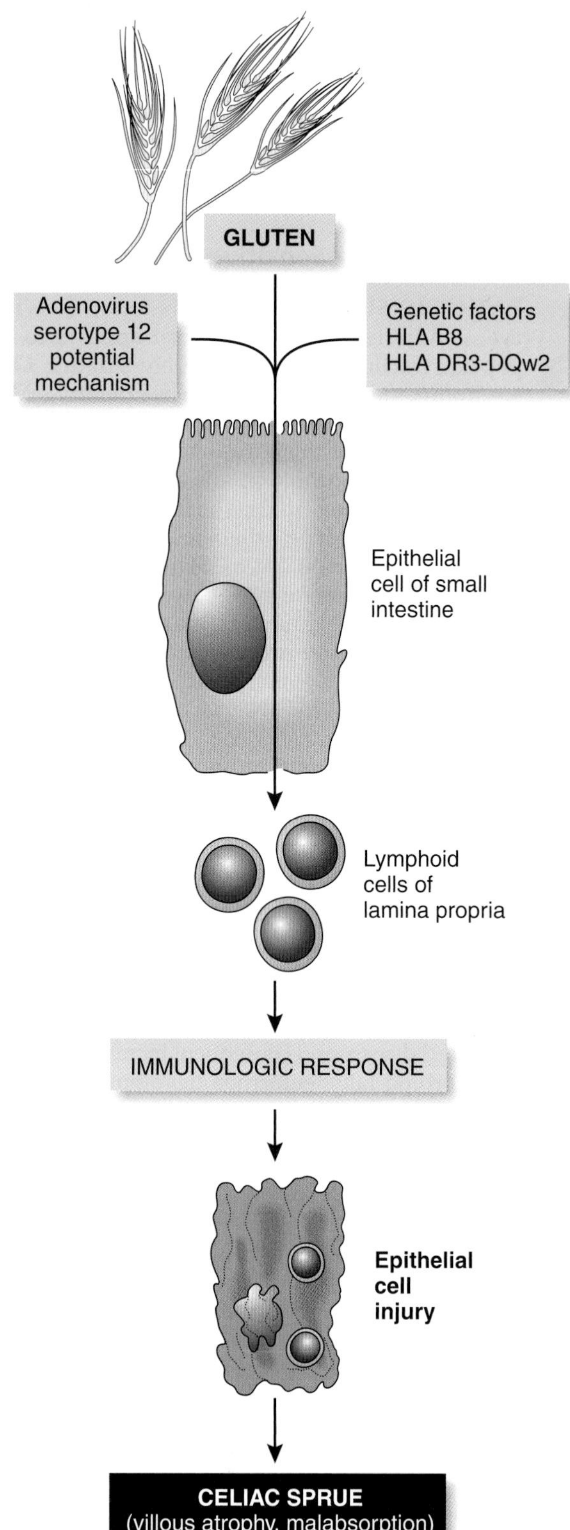

FIGURE 11-28. Proposed mechanism of the pathogenesis of celiac disease. HLA, human leukocyte antigen.

present in the surface epithelium (Fig. 11-29A and B), but in the GSE, these T cells may increase to the point where they outnumber the surface epithelial cells.

Surface epithelial cells are damaged and lose their brush border. This damage shortens their life span, so that mitotic activity in the crypts increases to compensate for the increased cell loss. As a result, hyperplasia of the crypts creates deeper crypts, even as villi decrease in height (Fig. 11-30). Eventually, a flat mucosa may result, but there are a series of gradations between total loss of villi and those of normal height. These changes are most prominent in the proximal small intestine where the most intense gluten exposure occurs; the distal ileum is only rarely involved. In severe cases, the surface area of the small intestine available for absorbing nutrients is greatly reduced.

There is evidence that patients with chronic GSE have an increased risk for primary intestinal T-cell lymphoma and small intestinal adenocarcinoma, but the magnitude of this risk is unclear.

Tropical Sprue

Affected locations are the Indian subcontinent, portions of Southeast Asia, Central America, and the Caribbean. Tropical sprue can develop both in residents and in visitors to the area. Evidence supports a complex bacterial etiology in that broad-spectrum antibiotics are effective in alleviating the condition. The exact nature of the causative agent(s) is uncertain.

The entire small intestine, including the ileum, is involved. The histologic appearance is very similar to that of GSE; however, intraepithelial lymphocytes are more prominent in the crypts than in the villus tips. A completely flat mucosa is less common than in GSE.

Severe folate and B_{12} deficiency may occur, the latter reflecting ileal involvement; this effect may lead to megaloblastic change.

Whipple Disease

Although this disease is uncommon, it is important to recognize this process, which also presents as malabsorption. The causative actinobacterium was identified only many years after the disease was first described. Villi are enlarged and bulbous, owing to massive numbers of bacteria within macrophages, which are unable to degrade the organisms. These macrophages take on a foamy appearance (Fig. 11-31A to D) when the PAS stain is employed. This time-honored method of establishing the diagnosis of the disease is being replaced by specific polymerase chain reaction (PCR) testing for the causative organism. Extraintestinal manifestations are common and affect the heart, joints, lymph nodes, and brain. Because of the CNS involvement, these patients may first present with neuropsychiatric symptoms. The disease responds dramatically to antibiotic therapy.

Giardiasis

The causative agent is *Giardia lamblia.* Symptoms of *G. lamblia* infection (giardiasis) may include severe watery diarrhea as well as abdominal discomfort with nausea and vomiting. Malabsorption can occur. Infection usually occurs after drinking from unprotected water sources. *Giardia* spores are extremely hardy, and person-to-person transmission can occur, particularly among children in day care centers. The trophozoites can be identified in duodenal fluid or stool, but they are often first identified in a duodenal biopsy. Although the organisms have a characteristic pear shape when seen in fluids, they tend to be oriented in profile as sickle or triangular shapes in biopsies (Fig. 11-32A and B). *Giardia* are usually very numerous, adheres to the epithelial surface, and do not invade. The underlying mucosa is often completely normal or may show mild nonspecific inflammatory changes, including a slight increase in lymphocytes.

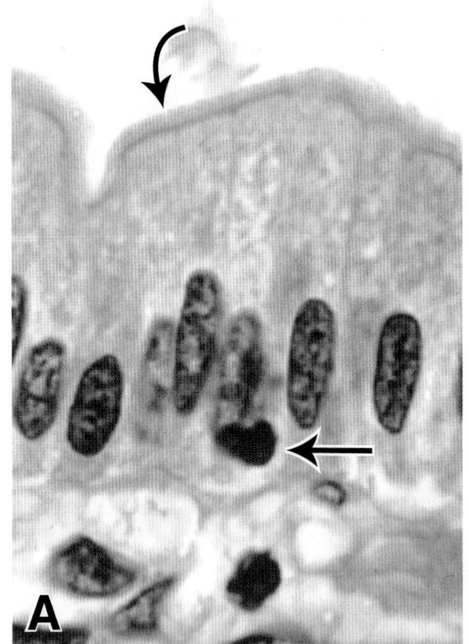

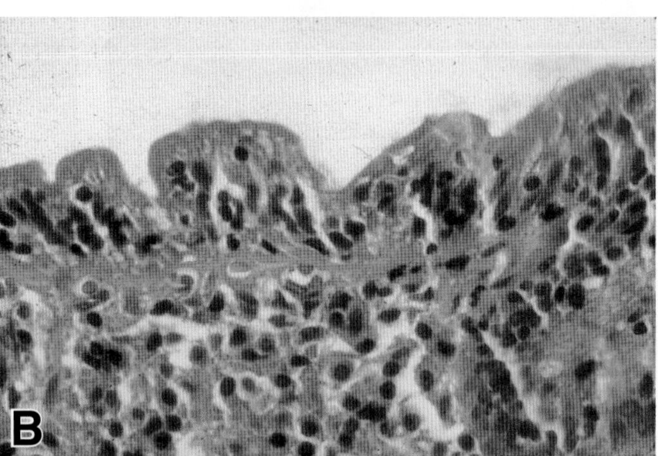

FIGURE 11-29. Small intestine in celiac disease. A. High-magnification view of small intestine surface epithelium; note the **brush border** (*curved arrow*) and intraepithelial lymphocyte (*arrow*). **B.** The surface epithelium in **celiac disease**: the epithelial height is reduced; the brush border is destroyed, and intraepithelial lymphocytes are numerous.

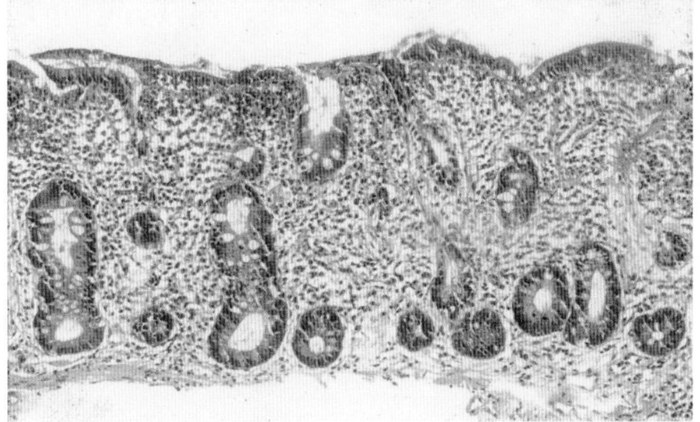

FIGURE 11-30. Classic advanced celiac disease: villi are no longer visible, crypts are taller than normal, and a lymphoplasmacytic infiltrate expands the lamina propria. Even at low power, damage to the surface epithelium is evident.

Small Bowel Bacterial Overgrowth

In this condition, there is an overgrowth of colonic-type anaerobic bacteria in the small bowel. Conditions interfering with overall gut motility, such as diabetes, scleroderma, and pseudo-obstruction, can lead to the syndrome. The term "blind loop syndrome" may be used if the stasis is because of an anatomic defect, such as small bowel diverticula or prior surgery. The mucosa may appear to be normal or show varying degrees of patchy nonspecific inflammation. It is thought that deconjugation of bile salts by the bacteria or their use of micronutrients is the major contributing pathogenic factor. This and the other multiple causes of malabsorption are depicted in Figure 11-33.

INTESTINAL ISCHEMIA

Impaired intestinal blood flow for any reason can cause ischemic bowel disease. The most common type of ischemic bowel disease is acute intestinal ischemia, most often related to occlusion of the superior mesenteric artery, which causes injury ranging from mucosal necrosis to transmural bowel infarction. A lesser number of cases result from vasculitis. Volvulus, intussusception, and incarceration of the intestine in a hernial sac may all lead to arterial as well as venous occlusion. Chronic intestinal ischemia syndromes are less common and generally require severe compromise of two or more major arteries, usually by atherosclerosis.

Intestinal ischemic necrosis may also occur in the absence of vascular occlusion and is more common than that caused by occlusive disease. It is seen in hypoxic patients with shock from a variety of causes, including hemorrhage, sepsis, and acute myocardial infarction. In shock, blood flow redistributes to favor the brain and other vital organs, and patients have often received α-adrenergic agents, which further shunt blood away from the intestine. Drastically lowered perfusion pressure produces arteriolar collapse, thereby aggravating the ischemia.

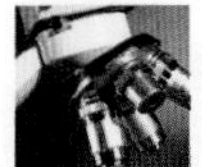

PATHOLOGY: Infarcted bowel is edematous and diffusely purple (Fig. 11-34). The demarcation between the infarcted bowel and normal tissue is usually sharp, although venous occlusion may lead to a more diffuse appearance. Hemorrhage is prominent in the mucosa and submucosa, especially in venous occlusion (e.g., mesenteric vein thrombosis). The mucosal surface shows irregular wide areas of sloughing, and the wall becomes thin and distended. Bubbles of gas (pneumatosis) may be present in the bowel wall and mesenteric veins. The serosal surface is cloudy and covered by an inflammatory exudate.

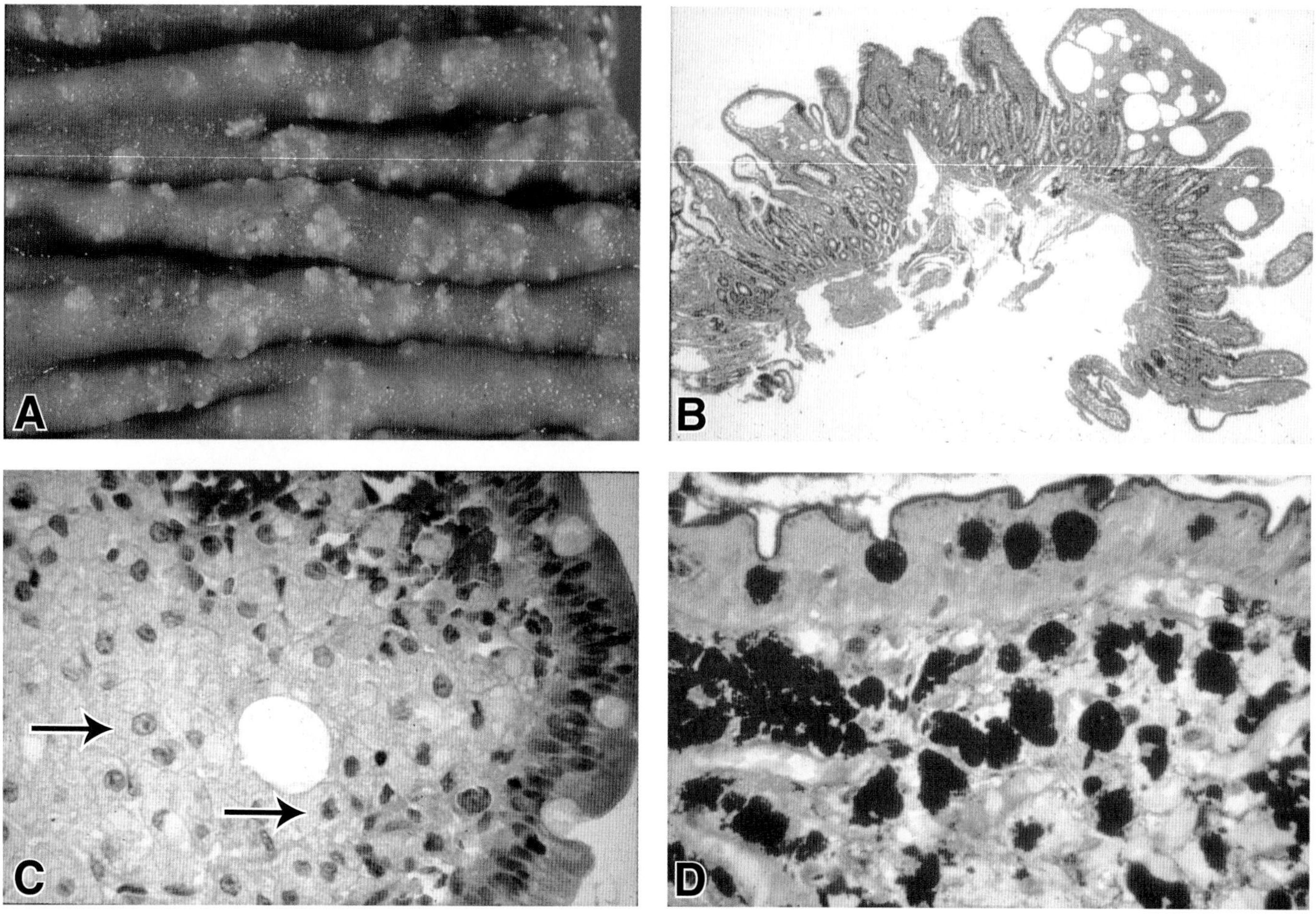

FIGURE 11-31. **Whipple disease. A.** The gross specimen showing white elevated areas; these are due to lipid collecting in the damaged mucosa. **B.** At low magnification, the villi are short and club shaped; the large cystic-appearing areas represent fat trapped owing to compression of mucosal lymphocytes. **C.** The lamina propria contains abundant foamy macrophages (*arrows*). **D.** The partially digested bacteria in these macrophages impart strong periodic acid–Schiff positivity.

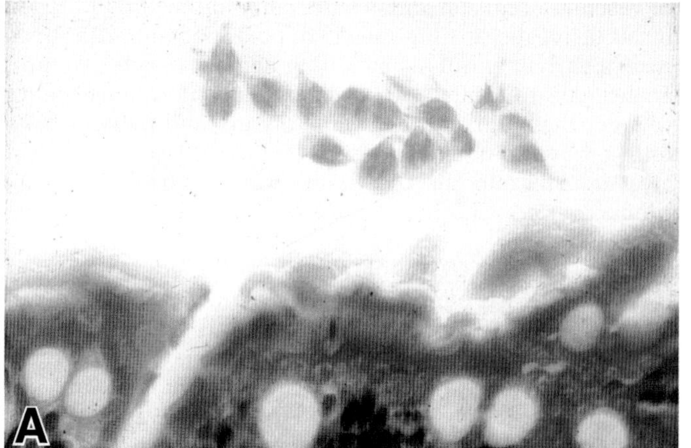

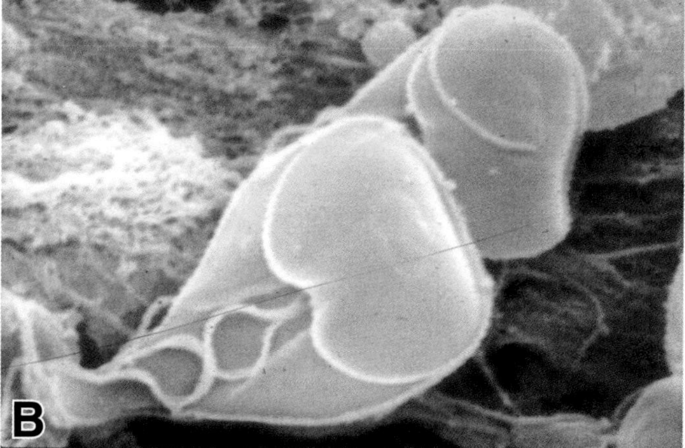

FIGURE 11-32. **Giardiasis. A.** A group of ***Giardia*** is seen just above the surface epithelium in this jejunal biopsy. **B.** A single trophozoite from this area is seen here by scanning electron microscopy.

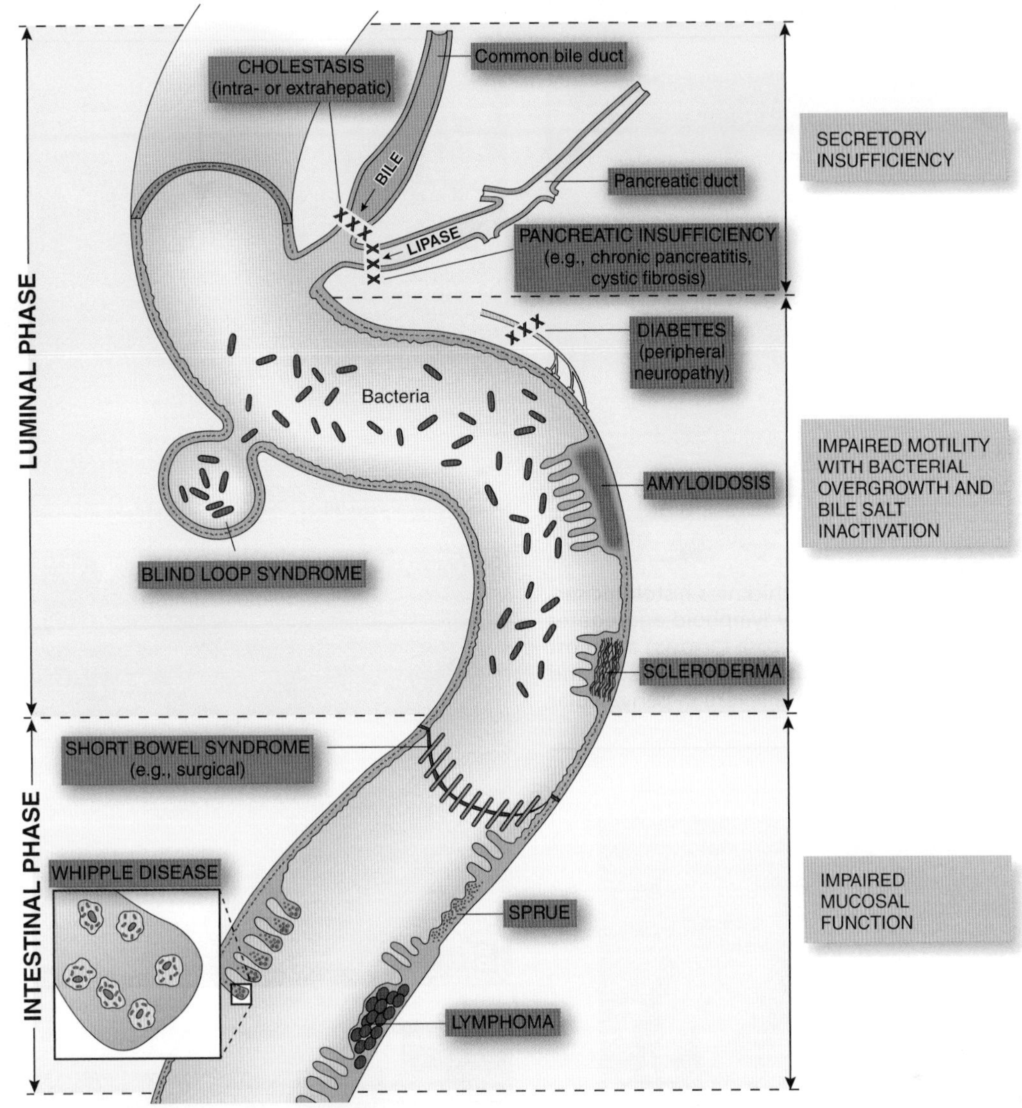

LUMINAL PHASE

CHOLESTASIS
(intra- or extrahepatic)

Common bile duct

BILE

SECRETORY
INSUFFICIENCY

Pancreatic duct

LIPASE

PANCREATIC INSUFFICIENCY
(e.g., chronic pancreatitis,
cystic fibrosis)

DIABETES
(peripheral
neuropathy)

Bacteria

IMPAIRED MOTILITY
WITH BACTERIAL
OVERGROWTH AND
BILE SALT
INACTIVATION

AMYLOIDOSIS

BLIND LOOP SYNDROME

SCLERODERMA

INTESTINAL PHASE

SHORT BOWEL SYNDROME
(e.g., surgical)

WHIPPLE DISEASE

IMPAIRED
MUCOSAL
FUNCTION

SPRUE

LYMPHOMA

FIGURE 11-33. The causes of malabsorption.

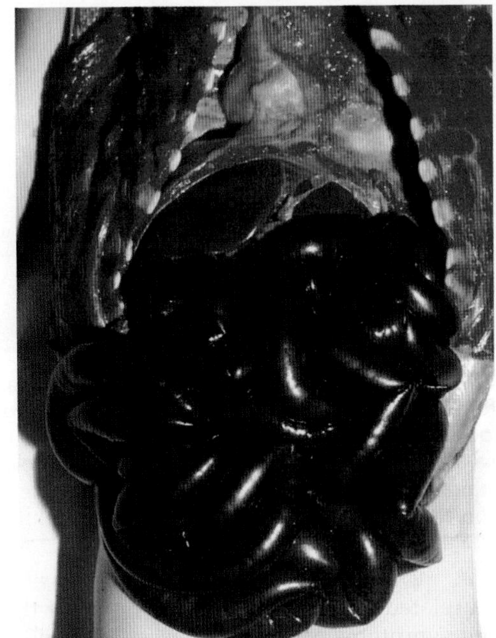

FIGURE 11-34. Infarcted small bowel at autopsy of an infant who died after volvulus had occluded the superior mesenteric artery. The entire small bowel is dilated, hemorrhagic, and necrotic.

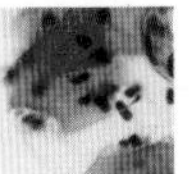

CLINICAL FEATURES: Symptoms of acute ischemia include abdominal pain, which begins abruptly, often with bloody diarrhea, hematemesis, and shock. In untreated cases, perforation is frequent. As infarction progresses, systemic symptoms become more severe.

Atherosclerotic narrowing of major splanchnic arteries leads to chronic intestinal ischemia. As in the heart, it causes intermittent abdominal pain, called intestinal (abdominal) angina. The pain usually starts within a half hour of eating and lasts for a few hours. Frank intestinal infarction may be heralded by abdominal angina. Recurrent abdominal pain may also reflect pressure on the celiac axis from the surrounding structures, called the **celiac compression syndrome**.

CROHN DISEASE

Crohn disease can involve any part of the gastrointestinal tract, but the small intestine, in particular the terminal ileum, is its main target. This disorder is transmural and patchy and is marked by chronic inflammation, lymphoid aggregates, and often granulomas (Fig. 11-35). Its etiology remains unknown, but information concerning genetic associations has been accumulating rapidly. Of note, the "fat wrapping" (Fig. 11-36A), which is a favorite sign of the disease for surgeons, is best seen

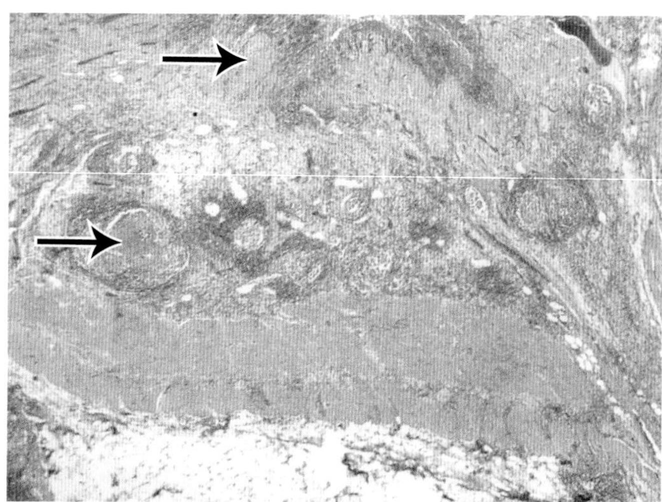

FIGURE 11-35. Crohn disease. This full-thickness histologic section showing transmural involvement by lymphoid aggregates and granulomas. The mucosa and submucosa (*arrows*) are most severely affected, but the infiltrate also involves muscle and mesentery. Note the tendency to be more severe in perivascular areas. See also Figure 11-48.

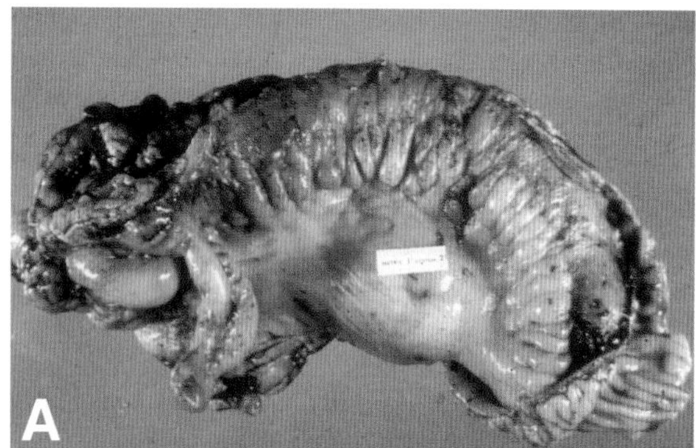

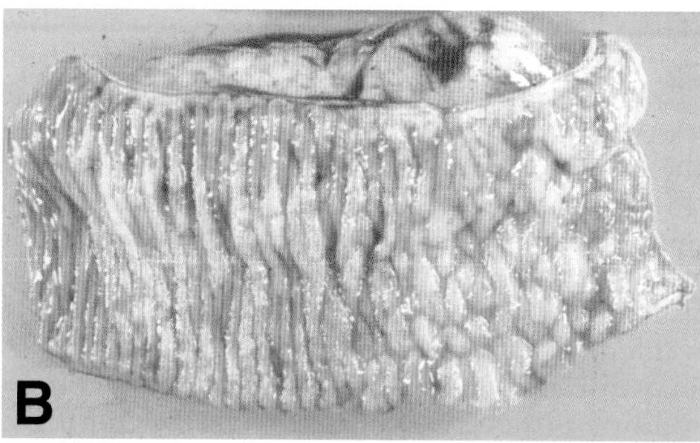

FIGURE 11-36. Small intestine in crohn disease A. Fat wrapping is a manifestation of transmural involvement but is not always evident. **B.** The cobblestoning is a result of the patchy nature of **Crohn** disease (see also Fig. 11-47 for a linear ulcer).

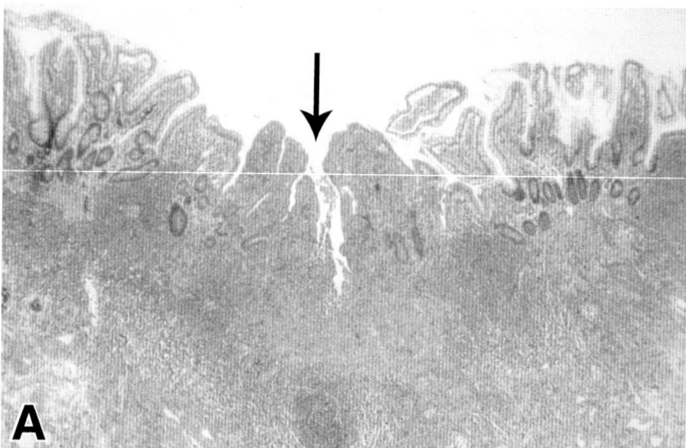

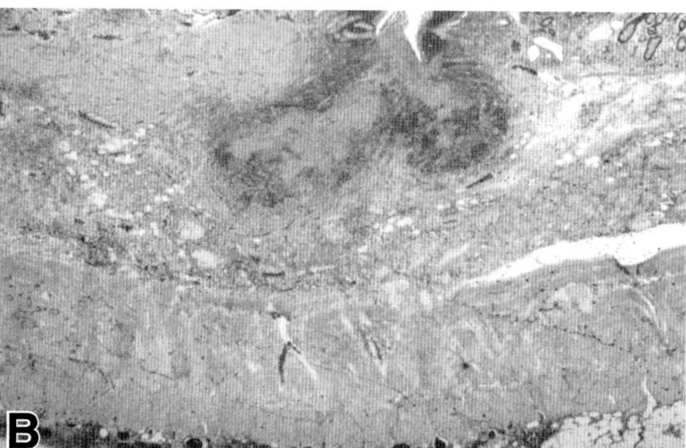

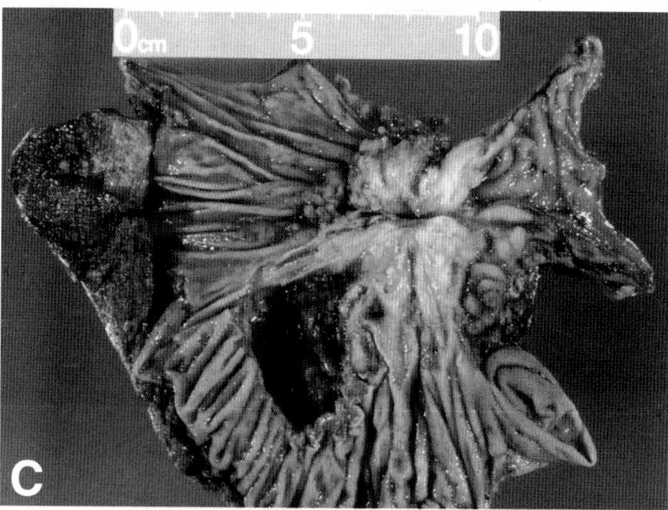

FIGURE 11-37. Intestinal fissuring in crohn disease A. A small **fissure ulcer**, knife-like (*arrow*), often starts over a lymphoid aggregate. **B.** The process continues, causing a fissure extending into the submucosa and beyond, ultimately penetrating the bowel wall. **C.** A **fistula** may result from such transmural involvement. Here, an ileocolonic fistula has resulted.

in the small intestine and is a result of transmural disease. Likewise, the phenomenon of "cobblestoning" (Fig. 11-36B) and the characteristic linear ulcers are also best observed within the small intestine. Transmural involvement with subsequent luminal narrowing often produces obstructive symptoms related to the small intestine, one of the major debilitating symptoms of Crohn disease. Likewise, intestinal fistulas (Fig. 11-37A to C) between loops of intestine are often a major clinical problem. See section on colon (below) for additional details.

INFECTIONS AND TOXINS

Infectious diarrhea is particularly lethal in underdeveloped countries and in infants. In countries with poor sanitation, the death toll from childhood diarrhea is staggering: 750,000 children under 5 years of age die annually of diarrhea, over 80% of them in Africa and Southeast Asia.

The small bowel normally contains few bacteria (usually $<10^4$/mL), mostly bacilli such as lactobacilli. These organisms travel in the food stream and ordinarily do not colonize the small intestine. Infectious diarrhea is caused by bacterial colonization (e.g., with toxigenic strains of *Escherichia coli* and *Vibrio cholerae*). The most significant problem in infectious diarrhea is increased intestinal secretion, stimulated by bacterial toxins and enteric hormones. Decreased absorption and increased peristaltic activity contribute less to the diarrhea.

The colon harbors abundant bacteria, at concentrations seven orders of magnitude greater than in the small intestine. Anaerobic bacteria in the colon (e.g., *Bacteroides* and *Clostridium* species) outnumber aerobic organisms 1000-fold. With the more rapid transit of intestinal contents during diarrhea, the flora is shifted to more aerobic populations, including *E. coli*, *Klebsiella*, and *Proteus*. Moreover, offending organisms themselves become conspicuous, and pathogens of the small intestine such as *V. cholerae* may be the major isolate in the stool.

Agents of infectious diarrhea are classified into **toxigenic** (i.e., producing diarrhea by elaborating toxins) or as adherent or invasive bacteria (Table 11-1 lists reaction patterns).

Table 11-1

Histologic Patterns of Bacterial Infections of the Gastrointestinal Tract

Minimal inflammatory changes	*Vibrio cholerae* Toxigenic *Escherichia coli* *Neisseria* sp.
Acute self-limited colitis	*Shigella* *Campylobacter jejuni* *Aeromonas* *Salmonella* *Clostridium difficile*
Pseudomembranous pattern	*C. difficile* *Shigella* Enterohemorrhagic *E. coli*
Granulomas	*Yersinia* sp. *Mycobacterium bovis* *Mycobacterium avium-intracellulare* *Actinomycosis*
Histiocytic	Whipple disease (*Tropheryma whippelii*) *M. avium-intracellulare*
Lymphohistiocytic	*Lymphogranuloma venereum*
Architectural distortion	*Salmonella typhimurium* *Shigella*

Toxigenic Diarrhea

The prototypical organisms that cause diarrhea by secreting toxins are *V. cholerae* and toxigenic strains of *E. coli*.

The characteristics of toxigenic diarrhea are as follows:

- Damage to the intestinal mucosal is minimal or absent.
- The organism remains on the mucosal surface, where it secretes its toxin.
- Fluid secreted into the small intestine causes watery diarrhea, which can lead to dehydration, particularly in the case of cholera.

Toxigenic *E. coli*

Toxigenic E. coli gives rise to diarrhea in underdeveloped tropical areas and, probably, causes most "traveler's diarrhea" among visitors to such regions. The infection is acquired from contaminated water and food. Many people in Latin America, Africa, and Asia are asymptomatic carriers of the infection. Nonimmune people (local children or travelers from abroad) develop diarrhea when they encounter the organism. Toxigenic strains produce diarrhea by adhering to the intestinal mucosa and elaborating one or more of at least three enterotoxins that cause secretory dysfunction of the small bowel. One of the enterotoxins elaborated by *E. coli* is structurally and functionally similar to cholera toxin, and another acts on guanylyl cyclase. Toxigenic *E. coli* produces no distinctive macroscopic or light-microscopic alterations in the intestine but results in an acute, self-limited diarrheal illness, with watery stools lacking neutrophils and erythrocytes. In severe cases, fluid and electrolyte loss can lead to extreme dehydration and even death.

Cholera

Cholera is a severe diarrheal illness caused by the enterotoxin of *V. cholerae*, an aerobic, curved, Gram-negative rod. The organism proliferates in the lumen of the small intestine and causes profuse watery diarrhea, rapid dehydration, and (if fluids are not restored) shock and death within 24 hours of the onset of symptoms.

Cholera is a worldwide public health problem, affecting an estimated 3 to 5 million people per year. It is acquired by ingesting *V. cholerae*, mainly in contaminated food or water. Epidemics spread readily in areas where human feces pollute the water supply. Shellfish and plankton may serve as a natural reservoir for the organism, and shellfish ingestion accounts for most of the sporadic cases in the United States.

Bacteria cause diarrhea by elaborating a potent exotoxin, **cholera toxin**, which is composed of A and B subunits. The latter binds to GM_1 ganglioside in the enterocyte cell membrane. The A subunit then enters the cell, where it activates adenylyl cyclase. The consequent rise in cell cAMP causes massive secretion of sodium and water by the enterocyte into the intestinal lumen (Fig. 11-38). Most fluid secretion occurs in the small bowel, where there is a net loss of water and electrolytes. *V. cholerae* causes little visible alteration in the affected intestine, which appears grossly normal or only slightly hyperemic.

Untreated cholera has a 50% mortality rate. Replacing lost salts and water is a simple, effective treatment, often achievable by oral rehydration with preparations of salt, glucose, and water. The illness subsides spontaneously in 3 to 6 days,

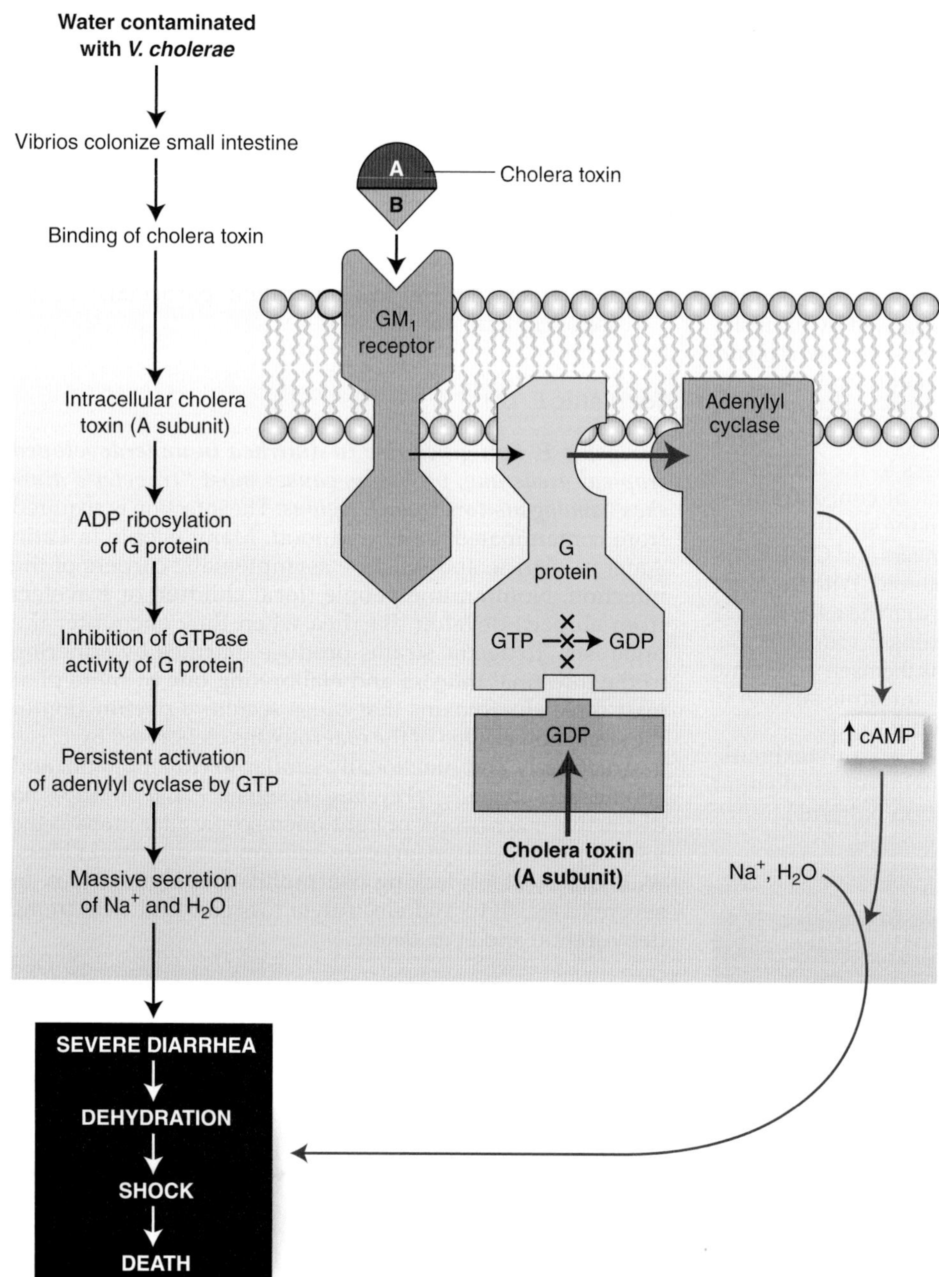

FIGURE 11-38. Cholera. Infection comes from water contaminated with *Vibrio cholerae* or food prepared with contaminated water. *Vibrios* traverses the stomach, enter the small intestine, and propagate. Although they do not invade the intestinal mucosa, *Vibrio* elaborates a potent toxin that induces a massive outpouring of water and electrolytes. Severe diarrhea ("rice water stool") leads to dehydration and hypovolemic shock. ADP, adenosine diphosphate; cAMP, cyclic adenosine monophosphate; GDP, guanosine diphosphate; GTP, guanosine triphosphate; Na^+, sodium ion.

a period that can be shortened by antibiotic therapy. Infection with *V. cholerae* confers long-term protection from recurrent illness, but available vaccines have limited effectiveness.

Enteroinvasive Bacteria

Among these invasive organisms, *Shigella*, *Salmonella*, and certain strains of *E. coli*, *Yersinia*, and *Campylobacter* are the most widely recognized. Invasive organisms tend to infect the distal ileum and colon, whereas toxigenic bacteria mainly involve the upper intestinal tract. The mechanisms by which invasive bacteria produce diarrhea are uncertain. Enterotoxins have been identified, but their role in causing diarrhea is not established. Mucosal invasion by bacteria increases synthesis of prostaglandins in affected tissues, and inhibitors of prostaglandin synthesis seem to block fluid secretion. Possibly, the damaged mucosa cannot absorb fluid from the lumen.

Shigella

Shigellosis is caused by any of the four species of the genus *Shigella.* The infection mainly affects the colon, although the terminal ileum is occasionally involved. A granular and hemorrhagic mucosa displays many shallow serpiginous ulcers. Inflammation is especially severe in the sigmoid colon and rectum, but is usually superficial. In the early stage, neutrophils accumulate in damaged crypts (crypt abscesses), similarly to those seen in ulcerative colitis (see below); the lymphoid follicles of the mucosa break down to form ulcers. Unlike ulcerative colitis, signs of chronicity are not present. As infection recedes, ulcers heal, and the mucosa returns to normal.

Typhoid Fever

Typhoid fever (*Salmonella typhi* enteritis) is uncommon in the industrialized world but is still a problem in underdeveloped countries. Necrosis of lymphoid tissue, mainly in the terminal ileum, leads to scattered ulcers. Infection of Peyer patches results in oval ulcers, in which the longer dimension is in the longitudinal axis of the intestine. Occasionally, lymphoid follicles in the large bowel or the appendix are ulcerated. The base of the ulcer contains black necrotic tissue mixed with fibrin.

Early lesions of typhoid fever show large basophilic macrophages filled with typhoid bacilli, erythrocytes, and necrotic debris. Necrosis of lymphoid follicles becomes confluent, and mucosal ulceration follows. Similar lymphoid hyperplasia and necrosis are seen in regional lymph nodes. Within a week of the acute symptoms, ulcers heal completely, leaving little fibrosis or other sequelae. Intestinal hemorrhage and perforation, principally in the ileum, are the most feared complications of typhoid fever and tend to occur in the third week and during convalescence.

Nontyphoidal Salmonellosis

Formerly known as **paratyphoid fever**, enteritis caused by *Salmonella* strains other than *S. typhi* is generally far less serious than typhoid fever. The principal target is the ileum, but minor involvement of the colon may also occur. Organisms invade the mucosa, which shows mild ulceration, edema, and infiltration with neutrophils. Hematogenous dissemination from the intestine may carry infection to the bones, joints, and meninges. People with sickle cell disease tend to develop *Salmonella* osteomyelitis, possibly because phagocytosis of products of hemolysis prevents further cellular ingestion of the organisms and allows their dissemination through the bloodstream.

Escherichia coli

Enteroinvasive, enteroadherent, and enterohemorrhagic strains of *E. coli* may uncommonly cause bloody diarrhea similar to shigellosis and are a prominent cause of traveler's diarrhea. Certain strains of *E. coli*, particularly serotype 0157:H7, produce *Shigella*-like toxins, but the role of these proteins in the pathogenesis of the enterocolitis is not understood. Serotype 0157:H7 has also been implicated in the hemolytic-uremic syndrome in children.

Yersinia

Yersinia enterocolitica and *Yersinia pseudotuberculosis* are transmitted by pets or contaminated food, and infection is most common in young children. *Yersinia* infection causes diarrhea, cramps, and fever and lasts 1 to 3 weeks. Peyer patches are hyperplastic, with acute ulceration of overlying mucosa. A fibrinopurulent exudate covering the ulcers often contains many organisms.

In addition to causing enterocolitis, *Yersinia* produces acute mesenteric adenitis and right lower quadrant pain. It may so resemble appendicitis that infected children have mistakenly been taken to laparotomy for *Yersinia* infection. Lymph nodes show epithelioid granulomas with central necrosis in the case of *Y. pseudotuberculosis*. The ileum and appendix may contain similar granulomas, imparting an appearance that resembles that of Crohn disease.

Adults, who are less susceptible to *Yersinia* infection than are children, suffer acute diarrhea, often followed within a few weeks by erythema nodosum, erythema multiforme, or polyarthritis. Patients with chronic debilitating diseases may develop *Yersinia* bacteremia, which is most resistant to antibiotic treatment. Interestingly, people with thalassemia are particularly susceptible to *Y. enterocolitica* infection. Identification by culture can be difficult, but PCR analysis is effective.

Campylobacter jejuni

Campylobacter jejuni is one of the most common causes of bacterial diarrhea, with a higher incidence than that of nontyphoidal *Salmonella* and *Shigella* in some U.S. studies. In a report from Great Britain, *Campylobacter* caused half of cases of bacterial diarrhea. Humans contract the disease mainly by contact with infected domestic animals or by eating poorly cooked or contaminated food. The histologic appearance is similar to that of *Shigella* infection. Adults usually recover in less than a week.

Food Poisoning

STAPHYLOCOCCUS AUREUS: S. aureus is a common cause of food poisoning. Symptoms result from eating food contaminated with *Staphylococcus* strains that make an exotoxin that damages gastrointestinal epithelium. Severe vomiting and abdominal cramps occur within 6 hours of ingesting the toxin and are often followed by diarrhea. Most patients recover in 1 to 2 days.

CLOSTRIDIUM PERFRINGENS: This bacterium produces an enterotoxin that causes vomiting and diarrhea. The organism is anaerobic but tolerates exposure to air for up to 3 days. Enterotoxin activity is maximal in the ileum. In most cases, watery diarrhea and severe abdominal pain begin 8 to 24 hours after ingestion of contaminated food and last about 1 day.

Rotavirus and Norwalk Virus

ROTAVIRUS: Rotavirus infection is a common cause of infantile diarrhea, accounting for about half of cases of acute diarrhea in hospitalized children younger than 2 years. Rotavirus has been demonstrated in duodenal biopsy specimens. It is associated with injury to the surface epithelium and impaired intestinal absorption for periods of up to 2 months.

NORWALK VIRUSES: These highly infectious agents account for one third of the epidemics of viral gastroenteritis in the United States. There have been a number of notorious outbreaks on cruise ships. The virus targets the upper small intestine, causing patchy mucosal lesions and malabsorption. Vomiting and diarrhea are usual, but symptoms resolve within 2 days.

Other viruses implicated as etiologic agents of infective diarrhea include echovirus, coxsackievirus, cytomegalovirus, adenovirus, and coronavirus.

NEOPLASMS

Despite the length and large surface area of the small intestine, primary neoplasms of the small intestine are less common than are those in the esophagus, stomach, or colon.

Benign Neoplasms

Small Bowel Adenomas

Small bowel adenomas resemble those of the colon, they are, however, far less common. Unlike the colonic lesions, these adenomas are not frequent precursors of adenocarcinoma. They occur sporadically and are also seen commonly in FAP.

Peutz–Jeghers Polyps

Polyps in this syndrome may occur anywhere in the GI tract but are most common in the small intestine. They have a characteristic gross and microscopic (Fig. 11-39A and B) appearance. Bland-appearing small intestinal epithelium, often with an unusual architectural arrangement, is intermixed with large arborizing branches of smooth muscle. This autosomal dominant disorder is characterized by buccal pigmentation and macular lesions on the lips, hands, feet, and genitals. Most patients have mutations in the *LKB1* tumor suppressor gene on chromosome 19p13.3. There is an increased risk for cancer, largely outside the gastrointestinal tract, involving the testis, ovary, uterus, or pancreas.

Malignant Tumors

Adenocarcinoma

Adenocarcinomas resemble their colonic counterparts but are much less frequent. They occur most often proximally, particularly in the duodenum. They can be polypoid, ulcerated, or manifest a constricted napkin ring appearance. There is a much greater (80-fold) risk of small bowel adenocarcinoma in patients with Crohn disease or celiac disease. In the former, the tumors arise distally in inflamed intestine. These tumors are also increased in FAP and Peutz–Jeghers syndrome.

Metastases

Secondary carcinomas of the small intestine are about as common as are primary adenocarcinomas. Metastases from melanomas and tumors of the lung, breast, colon, and kidney are the most frequent.

Gastrointestinal Stromal Tumors

The small intestine is second to the stomach in the incidence of these tumors. However, those arising in the small intestine are more likely to behave aggressively. They frequently have a deep central ulceration, which can cause severe bleeding. These GISTs tend more to be composed of spindled cells than do gastric GISTs, which often have areas with an epithelioid appearance.

Neuroendocrine Tumors (Carcinoid Tumors)

As noted above, the term **neuroendocrine tumors (NETs)** has largely replaced "carcinoid" in designating these tumors All NETs are considered malignant, but they vary greatly in their metastatic potential. The gastrointestinal tract is the most common site for NETs (the bronchus being the next most common site). In addition to the site of origin, the size, depth of invasion, hormonal responsiveness, and the presence or absence of function are major indicators of likely aggressiveness. The appendix is the most common GI site of origin, followed by the rectum; tumors in these locations are usually innocuous. NETs of the ileum are mostly small but are often aggressive.

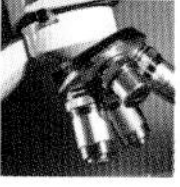

PATHOLOGY: Small NETs usually present as submucosal nodules covered by intact mucosa. Larger tumors may grow in polypoid, intramural, or annular patterns and often undergo secondary ulceration. Cut surfaces are firm and white to yellow. As they enlarge, NETs invade the muscular coat and penetrate the serosa, often causing conspicuous desmoplasia, which can lead to peritoneal adhesions, kinking of the bowel, and possible intestinal ob-

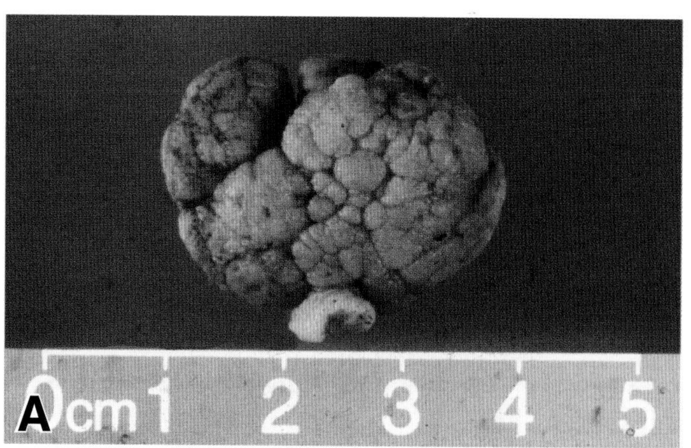

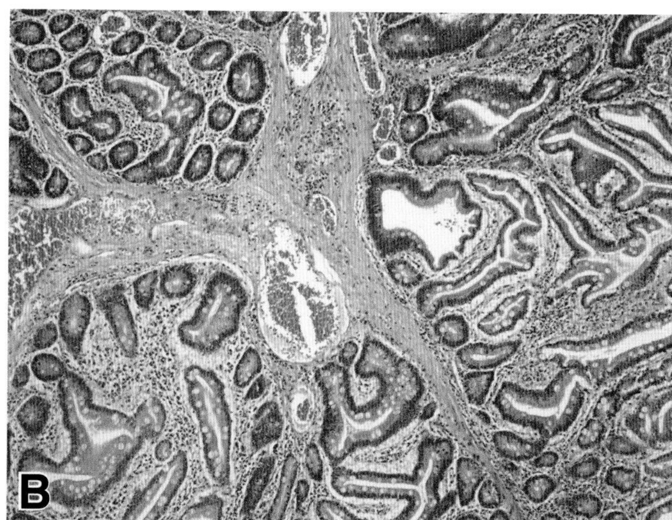

FIGURE 11-39. Peutz-Jeghars Polyps. A. This polyp has a characteristic striking bosselated appearance. **B.** The histology is characterized by arborizing bundles of smooth muscle. The epithelium and glands between closely resemble the bland appearance of their normal counterparts but form an unusual architectural configuration.

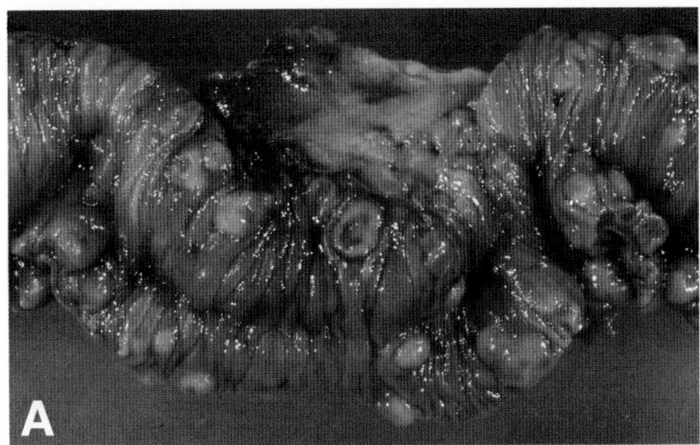

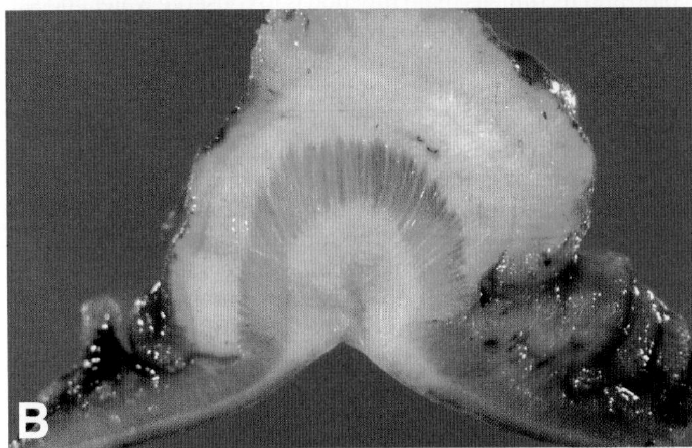

FIGURE 11-40. Ileal NETS. **A. Ileal neuroendocrine tumors** are frequently multiple, producing several mucosal-covered pale yellow tumors. **B.** The frequent characteristic "knuckling" of the intestinal wall is because of the brisk fibrous response to the invading tumor.

struction. Ileal NETs are multiple in about 40% of cases (Fig. 11-40A and B).

Small, round cells in NETs form nests, cords, and rosettes. Occasional gland-like structures are also seen (hence the term "carcinoid"). Nuclei are remarkably regular, and mitoses are rare. By electron microscopy, the abundant eosinophilic cytoplasm contains neurosecretory-type granules. Despite their bland appearance, jejunal and ileal tumors behave more aggressively than do similar-appearing NETs originating at other sites.

When these tumors metastasize to regional lymph nodes, they may produce a bulky mass far larger than the primary tumor. Subsequent hematogenous spread is reflected in metastases at distant sites, particularly the liver. Patients occasionally present with a huge amount of metastatic NETs in the liver, all due to a small, clinically silent primary tumor in the ileum.

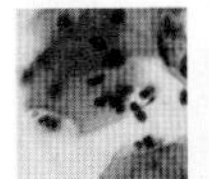

CLINICAL FEATURES: Carcinoid syndrome occurs in a small percentage of patients with NETs. It is a unique but uncommon clinical condition caused by the release of active tumor products, notably serotonin. *Classic symptoms include diarrhea (often the most distressing symptom), episodic flushing, bronchospasm, cyanosis, telangiectasia, and skin lesions.* The metabolic product of serotonin, namely, 5-hydroxyindoleacetic acid (5-HIAA), is the basis for a urine test for carcinoid. In half of the patients, high levels of serotonin in the heart result in the formation of fibrous plaques on tricuspid and pulmonic valves, the endocardium of the right-sided cardiac chambers, the vena cava, the coronary sinus, and the pulmonary artery. Valvular distortion leads to pulmonic stenosis and tricuspid regurgitation.

Lymphoma

Several types of lymphoma occur in the small intestine (see Chapter 18): Burkitt lymphoma, large B-cell lymphoma ("Western" lymphoma), and enteropathy-associated intestinal T-cell lymphoma (EATL).

Burkitt lymphoma develops mainly in the terminal ileum of children, with males predominating. The tumors form bulky masses. In many cases, Epstein–Barr virus can be detected. The disorder can be seen in young adults who suffer immunodeficiency and some are HIV positive. **Diffuse large B-cell lymphoma** often presents as a large luminal mass in an older adult and tends to be quite aggressive. **EATL** complicates celiac disease. Severe malnutrition despite adherence to a gluten-free diet, often heralds its onset. EATL has the worst prognosis of the intestinal lymphomas.

The Appendix

The appendix is a true diverticulum of the cecum. Its microscopic structure is the same as that of the colon from which it arises, although the submucosal lymphoid tissue is particularly robust, especially in childhood.

APPENDICITIS

The most important disease of the appendix is acute appendicitis (Fig. 11-41). This may occur at any age, but children and adults over 60 years are most affected. The familiar presenting sign is right lower quadrant pain, which, if not treated, is followed by signs of peritoneal inflammation. Treatment is surgical removal or antibiotic therapy. The genesis of appendicitis remains largely mysterious. In many patients, there appears to be luminal obstruction by lumps of fecal concretions known as fecaliths. However, these are often not present. On occasion, a specific infectious agent is identified, such *Yersinia*, *Actinomyces*, or *Campylobacter*. In some children, a tangle of pinworms (*Enterobius vermicularis*) may contribute to luminal obstruction.

However, in most cases, there is no apparent specific infectious agent. There is often mucosal erosion or ulceration, followed by a transmural infiltrate of neutrophils.

Granulomatous appendicitis may represent involvement by Crohn disease (see above) or an infectious agent. However, most granulomas involving the appendix involve neither of these entities and are of unknown cause and significance.

A **mucocele** is a distended appendix filled with mucinous material. Rarely, these are due to inflammation causing focal luminal obstruction. More commonly, a dilated mucin-filled appendix reflects a neoplastic process (see below).

APPENDICEAL NEOPLASMS

Appendiceal Neuroendocrine Tumors

NETs are common in the appendix. Most of these are small and benign and are found incidentally at the time of appendectomy. Small (<1.5 cm) NETs of the appendix are of no

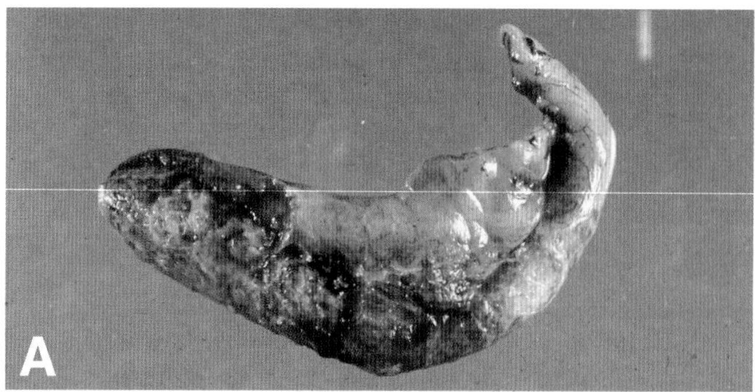

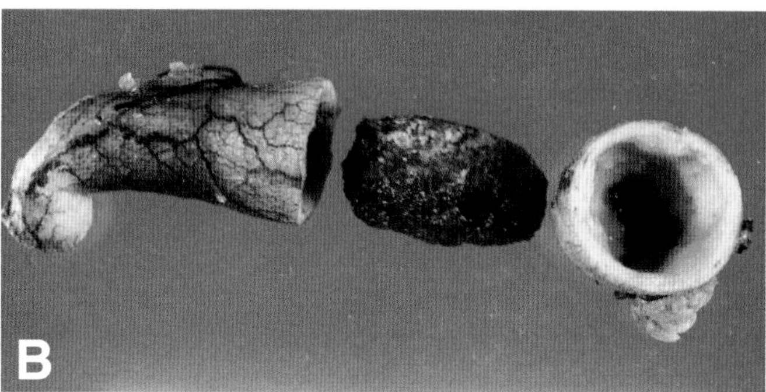

FIGURE 11-41. Acute appendicitis. A. The distal appendix is dilated, congested, and partly covered by fibrin (arrow) in this case of **appendicitis. B.** The lumen in this case of appendicitis was dilated owing to a large **fecalith**. 61B From Mitros FA. *Atlas of Gastrointestinal Pathology*. New York, NY: Gower Medical Publishing, 1988. Copyright Lippincott Williams & Wilkins.

clinical significance. Tumors between 1 and 2 cm in diameter show a low rate of metastasis (about 1%). Larger lesions are increasingly aggressive.

Epithelial Tumors

Epithelial tumors are the most clinically important neoplasms of the appendix. They dilate the lumen and expand its length, resulting in mucoceles. However, a better descriptive term is **cystadenoma** or **mucinous tumor**. The neoplastic epithelial lining of these lesions is usually well differentiated (Fig. 11-42A and B); they can invade and penetrate the wall of the appendix. When this happens, abundant mucin may fill the peritoneal cavity, causing a lesion known as **pseudomyxoma peritonei**. Rarely, frank adenocarcinomas are described.

The Large Intestine

ANATOMY

The large intestine is the portion of the gut from the ileocecal valve to the anus. It is 90 to 125 cm long in adults and includes the colon and rectum. Its main function is to conserve water and salt and to store and dispose of waste material in the form of feces.

The large intestine has six regions, distally from the ileocecal valve: (1) cecum, (2) ascending colon, (3) transverse colon, (4) descending colon, (5) sigmoid colon, and (6) rectum. The bend between the ascending and transverse colon in the right upper quadrant is the **hepatic flexure** and that between the transverse and descending segments in the left upper quadrant is the **splenic flexure**. The lumen progressively narrows from the cecum to the sigmoid colon. Like the small intestine, the colon has outer longitudinal and inner circular muscle coats. However, in the colon, the longitudinal muscle has three separate bundles, the **taeniae coli**. Evaginations of the colonic wall between taeniae, the **haustra**, appear as external sacculations. The ileocecal valve is a sphincter that regulates the flow of intestinal contents into the cecum. However, it is an incompetent sphincter, and reflux of cecal contents into the ileum is usual. The external anal sphincter is the major mechanism by which bowel continence is maintained.

The colonic mucosa is flat and punctuated by numerous pits, the **crypts of Lieberkühn**. The surface epithelium is primarily simple columnar cells with occasional goblet cells. The crypts mostly contain goblet cells, except at their bases, where a few undifferentiated cells and a variety of neuroendocrine cells are located. The lamina propria contains lymphocytes, plasma cells, macrophages, and fibroblasts, plus occasional

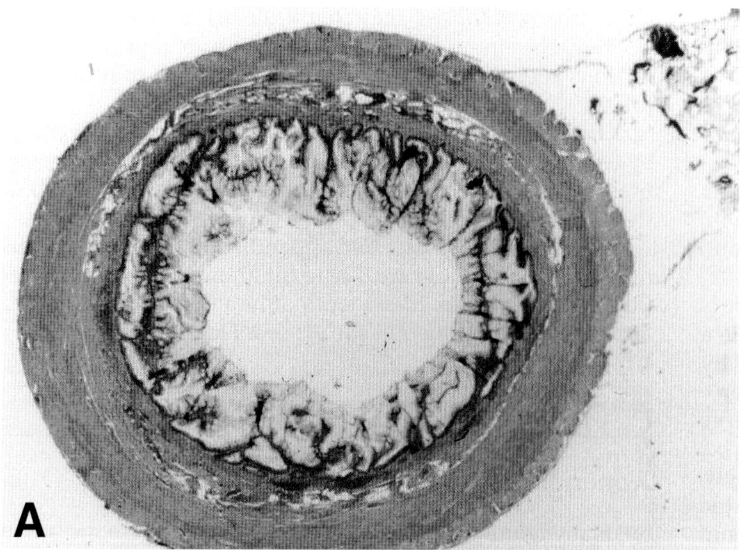

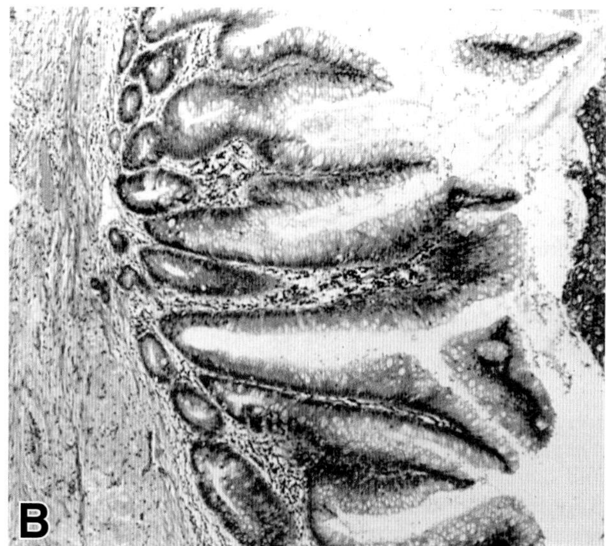

FIGURE 11-42. Mucinous tumor of the appendix. A. The neoplasm encircles the entire lumen. **B.** At higher power, its peculiar villous configuration is appreciated.

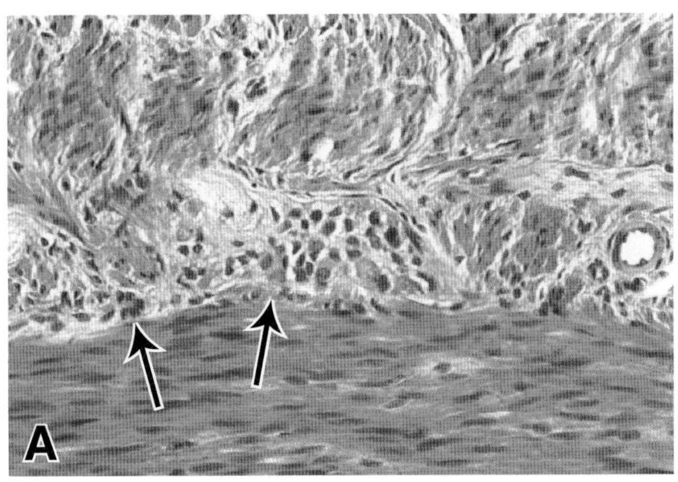

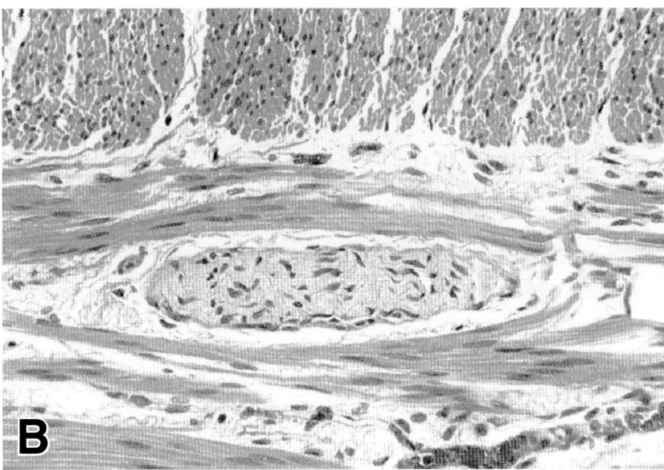

FIGURE 11-43. Hirschsprung disease. A. A photomicrograph of ganglion cells in the wall of a normal rectum (*arrows*). **B.** A rectal biopsy specimen from a patient with Hirschsprung disease showing a nonmyelinated nerve in the mesenteric plexus and an absence of ganglion cells.

eosinophils. Lymphoid aggregates traverse the muscularis mucosae and extend into the submucosa. The submucosa is similar to that in the small intestine, but lymphatic channels are far less prominent. Colonic lymphatics drain into paracolic nodes in the mesenteric fat, intermediate nodes along the colic blood vessels, and central nodes near the aorta. Parasympathetic and sympathetic innervations terminate in Meissner submucosal and Auerbach myenteric plexuses.

CONGENITAL DISORDERS

Hirschsprung Disease

In Hirschsprung disease, dilation of the colon is caused by defective colorectal innervation: ganglion cells are absent beginning in the internal anal sphincter and extending proximally for variable lengths (Fig. 11-43). In 10% of cases, the whole colon is aganglionic; rarely, the small intestine is also involved. Hirschsprung disease affects 1 in 5,000 live births; 80% of patients are male except in long-segment disease, in which the male to female ratio is equal.

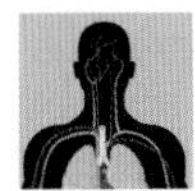

PATHOPHYSIOLOGY: The developmental sequence that leads to innervation of the colon is interrupted in Hirschsprung disease. The normal caudal migration of cells from the neural crest to the intramural ganglion cells is aborted. Because the internal anal sphincter is at the far end of this migration, the aganglionic segment always starts there. It may extend variably proximally, depending on where primitive neuroblast migration halts. The aganglionic rectum and sometimes the adjacent colon are permanently contracted; hence, fecal contents cannot readily enter the stenotic area. The proximal bowel becomes dilated because of functional distal obstruction.

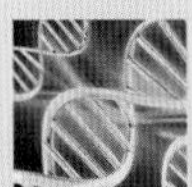

MOLECULAR PATHOGENESIS: Most cases of Hirschsprung disease are sporadic, but 10% are familial. Half of familial cases, and 15% of sporadic ones, reflect inactivating mutations of the *RET* receptor tyrosine kinase gene on chromosome 10q (see MEN2 syndrome, Chapter 19).

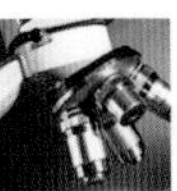

PATHOLOGY: The large intestine in Hirschsprung disease has a constricted and spastic aganglionic segment. Proximal to this area, the bowel is very dilated. Definitive diagnosis requires a demonstration of the absence of ganglion cells on rectal biopsy (Fig. 11-43B). There is also a striking increase in nonmyelinated cholinergic nerve fibers in the submucosa and between muscle coats (neural hyperplasia).

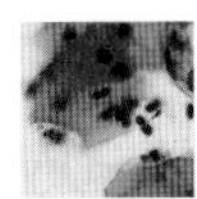

CLINICAL FEATURES: ***Hirschsprung disease is the most common cause of congenital intestinal obstruction.*** Typically, newborns show delayed passage of meconium and vomiting in the first few days of life. In some cases, complete intestinal obstruction may require immediate surgical relief. Children whose involved rectal segments are short may experience only partial obstruction, constipation, abdominal distention, and recurrent fecal impactions. Hirschsprung disease is treated by surgical removal of the aganglionic segment and reconstruction.

Pseudomembranous Colitis

Pseudomembranous colitis is a generic term for an inflammatory disease of the colon that is characterized by **exudative mucosal plaques**. It is most often caused by *C. difficile* as a result of antibiotic therapy. Virtually, all antibiotics have been implicated, although some have been associated with a higher risk. Hospitalization is another major risk factor.

C. difficile is transmitted via the fecal–oral route and is ingested in vegetative form or as spores. When normal protective gut florae are killed by antibiotics, the more resistant *C. difficile* can gain a foothold and begin producing its toxins, namely, toxins A and B. Toxin A activates and recruits inflammatory mediators, whereas toxin B is directly cytotoxic. *C. difficile* is not invasive and mediates damage solely via production of toxins.

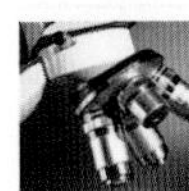

PATHOLOGY: Pseudomembranous colitis features raised yellowish plaques up to 2 cm that adhere to the underlying mucosa (Fig. 11-44). The intervening mucosa is congested and edematous, but

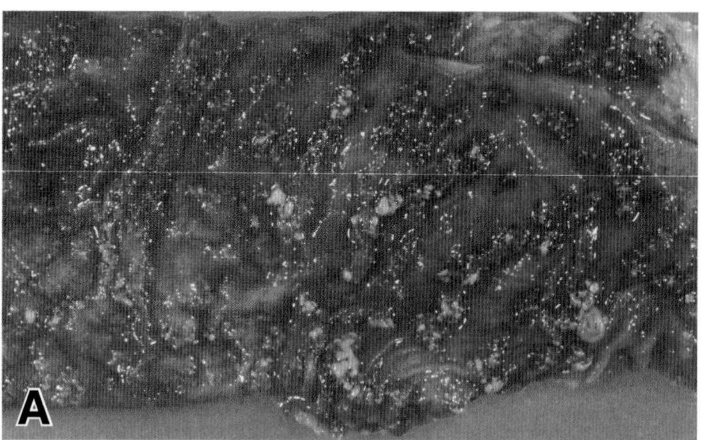

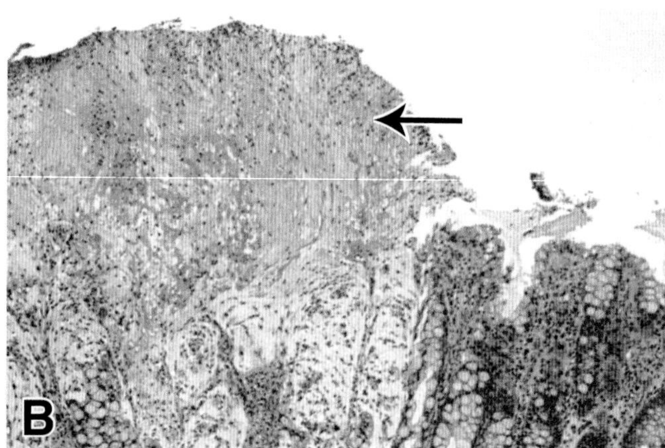

FIGURE 11-44. Pseudomembranous colitis. A. The colon showing variable involvement ranging from erythema to yellow-green areas of pseudomembrane. **B.** Microscopically, the pseudomembrane (*arrow*) consists of fibrin, mucin, and inflammatory cells (largely neutrophils).

not ulcerated. In severe cases, plaques coalesce into extensive pseudomembranes. Superficial epithelial necrosis is believed to be the initial pathologic event. Colonic crypts then become disrupted and expanded by mucin and neutrophils. The pseudomembrane consists of debris from necrotic epithelial cells, mucus, fibrin, and neutrophils. In milder cases, well-formed pseudomembranes may be absent, and the pathology is subtler, with focal damage to the surface epithelium.

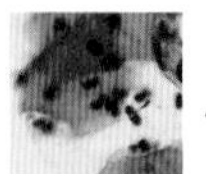

CLINICAL FEATURES: Antibiotic-associated *C. difficile* infections are virtually always accompanied by mild-to-moderate watery diarrhea, but the disorder does not usually progress to colitis. In patients with pseudomembranous colitis, fever, leukocytosis, and abdominal cramps are superimposed on a severe diarrhea that can be bloody. In some cases, the disease can progress to fulminant colitis, which can lead to serious complications, such as colonic perforation, toxic megacolon, and death.

The diagnosis is usually made by identifying toxins in stool by cytotoxin assay, immunoassay, or molecular methods. *C. difficile* infections are treated with antibiotics (metronidazole or vancomycin) and supportive fluid and electrolyte therapy. Treatment for patients with multiple recurrences is replenishment of normal gut flora with a **"fecal transplant."**

Neonatal Necrotizing Enterocolitis

Necrotizing enterocolitis is one of the most common acquired surgical emergencies in newborns. It is particularly common in premature infants after oral feeding and is likely related to an ischemic event involving the intestinal mucosa. This event is followed by bacterial colonization, usually with *C. difficile*, which is found in the stool of up to 50% of neonates. Lesions vary from those typical of pseudomembranous enterocolitis to gangrene and perforation of the bowel.

DIVERTICULAR DISEASE

Diverticular disease covers two entities: **diverticulosis** and its inflammatory complication, **diverticulitis**.

Diverticulosis

Diverticulosis entails acquired herniation of the mucosa and submucosa through the muscularis propria. It is common in Western societies where it increases in frequency with age. In Asia, Africa, and underdeveloped countries, the condition is infrequent. Western diets, which are rich in meat and refined carbohydrates, lack dietary residue, leading to sustained bowel contraction and thus increased intraluminal pressure. Such pressure may lead to herniation of the mucosa and submucosa of the colon. In addition to pressure, defects in the colon wall are required. The circular muscle of the colon is interrupted by connective tissue clefts at the sites of penetration by the nutrient vessels that supply the submucosa and mucosa. In older people, this connective tissue loses its resilience and thus its resistance to the effects of increased intraluminal pressure.

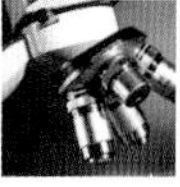

PATHOLOGY: True diverticula involve all layers of the intestinal wall. In diverticulosis, the structures are actually pseudodiverticula, in which only the mucosa and submucosa are herniated through the muscle layers. The sigmoid colon is affected in 95% of cases, but diverticulosis can affect any segment of the colon, including the cecum. Diverticula vary in number from a few to hundreds. They measure up to 1 cm and are connected to the intestinal lumen by necks of varying length and caliber. Diverticula are characteristically seen as flask-like structures that extend from the lumen through the muscle layers (Fig. 11-45). Their walls are continuous with the surface mucosa and thus have epithelium *and* submucosa. The outer base is formed by serosal connective tissue.

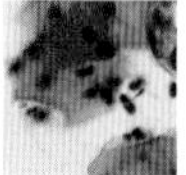

CLINICAL FEATURES: ***At least 80% of persons with diverticulosis are symptom free.*** Symptomatic patients complain of episodic colicky abdominal pain. Both constipation and diarrhea, sometimes alternating, may occur, and flatulence is common. Chronic blood loss may lead to anemia.

Diverticulitis

Of patients with diverticulosis, 10% to 20% will develop diverticulitis at some point. Acute diverticulitis is thought

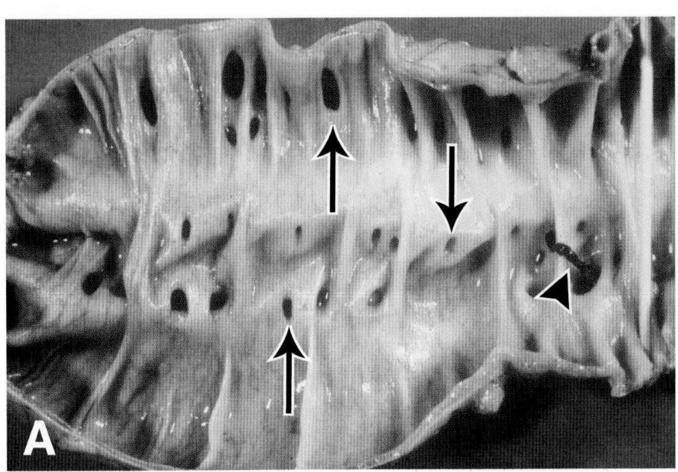

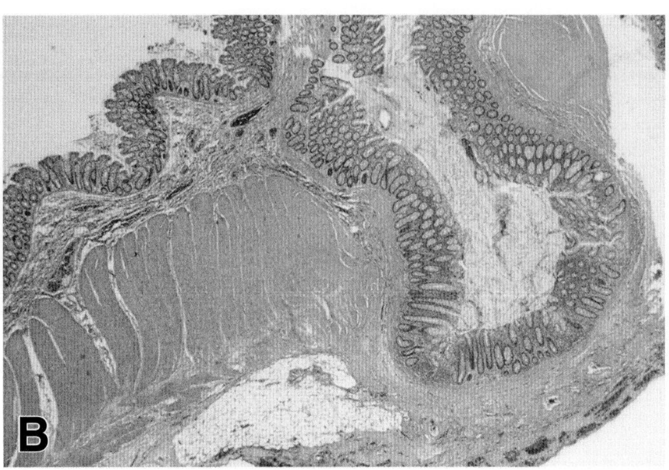

FIGURE 11-45. Diverticulosis of the colon. A. The mouths of numerous diverticula are seen between the taenia (*arrows*). There is a blood clot seen protruding from the mouth of one of the diverticula (*arrowhead*). This was the source of massive gastrointestinal bleeding. **B.** Sections showing mucosa including muscularis mucosa and submucosa, which have herniated through a defect in the bowel wall, producing a diverticulum.

to be precipitated by irritation from retained fecal material. Inflammation of the diverticulum can eventually precipitate rupture. Beyond this acute episode, chronic diverticular disease may develop from a combination of abnormal colonic motility, visceral hypersensitivity, imbalance among intestinal flora (called dysbiosis), and chronic inflammation; all lead to an irritable bowel-like syndrome.

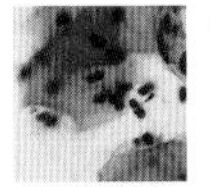

PATHOLOGY: Inflammation of the wall of the diverticulum leads to perforation and the release of fecal bacteria into peridiverticular tissues. The resulting abscess is usually contained in the appendices epiploicae and pericolonic adipose tissue. Infrequently, free perforation results in generalized peritonitis. In response to repeated episodes of diverticulitis, fibrosis may constrict the bowel lumen, causing obstruction. Fistulas may form between the colon and adjacent organs, including the bladder, vagina, small intestine, and skin of the abdomen.

CLINICAL FEATURES: The most common symptoms of acute diverticulitis, which usually occur after perforation, are persistent lower abdominal pain and fever. Changes in bowel habits, from diarrhea to constipation, are frequent. Dysuria indicates bladder irritation. Most patients have left lower quadrant tenderness and, often, a palpable mass in that area. Leukocytosis is the rule. Antibiotics and supportive measures usually alleviate acute diverticulitis, but 20% of patients eventually require surgery. Medical management to prevent subsequent attacks and chronic diverticular disease includes high-fiber diet; long-term, cyclical antibiotic therapy, anti-inflammatory medication (mesalamine); and, potentially, probiotics.

INFLAMMATORY BOWEL DISEASE

The term IBD encompasses **Crohn disease** and **ulcerative colitis**. These two disorders have certain common features but usually differ enough to be clearly distinguishable. Cases that cannot be distinguished are labeled **indeterminate colitis**.

Both Crohn disease and ulcerative colitis show histologic features of chronicity, including architectural glandular distortion; chronic inflammation, with or without active neutrophilic inflammation; and metaplasia. Extraintestinal complications of IBD are more common with Crohn disease but also occur in ulcerative colitis (Fig. 11-46). Although their precise causes are unknown, epidemiologic, clinical, and animal studies suggest that mucosal injury accrues from altered immune responses and abnormal interactions of bacteria with intestinal epithelia.

CROHN DISEASE

Crohn disease mainly affects the distal small intestine but may involve any part of the digestive tract and even extraintestinal tissues. The colon, particularly the right colon, is often affected.

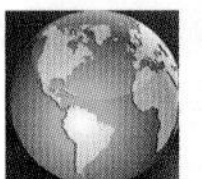

EPIDEMIOLOGY: Crohn disease has a worldwide incidence of 0.7 to 14.6 per 100,000 but is more common in developed countries. Its incidence has increased dramatically in the past 30 years, probably owing to a combination of factors related to adoption of a "Western lifestyle." Age distribution is bimodal, with a peak in adolescents or young adults and a second smaller peak in the 50s and 60s. It is most common in people of European origin, with a considerably higher frequency among Ashkenazi Jews. Males predominate among children, but in adults, there is a slight female predominance. Smokers are at an increased risk of developing Crohn disease and of having more severe disease, compared with nonsmokers.

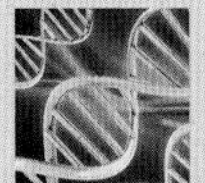

MOLECULAR PATHOGENESIS: The cause of Crohn disease is not known. The leading theories involve a combination of a genetically susceptible host, defective mucosal barrier, intestinal dysbiosis (altered intestinal flora), or inadequate/inappropriate immune response. Genome-wide association studies suggest that alterations in innate and adoptive immunity and autophagy play a role in disease susceptibility. These defects

Uveitis, scleritis, episcleritis
Aphthous stomatitis
Chronic bronchitis
Bronchiectasis
Ankylosing spondylitis
Sclerosing cholangitis
Cholelithiasis
Pancreatitis
Erythema nodosum
Nephrolithiasis
Anemia
Malnutrition
Hyperhomo-cysteinemia
Osteopenia/osteoporosis
Arthritis
Pyoderma gangrenosum

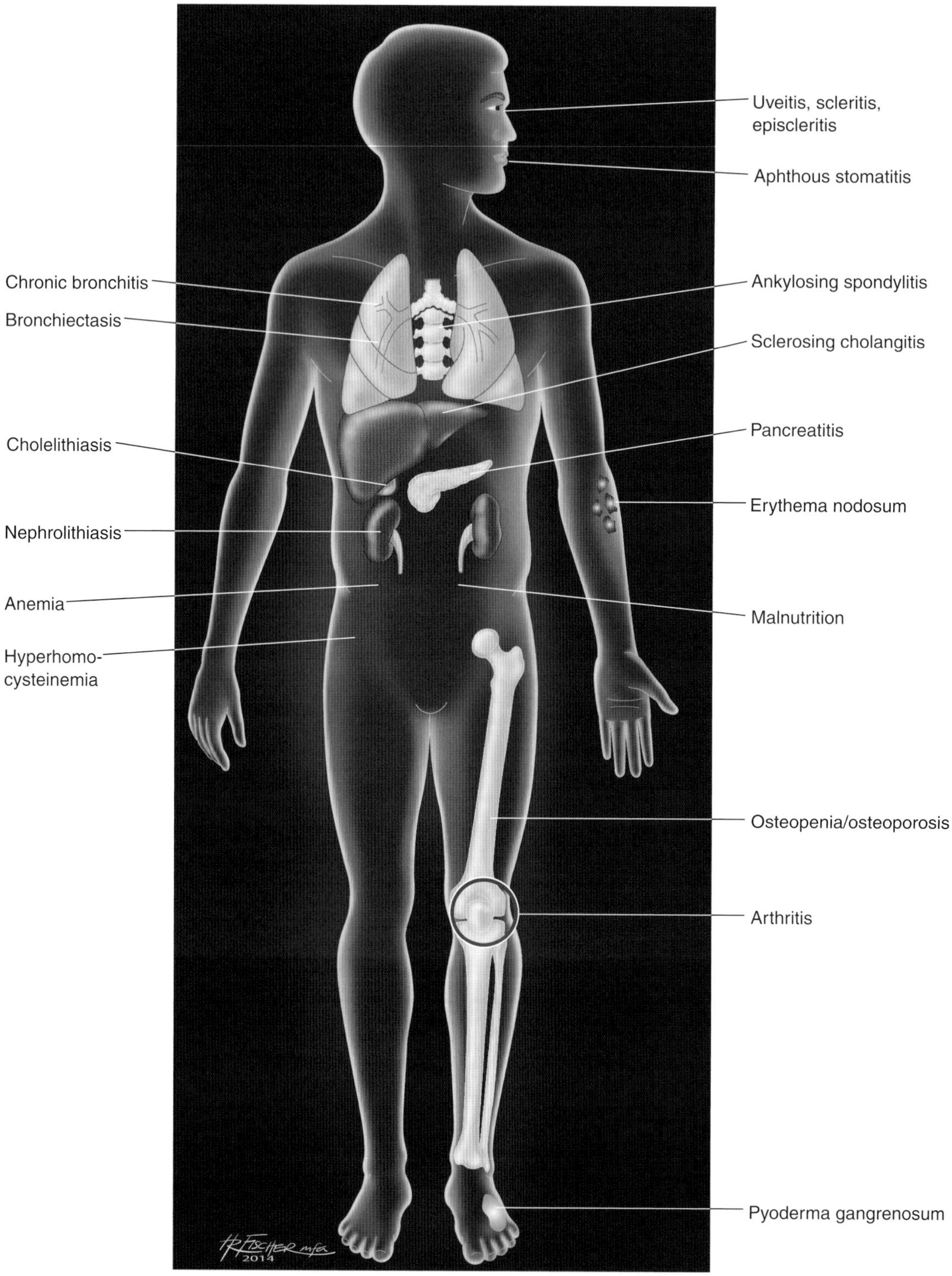

FIGURE 11-46. Systemic complications of inflammatory bowel disease. These conditions are more common with Crohn disease but may also be seen in ulcerative colitis.

imply problems in the recognition and handling of intracellular bacteria. The T-cell response (adaptive immune system) in Crohn disease involves T_H1, which is mediated by IL-12, IFN-γ, and TNF.

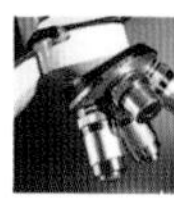

PATHOLOGY: Two key features of Crohn disease differentiate it from other GI inflammatory diseases: (1) Inflammation usually involves all layers of the bowel wall and is thus referred to as **transmural**. (2) Intestinal involvement is discontinuous; areas of inflammation are separated by apparently normal intestine (skip lesions).

Crohn disease may involve different parts of the bowel singly or in combination. It affects the ileum and cecum in half of cases, only the small intestine in 30%, and only the colon in 20%. Less commonly, the disease affects the duodenum, stomach, and esophagus, as focal acute inflammation with

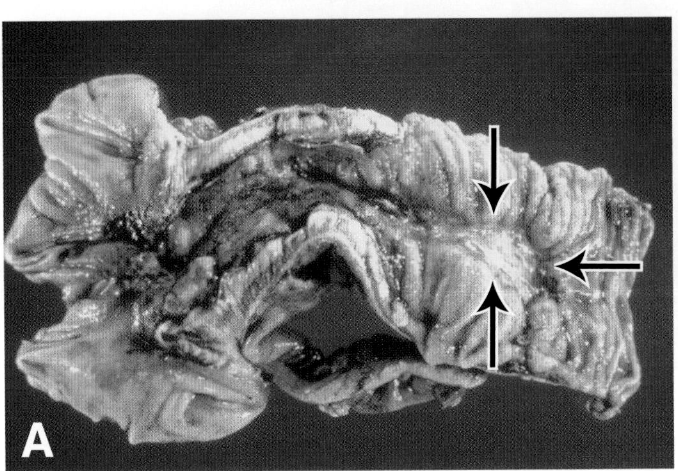

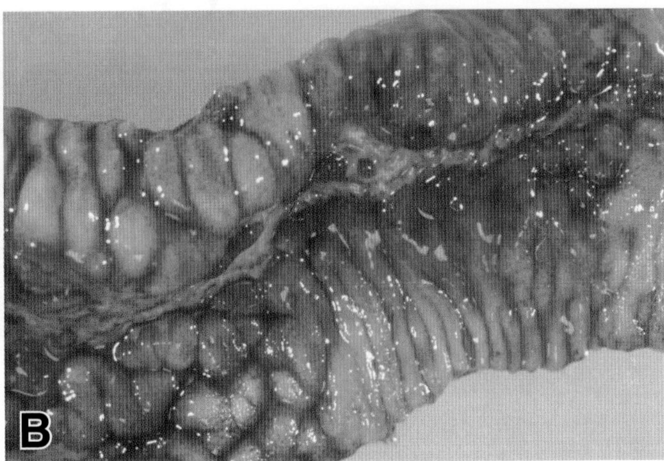

FIGURE 11-47. Crohn disease. A. The terminal ileum showing striking thickening of the wall of the distal portion with distortion of the ileocecal valve. A longitudinal ulcer is present (*arrows*). **B.** Another longitudinal ulcer is seen in this segment of ileum. The large rounded areas of edematous damaged mucosa give a "cobblestone" appearance to the involved mucosa. A portion of the mucosa to the lower right is uninvolved.

or without granulomas. In women with anorectal disease, inflammation may spread to the external genitalia.

The pathology of Crohn disease is highly variable. The bowel and adjacent mesentery are thickened and edematous. Mesenteric fat often surrounds the bowel (the so-called **creeping fat**). Mesenteric lymph nodes are frequently enlarged, firm, and matted together. The intestinal lumen is narrowed by edema in early cases and by a combination of edema and fibrosis in long-standing disease. Nodular swelling, fibrosis, and mucosal ulceration lead to a "**cobblestone**" appearance (Fig. 11-47). In early cases, ulcers have either an aphthous or a serpiginous appearance; later, they become deeper and appear as linear clefts or fissures (Fig. 11-47B).

There are thickening, edema, and fibrosis of all bowel layers. Involved loops are often adherent and fistulas may form between such segments. Most fistulas end blindly and form abscess cavities in the peritoneum, mesentery, or retroperitoneal structures. Lesions in the distal rectum and anus may create perianal fistulas, a well-known presenting feature.

Crohn disease is mainly a chronic inflammatory process. Early in the disease, inflammation may be confined to the mucosa and submucosa. Small, superficial mucosal ulcers (aphthous ulcers) are seen, as are mucosal and submucosal edema and infiltrates of lymphocytes, plasma cells, eosinophils, and macrophages. Mucosal architecture is abnormal, often showing regenerative changes in crypts and villous distortion. Pyloric metaplasia and Paneth cell hyperplasia are common in the small and large intestines. Later, long, deep, fissure-like ulcers, vascular hyalinization, and fibrosis appear.

Lymphocytes form aggregates throughout the wall, and the muscularis mucosae and nerves of the submucosal and myenteric plexuses all proliferate (Fig. 11-48). Discrete, noncaseating granulomas may be present, mostly in the submucosa (Fig. 11-48B). These resemble those of sarcoidosis, with focal aggregates of epithelioid cells, surrounded by a rim of lymphocytes. Multinucleated giant cells may be present. The centers of the granulomas usually have hyaline material but only rarely necrosis.

Discrete granulomas strongly suggest Crohn disease, but their absence does not exclude the diagnosis because they are present in less than half of cases.

The pathologic features of Crohn disease are summarized in Figure 11-49.

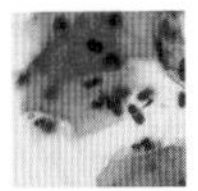

CLINICAL FEATURES: The clinical manifestations and natural history of Crohn disease are highly variable and reflect the diversity of anatomic sites affected. The most common symptoms are abdominal pain and diarrhea, with passage of blood and/or mucus. Recurrent fever is frequent. If it mainly involves the ileum and cecum, its sudden onset may mimic appendicitis, with right lower quadrant pain, intermittent diarrhea, fever, and a tender right lower quadrant mass. When the small intestine is diffusely involved, malabsorption and malnutrition tend to be major features. Colonic involvement produces **diarrhea** and sometimes **colonic bleeding**. In a few patients, the major site of involvement may be the anorectal region, and recurrent anorectal fistulas may be the presenting sign.

There are many extraintestinal manifestations and associated disorders in Crohn disease (Fig. 11-46). Small bowel cancer occurs at least threefold more commonly in patients with the malady. The risk of colorectal cancer is also higher, more in patients with extensive involvement of the colon, a family history of colorectal cancer, or sclerosing cholangitis.

There is no known cure for Crohn disease. Corticosteroids, sulfasalazine, metronidazole, azathioprine, 6-mercaptopurine, methotrexate, and anti–TNF-α antibodies, such as infliximab, may suppress the inflammatory reaction. However, these medications put patients at increased risk for opportunistic infections.

Surgical resection of obstructed or severely involved portions of intestine and drainage of abscesses caused by fistulas are required in some cases. Recurrence and the need for repeated resections occasionally create short-bowel syndrome.

Ulcerative Colitis

Ulcerative colitis is chronic, superficial inflammation of the colon and rectum.

The disorder is characterized by chronic diarrhea and rectal bleeding, with episodic exacerbations and remissions.

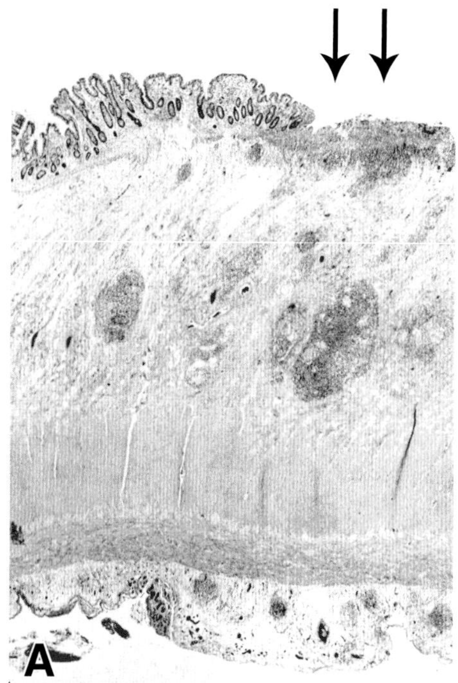

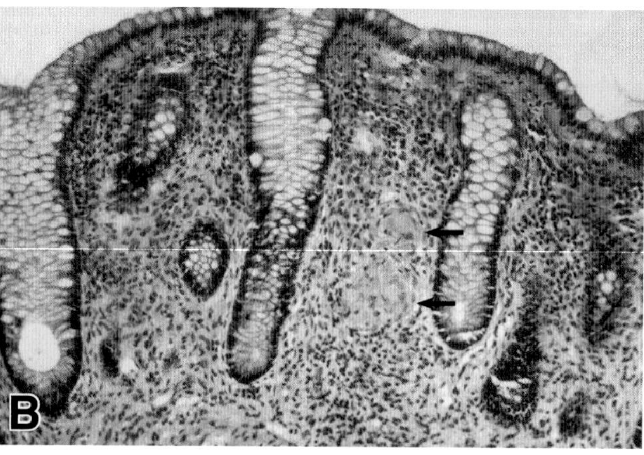

FIGURE 11-48. **Crohn disease. A.** The colon involved with Crohn disease showing an area of mucosal ulceration (*arrows*), an expanded submucosa with lymphoid aggregates, and numerous lymphoid aggregates in the subserosal tissues immediately adjacent to the muscularis propria. **B.** A mucosal biopsy in Crohn disease showing a small epithelioid granuloma (*arrows*) between two intact crypts.

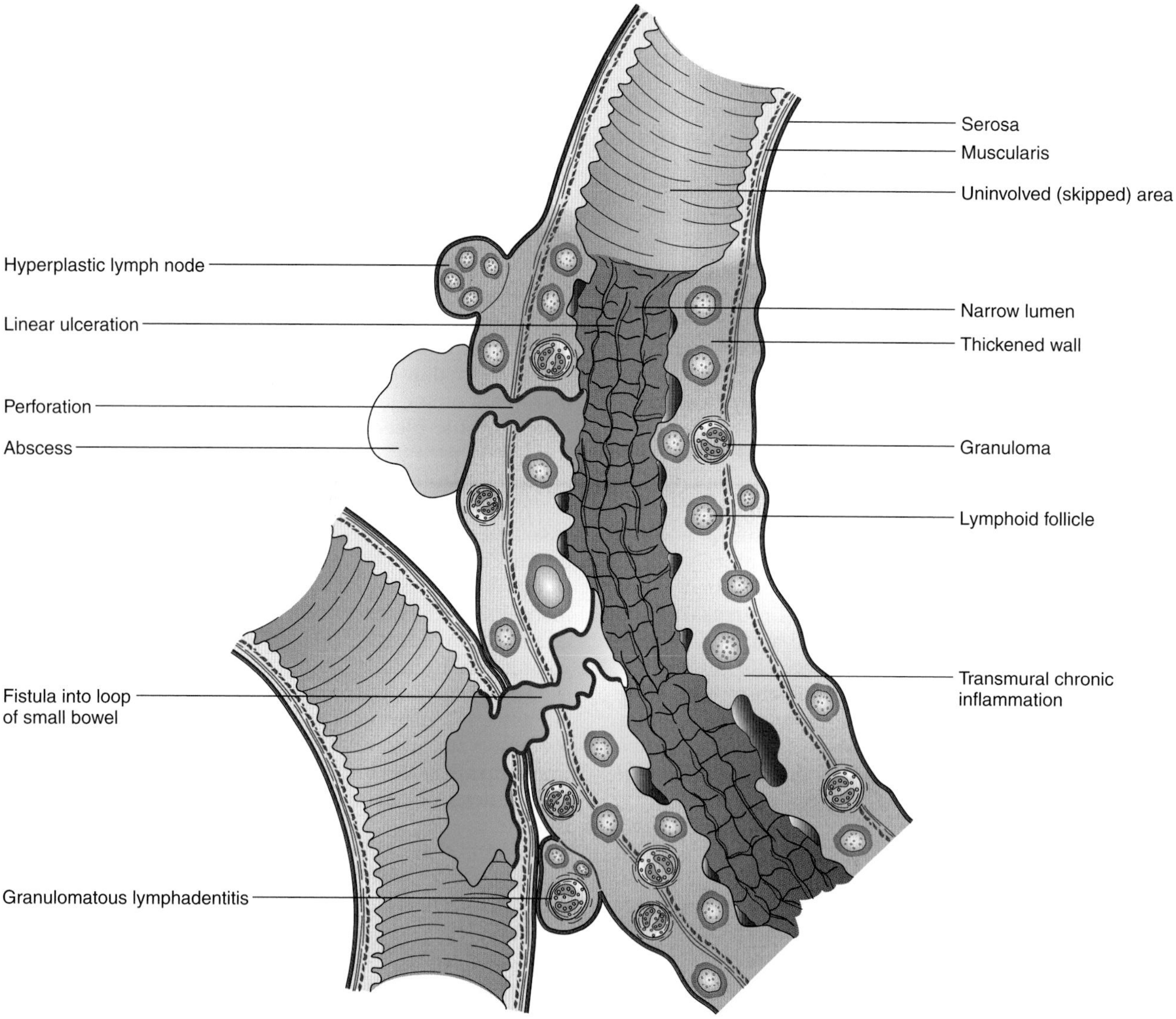

Serosa
Muscularis
Uninvolved (skipped) area
Hyperplastic lymph node
Linear ulceration
Narrow lumen
Thickened wall
Perforation
Abscess
Granuloma
Lymphoid follicle
Fistula into loop of small bowel
Transmural chronic inflammation
Granulomatous lymphadentitis

FIGURE 11-49. **Crohn disease.** A schematic representation of the major features of Crohn disease in the small intestine.

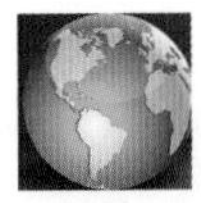

EPIDEMIOLOGY: Worldwide, the incidence ulcerative colitis ranges from 1.5 to 24.5 per 100,000 and occurs more often in developed countries. Similar to Crohn disease, its incidence is increasing in countries that adopt "Western" lifestyles, suggesting that environmental factors contribute to the pathogenesis of the disease. It also has a bimodal age distribution, with a peak from 15 to 30 years and another between 50 and 70. In the United States, whites are affected more than blacks. Smoking seems to inhibit the development of ulcerative colitis, but ex-smokers are also at an increased risk. People with a family history of IBD have a higher risk of developing ulcerative colitis, although this relationship is not as strong as that in Crohn disease.

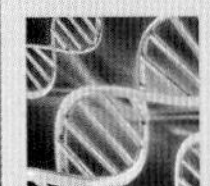

MOLECULAR PATHOGENESIS: ***The cause of ulcerative colitis is unknown.*** Leading theories suggest that genetically predisposed individuals develop dysregulated mucosal immune responses to gut flora, leading to bowel inflammation. Over 40 susceptibility loci are associated with ulcerative colitis, and half overlap with those for Crohn disease. Some encode proteins involved in epithelial cell adhesion and so perhaps contribute to mucosal barrier dysfunction. The T-cell response in ulcerative colitis is T_H2 dominant and mediated by natural killer T cells. This combination of factors produces mucosal hyperresponsiveness to commensal bacteria and an exaggerated immune response, causing chronic inflammation and damage.

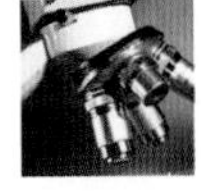

PATHOLOGY: Major pathologic features of ulcerative colitis that help to differentiate it from other inflammatory conditions, particularly Crohn disease, are as follows:

- **Ulcerative colitis is diffuse.** It begins in the distal rectum and extends proximally for a variable distance (Fig. 11-50). Isolated rectal involvement is termed **ulcerative proctitis**, whereas extension to the splenic flexure is called **proctosigmoiditis** or **left-sided colitis**. If the entire colon is involved, it is known as **pancolitis**. The disease is confluent without skip lesions. Sparing of the rectum is possible but should raise the possibility of Crohn disease.

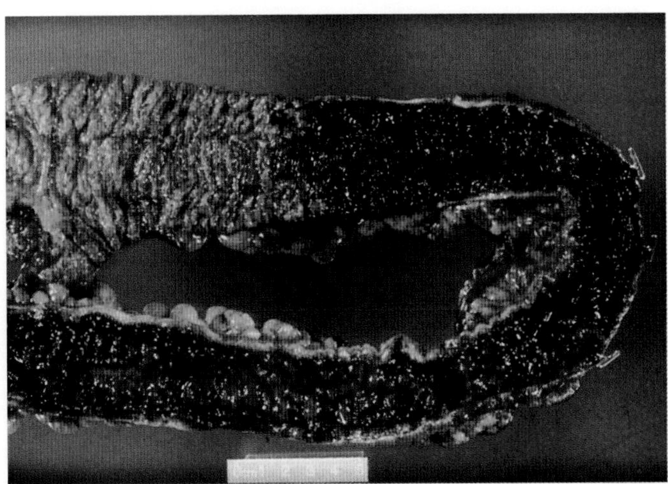

FIGURE 11-50. Ulcerative colitis. Prominent erythema and ulceration of the colon begins in and are most severe in the rectosigmoid area and extend into the ascending colon.

- **Inflammation in ulcerative colitis is limited to the colon and rectum.** If the cecum is affected, the disease ends at the ileocecal valve, although minor inflammation of the adjacent ileum (**backwash ileitis**) sometimes occurs.
- **Ulcerative colitis is a mucosal disease.** Deeper layers are involved mainly in infrequent fulminant cases and are usually associated with toxic megacolon.

This morphologic sequence of ulcerative colitis may develop rapidly or it may take years.

EARLY COLITIS: Early in the disease, the mucosal surface is raw, red, and granular. It is frequently covered with a yellowish exudate and bleeds easily. Later, small superficial ulcers or erosions may appear. These occasionally coalesce into irregular, shallow, ulcerated areas that seem to surround islands of intact mucosa.

The histology of early ulcerative colitis correlates with colonoscopic appearances and includes (1) mucosal congestion, edema, and tiny hemorrhages; (2) diffuse chronic inflammation in the lamina propria (Fig. 11-51); and (3) damage and distortion of colorectal crypts, which are often surrounded and infiltrated by neutrophils (cryptitis). Neutrophils in the crypts and suppurative necrosis of crypt epithelium cause crypt abscesses (dilated crypts filled with neutrophils) (Fig. 11-51B).

PROGRESSIVE COLITIS: As the disease progresses, mucosal folds are lost (atrophy). Lateral extension and coalescence of crypt abscesses can undermine the mucosa, leaving areas of ulceration adjacent to hanging fragments of mucosa. Such mucosal excrescences are inflammatory polyps. Tissue repair accompanies tissue destruction, and granulation tissue develops in denuded areas. Importantly, the strictures characteristic of Crohn disease are absent. In late stages, crypts may appear tortuous, branched, and shortened (Fig. 11-51C), with diffuse mucosal atrophy.

ADVANCED COLITIS: In long-standing cases, the large bowel is often shortened, especially on the left side. Mucosal folds are indistinct and are replaced by a granular or smooth mucosal pattern. In advanced ulcerative colitis, mucosal atrophy and chronic inflammation are present in the mucosa and superficial submucosa. Paneth cell metaplasia is common.

The pathologic features of ulcerative colitis are summarized in Figure 11-52.

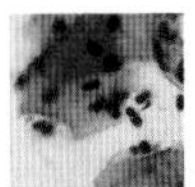

CLINICAL FEATURES: The clinical course and manifestations are quite variable. Most patients have intermittent attacks, with partial or complete remissions in between. A few (<10%) have a very long remission (several years) after their first attack. Some 20% have continuous symptoms without remission.

MILD COLITIS: Half of patients with ulcerative colitis have mild disease. Their major symptom is rectal bleeding, sometimes with **tenesmus** (rectal pressure and discomfort). In these patients, disease is usually limited to the rectum but may extend to the distal sigmoid colon. Extraintestinal complications are uncommon. In most patients in this category, the disease remains mild throughout their lives.

MODERATE COLITIS: About 40% of patients have moderate disease. They usually have episodic loose bloody stools, crampy abdominal pain, and often low-grade fever, lasting days or weeks. Anemia is commonly caused by chronic fecal blood loss.

SEVERE COLITIS: About 10% of patients have severe or fulminant disease. The disease may begin this way, but more often severe colitis supervenes during a flare of activity. Patients have many (sometimes >20) bloody bowel movements daily,

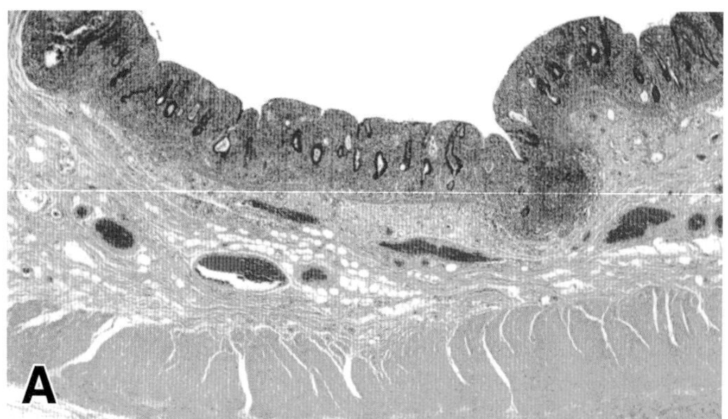

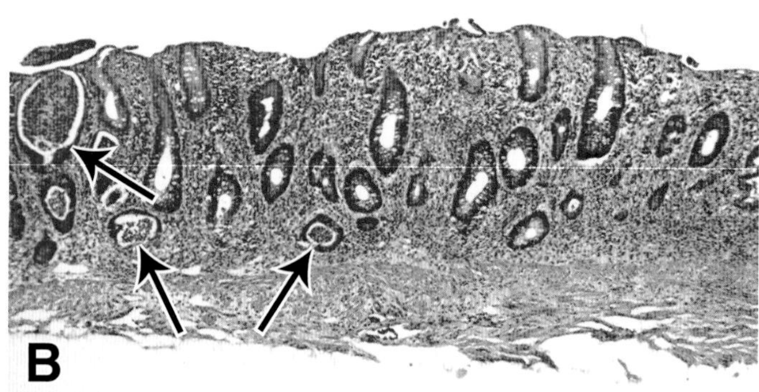

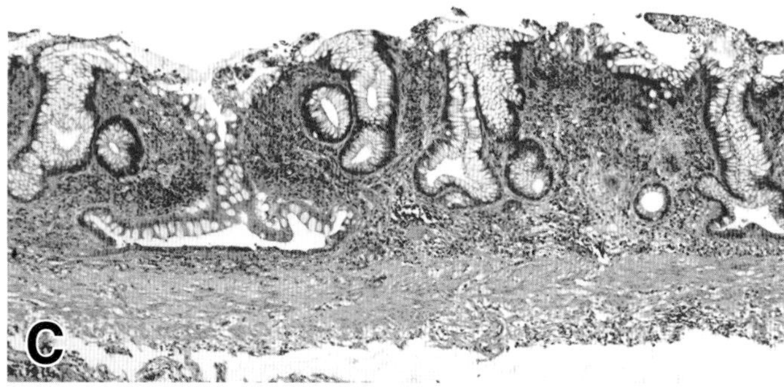

FIGURE 11-51. Ulcerative colitis. A. A full-thickness section of colon resected for ulcerative colitis showing inflammation affecting the mucosa with sparing of the submucosa and muscularis propria. **B.** A mucosal biopsy from a patient with active ulcerative colitis showing expansion of the lamina propria and several crypt abscesses (*arrows*). **C.** Chronic ulcerative colitis showing significant crypt distortion and atrophy.

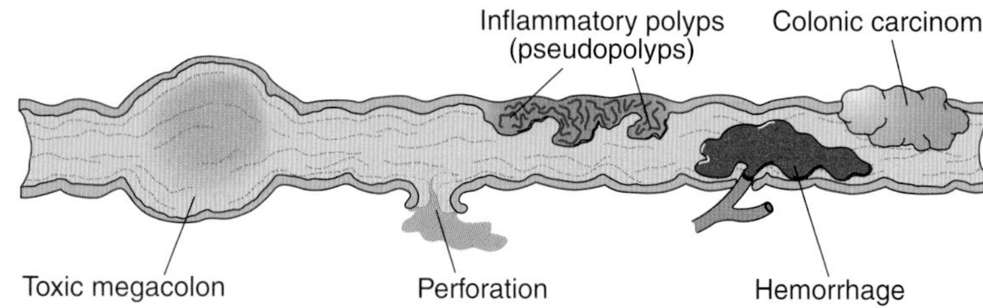

FIGURE 11-52. Ulcerative colitis. A schematic representation of the major features of ulcerative colitis in the colon.

often with fever and other systemic symptoms. Blood and fluid loss rapidly lead to anemia, dehydration, and electrolyte depletion. Massive hemorrhage may be life-threatening. Toxic megacolon refers to extreme dilation of the colon that carries a high risk for perforation and is particularly dangerous may supervene.

The medical treatment of ulcerative colitis depends on the sites involved and the severity of the inflammation. The 5-aminosalicylate–based compounds (e.g., mesalazine) are mainstays of treatment for patients with mild-to-moderate disease. Corticosteroids and immunosuppressive/immunoregulatory agents (azathioprine, cyclosporine, or anti–TNF-α agents) are used in patients with severe and refractory disease. There may be some benefit of fecal transplant in patients with refractory disease.

Table 11-2 *compares the pathologic features of Crohn disease and ulcerative colitis.*

Ulcerative Colitis and Colorectal Cancer

Patients with long-standing ulcerative colitis have a much higher risk of colorectal cancer than does the general population. Colorectal epithelial dysplasia is a precursor to colorectal carcinoma, particularly when high grade. The magnitude of this increased risk is greater if the entire colon is involved. In cases where inflammation is limited to the rectum, the risk of colorectal cancer is similar to that of the general population. After 10 years with ulcerative colitis, the chances for colorectal cancer are estimated to be 2%, 8% after 20 years, and 18% after 30 years. Patients with ulcerative colitis who develop primary sclerosing cholangitis are at a higher risk of dysplasia and colorectal cancer.

POLYPS OF THE COLON AND RECTUM

A gastrointestinal polyp is a mass that protrudes into the gut lumen. Polyps are classified by their attachment to the bowel wall (e.g., sessile or pedunculated with a discrete stalk), their histology (e.g., hyperplastic or adenomatous), and their neoplastic potential (i.e., benign or malignant). By themselves, polyps are not usually symptomatic, and their clinical importance lies in their potential for malignant transformation.

Table 11-2

Comparison of the Pathologic Features in the Colon of Crohn Disease and Ulcerative Colitis

Lesion	Crohn Disease	Ulcerative Colitis
Macroscopic		
Thickened bowel wall	Typical	Uncommon
Luminal narrowing	Typical	Uncommon
"Skip" lesions	Common	Absent
Right colon predominance	Typical	Absent
Fissures and fistulas	Common	Absent
Circumscribed ulcers	Common	Absent
Confluent linear ulcers	Common	Absent
Inflammatory polyps	Absent	Common
Microscopic		
Transmural inflammation	Typical	Rare
Submucosal fibrosis	Typical	Absent
Fissures	Typical	Rare
Granulomas	Common	Absent
Crypt abscesses	Typical	Typical

Hyperplastic Polyps

Hyperplastic polyps are small, sessile mucosal protrusions with exaggerated crypt architecture. They are the most common polyps of the colon, especially in the rectum. Hyperplastic polyps are present in 40% of rectal specimens in people younger than 40 years and in 75% of older people. They are more common in colons with adenomatous polyps and in populations with high rates of colorectal cancer. Hyperplastic polyps are thought to be caused by defective proliferation and maturation of normal epithelium. Thus, cell proliferation occurs at the base of the crypt, and upward migration of the cells is slowed. The epithelial cells differentiate and acquire absorptive characteristics lower in the crypts and persist at the surface longer than do normal cells.

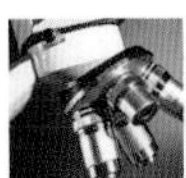

PATHOLOGY: Hyperplastic polyps are small, sessile, raised mucosal nodules, up to 0.5 cm, but occasionally larger (Fig. 11-53A). They are almost always multiple. The crypts of hyperplastic polyps are elongated and show relatively normal crypt bases. The epithelium in the upper third of the crypts contains hyperplastic goblet and mucinous cells and absorptive cells. Dysplasia is absent, and the polyps display a serrated contour and tufted surface (Fig. 11-53B).

Sessile Serrated Adenomas

These polyploidy lesions typically arise in the right colon and show hypermethylation of the promoter for the mismatch repair enzyme, *MLH1*, mutations in *BRAF*, and a high incidence of microsatellite instability. **The carcinomas that arise from sessile serrated adenomas tend to be bulky, mucinous, and right sided. Because of their malignant potential, these polyps should be entirely resected.**

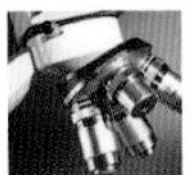

PATHOLOGY: Serrated adenomas are sessile or flat. They may appear as misshapen, abnormal mucosal folds and often have abundant adherent mucin (Fig. 11-54A). The lesions are usually larger than 1 cm. They exhibit irregular, asymmetric cell proliferation, in which cells may divide anywhere along the crypt. Intermixed goblet and mucin cells extend to the base. Some crypt bases are dilated with abundant mucin, whereas others show boot-, "L"-, or inverted "T"-shaped crypts (Fig. 11-54B). These adenomas may develop low- to high-grade dysplasia (Fig. 11-54C) and, eventually, invasive carcinoma.

Traditional Serrated Adenomas

These polyps are much less common than hyperplastic polyps or sessile serrated adenomas. Diverse molecular abnormalities include *BRAF* mutations and *KRAS* mutations, and some show a CpG island methylation of the promoter for *MGMT* (see Chapter 4). Like sessile serrated adenomas, these polyps should be entirely removed because of their malignant potential.

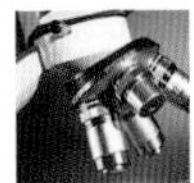

PATHOLOGY: Traditional serrated adenomas typically display tubulovillous or villous architecture. Lining epithelial cells have abundant eosinophilic cytoplasm, with an elongated nucleus and open or

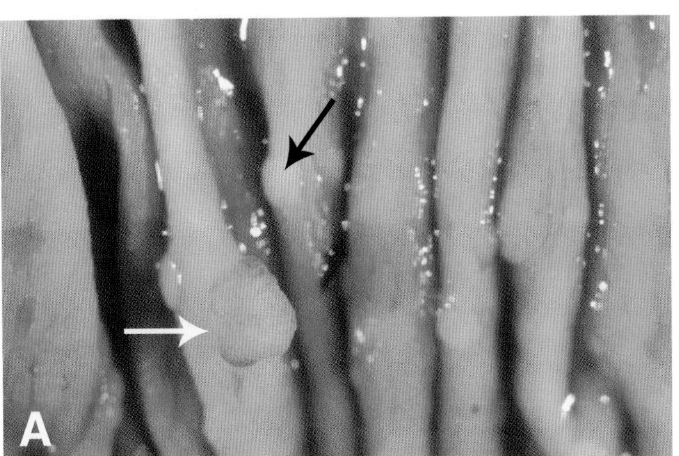

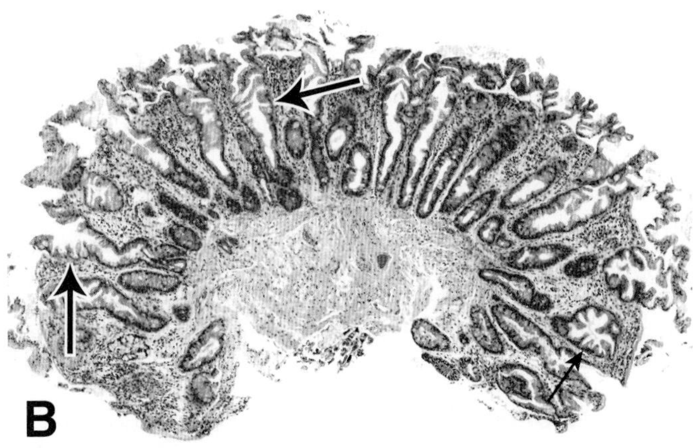

FIGURE 11-53. Hyperplastic polyp. A. This hyperplastic polyp is small, sessile, and pale (*black arrow*). The larger adjacent polyp (*white arrow*) is an adenoma. **B.** Microscopically, there is a "sawtooth" appearance to the surface (*arrows*) with relatively normal-appearing crypt bases.

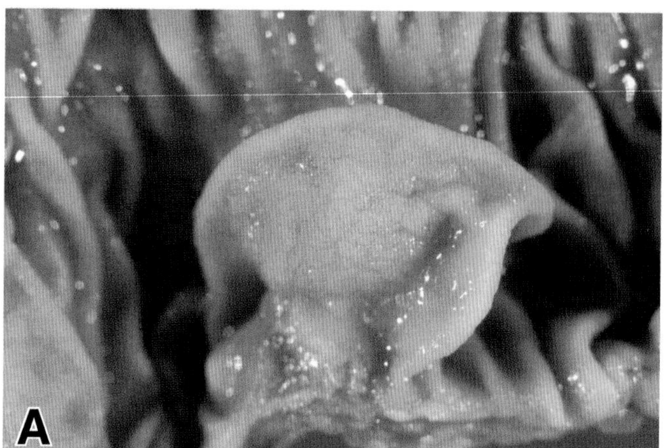

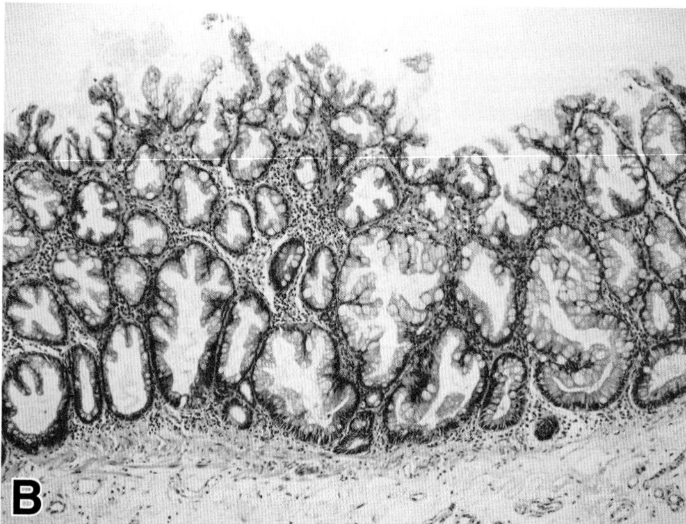

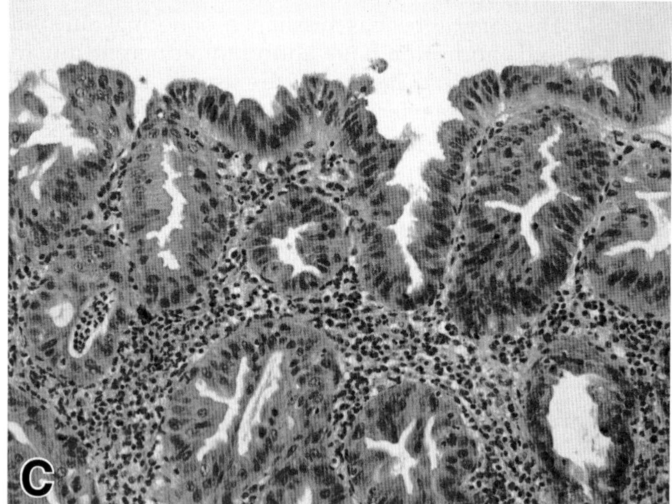

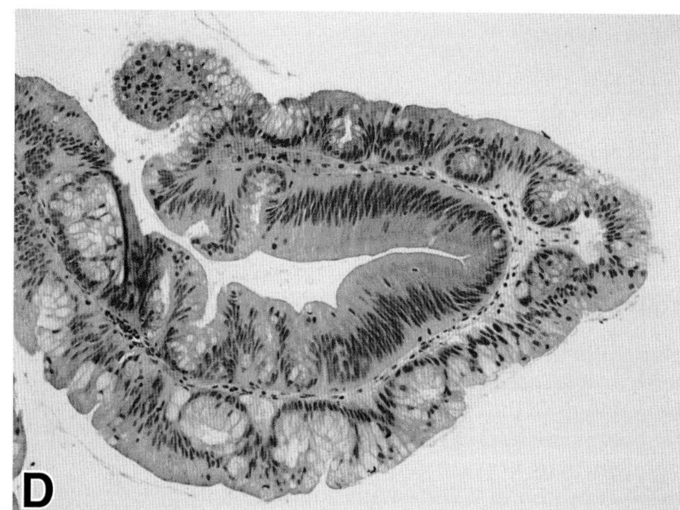

FIGURE 11-54. Premalignant serrated polyps. A. Sessile serrated adenoma. The gross appearance is often that of an enlarged flattened mucosal fold. **B. Sessile serrated adenoma.** Microscopically, the abnormal proliferation of goblet cells gives the crypts a serrated appearance down to the bases, causing the bases to become dilated with abundant mucin and the characteristic formation of boot-, "L"-, or inverted "T"-shaped crypts. **C. Sessile serrated adenoma** with cytologic high-grade dysplasia. **D. Traditional serrated adenoma.** The most characteristic feature of this polyp type is formation of ectopic crypts, often with a villous architecture and lining epithelial cells with abundant eosinophilic cytoplasm.

hyperchromatic chromatin. The most characteristic feature of these polyps is the formation of ectopic crypts (Fig. 11-54D).

Adenomatous Polyps

Adenomatous polyps (tubular adenomas) are neoplasms of colonic epithelium. They are composed of neoplastic epithelial cells that have migrated to the surface and accumulated beyond the needs for replacement of the cells sloughed into the lumen.

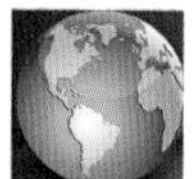

EPIDEMIOLOGY: Adenomatous polyps occur most often in industrialized countries. As with diverticular disease, the only known consistent environmental difference between high-risk and low-risk populations is a "Western" diet. After age 50, the incidence of adenomas rises rapidly; in the United States, at least one adenomatous polyp is present in half of the adult population. This proportion reaches greater than two thirds among those older than 65. Smoking, obesity, and a family history of colon adenomas or carcinoma increase the risk for the development of adenomas.

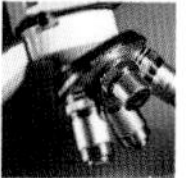

PATHOLOGY: Almost half of adenomatous polyps in the United States are in the rectosigmoid colon. The remaining half are evenly distributed throughout the rest of the colon. Adenomas vary from barely visible nodules, small, pedunculated adenomas, or large, sessile (flat) lesions. They are classified by architecture into tubular, villous, and tubulovillous types. These polyps are the usual precursors to colon cancer, and their epithelium is by definition dysplastic.

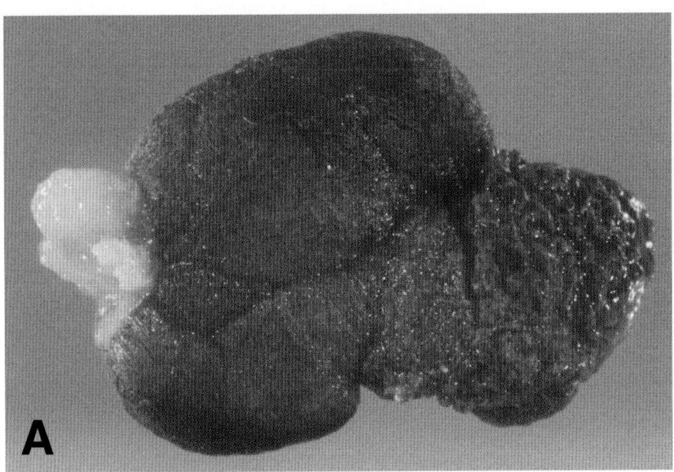

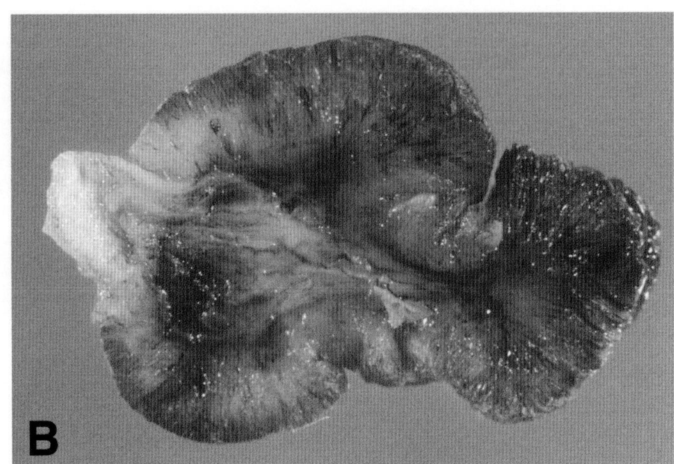

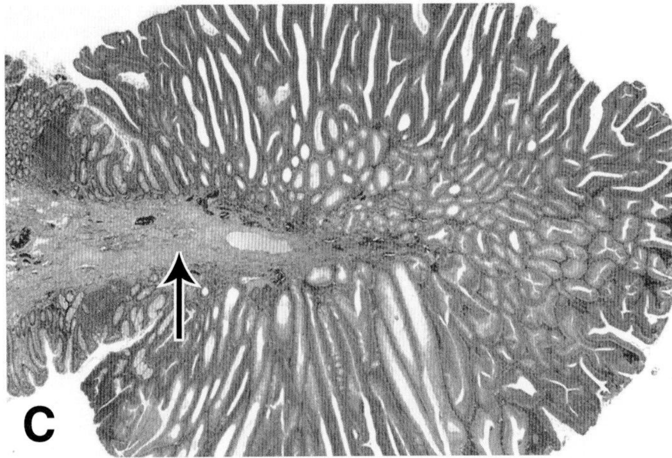

FIGURE 11-55. Tubular adenoma of the colon. A. The adenoma showing a characteristic stalk and bosselated surface. **B.** The bisected adenoma showing the stalk covered by the adenomatous epithelium. The ashen white color is cautery at the polypectomy resection margin from the polypectomy. **C.** Microscopically, the adenoma showing a repetitive pattern that is largely tubular. The stalk (*arrow*), which is in continuity with the submucosa of the colon, is not involved and is lined by normal colonic epithelium.

TUBULAR ADENOMAS: These lesions represent two thirds of large bowel adenomas. They are typically bosselated-surfaced lesions, less than 2 cm, often with a stalk (pedunculated, Fig. 11-55). Some tubular adenomas, particularly the smaller ones, may be sessile (flat).

Tubular adenomas show closely packed epithelial tubules, which may be uniform or irregular and excessively branched (Fig. 11-55C). Tubular adenomas display at least low-grade epithelial dysplasia and, occasionally, high-grade dysplasia, with increased nuclear pleomorphism and complex architecture. High-grade dysplasia can progress to invasive adenocarcinoma, the diagnosis of which requires neoplastic glands below the muscularis mucosae (Fig. 11-56). As long as dysplasia is confined to the mucosa, the lesion is cured by complete polypectomy.

The risk of invasive carcinoma correlates with the size of the adenoma. Only 1% of tubular adenomas less than 1 cm have invasive cancer at the time of resection; of those 1 to 2 cm, 10% harbor malignancy; of those greater than 2 cm, 35% are malignant. Small flat adenomas may be missed during conventional endoscopy and thus have a high risk of progression to cancer.

VILLOUS ADENOMAS: These polyps constitute one tenth of colonic adenomas and are found mainly in the rectosigmoid region. They are typically large, broad-based, elevated lesions with shaggy, cauliflower-like surfaces (Fig. 11-57A). However, they can be small and pedunculated. Most exceed 2 cm, some may reach 10 to 15 cm. Villous adenomas are composed of thin, tall, fingerlike processes that resemble the villi of the small intestine. They are lined externally by neoplastic epithelial cells and are supported by a core of normal lamina propria (Fig. 11-57B).

Dysplasia in villous adenomas resembles that in tubular adenomas. However, villous adenomas contain foci of carcinoma more often than do tubular adenomas. In villous adenomas under 1 cm, the risk of cancer is 10 times higher than that for tubular adenomas of comparable size. More than one third of all resected villous adenomas contain invasive cancer.

TUBULOVILLOUS ADENOMAS: Many adenomatous polyps have both tubular and villous features. Polyps with 25% to 75% villous architecture are "**tubulovillous**." These tend to be intermediate in distribution and size between tubular and villous forms, with one third being greater than 2 cm. Tubulovillous polyps are also intermediate between tubular and villous adenomas in the risk of invasive carcinoma.

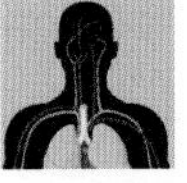

PATHOPHYSIOLOGY: The precursor to colorectal carcinoma is dysplasia, usually in the form of an adenoma. The pathogenesis of adenomas of the colon and rectum involves neoplastic alteration of crypt epithelial homeostasis, with (1) diminished apoptosis, (2) persistent cell replication, and (3) failure of epithelial cells to mature and differentiate as they migrate toward crypt surfaces. Normally, DNA synthesis stops when cells reach the upper one third of crypts, after which they mature, migrate to the surface, and then are sloughed into the lumen. Adenomas represent focal disruption of this orderly sequence in that epithelial cells may proliferate throughout the entire depth of the crypt. Mitotic figures are present along the entire length of the

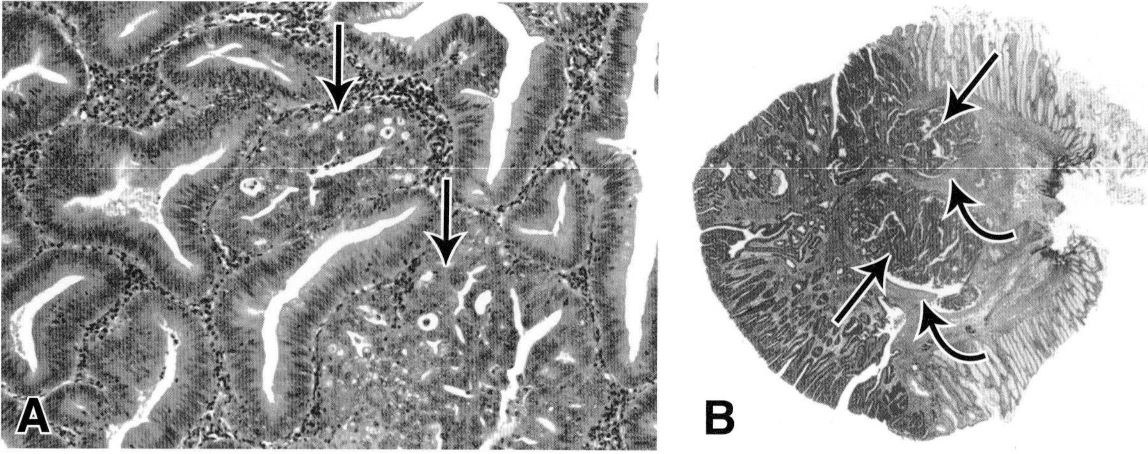

FIGURE 11-56. Adenocarcinoma arising in a pedunculated adenomatous polyp. A. Both low-grade dysplasia and high-grade dysplasia are present. The former is characterized by elongated, hyperchromatic, pseudostratified nuclei. The latter is characterized by a cribriform pattern and increased nuclear pleomorphism (*arrows*). **B.** Trichrome stain showing tumor invading (*arrows*) the stalk (*blue; curved arrows*). Because there was a margin of resection of over 1 mm, polypectomy was sufficient therapy.

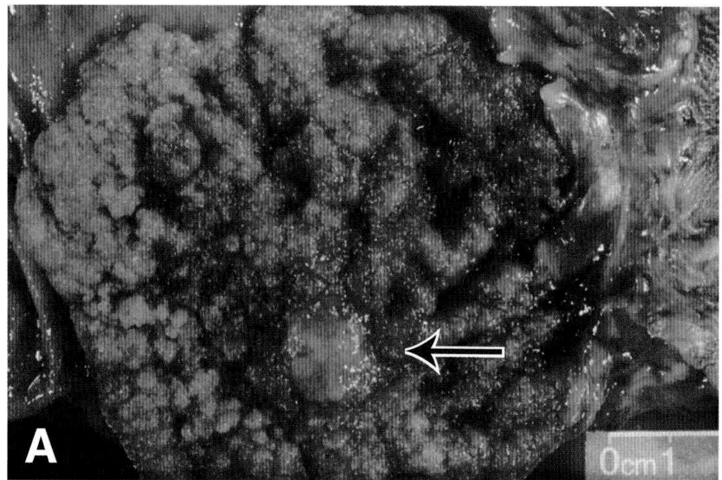

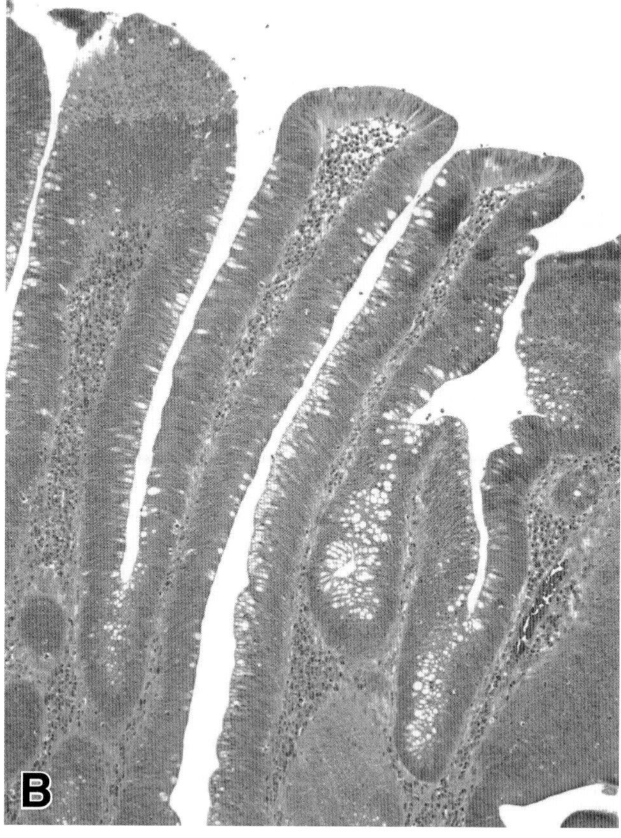

FIGURE 11-57. Villous adenoma of the colon. A. The colon contains a large, broad-based, elevated lesion that has a cauliflower-like surface. A firm area near the center of the lesion (*arrow*) proved on histologic examination to be an adenocarcinoma. **B.** Microscopic examination showing fingerlike processes with fibrovascular cores lined by low-grade dysplastic epithelium.

crypt and on the mucosal surface of adenomas. As the lesion evolves, the proliferation rate exceeds that of sloughing, and cells accumulate in upper crypts and on the surface.

Familial Adenomatous Polyposis

Also called adenomatous polyposis coli (APC), FAP accounts for less than 1% of colorectal cancers. It is caused by a heritable, germline mutation in the *APC* gene on the long arm of chromosome 5 (5q21-22) (see below). Most cases are familial, but 30% to 50% reflect new mutations. FAP is characterized by hundreds to thousands of adenomas carpeting the colorectal mucosa, sometimes throughout its entire length, but particularly in the rectosigmoid region (Fig. 11-58). These are mostly tubular adenomas, but tubulovillous and villous adenomas may also be present. Microscopic adenomas, sometimes involving a single crypt, are numerous. A few polyps are usually already present by age 10, but symptoms generally begin by age 36. By this time, cancer is often already present. Carcinoma of the colon and rectum is inevitable in FAP patients, with the mean

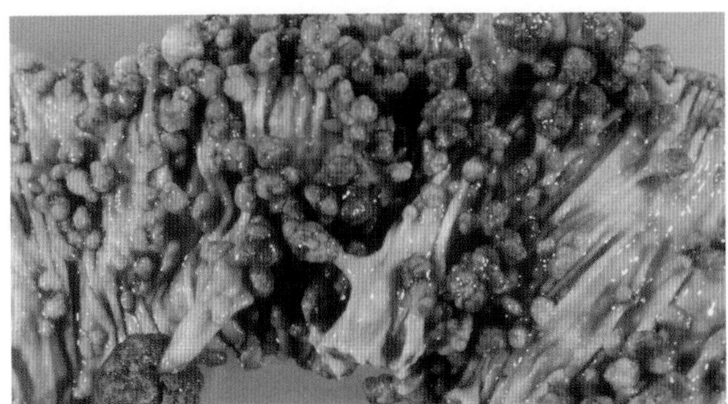

FIGURE 11-58. Familial polyposis. The colon contains thousands of adenomatous polyps with several exceeding 1 cm in diameter.

age of onset at 40 years. Total colectomy before the onset of cancer is curative, but some patients may also have tubular adenomas in the small intestine and stomach, and these have the same malignant potential as those in the colon.

FAP mutations are found in only three fourths of familial cases. Some FAP mutation-negative patients have mutations in *MYH* (a rare, autosomal recessive, polyposis syndrome that clinically overlaps FAP).

Colorectal Adenocarcinomas

In Western societies, colorectal cancer is the third most common cause of cancer and the second leading cause of cancer death. There is a marked geographic difference in the incidence of this cancer, with rates differing by 10-fold between developing and developed countries. This difference is largely attributed to environmental factors because countries that more recently adopted "Western" diets and lifestyles have seen marked increases in colorectal cancer rates. Moreover, people who migrate from low-incidence regions to high-incidence regions develop these cancers at rates similar to the latter region. The term "colorectal" is used because cancers of the colon and rectum share certain biologic features, but there are also differences between them. For instance, colon cancer rates are about equal between men and women, but rectal cancer shows a slight male predominance. The two tumors are also treated differently.

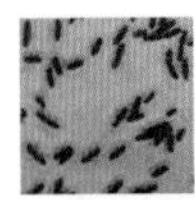

ETIOLOGIC FACTORS: Factors that lead to the development of adenomatous polyps favor colorectal cancer as well. There are several modifiable and nonmodifiable risk factors (see below). Although no one feature of a "Western" lifestyle is identified as causative, multiple factors contribute to a higher incidence of colon cancer. Diet seems to have the greatest impact—either via a direct effect or because of its influence on altering gut flora.

Risk Factors for Colorectal Carcinoma

AGE: Increasing age is probably the single most important risk factor for colorectal cancer in the general population. The risk is low (but not zero) before age 40. It then increases steadily to age 50, after which it doubles each decade.

PRIOR COLORECTAL CANCER: Patients with one colorectal cancer are at increased risk for a subsequent tumor. In fact, 5% to 10% of patients treated for colorectal cancer develop a second such malignancy. Moreover, 2% to 5% of those with a new colorectal cancer have another simultaneous (synchronous) colorectal primary cancer.

ULCERATIVE COLITIS AND CROHN DISEASE: These chronic inflammatory diseases increase colorectal cancer risk in proportion to their duration and extent of large bowel involvement.

GENETIC FACTORS: The risk of colorectal cancer is increased in relatives of patients with the disease, suggesting a genetic contribution to tumorigenesis. People with two or more first- or second-degree relatives with colorectal cancer constitute 20% of all patients with this tumor. Some 5% to 10% of colorectal cancers are inherited as autosomal dominant traits, the most common syndrome being hereditary nonpolyposis colorectal carcinoma (HNPCC or Lynch syndrome [see below]).

DIET: Consumption of animal products, including fat, cholesterol, and protein, parallels the incidence of colorectal cancer. Diets low in fruits, vegetables, and whole grains (fiber) have also been implicated in colorectal carcinogenesis. The reasons for this finding are not entirely clear, but may be related to an effect on gut flora and stool transit time.

PHYSICAL ACTIVITY AND OBESITY: These factors combined are thought to account for up to one third of colorectal cancers. Although not well understood, physical inactivity decreases gut motility. Obesity increases the levels of circulating estrogens and decreases insulin resistance, factors that are believed to influence cancer risk.

CIGARETTE SMOKING AND ALCOHOL: Cigarette smoking has been reported to be an independent risk factor for colon cancer. Chronic alcoholism has also been reported to increase the risk for colorectal cancer although the putative association merits further study.

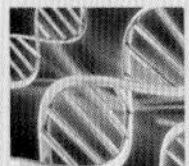

MOLECULAR PATHOGENESIS: In 85% of cases of colorectal carcinoma, it is estimated that at least 8 to 10 mutational events must accumulate before an invasive cancer with metastatic potential develops. This process is initiated in histologically normal mucosa, proceeds through an adenomatous precursor stage, and ends as invasive adenocarcinoma (see Chapter 4).

The most important mutational events involve the following (Fig. 11-59A):

- ***APC* gene:** As noted above, germline mutations in the adenomatous polyposis coli (APC) tumor suppressor gene lead to familial adenomatous polyposis. ***APC is also somatically mutated in 70% to 80% of sporadic colorectal cancers.*** Normal APC is a negative regulator of β-catenin. It binds β-catenin and causes its phosphorylation, followed by ubiquitination and proteasomal degradation. Mutant APC allows β-catenin to accumulate in the nucleus, where it is a transcriptional activator of key proliferation genes (e.g., *cyclin D1* and *MYC*). Some tumors with normal *APC* have mutations in the **β-*catenin* gene** itself. *APC* mutations in normal colonic mucosa precede the development of sporadic adenomas. Thus, *APC* is central to the early development of most colorectal neoplasms.
- *KRAS:* Activating mutations of the *KRAS* proto-oncogene occur early in tubular adenomas of the colon.
- ***DCC* gene:** A putative tumor suppressor gene, deleted in colon cancer (*DCC*), is located on chromosome 18 and is often missing in colorectal cancers.
- *TP53:* Mutations in p53 facilitate the transition from adenoma to the most common type of adenocarcinoma and are late events in colon carcinogenesis.

In 15% of colorectal cancers, the process of **DNA mismatch repair** (MMR; see Chapter 4) is impaired, leading to deficient repair of spontaneous replication errors, particularly in regions with simple repetitive sequences (microsatellites).

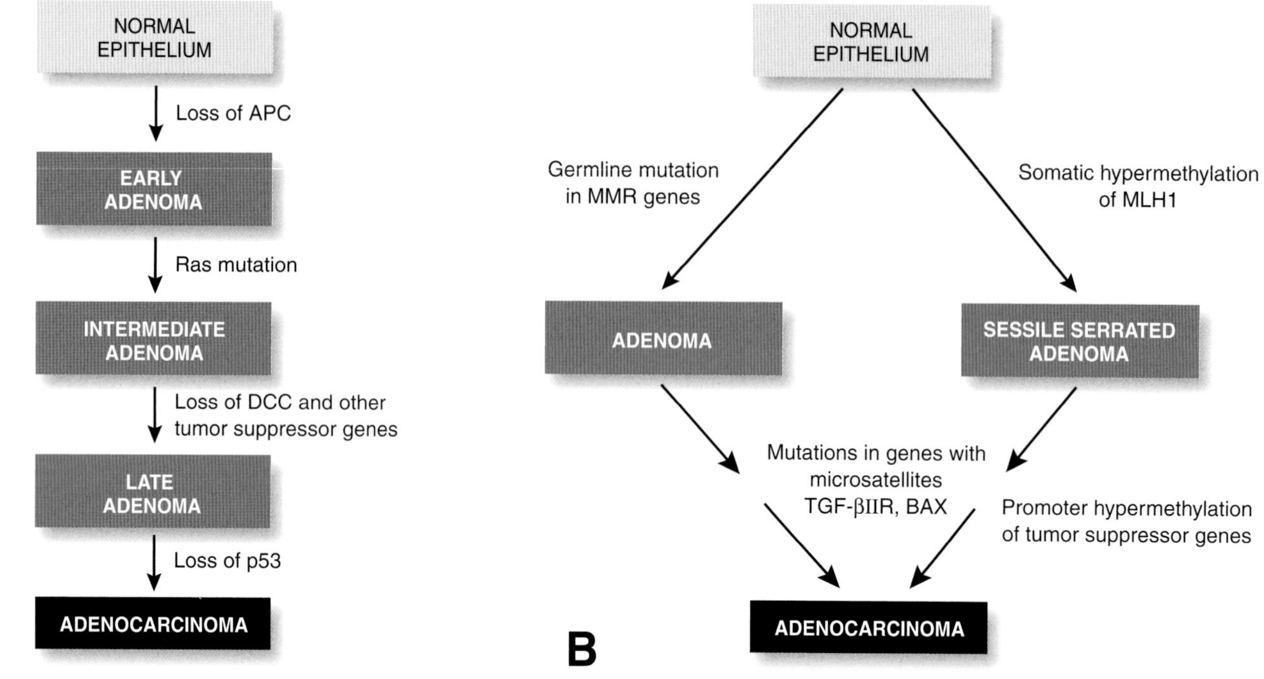

FIGURE 11-59. Model of some of the genetic alterations involved in colonic carcinogenesis. A. The tumor suppressor pathway. **B.** The mismatch repair (MMR) defect pathway. APC, adenomatous polyposis coli; BAX, BCL2-associated X protein; DCC, deleted in colon cancer; MLH1, MutL homolog-1; TGF-βIIR, transforming growth factor-β_2 receptor.

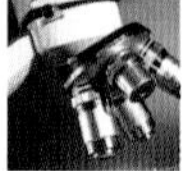

PATHOLOGY: ***The large majority of colorectal cancers are adenocarcinomas that resemble their counterparts elsewhere in the digestive tract.*** They tend to be polypoid and ulcerating or infiltrative, and may be annular and constrictive (Fig. 11-60). Polypoid cancers are more common in the right colon, particularly the cecum, where the large lumen allows unimpeded intraluminal growth. Annular constricting tumors occur more often in the distal colon. Tumors often ulcerate, regardless of growth pattern.

About 15% of colon cancers secrete abundant mucin and are called **mucinous** adenocarcinomas. The degree of differentiation influences the prognosis; better-differentiated tumors tend to have a more favorable outlook.

Colon cancers can spread by direct extension or vascular invasion. Serosal connective tissue offers little resistance to tumor spread, and cancer cells are often seen in the pericolorectal fat far from the primary site. The peritoneum is occasionally involved, in which case there may be multiple deposits throughout the abdomen.

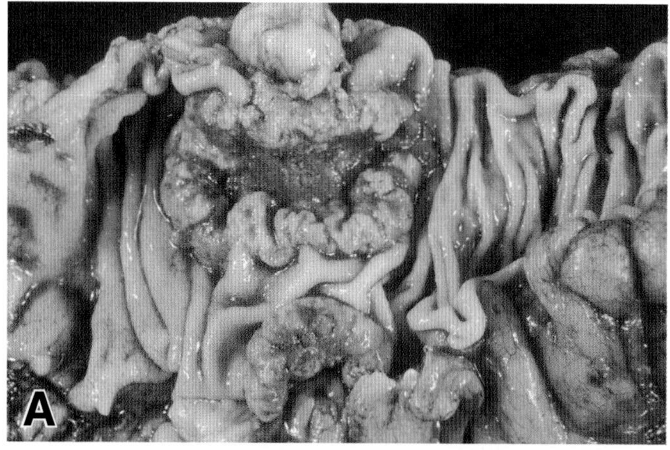

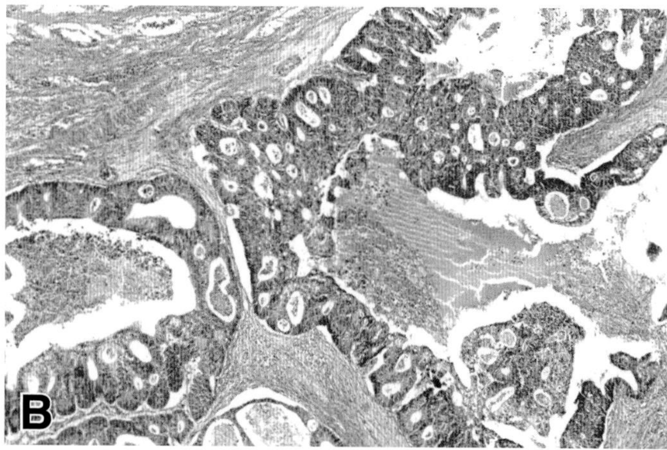

FIGURE 11-60. Adenocarcinoma of the colon. A. A resected colon showing an ulcerated mass with enlarged, firm, rolled borders. **B.** Microscopically, this colon adenocarcinoma consists of moderately differentiated glands with a prominent cribriform pattern and frequent central necrosis.

Colorectal cancer invades lymphatic channels and initially involves lymph nodes immediately below the tumor. The liver is the most common metastatic organ site, but the tumor may spread widely. The prognosis of colorectal cancer is more closely related to tumor extension through the large bowel wall than to its size or histopathology.

Staging of these tumors uses the *t*umor, *l*ymph nodes, and *m*etastasis (TNM) system (see Chapter 4). T1 tumors invade the submucosa; T2 tumors infiltrate into, but not through, the muscularis propria; T3 tumors invade pericolorectal soft tissue; and T4 tumors penetrate the serosa (T4a) or involve adjacent organs (T4b). N reflects the presence or absence of lymph node metastases, and M the presence or absence of distant metastases.

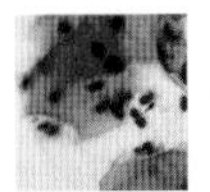

CLINICAL FEATURES: Initially, colorectal cancer is clinically silent. As the tumor grows, the most common sign is **fecal occult blood,** particularly when the tumor is in the proximal colon. Both occult blood and **bright red blood** in the feces may occur if a lesion is located in the distal colorectum.

Cancers on the left side of the colon, where the lumen is narrow and feces are more solid, often constrict the lumen and produce **obstructive symptoms**. These include changes in bowel habits and abdominal pain. Colorectal cancers sometimes **perforate** early and cause peritonitis. By contrast, right-sided cancers may grow large without causing obstruction, especially in the cecum where the lumen is large and fecal contents are liquid. As a result, right-sided tumors can lead to asymptomatic chronic bleeding. **Iron-deficiency anemia** is often the first indication of colorectal cancer.

A positive test for fecal occult blood predicts the presence of a cancer or an adenoma in 50% of cases. Periodic fiberoptic colonoscopy and testing for occult blood in feces can detect tumors at early stages and have improved survival in colorectal cancer.

Resection is the only curative treatment for colorectal cancer. Small polyps are easily removed endoscopically; large lesions require segmental resection.

Hereditary Nonpolyposis Colorectal Cancer (Lynch Syndrome)

HNPCC is an autosomal dominant inherited disease that accounts for 3% to 5% of colorectal cancers.

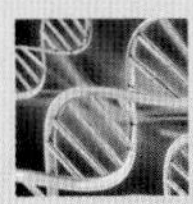

MOLECULAR PATHOGENESIS: Lynch syndrome is caused by germline mutations in a DNA mismatch repair (*MMR*) gene. Usually, human MutS homolog-2 (*hMSH2*) on chromosome 2p and human MutL homolog-1 (*hMLH1*) on chromosome 3p are affected (Fig. 11-59 B). HNPCC features a germline mutation in one allele of one *MMR* gene. The fact that one allele is mutated hinders repair of any second sporadic mutation in the other allele (somatic "second hit"; see Chapter 4). Thereafter, repair of spontaneous replication errors is ineffective. Widespread genomic instability results, particularly in simple repetitive sequences (microsatellites), which are particularly prone to replication errors. Thus, genes that regulate growth and differentiation, and other mismatch repair genes, are disabled by unrepaired mutations.

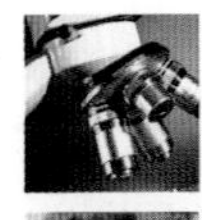

PATHOLOGY AND CLINICAL FEATURES: Lynch syndrome tumors are more often of the mucinous, signet ring cell type and solid (medullary) variety than are sporadic tumors, with many intratumor lymphocytes and Crohn-like lymphocytic reactions. HNPCC patients tend to (1) present with cancer at a young age; (2) have few adenomas (hence "nonpolyposis"); (3) develop tumors proximal to the splenic flexure (70%); (4) have multiple synchronous or metachronous colorectal cancers; and (5) develop extracolonic cancers, especially of the endometrium, ovary, stomach, small intestine, urinary tract, pancreas, hepatobiliary tract, skin, and CNS.

OTHER TUMORS OF THE LARGE INTESTINE

Colonic Mesenchymal Tumors

Mesenchymal tumors arising from tissues normally in the colon include lipoma, liposarcoma, neurofibroma, ganglioneuroma, peripheral nerve sheath tumors, leiomyoma, leiomyosarcoma, vascular tumors, and GISTs (see above). Of these, the most common are submucosal lipomas and leiomyomas.

Colonic Neuroendocrine Tumors

These tumors were also called carcinoid tumors (see above). Half of colorectal NETs have metastasized by the time they are discovered.

Large Bowel Lymphomas

Primary lymphoma of the colorectum is uncommon. It may be seen as (1) segmental mucosal involvement, (2) diffuse polypoid lesions, or (3) a mass extending beyond the colorectum. Symptoms are similar to those of other intestinal cancers, but the diffuse polypoid form may resemble inflammatory or adenomatous polyps. Most colonic lymphomas are tumors of B cells.

The Anus

The anal canal extends from the level of the pelvic floor to the proximal margin of the anal verge. It is about 4 cm long and is divided into three parts, based on its lining epithelium: the colorectal zone (lined by glandular mucosa), the transition zone (varying, transitional mucosa), and the distal zone (lined by squamous mucosa). The dentate (pectinate) line (formed by the anal valves, roughly midway through the anal canal) is easily identified, and the superior border of the anal canal may be defined as 2 cm above this line.

BENIGN LESIONS OF THE ANAL CANAL

Hemorrhoids

They result from downward displacement of the anal cushions. Internal hemorrhoids arise from the superior hemorrhoidal plexus above the dentate (pectinate) line. They are covered by rectal or transitional mucosa. External hemorrhoids originate from the inferior hemorrhoidal plexus below that line and are covered by squamous mucosa. ***Hemorrhoids affect at least 5%***

of people in Western countries (likely a gross underestimate because most people treat themselves for this condition). They are most common in whites between ages 45 and 65 years. Pregnancy is another risk factor, presumably related to increased abdominal pressure.

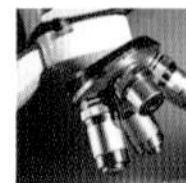

PATHOLOGY: Hemorrhoids are dilated vascular spaces with excess smooth muscle in their walls. Hemorrhage and thrombosis are common.

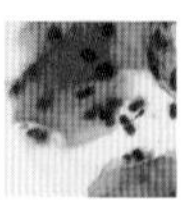

CLINICAL FEATURES: Hemorrhoids cause painless rectal bleeding associated with bowel movements. Whereas chronic blood loss may lead to **iron-deficiency anemia**, other causes must be ruled out before it is attributed to hemorrhoidal bleeding. **Rectal prolapse** is common and causes perineal irritation or anal itching. Prolapsed hemorrhoids may become irreducible and result in painful, strangulated hemorrhoids. **Thrombosed** external hemorrhoids are exquisitely painful and require evacuation of the offending clots. Hemorrhoids are treated with dietary and lifestyle modifications aimed at improving the quality of stools and reducing straining on the toilet. Medical and surgical interventions are also available.

Anal Condylomata Acuminata (Anal Warts)

These lesions are typically benign but may potentially develop into squamous cancers.

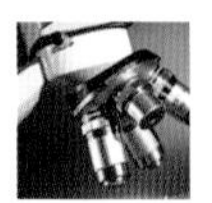

PATHOLOGY: Condylomata have a cauliflower-like growth pattern of papillary excrescences lined by squamous epithelium, which is often hyperkeratotic. The squamous cells show characteristic koilocytic change, having enlarged nuclei with irregular nuclear contours, often binucleated, with perinuclear cytoplasmic clearing. These can develop dysplasia—graded mild, moderate, or severe, similarly to the grading scheme in the cervix (see Chapter 16).

MALIGNANT TUMORS OF THE ANAL CANAL

Anal Canal Squamous Cell Carcinomas

These cancers, although increasing in frequency, are relatively uncommon. They are more common in women than in men, and their incidence is 1.4 per 100,000. In the highest-risk group, homosexuals who practice anal-receptive intercourse, the incidence approaches 35 per 100,000.

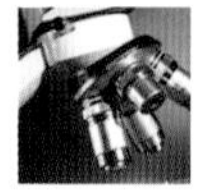

PATHOLOGY: Anal cancers have various histologic patterns although they are simply classified as **squamous cell carcinomas. Bowen disease of the anus** is squamous carcinoma in situ. Anal cancers spread directly into the surrounding tissues, including internal and external sphincters, perianal soft tissues, the prostate, and the vagina.

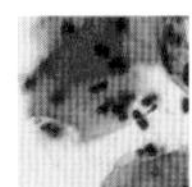

CLINICAL FEATURES: The major risk factor for anal squamous cell carcinoma is infection with HPV. Other risk factors include HIV infection, immunosuppression in organ transplantation, the presence of an immune disorder, and smoking.

PERITONITIS

Bacterial Peritonitis

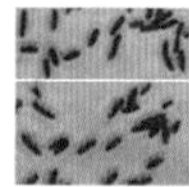

ETIOLOGIC FACTORS

PERFORATION: ***The most common cause of bacterial peritonitis is perforation of an abdominal viscus*** (e.g., an inflamed appendix, peptic ulcer, or colon diverticulum). Peritonitis results in an acute abdomen, with severe abdominal pain and tenderness. Nausea, vomiting, and a high fever are usual. In severe cases, generalized peritonitis, paralytic ileus, and septic shock ensue. Often, the perforation is "walled off," in which case a peritoneal abscess results.

SPONTANEOUS BACTERIAL PERITONITIS: Sometimes, peritoneal infection lacks a clear cause. ***Such spontaneous bacterial peritonitis occurs most often in adults with cirrhosis complicated by portal hypertension and ascites*** (see Chapter 12). Enteric organisms, mainly Gram-negative bacilli, appear to move from the gut to mesenteric lymph nodes. From there, they seed the ascitic fluid, where phagocytic and antibacterial activities are low.

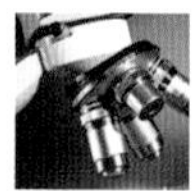

PATHOLOGY: Grossly, bacterial peritonitis resembles purulent infection elsewhere. A fibrinopurulent exudate covers the surface of the intestines. When it organizes, fibrinous and fibrous adhesions form between loops of bowel, which then adhere to each other. Such adhesions may eventually be lysed, or they may lead to **volvulus** and **intestinal obstruction**. Bacterial salpingitis, usually caused by gonococcus, may terminate in pelvic peritonitis and adhesions. This occurrence defines **pelvic inflammatory disease** (see Chapter 16).

NEOPLASMS OF THE PERITONEUM

Malignant Peritoneal Mesotheliomas

One quarter of mesotheliomas arise in the peritoneum. ***Like pleural mesotheliomas, some of these malignant tumors are associated with exposure to asbestos, whereas many are idiopathic.*** Pathologic characteristics of peritoneal mesotheliomas are identical to those of their pleural counterparts (see Chapter 10).

Primary Peritoneal Carcinomas

Primary peritoneal carcinomas present as tumor masses involving the omentum and peritoneum. They are morphologically identical to serous carcinomas of the ovary, except that in primary peritoneal carcinomas, the ovaries are normal.

Metastatic Carcinomas

Ovarian, gastric, and pancreatic carcinomas are particularly likely to seed the peritoneum, but any intra-abdominal malignancy can spread to the peritoneum.

12 The Liver and Biliary System

Arief A. Suriawinata ▪ Swan N. Thung

LEARNING OBJECTIVES

- Correlate the structure and specific function of cells found within the liver lobule with the metabolic functions of the liver.
- Compare and contrast the etiologic agents, pathogenesis, and clinical course of viral hepatitis.
- Distinguish between type I and type II autoimmune hepatitis.
- Describe the progressive stages of alcoholic liver disease.
- Discuss the risk factors for and the pathogenesis of nonalcoholic fatty liver disease.
- Describe the pathogenesis of cirrhosis and correlate it with the pathologic and clinical features of the disease process.
- Describe the pathogenesis of the most common heritable disorders associated with cirrhosis.
- Differentiate between primary (genetic) and secondary iron overload syndromes in terms of iron storage dysregulation.
- Describe the histologic patterns and agents associated with drug-induced liver disease.
- Correlate the clinical consequences of liver failure with the pathogenesis of the disease process.
- Describe the causes and consequences of portal hypertension.
- Discuss different mechanisms of defective bilirubin metabolism.
- Differentiate intrahepatic and extrahepatic cholestasis.
- Differentiate the pathogenesis and clinical course of primary biliary cirrhosis and sclerosing cholangitis.
- List the distinguishing features of benign and malignant hepatic neoplasms.
- Describe the pathophysiology of cholelithiasis.
- Differentiate the pathologic findings and clinical consequences of acute and chronic cholecystitis.
- Describe carcinomas associated with the liver, gallbladder and bile ducts.

STRUCTURE OF THE LIVER AND THE BILIARY SYSTEM

The liver, located in the right upper quadrant of the abdomen, just below the diaphragm, has two lobes, a larger **right lobe** and a smaller **left lobe**, which meet at the level of the gallbladder bed. The **gallbladder** lies inferiorly in a fossa of the right hepatic lobe and extends a little below the inferior margin of the liver.

The liver has a dual blood supply: (1) the **hepatic artery**, a branch of the celiac axis; and (2) the **portal vein**, formed where the splenic and superior mesenteric veins join. The **hepatic veins** empty into the inferior vena cava, which is partly surrounded by the posterior surface of the liver. Hepatic lymphatics drain mainly into the porta hepatis and celiac lymph nodes.

The right and left hepatic ducts merge to form the **hepatic duct**, which joins the cystic duct from the gallbladder to form the **common bile duct**. The latter meets the pancreatic duct immediately before emptying into the duodenum. It terminates in the ampulla of Vater, where its lumen is guarded by the sphincter of Oddi.

Liver lobules are polyhedral (Figs. 12-1 and 12-2), classically depicted as hexagons. **Portal triads** (or portal tracts) are peripheral, at the angles of the polygon, and contain

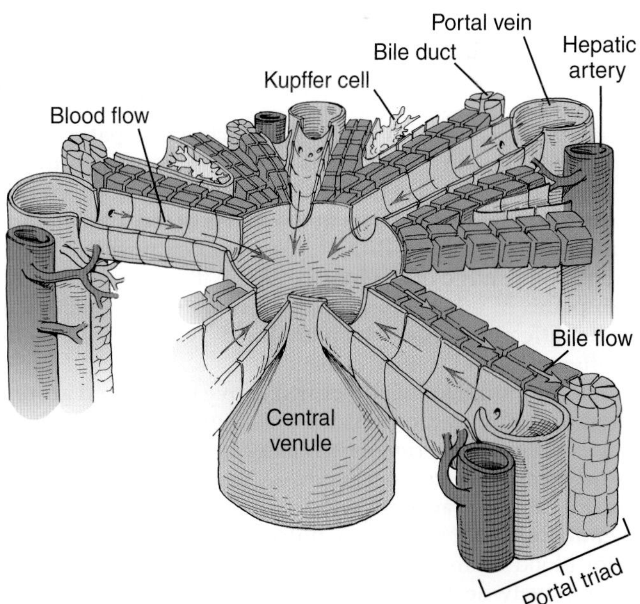

FIGURE 12-1. Microanatomy of the liver. The classic lobule is composed of portal triads, hepatic sinuses, a terminal hepatic venule (central venule), and associated plates of hepatocytes. *Red arrows* indicate the direction of sinusoidal blood flow. *Green arrows* show the direction of bile flow. (From Ross MH, Pawlina W. *Histology: A Text and Atlas*, 6th ed. Philadelphia: Lippincott Williams & Wilkins, 2011: 636.)

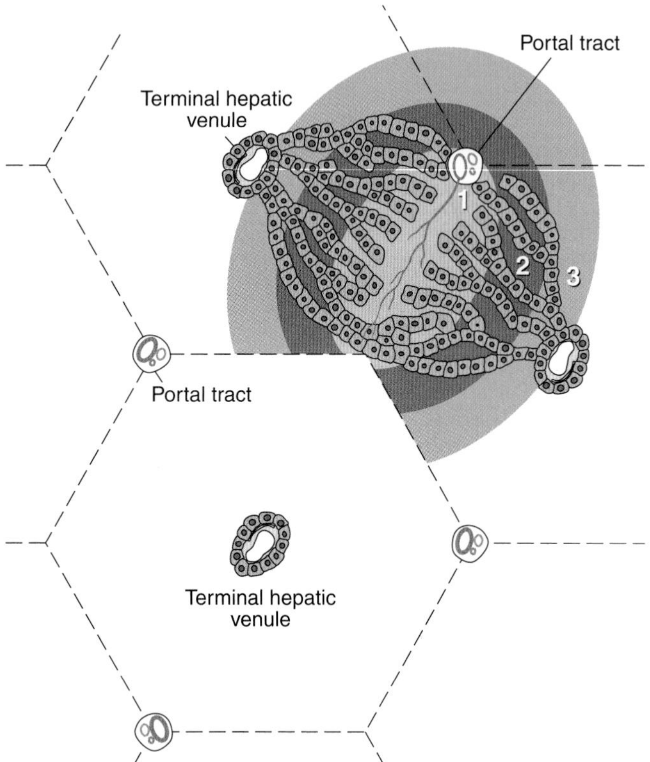

FIGURE 12-2. Morphologic and functional concepts of the liver lobule. In the classic *morphologic* liver lobule, the periphery of the hexagonal lobule is anchored in the portal tracts, and the terminal hepatic venule is in the center. The *functional* liver lobule is an acinus derived from the gradients of oxygen and nutrients in the sinusoidal blood. In this scheme, the portal tract, with the richest content of oxygen and nutrients, is in the center (zone 1). The region most distant from the portal tract (zone 3) is poor in oxygen and nutrients and surrounds the terminal hepatic venule. Zone 2 is intermediate in location between zones 1 and 3.

intrahepatic branches of the (1) **bile ducts**, (2) **hepatic artery**, and (3) **portal vein**. Portal tracts are invested by the **limiting plate**, a layer of adjacent hepatocytes. The **central venule (terminal hepatic venule)** is at the center of the lobule. Radiating from it are **one-cell-thick plates of hepatocytes**, which extend to the edge of the lobule, where they are continuous with plates of other lobules. Between plates of hepatocytes are **hepatic sinusoids**, which are lined by endothelial cells, Kupffer cells, and stellate cells.

The structural lobule described above is arranged around a central venule and reflects the histologic appearance of the liver. ***However, a functional unit can be conceptualized with the portal tract* at the center** (Fig. 12-2). Such a construct reflects the **functional gradients** within lobules and is termed the **liver acinus**. That is, oxygen, nutrients, and so on, delivered by the blood are most concentrated near the portal tracts, then progressively decline as hepatocytes extract these materials from the blood going through the sinusoids toward the central venule. Such a construct allows for concentric functional zones. **Zone 1** is the most highly oxygenated zone, around portal tracts. **Zone 3** surrounds central venules and is poor in oxygen. **Zone 2** is intermediate and midlobular. Ischemic injury usually affects zone 3 first. The differences between hepatocytes in the acinus are not limited to the blood flow to which they are exposed but are also heterogeneous with respect to metabolism, independent of oxygenation. In particular, toxic injury is often prominent in zone 3, the cells of which are enriched in enzymes that perform drug detoxification and biotransformation. However, for convenience, pathologic changes in the liver are usually designated in relation to the classic histologic lobule. For example, centrilobular necrosis describes a lesion around central venules, and periportal fibrosis occurs at the periphery of the classic lobule. Yet, functionally, these changes occur in zones 3 and 1, respectively.

FUNCTIONS OF THE LIVER

The liver, through its hepatocytes, performs metabolic, synthetic, storage, catabolic, and excretory functions.

METABOLIC FUNCTIONS: The liver is a center of **glucose homeostasis** and responds rapidly to fluctuations in blood glucose levels. Free fatty acids are taken up by the liver and oxidized to produce energy or are converted to triglycerides and secreted as **lipoproteins** to be used elsewhere.

SYNTHETIC FUNCTIONS: Most plasma proteins are synthesized in the liver. **Albumin** is the main source of plasma oncotic pressure; in chronic liver disease decreased albumin causes edema and ascites. Blood **clotting factors**, including prothrombin and fibrinogen, are produced by hepatocytes. Severe and often life-threatening bleeding may thus complicate liver failure. Hepatic endothelial cells manufacture **factors V and VIII**; as a result, hemophilia can be treated by liver transplantation. **Complement** and other "acute-phase reactants" (e.g., ferritin, C-reactive protein, and serum amyloid A) are also secreted by the liver. Numerous specific **binding proteins** (such as those for iron, copper, and vitamin A) are also secreted by the liver.

STORAGE FUNCTIONS: The liver stores glycogen, triglycerides, iron, copper, and lipid-soluble vitamins. Severe liver disease can result from excessive storage—for example, abnormal glycogen deposition in type IV glycogenosis, excess iron in hemochromatosis, and copper in Wilson disease.

CATABOLIC FUNCTIONS: The liver catabolizes many endogenous substances, such as hormones and serum proteins. As a result, in chronic liver disease, impaired elimination of estrogens causes feminization in men. The liver is also the principal **detoxifier of foreign compounds**, such as drugs, industrial chemicals, environmental contaminants, and, perhaps, products of intestinal bacterial metabolism.

Ammonia from amino acid metabolism is mainly removed by the liver. Serum ammonia increases in liver failure and is used as a marker for this condition.

EXCRETORY FUNCTIONS: The principal excretory product of the liver is **bile**, an aqueous mixture of conjugated bilirubin, bile acids, phospholipids, cholesterol, and electrolytes. Bile is a repository for the products of heme catabolism and is vital for fat absorption in the small intestine. Normal bile production is critical for eliminating environmental toxins, carcinogens, and drugs and their metabolites.

CAUSES AND EFFECTS OF LIVER INJURY: INTRODUCTION

Liver injury may be caused by hepatocyte destruction by viral infection or autoimmune effects (hepatitis), environmental agents such as alcohol (fatty liver or cirrhosis), or drugs and other toxic agents. Defects in the storage functions of the liver for iron and copper can also lead to hepatocyte injury either directly or through indirect mechanisms. Neoplastic disease of the liver may be primary, often the end product of chronic viral infection or, far more commonly represents metastatic tumors deposited in the liver. The result of such damage to the liver may be either acute liver failure or chronic injury, the latter resulting in cirrhosis. This condition is characterized by the destruction of normal liver architecture and impairment of vascular flow, resulting in hypertension in the portal circulation (portal hypertension). Defects in bile flow and metabolism may cause hyperbilirubinemia (increased concentration of bilirubin in the blood), expressed clinically as jaundice, with yellow skin and sclera and a host of systemic effects, as well as local injury to the liver itself.

HEPATITIS

Hepatitis (i.e., inflammation of the liver) results from viral infection or autoimmune processes. ***Infection of hepatocytes causes liver necrosis and inflammation and may be either acute or chronic.***

Acute Viral Hepatitis

The hallmark of acute viral hepatitis is liver cell death (Fig. 12-3). Within the hepatic lobule, scattered single-cell necrosis or death of small clusters of hepatocytes is seen. A few apoptotic liver cells appear as small, deeply eosinophilic bodies (**acidophilic bodies**), sometimes with pyknotic nuclei. Acidophilic bodies are characteristic of viral hepatitis but are also seen in many other liver diseases. In acute viral hepatitis, many liver cells show varying degrees of hydropic swelling and differences in size, shape, and staining properties. Concomitantly, regenerative liver cells may have larger nuclei and basophilic cytoplasm. The resulting irregular liver cell plates are described as **lobular disarray**.

Mononuclear cells, mostly lymphocytes, infiltrate lobules diffusely, surround individual necrotic liver cells, and accumulate in areas of focal necrosis. Macrophages may be prominent, whereas sparse eosinophils and polymorphonuclear leukocytes are not uncommon. Characteristically, lymphocytes infiltrate between the wall of the central vein and the liver cell plates. Mononuclear inflammatory cells also accumulate within portal tracts. Sometimes, lymphocytes in portal tracts form follicles, particularly in hepatitis C. The limiting plate of hepatocytes around the portal tracts is usually intact. Cholestasis (visible bile in canaliculi) is common. Clinically, this may be expressed as jaundice in the patient. If severe, it is called **cholestatic hepatitis**, in which many liver cells are arrayed around dilated bile canaliculi, giving an acinar or glandular appearance. Lumens of dilated canaliculi may contain large bile plugs (Fig. 12-4). These changes are gradually reversed when recovery occurs and normal hepatic architecture is completely restored.

Confluent hepatic necrosis reflects a particularly severe form of acute hepatitis and is characterized by death of many hepatocytes in a geographical distribution. In extreme cases, almost all liver cells in a lobule die (**massive hepatic necrosis**). The most common viral cause is acute hepatitis B; only rarely does confluent hepatic necrosis result from infection with other hepatotropic viruses. The lesions are not unique to viral hepatitis but may also occur after exposure to hepatotoxic chemicals and in autoimmune hepatitis (see below). Unlike most common forms of acute viral hepatitis, in which liver cell necrosis appears to be random and patchy, confluent hepatic necrosis typically affects whole regions of lobules The lesions of confluent hepatic necrosis, in order of increasing severity, are termed bridging necrosis, submassive necrosis, and massive necrosis (Fig. 12-5).

In the case of submassive necrosis, entire lobules die, an effect that may rapidly proceed to hepatic failure, defined clinically as **fulminant hepatitis**. Massive hepatic necrosis is both rare and almost invariably fatal. The liver is shrunken to as little as 500 g (one third of normal weight). The capsule is wrinkled, with mottled, soft, and flabby red-tan parenchyma. Virtually, all hepatocytes are dead (Fig. 12-6), and only the collagenous frameworks remain. Liver transplantation is a mainstay of therapy.

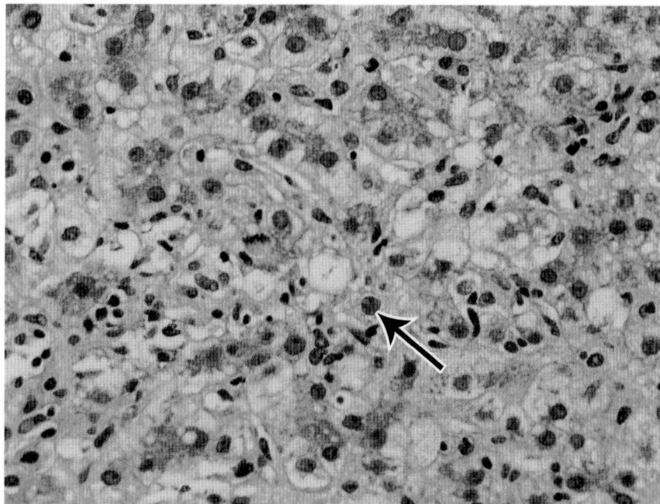

FIGURE 12-3. Acute viral hepatitis. Disarray of liver cell plates, swollen (ballooned) hepatocytes, and an infiltrate of lymphocytes and scattered mononuclear inflammatory cells. The remnants of apoptotic hepatocytes have been extruded into the sinusoids, where they appear as acidophilic bodies (*arrow*).

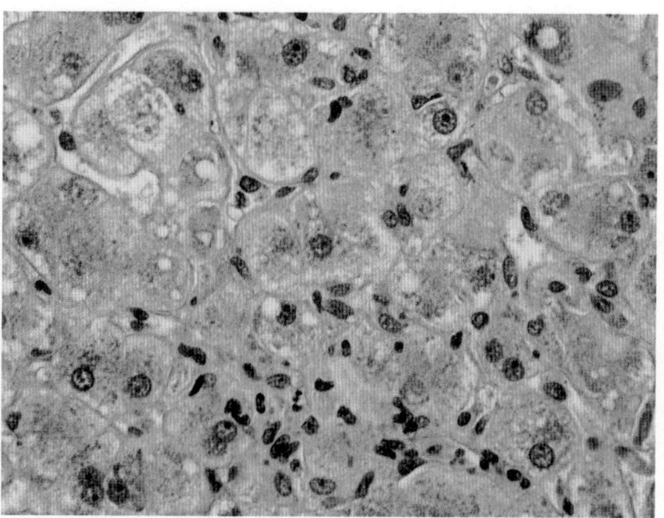

FIGURE 12-4. Cholestasis. Hepatocytes are swollen and bile stained (feathery degeneration).

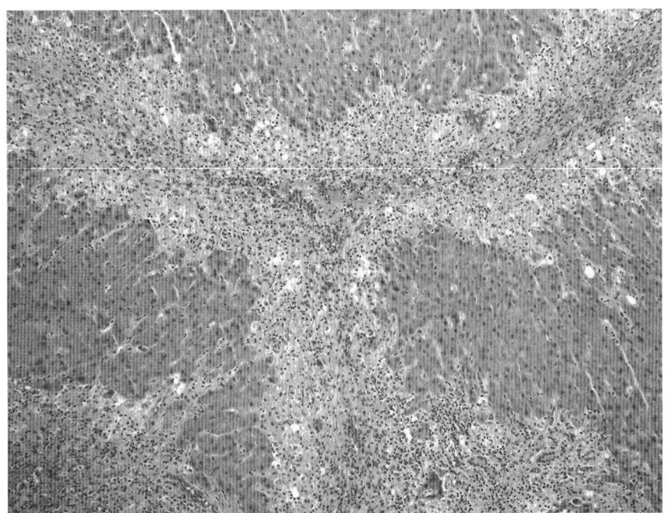

FIGURE 12-5. Confluent hepatic necrosis. Hemorrhagic zones of necrosis bridge adjacent central veins and portal tracts (bridging necrosis).

The Morphology of Chronic Hepatitis

The morphologic spectrum of chronic hepatitis ranges from mild portal inflammation with little or no liver cell necrosis to widespread inflammation, necrosis, and fibrosis, eventuating in cirrhosis (Fig. 12-7).

PORTAL TRACT LESIONS: In chronic hepatitis, portal tracts are variably infiltrated by lymphocytes, plasma cells, and macrophages (Fig. 12-7). These expanded portal tracts often show mild-to-severe proliferation of bile ductules, which is a nonspecific response to chronic liver injury. In the case of chronic hepatitis C, lymphoid aggregates or follicles with reactive centers are often present.

PIECEMEAL NECROSIS: Piecemeal necrosis is focal inflammatory destruction of the limiting plate of hepatocytes. A periportal chronic inflammatory infiltrate creates an irregular border between portal tracts and the lobular parenchyma (Fig. 12-7A).

INTRALOBULAR LESIONS: Focal necrosis and parenchymal inflammation typify chronic hepatitis. Scattered acidophilic bodies and enlarged Kupffer cells are common (Fig. 12-3). In chronic hepatitis B, scattered hepatocytes may show a large granular cytoplasm with abundant HBsAg (**ground-glass hepatocytes**).

PERIPORTAL FIBROSIS: Progressive loss of periportal hepatocytes by piecemeal necrosis leads to the deposition of collagen, giving portal tracts a stellate (star-shaped) appearance. In time, fibrosis may join adjacent portal tracts or approach the central vein, ultimately developing into cirrhosis (Fig. 12-7B).

VIRAL HEPATITIS: CAUSATIVE AGENTS

Worldwide, more than 500 million people are infected with hepatotropic viruses, which place them at great risk for hepatocellular carcinoma (HCC). Many viruses and other infectious agents can produce hepatitis and jaundice (Table 12-1), but in the industrialized world, more than 95% of cases of viral hepatitis are caused by hepatitis A, B, C, D, and E viruses (HAV, HBV, etc.)

Hepatitis A Virus

Hepatitis A virus (HAV) is a small RNA-containing enterovirus of the picornavirus family (which includes polio virus). It mainly replicates in hepatocytes, but gastrointestinal epithelial cells may also be infected. Infectious virus progenies are shed into the bile and present in the feces. Because HAV is not directly cytopathic, hepatic injury has been attributed to the immunologic reaction against virally infected hepatocytes.

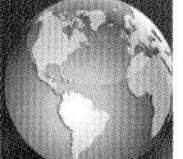

EPIDEMIOLOGY: The only reservoir for HAV is acutely infected people, so transmission is mostly from person to person by the fecal–oral route. Epidemics of hepatitis A occur in crowded and unsanitary conditions, such as exist in warfare, or by fecal contamination of water and food. Edible shellfish in contaminated waters

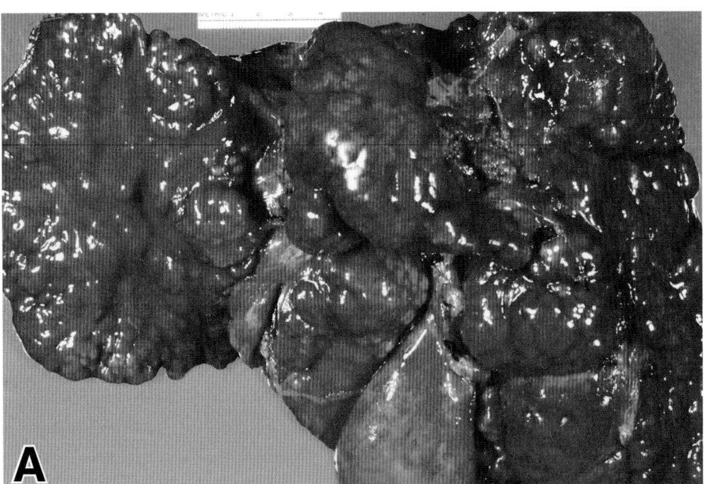

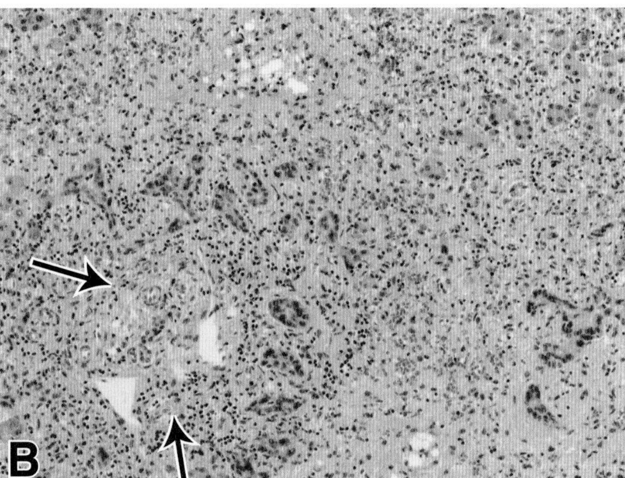

FIGURE 12-6. Massive hepatic necrosis. A. The liver is soft and reduced in size and shows a mottled, yellowish surface ("acute yellow atrophy"). **B.** Complete loss of the hepatocytes. The framework of the lobule has collapsed. The portal tracts (*arrows*) are expanded and contain ductular reaction.

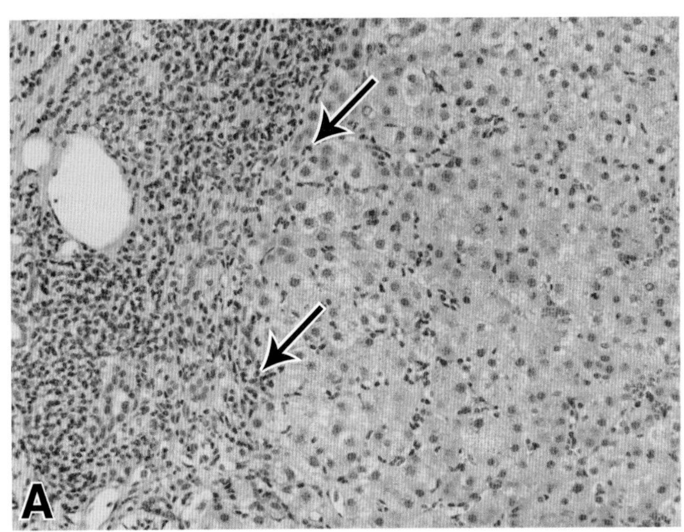
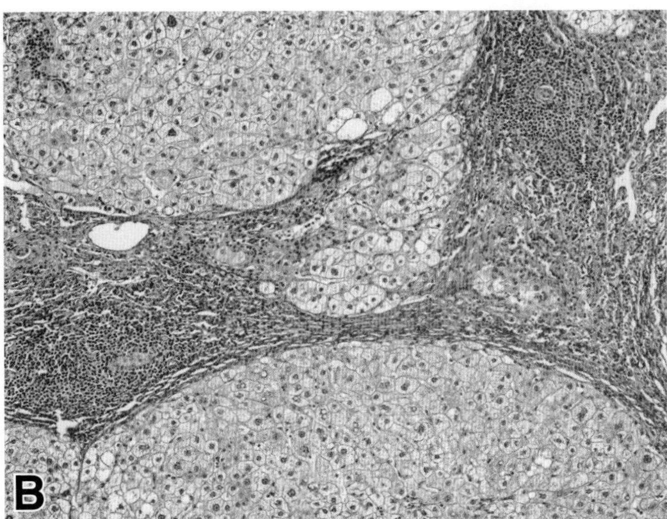

FIGURE 12-7. Severe chronic hepatitis. A. Mononuclear inflammatory infiltration in an expanded portal tract (*left*). Interface hepatitis is penetration of inflammation to the limiting plate and surrounds groups of hepatocytes at the border of the portal tract (*arrows*). **B. Chronic hepatitis with cirrhosis.** A liver from a patient with long-standing chronic hepatitis C showing lymphocytic aggregates, bridging fibrosis, and nodular transformation.

concentrate the virus and may transmit infection if they are not adequately cooked.

In industrialized countries, which have low rates of infection, most cases of hepatitis A are seen in older children and adults. By contrast, in less developed regions, where the disease is endemic, most of the population is infected before 10 years of age.

In the United States, about 10% of the population younger than 20 years show serologic evidence of previous HAV infection, indicating that ***most HAV infections are anicteric, that is, they do not produce visible jaundice.*** Hepatitis A is common in day care centers, among international travelers, and in men who have sex with men. However, no source is identified in about half of cases. Hepatitis A vaccination confers long-term protection from the disease, and universal vaccination programs have significantly reduced the incidence of acute hepatitis A in the United States.

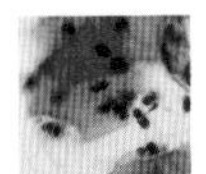

CLINICAL FEATURES: After an incubation period of 3 to 6 weeks (mean, about 4 weeks), HAV-infected patients develop nonspecific symptoms, including fever, malaise, and anorexia. Concomitantly, liver injury is evidenced by a rise in serum aminotransferases (Fig. 12-8). Aminotransferase levels begin to decline, usually 5 to 10 days later. The period of viremia is also short, occurring early in the disease, at which time jaundice may appear. It remains

Table 12-1

Infectious Agents That Cause Hepatitis

Hepatitis A virus	Herpes simplex virus
Hepatitis B virus ± Hepatitis D virus	Cytomegalovirus
Hepatitis C virus	Enteroviruses other than hepatitis A virus
Hepatitis E virus	
Yellow fever virus	Leptospires (leptospirosis)
Epstein–Barr virus (infectious mononucleosis)	*Entamoeba histolytica* (amebic hepatitis)
Lassa, Marburg, and Ebola viruses	

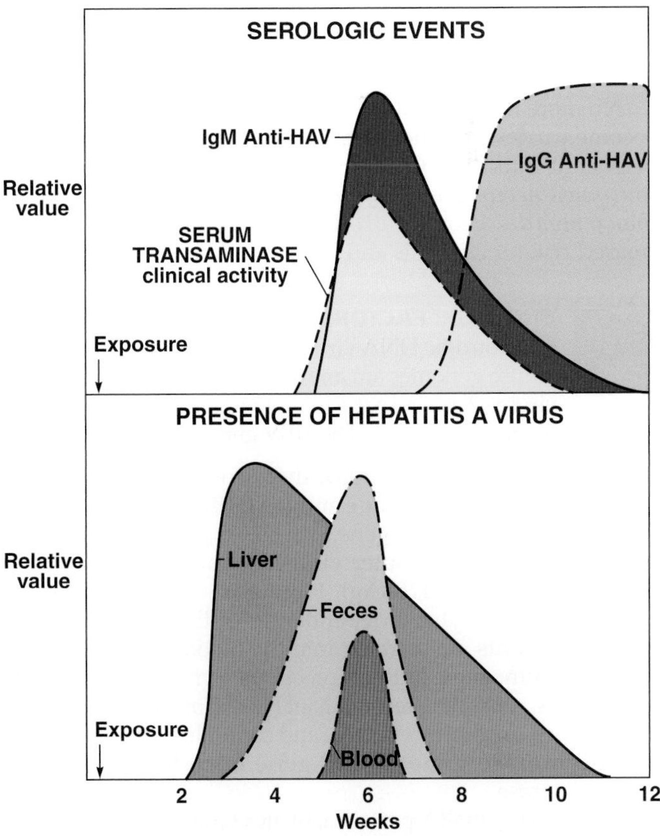

FIGURE 12-8. Typical serologic events associated with hepatitis A virus (HAV). Ig, immunoglobulin.

evident for an average of 10 days but may persist for more than a month. Aminotransferase levels generally return to normal by the time jaundice has disappeared. ***Hepatitis A never becomes chronic. There is no carrier state, and infection provides lifelong immunity.*** Fulminant hepatitis is rare, and virtually, all patients recover without sequelae.

Hepatitis B

Unlike hepatitis A, hepatitis B infection is a major cause of acute and, more significantly, chronic liver disease. More than 350 million chronic carriers of HBV in the world constitute an enormous reservoir of infection. Carrier rates of chronic infection vary from 0.3% (the United States and Western Europe) to 20% (Southeast Asia, Sub-Saharan Africa, Oceania, and the Pacific and Amazon basins), depending on the rate of primary infection. In endemic areas, high carrier rates are sustained by vertical transmission from carrier mothers to newborns. **The use of a protective vaccine has drastically lowered the incidence of HBV in the United States, where vaccination is common.** In the industrialized world, chronic HBV carriers are most common among male homosexuals and IV drug users. ***Infectious virus is only present in blood, saliva, and semen.*** Most cases of hepatitis B are now transmitted by intimate contact, which transfers virus through breaks in the skin or mucous membranes. Anal sexual contact is thus an important mode of transmission.

Rarely, acute hepatitis B can be a fulminant disease that is associated with massive liver cell necrosis. However, most adult patients have acute, self-limited hepatitis B, similar to that produced by HAV, which is usually followed by complete recovery and lifelong immunity. Symptoms of hepatitis B are largely similar to those of hepatitis A, but acute hepatitis B tends to be somewhat more severe, and its incubation period is much longer.

No more than 10% of people infected with HBV as adults become carriers, but neonatal hepatitis B generally leads to persistent infection. ***Chronic hepatitis is characterized by continued necrosis and inflammation in the liver for more than 6 months.*** People with chronic HBV infection are at increased risk for cirrhosis and hepatocellular carcinoma.

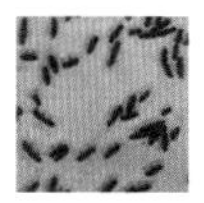

ETIOLOGIC FACTORS: Hepatitis B virus (HBV) is a hepatotropic DNA virus of the **hepadnavirus** group, whose genomes are among the smallest of all known viruses. The viral particle is a 42-nm sphere (*Dane particle*) that contains the viral DNA. The HBV genome has four genes.

- **Core (*C*) gene:** The core of the virus contains the **core antigen (HBcAg)** and the **e antigen (HBeAg)**, both of which are products of the *C* gene.
- **Surface gene:** The outer viral coat contains **hepatitis B surface antigen (HBsAg)**. HBsAg is synthesized by infected hepatocytes independently of the viral core, and vast amounts are secreted into the blood. These particles are immunogenic but not infectious. Synthetic hepatitis B vaccines, containing recombinant HBsAg or its immunogenic epitopes, are highly effective and confer lifelong immunity.
- **Polymerase gene:** The *P* gene encodes viral DNA polymerase.
- ***X* gene:** The small X protein activates viral transcription and probably plays a role in HBV-related hepatocarcinogenesis associated with chronic HBV infection.

The antigens produced by the virus and the antibody response to them are of diagnostic and prognostic significance (Fig. 12-9).

HBsAg is the first marker to appear in the serum of patients with acute hepatitis B. It appears 1 to 8 weeks after exposure and disappears from the blood during convalescence in those patients who recover rapidly. Simultaneously with, or shortly thereafter, HBsAg disappears, and serum antibody to HBsAg (anti-HBs) becomes detectable. Its appearance heralds complete recovery and provides lifelong immunity.

HBcAg (core antigen) is not seen in blood of persons with acute hepatitis B, but antibody to HBcAg (anti-HBc) appears shortly after HBsAg. Antibody to HBcAg serves only as a marker of prior HBV infection.

HBeAg circulates before the onset of clinical disease and after the appearance of HBsAg. It generally disappears within about 2 weeks, whereas HBsAg is still present. Serum HBeAg correlates with a period of intense viral replication and, hence, maximal infectivity of the patient. Anti-HBe antibody appears shortly after the antigen disappears and is detectable up to 2 years or more after the hepatitis resolves. Most patients with chronic infection remain positive for serum HBeAg, but they may seroconvert during the symptomatic phase of chronic infection.

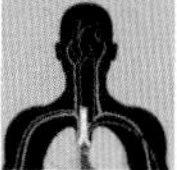

PATHOPHYSIOLOGY: Hepatitis B virus is not directly cytopathic. Asymptomatic chronic carriers of the virus, who have large loads of the infectious agent in the liver, remain asymptomatic for years in a state of immune tolerance, without functional or biochemical evidence of liver cell injury. Cytotoxic ($CD8^+$) T lymphocytes (CTLs) that target multiple HBV epitopes cause most of the destruction of hepatocytes and consequent clinical liver disease. Target viral antigens are expressed on the surface of infected hepatocytes, where they are recognized by $CD8^+$ cells. These CTLs, in turn, kill infected hepatocytes.

Three phases of chronic hepatitis B are recognized:

1. **Immune tolerant phase:** Patients in this phase have very high HBV DNA levels but little significant hepatocellular inflammation or necrosis. Serum aminotransferase levels are normal. This phase may last for decades and is common among those who acquired HBV by vertical transmission as neonates. HBV DNA integrates into cellular DNA. Patients in this phase are at increased risk for hepatocellular carcinoma (HCC).
2. **Immune active phase:** This phase is characterized by HBV viremia, liver cell necrosis, and elevated serum aminotransferases. Portal-based inflammatory infiltrates and hepatocyte necrosis are seen. Significant liver injury, cirrhosis, and HCC tend to develop in this phase. Antiviral therapy is often initiated in the immune active phase.
3. **Inactive phase:** In the inactive phase, serum aminotransferases are normal, and blood levels of HBV DNA are low. These people are "asymptomatic carriers" and are at very low risk of progression to cirrhosis or HCC. However, they may revert to immune active disease and thus require long-term follow-up. A recovery phase does not generally occur.

In some chronic HBV carriers, HBsAg–anti-HBs complexes circulate in the blood. Thus, these patients produce antibody but do not clear the viral antigen from the circulation. Such circulating immune complexes may lead to **extrahepatic** complications, including a serum sickness–like syndrome (fever, rash, urticaria, and acute arthritis), polyarteritis, glomerulonephritis, and cryoglobulinemia. In fact, one third to one half

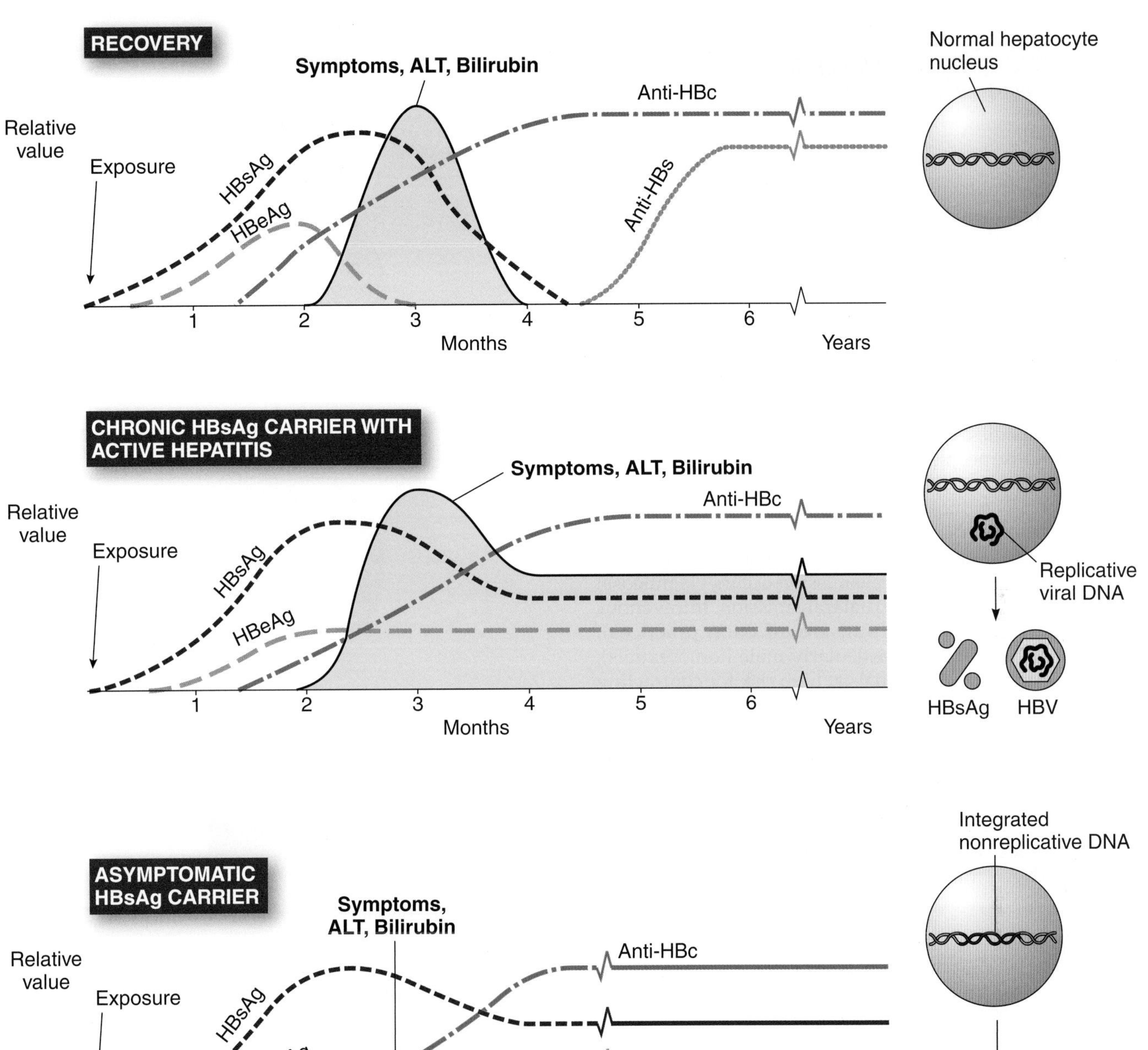

FIGURE 12-9. Typical serologic events in three distinct outcomes of hepatitis B. *Top panel.* In most cases, the appearance of antibody to hepatitis B surface antigen (HBsAg; anti-HBs) ensures complete recovery. Viral DNA disappears from the nucleus of the hepatocyte. *Middle panel.* In about 10% of cases of hepatitis B, HBs antigenemia is sustained for longer than 6 months, owing to the absence of anti-HBs. Patients in whom viral replication remains active, as evidenced by sustained high levels of HBeAg in the blood, develop active hepatitis. In such cases, the viral genome persists in the nucleus but is not integrated into host DNA. *Lower panel.* Patients in whom active viral replication ceases or is attenuated, as reflected in the disappearance of HBeAg from the blood, become asymptomatic carriers. In these individuals, fragments of the hepatitis B virus (HBV) genome are integrated into the host DNA, but episomal DNA is absent. ALT, alanine aminotransferase; anti-HBc, antibody to hepatitis B core antigen; HBeAg, hepatitis B e antigen.

of patients with polyarteritis nodosa are HBV carriers. Again, chronic hepatitis B is associated with a significant risk of liver cancer (see below). ***The possible outcomes of infection with HBV are summarized in*** Figures 12-9 and 12-10.

Hepatitis C

The most important consequences of HCV infection relate to chronic disease. Despite complete recovery from clinical and biochemical acute liver disease, 85% of patients develop chronic hepatitis (Fig. 12-11). The disorder is mild in most patients for at least 10 years and often for 20 years or more. Cirrhosis develops in 20% of people chronically infected with HCV for 10 to 30 years. ***Of patients with cirrhosis, up to 5% per year develop HCC.*** The incidence of new cases of acute HCV infection in the United States has fallen from 230,000 annually in the 1980s to 16,000 now, a drop of 93% likely because of the screening of blood supply for anti-HCV antibodies. However, mortality due to hepatitis C is increasing because people infected long ago are aging. The recent development of drugs that cure hepatitis C in a matter of weeks should drastically reduce the prevalence of the disease.

HCV infection is transmitted by contact with infected blood through direct percutaneous exposure to blood or unsafe injection practices. Less efficient transmission occurs via mucosal routes, such as vertical and sexual transmission. Intravenous drug abuse (especially with unsafe injection practices), high-risk sexual behavior (particularly male homosexuals), and alcoholism place individuals at high risk for contracting infection with HCV. Transmission from infected mothers to newborn babies is infrequent (2.7% to 8.4%) but is four to five times more common in women coinfected with HIV.

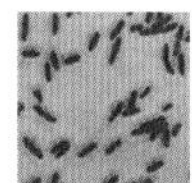

ETIOLOGIC FACTORS: Hepatitis C virus (HCV) is an enveloped flavivirus. Its single-stranded RNA genome of 9,600 bases encodes one transcript. This mRNA is translated into a polyprotein of about 3,000 amino acids, which is cleaved into three structural proteins (one core and two envelope proteins) and six nonstructural proteins. Short untranslated regions at the end of the genome are required for replication.

The virus is genetically unstable, leading to the existence of multiple genotypes and subtypes. Six different but related HCV genotypes are known, which respond differently to antiviral therapy. Types 1, 2, and 3 are most common (about 75% in the United States and Western Europe). In an individual patient, many mutant HCVs arise, which likely accounts for several features of infection, including (1) the inability of anti-HCV antibodies to clear the infection, (2) persistent and relapsing infection in the chronic hepatitis phase, and (3) lack of progress in developing a vaccine.

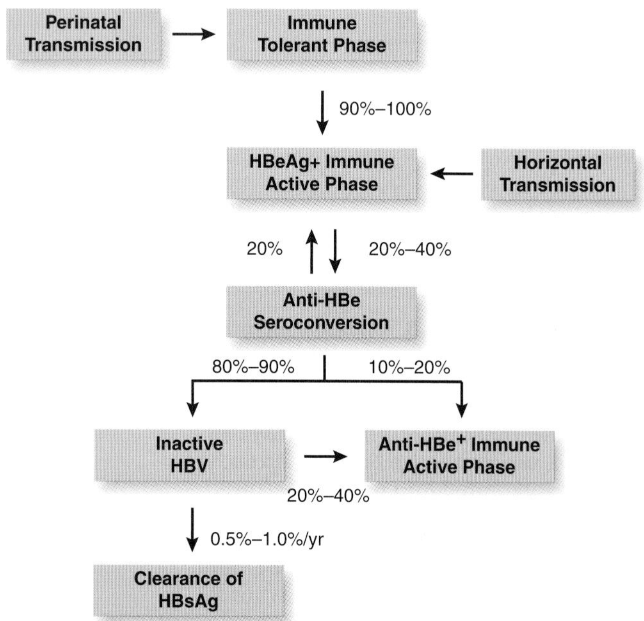

FIGURE 12-10. Outcomes of infection with the hepatitis B virus (HBV). HBeAg, hepatitis B e antigen.

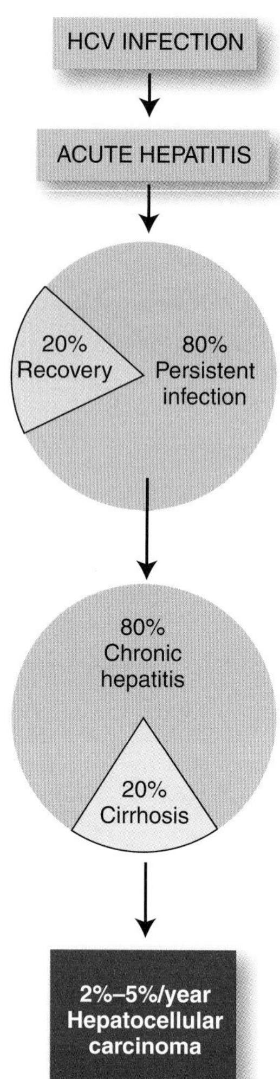

FIGURE 12-11. Outcomes of infection with the hepatitis C virus (HCV).

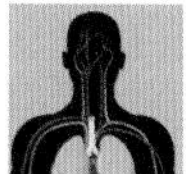

PATHOPHYSIOLOGY: HCV is not directly cytopathic, and many chronic HCV carriers have no liver cell injury. Despite active humoral and cellular immune responses against all viral proteins, most patients have persistent viremia. ***Liver cell injury probably reflects CTL killing of virus-infected hepatocytes.*** HCV persistence is not well understood. The high level of virus genome mutation (see above) and defects in HCV-specific cellular immunity probably contribute.

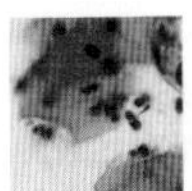

CLINICAL FEATURES: The incubation period of hepatitis C is similar to that of hepatitis B. Serum aminotransferases (Fig. 12-12) usually rise in 4 to 12 weeks after exposure (range, 2 to 26 weeks). Within 1 to 3 weeks of infection, HCV RNA circulates in the blood. Anti-HCV antibodies usually appear 7 to 8 weeks after infection and persist during the chronic phase. Acute hepatitis C is mild or asymptomatic in most people; only 10% to 20% develop jaundice. About 20% of HCV patients spontaneously clear the virus. Fulminant acute hepatitis, if it occurs at all, is rare. Even in the absence of elevated aminotransferases or significant risk factors for progression, patients can present with significant fibrosis and even cirrhosis. Liver biopsy is vital to estimating the risk of clinical progression.

Extrahepatic manifestations of hepatitis C are common and include mixed cryoglobulinemia, a systemic vasculitis caused by deposition of circulating immune complexes in the microvasculature. The skin (leukocytoclastic vasculitis), salivary glands (sicca syndrome), nervous system (mononeuritis multiplex), and kidney (membranoproliferative glomerulonephritis) may be affected. Non-Hodgkin B-cell lymphomas are more common in patients with chronic hepatitis C.

Table 12-2 ***compares the major features of the common forms of viral hepatitis.***

Table 12-2

Comparative Features of the Common Forms of Viral Hepatitis

	Hepatitis A	Hepatitis B	Hepatitis C
Genome	RNA	DNA	RNA
Incubation period	3–6 weeks	6 weeks–6 months	7–8 weeks
Transmission	Oral	Parenteral	Parenteral
Blood	No	Yes	Yes
Feces	Yes	No	No
Vertical	No	Yes	5%
Fulminant	Very rare	Yes	Rare hepatic necrosis
Chronic hepatitis	No	10%	80%
Carrier state	No	Yes	Yes
Liver cancer	No	Yes	Yes

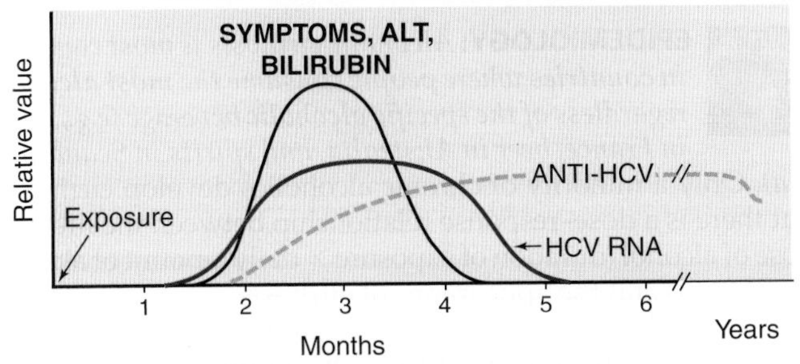

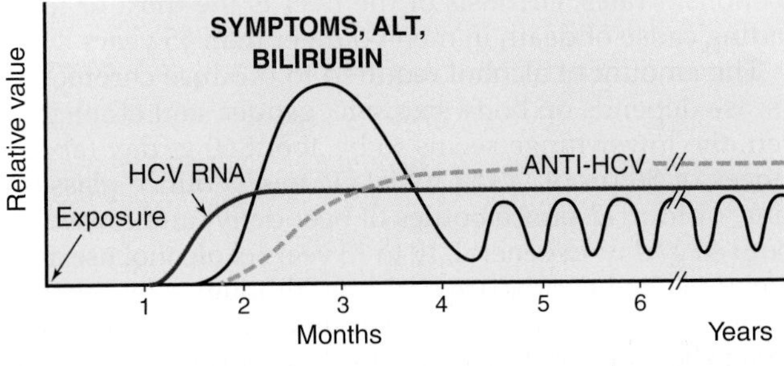

FIGURE 12-12. Clinical course of hepatitis C virus (HCV). Typical serologic events in two distinct outcomes. *Top panel.* About 20% of the patients with acute hepatitis C have a self-limited infection that resolves in a few months. Anti-HCV appears at the end of the clinical course and persists. *Bottom panel.* The remaining patients with hepatitis C develop chronic illness, with exacerbations and remissions of clinical symptoms. The development of anti-HCV does not affect the clinical outcome. Chronic hepatitis often eventuates in cirrhosis. ALT, alanine aminotransferase.

Hepatitis D

Assembly of hepatitis D virus (HDV) in the liver requires HBsAg to be present. Therefore, infection with HDV is limited to people who are also infected with HBV. The two infections may be simultaneous (coinfection), or HDV infection may follow HBV infection (superinfection). HDV and HBsAg are cleared together, and the clinical course is usually similar to that for the usual acute hepatitis B. However, in some patients, coinfection with HDV leads to severe, fulminant, and often fatal hepatitis, particularly in intravenous drug abusers. ***Superinfection of an HBV carrier with HDV typically increases either the probability of developing or the severity of existing chronic hepatitis.***

Hepatitis E

Hepatitis E is most often a self-limited, acute, icteric disease similar to hepatitis A. The virus occurs as four related genotypes that differ in epidemiologic and clinical characteristics. Genotypes 1 and 2 account for more than half of cases of acute viral hepatitis in young to middle-aged people in the poorer regions of the world. Large epidemics are associated with heavy rains in areas with inadequate sewage disposal. HEV infection may be transmitted via several routes: waterborne; zoonotic associated with eating raw or undercooked meat of infected wild animals such as pig, boar, or deer; and parenteral and vertical transmission. Genotype 3 is predominantly a zoonotic infection of pigs transmitted to humans by the consumption of undercooked pork products, predominantly pork and pork liver sausage. The virus is common in European swine herds, and more than 15% of Europeans have antibodies to the virus, most often as a result of silent infections. However, debilitated, elderly, or post-transplant patients may develop chronic hepatitis. Blood products may also transmit the virus and pose a particular risk to such patients.

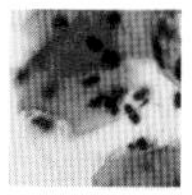

CLINICAL FEATURES: The incubation period for HEV is 35 to 40 days. In genotypes 1 and 2 infection, jaundice, hepatomegaly, fever, and arthralgias are common and usually resolve within 6 weeks, with 1% to 12% mortality. Like hepatitis A, clinical illness from hepatitis E is far more common in adults than in children; in the latter, infection is often subclinical. The disease is very dangerous in pregnant women, in whom mortality may reach 20% to 40%. Chronic disease and carrier states are unknown in immunocompetent patients, but immunocompromised people may develop chronic hepatitis E. Although, as noted, most infections with genotype 3 virus are asymptomatic in immunocompetent persons, there is growing concern that all genotypes of HEV may be associated with extrahepatic neurologic disease, in particular Guillain–Barré syndrome. A successful vaccine against HEV infection has been developed and successfully tested in phase II clinical trials but is not yet licensed in the United States.

Other Human Hepatitis Viruses Remain Conjectural

Hepatitis G virus (HGV), now more commonly referred to as GB virus C (GBV-C), is a lymphotropic flavivirus discovered in 1995 in relation to HCV infection. HGV infection by itself does not cause any known disease.

AUTOIMMUNE HEPATITIS

Autoimmune hepatitis is a severe type of chronic hepatitis associated with circulating autoantibodies and elevated serum immunoglobulins. The disorder may appear at any age; 70% of cases occur in women. In the United States, autoimmune hepatitis affects up to 200,000 people and accounts for 6% of liver transplants.

PATHOPHYSIOLOGY: There are two types of autoimmune hepatitis:

- **Type I** disease is more common (80% of cases) and features antinuclear and anti–smooth muscle antibodies. Some 70% of cases occur in women younger than 40 years, among whom one third have other autoimmune diseases, including thyroiditis, rheumatoid arthritis, and ulcerative colitis. Of patients with type I autoimmune hepatitis, 25% present with cirrhosis, indicating that the disease usually has had a prolonged asymptomatic course prior to diagnosis. There are antibodies against many cytosolic enzymes, but the hepatocyte membrane asialoglycoprotein receptor is the main candidate target for antibody-dependent cell-mediated cytotoxicity (ADCC). The HLA-*DRB1* gene confers particular susceptibility to type I autoimmune hepatitis. Some patients may present with a poorly characterized "overlap syndrome," with mixed clinical and histologic features of autoimmune hepatitis and either primary biliary cholangitis (PBC) or primary sclerosing cholangitis (PSC) (see below).
- **Type II** autoimmune hepatitis occurs mainly in children who are 2 to 14 years old. Antibodies against the liver and kidney microsomes (anti-LKM) are characteristic. However, the key autoantigen is a P450-type drug-metabolizing enzyme (CYP 2D6). These patients often have other autoimmune diseases (e.g., type I diabetes and thyroiditis). Genetic determinants of type II disease are not defined.

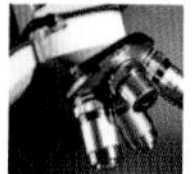

PATHOLOGY: Autoimmune hepatitis basically resembles acute and chronic viral hepatitis histologically, but lobular inflammation and necrosis are more pronounced. The inflammatory infiltrate is rich in plasma cells, an important diagnostic feature. Confluent hepatic necrosis may be seen in severe acute cases.

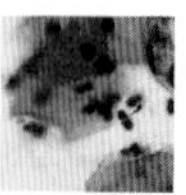

CLINICAL FEATURES: Autoimmune hepatitis can arise insidiously, with fatigue and mild right upper quadrant discomfort. Often, there is a personal or family history of autoimmunity. With time, aminotransferase levels rise markedly and may exceed 1,000 IU/mL. Marked hyperglobulinemia is common. In severe cases, jaundice, hepatic synthetic dysfunction, and even liver failure ensue, but the condition rarely presents as fulminant disease. Untreated, autoimmune hepatitis often progresses to cirrhosis. Autoimmune hepatitis usually responds to combinations of corticosteroids and immunosuppressants, such as azathioprine. Although patients whose disease progresses to cirrhosis may receive liver transplants, autoimmune hepatitis recurs in up to 20% of patients.

ALCOHOLIC LIVER DISEASE

The harmful effects of excess alcohol (ethanol, ethyl alcohol) consumption have been recognized almost since the dawn of recorded history. Ethanol is now seen as a hepatotoxin that acts both directly and indirectly.

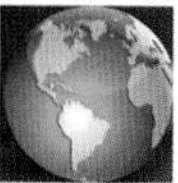

EPIDEMIOLOGY: ***Alcoholic cirrhosis is most common in countries where people consume the most alcohol, regardless of the specific alcoholic beverage (e.g., wine in France, beer in Australia, and spirits in Scandinavia).*** Only a minority of chronic alcoholics develop cirrhosis, but there is a dose–response relationship between the lifetime dose of alcohol (duration of exposure × daily amount of alcohol consumed) and the appearance of cirrhosis.

About 10% of men and 5% of women in the United States abuse alcohol. In some countries, this figure is much higher. ***Some 15% of alcoholics develop cirrhosis; many of them die due to hepatic failure or from extrahepatic complications of cirrhosis.*** In many urban areas of the United States with high alcoholism rates, cirrhosis of the liver is the third or fourth leading cause of death in men younger than 45 years.

The amount of alcohol required to produce chronic liver disease depends on body size, age, gender, and ethnicity. In men, the lower range seems to be about 60 g/day (about 6 ounces of 86 proof [43%] whiskey, four 5-ounce glasses of wine, or four 12-ounce bottles of beer daily) and for women about 40 g/day. In general, 10 to 15 years of alcohol use at this level is needed to produce cirrhosis, although a few cirrhotic patients give shorter histories. For unknown reasons, women seem to be more predisposed to the harmful effects of alcohol, perhaps because they metabolize alcohol differently and have lower body masses.

The epidemiology of alcoholic liver disease is complicated by its association with the hepatotropic viruses. HBV seropositivity is two- to fourfold more common in alcoholics than in control populations. The prevalence of anti-HCV antibodies is up to 10% among alcoholics and is even higher among alcoholics with chronic liver disease. People who abuse alcohol and also have hepatitis C are more likely to develop liver disease than their uninfected counterparts.

Ethanol Metabolism

Ethanol is rapidly absorbed from the stomach and eventually distributed in body water space. Between 5% and 10% is excreted unchanged, mostly in the urine and expired breath. The remaining 90% is metabolized by the liver to acetaldehyde and acetate, largely by cytosolic **alcohol dehydrogenase (ADH)**. The mixed-function oxidase in the **microsomal ethanol-oxidizing system** is a minor metabolic pathway for alcohol. Clearance of alcohol from the body, unlike most drugs, is linear—that is, a fixed quantity is metabolized per unit time. Roughly, for the average man, 7 to 10 g of alcohol is eliminated per hour. However, because the microsomal pathway (see above) is upregulated in chronic alcoholics, they metabolize ethanol more rapidly, as long as they do not suffer from active liver disease.

Alcoholic Liver Disease

Alcoholic liver disease spans three major morphologic and clinical entities, namely, **fatty liver, acute alcoholic hepatitis,** and **cirrhosis**. These lesions usually occur in sequence, but they may coexist in any combination and seem to be independent entities.

Fatty Liver

MOLECULAR PATHOGENESIS: Virtually, all chronic alcoholics, regardless of their pattern of drinking, accumulate fat in hepatocytes (**steatosis**). The relative contributions of different metabolic pathways to steatosis may depend on the amount of alcohol consumed, dietary lipid content, body stores of fat, hormonal status, and other variables. ***Still, accumulation of fat clearly depends on alcohol intake because it is fully and rapidly reversible if alcohol ingestion stops.***

Dietary fat, as chylomicrons and free fatty acids, is transported to the liver, where it is taken up by hepatocytes. Triglycerides are then hydrolyzed to free fatty acids. These, in turn, undergo β-oxidation in mitochondria or are converted by the endoplasmic reticulum to triglycerides. These newly synthesized triglycerides are secreted as lipoproteins or are retained for storage.

Most of the fat deposited in the liver after chronic alcohol consumption is from the diet. Ethanol increases lipolysis and thus delivery of free fatty acids to the liver. Within hepatocytes, ethanol (1) increases fatty acid synthesis, (2) decreases mitochondrial oxidation of fatty acids, (3) raises triglyceride production, and (4) impairs release of lipoproteins. Collectively, these metabolic consequences produce a fatty liver.

PATHOLOGY: In the setting of high alcohol intake, the liver becomes yellow and enlarged, sometimes to as much as three times its normal weight. This increased weight reflects not only fat accumulation but also that of protein and water. The extent of visible fat accumulation varies from minute droplets scattered in the cytoplasm of a few hepatocytes to distention of the entire cytoplasm of most cells by coalesced droplets (Fig. 12-13). In the latter case, liver cells may be barely recognizable as such and resemble adipocytes, with their cytoplasm distended by a clear area and their nuclei flattened and displaced to the periphery of the cell.

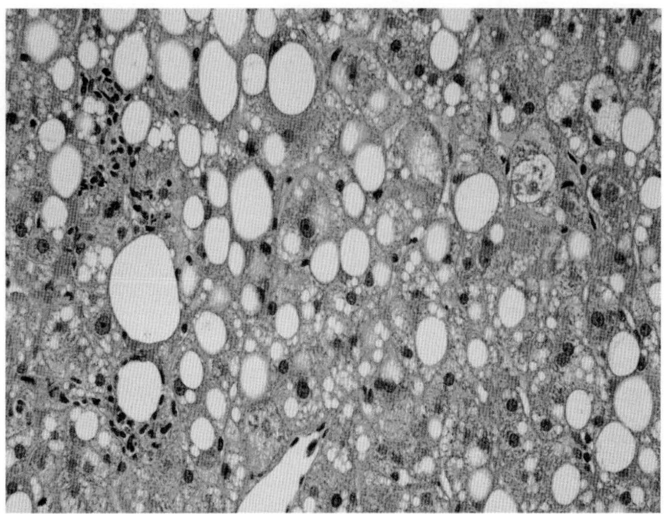

FIGURE 12-13. Alcoholic fatty liver. The cytoplasm of almost all of the hepatocytes distended by fat that displaces the nucleus to the periphery.

Chronic ethanol ingestion elicits pronounced hepatic functional alterations. Liver mitochondria show decreased rates of substrate oxidation (e.g., of fatty acids) and impaired ATP formation. The activity of cytochrome P450–dependent mixed-function oxidases is increased, resulting in the enhancement of the metabolism of a variety of drugs. ***This increased microsomal function also augments metabolism of hepatic toxins, thus exaggerating the danger of agents such as acetaminophen, in which it is the drug's metabolic products that are most toxic.*** Whereas chronic alcohol consumption promotes microsomal functions, acute alcohol ingestion that leads to high blood levels inhibits mixed-function oxidases and acutely reduces the rate of clearance of drugs from the body.

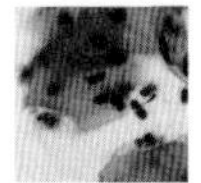

CLINICAL FEATURES: Patients with uncomplicated alcoholic fatty liver have surprisingly few symptoms of liver disease. Despite the striking morphologic change in the liver, alcoholic fatty liver is fully reversible and does not by itself progress to more severe disease. The best treatment for fatty liver because of alcohol is simply abstinence. ***Fatty liver, although characteristic of alcoholism, is not limited to it. Fatty liver may also be seen in nonalcoholic fatty liver disease (NAFLD; see below), hepatitis C, after certain drugs, obesity, and in many other conditions.***

Alcoholic Hepatitis

Alcoholic hepatitis is characterized by (1) hepatocyte necrosis, mainly in the central zone; (2) cytoplasmic hyaline inclusions within hepatocytes (Mallory-Denk bodies); (3) an acute inflammatory infiltrate in the lobule, and (4) perivenular fibrosis (Fig. 12-14). **The pathogenesis of alcoholic hepatitis is a mystery.** Alcoholics may have mild fatty liver for many years and, without any change in drinking habits, suddenly develop acute alcoholic hepatitis. It may be that long-standing, subclinical alcoholic hepatitis precedes clinically overt hepatitis. Nevertheless, the often-explosive presentation of alcoholic

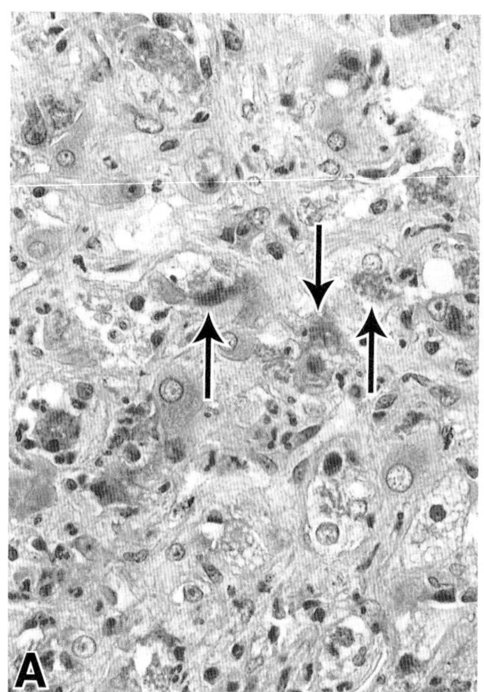

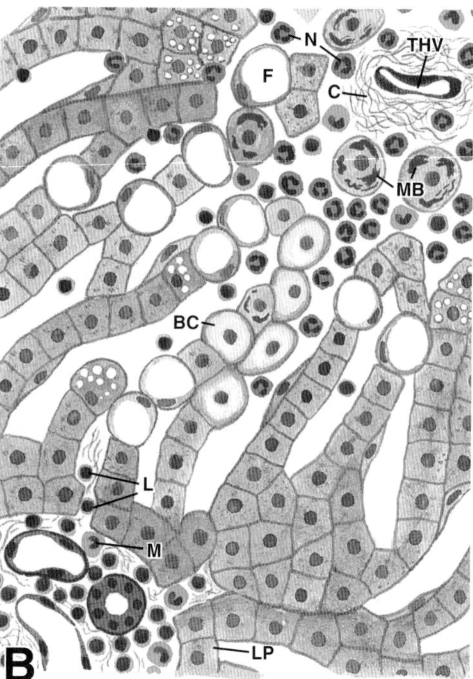

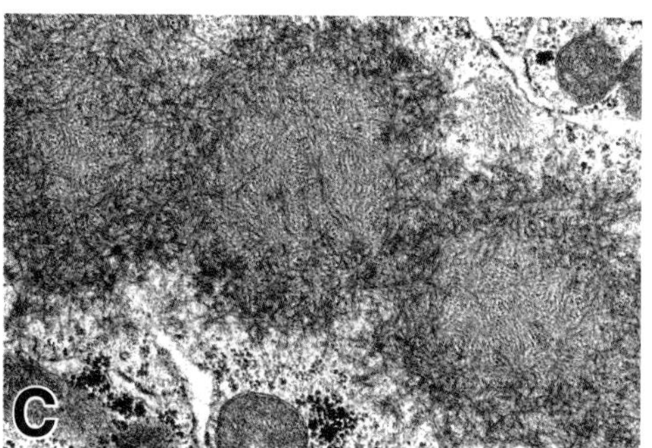

FIGURE 12-14. Alcoholic hepatitis. A. Necrosis and degeneration of hepatocytes, Mallory–Denk bodies (MB) (eosinophilic inclusions) in the cytoplasm of injured hepatocytes (*arrows*) and infiltration by neutrophils. **B. Schematic representation of the major pathologic features of alcoholic hepatitis.** The lesions are predominantly centrilobular and include necrosis and loss of hepatocytes, ballooned cells (BC), and MB in the cytoplasm of damaged hepatocytes. The inflammatory infiltrate consists predominantly of neutrophils (N), although a few lymphocytes (L) and macrophages (M) are also present. The central venule, or terminal hepatic venule (THV), is encased in connective tissue (C) (central hyaline sclerosis. Fat-laden hepatocytes (F) are evident in the lobule. The portal tract displays moderate chronic inflammation, and the limiting plate (LP) is focally breached. **C. Ultrastructure of MB.** Dense, interwoven bundles of cytokeratin filaments are in the cytoplasm of hepatocytes.

hepatitis suggests that some environmental or physiologic cofactor is involved, although none has been identified.

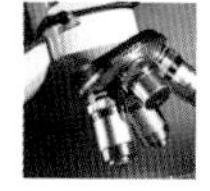

PATHOLOGY: Typically, in alcoholic hepatitis, the hepatic architecture is intact. Hepatocytes show variable hydropic swelling, giving them a heterogeneous appearance. Isolated necrotic liver cells or clusters of them have pyknotic nuclei and show karyorrhexis. Scattered hepatocytes contain **Mallory-Denk bodies (alcoholic hyaline)** (Fig. 12-14). These cytoplasmic inclusions are more common in visibly damaged, swollen hepatocytes and appear as irregular skeins of eosinophilic material or as solid eosinophilic masses, often perinuclearly. They are aggregates of intermediate (cytokeratin) filaments (Fig. 12-14C). The damaged, ballooned hepatocytes, particularly those with Mallory bodies, are surrounded by neutrophils. A more diffuse, intralobular inflammatory infiltrate is also present. Mallory-Denk bodies are characteristic of, but not specific for, alcoholic liver disease because they may also be present in nonalcoholic steatohepatitis (NASH), chronic cholestatic syndromes, Wilson disease (WD), and HCC. Mild-to-severe cholestasis is seen in up to one third of cases. Alcoholic hepatitis is usually, but not always, superimposed on an existing fatty liver, although there is no evidence that fat accumulation predisposes or contributes to the development of alcoholic hepatitis.

Collagen deposition is always seen in alcoholic hepatitis, especially around central veins (terminal hepatic venules). Chronic alcohol exposure activates hepatic stellate cells to deposit intrasinusoidal collagen. In severe cases, venules and perivenular sinusoids are obliterated and surrounded by dense fibrous tissue to yield **central hyaline sclerosis** (Figs. 12-14). This condition is often associated with noncirrhotic portal hypertension.

Portal tracts in alcoholic hepatitis are highly variable. Some are virtually normal, whereas others are enlarged, with a mononuclear infiltrate and proliferated bile ductules. The altered portal tracts often show spurs of fibrous tissue that penetrate the lobules.

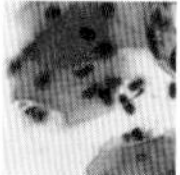

CLINICAL FEATURES: Patients with alcoholic hepatitis have malaise and anorexia, fever, right upper quadrant abdominal pain, and jaundice. Leukocytosis is common. Serum aminotransferases, particularly AST, are moderately elevated but not as high as in viral hepatitis: AST usually remains under 400, and the AST to ALT ratio is typically 2:1. Serum alkaline phosphatase is usually increased. In severe cases, a prolonged prothrombin time often portends an ominous prognosis.

The outlook in patients with alcoholic hepatitis reflects the severity of liver cell injury. In some patients, the disease progresses rapidly to hepatic failure and death. Mortality in the acute stage of alcoholic hepatitis remains at about 10%. Most of those who abstain from alcohol after recovery from acute alcoholic hepatitis recover. However, of those who continue to drink, up to 70% ultimately develop cirrhosis. There is no specific treatment for acute alcoholic hepatitis. Corticosteroids improve short-term mortality and thus are often given if there is no infection or renal failure. Nutritional therapy can be beneficial.

Alcoholic Cirrhosis

In about 15% of alcoholics, hepatocellular necrosis, fibrosis, and regeneration eventually lead to formation of fibrous septa around hepatocellular nodules (Fig. 12-15). The other lesions of alcoholic liver disease—fatty liver and acute or persistent alcoholic hepatitis—are often seen in conjunction with cirrhosis (see below). Activated hepatic stellate cells in the sinusoids, which produce perisinusoidal collagen, probably contribute to the development of cirrhosis. The prognosis in cases of established alcoholic cirrhosis is much better in those who abstain from alcohol. Nevertheless, many patients progress to end-stage liver disease, and alcoholic liver disease is a common indication for liver transplantation.

NONALCOHOLIC FATTY LIVER DISEASE

NAFLD closely resembles alcoholic liver disease and includes diverse liver injuries, from simple steatosis, with or without associated hepatitis to nonalcoholic steatohepatitis (NASH), to bridging fibrosis and cirrhosis. Risk factors for NAFLD include obesity, type 2 diabetes mellitus, hyperlipidemia, and metabolic syndrome. About half of people with both morbid obesity and diabetes have NASH; about 20% of these will develop cirrhosis.

NASH overlaps alcoholic liver disease histologically, with steatosis, lobular and portal inflammation, hepatocyte necrosis, Mallory-Denk bodies, and fibrosis. As in alcoholic liver disease, centrilobular fibrosis is common. If cirrhosis develops, steatosis often disappears. ***Thus, NASH is the likely cause of many cases of the so-called cryptogenic cirrhosis.***

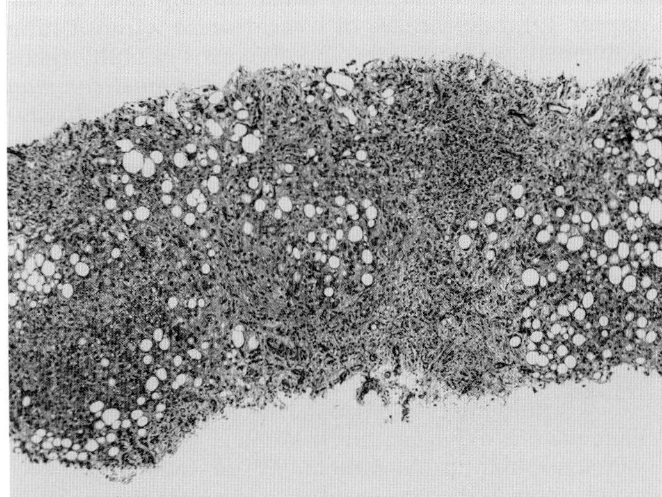

FIGURE 12-15. Micronodular cirrhosis. Cirrhotic liver from a chronic alcoholic. Note the small, regenerative nodules of parenchyma and fatty change.

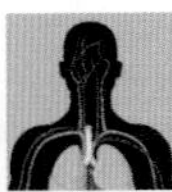

PATHOPHYSIOLOGY: The pathogenesis of NAFLD and NASH may overlap that of alcoholic hepatitis. In most cases, insulin resistance is associated with increased hepatic mitochondrial oxidation of free fatty acids, increased oxidative stress, and lipid peroxidation. Progression to cirrhosis is often insidious, and many patients remain asymptomatic, with only moderate increases in serum liver enzyme activities.

NAFLD is considered the hepatic manifestation of the metabolic syndrome, which consists of abdominal obesity, dyslipidemia, insulin resistance, and hypertension (see Chapter 19). Weight reduction, including that via bariatric surgery, tends to improve NAFLD and NASH, but no definitive treatment is yet available.

CIRRHOSIS

Cirrhosis is defined as the destruction of normal liver architecture by fibrous bands around regenerative nodules of hepatocytes. It is the eighth leading cause of death in the United States and the 13th globally. The morphologic pattern invariably results from persistent liver cell necrosis. Advanced cases of cirrhosis all tend to have a similar appearance, and the cause often can no longer be ascertained by morphologic examination alone. In earlier stages, on the other hand, features characteristic of an inciting pathogenic insult may be evident. For example, fat and Mallory bodies are typical of alcoholic liver injury, whereas chronic inflammation and periportal necrosis are prominent in chronic viral hepatitis.

The pathogenesis of cirrhosis involves death and regeneration of hepatocytes, extracellular matrix deposition by activated hepatic stellate cells, and resulting alterations in hepatic vascular architecture.

Early in the evolution of cirrhosis, the **micronodular** type (Fig. 12-15) is characterized by small, uniform nodules separated by thin fibrous septa. At the other end, ordinarily late in the disease, is **macronodular cirrhosis** (Fig. 12-16), with grossly visible, coarse, irregular nodules, mirrored histologically by large nodules that vary in size and shape and are encircled by similarly variably broad bands of connective tissue. ***Between these extremes are many cases with features of both. In practice, the different appearances of cirrhosis are less important than their etiologies.***

If the underlying cause of cirrhosis is removed, functional and structural improvement may occur, although complete regression is unlikely.

MICRONODULAR CIRRHOSIS (Laennec cirrhosis): Nodules in micronodular cirrhosis usually measure less than 3 mm, scarcely larger than a lobule (Fig. 12-15). They show no landmarks of lobular architecture, such as portal tracts or central venules. Connective tissue septa separating nodules are usually thin, but irregular focal collapse of parenchyma may lead to wider septa. In its active stages, mononuclear inflammatory cells and proliferated bile ductules are found in the septa. ***The prototypical cause of micronodular cirrhosis is alcoholic injury, but other etiologies may also be responsible.***

MACRONODULAR CIRRHOSIS: Macronodular cirrhosis is classically due to chronic hepatitis. Broad connective tissue septa (Fig. 12-16) show elements of preexisting portal tracts, mononuclear inflammatory cells, and proliferated bile ductules. After the passage of time, micronodular cirrhosis can become macronodular, with continued regeneration and expansion of existing nodules, especially in alcoholics who stop drinking.

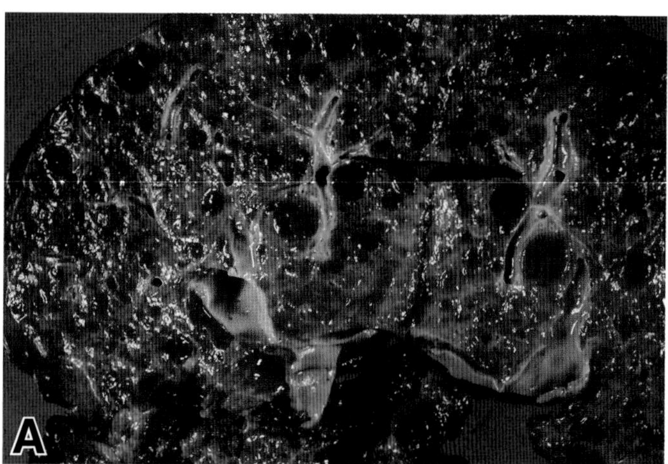

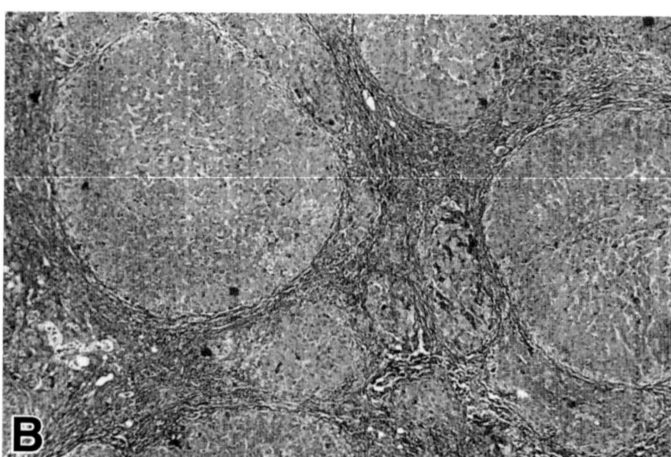

FIGURE 12-16. **Macronodular cirrhosis. A.** The liver is misshapen, and the cut surface reveals irregular nodules and connective tissue septa of varying width. **B.** Nodules of varying size and irregular fibrous septa.

The diseases associated with cirrhosis are listed in Table 12-3. They have little in common, except that they all entail persistent liver cell necrosis. Most cases of cirrhosis are attributable to alcoholism and chronic viral hepatitis. In some 15% of cases, etiologies remain unknown and are labeled **cryptogenic cirrhosis**. As noted above, nonalcoholic steatohepatitis (NASH) is now felt to account for a significant proportion of cryptogenic cirrhosis.

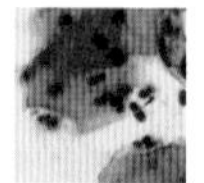

CLINICAL FEATURES: Cirrhosis invariably is associated with complications secondary to parenchymal liver failure, endocrine abnormalities, and portal hypertension. Decompensated cirrhosis leads to a life expectancy as low as 2 years, whereas that of compensated cirrhosis is 10 to 13 years. Portal hypertension results in bleeding, gastroesophageal varices, ascites, splenomegaly, and hepatorenal syndrome. Gynecomastia, testicular atrophy, and vascular "spiders" reflect endocrine disturbances. Liver failure features jaundice, coagulopathy, hepatic encephalopathy, and elevated blood ammonia.

Table 12-3

Major Causes of Cirrhosis
Alcoholic liver disease
Nonalcoholic fatty liver disease
Chronic hepatitis
Chronic viral hepatitis
Autoimmune hepatitis
Drugs
Biliary disease
Extrahepatic biliary obstruction
Primary biliary cirrhosis
Primary sclerosing cholangitis
Metabolic disease
Hemochromatosis
Wilson disease
α_1-Antitrypsin deficiency
Tyrosinemia
Glycogen storage disease
Hereditary fructose intolerance
Hereditary storage diseases
Galactosemia
Cryptogenic

HERITABLE DISORDERS ASSOCIATED WITH CIRRHOSIS

A number of inherited disorders ultimately result in liver damage and cirrhosis. Diseases resulting in excess deposition of abnormally folded proteins α1-AT or of metals (copper and iron) result in cirrhosis.

α_1-Antitrypsin Deficiency

α_1-AT deficiency is an autosomal recessive disease that was initially described as a cause of emphysema (see Chapter 10). Later, cases of liver disease without lung involvement were reported. Involvement of both organs is now recognized. ***α_1-AT deficiency is the most common genetic liver disease and the most common genetic disease treated by liver transplantation.*** Although it occurs in 1 in 2,000 live births, only 10% to 15% of those affected develop liver disease.

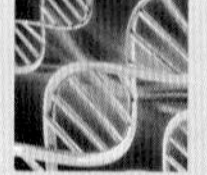

MOLECULAR PATHOGENESIS: α_1-AT is a serine protease inhibitor (serpin) secreted largely in the liver, which inactivates neutrophil elastase. Both pulmonary and hepatic disorders are caused by inadequate α_1-AT secretion by the liver. PiZ is the most common mutant α_1-AT protein (95% of cases) and is retained within the hepatocyte ER, where it folds abnormally. Insoluble aggregates of the mutant protein cannot be exported or degraded and accumulate, thereby damaging the cell.

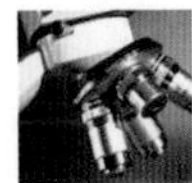

PATHOLOGY: Hepatocytes in patients with α_1-AT deficiency contain faintly eosinophilic, PAS-positive cytoplasmic droplets which contain amorphous material within dilated ER cisternae. The disease often presents with chronic hepatitis, which terminates in cirrhosis. α_1-AT deficiency may also cause hepatitis in the newborn (see below). Micronodular cirrhosis develops by the age of 2 to 3 years in these children and may ultimately become macronodular.

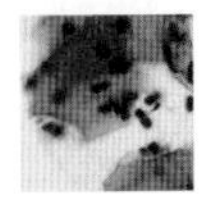

CLINICAL FEATURES: Liver disease in α_1-AT deficiency varies from rapidly fatal neonatal hepatitis to no hepatic dysfunction at all. ***Of infants with the ZZ genotype—who are susceptible to the development of clinical disease—10% have neonatal cholestatic jaundice (conjugated hyperbilirubinemia).*** Most infants recover within 6 months, but 10% to 20% develop permanent liver disease. Children with cirrhosis usually die before 10 years of age from hepatic failure or other complications of the disease. However, liver transplantation is curative. Some patients are asymptomatic until early adulthood, when symptoms of cirrhosis may be the initial complaint. ***Cirrhosis in α_1-AT deficiency is prone to a high incidence of HCC.***

Wilson Disease Is an Inherited Disorder of Copper Metabolism

WD is an autosomal recessive disease in which excess copper is deposited in the liver and brain (Fig. 12-17). In all, 1 in 150 to 180 people is a carrier, and 1 in 30,000 children develop clinical disease.

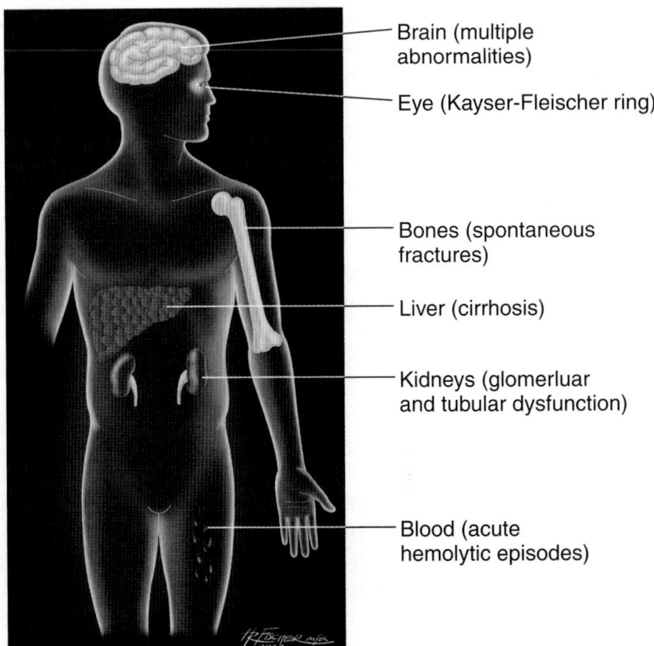

FIGURE 12-17. Wilson disease. The organs principally affected in Wilson disease.

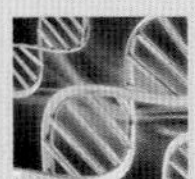

MOLECULAR PATHOGENESIS: Dietary copper intake usually exceeds the body's needs, the excess being excreted by the liver into the bile. Copper is normally bound to ceruloplasmin in hepatocytes and then secreted into the blood. The gene for WD, namely, *ATP7B* on chromosome 13, codes for an ATP-dependent, transmembrane cation channel, which transports copper within hepatocytes before it is excreted. ***Mutations in ATP7B impair copper transport. Both biliary copper excretion and incorporation into ceruloplasmin are deficient.*** In WD, serum ceruloplasmin levels are very low, a deficiency thought to be caused by hepatic copper overload. Excess copper is toxic to hepatocytes, which die and release their copper into the blood. The copper is then deposited in extrahepatic tissues. The central role of the liver in WD is underscored by the fact that liver transplantation is curative.

Just how excess copper injures cells is unclear. However, copperopper can replace iron in the Fenton reaction to convert hydrogen peroxide into hydroxyl radicals (see Chapter 1).

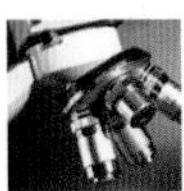

PATHOLOGY: ***In WD, the liver progresses from mild-to-severe chronic hepatitis. Cirrhosis may develop rapidly, even in childhood.*** Features of severe hepatocyte injury and steatosis may be seen. Hepatocytes often contain Mallory-Denk bodies, and cholestasis is common. Initially, cirrhosis is micronodular, but in time, it becomes macronodular.

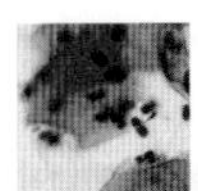

CLINICAL FEATURES: In half of patients with WD, some symptoms are shown by adolescence. The rest usually become ill early in adulthood, although WD can present later. Initial symptoms reflect chronic liver disease in about half of patients, one third are first seen with neurologic complaints, and about 10% have psychiatric illnesses.

LIVER: Liver-related symptoms are nonspecific at first and may progress to chronic liver disease indistinguishable from that of other forms of chronic hepatitis. Eventually, chronic hepatitis and cirrhosis result in jaundice, portal hypertension, and hepatic failure.

BRAIN AND EYE: Neurologic disease begins with mild incoordination and tremors. If untreated, dysarthria and dysphagia appear, followed by disabling dystonia and spasticity. Ocular manifestations invariably accompany neurologic disease. **Kayser–Fleischer rings** are golden brown, bilateral corneal discolorations around the edge of the iris that obscure its muscular pattern (Fig. 12-18). They represent copper deposited in Descemet membrane.

Treatment of WD prevents copper accumulation in tissues and removes copper already deposited. Copper-chelating agents, trientine and D-penicillamine, augment urinary copper excretion. Treatment often reverses central nervous system (CNS) dysfunction and liver disease. Presymptomatic patients are maintained with zinc, which blocks intestinal absorption of copper. Liver transplantation is curative for WD.

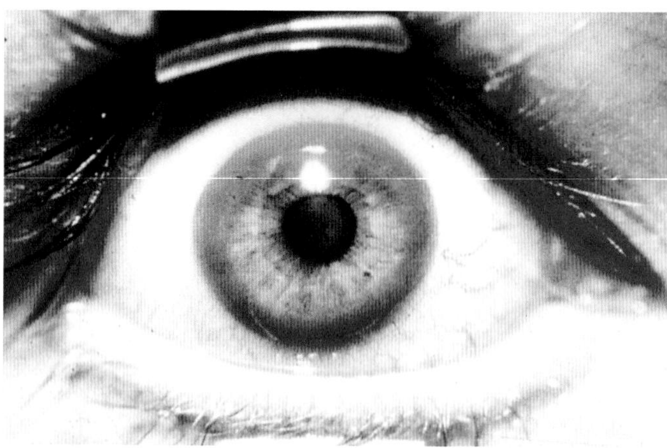

FIGURE 12-18. Kayser–Fleischer ring. The deposition of copper in the Descemet membrane is reflected in a peripheral brown color, which obstructs the view of the underlying iris.

REGULATION OF IRON METABOLISM: INTRODUCTION

One of the functions of the liver is the regulation of iron in the body, both heme in the red cell and iron storage in general. Deficiencies in heme synthesis lead to a set of diseases designated porphyria; deficiencies in heme degradation are associated with bilirubinemia and jaundice, as discussed below. Storage of excessive iron causes hemochromatosis.

THE PORPHYRIAS

Porphyrias, either acquired or inherited, are caused by deficiencies in heme biosynthesis and are characterized by accumulation of porphyrin intermediates. Porphyrias are divided into hepatic and erythropoietic porphyrias, based on where the defective heme metabolism and the accumulation of porphyrins and their precursors occur. Genetic porphyrias are heterogeneous, usually with unique mutations in individual families.

Hepatic porphyrias are inherited as autosomal dominant traits and are often precipitated by administration of drugs, sex hormones, starvation, hepatitis C, HIV infection, and alcohol consumption. The liver shows variable steatosis, hemosiderosis, fibrosis, and cirrhosis. Needle-shaped cytoplasmic inclusions may be present.

ACUTE INTERMITTENT PORPHYRIA: This is the most common genetic porphyria and reflects a deficiency of porphobilinogen deaminase activity in the liver. Only 10% of gene carriers show clinical symptoms, which generally affect young adults. Colicky abdominal pain and neuropsychiatric symptoms predominate.

PORPHYRIA CUTANEA TARDA: This disorder is the most frequent clinical porphyria. It may be acquired or inherited as an autosomal dominant trait and is characterized by deficient uroporphyrinogen decarboxylase activity. Typical patients are middle aged or elderly, with cutaneous photosensitivity and liver disease with hepatic iron overload.

Other inherited porphyrias, termed **erythropoietic porphyrias** and **congenital erythropoietic porphyrias**, are caused by enzyme deficiencies in erythrocytes. They are characterized by cutaneous photosensitivity and, occasionally, liver disease.

IRON OVERLOAD SYNDROMES

Excessive iron accumulates in the body (siderosis) in two major groups of iron overload syndromes, divided on the basis of etiology. **Hereditary hemochromatosis (HH)** is caused by a common genetic alteration in the control of intestinal iron absorption. ***Secondary iron overload complicates certain hematologic disorders, such as ineffective erythropoiesis caused by sickle cell anemia, thalassemia major, and other anemias.*** The excess iron derives from hemolysis or transfused blood. Secondary iron overload alone rarely causes liver disease.

Body Iron Storage

The normal total body content of iron is 3 to 4 g. Most of this (about 2.5 g) is bound up in hemoglobin. Iron normally enters the body by being absorbed through the duodenal mucosa. ***There is no mechanism for iron excretion, and keeping body iron within acceptable limits requires strict control of intestinal iron uptake.*** The mechanisms for the control of normal iron metabolism are reviewed in Figure 12-19.

Several principal proteins control this process:

- **Hepcidin:** Hepcidin level is central to iron homeostasis. This peptide is manufactured and exported by the liver. The protein blocks transit of iron through enterocytes to the blood and inhibits its secretion from stores in hepatocytes and macrophages. It does this by binding the main iron export channel in these cells, **ferroportin**, and promoting its degradation. Hepcidin synthesis is stimulated when body iron stores are sufficient and is downregulated when the body needs more iron. Upregulation of synthesis requires a group of proteins, such as transferrin receptor-2 (TfR2), hemojuvelin, and HFE, the product of the High Iron Fe (*HFE*) gene. In renal failure, hepcidin is not eliminated efficiently, and its levels are generally elevated.
- **Ferroportin:** This protein is the obligatory iron channel in cells. It is required for cells (mainly enterocytes, hepatocytes, and macrophages) to export iron or to transport it through the cell. Hepcidin inhibits ferroportin function by displacing iron from it, thereby causing the hepcidin–ferroportin complex to be internalized and degraded.
- **Transferrin (Tf):** The principal form of the Tf molecule is the main iron carrier in the blood. One Tf molecule binds two Fe^{3+} ions. Tf also mediates iron uptake by cells via its main receptor (TfR1). Normal plasma iron ranges from 80 to 100 mg/dL, and Tf is ordinarily about 33% saturated. A small amount of free iron—not bound by Tf—also circulates normally. In times of huge iron excess, free iron may be the predominant form of iron in the blood.
- **Ferritin:** This multimeric protein is responsible for storing iron within cells and is present in every cell type. It binds the ferric (Fe^{3+}) form of iron to form a complex called **hemosiderin**, thereby preventing the stored iron from generating free radical species via the Fenton reaction (see Chapter 1). Blood ferritin levels generally reflect the status of the body's iron stores: low serum ferritin is an indicator of iron deficiency. High ferritin levels occur when the body has large amounts of stored iron. Iron is ordinarily stored in macrophages and hepatocytes bound to **ferritin**.

Iron Entry Into Cells

Under normal circumstances, the main iron portal of entry into enterocytes is a cell membrane channel referred to as divalent metal transporter 1 (DMT-1). Other cells generally admit iron via a different receptor-mediated pathway: Tf-bound iron is recognized by TfR1 and internalized. Free iron (not bound by Tf) enters cells differently, via poorly understood mechanisms. ***It is this pathway, by which unbound iron enters cells, that allows intracellular iron accumulation when regulatory mechanisms malfunction (see below).***

Hereditary Hemochromatosis

Toxic iron accumulation in HH is harmful to parenchymal cells, particularly of the liver, heart, and pancreas. ***The clinical hallmarks of advanced HH are cirrhosis, diabetes, skin pigmentation, and cardiac failure.*** HH is the most common inherited metabolic disorder in whites. It manifests most often in patients aged 40 to 60 years. Men are affected 10 times as often as women, probably because women lose iron by menstruation. However, postmenopausal women may also develop HH. Because maximal daily iron absorption is about 4 mg, hemochromatosis develops over years.

Iron Metabolism in Hereditary Hemochromatosis

MOLECULAR PATHOGENESIS: There are several different forms of HH, all related to failure of hepcidin synthesis. In most cases, the *HFE* gene is mutated. A particular mutation (C282Y), when present in both alleles of the *HFE* gene, is responsible for HH in 90% of patients. Rarer forms of hemochromatosis are caused by mutations in other genes that control hepcidin expression, such as TfR2 and hemojuvelin. Rarely, the hepcidin gene itself (*HAMP*) is mutated.

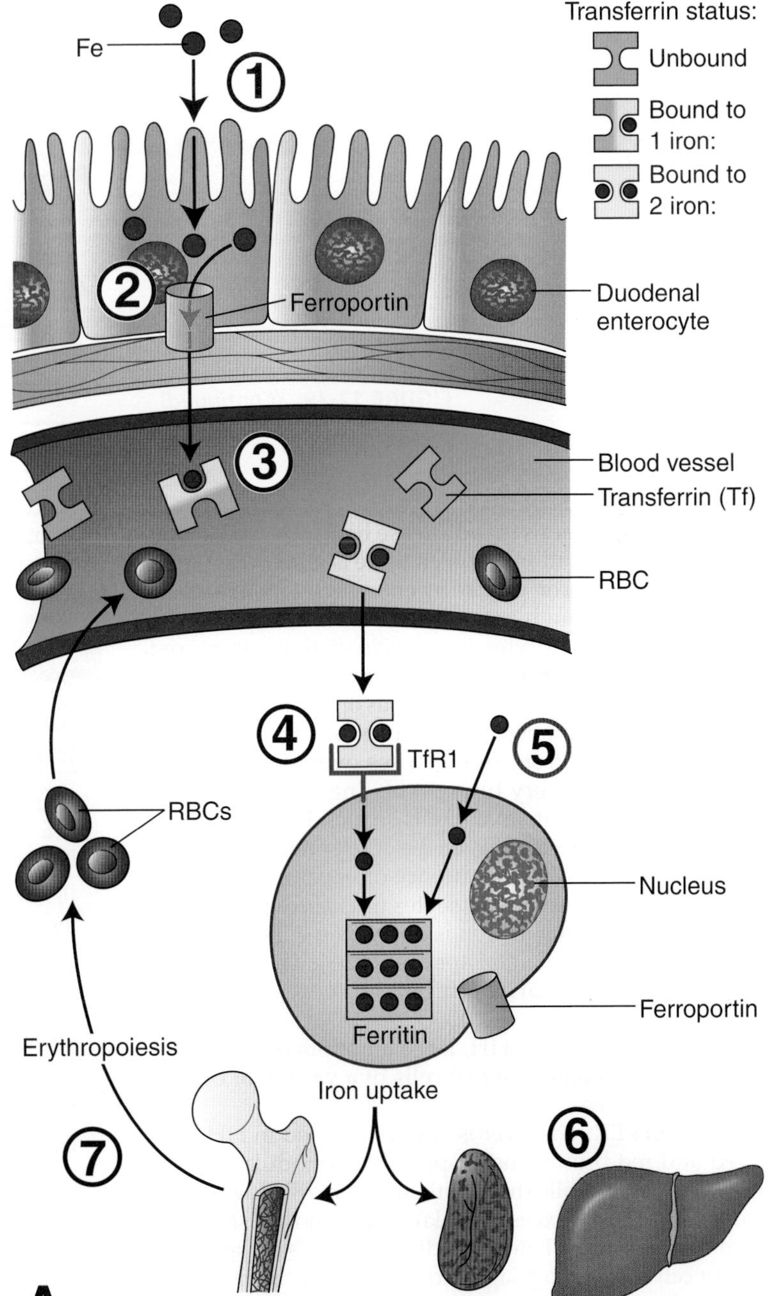

FIGURE 12-19. Normal iron metabolism and the role of hepcidin in its regulation. A. Iron absorption and utilization. (*1*) Iron enters duodenal enterocytes. These cells have a specific transporter that mediates iron entry. (*2*) Iron traverses enterocytes on its way to the circulation. Once in enterocyte cytosol, iron is exported by a specific channel, ferroportin, which mediates iron export in enterocytes and other cells. (*3*) Having traversed the enterocytes, Fe^{3+} binds to Tf, the principal means by which iron circulates. (Some free iron, i.e., iron not bound to Tf, circulates in normal circumstances.) (*4*) Tf is recognized by a receptor (TfR1) on cells that are engaged in iron uptake. It is stored bound to ferritin. (*5*) A small amount of iron enters cells as free iron, unbound to Tf. It, too, is stored as ferritin. (*6*) Excess iron supplies are stored in macrophages and hepatocytes. (*7*) Cells in the bone marrow incorporate iron into hemoglobin for use in erythrocytes. **B.** Hepcidin regulation of iron uptake. (*1*) Hepcidin is produced by hepatocytes and exported into the circulation. (*2*) The duodenum, the principal portal of iron entry into the body, is a key site of hepcidin action. (*3*) If hepcidin is present, it binds ferroportin. This has two consequences. First, iron is denied access to ferroportin and thus cannot be exported. Second, hepcidin binding causes the hepcidin–ferroportin complex to be internalized and degraded. (*4*) The sequence is illustrated here for enterocytes but applies comparably to the other cells that store and export iron, such as macrophages and hepatocytes. Tf, transferrin.

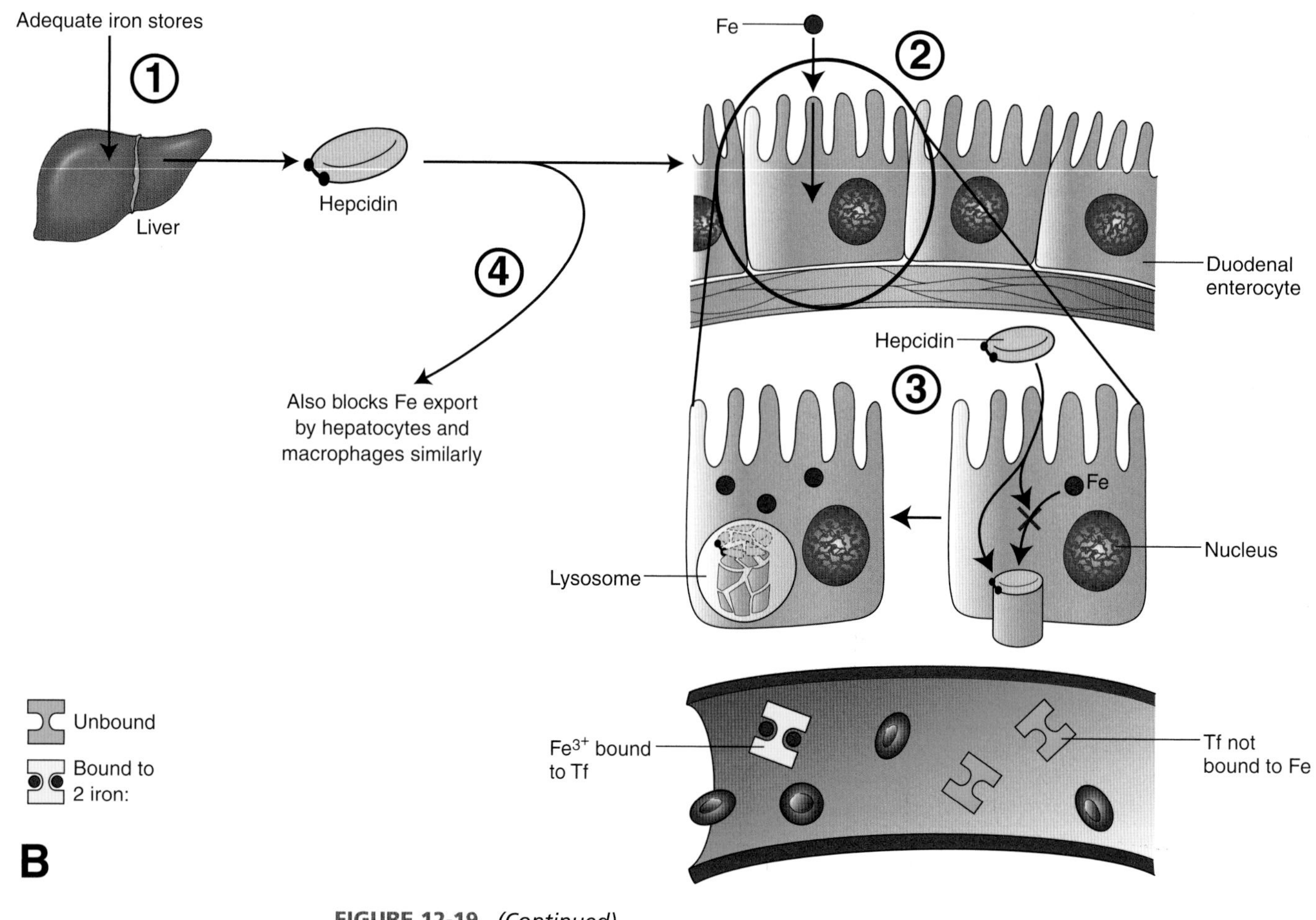

FIGURE 12-19. *(Continued)*

PATHOPHYSIOLOGY: At the center of HH is hepcidin. Mutations that decrease hepcidin production mimic a situation in which there is insufficient iron. As a result, iron uptake by enterocytes increases. As well, iron transit through enterocytes, and iron export from macrophages and hepatocytes, into the circulation is increased because hepcidin is not present to mediate downregulation of the ferroportin exporter. The exporter thus operates unchecked. The combination of enhanced iron absorption through the gut and increased export from storage sites overwhelms the Tf system and results in very high circulating free iron levels. Massive influx of iron into many cells ensues. In hepatocytes, this flood of free iron exceeds even the accelerated iron export (see above) that occurs in the absence of hepcidin-mediated inhibition of ferroportin. Hepatocytes thus accumulate iron, and as noted in Chapter 1, iron is a key factor in cell injury mediated by reactive oxygen species (ROS). The causes of iron overload are summarized in Table 12-4.

PATHOLOGY: In HH, large amounts of iron accumulate in parenchymal cells of a variety of organs and tissues.

LIVER: The liver is always affected in HH. It is enlarged and red brown and displays micronodular cirrhosis. Hepatocytes and bile duct epithelium are filled with iron granules (Fig. 12-20). Excess cellular iron is mostly stored in lysosomes as ferric iron. Late in the disease, iron is conspicuous in Kupffer cells, owing to phagocytosis of necrotic hepatocytes. Within the fibrous septa, iron is prominent in bile ductules and macrophages. Eventually, as with other forms of micronodular cirrhosis, macronodular cirrhosis supervenes.

Table 12-4

Causes of Iron Overload

Causes of Iron Overload
Increased iron absorption
Hereditary hemochromatosis
HFE associated: C282Y and H63D homozygotes and C282/H63D heterozygotes
Hemochromatosis associated with mutations in transferrin receptor-2 (TfR2) and ferroportin
Juvenile hemochromatosis: mutations in hemojuvelin and hepcidin
Chronic liver disease (e.g., alcoholic liver disease)
Iron-loading anemias
Porphyria cutanea tarda
Dietary iron overload; excess medicinal iron
Parenteral iron overload
Multiple blood transfusions
Injectable medicinal iron

HFE, High Iron Fe protein. Product of *HFE* gene .

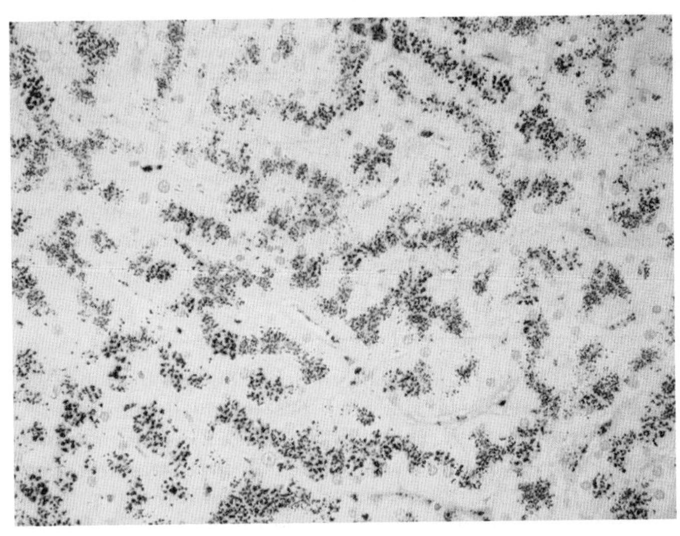

FIGURE 12-20. Hemochromatosis. Perl iron stain demonstrating marked iron (*blue*) in hepatocytes along the bile canaliculi.

SKIN: In HH, the skin is pigmented, but iron deposits in the skin in only half of patients. Most patients have increased melanin in the basal melanocytes.

PANCREAS: Diabetes secondary to the deposition of iron in the pancreas is common in HH. The organ is rust colored and fibrotic. Exocrine and endocrine cells have excess iron, and there is cell loss in both acini and islets of Langerhans. The combination of pigmented skin and glucose intolerance in HH is called **bronze diabetes**.

HEART: Congestive heart failure is a frequent cause of death in HH. Myocardial fibers contain iron pigment, more extensively in ventricles than in atria. Cardiac myocyte necrosis and resulting interstitial fibrosis are common.

ENDOCRINE SYSTEM: Many endocrine glands are affected in HH, including the pituitary, adrenal, thyroid, and parathyroid glands. Except for the pituitary, in which the release of gonadotropins is impaired, tissue damage does not occur in these organs.

JOINTS: About half of patients with HH show arthropathy, which is worst in the fingers and hands. HH arthritis affecting larger joints, such as the knee, can be disabling.

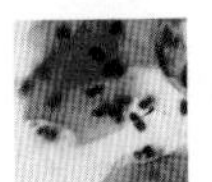

CLINICAL FEATURES: HH generally becomes symptomatic in midlife. The liver disease usually progresses slowly, but one fourth of untreated patients eventually die in hepatic coma or from gastrointestinal hemorrhage. Cirrhosis may lead to HCC; the 10-year cumulative chance of liver cancer reaches 30%. Treatment of HH involves removal of iron from the body, most effectively by repeated phlebotomy. Without treatment, 10-year survival with HH is only 6%.

DRUG-INDUCED LIVER INJURY

Drug-induced liver injury can mimic nearly any type of liver disease, with severity ranging from asymptomatic elevations of transaminases to acute liver failure. ***In fact, drugs are the most common cause of acute liver failure in the United States.*** Drugs cause injury in either **predictable** or **unpredictable** patterns. The former refers to drugs that cause liver injury in a dose-dependent manner (e.g., carbon tetrachloride; phalloidin, the toxin of the mushroom *Amanita phalloides*; and the analgesic acetaminophen). Unpredictable injury occurs with low frequency, irrespective of dose and without obvious predisposition **(idiosyncratic reaction)**.

Most drug reactions are unpredictable and seem to represent idiosyncratic events. This type of hepatotoxicity is presumed to occur in people with metabolic or genetic predispositions. In them, injury may reflect unusual sensitivity to a dose-related side effect. By contrast, some drugs or their metabolites may trigger immunologic reactions in the liver (autoimmune hepatitis). ***There is no specific test to predict or diagnose idiosyncratic drug-induced hepatotoxicity.***

Histologic Patterns of Drug-Induced Liver Disease

Drug toxicities span nearly the whole gamut of pathologies seen in non–drug-induced liver diseases. However, individual drugs usually have characteristic patterns of liver toxicity. Such patterns include zonal hepatocellular necrosis, cholestasis, acute or chronic hepatitis, and fatty liver.

Zonal Hepatocellular Necrosis

Toxic doses of acetaminophen *predictably* cause centrilobular necrosis, although very high doses can lead to panlobular necrosis. This zonal pattern probably reflects the greater activity of drug-metabolizing enzymes in the central zones. Other classic agents that produce such injury are carbon tetrachloride and phalloidin. In affected zones, hepatocytes show coagulative necrosis, hydropic swelling, and variable small droplet fat. Inflammation is sparse. Patients either die in acute hepatic failure or recover without sequelae. ***Acetaminophen-induced hepatotoxicity is the most common cause of acute liver failure in the United States and is frequently seen in suicidal gestures. Symptomatic patients invariably present soon after an ingestion.***

Cholestasis

Injury to intralobular and interlobular bile ducts is a common, unpredictable reaction to drugs. When it occurs, bile accumulates in hepatocytes and canaliculi. It is called *pure cholestasis* (Fig. 12-21) if there is no inflammation. Drugs that cause pure cholestasis include estrogens, androgens, and several antibiotics (e.g., sulfamethoxazole). If cholestasis is accompanied by inflammation, the term **cholestatic hepatitis** is used.

Acute and Chronic Hepatitis

Inflammatory reactions are common in many *unpredictable* hepatotoxic drug reactions. All of the features of acute viral hepatitis can occur after exposure to a wide variety of drugs (e.g., isoniazid and antibiotics). The inflammation is a general response to cell injury and necrosis, such as is seen in viral or autoimmune hepatitis. ***The entire range of acute liver injury, from mild anicteric hepatitis to rapidly fatal massive hepatic necrosis, is encountered.*** Typically, drug-induced hepatitis and liver enzyme elevations associated with it resolve when the offending drug is withdrawn. If exposure continues, chronic hepatitis and even cirrhosis may develop. Sometimes, inflammation may reflect **drug-induced autoimmune hepatitis** (e.g., nitrofurantoin), either as an immune response to the drug or by unmasking classic autoimmune hepatitis. The presence

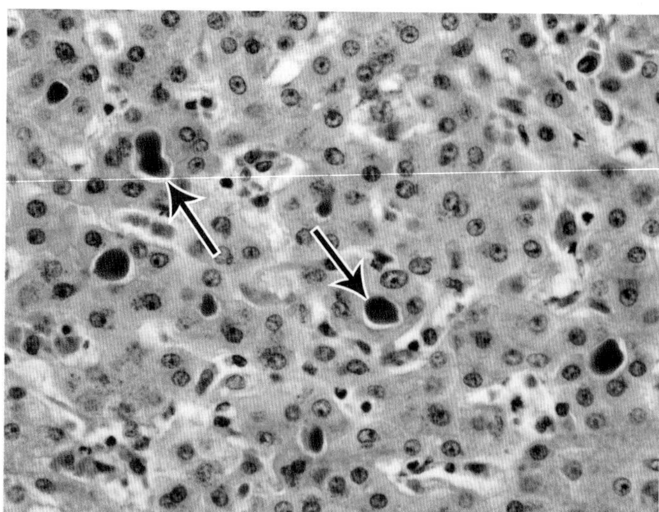

FIGURE 12-21. Bile stasis. The liver from a patient with drug-induced cholestasis showing prominent bile plugs in dilated bile canaliculi (*arrows*). In the absence of inflammation, this lesion may be termed *pure cholestasis.*

of eosinophils in the inflammatory infiltrate suggests such a drug reaction. ***An inflammatory infiltrate, regardless of its composition, is not specific for drug-associated hepatotoxicity.***

Fatty Liver

Accumulation of triglycerides within hepatocytes (i.e., hepatic steatosis or fatty liver) generally occurs in a predictable manner. Although there may be substantial overlap, two morphologic patterns are recognized: macrovesicular and microvesicular steatosis.

Macrovesicular steatosis is itself clinically inconsequential and appears similar to that seen in alcoholic steatosis. In addition to its association with chronic ethanol ingestion, macrovesicular fat results from accidental exposure to direct hepatotoxins, such as carbon tetrachloride. Corticosteroids and some antimetabolites, such as methotrexate, may also cause macrovesicular steatosis. Unlike macrovesicular steatosis, microvesicular fatty liver is often associated with severe and, sometimes fatal, liver disease. Small fat vacuoles are dispersed throughout the cytoplasm of hepatocytes, and the nucleus retains its central position.

REYE SYNDROME: This now rare acute disease of children is characterized by microvesicular steatosis, hepatic failure, and encephalopathy. Symptoms usually begin after a febrile illness, such as influenza or varicella infection, and often correlate with aspirin administration. Because the use of aspirin has declined in children, Reye syndrome has become uncommon.

Vascular Lesions

Occlusion of hepatic veins (**Budd–Chiari syndrome**; see below) may follow the use of oral contraceptives, perhaps because they induce hypercoagulability in some people. **Peliosis hepatis** is a peculiar hepatic lesion with cystic, blood-filled cavities that are not lined by endothelial cells. Anabolic sex steroids, contraceptive steroids, and the antiestrogen tamoxifen sometimes produce this lesion.

Mass Lesions and Altered Hepatic Morphology

Hepatocellular adenoma, usually induced by exogenous steroids, and **hemangiosarcoma**, caused by intravenous administration of the radioactive contrast agent thorium dioxide dye (no longer used), are among the very few mass lesions caused by drugs. Chronic exposure to inorganic arsenic, usually in insecticides, and occupational inhalation of vinyl chloride have also been linked to hepatic angiosarcomas.

HEPATIC FAILURE

Hepatic failure is the clinical syndrome that occurs when the liver cannot sustain its vital activities. It may develop acutely, mostly because of viral hepatitis or toxic exposure, or appear as chronic liver diseases, such as chronic viral hepatitis or cirrhosis. Advances in supportive care have improved survival in acute hepatic failure, but mortality for this condition without liver transplantation exceeds 50%. The consequences of hepatic failure are depicted in Figure 12-22. Symptoms include jaundice, hepatic encephalopathy, coagulation defects, steroid hormone imbalance, and portal hypertension.

Hyperbilirubinemia Refers to Inadequate Clearance of Bilirubin by the Liver

Hyperbilirubinemia resulting in jaundice in hepatic failure is mostly conjugated, although unconjugated bilirubin levels also tend to increase (as described below). On occasion, increased erythrocyte turnover may add to unconjugated hyperbilirubinemia, thereby aggravating the jaundice.

Hepatic Encephalopathy

Altered mental status is common in patients with acute liver failure and portal hypertension (see below).

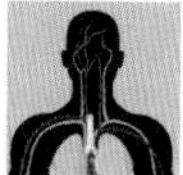

PATHOPHYSIOLOGY: No one factor explains the clinical syndrome of hepatic encephalopathy. Because of hepatocyte dysfunction and/or structural or functional vascular shunts, harmful compounds absorbed from the intestine escape hepatic detoxification. **Portal–systemic encephalopathy** is particularly evident after surgical construction of a portal–systemic anastomosis (portal vein to inferior vena cava or its equivalent).

Among the several toxic compounds implicated in hepatic encephalopathy are ammonia, γ-aminobutyric acid, and a variety of mercaptans. Failure of the liver to detoxify such substances leads to alterations in brain neurotransmission and osmolality.

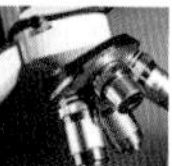

PATHOLOGY: Cerebral edema is the major cause of death in most patients with hepatic encephalopathy. It often coincides with uncal and cerebellar herniation. This edema is a specific lesion associated with hepatic coma, although the precise mechanism is obscure.

Coagulation Defects

In liver failure, impaired synthesis of coagulation factors and thrombocytopenia lead to poor hemostasis. The clotting

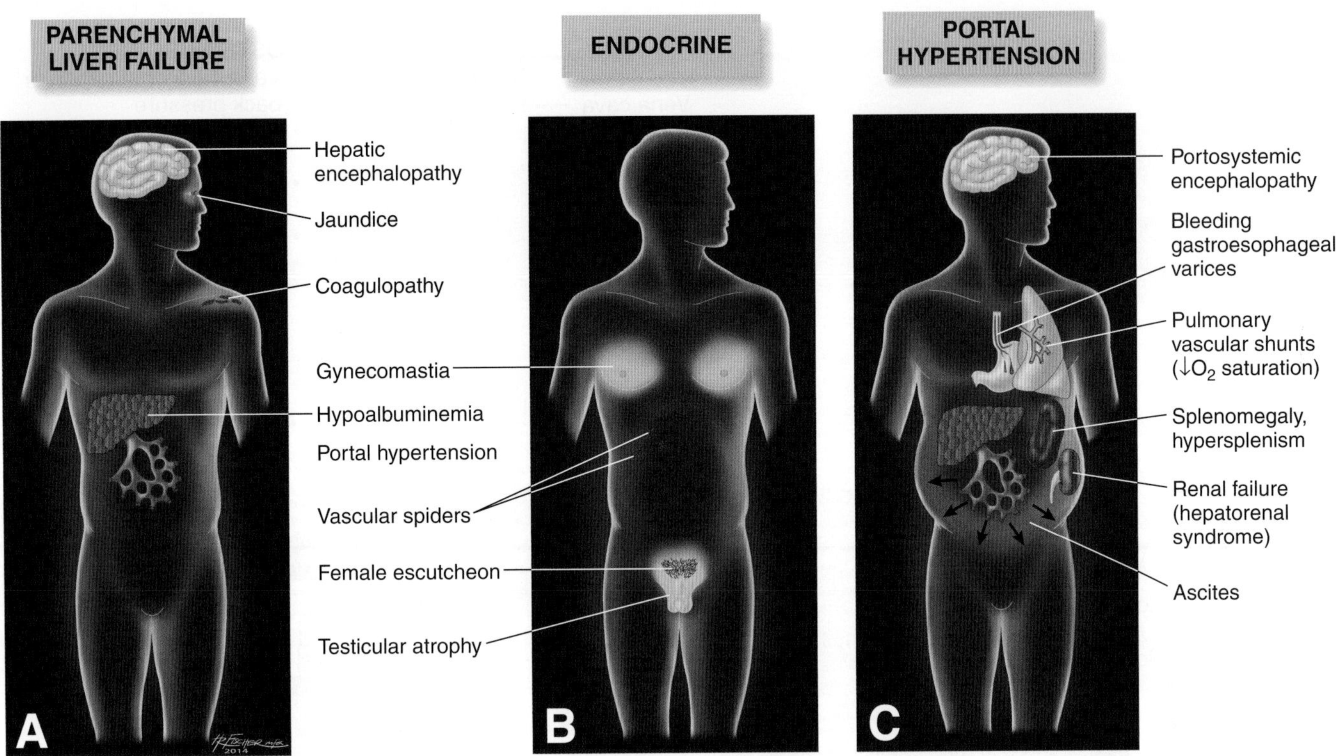

FIGURE 12-22. Complications of cirrhosis and hepatic failure. Clinical features related to **(A) parenchymal liver failure, (B) endocrine disturbances,** and **(C) portal hypertension.** There is considerable overlap of these clinical features with regard to their pathogeneses.

factors—fibrinogen, prothrombin, and factors VII, IX, and X—are reduced, thus reflecting generalized impairment of hepatic protein synthesis.

Thrombocytopenia (<80,000/μL) is common in hepatic failure, as are qualitative defects in platelet function. Hypersplenism, bone marrow depression, and failure of thrombopoietin synthesis decrease circulating platelet levels. Products of liver cell necrosis and release of tissue factor may lead to activation of the coagulation cascade and result in a DIC–like state.

Hypoalbuminemia

Impaired hepatic albumin synthesis causes hypoalbuminemia. This is an important factor in the pathogenesis of edema and ascites that often complicate chronic liver disease.

Steroid Hormone Imbalance

In men, **hyperestrogenism** results from reduced estrogen catabolism and conversion of weak androgens to estrogen in chronic liver failure. This effect leads to **gynecomastia**, a female body habitus and female distribution of pubic hair (female escutcheon). Vascular effects of hyperestrogenism are common and include **spider angiomas** in the drainage territory of the superior vena cava (upper trunk and face) and **palmar erythema**. In addition, a direct toxic action of alcohol on gonadal function independent of chronic liver disease occurs in both male and female alcoholics.

PORTAL HYPERTENSION OFTEN RESULTS FROM LIVER FAILURE

The portal vein carries the major venous drainage from the gastrointestinal tract, pancreas, and spleen to the liver, accounting for two thirds of the liver's blood flow but less than half of its total oxygen supply. The remainder is supplied by the hepatic artery. ***Portal hypertension is either an absolute increase in portal venous pressure or an increase in the pressure gradient between the portal vein and the hepatic vein.*** Obstruction to blood flow somewhere in the portal circuit is responsible. Increased portal pressure causes opening of **portal–systemic collateral channels**, bleeding from gastroesophageal varices, ascites, splenomegaly, and renal and pulmonary disease (Fig. 12-22). Increased resistance to portal blood outflow is the basis for diagnosing portal hypertension (Fig. 12-23). This increase in resistance can originate in one of the following three areas:

1. **Sinusoidal (intrahepatic):** Injury to sinusoids leads to sinusoidal, or intrahepatic, portal hypertension. In the Western world, cirrhosis is the most common cause of all forms of portal hypertension. In cirrhosis, fibrosis produces obstruction of intrahepatic sinusoids, thereby impeding the inflow of portal blood. The result is increased pressure in the portal vein. Intrahepatic portal hypertension is usually caused by cirrhosis.

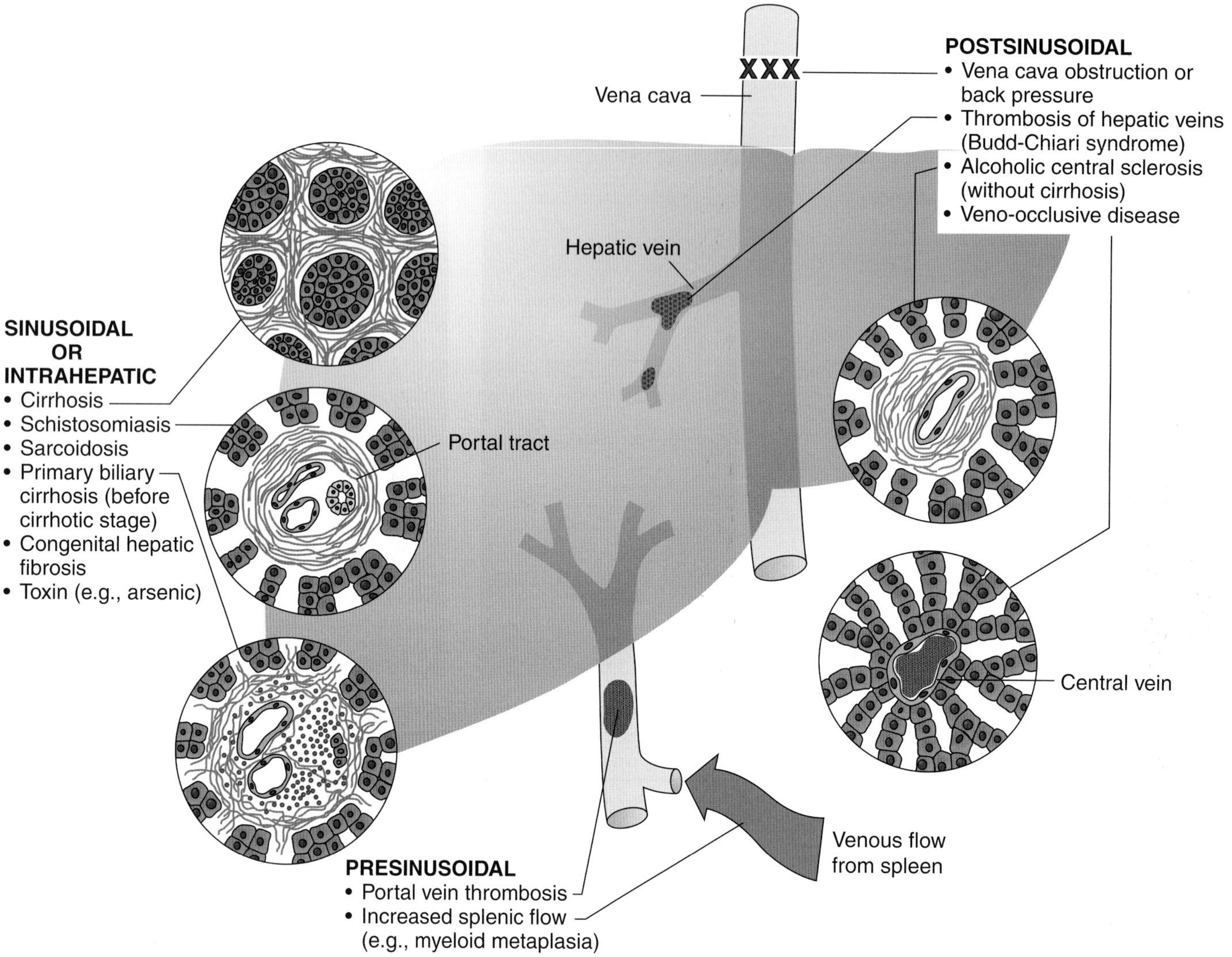

Vena cava
XXX
POSTSINUSOIDAL
• Vena cava obstruction or back pressure
• Thrombosis of hepatic veins (Budd-Chiari syndrome)
• Alcoholic central sclerosis (without cirrhosis)
• Veno-occlusive disease
Hepatic vein
SINUSOIDAL OR INTRAHEPATIC
• Cirrhosis
• Schistosomiasis
• Sarcoidosis
• Primary biliary cirrhosis (before cirrhotic stage)
• Congenital hepatic fibrosis
• Toxin (e.g., arsenic)
Portal tract
Central vein
Venous flow from spleen
PRESINUSOIDAL
• Portal vein thrombosis
• Increased splenic flow (e.g., myeloid metaplasia)

FIGURE 12-23. Causes of portal hypertension.

2. **Presinusoidal:** Resistance to blood flow in the extrahepatic portal vein (e.g., thrombotic occlusion) is known as **presinusoidal portal hypertension**.
3. **Postsinusoidal:** If the point of resistance is in the hepatic veins, venules, or cardiac circulation, **postsinusoidal portal hypertension** may result. This can occur if blood flow in the hepatic veins is impeded, as in **Budd–Chiari syndrome** or congestive heart failure.

PATHOPHYSIOLOGY: Intrahepatic portal hypertension, such as occurs in cirrhosis, offers the best paradigm for understanding the pathogenesis of portal hypertension. As fibrosis develops, sinusoids become increasingly disordered. Regenerative nodules in the cirrhotic liver impinge on the hepatic veins, thereby obstructing blood flow beyond the lobules. The small portal veins and venules are trapped, narrowed, and often obliterated by scarring of the portal tracts. Blood flow through the hepatic artery is increased, and small arteriovenous communications open. In this way, arterial blood flow increases and adds to portal hypertension as a result of obstruction of blood flow distal to the sinusoid. The increase in portal pressure opens vascular shunts that decompress the portal circuit. Although ostensibly valuable, these shunts are a mixed blessing because they cause complications such as bleeding varices and encephalopathy.

Worldwide, hepatic schistosomiasis is a major cause of intrahepatic portal hypertension. Granulomatous inflammatory reaction to parasitic ova in the intrahepatic portal venules interferes with sinusoidal blood flow. **Idiopathic portal hypertension**, also called **noncirrhotic portal hypertension**, refers to occasional cases of intrahepatic portal hypertension with splenomegaly in the absence of demonstrable intrahepatic or extrahepatic disease. Known causes of idiopathic portal hypertension are chronic exposure to copper, arsenic, and vinyl chloride.

Portal Vein Thrombosis

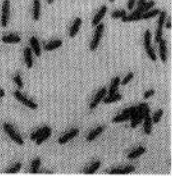

ETIOLOGIC FACTORS: Portal vein thrombosis occurs most often in the setting of cirrhosis. Other causes include tumors, infections, hypercoagulability states, pancreatitis, and surgical trauma.

Postsinusoidal Portal Hypertension

Budd–Chiari Syndrome

Budd–Chiari syndrome is a congestive disease of the liver caused by occlusion of the hepatic veins and their tributaries.

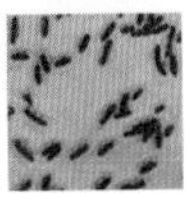

ETIOLOGIC FACTORS: Hepatic vein thrombosis is the main cause of Budd–Chiari syndrome; it may occur in diverse diseases, such as myeloproliferative neoplasms (especially polycythemia vera), hypercoagulable states associated with malignancies, use of oral contraceptives, pregnancy, bacterial infections, paroxysmal nocturnal hemoglobinuria, metastatic and primary tumors in the liver, and surgical trauma. In 20% of cases, there is no clear cause. Thrombi form most often in the large hepatic veins, near their exit from the liver, and in the intrahepatic part of the inferior vena cava. Increased venous back-pressure from severe congestive heart failure, tricuspid stenosis, or regurgitation or constrictive pericarditis may mimic the syndrome.

Hepatic veno-occlusive disease, a variant of Budd–Chiari syndrome, is caused by hepatic sinusoidal injury that results in occlusion of the centrilobular hepatic sinusoids, central venules, and small branches of the hepatic veins. This disorder is most often traced to ingestion of toxic pyrrolizidine alkaloids in plants of the *Crotalaria* and *Senecio* genera, which are used in "bush teas." It is also seen in patients given certain antineoplastic agents, after hepatic irradiation and after bone marrow transplantation, possibly as a manifestation of graft-versus-host disease.

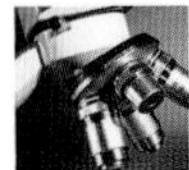

PATHOLOGY: In the acute stage of **hepatic vein thrombosis**, the liver is swollen and tense. Its cut surface is mottled and oozes blood (Fig. 12-24A). In the chronic stage, the cut surface is paler, and the liver is firm, owing to an increase in connective tissue. The hepatic veins have thrombi in varying stages of evolution, from recent clots to well-organized thrombi that have been canalized.

In the acute stage of both Budd–Chiari syndrome and veno-occlusive disease, the sinusoids of the central zone are dilated and packed with erythrocytes (Fig. 12-24B). Liver cell plates are compressed, with hemorrhage and necrosis of centrilobular hepatocytes. In long-standing venous congestion, fibrosis of the central zone may radiate to more peripheral portions of the lobules (Fig. 12-24C). Sinusoids are dilated, and central to midzonal hepatocytes show pressure atrophy. Eventually, **reverse lobulation** occurs, with connective tissue septa linking adjacent central zones to form nodules with a single central portal tract. This fibrosis is usually not severe enough to justify a label of cirrhosis.

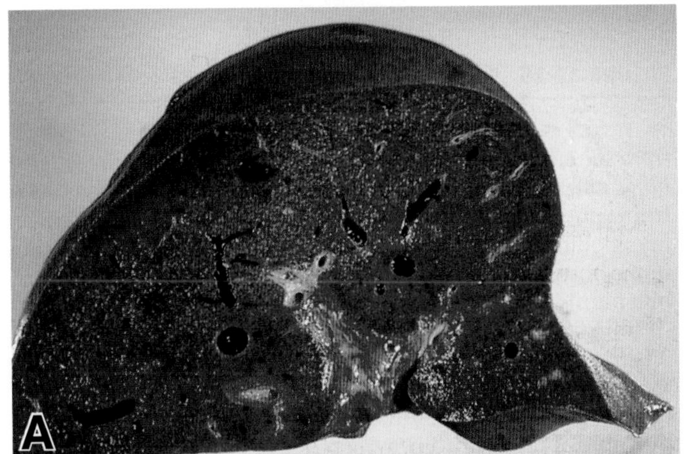

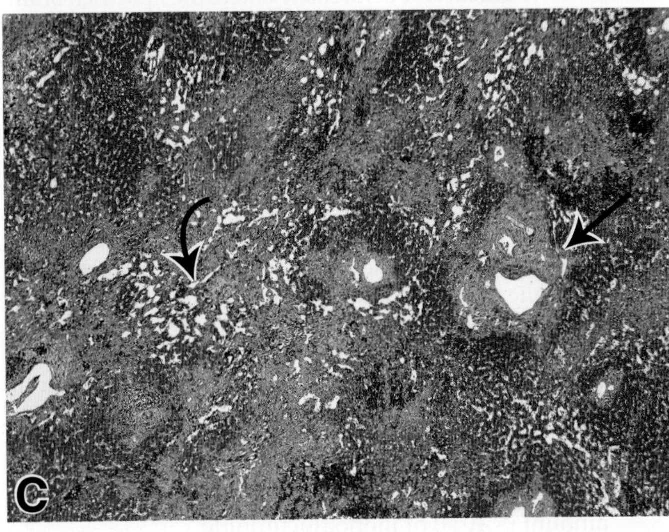

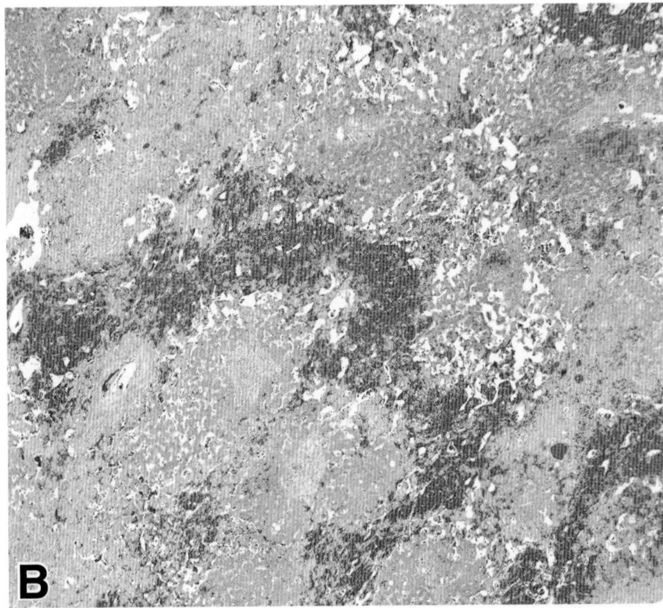

FIGURE 12-24. Budd–Chiari syndrome. A. The cut surface of the liver from a patient who died of Budd–Chiari syndrome showing thrombosis of the hepatic veins and diffuse congestion of the parenchyma. **B.** Liver parenchyma from a patient with **acute Budd–Chiari syndrome** revealing centrilobular necrosis and hemorrhage. **C. Chronic Budd–Chiari syndrome.** Cirrhosis has developed with bridging fibrosis emanating from the central venules rather than the portal tracts. Note the dilated sinusoids (*curved arrow*) and intact portal tract (*arrow*).

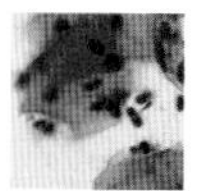

CLINICAL FEATURES: Complete thrombosis of the hepatic veins presents as an acute illness, with abdominal pain, enlargement of the liver, ascites, and mild jaundice. Acute hepatic failure and death often follow quickly. Most often, the obstruction of the hepatic venous circulation is incomplete, and similar symptoms persist for periods from a month to a few years. More than 90% of patients with Budd–Chiari syndrome develop ascites, usually severe, and splenomegaly is common. Typically, serum bilirubin and aminotransferase activities increase only modestly. Most patients eventually die in hepatic failure or from complications of portal hypertension. Liver transplantation is usually curative.

Effects of Portal Hypertension

Varices

Esophageal varices are the most important complication of portal hypertension. They arise when collateral portal–systemic vascular channels open to relieve pressure in the portal circuit. One of the most common causes of death in patients with disorders associated with portal hypertension is exsanguinating upper gastrointestinal hemorrhage from **bleeding esophageal varices** (see Chapter 11). There is no simple correlation between the magnitude of the portal venous pressure and the risk of variceal bleeding, but that risk does rise with increasing size of the varices. Back-pressure in the portal vein also dilates its tributaries, including the inferior hemorrhoidal veins, which become dilated and tortuous **(anorectal varices)**. Collateral veins radiating about the umbilicus produce a pattern known as **caput medusae**. Bleeding esophageal varices portend a poor prognosis: acute mortality may be as high as 40%. In patients with cirrhosis who have survived one episode of variceal bleeding, long-term survival is unlikely because the chances of rebleeding or worsening liver failure are high.

Splenomegaly

The spleen in portal hypertension enlarges progressively and often causes **hypersplenism**, a condition that decreases life span and consequently reduces levels in the circulation of all formed elements of the blood (pancytopenia). Hypersplenism is attributed to a prolonged transit time through the hyperplastic spleen.

Ascites

Ascites is accumulation of fluid in the peritoneal cavity. It often accompanies portal hypertension, and the amount of fluid may be so great (often many liters) that it distends the abdomen and interferes with breathing. The onset of ascites in cirrhosis is associated with a poor prognosis. The pathogenesis of ascites is illustrated in Figure 12-25.

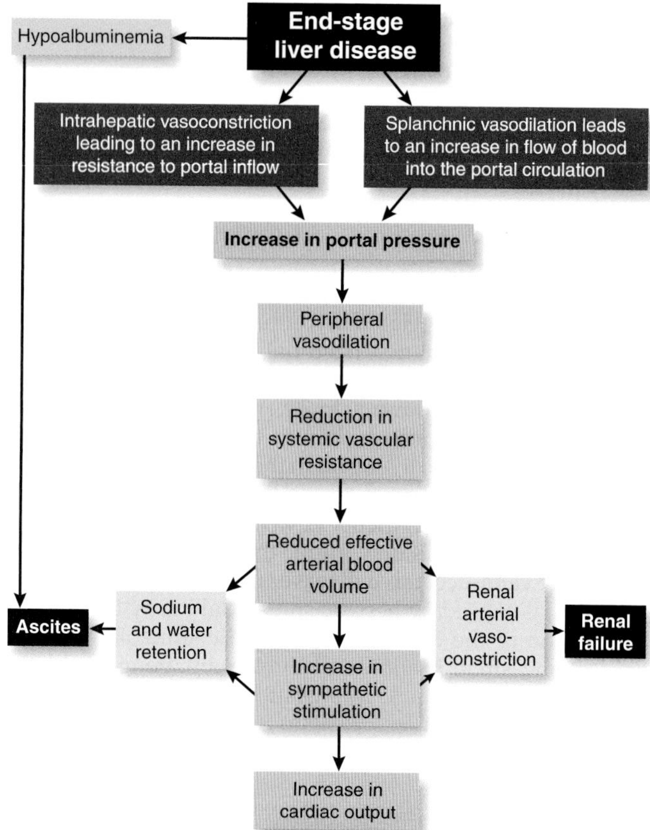

FIGURE 12-25. Pathogenesis of ascites.

BILIRUBIN METABOLISM AND MECHANISMS OF JAUNDICE

Bilirubin and Heme Catabolism

The liver is critical to the excretion of the products of heme catabolism via its major excretory product, namely, bile. About 80% of this heme comes from senescent erythrocytes, removed from the circulation by mononuclear phagocytes of the spleen, bone marrow, and liver. The remainder of the heme comes from other sources, including cytochrome P450 isoenzymes, myoglobin, and premature breakdown of erythroid progenitors in the bone marrow. Heme is converted to bilirubin, the major bile pigment, via an enzymatic process within macrophages.

Bilirubin dissolves poorly in water and in the circulation; it is transported bound to albumin. Albumin in the blood and extracellular space is a large reservoir for binding bilirubin, ensuring a low extracellular concentration of free (unbound) bilirubin. Free bilirubin, which is not bound to albumin or conjugated to glucuronic acid, easily enters the lipid-rich brain, where it is very toxic. High concentrations in newborns cause irreversible brain injury, termed **kernicterus**.

Transfer of bilirubin from blood to the bile involves the following four steps:

1. **Uptake:** The albumin–bilirubin complex is dissociated when it reaches hepatocytes, and bilirubin is transported across the plasma membrane. Transporter proteins facilitate mostly passive uptake by hepatocytes.
2. **Binding:** Once inside hepatocytes, bilirubin binds to cytosolic proteins, known collectively as **glutathione S-transferases** (also termed *ligandin*).
3. **Conjugation:** Bilirubin is converted to a water-soluble glucuronic acid conjugate for excretion. This is done in the endoplasmic reticulum (ER), where the uridine diphosphate-glucuronyl transferase (UGT) system attaches glucuronic acid to bilirubin. The process yields mostly water-soluble bilirubin diglucuronide and a small amount (<10%) of monoglucuronide.

4. **Excretion:** Conjugated bilirubin diffuses through the cytosol to bile canaliculi and is excreted into the bile by an energy-dependent carrier-mediated process. This is the rate-limiting step in the transhepatic transport of bilirubin. Bile acids, the primary end product of cholesterol that is synthesized predominantly by centrilobular hepatocytes, are also excreted into the bile.

Conjugated bilirubin enters the small intestine as part of mixed micelles but is not absorbed there. It remains intact until it reaches the distal small bowel and colon, where it is hydrolyzed by bacterial flora into free (unconjugated) bilirubin, which is reduced to a mixture of pyrroles, collectively called **urobilinogen**. Most urobilinogen is excreted in feces, but a small amount is absorbed in the terminal ileum and colon, returned to the liver, and re-excreted into the bile. Bile acids are also reabsorbed in the terminal ileum and salvaged by the liver. This recycling process is called the **enterohepatic circulation of bile**. Some urobilinogen escapes reabsorption by the liver, reaches the systemic circulation, and is excreted in the urine.

Overproduction of bilirubin (**hyperbilirubinemia** occurring with blood concentrations greater than 1.0 mg/dL) interferes with its hepatic uptake or intracellular metabolism. This process results in **jaundice** or **icterus** (i.e., yellow coloration of the skin and sclerae apparent when circulating bilirubin levels exceed 2.5 to 3.0 mg/dL). **Cholestatic jaundice** is the histologic appearance of hyperbilirubinemia associated with **cholestasis**, the pathologic plugging of dilated bile canaliculi with inspissated bile. In such cases, bile pigment becomes visible in hepatocytes. Many conditions are associated with hyperbilirubinemia (Fig. 12-26).

Unconjugated Hyperbilirubinemia

Increased production of free bilirubin results from enhanced destruction of erythrocytes (e.g., hemolytic anemia) or ineffective erythropoiesis. Hyperbilirubinemia from uncomplicated hemolysis is mainly unconjugated bilirubin, whereas parenchymal liver disease predominantly causes elevation of conjugated bilirubin (although there may also be some degree of increase in unconjugated bilirubin). Unconjugated hyperbilirubinemia is of little clinical significance in adults but can cause kernicterus with catastrophic brain damage in newborns (see Chapter 5). Generalized liver injury (such as that caused by viral hepatitis or certain drugs) may interfere with the net uptake of bilirubin by liver cells, also resulting in unconjugated hyperbilirubinemia. Generalized liver injury resulting from viral infection or certain drugs may interfere with net uptake of bilirubin by liver cells and hence cause mild unconjugated hyperbilirubinemia.

Decreased Bilirubin Conjugation

Several inherited syndromes affecting the level of UGT activity decrease bilirubin conjugation.

- **Crigler–Najjar syndrome type I** is a rare recessive disease in which patients totally lack hepatic uridine glucuronyl transferase (UGT) activity.
- **Crigle–Najjar syndrome type II** is milder, with a partial deficiency of the enzyme. The former disease was invariably fatal before the advent of phototherapy and liver transplantation in patients suffering from chronic severe unconjugated hyperbilirubinemia in early childhood. Type II disease patients almost always develop normally, although some do show neurologic changes resembling kernicterus.
- **Gilbert syndrome** is a common inherited condition resulting from inactivating *UGT* gene promoter mutations. The reduced level of UGT is generally without clinical import in otherwise healthy individuals. Mild hemolysis, which also tends to increase bilirubin levels, occurs in more than half of persons with Gilbert syndrome, but the mechanism is unclear.

Mutations in Multidrug Resistance Proteins

MRPs mediate transmembrane transport of organic ions, including conjugated bilirubin, bile acids, and phospholipids. Mutations in genes encoding these proteins, or in other canalicular transporters, impair hepatocellular secretion of bilirubin glucuronides and other organic anions into canaliculi. The spectrum of resultant diseases varies from innocuous to lethal. **Dubin–Johnson syndrome** is caused by mutations in *ABCC2/MRP2* gene. It is a benign, autosomal recessive disease characterized by chronic conjugated hyperbilirubinemia and conspicuous deposition of dark pigment in the liver. Clinical symptoms are usually mild, with slight intermittent jaundice and vague nonspecific complaints. Dark urine is present in half of those affected. **Rotor syndrome** is an extremely rare autosomal recessive condition that is similar to Dubin–Johnson syndrome but without liver pigmentation.

Jaundice, Sepsis, and Neonatal Hyperbilirubinemia

Severe conjugated hyperbilirubinemia may occur in sepsis caused by either Gram-positive or Gram-negative bacteria. In such situations, serum alkaline phosphatase and cholesterol levels are usually low, suggesting a defect in excretion of conjugated bilirubin. Liver pathology is nonspecific and includes mild canalicular cholestasis and slight fat accumulation. Portal tracts may contain excess inflammatory cells and variable bile ductule proliferation. Occasionally, dilated ductules are filled with inspissated bile.

Neonatal hyperbilirubinemia occurs in the absence of any specific disorder. Hepatic clearance of bilirubin in the fetus is minimal; hepatic uptake, conjugation, and biliary excretion are all much lower than in children and adults. Liver UGT activity is less than 1% of that in adults, and ligandin levels are low. Fetal bilirubin levels are low because bilirubin crosses the placenta and is conjugated and excreted by the mother's liver.

The liver of newborns becomes responsible for clearing bilirubin before the conjugation and excretion are fully developed. Moreover, increased erythrocyte destruction in the postnatal period adds to the liver's duties in the newborn. ***Thus, 70% of normal infants have transient unconjugated hyperbilirubinemia.*** Such physiologic jaundice is more pronounced in premature infants because liver clearance of bilirubin is less developed, and red blood cell turnover is greater than in term infants. When hepatic bilirubin-conjugating capacity reaches adult levels, about 2 weeks after birth, serum bilirubin levels rapidly decline to adult values. Absorption of light by unconjugated bilirubin

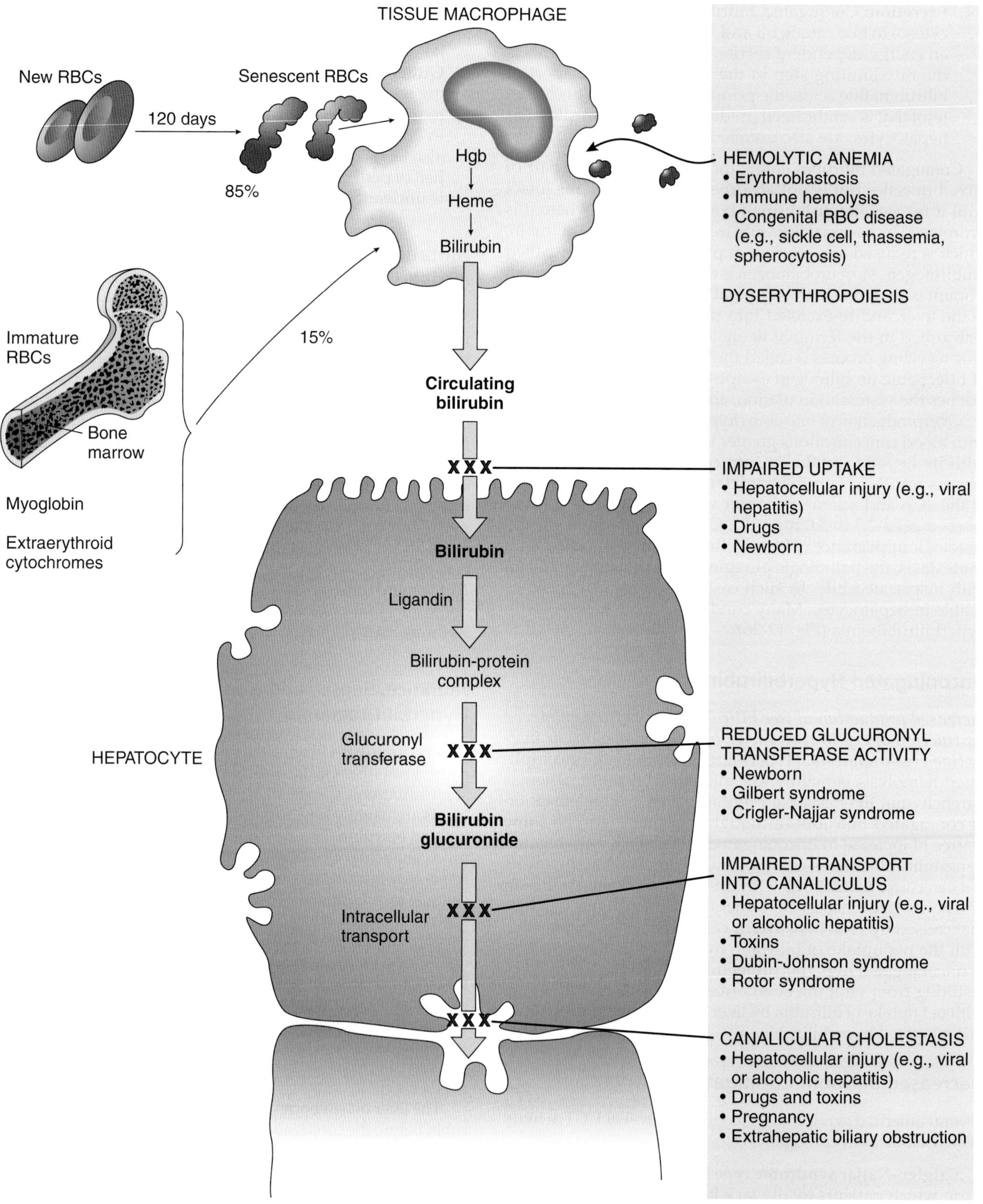

FIGURE 12-26. Mechanisms of hyperbilirubinemia at the level of the hepatocyte. Bilirubin is derived principally from the senescence of circulating red blood cells (RBCs), with a smaller contribution from the degradation of erythropoietic elements in the bone marrow, myoglobin, and extraerythroid cytochromes. Hyperbilirubinemia and jaundice result from overproduction of bilirubin (hemolytic anemia), dyserythropoiesis, impaired bilirubin uptake, or defects in its hepatic metabolism. The locations of specific blocks in the metabolic pathway of bilirubin in the hepatocyte are illustrated. Hgb, hemoglobin.

generates water-soluble bilirubin isomers. ***Thus, phototherapy is now routinely used to treat neonatal jaundice.***

Cholestasis

Cholestasis is pathologic plugging of dilated bile canaliculi by inspissated bile. Bile pigment, which is normally invisible, is also seen in hepatocytes. Functionally, cholestasis represents decreased bile flow through the canaliculus and reduced secretion of water, bilirubin, and bile acids by hepatocytes. The inability to excrete bile acids into canaliculi raises serum and hepatocellular bile acid levels. As detergents, bile acids injure cells by both detergent action and direct activation of apoptosis. They are thus potent hepatotoxins, and their accumulation within hepatocytes causes much of the hepatic injury and progression to cirrhosis associated with cholestasis. Elevation of serum bile acids is the likely cause of severe itching (**pruritus**) associated with cholestasis.

Clinical diagnosis depends on the accumulation of materials in the blood that are normally transferred to the bile, including bilirubin, cholesterol, and bile acids, and elevated blood activities of certain enzymes, typically alkaline phosphatase. Cholestasis caused by intrinsic liver disease is **intrahepatic cholestasis,** whereas cholestasis caused by obstruction of large bile ducts is termed **extrahepatic cholestasis**.

The extrahepatic biliary system may be obstructed by gallstones lodged in the common bile duct, cancers of the bile duct or surrounding tissues (pancreas or ampulla of Vater), external compression by enlarged neoplastic lymph nodes in the porta hepatis (as in lymphoma), benign strictures postoperative scarring or primary sclerosing cholangitis [PSC], and congenital extrahepatic biliary atresia (Fig. 12-27).

PATHOPHYSIOLOGY: Several mechanisms of cholestasis have been proposed.

DAMAGE TO CANALICULAR PLASMA MEMBRANES: The canalicular plasma membrane is the site of sodium (and therefore fluid) secretion into the bile. Alterations in the canalicular membrane by drugs and other agents that can perturb its structure inhibit the Na^+/K^+-ATPase, decrease bile flow, and produce morphologic alterations.

ALTERED CONTRACTILE PROPERTIES OF THE CANALICULUS: Bile is propelled along the canaliculus by a peristalsis-like contractile activity of hepatocytes. Agents that interact with the pericanalicular actin microfilaments (e.g., cytochalasin and phalloidin) inhibit this peristalsis and may cause cholestasis.

ALTERATIONS IN CANALICULAR MEMBRANE PERMEABILITY: Agents that cause cholestasis, including estrogens and taurolithocholate, may allow back diffusion of bile components by making canalicular membranes more permeable, or "leaky."

PATHOLOGY: ***Cholestasis is characterized by the presence of brownish bile pigment within dilated canaliculi and in hepatocytes*** (Figs. 12-4 and 12-21). Canaliculi are enlarged. Bile accumulates in hepatocytes in large, bile-laden lysosomes. In both intrahepatic and extrahepatic cholestasis, bile pigment initially is centrilobular. When cholestasis persists, secondary morphologic abnormalities develop. Scattered necrotic hepatocytes probably reflect the toxicity of excess intracellular bile. Intrasinusoidal macrophages and Kupffer cells contain bile pigment and cellular debris. Whereas early cholestasis is limited almost entirely to the central zone, chronic cholestasis is also marked by bile plugs at the periphery of lobules.

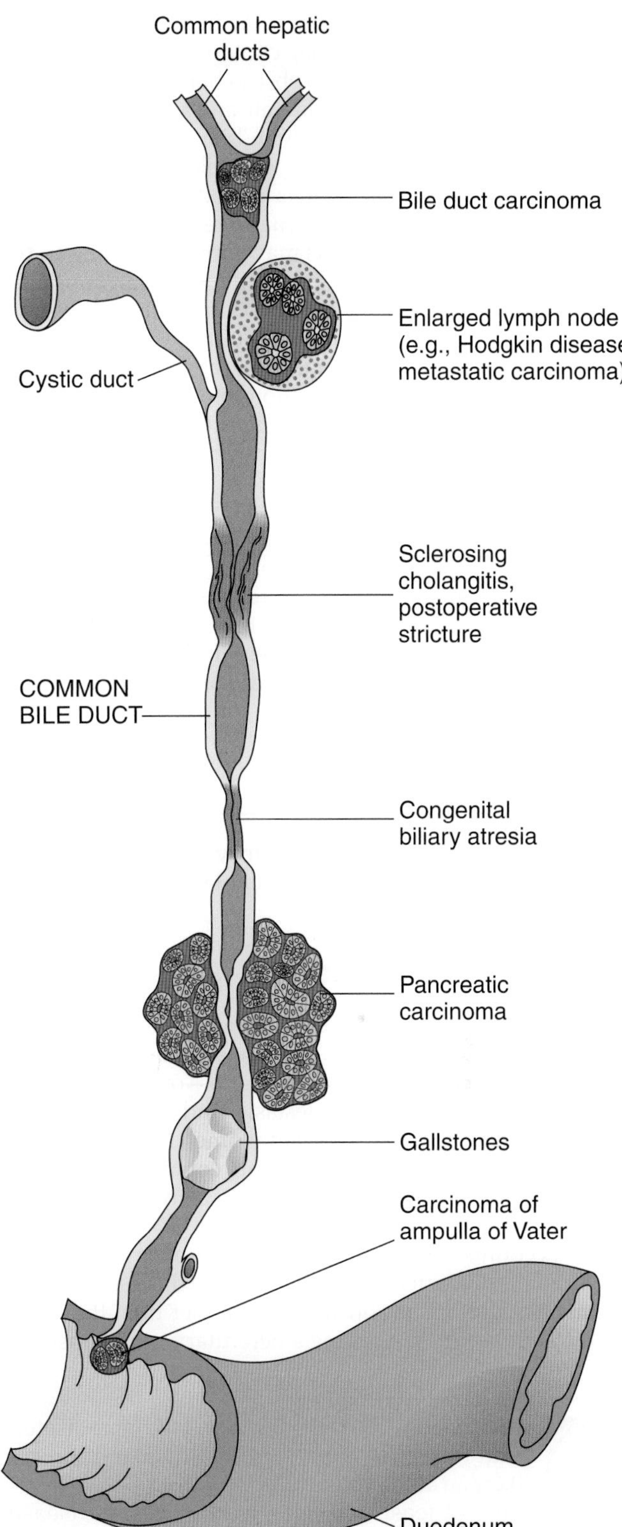

FIGURE 12-27. Major causes of extrahepatic biliary obstruction.

In **extrahepatic biliary obstruction**, the liver is swollen and bile stained. Prolonged obstruction suppresses bile secretion, causing the bile to become almost colorless ("white bile").

The liver, however, remains green. At first, edema in portal tracts accompanies centrilobular cholestasis, progressing to portal mononuclear infiltrates as obstruction persists. Tortuous and distended bile ductules proliferate and attract neutrophils. Damaged hepatocytes swollen with bile show (1) hydropic swelling, (2) diffuse impregnation with bile pigment, and (3) a reticulated appearance. This triad is termed **feathery degeneration** (Fig. 12-4). Cholestasis eventually reaches the periphery of the lobule. Dilated bile ducts may rupture, leading to **bile lakes**, which are focal, golden yellow deposits surrounded by degenerating hepatocytes. Infection of obstructed biliary passages often produces superimposed suppurative cholangitis, intraluminal pus, and even intrahepatic abscesses. Within bile ducts and ductules, biliary concretions may be conspicuous. If extrahepatic biliary obstruction is untreated, septa eventually extend between portal tracts of contiguous lobules to form **micronodular cirrhosis** (see above).

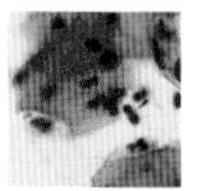

CLINICAL FEATURES: Whatever the cause, cholestasis usually presents with jaundice. **Pruritus** (itching) is common and can be severe and intractable. It may be caused by deposition of bile acids in the skin, but other bile components may play a role. Cholesterol accumulates in the skin to form **xanthomas. Malabsorption** may develop in cases of protracted cholestasis.

PRIMARY CHOLANGITIS

The two types of primary inflammatory disease of bile ducts (biliary cholangitis and sclerosing cholangitis) are both associated with autoimmunity.

Primary Biliary Cholangitis

PBC is an immune-mediated, chronic, progressive cholestatic disease in which intrahepatic bile ducts are destroyed (**nonsuppurative destructive cholangitis**). Loss of bile ducts leads to impaired bile secretion, cholestasis, and hepatic damage. PBC occurs mainly in middle-aged women (10:1 female predominance). The term *cirrhosis* in this context is somewhat misleading because it is actually a late complication of the disease.

PBC accounts for up to 2% of deaths from cirrhosis. Cases are sporadic, although the prevalence of the disease in families of patients with PBC is considerably higher than that in the general population, suggesting a hereditary predisposition.

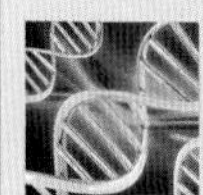

MOLECULAR PATHOGENESIS: PBC is associated with many immune abnormalities and thus is likely an autoimmune disease. Most (85%) patients have at least one other autoimmune disease (chronic thyroiditis, rheumatoid arthritis, scleroderma, Sjögren syndrome, or systemic lupus erythematosus). The *DRB1*008* family of major histocompatibility complex–encoded genes is associated with PBC.

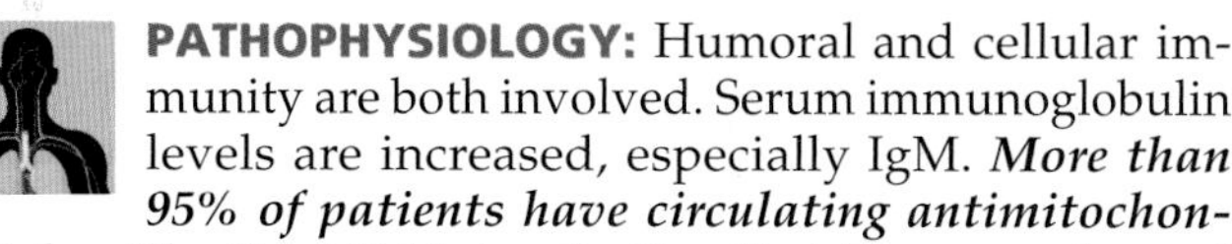

PATHOPHYSIOLOGY: Humoral and cellular immunity are both involved. Serum immunoglobulin levels are increased, especially IgM. ***More than 95% of patients have circulating antimitochondrial antibodies (AMAs), a finding that is commonly used to diagnose PBC.*** Autoantibodies bind epitopes associated with the mitochondrial pyruvate dehydrogenase complex. Despite their specificity, AMAs do not affect mitochondrial function and play no known role in the pathogenesis or progression of the disease. Other circulating autoantibodies are antinuclear, antithyroid, antiplatelet, antiacetylcholine receptor, and antiribonucleoprotein antibodies. The complement system is also chronically activated. The cells surrounding and infiltrating the sites of bile duct damage are mostly suppressor/cytotoxic ($CD8^+$) lymphocytes, suggesting that they mediate the destruction of the ductal epithelium.

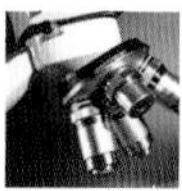

PATHOLOGY: Pathologic stages of PBC are (1) portal stage, (2) periportal stage, (3) septal stage, and (4) biliary cirrhosis (Fig. 12-28). Early PBC features a unique lesion, a **chronic destructive cholangitis** involving small- and medium-sized intrahepatic bile ducts and marked inflammation in portal areas. Epithelioid granulomas often occur in portal tracts and may impinge on the bile ducts. With disease progression, bile ducts are reduced in number, and ductular proliferation is evident in the periportal areas. Ultimately, destructive inflammation leads to the loss of small bile ducts. Collagenous septa extend from the portal tracts into the lobular parenchyma and begin to encircle some lobules. The end stage of PBC is cirrhosis, with a dark green, bile-stained, nodular liver and mainly portal-to-portal bridging fibrous septa.

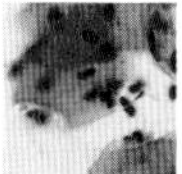

CLINICAL FEATURES: ***Some 90% to 95% of those afflicted with PBC are women, usually those who are 30 to 65 years old.*** Fatigue and pruritus are the most common initial symptoms, but many patients have no symptoms during the early stage of PBC. Some remain asymptomatic and appear to have an excellent prognosis; others ultimately develop advanced cirrhosis and its complications. The diagnosis of PBC is confirmed when a patient meets two of the following three criteria: (1) AMA titer of 1:40 or higher; (2) biochemical cholestasis, as indicated by elevated serum

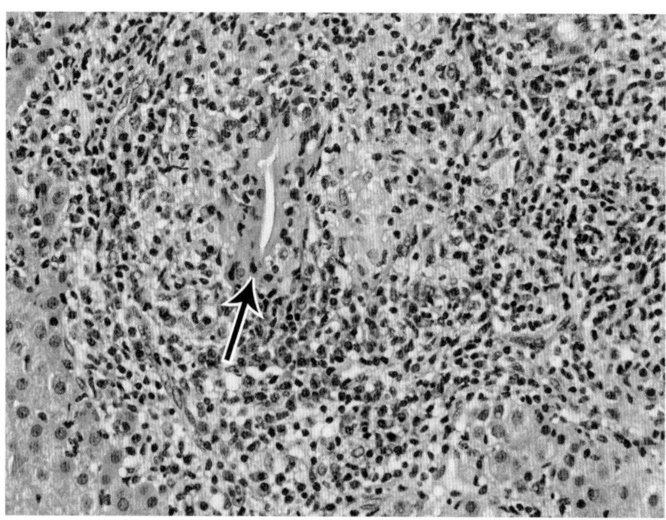

FIGURE 12-28. Florid duct lesion in primary biliary cirrhosis (PBC), stage I. A portal tract expanded by an inflammatory infiltrate consisting of lymphocytes, plasma cells, eosinophils, and macrophages. Florid duct lesion represents a damaged bile duct (*arrow*) by the inflammation.

alkaline phosphatase for at least 6 months; and (3) typical liver histology. Blood cholesterol levels increase strikingly, and an abnormal lipoprotein (lipoprotein-X) appears, a finding in many forms of chronic cholestasis. Cholesterol-laden macrophages accumulate in subcutaneous tissues, where they form localized lesions termed **xanthomas**. Impaired bile excretion into the intestine often causes severe **steatorrhea**, owing to fat malabsorption. Associated malabsorption of vitamin D and calcium eventuates in **osteomalacia** and **osteoporosis**. Those patients who develop cirrhosis die of liver failure or complications of portal hypertension. The course of PBC is usually indolent and may be as long as 20 to 30 years. Liver transplantation is highly effective in end-stage PBC.

Primary Sclerosing Cholangitis

PSC is a chronic cholestatic liver disease of unknown etiology, in which inflammation and fibrosis narrow and then obstruct intrahepatic and extrahepatic bile ducts. It usually occurs in men (70%), with a mean age of 40 years. PSC prevalence is 14 cases per 100,000 population. Progressive biliary obstruction typically leads to persistent obstructive jaundice, recurrent cholangitis, and eventually to secondary biliary cirrhosis.

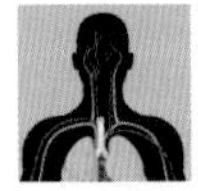

PATHOPHYSIOLOGY: ***The cause of PSC is unknown, but two thirds of patients also have ulcerative colitis.*** A few cases have been described in patients with Crohn disease of the colon. In one fourth of cases, no other disease is present. Genetic and immunologic factors are implicated in the pathogenesis of PSC. PSC can occur in families, sometimes associated with certain HLA haplotypes, including HLA B8. Hypergammaglobulinemia is common, as are circulating immune complexes and antineutrophil cytoplasmic antibodies (p-ANCA see Chapter 8), and complement activation by the classic pathway. Portal tracts contain an increased number of T cells.

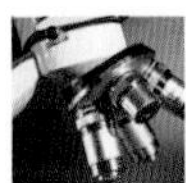

PATHOLOGY: In PSC, liver disease progresses from a portal stage, demonstrating periductal inflammation and "concentric, onion-skin" fibrosis in the portal tracts (Fig. 12-29A) to bridging fibrosis and end-stage biliary cirrhosis, a progression similar to that seen in PBC.

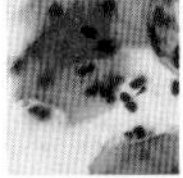

CLINICAL FEATURES: The median survival in symptomatic patients with PSC is 8 to 9 years. Asymptomatic patients have a better prognosis. Clinical presentations vary from asymptomatic elevations in cholestatic liver tests to symptoms of biliary obstruction, recurrent cholangitis, and evidence of end-stage liver disease. Infection may be followed by abscess formation. ***Cholangiocarcinoma develops in up to 20% of patients with PSC.*** Liver transplantation may be curative; however, PSC often recurs in the transplanted liver.

BENIGN TUMORS OF THE LIVER

Benign tumors of the liver are not an uncommon incidental finding but are most often of little clinical consequence. However, such tumors can sometimes result in catastrophic peritoneal bleeding.

Liver Adenomas

Once rare, these tumors became more common with oral contraceptive use. Lower dose estrogen and progesterone combinations have reduced the incidence of liver adenomas.

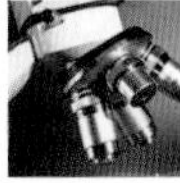

PATHOLOGY: Hepatocellular adenomas are usually solitary, sharply demarcated masses measuring up to 40 cm and weighing up to 3 kg. Multiple smaller adenomas are present in 25% of cases. If a liver has more than 10 adenomas, it is diagnosed as hepatocellular adenomatosis. These tumors are encapsulated and paler than nearby liver parenchyma. ***The neoplastic hepatocytes resemble normal hepatocytes but are not arrayed in a lobular architecture.*** Portal tracts and central venules are absent. The cells of adenomas may be very large and eosinophilic, or filled with glycogen or fat, which makes the cytoplasm appear clear or

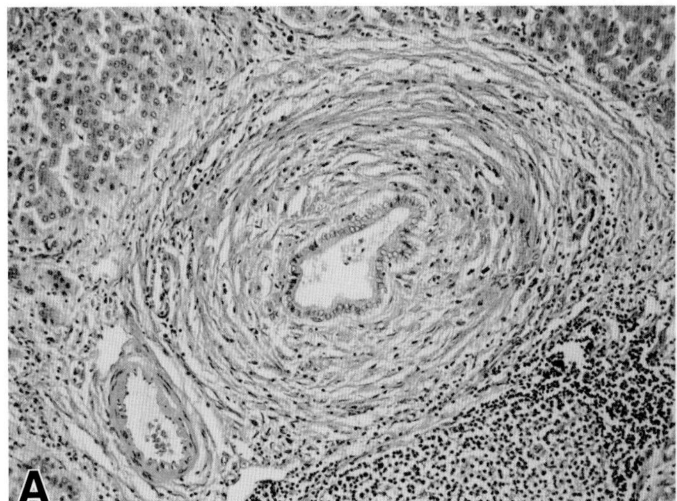

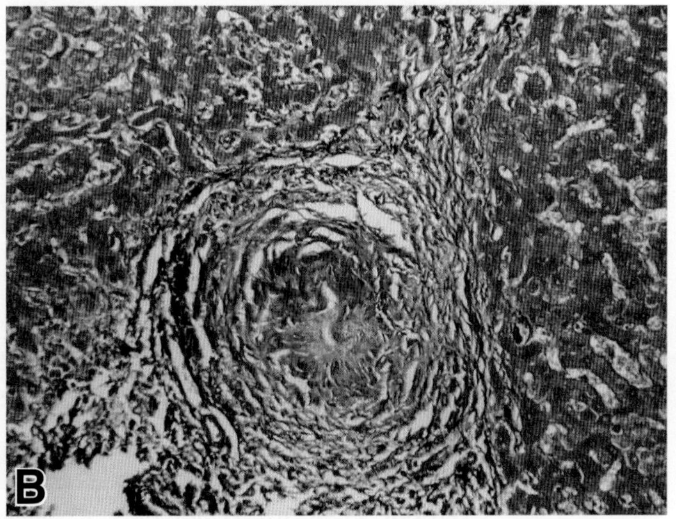

FIGURE 12-29. Primary sclerosing cholangitis (PSC). A. An inflamed portal tract with a dilated bile duct and "onion-skin" periductal fibrosis. **B.** A bile duct scar representing a destroyed bile duct in PSC (trichrome stain).

vacuolated. The presence of small arteries within the parenchyma suggests an adenoma as opposed to normal liver.

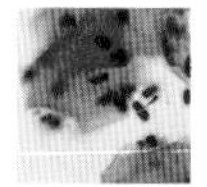

CLINICAL FEATURES: In about one third of patients with hepatic adenomas (particularly pregnant women who have used oral contraceptives), these tumors bleed into the peritoneal cavity and require immediate surgery. Even large adenomas may disappear if oral contraceptives are discontinued. Occasional liver adenomas have been reported in men who use anabolic steroids.

Hemangiomas

Benign hemangiomas in the liver occur at all ages and in both sexes. They are common, being present in up to 7% of autopsy livers. They are normally small and asymptomatic, although larger tumors may cause abdominal symptoms and even hemorrhage into the peritoneum. Grossly, hemangiomas are usually solitary and under 5 cm, but multiple hemangiomas and giant forms (>15 cm) have been described. They resemble cavernous hemangiomas found elsewhere.

Mesenchymal Hamartoma

Mesenchymal hamartoma is a benign liver tumor formed as a developmental malformation of liver mesenchyme. It shows large, serous fluid cysts surrounded by loose mesenchyme containing a mixture of bile ducts, hepatocyte cords, and clusters of vessels. The mesenchymal tissue consists of scattered stellate-shaped cells in a loose matrix. Complete surgical excision is curative.

MALIGNANT TUMORS OF THE LIVER

Primary malignant liver tumors, specifically hepatocellular carcinoma (HCC), were once uncommon, but now are an ever-increasing problem because of their association with chronic viral hepatitis. Nevertheless, metastatic liver tumors, often derived from primary disease in the gastrointestinal tract, are the most common cancers found in the liver.

Hepatocellular Carcinoma

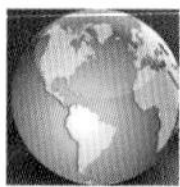

EPIDEMIOLOGY: Worldwide, HCC is probably the most common human cancer, demonstrating a striking geographical variability. In Western industrialized countries, HCC is uncommon, but its incidence has nearly doubled in the past 20 years, mostly in patients with chronic hepatitis C. In Sub-Saharan Africa, Southeast Asia, and Japan, HCC may occur up to 50 times more often. More than 85% of cases of HCC occur in countries with a high prevalence of chronic HBV infection. Most patients have had chronic hepatitis B for years, often after perinatal transmission from an infected mother to her newborn child. Persistent HBV infection is very dangerous, with up to a 200-fold increased risk for HCC. ***HCV is less common than HBV worldwide, but most cases of HCC in Europe, North America, and Japan are associated with hepatitis C.*** In the United States, HCV infection is present in about 50% of HCC. As with HCC in hepatitis B, most patients with HCV who develop HCC have underlying cirrhosis, and the cumulative occurrence of HCC in HCV-induced cirrhosis is as high as 70% after 15 years. Other causes of HCC showing substantial risk are hemochromatosis and α_1-AT deficiency. Aflatoxin B_1 a fungal food contaminant found most often in less developed countries is a potential risk factor found most often in contaminated grains and nut products. The incidence of liver cancer in humans correlates roughly with the dietary content of aflatoxin, but the connection remains problematic.

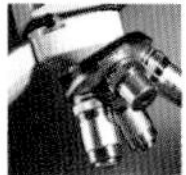

PATHOLOGY: HCCs are solitary or multiple soft, hemorrhagic tan masses (Fig. 12-30A). Occasionally, a green color indicates bile production. HCCs tend to grow into portal and hepatic veins, and they may extend from the latter into the vena cava and even the right atrium. The tumor may spread widely, but metastases favor the lungs and portal lymph nodes. HCCs range from so well differentiated as

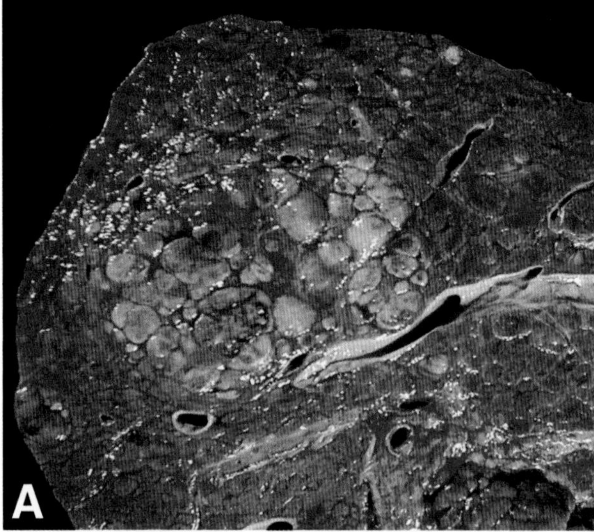

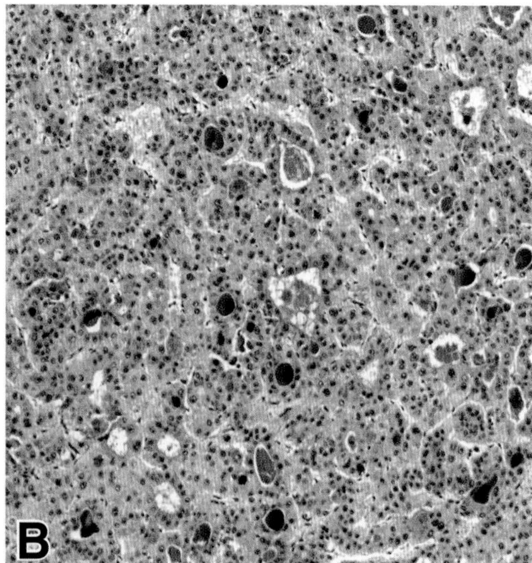

FIGURE 12-30. Hepatocellular carcinoma (HCC). A. Cross section of a cirrhotic liver showing a poorly circumscribed, nodular area of yellow, partially hemorrhagic HCC. **B.** In this moderately differentiated tumor, HCC cells are arranged in an acinar pattern and surround concretions of inspissated bile.

to be hard to distinguish from normal liver to anaplastic or undifferentiated neoplasms. In most cases, tumor cells are arranged in trabeculae or plates as in normal liver ("trabecular pattern"). These plates are separated by endothelium-lined sinusoids. In a "pseudoglandular (adenoid, acinar) pattern," malignant hepatocytes are arranged around a lumen, which may contain bile (Fig. 12-30B). Despite their resemblance to glands, these are not true glands, and the lesion should not be confused with cholangiocarcinoma or other adenocarcinomas. Neither histologic pattern carries a particular prognostic significance.

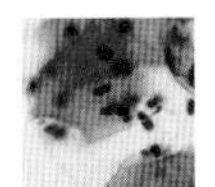

CLINICAL FEATURES: HCC usually presents as a painful and enlarging mass. If discovered at an advanced stage, the prognosis is dismal. Patients die of malignant cachexia, rupture of the tumor with catastrophic bleeding into the peritoneal cavity, or complications of cirrhosis. HCC may cause paraneoplastic syndromes (e.g., polycythemia, hypoglycemia, and hypercalcemia) owing to ectopic hormone production by the tumor. α-Fetoprotein (AFP) levels are often elevated, as in other benign and malignant liver diseases and some extrahepatic disorders.

If a small tumor is confined to one hepatic lobe, segmental resection can provide acceptable tumor-free survival rates. Ablative therapies (e.g., absolute alcohol injection, radiofrequency ablation, cryotherapy, and transarterial embolization) can slow tumor progression. In patients with cirrhosis and limited tumor burden, liver transplantation gives the best tumor-free survival.

Cholangiocarcinoma

Cholangiocarcinoma is a bile duct carcinoma that originates anywhere in the biliary tree, from large intrahepatic bile ducts at the porta hepatis to the smallest ducts at the edges of hepatic lobules. It occurs mainly in older people of both sexes, with an average age at presentation of 60 years. It may occur anywhere but is particularly common in parts of Asia where the liver fluke is endemic. The prognosis is usually dismal.

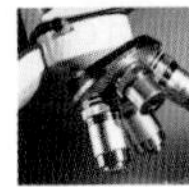

PATHOLOGY: Peripheral tumors or intrahepatic cholangiocarcinomas contain small cuboidal cells in ductular or glandular patterns (Fig. 12-31). They often show substantial fibrosis and thus may be confused with metastatic breast or pancreas carcinomas on liver biopsy.

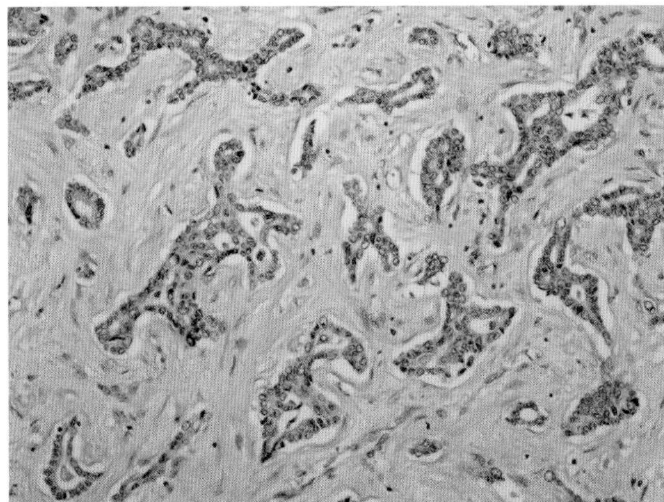

FIGURE 12-31. Cholangiocarcinoma. Well-differentiated neoplastic glands are embedded in a dense fibrous stroma.

Metastatic Cancer

Of all metastatic cancers, one third affect the liver, including one half of cancers of the gastrointestinal tract, breast, and lung. Metastatic disease is the most common malignancy in the liver. Pancreatic carcinoma, malignant melanoma, and hematologic malignancies also often metastasize the liver, but any tumor may do so.

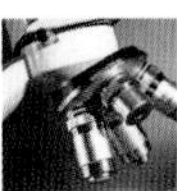

PATHOLOGY: The liver may have a single metastatic nodule or be almost replaced by metastases (Fig. 12-32). The weight of the organ may exceed 5 kg. ***Such metastases are the most common cause of massive hepatomegaly.*** Metastatic tumors can appear on the liver surface as umbilicated masses. Hepatic metastases tend to resemble their primary tumors but may be so poorly differentiated that a primary site cannot be determined.

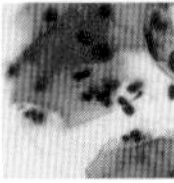

CLINICAL FEATURES: Metastatic cancers to the liver often present with weight loss. If the patient lives long enough, hepatic failure may ensue. Often, the first indication of a metastatic tumor is an unexplained increase in serum alkaline phosphatase. Most patients die within a year of diagnosis, but surgical resection of a solitary metastasis may be curative.

DISEASES OF THE GALLBLADDER

Anatomy

The gallbladder is a thin, elongated sac, about 8 cm long and about 50 mL in volume, which occupies a fossa on the inferior surface of the liver between the right and quadrate lobes. It originates from the same foregut diverticulum that gives rise to the liver. Its primary function is storage, concentration, and release of bile. The cystic duct is about 3 cm long and drains the gallbladder into the hepatic duct. It conducts dilute bile from the hepatic duct into the gallbladder, where it is concentrated and subsequently discharged into the common bile duct.

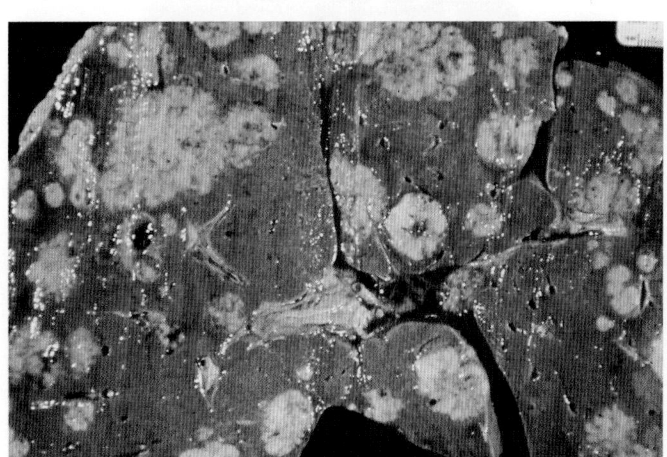

FIGURE 12-32. Metastatic carcinoma in the liver. The cut surface of the liver showing many firm, pale masses of metastatic colon cancer.

The gallbladder wall is composed of a mucous membrane, a muscularis and an adventitia. It is covered by a reflection of visceral peritoneum. The mucosa is thrown into folds and consists of columnar epithelium and a lamina propria of loose connective tissue. **Rokitansky–Aschoff sinuses** are mucosal diverticula that dip into the gallbladder wall.

CHOLELITHIASIS

Cholelithiasis refers to stones in the gallbladder lumen or in the extrahepatic biliary tree. In the industrialized countries, three quarters of gallstones are mainly **cholesterol**; the rest are **calcium bilirubinate** and **other calcium salts** (**pigment gallstones**). Pigment stones are more common in the tropics and Asia. Most gallstones are not radiopaque but are readily detected by ultrasonography. They are often asymptomatic but cause mild-to-severe pain (**biliary colic**) if they lodge in the cystic or common bile ducts.

Cholesterol Stones

Cholesterol stones measure up to 4 cm and may be round or faceted, yellow to tan, single or multiple (Fig. 12-33). They are mostly cholesterol, plus some calcium salts and mucin.

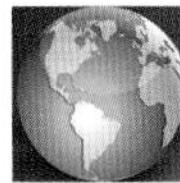

EPIDEMIOLOGY: Some 20% of American men and 35% of women older than 75 years have gallstones at autopsy. ***Premenopausal women develop cholesterol gallstones three times more often than do men. The incidence is highest in users of oral contraceptives and women with several pregnancies.***

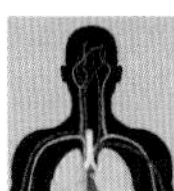

PATHOPHYSIOLOGY: Formation of cholesterol gallstones reflects the physicochemical qualities of bile and local factors in the gallbladder.

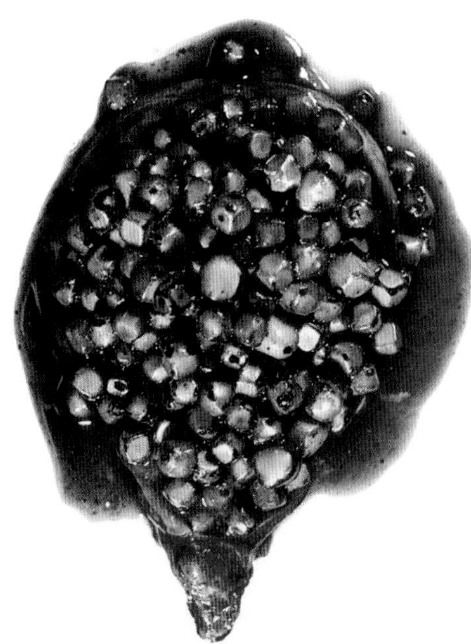

FIGURE 12-33. Cholesterol gallstones. The gallbladder has been opened to reveal numerous yellow cholesterol gallstones.

- **Bile formation in the liver:** Bile containing excess cholesterol or that is deficient in bile acids becomes supersaturated in cholesterol. Cholesterol then precipitates as solid crystals to form stones (**lithogenic bile**). Obesity increases hepatic cholesterol secretion even more, further supersaturating the bile with cholesterol.
- **Local factors in the gallbladder:** Biliary proteins can function as nuclei of crystallization, and hypersecretion of gallbladder mucus accelerates cholesterol precipitation from gallbladder bile.
- **Gallbladder motility:** Impaired gallbladder motor function results in stasis, causing bile sludging that progresses to macroscopic stones.

Estrogens increase hepatic secretion of cholesterol and decrease secretion of bile acids, perhaps explaining why women form cholesterol gallstones more often. Pregnancy magnifies these effects. Progesterone, the main hormone of pregnancy, inhibits discharge of bile from the gallbladder. The gallbladder empties more slowly, and the resulting stasis increases the opportunity for cholesterol crystals to precipitate. Similar mechanisms may also explain the increase in gallstones with oral contraceptive use.

Other major risk factors for cholesterol gallstones include increased biliary cholesterol secretion or decreased secretion of bile salts and lecithin or both.

Factors associated with **increased biliary cholesterol secretion** include:

- Increasing age
- Obesity
- Ethnicity (e.g., Native Americans, Chilean women, and some northern Europeans)
- Familial predisposition
- Diet high in calories and cholesterol
- Certain metabolic abnormalities associated with high blood cholesterol levels. ***Decreased secretion of bile salts and lecithin occurs in nonobese whites who develop gallstones.*** Disorders that interfere with enterohepatic circulation of bile acids (e.g., pancreatic insufficiency in cystic fibrosis or Crohn disease) also reduce bile acid secretion and favor gallstone formation.

Pigment Stones

Less common than the yellow/tan cholesterol stones are the so-called **pigment stones**, classified by their color and differing mode of pathogenesis.

Black Pigment Stones

Black pigment stones measure less than 1 cm and are irregular and glassy. They contain calcium bilirubinate, bilirubin polymers, calcium salts, and mucin.

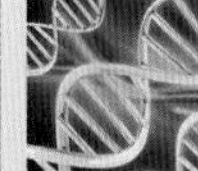

PATHOGENESIS: Black stones are more common in older or undernourished people. Chronic hemolysis, as in hemoglobinopathies, predisposes to the development of black pigment stones. Cirrhosis is also associated with a high incidence of black stones, either because it increases hemolysis or because of damage to liver cells. However, usually, no cause for the formation of black pigment stones is found.

Brown Pigment Stones

Brown pigment stones are spongy and laminated, containing calcium bilirubinate, cholesterol, and calcium soaps of fatty acids. Unlike other types of gallstones, they are more common in intrahepatic and extrahepatic bile ducts than in the gallbladder. ***Brown stones are almost always associated with bacterial cholangitis, for which Escherichia coli is the main cause.*** They are uncommon in Western countries but are not infrequent in Asia, where they are almost entirely seen in people infested with *Ascaris lumbricoides* or *Clonorchis sinensis*, helminths that may invade the biliary tract.

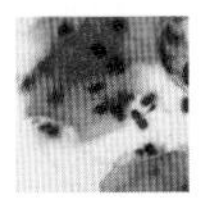

CLINICAL FEATURES: Gallstones in the gallbladder may remain "silent" for many years, and few patients die as a result of cholelithiasis itself. The 15-year cumulative probability that asymptomatic stones will lead to biliary pain or other complications is less than 20%. Laparoscopic cholecystectomy is the treatment of choice.

Most complications of cholelithiasis relate to gallstones obstructing the cystic or common bile ducts. Passage of a stone into the cystic duct often, but not always, causes severe biliary colic and may lead to acute cholecystitis. Repeated bouts of acute cholecystitis give rise to chronic cholecystitis, which may also result from the presence of stones alone. Gallstones entering the common duct (**choledocholithiasis**) may cause obstructive jaundice, cholangitis, and pancreatitis. They are the most common cause of acute pancreatitis in people who do not drink alcohol. In cystic duct obstruction, with or without acute cholecystitis, bile in the gallbladder is reabsorbed and replaced by a clear mucinous fluid secreted by gallbladder epithelium; the resulting **hydrops of the gallbladder (mucocele) is** characterized by a distended and palpable gallbladder, which may become secondarily infected.

ACUTE CHOLECYSTITIS

Acute cholecystitis is diffuse inflammation of the gallbladder, usually secondary to obstruction of the gallbladder outlet.

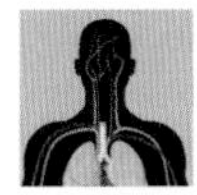

PATHOPHYSIOLOGY: *People with gallstones account for 90% of cases of acute cholecystitis.* The remaining cases (**acalculous cholecystitis**) are linked to sepsis, severe trauma, and infection of the gallbladder with *Salmonella typhosa*. Bacterial infection is usually a consequence of biliary obstruction rather than a primary event.

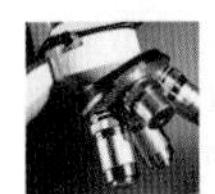

PATHOLOGY: In acute cholecystitis, the external surface of the gallbladder is congested and layered with a fibrinous exudate. The wall is thickened by edema, and the mucosa is fiery red or purple. Gallstones are usually found in the lumen, and one is often seen obstructing the cystic duct. Rarely, in **empyema of the gallbladder**, the cystic duct is completely obstructed, allowing bacteria to invade the gallbladder and distending the organ with cloudy, purulent fluid.

In the gallbladder wall, edema and hemorrhage are striking, with accompanying acute and chronic inflammation (Fig. 12-34). Suppuration in the wall often follows bacterial invasion. The mucosa shows focal ulcers or, in severe cases, widespread necrosis (**gangrenous cholecystitis**).

Perforation is a dreaded complication of bacterial infection. Bile leakage into the peritoneum can cause **bile peritonitis**.

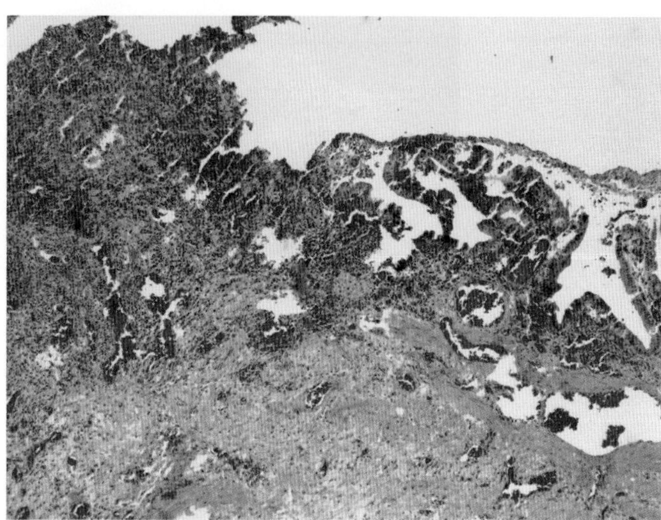

FIGURE 12-34. Acute cholecystitis. Gallbladder removed from a patient with acute cholecystitis demonstrating ulceration of the mucosa (*left*) and acute and chronic inflammation.

More often, inflammatory adhesions form a **pericholecystic abscess** and limit the spread of gallbladder contents after perforation. Erosion of gallbladder contents into a viscus may create a **cholecystenteric fistula**.

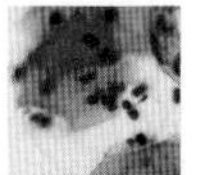

CLINICAL FEATURES: Right upper quadrant abdominal pain is usually the presenting symptom. Mild jaundice, caused by stones in, or edema of, the common bile duct, is seen in 20% of patients. The acute illness generally subsides within a week, but persistent pain, fever, leukocytosis, and shaking chills herald the progression of the disease and the need for cholecystectomy. As inflammation resolves, the gallbladder wall becomes fibrotic. Although the mucosa may heal, the function of the gallbladder remains impaired.

CHRONIC CHOLECYSTITIS

Chronic cholecystitis (i.e., persistent chronic inflammation) is the most common disease of the gallbladder. It is almost always associated with gallstones but may also result from repeated attacks of acute cholecystitis. In the latter case, the pathogenesis probably relates to chronic irritation and chemical injury to the gallbladder epithelium.

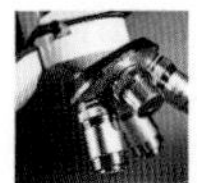

PATHOLOGY: The wall of a chronically inflamed gallbladder is thickened and firm (Fig. 12-35A), and its serosal surface commonly shows fibrous adhesions to surrounding structures, which are residues of previous episodes of acute cholecystitis. Gallstones are usually found within the lumen. The bile frequently contains gravel or sludge (i.e., fine precipitates of calculous material) with coliform organisms in about half of the cases. The mucosa tends to be focally ulcerated and atrophic but may be intact. The fibrotic wall is chronically inflamed throughout and penetrated by Rokitansky–Aschoff sinuses (Fig. 12-35B). Longstanding inflammation may lead to calcification of the gallbladder wall (**porcelain gallbladder**).

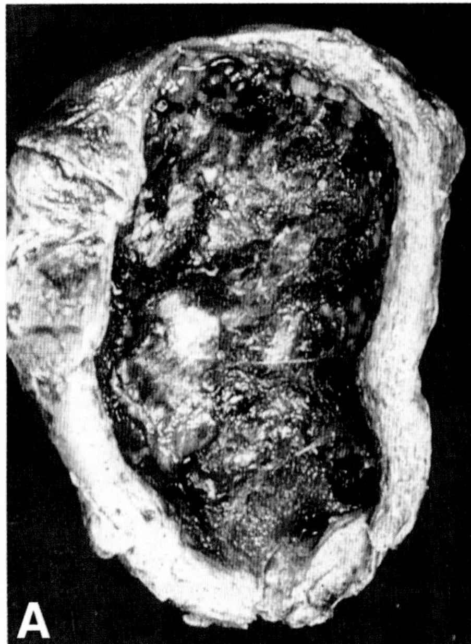

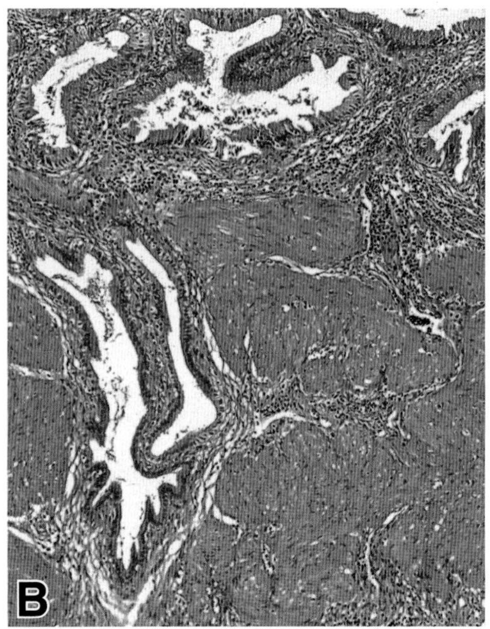

FIGURE 12-35. Chronic cholecystitis. A. The gallbladder is thickened and fibrotic. The lumen had contained several gallstones. **B.** The same specimen as in **A** showing chronic inflammation of the gallbladder and a sinus of Rokitansky–Aschoff extending into the muscularis.

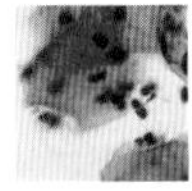

CLINICAL FEATURES: Many patients with chronic cholecystitis complain of nonspecific abdominal symptoms, but it is not at all clear that these are related to the gallbladder disease. On the other hand, pain in the right upper quadrant is typical and often episodic. The diagnosis is best made by ultrasound examination, which shows gallstones in a thick, contracted gallbladder. Cholecystectomy is curative.

TUMORS OF THE GALLBLADDER

Tumors of the gall bladder and bile ducts include both benign and malignant lesions. Of greatest clinical significance are malignant adenocarcinomas of the gallbladder and bile ducts.

Benign Tumors

Papillomas are the most common benign tumors of the gallbladder and may be single or multiple. They are associated with gallstones in 75% of cases. A combined proliferation of smooth muscle and Rokitansky–Aschoff sinuses is an **adenomyoma; it is adenomyomatous hyperplasia when it diffusely involves the gallbladder**. Similar benign tumors may occur in the bile ducts, where they may obstruct biliary flow and cause jaundice.

Adenocarcinoma

Adenocarcinoma of the gallbladder is not rare. It is found incidentally in 2% of patients who undergo cholecystectomy. Because this cancer is usually associated with cholelithiasis and chronic cholecystitis, it is much more common in women and in populations with a high incidence of cholelithiasis, such as Native Americans. Calcified (porcelain) gallbladders (see above) are particularly prone to developing gallbladder cancer.

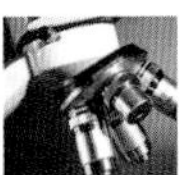

PATHOLOGY: Gallbladder carcinoma may occur anywhere in the gallbladder but most often involves the fundus. The tumor tends to be an infiltrative, well-differentiated adenocarcinoma. It is usually desmoplastic, and thus the gallbladder wall becomes thickened and leathery. Metastases occur via both lymphatic spread and direct extension into the liver, contiguous structures, and peritoneum.

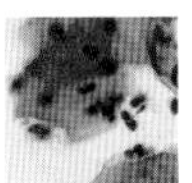

CLINICAL FEATURES: The symptoms of gallbladder carcinoma are like those of gallstone disease. However, by the time these tumors are symptomatic, they are almost always incurable; 5-year survival is less than 3%. For practical purposes, only those patients whose tumors are discovered incidentally during cholecystectomy are cured.

Carcinomas of the Bile Duct and Ampulla of Vater

Cancer of the extrahepatic bile ducts is almost always adenocarcinoma. It may occur anywhere along the duct, including the point where the right and left hepatic ducts join to form the common hepatic duct (hilar cholangiocarcinoma).

These tumors are less common than gallbladder cancer and affect both sexes comparably. Gallstones are often found in those affected, and there is an association with inflammatory diseases of the colon. As in carcinoma of the gallbladder, growth may be endophytic (into the lumen) or diffusely infiltrative. The prognosis is poor, but because symptoms arise early in the disease, the outcome is somewhat better than that for gallbladder cancer. **Adenocarcinomas of the ampulla of Vater** may also obstruct bile flow. They usually present as obstructive jaundice but occasionally as pancreatitis. Surgical treatment of cancer of the ampulla of Vater gives a 5-year survival rate of 35%.

13 The Exocrine Pancreas

David S. Klimstra ▪ Edward B. Stelow

LEARNING OBJECTIVES

- Describe the anatomic structure of the pancreas and its secretory ducts.
- Describe biochemical and physiologic mechanisms that protect acinar cells from damage by pancreatic enzymes.
- What are the commonly used serum markers of pancreatic damage?
- Describe common etiologies and pathophysiologic mechanisms associated with both acute and chronic pancreatitis.
- Describe the structure and formation of pancreatic pseudocysts.
- Describe the relationship between elevated serum IgG4 and a subtype of chronic pancreatitis.
- Describe the molecular pathogenesis of hereditary pancreatitis.
- What are the histopathologic features of chronic calcifying pancreatitis and groove pancreatitis?
- What are the clinical signs and symptoms of acute and chronic pancreatitis?
- What etiologies have been associated with infiltrating ductal adenocarcinoma of the pancreas?
- Name and describe the preneoplastic lesion associated with ductal carcinoma of the pancreas.
- What are the molecular features noted in the progression of pancreatic intraductal neoplasia to invasive disease?
- Describe the pathologic appearance and clinical features of ductal adenocarcinoma.
- Define Courvoisier sign and Trousseau syndrome in relation to pancreatic cancer.

ANATOMY AND PHYSIOLOGY

The pancreas is a mixed exocrine and endocrine gland, 10 to 15 cm long, and weighing 60 to 150 grams. It lies transversely in the upper abdomen, cradled between the loop of the duodenum and the hilum of the spleen (for discussion of diseases of the endocrine gland, see Chapter 19). It has three anatomic subdivisions:

- The **head** is in the concavity of the duodenum and extends to the superior mesenteric vessels, which pass through a groove immediately behind the organ.
- The **neck** connects the head to the distal portion of the gland.
- The **tail** constitutes the distal two thirds of the pancreas and extends to the hilum of the spleen.

Exocrine pancreatic secretions drain into the major ducts of Wirsung and Santorini, which join the common bile duct and empty into the duodenum through the ampulla of Vater. In a significant minority of individuals, these ducts remain separated by a septum and enter the duodenum independently. The ampulla is surrounded by a circular complex of smooth muscle fibers, the sphincter of Oddi, which controls passage of pancreatic juice and bile into the duodenum.

Exocrine tissue comprises 80% to 85% of the pancreas and contains acini lined by single layer of pyramidal cells. The cytoplasm of these cells is basophilic owing to abundant rough endoplasmic reticulum. The apical cytoplasm contains eosinophilic zymogen granules. Acinar cells synthesize some 20 different digestive enzymes, mostly in the form of inactive proenzymes. These enzymes include trypsin, chymotrypsin, amylase, lipase, and elastase, which are secreted upon neural and hormonal stimulation and are subsequently activated in the duodenum. Amylase and lipase are secreted in their active forms. The daily secretion of 1.5 to 3 L of pancreatic juice attests to the remarkable synthetic and secretory capacity of the exocrine pancreas.

The major endocrine diseases of the pancreas are discussed in Chapter 19.

CONGENITAL ANOMALIES

There are many anatomic variations in the major pancreatic ducts and their relationship to the common bile duct, most of which are considered normal and are rarely of clinical significance. Other developmental variations have clinical consequences and are, therefore, regarded as developmental defects.

PANCREAS DIVISUM: Pancreas divisum, the most common congenital anomaly, results from failure of the two embryonic pancreatic ducts to fuse, leading to retention of two separate ductal systems. Usually, the two lobes of the organ do fuse, so the abnormality is not evident unless the course of the pancreatic ducts is specifically defined. Chronic pancreatitis develops in up to 25% of people with pancreas divisum.

HETEROTOPIC PANCREAS: Pancreatic tissue occurring outside its normal location, mostly in the walls of the duodenum, stomach, and jejunum, is an incidental finding in up to 15% of autopsies. Infrequently, pancreatic neoplasms of various types arise in heterotopic tissue, most often infiltrating ductal adenocarcinoma.

ACUTE PANCREATITIS

Acute pancreatitis is not solely an inflammatory condition, but rather reflects myriad local, regional, and systemic changes seen with the release of these enzymes. For unknown reasons, the incidence of acute pancreatitis has increased in the past few decades.

The severity of acute pancreatitis varies greatly. At one end of the spectrum is a mild, self-limited disease, with acute inflammation and stromal edema, and little or no acinar cell necrosis. This is usually not associated with systemic manifestations of disease. At the other extreme is a severe, sometimes fatal, acute hemorrhagic pancreatitis with massive necrosis. In these cases, systemic manifestations such as shock, acute respiratory distress, acute renal failure, and disseminated intravascular coagulation may develop. The cause is a massive enzymatic leak from the gland, reflected in extremely high serum levels of amylase and lipase.

Repeated bouts of acute pancreatitis may lead to chronic pancreatitis, which is characterized by recurrent attacks of severe abdominal pain and progressive fibrosis and atrophy of the gland, culminating in pancreatic insufficiency. However, antecedent acute episodes are only appreciated clinically in half of cases of chronic pancreatitis.

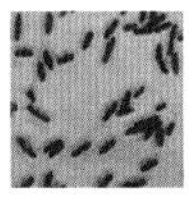

ETIOLOGIC FACTORS: **Acinar cell injury** and **duct obstruction** are the major causes of acute pancreatitis. These processes progress to inappropriate extracellular leakage of activated digestive enzymes and consequent autodigestion of pancreatic and extrapancreatic tissues. There may be some genetic predispositions to the development of acute pancreatitis (see section on "Chronic Pancreatitis").

ACTIVATED PANCREATIC ENZYMES: Inappropriate activation of pancreatic proenzymes occurs in all forms of pancreatitis. Acinar cells are shielded from the potentially destructive action of their digestive enzymes (proteases, nucleases, amylase, lipase, and phospholipase A) by three mechanisms:

- Enzymes are physically isolated from the cytosol by an intricate, intracellular, cavitary system of endoplasmic reticulum; Golgi complex; and zymogen granule membranes.
- Many digestive enzymes are synthesized as inactive forms (e.g., chymotrypsinogen, proelastase, prophospholipase, and trypsinogen).
- Specific enzyme inhibitors tend to protect the pancreas.

Inhibitors of proteolytic enzymes are present in many body fluids and tissues. The plasma protease inhibitors are α_1-antitrypsin, α_2-macroglobulin, C_1 esterase inhibitor, and pancreatic secretory trypsin inhibitor. Trypsin itself does not produce cell necrosis. Rather, it activates other pancreatic proenzymes, such as prophospholipase A_2 and proelastase, and so is central to the pathogenesis of acute pancreatitis.

SECRETION AGAINST OBSTRUCTION AND DUCT INSUFFICIENCY: The enzymes secreted by acinar cells are discharged into the ductal system and enter the duodenum. A small amount diffuses back into periductular extracellular fluid and eventually into plasma. Whenever lumina of pancreatic ducts are narrowed, easy outflow of exocrine secretions is impaired, and intraductal pressure and back diffusion across the ducts increase. This is suspected to cause inappropriate activation of digestive proenzymes. Heavy meals may induce the release of pancreatic secretagogues and so augment the production of pancreatic enzymes.

Gallstones sometimes obstruct pancreatic ducts, and 45% of patients with acute pancreatitis also have cholelithiasis. Conversely, the risk of acute pancreatitis in patients with gallstones is 25 times higher than that in the general population, and 5% of patients with gallstones develop acute pancreatitis. The reason for the association between pancreatitis and cholelithiasis is obscure. **Anatomic anomalies** (e.g., pancreas divisum) and **neoplasms** (ampullary and pancreatic tumors) can also lead to acute pancreatitis owing to duct insufficiency or obstruction, respectively.

ETHANOL: ***Chronic alcohol abuse accounts for one third of cases of acute pancreatitis, although only 5% to 10% of chronic alcoholics develop this complication.*** The pathogenesis of ethanol-induced pancreatitis (acute and chronic) is not well understood (see below). Ethanol per se does not cause significant injury to pancreatic acinar or duct cells.

Alcohol consumption may cause spasm or acute edema of the sphincter of Oddi, especially after an alcoholic binge. It also stimulates secretion from the small intestine, which triggers the exocrine pancreas to release pancreatic juice.

Idiopathic pancreatitis is the third most common form of the disease and accounts for 10% to 20% of cases.

Factors implicated in acute hemorrhagic pancreatitis are shown in Figure 13-1.

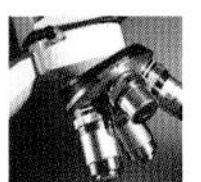

PATHOLOGY: In acute hemorrhagic pancreatitis, the pancreas is initially edematous and hyperemic. Within a day, pale, gray foci appear, rapidly becoming friable and hemorrhagic (Fig. 13-2A). In severe cases, most of the pancreas is converted into a large retroperitoneal hematoma, in which pancreatic tissue is barely recognizable. Yellow-white areas of fat necrosis appear around the pancreas, including in the adjacent mesentery (Fig. 13-2B). These nodules of necrotic fat have a pasty consistency that becomes firmer and chalk-like as more calcium and magnesium soaps are produced. Soap production reflects the interaction of cations with free fatty acids released by the action of activated lipase on triglycerides in fat cells. As a result, blood calcium may be depressed, sometimes to the point of causing neuromuscular irritability.

The most prominent microscopic findings in acute pancreatitis are acinar cell and fat necrosis, often with some degree of acute inflammation (Fig. 13-3). Necrosis is usually patchy and rarely involves the entire gland. Irregular fibrosis of the pancreas and occasionally calcification (i.e., chronic pancreatitis) result from healed acute pancreatitis.

PANCREATIC PSEUDOCYST: Half of patients who survive acute pancreatitis develop pancreatic pseudocysts, which are centered in peripancreatic tissues. Pseudocysts surrounded by connective tissue, display no epithelial lining, and contain degraded blood, inflammatory cells, debris, and fluid rich in pancreatic enzymes. Pseudocysts may enlarge to compress and even obstruct the duodenum or other structures. They may become secondarily infected and form abscesses. Rupture is a rare complication that leads to chemical or septic peritonitis.

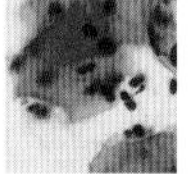

CLINICAL FEATURES: Patients with acute pancreatitis present with severe epigastric pain that is referred to the upper back, nausea, and vomiting. Within hours, catastrophic peripheral vascular collapse and shock may ensue. With sustained, shock, **acute respiratory distress syndrome,** and **acute renal failure** may occur within the first week. Early in the disease, pancreatic digestive enzymes from injured acinar cells enter the blood and

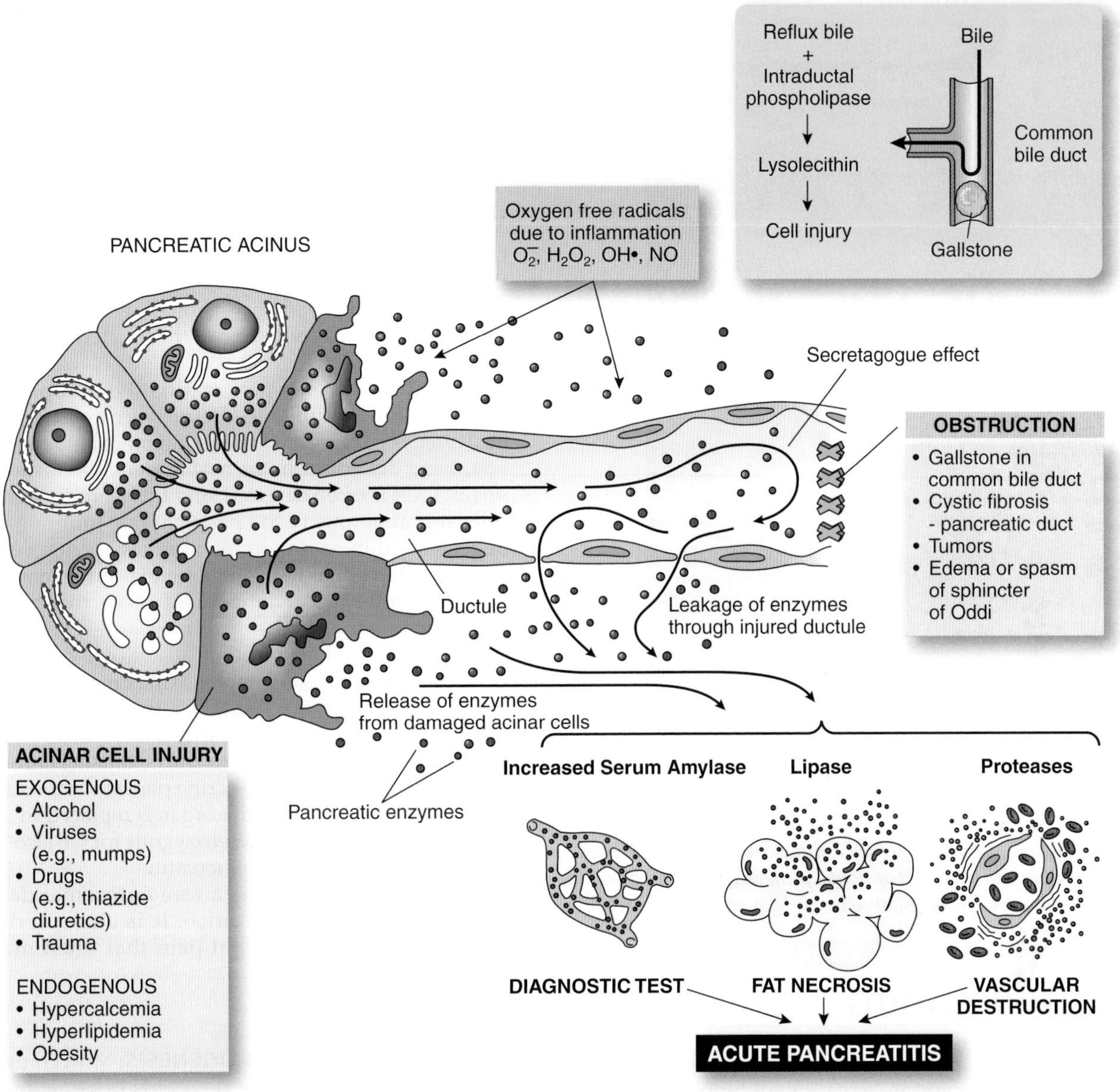

Reflux bile
+
Intraductal phospholipase
↓
Lysolecithin
↓
Cell injury

Bile
Common bile duct
Gallstone

PANCREATIC ACINUS

Oxygen free radicals due to inflammation
O_2^-, H_2O_2, OH•, NO

Secretagogue effect

OBSTRUCTION
- Gallstone in common bile duct
- Cystic fibrosis - pancreatic duct
- Tumors
- Edema or spasm of sphincter of Oddi

Ductule

Leakage of enzymes through injured ductule

Release of enzymes from damaged acinar cells

Pancreatic enzymes

ACINAR CELL INJURY

EXOGENOUS
- Alcohol
- Viruses (e.g., mumps)
- Drugs (e.g., thiazide diuretics)
- Trauma

ENDOGENOUS
- Hypercalcemia
- Hyperlipidemia
- Obesity

Increased Serum Amylase **Lipase** **Proteases**

DIAGNOSTIC TEST **FAT NECROSIS** **VASCULAR DESTRUCTION**

ACUTE PANCREATITIS

FIGURE 13-1. The pathogenesis of acute pancreatitis. Injury to the ductules or the acinar cells leads to the release of pancreatic enzymes. Lipase and proteases destroy tissue, thus causing acute pancreatitis. The release of amylase is the basis of a test for acute pancreatitis. H_2O_2, hydrogen peroxide; NO•, nitric acid; O_2^-, superoxide ion; OH•, hydroxyl radical.

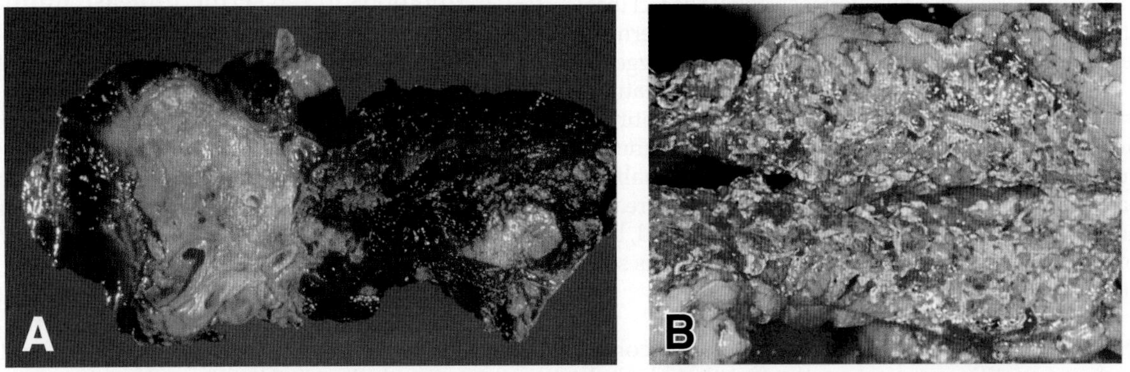

FIGURE 13-2. Acute hemorrhagic pancreatitis. A. Large areas of the pancreas are intensely hemorrhagic. **B.** The cut surface of the pancreas in a less severe case of acute pancreatitis, and at a somewhat later stage than in (A), showing numerous yellow-white foci of fat necrosis.

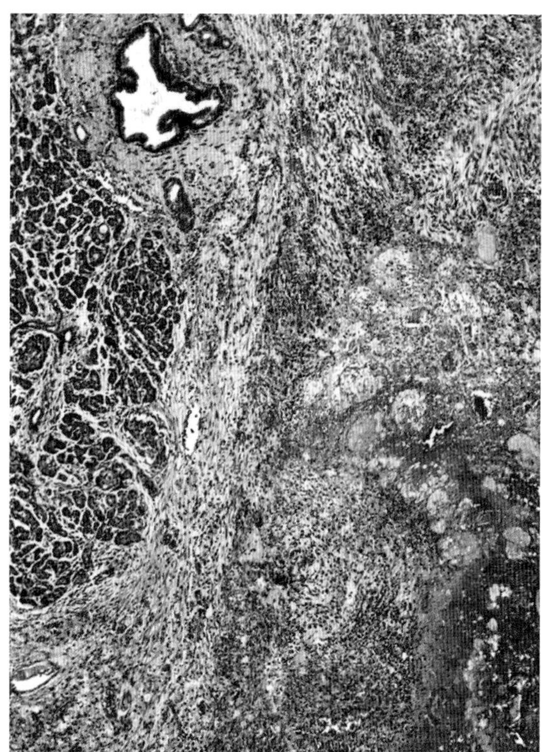

FIGURE 13-3. Acute hemorrhagic pancreatitis. A photomicrograph of the pancreas showing areas of acinar cell necrosis, hemorrhage, and fat necrosis (*lower right*). An intact lobule is seen on the left.

retroperitoneal area. ***Elevated serum amylase and lipase within 24 to 72 hours are diagnostic for acute pancreatitis.*** Infection of the pancreas with Gram-negative bacteria from the intestinal tract greatly increases mortality.

CHRONIC PANCREATITIS

Chronic pancreatitis features progressive destruction of pancreatic parenchyma and its replacement by fibrosis. The symptoms of chronic pancreatitis include recurrent or persisting abdominal pain or simply evidence of pancreatic exocrine or endocrine insufficiency.

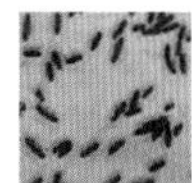

ETIOLOGIC FACTORS: Most factors that cause acute pancreatitis also cause chronic pancreatitis. The fact that chronic pancreatitis is often characterized by intermittent "acute" attacks with periods of quiescence suggests that it may evolve from repeated episodes of acute pancreatitis. However, half of patients give no history of acute pancreatitis.

Chronic alcoholism is the major cause of chronic pancreatitis, accounting for nearly 80% of adult cases. About half of asymptomatic alcoholics show abnormal results for pancreatic exocrine function tests. The role of alcohol is undisputed, but the mechanism by which it causes chronic pancreatitis is still debated (see below).

PATHOPHYSIOLOGY: The link between alcohol and pancreatitis may rest on the fact that alcohol is a pancreatic secretagogue. Hypersecretion of enzymes by acinar cells without increased fluid leads to precipitation of "protein plugs" in small pancreatic ducts. These deposits obstruct the small ducts, at first causing only mild acute pancreatitis. Resolution with fibrosis facilitates the development of more plugs, which grow and become the nidus for calcium carbonate stones. This sequence causes a vicious circle that increases the risk of developing more and worse acute pancreatitis. Nevertheless, only a minority of severe alcoholics develop clinical chronic pancreatitis. Additional factors associated with chronic pancreatitis include the following:

- **Obstruction or insufficiency of the pancreatic duct.**
- **Chronic injury to acinar cells** (e.g., in hemochromatosis) is associated with pancreatic fibrosis and atrophy.
- **Chronic renal failure** increases the incidence of acute and chronic pancreatitis.
- **Autoimmune chronic pancreatitis (lymphoplasmacytic sclerosing pancreatitis, duct-destructive chronic pancreatitis, etc.)** often occurs in association with other autoimmune and sclerosing disorders. In the best understood form disease, serum IgG4 is often elevated, and IgG4-producing plasma cells are numerous in the parenchyma. Immunoglobulin deposits within basement membranes are described. The presence of hypergammaglobulinemia and autoantibodies, including anti-nuclear antibodies (ANA), rheumatoid factor, antilactoferrin, and anticarbonic anhydrase, supports the suggestions of an autoimmune etiology.
- **Cystic fibrosis** (CF; see Chapter 5) may manifest as chronic pancreatitis. In patients with CF, intraductal secretions are abnormally viscid. Plugs of inspissated mucus obstruct cystically distended pancreatic ducts, causing chronic pancreatitis and, eventually, exocrine pancreatic insufficiency. In late stages of CF, the entire organ is replaced by adipose tissue. Some individuals heterozygous for CF also have an increased risk of chronic pancreatitis.
- **Hereditary pancreatitis** is a rare autosomal dominant disease with 80% penetrance. It is characterized by recurring severe abdominal pain that often manifests in childhood.

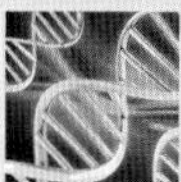

MOLECULAR PATHOGENESIS: Most commonly, hereditary disease develops because of point mutations that increase trypsin levels within the pancreas, largely owing to autoactivation of trypsinogen. Most forms of hereditary pancreatitis are caused by one of three point mutations in the **cationic trypsinogen** gene **(protease serine-1,** *PRSS1;* chromosome 7q). Mutations in the **serine protease inhibitor gene** (*SPINK1*) are also associated with the disease. ***About 40% of patients with hereditary pancreatitis later develop pancreatic ductal carcinomas.***

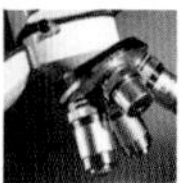

PATHOLOGY: By the time chronic pancreatitis is clinically evident, it is usually advanced. Chronic calcifying pancreatitis is the most common type of the disease and is associated with chronic alcoholism in over 90% of cases. The pancreas can be affected focally, segmentally, or diffusely. The parenchyma is firm, and the cut surface lacks the usual lobular appearance (Fig. 13-4A). The main pancreatic duct and its tributaries are commonly dilated, owing to obstruction by thick proteinaceous plugs, intraductal stones, or strictures. Pseudocysts or abscess formation are common.

Microscopically, large regions of the gland show irregular areas of fibrosis with loss of acinar, then ductal, and, eventually, endocrine parenchyma (Fig. 13-4B). Remaining pancreatic islets are embedded in the sclerotic tissue and may appear fused and enlarged until they too disappear. Some cases exhibit significant infiltration of adipose tissue into the gland, and the remaining islets may become suspended in the fat. Fibrotic areas show myofibroblasts and variable amounts of lymphocytes, plasma cells, and macrophages. Pancreatic ducts of all sizes contain variably calcified proteinaceous material, a finding more commonly associated with alcoholism. Ductal epithelium may be atrophic or hyperplastic and may show squamous metaplasia.

Groove or **paraduodenal pancreatitis** is a particular form of chronic pancreatitis that develops within the "groove" between the head of the pancreas, the common bile duct, and the duodenum; it usually develops in alcoholics. Because of the location of the disease, patients frequently develop jaundice (secondary to bile duct obstruction) or duodenal obstruction. Cystic changes are also common in this condition. Because the process only focally affects the pancreas, patients are often brought to surgery for a suspected pancreatic neoplasm.

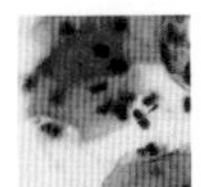

CLINICAL FEATURES: Half of patients with chronic pancreatitis have suffered repeated episodes of acute pancreatitis. One third of cases present with gradual onset of continuous or intermittent pain, with no acute attacks (Fig. 13-5). In some patients, chronic pancreatitis is initially painless but presents with diabetes or malabsorption. Once pancreatic calcifications are visible radiologically, most patients have diabetes or malabsorption or both. Conspicuous weight loss is common, and unrelenting epigastric pain, radiating to the back, may cripple the patient. Mortality is 3% to 4% per year, approaching 50% within 20 to 25 years. One fifth of patients die of complications of attacks of acute pancreatitis. The deaths from other causes relate particularly to alcohol-related disorders. Autoimmune pancreatitis often responds favorably to steroid therapy.

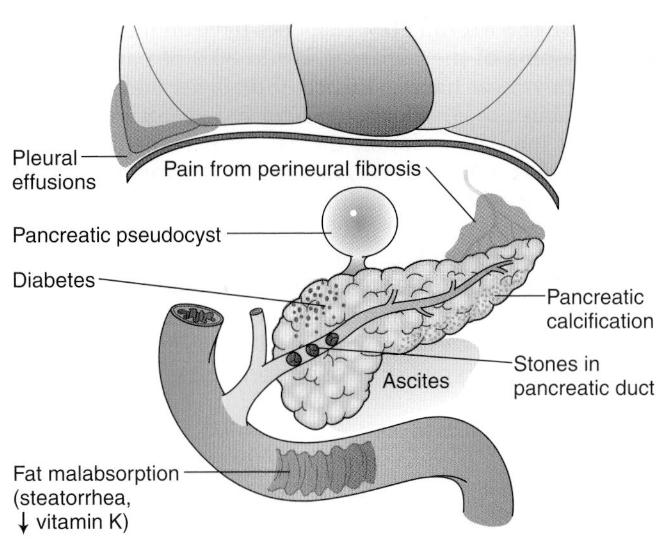

FIGURE 13-5. Complications of chronic pancreatitis.

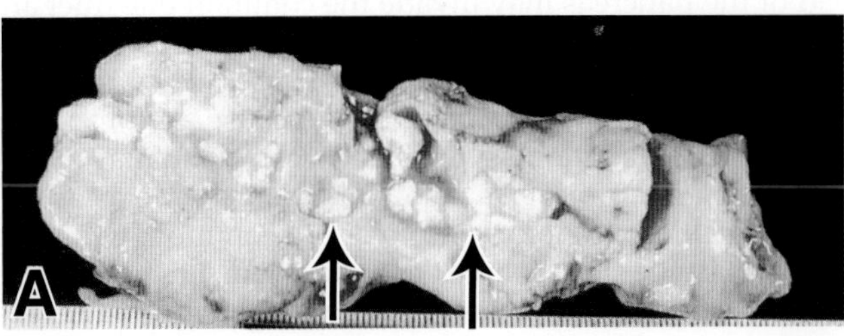

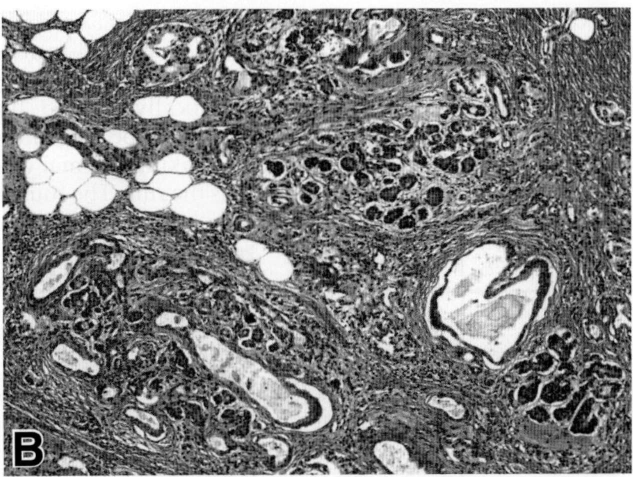

FIGURE 13-4. Chronic calcifying pancreatitis. A. The pancreas is shrunken and fibrotic, and the dilated duct contains numerous stones (*arrows*). **B.** Atrophic lobules of acinar cells are surrounded by dense fibrous tissue infiltrated by lymphocytes. The pancreatic ducts are dilated and contain inspissated proteinaceous material.

PANCREATIC EXOCRINE NEOPLASIA

Ductal Adenocarcinoma

Adenocarcinoma is the most common pancreatic malignancy and is often synonymous with "pancreatic cancer." It is the fourth most common cause of cancer death in American. The prognosis is dismal: a 5-year survival is less than 10%, and even the 20% of patients who can undergo surgical resection are rarely cured. The incidence of pancreatic cancer is increasing in many countries and has tripled in the United States over the past 50 years.

Over 54,000 new cases occur yearly in the United States, where it occurs 50% more often in Native Americans and blacks than in whites. Pancreatic cancer is a disease of late life, with a peak incidence in people over 60 years, although it may occur as early as the third decade. Males predominate (up to 3:1) at younger ages, but sex distribution equalizes in old age.

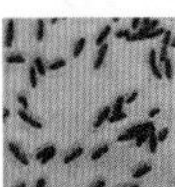

ETIOLOGIC FACTORS: The pathogenesis of pancreatic cancer is obscure. Epidemiologic studies implicate hereditary and environmental factors.

SMOKING: About 25% of pancreatic cancers are attributable to cigarette smoking; cigarette smoking increases pancreatic cancer risk two- to threefold, proportionate to the number of cigarettes smoked per day and the duration of smoking.

BODY MASS INDEX AND DIETARY FACTORS: Obesity and increased BMI are both risk factors. Diets high in meat (particularly grilled), fat, and nitrosamines may increase the risk of pancreatic cancer. High alcohol consumption (but not moderate drinking) increases the risk.

DIABETES MELLITUS: Diabetics have an increased risk for carcinoma of the pancreas. Up to 80% of patients with pancreatic cancer have evidence of diabetes mellitus at the time of cancer diagnosis. Patients with diabetes mellitus for 5 years or more have double the risk for pancreatic cancer.

CHRONIC PANCREATITIS: Chronic pancreatitis is a risk factor for pancreatic cancer, although conventional types (such as alcoholic pancreatitis) likely account for only few cases. Hereditary pancreatitis is more clearly linked to cancer.

FAMILIAL PANCREATIC CANCER: Hereditary factors play a role in pancreatic cancer risk, and several hereditary diseases are implicated (Table 13-1; also see Chapter 5). Increased risk is linked to non–Type O blood groups.

Table 13-1

Familial Cancer Syndromes and Relative Risk for Pancreatic Cancer

Syndrome	Chromosome	Gene Mutation	Relative Risk of Pancreatic Cancer
Peutz–Jeghers syndrome	19p13	*STK11/LKB1*	132-fold
Hereditary pancreatitis	7q35	*PRSS1*	50- to 80-fold
Familial atypical multiple mole melanoma syndrome	9p21	*P16 (CDKN2A)*	9- to 38-fold
Hereditary breast-ovarian cancer syndrome	13q12–13	*BRCA2*	3.5- to 10-fold
Hereditary nonpolyposis cancer syndrome	3p21, 2p22	*hMLH1, hMSH2*	Unknown

MOLECULAR PATHOGENESIS: Infiltrating ductal cancers exhibit a number of genetic alterations. Some of these occur in most cases; others are infrequent. A genetic tumor progression model is supported by morphologic findings of preneoplastic ductal proliferative lesions, called **pancreatic intraductal neoplasia (PanIN)**. PanINs are characterized by mucinous epithelium replacing the normal lining of the ducts. Early events, found in PanIN, include telomere shortening and mutational activation of the *KRAS* oncogene, which is mutated in up to 95% of ductal adenocarcinomas. Later in the sequence of neoplastic progression, mutational inactivation or deletion of tumor suppressor genes occurs. The sequence of abnormalities of the most common involved genes in the progression of PanIN to invasive carcinoma is shown in Figure 13-6. Overactivity or inappropriate expression of several growth factors and their receptors has been described, including EGF and its receptor (EGFR), TGF-β, FGF and its receptor (FGFR), and HER2/neu. BRCA2 is inactivated in 7% of pancreatic carcinomas, and a similar fraction loses DNA mismatch repair genes.

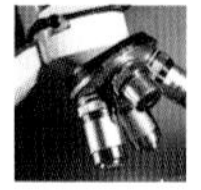

PATHOLOGY: Ductal adenocarcinoma may arise anywhere in the pancreas but is most common in the head (60% to 70%), followed by the body (10%) and tail (10% to 15%). Sometimes, the pancreas is diffusely involved. Tumors of the pancreatic head may cause biliary obstruction by compressing the common bile duct or ampulla of Vater. Classically, both the bile and pancreatic ducts are dilated ("double duct sign"). Ductal adenocarcinomas are usually firm, gray, poorly demarcated masses (Fig. 13-7A), which can be difficult to distinguish from surrounding areas of fibrosing chronic pancreatitis. Invasion of peripancreatic tissues and other local structures is common. Tumors of the head of the pancreas may invade the common bile duct and duodenal wall, and encasement of the superior mesenteric vessels is often found in unresectable cases. They may also obstruct the main pancreatic duct and cause atrophy of the body and tail. Carcinomas of the tail of the gland may extend into the spleen, transverse colon, or stomach. Metastases in the regional lymph nodes and liver are common. Other frequent metastatic sites include the peritoneum, lungs, adrenals, and bones; distant metastases and local spread render most cases unresectable.

Over 75% of infiltrating ductal adenocarcinomas are well to moderately differentiated (Fig. 13-7B), with well-formed individual tubular glands containing mucin-producing epithelial cells. Nuclear atypia may be focally marked, but some malignant glands may be so bland as to be difficult to distinguish from nonneoplastic ducts. Striking stromal desmoplasia around the neoplastic glands is the rule. The tumors

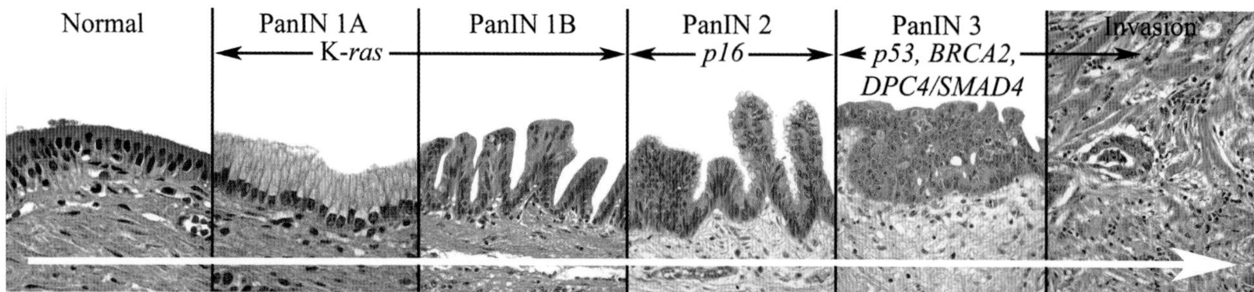

FIGURE 13-6. Pancreatic intraepithelial neoplasia (PanIN). From the left to the right, one proceeds from normal ductal epithelium to invasive carcinoma. Frequently mutated genes are shown when they are typically mutated within the spectrum of PanIN.

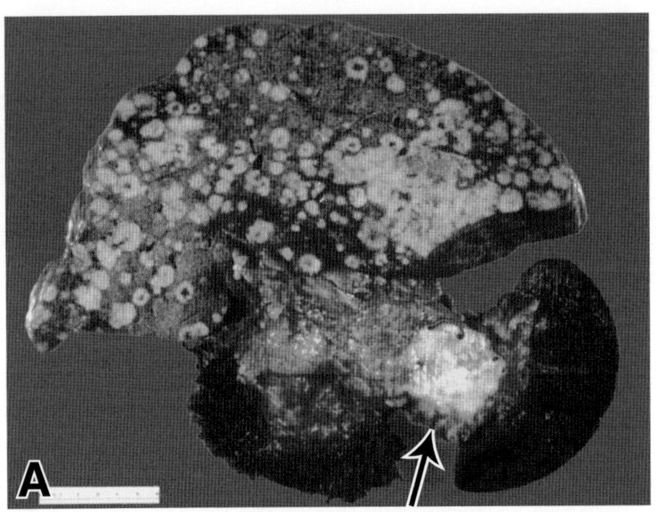

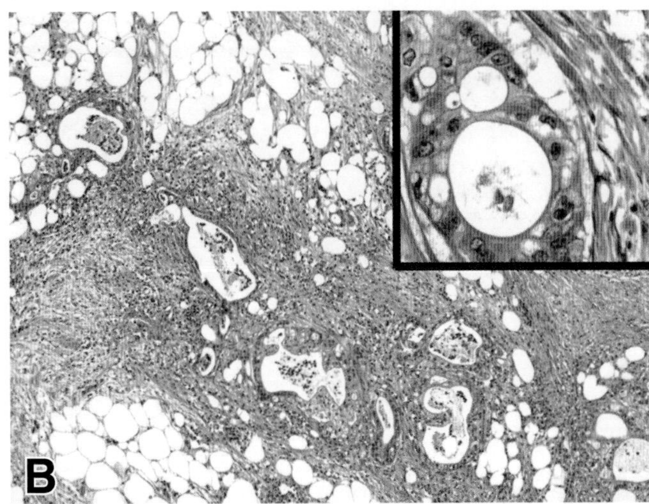

FIGURE 13-7. Infiltrating ductal adenocarcinoma of the pancreas. A. An autopsy specimen showing a large tumor in the tail of the pancreas (*arrow*) and extensive metastases in the liver. **B.** A section of the tumor revealing malignant glands infiltrating into adipose tissue with surrounding fibrous stroma. *Inset:* High-power image of a malignant gland.

are highly infiltrative and poorly circumscribed. Perineural invasion is a characteristic of these tumors and accounts for early and persistent pain.

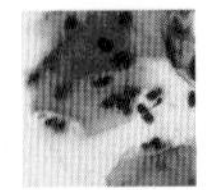

CLINICAL FEATURES: Patients with pancreatic cancer present with anorexia, conspicuous weight loss, and gnawing epigastric pain that often radiates to the back. Painless jaundice is seen in half of patients with cancer localized to the head of the pancreas. Early diagnosis of pancreatic cancer is unusual because the tumor is rarely symptomatic until it is advanced. Progressive deterioration almost invariably ensues, with intractable pain, cachexia, and death. Half of patients die within a year of diagnosis, and overall 5-year survival is less than 10%.

Courvoisier sign is an acute, painless gallbladder dilation accompanied by jaundice, owing to common bile duct obstruction by tumor. In about one third of patients, it may be the first sign of pancreatic cancer, but it does not identify potentially curable tumors.

Migratory thrombophlebitis (**Trousseau syndrome**, deep venous thrombosis) develops in 10% of patients with pancreatic cancer, especially when the tumor involves the body and tail of the pancreas The mechanisms underlying the hypercoagulable state that leads to migratory thrombophlebitis are not completely understood. However, (1) a serine protease synthesized and released by malignant tumor cells directly activates plasma factor X, and (2) tumor cells shed plasma membrane vesicles, tissue factor, and mucins, which have procoagulant activity.

The complications of pancreatic ductal carcinoma are shown in Figure 13-8.

Acinar Cell Carcinoma

Acinar cell carcinomas are rare (1% to 2% of pancreatic cancers) and recapitulate normal pancreatic acinar tissue, including the production of exocrine enzymes. These tumors usually develop in people in their 60s but on rare occasions also occur in children. Some patients show a characteristic paraneoplastic syndrome of subcutaneous fat necrosis, polyarthralgia, and peripheral eosinophilia, because of hypersecretion of massive amounts of lipase into the serum. The prognosis of acinar cell carcinoma is poor, but they are less rapidly fatal than are ductal adenocarcinomas. Acinar cell carcinomas are large and circumscribed and lack the desmoplastic stroma of ductal cancers. Microscopically, they are composed of uniform cells arranged in small acini and nests (Fig. 13-9).

Pancreatoblastoma

These uncommon tumors are usually seen in the first decade of life and may occur in the setting of Beckwith–Wiedemann syndrome. Serum α-fetoprotein levels may be elevated. Microscopically, tumors are composed of polygonal cells in solid

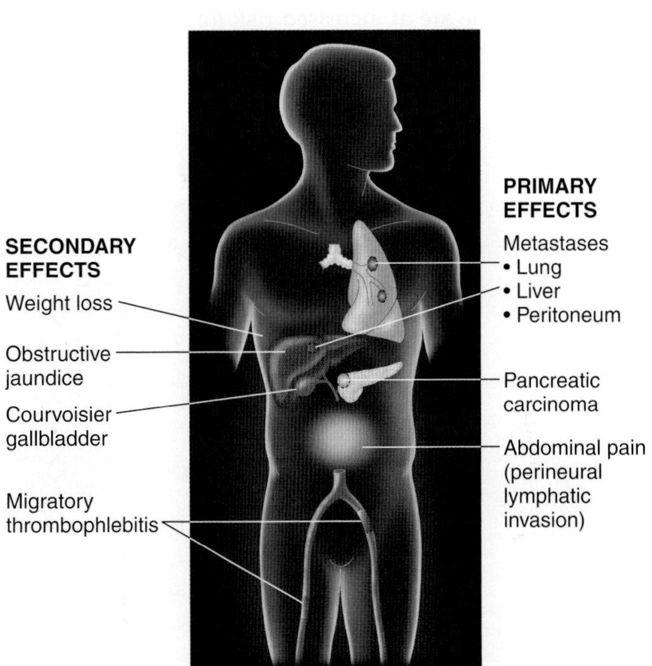

FIGURE 13-8. Complications of pancreatic ductal adenocarcinoma.

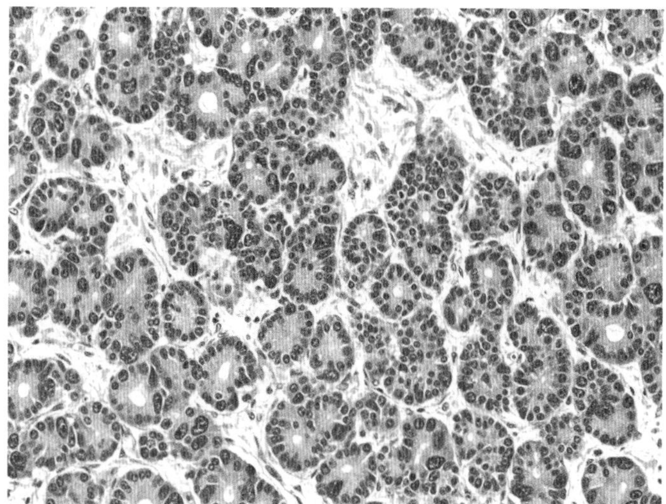

FIGURE 13-9. **Acinar cell carcinoma.** This malignant tumor is characterized by acinar formations reminiscent of normal pancreatic parenchyma.

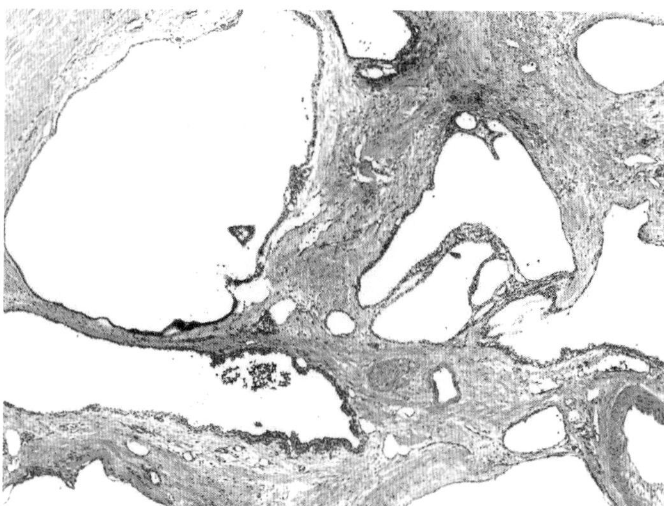

FIGURE 13-11. **Serous cystadenoma.** Cysts are embedded in a dense, fibrous stroma. The epithelial lining is composed of a single layer of glycogen-rich clear cells.

islands and acinar structures, with interspersed squamoid nests (Fig. 13-10). Acinar differentiation, with the production of exocrine enzymes, is consistently present, and some cases also have ductal or neuroendocrine differentiation. Lymph node or hepatic metastases occur in one third of patients and are associated with a poor prognosis. Surgery and chemotherapy can be curative in patients without metastatic disease.

Serous Cystic Neoplasm

Serous cystic neoplasms are composed of numerous small cystic structures that are uniformly lined by glycogen-rich cuboidal epithelium with marked cytoplasmic clearing (Fig. 13-11). They usually occur in adults, in the pancreatic body or tail. Females predominate (3:1). Patients with von Hippel–Lindau syndrome are at increased risk for its development, and tumors are often associated with inactivation of the *VHL* gene. Most such tumors are benign.

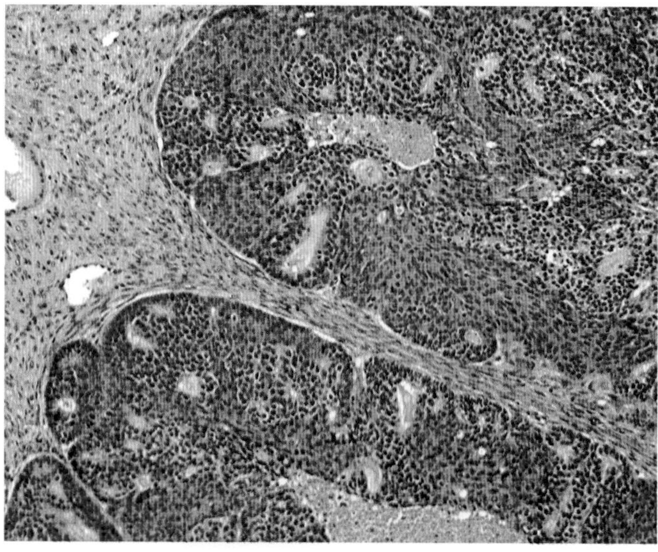

FIGURE 13-10. **Pancreatoblastoma.** There are spindle cell areas with scattered acinar structures.

Intraductal Papillary Mucinous Tumor

Intraductal papillary mucin-producing neoplasms (IPMNs) are composed of dilated pancreatic ducts (>5 mm) lined by neoplastic mucinous epithelium and filled with mucus. Numerous papillary projections extend into the duct lumen (Fig. 13-12). IPMNs most often arise in the head of the pancreas and are usually diagnosed in late adulthood, after being found incidentally or in patients with symptoms of

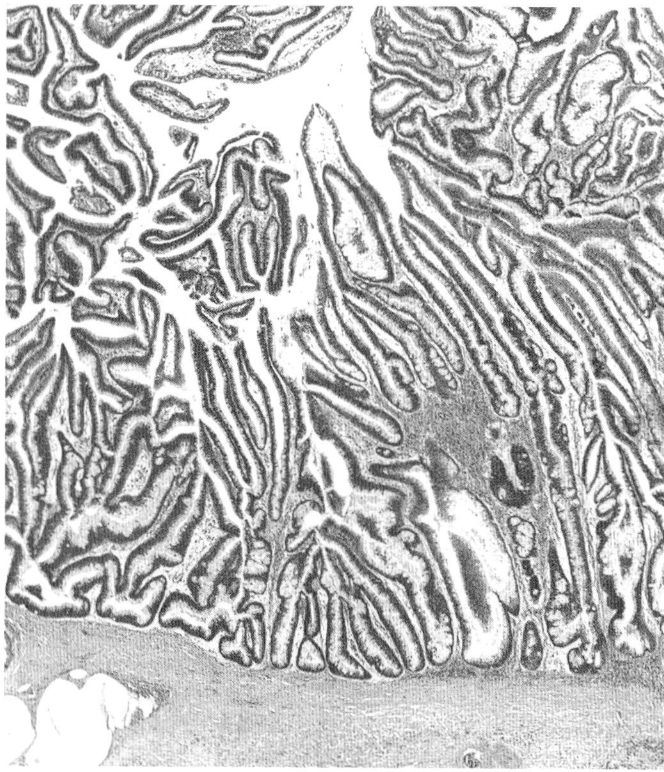

FIGURE 13-12. **Intraductal papillary mucinous neoplasm.** An exuberant papillary proliferation of tall mucin-secreting epithelium fills the pancreatic duct.

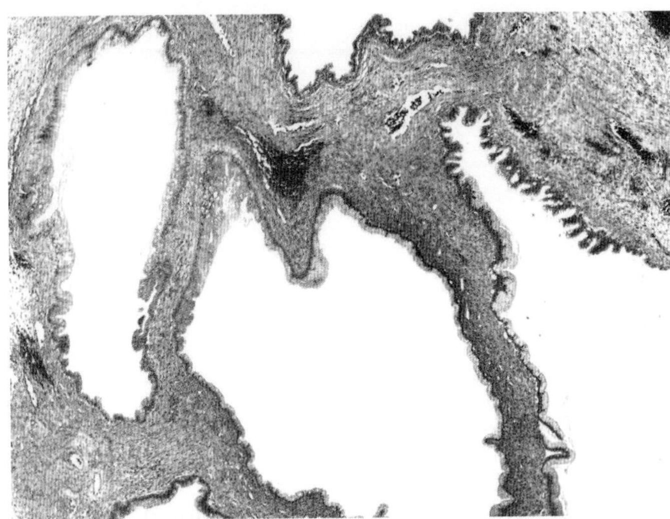

FIGURE 13-13. Mucinous cystic neoplasm. A mucin-rich epithelial lining of this cystic lesion rests on hypercellular, ovarian-like stroma.

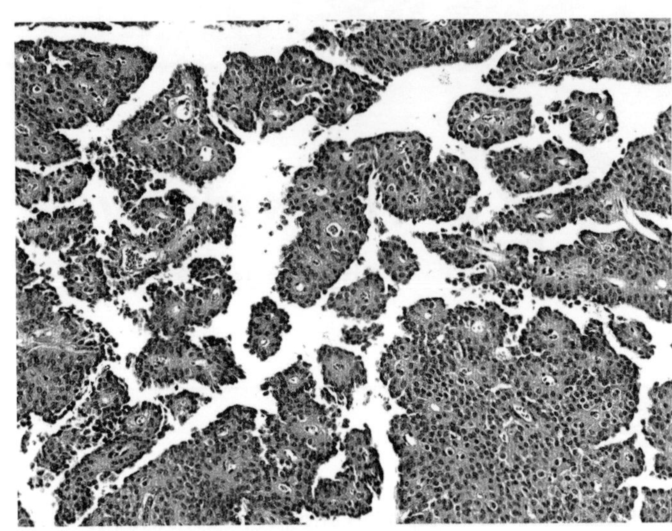

FIGURE 13-14. Solid pseudopapillary neoplasm. The tumor is composed of pseudopapillae with vascular cores.

chronic pancreatitis. A focus of invasive adenocarcinoma is found in up to one third of cases. Because they may harbor invasive carcinomas, larger tumors are often resected. The molecular pathogenesis of IPMNs involves many of the same genes altered in PanIN and pancreatic ductal adenocarcinoma.

Mucinous Cystic Neoplasm

Mucinous cystic neoplasm (MCN) is usually a multilocular cystic neoplasm lined by mucin-secreting epithelium with underlying cellular stroma (ovarian-like stroma) (Fig. 13-13). MCNs occur almost exclusively in middle-aged women. Tumors may reach 10 cm and do not communicate with the pancreatic duct system. They have a predilection for the pancreatic body and tail. Like IPMNs, these tumors may have varying degrees of epithelial atypia and are sometimes associated with invasive carcinoma. The prognosis of MCN (noninvasive) is excellent if it is completely removed. Molecular changes in MCNs are similar to those in PanIN and invasive pancreatic ductal adenocarcinoma.

Solid Pseudopapillary Neoplasm

Solid pseudopapillary neoplasms (SPNs) are solid and circumscribed, often with large cystically degenerated areas filled with blood and necrotic debris. The tumors are composed of monomorphic cells that form loose solid sheets and pseudopapillary structures (Fig. 13-14). The cell lineage of SPN is unclear, and most cases fail to express any of the characteristic immunohistochemical markers of ductal, acinar, or neuroendocrine differentiation. Most SPNs are very indolent and curable by surgical resection. Metastases, usually to the liver, occur in 10% of cases, and even those patients usually live for many years, underscoring the slow-growing nature of this neoplasm.

14 The Kidney

J. Charles Jennette

LEARNING OBJECTIVES

- Define the term nephron and list its constituent components.
- Discuss the function of podocytes, mesangial cells, and the glomerular basement membrane.
- Discuss the role of the basement membrane, foot processes, and slit diaphragm in selective renal filtration.
- Define renal congenital anomalies, including hypoplasia, ectopia, dysplasia, and horseshoe kidney.
- Differentiate between autosomal dominant and recessive polycystic kidney diseases in terms of pathogenesis and clinical features.
- Differentiate between the pathogenesis of nephrotic and nephritic syndromes in terms of pathogenesis, symptoms, and clinical features.
- Differentiate between immune complex- and ANCA-mediated glomerulonephritis.
- Define the terms proliferative and crescentic glomerulonephritis referring to the histologic appearance of affected glomeruli.
- What is the most common form of primary nephrosis in children and in adult?
- What is the most common cause of secondary nephrotic syndrome in adults?
- What renal diseases are commonly associated with rapidly progressive glomerulonephritis?
- Describe the light and electron microscopic histopathology of minimal-change disease.
- What are common primary and secondary etiologies of focal sclerosing glomerulosclerosis (FSGS)? What histopathologic changes are associated with variant forms of the disease?
- Describe the pathophysiology and histopathology associated with membranous glomerulonephritis.
- What are the characteristic glomerular lesions detected in diabetic nephropathy?
- What are the most common etiologies for renal amyloidosis?
- What are the major immunopathologic categories of membranoproliferative glomerulonephritis (MPGN)? Discuss the processes responsible for MPGN being associated with both nephrotic and nephritic diseases.
- Discuss the pathophysiology, histopathology, and clinical features of acute postinfectious glomerulonephritis.
- Discuss the pathologic and clinical manifestations of lupus nephritis. What is unique about class V disease?
- Discuss the etiology, pathophysiology, histopathology, and clinical presentation of IgA nephropathy.
- What is the most common clinical presentation of IgA nephropathy?
- Discuss the etiology and pathology of Alport syndrome and thin glomerular basement membrane disease.
- Describe the pathologic hallmark of anti-GBM glomerulonephritis detected by immunofluorescence microscopy. How does that differ from what is seen in renal immune complex deposition diseases?
- Discuss anti–glomerular basement membrane disease and Goodpasture syndrome.
- Discuss the pathophysiology of ANCA glomerulonephritis.
- Define systemic forms of ANCA vasculitis.
- Why is Henoch–Schönlein purpura closely related to a nephritic syndrome?
- Differentiate between typical hypertensive nephrosclerosis and malignant hypertensive nephropathy.
- By what mechanism do typical and atypical hemolytic–uremic syndrome (HUS) result in microangiopathic hemolytic anemia?
- Describe the histopathology associated with HUS.
- What are common etiologic factors in the production of renal infarcts?
- Differentiate between renal infarct and cortical necrosis. What are common causes of the latter?
- Differentiate between causes of prerenal, intrarenal, and postrenal acute kidney injury.
- Differentiate between the etiology and histology associated with acute ischemic and nephrotoxic acute tubular injury.
- Describe characteristic etiologies and histopathologic changes associated with acute and chronic pyelonephritis.
- What distinctive pattern of injury is associated with chronic tubulointerstitial nephritis?
- What drugs are most commonly associated with hypersensitivity nephritis?
- Describe the histopathology and clinical presentation of urate nephropathy.
- List types of renal stones and describe their etiology and pathophysiology.

- Describe the molecular abnormalities associated with Wilms tumor.
- Describe the histopathology and clinical presentation of Wilms tumor.
- Describe the molecular abnormalities associated with renal cell carcinoma.
- Describe the histopathology and clinical presentation of renal clear cell carcinoma.

ANATOMY

Each kidney consists of an outer cortex and an inner medulla. When a kidney is bisected, the medulla has approximately 12 pyramids, with their bases at the corticomedullary junction. A medullary pyramid and its overlying cortex constitute a **renal lobe**. A pyramid has an inner and an outer zone. The inner zone, the **papilla**, empties into a **calyx**, a funnel-shaped structure that conducts urine into the renal pelvis, which empties into the ureter. The gross and microscopic anatomy of the kidney is reviewed in Figure 14-1.

The **nephron** is the functional unit of the kidney and includes the glomerulus and its tubule, the latter terminating at a common collecting system (Fig. 14-1). The glomerulus is a

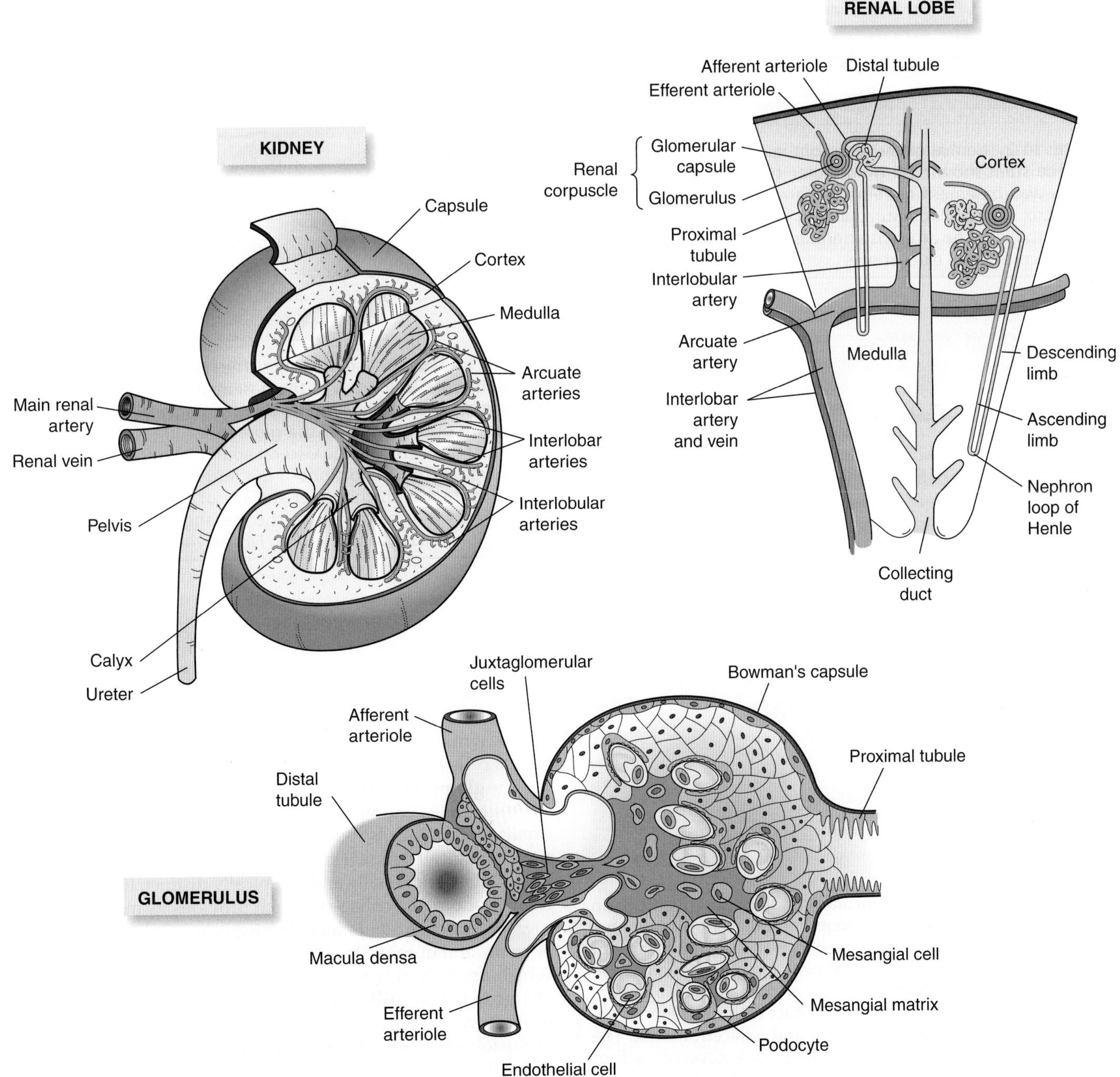

FIGURE 14-1. The gross and microscopic anatomy of the kidney.

specialized network of capillaries covered by epithelial cells called **podocytes** and supported by modified smooth muscle cells termed **mesangial cells** (Figs. 14-1, 14-2, 14-3, 14-4). As it enters the glomerulus, the afferent arteriole branches into

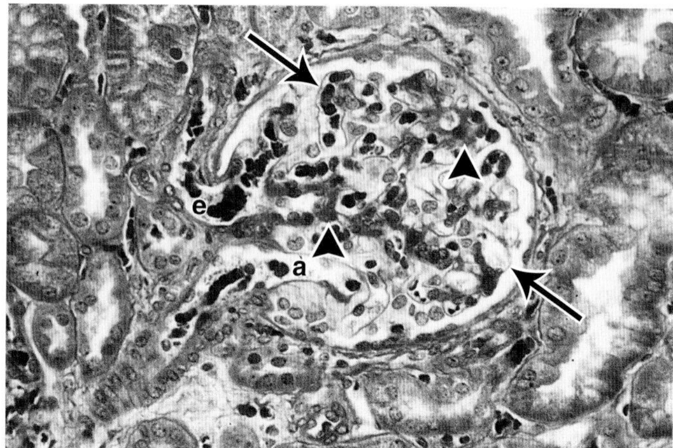

FIGURE 14-2. Normal glomerulus, light microscopy. The Masson trichrome stain showing a glomerular tuft with delicate blue capillary wall basement membranes (*arrows*), small amounts of blue matrix (*arrowheads*) surrounding mesangial cells, and the hilum on the left. The afferent arteriole (*a*) enters below, and the efferent arteriole (*e*) exits above.

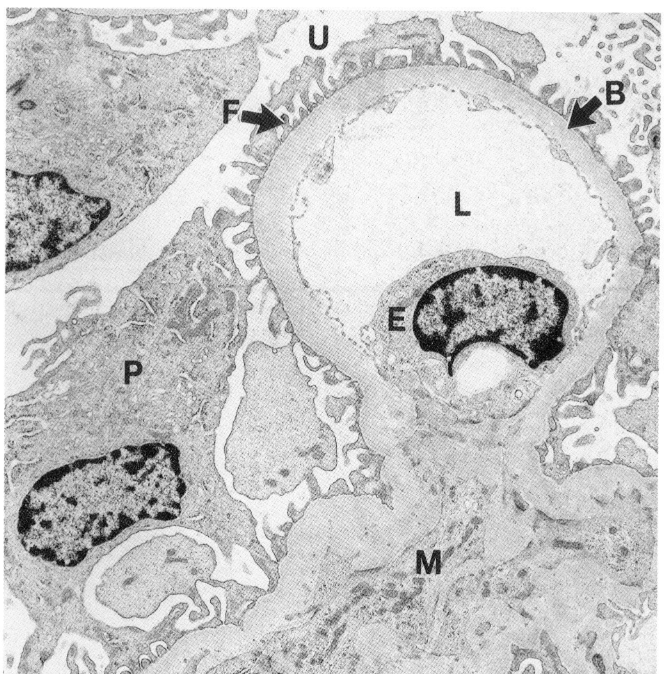

FIGURE 14-3. Normal glomerular capillary. In this electron micrograph of a single capillary loop and adjacent mesangium, the capillary wall portion of the lumen (L) is lined by a thin layer of fenestrated endothelial cytoplasm (shown at higher magnification in Fig. 14-5) that extends out from the endothelial cell body (E). The endothelial cell body is in direct contact with the mesangium, which includes the mesangial cell (M) and adjacent matrix. The outer aspect of the basement membrane (B) is covered by foot processes (F) from the podocyte (P) that line the urinary space (U). Compare this figure with Figures 14-4 and 14-5.

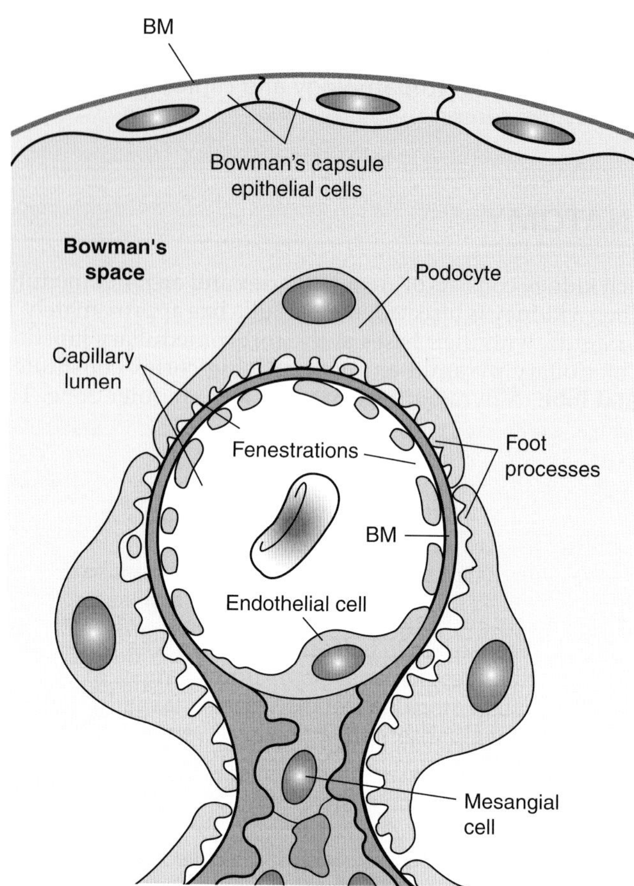

FIGURE 14-4. Normal glomerulus. The relationship of the different glomerular cell types to the basement membrane (BM) and mesangial matrix is illustrated using a single glomerular loop. The entire outer aspect of the glomerular BM (peripheral loop and stalk) is covered by the visceral epithelial cell (podocyte) foot processes. The outer portions of the fenestrated endothelial cell are in contact with the inner surface of the BM, whereas the central part is in contact with the mesangial cell and adjacent mesangial matrix. Compare with Figure 14-3.

capillaries, which form the convoluted glomerular tuft and eventually coalesce into the efferent arteriole that exits the glomerulus. Glomerular capillaries are lined by fenestrated endothelial cells lying on a basement membrane. The outer surface of this basement membrane is covered by podocytes. The Bowman space lies between the podocytes and the epithelial cells that line the Bowman capsule.

The **glomerular basement membrane** (GBM) (Figs. 14-3 and 14-5) separates endothelial cells from podocytes in peripheral capillary walls and also podocytes from the mesangium. Although morphologically similar to many other basement membranes, the GBM is functionally and chemically distinct. It is composed mainly of type IV collagen, which provides its major scaffolding. Other constituents include glycosaminoglycans, laminin, entactin, and fibronectin. The polyanionic glycosaminoglycans, which are rich in heparan sulfate, impart a strong negative charge to the GBM. This property allows (1) selective filtration of electrically neutral and cationic molecules and (2) relative exclusion of negatively charged molecules, such as albumin. The GBM also discriminates among molecules on the basis of size. The glomerular endothelial cell contains numerous 60- to 100-nm pores or fenestrations (Fig. 14-5), which permit passage

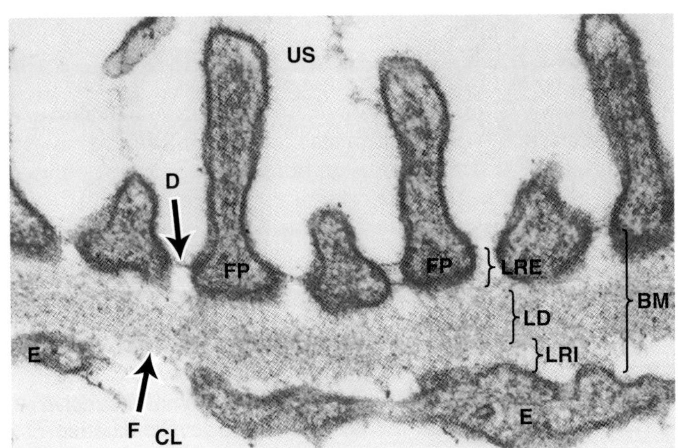

FIGURE 14-5. The glomerular filter. An electron micrograph illustrating the structures of the glomerular filter. Molecules that pass from the capillary lumen (CL) to the urinary space (US) traverse the fenestrations (F) of the endothelial cell (E), the trilaminar basement membrane (BM) (lamina rara interna [LRI], lamina densa [LD], and lamina rara externa [LRE]), and the slit pore diaphragm (D) that connects podocyte foot processes (FP).

of fluid, ions, and proteins (Fig. 14-4). Endothelial membrane proteins (e.g., adhesion molecules) and secretory products (e.g., prostaglandins and nitric oxide) play important roles in the pathogenesis of inflammatory and thrombotic glomerular diseases.

Podocytes rest on the outer aspect of the GBM and send cytoplasmic projections, **foot processes**, onto the lamina rara externa of the GBM (Fig. 14-5). Between adjacent foot processes is a thin membrane called the **slit diaphragm**, which is a modified adherens junction. Podocytes are the major glomerular barrier to protein loss in the urine. The mesangium is a cellular and matrix network that supports the glomerulus. Mesangial cells are modified smooth muscle cells situated in the center of the glomerular tuft between capillary loops.

The major segments of the tubule that arise from each glomerulus are the proximal tubule, loop of Henle, and distal tubule, which empties into the collecting duct.

The **juxtaglomerular apparatus** is located at the hilus of the glomerulus and consists of the following:

- **Macula densa**, a region of the thick ascending limb of the loop of Henle that has closely packed nuclei
- **Extraglomerular mesangial cells**, between the macula densa and the hilar arterioles
- **Terminal afferent arteriole** and **proximal efferent arteriole**, the wall of the afferent arteriole containing characteristic granular cells involved in the secretion of renin and angiotensin.

CONGENITAL AND INHERITED RENAL DISEASES

Congenital Anomalies

Renal Agenesis

Most infants born with bilateral renal agenesis are stillborn and have Potter sequence (see Chapter 5). Renal agenesis is often associated with other anomalies, especially elsewhere in the urinary tract or lower extremities. Unlike bilateral agenesis, unilateral renal agenesis is not serious if there are no associated anomalies because the contralateral kidney hypertrophies sufficiently to maintain normal renal function.

Renal Hypoplasia

Congenital hypoplastic kidneys are formed by six or fewer renal lobes (medullary pyramids with overlying cortex). Hypoplasia must be differentiated from small kidneys due to atrophy or scarring. A frequent variant of hypoplasia features enlargement of the insufficient glomeruli and thus is called **oligomeganephronia**. This enlargement indicates overwork of extant nephrons.

Renal Ectopia

The misplaced kidney is usually in the pelvis, owing to failure of the fetal kidney to migrate from the pelvis to the flank. One or both kidneys may be affected. In **simple ectopia**, the ureters drain into the appropriate side of the bladder. In **crossed ectopia**, the ectopic kidney is on the same side as its normal mate; the ectopic ureter crosses the midline and drains into the contralateral side of the bladder.

Horseshoe Kidney

In this anomaly, the kidneys are fused, usually at the lower poles (Fig. 14-6). This abnormality increases the risk for obstruction and renal infection (**pyelonephritis**) because the ureters are compressed as they cross over the junction between the two kidneys, when the organ is fused at the lower pole.

Renal Dysplasia

Renal dysplasia results from abnormal metanephric differentiation and has multiple genetic and somatic causes.

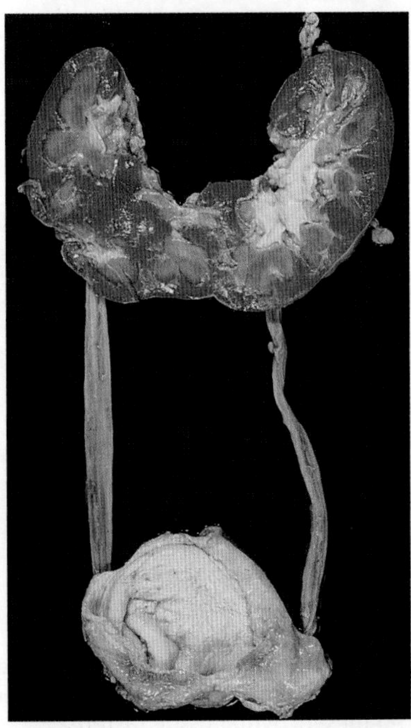

FIGURE 14-6. Horseshoe kidney. The kidneys are fused at the lower pole.

Many forms of dysplasia are accompanied by other urinary tract abnormalities, especially ones that cause obstruction of urine flow. This association suggests that obstruction to urine flow in utero can cause dysplasia. The histologic hallmark of renal dysplasia is undifferentiated tubules and ducts lined by cuboidal or columnar epithelium. These structures are surrounded by mantles of undifferentiated mesenchyme, which may contain smooth muscle and islands of cartilage (Fig. 14-7). Rudimentary glomeruli may be seen, and tubules and ducts may be cystically dilated. Renal dysplasia can be unilateral or bilateral, and the affected kidney may be quite large or very small.

Unilateral multicystic renal dysplasia is the most common cause of an abdominal mass in newborns and is adequately treated by removing the affected kidney. Bilateral aplastic dysplasia and diffuse cystic dysplasia cause oligohydramnios, the resultant Potter sequence, and life-threatening pulmonary hypoplasia (see Chapter 5).

Inherited Renal Diseases

Autosomal Dominant Polycystic Kidney Disease

ADPKD is the most common of a group of congenital diseases in which the renal parenchyma contains many cysts (Fig. 14-8). It affects 1 in 400 to 1 in 1,000 people in the United States, half of whom eventually develop end-stage renal failure. ADPKD is responsible for 5% of end-stage renal disease (ESRD) requiring dialysis or transplantation. Only diabetes and hypertension cause more ESRD than does ADPKD.

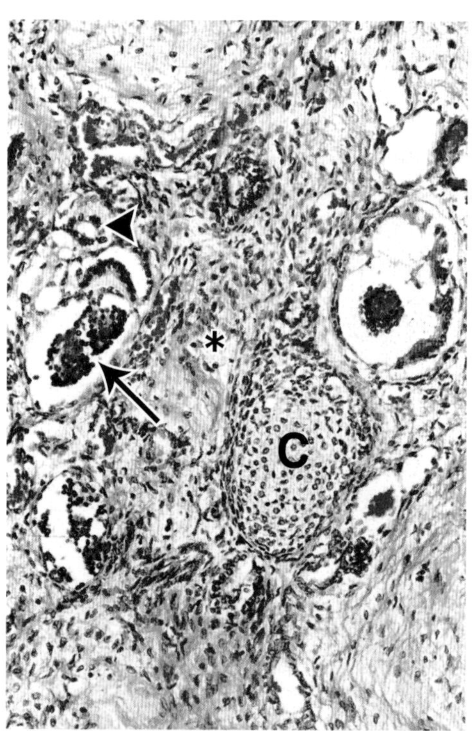

FIGURE 14-7. Renal dysplasia. Immature glomeruli (*arrow*), tubules (*arrowhead*), and cartilage (*C*) are surrounded by loose, undifferentiated mesenchymal tissue (*asterisk*).

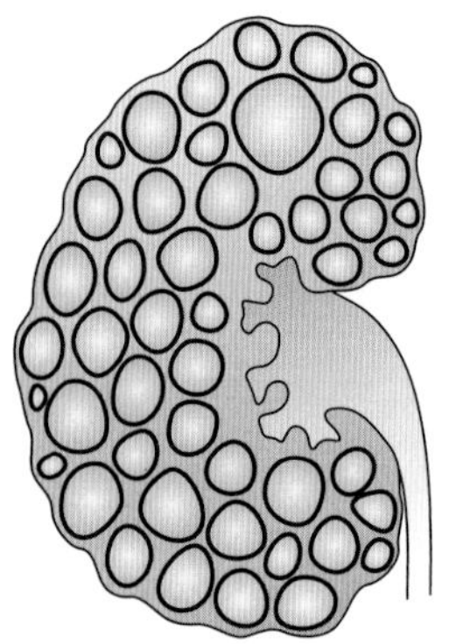

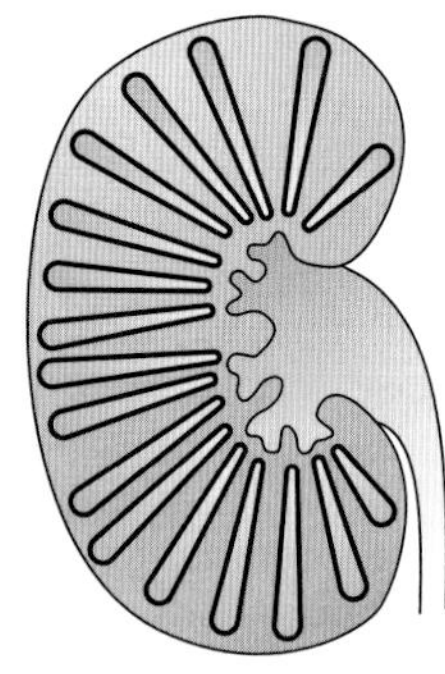

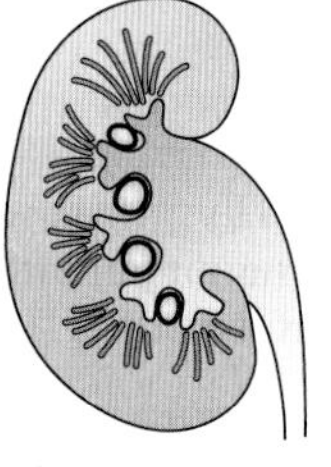

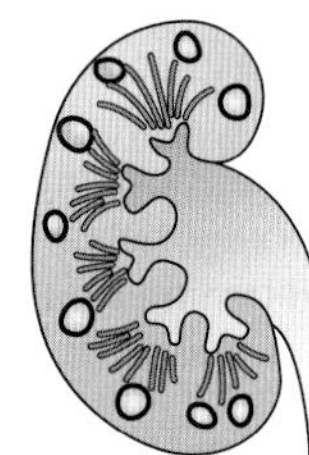

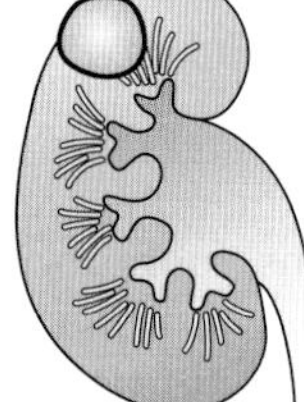

FIGURE 14-8. Cystic diseases of the kidney.

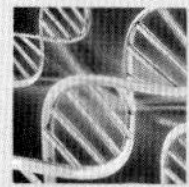

MOLECULAR PATHOGENESIS: Some 85% of ADPKD is caused by mutations in the polycystic kidney disease 1 gene (*PKD1*) and 15% by mutations in *PKD2*. The products of these genes, polycystin-1 and polycystin-2, are in the primary cilia of tubular epithelial cells and in cell–cell adhesion complexes. These structures sense the extracellular environment, including urine flow, thereby regulating intracellular calcium, tubule epithelial proliferation, cell polarity, and apoptosis. Defects in these proteins thus result in dysfunction of primary cilia (ciliopathy); they disrupt calcium signaling, cause disturbed cell polarity, and induce tubular epithelial cell proliferation. Cysts are believed to arise from a few tubular cells that proliferate abnormally. Because the cysts in ADPKD originate in fewer than 2% of nephrons, factors other than crowding of normal tissue by expanding cysts likely impair functional renal tissue. Apoptotic loss of renal tubules and accumulation of inflammatory mediators have been incriminated in the destruction of normal renal mass.

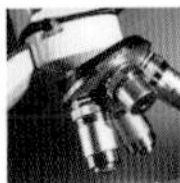

PATHOLOGY: The kidneys in ADPKD are both markedly enlarged and weigh up to 4,500 g (Fig. 14-9). The external contours are distorted by numerous cysts, as large as 5 cm, and are filled with a straw-colored fluid. These cysts are lined by cuboidal and columnar epithelium. They arise at any point along the nephron, including glomeruli, proximal tubules, distal tubules, and collecting ducts. Areas of normal renal parenchyma between the cysts undergo progressive atrophy and fibrosis as the disease advances with age.

Of the patients with ADPKD, one third also have **hepatic cysts**, whose lining resembles bile duct epithelium. Cysts occur in the spleen (10% of patients) and pancreas (5%) as well. **Cerebral aneurysms** occur in 20% of patients, and intracranial hemorrhage is the cause of death in 15% of patients with ADPKD.

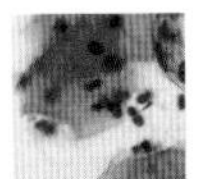

CLINICAL FEATURES: Most patients with ADPKD do not manifest clinically until the fourth decade of life, which is why this condition was once called adult polycystic kidney disease. Symptoms include a sense of heaviness in the loins, bilateral flank and abdominal pain, and abdominal masses. Hypertension is one of the earliest and most common manifestations. Eventually, hematuria, low-level proteinuria, and progressive renal insufficiency develop.

Autosomal Recessive Polycystic Kidney Disease

ARPKD is rare, occurring in about 1 in 10,000 to 40,000 live births. In the neonatal period, one quarter of these infants die, often because of pulmonary hypoplasia caused by oligohydramnios (Potter sequence) and because the large size of the kidneys impairs lung development and function. Children who survive the neonatal period have varying onset and rate of progression of renal insufficiency, as well as hepatic fibrosis and portal hypertension.

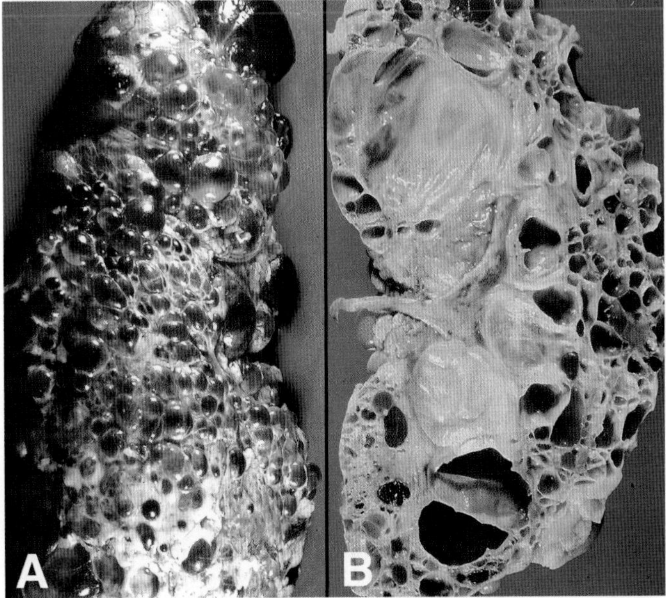

FIGURE 14-9. Autosomal dominant polycystic kidney disease. **A.** The kidneys are enlarged and studded with multiple fluid-filled structures. **B.** The parenchyma is almost entirely replaced by cysts of varying size.

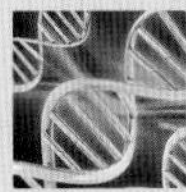

MOLECULAR PATHOGENESIS: ARPKD is caused by mutations in the *PKHD1* gene. The gene product, **fibrocystin**, is found in the primary cilia of the collecting ducts of the kidney, biliary ducts of the liver, and exocrine ducts of the pancreas. It appears to be involved in the regulation of cell differentiation, proliferation, and adhesion. Mutations of *PKHD1* also cause pancreatic cysts and hepatic biliary dysgenesis and fibrosis.

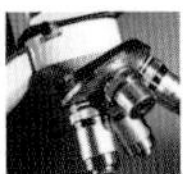

PATHOLOGY: Unlike ADPKD, the external kidney surface in ARPKD is smooth. The disease is invariably bilateral. The kidneys are often so large that delivery of the infant is impeded. The cysts are fusiform dilations of cortical and medullary collecting ducts and have a striking radial arrangement, perpendicular to the renal capsule (Fig. 14-10). Interstitial fibrosis and tubular atrophy are common, particularly in children in whom the disease presents later. As in ADPKD, the calyceal system is normal. The liver is usually affected by **congenital hepatic fibrosis,** with fibrous expansion of portal tracts and bile duct proliferation.

Nephronophthisis and Medullary Cystic Disease

Nephronophthisis is the most common genetic cause of end-stage renal disease (ESRD) in children and young adults.

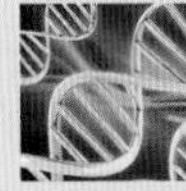

MOLECULAR PATHOGENESIS: Nephronophthisis and medullary cystic disease complex both cause pathologically similar progressive medullary tubulointerstitial disease. However, they have different genetic causes and inheritance. Nephronophthisis is autosomal recessive, with onset in infancy, childhood, or adolescence. It is caused by mutations in one of several *NPHP*-related genes, *NHP1* being the most common. Medullary cystic disease is autosomal dominant, with onset in adolescence and renal failure in adulthood. It is caused by defects in the *MCKD1* (mucin 1) gene or *MCKD2* gene (which codes for uromodulin).

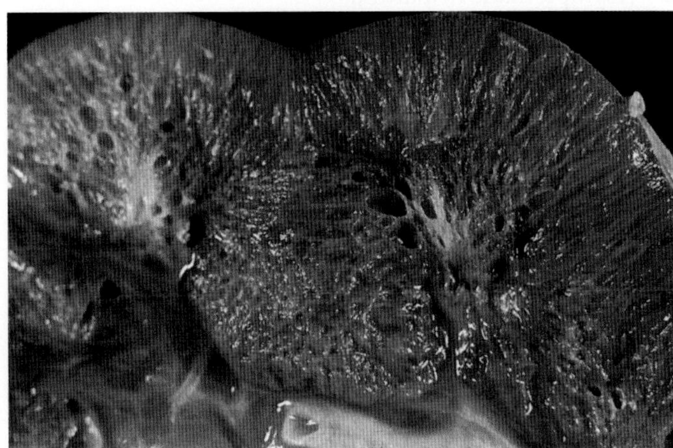

FIGURE 14-10. Autosomal recessive polycystic kidney disease. The dilated cortical and medullary collecting ducts are arranged radially, and the external surface is smooth.

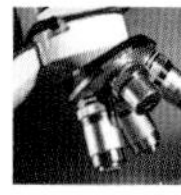

PATHOLOGY: The kidneys often, but not always, have multiple, variably sized cysts (up to 1 cm) at the corticomedullary junction (Fig. 14-8). These cysts arise from distal portions of the nephron. As corticomedullary cysts enlarge, the rest of the parenchyma becomes increasingly atrophic. Secondary glomerular sclerosis, interstitial fibrosis, and nonspecific inflammatory infiltrates dominate the late histologic picture.

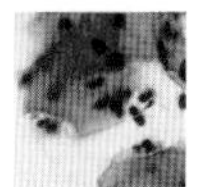

CLINICAL FEATURES: Patients present initially with deteriorating tubular function, such as impaired concentrating ability and sodium wasting, manifested as polyuria, polydipsia, and enuresis (bedwetting). Progressive azotemia and renal failure follow by the second decade. Medullary cystic disease is characterized by the onset of renal failure after the fourth decade and usually presents with polyuria. Hyperuricemia and gout may be accompanying findings.

ACQUIRED CYSTIC KIDNEY DISEASE

Simple cysts are usually incidental findings at autopsy and are rarely clinically symptomatic unless they are very large. They may be solitary or multiple and are usually found in the outer cortex, where they bulge the capsule. Multiple cortical and medullary cysts may form in the kidneys of patients with ESRD who are maintained on dialysis. After 5 years of dialysis, more than 75% of patients show bilateral cystic kidneys. The cysts are initially lined by flat-to-cuboidal epithelium, but hyperplastic and neoplastic epithelial proliferation may develop within 10 years of initiating dialysis. **Renal cell carcinoma (RCC)** develops in 5% of patients with acquired cystic disease (see below).

GLOMERULAR DISEASES

Many renal disorders are caused by injury to the glomerulus. Signs and symptoms of glomerular disease fall into one of the following categories:

- Asymptomatic proteinuria
- Nephrotic syndrome
- Asymptomatic hematuria
- Acute nephritic syndrome
- Rapidly progressive nephritic syndrome
- Chronic kidney injury
- End-stage renal disease (ESRD)

Nephrotic Syndrome

The nephrotic syndrome is characterized by hypoalbuminemia, edema, hyperlipidemia, and lipiduria (lipid in urine). Increased glomerular capillary permeability allows the loss of protein (notably albumin) from plasma into the urine (proteinuria).

Severe proteinuria causes the nephrotic syndrome (Fig. 14-11), but lower levels of proteinuria may be asymptomatic. Nephrotic syndrome results from **primary** glomerular diseases unrelated to a systemic disease, or it may be **secondary** to a systemic disease that affects other organs as well as the kidneys. Diabetic glomerulosclerosis is the most common cause of secondary nephrotic syndrome in adults. Table 14-1 lists the major causes and approximate frequency of the primary nephrotic syndrome in adults and children. Table 14-2 details selected pathologic features of some of these diseases (discussed below).

There are important differences in the rates of specific glomerular diseases that cause nephrotic syndrome in adults versus those in children. For example, minimal-change disease is responsible for most (70%) cases of primary nephrotic syndrome in children, but only 15% in adults. The primary glomerular diseases that most often cause primary nephrotic syndrome in adults are membranous glomerulonephritis (in whites and Asians) and focal segmental glomerulosclerosis in American blacks. Systemic diseases that involve the kidney, such as (most commonly) diabetes and also

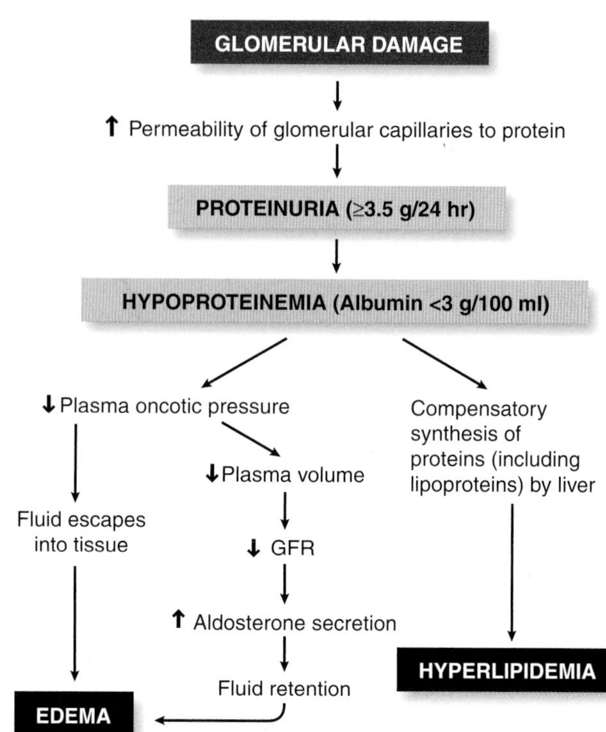

FIGURE 14-11. Pathophysiology of the nephrotic syndrome. GFR, glomerular filtration rate.

Table 14-1

Frequency of Causes for the Nephrotic Syndrome Induced by Primary Glomerular Diseases in Children and Adults

Cause	Children (%)	Adults (%)
Minimal-change disease	75	10
Membranous glomerulonephritis	5	30
Focal segmental glomerulosclerosis	10	35
Membranoproliferative glomerulonephritis	5	5
Other glomerular diseases[a]	5	20

[a]Includes many forms of mesangioproliferative and proliferative glomerulonephritis, such as immunoglobulin A nephropathy, which may cause nephritic and nephrotic features.

Table 14-2

Pathologic Features of Important Causes of the Nephrotic Syndrome

	Minimal-Change Disease	Focal Segmental Glomerulosclerosis	Membranous Glomerulonephritis	Membranoproliferative Glomerulonephritis
Light microscopy	No lesion	Focal and segmental glomerular consolidation	Diffuse global capillary wall thickening	Capillary wall thickening and endocapillary hypercellularity
Immunofluorescence microscopy	No immune deposits	No immune deposits	Diffuse capillary wall immunoglobulin	Diffuse capillary wall complement with or without immunoglobulin
Electron microscopy	No immune deposits	No immune deposits	Diffuse subepithelial deposits	Subendothelial dense deposits; intramembranous dense deposits (dense deposit disease)

amyloidosis and systemic lupus erythematosus, account for many cases of adult nephrotic syndrome in the United States. However, where chronic infectious diseases are common, immune complex membranoproliferative glomerulonephritis (MPGN) is a much more frequent cause of nephrotic syndrome.

Glomerulonephritis (Nephritic Syndrome)

Glomerulonephritis is characterized by decreased glomerular filtration rate (GFR), which causes elevated blood urea nitrogen and serum creatinine, oliguria, salt and water retention, hypertension, and edema. Hematuria may be microscopic or grossly visible, and proteinuria varies. Glomerular diseases associated with the nephritic syndrome are caused by inflammatory changes in glomeruli, including infiltration by leukocytes, hyperplasia of glomerular cells, and, in severe lesions, necrosis. Injury to glomerular capillaries results in spillage of protein and blood cells into the urine (proteinuria and hematuria, respectively). The inflammatory damage may also impair glomerular flow and filtration, resulting in renal insufficiency, fluid retention, and hypertension. Nephritic manifestations may (1) develop rapidly and result in reversible renal insufficiency (acute glomerulonephritis); (2) progress rapidly, with renal failure that resolves only with aggressive treatment (rapidly progressive glomerulonephritis); or (3) persist for years continuously or intermittently and proceed slowly to renal failure (chronic glomerulonephritis).

Some glomerular diseases tend to cause the nephrotic syndrome, whereas others lead to the nephritic syndrome (Table 14-3). However, except for minimal-change disease (which almost always causes nephrotic syndrome), all glomerular diseases may occasionally cause mixed nephritic and nephrotic manifestations. ***Renal biopsy evaluation is the only means of definitive diagnosis for most glomerular diseases, although clinical and laboratory data may be useful as presumptive evidence for a specific disease.***

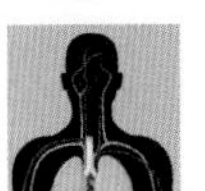

PATHOPHYSIOLOGY: Glomerulonephritis is often caused by immunologic mechanisms. Antibody- and cell-mediated immunity may both lead to glomerular inflammation, but three types of antibody-induced inflammation have been incriminated as the major pathogenetic processes in most forms of glomerulonephritis (Fig. 14-12). A less frequent cause of glomerulonephritis is dysregulation and uncontrolled activation of the alternative complement pathway. Major pathogenetic mechanisms responsible for glomerulonephritis are as follows:

Table 14-3

Tendencies of Glomerular Diseases to Manifest Nephrotic and Nephritic Features

Disease	Nephrotic	Nephritic
Minimal-change disease	++++	–
Membranous glomerulonephritis	+++	++
Focal segmental glomerulosclerosis	+++	++
Mesangioproliferative glomerulonephritis[a]	++	++
Membranoproliferative glomerulonephritis	++	++
Proliferative glomerulonephritis[a]	+	+++
Crescentic glomerulonephritis[a]	+	++++

[a]These histologic phenotypes can be caused by many categories of glomerular disease, including immunoglobulin A nephropathy, postinfectious glomerulonephritis, lupus glomerulonephritis, antineutrophil cytoplasmic autoantibody glomerulonephritis, anti–glomerular basement membrane glomerulonephritis, and C3 glomerulopathy.

- In situ immune complex formation
- Deposition of circulating immune complexes
- Antineutrophil cytoplasmic autoantibodies (ANCAs)
- Alternative pathway complement dysregulation

Immune complex formation in situ involves circulating antibodies binding to intrinsic antigens or foreign antigens within glomeruli. For example, anti-GBM autoantibodies bind a very specific epitope on the α4 chain of type IV collagen in GBMs. The resultant immune complexes in glomerular capillary walls attract leukocytes and activate complement and other humoral inflammatory mediators, resulting in inflammatory injury.

Circulating immune complexes may deposit in glomeruli and incite inflammation similar to that produced when immune complexes form in situ. For example, circulating antibodies can bind to antigens released into the blood by bacterial or viral infection to produce immune complexes. If these complexes escape phagocytosis, they can deposit in glomeruli and incite inflammation.

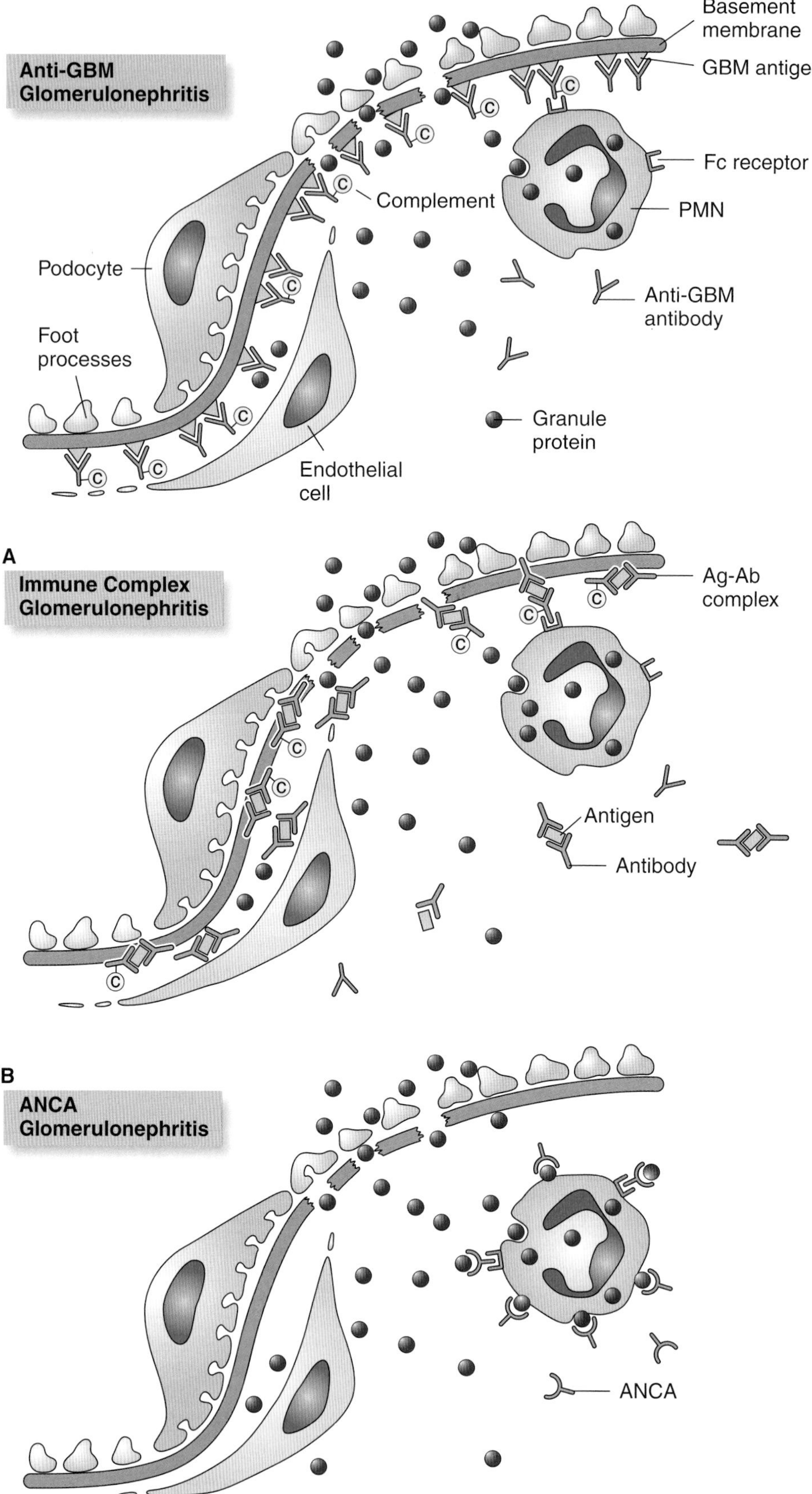

FIGURE 14-12. Antibody-mediated glomerulonephritis. A. Anti–glomerular basement membrane (GBM) antibodies cause glomerulonephritis by binding in situ to basement membrane antigens. This activates complement and recruits inflammatory cells. **B.** Immune complexes that deposit from the circulation also activate complement and recruit inflammatory cells. **C.** Antineutrophil cytoplasmic antibodies (ANCAs) cause inflammation by activating leukocytes by direct binding of the antibodies to the leukocytes and by Fc receptor engagement of ANCA bound to antigen. PMN, polymorphonuclear neutrophil; Ag-Ab complex, antigen–antibody complex.

Immunofluorescence microscopy detects immune complexes in glomeruli. Anti-GBM antibodies produce linear staining of GBMs (see above), whereas other immune complexes produce granular staining in capillary walls or mesangium or both.

Antineutrophil cytoplasmic autoantibodies (ANCA) cause severe glomerulonephritis with little or no glomerular Ig deposition. Such patients often have circulating autoantibodies specific for antigens in the cytoplasm of neutrophils, which activate these cells and so mediate glomerular inflammation. Most ANCAs are directed against myeloperoxidase (MPO-ANCA) or proteinase-3 (PR3-ANCA). Even minor stimulation of neutrophils and monocytes, such as by increased circulating levels of cytokines during viral infection, causes these inflammatory cells to express surface MPO and PR3, which then can interact with ANCAs. This binding activates neutrophils and causes them to adhere to microvascular endothelial cells, especially glomerular capillaries. In this location, they release products that promote vascular inflammation, including glomerulonephritis, arteritis, and venulitis. This inflammation is amplified by the release of factors from ANCA-activated neutrophils that activate the alternative complement pathway.

Formation of glomerular immune complexes in situ, deposition of immune complexes, and interaction of ANCAs with leukocytes all initiate glomerular inflammatory injury mediated by the attraction and activation of leukocytes (Fig. 14-12).

A fourth category of immune-mediated glomerulonephritis (**C3 glomerulopathy**) features dysregulation of the alternative complement pathway. This effect is caused by (1) the genetic absence or dysfunction of complement regulatory proteins (e.g., complement factor H, complement factor I), (2) autoantibodies that inhibit complement regulatory proteins, or (3) autoantibodies that stabilize the alternative pathway C3 convertase (C3 nephritis factor).

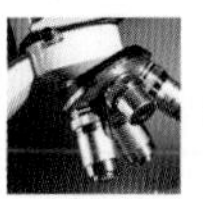

PATHOLOGY: ***Accurate pathologic diagnosis of glomerular diseases requires examination of renal tissue by light, immunofluorescence, and electron microscopy and integration of these findings with clinical information.*** Table 14-4 lists pathologic features useful in diagnosing glomerular diseases.

In general, pathologic features of acute inflammation, such as endocapillary and extracapillary hypercellularity (**proliferative glomerulonephritis**), leukocyte infiltration, and necrosis, are more common in disorders characterized mainly as nephritic than in those that are more typically nephrotic. **Glomerular crescent formation** (extracapillary proliferation) correlates with a more rapidly progressive course. Crescents are not specific for a particular cause of glomerular inflammation. They are, rather, markers of severe injury that result in extensive rupture of capillary walls, which allows inflammatory mediators to enter the Bowman space, where they stimulate macrophage infiltration and epithelial proliferation.

Table 14-4

Diagnostic Features of Glomerular Diseases

I. Light microscopic features
  A. Increased cellularity
    Infiltration by leukocytes (e.g., neutrophils, monocytes, macrophages)
    Proliferation of "endocapillary" cells (i.e., endothelial and mesangial cells)
    Proliferation of "extracapillary" cells (i.e., epithelial cells) (crescent formation)
  B. Increased extracellular material
    Localization of immune complexes
    Thickening or replication of GBM
    Increases in collagenous matrix (sclerosis)
    Insudation of plasma proteins (hyalinosis)
    Fibrinoid necrosis
    Deposition of amyloid
II. Immunofluorescence features
  A. Linear staining of GBM
    Anti-GBM antibodies
    Multiple plasma proteins (e.g., diabetic glomerulosclerosis)
    Monoclonal immunoglobulin chains
  B. Granular immune complex staining or complement staining alone
    Mesangium (e.g., IgA nephropathy)
    Capillary wall (e.g., membranous glomerulonephritis)
    Mesangium and capillary wall (e.g., lupus glomerulonephritis, C3 glomerulopathy)
  C. Irregular (fluffy) staining
    Monoclonal light chains (AL amyloidosis)
    AA protein (AA amyloidosis)
III. Electron microscopic features
  A. Electron-dense immune complex deposits or complement deposits
    Mesangial (e.g., IgA nephropathy)
    Subendothelial (e.g., lupus glomerulonephritis)
    Subepithelial (e.g., membranous glomerulonephritis)
  B. GBM thickening (e.g., diabetic glomerulosclerosis)
  C. GBM remodeling (e.g., membranoproliferative glomerulonephritis)
  D. Collagenous matrix expansion (e.g., focal segmental glomerulosclerosis)
  E. Fibrillary deposits (e.g., amyloidosis)

GBM, glomerular basement membrane; IgA, immunoglobulin A.

DISEASES PRESENTING AS NEPHROTIC SYNDROME

Minimal-Change Disease

Pathologically, Minimal-Change Disease Entails Effacement of Podocyte Foot Processes

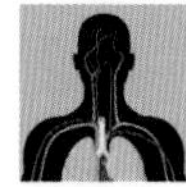

PATHOPHYSIOLOGY: The pathogenesis of minimal-change disease is unknown. The immune system may be involved: the disease may remit with corticosteroid treatment, and it may occur in association with an allergic disorder or a lymphoid neoplasm. The heavy proteinuria of minimal-change disease is accompanied by loss of polyanionic sites in the GBM and podocytes. This allows anionic proteins, especially albumin, to pass more easily across capillary walls.

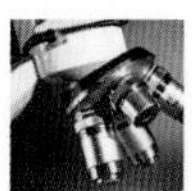

PATHOLOGY: ***Glomeruli in minimal-change disease appear essentially normal on light microscopy.*** Electron microscopy shows extensive **fusion of podocyte cell foot processes** (Figs. 14-13 and 14-14). This change occurs in almost all cases of nephrotic range proteinuria; it is not specific for minimal-change disease. Immunofluorescence studies for Ig and

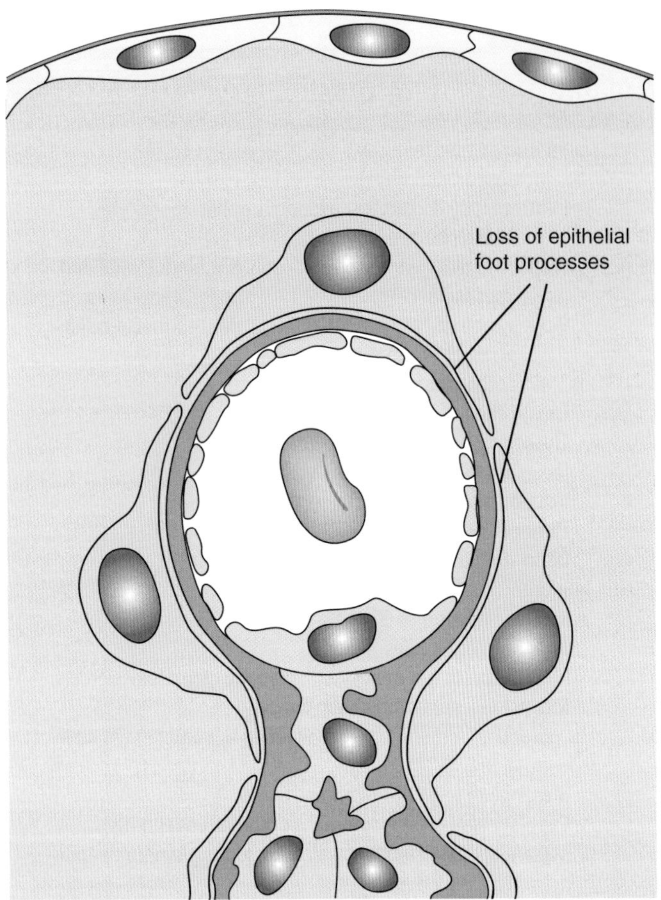

FIGURE 14-13. Minimal-change disease. This condition is characterized predominantly by epithelial cell changes, particularly effacement of foot processes. All other glomerular structures appear intact.

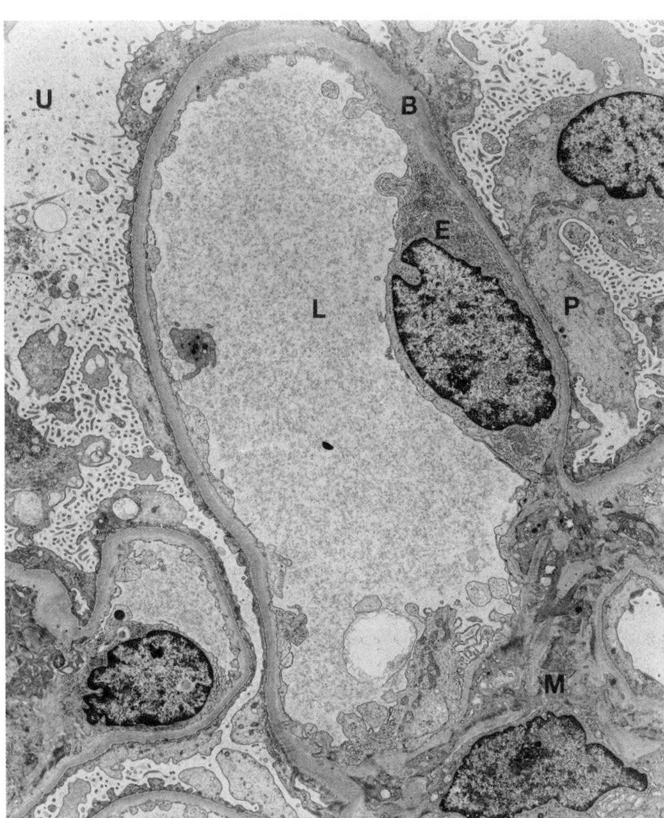

FIGURE 14-14. Minimal-change disease. In this electron micrograph, the podocyte (P) displays extensive effacement of foot processes and numerous microvilli projecting into the urinary space (U). Compare with Figure 14-3. B, basement membrane; E, endothelial cell; L, lumen; M, mesangial cell.

complement deposition are most often negative. Proteinuria leads to hypoalbuminemia, and a compensatory increase in lipoprotein secretion by the liver results in hyperlipidemia. A loss of lipoproteins through glomeruli causes lipids to accumulate in proximal tubular cells, reflected histologically as glassy (hyaline) droplets in tubular epithelial cytoplasm. Such droplets are not specific for minimal-change disease but are seen in any glomerular disease that causes nephrotic syndrome.

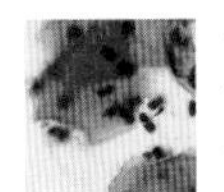

CLINICAL FEATURES: ***Minimal-change disease is responsible for 90% of nephrotic syndrome cases in children younger than 5, 50% in older children, and 15% in adults.*** In more than 90% of children and in fewer adults, proteinuria remits completely within 8 weeks of initiating corticosteroid therapy. If corticosteroids are withdrawn, most patients have intermittent relapses for up to 10 years. A minority of patients have only partial remission with corticosteroid therapy, and a smaller number are totally resistant and may develop azotemia. In such cases, the diagnosis of minimal-change disease may not be accurate, and focal segmental glomerulosclerosis may be present. In the absence of complications, the long-term outlook for patients with minimal-change disease is no different from that of the general population.

Focal Segmental Glomerulosclerosis

In FSGS, glomerular consolidation affects some (focal), but not all, glomeruli and initially involves only part of an affected glomerular tuft (segmental). Consolidated segments often show increased collagenous matrix (sclerosis; Fig. 14-15).

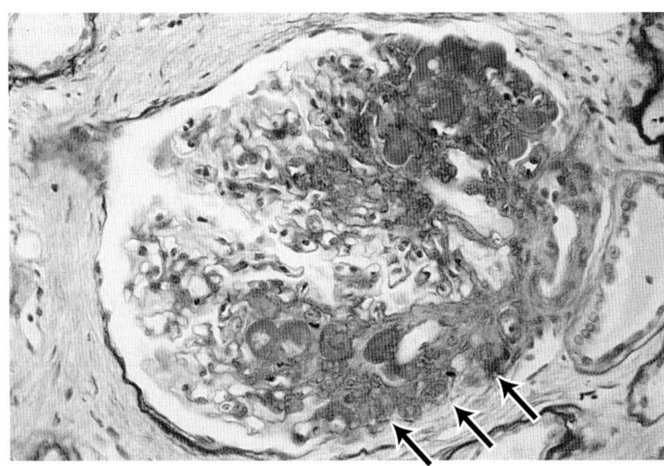

FIGURE 14-15. Focal segmental glomerulosclerosis. Periodic acid–Schiff (PAS) staining showing perihilar areas of segmental sclerosis and adjacent adhesions to the Bowman capsule (*arrows*).

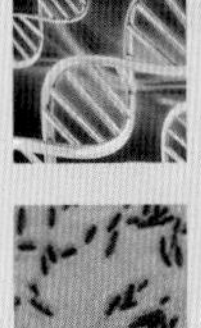

MOLECULAR PATHOGENESIS AND ETIOLOGIC FACTORS: FSGS may be idiopathic (primary) or secondary to several conditions (Table 14-5). Pathologic features and genetic evidence suggest that injury to podocytes may be common to all types of FSGS.

Several hereditary forms of FSGS reflect genetic abnormalities in podocyte proteins (e.g., podocin, nephrin, α-actinin-4, and TRPC6).

Congenital and acquired reductions in renal mass and excessive body mass (obesity) place adaptive stress on surviving nephrons. This strain appears to cause FSGS from overwork, with increased glomerular capillary pressure and filtration, and glomerular enlargement. Reduced blood oxygen (e.g., as in sickle cell disease or cyanotic congenital heart disease) also causes a similar pattern of glomerular injury. In all of these settings, glomerular enlargement reflects functional overwork, placing undue stress on podocytes because of their limited proliferative capacity.

Viruses, drugs, and serum factors are also implicated as causes of FSGS. Infection with HIV, especially in blacks, is associated with a variant of FSGS that displays a collapsing pattern of sclerosis (Fig. 14-16). Pamidronate, a drug used to treat osteolytic bone disease, causes collapsing FSGS in some patients probably by injuring podocytes. A serum permeability factor detected in some patients with FSGS and recurrence of the disease after renal transplantation suggests a systemic cause for the glomerular injury. Sequence variants in the gene encoding apolipoprotein 1 (*APOL1*), which provide protection against African sleeping sickness (trypanosomiasis), have been linked to FSGS in blacks; an ethnic group known to have a high incidence of FSGS and hypertension-related ESRD.

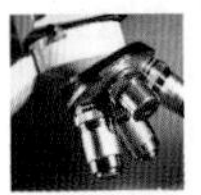

PATHOLOGY: Varying numbers of glomeruli show segmental obliteration of capillary loops by increased matrix or accumulation of cells or both. Insudation of plasma proteins and lipid gives lesions a glassy appearance, called **hyalinosis**. Adhesions to the Bowman capsule occur adjacent to sclerotic lesions. Uninvolved glomeruli may look entirely normal, although mild mesangial hypercellularity is occasionally present.

Table 14-5

Categories of Focal Segmental Glomerulosclerosis

Primary (idiopathic) focal segmental glomerulosclerosis (FSGS)
Secondary FSGS
Hereditary/genetic (e.g., mutations in podocyte genes)
Obesity (perihilar variant)
Reduced renal mass (perihilar variant)
Cyanotic congenital heart disease (usually perihilar variant)
Sickle cell nephropathy (usually perihilar variant)
Infection induced (e.g., HIV, collapsing variant)
Drug induced (e.g., pamidronate, collapsing variant)

Primary and secondary FSGS can have various histologic patterns of injury: perihilar, tip lesion, cellular, collapsing, not otherwise specified.

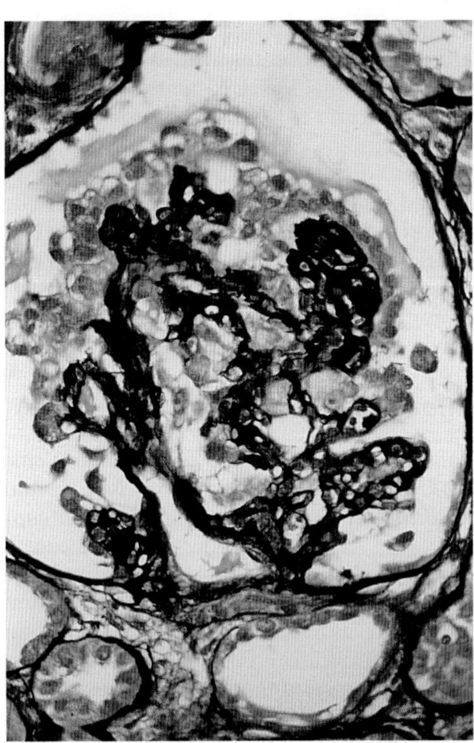

FIGURE 14-16. HIV-associated nephropathy. Silver staining showing a collapsing pattern of focal segmental glomerulosclerosis, with collapse of glomerular capillaries, increased matrix material (sclerosis), and hypertrophy of podocytes.

By electron microscopy, epithelial cell foot processes are diffusely effaced in FSGS, with occasional focal detachment or loss of podocytes from the GBM. Sclerotic segments show increased matrix material, wrinkling and thickening of basement membranes, and capillary collapse. Accumulation of electron-dense material in sclerotic segments represents insudative trapping of plasma proteins and corresponds to hyalinosis seen by light microscopy. ***Immune complexes are absent.*** However, irregular trapping of IgM and C3 occurs in the segmental areas of sclerosis and hyalinosis.

Several histologic variants of FSGS are recognized:

- **Perihilar sclerosis** in segments within glomeruli and in deep cortical (juxtamedullary) glomeruli (Fig. 14-15) is found in patients with reduced renal mass or obese patients.
- A **collapsing pattern** of sclerosis with hypertrophied and hyperplastic podocytes adjacent to sclerotic segments is typical of HIV-associated nephropathy, with IV drug abuse, and pamidronate therapy, and as an idiopathic process. This collapsing variant has a poor prognosis, and half of patients reach end-stage disease within 2 years.
- **Tip lesions** are characterized by sclerosis limited to glomerular segments adjacent to the origin of the proximal tubule. The variant is more likely to respond to steroid therapy than other forms of FSGS.
- **Cellular variants** of FSGS have prominent lipid-laden cells within the sites of glomerular consolidation.

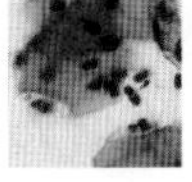

CLINICAL FEATURES: FSGS causes one third of primary nephrotic syndrome in adults and 10% in children. It is more common in blacks than in whites and is the leading cause of primary nephrotic syndrome in the former. For unknown reasons, its frequency has been increasing over the past few decades. Most often, asymptomatic proteinuria begins insidiously and progresses to the nephrotic syndrome. Many patients are hypertensive, and microscopic hematuria is frequent. Progress to ESRD after 5 to 20 years is frequent. Some, but not all, patients improve with corticosteroid therapy. Although renal transplantation is the preferred treatment for ESRD, FSGS recurs in one half of transplanted kidneys. Patients with FSGS due to obesity or reduced renal mass usually have a more indolent course, with lower levels of proteinuria. This variant benefits from treatment with angiotensin-converting enzyme (ACE) inhibitors or angiotensin receptor blockers (ARBs).

Membranous Glomerulonephritis

Membranous glomerulonephritis is a common cause of nephrotic syndrome in adults. It reflects the accumulation of subepithelial immune complexes in glomerular capillaries.

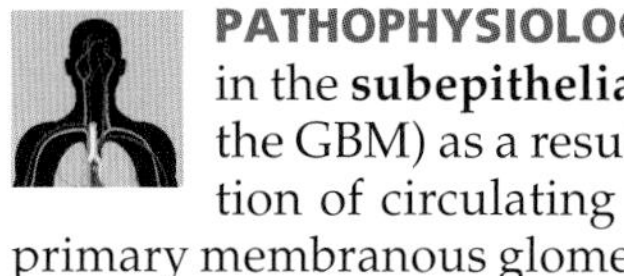

PATHOPHYSIOLOGY: Immune complexes localize in the **subepithelial zone** (between podocytes and the GBM) as a result of formation in situ or deposition of circulating complexes. Most patients with primary membranous glomerulonephritis exhibit circulating autoantibodies against PLA_2R, a podocyte transmembrane receptor. PLA_2R and anti-PLA_2R can be isolated from the immune complexes, supporting immune complex formation in situ. Sometimes, free antigens and antibodies cross the GBM independently to form subepithelial immune complexes. Secondary membranous glomerulonephritis is associated with autoimmune disease (SLE, autoimmune thyroid disease), certain infections (hepatitis B, malaria, and others), penicillamine therapy, and neoplastic diseases.

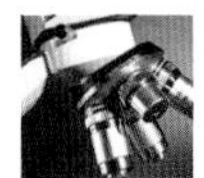

PATHOLOGY: In membranous glomerulonephritis, glomeruli are usually normocellular. Depending on the duration of the disease, capillary walls may be normal or thickened (Fig. 14-17). In intermediate disease stages, stains of basement membranes reveal multiple "spikes," which are projections of the basement membrane material around subepithelial immune complexes (Fig. 14-18).

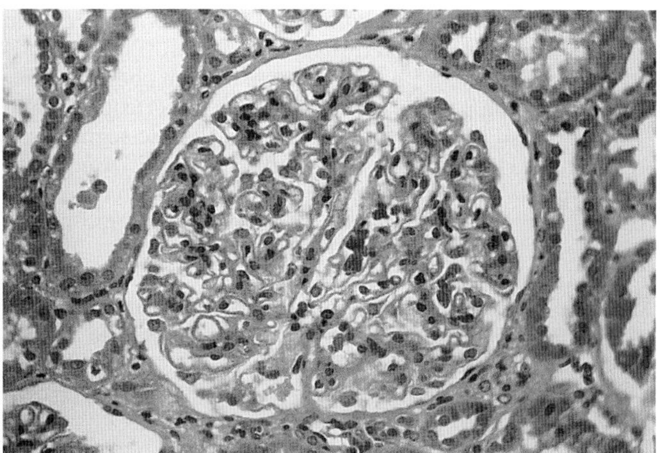

FIGURE 14-17. Membranous glomerulonephritis. The glomerulus is slightly enlarged and shows diffuse thickening of the capillary walls. There is no hypercellularity. Compare capillary walls to those shown in Figure 14-15.

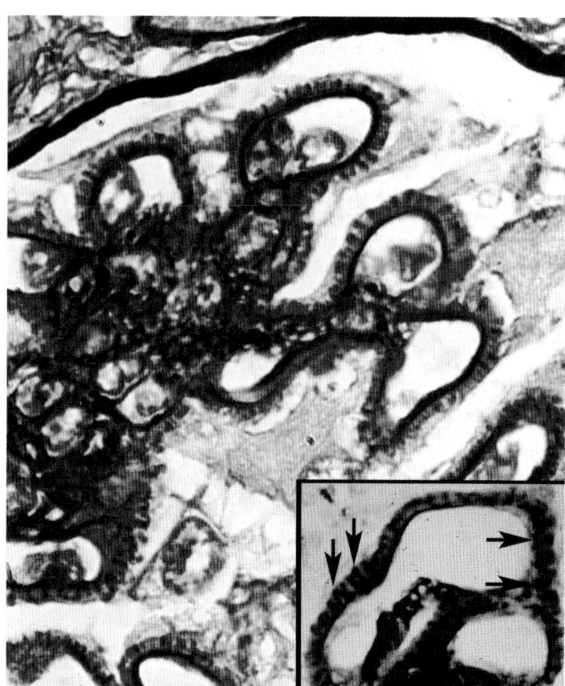

FIGURE 14-18. Membranous glomerulonephritis. Silver staining revealing multiple "spikes" diffusely distributed in the glomerular capillary basement membranes (*arrows*). This pattern corresponds to the stage II lesion illustrated in Figures 14-23 and 14-24. The appearance is produced by the deposition of silver-positive basement membrane material around silver-negative immune complex deposits.

As disease progresses, capillary lumens narrow, and glomerular sclerosis eventually ensues. Advanced membranous glomerulonephritis cannot be distinguished from other forms of chronic glomerular disease. Atrophy of tubules and interstitial fibrosis parallel the degree of glomerular sclerosis. Mesangial electron-dense deposits are rare in primary membranous glomerulonephritis but are more common in secondary disease (e.g., in lupus nephropathy).

By electron microscopy, immune complexes appear in capillary walls as electron-dense deposits (Fig. 14-19). The progressive ultrastructural changes caused by subepithelial immune complexes are divided into stages, as illustrated in Figure 14-19.

Immunofluorescence reveals diffuse granular staining of capillary walls for IgG and C3 (Fig. 14-20). There is intense staining for terminal complement components, including the membrane attack complex, which participate in inducing glomerular injury, especially to podocytes.

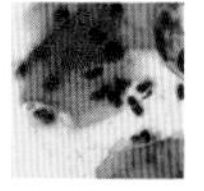

CLINICAL FEATURES: Membranous glomerulonephritis is the most common primary glomerular cause of nephrotic syndrome in white and Asian adults in the United States. The most common secondary glomerular cause is diabetic glomerulosclerosis. The course of membranous glomerulonephritis is highly variable. Spontaneous remission occurs in one fourth of patients within 20 years, and 10-year renal survival rate is greater than 65%. Patients with progressive renal failure are treated with corticosteroids or immunosuppressive drugs. The prognosis is better in children because of a higher rate of permanent spontaneous remission.

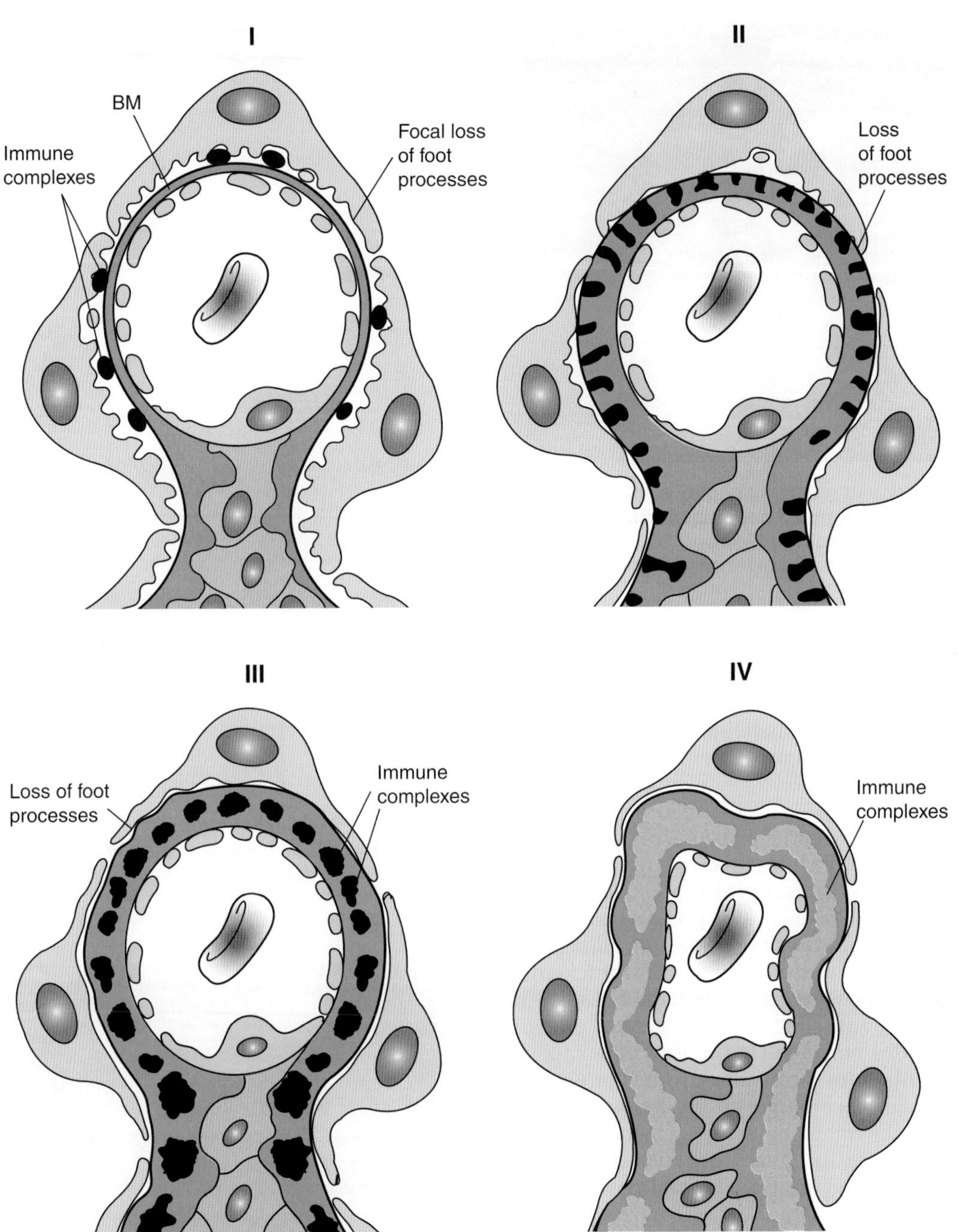

FIGURE 14-19. Membranous glomerulonephritis. This disease is caused by the subepithelial accumulation of immune complexes and the accompanying changes in the basement membrane (BM). Stage I exhibits scattered subepithelial deposits. The outer contour of the BM remains smooth. Stage II disease has projections (spikes) of BM material adjacent to the deposits. In stage III disease, newly formed BM has surrounded the deposits. With stage IV disease, the immune complex deposits lose their electron density, resulting in an irregularly thickened BM with irregular electron-lucent areas.

Membranous Lupus Glomerulonephritis

For a general discussion of lupus-associated glomerular disease, see lupus glomerulonephritis below. Characteristically, this disorder (lupus glomerulonephritis class V) is associated with immune complexes located in the subepithelial zone similar to the appearance of membranous glomerulonephritis (see above). This location of immune complexes predisposes to a nephrotic versus nephritic (inflammatory) presentation. Hence, this subtype of lupus-associated glomerular disease is best considered under nephrotic syndromes.

Diabetic Glomerulosclerosis

Diabetic glomerulosclerosis accounts for 40% of ESRD and thus is the leading cause of chronic renal failure in the United States.

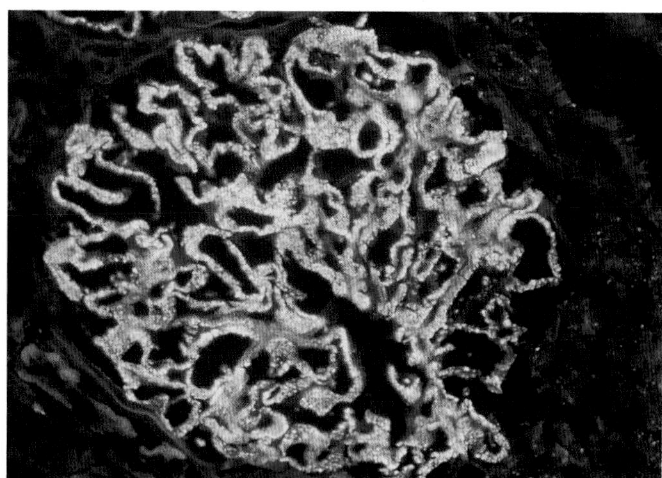

FIGURE 14-20. Membranous glomerulonephritis. Immunofluorescence microscopy showing granular deposits of immunoglobulin G outlining the glomerular capillary loops.

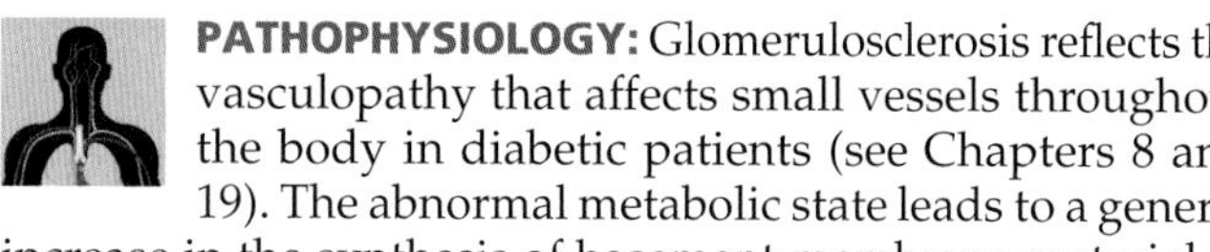

PATHOPHYSIOLOGY: Glomerulosclerosis reflects the vasculopathy that affects small vessels throughout the body in diabetic patients (see Chapters 8 and 19). The abnormal metabolic state leads to a general increase in the synthesis of basement membrane material in the microvasculature.

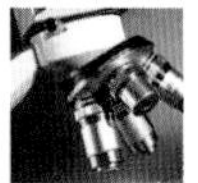

PATHOLOGY: The earliest lesions of diabetic glomerulosclerosis are glomerular enlargement, GBM thickening, and mesangial matrix expansion (Fig. 14-21). The numbers of podocytes decline. Mild mesangial hypercellularity may be present, along with the increase in mesangial matrix. Diffuse GBM thickening and mesangial matrix expansion are accompanied by sclerotic **Kimmelstiel–Wilson nodules** (Fig. 14-22). Insudated proteins form rounded nodules between (1) the Bowman capsule and the parietal epithelium ("capsular drops") or (2) subendothelial accumulations along capillary loops ("hyaline caps"). Tubular basement membranes are thickened. Sclerosing and insudative changes in afferent and efferent arterioles cause hyaline arteriolosclerosis. Generalized renal arteriosclerosis is also usually present. Vascular narrowing and reduced blood flow to the medulla predispose to papillary necrosis and pyelonephritis.

By electron microscopy, the basement membrane lamina densa may be 5- to 10-fold thicker. Mesangial matrix is increased, particularly in nodular lesions. By immunofluorescence, there is diffuse linear trapping of IgG, albumin, fibrinogen, and other plasma proteins in the GBM. This reflects nonimmunologic adsorption of these proteins to the thickened GBM, possibly owing to nonenzymatic glycosylation of GBM and plasma proteins.

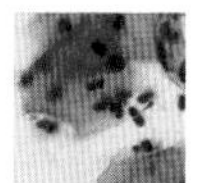

CLINICAL FEATURES: Glomerulosclerosis occurs in both type 1 and type 2 diabetes mellitus. Approximately 25% of such patients develop diabetic glomerulosclerosis. The earliest manifestation is microalbuminuria (slightly increased proteinuria). Overt proteinuria occurs between 10 and 15 years after the onset of diabetes and often becomes severe enough to cause the nephrotic syndrome. In time, diabetic glomerulosclerosis progresses to renal failure.

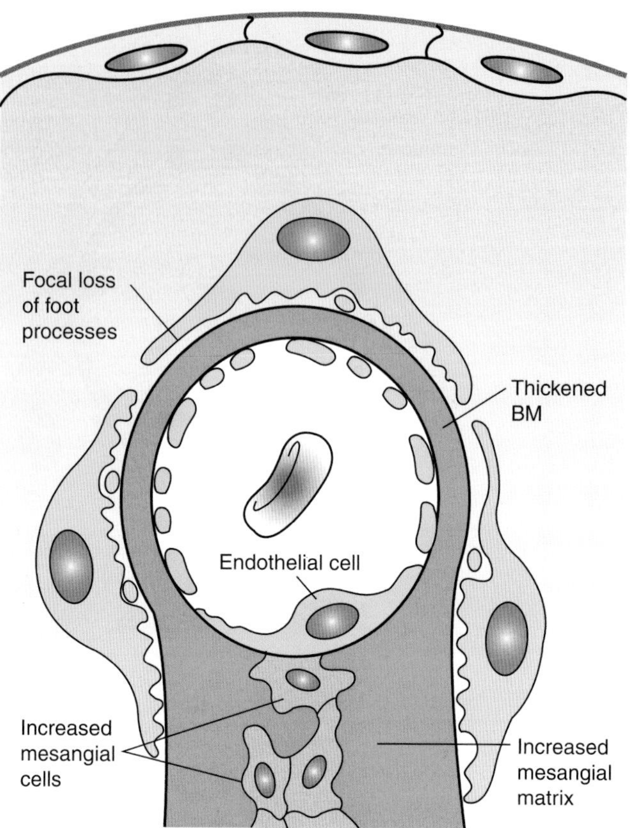

FIGURE 14-21. Diabetic glomerulosclerosis. The lamina densa of the glomerular basement membrane (BM) is thickened, and there is an increase in mesangial matrix material.

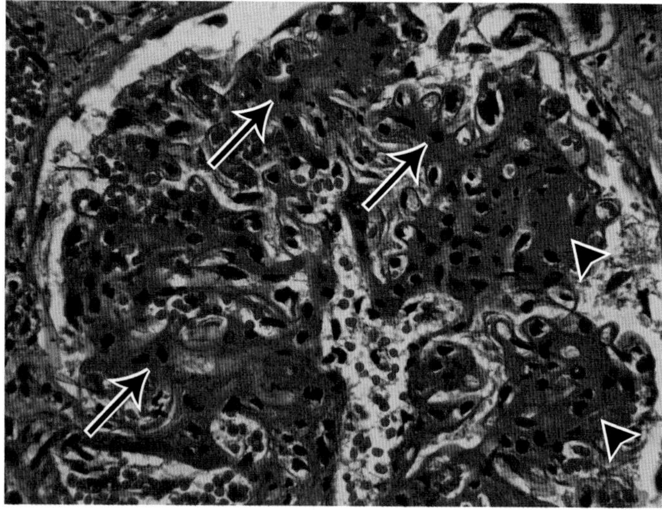

FIGURE 14-22. Diabetic glomerulosclerosis. There is a prominent increase in the mesangial matrix (*arrows*), forming several nodular lesions (*arrowheads*). Dilation of glomerular capillaries is evident, and some capillary basement membranes are thickened.

Amyloidosis

Renal disease is a frequent complication of AA serum amyloid A and AL Ig light-chain amyloidosis (see Chapter 7).

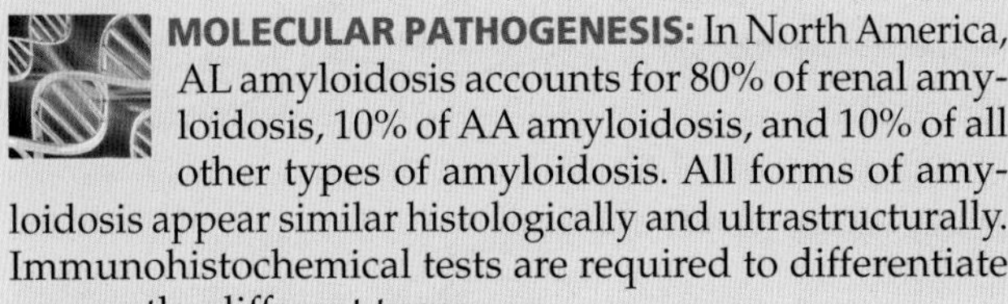

MOLECULAR PATHOGENESIS: In North America, AL amyloidosis accounts for 80% of renal amyloidosis, 10% of AA amyloidosis, and 10% of all other types of amyloidosis. All forms of amyloidosis appear similar histologically and ultrastructurally. Immunohistochemical tests are required to differentiate among the different types.

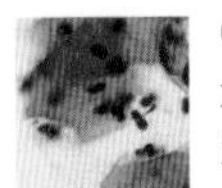

PATHOLOGY: Amyloid deposits are initially apparent in the mesangium but later extend into capillary walls and eventually obliterate capillary lumens (Figs. 14-23 and 14-24). Glomerular structure is completely destroyed in advanced amyloidosis, and glomeruli appear as large eosinophilic spheres.

By electron microscopy, amyloid is composed of nonbranching fibrils, about 10 nm in diameter. These are initially most abundant in the mesangium but often extend into capillary walls, especially in advanced cases (Fig. 14-24). Podocyte foot processes overlying the GBM are effaced.

CLINICAL FEATURES: Renal involvement is prominent in most cases of systemic amyloidosis. Proteinuria is often the initial manifestation and is nonselective (i.e., albumin and globulins are in the urine). Nephrotic syndrome occurs in 60% of patients.

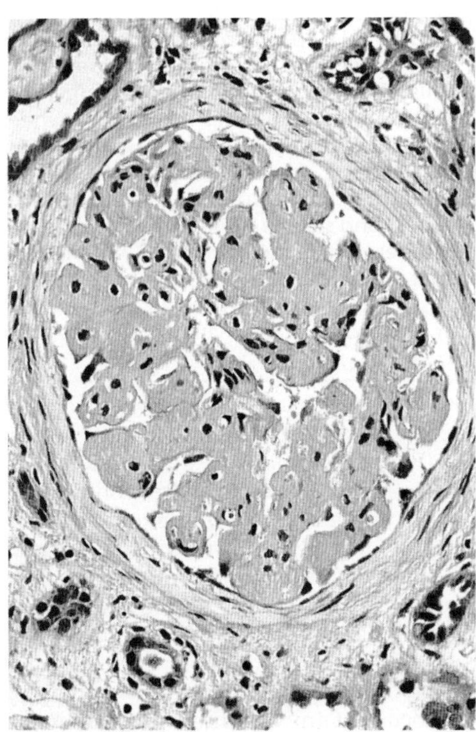

FIGURE 14-23. Amyloid nephropathy. Amorphous acellular material expands the mesangial areas and obstructs the glomerular capillaries. The deposits of amyloid may take on a nodular appearance, somewhat resembling those of diabetic glomerulosclerosis (see Fig. 14-27). However, amyloid deposits are not periodic acid–Schiff positive and are identifiable by Congo red staining.

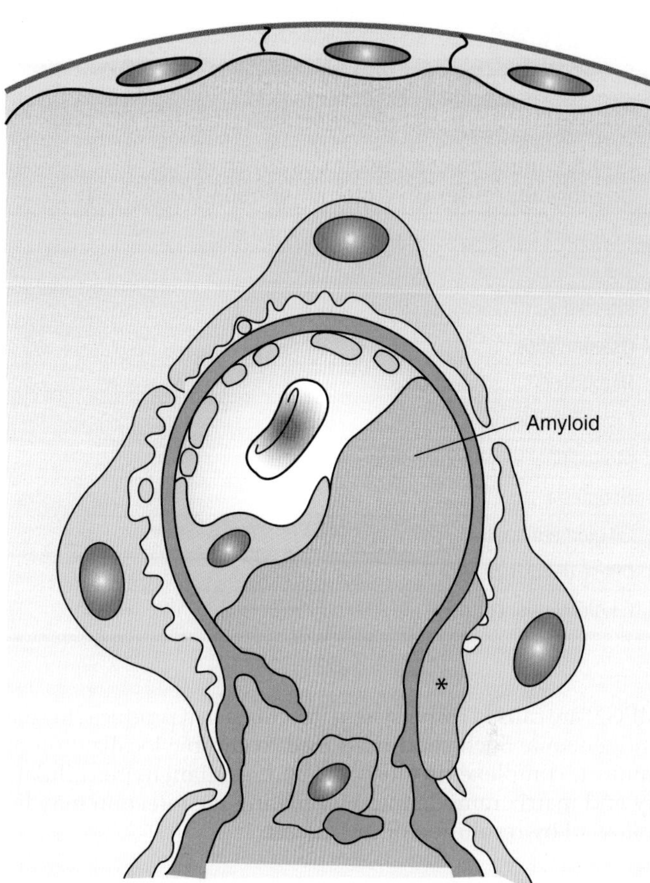

FIGURE 14-24. Amyloid nephropathy. This disorder is initially associated with the accumulation of characteristic fibrillar deposits in the mesangium. These inert masses, which are fibrillar by electron microscopy, extend along the inner surface of the basement membrane, frequently obstructing the capillary lumen. Focal extension of amyloid through the basement membrane (*asterisk*) may elevate the epithelial cell.

DISEASES PRESENTING AS BOTH NEPHROTIC AND NEPHRITIC SYNDROMES

Membranoproliferative Glomerulonephritis

MPGN is a pattern of glomerular inflammation that is characterized by hypercellularity and capillary wall thickening and reflects multiple etiologies. It may manifest as nephrotic or nephritic syndromes, or a combination of both.

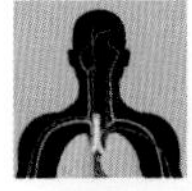

PATHOPHYSIOLOGY: MPGN is characterized by deposits in the mesangium and subendothelial zone of capillary walls that contain immune complexes or activated complement without immunoglobulins. Subepithelial deposits may also occur. The two major categories are immune complex and C3 MPGN (Table 14-6). The nephritogenic antigens in immune complex MPGN are usually unknown but may be related to infectious or autoimmune conditions (Table 14-6). C3 glomerulopathy is discussed in the next section.

Unlike the pathogens of acute postinfectious glomerulonephritis (see below), those associated with immune complex

Table 14-6

Classification of Membranoproliferative Glomerulonephritis

Primary immune complex (idiopathic) membranoproliferative glomerulonephritis (MPGN)
Secondary Immune Complex MPGN caused by:
Subacute bacterial endocarditis
Infected ventriculoatrial shunt
Osteomyelitis
Hepatitis C virus infection
Cryoglobulinemia
Monoclonal immunoglobulins
Neoplasia
C3 glomerulopathy
Dense deposit disease
C3 glomerulonephritis

MPGN are caused by persistent infections that produce chronic antigenemia. Such conditions lead to chronic localization of immune complexes in glomeruli and resultant hypercellularity and matrix remodeling. Eliminating the infection may be followed by resolution of the disease.

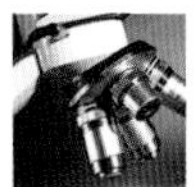

PATHOLOGY: Glomeruli in MPGN are diffusely enlarged, with florid mesangial cell proliferation and infiltration of macrophages. The resultant glomerular lobular distortion ("hypersegmentation"; Fig. 14-25) was once called **lobular glomerulonephritis**. Of these patients, 20% have crescents, usually involving only a minority of glomeruli. Capillary walls are thickened, and silver stains show a doubling or complex replication of GBMs.

Electron microscopy reveals thickening and replication of GBMs. This finding probably follows endothelial cell activation, as well as extension of mesangial cytoplasm into the subendothelial zone. Deposition of new basement membrane material between the mesangial cytoplasm and endothelial cell is noted (Figs. 14-26 and 14-27). Subendothelial and mesangial electron-dense deposits, corresponding to immune complexes or complement, are the likely stimuli for these events. Immunofluorescence microscopy shows granular deposition of immunoglobulins and complement in glomerular capillary loops and mesangium in immune complex MPGN and complement alone in C3 glomerulopathy.

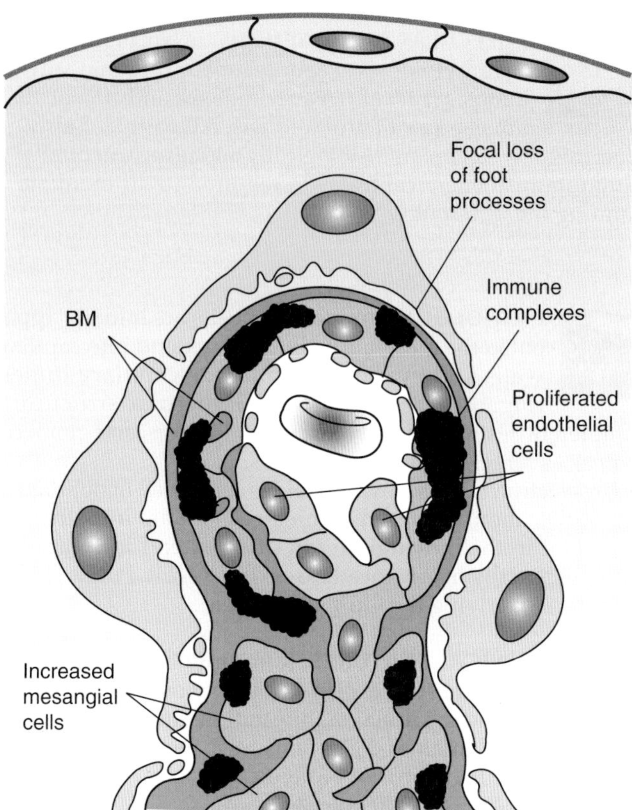

FIGURE 14-26. Type I membranoproliferative glomerulonephritis. In this disease, the glomeruli are enlarged. Hypercellular tufts and narrowing or obstruction of the capillary lumens are seen. Large subendothelial deposits of immune complexes extend along the inner border of the basement membrane (BM). The mesangial cells proliferate and migrate peripherally into the capillary. BM material accumulates in a linear manner parallel to the BM in a subendothelial position. The interposition of mesangial cells and BM between the endothelial cells and the original BM creates a double-contour effect. The accumulation of mesangial cells and stroma in the tufts narrows the capillary lumen. The proliferation of mesangial cells and the accumulation of BM material also widen the mesangium. The entire process leads progressively to lobulation of the glomerulus. Note the proliferation of endothelial cells and focal effacement of foot processes.

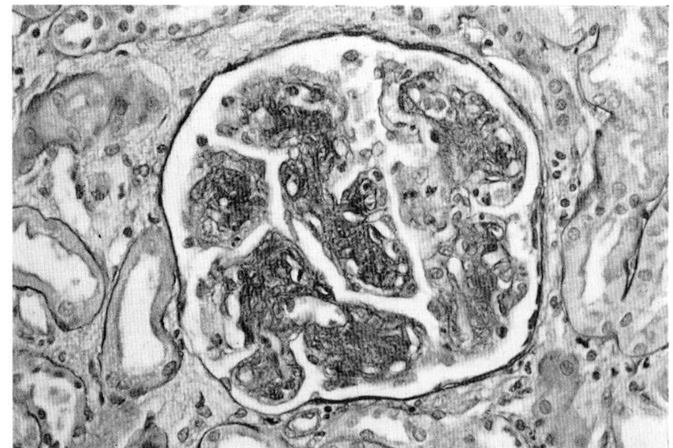

FIGURE 14-25. Type I membranoproliferative glomerulonephritis. The glomerular lobulation is accentuated. Increased cells and matrix in the mesangium and thickening of capillary walls are noted.

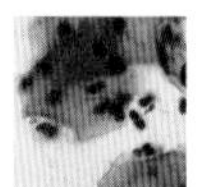

CLINICAL FEATURES: Immune complex MPGN can occur at any age but is most frequent in older children and young adults. MPGN accounts for 5% of primary nephrotic syndrome in children and adults in the United States. Immune complex MPGN occurs much more commonly in countries where chronic infections are more prevalent. The disease is usually persistent and slowly progressive. After 10 years, half of patients reach ESRD.

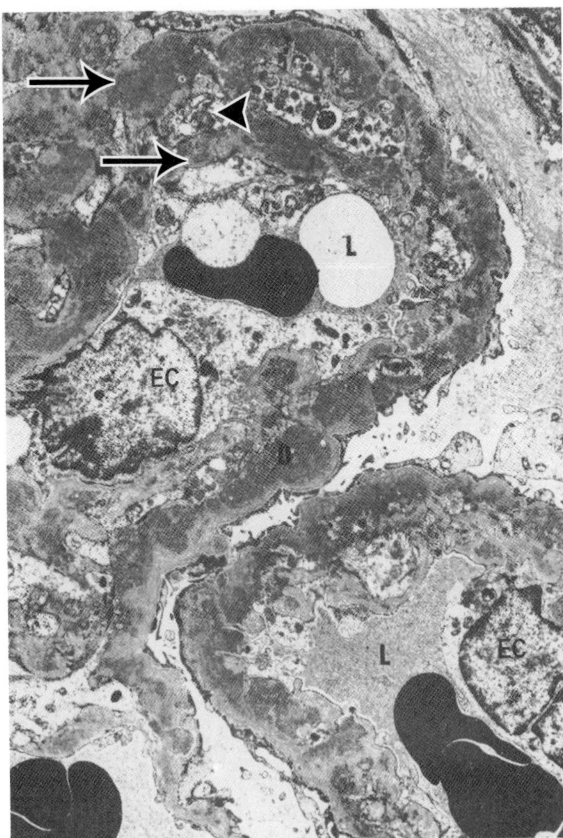

FIGURE 14-27. **Type I membranoproliferative glomerulonephritis.** An electron micrograph demonstrating a double-contour basement membrane (*arrows*), with mesangial interposition (*arrowhead*) and prominent subendothelial deposits. EC, endothelial cell; L, capillary lumen.

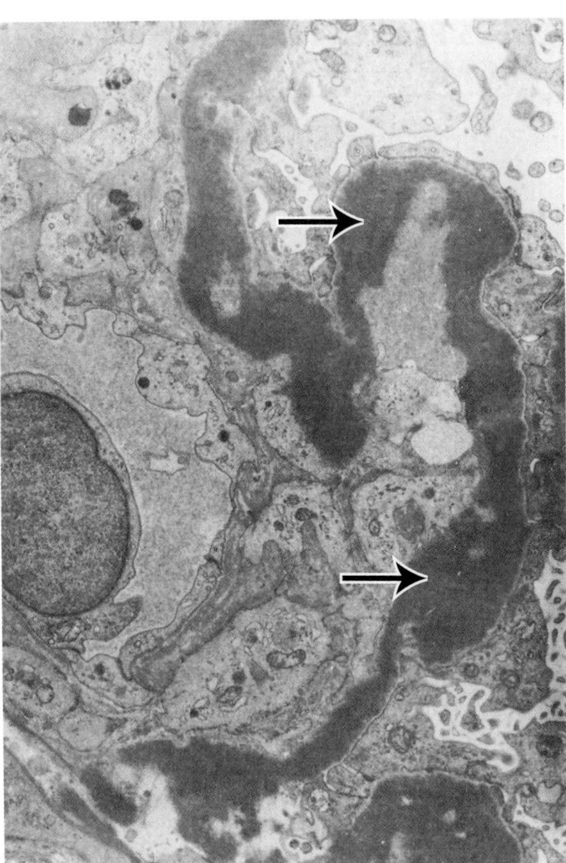

FIGURE 14-28. **C3 glomerulopathy (dense deposit disease).** An electron micrograph demonstrating thickening of the basement membrane with intramembranous dense deposits (*arrows*).

C3 Glomerulopathy

C3 glomerulopathy is a rare glomerulonephritis caused by complement dysregulation. It includes **dense deposit disease** (formerly called *type II MPGN*) and **C3 glomerulonephritis** (including a variant with an MPGN pattern).

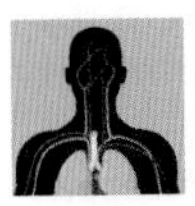

PATHOPHYSIOLOGY: The extensive glomerular localization of complement *without* immunoglobulin indicates that complement activation is a major mediator of the structural and functional abnormalities of C3 glomerulopathy. Deficient or ineffective regulatory factors of the alternative pathway of complement (e.g., complement factor H and complement factor I) that results from gene mutations or autoantibodies cause C3 glomerulopathy. Some patients have an IgG autoantibody, **C3 nephritic factor**, which stabilizes activated C3 convertase (C3bBb), thereby prolonging C3 activation.

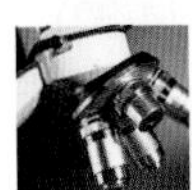

PATHOLOGY: The two pathologic types of C3 glomerulopathy are **dense deposit disease** and **C3 glomerulonephritis**. C3 glomerulopathy histologically resembles immune complex MPGN, with capillary wall thickening and increased cellularity. The distinctive pathologic feature of dense deposit disease is a ribbon-like zone of increased density in the center of a thickened GBM and in the mesangial matrix (Fig. 14-28). In addition, there are areas of density in peritubular capillary membranes and arteriolar elastic laminae.

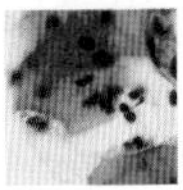

CLINICAL FEATURES: C3 glomerulopathy is rare ($<5/10^6$), and 80% of patients are children. Patients usually present with proteinuria (often nephrotic range), hematuria, hypertension, and impaired renal function. Hypocomplementemia, with low C3 and normal C4, is common. The prognosis is grim because 40% reach ESRD within 10 years.

Nonfibrillary Monoclonal Immunoglobulin Deposition

Ig deposition may be in GBMs, glomerular mesangial matrix, capillary walls, and tubular basement membranes. The underlying B-cell dyscrasia may be occult, or there may be overt multiple myeloma or lymphoma. Unlike the deposits of AL amyloid, those of Ig deposition do not form fibrils or stain with Congo red. The two major phenotypes are (1) nodular sclerosing glomerular disease with granular deposits by electron microscopy and (2) proliferative (or membranoproliferative) glomerulonephritis with homogeneous dense deposits. Monoclonal Ig deposition disease with nodular sclerosis usually manifests clinically as nephrotic syndrome, whereas proliferative glomerulonephritis with monoclonal Ig often presents as mixed nephritic and nephrotic syndrome.

DISEASES PRESENTING AS NEPHRITIC SYNDROME

Acute Postinfectious Glomerulonephritis

This disease features complement-rich immune complex deposits in glomeruli.

PATHOPHYSIOLOGY: Nephritogenic strains of group A streptococci or staphylococci are the usual cause of acute postinfectious glomerulonephritis. This condition reflects deposition in glomeruli of immune complexes containing antibody plus bacterial antigens. Poststreptococcal glomerulonephritis occurs with a 9- to 14-day latent period between antigen exposure and glomerulonephritis. Immune complexes can form in the circulation and deposit in glomeruli, or they may form in situ when bacterial antigens trapped in glomeruli bind to circulating antibodies. Potential instigating streptococcal antigens include glyceraldehyde phosphate dehydrogenase and cationic proteinase exotoxin B. Both enzymes can localize in glomerular capillary walls and activate complement even without antibodies. Alternatively, nephritogenic bacteria may release factors that activate complement without requiring immune complex formation. Such an event could explain the absence of Ig in some glomerular deposits.

Extensive complement activation nearly always accompanied by hypocomplementemia, as well as activation of other humoral and cellular inflammatory mediators, produces glomerular inflammation. The inflammatory mediators attract and activate neutrophils and macrophages and stimulate mesangial and endothelial cell proliferation. ***These effects result in marked glomerular hypercellularity, which defines acute diffuse proliferative glomerulonephritis.***

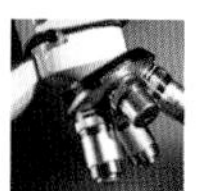

PATHOLOGY: The acute phase begins 1 to 2 weeks after the onset of the nephritogenic infection and resolves in more than 90% of patients after several weeks. In the acute phase, glomeruli are diffusely enlarged and hypercellular (Fig. 14-29), with proliferation of endothelial and mesangial cells (Fig. 14-30) and infiltration by neutrophils and macrophages. Crescents are uncommon.

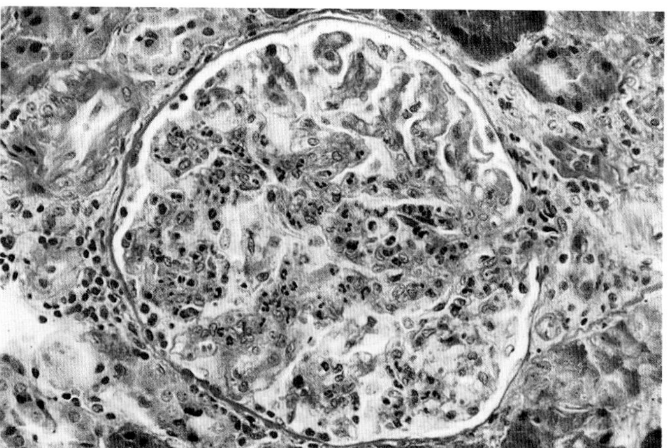

FIGURE 14-29. Acute poststreptococcal glomerulonephritis. A glomerulus of a patient who developed glomerulonephritis after a streptococcal infection contains many neutrophils (Masson trichrome stain).

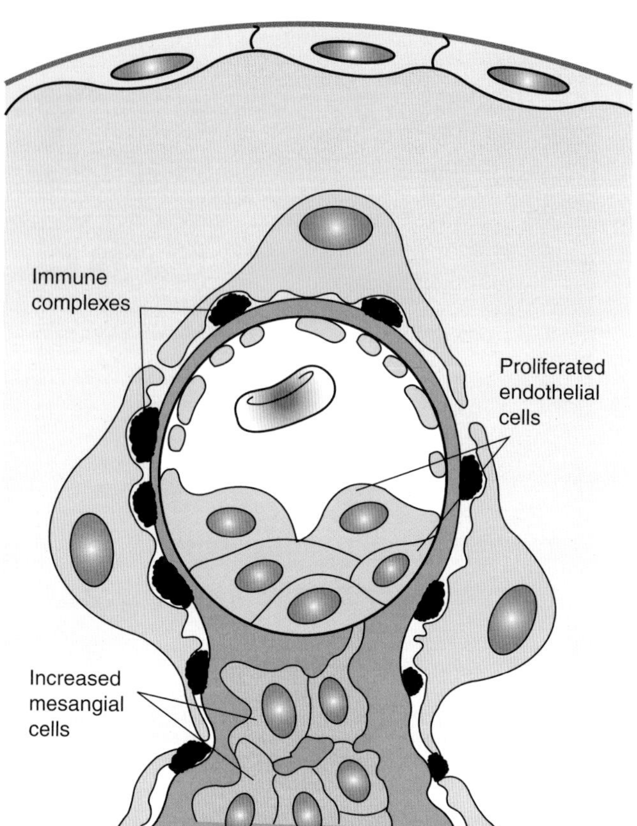

FIGURE 14-30. Postinfectious glomerulonephritis. Accumulation of numerous subepithelial immune complexes as hump-like structures is a characteristic feature. Less prominent subendothelial immune complexes are associated with endothelial cell proliferation and are related to increased capillary permeability and narrowing of the lumen. Frequently, proliferation of mesangial cells and a thickened mesangial matrix (BM) result in widening of the stalk and conspicuous trapping of immune complexes. BM, basement membrane.

During resolution, neutrophils and endothelial hypercellularity disappears first. Mesangial hypercellularity and matrix expansion remain, but all of these changes resolve completely in most patients after several months.

Ultrastructurally, acute postinfectious glomerulonephritis shows distinctive **subepithelial dense deposits** shaped like **"humps,"** which are on the epithelial side of the GBM (Figs. 14-30 and 14-31). These are invariably accompanied by mesangial and subendothelial deposits that are probably more important in pathogenesis, by virtue of their proximity to inflammatory mediator systems in the blood. Granular deposits of C3, with or without Ig, are observed by immunofluorescence in capillary walls, corresponding to the humps (Fig. 14-32).

CLINICAL FEATURES: Although declining in frequency, acute postinfectious glomerulonephritis is still one of the most common childhood renal diseases. Primary infection involves the pharynx (pharyngitis) or, especially in hot and humid environments, the skin (pyoderma). The nephritic syndrome begins abruptly with oliguria, hematuria, facial edema, and hypertension. Serum C3 levels

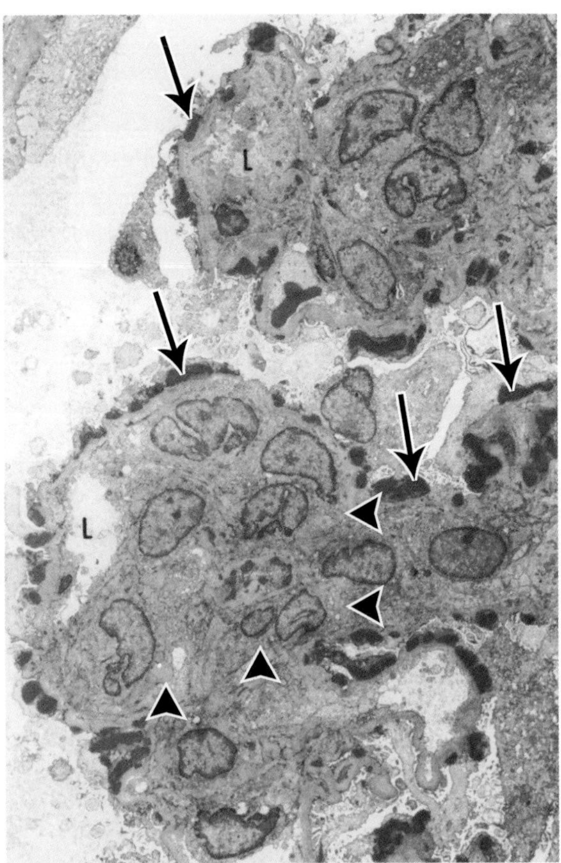

FIGURE 14-31. Acute postinfectious glomerulonephritis. An electron micrograph demonstrating numerous subepithelial humps (*arrows*) and mesangial hypercellularity (*arrowheads*). The capillary lumina (L) are markedly narrowed.

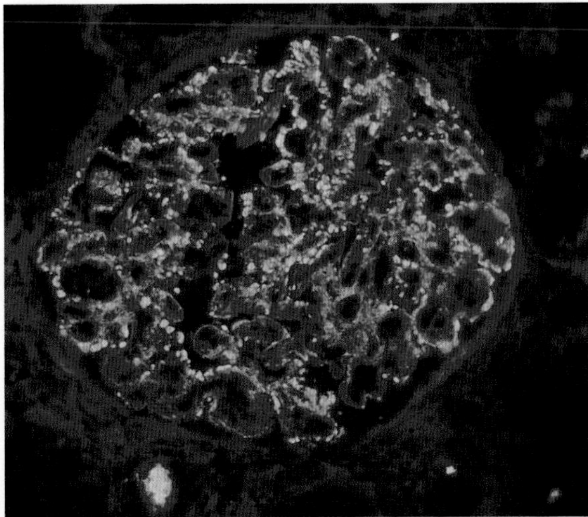

FIGURE 14-32. Acute postinfectious glomerulonephritis. An immunofluorescence micrograph demonstrating granular staining for C3 in capillary walls and the mesangium.

are lower during the acute syndrome but return to normal within 1 to 2 weeks. Overt nephritis resolves after several weeks, although hematuria and especially proteinuria may persist for several months. A few patients have an abnormal urinary sediment for years after the acute episode, and rare patients (particularly adults) develop progressive renal failure.

Lupus Glomerulonephritis

Nephritis is one of the most common complications of systemic lupus erythematosus (SLE) (see Chapter 3). Immune complexes in the mesangium cause less inflammation than subendothelial immune complexes. The latter are more exposed to cellular and humoral inflammatory mediators in blood and are, therefore, more likely to initiate inflammation. Subepithelial localization of immune complexes causes proteinuria but does not stimulate overt glomerular inflammation.

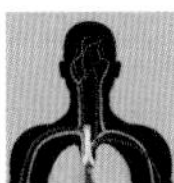

PATHOPHYSIOLOGY: Nephritogenic immune complexes may localize in glomeruli by deposition from the circulation or formation in situ or both. Circulating immune complexes containing high-avidity antibodies deposit in subendothelial and mesangial zones; low-affinity antibodies form immune complexes in situ in the subepithelial zone. Immune complexes formed in situ may involve antigens, such as double-stranded DNA and nucleosomes. These antigens accumulate on GBMs or in mesangial matrix through charge interactions. Glomerular immune complexes activate complement and initiate inflammation. Complement activation often causes hypocomplementemia. Immune complexes also localize in the renal interstitium, walls of interstitial vessels, and tubular basement membranes, where they may produce the tubulointerstitial inflammation.

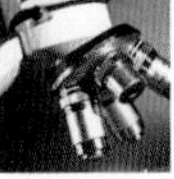

PATHOLOGY: The pathologic and clinical manifestations of lupus nephritis vary with the diverse patterns of immune complex accumulation in different patients (outlined in Table 14-7) and in the same patient over time (Fig. 14-33).

By immunofluorescence, subepithelial complexes are granular; subendothelial deposits may be granular or bandlike. The immune complexes often stain most intensely for IgG, but IgA and IgM are also almost always present; C3, C1q, and other complement components are typically observed. Granular staining along tubular basement membranes and interstitial vessels occurs in more than half of patients.

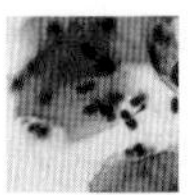

CLINICAL FEATURES: Renal disease develops in 70% of patients with SLE and is often the major cause of morbidity and mortality. The clinical manifestations and prognosis of renal dysfunction vary (Table 14-7), depending on the pathology of the underlying renal disease. ***Renal biopsy specimens from patients with lupus are used to assess disease category, activity, and chronicity.*** Class III and class IV lupus nephritis (Table 14-7) have the poorest prognosis and are treated most aggressively, usually with high doses of corticosteroids and immunosuppressive drugs. Fewer than 20% of patients with class IV disease reach ESRD within 5 years.

Immunoglobulin A Nephropathy

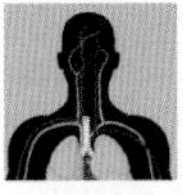

PATHOPHYSIOLOGY: Deposition of IgA1-dominant immune complexes is the cause of IgA nephropathy. IgA1, but not IgA2, has a hinge region that contains *O*-linked carbohydrates. Patients with IgA nephropathy have increased levels of IgA1 molecules that have fewer terminal galactose residues. The poorly O-galactosylated IgA1 provokes the production of IgG and

Table 14-7

Pathologic and Clinical Features of Lupus Nephritis

Location of Immune Lupus Nephritis Class	Location of Immune Clinical Complexes	Clinical Manifestations
I: Minimal mesangial	Mesangial	Mild hematuria and proteinuria
II: Mesangial proliferative	Mesangial	Mild hematuria and proteinuria
III: Focal	Mesangial and subendothelial	Moderate nephritis
IV: Diffuse	Mesangial and subendothelial	Severe nephritis
V: Membranous	Subepithelial and mesangial	Nephrotic syndrome
VI: Chronic sclerosing	Variable	Chronic renal failure

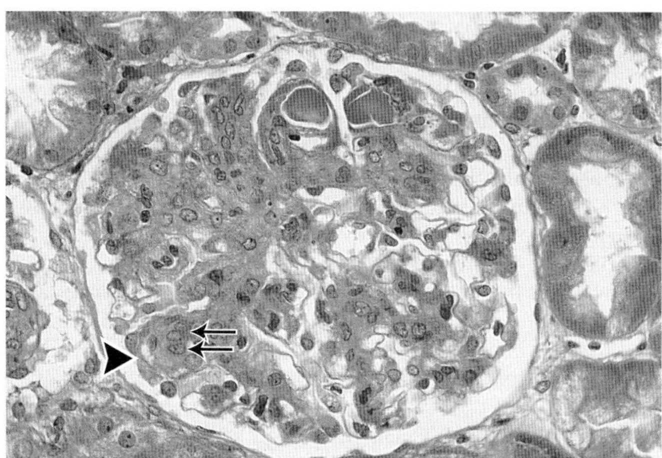

FIGURE 14-33. Proliferative lupus glomerulonephritis. Segmental endocapillary hypercellularity (*arrows*) and thickening of capillary walls (*arrowhead*) are present.

IgM autoantibodies, which react with the IgA1 hinge region. The reaction of the two results in circulating IgA1-containing immune complexes. Mesangial accumulation may entail several mechanisms. The poorly galactosylated IgA1 may be inefficiently cleared from the circulation and tend to aggregate, leading to mesangial trapping of both aggregates and immune complexes. IgA-containing immune complexes in the mesangium activate complement by the alternative pathway as demonstrated by the presence of C3 and properdin, but not C1q and C4. Mucosal exposure to viral, bacterial, or dietary antigens stimulates IgA-dominant immune responses. This circumstance may explain the propensity for ***respiratory or gastrointestinal infections to trigger exacerbations of IgA nephropathy.***

PATHOLOGY: Immunofluorescence microscopy is essential for the diagnosis of IgA nephropathy. Mesangial immunostaining for IgA is more intense than staining for IgG or IgM (Fig. 14-34). This is almost always accompanied by staining for C3. IgA deposited in the glomerular capillary wall (in addition to the mesangium) may be present in more severe cases and suggests a less favorable prognosis.

Depending on the severity and duration of the disease, a continuum of histologic findings is seen in IgA nephropathy, from (1) no discernible light microscopic changes to (2) focal or diffuse mesangial hypercellularity to (3) focal or diffuse proliferative glomerulonephritis (Fig. 14-35) to (4) chronic sclerosing glomerulonephritis. At the time of initial diagnosis of IgA nephropathy, focal proliferative glomerulonephritis is the most frequent manifestation. Crescents are not common, except in unusually severe cases.

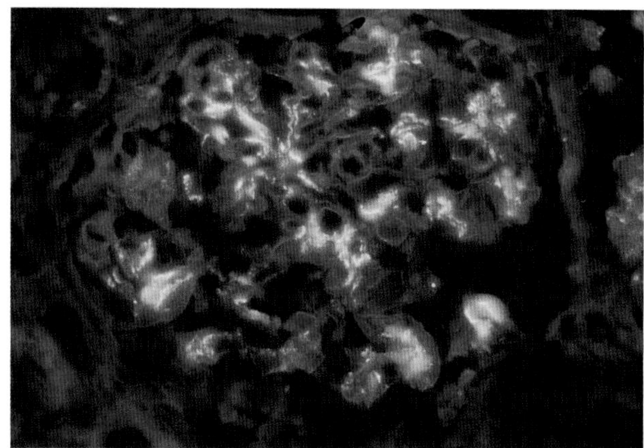

FIGURE 14-34. Immunoglobulin A (IgA) nephropathy. An immunofluorescence micrograph showing deposits of IgA in the mesangial areas.

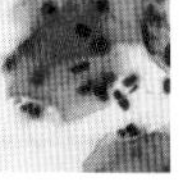

CLINICAL FEATURES: ***IgA nephropathy is the most common form of glomerulonephritis in developed countries.*** It accounts for 10% of cases in the United States, 20% in Europe, and 40% in Asia. IgA nephropathy is common in Native Americans and rare in blacks. It occurs most

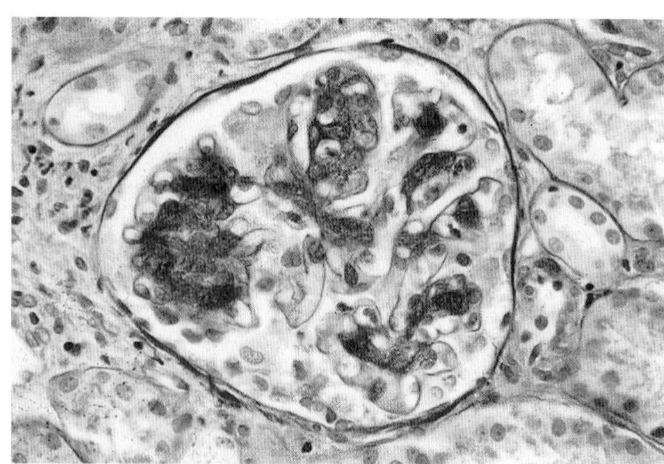

FIGURE 14-35. Immunoglobulin A nephropathy. Segmental mesangial hypercellularity and matrix expansion caused by the mesangial immune deposits (periodic acid–Schiff stain).

often in young men, with a peak age of 15 to 30 years at diagnosis. Clinical presentations vary; 40% of patients have asymptomatic microscopic hematuria, 40% have intermittent gross hematuria, 10% have nephrotic syndrome, and 10% have renal failure. The disease rarely resolves completely but may follow an episodic course, with exacerbations often coinciding with upper respiratory tract infections. IgA nephropathy is slowly progressive, and 20% of patients reaching end-stage renal failure after 10 years.

Hereditary Nephritis (Alport Syndrome)

Hereditary nephritis is a proliferative and sclerosing glomerular disease, often accompanied by defects of the ears or the eyes. It results from mutations in type IV collagen. In Alport syndrome, a hereditary hearing deficit accompanies nephritis.

MOLECULAR PATHOGENESIS: Several genetic mutations are responsible for the molecular defects in the GBM that lead to the renal lesions of hereditary nephritis. The most common, accounting for 85% of hereditary nephritis, is X linked and is caused by a mutation in the gene for the α5 chain of type IV collagen (*COL4A5*). An autosomal recessive form of hereditary nephritis is caused by mutations in *COL4A3* and *COL4A4*. Patients with hereditary nephritis who have renal transplants are at risk for developing antibodies to allograft GBMs.

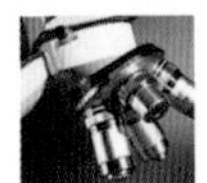

PATHOLOGY: Early glomerular lesions of hereditary nephritis show mild mesangial hypercellularity and matrix expansion. Renal disease progression is associated with increasing focal and eventually diffuse glomerular sclerosis. Tubular atrophy, interstitial fibrosis, and foam cells in tubules and interstitium accompany advanced glomerular lesions. Electron microscopy discloses an irregularly thickened GBM with splitting of the lamina densa into interlacing lamellae that surround electron-lucent areas (Fig. 14-36).

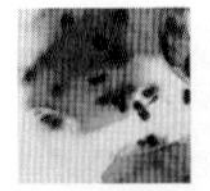

CLINICAL FEATURES: Hematuria develops early in boys with X-linked hereditary nephritis. Proteinuria and progressive renal failure usually follow in the second to fourth decades of life. In females, the X-linked disease is generally milder, with the rate of progression varying substantially.

Thin Glomerular Basement Membrane Nephropathy

This hereditary condition, also called **benign familial hematuria**, often presents as asymptomatic microscopic hematuria, with occasional intermittent gross hematuria. This disease and IgA nephropathy are common diagnostic considerations in patients with asymptomatic glomerular hematuria. Patients with thin basement membrane nephropathy usually do not develop renal failure or substantial proteinuria. By light microscopy, glomeruli are unremarkable. Electron microscopy shows reduced thickness of the GBM (150 to 300 nm; normal is 350 to 450 nm). The most common mode of inheritance is autosomal dominant. Heterozygous mutations in *COL4A3* and *COL4A4* genes lead to thin basement membrane disease, and homozygous ones give rise to Alport syndrome.

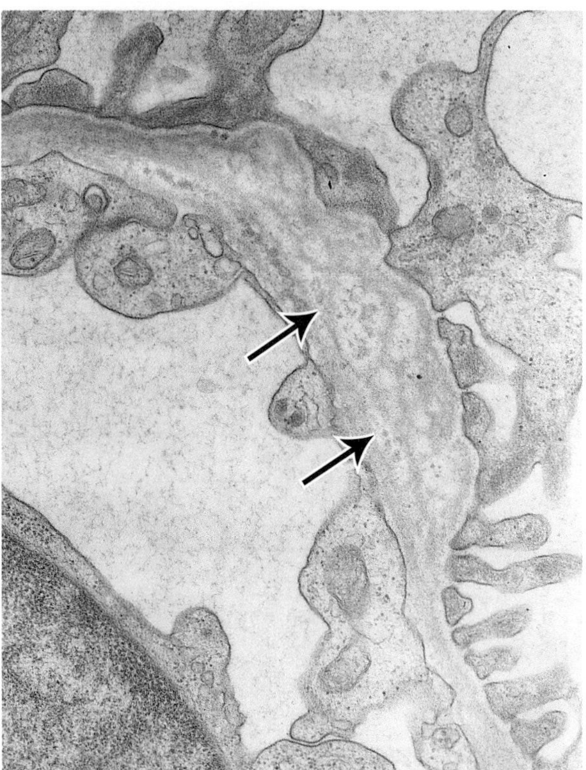

FIGURE 14-36. Hereditary nephritis (Alport syndrome). The lamina densa of the glomerular basement membrane is laminated (*arrows*) rather than forming a single dense band (compare this electron micrograph with Fig. 14-5).

AGGRESSIVE GLOMERULONEPHRITIS

Anti–Glomerular Basement Membrane Glomerulonephritis

Anti-GBM antibody disease is an uncommon but aggressive glomerulonephritis that may only affect the kidneys. It may also be combined with pulmonary hemorrhage, in which case it is **Goodpasture syndrome**.

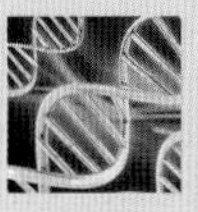

MOLECULAR PATHOGENESIS: ***Anti-GBM glomerulonephritis is mediated by an autoimmune response to type IV collagen in the GBM.*** The specific epitope is in the globular noncollagenous domain of the α3 chain of type IV collagen. Because the target antigen is also expressed on pulmonary alveolar capillary basement membranes, half of patients also have pulmonary hemorrhages and hemoptysis, sometimes severe enough to be life-threatening (Fig. 14-37). Anti-GBM antibodies or anti-GBM T cells or both may mediate the injury. The antibodies bind the autoantigens in situ, initiating acute inflammation by activating mediator systems, such as complement. Genetic susceptibility to anti-GBM disease is strongly associated with HLA-DRB1. Disease onset often follows viral upper respiratory tract infections, and pulmonary involvement appears to require synergistic injurious agents, such as cigarette smoke.

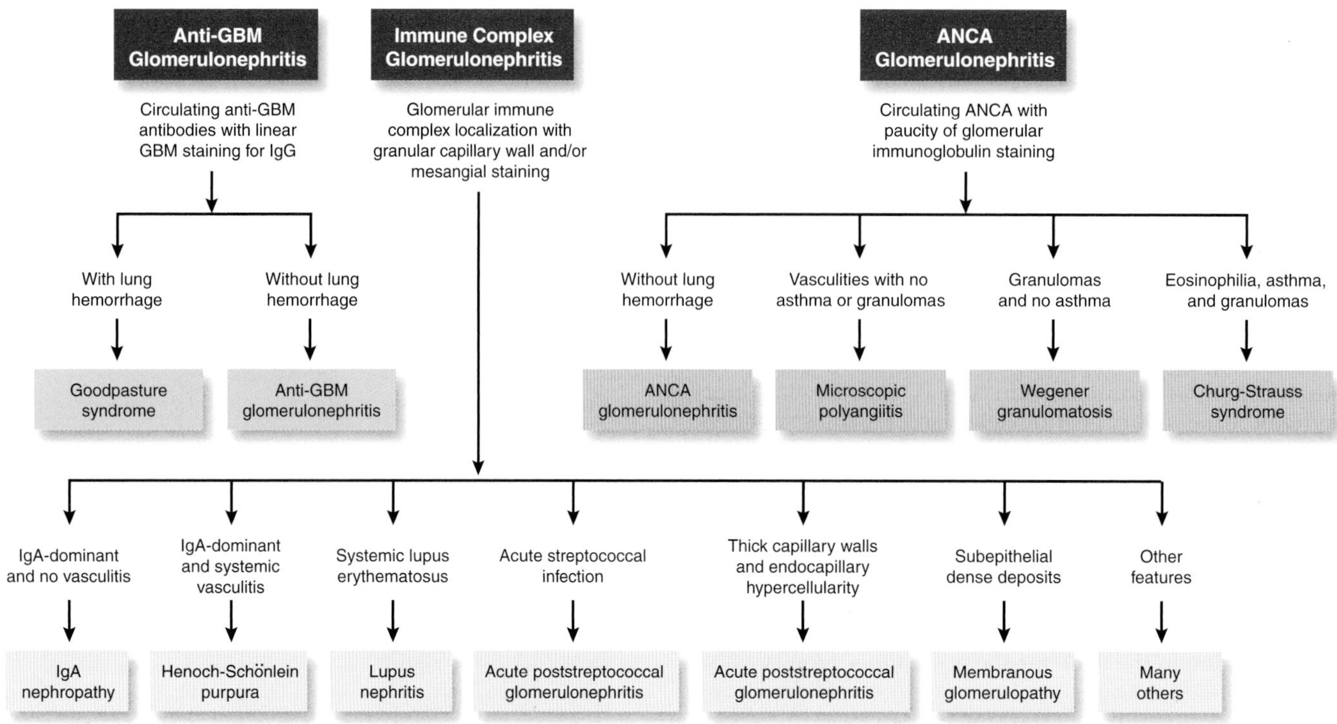

FIGURE 14-37. Algorithm demonstrating the integration of pathologic findings with clinical data to diagnose specific forms of primary or secondary glomerulonephritis. Note that an important initial categorization is as immune complex, anti–glomerular basement membrane (GBM), C3, or antineutrophil cytoplasmic autoantibody (ANCA) glomerulonephritis. Once this determination is made, more specific diagnoses depend on additional clinical or pathologic observations. Ig, immunoglobulin.

PATHOLOGY: *The pathologic hallmark of anti-GBM glomerulonephritis is diffuse linear GBM immunostaining for IgG, indicating autoantibodies bound to the basement membrane* (Fig. 14-38). This finding is not, however, entirely specific. More than 90% of patients with anti-GBM glomerulonephritis have glomerular crescents (**crescentic glomerulonephritis**) (Figs. 14-39 and 14-40), usually involving more than 50% of glomeruli. Focal glomerular fibrinoid necrosis is common. Involved lungs have marked intra-alveolar hemorrhage. By electron microscopy, GBMs show focal breaks, but no immune complex–type electron-dense deposits.

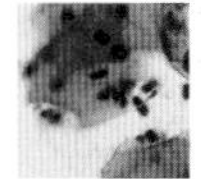

CLINICAL FEATURES: Anti-GBM glomerulonephritis typically presents with rapidly progressive renal failure and nephritic signs and symptoms. ***It accounts for 10% to 20% of rapidly progressive (crescentic) glomerulonephritis*** (Fig. 14-37; Table 14-8). Anti-GBM antibodies are detectable in 90% of patients. Treatment consists of high-dose immunosuppressive therapy and plasma exchange, which are most effective at an early stage of the disease. If ESRD develops, renal transplantation is successful with little risk of losing the allograft to recurrent glomerulonephritis if transplantation is done after anti-GBM antibodies have disappeared.

Antineutrophil Cytoplasmic Autoantibody Glomerulonephritis

ANCA glomerulonephritis is characterized by glomerular necrosis and crescents.

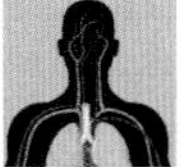

PATHOPHYSIOLOGY: ANCA glomerulonephritis patients show no evidence of glomerular deposition of anti-GBM antibodies or immune complexes. The discovery that 90% of patients with this pattern of glomerular injury have circulating ANCAs led to the demonstration that these autoantibodies cause the disease.

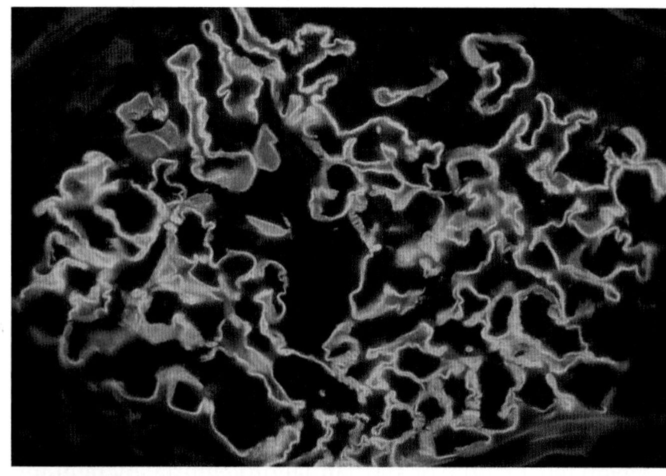

FIGURE 14-38. Anti–glomerular basement membrane (GBM) glomerulonephritis. Linear immunofluorescence for immunoglobulin G is seen along the GBM. Contrast this linear pattern of staining with the granular pattern of immunofluorescence typical for most types of immune complex deposition within capillary walls (see Fig. 14-32).

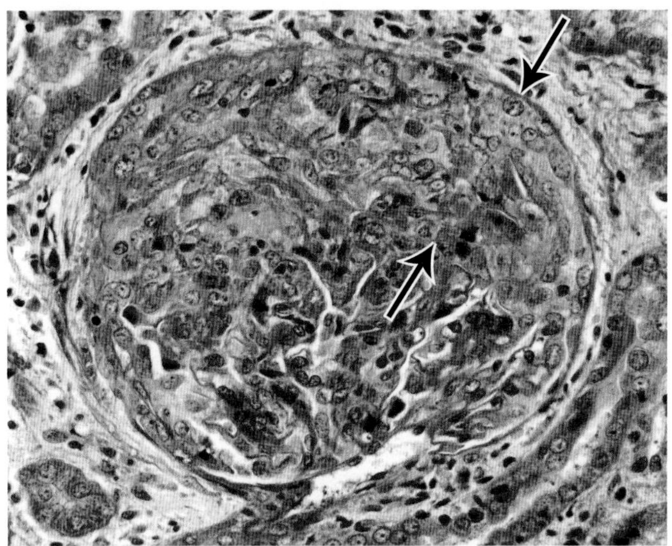

FIGURE 14-39. Crescentic anti–glomerular basement membrane glomerulonephritis. The Bowman space is filled by a cellular crescent (*between arrows*). The injured glomerular tuft is at the bottom (Masson trichrome stain).

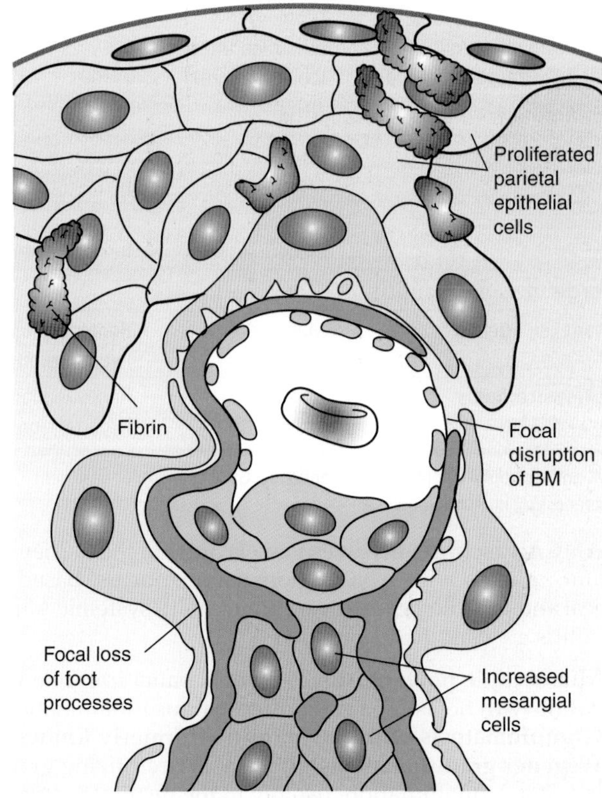

FIGURE 14-40. Crescentic (rapidly progressive) glomerulonephritis. A variety of pathogenic mechanisms cause crescent formation by disrupting glomerular capillary walls. This allows plasma constituents into the Bowman space, including coagulation factors and inflammatory mediators. Fibrin forms, and there is proliferation of parietal epithelial cells and influx of macrophages (not shown), resulting in crescent formation. BM, basement membrane.

Table 14-8

Frequency (%) of Immunopathologic Categories of Crescentic Glomerulonephritis in Different Age Groups

Category	Age (years) <20	20–64	>65
Anti–glomerular basement membrane	10	10	10
Immune complex	55	40	10
Antineutrophil cytoplasmic autoantibody	30	45	75
No evidence for the three categories above	5	5	5

Glomerulonephritis with crescents in more than 50% of glomeruli.

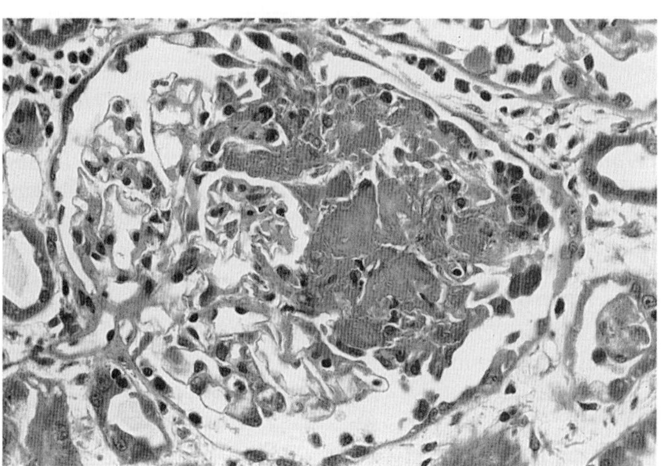

FIGURE 14-41. Antineutrophil cytoplasmic autoantibody glomerulonephritis. Segmental fibrinoid necrosis is illustrated. In time, this lesion stimulates crescent formation.

ANCAs are specific for cytoplasmic proteins in neutrophils and monocytes, usually myeloperoxidase (MPO-ANCA) or proteinase 3 (PR3-ANCA). These autoantibodies activate neutrophils to adhere to endothelial cells, release toxic oxygen metabolites, degranulate, and kill endothelial cells. Neutrophils activated by ANCAs also activate the alternative complement pathway, which further amplifies the inflammation.

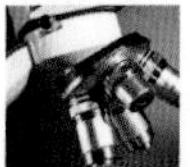

PATHOLOGY: More than 90% of patients with ANCA glomerulonephritis have glomerular necrosis (Fig. 14-41) and crescent formation (Fig. 14-42), often in more than half of glomeruli. There is little or no Ig or complement deposition, which distinguishes ANCA glomerulonephritis from anti-GBM and immune complex glomerulonephritis.

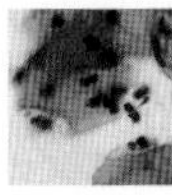

CLINICAL FEATURES: ANCA glomerulonephritis most commonly presents with rapidly progressive renal failure, with nephritic signs and symptoms. The disease accounts for 75% of rapidly progressive (crescentic) glomerulonephritis in patients older than 60 years,

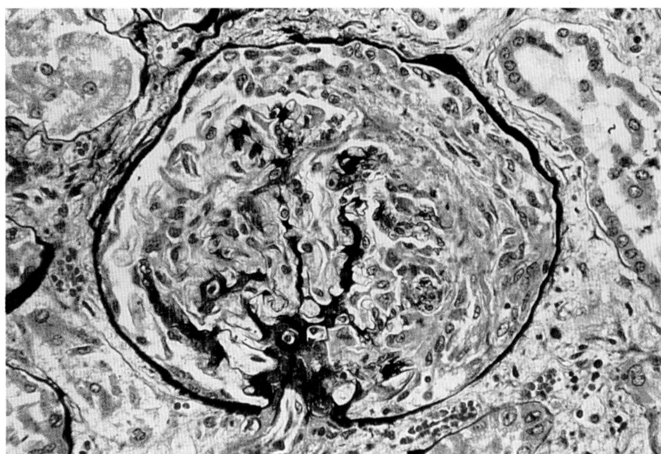

FIGURE 14-42. Antineutrophil cytoplasmic autoantibody glomerulonephritis. Silver staining showing focal disruption of glomerular basement membranes and crescent formation within the Bowman space.

45% in middle-aged adults, and 30% in young adults and children (Table 14-8). *In three fourths of patients with ANCA glomerulonephritis, systemic small vessel vasculitis is present (see below), which has many systemic manifestations, including pulmonary hemorrhage.* ANCA glomerulonephritis with pulmonary vasculitis causes **pulmonary–renal vasculitic syndrome** much more often than does Goodpasture syndrome. More than 80% of untreated patients with ANCA glomerulonephritis develop ESRD within 5 years. Immunosuppressive therapy reduces this to less than 20%. Once remission is induced with high-dose immunosuppression, patients are at risk for recurrent disease. The disease recurs in 15% of renal transplant recipients.

VASCULAR DISEASES

Renal Vasculitis

Many types of systemic vasculitis affect the kidney (Table 14-9). *In a sense, glomerulonephritis is a local form of vasculitis that involves glomerular capillaries.* Glomeruli may be the only site of vascular inflammation, or the renal disease may be a component of a systemic vasculitis (for additional details, see also Chapter 8).

Small Vessel Vasculitides

Small vessel vasculitis affects small arteries, arterioles, capillaries, and venules. Involvement of any of these can lead to glomerulonephritis. Other common manifestations include purpura, arthralgias, myalgias, peripheral neuropathy, and pulmonary hemorrhage. Immune complexes, anti–basement membrane antibodies, or ANCAs (Table 14-9) can cause small vessel vasculitides.

IgA vasculitis (Henoch–Schönlein purpura) is the most common childhood vasculitis. It is caused by vascular localization of immune complexes containing mostly IgA. The glomerular lesion is identical to that of IgA nephropathy.

Cryoglobulinemic vasculitis leads to proliferative glomerulonephritis, usually type I MPGN. By light microscopy, aggregates of cryoglobulins ("hyaline thrombi") are often seen within capillary lumens (see Chapter 18).

Table 14-9

Types of Vasculitis That Involve the Kidneys

Type of Vasculitis	Major Target Vessels in Kidney	Major Renal Manifestations
Small vessel vasculitis		
Immune complex vasculitis		
IgA vasculitis (Henoch–Schönlein purpura)	Glomeruli	Nephritis
Cryoglobulinemic vasculitis	Glomeruli	Nephritis
Anti-GBM vasculitis		
Goodpasture syndrome	Glomeruli	Nephritis
ANCA vasculitis		
Granulomatosis with polyangiitis (Wegener granulomatosis)	Glomeruli, arterioles, interlobular arteries	Nephritis
Microscopic polyangiitis	Glomeruli, arterioles, interlobular arteries	Nephritis
Eosinophilic granulomatosis with polyangiitis (Churg–Strauss syndrome)	Glomeruli, arterioles, interlobular arteries	Nephritis
Medium-sized vessel vasculitis		
Polyarteritis nodosa	Interlobar and arcuate arteries	Infarcts and hemorrhage
Kawasaki disease	Interlobar and arcuate arteries	Infarcts and hemorrhage
Large vessel vasculitis		
Giant cell arteritis	Main renal artery	Renovascular hypertension
Takayasu arteritis	Main renal artery	Renovascular hypertension

ANCA, antineutrophil cytoplasmic autoantibody; GBM, glomerular basement membrane; IgA, immunoglobulin A.

ANCA vasculitis involves vessels outside the kidneys in 75% of patients with ANCA glomerulonephritis. Based on clinical and pathologic features, patients with systemic ANCA vasculitis are classified as follows:

- **Microscopic polyangiitis**, if there is pauci-immune vasculitis with no asthma or granulomatous inflammation
- **Granulomatosis with polyangiitis (formerly known as Wegener granulomatosis)**, if there is necrotizing granulomatous inflammation, usually in the respiratory tract
- **Eosinophilic granulomatosis with polyangiitis (formerly known as Churg–Strauss syndrome)**, if there is eosinophilia and asthma

In addition to resulting in necrotizing and crescentic glomerulonephritis, ANCA vasculitides often entail necrotizing inflammation in other renal vessels, such as arteries, arterioles, and medullary peritubular capillaries.

Medium-Sized Vessel Vasculitis

Medium-sized vessel vasculitides affect arteries, but not arterioles, capillaries, or venules (see Chapter 8). The necrotizing arteritides, such as **polyarteritis nodosa**, which occurs mainly in adults, and **Kawasaki disease**, which principally afflicts young children, rarely cause renal dysfunction. However, they may involve renal arteries and result in pseudoaneurysm formation and renal thrombosis, infarction, and hemorrhage.

Large Vessel Vasculitis

Large vessel vasculitides, such as **giant cell arteritis** and **Takayasu arteritis**, affect the aorta and its major branches. These disorders may cause renovascular hypertension by involving the main renal arteries or the aorta at the origin of the renal arteries. Narrowing or obstruction of these vessels results in renal ischemia, which stimulates increased renin production and consequent hypertension (Table 14-9).

Hypertensive Nephrosclerosis

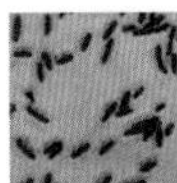

ETIOLOGIC FACTORS: Sustained systolic pressures greater than 140 mm Hg and diastolic pressures higher than 90 mm Hg define hypertension (see Chapter 8). Mild-to-moderate hypertension results in typical hypertensive nephrosclerosis. In fact, hypertensive nephrosclerosis is identified in about 15% of patients with the so-called "benign hypertension."

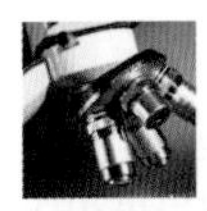

PATHOLOGY: The kidneys are atrophic and are usually affected bilaterally. Renal cortical surfaces are finely granular (Fig. 14-43), but coarser scars are occasionally present. On cut section, the cortex is thinned. Many glomeruli appear normal; others show varying degrees of ischemic change. Cells of the glomerular tuft are progressively lost, and collagen and matrix material are deposited within the Bowman space. Eventually, glomerular tufts are obliterated by a dense, eosinophilic globular scar, all inside the Bowman capsule. Tubular atrophy, owing to glomerular loss, is associated with interstitial fibrosis and chronic inflammation. Globally, sclerotic glomeruli and surrounding atrophic tubules are often clustered in focal subcapsular zones, with adjacent areas of preserved glomeruli and tubules (Fig. 14-44), which account for the granular surfaces of nephrosclerotic kidneys.

The pattern of change in renal blood vessels depends on vessel size. Intimas of arteries as small as arcuate arteries have fibrotic thickening, replication of the elastica-like lamina, and partial replacement of the muscularis with fibrous tissue. Interlobular arteries and arterioles may develop medial hyperplasia. Arterioles show concentric hyaline thickening of the wall, often with loss of smooth muscle cells or displacement to the periphery. This arteriolar change is termed **hyaline arteriolosclerosis**.

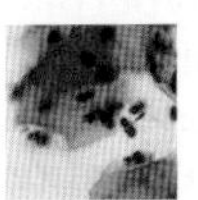

CLINICAL FEATURES: Although hypertensive nephrosclerosis does not usually impair renal function, some people with hypertension develop progressive renal failure, which may lead to ESRD. Because hypertension is so common, the relatively small percentage of hypertensive patients who develop renal insufficiency amounts to one third of patients with ESRD. ***Hypertensive nephrosclerosis is most prevalent and aggressive in blacks, among whom hypertension is the leading cause of ESRD.***

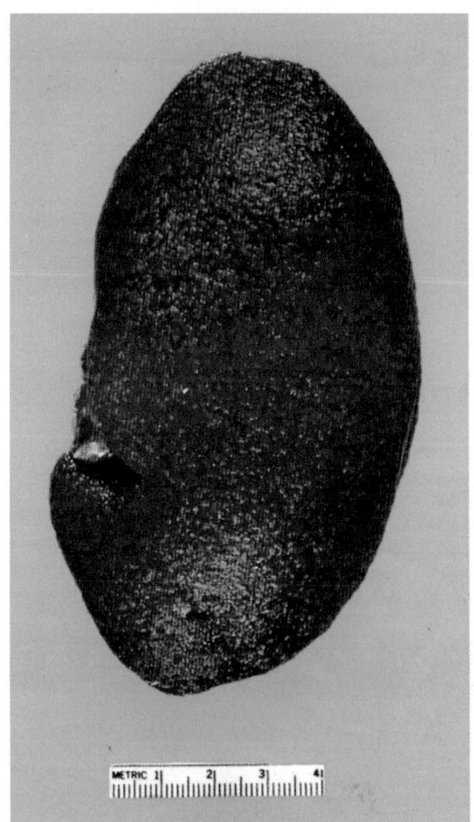

FIGURE 14-43. Hypertensive nephrosclerosis. The kidney is reduced in size, and the cortical surface exhibits fine granularity.

Malignant Hypertensive Nephropathy

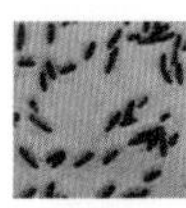

ETIOLOGIC FACTORS: No specific blood pressure defines malignant hypertension, but diastolic pressures greater than 130 mm Hg, retinal vascular changes papilledema (see Chapter 8), and renal functional impairment are usual criteria. There are prior histories of benign hypertension in half of patients, and many others have a background of chronic renal injury caused by many different diseases. Occasionally, malignant hypertension arises de novo in apparently healthy people, particularly young black men. The pathogenesis of the vascular injury may be explained by very high blood pressure, combined with microvascular vasoconstriction, causing endothelial injury as blood slams into narrowed small vessels. At such sites, plasma constituents leak into injured arteriolar walls (causing fibrinoid necrosis), into arterial intimas (edematous intimal thickening), and into the subendothelial zone of glomerular capillaries (consolidating glomeruli). At these sites of vascular injury, thrombosis can result in focal renal cortical necrosis (infarcts).

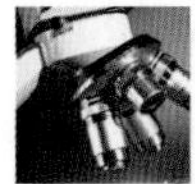

PATHOLOGY: Renal sizes in malignant hypertensive nephropathy vary from small to enlarged, depending on the duration of preexisting benign hypertension. The cut surface is mottled red and yellow, with occasional small cortical infarcts. Malignant hypertensive

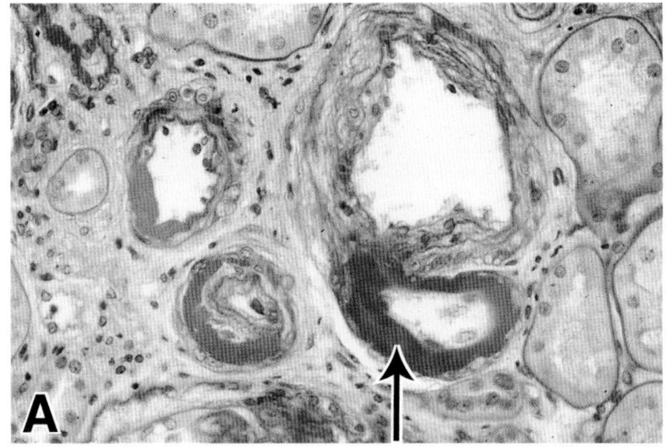

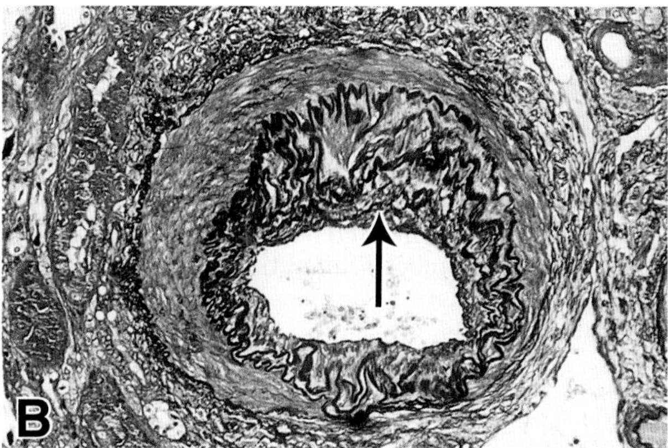

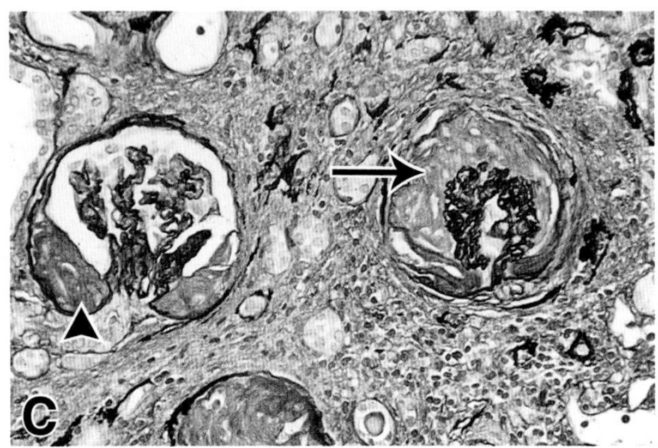

FIGURE 14-44. Hypertensive nephrosclerosis. A. Three arterioles with hyaline sclerosis (*arrow*) (periodic acid–Schiff stain). B. Arcuate artery with fibrotic intimal thickening causing narrowing of the lumen (*arrow*) (silver stain). C. One glomerulus with global sclerosis (*arrow*) and one with segmental sclerosis (*arrowhead*). Note also tubular atrophy, interstitial fibrosis, and chronic inflammation (silver stain).

nephropathy is often superimposed on hypertensive nephrosclerosis, with edematous (myxoid, mucoid) intimal expansion in arteries and fibrinoid necrosis of arterioles. Glomerular changes vary from capillary congestion to consolidation to necrosis (Fig. 14-45). Severe cases show thrombosis and focal ischemic cortical necrosis (infarction). These changes are identical to those seen in other forms of thrombotic microangiopathy (see below).

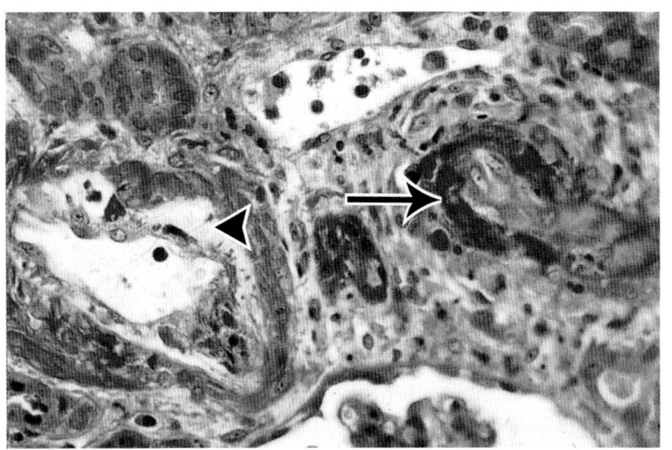

FIGURE 14-45. Malignant hypertensive nephropathy. Red fibrinoid necrosis (*arrow*) in the wall of the arteriole on the right and clear edematous expansion (*arrowhead*) in the intima of the interlobular artery on the left from a patient with malignant hypertension (Masson trichrome stain).

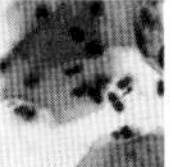

CLINICAL FEATURES: Malignant hypertension is more common in men than in women and typically occurs around the age of 40. Patients suffer headache, dizziness, and visual disturbances and may develop overt encephalopathy. Hematuria and proteinuria are frequent. Progressive renal deterioration develops if the condition persists. Aggressive antihypertensive therapy often controls the disease.

Renovascular Hypertension

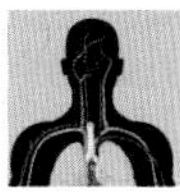

PATHOPHYSIOLOGY: Stenosis or total occlusion of a main renal artery produces hypertension that is potentially curable if the arterial lumen is restored. In patients with renal artery stenosis, hypertension reflects increased production of renin, angiotensin II, and aldosterone. Renal vein renin from an ischemic kidney is elevated, but it is normal in the contralateral kidney. Most (95%) cases are caused by atherosclerosis, which explains why this disorder is twice as common in men as in women, and mainly at older ages (average age, 55). Fibromuscular dysplasia and vasculitis are less common causes overall but are the most frequent etiology in children.

In **fibromuscular dysplasia**, the renal artery becomes fibrous and shows stenosis because of muscular hyperplasia. There are several patterns of renal artery involvement, namely, intimal fibroplasia, medial fibroplasia, perimedial fibroplasia, and periarterial fibroplasia. As the names imply, these disorders affect different layers of the artery, from the intima to the adventitia. Medial fibroplasia is the most common and accounts for two thirds of cases. This process creates areas of medial thickening alternating with areas of atrophy, producing a "string of beads" pattern in angiograms.

Hemolytic–Uremic Syndrome

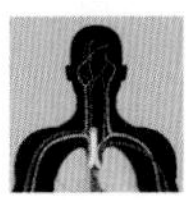

PATHOPHYSIOLOGY: HUS is a thrombotic microangiopathy. Endothelial damage allows plasma constituents to enter the intima of arteries walls of arterioles and the subendothelial zone of glomerular capillaries. As a result, narrowing of vessel lumens ischemia occurs. Passage of blood through vessels injured by HUS produces **microangiopathic hemolytic anemia (MAHA)** (see also Chapter 18). Thrombotic microangiopathies that resemble HUS and thrombotic thrombocytopenia (TTP) can also be caused by drugs, autoimmune diseases, and malignant hypertension (Table 14-10).

Typical postdiarrheal HUS features MAHA and acute renal failure, with little or no significant vascular disease outside the kidneys. ***Typical HUS is among the most common causes of acute renal failure in children.*** It is less common in adults. HUS occurs as isolated cases or in epidemics caused by food contaminated with enterohemorrhagic *Escherichia coli* (usually the O157:H7 strain).

Atypical HUS is unrelated to diarrhea and is caused by different mechanisms, including genetic abnormalities in complement regulatory proteins (mostly factor H but also factor I and membrane cofactor protein) or autoantibodies to complement regulatory proteins (anti–factor H) or both. Atypical HUS is more frequent in adults.

Table 14-10

Categories of Thrombotic Microangiopathy
Thrombotic thrombocytopenic purpura
Autoantibodies against ADAMTS13
Inherited deficiency in ADAMTS13
Typical hemolytic–uremic syndrome
E. coli
Shigella spp.
Pseudomonas spp.
Atypical hemolytic–uremic syndrome
Genetic mutation (e.g., factor H, factor I, membrane cofactor protein)
Autoantibodies to complement regulatory proteins (e.g., anti–factor H)
Drug-induced thrombotic microangiopathies
Mitomycin
Cisplatin
Cyclosporin
Tacrolimus
Anti-VEGF therapy
Autoimmune diseases
Systemic sclerosis (scleroderma)
Systemic lupus erythematosus
Antiphospholipid antibody syndrome
Malignant hypertension
Pregnancy and postpartum factors

VEGF, vascular endothelial growth factor.

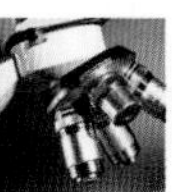

PATHOLOGY: The renal pathology of HUS is similar to that of malignant hypertensive nephropathy (see above), which is a form of thrombotic microangiopathy. The basic renal lesions are as follows:

- Arteriolar fibrinoid necrosis
- Arterial edematous intimal expansion
- Glomerular consolidation, necrosis, or congestion
- Vascular platelet-rich thrombosis

Electron microscopy of glomeruli shows electron-lucent expansion of the subendothelial zone (Figs. 14-46 and 14-47), owing to insudation of plasma proteins under injured endothelial cells. By fluorescence microscopy, fibrin and insudated plasma proteins are seen in injured vessel walls.

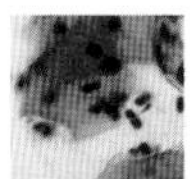

CLINICAL FEATURES: Patients with typical HUS present with hemorrhagic diarrhea and rapidly progressive renal failure. Even when dialysis is required, normal renal function usually returns within several weeks. However, impaired renal function may eventually reemerge after 15 to 25 years in more than half of patients. Atypical HUS is more frequent in adults and is not preceded by diarrhea. Its prognosis is worse than for typical HUS, often with multiple recurrences and more frequent progression to ESRD.

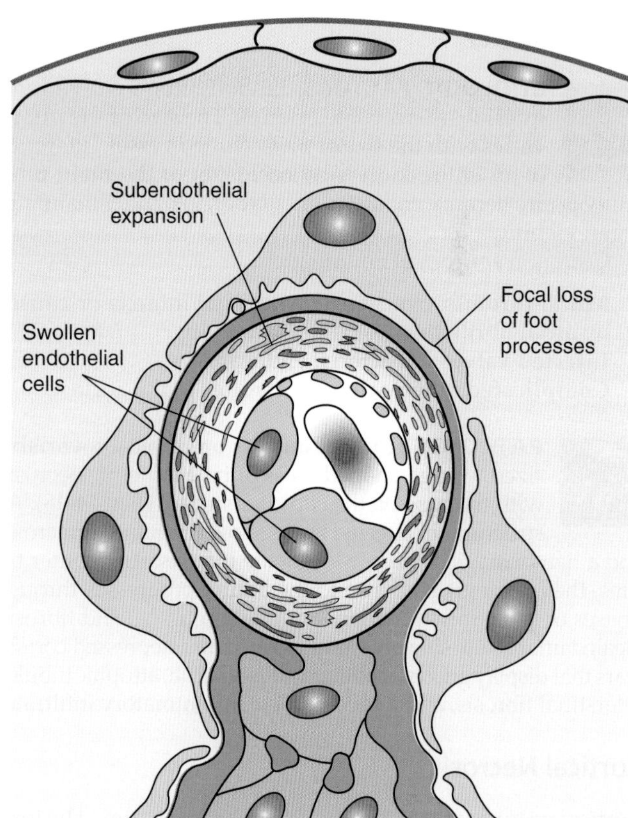

FIGURE 14-46. Hemolytic–uremic syndrome. A wide band of subendothelial expansion because of insudation of plasma proteins causes narrowing of the capillary lumen. Endothelial cell swelling also contributes to narrowing of the lumen.

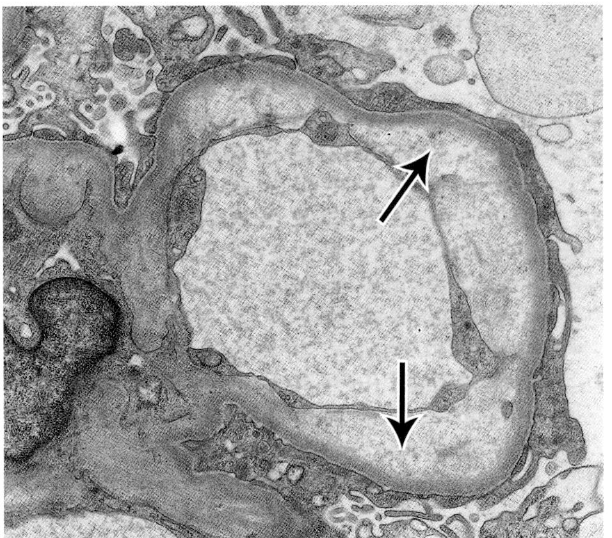

FIGURE 14-47. Thrombotic microangiopathy. An electron micrograph showing a wide band of lucent material in the subendothelial zone (*arrows*) corresponding to the subendothelial expansion, which causes marked narrowing of the lumen.

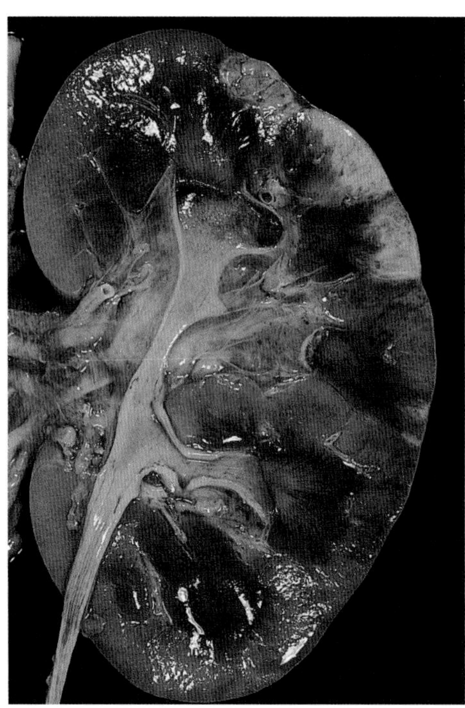

FIGURE 14-48. Renal infarcts. A bisected kidney showing three discrete areas of infarction characterized by marked pallor, which extends to the subcapsular surface.

Renal Infarcts

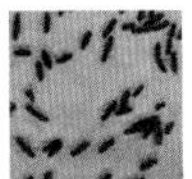

ETIOLOGIC FACTORS: Emboli often involve renal interlobar or arcuate arteries. The size of the infarct varies with the size of the occluded vessel. Infarction of an entire kidney by occlusion of the main renal artery is rare because collateral circulation generally maintains organ viability.

Common sources of emboli include:

- **Mural thrombi** overlying myocardial infarcts or caused by atrial fibrillation
- **Infected valves** in bacterial endocarditis
- **Complicated atherosclerotic plaques** in the aorta

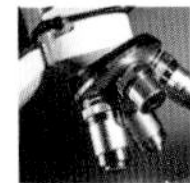

PATHOLOGY: Renal infarcts are typically variably sized, wedge-shaped areas of pale ischemic necrosis, with the base on the capsular surface (Fig. 14-48). All structures in affected zones show coagulative necrosis, and a hemorrhagic zone borders acute infarcts. As in other tissues, the histologic response to the infarct progresses through phases of acute inflammation, granulation tissue, and fibrosis. Healed infarcts are sharply circumscribed and depressed cortical scars that display ghosts of obliterated glomeruli, atrophic tubules, interstitial fibrosis, and a mild chronic inflammatory infiltrate.

Cortical Necrosis

Cortical necrosis affects all or part of the renal cortex. The term **infarct** applies if there is one area (or a few areas) of necrosis caused by arterial occlusion, but **cortical necrosis** implies more widespread ischemic necrosis.

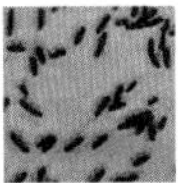

ETIOLOGIC FACTORS: Renal cortical necrosis can complicate any condition associated with hypovolemic or endotoxic shock, the classic situation being premature placental separation late in pregnancy (see Chapter 16).

The arterial blood to the medulla arises proximal to vessels supplying the outer cortex. Thus, occlusion of outer cortical vessels (e.g., by vasospasm, thrombi, or thrombotic microangiopathy) leads to cortical necrosis and spares the medulla.

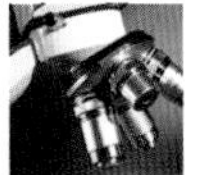

PATHOLOGY: Cortical necrosis varies from patchy to confluent (Fig. 14-49). In the most severely involved areas, all parenchymal elements exhibit coagulative necrosis. The proximal convoluted tubules are invariably necrotic, as are most of the distal tubules. In adjacent viable portions of the cortex, glomeruli and distal convoluted tubules are usually unaffected, but many proximal convoluted tubules may show ischemic injury, such as epithelial flattening or necrosis.

In the presence of extensive necrosis, the cortex is pale and diffusely necrotic, except for thin rims of viable tissue just beneath the capsule and at the corticomedullary junction. These are supplied by capsular and medullary collateral blood vessels, respectively.

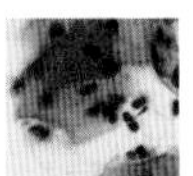

CLINICAL FEATURES: Severe cortical necrosis manifests as acute renal failure, which initially may be indistinguishable from that produced by acute tubular necrosis (ATN). Recovery is determined by the extent of the disease, but hypertension is common among survivors.

DISEASES OF TUBULES AND INTERSTITIUM

Acute kidney injury (AKI) produces a rapid rise in serum creatinine. It is classified as (1) **prerenal,** if caused by reduced

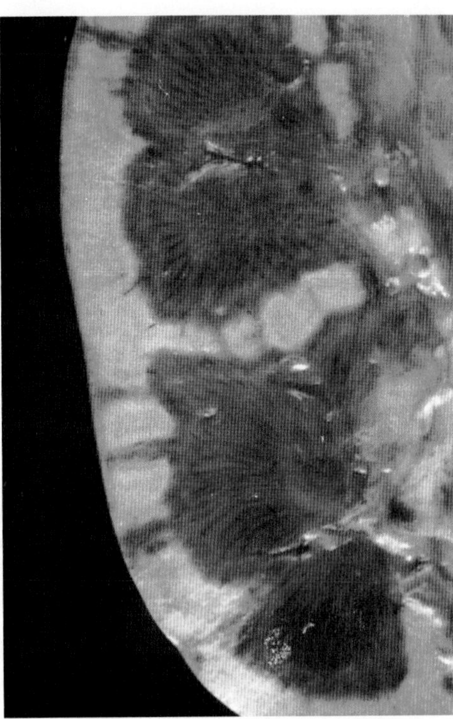

FIGURE 14-49. Renal cortical necrosis. The cortex of the kidney is pale yellow and soft owing to diffuse cortical necrosis.

Table 14-11

Causes of Acute Tubular Injury

Causes of Acute Tubular Injury
Ischemic prerenal acute renal failure or ischemic acute kidney injury
Massive hemorrhage
Septic shock
Severe burns
Dehydration
Prolonged diarrhea
Congestive heart failure
Volume redistribution (e.g., pancreatitis, peritonitis)
Nephrotoxin acute tubular injury
Antibiotics (e.g., aminoglycosides, amphotericin B)
Radiographic contrast agents
Heavy metals (e.g., mercury, lead, cisplatin)
Organic solvents (e.g., ethylene glycol, carbon tetrachloride)
Poisons (e.g., paraquat)
Heme protein cast nephropathies
Myoglobin (from rhabdomyolysis, e.g., with crush injury)
Hemoglobin (from hemolysis, e.g., with transfusion reaction)

blood flow to the kidneys; (2) **intrarenal,** if due to injury to the renal parenchyma; and (3) **postrenal,** if brought about by urinary tract obstruction. Intrarenal AKI is further categorized by the portion of the kidney that is mainly injured. These include **glomeruli**, **blood vessels**, **tubules** (e.g., ischemic acute tubular injury), or **interstitium** (acute tubulointerstitial nephritis). ***The most common cause for intrarenal AKI is ischemic acute tubular injury.***

Acute Tubular Injury

Ischemic AKI is severe, but potentially reversible, renal failure as a result of impaired tubular function caused by ischemia or toxic injury. ***If ischemia is severe enough to cause histologic tubular epithelial injury, it is considered intrarenal ischemic AKI.*** Extensive ischemia can result in overt necrosis of tubular epithelium, termed **acute tubular necrosis** (ATN).

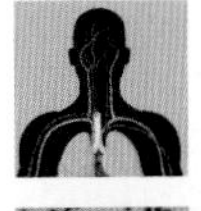

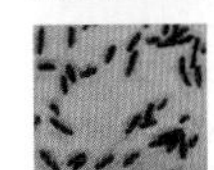

PATHOPHYSIOLOGY AND ETIOLOGIC FACTORS: Table 14-11 lists some causes of AKI due to acute tubular injury. The pathophysiology of ischemic AKI involves decreased glomerular filtration and tubular malfunction.

Ischemic acute tubular injury results from reduced renal perfusion, usually associated with hypotension. Tubular epithelial cells have a high metabolic rate and thus are particularly sensitive to oxygen deprivation, which rapidly depletes intracellular ATP. The kidneys are swollen, with a pale cortex and a congested medulla. Glomeruli and blood vessels are normal. Tubular injury is focal and is most pronounced in the proximal tubules and thick ascending limb of the loop of Henle, located in the outer medulla. The most frequent histologic abnormality is flattening (simplification) of tubular epithelial cells owing to sloughing of the apical cytoplasm into the urine. This process generates granular brown pigmented casts that can be detected by urinalysis. Widespread necrosis of tubular epithelial cells is uncommon, but simplification may be evident. By contrast, "necrosis" is subtle and appears as individual necrotic cells in some proximal or distal tubules. These single necrotic cells, plus a few viable cells, are shed into the tubular lumen, thereby focally denuding the tubular basement membrane (Fig. 14-50).

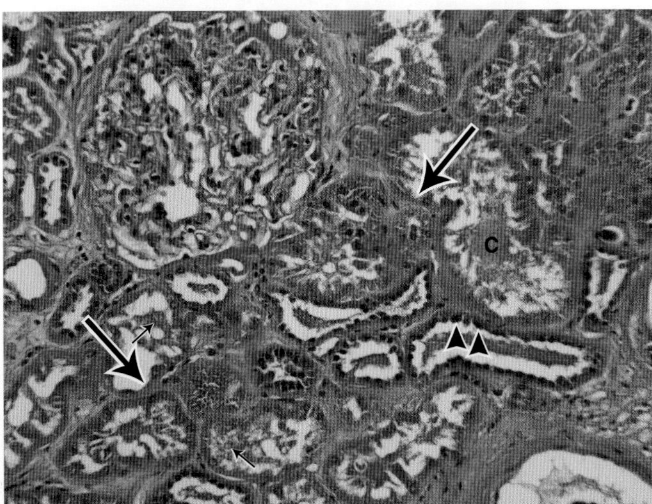

FIGURE 14-50. Ischemic acute tubular injury (ischemic acute kidney injury). Necrosis of individual tubular epithelial cells is evident both from focal denudation of the tubular basement membrane (*thick arrows*) and from the individual necrotic epithelial cells (*thin arrows*) present in some tubular lumina. Casts, the debris of dead tubular epithelium, fill many tubules (*C*). Some enlarged, regenerative-appearing epithelial cells are also present (*arrowheads*). Note the lack of significant glomerular or interstitial inflammation.

Nephrotoxic acute tubular injury is the term for chemical injury to epithelial cells. In addition to their sensitivity to ischemia, the metabolic needs of tubular epithelial cells make them susceptible to injury by toxins that perturb oxidative or other energy-producing pathways. At the same time, these cells absorb and concentrate toxins. Hemoglobin and myoglobin act as endogenous toxins that can induce acute tubular injury **(pigment nephropathy)** if they are present at high concentrations in the urine. Widespread necrosis of tubular epithelial cells is uncommon and appears as individual necrotic cells in some proximal or distal tubules. These single necrotic cells, plus a few viable cells, are shed into the tubular lumen, thus focally denuding the tubular basement membrane (Fig. 14-51).

Toxic acute tubular injury shows more extensive epithelial necrosis than is typical for ischemic injury (compare Figs. 14-50 and 14-51). However, toxic necrosis is largely limited to those tubular segments that are most sensitive to a particular toxin, usually the proximal tubule. In acute tubular injury caused by hemoglobinuria or myoglobinuria, many red-brown tubular casts are colored by heme pigments.

During the recovery phase of acute tubular injury, tubular epithelium regenerates, with mitoses, increased size of cells and nuclei, and cell crowding. Survivors eventually display complete restoration of normal renal architecture.

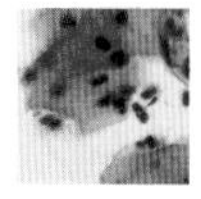

CLINICAL FEATURES: ***Ischemia is the leading cause of AKI.*** Rapidly rising serum creatinine, usually with decreased urine output (**oliguria**), is characteristic. Urinalysis shows degenerating epithelial cells and **"dirty brown" granular casts** (acute renal failure casts) with cell debris rich in cytochrome pigments.

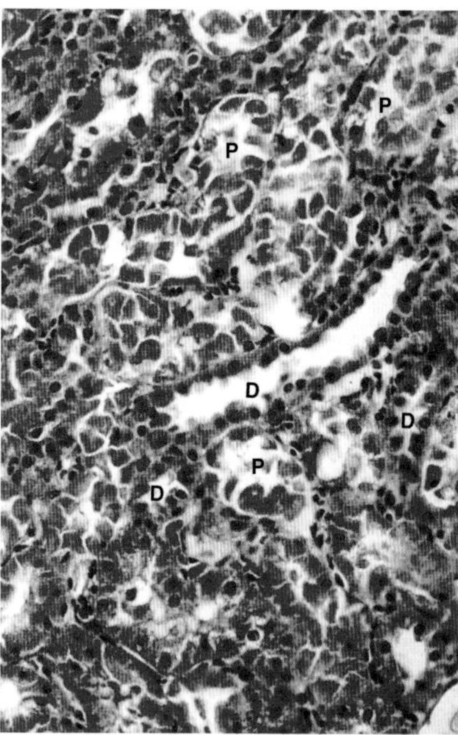

FIGURE 14-51. Toxic acute tubular necrosis caused by mercury poisoning. There is widespread necrosis of proximal tubular (P) epithelial cells, with sparing of distal and collecting tubules (D). Interstitial inflammation is minimal.

The duration of renal failure in patients with ischemic acute tubular injury depends on many factors, especially the nature and reversibility of the cause. Many patients develop uremia (azotemia, fluid retention, metabolic acidosis, and hyperkalemia), at least transiently, and may require dialysis. If the insult is removed immediately after injury begins, renal function may return within 1 to 2 weeks. However, recovery may take months.

Pyelonephritis

Acute Pyelonephritis

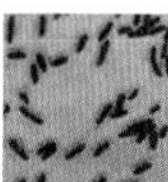

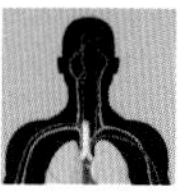

ETIOLOGIC FACTORS AND PATHOPHYSIOLOGY: Gram-negative bacteria from feces, mostly *E. coli*, cause 80% of acute pyelonephritis. **Uropathogenic *E. coli*** (see Chapter 6) have virulence factors that enhance their ability to not only infect the urinary tract but also produce pyelonephritis. Infection reaches the kidney by ascending through the urinary tract, a process that depends on several factors:

- Bacterial urinary infection
- Reflux of infected urine up the ureters into the renal pelvis and calyces
- Bacterial entry through the papillae into the renal parenchyma

These infections occur more commonly in females because they have short urethras and lack antibacterial prostatic secretions; sexual intercourse facilitates bacterial migration. Pregnancy predisposes to acute pyelonephritis for several reasons, including a high frequency of asymptomatic bacteriuria (10%), of which one quarter develops into acute pyelonephritis. Other causes include increased residual urine volume because high levels of progesterone make bladder musculature flaccid and less able to expel urine.

The bladder normally empties all but 2 to 3 mL of residual urine. Increased residual urine volume may further bacterial accumulation, for example, with prostatic obstruction or bladder atony because of neurogenic disorders, such as paraplegia or diabetic neuropathy. Diabetic glycosuria also facilitates infection by providing a rich bacterial growth medium.

Bacteria in bladder urine usually do not ascend to infect the kidneys. The ureter commonly inserts into the bladder wall at a steep angle (Fig. 14-52). Increased intravesicular pressure during micturition occludes the distal ureteral lumen and prevents urinary reflux. An anatomic abnormality, namely, a short passage of the ureter within the bladder wall, causes the ureter to insert more perpendicularly to the bladder mucosal surface. As a result, rather than occluding the lumen, micturition increases intravesicular pressure and pushes urine into the patent ureter. This reflux forces the urine into the renal pelvis and calyces.

The convexity of the simple papillae of central calyces tends to block reflux urine from entering the kidney (Fig. 14-52), but the concavity of peripheral compound papillae allows easier access. ***However, if pressure is prolonged, as in obstructive uropathy, all papillae are eventually vulnerable to retrograde entry of urine, allowing bacteria to access the renal interstitium and tubules.***

In addition to ascending through urine, bacteria and other pathogens can gain access to renal parenchyma through the bloodstream, resulting in **hematogenous pyelonephritis**. For example, in bacterial endocarditis, Gram-positive organisms, such as staphylococci, can spread from an infected valve and establish infection in the kidney. Hematogenous infections preferentially affect the cortex.

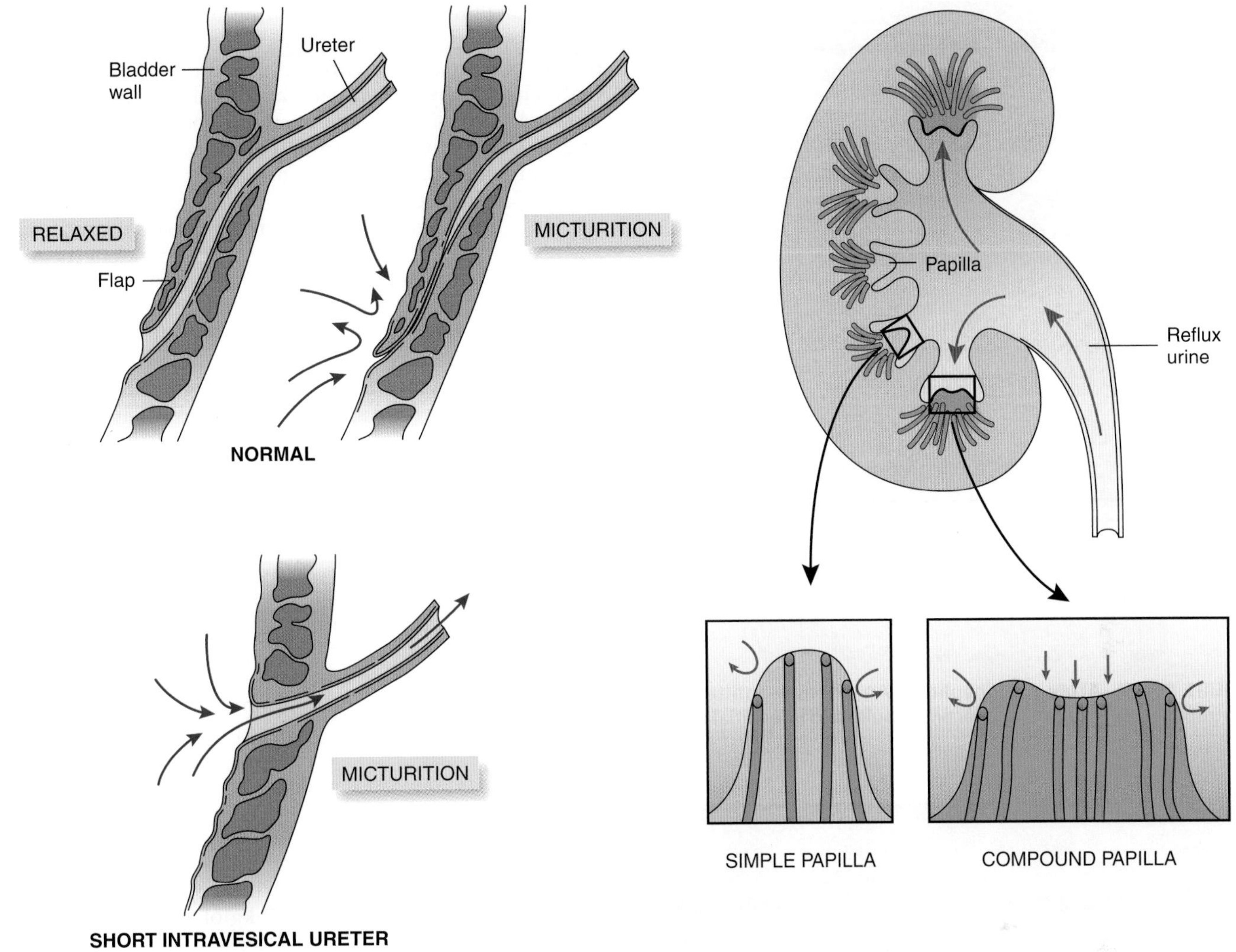

Bladder wall
Ureter
RELAXED
Flap
MICTURITION
NORMAL
Papilla
Reflux urine
SIMPLE PAPILLA
COMPOUND PAPILLA
MICTURITION
SHORT INTRAVESICAL URETER

FIGURE 14-52. Anatomic features of the bladder and kidney in pyelonephritis caused by ureterovesical reflux. In the normal bladder, the distal portion of the intravesical ureter courses between the mucosa and the muscularis, forming a mucosal flap. On micturition, the elevated intravesicular pressure compresses the flap against the bladder wall, occluding the lumen. People with a congenitally short intravesical ureter have no mucosal flap because the angle of entry of the ureter into the bladder approaches a right angle. Thus, micturition forces urine into the ureter. In the renal pelvis, simple papillae of the central calyces are convex and do not readily allow reflux of urine. By contrast, the peripheral compound papillae are concave and permit entry of refluxed urine.

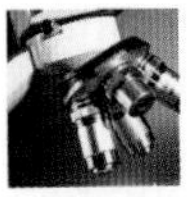

PATHOLOGY: The kidneys in acute pyelonephritis are swollen. They may have abscesses in the medulla if infection is ascending and in the cortex when it is hematogenous. The pelvic and calyceal urothelium tend to be hyperemic and covered by purulent exudate. The disease is often focal, and much of the kidney may be normal.

Most infections involve only a few papillary systems. The renal parenchyma, particularly the cortex, typically shows extensive focal destruction by inflammation, although vessels and glomeruli are often preferentially preserved. Infiltrates mainly contain neutrophils, which often fill tubules, especially collecting ducts (Fig. 14-53). In severe cases of acute pyelonephritis, necrosis of the papillary tips may occur (Fig. 14-54) or infection may extend beyond the renal capsule to cause a perinephric abscess.

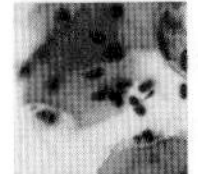

CLINICAL FEATURES: Symptoms of acute pyelonephritis include flank pain, costovertebral angle tenderness, fever, and malaise. Blood neutrophilia is common. Differentiating upper from lower urinary tract infections clinically is often difficult, but **leukocyte casts** in the urine suggest pyelonephritis.

Chronic Pyelonephritis

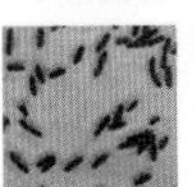

ETIOLOGIC FACTORS: Chronic pyelonephritis is caused by recurrent and persistent bacterial infection due to urinary tract obstruction or urine reflux or both.

In chronic pyelonephritis, medullary tissue and overlying cortex are preferentially injured by recurrent acute and chronic inflammation. Progressive atrophy and scarring ensue, leading to contraction or sloughing of involved papillary

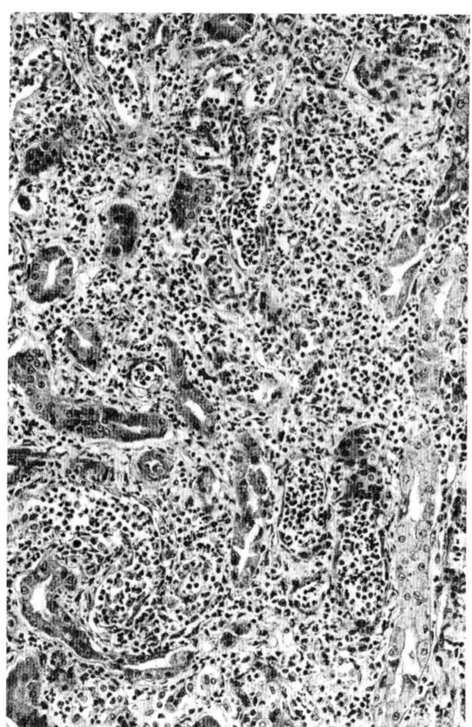

FIGURE 14-53. Acute pyelonephritis. An extensive infiltrate of neutrophils is present in the collecting tubules and interstitial tissue.

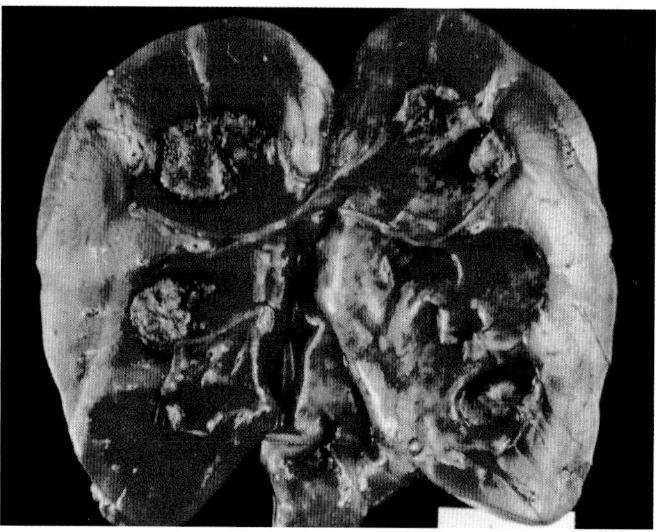

FIGURE 14-54. Papillary necrosis. The bisected kidney showing a dilated renal pelvis and dilated calyces secondary to urinary tract obstruction. The papillae are all necrotic and appear as sharply demarcated, ragged, yellowish areas.

tips and thinning of the overlying cortex. This process causes a distinctive gross appearance of broad depressed areas of cortical fibrosis and atrophy overlying a dilated calyx (**caliectasis**) (Fig. 14-55).

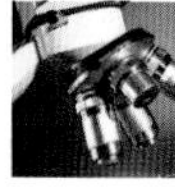

PATHOLOGY: The histologic appearance of chronic pyelonephritis is nonspecific. Many diseases cause chronic injury to the tubulointerstitial compartment and induce chronic interstitial inflammation, interstitial fibrosis, and tubular atrophy. Thus, chronic pyelonephritis is one of many etiologies, which result in a distinctive pattern of injury, called **chronic tubulointerstitial nephritis**. Only chronic pyelonephritis and analgesic nephropathy produce both caliectasis and overlying corticomedullary scarring. In obstructive uropathy, all of the calyces and the renal pelvis are dilated, and the parenchyma is uniformly thinned (Fig. 14-55). In cases associated with vesicoureteral reflux, the calyces at the poles of the kidney are preferentially expanded and are associated with overlying scars that indent the renal surface. The most characteristic (but not specific) tubular change is severe epithelial atrophy, with diffuse, eosinophilic, hyaline casts. Such tubules are "pinched-off" spherical segments, resembling colloid-containing thyroid follicles. This pattern, called **thyroidization**, results from breakup of tubules; residual segments form spherules (Fig. 14-56). Glomeruli may be uninvolved, show periglomerular fibrosis, or be sclerotic. Loss of most functioning nephrons sometimes leads to secondary FSGS. Fibrosis in arterial and arteriolar walls is common. There is marked scarring and chronic inflammation of the calyceal mucosa.

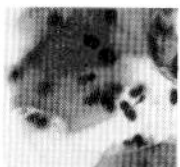

CLINICAL FEATURES: Most patients with chronic pyelonephritis have episodic symptoms of urinary tract infection or acute pyelonephritis, such as recurrent fever and flank pain. Some have a silent course until ESRD develops. Urinalysis shows leukocytes, and imaging studies reveal caliectasis and cortical scarring.

Analgesic Nephropathy

Analgesic nephropathy is a common cause of chronic tubulointerstitial disease. Patients with this nephropathy typically have taken a total of more than 2 kg of analgesics, often in combinations, such as aspirin and acetaminophen. The pathogenesis of analgesic nephropathy is not clear. Possibilities include direct nephrotoxicity or ischemic damage caused by drug-induced vascular changes or both.

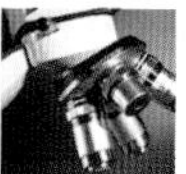

PATHOLOGY: Medullary injury with papillary necrosis occurs early in analgesic nephropathy. Atrophy, chronic inflammation, and scarring of the overlying cortex follow. The earliest histologic abnormality is a distinctive homogeneous thickening of capillary walls beneath the transitional epithelium of the urinary tract. Early parenchymal changes, which are confined to the papillae and inner medulla, consist of focal basement membrane thickening of tubules and capillaries, interstitial fibrosis, and focal coagulative necrosis. Necrotic areas eventually become confluent, first affecting the corticomedullary junction and then the collecting ducts. The necrotic foci contain few inflammatory cells. Eventually, the entire papilla becomes necrotic (**papillary necrosis**), often remaining in place as an amorphous mass.

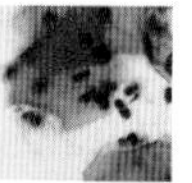

CLINICAL FEATURES: Signs and symptoms occur only late in analgesic nephropathy and include an inability to concentrate the urine, distal tubular acidosis, hematuria, hypertension, and anemia. Sloughing of necrotic papillary tips into the renal pelvis may result in colic as they pass through the ureters. Progressive renal failure often develops and eventuates in ESRD.

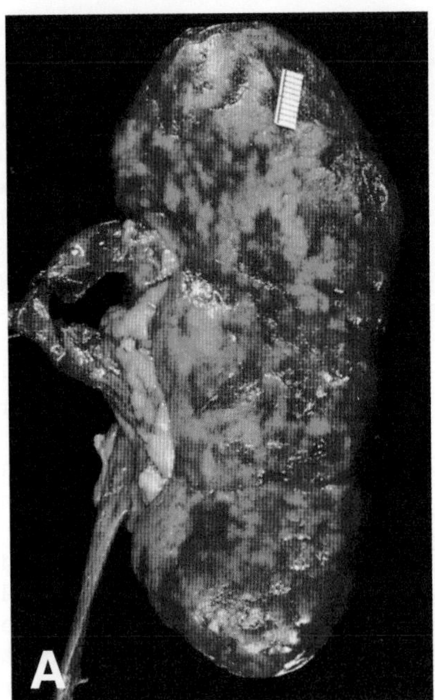

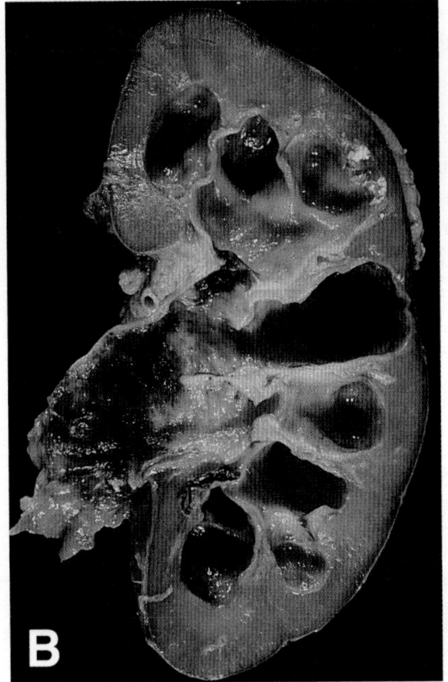

FIGURE 14-55. Chronic pyelonephritis. A. The cortical surface contains many irregular, depressed scars (reddish areas). **B.** There is marked dilation of calyces (caliectasis) caused by inflammatory destruction of papillae, with atrophy and scarring of the overlying cortex.

Drug-Induced (Hypersensitivity) Acute Tubulointerstitial Nephritis

PATHOPHYSIOLOGY: Acute drug-induced tubulointerstitial nephritis causes AKI. It entails infiltration by activated T cells and eosinophils, indicating a type IV cell-mediated immune reaction. The immunogen can be (1) the drug itself, (2) the drug bound to certain tissue components, (3) a drug metabolite, or (4) a tissue component altered by the drug. Drugs most commonly implicated include NSAIDs, diuretics, and certain antibiotics, especially β-lactam antibiotics (e.g., synthetic penicillins and cephalosporins).

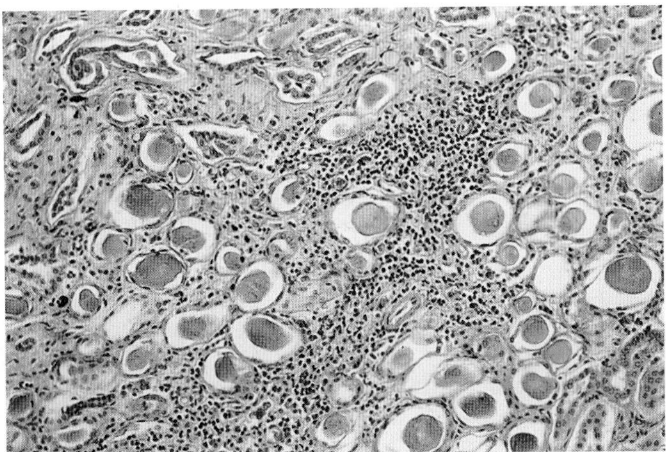

FIGURE 14-56. A light micrograph showing tubular dilation and atrophy. Many tubules contain eosinophilic hyaline casts resembling the colloid of thyroid follicles (so-called thyroidization). The interstitium is scarred and contains a chronic inflammatory cell infiltrate.

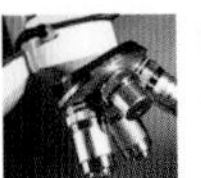

PATHOLOGY: Patchy cortical infiltration by lymphocytes and occasional eosinophils are typical. The medulla is usually less involved. Eosinophils tend to cluster, especially in tubular lumens and in the urine. Neutrophils are rare, and their presence should raise suspicion of pyelonephritis or hematogenous bacterial infection. There may be granulomatous foci, especially later in the disease. Proximal and distal tubules are focally invaded by white blood cells ("tubulitis").

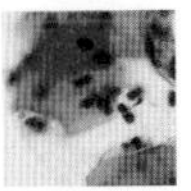

CLINICAL FEATURES: Acute tubulointerstitial nephritis usually presents as acute renal failure, typically about 2 weeks after a drug is started. Urinalysis shows erythrocytes, leukocytes (including eosinophils), and sometimes leukocyte casts. Tubular defects are common, including sodium wasting, glucosuria, aminoaciduria, and renal tubular acidosis. Systemic allergic symptoms, such as fever and rash, are often also present. Most patients recover fully within several weeks or months if the offending drug is discontinued.

Light-Chain Cast Nephropathy

Light-chain cast nephropathy refers to renal injury caused by monoclonal immunoglobulin light chains in the urine. These cause tubular epithelial injury and tubular casts.

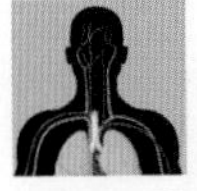

PATHOPHYSIOLOGY: As discussed above, multiple myeloma may produce AL amyloidosis, light-chain deposition disease, and light-chain cast nephropathy. The last is the most common kidney disease in patients with multiple myeloma. Glomeruli filter circulating light chains. However, at the acidic pH typical of urine, these light chains form casts by binding to Tamm–Horsfall glycoproteins, which are secreted by distal tubular epithelial cells. Renal dysfunction results from both the toxicity of free light chains for tubular epithelium and obstruction by the casts. The structure of light chain determines whether they induce light-chain cast nephropathy,

AL amyloidosis, or light-chain deposition disease. Occasional patients show several of these renal diseases.

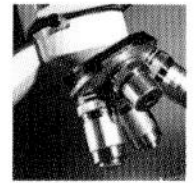

PATHOLOGY: Tubular lesions show many dense, brightly eosinophilic, and glassy (hyaline) casts in distal renal tubules and collecting ducts (Fig. 14-57). Casts that appear crystalline and exhibit fractures and angular borders may elicit foreign-body reactions. Interstitial chronic inflammation and edema typically accompany the tubular lesions. More chronic lesions show interstitial fibrosis and tubular atrophy. Focal calcium deposits (**nephrocalcinosis**) often occur in the fibrotic tubular interstitium.

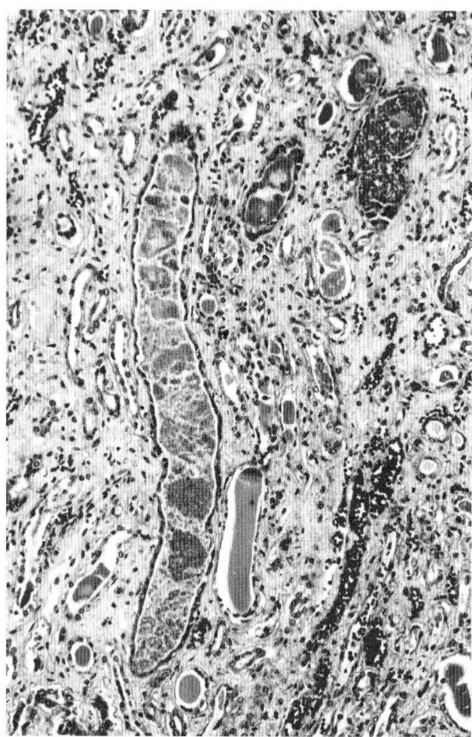

FIGURE 14-57. Light-chain cast nephropathy. A light micrograph showing numerous casts within tubular lumina.

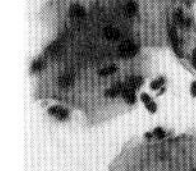

CLINICAL FEATURES: Light-chain cast nephropathy may manifest as acute or chronic renal failure. Proteinuria, predominantly of Ig light chains, is usually present, although not necessarily in the nephrotic range. Nephrotic range proteinuria in patients with multiple myeloma suggests AL amyloidosis or light-chain deposition disease rather than light-chain cast nephropathy.

Urate Nephropathy

Any condition that elevates blood levels of uric acid may cause urate nephropathy. The classic chronic disease in this category is primary gout (see Chapter 22).

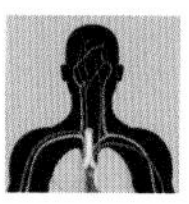

PATHOPHYSIOLOGY: In **chronic urate nephropathy** due to gout, crystalline monosodium urate deposits in the tubules and interstitium. In **tumor lysis syndrome**, blood uric acid suddenly increases as massive numbers of tumor cells die. Catabolism of huge amounts of purines from DNA released by necrotic tumor cells is responsible for hyperuricemia. The precipitation of uric acid crystals in the collecting ducts obstructs them and causes acute renal failure. Interference with uric acid excretion (e.g., chronic intake of certain diuretics) can also result in hyperuricemia. Chronic lead intoxication interferes with uric acid secretion by proximal tubules and results in **saturnine gout**.

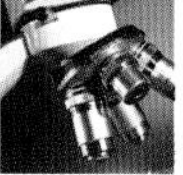

PATHOLOGY: In acute urate nephropathy, uric acid precipitates in collecting ducts and appears as yellow streaks in the papillae (Fig. 14-58A). The tubular deposits are amorphous after tissue processing, but birefringent crystals are visible in frozen sections (Fig. 14-58B). Tubules are dilated upstream of the obstruction. Uric acid crystals in collecting ducts may also elicit foreign-body reactions.

The pathogenesis of chronic urate nephropathy is similar to that of the acute form, but because the course is prolonged, more urate deposits in the interstitium, causing interstitial fibrosis and cortical atrophy. The **gouty tophus** is a focal accumulation of urate crystals surrounded by inflammatory cells, which may appear granulomatous and includes multinucleated giant cells. Uric acid stones account for 10% of **urolithiasis**; they occur in 20% of patients with chronic gout and 40% of those with acute hyperuricemia.

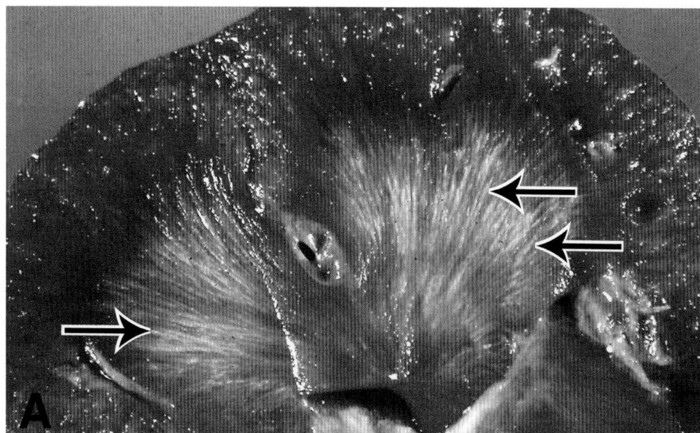

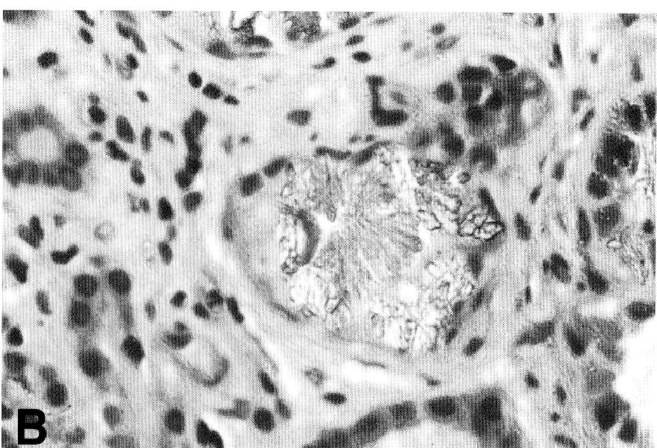

FIGURE 14-58. Urate nephropathy. A. Urate deposits appearing as golden streaks in the medulla (*arrows*). **B.** A frozen section demonstrating tubular deposits of uric acid crystals.

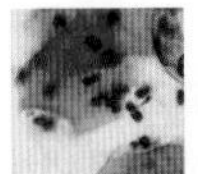

CLINICAL FEATURES: Acute urate nephropathy presents as acute renal failure; chronic urate nephropathy causes chronic renal tubular defects. Although histologic renal lesions occur in most patients with chronic gout, less than half experience significant renal functional impairment.

RENAL STONES (NEPHROLITHIASIS AND UROLITHIASIS)

Nephrolithiasis refers to stones within the renal collecting system, whereas **urolithiasis** describes stones elsewhere in the bladder or urinary tract. Calculi often form and accumulate in the renal pelvis and calyces. Stones vary in composition, depending on geography, metabolic alterations, and the presence of infection.

Renal stones are more common in men than in women. They vary in size from gravel (<1 mm) to large stones that dilate the entire renal pelvis. Although they may be well tolerated, in some cases, they result in severe hydronephrosis and pyelonephritis. They can also erode the mucosa and cause hematuria. Passage of a stone into the ureter brings on excruciating flank pain, termed **renal colic**. Larger kidney stones required surgical removal in the past, but ultrasonic disintegration (lithotripsy) and endoscopic removal are now effective.

A urinary stone is usually associated with increased blood levels and urinary excretion of its principal component. This is the case with uric acid and cystine stones. However, many patients with calcium stones have hypercalciuria without hypercalcemia. Mixed urate and calcium stones are common with hyperuricemia because urate crystals act as a nidus for the precipitation of calcium salts.

- **Calcium stones:** Most (75%) renal stones are calcium complexed with oxalate or phosphate. A mixture of these anions may occur, the former being more common in the United States. Calcium oxalate stones are hard and occasionally dark when covered by hemorrhage from the mucosa of the renal pelvis that has been injured by sharp calcium oxalate crystals. Calcium phosphate stones tend to be softer and paler.
- **Infection stones:** Infection, often with urea-splitting bacteria such as *Proteus* or *Providencia* spp., causes 15% of stones. The resulting alkaline urine favors magnesium ammonium phosphate (**struvite**) and calcium phosphate (**apatite**) precipitation. Such stones may be hard or soft and friable. Infection stones occasionally fill the pelvis and calyces to form a cast of these spaces, called a **staghorn calculus** (Fig. 14-59). Infection stones cause frequent complications, such as intractable urinary tract infection, pain, bleeding, perinephric abscess, and urosepsis.
- **Uric acid stones:** These stones occur in 25% of patients with hyperuricemia and gout, although most patients with uric acid stones have neither (**idiopathic urate lithiasis**). Urate stones are smooth, hard, and yellow and are usually less than 2 cm. Unlike calcium-containing stones, pure uric acid stones are radiolucent.
- **Cystine stones:** These account for only 1% of renal stones overall but are a significant fraction of childhood calculi. They occur only in hereditary cystinuria. Although composed only of cystine, they may be enveloped by a layer of calcium phosphate.

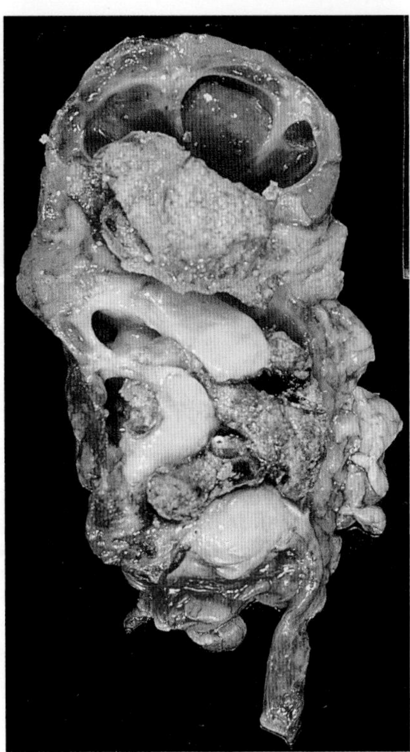

FIGURE 14-59. **Staghorn calculi.** The kidney showing hydronephrosis and stones that are casts of the dilated calyces.

OBSTRUCTIVE UROPATHY AND HYDRONEPHROSIS

Obstructive uropathy is caused by structural or functional abnormalities in the urinary tract that impede urine flow. It may cause renal dysfunction (obstructive nephropathy) and dilation of the collecting system (hydronephrosis). Urinary tract obstruction is detailed in Chapter 15.

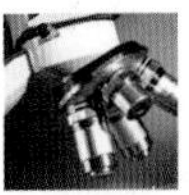

PATHOLOGY: The most prominent microscopic finding in early hydronephrosis is dilation of collecting ducts. This effect is followed by dilation of proximal and distal convoluted tubules. Eventually, the proximal tubules become widely dilated and are lost. Glomeruli are usually spared. Progressive dilation of the renal pelvis and calyces gives rise to renal parenchymal atrophy (Fig. 14-60). Hydronephrotic kidneys are more susceptible to pyelonephritis, adding injury to insult.

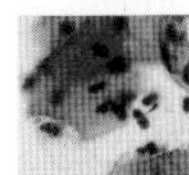

CLINICAL FEATURES: Bilateral acute urinary tract obstruction causes acute renal failure (**postrenal acute renal failure**), whereas unilateral obstruction is often asymptomatic. Many causes of acute obstruction are reversible; thus, prompt recognition is important. Left untreated, an obstructed kidney undergoes atrophy. If obstruction is bilateral, chronic renal failure ensues.

RENAL TRANSPLANTATION

Kidney transplantation is the treatment of choice for most patients with ESRD. The major obstacle is allograft rejection (see Chapter 3). However, the transplanted organ is also

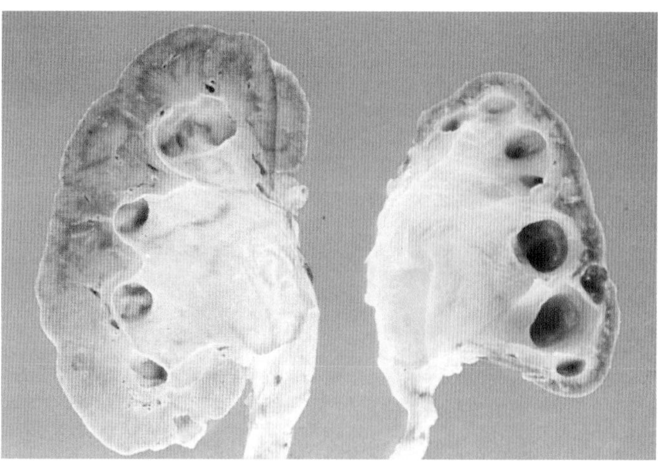

FIGURE 14-60. Hydronephrosis. Bilateral urinary tract obstruction has led to conspicuous dilation of the ureters, pelves, and calyces. The kidney on the right showing severe parenchymal atrophy.

susceptible to recurrence of the disease that destroyed the native kidneys and to nephrotoxicity from immunosuppressive drugs. Table 14-12 lists distinct, but often coexisting, patterns of renal allograft rejection.

Table 14-12

Categories of Renal Allograft Rejection

Category	Most Characteristic Lesion
Hyperacute antibody-mediated rejection	Neutrophils in peritubular capillaries, hemorrhage, and necrosis
Acute antibody-mediated rejection	
Acute antibody-mediated capillary rejection	Leukocytes and C4d in peritubular capillaries
Acute necrotizing transplant arteritis	Arterial fibrinoid necrosis
Acute T-cell–mediated rejection	
Acute tubulointerstitial rejection	Tubulitis (mononuclear leukocytes between epithelial cells of tubules) and interstitial activated lymphocytes
Acute endarteritis	Mononuclear leukocytes in arterial intima
Acute transplant glomerulitis	Mononuclear leukocytes in glomerular capillaries
Acute transplant arteritis	Acute transmural inflammation or necrosis
Chronic rejection	
Interstitial fibrosis and tubular atrophy	Tubular atrophy, interstitial fibrosis, interstitial chronic inflammatory cells, and thickening of peritubular capillary basement membranes
Chronic transplant arteriopathy	Arterial fibrotic intimal thickening
Chronic transplant glomerulopathy	Glomerular capillary wall thickening and glomerular basement membrane remodeling

BENIGN RENAL TUMORS

PAPILLARY RENAL ADENOMA: There is controversy as to whether any epithelial renal cell tumor should be considered benign. However, currently, neoplasms smaller than 5 mm with papillary or tubulopapillary growth patterns can be considered adenomas. Papillary renal adenomas occur more often with advancing age and are incidental autopsy findings in 40% of patients older than 70 years.

RENAL ONCOCYTOMA: This benign neoplasm accounts for 5% to 10% of primary renal tumors removed surgically. It derives from collecting duct intercalated cells. The cells are plump, with abundant, finely granular, acidophilic cytoplasm and round nuclei that lack atypia. The distinctive appearance of the tumor is because of abundant mitochondria in the cytoplasm. Oncocytomas are typically mahogany brown owing to mitochondrial lipochrome pigments. These tumors rarely metastasize.

MEDULLARY FIBROMA: Medullary fibromas (renomedullary interstitial cell tumors) are typically small (<0.5 cm in diameter), pale gray, and well circumscribed and are usually found in the midportion of medullary pyramids. They are composed of small stellate to polygonal cells in a loose stroma. Renal medullary fibromas are incidental findings in as many as half of all adult autopsies (Fig. 14-61).

ANGIOMYOLIPOMA: ***These tumors are strongly associated with tuberous sclerosis.*** Of patients with tuberous sclerosis, 80% have angiomyolipomas, but most patients with angiomyolipomas do not have tuberous sclerosis. These lesions are mixtures of well-differentiated adipose tissue, smooth muscle, and thick-walled vessels. Grossly, they are yellow and bosselated and may resemble renal cell carcinoma. However, they are always well encapsulated and lack necrosis.

MESOBLASTIC NEPHROMA: Mesoblastic nephromas are benign congenital neoplasms or hamartomas, usually found in the first 3 months of life. The lesions range from smaller than

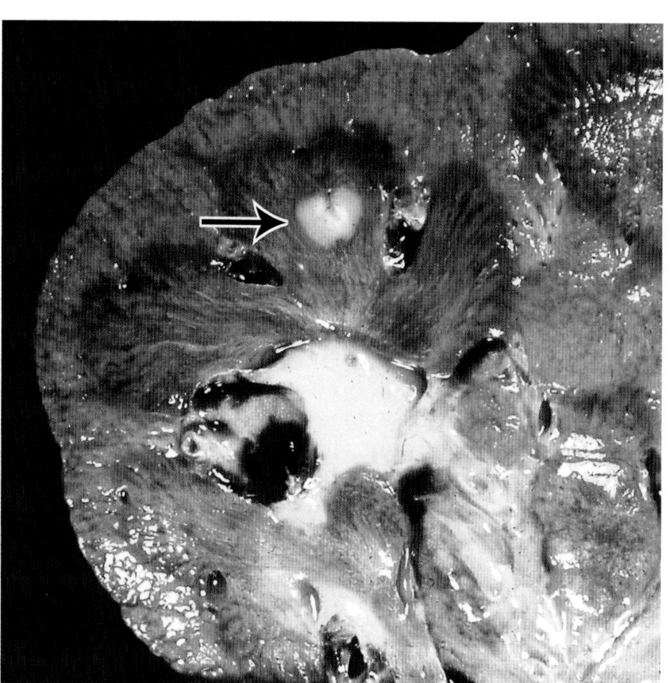

FIGURE 14-61. Medullary fibroma (arrow).

1 cm to larger than 15 cm and are composed of spindle cells of fibroblastic or myofibroblastic lineage. The tumor margins are usually irregular, with bands of cells interdigitating with adjacent renal parenchyma. Mesoblastic nephromas may recur if tumor tissue is left behind after surgical resection.

MALIGNANT TUMORS OF THE KIDNEY

Wilms Tumor (Nephroblastoma)

Wilms tumor is a malignancy of embryonal renal elements, including admixed blastema, stroma, and epithelium. Its incidence is 1 in 10,000, making it the most common abdominal solid tumor in children.

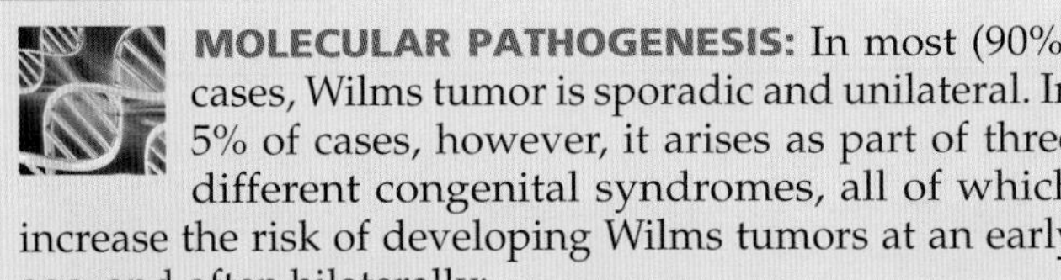

MOLECULAR PATHOGENESIS: In most (90%) cases, Wilms tumor is sporadic and unilateral. In 5% of cases, however, it arises as part of three different congenital syndromes, all of which increase the risk of developing Wilms tumors at an early age, and often bilaterally:

- **WAGR syndrome** (*W*ilms tumor, *a*niridia, *g*enitourinary anomalies, mental *r*etardation) is caused by a deletion on the short arm of chromosome 11 (11p13). Affected genes include the aniridia gene (*PAX6*) and **Wilms tumor gene 1 (*WT1*)**. Loss of one *WT1* allele leads to genitourinary anomalies. One third of children with WAGR develop Wilms tumor subsequent to loss of heterozygosity at the *WT1* I locus.
- **Denys–Drash syndrome (DDS)** is associated with Wilms tumor, intersexual disorders, and glomerular mesangial sclerosis. Mutations in the *WT1* gene in DDS are considered dominant negative mutations, possibly accounting for the fact that the DDS phenotype is far more severe than that of WAGR syndrome.
- **Beckwith–Wiedemann syndrome (BWS)** features Wilms tumor, overgrowth ranging from gigantism to hemihypertrophy, visceromegaly, and macroglossia.

WT1 is a tumor suppressor protein that regulates transcription of several other genes. Only 10% to 20% of sporadic Wilms tumors have *WT1* mutations. Thus, other genes besides *WT1* contribute to the genesis of sporadic Wilms tumors.

Nephrogenic rests (small foci of persistent primitive blastemal cells) are found in the kidneys of all children with syndromic Wilms tumors and in one third of sporadic cases. Given that such rests in the nontumorous kidney have the same somatic *WT1* mutations as are present in the tumors, these rests may represent clonal precursor lesions one or more steps along the pathway to tumor formation.

PATHOLOGY: Wilms tumors tend to be large when detected, with bulging, pale tan, cut surfaces enclosed by a thin rim of renal cortex and capsule (Fig. 14-62). Wilms tumors resemble normal fetal renal tissue (Fig. 14-63), including metanephric blastema, immature stroma (mesenchymal tissue), and immature epithelial elements. Most Wilms tumors contain all three elements in varying proportions. The blastema-like component contains small ovoid cells with scanty cytoplasm, in nests and trabeculae. The epithelial component appears as small tubular structures. Formations resembling immature glomeruli may sometimes be seen. The tumor stroma contains spindle cells, which are mostly undifferentiated but may show smooth muscle or fibroblast differentiation. Skeletal muscle is the most common heterotopic

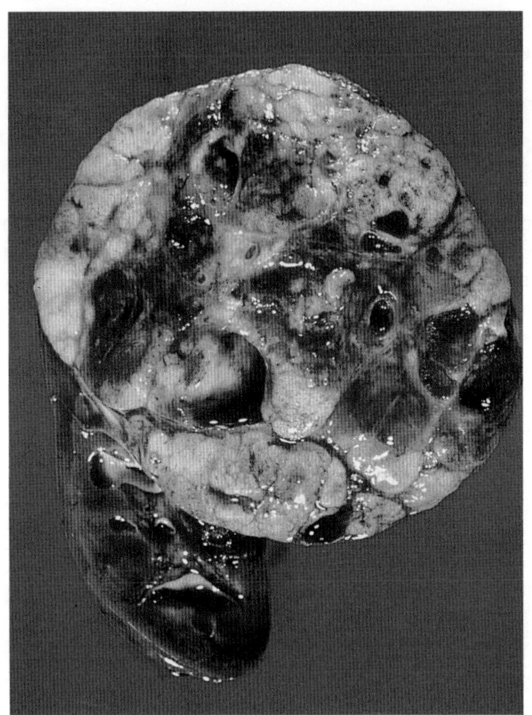

FIGURE 14-62. Wilms tumor. A cross section of a pale tan neoplasm attached to a residual portion of the kidney.

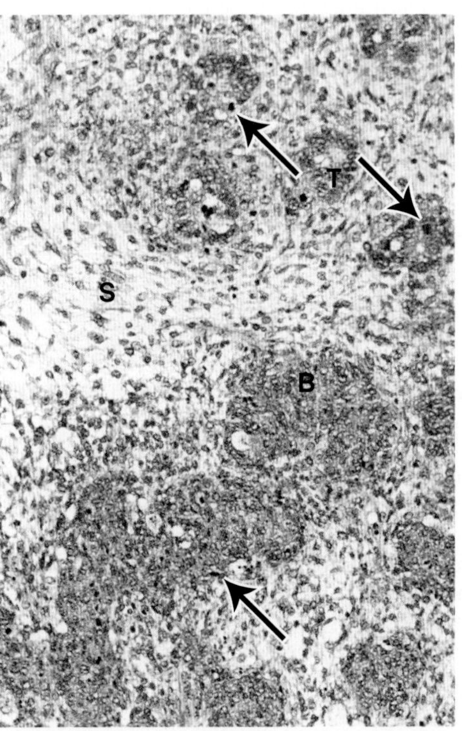

FIGURE 14-63. Wilms tumor (nephroblastoma), showing highly cellular areas composed of undifferentiated blastema (*B*), loose stroma (*S*) containing undifferentiated mesenchymal cells, and immature tubules (*T*). Note the many mitotic figures (*arrows*).

stromal element, although bone, cartilage, fat, or neural tissue is encountered occasionally.

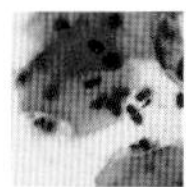

CLINICAL FEATURES: Wilms tumors represent 85% of pediatric renal neoplasms. They occur in 1 in 10,000 children, usually 1 to 3 years old, and 98% present before age 10. Familial cases usually show autosomal dominant inheritance. Most often, the diagnosis is made after recognition of an abdominal mass. Additional manifestations include abdominal pain, intestinal obstruction, hypertension, hematuria, and symptoms of traumatic tumor rupture. Chemotherapy and radiation therapy, plus surgical resection, provide long-term survival rates of 90%.

Renal Cell Carcinoma

RCC is a malignant neoplasm of renal tubular or ductal epithelial cells. It accounts for 80% to 90% of primary renal cancers. More than 30,000 cases occur each year in the United States.

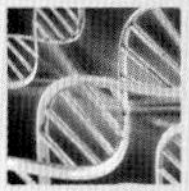

MOLECULAR PATHOGENESIS: Most RCCs are sporadic, but about 5% are inherited. Hereditary RCCs occur in the context of several syndromes including the following:

- **von Hippel–Lindau (VHL) syndrome** is an autosomal dominant cancer syndrome (see Chapter 5), with clear cell RCC (40% of cases of VHL disease) cerebellar hemangioblastomas, retinal angiomas, pheochromocytoma, and cysts in various organs.
- **Autosomal dominant RCC** is associated with defects in genes coding for Krebs cycle enzymes, including fumarate hydratase. The mutations are also associated with frequent formation of uterine fibroids (leiomyomas).
- **Hereditary papillary RCC**, an autosomal dominant inherited cancer, is characterized by multiple bilateral papillary tumors.

Hereditary RCCs tend to be multifocal and bilateral and appear in younger patients than do sporadic RCCs. A family history of RCC increases the risk for RCC four- to fivefold. ***In virtually all (98%) sporadic clear cell RCCs, one VHL allele is lost;* VHL *mutations occur in more than 50% of these tumors.*** Thus, loss of *VHL* tumor suppressor function plays a key role in clear cell RCC tumorigenesis. Abnormal *VHL* gene function causes the transcriptional regulatory molecule, hypoxia-inducible factor-α (HIF-α), to accumulate and upregulate proteins that activate kinase-dependent signaling pathways. Components of these pathways are targets for kinase inhibitors, and mTOR inhibitors have proven useful for treating RCC. Unlike clear cell RCC, hereditary papillary RCC and chromophobe RCC are not linked to *VHL.*

Tobacco, whether smoked or chewed, increases the risk of RCC; one third of RCCs are linked to tobacco use. Inherited and acquired renal cystic diseases may lead to RCC, especially papillary RCC. The cancer has also been tied to analgesic nephropathy.

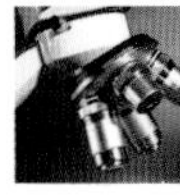

PATHOLOGY: The pathologic variants of RCC reflect differences in histogenesis and predict different outcomes. The most common histologic categories of RCC are shown in Table 14-13.

- **Clear cell RCC**, the most common type, arises from proximal tubular epithelial cells. It is typically yellow-orange, solid, or focally cystic, and focal hemorrhage and necrosis are common (Fig. 14-64). The removal of abundant cytoplasmic lipids and glycogen in tissue preparations accounts for the clear cytoplasm (Fig. 14-65). The cells are often arranged in round or elongated collections and are demarcated by a network of delicate vessels. Little cellular or nuclear pleomorphism is present.

Table 14-13

Categories of Renal Cell Carcinoma

Category	Frequency (%)
Clear cell type	70–80
Papillary type	10–15
Chromophobe type	5
Collecting duct type	1

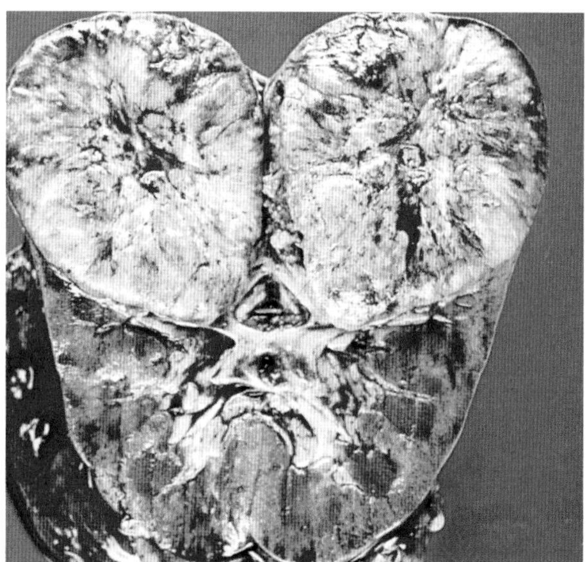

FIGURE 14-64. Clear cell renal cell carcinoma. The kidney contains a large irregular neoplasm with a variegated cut surface. Yellow areas correspond to lipid-containing cells.

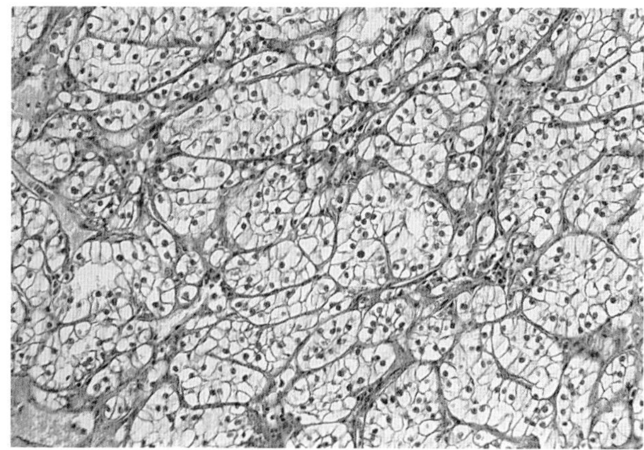

FIGURE 14-65. Clear cell renal cell carcinoma. Photomicrograph showing islands of neoplastic cells with abundant clear cytoplasm.

- **Papillary RCC** contains tumor cells on fibrovascular stalks. The cytoplasm may be eosinophilic or basophilic. These tumors arise from proximal tubular epithelial cells.
- **Chromophobe RCC** has a mixture of acidophilic granular cells and pale transparent cells with prominent cell borders, which impart a plant cell–like appearance. Chromophobe RCCs appear to arise from intercalated cells of the renal collecting ducts.

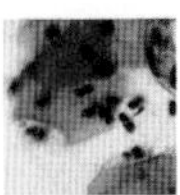

CLINICAL FEATURES: The incidence of RCC peaks in the sixth decade, and the tumor occurs twice as often in men as in women. ***Hematuria is the most common presenting sign, but incidental discoveries are common, mostly in imaging studies of the abdomen done for other reasons. The classic clinical triad of hematuria, flank pain, and a palpable abdominal mass occurs in fewer than 10% of patients.*** RCC is known as a "great mimic," and it produces ectopic hormones that may cause fever and paraneoplastic syndromes. For example, secretion of a PTH-like substance leads to symptoms of hyperparathyroidism, production of erythropoietin causes erythrocytosis, and RCC secretion of renin results in hypertension. Patients with RCC often come to medical attention because of symptoms from a metastasis.

The prognosis for RCC reflects tumor size, extent of invasion and metastasis, histologic type, and nuclear grade. ***Tumor stage is the single most important prognostic factor.*** If RCC remains inside the renal capsule, 5-year survival is 90%. This drops to 30% if there are distant metastases. The tumor spreads most frequently to the lungs and bones.

Renal medullary carcinomas are rapidly growing neoplasms that are usually associated with sickle cell disease.

Transitional Cell Carcinoma

Between 5% and 10% of primary kidney cancers are transitional cell carcinomas of the pelvis or calyces (see Chapter 15). These are morphologically identical to the more common transitional cell carcinomas of the urinary bladder and are associated with them in half of cases. Fewer than 5% of transitional cell carcinomas occur in the collecting system proximal to the bladder.

15 The Lower Urinary Tract and Male Reproductive System

Ivan Damjanov ▪ Peter A. McCue

LEARNING OBJECTIVES

- List the components of the male reproductive system and urinary tract.
- Describe the three components of the male urethra.
- List the three layers of transitional epithelium.
- Describe the structure of the testes and prostate.
- What are the most common causes of ureteral obstruction?
- What is the most common tumor of the renal pelvis and ureter? How does the term "field effect" apply to such tumors?
- Describe the etiology and histopathology of the following forms of cystitis: acute, chronic, interstitial, and malakoplakia.
- Describe the etiology, histopathology, and clinical significance of the following benign and metaplastic lesions of urothelium: Brunn buds and nests and cystic lesions including cystitis glandularis, squamous, and nephrogenic metaplasia.
- List important risk factors for bladder cancer.
- Describe the etiology, histopathology, and clinical significance of the following tumors of the bladder: exophytic and inverted papillomas, urothelial carcinoma in situ, PUNLMP, low-grade urothelial carcinoma, high-grade urothelial carcinoma, and invasive transitional cell carcinoma.
- List nonurothelial tumors of the bladder. What is their relationship to urachal remnants?
- Differentiate hypospadias, epispadias, phimosis, and priapism.
- Describe common non-neoplastic scrotal masses.
- Review common sexually transmitted diseases of the male reproductive system.
- Describe the histopathology of Peyronie disease.
- In terms of penile carcinoma, differentiate between carcinoma in situ, Bowen disease, erythroplasia of Queyrat, and Bowenoid papulosis.
- Describe cryptorchidism and the risks associated with this condition.
- Differentiate between hermaphroditism, female pseudohermaphroditism, and male pseudohermaphroditism.
- What are common pathologies observed in testicular biopsies of infertile males?
- List common infectious and noninfectious etiologies for orchitis.
- What genetic abnormalities and risk factors are associated with testicular tumors?
- Describe the origin, histopathology, and clinical consequences of intratubular testicular germ cell neoplasia (ITGCN).
- Differentiate between pure embryonal carcinomas, seminomas, and nonseminomatous germ cell tumors (NSGCTs) in terms of origin and histopathology.
- Differentiate between teratocarcinomas, yolk sac carcinomas, and choriocarcinomas in terms of origin and histopathology.
- Describe the characteristic histologic features of yolk sac tumors of childhood.
- Describe the classification and histopathology of gonadal stromal/sex cord tumors.
- Differentiate between the etiology of acute, chronic, and nonbacterial prostatitis.
- What are potential pathophysiologic mechanisms resulting in benign prostatic hyperplasia (BPH)?
- Describe the histopathology and clinical consequences of BPH.
- What are common molecular lesions associated with adenocarcinoma of the prostate?
- Describe commonly used screening and diagnostic paradigms used for the detection and evaluation of prostate cancer. What are the potential drawbacks?
- Differentiate between prostatic intraepithelial neoplasia (PIN) lesions and invasive prostatic adenocarcinoma in terms of histopathology.
- Briefly describe the Gleason grade group system as used in the grading of prostate adenocarcinoma.

LOWER URINARY TRACT

The ureters, urinary bladder, and urethra—collectively known as the lower urinary tract—constitute the outflow part of the urinary system (Fig. 15-1). In males, the lower urinary tract is closely related to the reproductive system.

Ureters

The ureters are paired tubes linking each renal pelvis to the bladder. The lowermost part of the ureters is obliquely embedded in the smooth muscular wall of the urinary bladder, which acts as sphincters known as the **ureterovesical valves**. These valves let urine pass downward into the bladder but not in the opposite direction (see also Chapter 14).

Urethra

The male urethra averages 20 cm long and has three parts: (1) **prostatic urethra**, traversing the prostate; (2) **membranous urethra**, penetrating the pelvic floor; and (3) **spongy or penile urethra**, in the central portion of the penis. The prostatic urethra contains ostia of the ejaculatory and prostatic ducts. The posterior part of the penile urethra, also called the **bulbous urethra**, receives secretions from the mucous bulbourethral (Cowper) glands. The anterior part of the penile urethra exhibits scattered mucus-secreting glands of Littré. The penile urethra terminates in the fossa navicularis, immediately proximal to the external orifice, or meatus, on the tip of the penis.

The female urethra is shorter, only 3 to 4 cm in length. It extends from its internal orifice at the urinary bladder to its external orifice in the vulva, directly below the clitoris. The wall of the female urethra also displays mucous glands.

Transitional Epithelium (Urothelium)

The urothelium has three epithelial zones. The **basal layer** lies on a basement membrane and contains cells that can divide and replace damaged superficial cells. Above the basal layer is the **intermediate zone**, which is composed of three to four layers of polygonal cells. Both basal and polygonal cells can flatten when the bladder dilates. The **superficial layer** consists of "umbrella cells," which are resistant to the urine that constantly bathes them.

Under the epithelium, the lamina propria incorporates mainly loose connective tissue, smooth muscle cells, and blood vessels. The muscularis mucosa is poorly developed and consists of thin discontinuous wisps of smooth muscle cells. Beyond the lamina propria lies a thick smooth muscle layer, covered by adventitia. Because the bladder, ureters, and urethra are retroperitoneal, they do not have an external serosa. Only part of the bladder dome has a serosal covering.

MALE REPRODUCTIVE SYSTEM

The male reproductive system includes the testis, epididymis, ductus (vas) deferens, seminal vesicles, prostate, and penis (Fig. 15-1).

Testes

Testes are paired oval organs measuring 4 cm in greatest dimension. Each is invested with a **tunica vaginalis**, a layer of mesothelial cells that covers the outer fibrous capsule of the testis, which is called the **tunica albuginea**. This capsule has internal septal ramifications that divide the testis into about 250 **lobules**. Each lobule consists of coiled seminiferous tubules and loose interstitial tissue containing blood vessels and Leydig interstitial cells.

Testicular arteries originate from the abdominal aorta and nourish the testes. The right internal spermatic vein empties into the inferior vena cava, whereas the left drains into the left renal vein. This anatomic difference has several clinical implications, as discussed below.

Spermatogenesis

These tubules are the principal functional unit of the testes. They contain seminiferous epithelium and **Sertoli cells**, which support spermatogenesis. Sertoli cells also secrete **inhibin**, which communicates with the pituitary to regulate the secretion of **gonadotropins** (i.e., follicle-stimulating hormone [FSH] and luteinizing hormone [LH]) (see Chapter 19). The interstitial spaces of the testis contain **Leydig cells**, the primary source of testosterone.

Hormonal stimuli increase the numbers of germ cells, primarily **spermatogonia**, which also begin differentiating into **primary spermatocytes**. Meiotic division of the diploid primary spermatocytes produces **secondary spermatocytes**, which carry a haploid number (23) of chromosomes. Secondary spermatocytes mature to **spermatids** and then to **spermatozoa**, which are discharged through the channels of the rete testis into the epididymal ducts.

The **epididymis** lies along the lateral–posterior aspect of the testis and extends into the ductus deferens. In the epididymis, spermatozoa are admixed with fluid secreted by epididymal lining cells and travel through the **vas deferens**, which empties its contents into the urethra. Finally, semen is ejaculated through the penile urethra as a mixture of spermatozoa in epididymal secretions and fluids made by **accessory glands**, namely, the seminal vesicles, prostate, Cowper bulbourethral glands, and urethral glands.

Prostate

The prostate contacts the posterior and inferior external layers of the urinary bladder, close to the rectum. Posteriorly, it is attached to **seminal vesicles**. Microscopically, it is a tubuloalveolar gland with a rich fibromuscular stroma. It develops under the influence of testosterone, which is essential for maintaining its production of seminal fluid.

Functionally, the prostate is organized into three distinct zones. The **transition zone** is around the prostatic urethra. The **central zone** sits slightly posterior and extends toward the seminal vesicles. The **peripheral zone** envelops the other zones and defines the boundaries of the gland. Precise anatomic boundaries of the zones are inapparent by light microscopy. However, the biologic discrimination between the zones is important, because most cancers arise in the peripheral zone, whereas hyperplasias generally originate in the transition zone.

The prostate lacks a true **capsule**. In some areas, there is a concentric band of fibromuscular tissue that blends into the adjacent glandular stroma. Thus, what constitutes capsular invasion by tumor is somewhat arbitrary. The lack of a well-defined capsule has implications in cancer staging for the surgeon and the pathologist.

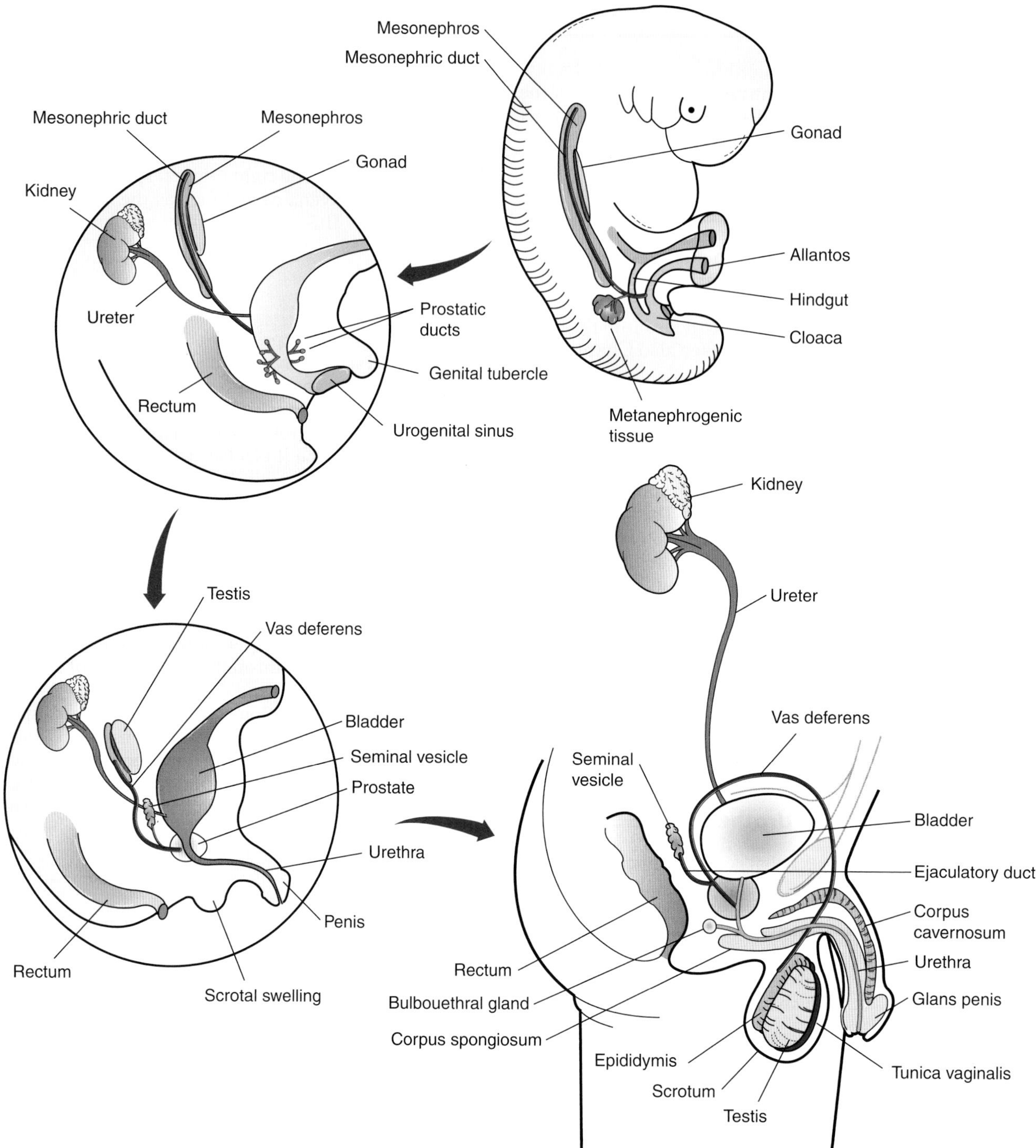

FIGURE 15-1. Embryologic development of the urinary tract and male reproductive system.

RENAL PELVIS AND URETER

Congenital Disorders

Developmental anomalies of the renal pelvis and ureters occur in 2% to 3% of all people. They do not usually cause clinical problems, but on occasion, may predispose to obstruction and urinary tract infections. The most significant developmental anomalies include agenesis, ectopia, duplications, obstructions, and dilations.

AGENESIS OF THE RENAL PELVIS AND URETERS: This rare anomaly always entails agenesis of the corresponding kidney. Unilateral agenesis is usually asymptomatic. Bilateral agenesis of the ureters and kidneys, a feature of **Potter syndrome**, is incompatible with extrauterine life (see Chapters 5 and 14).

ECTOPIC URETERS: Ureteric buds may develop at the wrong anatomic site during embryogenesis. The lower orifices of ectopic ureters can be found in many anomalous places, such as the midportion of the urinary bladder, seminal vesicles, urethra, or vas deferens.

DUPLICATIONS: Ureteral duplication is the most common congenital abnormality of the urinary system. Duplicate or multiple ureteric buds may originate on the side of the fetal bladder and may be unilateral, bilateral, complete, or partial. Usually, there are two parallel ureters, each with its own renal pelvis and separate vesical orifice. **Bifid ureters** (subdivided by a septum), **bifurcate ureters**, and many variations thereof may be encountered, but most are of no clinical significance.

URETERAL OBSTRUCTION: Obstructions can be traced to congenital **atresia** or abnormal **ureteral valves**. However, congenital **obstruction of the ureteropelvic junction (UPJ)**, which is the most common form of hydronephrosis in infants and children, is thought to be related to abnormal layering of smooth muscle cells and/or fibrous tissue replacing the smooth muscle cells at the UPJ. Urinary obstruction in these children is usually unilateral but is bilateral in 20% of cases. Obstruction is more common in boys than girls and is usually diagnosed during the first 6 months of life. Congenital UPJ obstruction is often associated with other urinary tract anomalies, including, in some cases, agenesis of the contralateral kidney.

DILATIONS OF THE RENAL PELVIS OR URETERS: Dilations of the renal pelvis or ureters that are localized are called **diverticula**. Generalized dilation of the entire ureter, **congenital megaureter**, may be unilateral or bilateral. Affected ureters are tortuous and lack peristalsis. The resulting stagnation of urine (**hydroureter**) is typically associated with progressive hydronephrosis, ultimately leading to renal failure.

Ureteritis and Ureteral Obstruction

Ureteritis, that is, an inflammation of the ureters, is a complication of descending infections from the kidneys or ascending infections from the bladder. Ureteritis is often associated with ureteral obstruction, which may be intrinsic or extrinsic (Fig. 15-2).

Intrinsic ureteral obstruction may be caused by calculi, intraluminal blood clots, fibroepithelial polyps, inflammatory strictures, amyloidosis, or tumors of the ureter.

Extrinsic causes of ureteral obstruction include the enlarged uterus during pregnancy, aberrant renal vessels to the lower pole of the kidney that cross the ureter, or endometriosis. Tumors that compress the ureters usually originate from the digestive tract and female genital tract and may compress the ureters by direct extension or through metastases to retroperitoneal lymph nodes.

Ureteral obstruction can also result from diseases of the urinary bladder, prostate, and urethra (e.g., bladder cancer near a ureteral orifice or bladder neck, neurogenic bladder, and prostatic hyperplasia or cancer). Proximal causes of ureteral obstruction tend to be unilateral, whereas more distal ones, such as prostatic diseases, lead to bilateral hydronephrosis, with the possibility of renal failure in untreated cases.

Idiopathic retroperitoneal fibrosis, a rare cause of ureteral obstruction, features dense fibrosis of retroperitoneal soft tissues and modest, nonspecific, chronic inflammation. On occasion, idiopathic retroperitoneal fibrosis is associated with systemic disease and is accompanied by inflammatory fibrosis in other areas. Some of these multisystemic cases are associated with elevated serum IgG4 and thus belong to the group of **IgG4-related diseases**. The fibrotic lesions are infiltrated with IgG4-positive plasma cells, which play a role in the genesis of fibrosis. The disease may respond to treatment with corticosteroids or immunosuppression. **Secondary retroperitoneal fibrosis** resembles the idiopathic form of the disease clinically and pathologically. It may evolve as a complication of surgery or radiation therapy, or as an adverse reaction to certain drugs, such as methysergide or β-adrenergic blockers.

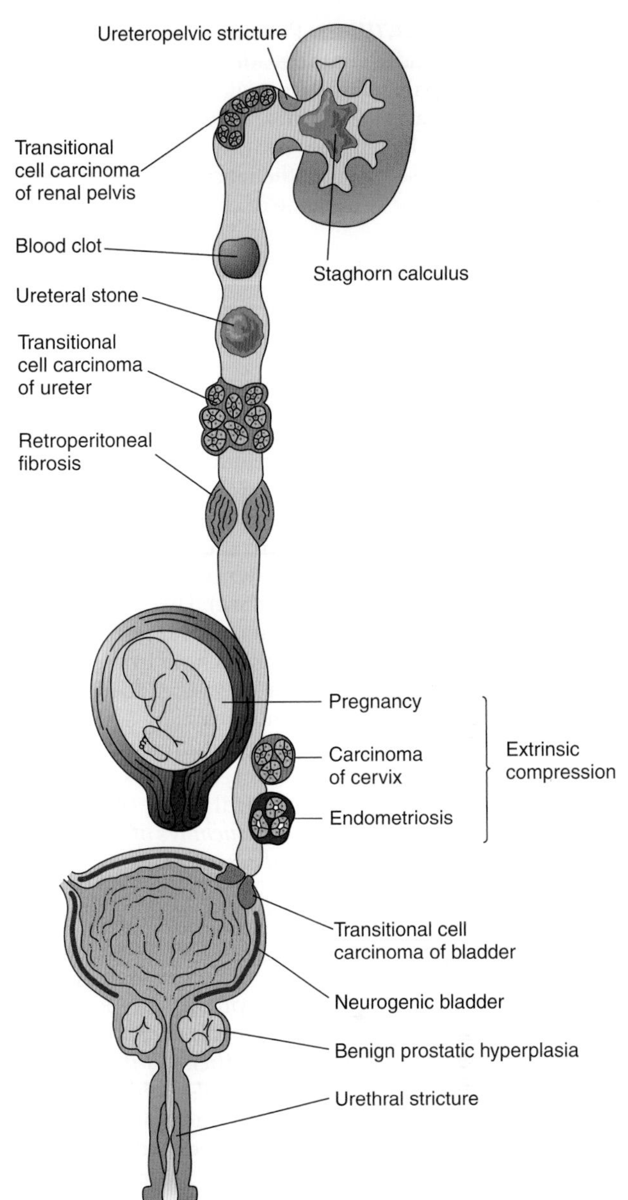

FIGURE 15-2. Most common causes of ureteral obstruction.

Tumors of the Renal Pelvis and Ureter

Tumors of the renal pelvis and ureter resemble those of the urinary bladder (see below) except that they are only one tenth as common. Most (>90%) are **urothelial (transitional) cell carcinomas**. Etiologies associated with such tumors of the renal pelvis and ureter are similar to those found in bladder cancer, suggesting a "field effect" in which the entire urothelial mucosa is a continuous "target organ." About 2% to 4% of tumors are bilateral, and almost half of treated patients develop subsequent urothelial bladder tumors.

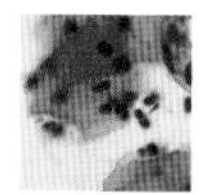

CLINICAL FEATURES: Patients most often present in their sixth and seventh decades with hematuria (80%) and flank pain (25%). Urothelial cell carcinoma of the ureter or renal pelvis requires radical nephroureterectomy. The entire ureter must be removed because of the high frequency of concurrent and subsequent urothelial carcinomas. Prognosis reflects the tumor stage at the time of diagnosis.

URINARY BLADDER

Congenital Disorders

Congenital developmental malformations of the urinary bladder include (1) bladder exstrophy, (2) diverticula, (3) urachal remnants, and (4) congenital vesicoureteral valve incompetence.

EXSTROPHY OF THE BLADDER: This malformation is characterized by the absence of the anterior bladder wall and part of the anterior abdominal wall. It occurs in 1 in 50,000 births. In some boys, it is associated with **epispadias** (i.e., incomplete formation of the penile urethra). This defect exposes the posterior bladder wall to the exterior and transforms the bladder into a cup-like organ that cannot hold urine. The posterior wall of the exstrophic bladder is exposed to mechanical injury and prone to frequent infection, causing squamous or glandular metaplasia. Exstrophy can be surgically repaired, but the metaplastic mucosa is at increased risk of bladder cancer, even 50 to 60 years after surgical repair of exstrophy.

DIVERTICULA: These saclike outpouchings of bladder wall are related to incomplete formation of muscular layers. They can be solitary or multiple. Urine retained inside such diverticula is commonly infected, which may lead to urinary stone formation. Congenital diverticula must be distinguished from **acquired vesical diverticula**, which typically occur in long-standing urinary tract obstruction as a result of prostatic hyperplasia.

URACHAL REMNANTS: The urachus is the fetal allantoic stalk connecting the bladder and umbilicus. If it persists and remains patent throughout, it forms a ***vesical–umbilical fistula****.* Incomplete regression of the urinary end, midportion, or umbilical end of the urachus leads to a **urachal diverticulum**, **umbilical–urachal sinus**, or **urachal cyst**, respectively. The columnar epithelium of urachal remnants may give rise to one third of bladder **adenocarcinomas**.

CONGENITAL VESICOURETERAL VALVE INCOMPETENCE: This anomaly results from an abnormal junction between the ureters and the urinary bladder. The condition is associated with **vesicoureteric reflux** (VUR) (for additional details, see Chapter 14). VUR is more common in young girls than boys and is often familial. In 75% of cases, the condition is asymptomatic, but it may lead to reflux pyelonephritis. Congenital VUR is distinguished from acquired VUR that occurs during pregnancy or with bladder hypertrophy.

Cystitis

Cystitis refers to an inflammation of the bladder. It may be acute or chronic and is the most common urinary tract infection. Cystitis often occurs in hospitalized patients, especially those who have had indwelling bladder catheters.

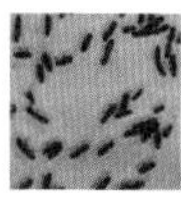

ETIOLOGIC FACTORS: *Cystitis is usually secondary to infection of the lower urinary tract.* Factors related to bladder infection include a patient's age and gender, the presence of bladder calculi, bladder outlet obstruction, diabetes mellitus, immunodeficiency, prior instrumentation or catheterization, radiation therapy, and chemotherapy. ***The risk of cystitis is greater in females because of a short urethra, especially during pregnancy.***

Coliform bacteria are the most common cause of cystitis, mostly *Escherichia coli*, *Proteus vulgaris*, *Pseudomonas aeruginosa*, and *Enterobacter* spp. Schistosomiasis is a common cause of cystitis in North Africa and the Middle East, where *Schistosoma haematobium* is endemic.

Iatrogenic cystitis is common after radiation therapy and chemotherapy. **Radiation cystitis** usually develops 4 to 6 weeks following radiation treatment of pelvic tumors and is most often seen in patients with uterine, rectal, or bladder cancer. Late consequences of radiation cystitis include extensive fibrosis, which may be transmural and incapacitating.

Drug-induced cystitis is most common after cyclophosphamide treatment, which typically produces hemorrhagic cystitis. Other cytotoxic drugs can also cause cystitis, but the injury is less prominent.

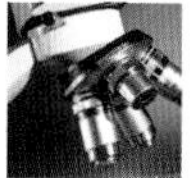

PATHOLOGY: Stromal edema, hemorrhage, and a neutrophilic infiltrate of variable intensity are typical of acute cystitis (Fig. 15-3). Focal petechial mucosal hemorrhages (**hemorrhagic cystitis**) are often seen in acute bacterial cystitis.

Acute cystitis that does not resolve progresses to chronic cystitis, characterized by an infiltrate of lymphocytes and plasma cell, and fibrosis of the lamina propria. Occasionally, an inflamed bladder mucosa contains lymphocytic follicles (**follicular cystitis**) or dense infiltrates of eosinophils (**eosinophilic cystitis**).

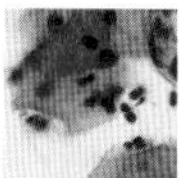

CLINICAL FEATURES: Virtually, all patients with acute or chronic cystitis complain of excessive urinary frequency, painful urination (**dysuria**), and lower abdominal or pelvic discomfort. The urine usually contains inflammatory cells, and the causative agent can be identified by culture. Most cases of acute cystitis respond well to treatment with antimicrobial agents. Recurrent and chronic cystitis often pose therapeutic problems.

Chronic Interstitial Cystitis

Chronic interstitial cystitis is persistent painful inflammation of the bladder in middle-aged women. It has no known cause and presents with suprapubic pain, an urge for frequent urination, hematuria, and dysuria. During cystoscopic dilation of the bladder, the mucosa typically develops hemorrhagic cracks and petechial hemorrhages. Urine cultures are almost always negative. In chronic stages of the disease, transmural inflammation of the bladder wall is occasionally associated with mucosal ulceration **(Hunner ulcer).** Chronic inflammation, including fibrosis and increased mast cells, is common in the mucosa and muscularis. Hunner ulcers feature intense acute inflammation. The disease is typically persistent and refractory to therapy.

Malakoplakia

Malakoplakia is an uncommon inflammatory disorder of unknown etiology. Originally described in the bladder, malakoplakia may be seen in many other sites. It occurs at all ages,

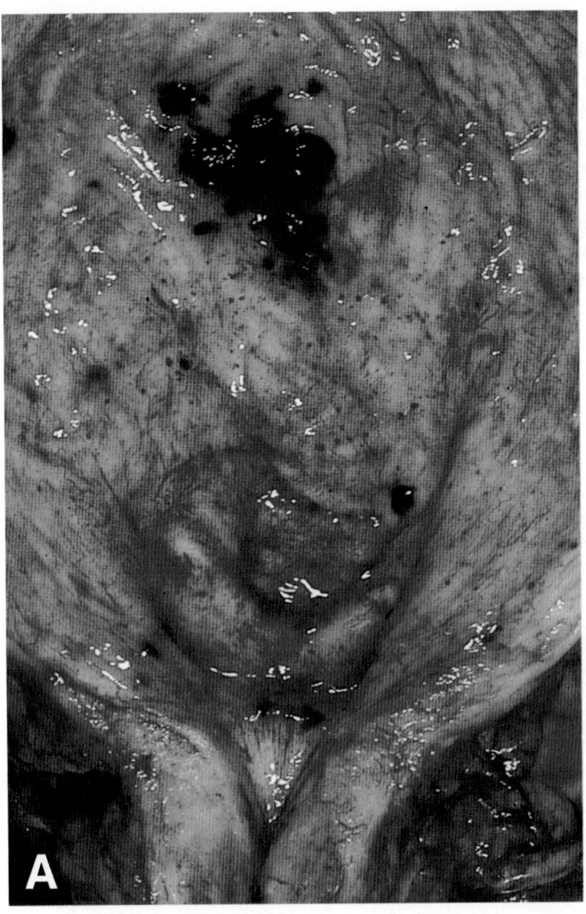

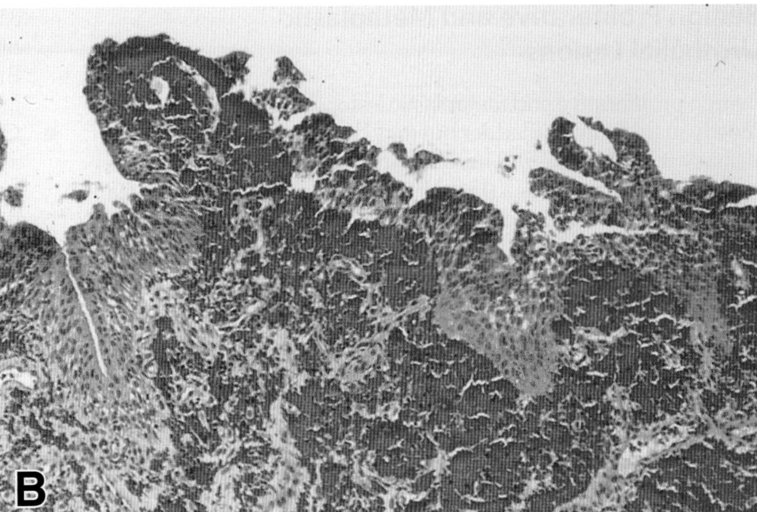

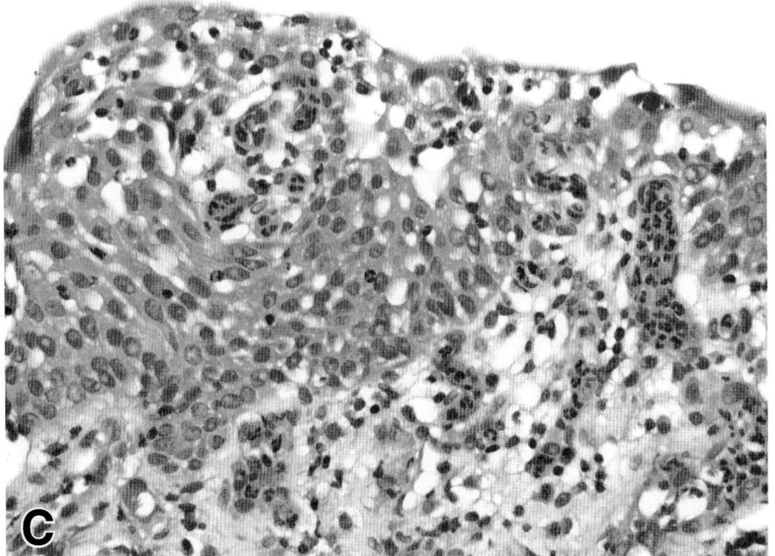

FIGURE 15-3. Acute cystitis. Cystitis was caused by an indwelling catheter. **A.** Several foci of hemorrhage are seen on the hyperemic bladder mucosa. **B.** Microscopic foci of mucosal hemorrhage. **C.** Acute cystitis. Polymorphonuclear leukocytes infiltrate the mucosa.

with a peak incidence in the fifth to seventh decades, and has a marked female preponderance.

Malakoplakia is often associated with urinary tract infection by *E. coli*, although a direct causal relationship is dubious. A clinical background of immunosuppression, chronic infections, or cancer is common.

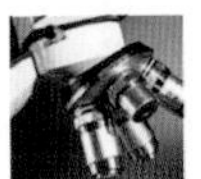

PATHOLOGY: Malakoplakia is characterized by soft, yellow plaques on the mucosal surface of the bladder. There is an intense infiltrate of chronic inflammatory cells mainly composed of large macrophages with abundant, eosinophilic cytoplasm containing PAS-positive granules (Fig. 15-4). Ultrastructurally, these granules are engorged lysosomes that contain fragments of bacteria, suggesting that malakoplakia may reflect an acquired defect in lysosomal degradation. Some of these macrophages have laminated, basophilic calcospherites, called **Michaelis–Gutmann bodies**, which represent calcium salt deposition in the enlarged lysosomes.

The clinical symptoms of malakoplakia of the bladder are indistinguishable from those of other forms of chronic cystitis. Treatment is ineffective.

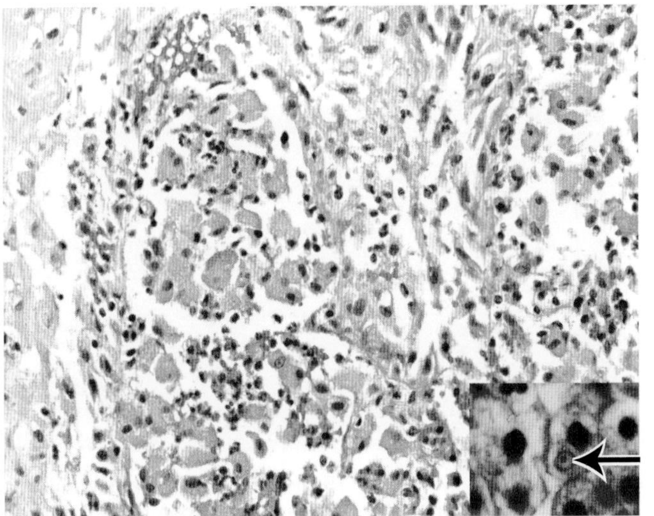

FIGURE 15-4. Malakoplakia. Inflammatory cells are mainly macrophages, with fewer lymphocytes. (*Inset*) A Michaelis–Gutmann body (*arrow*) is seen at high magnification.

Benign Proliferative and Metaplastic Urothelial Lesions

Benign proliferative and metaplastic lesions of urothelium occur mostly in the urinary bladder but may be found anywhere in the urinary tract (Fig. 15-5). These non-neoplastic lesions are characterized by hyperplasia (Fig. 15-5B) or combined hyperplasia and metaplasia. These lesions occur mostly in association with chronic inflammation due to urinary tract infections, calculi, neurogenic bladder, and (rarely) bladder exstrophy. They may also arise without a preexisting inflammatory condition.

- **Brunn buds** are bulbous invaginations of the surface urothelium into the lamina propria. They are found in over 85% of normal bladders and are considered normal variants of the urothelium (Fig. 15-5C). **Brunn nests** are similar to Brunn buds, but the urothelial cells are seen within the lamina propria, detached from the surface.
- **Cystic lesions of the urinary bladder (cystitis cystica)** appear as fluid-filled groups of cysts. Similar cysts can be seen in the urethra or ureter **(urethritis cystica and ureteritis cystica)** (Fig. 15-5C). Cystitis cystica is found in 60% of otherwise normal bladders. Histologically, all these lesions correspond to cystic Brunn nests, lined by normal urothelium. Transitional epithelium may undergo metaplasia into mucus-secreting epithelium, which is then diagnosed as **cystitis glandularis** (Fig. 15-5D).

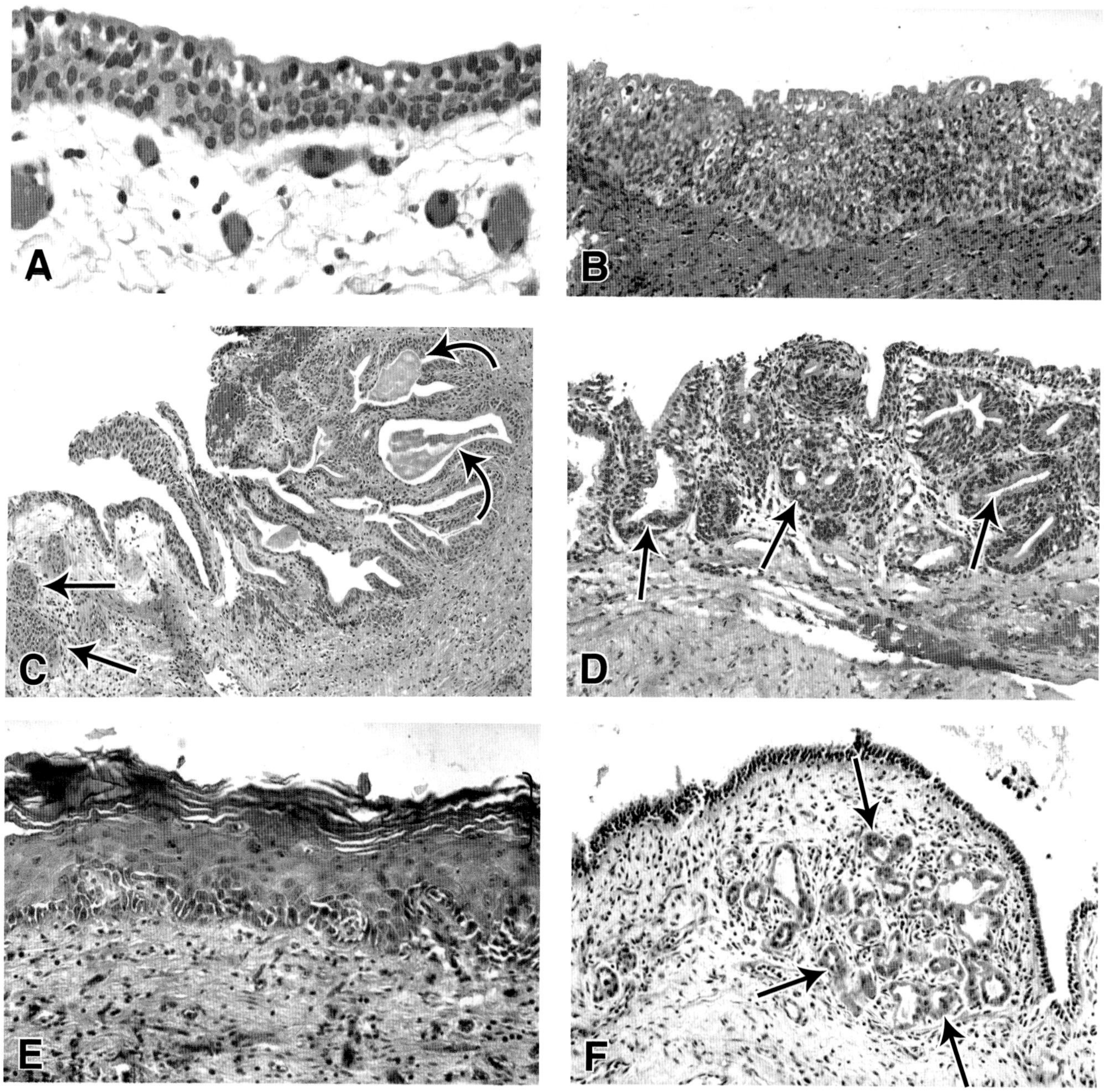

FIGURE 15-5. Proliferative and metaplastic changes of the urinary bladder. A. Normal bladder mucosa. B. Hyperplasia. Note the expansion of the normal 6 to 7 layers of urothelial cells. **C. Cystitis cystica.** Brunn nests (*straight arrows*) and cysts (*curved arrow*) protrude into the lamina propria. **D. Cystitis glandularis.** Metaplastic glandular mucosa is highlighted by the *arrows*. **E. Squamous metaplasia.** Note the keratinizing layer on the superficial epithelium (*bracket*). **F. Nephrogenic metaplasia** (*arrows*).

- **Squamous metaplasia** (Fig. 15-5E) is a reaction to chronic injury and inflammation and is particularly associated with calculi. It is seen in up to half of normal women and 10% of men.
- **Nephrogenic metaplasia** is a lesion caused by transformation of transitional epithelium to resemble renal tubules (Fig. 15-5F). It is most common in the urinary bladder but is also seen in the urethra and ureter. Many small tubules clustered in the lamina propria constitute a papillary exophytic nodule. The histogenesis is unclear, but some cases seem to result from implants of detached renal tubular cells carried downstream by urine. The lesion may produce tumor-like protrusions in the bladder, which may obstruct the ureters and require surgical treatment.

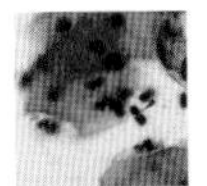

CLINICAL FEATURES: These proliferative and metaplastic urothelial lesions should not be confused with cancer. However, patients with such changes have a higher risk of urothelial bladder carcinoma and, in the case of cystitis glandularis, of **adenocarcinoma** as well. However, there is no evidence to suggest that these lesions themselves are preneoplastic.

Tumors of the Urinary Bladder

The most important aspects of bladder cancer are the following:

- The urinary bladder is the most common site of urinary tract tumors.
- They mostly occur in older patients (median, 65 years) and are rare in patients under age 50.
- Tumors are much more common in men than in women.
- Most tumors (90%) are urothelial malignant neoplasms (formerly called "transitional cell" cancers). Squamous cell cancers, adenocarcinomas, neuroendocrine malignancies, and sarcomas are rare.
- Tumors are often multifocal and can occur in any part of the urinary tract lined by transitional epithelium, from the renal pelvis to the posterior urethra.
- Local treatment is often followed by tumor recurrence.
- Tumor invasion into the muscularis propria markedly decreases the 5-year survival.

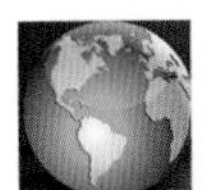

EPIDEMIOLOGY: Bladder cancer represents 7% of all new cancers in men and 2% in women. Bladder cancer shows significant geographic and sex differences throughout the world. The highest frequencies are among urban whites in the United States and Western Europe. It is less common in Japan and among American blacks.

A high incidence of bladder cancer in Egypt, Sudan, and some other African countries is caused by endemic schistosomiasis. Most of such cases are squamous cell carcinomas.

There is no genetic predisposition to bladder cancer, and no hereditary factors have been identified in the vast majority of cases.

The most important risk factors are as follows:

- Cigarette smoking (fourfold increased risk)
- Industrial exposure to azo dyes
- Infection with *S. haematobium* (in endemic regions)
- Drugs, such as cyclophosphamide and analgesics
- Radiation therapy (following cervical, prostate, or rectal cancer)

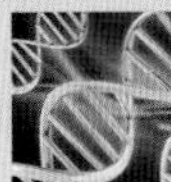

MOLECULAR PATHOGENESIS: ***Specific cytogenetic abnormalities occur in 50% of bladder cancers.*** These often include deletion of chromosome 9, 9p, 9q 11p, 13p, 14q, or 17p, as well as aneuploidy of chromosomes 3, 7, and 17. Deletions within 9p, which contains the **tumor suppressor gene *p16***, are consistent findings in low-grade papillary tumors and flat carcinomas in situ. Deletions in 17p, the site of the tumor suppressor gene ***TP53***, are often identified in invasive bladder cancers.

These genetic abnormalities suggest that cell cycle dysregulation caused by mutated *p53* allows propagation of genetically abnormal urothelial cells. Unregulated proliferation reflects accumulated mutations in cyclin-dependent kinase inhibitors (e.g., p16/INK4a) or deletion of the tumor suppressor gene *RB1* (Fig. 15-6).

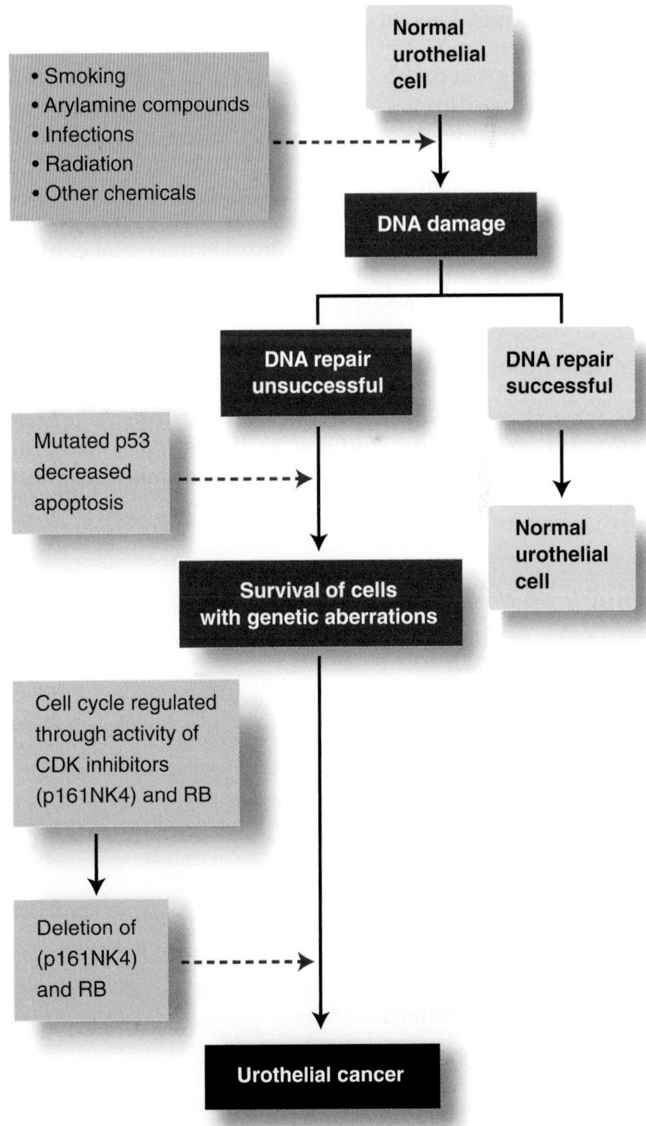

FIGURE 15-6. Hypothetical molecular model of urothelial neoplasms. The transition from normal urothelium to carcinoma occurs gradually in several steps.

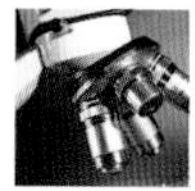

PATHOLOGY: Over 90% of all primary bladder tumors are epithelial tumors, mostly urothelial carcinomas (Table 15-1). Neoplastic urothelial lesions arising from the bladder mucosa comprise a spectrum. One end includes benign papillomas and low-grade exophytic papillary carcinomas. At the other end are invasive urothelial cell carcinomas and highly malignant tumors (Fig. 15-7). Other tumors are considerably less common.

Urothelial Papilloma

These papillomas are usually discovered incidentally in men aged 50 years or older, during cystoscopy for an unrelated condition or for painless hematuria. They represent less than 1% of bladder tumors and have two forms: classic exophytic papilloma and inverted papilloma.

Exophytic papilloma features papillary fronds lined by transitional epithelium, virtually indistinguishable from normal urothelium. On cystoscopy, most patients show single lesions 2 to 5 cm in diameter, but some tumors are multiple. Papillomas are generally considered benign, but some recur or progress to carcinoma, mandating regular follow-up. Most "recurrences" are new tumors that develop elsewhere in the urinary bladder.

Inverted papillomas are rare and typically present as nodular mucosal lesions, usually in the trigone area. The tumors are covered by normal urothelium, from which cords of transitional epithelium descend into the lamina propria. These lesions are most common in men in their sixth and seventh decades. Hematuria of recent onset is the usual clinical presentation. Inverted papillomas are benign tumors and are usually cured by simple excision.

Urothelial Carcinoma In Situ

This term is reserved for full-thickness lesions in which malignant changes are confined to the bladder mucosa. The involved urothelium is of variable thickness, with cellular atypia from the basal layer to the surface (Fig. 15-8). Atypia entails loss of nuclear polarity, nuclear irregularity, enlargement, hyperchromatism, and prominent nucleoli. *The basement membrane is intact, and there is no invasion into underlying stroma.*

One third of carcinomas in situ of the bladder are associated with subsequent invasive carcinoma. In turn, most invasive transitional cell carcinomas arise from carcinoma in situ rather than from papillary transitional cell cancers. Confined to the mucosal surface, in situ lesions most often appear as multiple, red, velvety, flat patches that often are near exophytic papillary transitional cell carcinomas (see below). Concurrent in situ cancers elsewhere in the bladder or ureters, urethra, and prostatic ducts are common. Carcinoma in situ is often multifocal at the time of discovery, or similar lesions may develop shortly thereafter. Tumors involving the bladder neck or the urethra may extend into the periurethral prostatic ducts.

Table 15-1

Tumors of Urinary Bladder

Tumors of Urinary Bladder
Urothelial Tumors
Urothelial cell papilloma
Exophytic papilloma
Inverted papilloma
Urothelial carcinoma in situ
Papillary urothelial neoplasm of low malignant potential
Papillary urothelial carcinoma, low grade[a]
Papillary urothelial carcinoma, high grade[a]
Invasive urothelial carcinoma
Other Malignant Tumors
Squamous cell carcinoma
Adenocarcinoma
Neuroendocrine (small cell) carcinoma
Carcinosarcoma
Sarcomas

[a]Papillary carcinomas may be invasive or noninvasive.

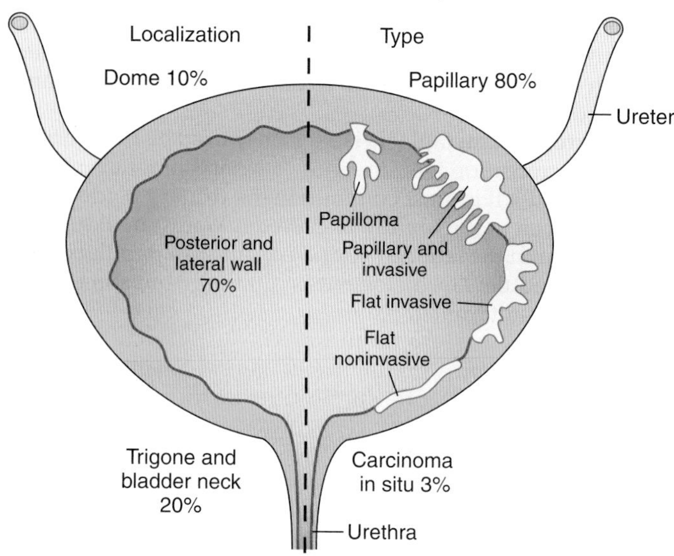

FIGURE 15-7. Urothelial neoplasms. Most tumors localize to the posterior and lateral walls; trigone and bladder neck are involved less often, and the dome least. Malignant tumors may be papillary or flat. Both flat and papillary tumors may be invasive or noninvasive. Benign transitional cell papillomas are rare.

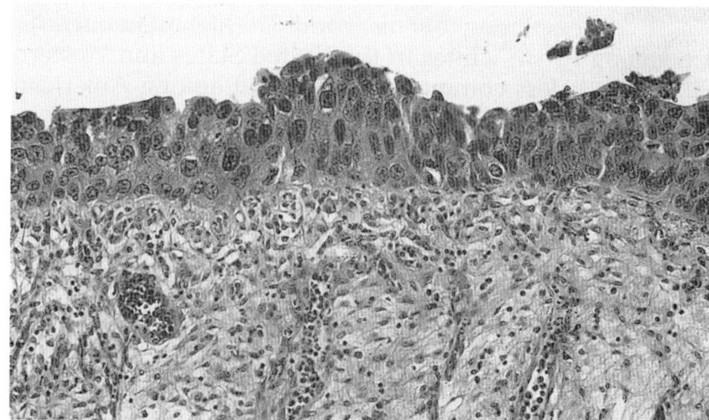

FIGURE 15-8. Urothelial carcinoma in situ. The urothelial mucosa showing nuclear pleomorphism and lack of polarity from the basal layer to the surface, without evidence of maturation.

Urothelial Carcinoma

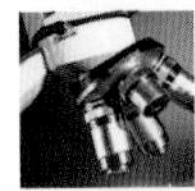

PATHOLOGY: Papillary cancer arises most frequently in the lateral or posterior bladder walls. Grossly, tumors may be small, delicate, low-grade papillary lesions limited to the mucosal surface, or larger, high-grade, solid masses that are invasive and ulcerated (Fig. 15-9).

Cancers are graded as papillary urothelial neoplasms of low malignant potential (PUNLMP) and papillary urothelial carcinomas, low grade and high grade. The latter may be invasive.

- **Papillary urothelial neoplasms of low malignant potential:** These papillary tumors resemble urothelial papillomas but show increased cellularity. They are considered intermediate between benign papillomas and low-grade papillary urothelial carcinomas. These lesions are usually larger than papillomas but lack architectural and cytologic atypia that are characteristic of low-grade carcinomas. PUNLMP may recur after resection or occasionally progress to higher grade tumors.
- **Low-grade papillary urothelial carcinoma:** Low-grade tumors have fronds lined by neoplastic urothelial epithelium with minimal architectural and cytologic atypia (Fig. 15-10A and B). The cells are moderately hyperchromatic with little nuclear pleomorphism and low mitotic activity. Papillae are long and delicate. Invasion of the lamina propria or the deep muscularis propria occurs in 10%.
- **High-grade papillary urothelial carcinoma:** These tumors show significant nuclear hyperchromasia and pleomorphism. The epithelium is disorganized (Fig. 15-10C and D), with mitoses in all layers. Approximately 80% of all high-grade tumors invade the lamina propria and, less often, the muscularis propria, or through the entire thickness of the bladder wall. Regional lymph nodes contain metastatic tumor in half of patients with these invasive tumors.
- **Invasive urothelial carcinoma:** These highly malignant tumors may evolve from papillary lesions or flat carcinomas in situ. In many cases, the nature of the initial lesion is unknown. Most, if not all, invasive carcinomas are high-grade tumors. The depth of invasion into the bladder wall, or beyond, determines the prognosis.

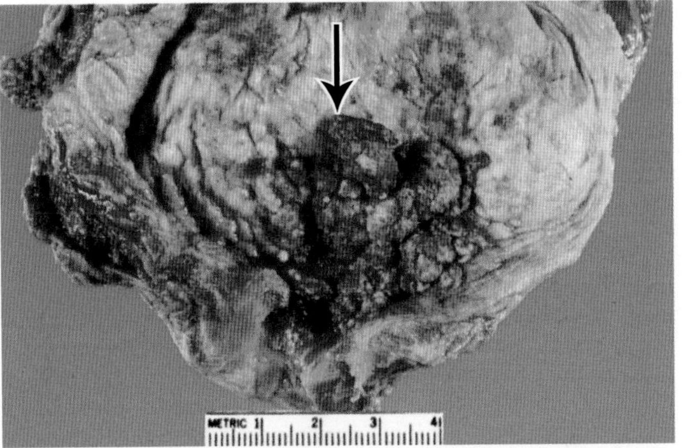

FIGURE 15-9. Urothelial carcinoma of the urinary bladder. A large exophytic tumor (*arrow*) is situated above the bladder neck.

Bladder cancers are staged according to the tumor node metastasis (TNM) system (Table 15-2). In order of decreasing frequency, metastases involve the regional and periaortic lymph nodes, liver, lung, and bone.

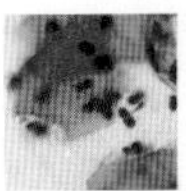

CLINICAL FEATURES: Urothelial carcinoma of the bladder typically manifests as sudden **hematuria** and, less often, **dysuria**. Cystoscopy reveals one or more tumors. At the time of presentation, 85% of tumors are confined to the urinary bladder; 15% show regional or distant metastases. Papillary lesions limited to the mucosa or lamina propria (stage T1) are commonly treated conservatively by transurethral resection. Radical cystectomy is done for patients whose tumors show muscle invasion and occasionally for advanced-stage tumors. In bladder cancer patients, the most common causes of death are uremia (from urinary outflow tract obstruction), extension into adjacent organs, and effects of distant metastases.

The probability of tumor extension and subsequent recurrence increases with the following:

- Increased tumor size
- High stage
- High grade
- Presence of multiple tumors
- Vascular or lymphatic invasion
- Urothelial dysplasia (including carcinoma in situ) at other sites in the bladder

The overall 10-year survival rate with noninvasive or superficially invasive low-grade urothelial tumors exceeds 95%, irrespective of the number of recurrences. Only 10% of low-grade tumors progress to higher grade tumors and thus a worse prognosis. Conservative treatment includes fulguration, intravesicular immunotherapy with BCG, or instillation of conventional chemotherapeutic agents. Invasive tumors or those refractory to conservative therapy are treated by cystectomy, possibly with adjuvant systemic chemotherapy. Tumors invading the bladder muscle have 25% to 30% overall mortality.

Recurrent or progressive disease is detected by cystoscopy and biopsy, or by less invasive techniques such as urinalysis for tumor markers, urine cytology, and cytogenic analysis of desquamated cells. Currently, aneuploidy for chromosomes 3, 7, and 17 and loss of 9p21 are detected.

Nonurothelial Bladder Cancers

Squamous cell bladder carcinomas develop in foci of squamous metaplasia, usually due to schistosomiasis. Bladder wall invasion is common by initial presentation, and prognosis is poor.

Adenocarcinomas are 1% of malignant bladder tumors. They derive from urachal epithelial remnants, foci of cystitis glandularis, or intestinal metaplasia. Most bladder adenocarcinomas are deeply invasive when they initially present and are not curable.

Neuroendocrine carcinoma, resembling small cell lung carcinoma, occurs uncommonly in the urinary bladder. It is highly malignant and has a poor prognosis.

Sarcomas of the bladder are rare. They are highly malignant, form bulky masses, and are often inoperable. **Leiomyosarcoma** is the most common form in adults.

Rhabdomyosarcoma, typically of the embryonal type, occurs mostly as **sarcoma botryoides** in children, as edematous, mucosal, polypoid masses resembling a cluster of grapes.

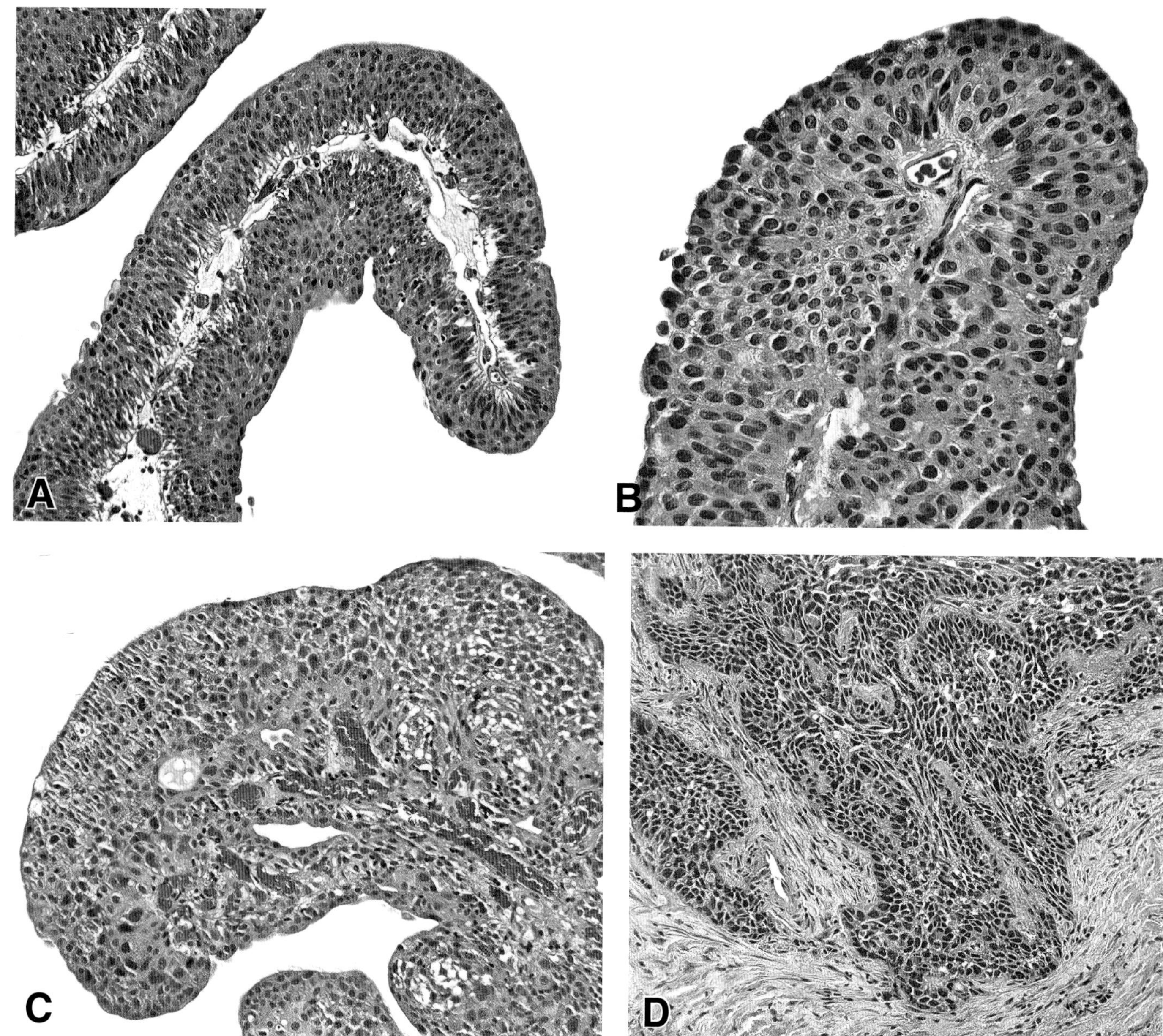

FIGURE 15-10. Urothelial tumors of the urinary bladder. A. Low-grade papillary urothelial carcinoma consists of exophytic papillae that have a central connective tissue core and are lined by slightly disorganized transitional epithelium. **B.** Low-grade papillary urothelial carcinoma at higher magnification showing mild architectural and cytologic atypia. **C.** High-grade papillary urothelial carcinoma displaying prominent architectural disorganization of the epithelium, which contains cells with pleomorphic hyperchromatic nuclei. **D.** Invasive high-grade papillary urothelial carcinoma consists of irregular nests of hyperchromatic cells invading into the muscularis.

Combined treatment with radiation therapy and chemotherapy has greatly increased survival rates.

PENIS, URETHRA, AND SCROTUM

Congenital Disorders of the Penis

Developmental anomalies of the penis include anomalies of the penile urethra and prepuce.

HYPOSPADIAS: ***This congenital anomaly features a urethra that opens on the underside (ventral) of the penis; the meatus is thus proximal to its normal location on the tip of the penis.*** It results from incomplete closure of the urethral folds of the urogenital sinus.

Hypospadias occurs in 1 in 350 male babies. Most cases are sporadic, but familial occurrence is known. It may be associated with other urogenital anomalies and complex, multisystemic, developmental syndromes. In 90% of cases, the meatus is located on the underside of the glans or the corona.

Table 15-2

TNM Staging of Urothelial Carcinoma of Urinary Bladder

T—Primary Tumor
T0 No grossly visible tumor
Ta Noninvasive papillary carcinoma
Tis Carcinoma in situ
T1 Invasion of the lamina propria
T2 Invasion of the muscularis propria
T2a Superficial invasion of the muscularis (inner half)
T2b Invasion of deep muscle (outer half)
T3 Invasion of the perivesical tissue
T4 Extravesical spread into adjacent organs or distant metastases
N—Regional Lymph Nodes
N0 No lymph node involvement
N1 Single lymph node metastasis
N2, N3 More lymph nodes involved
M—Distant Metastases
M0 No metastases
M1 Distant metastases

Less often, it occurs midshaft, in the scrotum or even in the perineum. Surgical repair is usually uncomplicated.

*EPISPADIAS: **In this rare congenital anomaly, the urethra opens on the upper side (dorsum) of the penis.*** In its most common form, the entire penile urethra is open along the whole shaft. Severe epispadias is sometimes associated with bladder exstrophy (Fig. 15-11). In its mildest form, the defect is limited to the glandular urethra. Surgical treatment of epispadias is more complicated than that of hypospadias.

*PHIMOSIS: **The orifice of the prepuce may be too narrow to allow retraction over the glans penis.*** Phimosis may be congenital or acquired. The latter is usually a consequence of recurrent infections or trauma of the prepuce in uncircumcised men. Circumcision is curative.

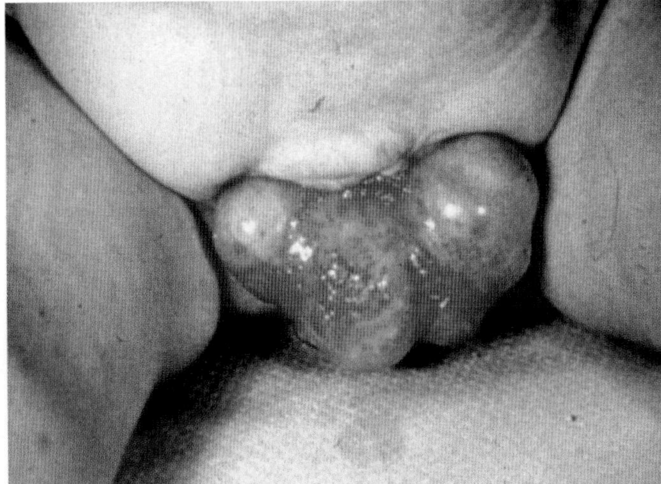

FIGURE 15-11. Exstrophy of the urinary bladder. From Weiss MA, Mills SE. *Atlas of Genitourinary Tract Diseases.* New York, NY: Gower Medical Publishers, 1988.

Scrotal Masses

Non-neoplastic scrotal masses and conditions that lead to scrotal swelling or enlargement often reflect abnormalities of testicular, epididymal, and scrotal development. Clinical problems related to these conditions are most often seen in children but may be found in adults (Fig. 15-12A to D).

HYDROCELE: This swelling reflects a collection of serous fluid in the scrotal sac between the two layers of the tunica vaginalis. Hydroceles are congenital or acquired.

Congenital hydrocele is the most common cause of scrotal swelling in infants and is often associated with inguinal hernia.

Acquired hydrocele in adults is caused by some other disease affecting the scrotum, such as infection, tumor, or trauma. The diagnosis is made by ultrasound or by transluminating the fluid in the cavity. Hydrocele is a benign condition that

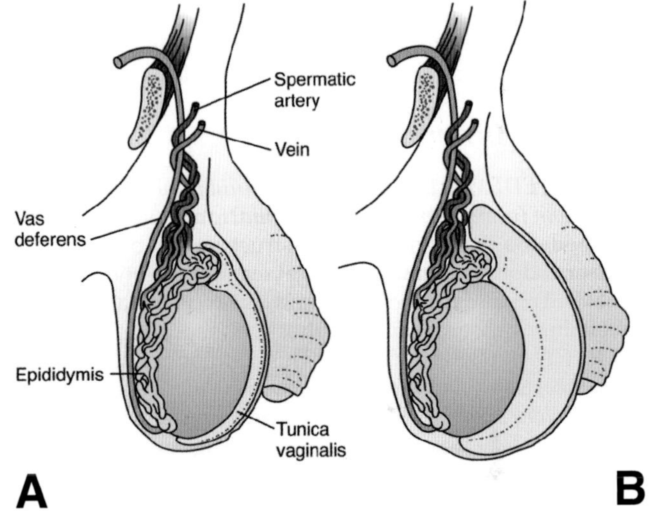

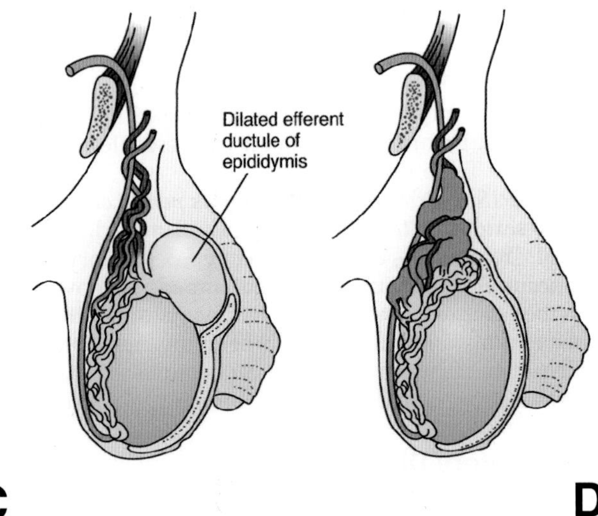

FIGURE 15-12. Scrotal masses. A. Normal testis and appendages. **B.** Hydrocele of tunica vaginalis. **C.** Spermatocele. **D.** Varicocele of spermatic cord veins.

disappears once the cause has been addressed. However, long-standing hydrocele may cause testicular atrophy or compress the epididymis, or the fluid may become infected and lead to **periorchitis**.

HEMATOCELE: ***Blood may accumulate between the layers of tunica vaginalis after trauma or hemorrhage into a hydrocele,*** or as a result of testicular tumors or infections.

SPERMATOCELE: ***This mass is a cyst formed from protrusions of widened efferent ducts of the rete testis or epididymis.*** It manifests as a hilar paratesticular nodule or a fluctuating mass filled with milky fluid. The cyst is lined by cuboidal epithelium that contains spermatozoa in various stages of degeneration.

VARICOCELE: ***This dilation of testicular veins appears as a nodularity on the lateral side of the scrotum.*** Most are asymptomatic and are considered a common cause of infertility and oligospermia. Testicular atrophy occurs only rarely and only in long-standing cases. Surgical ligation of the internal spermatic vein often improves reproductive function.

SCROTAL INGUINAL HERNIA: ***Intestinal protrusion into the scrotum through the inguinal canal is termed a scrotal hernia.*** The bowel may be repositioned, but if it remains untreated, such a hernia may cause adhesions or testicular atrophy. Hernias can only be repaired surgically.

Circulatory Disturbances

SCROTAL EDEMA: ***Lymph or serous fluid may accumulate in the scrotum from obstruction to lymphatic or venous drainage.*** **Lymphedema** from lymphatic obstruction can be caused by pelvic or abdominal tumors, surgical scars, or infections such as filariasis. **Transudation** of plasma is common in patients with heart failure, anasarca due to cirrhosis, or nephrotic syndrome.

ERECTILE DYSFUNCTION: This condition, also known as impotence, is *inability to achieve or maintain an erection sufficient for satisfactory sexual performance.* Its prevalence increases with age, from 20% at age 40 years to 50% by age 70.

Erection requires adequate filling of the penile corpora cavernosa and spongiosa with blood. Penile tumescence is the result of a complex interaction of mental, neural, hormonal, and vascular factors. Filling of these vascular spaces depends on nitric oxide (NO•)-mediated relaxation of vascular smooth muscle cells in the erectile cylinders. NO• release is related to cGMP so drugs that inhibit the phosphodiesterase that degrades cGMP (e.g., sildenafil [Viagra], vardenafil hydrochloride [Levitra], tadalafil [Cialis]) are used to treat erectile dysfunction. Disorders associated with erectile dysfunction are listed in Table 15-3.

PRIAPISM: Priapism is ***continuous penile erection unrelated to sexual excitation.*** Primary priapism is idiopathic and painful. Treatment is usually ineffective. Secondary priapism may occur in (1) pelvic diseases that impede outflow of blood from the penis (e.g., pelvic tumors or hematomas, thrombosis of pelvic veins, and infections); (2) hematologic disorders (e.g., sickle cell anemia, polycythemia vera, and leukemia); and (3) brain and spinal cord diseases (e.g., tumors and neurosyphilis).

Inflammatory Disorders

The most important inflammatory diseases of the penis are (1) sexually transmitted diseases (STDs); (2) nonspecific infections; (3) diseases of unknown etiology, such as balanitis xerotica obliterans; (4) dermatoses; and (5) dermatitis of the penile shaft and scrotum (Table 15-4).

Table 15-3

Erectile Dysfunctions

Neuropsychiatric
Psychiatric disorders (e.g., depression)
Spinal cord injury
Nerve injury during surgery (e.g., pelvic or perineal surgery)
Endocrine
Hypogonadism
Pituitary diseases (e.g., hyperprolactinemia)
Hypothyroidism, Cushing syndrome, Addison disease
Vascular
Diabetic microangiopathy
Hypertension
Atherosclerosis
Drugs
Antihypertensives
Psychotropic drugs
Estrogens, anticancer drugs, etc.
Idiopathic
"Performance anxiety"
Age-related "impotence"

Table 15-4

Inflammatory Lesions of the Penis

Sexually Transmitted Diseases
Herpes genitalis
Syphilis
Chancroid
Granuloma inguinale
Lymphogranuloma venereum
Human papillomavirus infections
Nonspecific Infectious Balanoposthitis
Bacterial, fungal, viral
Diseases of Unknown Etiology
Balanitis xerotica obliterans
Circinate balanitis
Plasma cell balanitis (Zoon balanitis)
Peyronie disease
Dermatitis Involving the Shaft of the Penis and Scrotum
Infectious (bacterial, viral, fungal)
Noninfectious (e.g., lichen planus, bullous skin diseases)

Sexually Transmitted Diseases

STDs (see Chapters 6 and 16) and lower urinary tract infections (Fig. 15-13) include the following:

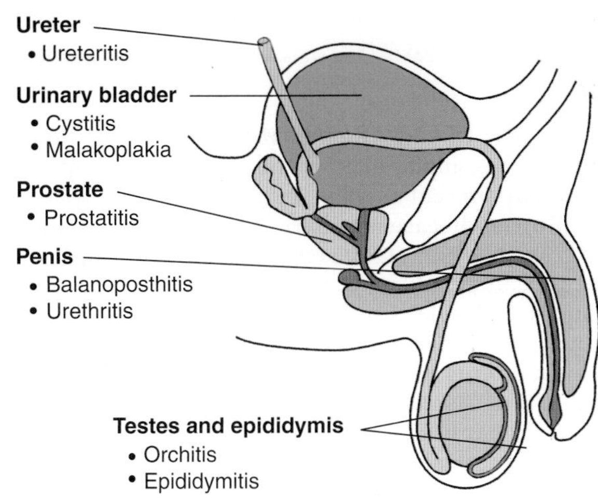

FIGURE 15-13. **Infections of the lower urinary tract and male reproductive system.**

- **Genital herpes** is most often caused by herpes simplex virus (HSV)-2 or, less commonly, by HSV-1. It is the most common STD affecting the glans and manifests typically as grouped vesicles that ulcerate and transform into crusts.
- **Primary syphilis**, caused by the spirochete, *Treponema pallidum*, may manifest as a solitary, soft ulcer (**chancre**), accompanied by palpable inguinal lymphadenopathy.
- **Chancroid** is caused by *Haemophilus ducreyi* and presents as a papule that transforms into a pustule and finally ulcerates. Shallow ulcers on the glans or the skin of the shaft are often associated with painful, suppurative, inguinal lymphadenitis.
- **Granuloma inguinale** is a tropical disease caused by *Calymmatobacterium granulomatis.* It appears as a raised ulcer with a copious chronic inflammatory exudate and granulation tissue. Such ulcers tend to enlarge and heal very slowly.
- **Lymphogranuloma venereum** is caused by *Chlamydia trachomatis.* It starts as a small, often innocuous, vesicle that ulcerates. The lesion is typically accompanied by tender enlargement of inguinal lymph nodes, which adhere to the skin and form sinuses draining pus and serosanguinous fluid.
- **Condyloma acuminatum** is caused by human papillomavirus type 6 or, less often, human papillomavirus type 11. It appears as flat-topped warts on the shaft (Fig. 15-14), small polyps on the glans and urethral meatus, or larger cauliflower-like tumors that may be confused with verrucous carcinoma.

Balanitis

In uncircumcised men, balanitis usually extends from the glans to the foreskin and is called **balanoposthitis**. Mostly, it is caused by bacteria, but it may also be produced by fungi in diabetics or immunosuppressed people. Balanitis typically reflects poor hygiene. Significant complications of chronic balanoposthitis are meatal stricture, phimosis, and paraphimosis.

BALANITIS XEROTICA OBLITERANS: This idiopathic chronic inflammatory condition is equivalent to lichen sclerosus of the vulva (see Chapter 16) and is characterized by fibrosis and sclerosis of subepithelial connective tissue. The affected portion of the glans is white and indurated. Fibrosis may constrict the urethral meatus or cause phimosis.

Peyronie Disease

This disorder is characterized by focal, asymmetric fibrosis of the penile shaft. During erections, the penis becomes curved and painful. Typically, it presents as an ill-defined induration of the penile shaft in a young or middle-aged

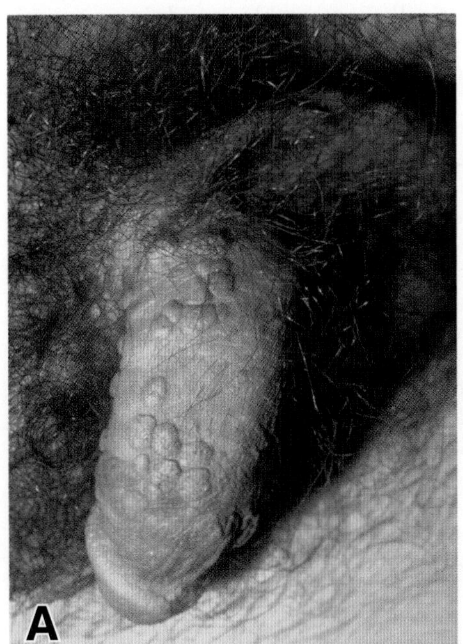

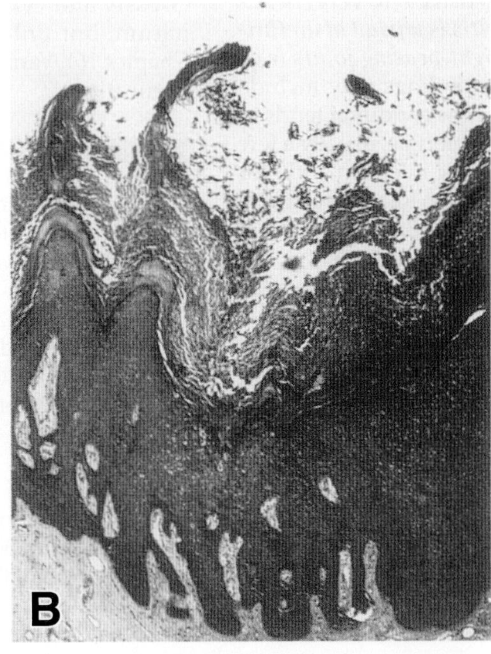

FIGURE 15-14. **Condylomata acuminata of the penis.** **A.** Raised, circumscribed lesions are seen on the shaft of the penis. **B.** Section of a lesion showing epidermal hyperkeratosis, parakeratosis, acanthosis, and papillomatosis.

man, with no change in the overlying skin. Microscopically, dense fibrosis is associated with sparse, chronic inflammation. Collagen focally replaces muscle in the septum of the corpus cavernosum.

Peyronie disease affects 1% of men over age 40. In most instances, it is mild and does not interfere with sexual function. Severe cases may be so incapacitating as to require surgery, but the outcome is not always satisfactory.

Urethritis

Urethritis refers to acute or chronic inflammation of the urethra.

SEXUALLY TRANSMITTED URETHRITIS: ***Urethritis presenting as urethral discharge is the most common sign of STDs in men.*** Women rarely notice distinct urethral discharge and usually complain of vaginal discharge.

Gonococcal and nongonococcal urethritis have an acute onset, related to recent sexual intercourse. The discharge is typically purulent and greenish yellow. Symptoms include redness and swelling, pain or tingling at the meatus of the urethra, and pain on micturition **(dysuria)** (see Chapters 6 and 16).

NONSPECIFIC INFECTIOUS URETHRITIS: ***Uropathogens such as E. coli and P. aeruginosa can cause urethritis.*** Typically, infection is associated with cystitis but may be caused by other diseases (e.g., prostatic hyperplasia or urinary stones).

Nonspecific infectious urethritis manifests clinically with urgency and a burning sensation during urination. Usually, there is no discharge, but men may express some milky fluid by "stripping" or "milking" the urethra.

URETHRAL CARUNCLES: ***Polypoid inflammatory lesions near the female urethral meatus cause pain and bleeding.*** They are idiopathic and occur only in women, mostly after menopause. Urethral prolapse and attendant chronic inflammation may be implicated.

Urethral caruncles present as 1- to 2-cm exophytic, often ulcerated, polypoid masses, at or near the urethral meatus. They show acutely and chronically inflamed granulation tissue and ulceration and hyperplasia of transitional cell or squamous epithelium.

REACTIVE ARTHRITIS (FORMERLY KNOWN AS REITER SYNDROME): ***Reactive arthritis is a triad of urethritis, conjunctivitis, and arthritis of weight-bearing joints (e.g., knee and intervertebral joints).*** Other findings may include balanitis, cervicitis, and skin eruptions. The condition tends to affect young adults with the HLA-B27 haplotype, usually a few weeks after chlamydial urethritis or enteric infection with, for example *Shigella, Salmonella, or Campylobacter.* Reactive arthritis may thus be an aberrant immune reaction to unknown microbial antigen(s). Symptoms usually disappear spontaneously in 3 to 6 months, but arthritis recurs in half of patients (See Chapter 22).

Tumors

Penile Cancer

Cancer of the penis originates from the squamous mucosa of the glans and contiguous urethral meatus or the prepuce and skin covering the penile shaft. It is uncommon in the United States but more frequent in underdeveloped countries. The tumor is virtually unknown in men circumcised at birth. HPV types 16 and 18 play a role in many penile cancers, and phimosis and cigarette smoking are risk factors.

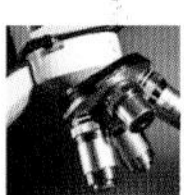

PATHOLOGY: Penile carcinoma may be preinvasive (in situ) or invasive.

SQUAMOUS CELL CARCINOMA IN SITU: Carcinoma in situ of the penis is similar to that in other sites (see Chapter 28). Grossly, it may present as Bowen disease or erythroplasia of Queyrat. **Bowen disease** is a sharply demarcated, erythematous, or grayish white plaque on the shaft. **Erythroplasia of Queyrat** appears as solitary or multiple, shiny, soft, erythematous plaques on the glans and foreskin. Both of these resemble **squamous cell carcinoma in situ** elsewhere. Progression to invasive squamous cell carcinoma is estimated to occur in less than 10% of cases.

Bowenoid papulosis of the penis is caused by HPV and affects young, sexually active men. In contrast to the solitary lesion of Bowen disease, Bowenoid papulosis appears as multiple brownish or violaceous papules. The lesions are sharply demarcated from normal epidermis, similar to HPV-induced warts. The altered epidermis shows some superficial stratification and maturation and may contain giant keratinocytes with multinucleated atypical nuclei. HPV type 16 can be demonstrated in 80% of patients, and type 18 is occasionally implicated. Virtually, all cases of Bowenoid papulosis regress spontaneously and do not progress to invasive carcinoma.

INVASIVE SQUAMOUS CELL CARCINOMA: The tumor presents as (1) an ulcer, (2) an indurated crater, (3) a friable hemorrhagic mass, or (4) an exophytic, fungating, papillary tumor. It usually involves the glans or prepuce and, less commonly, the penile shaft. Extensive destruction of penile tissue, including the urethral meatus, is seen when the tumor has been neglected. Microscopically, these are typically well-differentiated, focally keratinizing, squamous cell carcinomas. Invasive tumors usually have underlying dense, chronic inflammation. The tumor may invade deeply along the shaft and spread to inguinal lymph nodes, then to iliac nodes, and ultimately to distant organs.

VERRUCOUS CARCINOMA: Although it is cytologically benign, this tumor is a clinically malignant exophytic squamous cell carcinoma and verrucous carcinoma. Grossly and cytologically, it resembles **condyloma acuminatum**, but unlike the latter, it shows local invasion (see Chapter 16). Verrucous carcinoma rarely metastasizes. Surgery is curative.

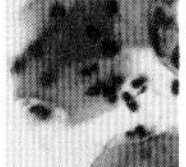

CLINICAL FEATURES: Most squamous cell cancers are confined to the penis at the time of presentation. Occult metastases to inguinal lymph nodes occur, but half of patients with enlarged regional lymph nodes do not have nodal metastases; reactive changes are as a result of tumor-associated inflammation.

Survival of patients with penile cancer is related to the clinical stage and, to a lesser degree, histologic grade of the tumor. Amputation of the penis is usually necessary. HPV infection is present in at least half of cases.

Scrotal Cancer

Squamous carcinoma of the scrotum typically affects men mostly in their 50s and 60s. At presentation, many tumors show invasion of the scrotal contents and metastases to regional nodes. Therapy is surgical excision. As in penile cancer, HPV has been often implicated.

TESTIS, EPIDIDYMIS, AND VAS DEFERENS

Cryptorchidism

Cryptorchidism, clinically known as* undescended testis, *is a congenital abnormality in which one or both testes are not in the scrotum. It is the most common urologic condition requiring surgical treatment in infants. The condition affects 5% of term male infants and 30% of those born prematurely. In the large majority of patients, testes descend into the scrotum in the first year of life. Thus, the prevalence of cryptorchidism from the end of the first year of life into adulthood is about 1%. It is bilateral in 30% of affected men.

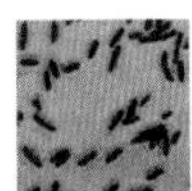

ETIOLOGIC FACTORS: Testicular maldescent is usually an idiopathic and isolated developmental disorder. It is rarely associated with other congenital anomalies.

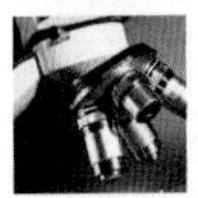

PATHOLOGY: Testicular descent may be arrested at any point from the abdominal cavity to the upper scrotum (Fig. 15-15). Cryptorchid testes are classified by their location as **abdominal, inguinal, or upper scrotal**. Rarely, the testes are located in unusual sites, such as the perineum or calf.

Cryptorchid testes are smaller than normal, even at an early age, and differences between the affected and unaffected testes increase with age. The testes are firm and show fibrosis.

The histology of cryptorchid testes varies with age. In infancy and early childhood, the seminiferous tubules in affected testes are smaller, with fewer than normal germ cells. Postpubertal testes also show decreased germ cells, and spermatogenesis is limited to a minority of tubules. Hyaline thickening of tubular basement membranes and prominent stromal fibrosis are observed (Fig. 15-16). Eventually, tubules lose all spermatogenic cells and are entirely hyalinized. **Orchiopexy** (surgical placement of a testis into the scrotum) done either in childhood or after puberty does not prevent loss of seminiferous epithelium and tubules; both untreated and repositioned testes lack all spermatogenesis in half of the cases.

A few adult cryptorchid testes (2%) contain atypical germ cells corresponding to carcinoma in situ.

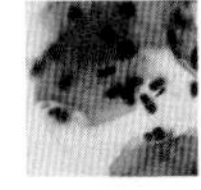

CLINICAL FEATURES: The clinical significance of undescended testes is that they entail increased incidences of **infertility** and **germ cell neoplasia**. All men with bilateral cryptorchid testes have **azoospermia** and are infertile. Unilateral cryptorchidism is associated with **oligospermia**, defined as a sperm count below 20 million/mL, in 40% of cases. Although oligospermia is a cause of reduced fertility, most men with one normal testis can father children. **Orchiopexy** (surgical placement of a testis into the scrotum) unless done prior to 1 year of age does not prevent a reduction in spermatogenesis in adulthood. For this reason, most urologists recommend the procedure be performed between 6 months and 1 year of age. ***Cryptorchidism is associated with a 20- to 40-fold increased risk for testicular cancer.*** Conversely, 10% of patients with germ cell neoplasia have cryptorchid testes. Intra-abdominal testes are at higher risk than those retained in the inguinal canal; in turn, inguinal testes are at higher risk than those high in the scrotum. A contralateral, normally descended testis is also at risk, about four times that in normal men. Unfortunately, orchiopexy does not eliminate the risk of cancer. However, if performed prior to puberty, the risk is substantially reduced.

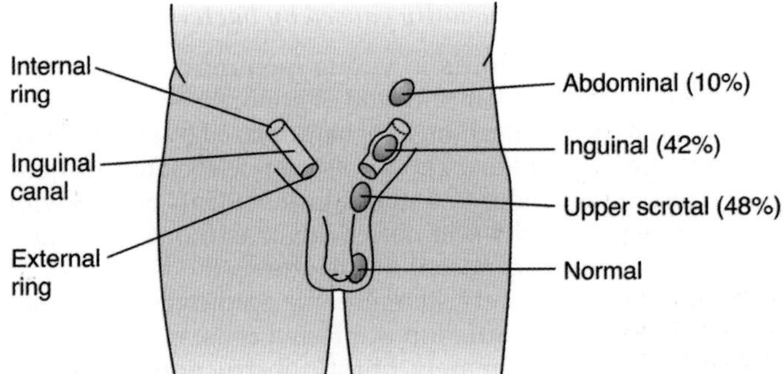

FIGURE 15-15. Cryptorchidism. In most instances, the testis has an upper scrotal location. It may also be retained in the inguinal canal and, rarely, in the abdominal cavity.

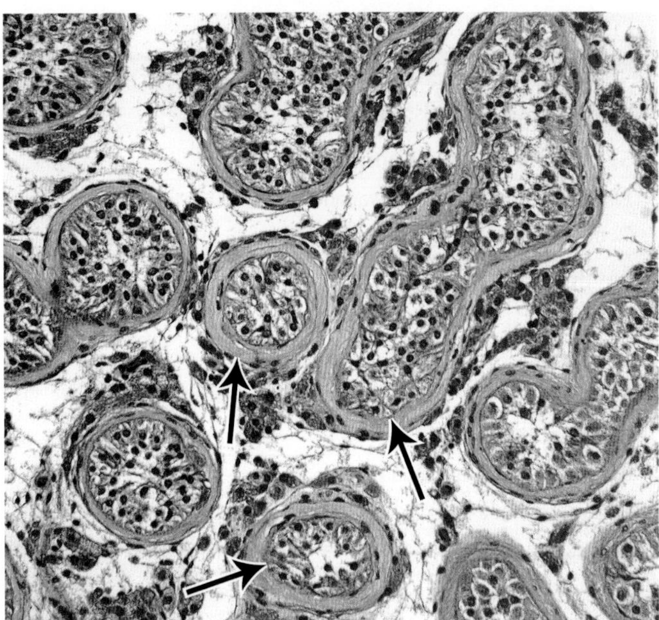

FIGURE 15-16. Cryptorchidism. The testis removed from a postpubertal man showing a markedly thickened hyalinized basement membrane (*arrows*) of seminiferous tubules, which show no signs of spermatogenesis.

Abnormalities of Sexual Differentiation

Disorders of gonadogenesis and formation of external genital organs, as well as development of secondary sex characteristics, can pertain to

- genetic sex (the presence or absence of X and Y chromosomes)
- gonadal sex (the presence or absence of testes or ovaries)
- genital sex (the appearance of external genital organs)
- psychosocial sexual orientation

Various conditions are listed in Table 15-5. Some of these, such as Klinefelter and Turner syndromes, are discussed in Chapter 5.

HERMAPHRODITISM: ***This rare developmental disorder is characterized by ambiguous genitalia in someone who exhibits both male and female gonads.*** Gonads may become ovotestes (combination of ovary and testis) or one gonad may

Table 15-5

Disorders of Sexual Differentiation
Sex Chromosomal Abnormalities
Klinefelter syndrome and its variants
Turner syndrome 46,XX males
Single-Gene Defects
Adrenogenital syndromes
Androgen insensitivity syndromes
Müllerian inhibitory substance deficiency
Prenatal Hormonal Effects
Exogenous hormones during pregnancy
Maternal hormone-producing tumors
Idiopathic Conditions
Hermaphroditism
Gonadal dysgenesis

be testis and the other ovary. Half of these patients have a female karyotype (46,XX). The others are genetic males (46,XY) or mosaics, or have a missing sex chromosome (45,X).

FEMALE PSEUDOHERMAPHRODITISM: ***Virilization of external genitalia may occur in genetic females (46,XX) who have normal ovaries and internal female genital organs.*** The vulva may fuse into scrotal folds, and clitoromegaly is common. This phenotype is most often seen in the adrenogenital syndrome (see Chapter 19).

MALE PSEUDOHERMAPHRODITISM: ***A spectrum of congenital disorders affects genetic males who have a normal 46,XY karyotype.*** The gonads are cryptorchid testes, but external genitalia appear feminine or ambiguously female with some virilization. Male pseudohermaphroditism occurs most often in **androgen insensitivity syndromes** caused by deficiency of the androgen receptor, also known as **testicular feminization syndrome.**

Male Infertility

Infertility is empirically defined as inability to conceive after 1 year of coital activity with the same sexual partner without contraception. Some 15% of couples are childless in the United States, but the true prevalence of infertility is difficult to assess because it is confounded by cultural and social issues. The male is infertile in 20% of couples, the female in 40%, and both partners in 20%. In the remaining 20% of infertile couples, no cause can be identified. The causes of male infertility are listed in Table 15-6 and are illustrated in Figure 15-17.

Table 15-6

Causes of Male Infertility
Supratesticular Causes
Disorders of the hypothalamic–pituitary–gonadal axis
Endocrine disease of the adrenal, thyroid; diabetes
Metabolic disorders
Major organ diseases (e.g., renal, hepatic, cardiopulmonary diseases)
Chronic infectious and debilitating diseases (e.g., tuberculosis, AIDS)
Drugs and substance abuse
Testicular Causes
Idiopathic: hypospermatogenesis or azoospermia
Developmental (cryptorchidism, gonadal dysgenesis)
Genetic disorders (e.g., Klinefelter syndrome)
Orchitis (immune and infectious)
Iatrogenic testicular injury (radiation, cytotoxic drugs)
Trauma of the testis and surgical injury
Environmental (possibly phytoestrogens)
Posttesticular Causes
Congenital anomalies of the excretory ducts
Inflammation and scarring of excretory ducts
Iatrogenic or posttraumatic lesions of excretory ducts

PATHOLOGY: Testicular biopsy may identify the causes of infertility:

- **Immaturity of seminiferous tubules** is seen in hypogonadotropic hypogonadism caused by pituitary or hypothalamic diseases. Seminiferous tubules show no spermatogenesis and resemble those of prepubertal testes.
- **Decreased spermatogenesis (hypospermatogenesis)** occurs in several systemic and endocrine diseases, including malnutrition and AIDS. Hypospermatogenesis is also found in cryptorchid testes and after vasectomy.
- **Germ cell maturation arrest** is usually idiopathic. It can occur at any stage of maturation.
- **Germ cell aplasia** ("Sertoli cells only" syndrome) is mostly idiopathic (Fig. 15-18).
- **Orchitis** is caused by viruses (e.g., mumps) or autoimmune diseases.
- **Peritubular and tubular fibrosis** may be related to congenital disorders such as cryptorchidism or to previous infection, ischemia, or radiation.

Epididymitis

- ***Epididymitis is the term for acute or chronic inflammation of the epididymis, usually caused by bacteria.***

Bacterial epididymitis in young men most often occurs in an acute form as a complication of gonorrhea or a sexually acquired *Chlamydia* infection. It is characterized by suppurative inflammation. In older men, *E. coli* from associated urinary tract infections is a more common culprit. Patients present with intrascrotal pain and tenderness, with or without associated fever. Epididymitis of recent origin shows the hallmarks of acute inflammation. Persistent chronic epididymitis is associated with the accumulation of plasma cells, macrophages, and lymphocytes; ultimately, fibrotic obstruction of infected ducts occurs. Gonorrheal epididymitis is a common cause of acquired male infertility.

Spermatic granulomas result from intense inflammatory responses to sperm outside their usual channels. Traumatic

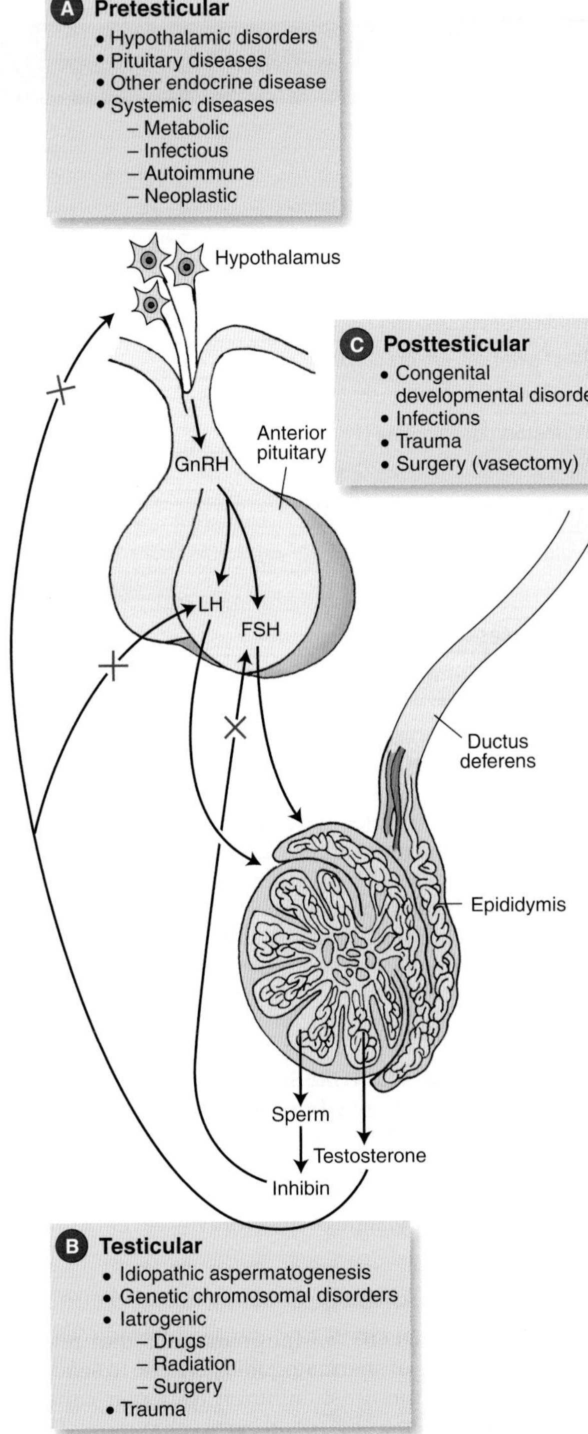

FIGURE 15-17. Causes of male infertility. A. Pretesticular infertility. **B.** Testicular infertility. **C.** Posttesticular (obstructive) infertility. FSH, follicle-stimulating hormone; GnRH, gonadotropin-releasing hormone; LH, luteinizing hormone.

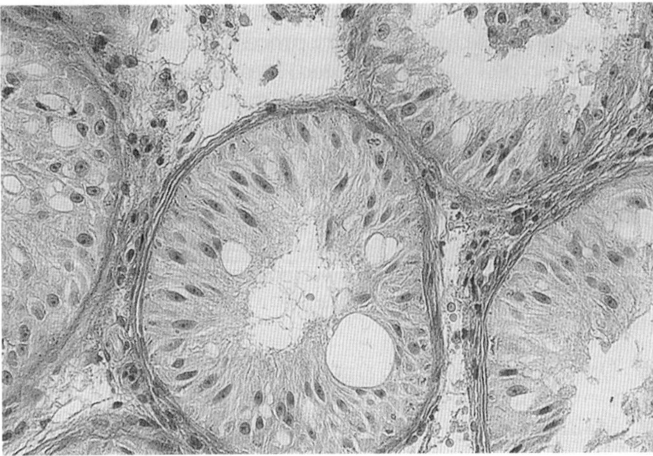

FIGURE 15-18. Germ cell aplasia–Sertoli cell only syndrome. The seminiferous tubules are lined by Sertoli cells and do not contain germ cells.

Orchitis

Orchitis refers to acute or chronic inflammation of the testis. It may occur as part of epididymo-orchitis, usually caused by ascending infection, or as isolated testicular inflammation. The latter is usually caused by hematogenous spread of pathogens but may be of autoimmune origin.

- **Mumps orchitis** occurs in 20% of men who develop mumps but is uncommon because of widespread immunization against the virus. Infection is characterized by testicular pain and gonadal swelling, most often unilateral. Interstitial inflammation leads to destruction and loss of seminiferous epithelium (Fig. 15-19).
- **Granulomatous orchitis** of unknown cause is a rare disorder of middle-aged men that presents acutely as painful testicular enlargement or insidiously as induration. It shows noncaseating granulomas, but neither organisms nor sperm remnants that might act as inciting agents are rupture of epididymal ducts may play a role. Patients present with scrotal pain and swelling, frequently for weeks or months. The epididymis contains a mixed inflammatory cell infiltrate with many sperm fragments and macrophages phagocytosing sperm. Inflammation eventually results in interstitial fibrosis, ductal obstruction, and infertility.

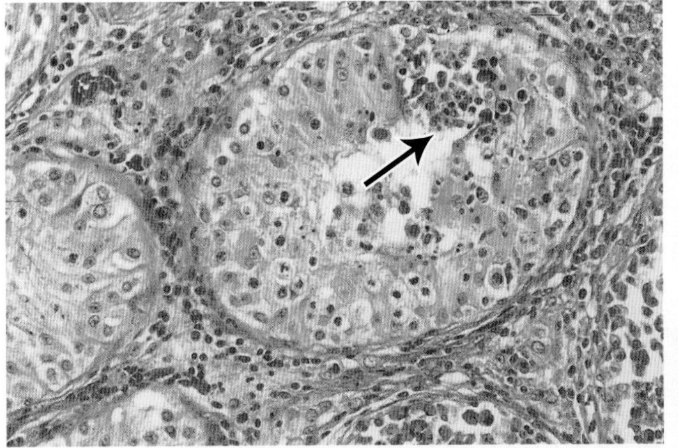

FIGURE 15-19. Viral orchitis. The interstitial spaces are infiltrated with mononuclear cells that spill focally into the lumen of seminiferous tubules (*arrow*). Note that the inflammation has interrupted normal spermatogenesis and that the seminiferous tubules do not contain sperm.

found. Variable numbers of seminiferous tubules are destroyed by the inflammatory process, which is considered to be a type IV (cell-mediated) hypersensitivity reaction.

- **Malakoplakia** of the testis has the same microscopic features and, presumably, the same histogenesis as malakoplakia elsewhere. It is typically related to *E. coli* infection.

Tumors of the Testis

Tumors of the testis account for less than 1% of all cancers in men. More than 90% of these tumors are characterized by the following:

- Diagnosis between 25 and 45 years of age
- Germ cell origin
- Malignancy
- Curable by a combination of surgery and chemotherapy
- Cytogenetic marker, isochromosome p12
- Metastasis first to periaortic abdominal lymph nodes

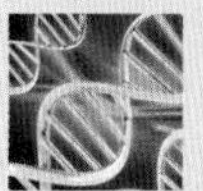

MOLECULAR PATHOGENESIS: The etiology of testicular tumors is not known. There is wide geographic and ethnic variation in the incidence of this cancer. For example, the neoplasms are five times more common among Americans of European descent than in those of African heritage. The only consistent cytogenetic abnormality is an additional fragment of chromosome 12 (isochromosome p12), found in 80% of germ cell tumors. As noted above, the only known risk factors are **cryptorchidism and gonadal dysgenesis**.

Malignant transformation of germ cells may occur during fetal development or in the peripubertal period; it involves spermatogonia that are stimulated to proliferate and differentiate into spermatocytes. Germ cell tumors progress through two pathways (Fig. 15-20). A carcinoma in situ stage consists of malignant germ cells located in the seminiferous tubules, which is termed **intratubular testicular germ cell neoplasia (ITGCN)**. This condition progresses to invasive carcinoma and accounts for most adult germ cell tumors. However, teratomas of prepubertal testes and yolk sac tumors of infancy apparently develop directly from germ cells without an in situ phase. Some migratory primordial germ cells may not find their way into the seminiferous tubules during fetal testicular organogenesis, but they eventually give rise to midline extragonadal germ cell tumors in the retroperitoneum, sacral region, anterior mediastinum, and the area near the pineal gland. Testicular tumors are classified histogenetically on the basis of their cell of origin into several groups (Table 15-7).

Intratubular Germ Cell Neoplasia

ITGCN represents a preinvasive form of germ cell tumors.

EPIDEMIOLOGY: ITGCN can be seen as (1) an isolated focal histologic change in 2% of cryptorchid testes or testicular biopsies performed for infertility, (2) widespread carcinoma in situ adjacent to almost all invasive germ cell tumors, and (3) lesions in 5% of contralateral testes in patients who had an orchiectomy for a testicular germ cell tumor.

Table 15-7

Testicular Tumors

Germ Cell Tumors—90%
Seminoma (40%)
Nonseminomatous germ cell tumors
Embryonal carcinoma (5%)
Teratocarcinoma (35%)
Choriocarcinoma (<1%)
Mixed germ cell tumors (15%)
Teratoma (1%)
Spermatocytic seminoma (1%)
Yolk sac tumor of infancy (2%)
Sex Cord Cell Tumors—5%
Leydig cell tumors (60%)
Sertoli cell tumors (40%)
Metastases—2%
Other Rare Tumors—3%

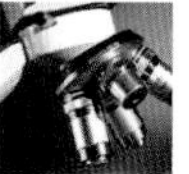

PATHOLOGY: ITGCN involves testes patchily, usually affecting less than 10% to 30% of tubules. Seminiferous tubules harboring this lesion have thick basement membranes and no sperm. The normal germ cells are replaced by neoplastic ones that are broadly attached to the basal lamina (Fig. 15-21). The tumor cells are larger than normal spermatogonia and have prominent central nuclei with finely dispersed chromatin and conspicuous nucleoli. Their cytoplasm is abundant and clear, with abundant glycogen.

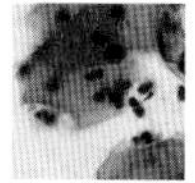

CLINICAL FEATURES: ITGCN is a precursor of invasive carcinoma, but the invasive tumor develops at an unpredictable pace. Half of men with ITGCN develop invasive cancer within 5 years and 70% in 7 years. The diagnosis of ITGCN on testicular biopsy is an indication for prophylactic orchiectomy.

Seminomas

EPIDEMIOLOGY: Malignant cells that retain the phenotype of spermatogonia give rise to **seminomas**. They are the most common testicular cancer and comprise up to 40% of all germ cell tumors. The peak incidence of seminomas is 30 to 40 years, and such tumors are not found before puberty, except in dysgenetic gonads.

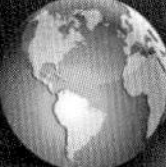

PATHOLOGY: Seminomas are solid, rubbery-firm, bosselated masses that are usually sharply demarcated from normal tissue, which may be compressed, atrophic, and fibrotic. On cross section, the tumors look lobulated and homogeneous tan or grayish yellow (Fig. 15-22). Areas of necrosis or hemorrhage are infrequent but may be seen in larger tumors.

Microscopically, seminomas resemble **ovarian dysgerminoma** (see Chapter 16). They feature a single population of uniform polygonal cells with central vesicular nuclei.

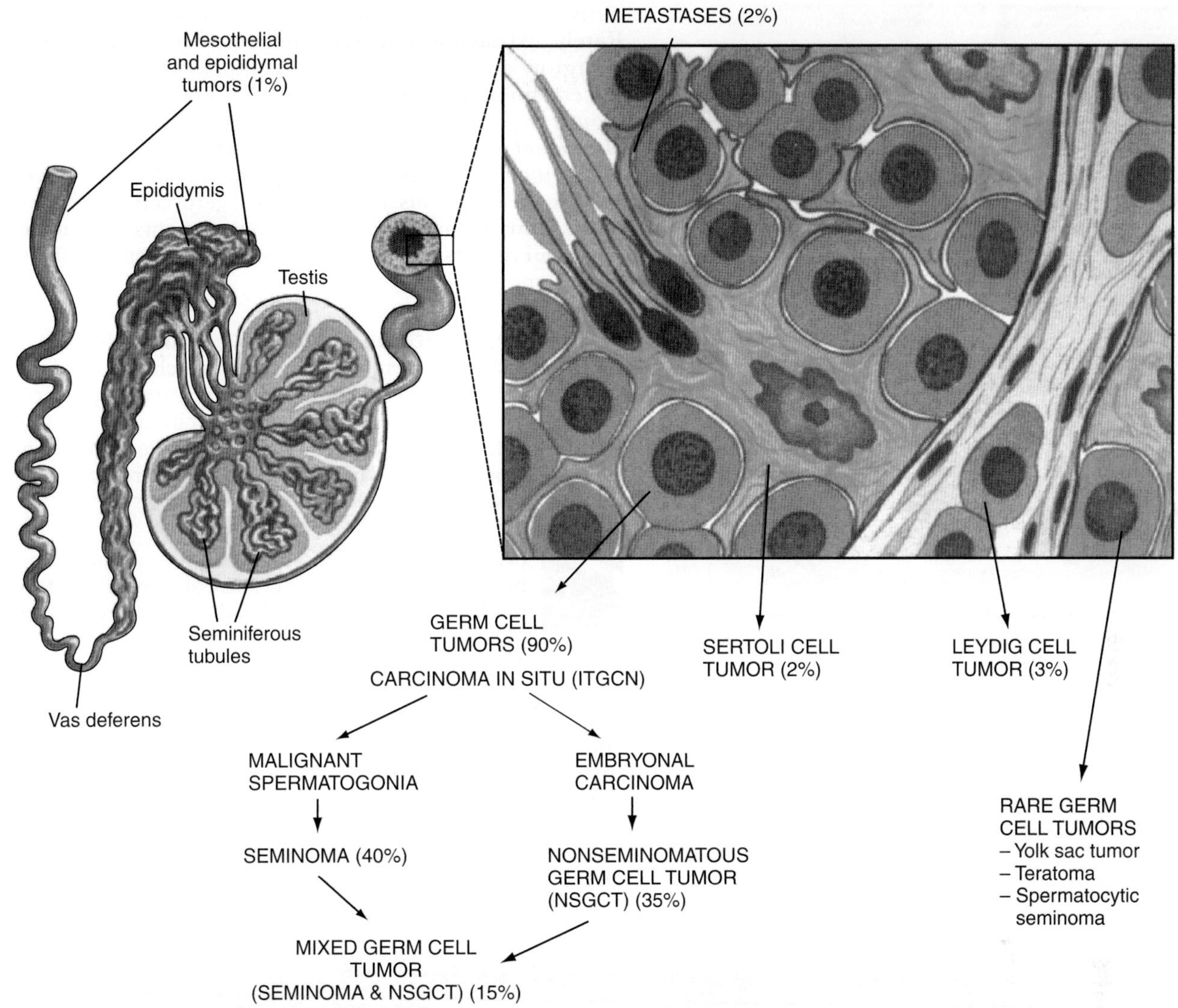

FIGURE 15-20. Tumors of the testis, epididymis, and related structures. Most testicular tumors originate from germ cells and are preceded by a carcinoma in situ stage known as intratubular germ cell neoplasia (ITGCN). Germ cell tumors of adult testes can be classified as seminomas (40%) or nonseminomatous germ cell tumors (NSGCTs) (35%). In 15% of cases, seminomatous elements are intermixed with NSGCT, forming mixed germ cell tumors. Some germ cell tumors (yolk sac tumor of childhood, childhood teratomas, and spermatocytic seminomas) develop without passing through a preinvasive ITGCN stage. Tumors originating from sex cord stromal cells (Leydig and Sertoli cell tumors) account for 5% of testicular tumors. Epididymal tumors, tumors of the mesothelial lining of the tunica vaginalis (adenomatoid tumors), and metastases are rare.

The ample cytoplasm may be eosinophilic or clear because it has considerable glycogen and some lipid. Cells grow in nests or sheets separated by fibrous septa, which are infiltrated with lymphocytes, plasma cells, and macrophages. Septa may also contain granulomas with giant cells. Tumor cells invade the testicular parenchyma and spread through seminiferous tubules into the rete testis. The epididymis is involved later in the disease, usually before spread to abdominal lymph nodes.

Seminoma cells express placental alkaline phosphatase (PLAP) on the plasma membrane. They also react with antibodies to c-Kit (CD117) and OCT3/OCT4, which are reliable markers for this tumor.

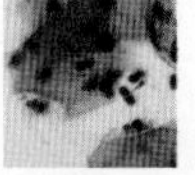

CLINICAL FEATURES: Seminomas are progressively growing scrotal masses that are often diagnosed while still curable by orchiectomy, with or without abdominal lymph node dissection. They are highly radiosensitive, and radiation therapy is important in treating tumors that are treated by surgery alone. Even in advanced stages of dissemination, chemotherapy can be curative. ***The cure rate for all histologic subtypes of seminoma is now over 90%.***

Nonseminomatous Germ Cell Tumors

Neoplastic germ cells in NSGCT can proliferate in an undifferentiated form, which resembles malignant embryonic cells and is termed **pure embryonal carcinoma**.

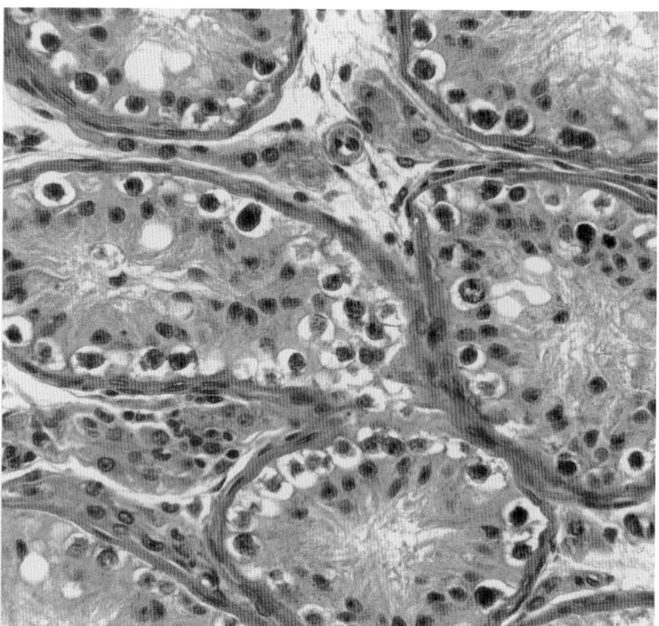

FIGURE 15-21. Intratubular germ cell neoplasia. The seminiferous tubules showing no signs of spermatogenesis but instead contain large atypical cells corresponding to intratubular carcinoma in situ.

In other cases, embryonal carcinoma cells differentiate into the three embryonic germ layers or extraembryonic tissues, which give rise to chorionic epithelium (cytotrophoblast and syncytiotrophoblast) and yolk sac–like epithelium. These complex tumors are composed of malignant undifferentiated embryonal cells, and their somatic and extraembryonic derivatives are **teratocarcinomas** or **malignant teratomas.** Rarely, extraembryonic components of teratocarcinomas overgrow and destroy all other components. Such tumors are classified as **yolk sac carcinoma** or **choriocarcinoma.** ***However, for clinical purposes, all germ cell tumors with embryonal carcinoma as their malignant stem cells are termed nonseminomatous germ cell tumors (NSGCTs), to distinguish them from seminomas.*** In 15% of cases, germ cell tumors have both seminoma and nonseminomatous elements. Such **mixed germ cell tumors** are treated clinically as nonseminomatous neoplasms.

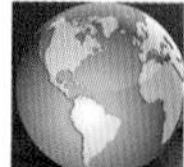

EPIDEMIOLOGY: NSGCTs constitute 55% of all testicular germ cell tumors, of which two thirds are teratocarcinomas, followed by mixed germ cell tumors and pure embryonal carcinomas. All other tumors of this group are extremely rare. Like seminomas, NSGCTs have a peak incidence in the third to fourth decades.

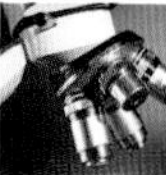

PATHOLOGY: NSGCTs vary in size and shape. They may be solid or partially cystic. Solid areas vary from white to yellow to red, indicating that they are composed of viable tumor cells, foci of necrosis, and hemorrhage, respectively (Fig. 15-23).

The histologic appearance of NSGCTs is highly variable (Fig. 15-24). Pure embryonal carcinomas display undifferentiated embryonal carcinoma cells that resemble the cells from preimplantation stage embryos (Fig. 15-24A). Because the tumor cells have little cytoplasm, their hyperchromatic, disproportionately large nuclei seem to overlap. Embryonal carcinoma cells may grow as broad solid sheets, cords, gland-like tubules and acini, and sometimes even papillary

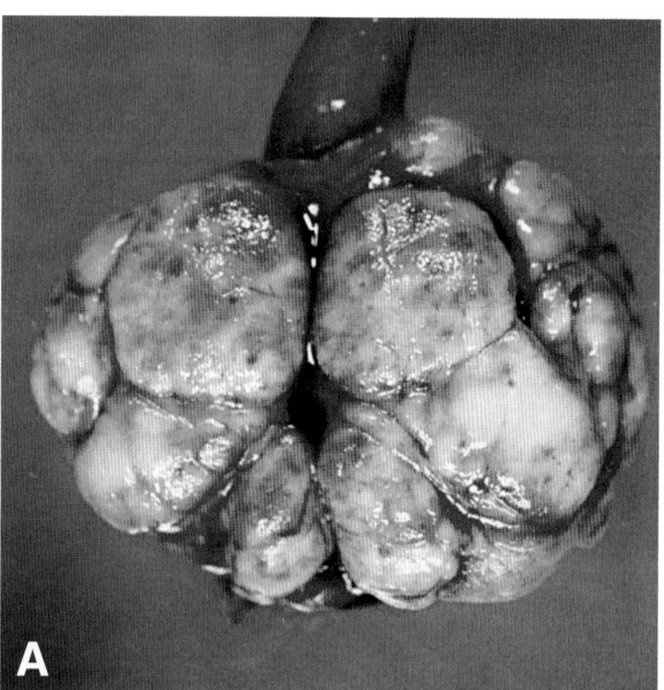

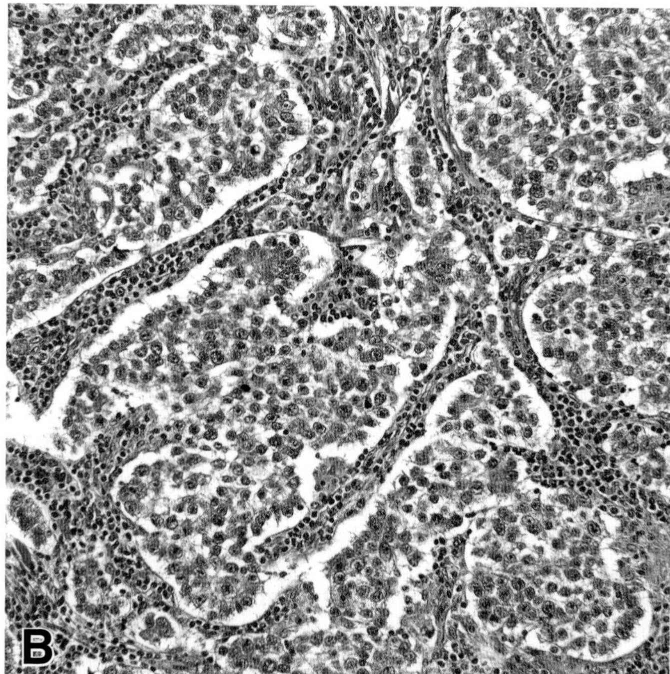

FIGURE 15-22. Seminoma. A. The cut surface of this nodular tumor is tan and bulging, suggesting that the tumor is firm and rubbery. **B.** Groups of tumor cells are surrounded by fibrous septa infiltrated with lymphocytes. Tumor cells have vesicular nuclei, which are much larger than the small round nuclei of the lymphocytes.

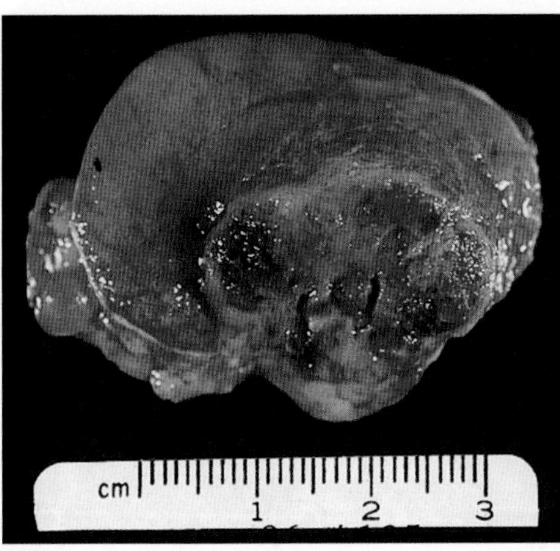

FIGURE 15-23. Nonseminomatous germ cell tumor of the testis. The cut surface of this small testicular tumor showing considerable heterogeneity, varying in color from white to dark red.

structures. Mitoses and apoptotic cells are common. Embryonal carcinomas invade the testis, epididymis, and blood vessels and metastasize to abdominal lymph nodes, lungs, and other organs. Like seminomas, these tumors react with antibodies to PLAP and OCT3/OCT4. Unlike seminomas and other tumors, they express cytokeratins and CD30, but not c-KIT (CD117).

Teratocarcinomas (malignant teratomas) feature differentiated somatic tissue. Thus, such nonseminomatous tumors have foci of embryonal carcinoma and other tissue types (Fig. 15-25). In most tumors, the malignancy resides in the embryonal carcinoma cells. Interestingly, when these cells metastasize, they can differentiate into somatic or extraembryonic tissues, in which case the metastatic tumor can resemble the original teratocarcinoma. In some cases, teratoma tissues mirror embryonic organs or embryonic tumors, such as neuroblastoma. These **immature teratomas** are also potentially malignant.

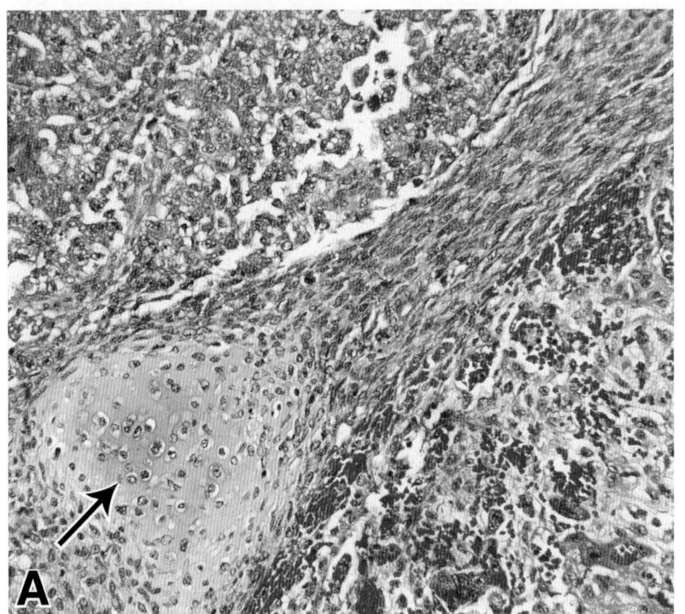

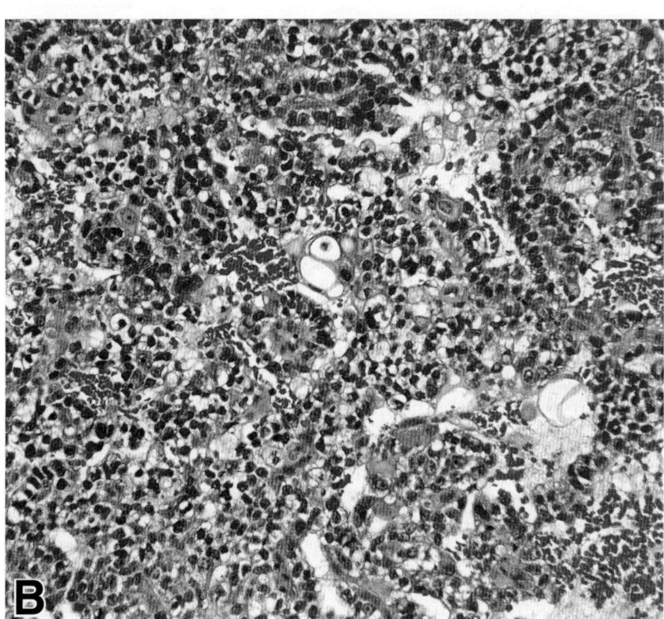

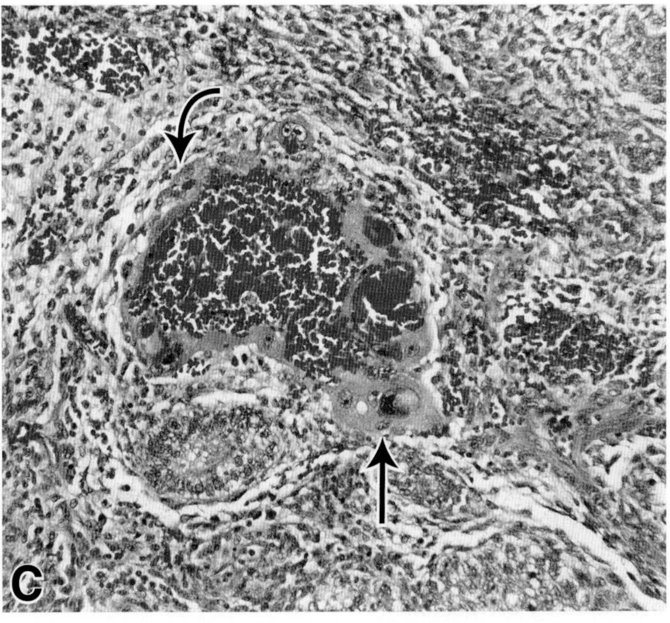

FIGURE 15-24. Nonseminomatous germ cell tumor (NSGCT). A. Somatic tissue of this tumor includes well-differentiated cartilage (*arrow*) and nondescript connective tissue separating the embryonal carcinoma (*upper left corner*) from the hemorrhagic choriocarcinoma (*right lower corner*). **B.** Yolk sac component consists of interlacing cords of epithelial cells surrounded by loose stroma resembling the early yolk sac. **C.** Choriocarcinoma component of the NSGCT consists of multinucleated syncytiotrophoblastic giant cells (*straight arrow*) and mononuclear cytotrophoblastic cells (*curved arrow*). Invasive growth of trophoblasts is usually associated with hemorrhage.

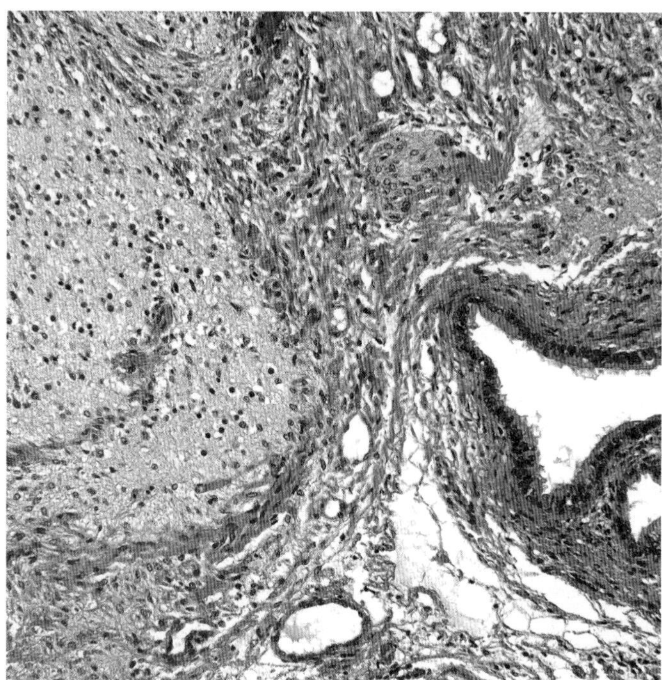

FIGURE 15-25. Teratoma. The tumor consists of neural tissue (*left*) connective tissue and smooth muscle cells (*midportion*) and glands lined by columnar epithelium (*right side of the picture*).

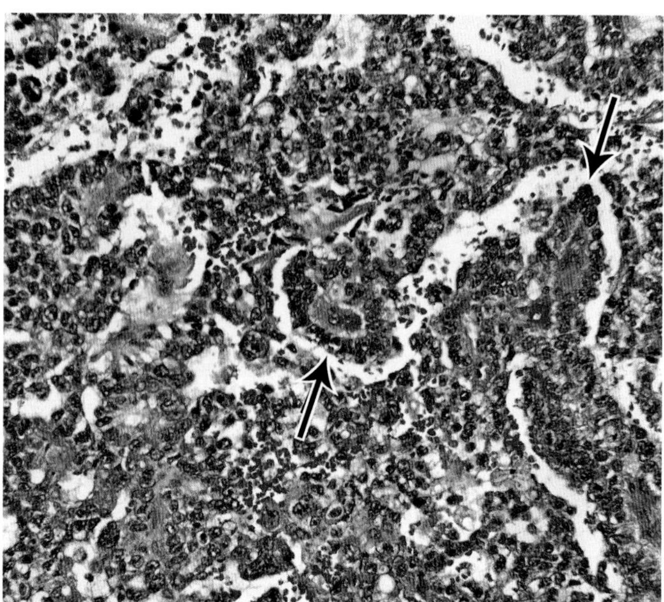

FIGURE 15-26. Yolk sac tumor. This childhood tumor is composed of interlacing strands of epithelial cells surrounded by loose connective stroma. The glomeruloid structures (Schiller–Duval bodies) are marked by *arrows*.

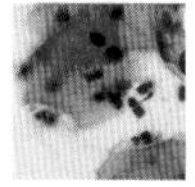

CLINICAL FEATURES: Most NSGCTs present as testicular masses. They tend to grow faster than seminomas and metastasize more readily and more widely. Hence, for some NSGCTs, metastases may be the first sign of the neoplasm.

Unlike seminomas, NSGCTs often contain yolk sac and syncytiotrophoblastic components. Yolk sac cells secrete α-fetoprotein (AFP), a fetal protein not normally found in the blood. Syncytiotrophoblast cells release hCG, a hormone of pregnancy that is not found in males. ***Elevated serum AFP or hCG is found in 70% of patients with NSGCTs and is thus a useful tumor marker.***

Treatment of NSGCT includes orchiectomy to remove the primary tumor, followed by platinum-based chemotherapy and, if indicated, surgical dissection of abdominal lymph nodes. Chemotherapy usually eliminates metastatic embryonal carcinoma cells, but differentiated tissues originating from them are resistant. ***Complete cures of NSGCTs are accomplished in over 90% of cases.***

Testicular Tumors in Prepubertal Boys

In the first 4 years of life, most testicular neoplasms are yolk sac tumors. Benign teratomas are the most common testicular tumor between the ages of 4 and 12 years.

YOLK SAC TUMORS: These neoplasms are composed of cells arranged into structures reminiscent of parts of the fetal yolk sac. The diagnosis is based on recognizing multiple microscopic tumor patterns and glomeruloid **Schiller–Duval bodies** (Fig. 15-26). These neonatal tumors resemble those of the yolk sac elements in NSGCTs. All such tumors secrete AFP into the serum. Yolk sac tumors of infancy and early childhood are considered malignant, but timely orchiectomy and removal of the tumor cure over 95% of patients.

TERATOMAS: These tumors of prepubertal testes are benign and are composed of mature somatic tissues. Orchiectomy and even testis-sparing surgery are curative.

Gonadal Stromal/Sex Cord Tumors

Gonadal stromal/sex cord tumors constitute 5% of testicular tumors.

LEYDIG CELL TUMORS: ***These are rare neoplasms composed of cells resembling interstitial (Leydig) cells of the testis.*** They can be hormonally active and secrete androgens or estrogens or both. Leydig cell tumors occur at any age, with distinct peaks in childhood and then in adults from the third to sixth decades.

PATHOLOGY: Leydig cell tumors vary from 1 to 10 cm and are circumscribed; some appear encapsulated. The cut surface is yellow to brown, and larger tumors have fibrous trabeculae, giving them a lobular appearance. Leydig tumor cells are uniform, with round nuclei and well-developed eosinophilic or vacuolated cytoplasm (Fig. 15-27). **Reinke crystals**—rectangular, eosinophilic, cytoplasmic inclusions—are characteristic of normal Leydig cells and are seen in 30% of tumors. Most (90%) Leydig cell tumors are benign, but it is difficult to predict their biologic behavior on histologic grounds.

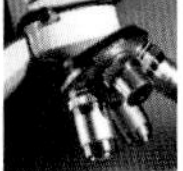

CLINICAL FEATURES: Androgenic effects of testicular Leydig cell tumors in prepubertal boys lead to precocious physical and sexual development. By contrast, feminization and gynecomastia are seen in some adults with this tumor. Either estrogen or testosterone levels may be elevated, but there is no characteristic pattern. All Leydig cell tumors in children and almost all tumors in adults are cured by orchiectomy.

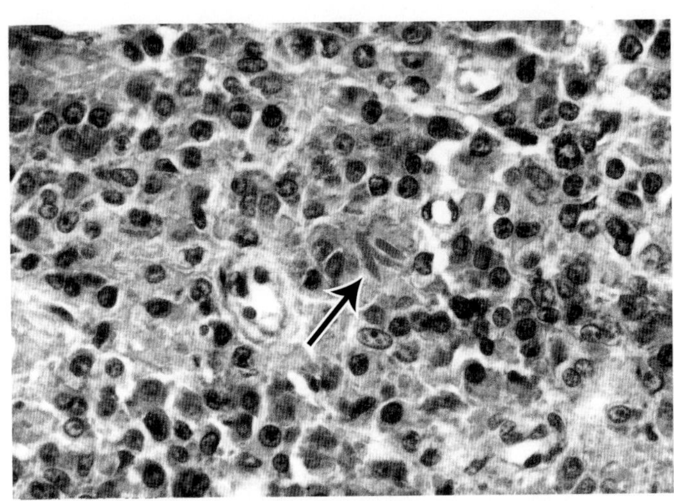

FIGURE 15-27. Leydig cell tumor. The tumor cells have uniform round nuclei and well-developed eosinophilic cytoplasm. Three cytoplasmic Reinke crystals are seen in the center of the field (*arrow*).

SERTOLI CELL TUMORS: Some testicular stromal sex cord tumors contain neoplastic Sertoli cells. Most (90%) are benign and produce few if any hormonal symptoms occur (Fig 15-28).

PROSTATE

Prostatitis

Prostatitis is the term for inflammation of the prostate. There are acute and chronic forms. Prostatitis is usually caused by coliform uropathogens, but often no etiology is found.

ACUTE PROSTATITIS: ***Typically, a complication of other urinary tract infections, acute prostatitis, results from the reflux of infected urine into the prostate.*** An acute inflammatory infiltrate is seen in prostatic acini and stroma. The inflammation causes intense discomfort on urination and is often associated with fever, chills, and perineal pain. Most patients respond well to antibiotics.

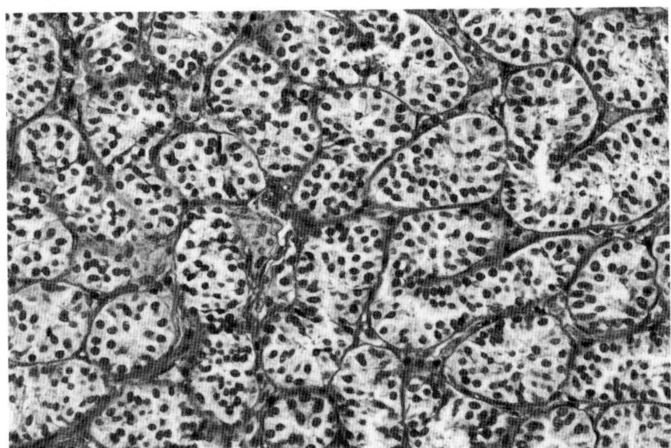

FIGURE 15-28. Sertoli cell tumor. The neoplastic cells are arranged in tubules surrounded by a basement membrane. These structures are reminiscent of seminiferous tubules devoid of germ cells.

CHRONIC BACTERIAL PROSTATITIS: ***This prolonged infection may or may not be preceded by an episode of acute prostatitis.*** Most patients complain of dysuria and burning at the urethral meatus. Suprapubic, perineal, and low back pain or discomfort and nocturia may be also present. The urine usually contains bacteria. In addition to reflux of urine, prostatic calculi and local prostatic duct obstruction may contribute to the development of chronic bacterial prostatitis. Infiltrates of lymphocytes, plasma cells, and macrophages are the rule. Prolonged antibiotic therapy is often, but not always, curative.

NONBACTERIAL PROSTATITIS: ***Sometimes in chronic prostatitis, no causative organism is identified.*** It is the most common form of inflammation in prostatic biopsies, in prostatectomy specimens, and at autopsy. Nonbacterial prostatitis typically affects men older than 50 years but can be seen at any age. In practice, this disorder is a diagnosis of exclusion. Microscopically, dilated glands are filled with neutrophils and foamy macrophages and are surrounded by chronic inflammatory cells. The condition may be asymptomatic or it may cause symptoms like those of chronic bacterial prostatitis. Usually, no specific therapy is available.

GRANULOMATOUS PROSTATITIS: In most cases, the cause of granulomatous prostatitis cannot be established. Rarely, this disease can be traced to specific causative agents, including *Mycobacterium tuberculosis*, BCG administration, or fungi such as *Histoplasma capsulatum*. Caseating or noncaseating granulomas are associated with localized destruction of prostatic ducts and acini and, in later stages, with fibrosis.

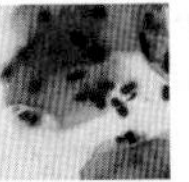

CLINICAL FEATURES: As indicated above, symptoms of chronic prostatitis are highly variable, and treatment may be ineffective. Most importantly, it may cause elevated serum prostate-specific antigen (PSA), a worrisome suggestion of prostatic malignancy (see below). Thus, the diagnosis is often made by biopsy done to exclude carcinoma.

Nodular Hyperplasia of the Prostate

Nodular prostatic hyperplasia, also called **benign prostatic hyperplasia (BPH)**, ***is a common disorder characterized clinically by obstruction of urinary outflow and pathologically by proliferation of glands and stroma.***

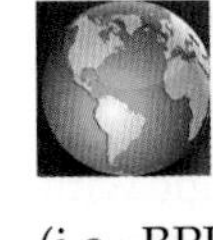

EPIDEMIOLOGY: BPH is most common in Western Europe and the United States and least frequent in Asia. Its prevalence in the United States is higher among blacks than among whites. Clinical prostatism (i.e., BPH severe enough to interfere with urination) peaks in the seventh decade. However, the prevalence of BPH is far greater at autopsy than is suggested by clinically apparent prostatism. In fact, 75% of men over age 80 have some degree of prostatic hyperplasia. The disorder is rare in men younger than 40 years.

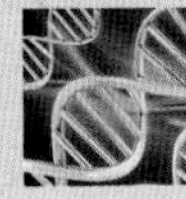

MOLECULAR PATHOGENESIS: The earliest histogenetic events in BPH remain unclear. Testosterone is necessary for prostatic development and the maintenance of secretory function.

The active androgen form is dihydrotestosterone (DHT), a product of the enzyme 5α-reductase. DHT binds nuclear receptors in glandular and stromal cells. In men, exogenous testosterone does not induce hyperplasia and does not stimulate atrophic glands. With aging, circulating testosterone levels decline in men with and without BPH. As well, no change in serum DHT is seen in men with BPH, although the ratio of circulating testosterone and DHT may be low. Conversely, drugs that block 5α-reductase (e.g., finasteride or dutasteride) reduce the size of the prostate in men with BPH. Prepubertal castration prevents the development of age-related BPH and completely protects against prostate cancer.

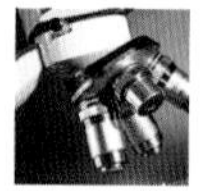

PATHOLOGY: Early nodular hyperplasia begins in the submucosa of the proximal urethra (**the transitional zone**). Enlarging nodules compress the centrally located urethral lumen and the more peripherally located normal prostate (Fig. 15-29). In well-developed BPH, the normal gland is actually limited to an attenuated rim of tissue beneath the capsule. Individual nodules are demarcated by enveloping fibrous pseudocapsules (Fig. 15-30B). Larger nodules may show focal hemorrhage or infarction.

In BPH, proliferation of epithelial cells of acini and ductules, smooth muscle cells, and stromal fibroblasts is all seen in variable proportions. Typical nodules contain variably sized hyperplastic prostatic acini randomly scattered throughout the stroma. The epithelial (adenomatous) component contains a double layer of cells, with tall columnar cells overlying a basal layer (Fig. 15-30C) and often showing papillary hyperplasia. Chronic inflammation and corpora amylacea (eosinophilic laminated concretions) are frequently seen within the acini. Nonspecific prostatitis is common in nodular hyperplasia. There is a dense intraglandular and periglandular infiltrate of lymphocytes, plasma cells, and macrophages, often with acute inflammatory cells and focal gland destruction. Squamous metaplasia of ductal epithelium at the periphery of infarcts is typical.

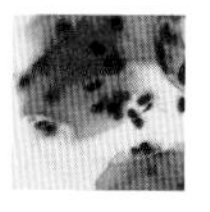

CLINICAL FEATURES: The symptoms of nodular hyperplasia result from compression of the prostatic urethra and consequent bladder outlet obstruction (Fig. 15-31). A history of decreased vigor of the urinary stream and increasing urinary frequency is typical. Rectal examination reveals a firm, enlarged, nodular prostate. If severe obstruction is prolonged, back-pressure results in hydroureter, hydronephrosis, and, ultimately, renal failure.

Treatment of BPH is either surgical or pharmacologic with drugs that block 5α-redutase. In addition, some patients receive α_1-adrenergic blockers to enhance urine flow. Transurethral radiofrequency ablation and cryotherapy are the surgical treatments of choice.

Adenocarcinoma of the Prostate

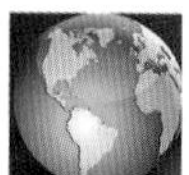

EPIDEMIOLOGY: ***In 1990, prostatic adenocarcinoma surpassed lung cancer to become the cancer most frequently diagnosed in American men.*** An estimated 160,000 new cases are diagnosed yearly in the United States. About 27,000 American men die annually from the tumor, a figure equivalent to that of colorectal carcinoma. Prostate cancer is largely a disease of elderly men; 75% of patients are 60 to 80 years of age. Autopsy studies confirm that the tumor is more common with advancing age. Prostate cancer is diagnosed at autopsy in 20% of men in their 40s and in 70% of men over age 70. American blacks have a rate twice as high as that of white Americans and suffer the highest prostate carcinoma–related death rates in the world. The risk is significantly increased in persons with first-degree relatives with prostate cancer. Many prostate cancers are so indolent (or latent) that they may never be clinically significant during the patient's lifetime. For this reason, the utility of screening for prostate cancer using blood PSA levels is controversial.

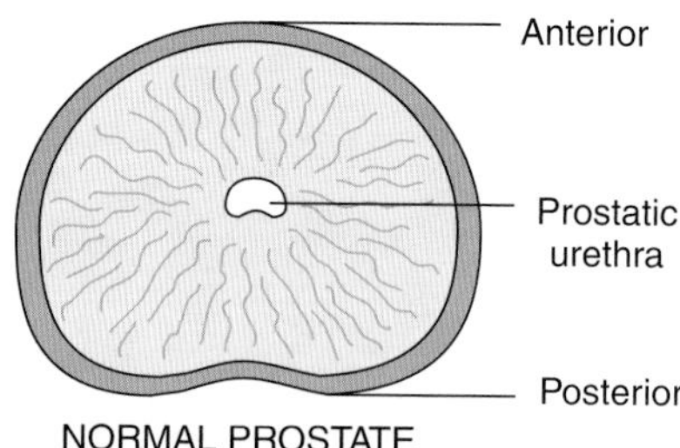

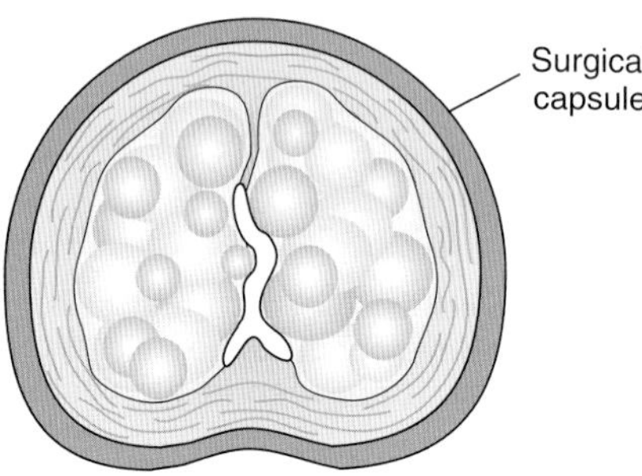

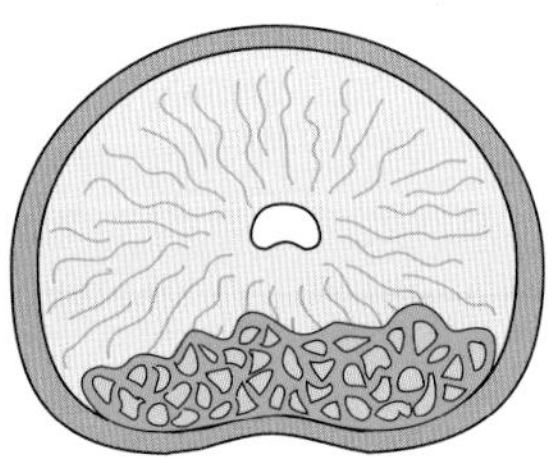

FIGURE 15-29. Normal prostate, nodular hyperplasia, and adenocarcinoma. In prostatic hyperplasia, which involves predominantly the periurethral part of the gland, the nodules compress and distort the urethra. The expansion of the central prostatic glands leads to compression of the peripheral parts and fibrosis, resulting in the formation of a so-called surgical capsule. Prostatic carcinoma usually arises from the peripheral glands, and compression of the urethra is a late clinical event.

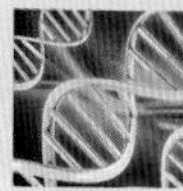

MOLECULAR PATHOGENESIS: Androgenic control of normal prostatic growth and the responsiveness of prostate cancer to castration and exogenous estrogens indicate a role for male hormones. However, patients with prostate cancer do not typically

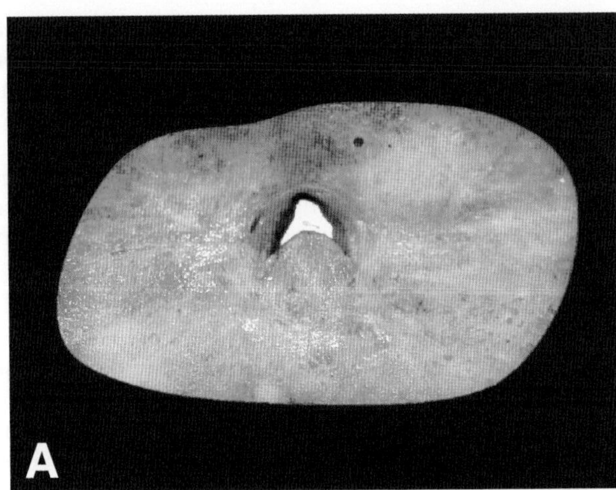

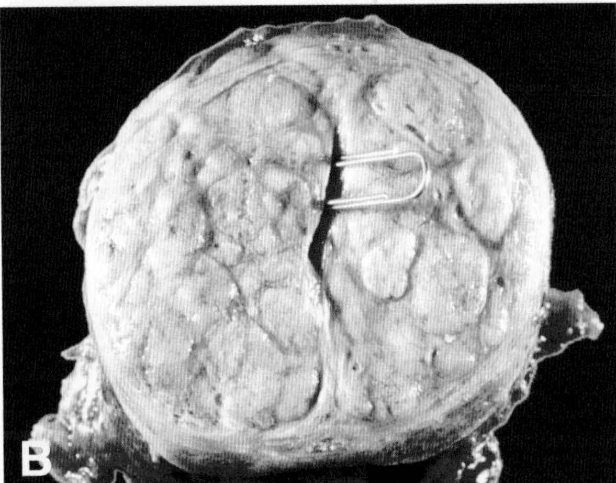

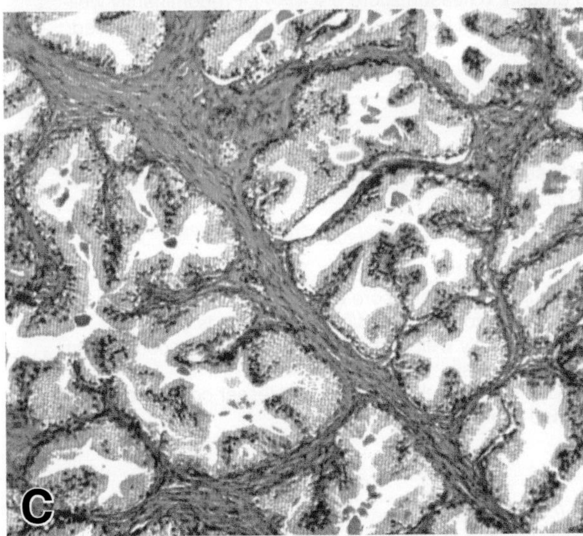

FIGURE 15-30. Nodular hyperplasia of the prostate. A. Normal prostate. **B.** The cut surface of a prostate enlarged by nodular hyperplasia showing numerous well-circumscribed nodules of prostatic tissue surrounded by pseudocapsules. The prostatic urethra (*paper clip*) has been compressed to a narrow slit. **C.** Hyperplastic prostate glands in nodular hyperplasia. The columnar epithelium lining the acini is composed of two cell layers: polarized clear cuboidal cells lining the acinar lumen and flattened basal cells interposed between the cuboidal acinar cells and the stroma. Hyperplastic cells line papillary projections protruding into the lumina of the acini.

have higher levels of circulating androgens. The androgen (*AR*) gene shows considerable variation in CAG repeats in exon 1. Men with fewer AR CAG repeats are at greater risk for developing prostate cancer. Advanced tumors frequently show somatic mutations that place the transcription factor gene *ETV1* under the control of the androgen-regulated TMPRSS2 promoter. Other cases show mutations or amplification in the androgen receptor gene, mutations or loss of the *PTEN* tumor suppressor gene, and defects in several additional loci. Somatic and germline mutations in the *BRCA2* and *ATM* DNA repair genes also occur.

There is consensus that intraductal dysplastic epithelial proliferation, termed **prostatic intraepithelial neoplasia (PIN)**, is a precursor lesion of prostatic adenocarcinoma. ***PIN describes prostatic ducts lined by cytologically atypical luminal cells and a concomitant decrease in basal cells.*** Nuclei of high-grade PIN are enlarged and show nucleoli and marked crowding (Fig. 15-32). High-grade PIN may precede invasive cancer by up to two decades, and the severity increases with increasing age.

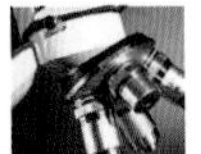

PATHOLOGY: Adenocarcinomas account for the vast majority of all primary prostatic tumors. They are commonly multicentric and located in the peripheral zones in over 70% of cases. The cut surface of a carcinomatous prostate shows irregular, yellow-white, indurated subcapsular nodules.

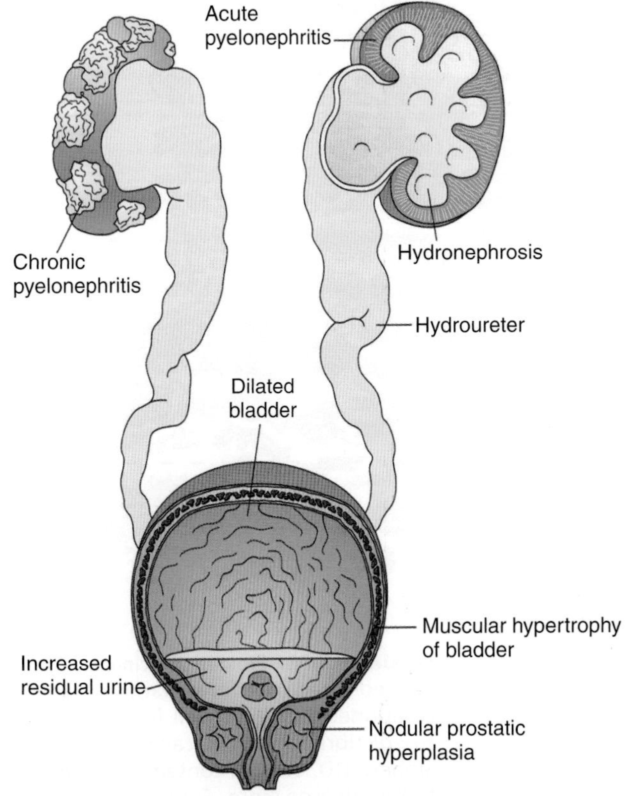

FIGURE 15-31. Complications of nodular prostatic hyperplasia.

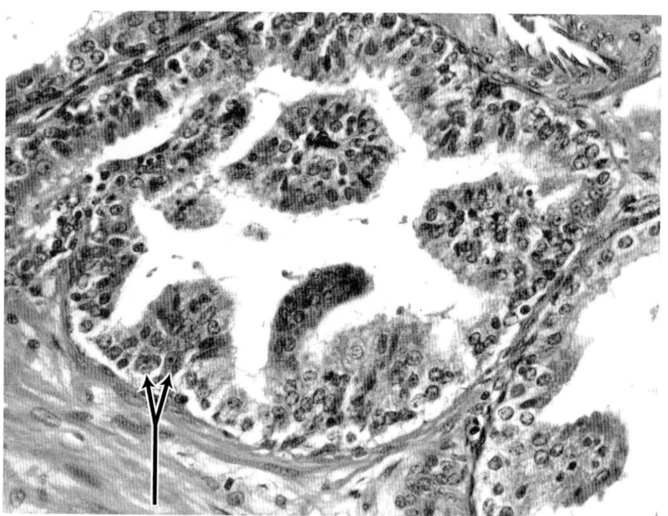

FIGURE 15-32. High-grade prostatic intraepithelial neoplasia. The large duct in the center is lined by atypical cells with enlarged nuclei and prominent nucleoli (*arrows*).

HISTOLOGIC FEATURES OF INVASIVE CARCINOMA: Most prostatic adenocarcinomas are of acinar origin and feature small- to medium-sized glands that lack organization and infiltrate the stroma. Well-differentiated tumors show uniform medium-sized or small glands (Fig. 15-33), lined by a single layer of neoplastic epithelial cells. Malignant acini have no basal cells, and no longer grow in lobular patterns. Progressive loss of differentiation of prostatic adenocarcinomas is characterized by the following:

- Increasing variability of gland size and configuration
- Papillary and cribriform patterns
- Rudimentary (or no) gland formation, with only solid cords of infiltrating tumor cells
- Uncommonly, a prostate cancer is composed of small undifferentiated cells growing individually or in sheets, without evidence of any structural organization.

CYTOLOGIC FEATURES: The prominence of pleomorphic and hyperchromatic nuclei is highly variable. One or two conspicuous nucleoli in a background of chromatin clumped near the nuclear membrane are the most frequent nuclear feature. The cytoplasm stains slightly eosinophilic or may be so

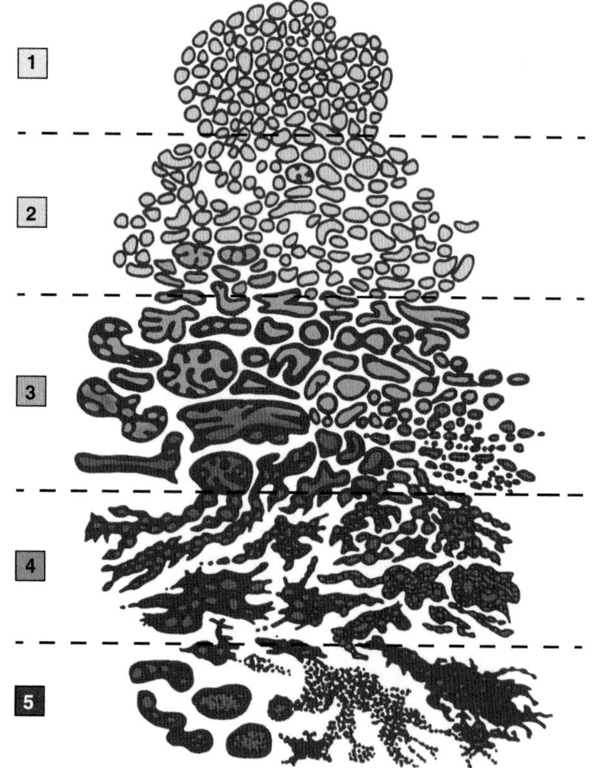

GLEASON GRADE GROUPS

Grade group 1 (Gleason score 3 + 3 = 6): Only individual discrete well-formed glands

Grade group 2 (Gleason score 3 + 4 = 7): Predominantly well-formed glands with lesser component of poorly formed/fused/cribriform glands

Grade group 3 (Gleason score 4 + 3 = 7): Predominantly poorly formed/fused/cribriform glands with lesser component of well-formed glands[a]

Grade group 4 (Gleason score 8):
- Only poorly formed/fused/cribriform glands *or*
- Predominantly well-formed glands and lesser component lacking glands[b]
- Predominantly lacking glands and lesser component of well-formed glands[b]

Grade group 5 (Gleason score 9–10): Lack of gland formation (or with necrosis) with or without poorly formed/fused/cribriform glands[a]

FIGURE 15-33. Prostatic carcinoma. Gleason grading system. [a]For cases with >95% poorly formed/fused/cribriform glands or lack of glands on a core or at radical prostatectomy, the component of <5% well-formed glands is not factored into the grade. [b]Poorly formed/fused/cribriform glands can be a more minor component. Table from Epstein JI, Zelefsky MJ, Sjoberg DD, et al. A contemporary prostate cancer grading system: a validated alternative to the Gleason score. *Eur Urol*. 2016;69(3):428-435.

vacuolated that it simulates clear cells of renal cell carcinoma. Cell borders are distinct in better-differentiated tumors but are not well demarcated in poorly differentiated ones.

GRADING: Prostatic adenocarcinoma is most commonly classified according to the **Gleason grading system** (Figs. 15-33 and 15-34), which is based on five histologic patterns of tumor gland formation and infiltration.

Recognizing the high frequency of mixed tumor patterns, the Gleason scores are combined into grades based on the prominent pattern and that of the minority pattern. The best-differentiated tumors constitute group 1 (Gleason score of 3 + 3 = 6; sums of 2–5 are not used in clinical practice). The most poorly differentiated cancers are defined as group 4 (Gleason score 4 + 4 = 8). Group 2 (Gleason 3 + 4 = 7) and group 3 (Gleason 4 + 3 = 7) are intermediate. Combined with tumor stage, Gleason grade groups have prognostic value; lower scores correlate with better prognoses.

INVASION AND METASTASIS: The high frequency of invasion of the prostatic capsule by adenocarcinoma reflects the tumor's subcapsular site of origin. Perineural tumor invasion within the prostate and in adjacent tissues is usual. Because peripheral nerves are devoid of perineural lymphatic channels, this mode of invasion represents contiguous spread of the tumor along a tissue space that offers a plane of low resistance.

The seminal vesicles are almost always involved by direct extension of prostate cancer. The earliest metastases occur in the obturator lymph nodes and then proceed to iliac and periaortic lymph nodes. Metastases to the lung reflect further lymphatic spread through the thoracic duct and dissemination from the prostatic venous plexus to the inferior vena cava. Bony metastases, particularly to the vertebral column, ribs, and pelvic bones, are common. They are painful and difficult to manage.

CLINICAL FEATURES: Current screening programs for prostate cancer that use digital rectal examination in combination with serum PSA levels are controversial. PSA is a glycoprotein produced by the prostate. It is a serine protease involved in liquifying seminal ejaculate and maintains a baseline serum level in men. Serum levels are increased by prostate inflammation, hypertrophy (prostatic volume), and neoplasia. Because most prostate cancers are asymptomatic, PSA screening combined with transrectal needle biopsy under ultrasound guidance is the most common detection method. Uncommonly, patients with prostate cancer present with bladder outlet obstruction or symptoms referable to metastatic tumor. High-resolution MRI of the prostate shows promise for cancer detection.

At present, guidelines for prostate cancer screening are in flux. Although widespread screening leads to more cancer diagnoses and treatment, it comes with side effects and quality of life issues. Given that several large epidemiologic studies report conflicting results with regard to the benefit of active prostate cancer therapy, the high frequency of side effects that occur with aggressive screening and treatment (e.g., incontinence and impotence) cannot be ignored. To this end, the U.S. Preventive Service Task Force (USPSTF) was convened to examine the relevant published literature. It concluded that there was insufficient evidence to recommend routine prostate cancer screening (and, by default, therapy). This position remains controversial. Other national organizations such as the American College of Physicians and the American Urological Association have adopted less extreme guidelines, recommending individualized patient evaluation and selective screening.

The principles of clinical staging (TNM) of prostate cancer are shown in Figure 15-35. Metastases are found in lymph nodes, bones, lung, and liver, in order of decreasing frequency.

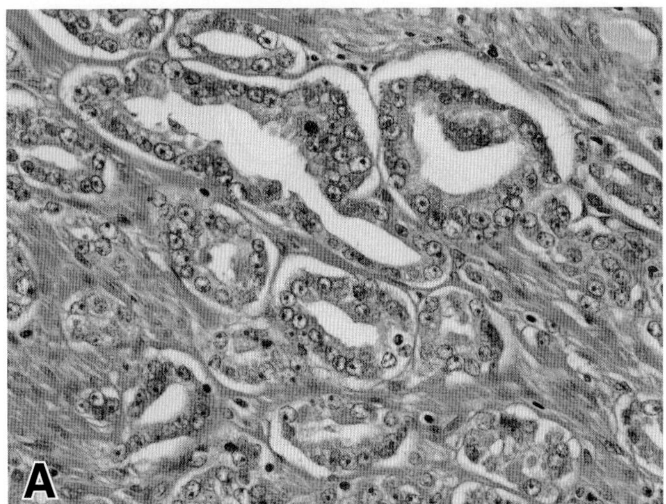

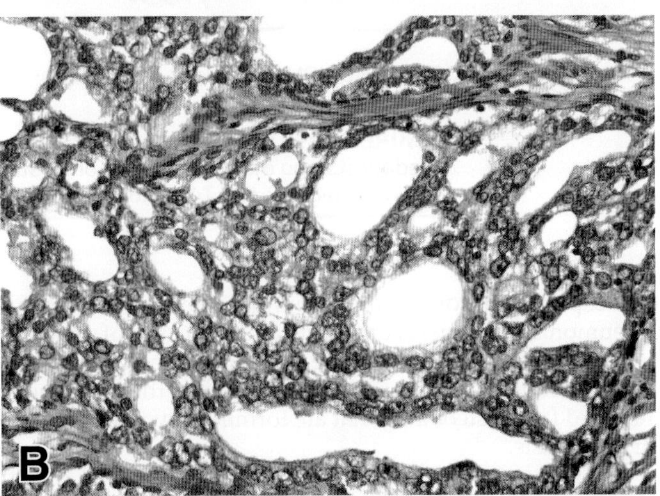

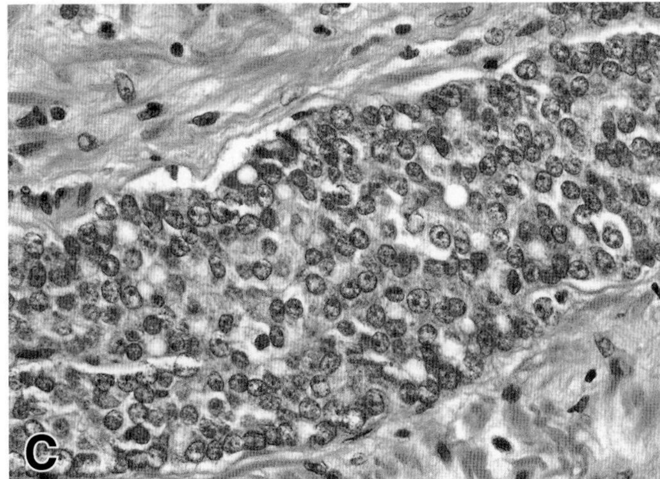

FIGURE 15-34. Gleason grading system. **A.** Gleason grade 1. **B.** Gleason grade 3. **C.** Gleason grade 5.

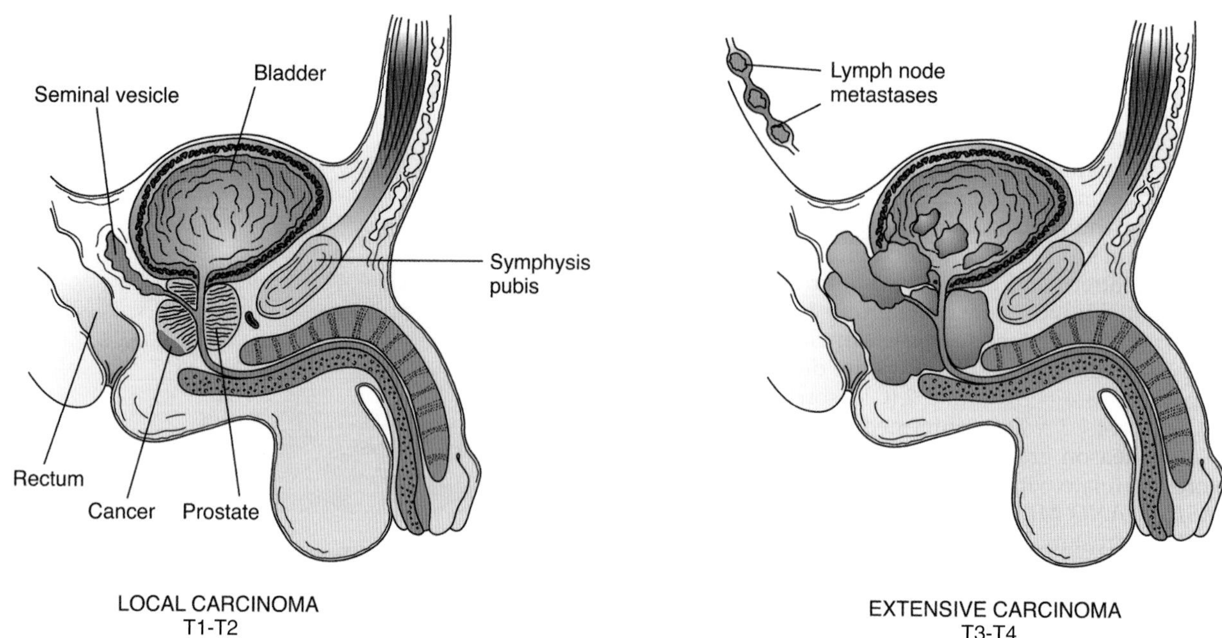

FIGURE 15-35. Staging of prostatic carcinoma. Tumor node metastasis system is most widely used for staging of prostate carcinoma. Stage T1 and T2 tumors are localized to the prostate, whereas stage T3 and T4 tumors have spread outside the prostate.

Widespread tumor dissemination (carcinomatosis), with pneumonia or sepsis, is the most common cause of death.

Serum alkaline phosphatase levels are elevated in patients with osteoblastic bony metastases because this enzyme is released from osteoblasts that are forming new bone at a site of metastasis.

Therapy for prostate cancer is highly controversial, owing to recent studies that suggest that many tumors may best be left alone. There is considerable difficulty in distinguishing between the tumors that are likely to benefit from treatment and those that are not. However, treatment generally depends on tumor stage. Patients with stage T1 and T2 cancers are treated by radical prostatectomy, radiofrequency ablation, cryogenic procedures, or radiation therapy. Radiation therapy may be either external beam or implanted radioactive seeds (brachytherapy). In stage T3 tumors, radiation therapy combined with androgen deprivation therapy is the treatment of choice, acknowledging that half of these patients have occult pelvic lymph node metastases (and possibly further systemic dissemination), which cannot be cured by surgical means. Patients with low-grade, low-volume tumors may opt to be managed by active surveillance only.

For patients with metastatic disease or whose tumors progress clinically, traditional chemotherapy combined with androgen deprivation is the main strategy. Bone metastases are treated with local radiation, bisphosphonates, and supplements of calcium and vitamin D.

The 5-year survival rates depend on stage and Gleason group (Fig. 15-33). Using staging data, survival is as follows: stages T1 and T2, 90%; stage T3, 40%; and stage T4, 10%.

16 The Female Reproductive Tract

George L. Mutter[1] ▪ Jaime Prat[1] ▪ David A. Schwartz[2]

LEARNING OBJECTIVES

- Describe the organ systems that comprise the female reproductive tract.
- Differentiate the histologic changes of menstrual, proliferative, and secretory phases of the menstrual cycle.
- Define the term "anovulatory bleeding" and describe the most common etiologic factor responsible for the condition.
- Describe the most common origin of and organs affected by ascending genital infections.
- List the most common sexually transmitted infections and describe their pathologic features.
- Distinguish between the etiologies and pathogenesis of cervicitis, salpingitis, and pelvic inflammatory disease.
- Discuss the role of HPV infection and its associated lesions in the female genital tract.
- Distinguish between vulvar classic VIN and differentiated VIN (dVIN) in terms of etiology and pathogenesis.
- Compare Paget disease of the breast with vulvar Paget disease.
- Compare and contrast the histopathology of acute and chronic cervicitis.
- Distinguish between LSIL, HSIL, superficially invasive, and deeply invasive squamous cell carcinoma of the cervix.
- Describe the importance of the cervical transition zone.
- Distinguish endocervical adenocarcinoma from squamous cell carcinoma of the cervix.
- Discuss the pathology and clinical features of salpingitis. Why is the condition associated with ectopic pregnancy?
- Discuss the relationship between serous tubal intraepithelial carcinoma, ovarian carcinoma, and *BRCA* mutations.
- Outline the etiology and pathogenesis of polycystic ovary syndrome.
- Describe common benign and borderline epithelial tumors of the ovary.
- Distinguish between the major types of malignant epithelial tumors of the ovary.
- List and describe germ cell tumors of the ovary.
- List and describe sex cord/stromal tumors of the ovary.
- Describe acute and chronic endometritis, pyometra, and adenomyosis.
- Differentiate between type I and type II forms of endometrial adenocarcinoma.
- Define the term "endometriosis" and list theories of its etiology.
- Compare and contrast benign and malignant smooth muscle tumors of the uterus.
- Compare the endometrium of pregnancy to that of the nongravid endometrium.
- Review the anatomy and histology of the placenta.
- Define the terms "placenta previa" and "placenta accreta."
- Compare and contrast dizygotic and monozygotic twinning in terms of placental structure.
- List common abnormalities of umbilical cord insertion.
- Discuss maternal and fetal responses to placental infections.
- Distinguish between fetal thrombotic vasculopathy and hemorrhagic endovasculopathy.
- Define the term "abruptio placentae" and discuss its clinical features.
- List the causes of uteroplacental malperfusion.
- Distinguish between preeclampsia and eclampsia and discuss their pathophysiology.
- List the factors associated with spontaneous abortions.

ANATOMY

Vulva

The vulva comprises the mons pubis, labia majora and minora, clitoris, and vestibule. At puberty, the mons pubis and lateral borders of the labia majora acquire increased subcutaneous fat and grow coarse hair. Sebaceous and apocrine glands in these regions develop concomitantly. The paired external openings of the paraurethral glands (Skene glands) flank the urethral meatus. Bartholin glands, posterolateral to the introitus, are branching, mucus-secreting, tubuloalveolar glands drained by a short duct lined by transitional epithelium. In addition, microscopic mucous glands are scattered throughout the area bounded by the labia minora. Inguinal and femoral lymph nodes provide primary lymph drainage routes, except for the clitoris (the homolog of the penis), which shares the lymphatic drainage of the urethra.

[1] The Female Reproductive System and Peritoneum.
[2] The Pathology of Pregnancy.

Vagina

The vagina extends from the uterus to the vestibule of the vulva and is lined by hormone-responsive squamous epithelium. Estrogens stimulate and progestins inhibit vaginal epithelial proliferation and maturation. Thus, in the secretory phase of the menstrual cycle or during pregnancy, when progesterone levels are high, intermediate cells, rather than superficial ones, predominate in vaginal smears. Maturing epithelial cells accumulate glycogen, giving their cytoplasm a clear appearance. Lymphatics from the vaginal vault and upper vagina join branches from the cervix, to drain into pelvic and then into para-aortic nodes. The lower vagina drains into inguinal and femoral nodes.

Cervix

The cervix is the inferior part of the uterus that connects the corpus to the vagina (Fig. 16-1). Its exposed portion (the **exocervix, ectocervix**, or **portio vaginalis**) protrudes into the upper vagina and is covered by glycogen-rich squamous epithelium.

The **endocervix** is the canal that leads to the endometrial cavity. It features longitudinal mucosal ridges made of fibrovascular cores lined by a single layer of mucinous columnar cells. Occasionally, retention of mucous in an endocervical produces cystic dilations of these glands, termed **nabothian cysts**. The **external os** is the *macroscopic* junction between the exocervix and endocervix. The **squamocolumnar junction** is the *microscopic* junction of the squamous and mucinous columnar epithelia. The area between the endocervix and endometrial cavity is called the **isthmus** or **lower uterine segment**.

The exocervix remodels continuously throughout life. During embryonic development, upward migration of squamous cells meets columnar epithelium of the endocervix to form the initial squamocolumnar junction (Fig. 16-2). In some young women, this "original" squamocolumnar junction is located at the internal os.

The area between the distalmost squamocolumnar junction and the external os is called the **transformation zone**. Immature squamous epithelium of this zone displays progressive nuclear maturation and increasing amounts of glycogen-free cytoplasm toward the surface. Colposcopy (examination of the cervix using a magnifying device, the colposcope) shows a thin white membrane, which eventually becomes thicker and whiter as the squamous epithelium matures (Figs. 16-2 and 16-3). As cells accumulate glycogen, they become indistinguishable from normal squamous epithelium lining the exocervix. Importantly, the transformation zone is the site of cervical squamous carcinoma (see below).

Examination of the transformation zone by iodine staining is the basis of the **Schiller iodine test**. Normal mature (glycogen-rich) squamous cells lining the exocervix stain with iodine, and the exocervix appears mahogany brown. If they are immature (glycogen poor), no iodine staining occurs, and the exocervix is pale.

Ovaries

The ovaries are paired organs that flank the uterus. They are attached to the posterior surface of the broad ligament by a peritoneal fold, the mesovarium.

The ovary is covered by a single layer of epithelial cells, confusingly termed "germinal epithelium," which is continuous with the peritoneum. Beneath this, the most superficial layer of the ovarian cortex consists of dense connective tissue, the tunica albuginea. The body of the ovary (the cortex and medulla) is composed of a mesenchymal stroma containing

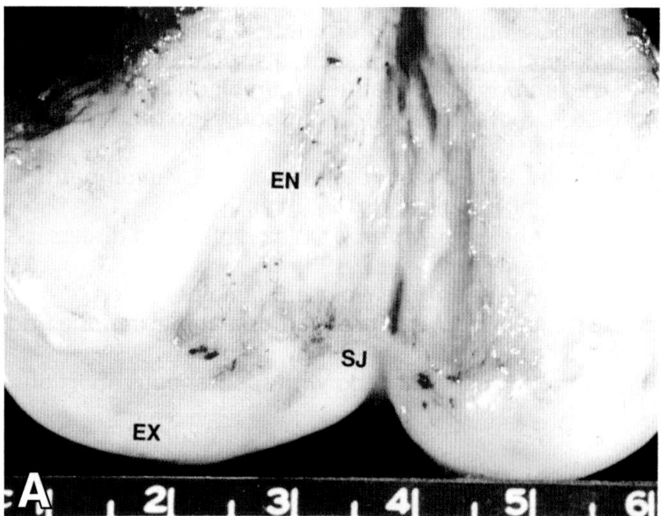

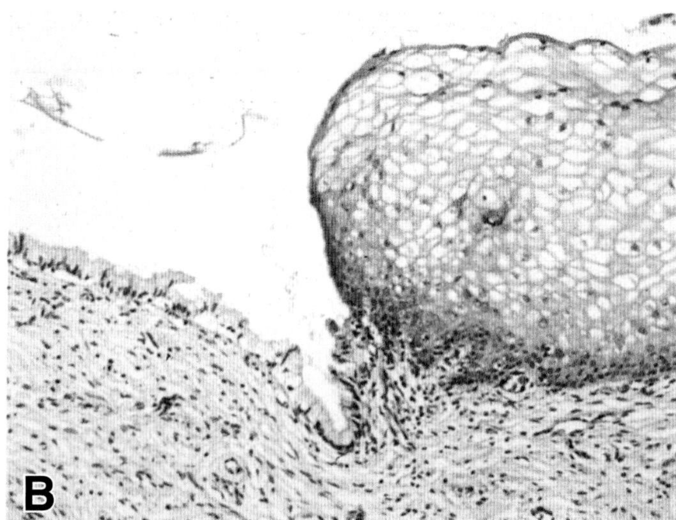

FIGURE 16-1. Anatomy of the cervix. A. The cervix has been opened to show the endocervix (EN), squamocolumnar junction (SJ), and exocervix (EX). The thick layer of squamous cells covering the EX accounts for its white color. **B.** A microscopic view of the SJ. The EN is lined by a single layer of columnar mucus-producing cells that abruptly meets the EX lined by mature squamous cells. *Note:* In specimens in which the SJ is on the ectocervix or in the endocervical canal, the region between it and the external os is called the *transformation zone* (see Fig. 16-2).

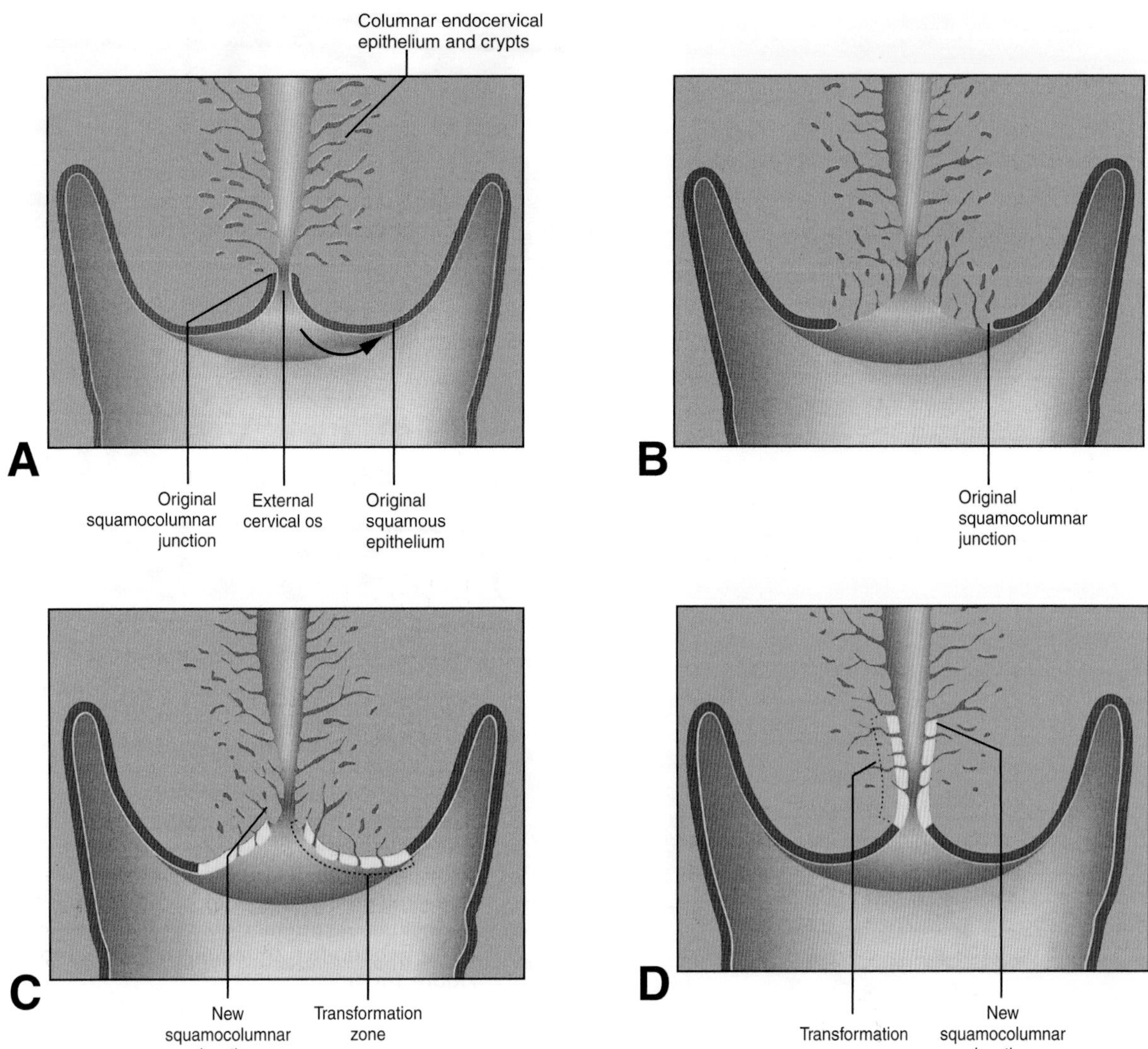

FIGURE 16-2. The transformation zone of the cervix. A. Prepubertal cervix. The squamocolumnar junction is situated at the external cervical os. The arrow shows the direction of the movement that takes place as a result of the increase in bulk of the cervix during adolescence. **B. The process of eversion.** On completion, endocervical columnar tissue lies on the vaginal surface of the cervix and is exposed to the vaginal environment. **C. Postadolescent cervix.** The acidity of the vaginal environment is one of the factors that encourages squamous metaplastic change, replacing the exposed columnar epithelium with squamous epithelium. **D. Postmenopausal cervix.** At this time, cervical inversion occurs. This phenomenon is the reverse of eversion, which was so important in adolescence. The transformation zone is now drawn into the cervical canal, often making it inaccessible to colposcopic examination. Data from Robboy SJ, Anderson MC, Russell P, eds. *Pathology of the Female Reproductive Tract*. London: Churchill-Livingstone, 2002:111-112, 140, 147, 167, 203, 248, 322, 354.

spindle-shaped fibroblast-like cells and scattered bundles of smooth muscle cells. **The cortical region contains the primary germ cells and developing follicles.** The inner medulla of the cortex is highly vascular and contains hilus cells, which are similar to testicular Leydig cells.

Ovaries appear early in fetal life as swellings of the genital ridges. At the 19th gestational day, germ cells migrate from the primitive yolk sac to the gonads and multiply by mitotic division. By the 40th day, ovaries and testes are histologically distinct. Toward the third trimester of fetal life, germ cells stop multiplying and instead continue to develop by meiosis. Of 1 million primordial follicles present at birth, only 70% remain by puberty, and fewer than 15% persist to age 25 years. Only some 450 ova are actually shed during a woman's average 35-year reproductive lifetime.

The ovarian cortical stromal fibroblast-like cells give rise to granulosa and theca cells, which form a functional unit about each ovum (theca interna and theca externa). The complex of a germ cell and supporting granulosa cells is known first as a **primordial follicle**. During the reproductive period, a dominant follicle develops every month into a **Graafian follicle**, which then ruptures during ovulation. Ovulation itself is

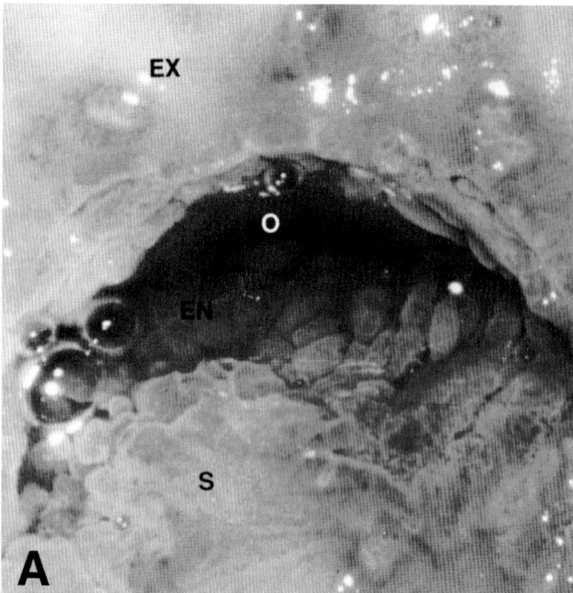

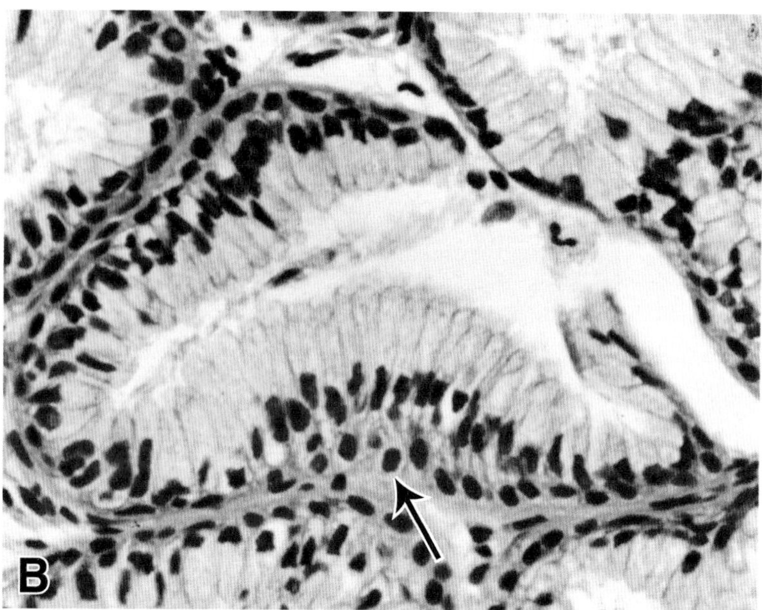

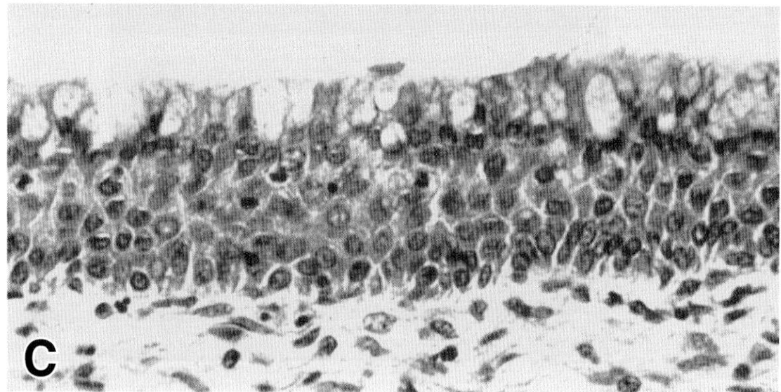

FIGURE 16-3. Squamous metaplasia in the transformation zone. A. In this colposcopic view of the cervix, a white area of metaplastic squamous epithelium (S) is situated between the exocervix (EX) and the mucinous endocervix (EN), which terminates at the internal os (O). **B.** In the early stages of squamous metaplasia of the transformation zone, the reserve cells, which normally constitute a single layer, begin to proliferate (*arrow*). **C.** At a later stage, the proliferating reserve cells displace the glandular epithelium. As a final step, the metaplastic cells mature into glycogen-rich squamous cells, resembling those in Figure 16-1B.

often associated with mild cramping pain, which, if severe, is called **mittelschmerz**, or mid-cycle pain. After ovulation, the follicle granulosa cells luteinize, with hypertrophy and lipid accumulation. They then secrete progesterone in addition to estrogens. The collapsed follicle turns bright yellow and becomes the **corpus luteum** (yellow body).

Ovarian stromal cells, including the hilus cells, and those resembling luteinized cells of the theca interna, both respond to pituitary hormones. These specialized cells secrete both androgens and estrogens, which stimulate proliferation in end organs (e.g., uterus). They inhibit hypothalamic function by negative feedback loops.

Fallopian Tubes

The fallopian tubes extend from the uterine fundus to the ovaries. An interstitial portion, the **isthmus**, lies within the cornua of the uterus and connects the uterine cavity with the straight portion of the tube. As the tube extends to the ovary, it increases in diameter to form the **ampulla**, which merges with the **infundibulum**. The fimbriated end opens like the bell of a trumpet and has fingerlike extensions that envelop the ovary. The lining cells are ciliated and are important in the transport of ova.

Uterus

The uterine corpus (body) is smaller than the cervix at birth and during childhood but increases rapidly in size after puberty. The endometrium is composed of glands and stroma. It is thin at birth, consisting of a continuous surface of cuboidal epithelium, which dips to line a few sparse tubular glands. After puberty, the endometrium thickens. The superficial two thirds, the "zona functionalis," responds to hormones and is shed with each menstrual phase. The deepest third, the basal layer, is the germinative portion that regenerates a new functional zone with each cycle.

The endometrium is supplied with arteries that branch into two types of vessels. The basal arteries supply the basal endometrium, and the spiral arteries nourish the superficial two thirds.

THE MENSTRUAL CYCLE

Normal uterine endometrium undergoes sequential changes that support the growth of implanted fertilized ova (Fig. 16-4). If conception does not occur, the endometrium is shed, after which it is regenerated to support a fertilized ovum in the next cycle.

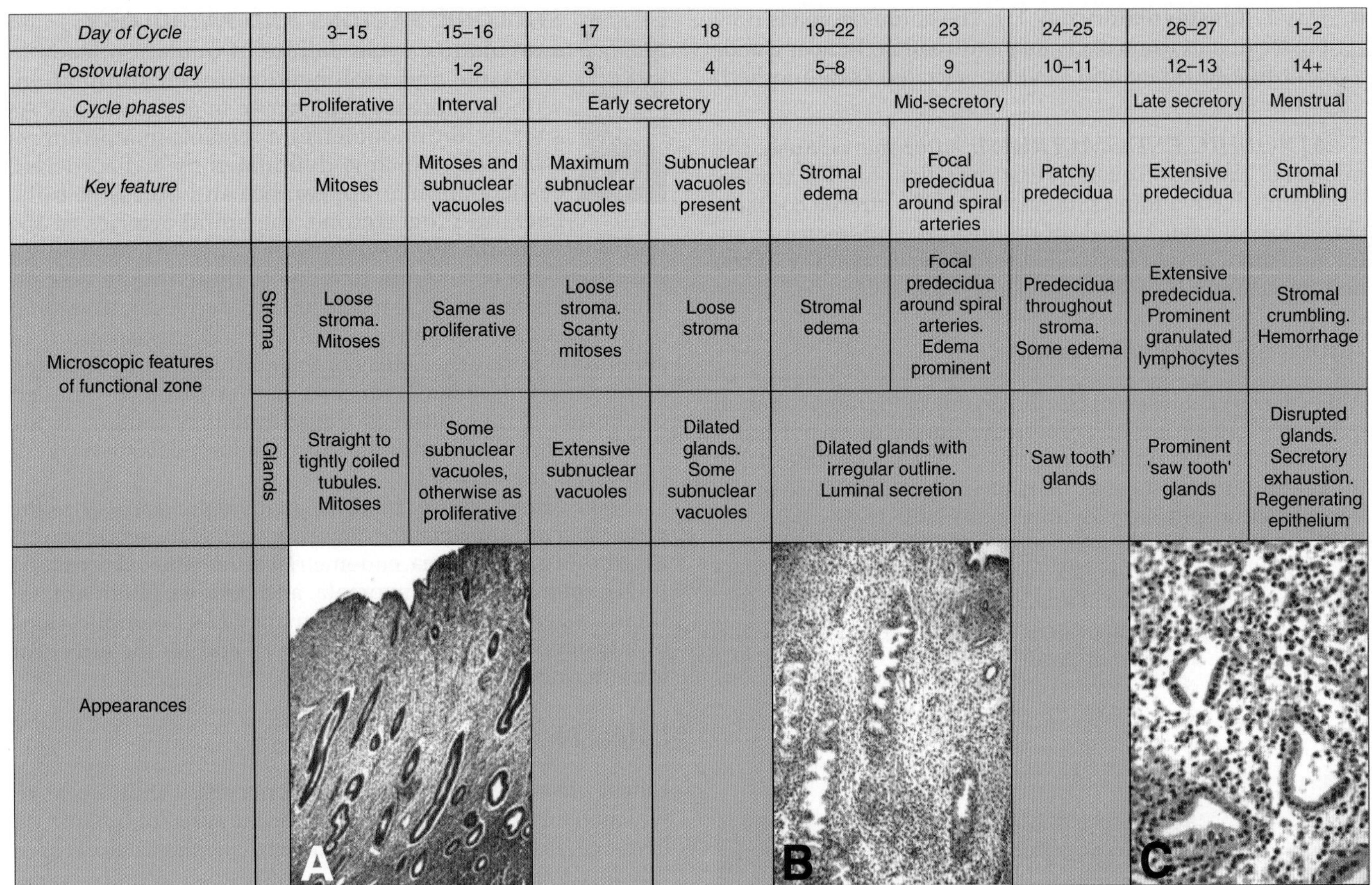

Day of Cycle		3–15	15–16	17	18	19–22	23	24–25	26–27	1–2
Postovulatory day			1–2	3	4	5–8	9	10–11	12–13	14+
Cycle phases		Proliferative	Interval	Early secretory		Mid-secretory			Late secretory	Menstrual
Key feature		Mitoses	Mitoses and subnuclear vacuoles	Maximum subnuclear vacuoles	Subnuclear vacuoles present	Stromal edema	Focal predecidua around spiral arteries	Patchy predecidua	Extensive predecidua	Stromal crumbling
Microscopic features of functional zone	Stroma	Loose stroma. Mitoses	Same as proliferative	Loose stroma. Scanty mitoses	Loose stroma	Stromal edema	Focal predecidua around spiral arteries. Edema prominent	Predecidua throughout stroma. Some edema	Extensive predecidua. Prominent granulated lymphocytes	Stromal crumbling. Hemorrhage
	Glands	Straight to tightly coiled tubules. Mitoses	Some subnuclear vacuoles, otherwise as proliferative	Extensive subnuclear vacuoles	Dilated glands. Some subnuclear vacuoles	Dilated glands with irregular outline. Luminal secretion		`Saw tooth' glands	Prominent 'saw tooth' glands	Disrupted glands. Secretory exhaustion. Regenerating epithelium
Appearances		A				B			C	

FIGURE 16-4. **Main histologic features of the endometrial phases of the normal menstrual cycle. A.** Proliferative phase. Straight tubular glands are embedded in a cellular monomorphic stroma. **B.** Secretory phase, day 24. Dilated tortuous glands with serrated borders are situated in a predecidual stroma. **C.** Menstrual endometrium. Fragmented glands, dissolution of the stroma, and numerous neutrophils are evident. Data from Robboy SJ, Anderson MC, Russell P, eds. *Pathology of the Female Reproductive Tract*. London: Churchill-Livingstone, 2002:111-112, 140, 147, 167, 203, 248, 322, 354.

MENSTRUAL PHASE: Without a blastocyst to secrete human chorionic gonadotropin (hCG), ovarian granulosa and theca cells degenerate, and progesterone levels fall. The endometrium becomes desiccated, spiral arteries collapse, and the stroma disintegrates. Menses composed of about 35 mL of blood start at day 28 and last 3 to 7 days. The denuded surface is then regenerated by extension of the residual glandular epithelium (Fig. 16-4C).

PROLIFERATIVE PHASE: The endometrium is under estrogenic stimulation during days 3 to 15 of the menstrual cycle. Tubular to coiled glands in the functional zone are evenly distributed and supported by a cellular stroma (Fig. 16-4A). Glands are narrow early in the proliferative phase but coil and increase slightly in caliber over time. Columnar cells lining the glands increase from one layer in thickness to a mitotically active pseudostratified epithelium. The glands secrete a watery alkaline fluid that facilitates passage of sperm through the endometrium into the fallopian tubes. The stroma is also mitotically active. Spiral arteries are narrow and inconspicuous.

SECRETORY PHASE: Ovulation occurs about 14 days after the last menstrual period. The Graafian follicle that discharged its ovum becomes a corpus luteum. Granulosa cells of the corpus luteum secrete progesterone, which transforms the endometrium from a proliferative to a secretory state (Fig. 16-4B).

- **Days 17 to 19 (postovulatory days 3 to 5):** Endometrial glands enlarge, dilate, and become more coiled. The lining cells develop abundant and prominent, glycogen-rich, subnuclear vacuoles (day 17). Over the next several days, these cells produce copious secretions that support the zygote (fertilized ovum) as it develops chorionic villi capable of invading the endometrium.
- **Days 20 to 22 (postovulatory days 6 to 8):** The endometrium displays prominent stromal edema. Glands are dilated and more tortuous.
- **Day 23 (postovulatory day 9):** Stromal cells surrounding spiral arteries enlarge and exhibit large vesicular nuclei and abundant eosinophilic cytoplasm ("vascular cuffing"). With time, these cells become more extensively distributed until they fill the functional zone. They are precursors of the decidual cells of pregnancy and are referred to as "predecidua."

- **Day 27 (postovulatory day 13):** The entire stroma is now predecidualized and ready for menstruation. Tubular glands continue to dilate and develop serrated (saw-toothed) borders.

ATROPHIC ENDOMETRIUM: After menopause, the number of glands and quantity of stroma diminish. The remaining glands have a thin epithelium, and the stroma contains abundant collagen. Glands of the atrophic endometrium are often dilated, a condition called **senile cystic atrophy of the endometrium**.

Abnormal Uterine Bleeding

Abnormal (dysfunctional) bleeding is one of the most common gynecologic disorders of reproductive-aged women but is still poorly understood. Importantly, the causes usually lie outside the uterus, and most cases are related to a disturbance of the hypothalamic–pituitary–ovarian axis (Table 16-1).

Anovulatory bleeding, the most common form of dysfunctional bleeding, is a complex syndrome of many causes that manifests as the absence of ovulation during the reproductive years. It occurs most often at either end of reproductive life (i.e., menarche and menopause).

Table 16-1

Causes of Abnormal Uterine Bleeding (Including Uterine and Extrauterine Causes)

Newborn	Maternal Estrogen
Childhood	Iatrogenic (trauma, foreign body, infection of vagina)
	Vaginal neoplasms (sarcoma botryoides)
	Ovarian tumors (functional)
Adolescence	Hypothalamic immaturity
	Psychogenic and nutritional problems
	Inadequate luteal function
Reproductive age	Anovulatory
	Central: psychogenic, stress
	Systemic: nutritional and endocrine disease
	Gonadal: functional tumors
	End-organ: benign endometrial hyperplasia
	Pregnancy: ectopic, retained placenta, abortion, mole
	Ovulatory
	Organic: neoplasia, infections (PID), leiomyomas
	Polymenorrhea: short follicular or luteal phases
	Iatrogenic: anticoagulants, IUD
Menopause	Irregular shedding
Postmenopause	Carcinoma, EIN, benign hyperplasias, polyps, leiomyomata

EIN, endometrial intraepithelial neoplasia; IUD, intrauterine device; PID, pelvic inflammatory disease.

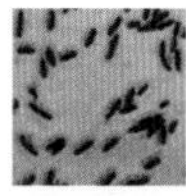

ETIOLOGIC FACTORS AND PATHOLOGY: In an anovulatory cycle, failure of ovulation leads to excessive and prolonged estrogen stimulation, without a postovulatory rise in progesterone. As a result, the endometrium remains in a proliferative state, which is dominated by a disordered, cystic glandular appearance and excessive bulk. Lacking progesterone, the spiral arteries of the endometrium do not develop normally. "Breakthrough bleeding" can occur from damage to these fragile vessels. Thrombosis causes local tissue breakdown resembling that of menstrual endometrium, resulting in bleeding out of synchrony with other areas of the endometrium. Elevated estrogen levels usually decline, either through delayed ovulation or involution of the stimulatory follicle. If the decline is rapid, the endometrium undergoes a heavy synchronized menstrual flow.

Some causes of menstrual irregularity are intrinsic to the uterus and are not considered dysfunctional. These include (1) growths (e.g., carcinoma, endometrial intraepithelial neoplasia [EIN], submucosal leiomyomata, and polyps), (2) inflammation (e.g., endometritis), (3) pregnancy (e.g., complications of intrauterine or ectopic pregnancy), and (4) the effects of intrauterine devices (IUDs).

Luteal Phase Defects

Luteal phase defect results in an abnormally short cycle, in which menses occur 6 to 9 days after the surge of luteinizing hormone (LH) associated with ovulation. It occurs when a corpus luteum develops improperly or regresses prematurely. Luteal phase defects are responsible for 3% of cases of infertility and must be considered in assessing infertility abnormal uterine bleeding. A biopsy showing an endometrium over 2 days out of synchrony with the chronologic day of the menstrual cycle confirms the diagnosis.

GENITAL INFECTIONS

Infectious diseases of the female genital tract are common and are caused by many organisms (Table 16-2).

Bacterial Infections

Gonorrhea is caused by *Neisseria gonorrhoeae* (also called **gonococcus**), a fastidious, Gram-negative diplococcus. Except for perinatal transmission, spread is almost always by sexual intercourse. Infected people who are asymptomatic are a significant reservoir of infection. A million cases of gonorrhea occur yearly in the United States. The infection is a frequent cause of acute salpingitis and pelvic inflammatory disease (PID) (Fig. 16-5).

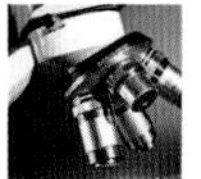

PATHOLOGY: Gonorrhea begins in the mucous membranes of the urogenital tract. Bacteria attach to surface cells, after which they invade superficially and provoke acute inflammation. The disease is a suppurative infection, eliciting a vigorous acute inflammatory response, with copious pus and frequent submucosal abscesses. Smears of pus reveal numerous neutrophils, often containing phagocytosed bacteria. If untreated, the inflammation becomes chronic, with macrophages and lymphocytes predominant.

Table 16-2

Infectious Diseases of the Female Genital Tract

Organism	Disease	Diagnostic Feature
Sexually Transmitted Diseases		
Gram-negative rods and cocci		
Calymmatobacterium granulomatis	*Granuloma inguinale*	Donovan body
Gardnerella vaginalis	*Gardnerella infection*	Clue cell
Haemophilus ducreyi	Chancroid (soft chancre)	
Neisseria gonorrhoeae	Gonorrhea	Gram-negative diplococcus
Spirochetes		
Treponema pallidum	Syphilis	Spirochete
Mycoplasmas		
Mycoplasma hominis	Nonspecific vaginitis	
Ureaplasma urealyticum	Nonspecific vaginitis	
Rickettsiae		
Chlamydia trachomatis types D–K	Various forms of pelvic inflammatory disease (PID)	
Chlamydia trachomatis type L_{1-3}	Lymphogranuloma venereum	
Viruses		
Human papillomavirus	Condyloma acuminatum/planum Neoplastic potential	Koilocyte
Types 6, 11, 40, 42, 43, 44, 57	Low risk	Low-grade squamous intraepithelial lesion
Types 16, 18, 31, 33, 35, 39, 45, 51, 52, 56, 58, 66	High risk	High-grade squamous intraepithelial lesion
Herpes simplex type 2	Herpes genitalis	Multinucleated giant cell with intranuclear homogenization and inclusion bodies
Cytomegalovirus	Cytomegalic inclusion disease	Bulbous intranuclear inclusion body
Molluscum contagiosum	Molluscum infection	Molluscum body
Protozoa		
Trichomonas vaginalis	Trichomoniasis	Trichomonad
Selected Nonsexually Transmitted Diseases		
Actinomyces and related organisms		
Actinomyces israelii	PID (one of many organisms)	Sulphur granules
Mycobacterium tuberculosis	Tuberculosis	Necrotizing granulomas
Fungi		
Candida albicans	Candidiasis	*Candida* sp.

CLINICAL FEATURES: In one half of infected women, gonorrhea remains asymptomatic. When symptomatic, infected women initially exhibit endocervicitis, with vaginal discharge or bleeding. Urethritis presents as dysuria rather than as a urethral discharge. The organisms ascend through the cervix and endometrial cavity, where they cause **acute endometritis**. They then attach to mucosal cells in the fallopian tube and elicit acute inflammation, which is confined to the mucosal surface and produces both acute and chronic salpingitis. Fallopian tubes swell with pus, causing acute abdominal pain. Infection may then spread to the ovary, sometimes causing a **tubo-ovarian abscess**. Involvement of pelvic and abdominal cavities leads to subdiaphragmatic and pelvic abscesses. Systemic complications of gonorrhea include septicemia and septic arthritis. At all sites of infection, the organisms induce purulent inflammatory reactions that rarely resolve completely. Dense fibrous adhesions often remain; they distort and destroy the plicae of the fallopian tube and frequently leading to sterility. Adhesions increase the risk for tubal pregnancy. Neonatal infections, derived from the birth canal of a mother with gonorrhea, usually manifest as conjunctivitis, although disseminated infections occur occasionally. Neonatal gonococcal conjunctivitis has been largely eliminated in developed countries by routine instillation of antibiotics into the conjunctiva at birth.

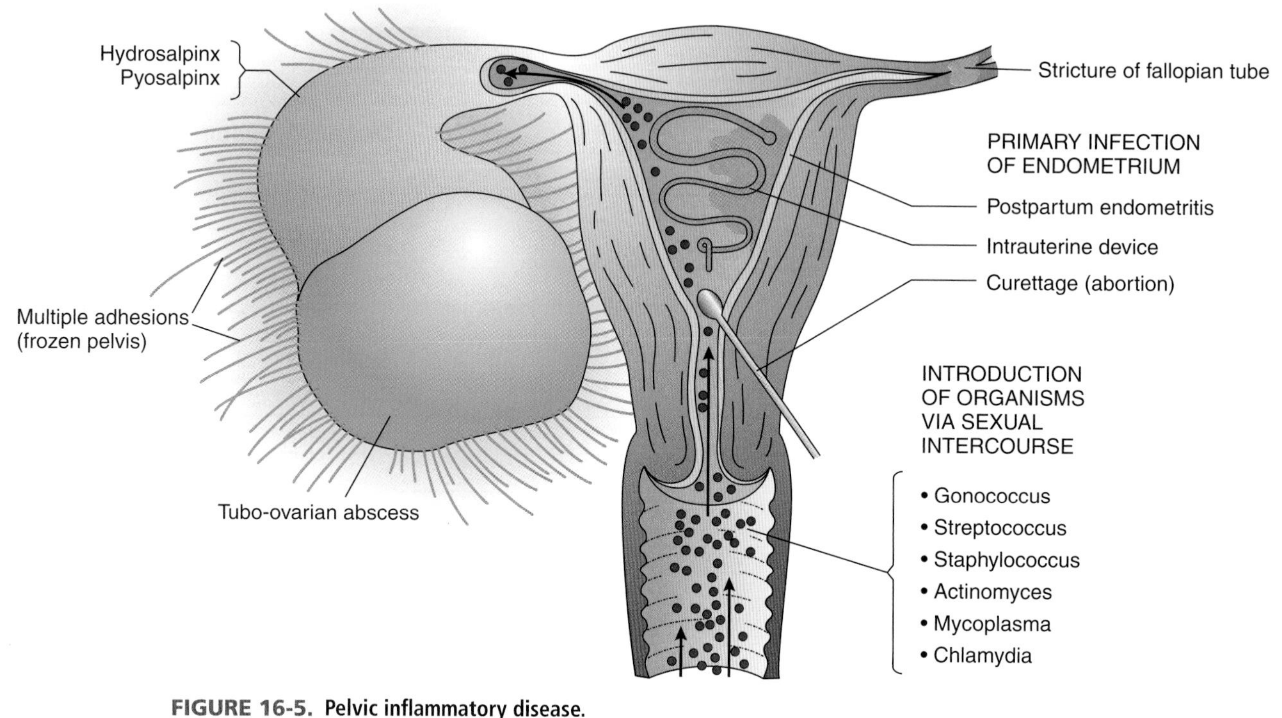

FIGURE 16-5. Pelvic inflammatory disease.

Syphilis

Syphilis (lues) is a chronic, sexually transmitted, systemic infection caused by the spirochete *Treponema pallidum*. Spread is via sexual contact with an infected person or transplacental spread (congenital syphilis).

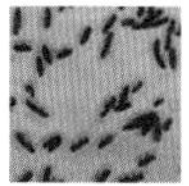

ETIOLOGIC FACTORS AND PATHOPHYSIOLOGY: *T. pallidum* is very fragile and is killed by soap, antiseptics, drying, and cold. Person-to-person transmission requires direct contact between a rich source of spirochetes, for example, an open lesion or abraded skin of the genital organs, rectum, mouth, fingers, or nipples. The organisms reproduce at the site of inoculation, pass to regional lymph nodes, gain access to systemic circulation, and disseminate throughout the body. Although *T. pallidum* induces an inflammatory response and is taken up by phagocytic cells, it persists and proliferates. Chronic infection and inflammation cause tissue destruction, sometimes for decades. Untreated, syphilis persists, often waxing and waning, through three stages (Fig. 16-6).

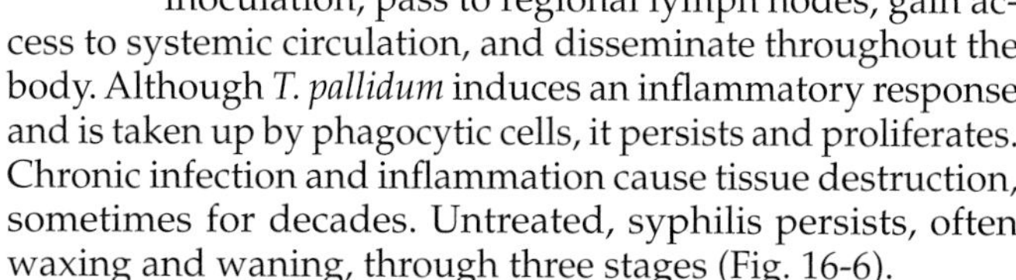

- The **primary stage** features a **chancre** that usually appears after about 3 weeks at the portal of bacterial entry. Chancres, as well as the lesions of the other stages of syphilis, show a characteristic **"luetic vasculitis,"** characterized by endothelial cell proliferation and swelling, with vessel walls thickened by lymphocytes and fibrosis. Clinically, it is a painless, indurated papule, 1 cm to several centimeters in diameter, surrounded by an inflammatory cuff that breaks down to form an ulcer. The lesion may persist for 2 to 6 weeks, after which it heals spontaneously.
- **Secondary syphilis** appears after a latent period of several weeks to months and features low-grade fever, headache, malaise, lymphadenopathy, skin rash, and highly infectious lesions called **condylomata lata** (syphilitic warts) on the perineum and vulva (Fig. 16-7). These secondary lesions heal after 2 to 6 weeks, and symptoms disappear spontaneously.
- The **tertiary stage** develops any time thereafter and may entail severe damage to the cardiovascular system or CNS. ***Damage to, and scarring of, the ascending aorta (syphilitic aortitis) commonly leads to dilation of the aortic ring, separation of the valve cusps, and regurgitation of blood through the aortic valve (aortic insufficiency).*** **Neurosyphilis** results from slow progressive infection of the meninges, cerebral cortex, spinal cord, cranial nerves, or eyes.
- **Congenital syphilis** occurs when the organism disseminates in fetal tissue and is discussed under the "Pregnancy and the Placenta" sections (see below).

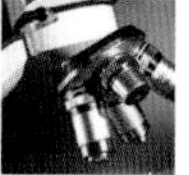

PATHOLOGY: The hallmark of syphilis in biopsy specimens is a dense inflammatory infiltrate composed of lymphocytes and plasma cells, particularly adjacent to blood vessels. The more advanced stages of disease show greater obliterative endarteritis and subsequent tissue destruction.

Granuloma Inguinale

Granuloma inguinale is caused by *Calymmatobacterium granulomatis*, a sexually transmitted, Gram-negative, encapsulated rod. The disease occurs with equal frequency in women and men. The disease occurs principally in tropical countries and is uncommon in the United States.

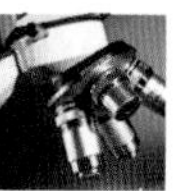

PATHOLOGY: The primary lesion begins as a painless, ulcerated nodule involving genital, inguinal, or perianal skin. The organisms invade through skin abrasions and spread initially by direct extension, destroying

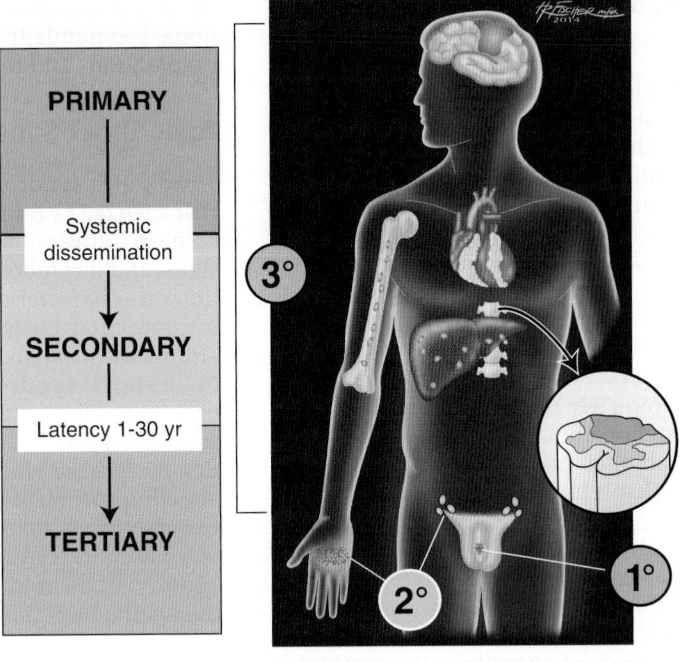

FIGURE 16-6. Clinical characteristics of the various stages of syphilis.

skin and underlying tissues. Extensive local spread and lymphatic permeation occur later. Vacuolated macrophages teem with characteristic intracellular bacteria (**Donovan bodies**). The organism, best seen with the Wright stain, resembles a closed safety pin. Hyperplasia of overlying squamous epithelium may be so exuberant as to be misinterpreted as a squamous cell carcinoma. Relapses after antibiotic therapy are common.

Chancroid

Chancroid, also called **soft chancre**, is caused by *Haemophilus ducreyi*, a Gram-negative bacillus. It is rare in the United States but is common in underdeveloped countries.

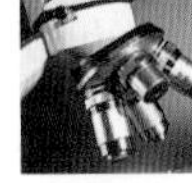

PATHOLOGY: Single or sometimes multiple small, vesiculopustular lesions appear on the cervix, vagina, vulva, or perianal region 3 to 5 days after sexual contact with an infected partner. At this stage, microscopic examination shows granulomatous inflammation. The lesion may rupture to form a painful, purulent ulcer that bleeds easily. Inguinal lymphadenopathy, fever, chills, and malaise may occur. A major complication is scarring during the healing phase, which may cause urethral stenosis.

Gardnerella

Sexual transmission of *Gardnerella vaginalis*, a Gram-negative coccobacillus, causes many cases of "nonspecific vaginitis." Because the organism does not penetrate the mucosa, it causes no inflammation, and biopsies appear normal. A wet mount specimen of a vaginal discharge or a Papanicolaou-stained smear (Pap smear) can identify the bacteria. **Clue cells**, namely, squamous cells covered by coccobacilli, are pathognomonic.

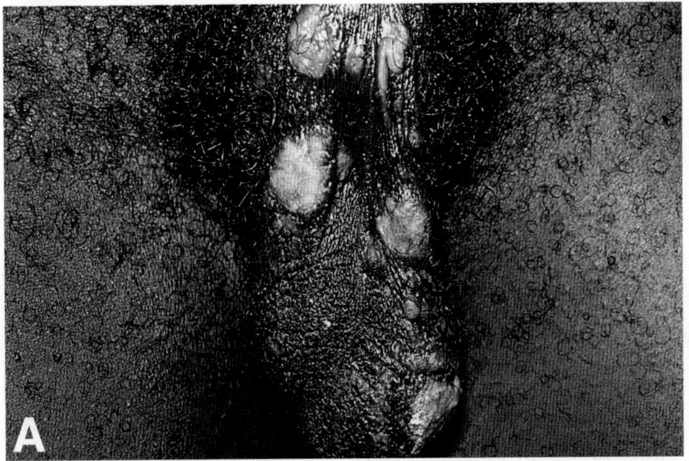

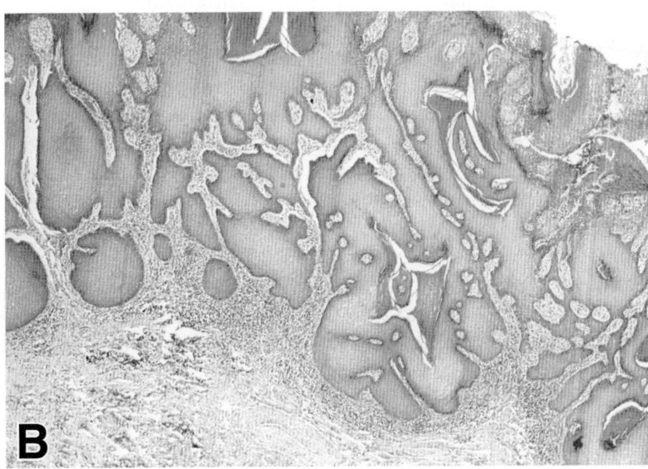

FIGURE 16-7. Condylomata lata in secondary syphilis. A. Whitish plaques are seen on the vulva and perineum. **B.** A photomicrograph showing papillomatous hyperplasia of the epidermis with underlying chronic inflammation.

Mycoplasma and Chlamydial Infections

Mycoplasma

Mycoplasma are minute pleomorphic organisms that have no cell wall. They are common oropharyngeal and urogenital tract commensals and colonize the lower genital tract through sexual contact. *Ureaplasma urealyticum* can be isolated from the lower genital tract in 40% of healthy women. It may cause infertility, may generate adverse effects on pregnancy, and can precipitate perinatal infections. *Mycoplasma hominis* is found in the lower genital tract of 5% of healthy women and causes a small proportion of cases of symptomatic cervicitis and vaginitis. *M. hominis* is often isolated in association with *G. vaginalis* or *Trichomonas vaginalis* infection. Although the role of mycoplasma in genital tract infections is not completely understood, the organisms are encountered in pelvic inflammatory disease (PID), acute salpingitis, spontaneous abortion, and puerperal fever. Affected tissue is usually unremarkable histologically.

Chlamydia

Chlamydia trachomatis is a common, venereally transmitted, Gram-negative, intracellular rickettsia. *C. trachomatis* causes several disorders in women, men, and infants. It has been found in the genital tracts of about 8% of asymptomatic women and 20% of women with symptoms of lower genital tract infection. Chlamydial disease is easily confused with gonorrhea because the symptoms of both diseases are similar.

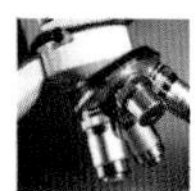

PATHOLOGY: The cervical mucosa is severely inflamed, and endocervical and metaplastic squamous cells contain small inclusion bodies. Cytologically, perinuclear intracytoplasmic inclusions with distinct borders and intracytoplasmic **coccoid bodies** are seen. Complications include ascending infection of the endometrium, fallopian tube, and ovary, which may result in tubal occlusion and infertility. Chlamydia may also infect Bartholin glands and cause acute urethritis. Infants delivered vaginally to infected mothers are prone to develop conjunctivitis, otitis media, and pneumonia.

Lymphogranuloma Venereum

Lymphogranuloma venereum is a venereal infection of men and women, endemic in tropical countries. It is caused by a form of *C. trachomatis*, serotypes L1 through L3.

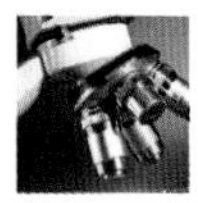

PATHOLOGY: After a few days to a month, a small painless vesicle forms at the site of inoculation. It heals rapidly and is often not even noticed. In the second stage, inguinal lymph nodes become enlarged and may rupture to form suppurative fistulas. Perirectal lymph nodes in women become matted and painful. In untreated patients, a third stage may appear after latency lasting several years. In this phase, scarring causes lymphatic obstruction, resulting in genital elephantiasis and rectal strictures. Infected tissues in the second and third stages show necrotizing granulomas and neutrophilic infiltrates. Inclusion bodies within macrophages may also be seen.

Trichomoniasis

T. vaginalis is a large, pear-shaped, flagellated protozoan that often causes vaginitis. It is transmitted sexually, and 25% of infected women are asymptomatic carriers. Infection causes a heavy, yellow-gray, thick, foamy discharge with severe itching, dyspareunia (painful intercourse), and dysuria (painful urination). The motile trichomonads are identified on wet mount preparations and may also be demonstrated in Pap smears.

Toxic Shock Syndrome

Toxic shock syndrome is an acute, sometimes fatal disorder characterized by fever, shock, and a desquamative erythematous rash. In addition, vomiting, diarrhea, myalgias, neurologic signs, and thrombocytopenia are common. Pathologic alterations are characteristic of shock, and lesions of disseminated intravascular coagulation are usually prominent. Certain strains of *Staphylococcus aureus* release an exotoxin called **toxic shock syndrome toxin-1**, which impairs the ability of mononuclear phagocytes to clear other potentially toxic substances, such as endotoxin. Toxic shock syndrome was first recognized when long-acting tampons were introduced, allowing sufficient time for the staphylococci to proliferate. Contraceptive "sponges" were also associated. The incidence of toxic shock syndrome has decreased markedly since recognition of the role of tampons in promoting colonization of the vagina by *S. aureus*.

Polymicrobial Infections

Cervicitis

Inflammation of the cervix is common and is related to constant exposure to bacterial flora in the vagina. Acute and chronic cervicitis are caused by many organisms, particularly endogenous vaginal aerobes and anaerobes, *Streptococcus*, *Staphylococcus*, and *Enterococcus*. Other specific organisms include *C. trachomatis*, *N. gonorrhoeae*, and, occasionally, herpes simplex type 2. Some agents are sexually transmitted; others may be introduced by foreign bodies, such as residual fragments of tampons and pessaries.

Salpingitis

Salpingitis refers to an inflammation of the fallopian tubes, typically due to infections that ascend from the lower genital tract. The most common causative organisms are *N. gonorrhoeae*, *Escherichia coli*, *Chlamydia*, and *Mycoplasma*. Most infections are polymicrobial. Acute episodes of salpingitis (particularly if due to chlamydia) may be asymptomatic. A fallopian tube damaged by prior infection is very susceptible to reinfection.

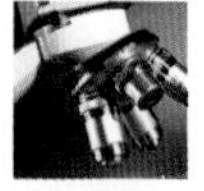

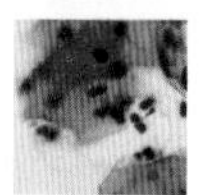

PATHOLOGY AND CLINICAL FEATURES: Acute salpingitis is characterized by neutrophil infiltration, edema, and congestion of mucosal folds (plicae). In chronic salpingitis, the inflammatory infiltrate is mainly lymphocytes and plasma cells; edema and congestion are usually minimal. In late stages, the fallopian tube may seal and become distended with pus (**pyosalpinx**) or a transudate (**hydrosalpinx**). In severe chronic salpingitis, dense adhesions cause the end of the tube to become blunted and clubbed. A blocked lumen may lead to hydrosalpinx or pyosalpinx. The damage wrought by chronic salpingitis may also impair tubal motility and passage of sperm, resulting in **infertility**. Chronic salpingitis is a common cause of **ectopic pregnancy** because adherent mucosal plicae create pockets in which ova are entrapped.

The fallopian tube allows infections from the lower genital tract to ascend to the peritoneal cavity, leading to peritonitis and PID. The adjacent ovary may also be involved, sometimes as a **tubo-ovarian abscess**.

Pelvic Inflammatory Disease

PID is an infection of pelvic organs caused by extension of one of several microorganisms above the uterine corpus (Fig. 16-5). Ascending infection results in bilateral acute salpingitis, pyosalpinx, and tubo-ovarian abscesses. ***N. gonorrhoeae and Chlamydia are the main organisms responsible for PID, but most infections are polymicrobial.***

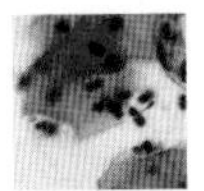

CLINICAL FEATURES: Patients with PID typically present with lower abdominal pain. Physical examination reveals bilateral adnexal tenderness and marked discomfort when the cervix is manipulated (chandelier sign). Complications of PID include (1) rupture of a tubo-ovarian abscess, which may result in life-threatening peritonitis; (2) infertility from scarring of the healed tubal plicae; (3) increased rates of ectopic pregnancy; and (4) intestinal obstruction from fibrous bands and adhesions.

Nonsexually Transmitted Genital Infections

Tuberculosis

Mycobacterium tuberculosis may infect any part of the female genital tract. Salpingitis resulting from hematogenous dissemination from the respiratory tract is the usual initial lesion. Half of cases are complicated by tuberculous endometritis. Genital tuberculosis occurs in 1% of infertile women in the United States and in over 10% of such women in less developed countries. Detecting acid-fast bacilli (AFB) confirms the diagnosis.

Candidiasis

In all, 10% of women are asymptomatic carriers of fungi in the vulva and vagina, *Candida albicans* being the most common offender. Only 2% present with clinically apparent candidal vulvovaginitis. However, the risk is greatly increased by diabetes mellitus, oral contraceptive use, and pregnancy. Untreated infections wax and wane, often disappearing after delivery.

Viral Infections

Human Papillomavirus

HPV is a DNA virus that infects genital skin and mucosal surfaces to produce wartlike lesions referred to as **condylomata acuminatum** or flat ones known as **squamous intraepithelial lesions (SILs)**. HPV is associated with many different types of cancer in the female reproductive tract. Over 100 HPV serotypes are known, one third of which cause genital tract lesions. The median time from infection to first detection of HPV is 3 months. About 20 million people are currently infected with HPV. In the United States, genotypes 6 and 11 account for over 80% of visible condylomata. HPV genotypes 16, 18, and 31 and a number of additional types are associated with a high risk for the development of squamous cell carcinoma in the female lower genital tract, as well as anal and oropharyngeal cancers in both sexes.

Most cases of HPV are diagnosed by a cervical Pap smear. However, false positives and indeterminate results (ASCUS, atypical squamous cells of unknown significance) occur. Additionally, many women are exposed to HPV infections that result in an abnormal Pap smear, but will be cleared by the host immune response and not progress to cancer. Recent tests directly detect HPV DNA and can determine whether high-risk genotypes are present. Treatment is based on the histology of lesions (low grade vs. high grade), which predicts those at greatest risk for progression to cancer and, if available, the HPV genotype.

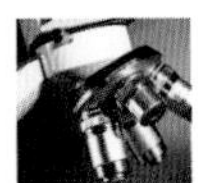

PATHOLOGY: Lesions in the vulva, perianal region, perineum, vagina, and cervix caused by HPV infection are separated into low and high grades, based on the appearance of the affected epithelium, which may be flat or exophytic. **The terms *low-grade (LSILs) or high-grade (HSILs) are based on the corresponding infecting viral subtype and the risk of progression to invasive squamous cell carcinoma*.** The warty form of low-grade squamous intraepithelial lesion (LSIL) is known as condylomata acuminatum. Acuminate warts are generally caused by low cancer risk viral subtypes and may present as papules, plaques, or nodules, which eventually become spiked or cauliflower-like excrescences (Fig. 16-8A). LSIL is characterized by koilocytes (from the Greek *koilos* for "hollow"), epithelial cells with a perinuclear halo, and a wrinkled nucleus bearing HPV particles (Fig. 16-8B). Viral DNA typically remains episomal. Extensive viral replication causes cytoplasmic injury, which results in koilocytosis (Fig. 16-8C). High-grade squamous intraepithelial lesions (HSILs) are discussed with diseases of the vulva and cervix below.

Herpesviruses

Herpes simplex type 2 is a large double-stranded DNA virus that commonly causes sexually transmitted genital infections. After an incubation period of 1 to 3 weeks, small vesicles develop on the vulva and erode into painful ulcers. Similar lesions occur in the vagina and cervix. Epithelial cells adjacent to intraepithelial vesicles show ballooning degeneration, and many contain large nuclei with eosinophilic viral inclusions.

Herpesvirus infections typically follow a relapsing, remitting course. Although latent, the virus resides in spinal (sacral) ganglia. If the virus reactivates during pregnancy, passage through the birth canal results in transmission to the newborn infant, often with fatal consequences. Active vaginal herpetic lesions at the time of delivery are, therefore, an indication for cesarean delivery.

Cytomegalovirus

CMV is a ubiquitous double-stranded DNA virus belonging to the Herpesvirus family. More than 80% of people over the age of 35 have antibodies to CMV. Several lines of evidence suggest that many cases are sexually transmitted: (1) seroprevalence of CMV has risen in young adults, (2) the virus is recovered more often from cervical secretions and semen than from any other body sites, and (3) viral titers in semen are 100,000 times higher than in urine. Although CMV only rarely causes genital infections in women, infection of the endometrium may result in spontaneous abortion or infection of the newborn. Infected cells exhibit characteristic large, eosinophilic, intranuclear inclusions, and, occasionally, cytoplasmic inclusions.

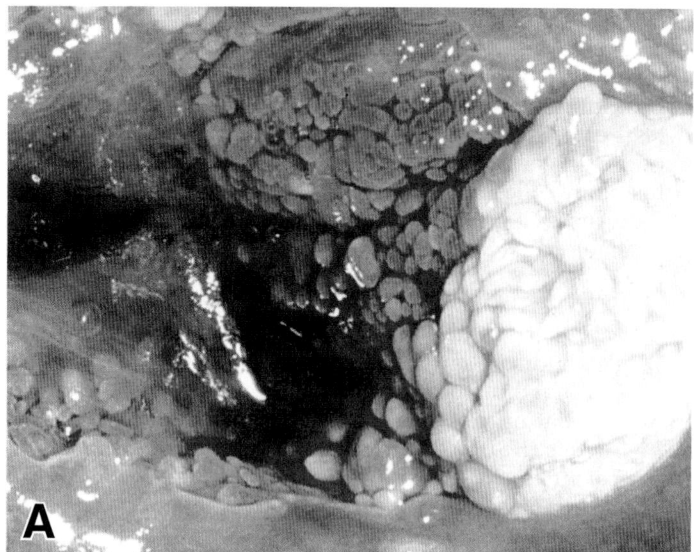

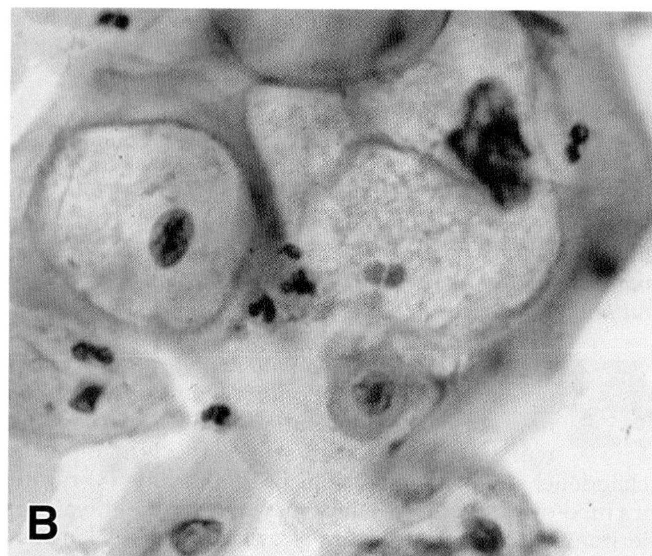

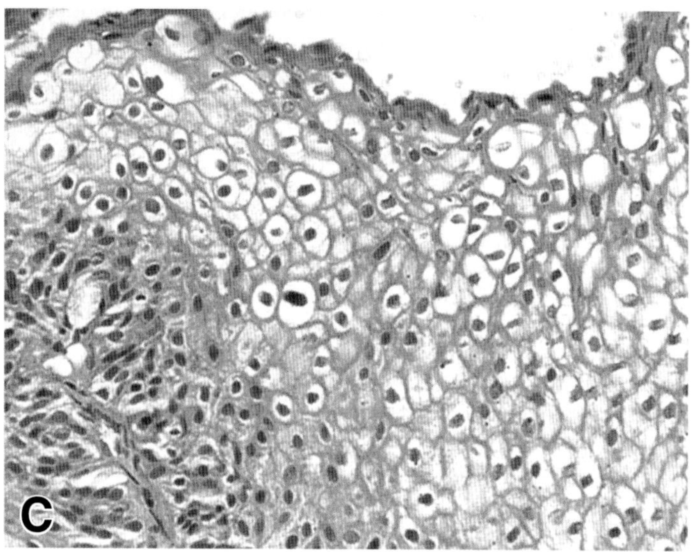

FIGURE 16-8. Human papillomavirus–induced condylomatous infections. A. Condyloma acuminatum on the cervix, visible with the naked eye as cauliflower-like excrescences. **B.** A cervical smear contains characteristic koilocytes, with a perinuclear halo and a wrinkled nucleus that contains viral particles. **C.** Biopsy of the condyloma showing koilocytes with perinuclear halos and significant nuclear pleomorphism and altered chromatin density.

Vulva

CYSTIC LESIONS

BARTHOLIN DUCT CYST: The paired Bartholin glands produce a clear mucoid secretion that continuously lubricates the vestibular surface. The ducts are prone to obstruction and consequent cyst formation. Cyst infection may lead to abscess formation. Bartholin gland abscess was formerly associated with gonorrhea, but staphylococci, chlamydia, and anaerobes are now more frequently the cause. Treatment consists of incision, drainage, marsupialization, and appropriate antibiotics.

FOLLICULAR CYSTS: Follicular cysts recapitulate the most distal portion of the hair follicle. Also called **epithelial inclusion cysts** or **keratinous cysts**, follicular cysts frequently appear on the vulva, especially the labia majora. They contain a white cheesy material and typically are lined by stratified squamous epithelium.

MUCINOUS CYSTS: Vulvar mucinous glands occasionally become obstructed and develop cysts. Mucinous columnar cells line the cyst and may become infected.

DERMATOSES

Vulvar Acute Dermatitis

The most common endogenous types of acute dermatitis are **atopic (hypersensitivity) dermatitis** and **seborrheic dermatitis**, seen as a scaly macular eruption. Dermatitides with exogenous causes include irritant dermatitis (e.g., urine on the vulvar skin) and contact allergic dermatitis and are manifest as either acute or chronic dermatitis.

Vulvar Chronic Dermatitis

Vulvar chronic dermatitis follows many diseases that are clinically pruritic and thus subject to repeated scratching in their active phase. These include lichen planus, psoriasis, and lichen sclerosus (see Chapter 20). The skin is thickened and white, with exaggerated markings ("lichenification") as a result of marked hyperkeratosis. Scaling is generally present, and excoriations as a result of recent scratching are often seen.

LICHEN SCLEROSUS: Lichen sclerosus is an inflammatory disease associated with autoimmune disorders, such as vitiligo, pernicious anemia, and thyroiditis. An autoimmune etiology of lichen sclerosus is further suggested by the presence of activated T cells in the dermis.

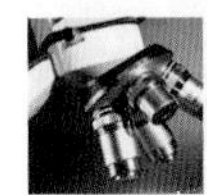
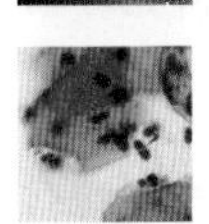

PATHOLOGY AND CLINICAL FEATURES: The condition is characterized by white plaques and atrophic skin, with a parchment-like or crinkled appearance and, occasionally, marked contracture of vulvar tissues (Fig. 16-9A). Hyperkeratosis, loss of rete ridges, epithelial thinning with flattening of rete pegs, cytoplasmic vacuolation of the basal layer, and a homogeneous, acellular zone in the upper dermis are seen (Fig. 16-9B). A band of lymphocytes with few plasma cells typically underlies this layer. The disease develops insidiously and is progressive, often causing itching and dyspareunia. ***Women with symptomatic lichen sclerosus have a 15% chance of developing squamous cell carcinoma.***

MALIGNANT TUMORS AND PREMALIGNANT CONDITIONS

Vulvar Intraepithelial Neoplasia

Vulvar carcinoma, mostly squamous cell carcinoma, accounts for 3% of all female genital cancers and occurs mainly in women over age 60. These tumors are divided into keratinizing squamous cell carcinomas unrelated to HPV, termed **differentiated VIN (dVIN) or VIN simplex** (>70% of cases), and warty or basaloid carcinomas associated with high-risk genotypes of HPV (<25% of cases). LSILs include flat condylomas and bland flat lesions that rarely exhibit diagnostic koilocytes. HSILs (formerly known as VIN usual type or "classic VIN") include warty and basaloid types of lesions.

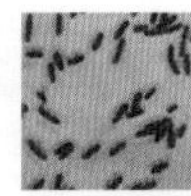
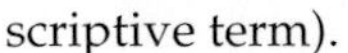

ETIOLOGIC FACTORS AND CLINICAL FEATURES: Keratinizing squamous carcinomas frequently develops in older women (mean age, 76 years), sometimes in the context of long-standing lichen sclerosus. The precursor lesion is dVIN (Fig. 16-10A), which carries a high risk for cancer development. These cancers develop as nodules or masses in a background of **"leukoplakia"** (*white plaques,* a nonspecific, descriptive term).

By contrast, the less common HPV-associated warty and basaloid carcinomas are preceded by **classic VIN** (Fig. 16-10B), which is typically associated with **HPV-16** infection. Since 1980s, there has been a 5- to 10-fold increase in classic VIN in women under age 40. Nevertheless, HPV-associated VIN lesions have a low risk of progression to invasive cancer (6%), except in older or immunosuppressed women.

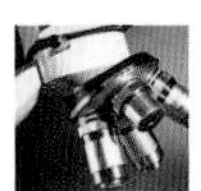

PATHOLOGY: VIN reflects a spectrum of neoplastic changes from minimal-to-severe cellular atypia with differing pathogenesis as described above. These lesions may be single or multiple, and macular, papular, or plaque like. Histologic grades of VIN I, VIN II, and VIN III correspond to mild, moderate, and severe dysplasia, respectively. However, grade III (which includes squamous cell carcinoma in situ [CIS]) is by far the most common. As in comparable lesions in the cervix (see below), criteria used in establishing the grade of classic VIN include (1) nuclear size and atypia, (2) number and severity of atypical mitoses, and (3) loss of cytoplasmic differentiation toward the epithelial surface.

Keratinizing squamous cell carcinomas usually follow the precursor lesion dVIN. Two thirds of larger tumors are exophytic, and the remainder are ulcerative and endophytic. The tumor is composed of invasive nests of malignant squamous epithelium with central keratin pearls. The tumors grow slowly, extending to contiguous skin, vagina, and rectum. They

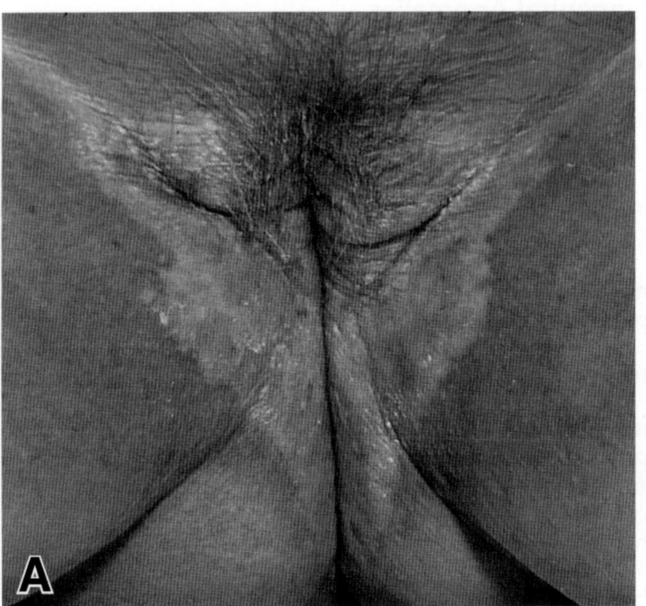

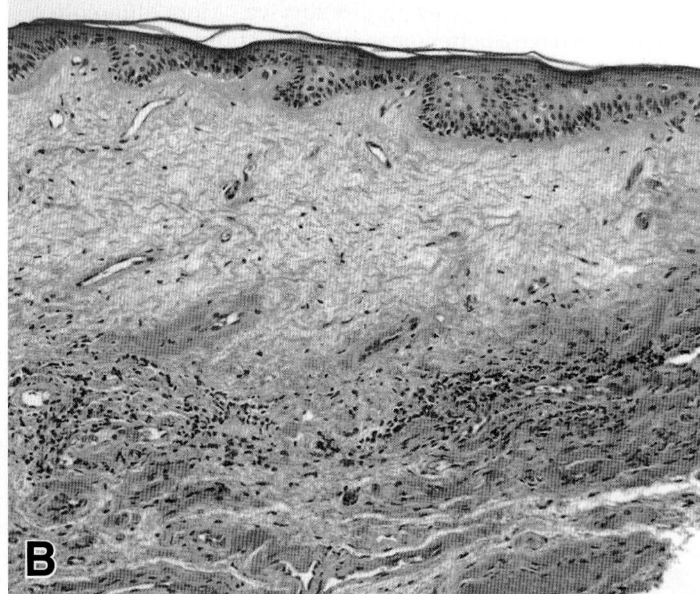

FIGURE 16-9. Lichen sclerosus of vulva. A. The sharply demarcated white lesion affects the vulva and perineum. **B.** The epidermis is thin and exhibits hyperkeratosis and a lack of the normal rete pattern. The dermis displays an acellular, homogeneous zone overlying a mild chronic inflammatory infiltrate.

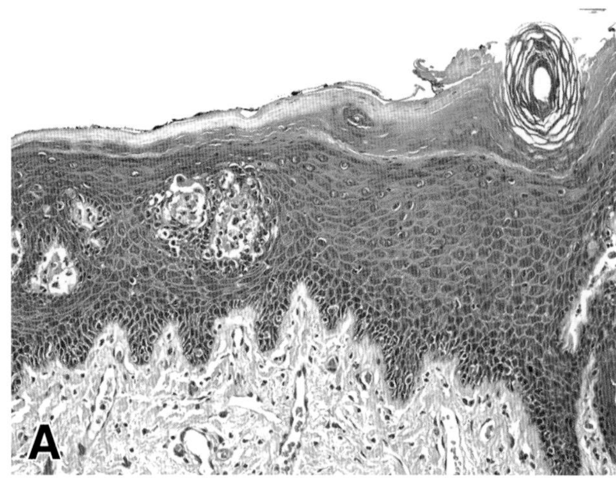

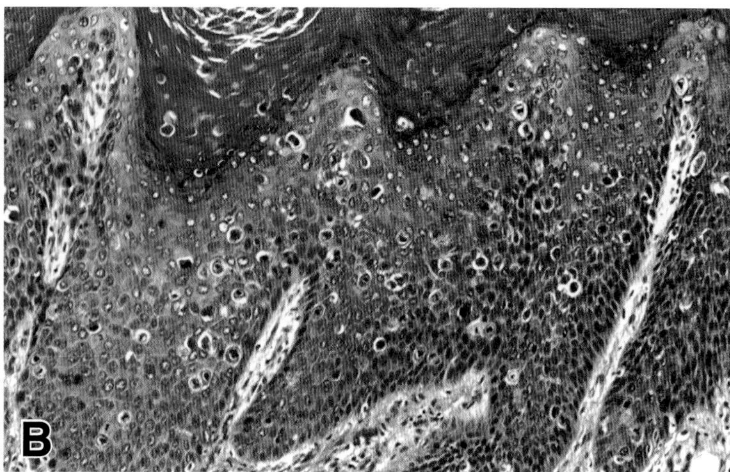

FIGURE 16-10. Vulvar intraepithelial neoplasia (VIN). A. Differentiated VIN is not associated with human papillomavirus (HPV) and demonstrates atypia accentuated in the basal and parabasal layers. There is striking epithelial maturation in the superficial layers. **B.** Classic VIN is caused by HPV and includes features of full-thickness atypia, numerous mitoses, and often, as in this example, hyperkeratosis.

metastasize initially to superficial inguinal lymph nodes and then to deep inguinal, femoral, and pelvic lymph nodes. dVIN shows severe nuclear atypia of the basal layer with striking epithelial maturation in the superficial layers (Fig. 16-10A). Superficial keratinocytes contain rounded nuclei with enlarged nucleoli, ample eosinophilic cytoplasm, and prominent intercellular bridges. Rete pegs often contain keratin pearls.

PATHOLOGY: Most patients with VIN present with vulvar itching and burning. Raised, well-defined skin lesions of variable sizes may be pink, red, brown, or white. The prognosis for patients with vulvar cancer is generally good, with 70% overall 5-year survival. Tumor grade, size, location, and, most importantly, the number of lymph node metastases predict survival. More differentiated tumors have a better mean survival, approaching 90% if nodes do not contain metastases.

Malignant Melanoma

Although uncommon, malignant melanoma is the second most frequent cancer of the vulva (5%). It occurs in the sixth and seventh decades but is occasionally found in younger women. It has biologic and microscopic characteristics of melanoma occurring elsewhere in the body. Vulvar melanoma tends to be highly aggressive, and the prognosis is poor.

Extramammary Paget Disease

The disorder usually occurs on the labia majora in older women. Women with Paget disease of the vulva complain of pruritus or a burning sensation for many years.

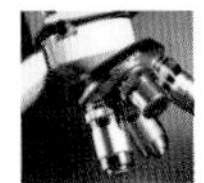

PATHOLOGY: The lesion is large, red, moist, and sharply demarcated. Diagnostic cells (Paget cells) may arise in the epidermis or epidermally derived adnexae. They have pale, vacuolated cytoplasm (Fig. 16-11), with abundant glycosaminoglycans. The cells stain with periodic acid–Schiff (PAS) and mucicarmine and express carcinoembryonic antigen (CEA). They appear as large single cells or, less often, as clusters of cells that lack intercellular bridges and are usually confined to the epidermis. Unlike Paget disease of the breast, which is almost always associated with underlying duct carcinoma, extramammary Paget disease is only rarely associated with carcinoma of the skin adnexae. Metastases occur rarely, so treatment requires only wide local excision or simple vulvectomy.

Vagina

NONNEOPLASTIC CONDITIONS

Congenital Anomalies

Congenital absence of the vagina is generally associated with anomalies of the uterus and urinary tract. If there is a functional uterus, the absence of a vagina may lead to the accumulation of menstrual blood in the uterus.

Septate vagina results from failure of embryonic Müllerian ducts to fuse properly, and the resulting median wall does not resorb.

Vaginal atresia and imperforate hymen prevent the vaginal embryonic lining from maturing from Müllerian to squamous epithelium, which can cause vaginal adenosis (see below).

Diminished Estrogen Stimulation

Atrophic vaginitis is thinning and atrophy of the vaginal epithelium. The thinned epithelium is a poor barrier to infections or abrasions. The condition occurs most commonly in postmenopausal women with low estrogen levels. Dyspareunia and vaginal spotting are common symptoms.

Vaginal Adenosis

In vaginal adenosis, the glandular epithelium that normally lines the embryonic vagina fails to be replaced during fetal life by squamous epithelium. The now discontinued use of diethylstilbestrol (DES) to prevent miscarriages in women

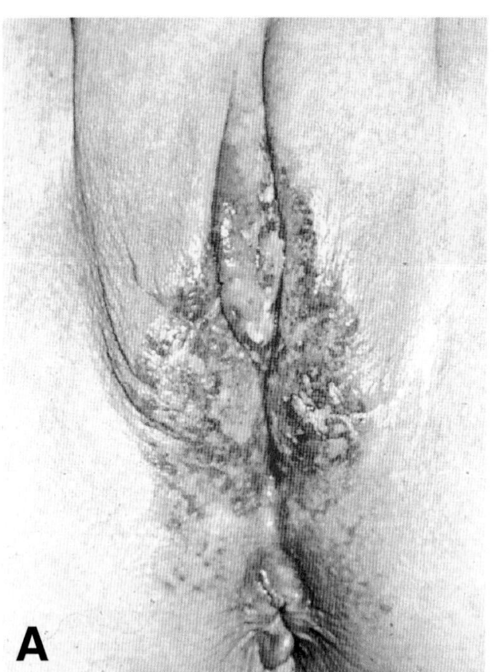

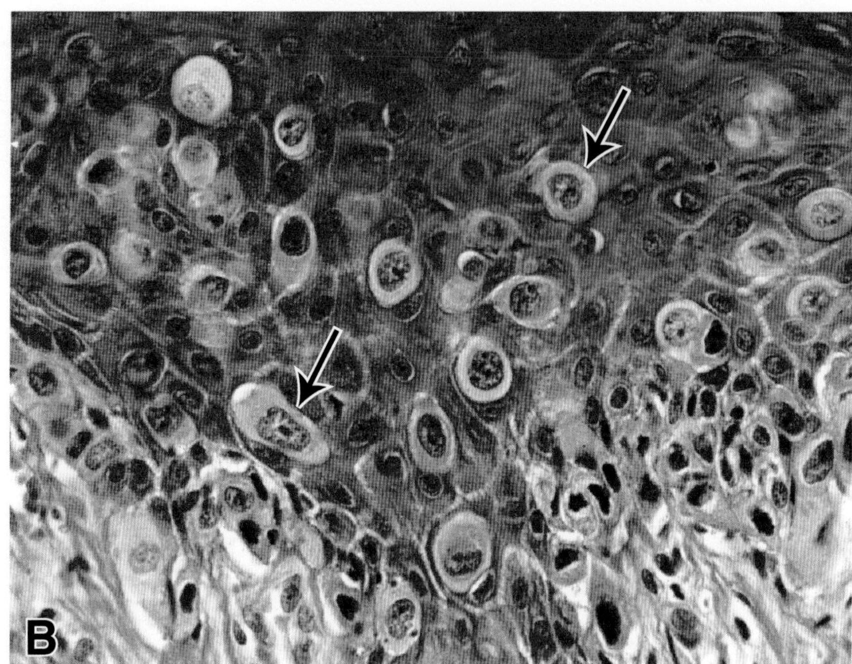

FIGURE 16-11. Paget disease of the vulva. A. The lesion is red, moist, and sharply demarcated. **B.** Individual Paget cells (*arrows*), characterized by an abundant pale cytoplasm, infiltrate the epithelium, and are interspersed among normal keratinocytes.

in the 1970s, led to a substantial increase in this disorder in daughters of those women.

Rare cases of **clear cell adenocarcinoma** of the vagina have also occurred in the young daughters of women treated with DES although, currently essentially, all cases of this rare tumor occur in postmenopausal women and are not associated with DES use. Clear cell adenocarcinomas are almost invariably curable when small and asymptomatic, but in more advanced stages, may spread by hematogenous or lymphatic routes.

MALIGNANT TUMORS OF THE VAGINA

Primary malignant tumors of the vagina are uncommon, constituting about 2% of all genital tract tumors. **Most (80%) vaginal malignancies represent metastatic spread.** The most common symptoms are vaginal discharge and bleeding during coitus, but advanced tumors may cause pelvic or abdominal pain and edema of the legs. Tumors confined to the vagina are usually treated by radical hysterectomy and vaginectomy.

Squamous Cell Carcinoma

This tumor is generally a disease of older women, with peak incidence between the ages of 60 and 70. It is most common in the anterior wall of the upper third of the vagina, where it usually grows as an exophytic mass. High-grade **vaginal intraepithelial lesion** (vaginal HSIL), a term that replaces both "vaginal dysplasia" and "carcinoma in situ," frequently precedes invasive carcinoma. Vaginal squamous cell carcinoma may develop some years after cervical or vulvar carcinoma, suggesting a carcinogenic field effect in the lower genital tract, that is related to HPV infection. Prognosis is related to the extent of tumor spread at the time of discovery. Five-year survival in patients with tumors confined to the vagina (stage I) is 80%, whereas it is only 20% for those with extensive spread (stages III/IV).

Rhabdomyosarcoma

This tumor typically consists of confluent polypoid masses resembling a bunch of grapes and hence may be called "sarcoma botryoides" (from the Greek *botrys* for "grape cluster") (Fig. 16-12). It occurs almost exclusively in girls under 4 years. It arises in the lamina propria of the vagina and consists of primitive spindle rhabdomyoblasts (Fig. 16-12C), some of which show cross-striations. The tumor is usually detected because of spotting on the child's diaper. Tumors under 3 cm in greatest dimension tend to be localized. Even in advanced cases, half of patients survive with radical surgery and chemotherapy.

Cervix

CERVICITIS

Inflammation of the cervix is common and is related to constant exposure to bacterial flora in the vagina. Acute and chronic cervicitis are caused by many organisms, particularly endogenous vaginal aerobes and anaerobes (see above).

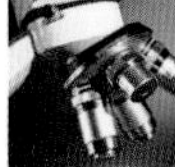

PATHOLOGY: In **acute cervicitis**, the cervix is grossly red, swollen, and edematous, with copious pus "dripping" from the external os. Microscopically, the tissues exhibit extensive acute inflammation and stromal edema.

Chronic cervicitis is more common. The cervical mucosa is hyperemic and may show true epithelial erosions.

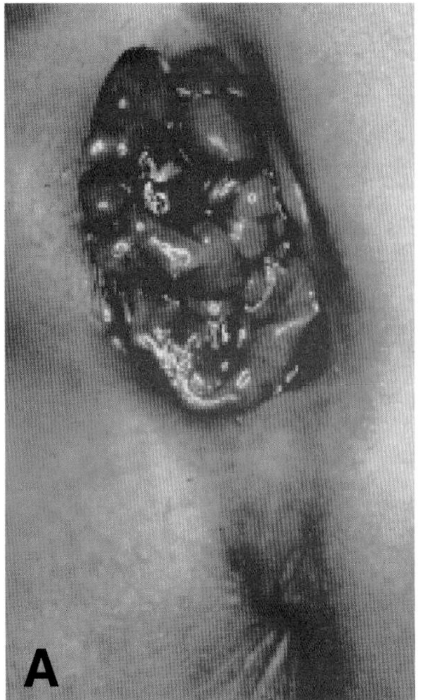

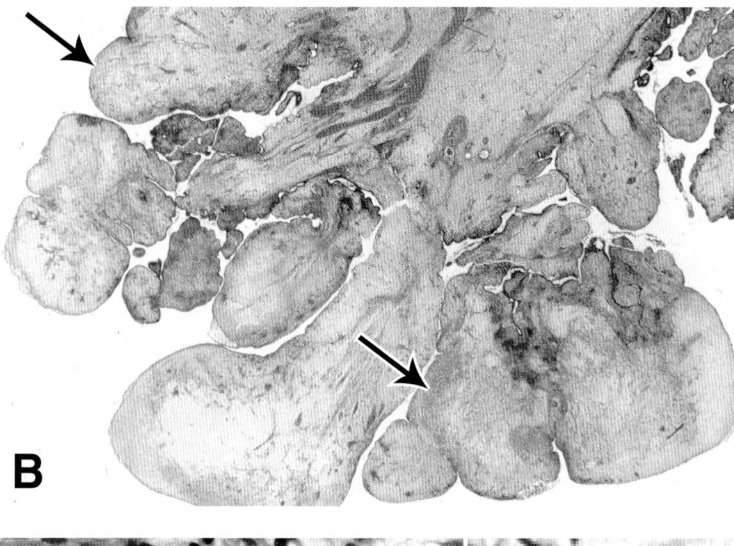

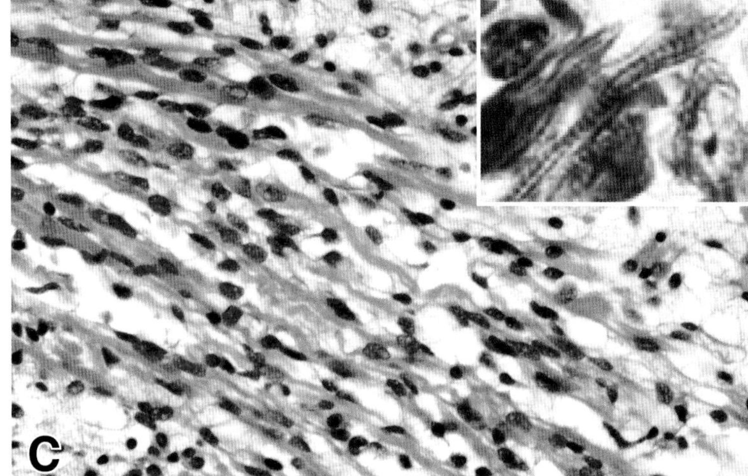

FIGURE 16-12. Embryonal rhabdomyosarcoma (sarcoma botryoides) of vagina. A. The grapelike tumor protrudes through the introitus. **B.** A section of the tumor showing a dense layer of neoplastic stroma termed "the cambium layer" (*arrows*) beneath the surface epithelium of the vagina. A loose neoplastic stroma is present beneath the cambium layer. **C.** The tumor cells are composed of elongated, primitive rhabdomyoblasts, with cross-striations seen at high magnification in the *inset*.

The stroma is infiltrated, principally by lymphocytes and plasma cells. Metaplastic squamous epithelium of the transformation zone may extend into endocervical glands, forming clusters of squamous epithelium, which must be differentiated from carcinoma.

BENIGN TUMORS AND TUMOR-LIKE CONDITIONS OF THE CERVIX

Endocervical Polyps

Endocervical polyps are the most common cervical growths (Fig. 16-13). They appear as single smooth or lobulated masses, usually under 3 cm in greatest dimension. They typically manifest as vaginal bleeding or discharge. The lining epithelium of the polyp is mucinous, with variable squamous metaplasia, but may feature erosions and granulation tissue if women are symptomatic. Simple excision or curettage is curative. Cancer rarely arises in an endocervical polyp (0.2% of cases).

Microglandular Hyperplasia

This benign condition shows closely packed vacuolated glands that lack intervening stroma and are mixed with a neutrophilic infiltrate. This disorder may be confused with well-differentiated adenocarcinoma (see below). Microglandular hyperplasia is usually asymptomatic, and because it is typically associated with progestin stimulation, it usually occurs during pregnancy, in the postpartum period, and in women taking oral contraceptives.

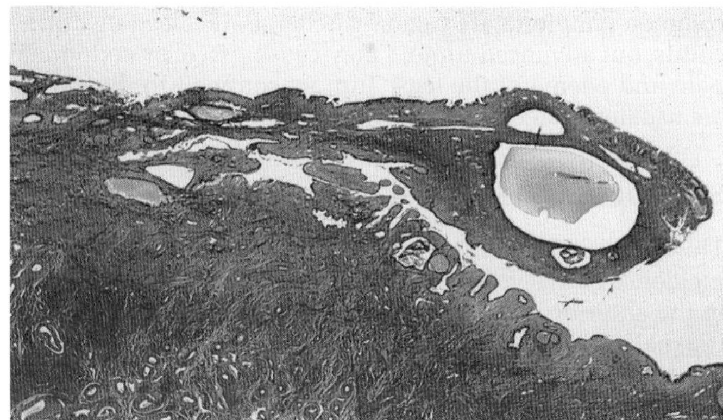

FIGURE 16-13. Endocervical polyp. An epithelial lining covers a fibrovascular core. Reprinted with permission from Stanley J, Robboy MD; Gynecologic Pathology Associates. Durham and Chapel Hill, NC.

Leiomyomas

Benign smooth muscle tumors of the cervix (leiomyomas) can prolapse into the endocervical canal and cause uterine contractions and pain, resembling the early phases of labor. The microscopic appearance is similar to that of uterine leiomyomas (see below).

SQUAMOUS CELL NEOPLASIA

Fifty years ago, cervical cancer was the leading cause of cancer death in American women. The introduction and widespread use of cytologic screening decreased cervical cancer by 50% to 85% in Western countries. It is now the sixth most common female cancer in the United States, and mortality has fallen by 70%. Worldwide, however, cervical cancer remains the second most common cancer in women.

Squamous Intraepithelial Lesions

SILs of the cervix are the consequence of infection with HPV and are designated as low grade (LSILs) or high grade (HSILs) based on the viral subtype and the risk of progression to invasive squamous cell carcinoma (Figs. 16-14 and 16-15).

The disease spectrum is primarily driven by the nature of the infecting virus, with each class demonstrating its own

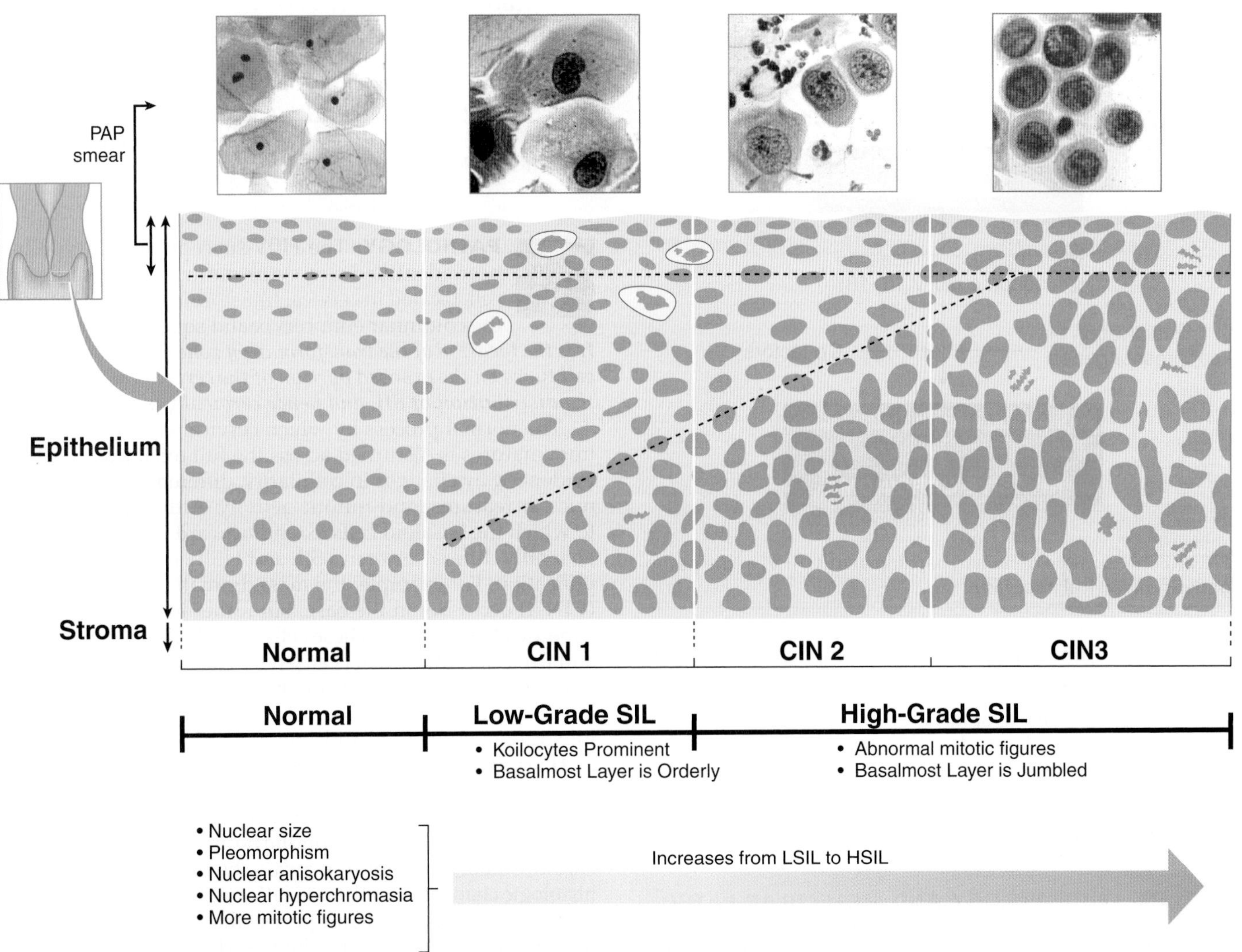

FIGURE 16-14. The Bethesda system for designation of premalignant cervical disease as squamous intraepithelial lesions (SILs). This chart integrates multiple aspects across the normal–LSIL (low-grade squamous intraepithelial lesion) and LSIL–HSIL (high-grade squamous intraepithelial lesion) interfaces, which correspond to therapeutic thresholds. It lists the qualitative and quantitative features that distinguish low cancer risk (LSIL) from high cancer risk (HSIL) lesions, which are generally caused by different subtypes of human papillomavirus. It also illustrates approximate counterparts for the legacy cervical intraepithelial neoplasia (CIN) system, which was based on a model of continuous progression rather than dichotomous viral subtypes. Finally, the scheme illustrates the corresponding cytologic smear resulting from exfoliation of the most superficial cells, indicating that even in the mildest disease state, abnormal cells reach the surface and are shed. Data from Robboy SJ, Anderson MC, Russell P, eds. *Pathology of the Female Reproductive Tract*. London: Churchill-Livingstone, 2002: 111-112, 140, 147, 167, 203, 248, 322, 354.

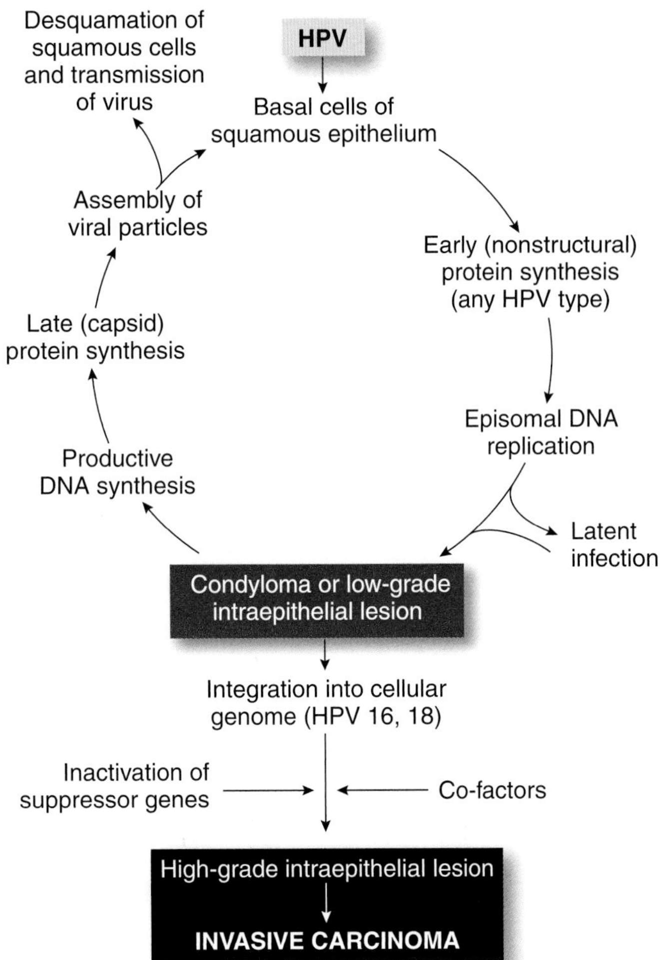

FIGURE 16-15. Role of human papillomavirus (HPV) in the pathogenesis of cervical neoplasia.

disease spectrum. The grades of SIL compared to older terminology are as follows:

- LSIL: CIN-1: mild dysplasia
- HSIL: CIN-2, moderate dysplasia; CIN-3, severe dysplasia, carcinoma in situ

LSIL rarely progresses in severity and commonly disappears. HSIL tends to progress and requires treatment.

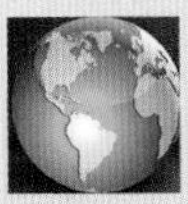

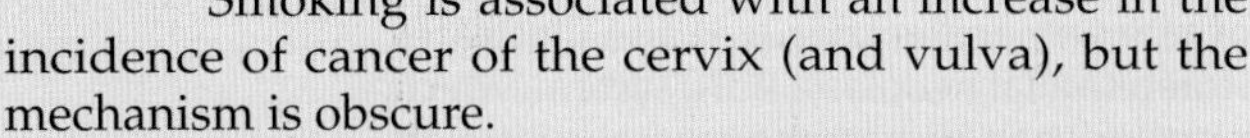

EPIDEMIOLOGY AND MOLECULAR PATHOGENESIS: Cervical cancer usually manifests in women aged 40 to 60 years (mean 54), but SIL generally occurs before age 40. ***The critical factor is HPV infection, which correlates with multiple sexual partners and early age at first coitus.*** Thus, SIL is essentially a **sexually transmitted disease**. Smoking is associated with an increase in the incidence of cancer of the cervix (and vulva), but the mechanism is obscure.

In LSIL, HPV is episomal and replicates freely to cause cell death. Huge numbers of virus must accumulate in the cytoplasm before the cell becomes visible as a koilocyte. In most cases of HSIL, viral DNA integrates into the cell genome. Proteins encoded by HPV-16, namely, E6 and E7 genes bind and inactivate p53 and Rb proteins, respectively, and mitigate their tumor suppressor functions (see Chapter 4). Once HPV integrates into host DNA, copies of intact virus do not accumulate; for this reason, koilocytes are absent in many cases of HSIL and all invasive cancers (Fig. 16-15).

As noted above, roughly 85% of LSIL lesions have low-risk HPV. Genital warts (condylomata acuminata) of the cervix often exhibit HPV-6 or HPV-11, both considered low-risk HPV types. By contrast, cells in HSIL usually contain HPV types 16, 18, 31, 33, 35, 39, 45, 51, 52, 56, 58, 59, and 68. **HPV types 16 and 18** are found in 70% of invasive cancers; other high-risk types account for another 25%.

Hormonally induced eversion of the cervix and an acidic vaginal environment encourage the development of the transformation zone. Without HPV, benign squamous metaplasia is the eventual outcome. But in the presence of HPV or other carcinogenic agents, transformation zone stem cells are diverted into SIL and may progress to invasive carcinoma.

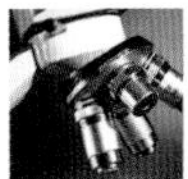

PATHOLOGY: The HPV-susceptible cell type has been identified as a cytokeratin 7–expressing stem cell, located in cervical transformation zone between the columnar endocervix and squamous exocervix. ***It is the location of the transformation zone and its component cell types on the exposed portion of the cervix that determines the distribution of SIL and hence cervical cancer.***

The normal process by which cervical squamous epithelium matures is disturbed across the full thickness of SIL, as evidenced by changes in cellularity, differentiation, polarity, nuclear features, and mitotic activity. Although the height to which the basaloid cells extend upward in the epithelium generally differs between LSIL and HSIL, this is an oversimplification. For example, the most dramatic changes in **LSIL (CIN-1)** occur not in the base, but rather in koilocytes of the superficial epithelium. These cells show ballooned cytoplasm and irregular large nuclei caused by episomal viral propagation within differentiated squamous cells, which are absent in the base. Features in the basal region related to genomic integration of virus in propagating basal cells are prominent in **HSIL (CIN-2/CIN-3)**. These include disorganization of basal cell alignment along the basement membrane and nuclear changes that persist as cells are pushed upward in the epithelium. Abnormal mitotic figures, pathognomonic of chromosomal aneuploidy, may also be present in HSILs. The histologic changes of LSIL and HSIL are shown in Figure 16-16.

Because abnormal cells are present throughout the epithelium in women with SIL, they are shed into the Pap smear. Nuclear abnormalities and the degree of cytoplasmic differentiation in exfoliated abnormal cells identify LSIL and HSIL. Definitive classification is best made in a histologic specimen, where the full epithelium can be assessed. Mosaicism (irregular surface resembling inlaid woodwork) and vascular punctuation are two patterns most often seen in on colposcopic examination HSIL.

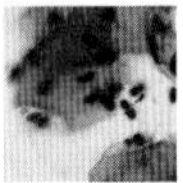

CLINICAL FEATURES: The mean age at which women develop SIL has declined over the past few decades and is now 25 to 30 years. Overall, 70% of cases of LSIL regress, 6% progress to HSIL, and less than 1% become invasive cancer. ***If untreated, 10% to 20% of cases of HSIL progress to invasive carcinoma.***

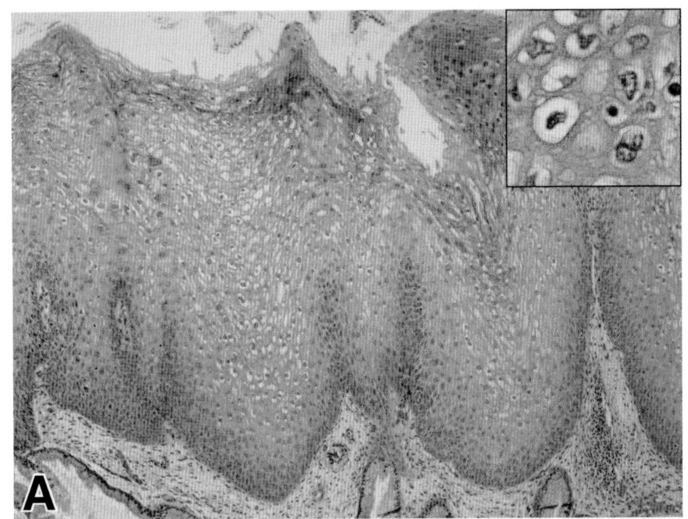

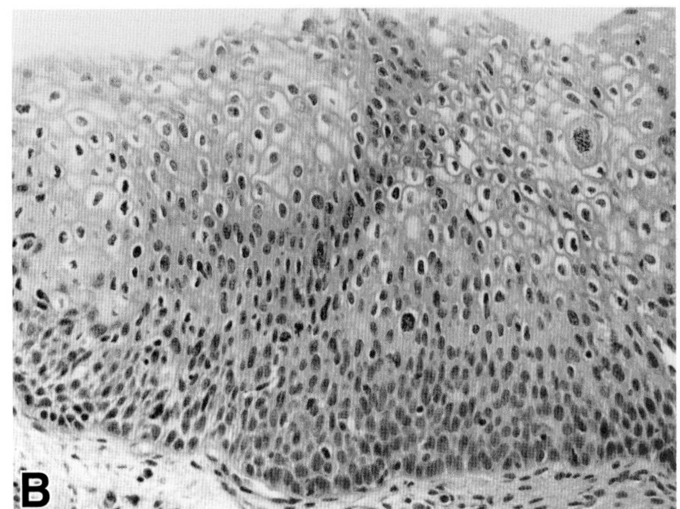

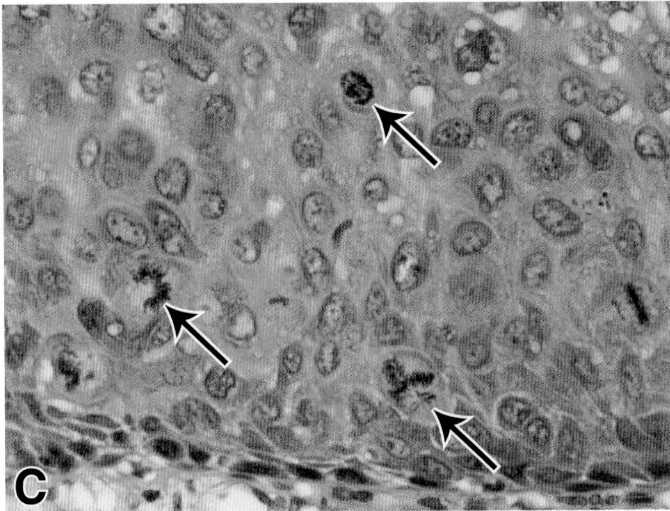

FIGURE 16-16. Cervical squamous intraepithelial lesions (SILs). **A.** Low-grade SIL (LSIL/CIN-1): The cervical epithelium showing pronounced vacuolated koilocytes (*inset*) in the upper epithelium and a thin basal zone that maintains polarity against the basement membrane. **B.** High-grade SIL (HSIL/CIN-2/-3): Basal cells with integrated HPV proliferate as neoplastic clones through the entire epithelium. Basal cells are disorganized and extend upward to a higher level without differentiation. Koilocytes may occur but are infrequent. **C.** Atypical mitoses (*arrows*) in this HSIL indicating an aneuploid genotype, seen with high-risk viruses. Horseshoe, multipolar, and unequal metaphases are seen. CIN, cervical intraepithelial neoplasia.

Biopsy is indicated when SIL is discovered on Pap smear. Targeted cervical biopsies may be visually directed by colposcopy, or the entire transformation zone can be removed by a wire "loop" electrosurgical excision procedure (LEEP). Women with LSIL are often followed conservatively (i.e., repeated Pap smears plus close follow-up), although some gynecologists advocate local ablative treatment. High-grade lesions are treated by ablation methods, determined by their anatomic distribution. LEEP may be sufficient, if the margins are negative. Cervical conization (removal of a cone of tissue around the external os), cryosurgery, and (rarely) hysterectomy may also be done. Follow-up smears and clinical examinations should continue for life because vaginal or vulvar squamous cancer may develop later.

Superficially Invasive Cervical Cancer

Stromal invasion by squamous carcinoma usually arises from overlying HSIL.

The earliest recognizable invasive changes are small irregular epithelial buds emanating from the base of HSILs, previously called "microinvasive" (Fig. 16-17). These small (<1 mm) tongues of neoplastic epithelial cells do not affect the prognosis of HSILs; hence, they can be treated with conservative surgery.

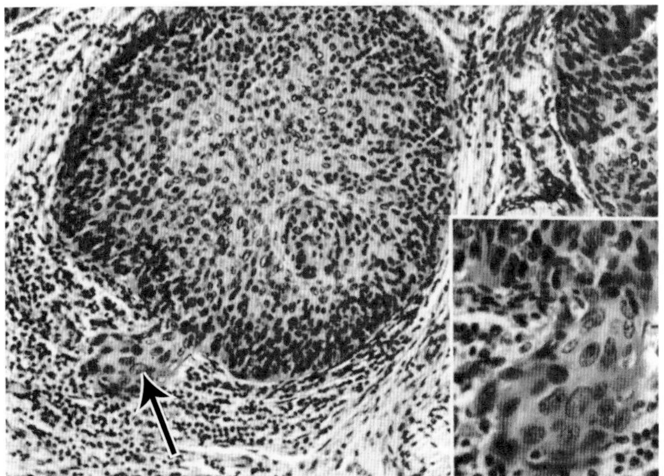

FIGURE 16-17. Early ("microinvasive") stromal invasion in a superficially invasive squamous cell carcinoma. Section of the cervix showing that high-grade squamous intraepithelial lesion in an endocervical gland has broken through the basement membrane (*arrow*) to invade the stroma. (*Inset*) A higher power view of the early invasive focus.

Invasive Squamous Cell Carcinoma

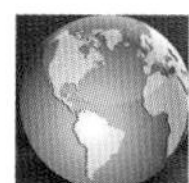

EPIDEMIOLOGY: Squamous cell carcinoma is by far the most common type of cervical cancer. In the United States, roughly 12,000 new cases occur annually, which is less than either endometrial or ovarian cancer. However, in underdeveloped areas, where cytologic screening is less available, cervical cancer is still a major cause of cancer death. The HPV vaccine decreases individual risk of cervical cancer by 97%.

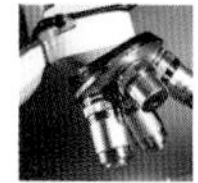

PATHOLOGY: Early stages of cervical cancer are often poorly defined, granular, eroded lesions or nodular, and exophytic masses. If the tumor resides mainly within the endocervical canal, it can be an endophytic mass that infiltrates stroma and causes diffuse enlargement and hardening of the cervix. Most tumors are nonkeratinizing, with solid nests of large malignant squamous cells and no more than individual cell keratinization. A few cancers show nests of keratinized cells in concentric whorls, the so-called keratin pearls. The least common, and most aggressive, tumor is small cell carcinoma. It consists of infiltrating masses of small, cohesive, nonkeratinized, malignant cells and has the worst prognosis.

Cervical cancer spreads by direct extension or through lymphatic vessels (Fig. 16-18) and only rarely by the hematogenous route. Local extension into surrounding tissues (parametrium, stage IIIB) may result in **ureteral compression** and cause clinical complications of hydroureter, hydronephrosis, and renal failure, the most common cause of death (50% of patients). Bladder and rectal involvement (stage IVA) may lead to fistula formation. Lymphatic metastases are seen in paracervical, hypogastric, and external iliac nodes.

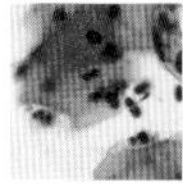

CLINICAL FEATURES: In early stages of cervical cancer, patients complain most often of vaginal bleeding after intercourse or douching. With more advanced tumors, symptoms are related to the route and degree of spread. The Pap smear remains the most reliable screening test for detecting cervical cancer.

The anatomic stage of cervical cancer is the best predictor of survival. Radical hysterectomy is favored for localized tumor, especially in younger women; radiation therapy or combinations of the two are used for more advanced tumors.

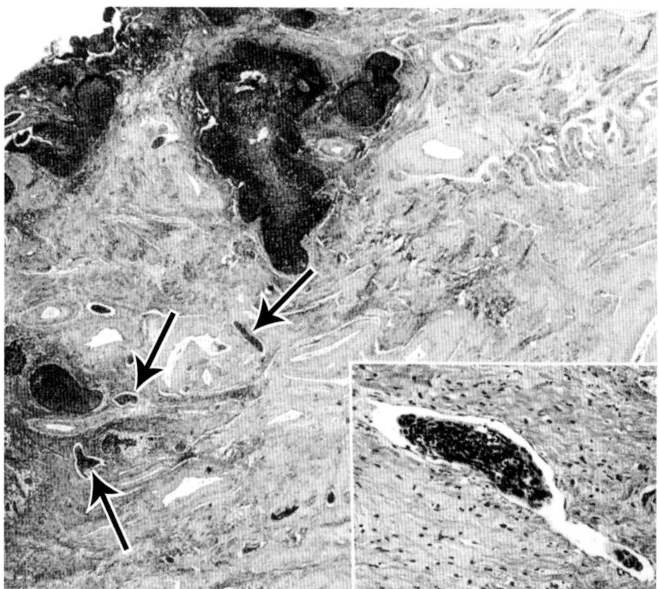

FIGURE 16-18. Squamous cell cancer of the cervix with lymphatic invasion. Low magnification showing a squamous cell carcinoma that has invaded the stroma and permeated the lymphatics (*arrows*). (*Inset*) A high-power view of lymphatic invasion.

Endocervical Adenocarcinoma

The incidence of cervical adenocarcinoma has increased recently, with a mean age of 56 years at presentation. Most tumors are of endocervical cell (mucinous) type, but the various subtypes have little bearing on overall survival. Adenocarcinoma shares epidemiologic factors with squamous carcinoma of the cervix and spreads similarly. It is often associated with adenocarcinoma in situ and contains HPV types 16 or 18.

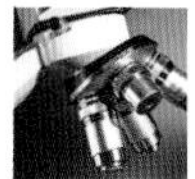

PATHOLOGY: *ADENOCARCINOMA IN SITU:* Also called **cervical glandular intraepithelial neoplasia**, this lesion generally arises at the squamocolumnar junction and extends into the endocervical canal. It displays tall columnar cells with eosinophilic or mucinous cytoplasm, sometimes resembling goblet cells. The pattern of spread and involvement of endocervical glands resemble those of cervical SIL. Adenocarcinoma in situ typically is intraepithelial, maintaining normal endocervical gland architecture. The neoplastic cells show slight enlargement, atypical hyperchromatic nuclei, increased nuclear to cytoplasmic ratio, and variable mitoses. Squamous HSIL occurs in 40% of cases of adenocarcinoma in situ.

INVASIVE ADENOCARCINOMA: This tumor typically presents as a fungating polypoid (Fig. 16-19A) or papillary mass. Exophytic tumors often have a papillary pattern (Fig. 16-19B), whereas endophytic ones display tubular or glandular patterns. Poorly differentiated tumors are predominantly composed of solid sheets of cells.

Adenocarcinoma of the endocervix spreads by local invasion and lymphatic metastases, but overall survival is somewhat worse than for squamous carcinoma. Treatment is similar to that for squamous carcinoma.

Fallopian Tube

SALPINGITIS

Refer to polymicrobial genital infections above.

FALLOPIAN TUBE TUMORS

Thorough evaluation of the fallopian tube in women at heightened hereditary risk for "ovarian" cancer (*BRCA* mutation) has shown that many resultant cancers arise in the tubal fimbria as **serous tubal intraepithelial carcinoma** (STIC). The tubal fimbria has also been shown to be an early site of involvement of some sporadic (nonhereditary) serous adenocarcinomas. STIC lesions are physically small, often grossly inapparent, and composed of mitotically active regions of atypical epithelium expressing mutant *TP53*.

Fallopian tube involvement by metastases or implants from adjacent ovarian and uterine neoplasms also occurs. Most primary malignancies are adenocarcinomas, with a peak incidence among 50- to 60-year-olds.

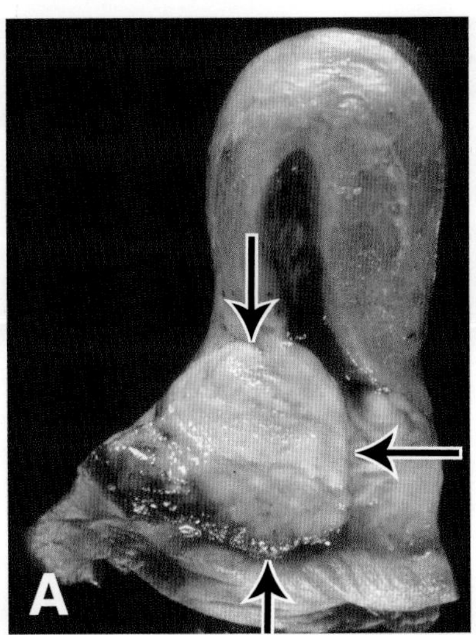

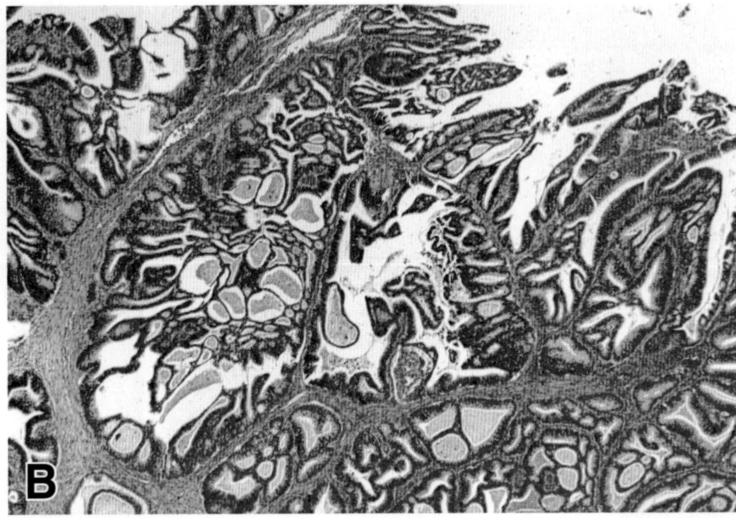

FIGURE 16-19. Endocervical adenocarcinoma. A. The endocervical tumor appears as a polypoid mass (*arrows*). **B.** Microscopic view of endocervical adenocarcinoma showing a papillary pattern of growth.

Ovary

CYSTIC LESIONS OF THE OVARIES

Ovarian cysts usually arise from invaginated surface epithelium (**serous cysts**) and are the most common cause of enlarged ovaries. Almost all of the rest derive from ovarian follicles.

Follicle Cysts

Ovarian follicle cysts are thin-walled, fluid-filled structures lined internally by granulosa cells and externally by theca interna cells. They occur at any age up to menopause, are unilocular, and may be single, multiple, unilateral, or bilateral. They arise from ovarian follicles and are probably related to abnormalities in pituitary gonadotropin release.

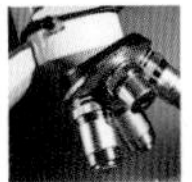

PATHOLOGY: Follicle cysts rarely exceed 5 cm. In an unstimulated state, the granulosa cells of the cyst have uniform, round nuclei, and little cytoplasm. Thecal cells are small and spindle shaped. Occasionally, the layers may be luteinized, and the lumen contains fluid high in estrogen or progesterone. If the cyst persists, hormonal output can cause precocious puberty in a child and menstrual irregularities in an adult. The only significant complication is mild intraperitoneal bleeding.

Corpus Luteum Cysts

A corpus luteum cyst results from delayed resolution of a corpus luteum's central cavity. Continued progesterone synthesis by the luteal cyst leads to menstrual irregularities. Rupture of a cyst can cause mild hemorrhage into the abdominal cavity. A corpus luteum cyst is typically unilocular, 3 to 5 cm in size, with a yellow wall. Cyst contents vary from serosanguinous fluid to clotted blood. Microscopic examination shows numerous large, luteinized granulosa cells. The condition is self-limited.

Theca Lutein Cysts

Theca lutein cysts, also called *hyperreactio luteinalis*, are often multiple and bilateral. They are associated with high levels of circulating gonadotropin (as is the case in pregnancy, hydatidiform mole, choriocarcinoma, or exogenous gonadotropin therapy) or physical impediments to ovulation (dense adhesions and cortical fibrosis). Excessive gonadotropin levels result in exaggerated stimulation of the theca interna and extensive cyst formation.

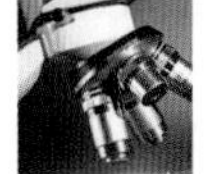

PATHOLOGY: Multiple thin-walled cysts filled with clear fluid and a markedly luteinized layer of theca interna replace both ovaries. Ovarian parenchyma shows edema and foci of luteinized stromal cells. Intra-abdominal hemorrhage caused by torsion or rupture of the cyst may require surgical intervention.

POLYCYSTIC OVARY SYNDROME

Polycystic ovary syndrome (Stein–Leventhal syndrome) reflects (1) excess secretion of androgenic hormones, (2) persistent anovulation, and (3) many small subcapsular ovarian cysts. It was first described as a syndrome of **secondary amenorrhea, hirsutism, and obesity,** but clinical presentations are now known to be far more variable and include amenorrheic women who appear otherwise normal and, even rarely, have ovaries lacking polycystic features. ***This condition is a common cause of infertility: up to 7% of women experience polycystic ovary syndrome.***

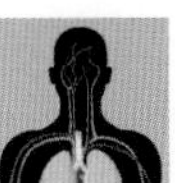

PATHOPHYSIOLOGY: Polycystic ovary syndrome is a state of functional ovarian hyperandrogenism with elevated levels of LH. Increased LH probably results from, rather than causes ovarian dysfunction (Fig. 16-20).

1. The central abnormality is thought to be increased ovarian production of androgens, although adrenal hypersecretion of androgens may also occur. The rate-limiting enzyme in androgen biosynthesis, cytochrome $P450_{c17}\alpha$ (17α-hydroxylase), is abnormally regulated.

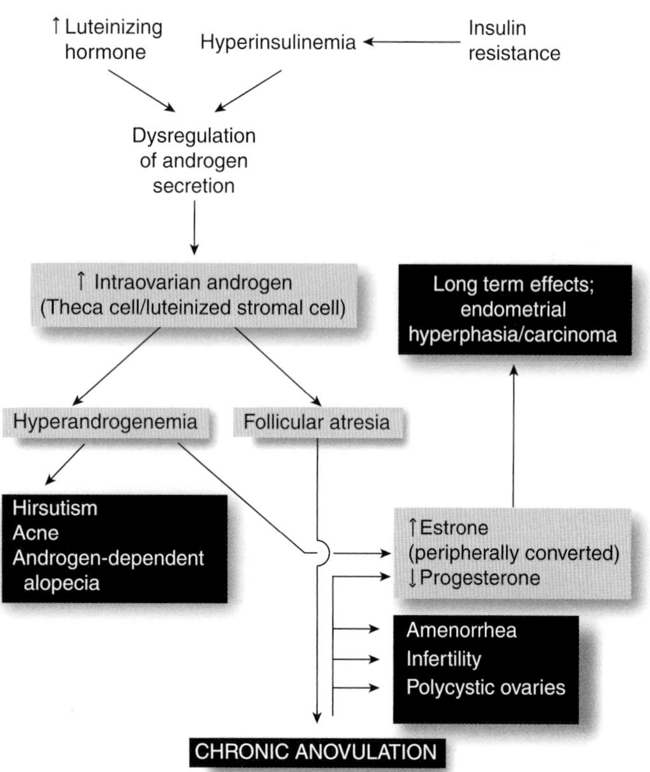

FIGURE 16-20. Pathogenesis of polycystic ovary syndrome.

2. Excess ovarian androgens act locally to cause (1) premature follicular atresia, (2) multiple follicular cysts, and (3) a persistent anovulatory state. Impaired follicular maturation results in decreased secretion of progesterone. Peripherally, hyperandrogenism leads to hirsutism, acne, and male-pattern (androgen-dependent) alopecia. Affected patients may have high serum levels of androgens, such as testosterone, androstenedione, and dehydroepiandrosterone sulfate. However, there are individual variations, and some patients have normal androgen levels.
3. Excess androgens are converted to estrogens in peripheral adipose tissue, an effect that is exaggerated by obesity. Acyclic estrogen production and progesterone deficiency increase pituitary secretion of LH.
4. Women with polycystic ovary syndrome exhibit marked peripheral insulin resistance, out of proportion to the degree of obesity. The mechanism appears to involve a post–insulin-receptor defect, possibly related to decreased expression of a glucose transporter. In any event, the resulting hyperinsulinemia seems to contribute to increased ovarian hypersecretion of androgens and direct stimulation of pituitary LH production.

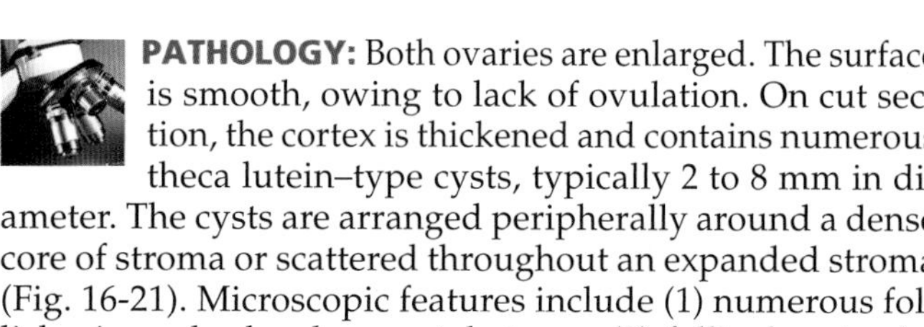

PATHOLOGY: Both ovaries are enlarged. The surface is smooth, owing to lack of ovulation. On cut section, the cortex is thickened and contains numerous theca lutein–type cysts, typically 2 to 8 mm in diameter. The cysts are arranged peripherally around a dense core of stroma or scattered throughout an expanded stroma (Fig. 16-21). Microscopic features include (1) numerous follicles in early developmental stages; (2) follicular atresia; (3) increased stroma, occasionally with luteinized cells (hyperthecosis); and (4) features of anovulation (thick, smooth capsule and absence of corpora lutea and corpora albicantiae). Many subcapsular cysts show thick zones of theca interna, in which some cells may be luteinized.

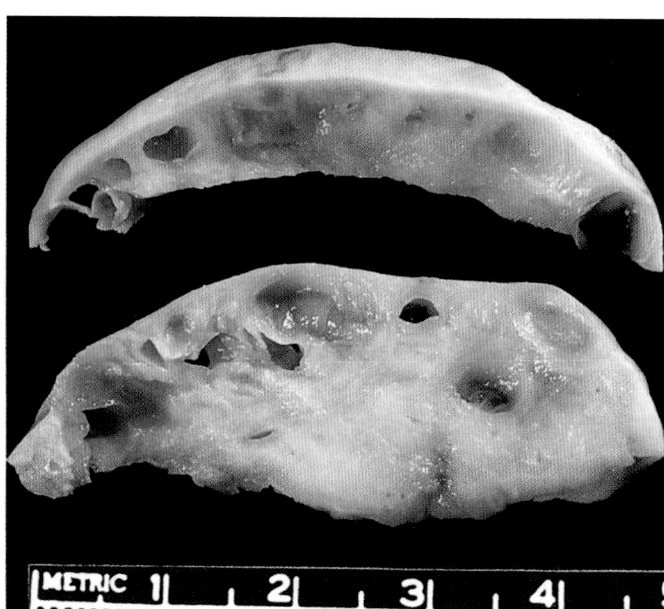

FIGURE 16-21. Polycystic disease of the ovary. Cut sections of an ovary showing numerous cysts embedded in a sclerotic stroma.

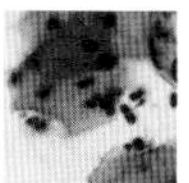

CLINICAL FEATURES: ***Some three quarters of women with anovulatory infertility have polycystic ovary syndrome.*** Patients are typically in their 20s and complain of early obesity, menstrual problems, and hirsutism. Half of women with polycystic ovary syndrome are amenorrheic, and most others have irregular menses. Only 75% are actually infertile, indicating that some do occasionally ovulate. Unopposed acyclic estrogen activity increases the incidence of endometrial hyperplasia and adenocarcinoma.

Treatment of polycystic ovary syndrome targets two common problems in reproductive endocrinology—hirsutism and anovulation. Therapy is mostly hormonal and seeks to interrupt the constant excess of androgens.

STROMAL HYPERTHECOSIS

Stromal hyperthecosis refers to focal luteinization of ovarian stromal cells. These stromal cells are often functional and cause **virilization**. The condition is most common in postmenopausal women and, in a microscopic form, is found in one third of postmenopausal ovaries.

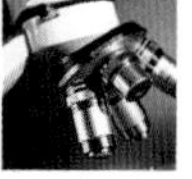

PATHOLOGY: If stromal hyperthecosis is detected clinically, usually owing to masculinizing signs, both ovaries may be enlarged, sometimes up to 8 cm in greatest dimension. The serosa is smooth, and the cut surface is homogeneous, firm, and brown to yellow. Single nests or nodules of luteinized stromal cells with deeply eosinophilic, often vacuolated cytoplasm, are seen in the cortex or medulla. Luteinized cells have a large central nucleus and a prominent nucleolus, features shared with all hormonally active stromal cells in the ovary.

OVARIAN TUMORS

There are many types of ovarian tumors. Some are benign, whereas others are borderline or malignant. About two thirds occur in reproductive-aged women; less than 5% develop in children. Approximately 80% of ovarian tumors are benign. Almost 90% of malignant and borderline tumors are diagnosed after the age of 40 years. Ovarian cancer is the second most frequent gynecologic malignancy (after endometrial cancer) and carries a higher mortality rate than all other female genital cancers combined. These neoplasms are difficult to detect at a curable stage, in over three fourths of patients, the tumor has spread to the pelvis or abdomen at the time of diagnosis. Approximately 22,000 new cases of ovarian cancer are diagnosed each year in the United States, and more than 14,000 women die from the disease. The lifetime risk of developing ovarian cancer is 2%. Although half of ovarian cancers occur in women older than 63 years, they may arise in younger women, most often those with a family history of the disease.

Ovarian tumors are classified by the ovarian cell type of origin (Fig. 16-22). Most are **epithelial tumors** (75%) that arise directly or indirectly from Müllerian epithelium. Other important groups are germ cell tumors (15%), sex cord/stromal tumors (5%), and tumors metastatic to the ovary (5%). In the Western world, common tumors account for about 90% of ovarian malignancies, serous adenocarcinoma being the most common.

Epithelial Tumors

Tumors of epithelial origin are broadly classified, according to cell proliferation, degree of nuclear atypia, and the presence or absence of stromal invasion as being (1) **benign,** (2) of **borderline tumor (BOT)** or tumor of low malignant potential (LMP), and (3) **malignant** (Fig. 16-22).

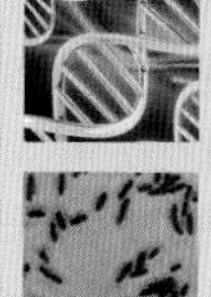

MOLECULAR PATHOGENESIS AND ETIOLOGIC FACTORS: Common epithelial neoplasms are apparently related to repeated disruption and repair of the epithelial surface resulting from cyclic or "incessant" ovulation. Thus, tumors occur most often in nulliparous women and least often in women in whom ovulation has been suppressed (e.g., by pregnancy or oral contraceptives). Persistent, high concentrations of pituitary gonadotropins after menopause may stimulate surface epithelial cells, thereby promoting the accumulation of genetic changes and consequent carcinogenesis.

Some 10% of patients with high-grade serous carcinoma (HGSC) have a family history of ovarian cancer. If a first-degree relative had ovarian cancer, a woman's risk of developing ovarian cancer is increased 3.5-fold. Women

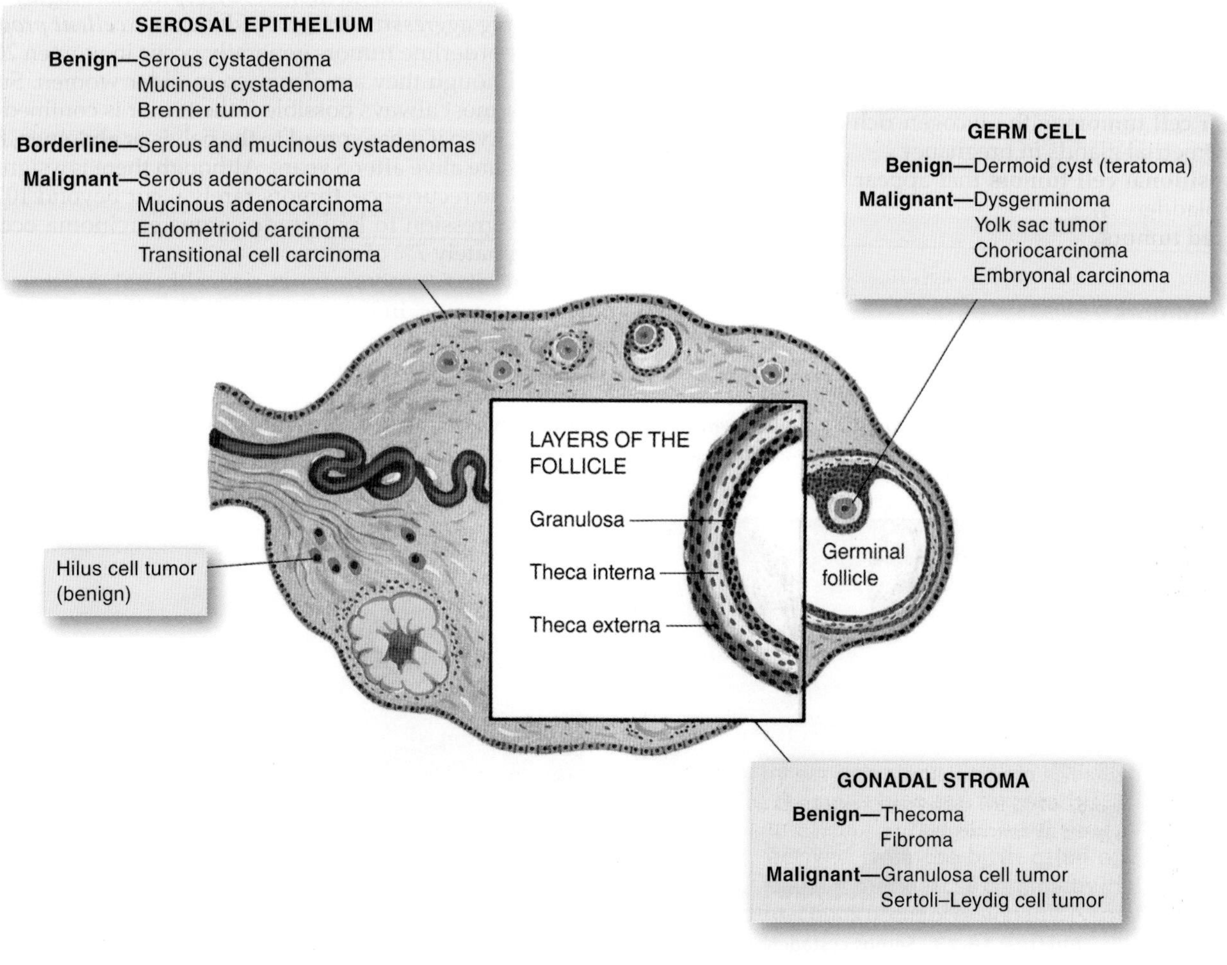

SEROSAL EPITHELIUM
Benign—Serous cystadenoma
Mucinous cystadenoma
Brenner tumor
Borderline—Serous and mucinous cystadenomas
Malignant—Serous adenocarcinoma
Mucinous adenocarcinoma
Endometrioid carcinoma
Transitional cell carcinoma

GERM CELL
Benign—Dermoid cyst (teratoma)
Malignant—Dysgerminoma
Yolk sac tumor
Choriocarcinoma
Embryonal carcinoma

LAYERS OF THE FOLLICLE
Granulosa
Theca interna
Theca externa

Germinal follicle

Hilus cell tumor (benign)

GONADAL STROMA
Benign—Thecoma
Fibroma
Malignant—Granulosa cell tumor
Sertoli–Leydig cell tumor

FIGURE 16-22. Classification of ovarian neoplasms based on cell of origin.

with a history of ovarian carcinoma are also at greater risk for breast cancer and vice versa. Defects in repair genes implicated in hereditary breast cancers, namely, *BRCA1* and *BRCA2*, are also incriminated in familial ovarian cancers. *BRCA1* and *BRCA2* mutations increase the risk 30- and 10-fold, respectively. Tumors arising in patients with germline *BRCA1* or *BRCA2* mutations are almost invariably of a high-grade serous type. Women with *BRCA1* mutations tend to develop ovarian cancers at younger ages than those who develop sporadic ovarian tumors, but *BRCA1*-related tumors have better prognoses. As is the case with endometrial carcinoma, women with hereditary nonpolyposis colon cancer (HNPCC, Lynch syndrome) are also at a greater risk for ovarian cancer.

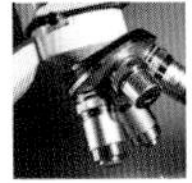

PATHOLOGY: Common epithelial tumors, particularly serous carcinomas, are thought to arise from ovarian surface epithelium (mesothelium) or serosa derived from the Müllerian ducts, the origin of the fallopian tubes, uterus, and vagina. As the ovary develops, the surface epithelium may extend into the ovarian stroma to form glands and cysts, and in some cases, these inclusion cysts become neoplastic.

In order of decreasing frequency, the epithelial tumors are:

- **Serous tumors** that resemble (and may derive from) fallopian tube epithelium
- **Mucinous tumors** that mimic the mucosa of the endocervix
- **Endometrioid tumors** that are similar to the glands of the endometrium
- **Clear cell tumors** with glycogen-rich cells that resemble endometrial glands in pregnancy
- **Transitional cell tumors** that appear like the mucosa of the bladder
- **Mixed tumors**

Benign Tumors

Cystadenomas

Common benign epithelial tumors (cystadenomas) are almost always cystic serous or mucinous adenomas and generally arise in women 20 to 60 years old. These tumors are frequently large, often 15 to 30 cm in diameter. Some, particularly mucinous ones, reach massive proportions, exceeding 50 cm in diameter, and may mimic the appearance of a term pregnancy. Serous cystadenomas tend to be unilocular (Fig. 16-23). By contrast, **mucinous tumors** usually show hundreds of small cysts (locules) (Fig. 16-24). Unlike their malignant counterparts, benign ovarian epithelial tumors tend to have thin walls and lack solid areas. A single layer of tall columnar epithelium lines the cysts. Papillae, if present, have a fibrovascular core covered by a layer of tall columnar epithelium identical to the cyst lining.

Transitional Cell Tumor (Brenner Tumor)

The typical Brenner tumor is benign and occurs at all ages. Half of cases present in women over the age of 50. Size varies from microscopic foci to masses 8 cm or more in diameter. Brenner tumors are adenofibromas, typically showing solid nests of transitional-like (urothelium-like) cells encased in a dense, fibrous stroma (Fig. 16-25). Epithelial nests are often cavitated, and the most superficial epithelial cells may exhibit mucinous differentiation. Borderline and proliferating tumors occur but are uncommon.

Borderline Tumors (Tumors of Low Malignant Potential)

"Borderline tumors" are a group of ovarian tumors characterized by epithelial cell proliferation and nuclear atypia but not destructive stromal invasion. Despite histologic features suggesting aggressiveness, they share an excellent prognosis. Serous borderline tumors generally occur in women 20 to 50 years although they are also seen in older women. Surgical cure is almost always possible if the tumor is confined to the ovaries. Even if it has spread to the pelvis or abdomen, 80% of patients are alive after 5 years. Although there is a significant rate of late recurrence, tumors rarely recur beyond 10 years. Late progression to low-grade serous carcinoma occurs in approximately 7% of cases.

Borderline tumors vary in size, although mucinous ones may be gigantic. In serous tumors of borderline malignancy, papillary projections, ranging from fine and exuberant to grapelike clusters arising from the cyst wall, are common (Fig. 16-26). These structures resemble papillary fronds in benign cystadenomas, but they show (1) epithelial stratification, (2) moderate nuclear atypia, (3) mitotic activity. Similar

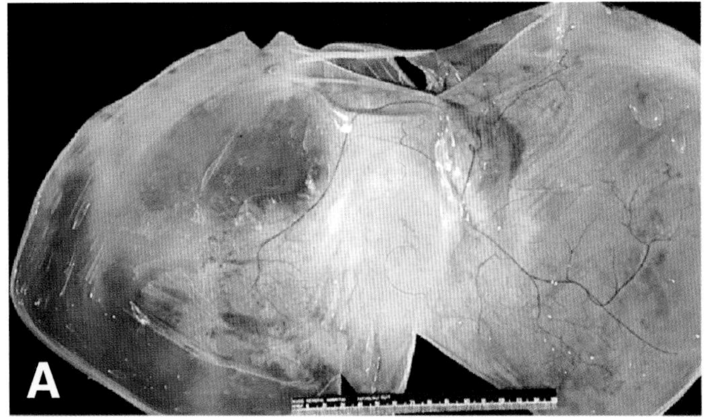

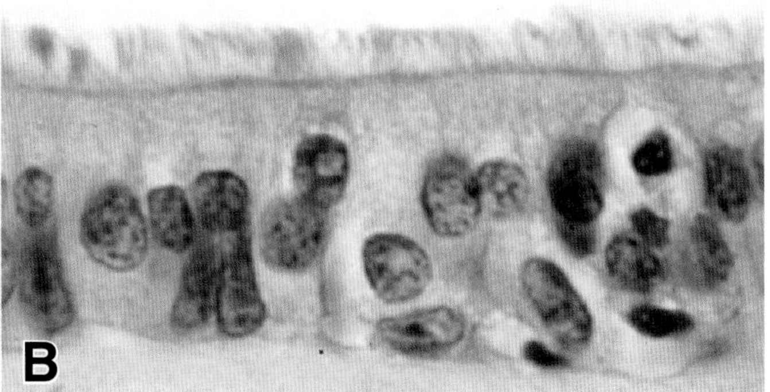

FIGURE 16-23. Serous cystadenoma of the ovary. A. Gross appearance of serous cystadenoma of the ovary. The fluid has been removed from this huge unilocular serous cystadenoma. The wall is thin and translucent. **B.** On microscopic examination, the cyst is lined by a single layer of ciliated tubal-type epithelium.

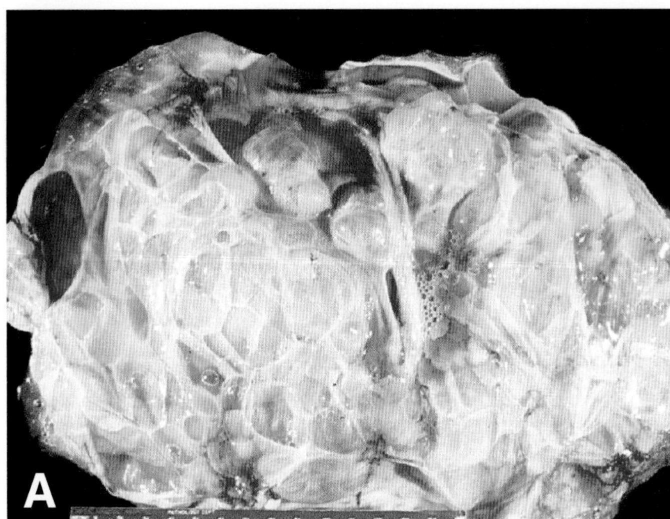

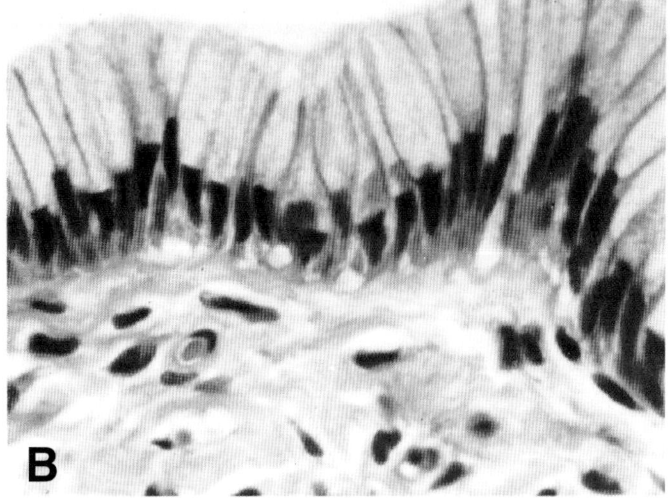

FIGURE 16-24. Mucinous cystadenoma of the ovary. A. The tumor is characterized by numerous cysts filled with thick, viscous fluid. **B.** A single layer of mucinous epithelial cells lines the cyst.

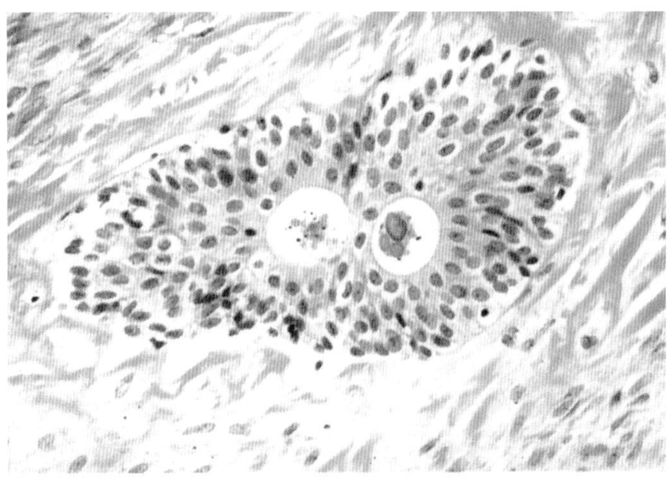

FIGURE 16-25. Brenner tumor. A nest of transitional-like cells is embedded in a dense, fibrous stroma.

criteria apply to borderline mucinous tumors, although papillary projections are less conspicuous. ***By definition, the presence of more than focal microinvasion (i.e., discrete nests of epithelial cells <5 mm into the ovarian stroma) identifies a tumor as low-grade invasive serous carcinoma, rather than a borderline tumor.***

Malignant Epithelial Tumors

Ovarian carcinomas are most common in women 40 to 60 years old and are rare under the age of 35. Based on light microscopy and molecular genetics, they are classified into five main subtypes (Table 16-3), which, in descending order of frequency, are high-grade serous carcinomas (>70%), endometrioid carcinomas (10%), clear cell carcinomas (10%), mucinous carcinomas (3% to 4%), and low-grade serous carcinomas (<5%).

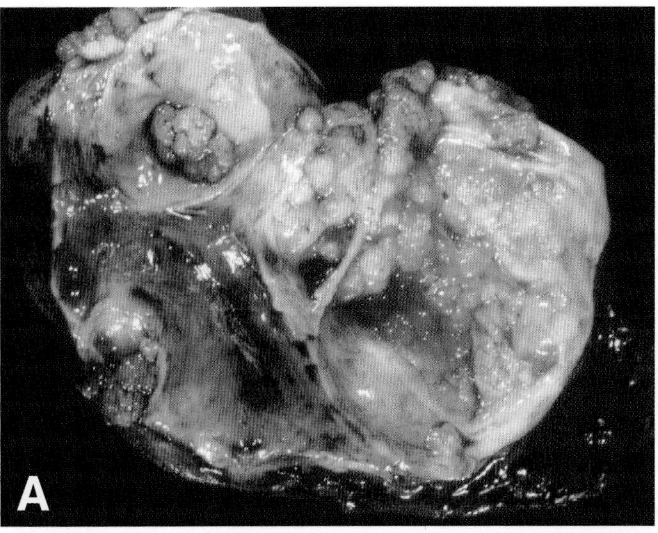

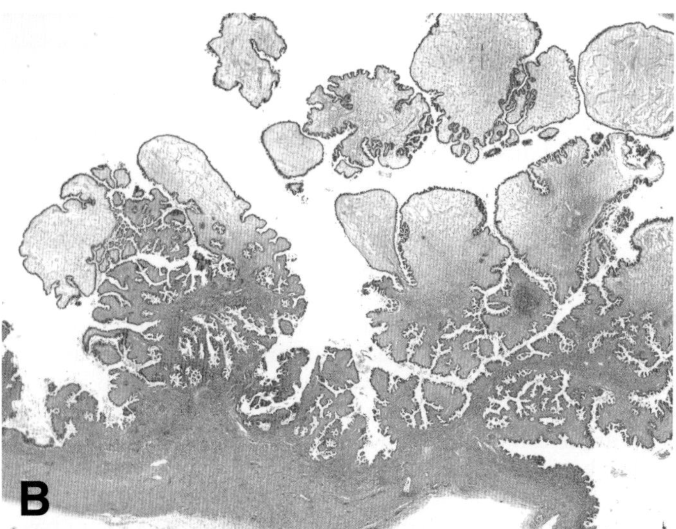

FIGURE 16-26. Serous cystic borderline tumor. A. The inner surface of the cysts is partly covered by closely packed papillae (endophytic growth). **B.** Microscopic view of the papillary tumor. The papillae show hierarchical and complex branching without stromal invasion. Some papillae have fibroedematous stalks.

Table 16-3

Main Subtypes of Ovarian Carcinoma

	Low-Grade Serous	High-Grade Serous	Clear Cell	Endometrioid	Mucinous
Usual stage at diagnosis	Early or advanced	Advanced	Early	Early	Early
Presumed tissue of origin/precursor lesion	Serous borderline tumor	Fallopian tube or tubal metaplasia in inclusions of ovarian surface epithelium	Endometriosis, adenofibroma	Endometriosis, adenofibroma	Adenoma–border-line-carcinoma se-quence; teratoma
Genetic risk	unknown	BRCA1/2	unknown	HNPCC	unknown
Significant molecu-lar abnormalities	BRAF or K-ras	p53 and pRb pathways	HNF-1β	PTEN, β-catenin, K-ras MI	K-ras
Proliferation	Low	High	Low	Low	Intermediate
Response to primary chemotherapy	26%–28%	80%	15%	unknown	15%
Prognosis	Favorable	Poor	Intermediate	Favorable	Favorable

HNF-1β, hepatocyte nuclear factor-1β; HNPCC, hereditary nonpolyposis colon cancer.

Serous Adenocarcinoma

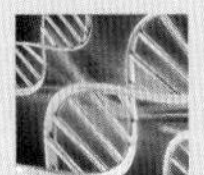

MOLECULAR PATHOGENESIS: ***Low- and high-grade serous carcinomas are fundamentally different tumors.*** Low-grade tumors are frequently associated with serous borderline tumors and have mutations of *KRAS* or *BRAF* oncogenes. By contrast, high-grade serous carcinomas appear to arise de novo without identifiable precursor lesions. They have a high frequency of mutations in *p53*, but not in *KRAS* or *BRAF*. Carcinomas arising in patients with germline *BRCA1* or *BRCA2* mutations (hereditary ovarian cancers) are almost invariably of the high-grade serous type and commonly have *p53* mutations. A significant number of *BRCA1*- or *BRCA2*-related tumors arise in the epithelium of the fimbriated end of the fallopian tube, suggesting that at least some sporadic high-grade ovarian and "primary" peritoneal serous carcinomas may actually develop from the distal fallopian tube and "spill over" onto adjacent tissues.

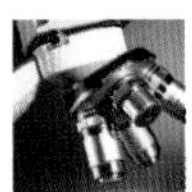

PATHOLOGY: Low-grade serous carcinomas are characterized by irregular invasion of the ovary by small nests of tumor cells with variable desmoplasia (Fig. 16-27). Nuclear uniformity is the principal criterion for distinguishing between low- and high-grade serous carcinomas. Low-grade serous carcinomas rarely progress to high-grade tumors. Psammoma bodies are often present.

High-grade serous carcinomas (often called "cystadenocarcinoma") are mainly solid, multinodular masses, usually with necrosis and hemorrhage (Fig. 16-28A). Once a tumor has reached 10 to 15 cm, it has often spread beyond the ovary and seeded the peritoneum. High-grade serous cancers typically show obvious stromal invasion. Most tumors have a high nuclear grade, irregularly branching, highly cellular papillae with little or no stromal support, and slitlike glandular lumens within more solid areas (Fig. 16-28B). The mitotic rate is very high.

Mucinous Adenocarcinoma

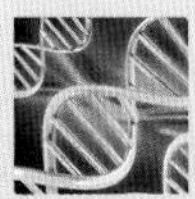

MOLECULAR PATHOGENESIS: Mucinous ovarian tumors are often heterogeneous. Benign, borderline, noninvasive, and invasive malignant components may coexist within the same tumor.

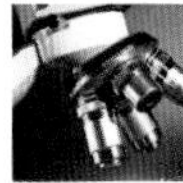

PATHOLOGY: Mucinous carcinomas are usually large, unilateral, multilocular, or unilocular cystic masses containing mucinous fluid. They often include papillary and solid areas that may be soft and mucoid or firm, hemorrhagic, and necrotic. Because these tumors are bilateral in only 5% of cases, finding bilateral or unilateral mucinous tumors smaller than 10 cm raises suspicion of metastatic mucinous carcinoma from the gastrointestinal tract or elsewhere.

Endometrioid Adenocarcinoma

Endometrioid adenocarcinoma histologically resembles its endometrial counterpart (Fig. 16-29A). It may have areas of squamous differentiation and is second only to serous adenocarcinoma in frequency, comprising 10% of all ovarian cancers. These tumors occur most commonly after menopause. Up to one half of these ovarian cancers are bilateral, and, at diagnosis, most tumors are confined either to the ovary or within the pelvis.

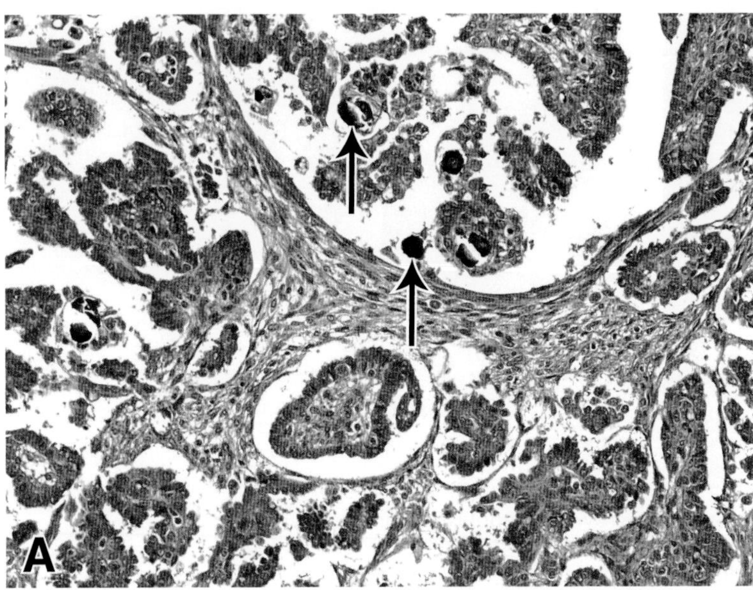

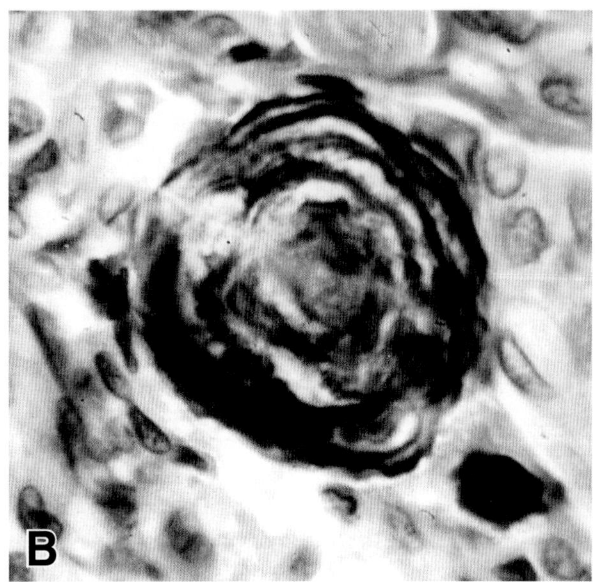

FIGURE 16-27. Low-grade serous carcinoma. A. The nests of tumor cells are disorderly distributed and appear surrounded by clefts. In contrast to high-grade serous carcinoma, the nuclei are low grade. Psammoma bodies (*arrows*) are seen. **B.** A higher power view showing the laminated structure of a psammoma body.

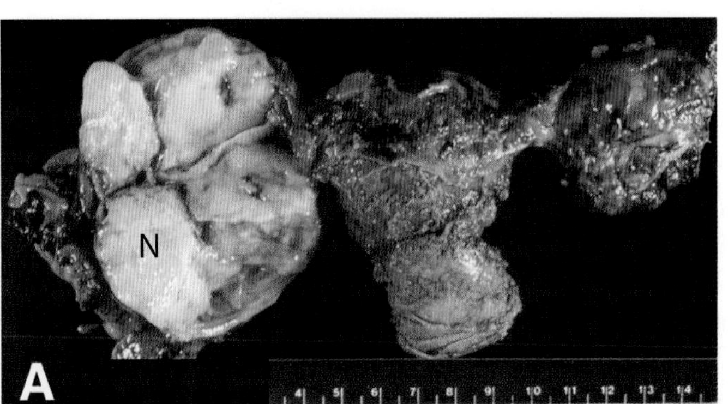

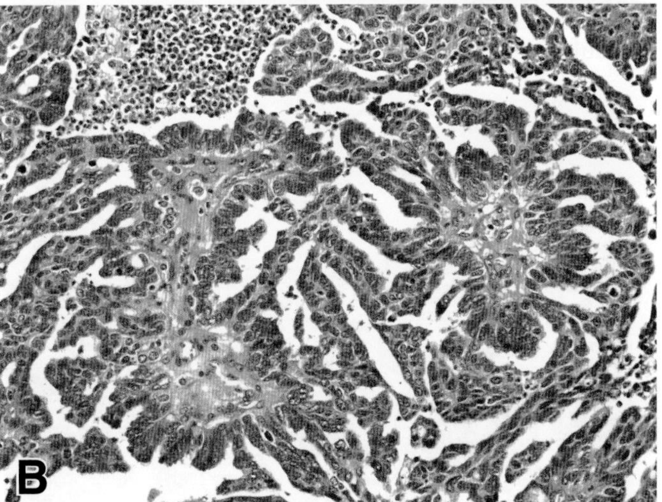

FIGURE 16-28. High-grade serous cystadenocarcinoma. A. In addition to cysts (*left*), the ovary is enlarged by a solid tumor that exhibits extensive necrosis (N). **B.** Microscopic examination showing complex papillae, lined by atypical nuclei, forming glomeruloid structures.

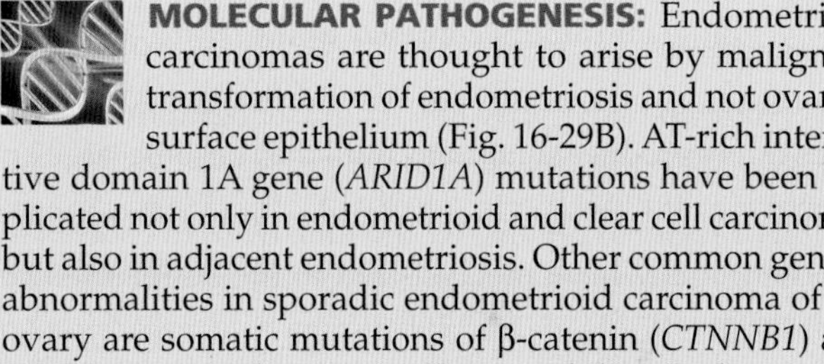

MOLECULAR PATHOGENESIS: Endometrioid carcinomas are thought to arise by malignant transformation of endometriosis and not ovarian surface epithelium (Fig. 16-29B). AT-rich interactive domain 1A gene (*ARID1A*) mutations have been implicated not only in endometrioid and clear cell carcinomas but also in adjacent endometriosis. Other common genetic abnormalities in sporadic endometrioid carcinoma of the ovary are somatic mutations of β-catenin (*CTNNB1*) and *PTEN* genes and microsatellite instability. Endometrioid borderline tumors also have β-catenin mutations.

PATHOLOGY: Endometrioid carcinomas vary from 2 cm to more than 30 cm. Most are largely solid with areas of necrosis, although they may be cystic. Endometrioid tumors are graded like their endometrial counterparts. Some 20% of patients with endometrioid carcinoma of the ovary also harbor an endometrial cancer. As with all malignant epithelial tumors of the ovary, prognosis depends on the stage at which it presents.

Clear Cell Adenocarcinoma

This enigmatic ovarian cancer is closely related to endometrioid adenocarcinoma and often occurs in association with endometriosis (Fig. 16-30A). It constitutes 5% to 10% of all ovarian cancers, usually occurring after menopause. Roughly half of clear cell carcinomas carry *ARID1A* mutations and lack BAF250 protein. Although patients typically present with stage I or II disease, clear cell carcinomas have a poor prognosis compared with other low-stage ovarian carcinomas. Tumors range in size from 2 to 30 cm, and 40% are bilateral. Most are partially cystic and show necrosis and hemorrhage in the solid areas.

Clear cell ovarian adenocarcinomas resemble their counterparts in the vagina and have sheets or tubules of malignant

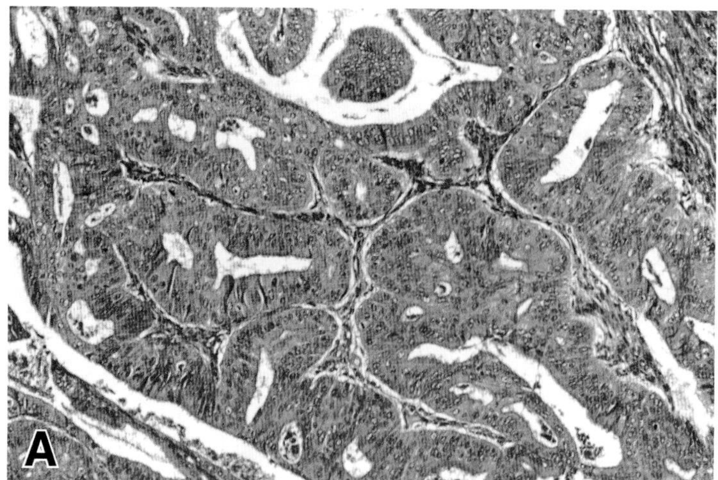

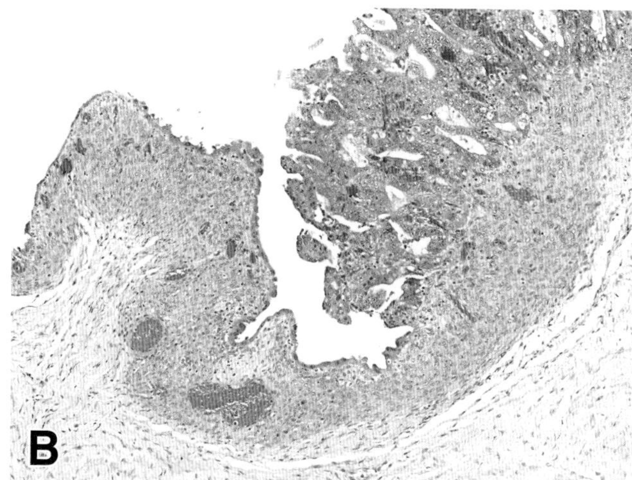

FIGURE 16-29. Endometrioid adenocarcinoma. A. The crowded neoplastic glands are lined by stratified non–mucin-containing epithelium. Nuclear atypia is moderate to severe. **B.** Endometrioid adenocarcinoma (*right*) arising in endometriosis. Note the stromal cells of endometriosis.

cells with clear cytoplasm (Fig. 16-30B). The clinical course parallels that of endometrioid carcinoma.

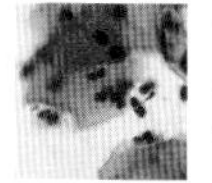

CLINICAL FEATURES: Most ovarian tumors do not secrete hormones. However, the cancer antigen, CA-125, is detectable in the serum in about half of epithelial tumors confined to the ovary and about 90% that have spread. The specificity of this test is highest when combined with transvaginal ultrasonography. Ovarian masses rarely produce symptoms until they become large and distend the abdomen to cause pain, pelvic pressure, or compression of regional organs. By the time ovarian cancers are diagnosed, many have metastasized to (i.e., implanted on) the surfaces of the pelvis, abdominal organs, or bladder. Ovarian tumors have a tendency to implant in the peritoneal cavity on the diaphragm, paracolic gutters, and omentum. Lymphatic spread preferentially involves para-aortic lymph nodes near the origin of the renal arteries and, to a lesser extent, the external iliac (pelvic) or inguinal lymph nodes. In addition to local symptoms, metastatic cancers often cause ascites, weakness, weight loss, and cachexia.

Survival in patients with malignant ovarian tumors is generally poor. The most important prognostic index is the surgical stage of the tumor at the time of detection (Table 16-4).

Germ Cell Tumors

Tumors derived from germ cells make up 15% of ovarian tumors. In adult women, ovarian germ cell tumors are virtually all benign (mature cystic teratoma and dermoid cyst), but in children and young adults aged 15 years or younger, 15% to 30% are cancerous. ***In children, germ cell tumors are the most common ovarian cancer (60%); they are rare after menopause.***

Neoplastic germ cells may differentiate along several lines (Fig. 16-31):

- **Dysgerminomas** are composed of neoplastic germ cells, similar to oogonia of fetal ovaries.
- **Teratomas** differentiate toward somatic (embryonic or adult) tissues.

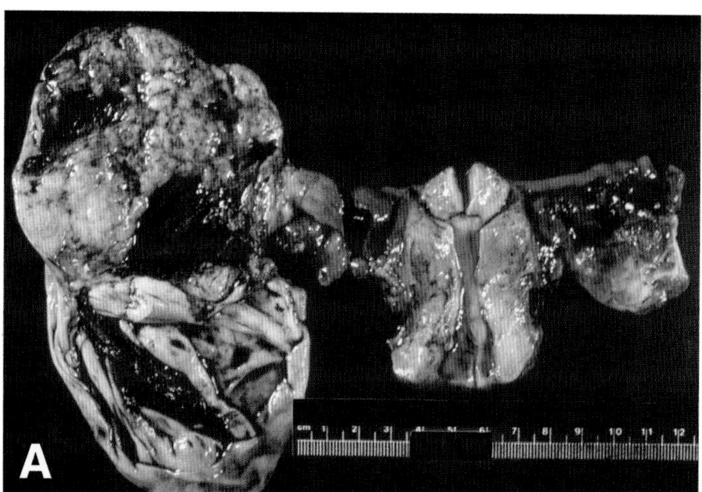

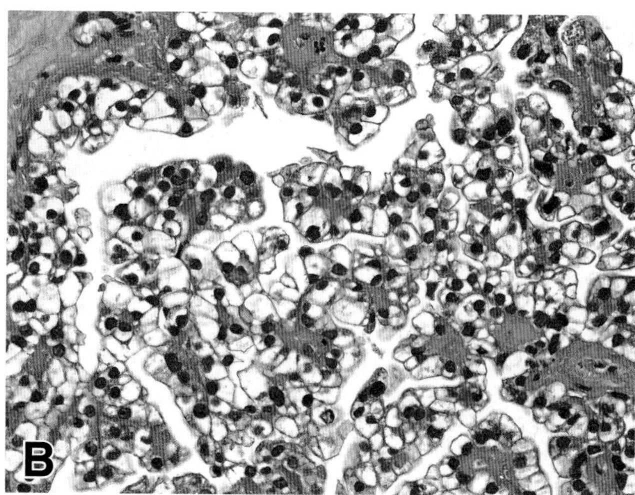

FIGURE 16-30. Clear cell adenocarcinoma. A. Clear cell adenocarcinoma arising as an ovarian mass in a large, hemorrhagic endometriotic cyst. **B.** The clear cells are polyhedral and have eccentric, hyperchromatic nuclei without prominent nucleoli.

Table 16-4

FIGO (2012) Staging of Cancer of the Ovary, Fallopian Tube, and Peritoneum

Stage	Anatomic Distribution
Stage I	Tumor confined to ovaries or fallopian tube(s)
IA	Tumor limited to one ovary (capsule intact) or fallopian tube Surface free of tumor and washings negative
IB	Tumor limited to both ovaries (capsules intact) or fallopian tubes Surface free of tumor and washings negative
IC	Tumor limited to one or both ovaries or fallopian tubes, with any of the following:
IC1	Surgical spill intraoperatively
IC2	Capsule ruptured before surgery or tumor on ovarian or fallopian tube surface
IC3	Malignant cells in the ascites or peritoneal washings
Stage II	Tumor involves one or both ovaries or fallopian tubes with pelvic extension (below pelvic brim) or primary peritoneal cancer
IIA	Extension and/or implants on the uterus and/or fallopian tubes and/or ovaries
IIB	Extension to other pelvic intraperitoneal tissues
Stage III	Cytologically or histologically confirmed spread to the peritoneum outside the pelvis and/or metastasis to the retroperitoneal lymph nodes
IIIA	Metastasis to the retroperitoneal lymph nodes with or without microscopic peritoneal involvement beyond the pelvis
IIIA1	Positive retroperitoneal lymph nodes only (cytologically or histologically proven)
IIIA1 (i)	Nodal metastasis ≤10 mm in greatest dimension
IIIA1 (ii)	Nodal metastasis >10 mm in greatest dimension
IIIA2	Microscopic extrapelvic (above the pelvic brim) peritoneal involvement with or without positive retroperitoneal lymph nodes
IIIB	Macroscopic peritoneal metastases beyond the pelvic brim ≤2 cm in greatest dimension with or without positive retroperitoneal nodes
IIIC	Macroscopic peritoneal metastases beyond the pelvic brim >2 cm in greatest dimension with or without positive retroperitoneal nodes
Stage IV	Distant metastasis excluding peritoneal metastases
IVA	Pleural effusion with positive cytology
IVB	Metastases to extra-abdominal organs (including inguinal lymph nodes and lymph nodes outside abdominal cavity)

FIGO, International Federation of Gynecology and Obstetrics.

- **Yolk sac tumors** form extraembryonic endodermal and mesenchymal tissue.
- **Choriocarcinomas** feature cells similar to those covering the placental villi.

Germ cell tumors in infants tend to be solid and immature (e.g., yolk sac tumor and immature teratoma). Tumors in young adults show greater differentiation, as in mature cystic teratoma. Malignant germ cell tumors in women older than 40 years usually result from transformation of a component of a benign cystic teratoma.

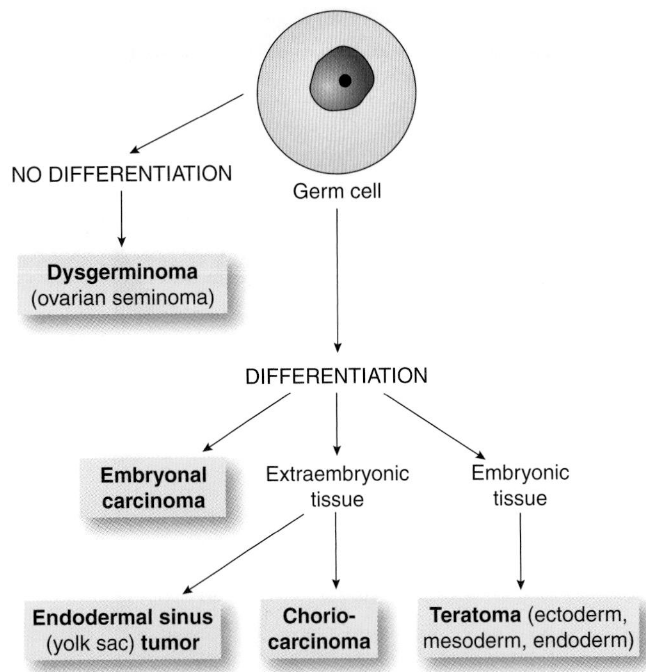

FIGURE 16-31. Classification of germ cell tumors of the ovary.

Malignant germ cell tumors are very aggressive. Solid ovarian germ cell tumors were once always fatal, but now, over 80% of patients survive with chemotherapy.

Benign Tumors

Mature Teratoma (Mature Cystic Teratoma and Dermoid Cyst)

Mature teratomas accounts for one fourth of all ovarian tumors, with a peak incidence in the third decade. Mature teratomas develop by **parthenogenesis**. Haploid (postmeiotic) germ cells endoreduplicate to give rise to diploid genetically female tumor cells (46,XX).

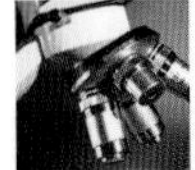

PATHOLOGY: Mature teratomas are cystic, and almost all contain skin, sebaceous glands, and hair follicles (Fig. 16-32). Half have smooth muscle, sweat glands, cartilage, bone, teeth, and respiratory epithelium. Other tissues, like gut, thyroid, and brain, are seen less often. If present, nodular foci in the cyst wall ("mammary tubercles" or "Rokitansky nodules") contain tissue elements of all three germ cell layers: (1) ectoderm (e.g., skin and glia), (2) mesoderm (e.g., smooth muscle, and cartilage), and (3) endoderm (e.g., respiratory epithelium).

Very few (1%) dermoid cysts become malignant. These cancers usually occur in older women and correspond to the tumors that arise in other differentiated tissues of the body. Three fourths of cancers that arise in dermoid cysts are squamous cell carcinomas. The remainder are carcinoid tumors, basal cell carcinomas, thyroid cancers, and others. Rarely, functional gut derivatives may cause carcinoid syndrome. The prognosis of patients with malignancies in mature cystic teratoma is related largely to the stage of the cancer.

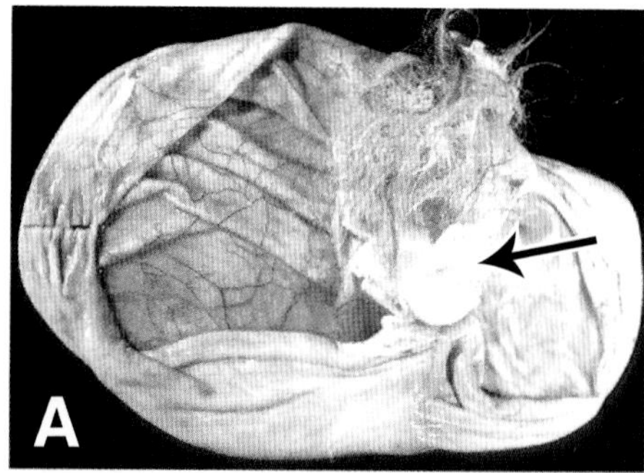

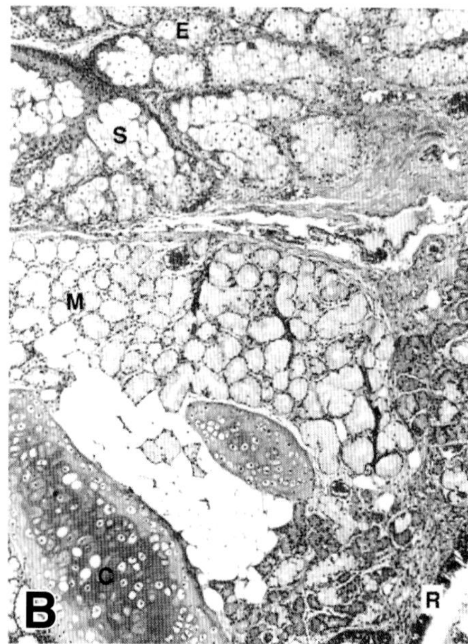

FIGURE 16-32. Mature cystic teratoma of the ovary. A. A mature cystic teratoma has been opened to reveal a solid knob (*arrow*) from which hair projects. **B.** A photomicrograph of the solid knob showing epidermal and respiratory components. Tissue resembling the skin exhibits an epidermis (*E*) with underlying sebaceous glands (*S*). The respiratory tissue consists of mucous glands (*M*), cartilage (*C*), and respiratory epithelium (*R*).

Struma ovarii is a cystic lesion with mainly thyroid tissue (5% to 20% of mature cystic teratomas). Rarely, hyperthyroidism has occurred with struma ovarii.

Malignant Tumors

Dysgerminoma

Dysgerminoma, the ovarian counterpart of testicular seminoma, is composed of primordial germ cells. It accounts for less than 2% of ovarian cancers in all women, but constitutes 10% in women younger than 20 years. Most patients are between 10 and 30 years of age. The tumors are bilateral in 15% of cases.

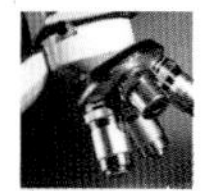

PATHOLOGY: Dysgerminomas are often large and firm and have a bosselated external surface. The cut surface is soft and fleshy. They contain large nests of monotonously uniform tumor cells that have clear glycogen-filled cytoplasm and irregularly flattened central nuclei (Fig. 16-33). Fibrous septa containing lymphocytes traverse the tumor.

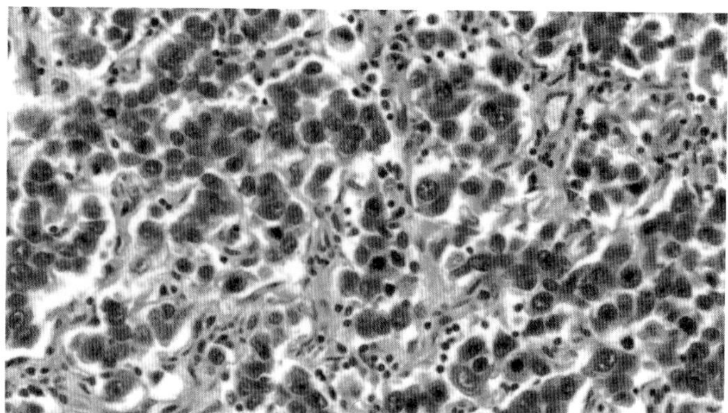

FIGURE 16-33. Dysgerminoma. The neoplastic germ cells are distributed in nests separated by delicate fibrous septa. The stroma contains lymphocytes.

Dysgerminomas are treated surgically; 5-year survival for patients with stage I tumor approaches 100%. Because the tumor is highly radiosensitive and also responsive to chemotherapy, even higher stage tumors have 5-year survival rates exceeding 80%.

Immature Teratoma

Immature teratomas of the ovary contain elements derived from the three germ layers. However, unlike mature cystic teratomas, immature teratomas contain embryonal tissues. These tumors comprise 20% of malignant tumors at all sites in women under the age of 20 but become progressively less common in older women.

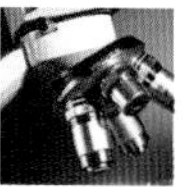

PATHOLOGY: Immature teratomas are predominantly solid and lobulated, with numerous small cysts. Solid areas may contain grossly recognizable immature bone and cartilage. Multiple tumor components are usually seen, including those differentiating toward neural tissue (neuroepithelial rosettes and immature glia), glands, and other structures found in mature cystic teratomas. Grading is based on the amount of immature tissue present. Metastases of immature teratomas are composed of embryonal, usually stromal, tissues. By contrast, rare metastases of mature cystic teratomas resemble epithelial adult-type malignancies.

Survival reflects tumor grade. Well-differentiated immature teratomas have a good prognosis, but high-grade tumors (mainly embryonal tissue) are often lethal.

Yolk Sac Tumor (Primitive Endodermal Tumor)

Yolk sac tumors are highly malignant tumors of women under the age of 30 that histologically resemble mesenchyme of the primitive yolk sac. They are the second most common malignant germ cell tumors and are almost always unilateral.

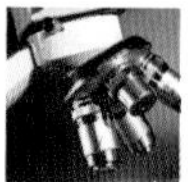

PATHOLOGY: Yolk sac tumors are large and exhibit extensive necrosis and hemorrhage. Several patterns are seen. The most common is a reticular, honeycombed structure of communicating spaces lined by primitive epithelial cells. They display glycogen-rich, clear cytoplasm, and large hyperchromatic nuclei (primitive endoderm). Glomerular or **Schiller–Duval bodies** (Fig. 16-34A) are found sparingly in a few tumors but are characteristic. They consist of papillae that protrude into a space lined by tumor cells, resembling the glomerular Bowman space. The

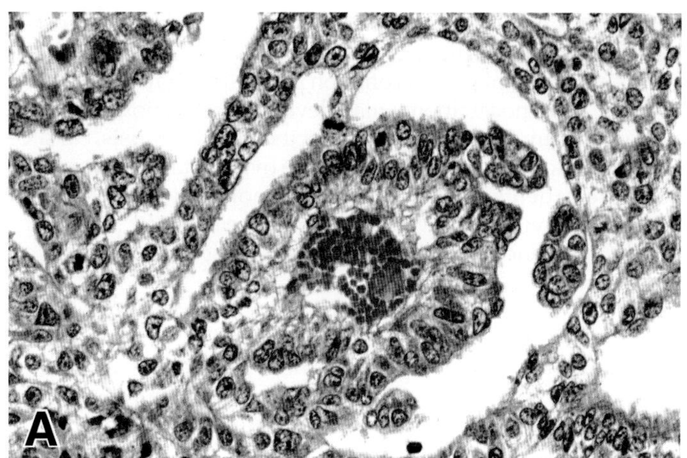

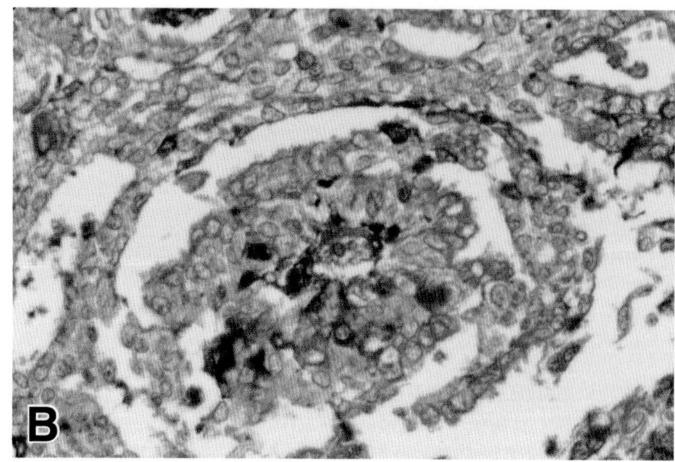

FIGURE 16-34. Yolk sac tumor of the ovary. A. Glomeruloid Schiller–Duval body that resembles the endodermal sinuses of the rodent placenta and consists of a papilla protruding into a space lined by tumor cells. **B.** Strong immunoreaction for α-fetoprotein.

papillae are covered by a mantle of embryonal cells and contain a fibrovascular core and a central blood vessel.

Detection of α-fetoprotein in the blood (Fig. 16-34B) is useful for diagnosis and for monitoring the effectiveness of therapy. Although once uniformly fatal, 5-year survival with chemotherapy for stage I yolk sac tumors now exceeds 80%.

Choriocarcinoma

Choriocarcinoma of the ovary is a rare tumor that mimics the epithelial covering of placental villi, namely, cytotrophoblast and syncytiotrophoblast. If it arises before puberty or together with another germ cell tumor, it is most likely of germ cell origin. Young girls may show precocious sexual development, menstrual irregularities, or rapid breast enlargement. In reproductive-aged women, however, it may also be a metastasis from an intrauterine gestational tumor.

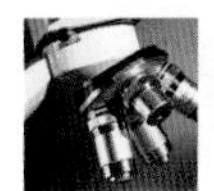

PATHOLOGY: Choriocarcinoma is unilateral, solid, and widely hemorrhagic. Microscopically, it shows a mixture of malignant cytotrophoblast and syncytiotrophoblast (see placenta, choriocarcinoma, below). The syncytial cells secrete hCG, which accounts for the frequent finding of a positive pregnancy test. Bilateral theca lutein cysts, a result of hCG stimulation, may also be found. Serial serum hCG determinations are useful both for diagnosis and follow-up. The tumor is highly aggressive but responds to chemotherapy.

Sex Cord/Stromal Tumors of the Ovary

Tumors of sex cord and stroma originate from either primitive sex cords or mesenchymal stroma of developing gonads. They represent 10% of ovarian tumors, vary from benign to low-grade malignant, and may differentiate toward female (granulosa and theca cells) or male (Sertoli and Leydig cells) structures.

Benign Tumors

Fibroma

Fibromas account for 75% of all stromal tumors and 7% of all ovarian tumors. They occur at all ages, peaking in the perimenopausal period, and are almost always benign.

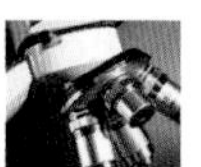

PATHOLOGY: Tumors are solid, firm, and white. The cells resemble the stroma of the normal ovarian cortex, being well-differentiated spindle cells, with variable amounts of collagen. Half of the larger tumors are associated with ascites and, rarely, with ascites and pleural effusions **(Meigs syndrome)**.

Thecoma

Thecomas are functional ovarian tumors of postmenopausal women and are almost always benign. They are closely related to fibromas, but additionally contain varying amounts of steroidogenic cells, which, in many cases, produce estrogens or androgens.

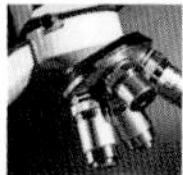

PATHOLOGY: Thecomas are solid tumors, mostly 5 to 10 cm in diameter. The cut section is yellow, owing to the many lipid-laden theca cells, which are large and oblong to round, with lipid-rich vacuolated cytoplasm (Fig. 16-35). Bands of hyalinized collagen separate nests of theca cells.

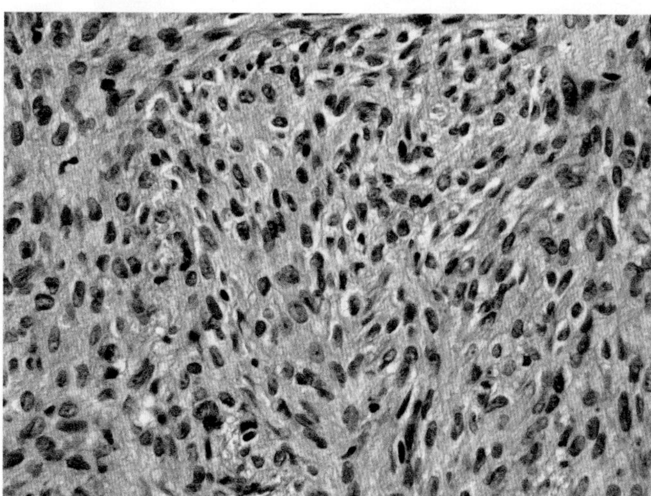

FIGURE 16-35. Thecoma of the ovary. Oblong cells are invested by collagen. The cytoplasm contains lipid.

Because they produce estrogen, thecomas in premenopausal women may cause irregular menstrual cycles and breast enlargement. Endometrial hyperplasia and cancer are well-recognized complications.

Malignant Tumors

Granulosa Cell Tumor

Granulosa cell tumors are the prototypical functional neoplasms of the ovary associated with estrogen secretion. They should be considered malignant because of their potential for local spread and the rare occurrence of distant metastases.

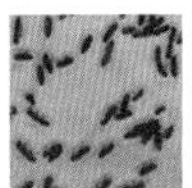

ETIOLOGIC FACTORS: Most granulosa cell tumors occur after menopause (adult form) and are unusual before puberty. A juvenile form in children and young women has distinct clinical and pathologic features (hyperestrinism and precocious puberty). Development of granulosa cell tumors is linked to the loss of oocytes. Oocytes appear to regulate granulosa cells, and tumorigenesis occurs when follicles are disorganized or atretic.

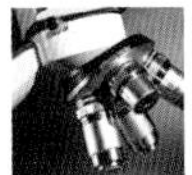

PATHOLOGY: Adult-type granulosa cell tumors, like most ovarian tumors, are large and focally cystic to solid. The cut surface shows yellow areas, owing to lipid-rich luteinized granulosa cells, white zones of stroma, and focal hemorrhages (Fig. 16-36). Granulosa cell tumors show diverse growth patterns. Random nuclear arrangement about a central degenerative space (**Call–Exner bodies**) gives a characteristic follicular pattern (Fig. 16-36B). Tumor cells are typically spindle shaped and have a cleaved, elongated nucleus (coffee-bean appearance). They secrete **inhibin**, a protein that suppresses pituitary release of follicle-stimulating hormone (FSH). These tumors can often express **calretinin**, a neuronal protein, which suggests possible neural differentiation or derivation for these neoplasms.

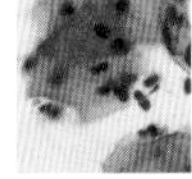

CLINICAL FEATURES: ***Three fourths of granulosa cell tumors secrete estrogens.*** Thus, endometrial hyperplasia is a common presenting sign. Endometrial adenocarcinoma may develop if a functioning granulosa cell tumor remains undetected. At diagnosis, 90% of granulosa cell tumors are within the ovary (stage I). Over 90% of these patients survive 10 years. Tumors that have extended into the pelvis and lower abdomen have a poorer prognosis. Late recurrence 5 to 10 years after surgical removal is not uncommon and is usually fatal.

Sertoli–Leydig Cell Tumors

Ovarian Sertoli–Leydig cell tumors (**arrhenoblastoma** or **androblastoma**) are rare androgen-secreting mesenchymal neoplasms of low malignant potential that resemble embryonic testis. Tumor cells typically secrete weak androgens (dehydroepiandrosterone), so they are usually quite large before patients complain of masculinization. Sertoli–Leydig cell tumors occur at all ages but are most common in young women of childbearing age.

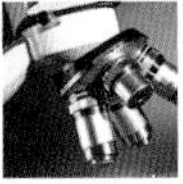

PATHOLOGY: Sertoli–Leydig cell tumors are unilateral, usually 5 to 15 cm, and tend to be lobulated, solid, and brown to yellow. They vary from well to poorly differentiated, and some contain heterologous elements (e.g., mucinous glands and, rarely, even cartilage). Large Leydig cells have abundant eosinophilic cytoplasm and a central round to oval nucleus with a prominent nucleolus. Tumor cells are embedded in a sarcomatoid stroma. (The stroma, in some areas, often differentiates into immature solid tubules of embryonic Sertoli cells.)

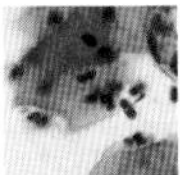

CLINICAL FEATURES: Nearly half of all patients with Sertoli–Leydig cell tumors exhibit signs of virilization, hirsutism, male escutcheon, enlarged clitoris, and deepened voice. Initial signs are often

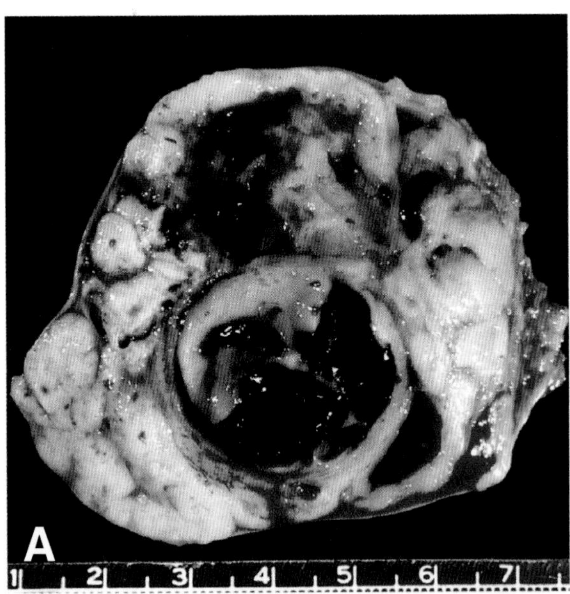

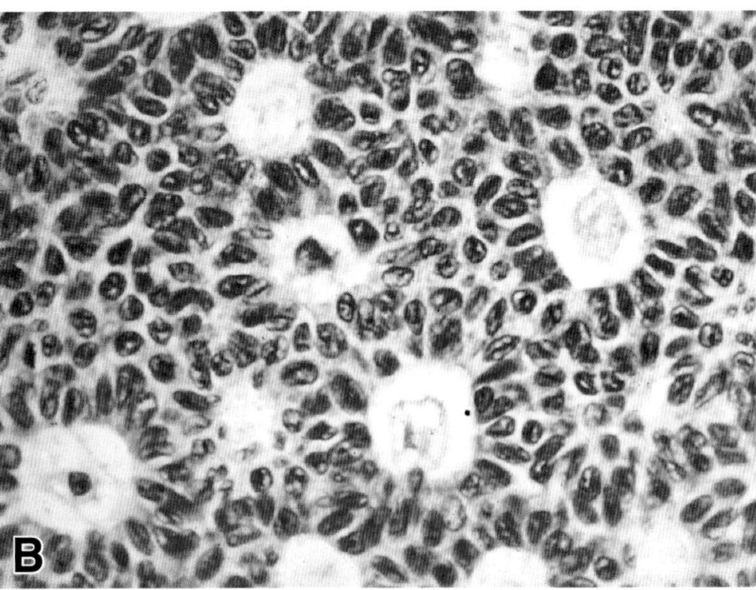

FIGURE 16-36. Granulosa cell tumor of the ovary. A. Cross section of the enlarged ovary showing a variegated solid tumor with focal hemorrhages. The yellow areas represent collections of lipid-laden luteinized granulosa cells. **B.** The orientation of tumor cells about central spaces results in the characteristic follicular pattern (Call–Exner bodies).

defeminization, manifested as breast atrophy, amenorrhea, and loss of hip fat. Once the tumor is removed, these signs disappear or lessen. Well-differentiated tumors are virtually always cured by surgical resection, but poorly differentiated ones may metastasize.

Steroid Cell Tumor

Steroid cell tumors of the ovary, also called **lipid cell** or **lipoid cell tumors**, are composed of cells that resemble lutein cells, Leydig cells, and adrenal cortical cells. Most steroid cell tumors are hormonally active, usually with androgenic manifestations. Some secrete testosterone; others synthesize weaker androgens. **Hilus cell tumor** is a specialized form of steroid cell tumor that is typically a benign neoplasm of Leydig cells. It arises in the hilus of the ovary, usually after menopause. Because it secretes testosterone, the most potent of the common androgens, masculinizing signs are frequent (75%), even with small tumors. Most hilus cell tumors contain "crystalloids of Reinke" (rodlike cytoplasmic structures).

Tumors Metastatic to the Ovary

About 3% of cancers found in the ovaries arise elsewhere, mostly in the breast, large intestine, endometrium, and stomach, in descending order. These tumors vary from microscopic lesions to large masses. Those from the breast are usually minute and are seen in 10% of ovaries removed prophylactically in cases of advanced breast cancer. Metastatic tumors large enough to cause symptoms most often originate in the colon. Commonly, the tumor cells stimulate ovarian stroma to differentiate into hormonally active cells (luteinized stromal cells), leading to androgenic and, sometimes, estrogenic symptoms.

Krukenberg tumors are metastases to the ovary that are composed of nests of mucin-filled "signet-ring" cells in a cellular stroma derived from the ovary. The stomach is the primary site in 75% of cases, and most of the rest are from the colon.

Bilateral ovarian involvement and multinodularity suggest a metastatic carcinoma, and both ovaries are grossly involved in 75% of cases. Even an ovary that appears uninvolved grossly may contain surface implants or minute foci of tumor within the parenchyma. Thus, when metastasis to one ovary is documented, the other should also be removed.

Peritoneum

The peritoneum is a nearly continuous membrane that lines the peritoneal cavity and separates viscera from the abdominal wall. In men, the peritoneum is a closed system. In women, it is an "open system" interrupted in the pelvis by the fallopian tubes, which provide a final conduit for transmission of pathogens and chemicals from the genital tract to the peritoneal cavity.

The cells that line the peritoneal cavity and those that form the serosa of the ovary are both of celomic epithelial origin. ***Thus, it is not clear whether tumors and tumor-like lesions of the peritoneum and ovary (i.e., Müllerian epithelial lesions) are the same entity in both locations.***

Many inflammatory lesions involve the peritoneum. Granulomatous peritonitis develops as a response to foreign materials, such as sutures, surgical glove powder, or contrast media. Exposure to intestinal contents after perforation (e.g., in Crohn disease or diverticulitis), rupture of a mature cystic teratoma (dermoid cyst) of the ovary, and, of course, tuberculosis can also cause peritoneal inflammation. Reactive mesothelial proliferation occurs with the slightest irritation. Peritonitis is discussed in Chapter 11.

MESOTHELIAL TUMORS

Mesothelial tumors range from benign to multicentric aggressive malignancies.

Well-Differentiated Papillary Mesotheliomas

Well-differentiated papillary mesotheliomas are rare in reproductive-aged women. They are typically asymptomatic and usually found incidentally at operation. These tumors are solitary, small, broad-based, wartlike polypoid or nodular excrescences, with a single layer of small bland cuboidal cells covering thick papillae. They often resemble serous epithelial tumors of the ovary, but are treated differently.

Diffuse Peritoneal Malignant Mesotheliomas

These tumors arise from peritoneal mesothelium. They are rare in women and constitute only a small proportion of all malignant mesotheliomas, most of which are pleural. They must be distinguished from serous adenocarcinomas, including those arising from the peritoneal surface itself and those metastatic from the ovary, because they are treated differently and have much different survival rates. Most patients are middle aged or postmenopausal with nonspecific symptoms such as ascites, abdominal discomfort, digestive disturbances, and weight loss. Unlike pleural tumors, asbestos exposure is uncommon in women with peritoneal mesothelioma, although such tumors have been reported.

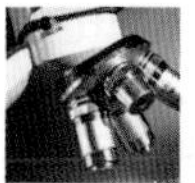

PATHOLOGY: Diffuse malignant mesothelioma extensively involves and thickens the peritoneum and serosa of the various abdominal and pelvic organs. It has a tubulopapillary to solid pattern. Unlike pleural mesothelioma, the sarcomatoid type is rare. The epithelial variant displays polygonal or cuboidal neoplastic cells with abundant cytoplasm. Thrombomodulin, calretinin, wt-1, cytokeratin 5/6, and HBME-1 are markers of malignant mesothelioma, whereas CA-125, CEA, and estrogen and progesterone receptors (ER and PR) are markers of ovarian epithelial tumors. No effective treatment is available.

SEROUS TUMORS (PRIMARY AND METASTATIC)

Unlike the ovary, which features a wide range of tumors, serous tumors are virtually the only type found in the peritoneum. Mucinous tumors in the peritoneum are metastases from a primary cancer of the appendix or ovary.

Serous Tumors of Borderline Malignancy

Most serous borderline tumors in the peritoneum are metastases from the ovary, but some may be primary in the peritoneum. In the latter case, serous peritoneal tumors without invasion are usually benign; those that are invasive carry a worse prognosis. The pathology is similar to tumors of the ovary.

Serous Adenocarcinoma

The frequency of serous adenocarcinoma arising de novo in the peritoneum is estimated as 10% of its counterpart in the ovary. The mean age of women with this tumor is 50 to 65 years. The diagnosis of a primary peritoneal tumor requires demonstration of normal ovaries. Abdominal pain and ascites are frequent presentations. Like ovarian cancer, serous adenocarcinoma primarily in the peritoneum may have a familial basis and can metastasize to distant locations.

PSEUDOMYXOMA PERITONEI

Pseudomyxoma peritonei is the accumulation of jellylike mucus in the pelvis or peritoneum. Previously interpreted as spread from mucinous ovarian tumors, pseudomyxoma peritonei is now understood to derive largely from mucus-producing adenocarcinomas of the appendix.

Uterus

CONGENITAL ANOMALIES OF THE UTERUS

Congenital anomalies of the uterus are rare.

- **Congenital absence of the uterus (agenesis)** reflects failure of Müllerian ducts to develop. Because elongation of these ducts during embryonic life requires the Wolffian ducts as guides, uterine agenesis is almost always accompanied by other urogenital tract anomalies and agenesis of the vagina and fallopian tubes.
- **Uterus didelphys** is a double uterus, owing to failure of the two Müllerian ducts to fuse in early embryonic life. A double vagina commonly accompanies this anomaly.
- **Uterus duplex bicornis** is a uterus with a common fused wall between two distinct endometrial cavities. The common wall between the apposed Müllerian ducts fails to degenerate to form a single uterine cavity.
- **Uterus septus** is a single uterus with a partial septum, secondary to incomplete resorption of the wall of the fused Müllerian ducts. These patients have an increased risk for habitual abortion.
- **Bicornuate uterus** refers to a uterus with two cornua (horns) and a common cervix. Didelphic and bicornuate uterine fusion defects increase the risk of premature birth only slightly.

Conditions of the Endometrium

Endometritis

Endometritis refers to an abnormal inflammatory infiltrate in the endometrium. It must be distinguished from the normal presence of neutrophils during menstruation and mild lymphocytic infiltrates at other times. In most cases of endometritis, the findings are nonspecific and rarely point to a specific cause.

ACUTE ENDOMETRITIS: This condition is defined as the abnormal presence of polymorphonuclear leukocytes in the endometrium. Most cases result from an ascending infection from the cervix after the usually impervious cervical barrier is compromised by abortion, delivery, or medical instrumentation.

CHRONIC ENDOMETRITIS: Although lymphocytes and lymphoid follicles occur occasionally in a normal endometrium, plasma cells in the endometrium are diagnostic of chronic endometritis. The disorder is associated with IUDs, PID, and retained products of conception after an abortion or delivery. Patients usually complain of bleeding or pelvic pain or both. The condition is generally self-limited.

PYOMETRA: Defined as pus in the endometrial cavity, pyometra is associated with gross anatomic defects, such as fistulous tracts between bowel and uterine cavity, bulky or perforating malignancies, or cervical stenosis. Long-standing pyometra may rarely be associated with the development of endometrial squamous cell cancer.

ADENOMYOSIS

Adenomyosis is the presence of endometrial glands and stroma within the myometrium. Pain, dysmenorrhea, or menorrhagia correlate with adenomyosis if the glands are 1 mm or more beneath the endometrial myometrial junction; more severe symptoms occur as glands penetrate more deeply into the myometrium. Pain is present as foci of adenomyosis enlarge when blood is entrapped during menses. One fifth of all uteri surgically removed show some adenomyosis.

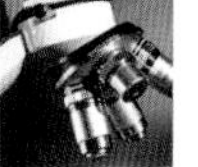

PATHOLOGY: The uterus may be enlarged. The myometrium discloses small, soft, tan areas, some of which are cystic. Microscopic examination shows glands lined by proliferative to inactive endometrium and surrounded by endometrial stroma with varying degrees of fibrosis.

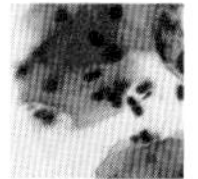

CLINICAL FEATURES: Many patients with adenomyosis are asymptomatic, although pelvic pain, dysfunctional uterine bleeding, dysmenorrhea, and dyspareunia are common. These symptoms appear in parous women of reproductive age and regress after menopause.

ENDOMETRIAL TUMORS

Endometrial Polyps

Polyps occur mostly in the perimenopausal period and not before menarche. They are monoclonal outgrowths of endometrial stromal cells that are altered by chromosomal translocation, with secondary induction of polyclonal glandular elements. Stroma and glands of endometrial polyps respond poorly to hormonal stimulation and do not slough upon menstruation.

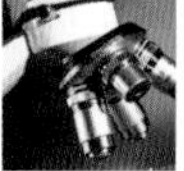

PATHOLOGY: Most endometrial polyps arise in the fundus, but they can be found anywhere within the endometrium. They vary from several millimeters to growths filling the entire endometrial cavity. Most are solitary, but 20% are multiple. Polyp cores are composed of (1) endometrial glands, often cystically dilated and hyperplastic; (2) fibrous endometrial stroma; and (3) thick-walled, coiled, dilated blood vessels, derived from a straight artery that normally would have supplied the basal zone of the endometrium. Cores are covered by endometrial epithelium, usually out of cycle from adjacent normal endometrium.

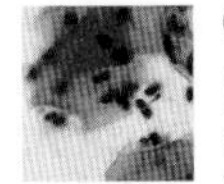

CLINICAL FEATURES: Endometrial polyps typically present with intermenstrual bleeding, owing to surface ulceration or hemorrhagic infarction. Because bleeding in an older woman may indicate endometrial cancer, this sign must be thoroughly evaluated. Endometrial polyps are not ordinarily precancerous, although up to 0.5% harbor adenocarcinoma.

Endometrial Hyperplasia

The 2014 WHO classification of endometrial hyperplasias divides lesions into etiologic subgroups based on cancer risk and treatment options. **Nonatypical endometrial hyperplasia** is a functionally normal endometrium that responds to an abnormal hormonal state of excess estrogen; **endometrial intraepithelial neoplasia (EIN)**, also called **atypical endometrial hyperplasia** features mutated precancerous cells that grow as a neoplastic clone.

Nonatypical Hyperplasia

Nonatypical endometrial hyperplasia is a spectrum of changes, dependent upon the duration and dose of estrogen exposure. ***It is characterized by diffuse architectural and randomly distributed cytologic change.*** The earliest ones are isolated cystic expansion of scattered proliferative glands without a substantial change in gland density, often designated **persistent proliferative** or **disordered proliferative** endometrium. Morphologic transition to nonatypical endometrial hyperplasia occurs when gland density becomes irregular throughout, with some regions having more glands than stroma. Glands are irregularly distributed and punctuated by cysts, creating a variably increased ratio of glands and stroma. Cytologic change, when it occurs, is most often metaplastic and distributed in random manner. Sudden loss of estrogen leads to massive shedding with attendant heavy menses. Adenocarcinoma develops in 1% to 3% of cases.

Endometrial Intraepithelial Neoplasia

EIN (also termed "atypical hyperplasia") is a monoclonal neoplastic growth of genetically altered cells that are associated with a greatly increased risk of becoming endometrioid type of endometrial adenocarcinoma (Fig. 16-37). EIN is composed of crowded aggregates of cytologically altered tubular or slightly branching glands. Within the lesion, the area of glands exceeds that of stroma. Residual normal glands may be adjacent to or admixed with EIN. Thirty-seven percent of patients with EIN will develop adenocarcinoma, almost always of the endometrioid type. EIN lesions begin at a single point and then expand centripetally as proliferating neoplastic glands that displace and separate normal glands. Diagnostic features of EIN include alterations in nuclear size, shape, and texture and changes in cytoplasmic differentiation. Malignant transformation is evident when glands develop solid, cribriform, or mazelike patterns characteristic of adenocarcinoma. Hysterectomy is the therapy of choice in women who do not desire future pregnancy.

Endometrial Adenocarcinoma

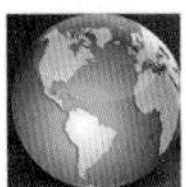

EPIDEMIOLOGY: Endometrial carcinoma is the fourth most frequent cancer in American women and the most common gynecologic cancer (Table 16-5). It caused 11,000 deaths in the United States in 2017 (2% of all cancers in women). The incidence of this cancer was stable from 1950 to 1970, but by 1975, it had increased by 40%, possibly related to the use of estrogens for easing symptoms of menopause. By 1985, the rates had returned nearly to 1950 levels, a trend that correlated with the use of lower doses of estrogen, incorporation of progestins (estrogen antagonists) into estrogen replacement regimens, and increased surveillance of women treated with estrogens.

The incidence of endometrial cancer varies with age, from 12 cases per 100,000 women at age 40- to 7-fold higher in 60-year-olds. Three quarters of women with endometrial cancer are postmenopausal with a median age at diagnosis of 63 years.

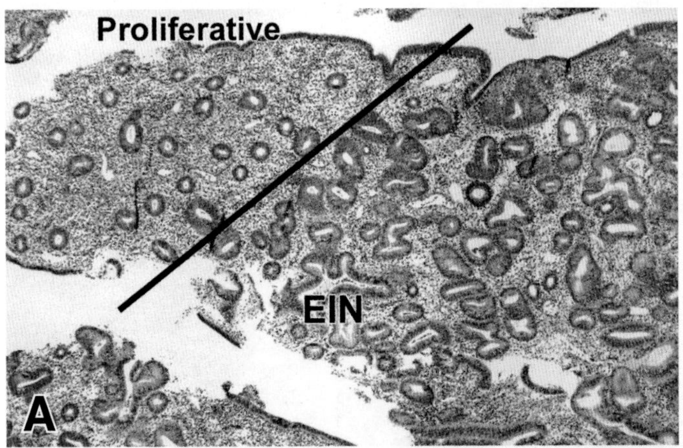

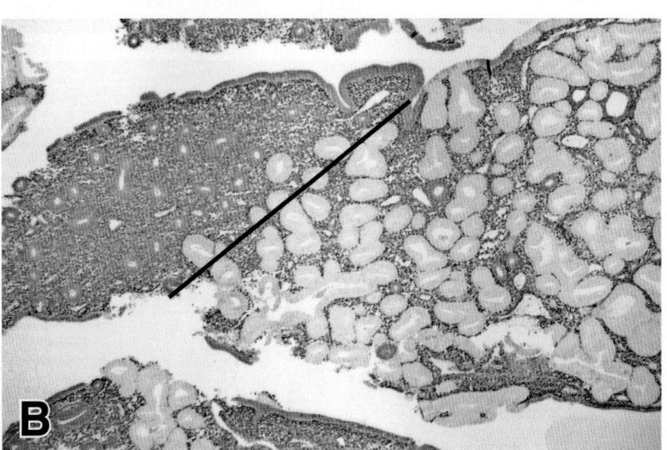

FIGURE 16-37. Endometrial intraepithelial neoplasia (EIN; atypical endometrial hyperplasia). A. Tight clusters of cytologically altered neoplastic endometrial glands with abundant cytoplasm and rounded nuclei (*right*) are offset from the background endometrium (*left*) in this geographic focus of EIN. Measurement across the perimeter of this aggregate of individual tubular glands exceeds 1 mm, and features of adenocarcinoma such as cribriform, mazelike, or solid architecture are lacking. **B.** Glands affected by EIN showing loss of PTEN expression by immunohistochemistry (loss of brown staining).

Table 16-5

Clinicopathologic Features of Endometrial Carcinoma

	Type I: Endometrioid Carcinoma	Type II: Serous Carcinoma
Age	Premenopausal and perimenopausal	Postmenopausal
Unopposed estrogen	Present	Absent
Hyperplasia precursor	Present	Absent
Grade	Low	High
Myometrial invasion	Superficial	Deep
Growth behavior	Stable	Progressive
Genetic alterations	Microsatellite instability, PTEN, PIK3CA, β-catenin	p53 mutations, loss of heterozygosity

Endometrial carcinoma is broadly grouped into two histologic types (Fig. 16-38 and Table 16-5). **Type I tumors** (about 80%) are endometrioid carcinomas, which often arise from EIN precursors and are associated with estrogenic stimulation, occur mainly in postmenopausal women. The tumors are associated with obesity, hyperlipidemia, anovulation, infertility, and late menopause. Most endometrioid carcinomas are confined to the uterus and follow a favorable course. By contrast, **type II tumors** (about 10%) are nonendometrioid, largely papillary serous carcinomas, arising occasionally in endometrial polyps. A preinvasive form of disease, serous endometrial intraepithelial carcinoma (serous EIC, not to be confused with EIN) can metastasize to the peritoneum by exfoliation and surface spread. Although serous EIC can exhibit malignant behavior, it is not generally considered a precancerous lesion. Risk factors for type II tumors are similar to those for type I but are not generally associated with hyperplasia. However, type II tumors readily invade the myometrium and vascular spaces and are highly lethal. The molecular alterations of endometrioid (type I) carcinomas are different from those of the nonendometrioid (type II) carcinomas.

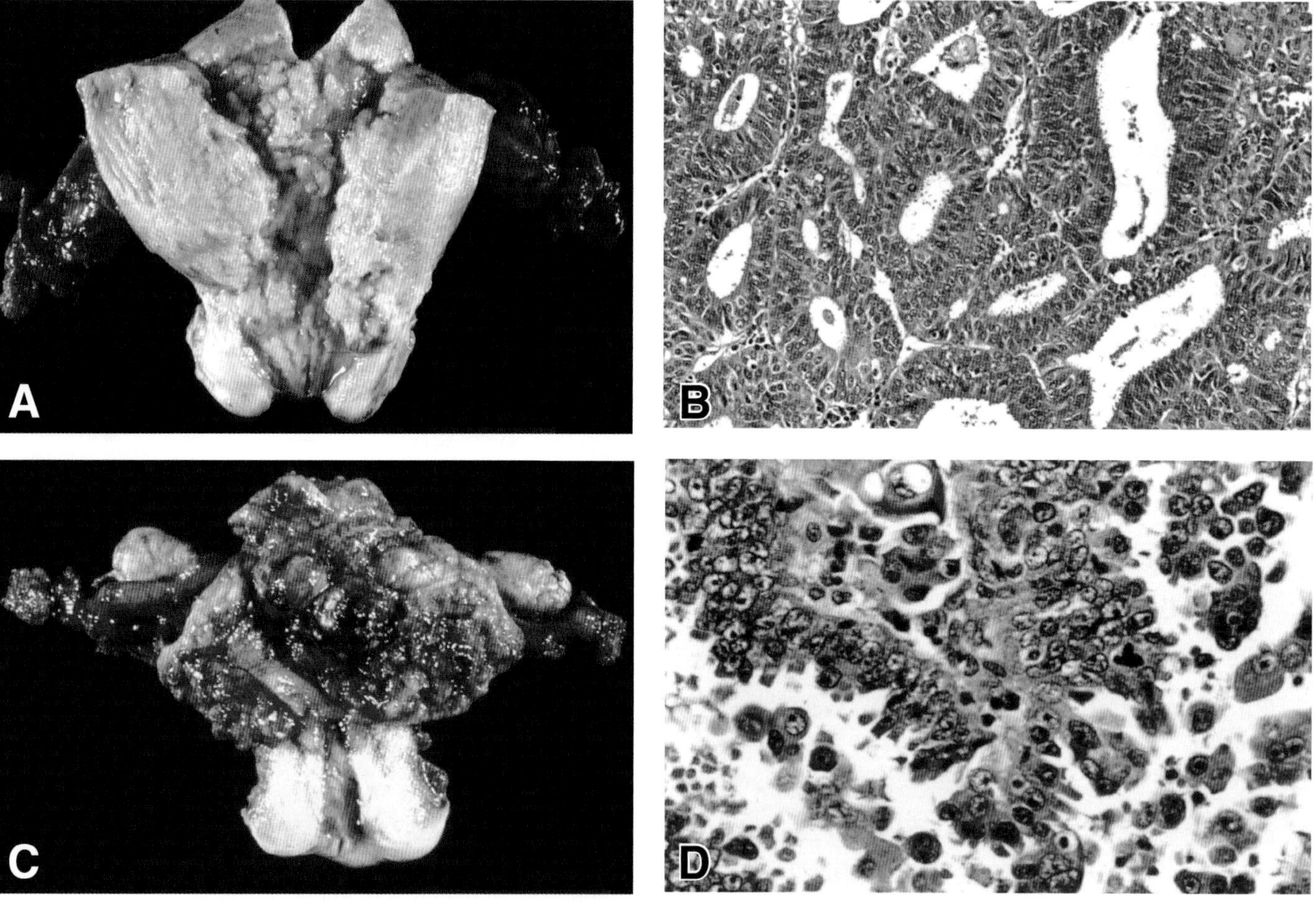

FIGURE 16-38. Adenocarcinoma of the endometrium. A, B. Endometrioid carcinoma. Polypoid tumor with only superficial myometrial invasion. Well-differentiated (grade 1) adenocarcinoma. The neoplastic glands resemble normal endometrial glands. **C, D. Nonendometrioid carcinoma.** Large hemorrhagic and necrotic tumor with deep myometrial invasion. Serous carcinoma (severe cytologic atypia) exhibiting stratification of anaplastic tumor cells and abnormal mitoses.

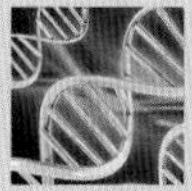

MOLECULAR PATHOGENESIS: Endometrial cancer occurs in association with a higher incidence of both breast and ovarian cancer in closely related women, suggesting a genetic predisposition.

Over 90% of type II nonendometrioid carcinomas have p53 mutations, and 80% lose estrogen and progesterone receptors. Type I tumors show a stepwise accumulation of mutation, the most common being inactivation of the tumor suppressor *PTEN*, which is inactivated in up to two thirds of cases.

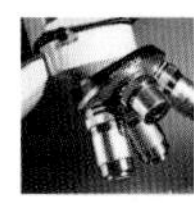

PATHOLOGY: Endometrial cancer grows in diffuse or exophytic patterns (Fig. 16-38). Regardless of its site of origin, the tumor often tends to involve multiple areas. Large tumors are usually hemorrhagic and necrotic.

ENDOMETRIOID ADENOCARCINOMA OF THE ENDOMETRIUM: The FIGO system divides this tumor into three grades depending on the ratio of glandular and solid elements, the latter signifying poorer differentiation.

- **Grade 1:** Well differentiated; almost only neoplastic glands, with minimal (<5%) solid areas
- **Grade 2:** Moderately differentiated; 5% to 50% of malignant epithelium forms glands
- **Grade 3:** Poorly differentiated; large (>50%) areas of solid tumor

Nuclei of endometrial adenocarcinoma range from bland to markedly pleomorphic, usually with prominent nucleoli. Mitoses are abundant and may be abnormal in less differentiated tumors. Tumor cells that grow in solid sheets are generally poorly differentiated.

Additional variants of endometrial carcinoma demonstrate squamous cells as well as glands (**well and poorly differentiated endometroid adenocarcinoma with squamous differentiation**). A **secretory type** with subnuclear glycogen-containing vacuoles occurs.

OTHER TYPES (NONENDOMETRIOID) OF ENDOMETRIAL CARCINOMA: Nonendometrioid types of endometrial carcinoma are less common. They are aggressive as a group, and histologic grading is not clinically useful or separately diagnosed because all cases are considered high grade. The most common is **serous adenocarcinoma**, which histologically resembles, and behaves like, serous adenocarcinoma of the ovary (see below) (Fig. 16-38D). It often shows transtubal spread to peritoneal surfaces.

Most endometrial carcinomas arise in the uterine corpus, but a small proportion originate in the lower uterine segment (isthmus). These tumors often occur in women under the age of 50 and are often high grade and deeply invasive.

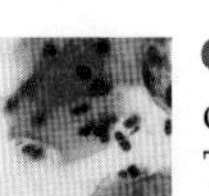

CLINICAL FEATURES: Endometrial cancers usually occur in perimenopausal or postmenopausal women. The chief complaint is commonly abnormal uterine bleeding, especially in the early stages of tumor growth confined to the endometrium. Unfortunately, cervicovaginal cytologic screening does not efficiently detect early endometrial cancer. Transvaginal ultrasound is valuable diagnostically in postmenopausal patients in whom an endometrium greater than 5 mm thickness is considered highly suspicious. Unlike cervical cancer, endometrial cancer may bypass pelvic lymph nodes and spread directly to para-aortic nodes. Patients with advanced cancers may also have pulmonary metastases (40% of cases with metastases).

Women with well-differentiated cancers confined to the endometrium are usually treated by simple hysterectomy. Survival in endometrial carcinoma depends on stage and type. Actuarial survival for all patients with endometrial cancer following treatment is 80% after 2 years, decreasing to 65% after 10 years. Tumors that have penetrated the myometrium or invaded lymphatics are more likely to have spread beyond the uterus.

ENDOMETRIOSIS

Endometriosis is the presence of benign endometrial glands and stroma outside the uterus. It afflicts 5% to 10% of women of reproductive age and regresses after natural or artificial menopause. The mean age at diagnosis is the late 20s to early 30s, although it may appear any time after menarche. Sites most frequently involved are the ovaries (>60%), other uterine adnexa (uterine ligaments, rectovaginal septum, and pouch of Douglas), and the pelvic peritoneum. Endometriosis can be even more widespread and, occasionally, affects the cervix, vagina, perineum, bladder, and umbilicus. Even pelvic lymph nodes may contain foci of endometriosis. Rarely, distant areas such as lungs, pleura, small bowel, kidneys, and bones contain lesions.

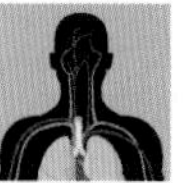

PATHOPHYSIOLOGY: The pathogenesis of endometriosis is uncertain. Several theories, not necessarily mutually exclusive, are proposed:

- **Transplantation** of endometrial fragments to ectopic sites
- **Metaplasia** of the multipotential celomic peritoneum
- **Induction** of undifferentiated mesenchyme in ectopic sites to form lesions after exposure to substances released from shed endometrium

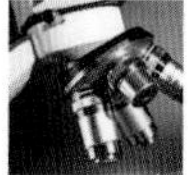

PATHOLOGY: The earliest lesions of endometriosis may be yellow-red stains, reflecting breakdown of blood products. Red lesions, which also occur early in the disease, are actively growing foci of endometriosis (Fig. 16-39). Operative specimens usually contain black lesions that show some degree of resolution. Small foci on the ovary and peritoneal surfaces are called "mulberry" nodules. With repeated cycles of hemorrhage and subsequent fibrosis, affected surfaces may scar and become grossly brown ("powder burns"). Over time, fibrous adhesions may become more pronounced and lead to complications, such as intestinal obstruction. Repeated hemorrhage in the ovaries may turn endometriotic foci into cysts up to 15 cm in diameter, which contain inspissated, chocolate-colored material ("chocolate cysts").

Endometriosis is characterized by ectopic normal endometrial glands and stroma (Fig. 16-39). Occasionally, healed foci may contain only fibrous tissue and hemosiderin-laden macrophages, which by themselves are not diagnostic. Immunohistochemical demonstration of CD-10 can be diagnostic.

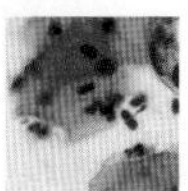

CLINICAL FEATURES: Symptoms of endometriosis depend on where implants are located. Dysmenorrhea, caused by implants on uterosacral ligaments, is common. Lesions swell just before or during

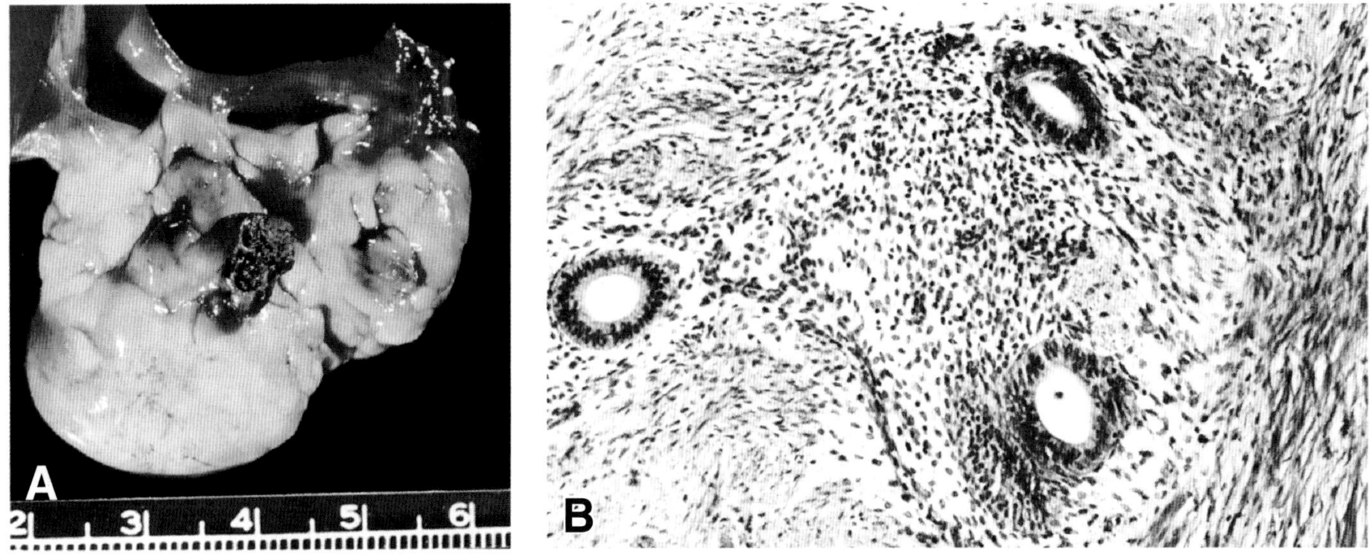

FIGURE 16-39. Endometriosis. A. Implants of endometriosis on the ovary appear as red-blue nodules. **B.** A microscopic section showing endometrial glands and stroma in the ovary.

menstruation, producing pelvic pain. Half of women with dysmenorrhea have endometriosis. Other symptoms include dyspareunia and cyclical abdominal pain.

Infertility is the primary complaint in one third of women with endometriosis (Fig. 16-40). The hormonal milieu in a woman who does not achieve pregnancy encourages the development of endometriosis. In turn, once endometriosis develops, it contributes to the infertile state, and a vicious circle is established. Conversely, pregnancy may alleviate the disease. Conservative surgery allows many women with endometriosis to become pregnant.

Malignant transformation occurs in about 1% to 2% of cases of endometriosis. Clear cell and endometrioid tumors are the most frequent forms.

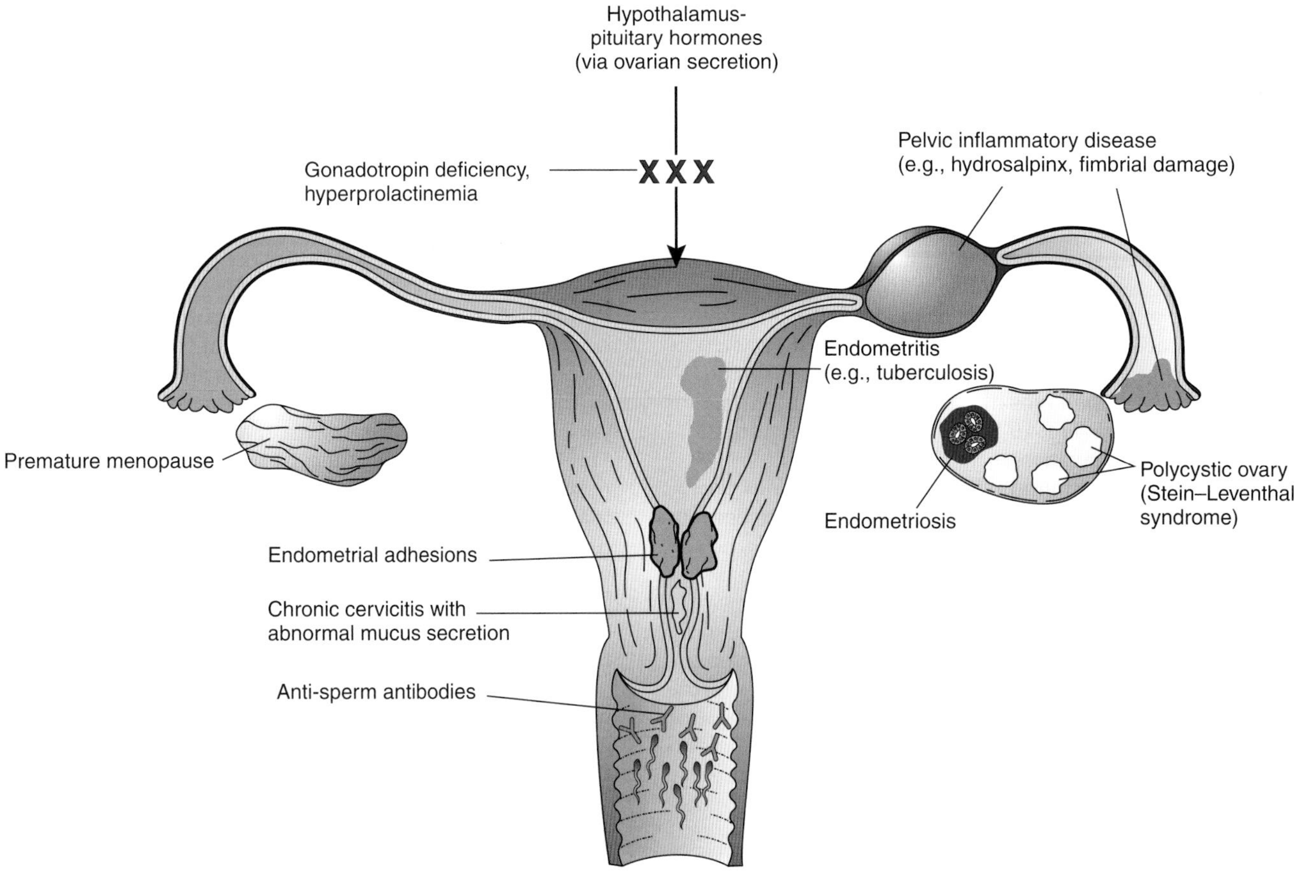

FIGURE 16-40. Causes of acquired infertility.

OTHER TUMORS OF THE UTERUS

Endometrial Stromal Tumors

Some endometrial stromal tumors are pure sarcomas; in others, sarcomatous (stromal) and epithelial elements are intermingled. The nomenclature of these tumor types, the spectrum of their histologic components, and the correlation of each tumor type with its potential for malignant behavior are presented in Table 16-6.

Leiomyomas

Leiomyomas are benign tumors of smooth muscle origin and are colloquially known as "myomas" or "fibroids." Including minute tumors, leiomyomas occur in 75% of women over age 30. They are rare before age 20, and most regress after menopause. Although often multiple, each tumor is monoclonal. Estrogen promotes their growth but does not initiate them.

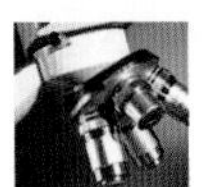

PATHOLOGY: Grossly, leiomyomas are firm, pale gray, whorled and without encapsulation (Figs. 16-41 and 16-42). They vary from 1 mm to large tumors over 30 cm in diameter. Their cut surface bulges, and borders are smooth and distinct from neighboring myometrium. Most uterine leiomyomas are intramural, but some are submucosal, subserosal, or pedunculated. The tumors show little mitotic activity (<4 mitoses per 10 high-power fields), lack nuclear atypia, and geographical necrosis and have little or no malignant potential. A **"mitotically active leiomyoma"** is one that shows brisk mitotic activity but is relatively small, is sharply demarcated from adjacent normal myometrium, and lacks both necrosis and significant cellular atypia. It is usually benign. Mutations of *MED12*, a subunit of a transcriptional regulator, occurs in 70% of leiomyomas.

Microscopically, leiomyomas exhibit interlacing fascicles of uniform spindle cells containing elongated nuclei with

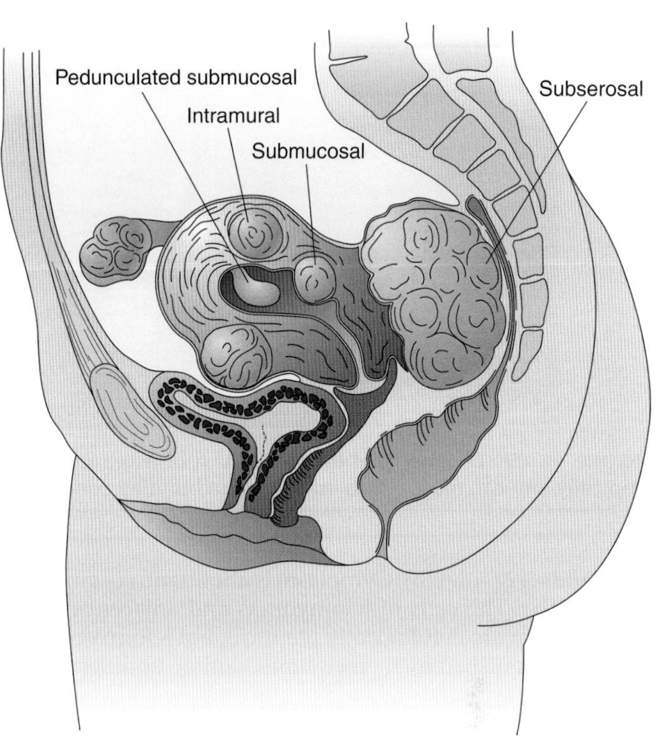

FIGURE 16-41. Leiomyomas of the uterus. The leiomyomas are intramural, submucosal (a pedunculated one appearing in the form of an endometrial polyp), and subserosal (one compressing the bladder and the other the rectum).

Table 16-6

Nomenclature of Uterine Tumors

Tumor	Epithelium	Stroma	Clinical Behavior
Epithelium and Stroma			
Endometrial polyp	Polyclonal benign	Neoplastic	Benign
Nonatypical endometrial hyperplasia	Polyclonal benign	Polyclonal benign	Benign
Endometrial intraepithelial neoplasia	Neoplastic	—	Premalignant
Endometrial adenocarcinoma	Neoplastic	—	Malignant
Endometrial stromal nodule	—	Neoplastic	Benign
Endometrial stromal sarcoma	—	Neoplastic	Low-grade malignant
Undifferentiated sarcoma	—	Neoplastic	Malignant
Adenosarcoma	Unknown	Neoplastic	Low-grade malignant
Carcinosarcoma	Neoplastic	Neoplastic, transformed epithelial cells	Malignant
Smooth Muscle			
Leiomyoma	—	Neoplastic	Benign
Cellular leiomyoma	—	Neoplastic	Benign
Intravenous leiomyomatosis	—	Neoplastic	Locally aggressive
Leiomyosarcoma	—	Neoplastic	Malignant

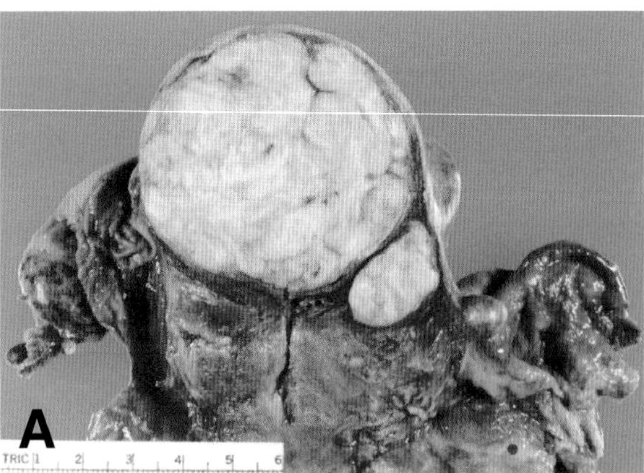

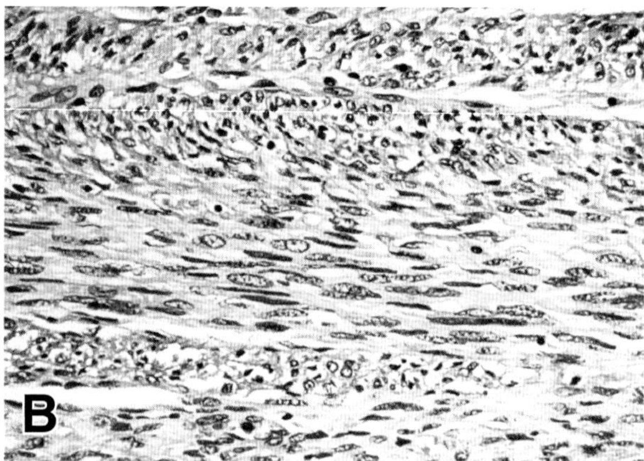

FIGURE 16-42. Leiomyoma of the uterus. A. A bisected uterus displaying a prominent, sharply circumscribed, fleshy tumor. **B.** Microscopically, smooth muscle cells intertwine in bundles, some of which are cut longitudinally (elongated nuclei) and others transversely.

blunt ends (Fig. 16-42B). Cytoplasm is abundant, eosinophilic, and fibrillar. The cells of leiomyomas and adjacent normal myometrium are cytologically identical, but leiomyomas are easily distinguished by their circumscription, nodularity, and denser cellularity.

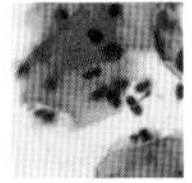

CLINICAL FEATURES: Submucosal leiomyomas may cause bleeding, owing to ulceration of thinned, overlying endometrium, or become pedunculated and protrude through the cervical os, eliciting cramping pains. Many intramural leiomyomas are symptomatic because of their sheer bulk, and large ones may interfere with bowel or bladder function or cause dystocia in labor. Pedunculated leiomyomas on the uterine serosa may interfere with the function of neighboring viscera. Leiomyomas may also infarct and become painful if they undergo torsion.

Leiomyomas usually grow slowly but occasionally enlarge rapidly during pregnancy. Large symptomatic leiomyomas are removed by myomectomy or hysterectomy. Ablation by arterial thrombosis has also been used.

Leiomyosarcomas

Leiomyosarcoma is a smooth muscle malignancy whose incidence is 1 in 1,000 of its benign counterpart. It accounts for 2% of uterine cancers. Its pathogenesis is uncertain, but at least some appear to arise within leiomyomas. Women with leiomyosarcomas are on average more than a decade older (age above 50) than those with leiomyomas, and the malignant tumors are larger (10 to 15 cm vs. 3 to 5 cm) (Fig. 16-43A).

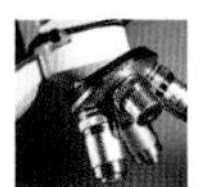

PATHOLOGY: Leiomyosarcoma should be suspected when an apparent leiomyoma is soft, shows areas of necrosis on gross examination, has irregular borders (invasion of adjacent myometrium), or fails to protrude above the surface when cut. Evidence that a uterine smooth muscle tumor is a leiomyosarcoma includes (1) the presence of geographical necrosis with a sharp transition from viable tumor (Fig. 16-43B); (2) 10 or more mitoses per 10 high-power fields (Fig. 16-43C), if the tumor is more than 5 cm in diameter; (3) 5 or more mitoses per 10 HPFs, in association with geographical necrosis and diffuse cytoplasmic/nuclear atypia; and (4) myxoid and epithelioid smooth muscle tumors with 5 or more mitoses per 10 HPFs.

Nearly half of recurrences first present in the lung, and 5-year survival is 20%

Pregnancy

Pregnancies can be affected by placental abnormalities such as abnormal placental size, shape, membranes masses, infarcts, and hematomas. Abnormalities in the cord, including length and point of placental insertion, are also important indicators of potential disease. Infectious and vascular disease of the placenta are of particular importance, as are hypertensive disease of the mother that results from abnormalities in the placental vasculature.

ENDOMETRIUM OF PREGNANCY

The corpus luteum of pregnancy requires continuous stimulation by hCG secreted by the placental trophoblast of the developing embryo. Trophoblast begins to develop at about day 23 of pregnancy. Under hCG stimulation, the corpus luteum increases its progesterone output, stimulating secretion of fluid by endometrial glands. In the hypersecretory endometrium of pregnancy, highly dilated glands are lined by cells with abundant glycogen. These features can persist for up to 8 weeks after delivery.

The hypersecretory response may be exaggerated with intrauterine pregnancy, ectopic pregnancy, or trophoblastic disease. Glandular cell nuclei may enlarge and appear bulbous and polyploid, owing to DNA replication without cell division. These nuclei protrude beyond the apparent cellular cytoplasmic limits into the gland lumen, an appearance referred to as the **Arias-Stella phenomenon** (Fig. 16-44). Enlarged nuclei are polyploid rather than aneuploid, a condition sometimes seen in adenocarcinoma.

PLACENTAL ANATOMY

The placenta includes the **placental disc, umbilical cord,** and **extraplacental membranes** (Fig. 16-45). It is a flattened discoid organ with two surfaces. The fetus faces one aspect **(fetal** or **chorionic surface),** which is covered by membranes, the **amnion** and **chorion**. These contain the **amniotic fluid** that surrounds the fetus. The opposite surface is the **maternal surface** (or the **decidual surface**, because the endometrium becomes decidualized during pregnancy).

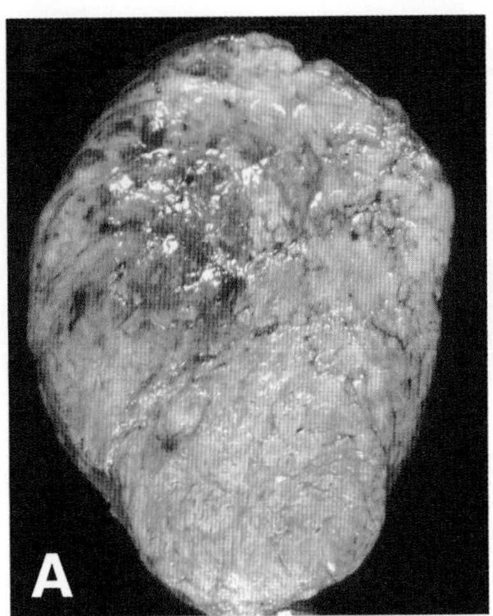

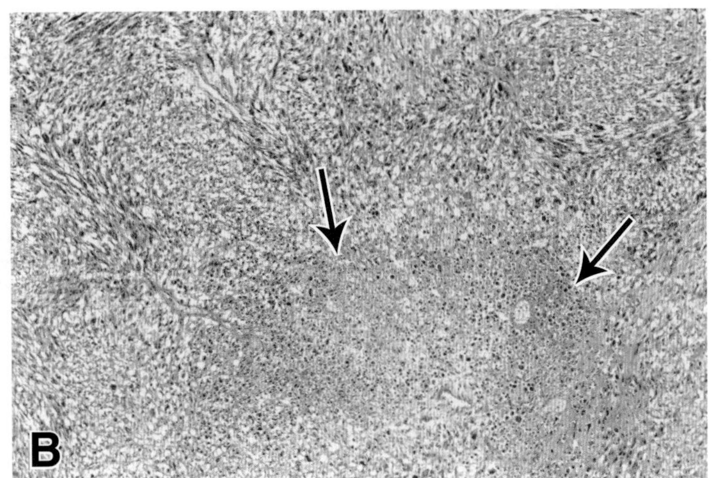

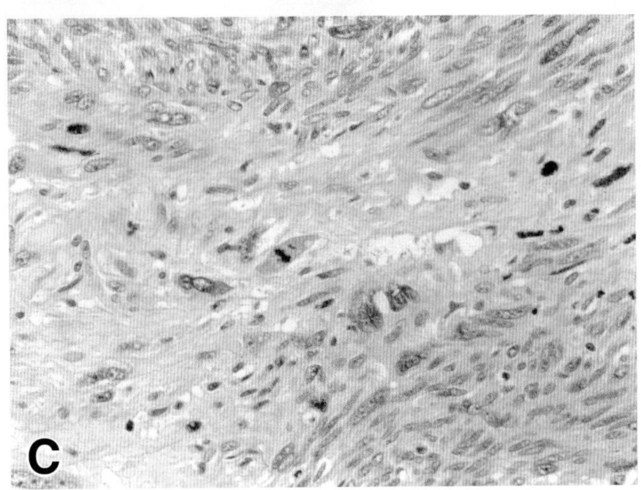

FIGURE 16-43. Leiomyosarcoma of the uterus. **A.** The uterus has been opened to reveal a large, soft leiomyosarcoma with extensive necrosis that replaces the entire myometrium. **B.** A zone of coagulative tumor necrosis (*arrows*) appears demarcated from the viable tumor. **C.** The tumor showing considerable nuclear atypia and abundant mitotic activity.

Fetal blood enters the placenta through two umbilical arteries that spiral around an umbilical vein. The umbilical cord inserts into the chorionic surface on the placenta. The major branches of the umbilical arteries and vein then branch along the surface of the disc and penetrate into the placental disc to form the chorionic villous tree. These villous trunks progressively subdivide into smaller branches, ending in the terminal (or, tertiary) villi, where oxygen and nutrient transport occurs. At term, the terminal villi constitute 40% of the villous volume and 60% of villous cross sections.

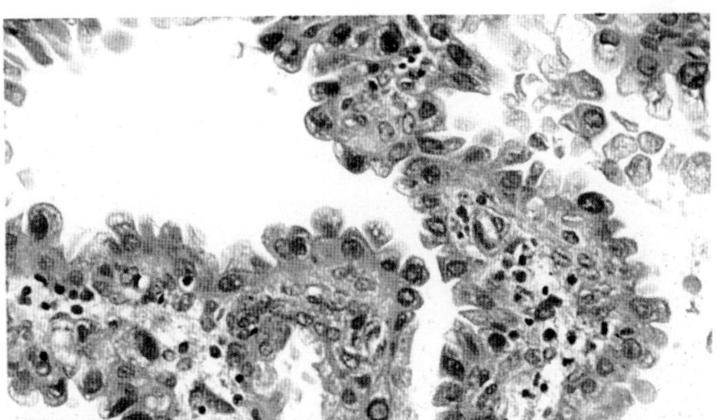

FIGURE 16-44. Arias-Stella reaction of pregnancy associated with human chorionic gonadotropin stimulation. A section of endometrium showing enlarged, bulbous nuclei that protrude into the gland lumen.

The **decidua** forms the border between fetal villous trees and the underlying uterus. The decidua contains small uterine arteries (**spiral arterioles**), which supply the placenta with maternal blood (Fig. 16-46). These arteries undergo a series of **remodeling** changes that decrease vascular resistance to uterine blood flow and support the developing placenta and fetus. Each spiral arteriole delivers maternal blood to the center of an anatomic subunit of the placenta, the **cotyledon**. Maternal blood entering the placental disc is no longer confined to a vessel, but instead occupies a cavity, the **intervillous space**, where it exchanges oxygen and nutrients. Importantly, the maternal and fetal circulations in the placenta are entirely separate systems.

The terminal villus is the functional unit of exchange of the placenta. The chorionic villous tree is covered by the trophoblastic layer. It consists of an inner layer of **cytotrophoblast (Langhans cells)**, a middle layer of **intermediate trophoblast**, and an outer layer of **syncytiotrophoblast**. The villous stroma is loose mesenchyme containing embryonal macrophages, termed **Hofbauer cells**. In the third trimester, syncytiotrophoblast nuclei aggregate to form multinuclear protrusions (**syncytial knots**). In other areas along the villous surface, syncytium between the knots becomes markedly attenuated. At these points, the trophoblastic cytoplasm comes into direct contact with the endothelium of the fetal capillaries to form the **vasculosyncytial membrane**. These specialized zones facilitate gas and nutrient transfer across the placenta.

In addition to releasing waste and absorbing oxygen and nutrients, the villi are hormonally active. The syncytiotrophoblast secretes **human chorionic gonadotropin (hCG)**, which prevents

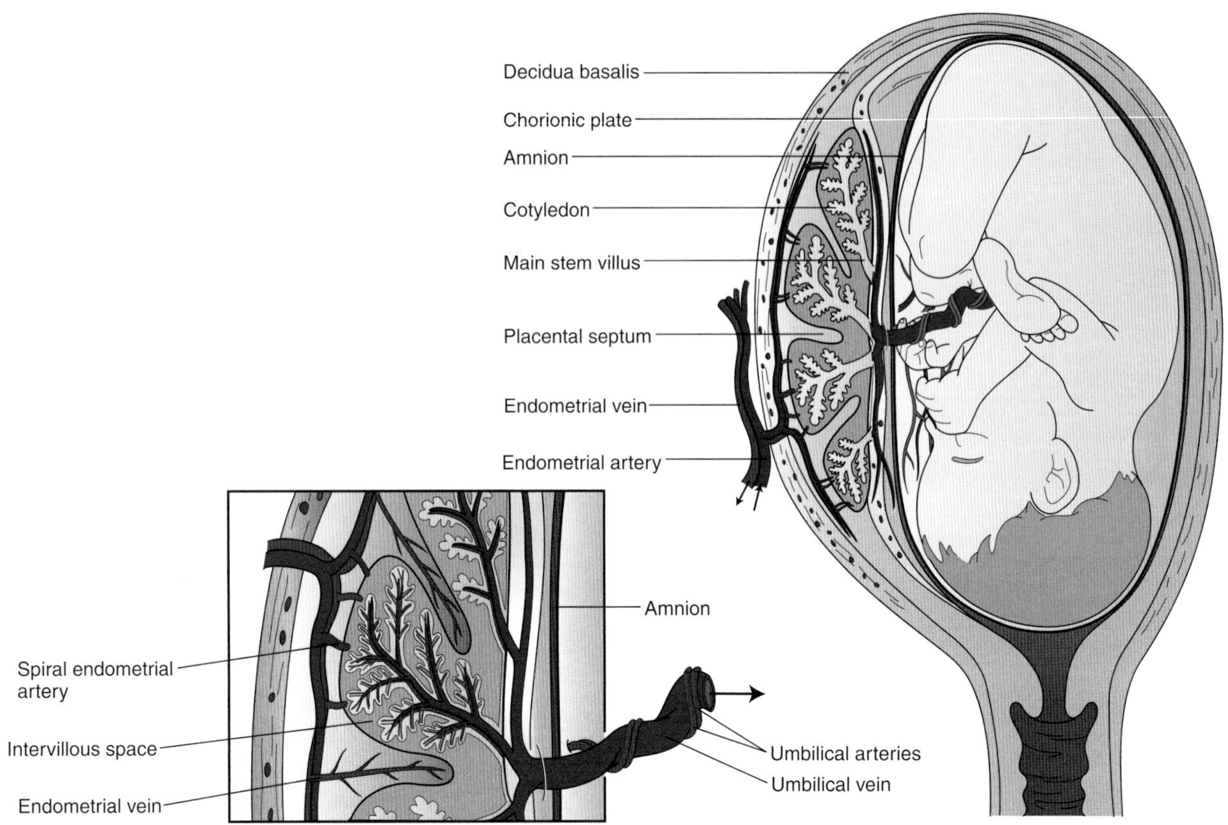

FIGURE 16-45. Modern diagram of the pregnant uterus, including fetus, placenta, and circulation.

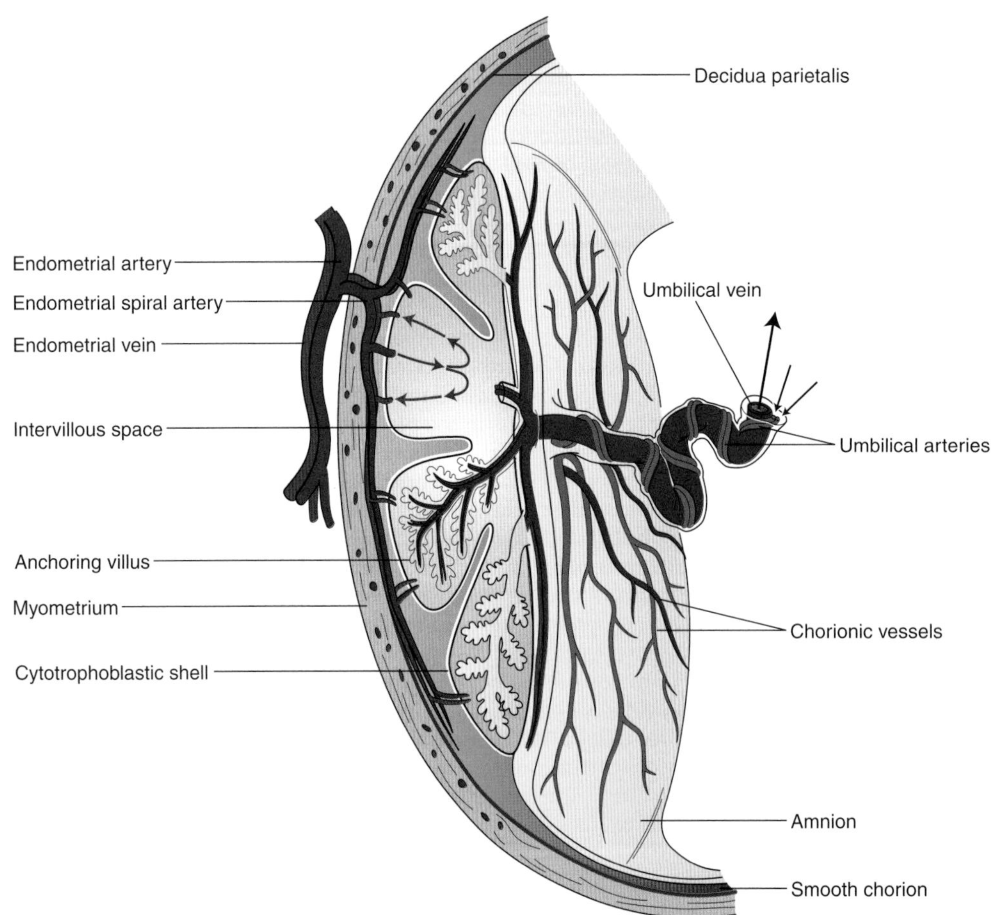

FIGURE 16-46. Cross-sectional diagram of the placenta and its circulation.

degeneration of the corpus luteum. It also secretes **progesterone** to maintain the integrity of the decidua, and **human placental lactogen (HPL)**, which raises maternal glucose levels and so assists in adequate fetal nutrition.

PLACENTAL IMPLANTATION

The placenta is normally implanted in the uterine wall above the internal cervical os. It may implant at the lower portion of the uterus and either partially or completely cover the internal os, a condition termed **placenta previa** (0.3% to 1% of pregnancies). Risk factors include smoking, increased age, multiple prior pregnancies, previous cesarean births, and prior abortions. Placenta previa must be recognized before delivery to avoid the fetus being delivered through its own placenta, risking life-threatening hemorrhage. Placenta previa is one of the most frequent causes of third-trimester bleeding and entails a high risk of abruption, postpartum hemorrhage, prolapsed umbilical cord, fetal malpresentation, intrauterine growth restriction, and fetal and perinatal mortality. Placenta previa is often associated with another abnormal condition, **placenta accreta** (partial or total lack of the decidual layer, see below), in which case it is **placenta previa accrete**.

MULTIPLE GESTATIONS

Slightly less than 1% of normal pregnancies yield dizygotic or monozygotic twins.

DIZYGOTIC TWINS: Fertilization of two separate ova results in genetically different twins, of the same or opposite sex. Dizygotic twinning has a strong hereditary component, which is limited to the maternal side. This type of twinning and multiple gestations occur more commonly in women who have used hormones to induce ovulation artificially or who have been impregnated after in vitro fertilization.

Separate placentas develop when two fertilized ova implant apart from one another. If they implant near each other, the two placentas show varying degrees of fusion and may appear to be one. If the ova implant apart, there are discrete conceptuses, each placenta having its own amniotic sac. In cases when the placentas fuse, the membranes between the two fetuses display two amnions and two chorions (diamnionic, dichorionic gestation).

MONOZYGOTIC TWINS: Early division of a single fertilized ovum results in genetically identical twins of the same sex. If a fertilized ovum divides within 2 days of fertilization, before the trophoblast has differentiated, two separate embryos develop, each with its own placenta and amniotic sac (dichorionic, diamniotic twinning). Hence, dichorionic placentas may be either monozygotic or dizygotic, whereas monochorionic placentas are always monozygotic. If division occurs from the third to eighth days after conception, the trophoblast (but not the amniotic cavity) has already differentiated. A single placenta with two amniotic sacs develops (monochorionic, diamniotic twinning). A monochorionic, monoamniotic placenta is formed if division occurs between the 8th and 13th day after conception because the amniotic cavity has already developed. Incomplete separation of monozygous twins results in **conjoint (formerly Siamese) twins** within a monoamniotic, monochorionic placenta (Fig. 16-47).

ECTOPIC PREGNANCY

Ectopic pregnancy is implantation of a fertilized ovum outside the endometrium. The frequency of ectopic pregnancy in the United States has increased threefold, to 1.5% of live births, during the past two decades, although mortality has sharply declined. **Over 95% of such pregnancies are in the fallopian tube, mostly in the distal and middle thirds.**

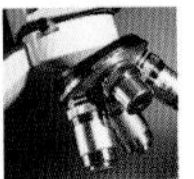

PATHOLOGY: Ectopic pregnancy results when passage of a conceptus along a fallopian tube is impeded, for example, by mucosal adhesions or abnormal tubal motility owing to inflammatory disease or endometriosis. The trophoblast readily penetrates the tubal mucosa and musculature. Blood from the tubal implantation site enters the peritoneum, causing abdominal pain. Ectopic pregnancy is also associated with anomalous uterine bleeding after a period of amenorrhea and Arias-Stella cells in the endometrium. The thin tubal wall usually ruptures by the

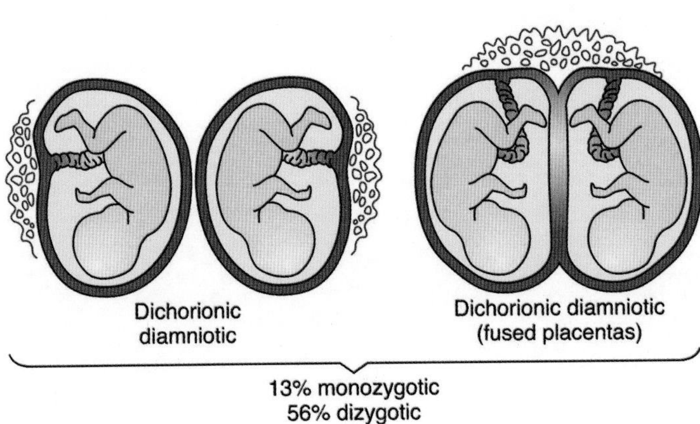

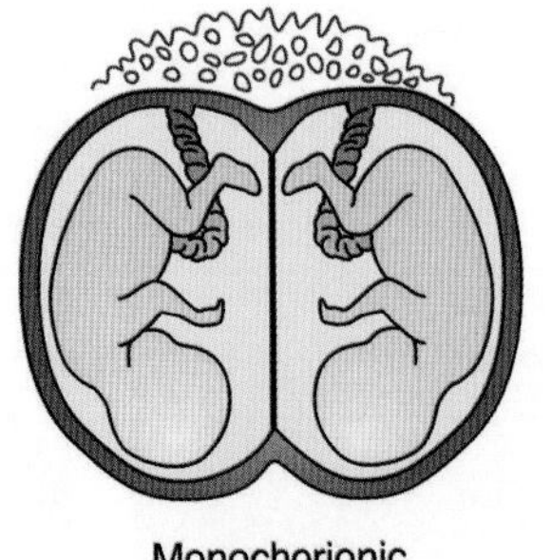

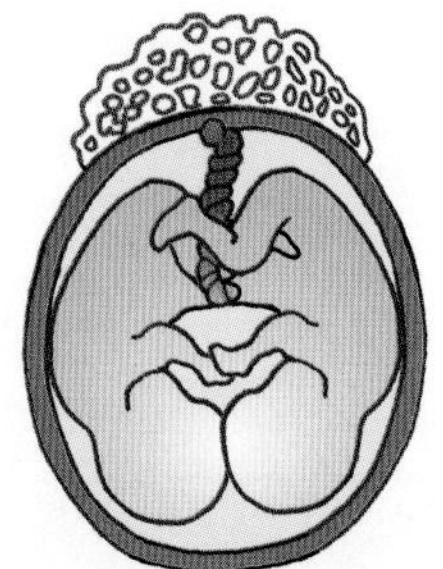

FIGURE 16-47. Placental structure in twin pregnancies. The percentages in the figure refer to the proportion of total twin pregnancies (100%) accounted for by each variant.

12th week of gestation. ***Tubal rupture is life-threatening because it can lead to rapid exsanguination.***

Rupture of the tube's interstitial portion produces greater intra-abdominal hemorrhage than rupture in other locations because the vasculature there is richer, and rupture occurs later in gestation. In the isthmus, the tube ruptures early (within the first 6 weeks) because its thick muscular wall does not allow much distention. Tubal pregnancies in the ampulla tend to be of longer duration because the distensible tubal wall can accommodate a growing pregnancy for a longer time.

Ectopic pregnancy must be treated promptly with surgery or chemotherapy. Administration of methotrexate terminates ectopic pregnancy and is used when the conceptus is smaller than 4 cm.

ABNORMALITIES OF THE UMBILICAL CORD

At term, the umbilical cord normally measures 35 to 100 cm in length. Abnormally, short umbilical cords are associated with increased perinatal mortality, intrauterine fetal distress, and intrauterine growth restriction. The point of insertion of the cord is usually at or near the center of the placental disc, but 7% show a **marginal insertion**, at the placenta's edge. About 1% of umbilical cords insert into the membranes, called a **velamentous** or **membranous insertion**. Velamentous and marginal cord insertions are often seen in spontaneous abortions and fetuses with congenital anomalies. A serious potential complication of velamentous vessels is **vasa previa**, a condition in which fetal vessels either cross or are near the internal os.

INFECTIONS IN PREGNANCY

Chorioamnionitis

Infectious organisms, almost exclusively bacteria, can ascend from the maternal birth canal, pass through the cervical os, and infect the decidua and placental tissues, the amniotic fluid, and, potentially, the fetus.

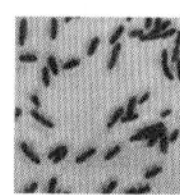

ETIOLOGIC FACTORS: Acute chorioamnionitis is usually caused by bacteria that are normally present in the maternal cervicovaginal canal. The most common bacterial causes of chorioamnionitis are group B *Streptococcus* sp., *E. coli*, *Enterococcus*, other streptococcal species, *Staphylococcus* sp., Gram-negative bacilli, *Bacteroides*, *M. hominis*, and *Ureaplasma*.

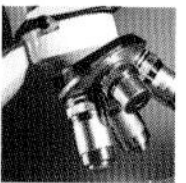

PATHOLOGY: Upon reaching the uterine cavity, bacteria elicit a **maternal inflammatory response (MIR)**. Maternal neutrophils circulating in the intervillous space migrate upward toward the fetal surface, or chorionic plate, resulting in **acute subchorionitis**. The neutrophils then migrate up from the subchorion into the chorion. Maternal neutrophils are recruited from the decidual blood vessels and enter the chorion of the extraplacental membranes (Fig. 16-48A). Maternal neutrophil infiltration of either the chorion of the placenta or its membranes is termed **acute chorioamnionitis**. Maternal inflammatory cells can also migrate from the decidual and spiral arteries into the decidua underlying the extraplacental membranes or the placental disc to cause **acute deciduitis**. Deciduitis may be so severe as to cause necrosis of the decidua (**necrotizing deciduitis**)

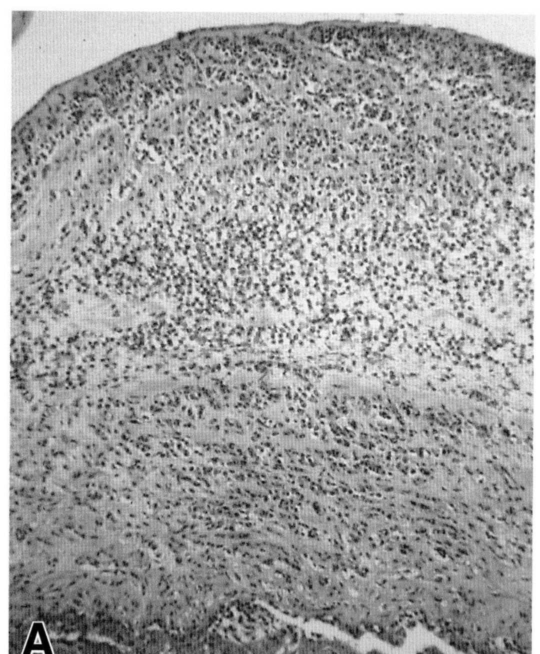

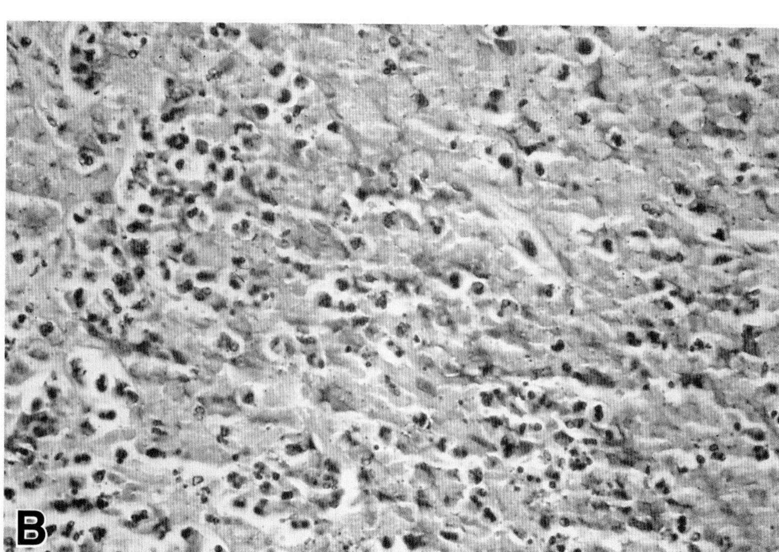

FIGURE 16-48. Maternal inflammatory responses to ascending infection. A. Acute chorioamnionitis (maternal inflammatory response [MIR]). The chorion contains numerous acute inflammatory cells, recruited from the maternal intervillous space. **B. Acute necrotizing deciduitis (MIR).** The decidua contains numerous inflammatory cells of maternal origin and is necrotic.

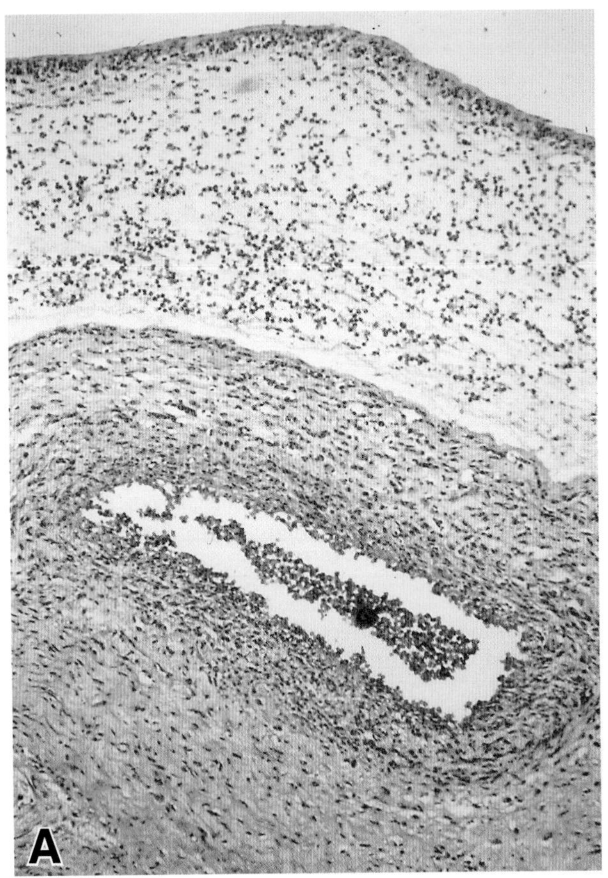

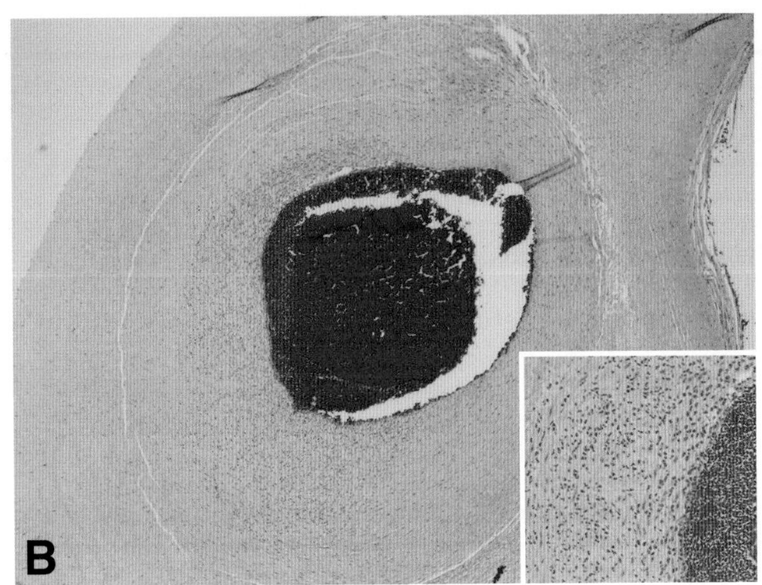

FIGURE 16-49. Fetal inflammatory responses (FIRs) to ascending infection. A. Acute chorionic vasculitis (FIR). The wall of this large chorionic plate blood vessel is infiltrated by fetal neutrophils. The overlying chorion showing acute chorioamnionitis. **B. Acute funisitis (FIR).** The muscular wall of this umbilical vessel contains numerous fetal inflammatory cells (*inset:* higher magnification).

(Fig. 16-48B), or it can form small collections of neutrophils (**decidual microabscesses**). Because the maternal spiral arteries, which supply the placenta with oxygenated maternal blood, are in the decidua, decidual infection can threaten the pregnancy.

A fetal inflammatory response (FIR) may also develop. Acute chorionic vasculitis, a component of FIR, occurs when fetal neutrophils migrate from the fetal bloodstream into the walls of the large chorionic plate vessels (branches of the umbilical cord vessels) at the surface of the placental disc (Fig. 16-49A). Fetal neutrophils also migrate from the lumen of the umbilical cord blood vessels into the muscular vessel walls, resulting in a vasculitis of the cord vessels termed **acute funisitis** (Fig. 16-49B). Fetal neutrophils can migrate completely through umbilical vessel walls and infiltrate the mesenchyme (Wharton jelly). Cerebral palsy is statistically associated with severe FIR, but not with mild-to-moderate MIR (see below).

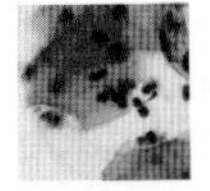

CLINICAL FEATURES: Acute chorioamnionitis (10% of placentas) can cause preterm labor, premature rupture of membranes, and fetal and neonatal infections, with subsequent FIR and intrauterine hypoxia. The mother may have fever, uterine tenderness, and foul-smelling or cloudy amniotic fluid. Major risks are postpartum endometritis and pelvic sepsis with venous thrombosis.

In preterm, low-birth-weight (<2,500 g) infants, especially very low weight (<1,500 g), acute chorioamnionitis often leads to severe neurologic disease, stillbirth, neonatal sepsis, and death. However, it can also cause morbidity in full-term infants. The risks of chorioamnionitis to the fetus include (1) pneumonia after inhalation of infected amniotic fluid; (2) skin or eye infections from direct contact with organisms in the fluid; and (3) neonatal gastritis, enteritis, or peritonitis from ingestion of infected fluid.

Amniotic Infection

Amniotic Fluid

Amniotic fluid is initially formed as a transudate of maternal fluids, but later a combination of the amnion, fetal lungs, and kidneys contributes to its formation. The fetus also inhales and exhales amniotic fluid during breathing movements before birth.

Intra-Amniotic Infection

Although amniotic fluid is normally sterile, it can be seeded with bacteria. Thus, microorganisms can gain a portal of entry into the fetus, most frequently the respiratory tract, from which they can enter the bloodstream and disseminate to other fetal organs. These infants can be born with "congenital" or early-onset neonatal infections, including pneumonia, sepsis, and meningitis. Placentas of these infants typically demonstrate acute chorioamnionitis, often with a component of FIR. Amniotic infections can portend a serious or fatal outcome for the neonate.

Infection of the Chorionic Villi

Villitis is an inflammatory infiltrate involving the chorionic villi. Microorganisms in the maternal blood, usually viruses, or less commonly bacteria, can gain access to the placenta. Villitis is sometimes of unknown etiology. Potential agents include (1) bacteria (*Listeria*, *T. pallidum*, *M. tuberculosis*, *Mycoplasma* sp., and *Chlamydia* sp.), (2) viruses (rubella, cytomegalovirus, and herpes), (3) parasites and protozoa (*Toxoplasma* sp. and *Trypanosoma cruzi*) and, (4) fungi (*Candida* sp.). Villitis can interfere with oxygen transport to the fetus, and transmission of the etiologic agent through the villi can infect the fetus.

Infections of the Fetus

Cytomegalovirus

Cytomegalovirus (CMV) is one of the TORCH agents (see Chapter 5) that can cause congenital infection in a newborn. Dangerous intrauterine infection can occur when the mother acquires a primary (first-time) infection while pregnant. Less dangerous to the infant is reactivation of latent maternal CMV infection during pregnancy. In Western nations, 8% of women develop a primary viral infection during pregnancy, of which one half will transmit the virus to their fetus. In developing nations and in poorer socioeconomic groups, congenital CMV infections are less common because those women most likely were exposed to CMV previously.

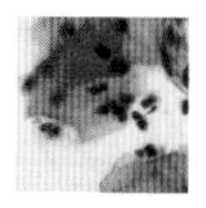

CLINICAL FEATURES: Among fetuses infected with CMV, one fourth are born with clinical symptoms. Some 5% to 10% of neonates will not have symptoms at birth but will subsequently develop hearing loss, visual impairment, and mental retardation. In more severe cases, generalized infections of the infant can occur, including low birth weight, microcephaly, seizures, and skin manifestations. Multiorgan dissemination is characterized by cerebral abnormalities, splenomegaly, and hepatitis. Occasionally, congenital CMV may be lethal for the infant.

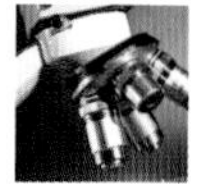

PATHOLOGY: CMV enters the placenta from maternal blood and results in chronic villitis. Endothelial infection causes cellular swelling, luminal occlusion, endothelial necrosis, and, eventually, vascular destruction. These effects result in thrombosis, ischemic villous necrosis, and, eventually, avascular villi with villous scarring (fibrosis). Villous stromal macrophages (Hofbauer cells) may be increased. Remote CMV infection can be reflected in villous microcalcifications. When CMV infection occurs near the time of delivery, characteristic intranuclear and intracytoplasmic inclusions of CMV may be identifiable (Fig. 16-50), but they are rare or absent in cases of remote intrauterine infection.

Congenital Syphilis

During pregnancy, the syphilitic treponeme disseminates in fetal tissues, which are injured by the proliferating organisms and accompanying inflammatory response. Fetal infection produces stillbirth, neonatal illness, or death or progressive postnatal disease.

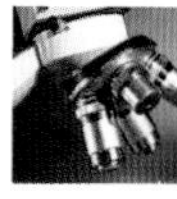

PATHOLOGY: Lesions of congenital syphilis are identical to those of adult disease. Infected tissues show a chronic inflammatory infiltrate of lymphocytes and plasma cells and endarteritis obliterans.

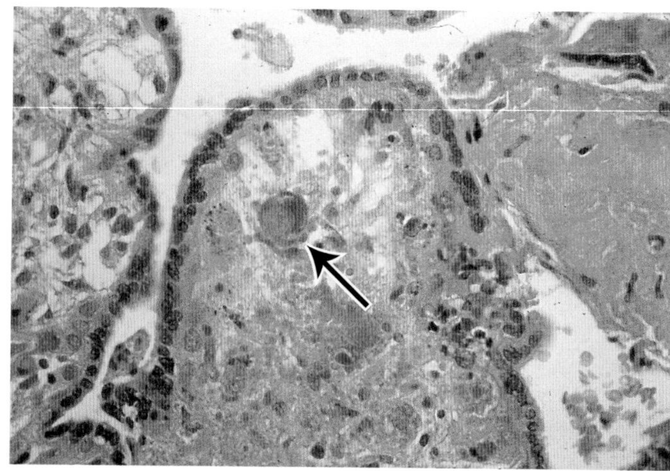

FIGURE 16-50. Chronic villitis caused by cytomegalovirus (CMV). The villi are infiltrated by chronic inflammatory cells. An enlarged cell with a CMV inclusion is present (*arrow*).

Virtually, any tissue can be affected, but the skin, bones, teeth, joints, liver, and CNS are characteristically involved (see Chapter 5).

Listeria

Listeriosis is a potentially serious infection most commonly acquired by eating food contaminated with the bacillus, *Listeria monocytogenes*. Common sources of infection are unpasteurized milk products, such as some soft cheeses and uncooked luncheon meats. Pregnant women and their infants are at increased risk for *listeriosis*. The bacteria can circulate in the maternal blood and infect the placenta and the fetus, causing miscarriage, stillbirth, and premature delivery. In infants, *Listeria* infection is characterized by granulomatous rash and pyogenic granulomas throughout the body. *Listeria* is also responsible for 5% of cases of neonatal meningitis.

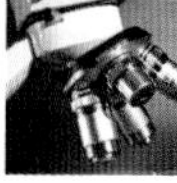

PATHOLOGY: Placentas infected with *Listeria* contain numerous microabscesses that destroy villi and produce an acute intervillositis. Necrotizing chorioamnionitis and severe funisitis are frequent.

Toxoplasma

Toxoplasma gondii, a cat parasite, is a protozoan found in the urine of infected animals. Infections acquired by the fetus early in pregnancy are more likely to be severe than those acquired later.

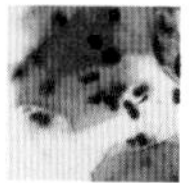

CLINICAL FEATURES: The classic triad of congenital toxoplasmosis, namely, hydrocephalus, intracranial calcifications, and chorioretinitis, is well known but does not occur in most infants infected in utero. Severe manifestations of congenital toxoplasmosis include encephalitis, multiple organ infection, epilepsy, mental retardation, blindness, and stillbirth.

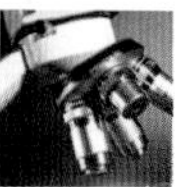

PATHOLOGY: Characteristic cysts of *Toxoplasma* can be present in the subamnionic connective tissue, chorionic villi, trophoblast, and umbilical cord. Like syphilis and CMV, Hofbauer cell hyperplasia can also occurs in toxoplasmosis. In some cases, thrombosis of placental blood vessels takes place, with or without calcification.

Erythrovirus (Parvovirus B19)

Erythrovirus, formerly called parvovirus B19, is a DNA virus that causes ecthyma infectiosum, a benign disease with fever and rash in children. If a pregnant woman becomes infected, the risk for stillbirth rises, especially if the infection occurs in the first and second trimesters. Mothers transmit the agent to their fetus in 30% of cases of acute maternal infection. The virus produces distinctive ground-glass intranuclear inclusions, termed "lantern cells," which are most evident in nucleated fetal red blood. Placentas are typically enlarged, and villi are edematous. Newborns tend to be hydropic and anemic and may have cardiac involvement.

Human Immunodeficiency Virus

If a woman infected with HIV becomes pregnant, her infant can become infected via three major routes. The virus can cross the placenta; it can infect the newborn at the time of delivery; or infection can be transmitted through breastfeeding. Risk factors for transmission of HIV from a mother to her fetus are shown in Table 16-7.

VASCULAR DISORDERS OF THE PLACENTA

Fetal Thrombotic Vasculopathy

Thrombosis occurring anywhere in the circulation of the placenta is called FTV and indicates an unfavorable intrauterine environment for the fetus. Clots can develop either in the arterial or in venous circulation of the placenta and umbilical cord, although the venous circulation is most often affected. Risk factors for development of FTV include villitis and disorders of coagulation, particularly hypercoagulable syndromes (see Chapter 18). A variety of poor outcomes are associated with FTV, including stillbirth, neonatal death, intrauterine growth restriction, and, in surviving infants, neurologic injury. FTV may occur with similar clots in fetal organs.

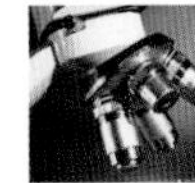

PATHOLOGY: Thrombi of varying ages are often seen in chorionic villous blood vessels. In cases of acute FTV, large thrombi may be present in the umbilical cord vessels or in the large-sized vessels of the chorionic plate. Microscopically, acute thrombi often involve smaller fetal vessels, including the secondary and tertiary villi. In chronic FTV, chorionic villi downstream from thrombosed vessels undergo progressive fibrosis, giving a distinctive appearance to clusters of scarred, **avascular villi** (Fig. 16-51). A thrombus can be incorporated into the vessel wall to form a mural thrombus, or **cushion defect**. Microcalcifications, stromal fibrosis, and deposition of hemosiderin result from degeneration of red blood cells.

FTV in the umbilical cord vessels can be catastrophic and can complicate abnormally long or excessively twisted cords, velamentous cord insertion, entanglement of the cord, and cord knots.

Table 16-7

Risk Factors for Perinatal Transmission of HIV

Maternal Factors
Low CD4+ lymphocyte counts (T cells)
High HIV-1 RNA levels (viral load)
Acute retroviral syndrome during pregnancy
Presence of coinfections (hepatitis C, bacterial vaginosis, CMV)
Injection drug use
Absence of antiretroviral therapy or prophylaxis
Absence of prenatal care
Obstetric Factors
Duration of placental membrane rupture and/or chorioamnionitis
Invasive procedures
Vaginal delivery
Infant Factors
Premature delivery
Breastfeeding

CD, cluster of differentiation; CMV, cytomegalovirus.

Hemorrhagic Endovasculopathy

HEV results from irreversible injury to the endothelial cells lining fetal blood vessels in the chorionic villi. It is associated with increased perinatal morbidity and mortality, neurologic impairment, and abnormalities of fetal growth and development. HEV often occurs together with other placental abnormalities, including fetal thrombotic vasculopathy, villitis of unknown etiology, villous fibrosis, infarcts, erythroblastosis, and meconium staining. Hypertensive disease of pregnancy is the only known risk factor.

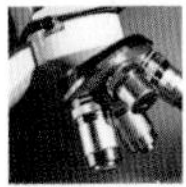

PATHOLOGY: HEV can affect any vessel in the chorionic villous tree. Extravasated fetal red blood cells extend from the lumen through the intimal lining and into the surrounding blood vessel wall, or the vessel wall may be necrotic. Red blood cells can be fragmented, and karyorrhexis of endothelial and nucleated red blood cells is common. HEV may accompany inflammatory infiltrates in the villi, in which case it is called **hemorrhagic villitis**.

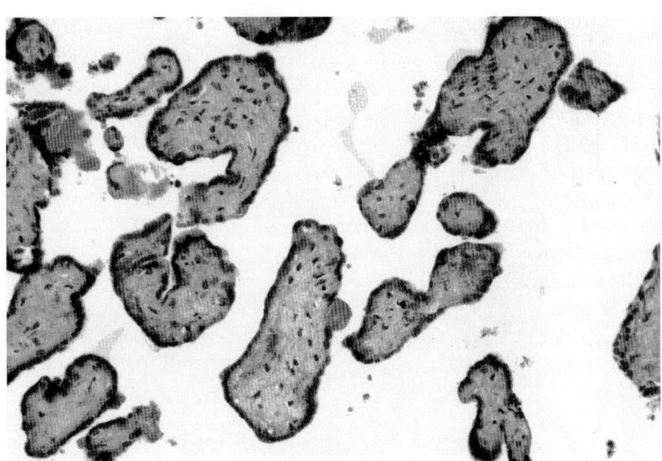

FIGURE 16-51. Avascular villi. The villous capillaries have been replaced by fibrous tissue as a result of a chronic thrombus in a larger upstream stem villus.

Abruptio Placentae

Retroplacental hematoma occurs between the basal plate of the placenta and the uterine wall and accounts for 8% of perinatal deaths. Hemorrhage derives from a ruptured maternal (spiral) artery or premature separation of the placenta. Retroplacental hemorrhage can be as a result of placental abruption (**abruptio placentae**), but in one third of cases, it occurs without clinical abruption. Although abruptio placentae are often the final dramatic consequence of a chronic placental disorder, most cases result from maternal vascular disease. Risk factors for retroplacental hematoma include maternal smoking, hypertensive disease of pregnancy, late maternal age, acute chorioamnionitis, uterine malformation, placenta previa, history of previous abruption, short umbilical cord, thrombophilia, multiparity, and cocaine use.

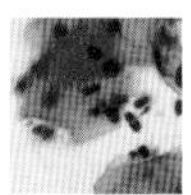

CLINICAL FEATURES: Abruptio placentae complicate 1% of pregnancies worldwide. Symptoms depend on the extent of abruption and include vaginal bleeding, uterine tenderness, abdominal or back pain, uterine tetanic contractions, fetal distress, maternal shock, hypofibrinogenemia, coagulopathy, and maternal or fetal death.

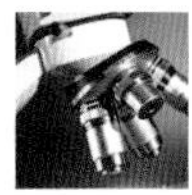

PATHOLOGY: Premature detachment of the placenta or rupture of a uterine blood vessel causes blood to accumulate between the placenta and the decidua basalis, forming a hematoma (Fig. 16-52). When a retroplacental hematoma is present for some time, the overlying villous tissue frequently shows ischemic infarction.

In the half of placental abruptions that are mild, neither the fetus nor the mother suffers ill consequences. However, many abruptions result in poor fetal outcomes, including neonatal shock from hypoxia and anemia, irreversible neurologic injury, and perinatal death.

In some cases, blood forces its way into the underlying myometrium, resulting in a **"Couvelaire uterus."** In such cases, mothers may develop anemia, coagulopathy, disseminated intravascular coagulation, adult respiratory distress syndrome (ARDS), shock, and death. Maternal death due to abruptio placentae is rare in developed nations (0.4 per thousand cases of abruption), but it continues to be an important cause of maternal death in the resource-poor regions of the world.

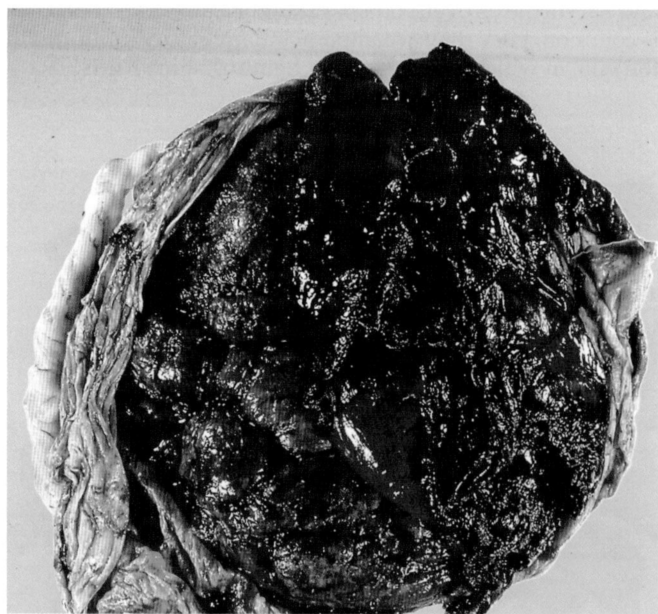

FIGURE 16-52. Retroplacental hematoma. The occurrence of a retroplacental hemorrhage such as this large hematoma may correlate with the presence of a clinical abruption.

Intervillous Thrombi

Rupture of a chorionic villous blood vessel causes blood to accumulate in the placenta and to form an intervillous thrombus or hematoma. Because the pressure of the fetal circulation in the placenta is higher than that of the maternal circulation, this represents a **fetomaternal hemorrhage.** Entry of fetal blood into the maternal circulation can have clinical implications if there are blood group incompatibilities between the fetus and mother. Small intervillous thrombi occur in up to 20% of full-term gestation placentas and are usually clinically insignificant. A larger thrombus or multiple thrombi cause fetal blood loss or hypoxia. Intervillous thrombi can develop as a result of preeclampsia or maternal thrombophilias, and when there is thrombosis in the maternal circulation.

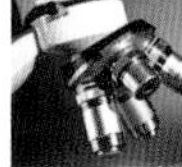

PATHOLOGY: Intervillous thrombi appear as well-demarcated red firm areas, much different from the surrounding spongy placental parenchyma. Hemorrhage compresses the surrounding villi. When intervillous thrombi occur remotely from the time of delivery, the rim of surrounding compressed villi display infarction or avascular scarring.

Placenta Accreta

Placenta accreta is caused by failure to form decidua. Normally, decidual endometrium separates the base of the placenta from the underlying uterine muscle. Placenta accreta occurs when the decidual layer is partially or totally absent, so that the villi are in direct contact with the underlying decidua or uterine muscle. In this case, the placenta does not separate normally from the uterine wall at the time of delivery, an event that may lead to life-threatening maternal hemorrhage. Risk factors for placenta accreta include placenta previa, prior cesarean births, advanced maternal age, high parity, and endometrial defects.

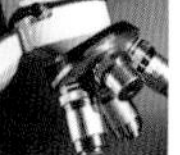

PATHOLOGY: Placenta accreta is classified according to the depth of myometrial invasion by the villi:

- **Placenta accreta** refers to attachment of villi to the surface of the uterine wall without further invasion (Fig. 16-53A).
- **Placenta increta** occurs when villi invade underlying myometrium, penetrating either superficially or deep into the myometrium (Fig. 16-53B).
- **Placenta percreta** describes villi penetrating the full thickness of the uterine wall. In some cases, placenta percreta penetrates through the uterine serosa and invades adjacent organs, such as the colon or urinary bladder; it can also result in uterine rupture.

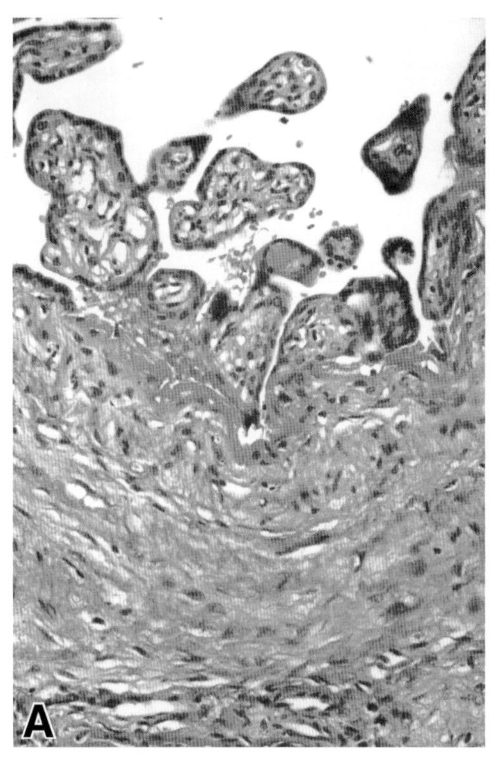

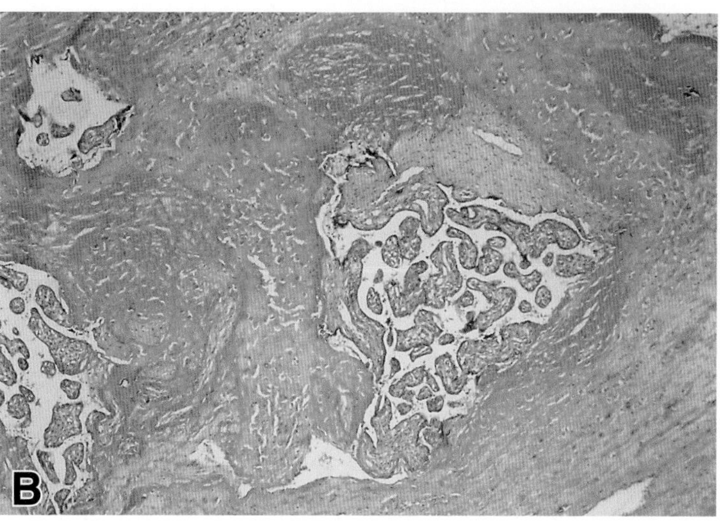

FIGURE 16-53. Placenta accretia and increta. A. Placenta accreta. Some of the chorionic villi (*top*) are in contact with the underlying muscle. The decidua is absent. **B. Placenta increta.** The chorionic villi have invaded deeply into the uterine wall.

CLINICAL FEATURES: Patients with placenta accreta can have a normal pregnancy and delivery. However, complications may occur during pregnancy, during delivery, or especially in the immediate postpartum period. Third-trimester bleeding is the most common presenting sign; substantial fragments of placenta may remain adherent after delivery and cause hemorrhage, endometritis, and disseminated intravascular coagulation. Bleeding often threatens the lives of both mother and baby and necessitate emergency hysterectomy.

Chronic Uteroplacental Malperfusion

Adequate oxygenation of the fetus during pregnancy requires that both fetal and maternal circulations between the uteroplacental and fetal structures operate properly. Chronic uteroplacental malperfusion and insufficiency are important causes of perinatal morbidity and mortality. They can result in stillbirth, neonatal death, preterm birth, intrauterine growth restriction, and, if the infant lives, neurologic damage. A large number of unrelated causes include villous hypoplasia, maternal floor infarction, massive perivillous fibrin deposition, diabetes, autoimmune diseases, villitis, placental infarcts, chronic abruption, fetal thrombotic vasculopathy, abnormally small or thin placentas, chorangiomas, large remote intervillous thrombi, and chronic umbilical cord abnormalities.

In cases of chronic uteroplacental malperfusion, terminal chorionic villi have a markedly increased number of vessels termed **chorioangiosis**. This endothelial proliferation increases the capillary surface area of the villi in the face of chronic intrauterine hypoxia. Additionally, **syncytiotrophoblast hyperplasia** may occur, in which case the syncytiotrophoblast forms prominent bulbous knots or folds, often bridging the intervillous space and touching the trophoblast of adjacent villi (Tenney–Parker change; Fig. 16-54).

Infarcts

Placental infarcts consist of an area of placental tissue that has undergone irreversible ischemic injury, owing to complete interruption of maternal vascular supply to the infarcted area. The most frequent causes of placental infarction are hemorrhage between the base of the placenta and the uterine wall (retroplacental hemorrhage and abruptio placentae) and occlusion or thrombosis of a uterine spiral artery.

Placental infarcts often accompany hypertensive diseases of pregnancy and are seen in association with preeclampsia, maternal thrombophilia, and cigarette smoking. Multiple infarcts,

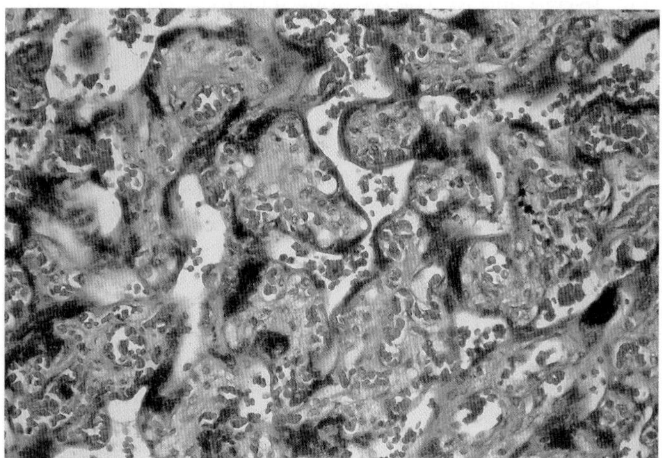

FIGURE 16-54. Tenney–Parker change (syncytiotrophoblast hyperplasia). The syncytiotrophoblast is knotted and hyperbasophilic and bridges the intervillous space to connect to adjacent villi. This is caused by chronic uteroplacental malperfusion of either maternal or fetal origin.

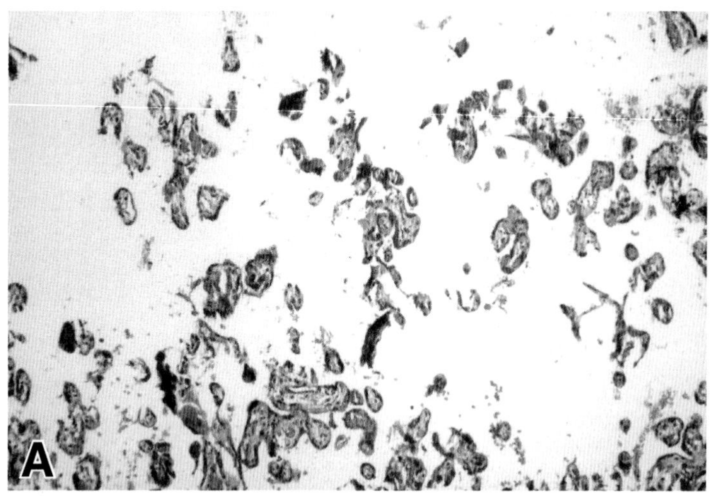

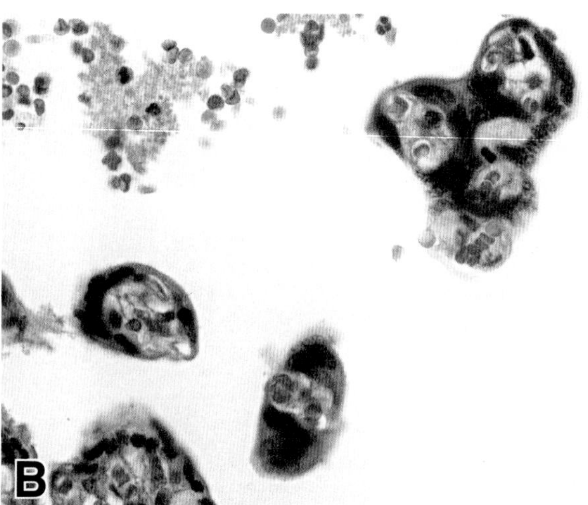

FIGURE 16-55. Villous hypoplasia. A. The diameter of the villi is decreased, resulting in an apparent increase in the intervillous space between villi. **B. High magnification of villous hypoplasia.** The characteristic features of chronic ischemia are present, including small, shrunken villi with stromal fibrosis and clumped trophoblast.

especially if they are large or in the central part of the placenta, can result in placental insufficiency and give rise to intrauterine growth restriction, neurologic injury, and perinatal death.

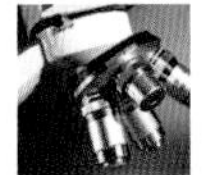

PATHOLOGY: Infarcts are dark red areas that are firmer than surrounding placental tissue. With increasing age, they become firmer, change in color from dark red to yellow and tan, and finally become white and more sharply delineated from the adjacent tissue.

Villous Hypoplasia

Villous hypoplasia (also called uneven accelerated maturation) results from chronic underlying disease of the spiral arterioles, including stenosis, fluctuating vasoconstriction, or, as occurs with preeclampsia, defective remodeling (see below). Decreased maternal perfusion of the intervillous space of the placenta gives rise to ischemic degeneration of chorionic villi (Fig. 16-55A and B). The resulting fetal hypoxia can produce stillbirth, neonatal death, intrauterine growth restriction, preterm birth, and neurologic injury in infants who survive.

Abnormal Fibrin Deposition

Small amounts of fibrin from the maternal circulation deposit in the placenta under normal conditions. **Rohr fibrin** is a necessary component of the basal plate of the placenta, where it faces the intervillous plate. **Nitabuch fibrin** is deposited in the deep part of the basal plate. A deficiency of Nitabuch fibrin is associated with placenta accreta.

Increased Perivillous Fibrin

Excess deposition of fibrin around villi can cause placental insufficiency by interfering with perfusion of the villi. Ischemic necrosis of the villi may eventuate (Fig. 16-56) and cause placental insufficiency.

Massive perivillous fibrin deposition (MPFD) can result in perinatal death. The cause of MPFD is unknown. The fibrin extends from the basal (decidual) part of the placenta up to the fetal (chorionic) surface. Dense fibrin fills the intervillous space and results in villous ischemic necrosis (Fig. 16-57). MPFD often brings on poor pregnancy outcomes.

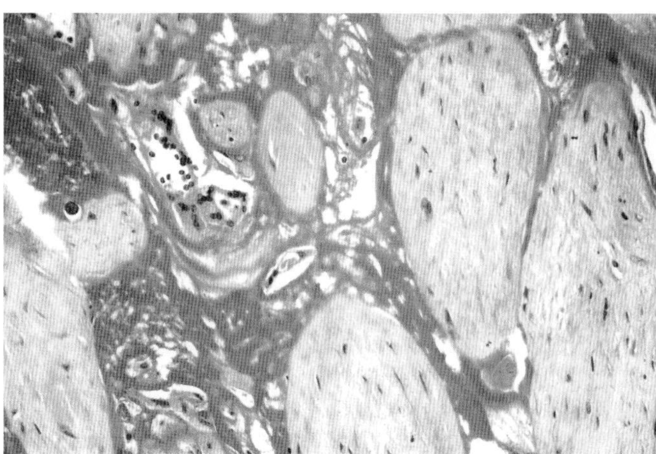

FIGURE 16-56. Increased villous fibrin. The fibrin has covered the chorionic villi, obstructed the intervillous space, and resulted in villous necrosis.

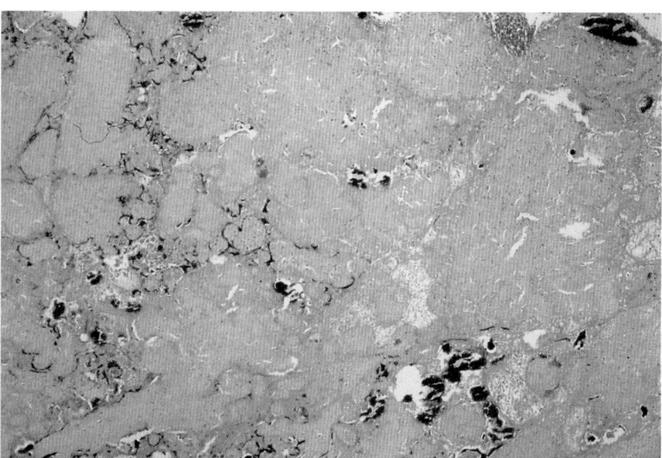

FIGURE 16-57. Massive perivillous fibrin deposition. Low magnification showing confluent villous necrosis and fibrin deposition in the intervillous space. The small, dark purple microcalcifications attest to the chronicity of this process.

Maternal floor infarction (MFI) is not a true infarct but shares some morphologic features with MPFD. Excessive fibrin extends confluently across the width of the placenta. It mainly affects the basal surface and decidua and extends upward to involve the villi. The floor of the placenta is firm, thickened, and often discolored tan yellow. Like MPFD, villi involved with MFI are embedded in dense fibrin and are necrotic. MFI has the same perinatal outcomes as does MPFD.

MATERNAL DISORDERS OF PREGNANCY

Preeclampsia and eclampsia define a syndrome of hypertension, proteinuria, and edema and, most severely, convulsions. Preeclampsia occurs in 6% of pregnant women in their last trimester, especially with their first child. If convulsive seizures appear, the syndrome is called eclampsia. Preeclampsia causes some 50,000 maternal deaths worldwide annually.

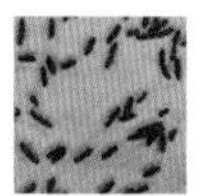

ETIOLOGIC FACTORS: Preeclampsia probably arises because of faulty remodeling of uterine spiral arteries that supply maternal blood to the placenta. Immunologic and genetic factors, as well as altered vascular reactivity, endothelial injury, and coagulation abnormalities, may also contribute. The characteristics of preeclampsia are as follows (Fig. 16-58A):

- Maternal blood flow to the placenta is markedly reduced because of ineffective remodeling of maternal spiral arteries of the decidua.
- Renal involvement contributes to hypertension and proteinuria.
- Disseminated intravascular coagulation may occur in preeclampsia.
- The risk of preeclampsia in a first pregnancy is manyfold higher than in subsequent pregnancies.
- Rarely, preeclampsia may not occur until the time of labor and delivery, or shortly thereafter (postpartum preeclampsia).
- Eclampsia is a cerebrovascular disorder characterized by seizures, worsening hypertension, and cerebral edema. It may precede other symptoms and does not necessarily evolve from preeclampsia.

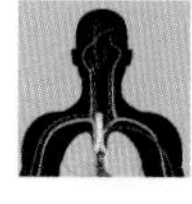

PATHOPHYSIOLOGY: Preeclampsia reflects reduced maternal blood flow to the uteroplacental unit because the spiral arteries of the uteroplacental bed never fully dilate.

Early in a normal pregnancy, fetal cytotrophoblast cells extend downward into the decidua and uterus. They invade the uterine spiral arteries and progressively replace the maternal-derived endothelium, medial elastic tissue, smooth muscle, and neural tissue. By the end of the second trimester, the normally narrow spiral arteries are dilated tubes lined by fetal-derived cytotrophoblast. This low-resistance arterial circuit supplies the increasing demands for oxygen and nutrients of the developing fetus.

Faulty cytotrophoblastic remodeling of the maternal uterine (spiral) arteries in early pregnancy (Fig. 16-58B) is believed to result from abnormal expression of integrins by the fetal-derived cytotrophoblast, as well as generalized apoptosis of the cytotrophoblast. This situation leads to limited invasion of the decidua and spiral arteries, in which case the spiral arteries cannot perfuse the growing fetus adequately. The resulting placental ischemia promotes release of cytokines such TNF-α and IL-6. Upregulation of placental antiangiogenic factors, such as vascular endothelial growth factor (VEGF) and soluble endoglin, may play a role in the onset of the clinical features of preeclampsia, including hypertension and proteinuria.

In preeclampsia, many spiral arteries escape invasion by trophoblastic tissue and so never dilate. The combination of vasoconstriction and structural changes in spiral arteries contributes to inadequate blood flow, placental ischemia, villous hypoplasia, and fetal hypoxia. The effectiveness of vasodilators in treating preeclampsia, including nitric oxide, prostacyclin (PGI_2), and endothelium-derived hyperpolarizing factor (EDHF), is further evidence for endothelial dysfunction in preeclampsia (Fig.16-58B).

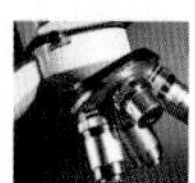

PATHOLOGY: ***Placental pathology usually precedes the clinical onset of maternal hypertension.*** Extensive placental infarction is seen in one third of women with severe preeclampsia, although it is often negligible in mild preeclampsia. Retroplacental hemorrhage or abruptio placentae occur in 15% and abnormally small placentas (<10th percentile) in 10% of cases (Fig. 16-52). Chorionic villi show signs of chronic maternal underperfusion, consisting of ischemically degenerated chorionic villi (villous hypoplasia; Fig. 16-55), fibrin (Fig. 16-56), increased placental site giant cells, syncytiotrophoblastic hyperplasia (Tenney–Parker change) (Fig. 16-54), and mural hypertrophy of membrane arterioles. The spiral arteries commonly show fibrinoid necrosis, clusters of lipid-rich macrophages, and a perivascular infiltrate of mononuclear cells; this constellation of findings is called **acute atherosis** (Fig. 16-59). These vessels are often thrombosed, resulting in focal placental infarcts.

Maternal kidneys in preeclampsia always exhibit glomerular changes. Glomeruli are enlarged, and endothelial cells are swollen, forming classic "bloodless" glomeruli of preeclampsia (glomerular endotheliosis). Fibrin accumulates between endothelial cells and the glomerular capillary basement membrane. Mesangial cell hyperplasia is the rule. These maternal renal changes are reversible with therapy or after delivery.

Fatal cases of eclampsia often show cerebral hemorrhages, ranging from petechiae to large hematomas. ***Liver abnormalities are present in 60% of women dying from preeclampsia,*** including periportal fibrin deposits and necrosis, lobular hemorrhage, and hepatic infarction.

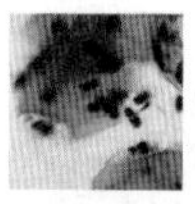

CLINICAL FEATURES: Preeclampsia usually begins insidiously after the 20th week of pregnancy, with excessive weight gain from fluid retention, increased maternal blood pressure, and proteinuria. As preeclampsia progresses from mild to severe, diastolic pressure persistently exceeds 110 mm Hg, proteinuria is greater than 3 g/day, and renal function declines. Disseminated intravascular coagulation (DIC) often supervenes. Preeclampsia is treated with antihypertensive and antiplatelet drugs, but definitive therapy requires removing the placenta. Eclampsia is treated with magnesium sulfate, which reduces cerebrovascular tone.

HELLP Syndrome

HELLP syndrome is a potentially fatal condition of pregnant women and their infants that most often follows the diagnosis of preeclampsia in the third trimester. Its name is an acronym for its major findings—*h*emolytic anemia, *e*levated *l*iver enzymes, and *l*ow *p*latelet count. It occurs in 0.2% to 0.6% of all pregnancies and in 4% to 12% of women with preeclampsia or eclampsia. Some 70% of cases occur antepartum, and 30% develop in the postpartum period.

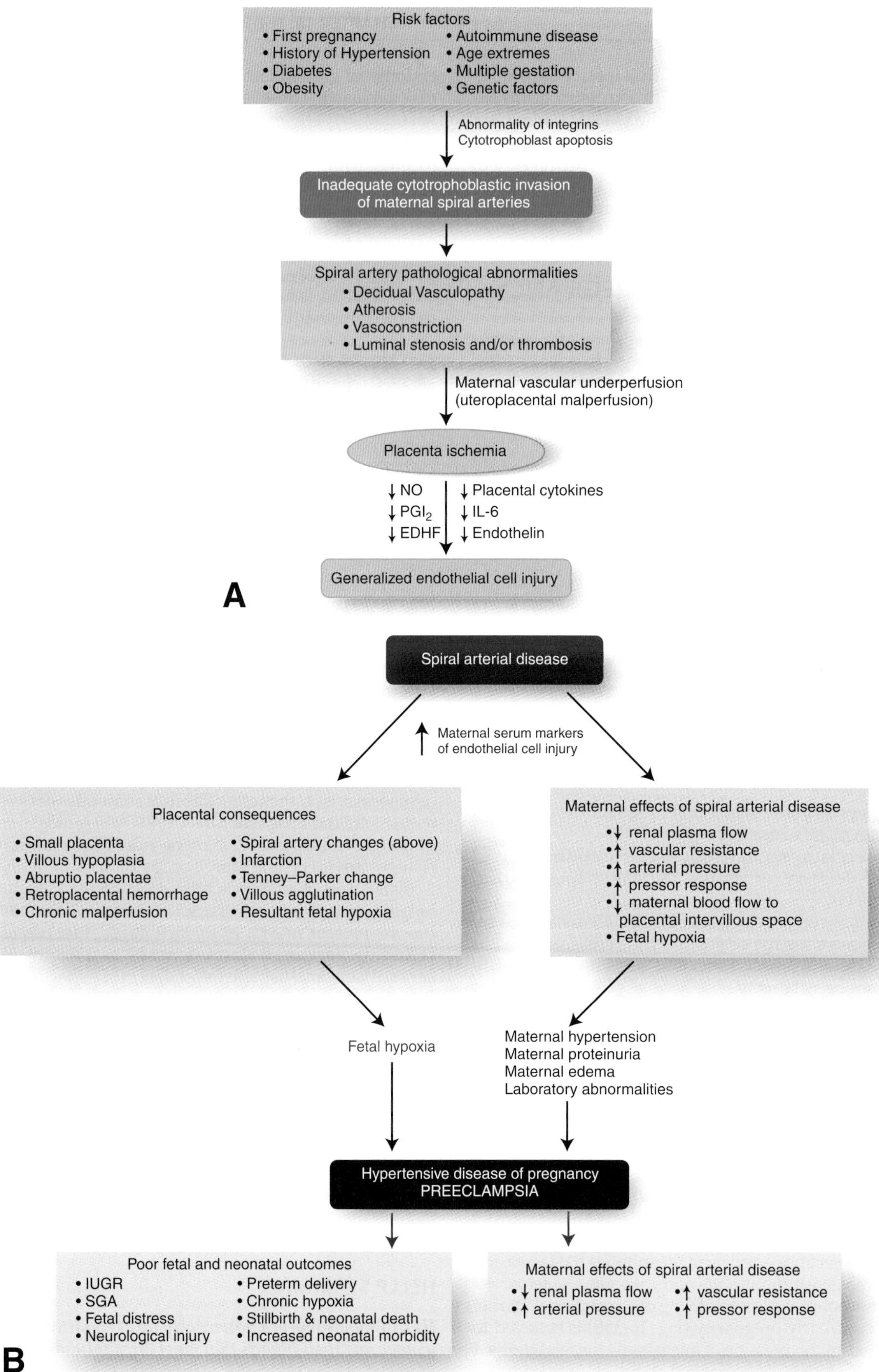

FIGURE 16-58. Pathogenesis of preeclampsia. A. Etiology of Preeclampsia B. Pathophysiology of Preeclampsia. EDHF, endothelium-derived hyperpolarizing factor; IL, interleukin; IUGR, intrauterine growth retardation; NO, nitric oxide; PGI_2, prostacyclin; SGA, small for gestational age.

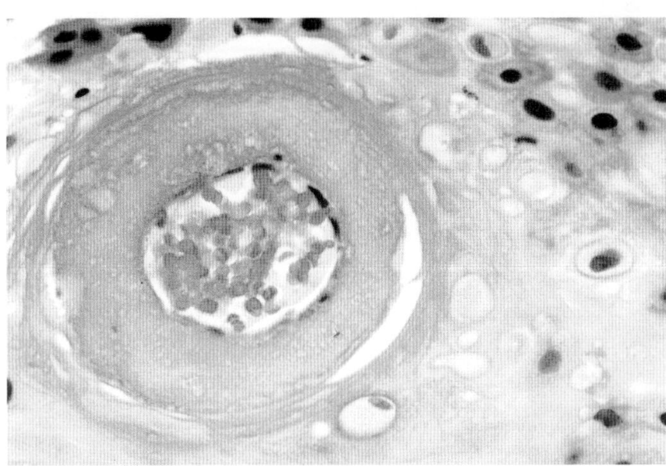

FIGURE 16-59. Decidual atherosis in preeclampsia. A small decidual artery showing fibrinoid thickening of the vessel wall.

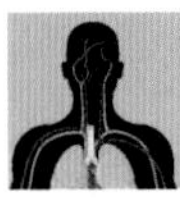

PATHOPHYSIOLOGY: The trigger for developing HELLP syndrome is unknown, but generalized activation of the coagulation cascade is thought to be the major problem. The syndrome is the final manifestation of an event that provokes microvascular endothelial damage and intravascular platelet activation. The latter causes vasospasm, platelet agglutination and aggregation, and further endothelial damage. Excessive platelet consumption results in DIC and microangiopathic anemia in 20% of women with HELLP syndrome. Obstruction of hepatic blood flow by fibrin deposits in the sinusoids gives rise to liver ischemia, resulting in periportal necrosis, and increased levels of liver enzymes. In severe cases, intrahepatic hemorrhage, subcapsular hematoma formation, or hepatic rupture occur. Additional complications include hemorrhage from DIC, pulmonary edema, placental abruption, ARDS, acute hepatorenal failure, and fetal death. The maternal mortality rate is 1%. Infant morbidity and mortality rates vary from 10% to 60%, depending on the severity of maternal disease.

PREGNANCY LOSS

Spontaneous Abortion

A pregnancy that ends with expulsion of a conceptus before the 20th week of gestation is called a spontaneous abortion, or miscarriage. Some 15% of recognized pregnancies abort spontaneously. An additional 30% of women abort without being aware that they were pregnant. Thus, about half of all pregnancies miscarry, making it the most common complication of early pregnancy. The most common symptom of spontaneous abortion is bleeding.

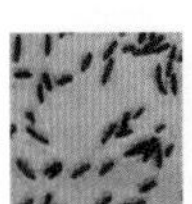

ETIOLOGIC FACTORS: Most spontaneous abortions occur before 12 weeks of gestation. Karyotypic anomalies are present in 50% of all spontaneous abortions, and in as many as 70% of those occurring before the 7th week of gestation. The principal factors responsible for later spontaneous abortion are:

- Infection early in pregnancy (e.g., *Listeria*, CMV, *Toxoplasma*, and coxsackievirus)
- Mechanical factors (e.g., uterine leiomyoma, septate uteri, and cervical incompetence)
- Endocrine factors (e.g., maternal diabetes, polycystic ovary, luteal phase defects, progesterone deficiency, and hypothyroidism)
- Immunologic factors
- Cigarette smoking
- Cocaine usage
- Congenital fetal malformations (e.g., neural tube defects)
- Chromosomal abnormalities
- Increasing maternal age
- Multiple gestation (e.g., twins, triplets, etc.)

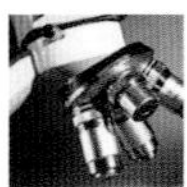

PATHOLOGY: An empty gestational sac with hydropic swelling of the chorionic villi (blighted ovum) suggests early fetal demise. The embryo may be grossly disorganized or show defects, such as spina bifida, anencephaly, or cleft palate. Chorionic villi may be histologically normal or show intravillous fibrosis or hydropic change. If infection preceded the miscarriage, there is often microscopic evidence of the infectious agent.

Recurrent Pregnancy Loss

Pregnancy loss is the most common complication of human pregnancy, affecting 10% to 15% of all human conceptions. For most fertile couples, miscarriage is a sporadic event, but 1% to 5% of fertile couples suffer from **recurrent pregnancy loss** (RPL; also termed **habitual abortion**).

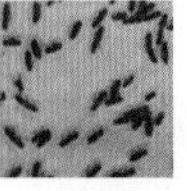

ETIOLOGIC FACTORS: The **antiphospholipid syndrome** accounts for 3% to 15% of recurrent pregnancy loss. Another important cause of RPL is **thrombophilia**, mostly **factor V Leiden** and **prothrombin G20210A** (factor II) mutations (see Chapter 18). In 4% of couples with RPL, there are chromosomal aberrations in one or both partners. Diverse endocrine factors can cause RPL, including hypothyroidism, polycystic ovary disease, diabetes, and inadequate production of progesterone. Anatomic conditions, such as cervical incompetence and uterine malformations, or immune factors are also involved in some cases. The latter include antithyroid autoantibodies and maternal immunization against male-specific minor histocompatibility (H-Y) antigens. Certain ovarian factors are risk factors for RPL, for example, luteal phase defects and advanced maternal age, with decreased ovarian reserve and decreased egg quality.

AMNIOTIC FLUID EMBOLISM

AFE is a rare, life-threatening obstetric emergency that results in an anaphylaxis-like syndrome. It occurs when amniotic fluid, fetal squamous cells, hair, vernix, and other amniotic materials enter the maternal circulation through the uterine veins in the decidual bed at the base of the placenta. Although maternal mortality has declined to 25%, it still accounts for 5% to 10% of maternal deaths in the United States. About 20% of infants die after their mothers develop AFE.

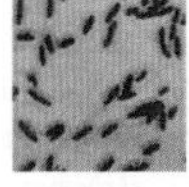

ETIOLOGIC FACTORS: The entry of amniotic fluid elements into the maternal bloodstream is thought to trigger the acute onset of symptoms of AFE. However, amniotic fluid cellular elements are not always identified in women with AFE, and they may be present in women

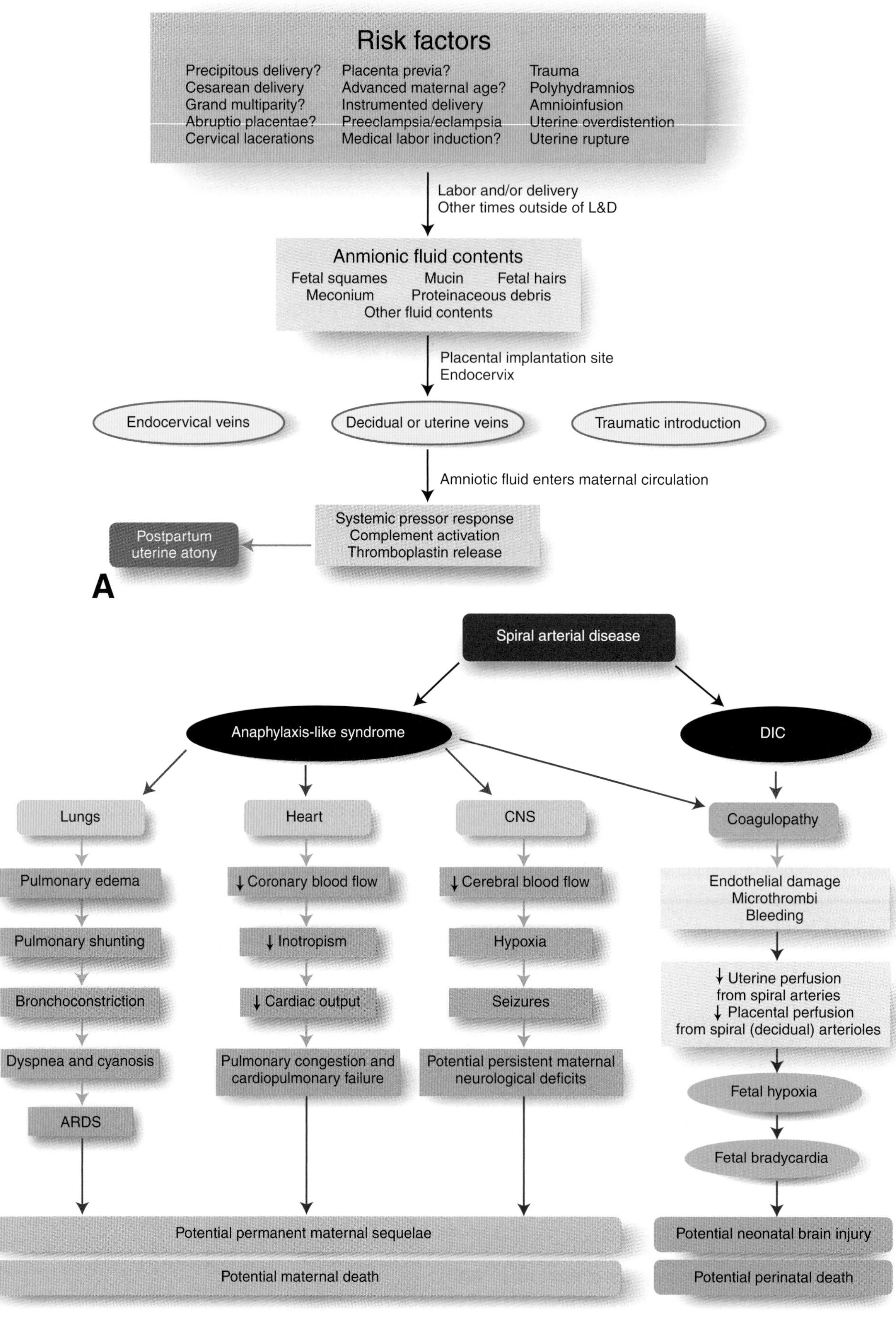

FIGURE 16-60. Current concepts of the pathophysiology of amniotic fluid embolism (anaphylactoid syndrome of pregnancy). **A.** Etiologic Factors in Amniotic Fluid Embolism **B.** Maternal and Fetal Systemic Effects of Amniotic Fluid Embolism. ARDS, adult respiratory distress syndrome; CNS, central nervous system; DIC, disseminated intravascular coagulation.

who do not develop the disorder. Amniotic fluid materials that enter the maternal bloodstream at the time of labor and delivery trigger an anaphylactic reaction or complement activation or both. The pathophysiology of amniotic fluid embolism is summarized in Figure 16-60.

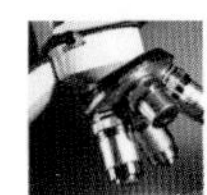

PATHOLOGY: In fatal cases of AFE, the lungs show diffuse alveolar damage (see Chapter10). Platelet-fibrin aggregates are present in pulmonary vessels, and increased megakaryocytes are often seen in alveoli, indicative of the onset of DIC. Distinctive fetal squamous epithelial cells are often present in both alveolar capillaries and larger blood vessels. Rarely, other fetal elements are present, including fetal hair.

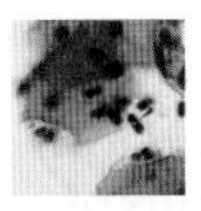

CLINICAL FEATURES: Initially, pulmonary arterial vasospasm, pulmonary hypertension, and elevation of right ventricular pressure cause hypoxia. Myocardial and pulmonary capillary damage ensue. Left heart failure and ARDS develop, further endangering the patient. Women surviving the first phase of AFE may develop a second phase, including uterine atony, hemorrhage, and DIC. A fatal consumptive coagulopathy is sometimes the initial presentation.

INTRAHEPATIC CHOLESTASIS OF PREGNANCY

ICP is the second leading cause of jaundice during pregnancy and may endanger the health of the fetus. The disorder occurs in only 1 or 2 women per 1,000 pregnancies, typically presenting as intense pruritus. ICP usually begins in the third trimester but can occur any time during pregnancy. It can result in fetal distress, spontaneous premature delivery, meconium aspiration syndrome, intrauterine fetal demise, and neonatal death.

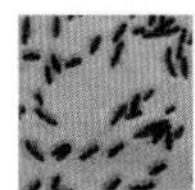

ETIOLOGIC FACTORS: The etiology of ICP is not known, but pregnancy hormones and genetic factors are probably involved. ICP most commonly occurs in the third trimester when maternal pregnancy hormone levels are at their highest; it occurs more often in multifetal pregnancies, which are associated with higher levels of hormones. Estrogens and glucuronides can cause cholestasis, and high-dose estrogen oral contraceptives can result in features of ICP in nonpregnant women.

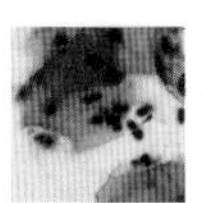

CLINICAL FEATURES: The most common maternal complaint is intense itching without a rash, most often involving the palms and soles. Levels of liver enzymes and serum bile acids can be elevated. Less common symptoms include jaundice, dark urine, right upper quadrant pain, and lighter stools. The risk of recurrence may be 90% in subsequent pregnancies.

17 The Breast

Anna Marie Mulligan ▪ Frances P. O'Malley

LEARNING OBJECTIVES

- Describe the components of the terminal duct lobular unit (TDLU).
- Correlate hormonal changes during the menstrual cycle with histologic changes in the TDLU.
- Describe changes in the breast that occur during pregnancy and the postpartum period.
- Differentiate between acute, periductal, and granulomatous mastitis.
- Summarize the current classification scheme for benign epithelial breast lesions, noting the associated risk of developing breast cancer.
- Describe the histopathology and clinical consequences of fibrocystic change.
- Differentiate between usual epithelial hyperplasia, atypical ductal hyperplasia, and low-grade ductal carcinoma in situ (DCIS).
- Differentiate between fibroadenomas and phyllodes tumors.
- What histopathologic characteristics differentiate benign from malignant phyllodes tumors?
- List several modifiable risk factors for sporadic breast cancer.
- Summarize the most common risk factors for familial breast cancer, including the pattern of inheritance, affected populations, and disease associations in both sexes.
- Differentiate between high-, intermediate-, and low-grade DCIS and microinvasive carcinoma in terms of histopathology.
- Describe the gross and histologic characteristics of Paget disease of the nipple.
- Differentiate between the clinical and histopathologic characteristics of atypical lobular hyperplasia and lobular carcinoma in situ.
- What is the most common receptor status of *BRCA1*-negative breast carcinomas?
- Differentiate between invasive ductal carcinoma of no special type and invasive lobular carcinoma in terms of histopathology and clinical presentation.
- List important prognostic factors in breast cancer staging.
- What is the significance of estrogen and progesterone receptor and HER2 status in the context of breast cancer prognosis and therapy?
- List the molecular subtypes of breast cancer and the likely prognosis for each.
- How are the molecular subtypes of breast cancer defined?
- Differentiate between physiologic, nonphysiologic, and pseudogynecomastia.
- List known risk factors for male breast cancer.

ANATOMY AND PHYSIOLOGIC CHANGES

The female breast is composed of skin, subcutaneous adipose tissue, and the functional component, which comprises ducts, lobules, and stroma. Collecting ducts, through which milk is secreted, open at the nipple. The nipple consists mainly of dense fibrous tissue mixed with smooth muscle. The latter gives the nipple its erectile capability and contributes to the expression of milk. Pigmentation increases in the nipple and areola at puberty and increases further during pregnancy. Stratified squamous epithelium that lines the nipple skin extends superficially into the collecting ducts before it transitions abruptly into glandular epithelium. The glands contain an inner luminal secretory epithelial cell layer and an outer myoepithelial cell layer.

Just beneath the nipple, collecting ducts dilate to form lactiferous sinuses, which subdivide into 15 to 25 lobes with segmental and subsegmental ducts. These terminate in the **terminal duct lobular unit (TDLU)**, where milk is made. The TDLU consists of (1) terminal ductules or acini, whose epithelium differentiates into secretory acini in pregnant or lactating glands; (2) intralobular collecting duct; and (3) specialized intralobular stroma (Figs. 17-1B and 17-2B).

The TDLU is a dynamic structure that changes cyclically during the menstrual cycle. These periodic alterations include epithelial proliferation and apoptosis, as well as changes in intralobular stroma. In the follicular phase of the menstrual cycle, terminal ducts are few in number and are lined by a simple, two-cell layer of epithelium surrounded by myoepithelium. After ovulation, mitoses increase in the luminal epithelium, as do acini and edema of the intralobular stroma. Myoepithelial cells become more prominent owing to cytoplasmic accumulation of glycogen. These changes may cause progressive fullness and tenderness of the breast. The TDLUs return to their follicular phase state during menses, when declining estrogen and progesterone levels cause apoptosis. At this time, lymphocytes infiltrate the intralobular stroma.

Full functional breast development occurs with the hormonal changes of pregnancy and lactation, during which time glandular tissue increases markedly (Fig. 17-1). Early in pregnancy, the TDLU grows rapidly and stromal vascularity and chronic inflammatory cells increase. In later pregnancy, lobular epithelial cells start to become vacuolated owing to increased secretion into distended lobular units. This vacuolation becomes more pronounced with lactation (Fig. 17-1C). At the end of lactation, the gland involutes dramatically, as pronounced cell death and tissue remodeling eventually return the breast to its prepregnancy state.

Fat increases as a percentage of total breast mass as a woman ages. In menopause, TDLUs atrophy, but large and intermediate-sized ducts persist (Fig. 17-1D). Fat predominates over fibrous tissue, but the latter typically cuffs the remaining ducts.

Outside of the TDLU, connective tissue and fat make up the bulk of the breast tissue. Mucopolysaccharides are also abundant in extracellular matrix, and a few lymphocytes, plasma cells, mast cells, and macrophages are present.

The breast is very vascular and contains a complex lymphatic network, draining mainly into axillary lymph nodes, with a minority communicating with internal mammary nodes.

DEVELOPMENTAL ABNORMALITIES

The most common anomaly of breast development is **supernumerary nipples,** or **polythelia**. This occurs with or without associated breast tissue (**polymastia**), which results from persistent epidermal thickenings. The extra nipples occur mostly along the milk line, which extends from the axilla to the groin, but other sites may rarely be involved. Congenitally **inverted nipple** is caused by a failure of nipple eversion during development, usually unilaterally.

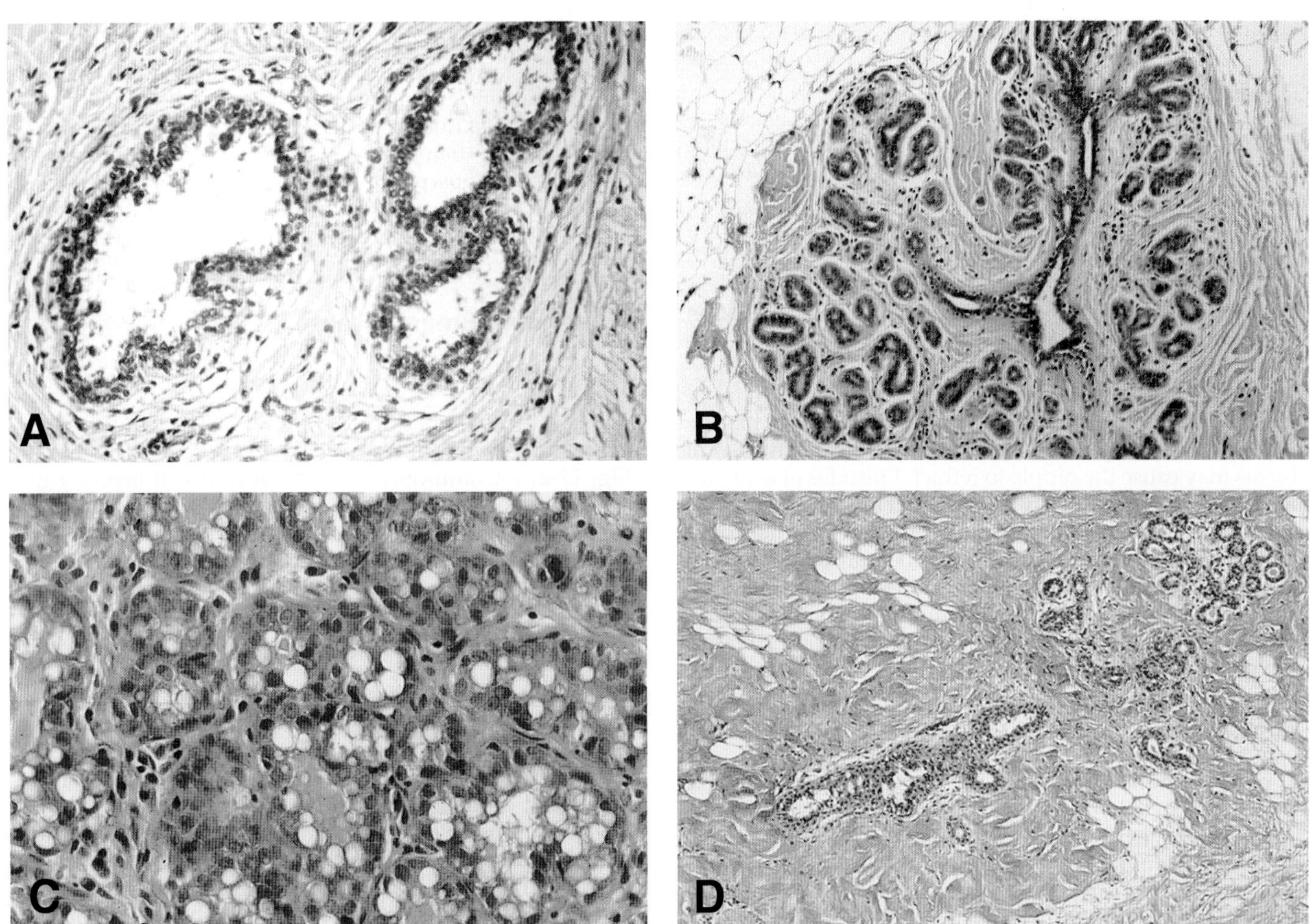

FIGURE 17-1. Normal breast architecture at various ages. A. Adolescent breast. Large and intermediate-size ducts are seen within a dense fibrous stroma. No lobular units are present. **B. Postpubertal breast.** The terminal duct lobular unit (TDLU) consists of small ductules arrayed around an intralobular duct. The two-cell–layered epithelium shows no secretory or mitotic activity. The intralobular stroma is dense and confluent with the interlobular stroma. **C. Lactating breast.** The TDLUs are conspicuously enlarged, with inapparent interlobular and intralobular stroma. The individual terminal ducts, now termed acini, show prominent epithelial secretory activity (cytoplasmic vacuolization). The acinar lumina contain secretory material. **D. Postmenopausal breast.** The TDLUs are absent. The remaining intermediate ducts and larger ducts are commonly dilated.

INFLAMMATORY DISEASES

Acute Mastitis

Acute mastitis is a common complication of breast feeding especially early in the postpartum period. The condition reflects bacterial infection, usually with *Staphylococcus* or *Streptococcus*. Patients have pain, swelling or redness, often with fever and malaise. Cracks in the skin or interruption in milk discharge predispose patients to bacterial infection.

Periductal Mastitis

Periductal mastitis is unrelated to lactation, age, or history of pregnancy. It presents with a painful subareolar mass and overlying erythema. The large majority of patients are cigarette smokers. Nipple ducts show keratinizing squamous metaplasia. A keratin plug can get trapped and result in duct rupture. Keratin debris spilling into the stroma then elicits a foreign body, chronic inflammatory response, which may become secondarily infected. Recurrences are common and can eventuate in fistulas. Surgical excision is curative.

Granulomatous Mastitis

Granulomatous inflammation (Fig. 17-3) of the breast can be caused by mycobacteria, parasites, fungi, or foreign material, such as silicone gel leakage from breast implants.

Duct Ectasia

Duct ectasia is common and is characterized by ductal dilation and periductal inflammation. It is accompanied by fibrosis of large and intermediate breast ducts, which contain inspissated material. Peri- or postmenopausal women are more likely to be symptomatic, complaining of a serous or bloody discharge, mass, or pain. As the disease progresses, duct wall fibrosis may cause the nipple to retract. Episodes of acute inflammation are occasionally complicated by abscess or sinus formation. Dilated ducts contain amorphous debris and foamy macrophages (Fig. 17-4). The lining epithelium and periductal stroma display inflammatory cells and foamy macrophages. Duct rupture incites a chronic inflammatory response, often with foreign body granulomas. Over time, fibrosis increases, with or without obliteration of ducts.

Fat Necrosis

Fat necrosis in the breast often presents as a hard mass and associated skin tethering, which in some patients may mimic carcinoma. Some patients report a history of trauma. Necrotic fat cells, acute inflammation, cholesterol clefts, and hemorrhage are evident early in the course of fat necrosis. Foamy macrophages and multinucleated giant cells that engulf lipid droplets then gradually accumulate (Fig. 17-5). With time, fibrosis and dystrophic calcification develop.

BENIGN EPITHELIAL LESIONS

Benign epithelial lesions are classified on the basis of their risk of subsequent cancer development.

- **Nonproliferative breast changes** (e.g., fibrocystic change) are not associated with increased risk.
- **Proliferative disease without atypia** (often classified simply as **proliferative breast disease**) entails a 1.5- to 2-fold increased risk of developing carcinoma over 5 to 15 years.
- **Proliferative lesions with atypia** involve even greater relative risk (four- to fivefold). Such patients require close clinical monitoring and may consider medical treatment options (e.g., estrogen antagonists).

Fibrocystic Change

FCC is a nonproliferative lesion that includes gross and microscopic cysts, apocrine metaplasia, mild epithelial hyperplasia, and an increase in fibrous stroma. The condition affects over one third of women 20 to 50 years old and then declines after menopause. Most women with FCC are asymptomatic, but some present with nodularity and, occasionally, pain. FCC is typically multifocal and bilateral.

The breast tissue in FCC consists grossly of firm fibrofatty tissue, within which multiple clear cysts ("blue dome" cysts) contain a dark, thin fluid (Fig. 17-2A). Cysts vary from 1 mm to several centimeters in size; they may lack epithelial lining or be lined by attenuated epithelium and myoepithelium (Fig. 17-2C). Their lining may include apocrine-type cells, which are large; exhibit abundant, granular, eosinophilic cytoplasm; and contain a basally located nucleus (Fig. 17-2D). Surrounding stroma is often sclerotic. Inflammation may be due to cyst rupture. Mild "usual" ductal hyperplasia (as discussed later) is frequent, with no more than 3 to 4 cell layers above the basement membrane (Fig. 17-2C). Acini are increased in number and size, are lined by columnar cells, and frequently contain calcifications.

Proliferative Breast Disease

Usual Epithelial Hyperplasia

Usual epithelial hyperplasia within ducts or lobules is typified by increased cellularity above the basement membrane (Fig. 17-2F). Commonly, more than four cell layers, often bridging across duct lumens, encompass luminal and basal epithelial cells. Usual epithelial hyperplasia does not show the characteristic alterations seen in atypical duct hyperplasia and low-grade ductal carcinoma in situ (DCIS) (as discussed later).

Sclerosing Adenosis

The lesions of SA vary from microscopic foci to masses that may be palpable; they may be mistaken for carcinoma in clinical and radiologic examinations. SA often calcifies and is sometimes targeted for core biopsies. The TDLU shows disordered epithelial, myoepithelial, and stromal components, resulting in distortion and expansion of lobules and obliteration of duct spaces (Fig. 17-6). However, a lobulocentric architecture is maintained. Immunohistochemistry can highlight the preservation of myoepithelial cells around distorted ducts in SA, thereby distinguishing the condition from invasive carcinoma.

Radial Scar/Complex Sclerosing Lesion

Radial scar is a benign sclerosing lesion that demonstrates a central fibroelastotic scar and peripheral radiating ducts and lobules. Larger lesions are sometimes seen mammographically

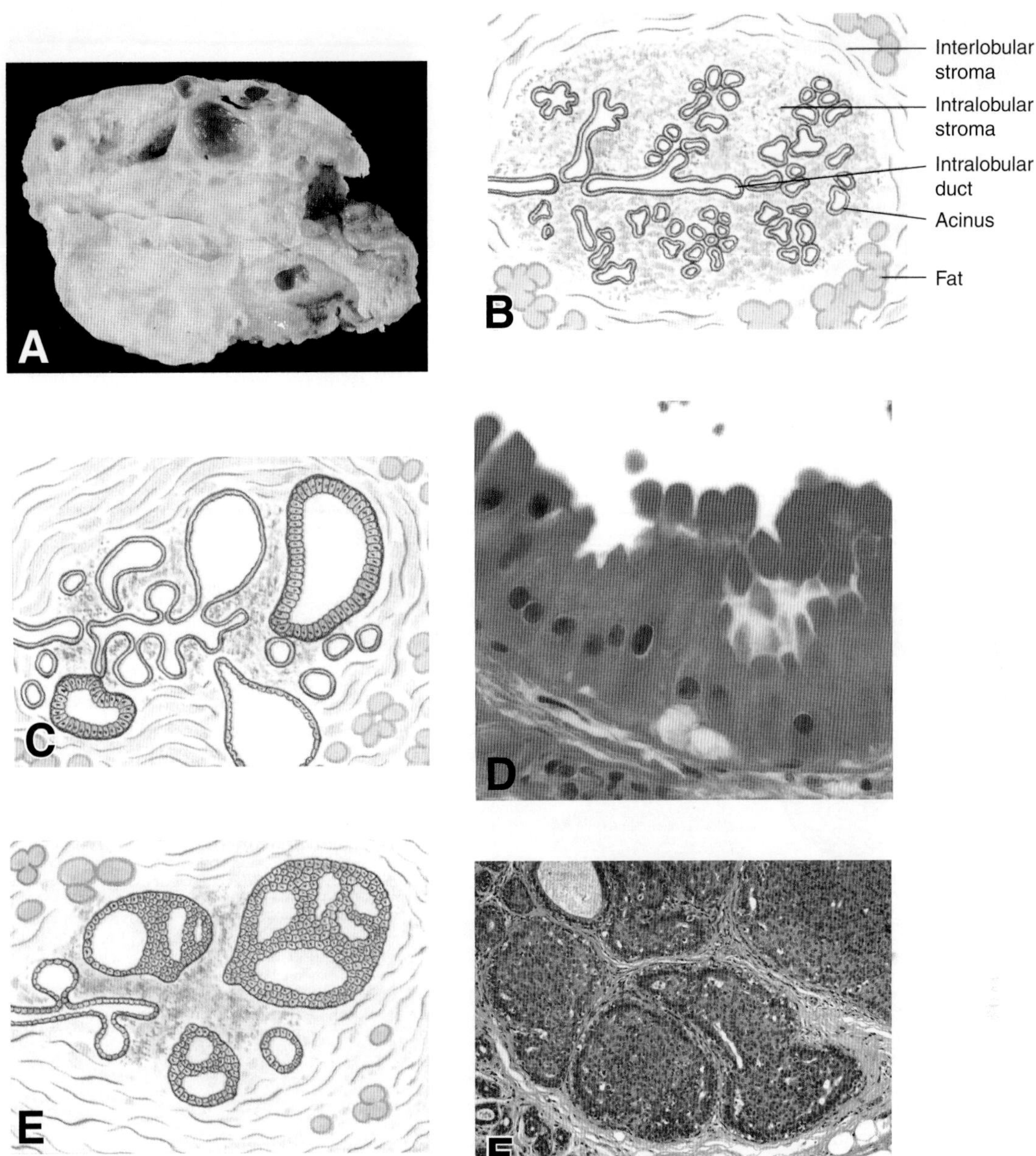

FIGURE 17-2. Fibrocystic change. A. Cysts of various sizes are dispersed in dense, fibrous connective tissue. Some of the cysts are large and contain old blood-tinged proteinaceous debris. **B. Normal terminal duct lobular unit. C. Nonproliferative fibrocystic change** combines cystic dilation of the terminal ducts with varying degrees of apocrine metaplasia of the epithelium and increased fibrous stroma. **D. Apocrine metaplasia.** Epithelial cells have apocrine features with eosinophilic cytoplasm. **E. Proliferative breast disease.** Terminal duct dilation and intraductal epithelial hyperplasia are present. **F. Florid epithelial hyperplasia of usual type.** The epithelium within the ducts proliferates and almost fills the duct lumen, and residual "secondary" spaces remain as peripheral slit-like spaces. Cytoplasmic borders are indistinct, and the nuclei appear round to oval and frequently overlap, resulting in a streaming pattern.

as stellate or spiculated structures with radiolucent central areas that may be difficult to distinguish from cancerous lesions. The entrapped and distorted small ducts are found within the central core (Fig. 17-7). At the edges, radiating ducts and lobules show diverse benign alterations. Occasionally, atypical hyperplasia or carcinoma may be present.

The lesion is associated with a twofold increase in breast cancer risk, which is even greater in women with coexisting proliferative disease, either with or without atypia. This increased risk pertains to both ipsilateral and contralateral breasts, indicating that radial scars are markers of generally increased susceptibility to breast cancer. Surgical excision is recommended.

Intraductal Papilloma

Papillomas are divided into central and peripheral types. Central papillomas arise in large lactiferous ducts and tend to be solitary. Peripheral papillomas originate in TDLUs and are usually multiple. Patients may present with a mass lesion or, often, a bloody nipple discharge. On mammography, central papillomas appear as well-circumscribed masses. Peripheral

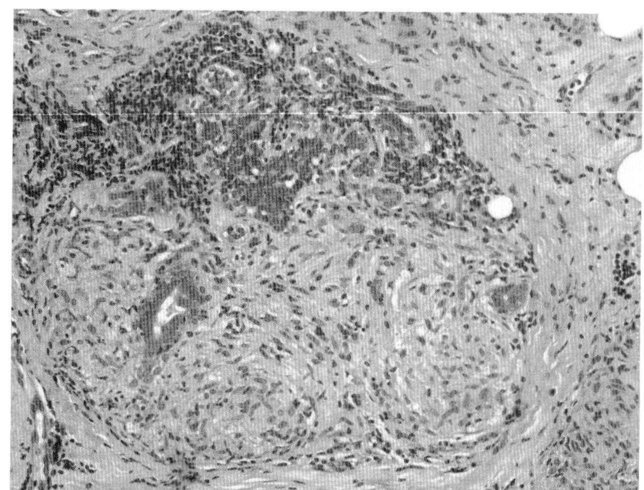

FIGURE 17-3. Breast lobule showing florid granulomatous inflammation characterized by collections of epithelioid histiocytes.

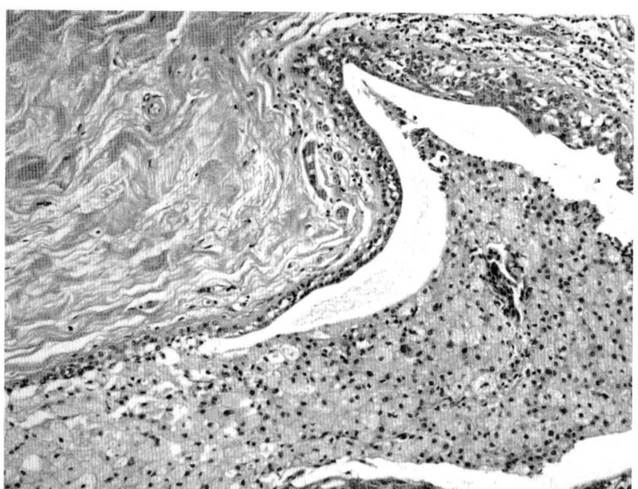

FIGURE 17-4. Duct ectasia. Dilated duct filled with foamy histiocytes. The duct epithelium is focally infiltrated by histiocytes, and chronic inflammation of the periductal stroma is present.

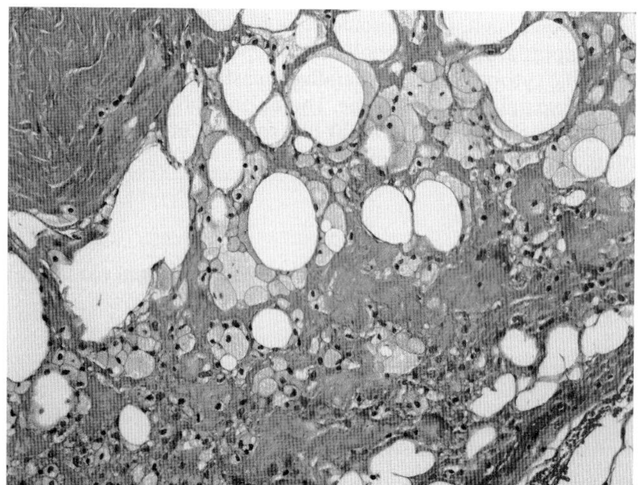

FIGURE 17-5. Fat necrosis. Necrotic fat cells with abundant foamy histiocytes.

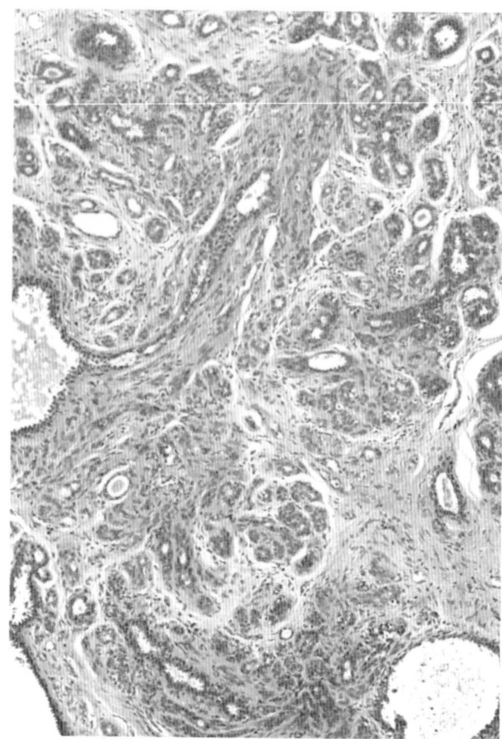

FIGURE 17-6. Sclerosing adenosis. This lesion is characterized by the proliferation of small, abortive, duct-like structures; myoepithelial cells expand and distort the lobule in which it arises. The lesion is well circumscribed, in contrast to a cancerous lesion.

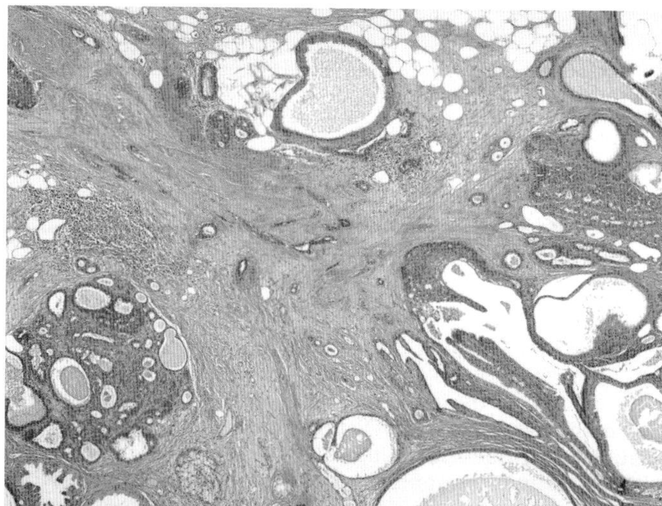

FIGURE 17-7. Radial scar. Angulated glands in a fibroelastotic center are surrounded by a radial distribution of benign ducts and apocrine cysts.

papillomas are often identified as clustered calcifications or small nodular masses.

Papillomas vary from microscopic foci to masses several centimeters across (Fig. 17-8A). Larger lesions frequently show foci of hemorrhage or necrosis. Dilated duct spaces contain multiple branching papillae with fibrovascular cores. These structures are lined by a layer of myoepithelium, on which one or more layers of epithelium lie (Fig. 17-8B). Florid epithelial hyperplasia of usual type or atypical ductal hyperplasia may

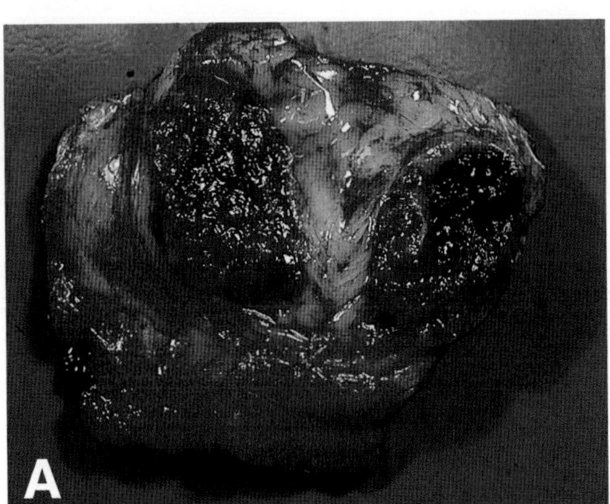

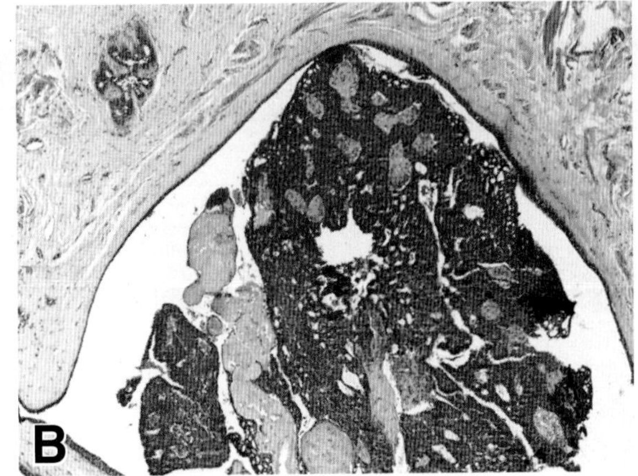

FIGURE 17-8. Intraductal papilloma. A. A large papillary mass is seen within dilated ducts. **B.** A photomicrograph shows a benign papillary growth in a subareolar duct.

be present. Papillomas often contain areas of apocrine change and, less often, those of squamous metaplasia. Sclerosis of papillae or duct walls is variable, but it may be marked and can entrap and distort benign epithelium at the periphery, mimicking an invasive process.

The relative risk of a concurrent or subsequent malignancy is twofold in patients with central papillomas and threefold if papillomas are peripheral; however, atypia within these lesions increases the risks five- and sevenfold, respectively. If a papilloma is found on core biopsy, excision is generally recommended because atypia or carcinoma may coexist in areas not sampled in the biopsy.

Proliferative Disease With Atypia

Atypical Ductal Hyperplasia

ADH is an intraductal epithelial proliferation with a dual population of low-grade neoplastic epithelial cells and benign cells. The benign lining may comprise normal cells or epithelial hyperplasia of usual type. The neoplastic population consists of monomorphic small cells that are evenly spaced, with well-defined cytoplasmic borders and round, hyperchromatic, uniform nuclei. These form architecturally complex structures, such as micropapillae, rigid bridges, bars, solid sheets, or cribriform arrays (Fig. 17-9). In cases where the duct is completely filled by neoplastic cells and two duct spaces extending at least 2 mm are involved, the lesion is considered low-grade ductal carcinoma in situ (DCIS, discussed later).

Half to two thirds of ADH lesions show alterations that overlap with low-grade DCIS. Common patterns of genetic alterations in proliferative breast lesions are summarized in Table 17-1.

In patients with ADH, the relative risk of subsequent breast cancer increases four- to fivefold. Hormonal therapy may be used to reduce the risk of developing breast cancer.

FIBROEPITHELIAL LESIONS

These masses arise from intralobular stroma and contain both stromal and epithelial elements.

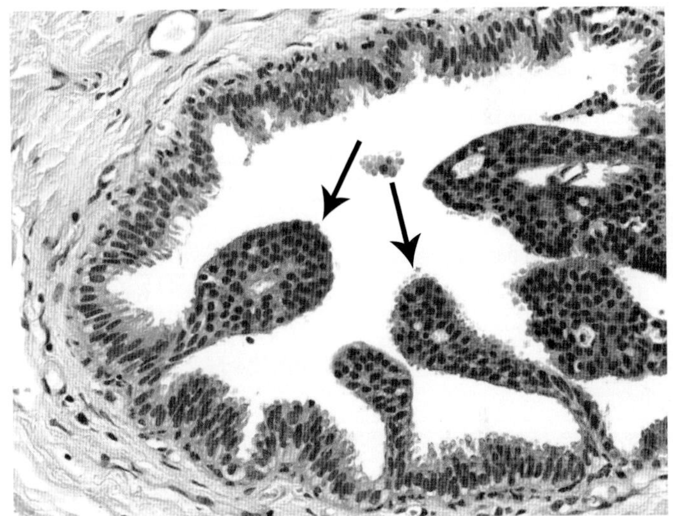

FIGURE 17-9. Atypical ductal hyperplasia. Micropapillae (*arrows*) project into the duct lumen and consist of cells with an increased nuclear-to-cytoplasmic ratio and nuclear hyperchromasia. Residual benign columnar cells are seen lining the duct.

Fibroadenoma

Fibroadenomas are common, mobile, painless breast lumps that most often affect 20- to 35-year-old women. Clinically silent lesions are particularly common and are usually identified by mammography. Lesions are typically well-defined solitary masses, which may be calcified. However, they can be multiple and bilateral, most often in Afro-Caribbean women.

Fibroadenomas are round or ovoid and rubbery (Fig. 17-10A) and are sharply demarcated from surrounding breast tissue. Most are less than 3 cm in size, but they can rarely be much larger (up to 20 cm) in young women or adolescents. Fibroadenomas have two components: stroma and epithelium (Fig. 17-10B). The stroma typically contains spindle cells and shows variable, but usually low, cellularity. With age, the stroma may become denser and calcify. The epithelial component is formed from normal TDLU constituents; epithelial

Table 17-1

Common Genetic Alterations Associated With Breast Lesions

Lesion Type	Other	Alteration
ADH	Loss	16q
	Gain	17p
Phyllodes tumors	Gain	1q
	Loss	13
Familial adenomatous polyposis	Mutation	*APC*, β-catenin
	Loss	5q
Familial breast cancer, high penetrance		*BRCA1, BRCA2*
	Li-Fraumeni	*TP53*
	Cowden	*PTEN*
	Hereditary diffuse gastric cancer	*CDH1*
	Peutz-Jeghers	*STK11*
Familial breast cancer, low penetrance	Ataxia telangiectasia	*ATM*
	Li-Fraumeni variant	*CHEK2*
Low-grade DCIS	Gain	1q
	Loss	16q
High-grade DCIS	Gain	17q, 8q, 5p
	Loss	11q, 14q, 8p, 13q
	Amplifications	17, 6, 8, 11
Encapsulated papillary carcinoma		LOH, 16q, 1q
Lobular neoplasia	Gain	1q, 6q
	Loss	16p, 16q (especially 16q22.1), 17p, 22q
Pleomorphic LCIS	Gains and losses	Same as lobular neoplasia
	Amplification	8q24, 17q12
	LOH	16q22.1, p53, *HER2, BRCA1*
Invasive ductal NST, low grade	Loss	16q
	Gain	1q, 16p
Invasive ductal NST, high grade		Heterogeneous and aneuploidy
Invasive lobular carcinoma	Loss	16q
	Gain	1q, 16p
Invasive lobular carcinoma, high grade		Same as invasive lobular carcinoma
	Amplification	8q24, 17q12, 20q13
Tubular carcinoma	Loss	16q (8p, 3p, 11q)
	Gain	1q, 16p
Medullary carcinoma	Mutations (acquired)	*TP53, BRCA1*
	Epigenetic inactivation	*BRCA1*
Micropapillary	Gain	8q, 17q, 20q
	Loss	6q, 13q
Metaplastic carcinoma	Mutations	*TP53*
Male breast cancer	Inherited mutations	*BRCA2*
	Acquired mutations	*TP53, PTEN, CHEK2*

ADH, atypical ductal hyperplasia; DCIS, ductal carcinoma in situ; LCIS, lobular carcinoma in situ; LOH, loss of heterozygosity; NST, no special type.

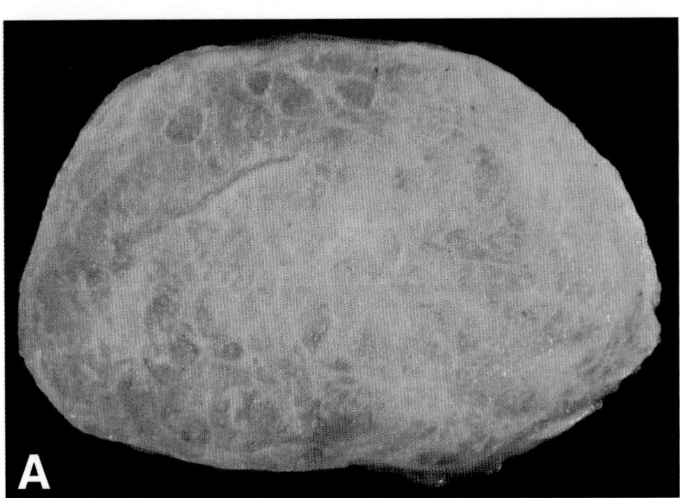

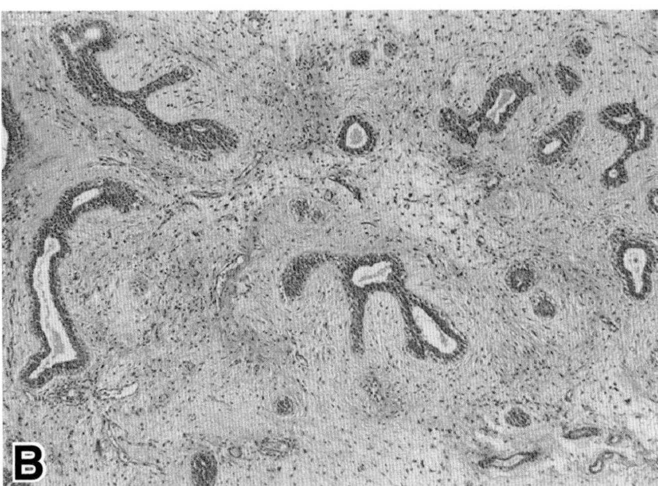

FIGURE 17-10. Fibroadenoma. A. Surgical specimen. This well-circumscribed tumor was easily enucleated from the surrounding tissue. The cut surface is characteristically glistening tannish-white and has a septate appearance. **B.** Microscopic section. Elongated epithelial duct structures are situated within a loose, myxoid stroma.

and myoepithelial layers are preserved. The relationship of the stroma to the epithelium is typically uniform throughout.

Fibroadenomas are surgically excised if they are of clinical or radiologic concern. They can, but do not often, recur. There is no increased risk of subsequent breast cancer.

Phyllodes Tumor

These lesions comprise less than 1% of breast tumors. They have epithelial and stromal components, the latter being neoplastic. They can occur at any age but are most common in the sixth decade. Phyllodes tumors present as rapidly growing breast masses and on mammograms appear well circumscribed or lobulated.

Lesions vary in size from a few centimeters across to 20 cm. **Benign** phyllodes tumors are sharply circumscribed. Their cut surfaces are firm, glistening, and grayish white. Clefts may be prominent. Malignant lesions often show infiltrative margins. On microscopy, fronds of hypercellular stroma can be observed to form leaf-like structures, which project into cystic spaces (Fig. 17-11). These spaces are lined by a dual layer of benign epithelium and myoepithelium. The stroma ranges from benign and hypercellular to frankly sarcomatous. Most phyllodes tumors are benign and have mild or moderately hypercellular stroma with mild cytologic atypia and few mitoses. In **malignant** phyllodes tumors, the stroma is hypercellular, with considerable pleomorphism, abundant mitoses (>10 per 10 HPFs), and stromal overgrowth. Malignant heterologous elements, such as bone, cartilage, or fat, may be present. Those tumors that are not clearly benign or malignant are called **borderline**.

The epithelium in phyllodes tumors appears to influence stromal growth. The tumors upregulate β-catenin activity and downstream effectors such as cyclin D1 via the Wnt pathway. Altered karyotypes may occur with malignant progression (Table 17-1).

The main risk of benign phyllodes tumors is local recurrence, which occurs 20% of the time, rather than metastasis. Metastases are rare overall, but up to 25% of high-grade malignant phyllodes tumors may disseminate. Only stromal components are seen in metastases. Axillary lymph node metastases are rare.

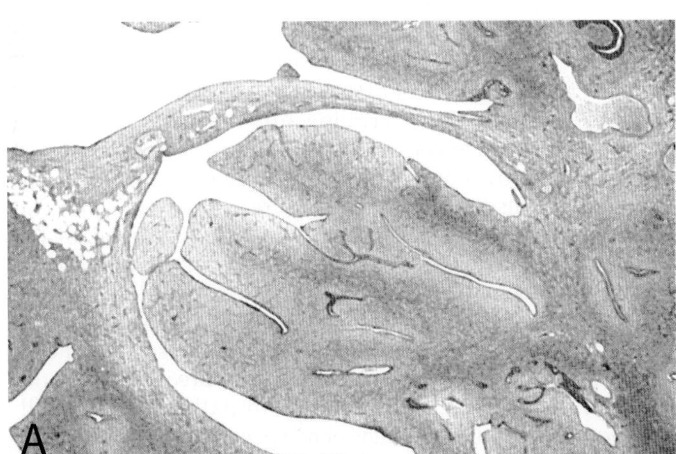

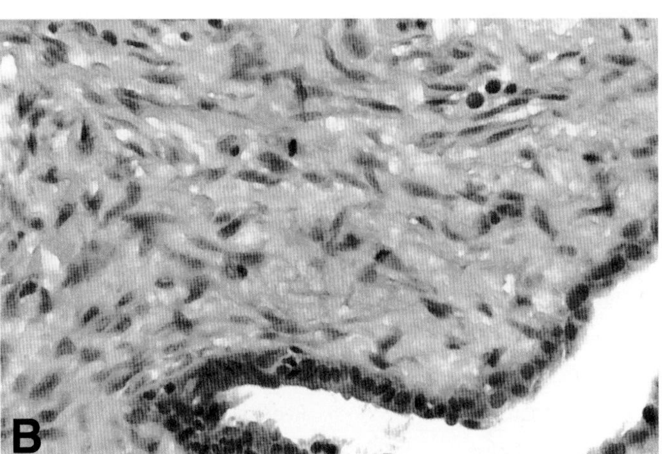

FIGURE 17-11. Phyllodes tumor. A. A polypoid tumor with a leaf-like pattern expands a duct. **B.** The stromal component adjacent to ductal epithelium is similar to a fibroadenoma but is more cellular. The residual ductal structure is benign.

STROMAL LESIONS

Stromal lesions arise from nonspecialized interlobular stroma. Mesenchymal lesions that occur outside the breast, such as lipomas or vascular tumors, can also occur in the breast. Uncommon stromal lesions specific to the breast are also found.

CARCINOMA OF THE BREAST

Breast cancer is the most common malignancy of women in the United States; its mortality in women is second only to lung cancer. The incidence of breast cancer has slowly increased over the past 50 years but has remained stable in the last decade. Women in the United States have a 1 in 8 lifetime risk of developing breast cancer. About 20% of women with breast cancer will die from it. Age-specific incidence rates increase dramatically after age 40 and plateau at 75 to 80 years. Breast cancer is uncommon before the age of 35 in all populations.

Breast cancer occurs four to five times more commonly in Western industrialized countries than in the developing world. The risk in daughters and granddaughters of women who migrated from countries of low incidence to Western countries increases with successive generations.

Widespread use of screening mammography in the 1980s led to a sharp increase in the proportion of diagnoses of noninvasive breast lesions (i.e., DCIS). The frequency of small invasive cancers has also increased. However, although widespread screening mammography greatly increased detection of early breast cancers, it has not appreciably decreased the incidence of late-stage breast cancers. Overall mortality has declined from 30% to 20%, and stage-specific mortality has also improved, mainly because of improved therapy.

Multiple risk factors for breast cancer have been identified, some of which cannot be modified and some of which are amenable to change (Table 17-2).

SPORADIC BREAST CANCER: Only about 25% of sporadic breast cancers have identifiable risk factors. Factors affecting the hormonal milieu modify breast cancer risk.

- The majority of breast cancers are stimulated by **estrogen.** Cumulative lifetime exposure to estrogen determines the level of this risk. Early menarche (younger than 11 years), late menopause, and older age at first term pregnancy increase the risk. Antiestrogens, including tamoxifen and aromatase inhibitors, decrease the development of estrogen receptor-positive (ER-positive) breast cancer. Oral contraceptives do not increase breast cancer risk, although hormone replacement therapy (HRT) increases it slightly, by 1.2 to 1.7 times.
- **Radiation** increases the risk of breast cancer, as documented in survivors of the atomic bomb and in women who received irradiation for Hodgkin lymphoma. Irradiation earlier in life (i.e., in childhood or adolescence) poses the greatest risk; exposure after the age of 40 years has not been shown to increase the incidence.
- **Total dietary fat** may increase the risk of breast cancer after menopause. However, the risk, if existent, is likely to be small.
- **Alcohol consumption** at high levels is associated with higher breast cancer rates.
- Postmenopausal women who are **overweight** or **obese** are at greater risk for breast cancer. Interestingly, obesity appears to have an opposite effect on breast cancer risk among premenopausal women.
- **Smoking.** Active smoking, particularly if begun at an early age and continuing for a long time, increases, by approximately 20%, the risk of developing breast cancer. This risk is strongly associated with a polymorphism at the *NAT2* gene site (*N*-acetyltransferase 2).
- Patients with **denser breasts** (i.e., ≥75% density) have a four- to fivefold greater risk of breast cancer. Mammographic breast density reflects the proportions of stroma and epithelium rather than fat in breasts.
- Prior breast biopsies showing **atypical hyperplasia** or **nonatypical proliferative breast disease** increase the relative risk of breast cancer 4 to 5 times and 1.5 to 2 times, respectively. Women with a previous incidence of breast cancer have a 10-fold increased risk of developing a second primary tumor in the ipsilateral or contralateral breast. Hormonal treatment with antiestrogens decreases this risk.

Table 17-2

Risk Factors for Breast Cancer Development

Not Modifiable	Modifiable
Age	Body mass index
BRCA germline mutations	Diet
Family history	Alcohol
Chest radiation	Exogenous estrogen
Race/ethnicity	Exercise
Height	Smoking
Age at menarche	Reproductive history
Age at menopause	Age at first full-term delivery
Breast density	Lactation
Atypia on prior breast biopsy	

FAMILIAL BREAST CANCER: The strongest association with increased risk for breast cancer is a family history of breast cancer at a young age in first-degree relatives. The risk is greater for bilateral breast cancer. Familial disease accounts for 10% of breast cancers. Two high-risk breast cancer susceptibility genes, *BRCA1* and *BRCA2,* account for 20% to 50% of familial tumors. Some inherited breast cancer susceptibility is part of more generalized familial cancer susceptibility syndromes (Table 17-1).

BRCA1 and *BRCA2* are tumor suppressor genes that display an autosomal dominant pattern of inheritance with variable penetrance. *BRCA1,* on chromosome 17q21, is involved in DNA repair, transcriptional regulation, chromatin remodeling, and protein ubiquitination. Germline mutations in *BRCA1* confer a lifetime breast cancer risk of between 37% and 85% by age 70 years, with over half of the cancers occurring before age 50. Carriers are also at significantly increased risk of other cancers, most notably ovarian cancer, with a lifetime risk of 15% to 40%. The incidence of cancers of the cervix, endometrium, fallopian tube, and stomach is elevated; prostate cancer is more common in male carriers. About 0.1% of the population has *BRCA1* germline mutations, but the rates are higher in Ashkenazi Jews and French Canadians. Breast cancers that develop in patients with germline mutations are typically high-grade ductal carcinomas of no special type (NST) (Fig. 17-12). In *BRCA1* carriers, the majority of cancers are negative for estrogen receptor (ER), progesterone receptor (PR), and human epidermal growth factor receptor 2 (HER2); in addition, p53 mutations are more common. Young age at onset is typical.

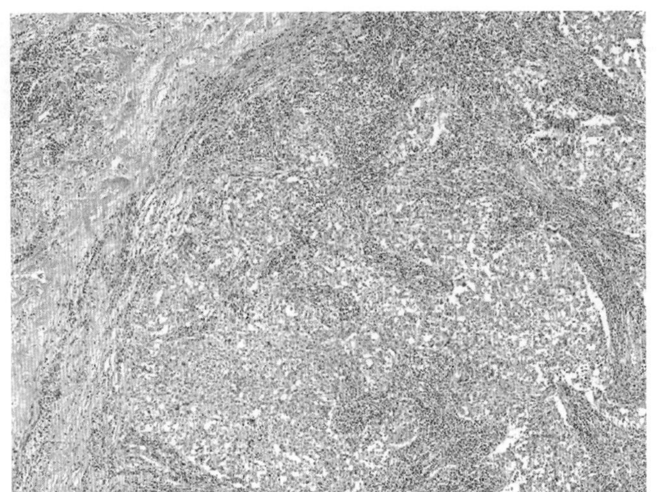

FIGURE 17-12. ***BRCA1*****-associated breast cancer.** High-grade invasive ductal carcinoma of no special type, characterized by pushing margins and a prominent lymphocytic infiltrate.

Germline mutations in *BRCA2*, located on chromosome 13q12, are associated with a 30% to 40% lifetime risk of developing breast cancer and an increased risk of ovarian cancer. Moreover, there is an increased incidence of uveal tract and skin melanomas and cancers of the pancreas and biliary tract. Male carriers of *BRCA2* mutations are also at risk of developing breast and prostatic cancers. Women mostly develop high-grade invasive ductal tumors of NST. *BRCA2*-related cancers are more commonly ER and PR positive than are BRCA1 cancers, but HER2 gene amplification is rare.

Ductal Carcinoma In Situ

Carcinoma of the breast may be **in situ** (confined by the gland's basement membrane) or **invasive**, in which the malignant cells have infiltrated through the basement membrane into adjacent breast stroma. Further subclassification is based on morphology, immunohistochemistry, and molecular profiling. Of women with biopsy-proven DCIS who received no further therapy, 20% to 30% subsequently developed invasive cancer.

DCIS identifies a heterogeneous group of lesions that vary in their architectural and cytologic features, as well as in their natural history. These abnormalities are considered nonobligate precursors of invasive carcinoma, the chance of progressing to invasion varying with the histologic subtype, grade, and extent. The incidence of DCIS has soared with the advent of widespread screening mammography in the mid-1980s. Once representing about 5% of breast cancers, it now accounts for 25% of breast cancers in screened populations. Unfortunately, this increased detection of DCIS has not been associated with a decreased incidence of advanced breast cancer.

In some cases, DCIS may be a precursor of invasive breast carcinoma. (1) DCIS is often seen together with invasive carcinomas. (2) In such cases, noninvasive and invasive diseases may show a similar cytologic appearance and nuclear grade. (3) DCIS and invasive carcinoma share distinct molecular and cytogenetic alterations. However, the mechanisms governing the progression of DCIS to invasive carcinoma are poorly understood.

Molecular analyses have shown differences in the numbers and types of chromosomal changes in low- and high-grade DCIS (Table 17-1). High-grade DCIS demonstrates similar molecular alterations to co-occurring invasive carcinoma. Low- and high-grade DCIS are therefore fundamentally distinct entities, and one does not necessarily evolve into the other. The same appears to be true for low- and high-grade invasive cancer.

DCIS predominantly involves ducts but can extend into lobules. It is characterized by a proliferation of malignant epithelial cells showing a range of histologic features (Fig. 17-13). Growth patterns may be cribriform, micropapillary, papillary, solid, and comedo types, and multiple architectural patterns

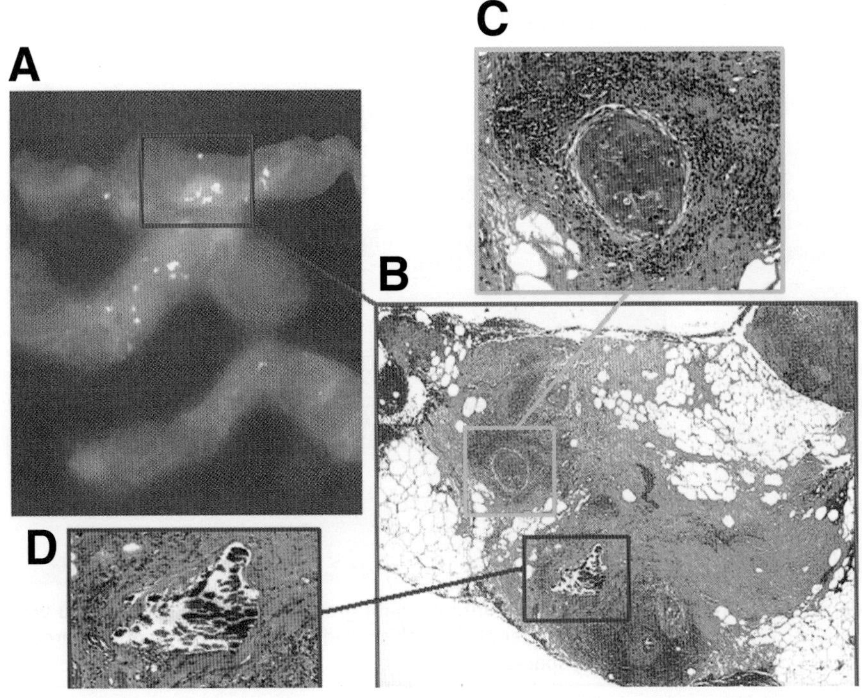

FIGURE 17-13. Ductal carcinoma in situ. A. Specimen radiograph of core biopsy shows linear and punctate atypical calcifications that are highly suspicious for cancer. **B.** Low-power photomicrograph showing high-grade in situ ductal carcinoma. **C.** High-power image of a duct expanded by in situ ductal carcinoma. **D.** High-power photomicrograph of tissue calcification.

can coexist in one lesion. The nuclear grade is prognostically more important.

- **High-grade DCIS** characterizes large, pleomorphic cells with marked variation in size and shape. The cells have abundant cytoplasm, irregular nuclei with prominent nucleoli and coarse chromatin. They proliferate rapidly. Intraductal necrosis is common (Fig. 17-14) and appears grossly as distended ducts with white necrotic material resembling comedos, hence the term **comedo necrosis** . The cellular necrotic debris often undergoes dystrophic calcification, which may be seen on mammography as linear, branching calcifications. Periductal chronic inflammation and formation of new vessels may be present. DCIS spreads through the duct system and often extends beyond clinically detected borders, making clear margins difficult to obtain.
- **Low-grade DCIS** is composed of uniform, small, and evenly spaced cells, with round, regular hyperchromatic nuclei (Fig. 17-15). Mitoses are infrequent. Micropapillary or cribriform growth predominates, and solid growth patterns are less common. Although necrosis is uncommon, foci of either punctate or comedo necrosis can be seen.
- **Intermediate-grade DCIS:** Intermediate-grade DCIS falls between high- and low-grade DCIS. Cells show moderate pleomorphism but maintain some degree of polarization (Fig. 17-16). Solid or cribriform growth is typical.
- **Microinvasive carcinoma:** This pattern is defined as one or more foci of invasive carcinoma, none of which exceed 1 mm in diameter (Fig. 17-17). ***This lesion typically occurs in the setting of high-grade DCIS.***

DCIS is distinguished from epithelial hyperplasia of usual type (see earlier discussion) because it most commonly lacks "basal" high-molecular-weight cytokeratin staining. Positive staining for myoepithelial cell markers (e.g., smooth muscle myosin heavy chain, calponin, and p63) confirms that the lesion is in situ and helps in cases with foci suspicious for microinvasion.

DCIS is most often visualized on mammography as calcifications. A small proportion of women present symptomatically with a mass lesion, a nipple discharge, or Paget disease of the nipple (see later discussion).

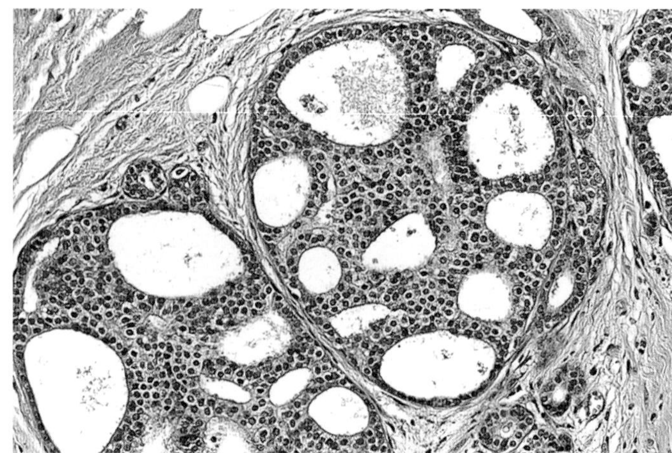

FIGURE 17-15. Ductal carcinoma in situ noncomedo type. A cribriform arrangement of tumor cells is evident.

DCIS is treated by surgical excision. Breast-conserving surgery is possible in many cases, and adjuvant radiation reduces the risk of recurrence. When tumors recur, they do so at the site of the previous surgery and are invasive carcinomas 50% of the time. Lymph node metastases are discovered in less than 1% of patients with DCIS. In all, the critical prognostic factors for patients with DCIS include lesion size, nuclear grade, presence of comedo necrosis, and margin status. Cancer-specific mortality is extremely low, with 1.0% to 2.6% dying from invasive cancer 8 to 10 years after the diagnosis of DCIS.

Paget Disease of the Nipple

In Paget disease of the nipple, malignant glandular cells penetrate the epidermis of the nipple and areola. It is invariably associated with underlying DCIS, with or without invasive ductal carcinoma. This disease is rare, occurring in 1% to 4% of breast cancers.

Paget disease presents as erythema or an eczematous change to the nipple and areola (Fig. 17-18A), sometimes with nipple retraction. Half of patients have palpable masses.

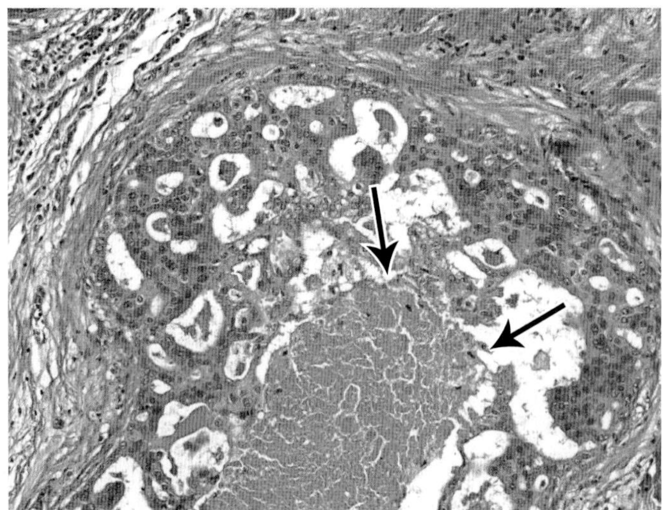

FIGURE 17-14. Ductal carcinoma in situ with comedo necrosis. Intraductal carcinoma with a cribriform architecture and central comedo necrosis (*arrows*).

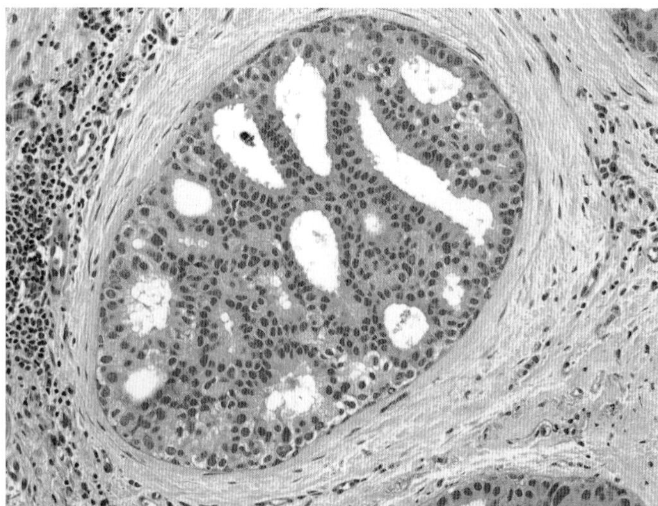

FIGURE 17-16. Intermediate-grade ductal carcinoma in situ with moderate nuclear pleomorphism and some polarization of cells around secondary spaces.

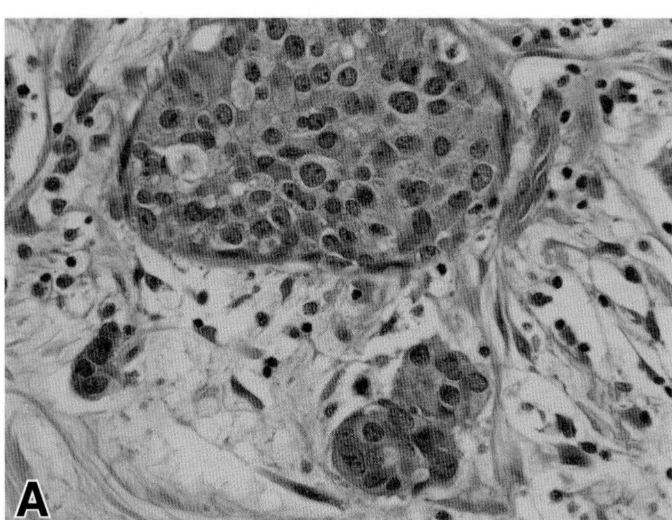

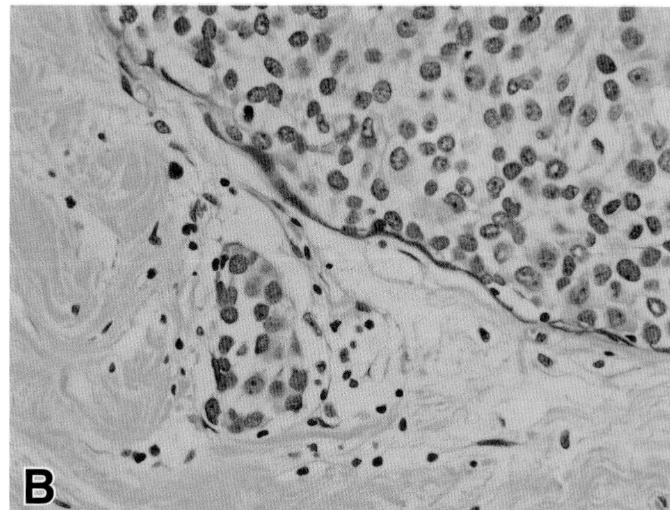

FIGURE 17-17. Ductal carcinoma in situ (**A**) with focus of microinvasive carcinoma. (**B**) Immunohistochemical staining with smooth muscle myosin heavy chain confirms the absence of a myoepithelial cell layer around the small stromal cluster.

Malignant glandular epithelial cells are present in the epidermis, singly or in small groups (Fig. 17-18B). They are large, have abundant cytoplasm that contains mucin globules and pleomorphic nuclei with prominent nucleoli. Paget cells genetically resemble underlying tumor cells in most of the cases. Prognosis is a function of the stage of the underlying breast cancer and not the presence of Paget cells.

Lobular Neoplasia

Both atypical lobular hyperplasia (ALH) and lobular carcinoma in situ (LCIS) reflect the same atypical proliferations of loosely cohesive epithelial cells, but they differ in terms of the risk of developing breast cancer (compare Fig. 17-19 and Fig. 17-20). Because LCIS is generally asymptomatic, its true incidence is unknown but is estimated at 1% to 4%. It is bilateral in up to 30% of patients and multicentric in 85% of them. Both ALH and LCIS are risk factors for the subsequent development of cancer. However, the cancers that develop are typically not at the same site as the initial lesions and may be in the contralateral breast. The risk of subsequent cancer is 3- to 5.5-fold for ALH and 7- to 10-fold for LCIS. At least some of the cases of LCIS are likely precursors to invasive carcinoma because (1) a disproportionately large number of

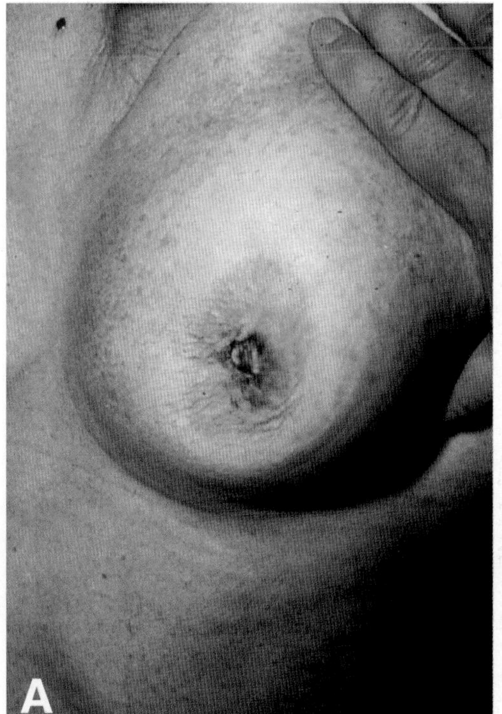

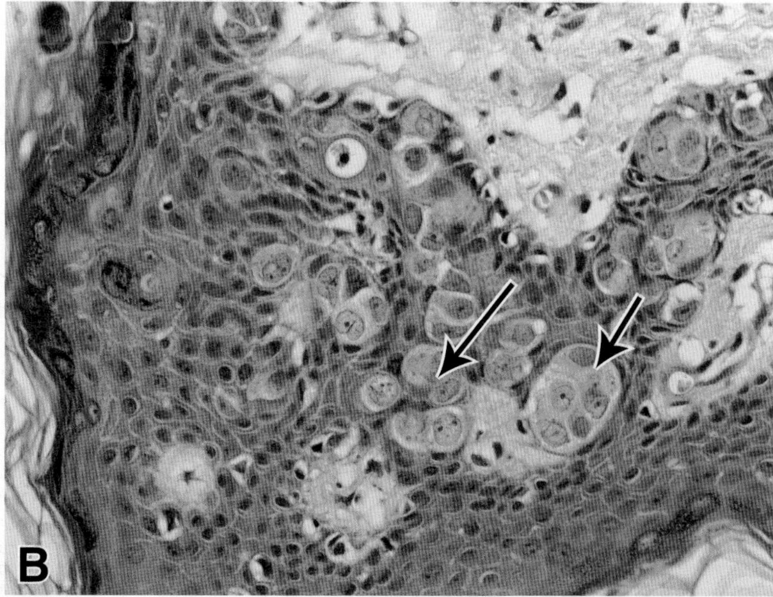

FIGURE 17-18. Paget disease of the nipple. A. An erythematous, scaly, and weeping "eczema" on the nipple. **B.** The epidermis contains clusters of ductal-type carcinoma cells that are larger and have more abundant pale cytoplasm (*arrows*) than surrounding keratinocytes.

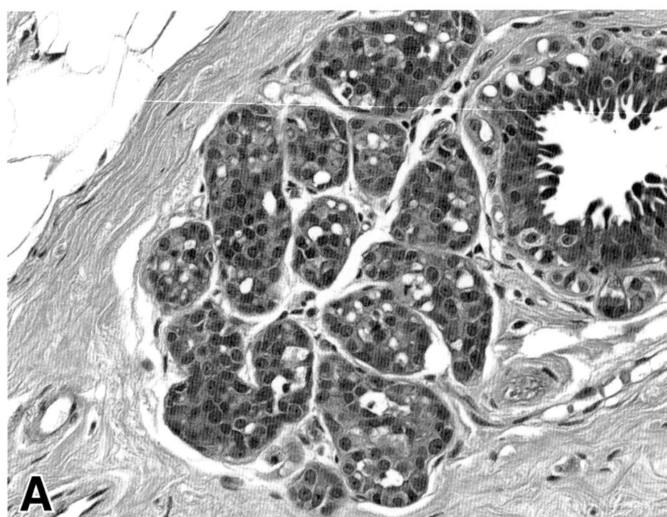

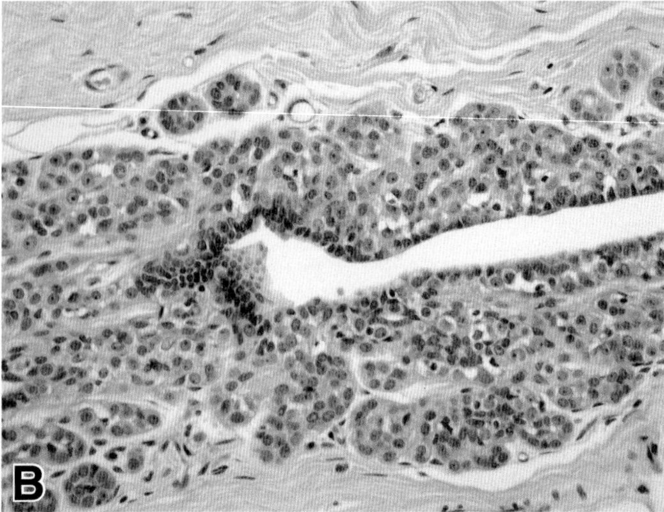

FIGURE 17-19. Lobular Neoplasia. A. Atypical lobular hyperplasia. There is minimal distention of the lobular acini by a uniform population of cells with intracytoplasmic lumina and round nuclei containing small nucleoli. **B. Pagetoid spread** of lobular neoplastic cells into the terminal duct. Here, the atypical cells lie beneath an attenuated surface layer of luminal epithelial cells.

tumors that develop are invasive lobular carcinomas, (2) two thirds of such tumors occur in the ipsilateral breast, and (3) coexistent LCIS and invasive lobular carcinomas often show the same genetic changes.

These studies have identified recurrent 16q22.1 loss in LCIS, ALH, and invasive lobular carcinoma, for which the target gene encodes E-cadherin (Table 17-1). This protein plays an essential role in cell adhesion and cell cycle regulation through the β-catenin/Wnt pathway. Patients with germline mutations in this gene are at high risk of developing lobular breast carcinoma and gastric signet ring cell carcinoma.

Lobular carcinoma in situ rarely appears grossly or with mammography. The cells of LCIS are monotonous and small, with round regular nuclei and minute nucleoli, although larger cells with conspicuous nucleoli occasionally dominate (Fig. 17-20). Cytoplasmic mucin vacuoles may be surrounded by a distinct halo. Unlike DCIS, the cells of LCIS do not form complex patterns but comprise solid clusters that pack and distend lobular acini. The growth pattern is loosely cohesive or dishesive. Gaps between individual cells reflect loss of cell–cell adhesion (see above). Pagetoid spread of lobular neoplastic cells is common in LCIS, where the cells track beneath ductal luminal epithelial cells.

Atypical lobular hyperplasia and LCIS are distinguished by the degree of filling and distention of acini. In LCIS, at least 50% of acini in a lobular unit are completely involved and distended by the atypical cell population, in contrast to less than 50% in ALH.

Distinguishing LCIS from low-grade solid DCIS may be difficult. The absence of immunostaining for E-cadherin in LCIS and ALH may help identify this distinction (Fig. 17-21) because DCIS cells retain cell membrane staining for E-cadherin.

The management of a patient with LCIS is controversial. For classic LCIS, many authorities would opt for no further surgical management. However, adjuvant hormonal therapy may be considered, and lifelong follow-up is required.

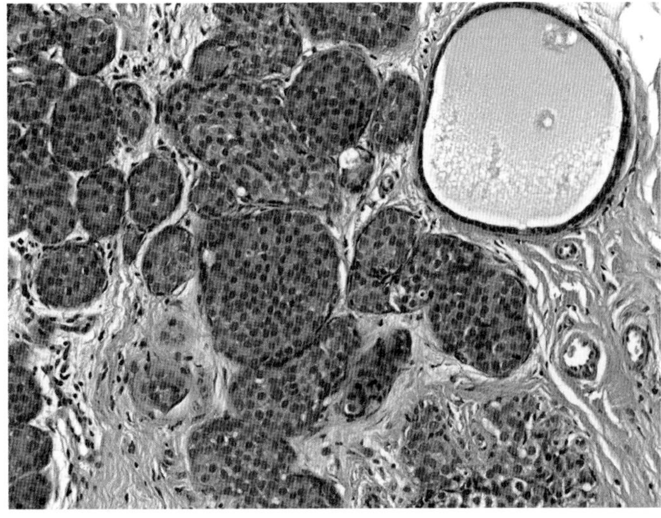

FIGURE 17-20. Lobular carcinoma in situ. The lumina of the terminal duct lobular units are distended by tumor cells, which exhibit round nuclei and small nucleoli. Cytoplasmic mucin vacuoles are present.

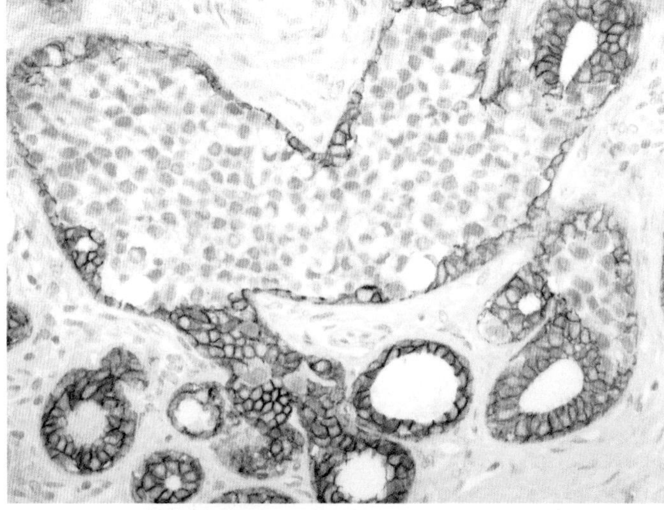

FIGURE 17-21. E-cadherin in lobular carcinoma in situ. Membranous E-cadherin expression is seen in residual luminal epithelial cells, but the lobular neoplastic cells should show loss of staining.

Invasive Breast Carcinoma

Breast cancer can occur anywhere in the breast but is most common in the upper outer quadrant. Patients most often have an ill-defined breast mass, which may be adherent to the skin or underlying muscle. Nonpalpable asymptomatic tumors are usually detected by mammography. These mostly appear radiologically as a spiculated mass or architectural distortion, with or without associated microcalcifications.

Most breast cancers are classified as carcinomas of no specific type (NST). The remainder are special types of carcinomas or have mixed morphologic features.

Ductal Carcinoma

Of invasive breast cancers, 50% to 70% fall in this category. These tumors are a heterogeneous group that do not show characteristics of a specific histologic type.

Ductal NST presents as irregular, dense masses on mammography or ultrasound (Fig. 17-22A). The tumors are usually moderately or poorly defined, are nodular or stellate, and have firm to hard cut surfaces (Fig. 17-22B). Tumor cells form trabeculae, sheets, nests, and glands (Fig. 17-22C). Nuclear pleomorphism and mitotic counts vary. High-grade lesions may show tumor necrosis. DCIS is present in up to 80% of cases and is typically of the same nuclear grade as the invasive component.

Most cases of ductal NST (75%) are ER and PR positive, and 15% are HER2 positive. Specific genetic lesions or alterations are associated with a particular histologic type or grade in some cases (Table 17-1). Overall, 35% to 50% of patients with ductal NST survive 10 years, differing according to grade, tumor and lymph node stage and the presence of lymphovascular invasion.

Lobular Carcinoma

Invasive lobular carcinoma is the second most common form of invasive breast cancer, accounting for 5% to 15% of all invasive cancers. Because stromal desmoplasia and fibrosis may be minimal, patients often have clinically silent disease grossly and by mammography. Lobular cancers characteristically show discohesive malignant epithelial cells, which infiltrate the stroma diffusely (Fig. 17-23). They often line up in a row and may show a periductal "targetoid" arrangement. They do not form ducts, but instead form solid sheets, trabeculae, or nests. Neoplastic cells typically contain intracytoplasmic lumina and eccentric nuclei and resemble the cells of LCIS.

Invasive lobular carcinoma is more often ER positive than is ductal NST, although high-grade lobular cancers may lack ER and overexpress HER2. E-cadherin expression is usually low or absent, reflecting biallelic loss of the tumor suppressor gene that encodes this protein. Patterns of genetic changes in invasive lobular carcinoma differ from those in ductal carcinomas (Table 17-1).

These cancers tend to spread to the peritoneum, retroperitoneum, ovary and uterus, leptomeninges, and gastrointestinal tract. Matched for grade and stage, their prognosis is similar to that of ductal NST cancers.

Uncommon Invasive Carcinomas

- **Tubular carcinomas** are well-defined stellate masses whose cells are composed of almost entirely open and angulated tubules, lined by a single layer of mildly atypical epithelial cells (Fig. 17-24A). Over 95% of tubular carcinomas are ER positive and HER2 negative. Lymph node metastases are rare, and patients with tubular carcinomas have an excellent prognosis.
- **Mucinous carcinomas** typically occur in older women. The cancers are well circumscribed, with a gelatinous texture. Low-grade malignant epithelial cells form acini, nests, or trabeculae, which appear to float in pools of extracellular mucin (Fig. 17-24B). The malignant epithelial cells do not invade the stroma directly. Most are ER positive and HER2 negative. Patients with pure mucinous carcinoma have an excellent prognosis.
- **Carcinomas with medullary features** are well circumscribed and soft and include all of the following: (1) grade two to three nuclei; (2) circumscribed, pushing margins; (3) syncytial growth pattern in more than 75% of the tumor; (4) a moderate or marked lymphoplasmacytic infiltrate; and (5) no tubule formation (Fig. 17-24C). Medullary cancers account for 2% to 3% of all breast cancers; are typically ER, PR, and HER2 negative ("triple negative"); and have characteristic patterns of genetic changes (see Table 17-1).

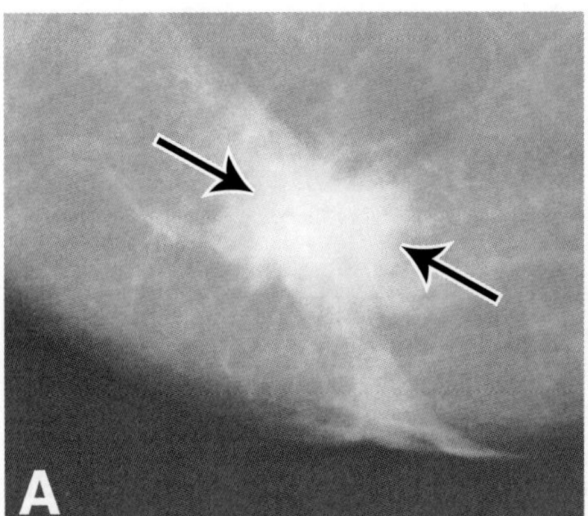

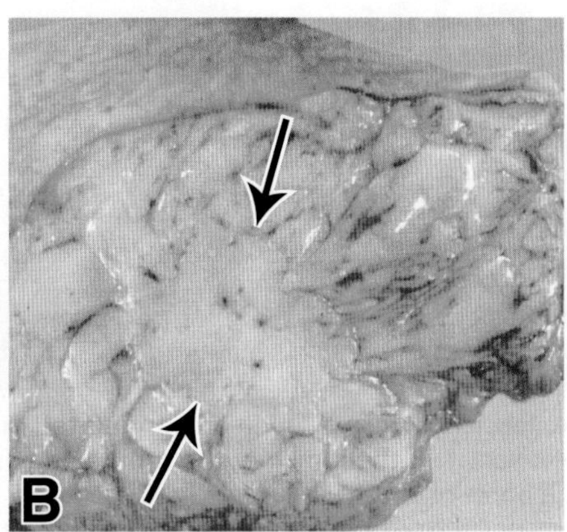

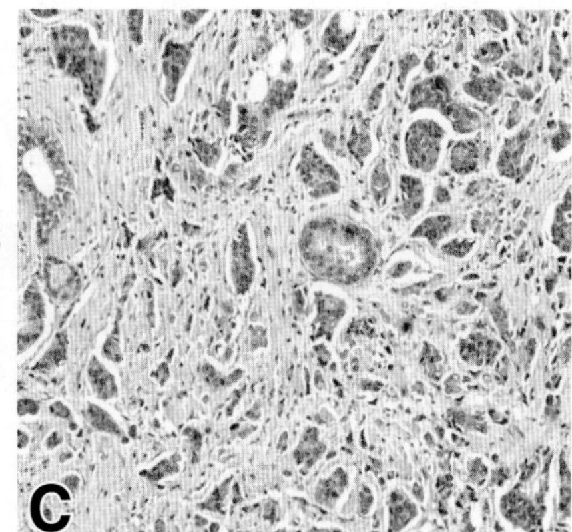

FIGURE 17-22. Carcinoma of the breast. A. Mammogram. An irregularly shaped, dense mass (*arrows*) is seen in this otherwise fatty breast. **B.** Mastectomy specimen. The irregular white, firm mass in the center (*arrows*) is surrounded by fatty tissue. **C.** Photomicrograph showing irregular cords and nests of invasive ductal carcinoma cells invading stroma.

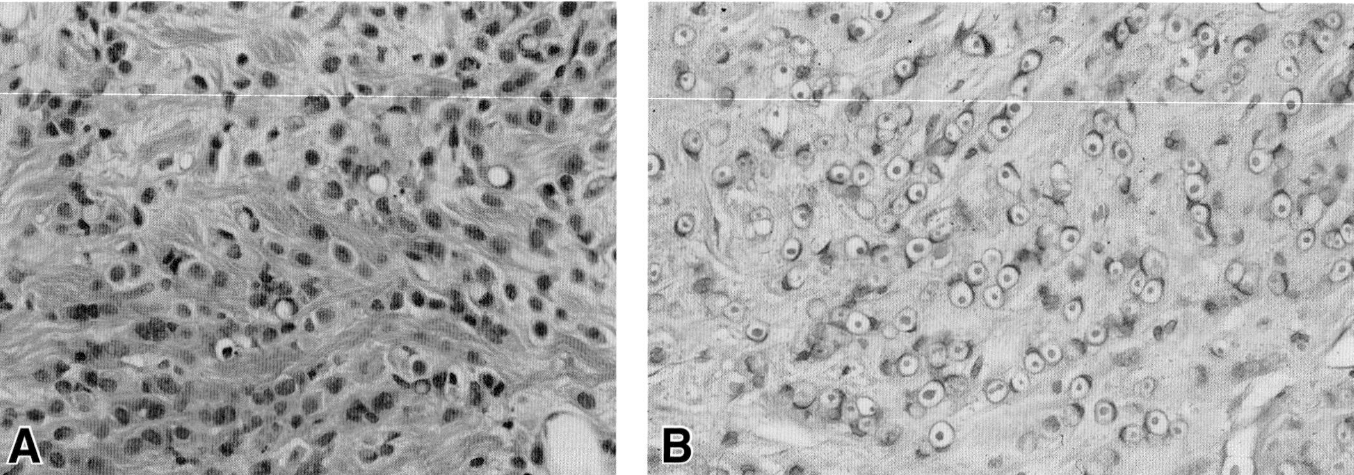

FIGURE 17-23. **Lobular carcinoma. A. Invasive lobular carcinoma.** In contrast to invasive ductal carcinoma, the cells of lobular carcinoma tend to form single strands that invade between collagen fibers in a diffuse pattern. The tumor cells are similar to those seen in lobular carcinoma in situ. **B. Signet ring carcinoma.** The tumor cells contain large amounts of clear mucin.

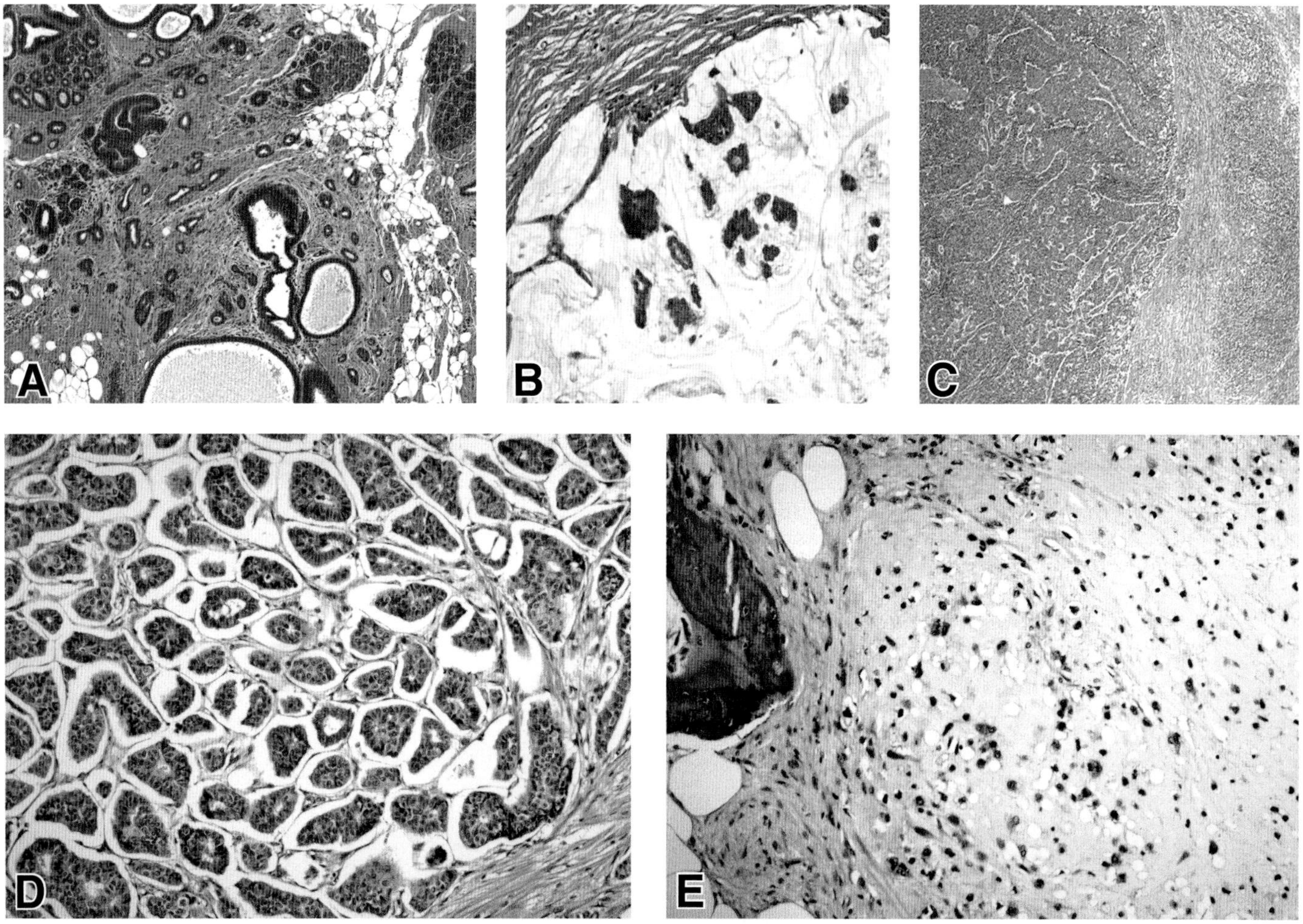

FIGURE 17-24. **Patterns of breast carcinoma. A. Tubular carcinoma.** Open and angulated malignant glands are dispersed between normal lobules and show extension into fat. A single layer of epithelium lines the tubules, and myoepithelial cells are absent. **B. Mucinous carcinoma.** Clusters of malignant cells float in large pools of extracellular mucin. **C. Medullary carcinoma.** The malignant cells are pleomorphic and grow in solid sheets, forming a blunt margin. There is no gland formation. Numerous mitoses are present. The tumor is surrounded by a dense lymphocytic infiltrate. **D. Micropapillary carcinoma.** Sponge-like pattern of empty spaces containing glands and small clusters of malignant epithelium. Focal serration of the outer borders of the glands is seen. **E. Metaplastic carcinoma.** Cartilaginous and osseous matrix in a metaplastic carcinoma with heterologous elements. Elsewhere, foci of poorly differentiated adenocarcinoma were seen.

- **Pure micropapillary carcinoma** occurs rarely, but micropapillary areas are more often admixed with ductal NST carcinoma. Malignant epithelial nests or acini are surrounded by a clear space (Fig. 17-24D). As micropapillary tumors invade lymphatic vessels and metastasize to lymph nodes readily, recognizing even a minor component of micropapillary carcinoma is important. The high frequency of lymph node metastases notwithstanding, it is unknown if micropapillary tumors have an inherently poorer prognosis. The large majority of micropapillary carcinomas are ER- and PR positive, and up to one third show HER2 positivity.
- **Metaplastic carcinomas** are heterogeneous tumors with malignant spindle cells, squamous cell carcinoma, or heterologous elements, such as bone or cartilage (Fig. 17-24E). Adenocarcinoma may be absent, but cytokeratin immunostains are at least focally present. These tumors typically cluster with the basal molecular subgroup on gene expression profiling (see below). Subtypes of this tumor have differing prognoses.

PROGNOSTIC FACTORS

Breast Cancer Staging

Breast cancer survival is strongly influenced by tumor stage, expressed as the TNM classification (tumor [T], regional lymph nodes [N], and distant metastasis [M]) (Table 17-3). Breast cancer spreads (1) by direct extension (e.g., to chest wall); (2) via lymphatics to axillary, internal mammary, and infra- and supraclavicular lymph nodes; and (3) hematogenously to distant sites. "Inflammatory breast cancer" has a particularly poor prognosis. This tumor features cutaneous edema, erythema, induration, and warmth and tenderness of overlying skin, resulting in an orange peel–like ("peau d'orange") appearance. Arm edema and pain may also occur, probably because of lymphatic obstruction by tumor. These findings correspond to tumor invasion of dermal lymphatic vessels.

Table 17-3

Pathologic Tumor Staging

pTis	Carcinoma in situ (ductal or lobar) or Paget disease without invasive carcinoma
pT1mic	Microinvasion (≤1 mm)
pT1a	Invasive tumor >1 mm but ≤5 mm
pT1b	Invasive tumor >5 mm but ≤1 cm
pT1c	Invasive tumor >1 cm but ≤2 cm
pT2	Invasive tumor >2 cm but ≤5 cm
pT3	Invasive tumor >5 cm
pT4	Edema or tumor ulcerating through skin or satellite skin nodules and/or chest wall invasion[a] or inflammatory breast carcinoma

[a]Does not include invasion of the pectoralis muscle.

Data from Edge SB, Byrd DR, Compton CC, et al., eds. *AJCC Cancer Staging Manual.* 7th ed. New York, NY: Springer; 2009.

Tumor Size

The prognosis of breast cancer varies with tumor size (T in the TNM protocol): patients with larger tumors show poorer survival. In assessing tumor size, only the invasive part is considered. Some locally advanced tumors are staged T4, based on skin or chest wall invasion, regardless of tumor size.

Lymph Node Status

The presence or absence of axillary lymph node metastases is a key prognostic indicator for patients with breast cancer. Axillary dissection risks significant postoperative morbidity (i.e., lymphedema and nerve damage), but sentinel lymph node (SLN) biopsy reduces this risk. This procedure requires injection of a dye or radioactive isotope and involves intraoperative lymphatic mapping of the draining or "sentinel" lymph node, the node most likely to contain breast cancer metastases. If it is negative, axillary dissection can safely be avoided. The actual impact of small metastases on the prognosis is small.

Distant Metastases

Distant metastases portend a poor prognosis. Breast cancers metastasize to bone, which is where metastatic disease presents in 25% of cases. Of women who die of breast cancer, 70% eventually develop bone involvement. Smaller percentages of patients have other metastases, usually to lung, liver, central nervous system, skin, and adrenal glands.

Tumor Grade

Histopathologic grading of breast tumors is one of the critical components of decision making. The Nottingham grading system, also called the modified Bloom and Richardson method, is the most widely used. It combines scores for tubule formation, nuclear pleomorphism, and mitotic count into a final grade of 1, 2, or 3 for low-, intermediate-, and high-grade carcinomas, respectively (Fig. 17-25). Patients with grade 1 tumors have a significantly better survival than those with grade 2 or grade 3 tumors.

Other Prognostic Features

- **Proliferative index and ploidy:** Tumors with a high proliferative index have worse prognoses than those with few mitoses. Several parameters are used to assess proliferation in breast cancers, including (1) mitotic index, assessed histologically; (2) the proportion of cells in the S phase of the cell cycle, determined by flow cytometry; (3) immunohistochemical staining for proteins (Ki67) expressed by actively proliferating cells; and (4) thymidine labeling index. Cell cycle analysis can also detect aneuploidy, which occurs in two thirds of breast cancers and confers a poorer prognosis. Notably, much of the prognostic impact of multigene predictor signatures (discussed below) comes from proliferation genes.
- **Estrogen and progesterone receptors:** Steroid receptor proteins are expressed by benign breast epithelium in 70% to 80% of breast cancers (ER > PR). ER and PR status is determined by immunohistochemistry, which uses antibodies to detect these nuclear receptors. Hormone receptor status is defined as positive when at least 1% of tumor cells stain (ie. are immunopositive). ER and PR estrogen and progesterone and stimulate cell growth. The greatest value

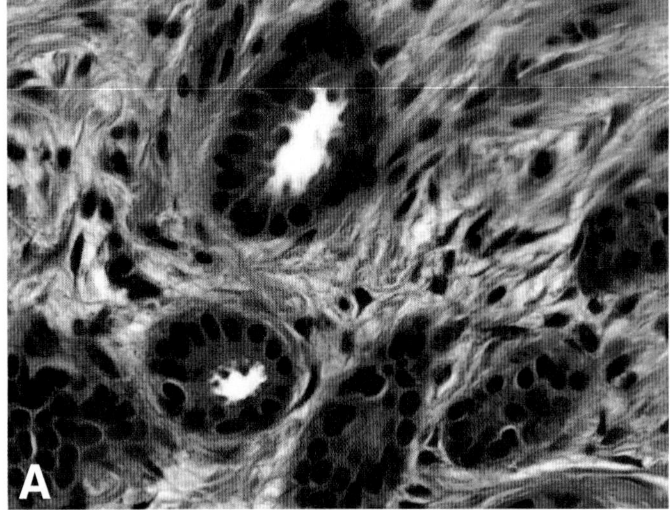

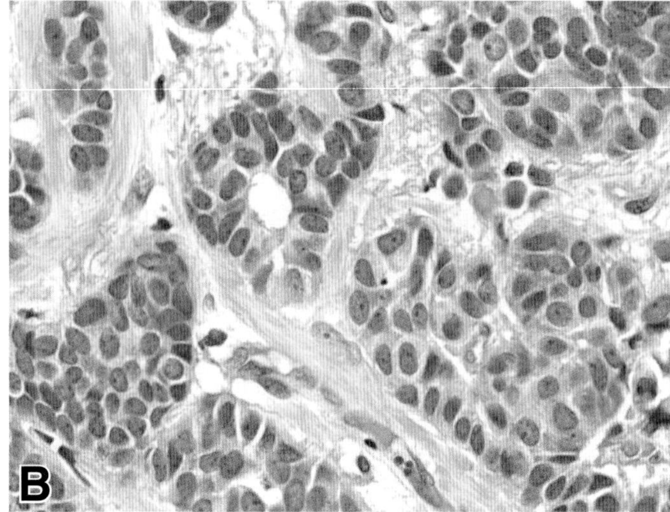

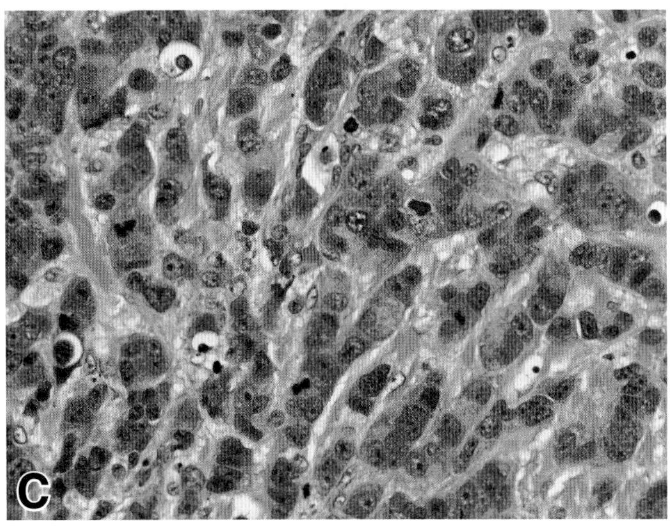

FIGURE 17-25. Tumor histologic grade. A. Low-grade invasive carcinoma showing good tubule formation, mild nuclear pleomorphism, and inconspicuous mitoses. **B. Moderately differentiated** carcinoma with less tubule formation, moderate nuclear pleomorphism, and variably prominent mitoses. **C. Poorly differentiated** carcinoma showing absent tubule formation, marked nuclear pleomorphism, and frequent mitotic figures.

of assessing hormone receptor status in breast cancer is its predictive ability. Patients with ER/PR-negative tumors are unlikely to respond to hormonal therapies with antiestrogens; on the other hand, patients with ER/PR-positive tumors show a greater probability of response.

- **HER2:** Overexpression or gene amplification (see Chapter 5) of HER2 occurs in 15% to 20% of newly diagnosed breast cancers. HER2 positivity is an adverse prognostic factor irrespective of lymph node status. However, these patients may be treated with monoclonal antibodies or tyrosine kinase inhibitors that target HER2. As with hormone receptor status, many patients who express HER2 show de novo or eventual resistance to such drugs. Immunohistochemistry detects cell membrane expression of the protein, and in situ hybridization identifies gene amplification (Fig. 17-26).

Molecular Subtypes

Microarray gene expression profiling and other techniques have identified a set of genes, an "intrinsic gene list," of which several molecular subgroups (Table 17-4) appear to predict clinical outcome and response to therapy.

- **Luminal A:** The luminal groups (A and B) are characterized by gene expression patterns similar to those of normal breast luminal epithelial cells, including low-molecular-weight cytokeratins 8/18, and ER and ER-associated genes. Luminal A tumors are typically of low grade and have an excellent prognosis.
- **Luminal B** tumors also express ER and ER-associated genes but are usually of higher grade than luminal A tumors. They exhibit higher proliferative indices and have a slightly worse prognosis than luminal A tumors.
- **HER2:** Tumors that overexpress HER2 are sometimes associated with ER negativity. These tumors behave aggressively, but targeting HER2 with an antibody, trastuzumab, has significantly increased patient longevity.
- **Basal-like cancers:** These highly aggressive tumors constitute 10% to 20% of invasive breast carcinomas. They are mainly ER and HER2 negative. Their name derives from their consistent expression of genes in the basal or myoepithelial cells of the breast, including high-molecular-weight cytokeratins 5/6, 14, and 17; caveolins 1 and 2; nestin; p63; and epidermal growth factor receptor (EGFR). These tumors are distinctive; are of high nuclear grade; and have many mitoses, pushing margins, central areas of necrosis or fibrosis, and a lymphocytic infiltrate. Cancers with medullary features and metaplastic carcinomas are typically basal-like. Most cancers arising in patients with germline *BRCA1* mutations are basal-like.

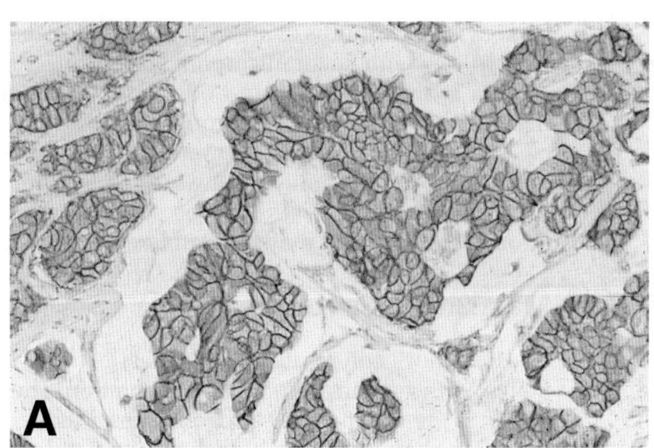

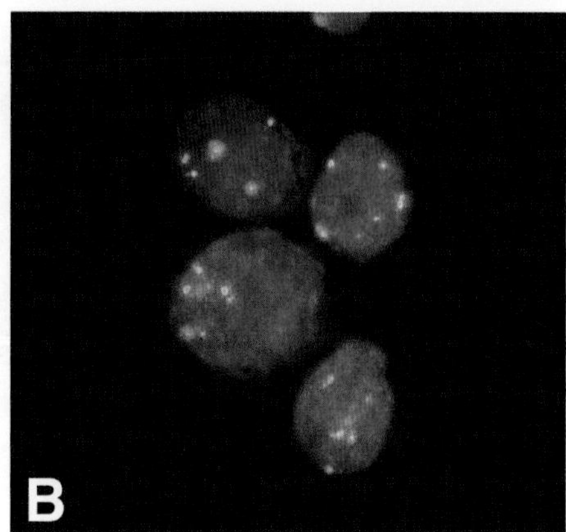

FIGURE 17-26. HER2/neu abnormalities in a breast cancer. A. Immunoperoxide staining of an invasive ductal carcinoma shows overexpression of the *HER2* (erbB-2) protein. **B.** Fluorescence in situ hybridization methodology identifies the gene copies of *HER2* (erbB-2) in cancer cells. The *HER2* probe is red, and a normal cell should have two copies. More than two copies indicates *HER2* gene amplification. The green probe identifies the centromeric region of chromosome 17.

Prognostic Assays

Although a large proportion of patients with breast cancer are treated with adjuvant chemotherapy, not all benefit from the therapy. In recent years, gene expression prognostic assays have been developed. Commercially available approaches quantify messenger RNA (mRNA) levels for a panel of genes. Analysis of respective gene expression levels leads to a prognostic score of potential use in guiding therapy. However, questions pertaining to the utility and degree of robustness of these different commercial products still exist. ***Importantly, in guiding treatment decisions and evaluating prognosis, these tools complement, but do not replace, histopathology and clinical analyses.***

Genetic analysis has demonstrated that breast cancers are markedly heterogeneous, and only a few gene mutations are actually present in a high percentage of tumors. These include *PTEN, PIK3CA,* and *TP53.* Analysis of matched primary and metastatic tumors shows that tumors are largely mosaics of subclones of cancer cells, and metastases may derive from genetically distinct subpopulations in the primary tumor (see Chapter 5).

THE MALE BREAST

Gynecomastia

Gynecomastia (Fig. 17-27) is benign enlargement of the male breast, with proliferation of ductal and stromal elements. It is due to decreased levels of androgens or increased estrogen effects. Breast enlargement resulting from adipose tissue is called **pseudogynecomastia**.

Physiologic gynecomastia occurs in most neonates owing to circulating maternal and placental estrogen and progesterone. Transient gynecomastia also affects over half of boys during puberty because estrogen production peaks earlier than that of testosterone. With increasing age, free testosterone decreases and adipose tissue expands, increasing the prevalence of breast enlargement.

Nonphysiologic gynecomastia results from the administration of certain drugs or disorders associated with low testosterone levels, high conversion of testosterone to estrogens, elevated estrogen levels, and increased sex hormone–binding globulin levels that lower free testosterone. It may occur in

Table 17-4

Molecular Subtypes of Breast Cancer

Molecular Subgroup	ER	PR	HER2	Proliferation Index	Other	Prognosis	Treatment
Luminal A	+	+	–	Low	CK8/18	Excellent	Hormonal
Luminal B	+	+	–/+	Moderate	CK8/18	Intermediate	Hormonal and chemotherapy
HER2+	–	–	+	High	AR	Poor	Trastuzumab Anthracyclines
Basal	–	–	–	Very high	CK5/6, CK14, vimentin, EGFR, c-kit	Poor	Platinum- and anthracycline-based chemotherapy PARP inhibitors

+, positive; –, negative; –/+, sometimes positive; AR, androgen receptor; ER, estrogen receptor; PARP, poly(adenosine diphosphate ribose) polymerase; PR, progesterone receptor.

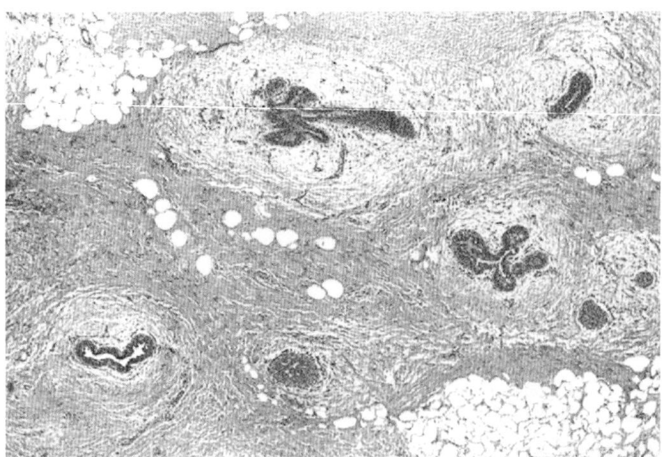

FIGURE 17-27. Gynecomastia. There is proliferation of branching, intermediate-sized ducts. The ductal epithelium is hyperplastic, and mitoses are present. A concomitant increase in the surrounding fibrous tissue causes a palpable mass.

patients with hyperthyroidism, cirrhosis, renal failure, and chronic lung disease. Certain hormone-producing tumors, including Leydig and Sertoli cell tumors, testicular germ cell tumors, and cancers of the liver and lung, may also result in gynecomastia. Drugs implicated in gynecomastia include digitalis, cimetidine, spironolactone, cannabis (marijuana), and tricyclic antidepressants.

Gynecomastia presents as a rubbery discrete mass or ill-defined area of induration that may display either a florid or fibrous phase (Fig. 17-27). The florid phase typically occurs early, within 6 months of onset. It is characterized by epithelial hyperplasia with flat or micropapillary architecture. Periductal stroma is hypercellular and edematous and demonstrates increased vascularity and chronic inflammation.

The fibrous phase is seen after 1 year or more. It lacks epithelial proliferation, and the stroma is more collagenous. Mixtures of both phases may be seen. Pseudoangiomatous stromal hyperplasia may be seen in either phase.

Male Breast Cancer

These tumors constitute 1% of breast cancers in the United States, with a mean age of 65 at presentation. The risk of breast cancer is greater in high-estrogen states. Men with Klinefelter syndrome have a 58-fold higher risk than normal men and an absolute risk of up to 3%. Male to female transsexuals following castration and high-dose estrogen and men treated with estrogen for prostate cancer are also at greater risk.

Some men with breast cancer have inherited germline mutations in *BRCA2* and show other gene mutation patterns that are similar to some observed in female breast cancers (see Table 17-1). Ionizing radiation has been implicated, being seen in Japanese men after nuclear fallout and in patients treated with therapeutic chest irradiation at a young age.

Most breast cancers in males are invasive carcinoma, NST; however, papillary carcinoma is disproportionately represented in men. Lobular carcinoma is rare. Ninety percent of cancers are ER- and PR positive. Androgen receptor positivity is frequently seen.

Most patients present with a painless lump. Nipple involvement, including retraction, discharge, or ulceration, is an early event. Paget disease is a presenting feature in 1% of affected men. Clinical management of breast cancer in male patients largely reflects results of clinical studies done in women.

18 Hematopathology

Riccardo Valdez ▪ Mary M. Zutter ▪ Shauying Li ▪ Alina Dulau Florea ▪ Bruce M. McManus ▪ Michael F. Allard ▪ Robert Yanagawa

LEARNING OBJECTIVES

- Differentiate between pluripotent hematopoietic stem cells, marrow-based progenitor cells, and blasts.
- Define and provide normal values for marrow cellularity.
- Define trilineage hematopoiesis, M:E ratio, and left shift.
- Explain the significance of polychromatophilia.
- Summarize the developmental pathways of T and B cells.
- Define the terms "microcytic," "normocytic," and "macrocytic" in reference to anemia. Provide examples of anemias for which the terms are characteristic.
- Under what circumstance is reticulocytosis an expected finding?
- What are characteristic signs and clinical symptoms of iron-deficiency anemia?
- Differentiate between anisocytosis, poikilocytosis, leukoerytroblastosis, acanthocytosis, spherocytosis, and elliptocytosis.
- What roles do folate and B12 play in megaloblastic anemias?
- Discuss the etiology and pathophysiology of α- and β-thalassemia.
- Summarize the major forms of hemoglobin found in infants, adults, and thalassemics.
- Discuss the genetic lesion found in carrier thalassemia, thalassemia trait, hemoglobin H disease, and hydrops fetalis.
- Discuss the etiology and pathophysiology associated with spherocytosis, elliptocytosis, and acanthocytosis.
- Under what conditions does G6PD deficiency result in hemolytic anemia?
- Discuss the clinical consequences of sickle cell disease.
- Differentiate between warm antibody, cold agglutinin, and cold hemolysins-mediated autoimmune hemolytic anemias.
- List conditions associated with microangiopathic hemolytic anemias.
- Discuss the etiologies and clinical findings associated with aplastic anemia and Fanconi anemia.
- Discuss the etiology, pathogenesis, and clinical findings associated with paroxysmal nocturnal hemoglobinuria.
- Differentiate between relative, absolute, primary, and secondary polycythemia.
- What conditions are likely to be associated with benign lymphocytosis, bone marrow plamacytosis, and lymphocytopenia?
- Differentiate between various causes of reactive lymph node hyperplasia.
- Differentiate between acute and chronic leukemia and lymphoma.
- Differentiate between the clinical findings and presentation of B-ALL and T-ALL.
- What are the common immunphenotypes of B-ALL and T-ALL?
- Describe the clinical findings and immunophenotype of B-cell chronic lymphocytic leukemia.
- List the most common mature B-cell lymphomas, stating the presumed cell of origin, distinctive features of immunophenotype, and clinical presentation.
- What is the cell of origin and clinical presentation of MALT lymphomas (MALTomas)?
- What characteristic genetic event defines most mantle cell lymphomas? What is a characteristic finding of their immunophenotype?
- Differentiate between sporadic, endemic, and immunodeficiency-associated Burkitt lymphoma. What is the relationship of c-MYC to this disease?
- Differentiate between MGUS and plasma cell lymphoma.
- What characteristic array of clinical findings is associated with plasma cell myeloma?
- Describe the etiology, immunophenotype, and clinical findings in adult T-cell leukemia/lymphoma.
- Differentiate between the characteristic clinical findings in mycosis fungoides and Sézary syndrome.
- Describe the histopathology of the subtypes of classic Hodgkin lymphoma and nodular lymphocyte-predominant Hodgkin lymphoma.
- What are the characteristic clinical findings in Hodgkin lymphoma?
- Distinguish between the immunophenotype and histopathology of nodular lymphocyte-predominant and classic Hodgkin disease.
- Outline common causes of neutropenia.
- Define the term "leukemoid reaction" and note common hematologic findings associated with it.

- Describe the characteristic karyotypic and molecular abnormalities associated with chronic myelogenous leukemia and explain how they are involved with disease etiology.
- Delineate the clinical phases and associated hematologic abnormalities of chronic myelogenous leukemia.
- Describe the characteristic genetic abnormalities and clinical findings associated with polycythemia vera and primary myelofibrosis.
- Differentiate between cutaneous and systemic mastocytosis in terms of molecular abnormalities and clinical findings.
- Define the general characteristics of myelodysplastic syndromes.
- What is the characteristic immunophenotype and clinical findings in acute myeloid leukemia?
- Define the clinical variants of Langerhans cell histiocytosis and describe the histopathology and clinical findings associated with them.
- Present an overview of the cellular and humoral components necessary for normal hemostasis.
- Present a stepwise overview of primary hemostasis, emphasizing the role of platelets.
- Present a stepwise overview of secondary hemostasis, describing how it interacts with primary hemostasis.
- What are critical factors that promote platelet adhesion and aggregation?
- Describe the components and function of the prothrombinase, Xase 1, and Xase 2 complexes.
- Describe the components and function of the anticoagulant complex.
- Describe critical components of the thrombolytic pathway.
- Describe major causes of thrombocytopenia.
- Describe the etiology, pathogenesis, and clinical consequences of idiopathic (immune) thrombocytopenic purpura (ITP).
- Describe the etiology, pathogenesis, and clinical consequences of thrombotic thrombocytopenic purpura (TTP).
- Describe important hereditary diseases of platelets.
- Differentiate between hemophilia A, hemophilia B, and von Willebrand disease in terms of genetics, hematologic abnormalities, and clinical presentation.
- Differentiate between the subtypes of vWD in terms of the molecular, biochemical, and functional presentation.
- What is the effect of vitamin K deficiency on humoral coagulation factors?
- What is the etiology and pathogenesis associated with DIC?
- What are common causes of thrombophilia?
- Describe the etiology, pathogenesis, and clinical findings associated with the antiphospholipid syndrome? What are lupus anticoagulants?

HEMATOPOIETIC STEM CELLS

Bone marrow consists of a complex network of solid cords containing stromal and hematopoietic cells, knitted together by extracellular matrix, which are separated by sinusoids. A semipermeable barrier between sinusoids and cords consists of an endothelial cell layer, a thin basement membrane, and an outer layer of interrupted reticular adventitial cells. The reticular adventitial cells branch extensively throughout the cords and help anchor stromal and hematopoietic cells. Bone marrow stromal cells include macrophages, endothelial cells, lymphocytes, and fibroblasts.

Pluripotent hematopoietic stem cells (HSCs) compromise a self-perpetuating pool in the bone marrow, in which self-renewal balances differentiation and exit (Fig. 18-1). The stem cells are admixed with progenitor and more mature hematopoietic cells, with HSCs representing only a small proportion of total hematopoietic cell mass. They are small, mononuclear, and difficult to identify by microscopy. HSCs are semidormant (noncycling) cells that differentiate to progenitor cells of specific lineages as needed.

Like stem cells, progenitor cells are small- to medium-sized mononuclear cells that resemble mature lymphocytes. In culture, they give rise to colonies of differentiated progeny. Progenitor cells, committed to red blood cell production ("burst-forming unit, erythroid" [BFU-E]), differentiate into a final progenitor cell (the "colony-forming unit, erythroid" [CFU-E]), which produces a small clone of mature erythroblasts in culture.

Granulocytic and monocytic cell lines also derive from a single progenitor cell. This cell, named the "colony-forming unit, granulocyte-monocyte" (CFU-GM), proceeds to a colony with both granulocytic and monocytic cells. As the cell matures, its progeny is increasingly committed to polymorphonuclear leukocytes (also termed "granulocytes") (CFU-G) or monocyte/macrophages (CFU-M). Eosinophils and basophils also have specific progenitor cells (CFU-Eo and CFU-Ba, respectively). Megakaryocytic progenitor cells (CFU-Meg) produce colonies in vitro consisting of four to eight megakaryocytes.

Hematopoiesis in the bone marrow responds to fluctuating needs for blood cells and maintains the size of the circulating blood cell mass. Growth factors mediate this responsiveness by regulating the rate of cellular proliferation, primarily in the progenitor cell compartment (Fig. 18-1). Deficiencies in one or more blood cell populations (e.g., postchemotherapy pancytopenia, especially neutropenia, ablative conditioning prior to bone marrow transplantation, and renal failure; see below) respond to treatment with several growth factors, including granulocyte-macrophage colony-stimulating factor (GM-CSF), granulocyte colony-stimulating factor (G-CSF), and erythropoietin (EPO). When released by renal interstitial peritubular cells in response to hypoxia, EPO activates erythroid progenitor cells. Progenitor cells mature into precursor cells, or **blasts**. Starting at the precursor stage, and continuing beyond, cells are morphologically recognizable in terms of their lineage. Maturation of precursor cells to mature cells entails progressive nuclear changes and cytoplasmic maturation to reflect cellular functions (e.g., oxygen carriage in red blood cells, cytotoxic enzymes in neutrophils). In parallel, lineage-related cell surface proteins/antigens appear. Such stage-specific antigens help to identify both cell types and stages of maturation.

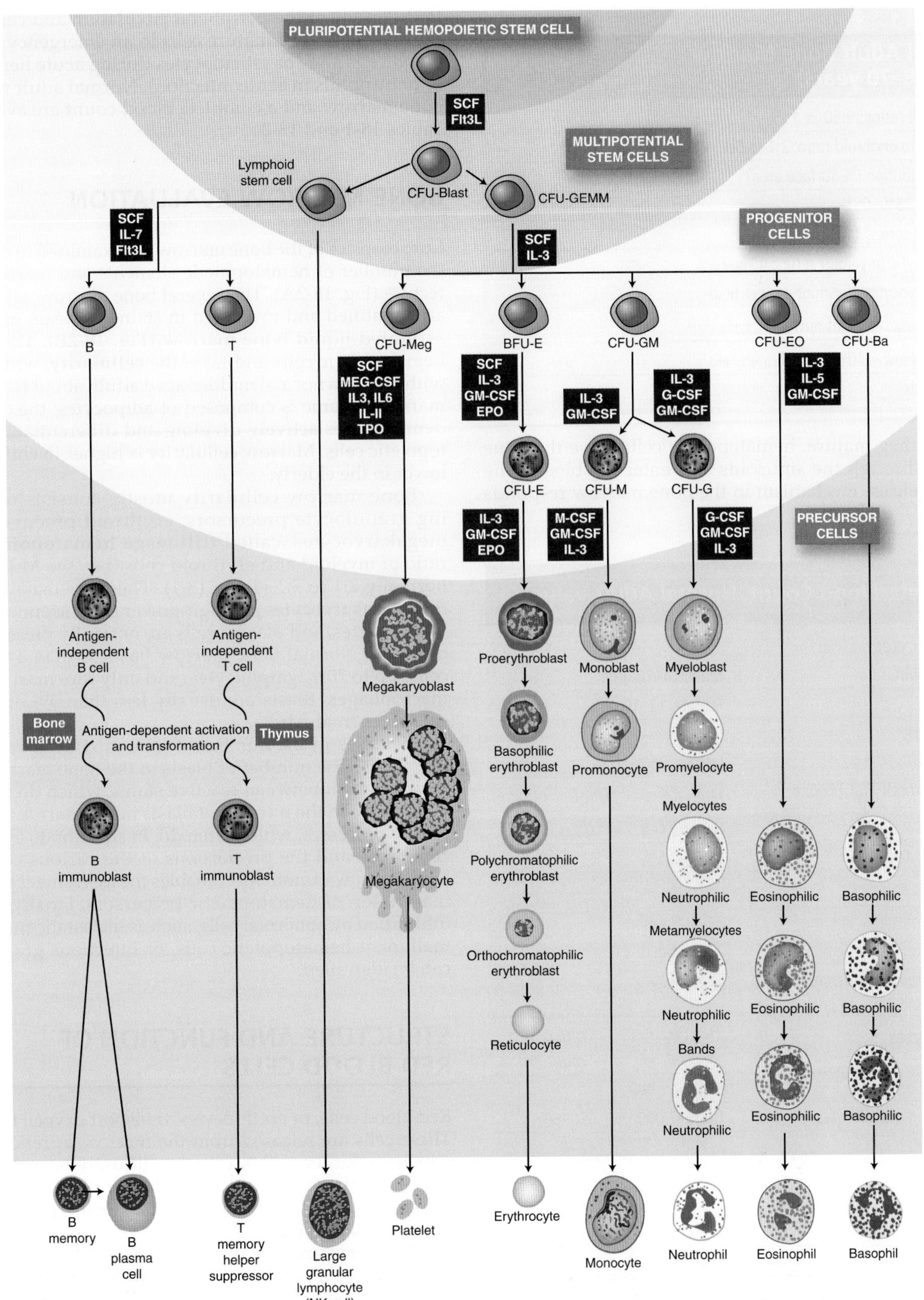

FIGURE 18-1. Cellular differentiation and maturation of the lymphoid and myeloid components of the hematopoietic system. Only the precursor cells (blasts and maturing cells) are identifiable by light microscopic evaluation of the bone marrow. BFU, burst-forming unit; CFU, colony-forming unit (Ba, basophils; E, erythroid; EO, eosinophils; G, polymorphonuclear leukocytes; GM, granulocyte-monocyte; M, monocyte/macrophages; Meg, megakaryocytic); CSF, colony-stimulating factor, G-CSF, granulocyte colony-stimulating factor; M-CSF, macrophage colony-stimulating factor; MEG-CSF, megakaryocyte colony-stimulating factor; EPO, erythropoietin; GM-CSF, granulocyte-macrophage colony-stimulating factor; IL, interleukin; NK, natural killer; SCF, stem cell factor; TPO, thrombopoietin.

Table 18-1

Normal Adult Bone Marrow (Age 18–70 years)
Fat to cell ratio: 50:50 ± 15%
Myeloid to erythroid ratio: 2:1 to 5:1
Cell distribution (% surface area)
Fat cells: 35%–65%
Erythroid series: 10%–20%
Granulocytic (myeloid) series: 40%–65%
Megakaryocytes: 2–5/high-power field
Plasma cells: <3% of nucleated cells
Lymphocytes: <20% of nucleated cells
No fibrosis

After they mature, hematopoietic cells leave the bone marrow through the sinusoids and enter the blood. The cellular release mechanism in the bone marrow responds to the needs of the peripheral circulation and can quickly provide a boost of mature cells in an emergency (e.g., red blood cells and/or reticulocytes during acute hemorrhage or neutrophils in acute infection). Normal adult values for bone marrow and a complete blood count are available in Tables 18-1 and 18-2.

Table 18-2

Complete Blood Count: Normal Adult Values		
Erythrocytes		
Hemoglobin	Male, 14–18 g/dL	
	Female, 12–16 g/dL	
Hematocrit	Male, 40%–54%	
	Female, 35%–47%	
Red blood cell (RBC) count	Male, 4.5–6 × 10^6/μL	
	Female, 4–5.5 × 10^6/μL	
Reticulocytes	0.5%–2.5%	
Indices		
Mean corpuscular volume	82–100 μm^3	
Mean corpuscular hemoglobin	27–34 pg	
Mean corpuscular hemoglobin concentration	32%–36%	
Leukocytes	*Absolute count/μL*	*Differential count (%)*
White blood cells	4,000–11,000	
Neutrophil granulocytes	1,800–7,000	50–60
Neutrophil bands	0–700	2–4
Lymphocytes	1,500–4,000	30–40
Monocytes	0–800	1–9
Basophils	0–200	0–1
Eosinophils	0–450	0–3
Platelets		
Quantitative normal value: 150,000–400,000/μL		
Qualitative estimation on smear: number of platelets/oil immersion field × 10,000 = estimated platelet count		
Normal ratio of RBC and platelets = 15:1 to 20:1		

BONE MARROW EVALUATION

Core biopsies of the bone marrow are examined to determine the number of hematopoietic elements and marrow architecture (Fig. 18-2A). The several bone marrow cell lineages are identified and evaluated in stained smears made from aspirated liquid bone marrow (Fig. 18-2B). The ratio of hematopoietic cells and fat is the **cellularity**, which varies with age. In a normal middle-aged adult, about half of bone marrow volume is composed of adipocytes; the other half demonstrates actively dividing and differentiating hematopoietic cells. Marrow cellularity is higher in children and lower in the elderly.

Bone marrow cellularity mostly consists of maturing granulocyte precursors, erythroid precursors, and megakaryocytes, called **trilineage hematopoiesis**. The ratio of myeloid and erythroid cells (i.e., the **M:E ratio**) is normally 2:1 to 5:1 (Table 18-1). There are usually two to five megakaryocytes per high-power field. Monocytic cells, lymphocytes, and plasma cells are normally present in low numbers. Normal bone marrow has less than 3% plasma cells, up to 20% lymphocytes, and only rare mast cells and macrophages. Blasts are usually less than 3% of marrow cells in normal adults.

Increases in the number of immature cells are termed **left shifts**. The number of blasts in the bone marrow helps to distinguish between reactive states, which do not show an increase in the number of blasts in the marrow and neoplastic processes, which often do. In addition to evaluating cellularity and the proportions of the various cell types, bone marrow examination enables the assessment of normal maturation of hematopoietic precursors. Finally, marrow infiltration by abnormal cells, such as metastatic tumor cells, malignant hematopoietic cells, or infectious granulomas, can be identified.

STRUCTURE AND FUNCTION OF RED BLOOD CELLS

Red blood cells, or erythrocytes, transport oxygen to tissues. These cells are released from the marrow as reticulocytes, which are larger and have more diffusely basophilic gray cytoplasm than mature RBCs. Reticulocytes still synthesize hemoglobin, and the ribosomes needed for this process impart **polychromatophilia**.

RBC membranes are attached to an underlying cytoskeletal network (Fig. 18-3), defects of which lead to abnormal red cell shape and shortened life span (see below). Transmembrane receptors, channels, and anchors for other membrane components insert into the lipid bilayer, as does the underlying cytoskeleton. The average life span of RBCs is 120 days. Changes in membrane proteins and phospholipids appear in aged red cells and are likely signals for their removal by mononuclear phagocytes.

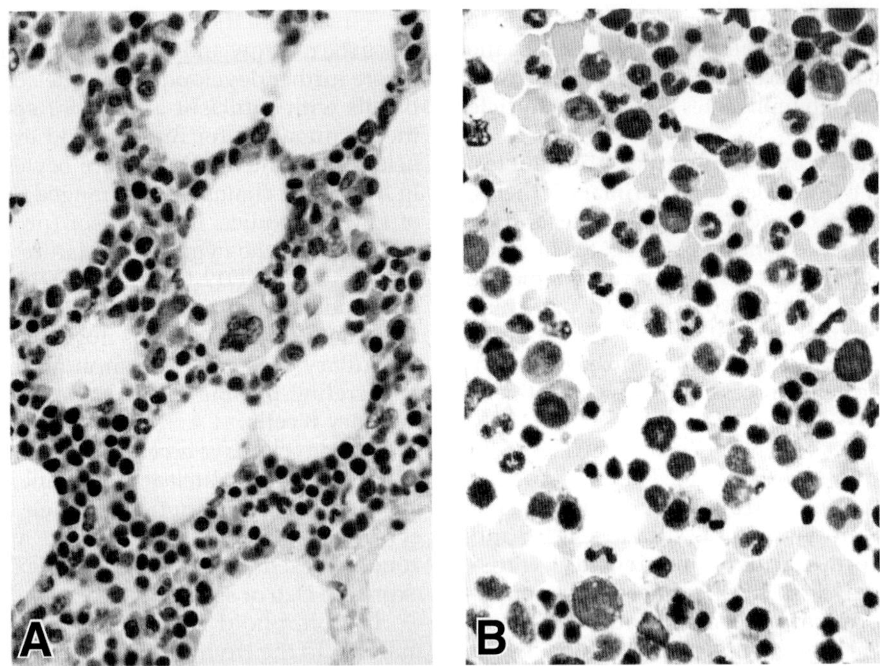

FIGURE 18-2. Normal bone marrow. A. Tissue section showing the normal relationship of cellular hematopoietic elements to fat cells, a normal myeloid to erythroid ratio (2:1) and a megakaryocyte in the center of the field (hematoxylin and eosin stain). **B.** Bone marrow aspirate smear from the same patient demonstrating normal hematopoietic elements in varying stages of differentiation (Wright-Giemsa stain).

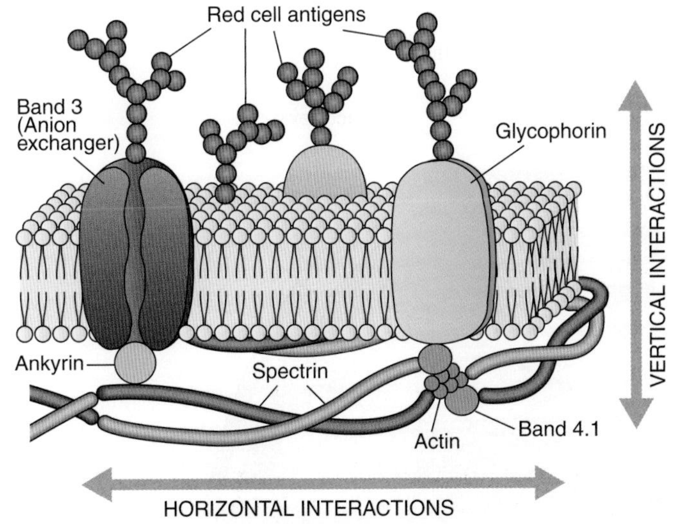

FIGURE 18-3. Structure of the erythrocyte plasma membrane. The membrane is stabilized by a number of interactions. The two vertical interactions are spectrin-ankyrin–band 3 and spectrin-protein 4.1–glycophorin. The two horizontal connections are spectrin heterodimers and spectrin-actin–protein 4.1.

STRUCTURE AND FUNCTION OF PLATELETS

Platelets are derived from megakaryocytes via the process of proplatelet formation and fragmentation. Thrombopoiesis requires the marrow microenvironment, plus stimulation by thrombopoietin (TPO). TPO is produced by the liver and binds the TPO receptor, c-Mpl, to stimulate megakaryocyte proliferation and differentiation. Mature megakaryocytes undergo proplatelet formation and fragmentation, which releases 1,000 to 4,000 anucleate platelets (see also "Hemostasis and Thrombosis" section below).

STRUCTURE AND FUNCTION OF LYMPH NODES AND LYMPHOCYTES

The lymphoid system consists of circulating T and B lymphocytes, natural killer cells (NK cells), and the secondary lymphoid organs, which mainly include the lymph nodes, spleen, and thymus. In addition to the tonsils in the oropharynx and nasopharynx (Waldeyer ring), aggregates of organized lymphoid tissue, known as mucosa-associated lymphoid tissue (MALT), are also present in extranodal sites, such as the gut, lungs, and skin. Peyer patches in the terminal ileum are a prototypic example of MALT.

All three major types of lymphocytes (T cells, B cells, and NK cells) develop from lymphoid stem cells in the bone marrow (Fig. 18-1). T cells mature and differentiate in the thymus. B cells undergo activation, transformation, and selection in the lymph nodes and spleen. NK cells do not go through a thymic or lymph node education phase, but rather are released into the peripheral circulation, where they appear as large granular lymphocytes. All lymphocyte development entails a tightly controlled sequence of gene expression and silencing. This process gives rise to sequential gain and loss of nuclear material and changes in the expression of cytoplasmic and surface antigens. Patterns of antigenic expression identify the lineage and maturation stage of normal and neoplastic lymphoid cells.

Lymphocytes from the circulation enter the lymph node cortex by migrating through the tall endothelial cells of the postcapillary venules in the **paracortex**. T cells tend to remain in the paracortex, whereas B lymphocytes home to the **follicle germinal centers**.

The B-cell–rich cortex contains two types of follicles: (1) immunologically inactive follicles, called **primary follicles**; and (2) immunologically active follicles, termed **secondary follicles**. Primary follicles are cohesive aggregates of small lymphocytes without well-defined germinal centers or mantle zones. Secondary follicles contain germinal centers, in which large noncleaved lymphocytes (**centroblasts**) mingle with small and larger lymphocytes with cleaved nuclei (**centrocytes**). Interdigitating dendritic cells process and present antigens to T lymphocytes (Fig. 18-4).

B-cell progenitor cells arise in the bone marrow (Fig. 18-5), where they are present in low numbers. They express the early B-cell surface antigens **CD10** (called common acute leukemia/lymphoma antigen [CALLA]) and **CD19**, and the nuclear enzyme **terminal deoxynucleotidyl transferase**. These cells largely lack CD20, a marker present at high levels on the more mature B-cell populations, and also do not show cell membrane Ig light (L) chains. B-cell progenitors increase in number during viral infections and in bone marrow recovery after chemotherapy or stem cell transplantation.

A fraction of the bone marrow–derived progenitor B cells leave the marrow and home to lymph node germinal centers, where further development and selection occurs. Specifically, B cells with sufficient affinity for specific antigens survive the germinal center reaction and eventually leave the follicle compartment. As B lymphocytes mature, the genes for Ig heavy (H) chains are rearranged, leading to the synthesis of IgM antibodies. In precursor (progenitor) B cells, IgM is expressed in the cytoplasm. Mature B cells express the pan B-cell antigens CD19, CD20, and CD22, together with surface Ig light and heavy chains. After activation and clonal expansion in germinal centers, B cells migrate to the B-cell–dependent medullary cords of the lymph nodes. There, they become Ig-secreting **plasma cells**, or they exit the lymph nodes as **memory B cells**.

Plasma cells have eccentric nuclei with clumped chromatin marginated at the nuclear membrane, traditionally described as "clock-face chromatin." In their abundant blue-purple cytoplasm, plasma cells often have a clear paranuclear clear zone, representing the Golgi complex. Plasma cells no longer express CD20 or surface Ig.

The lymphoid stem cells that migrate from the bone marrow to the thymus are exposed to a number of thymic hormones that induce sequential expression of pan T-cell surface antigens, such as CD2, CD3, CD5, CD7, CD4, or CD8 (Fig. 18-6). Recombination of T-cell receptor genes

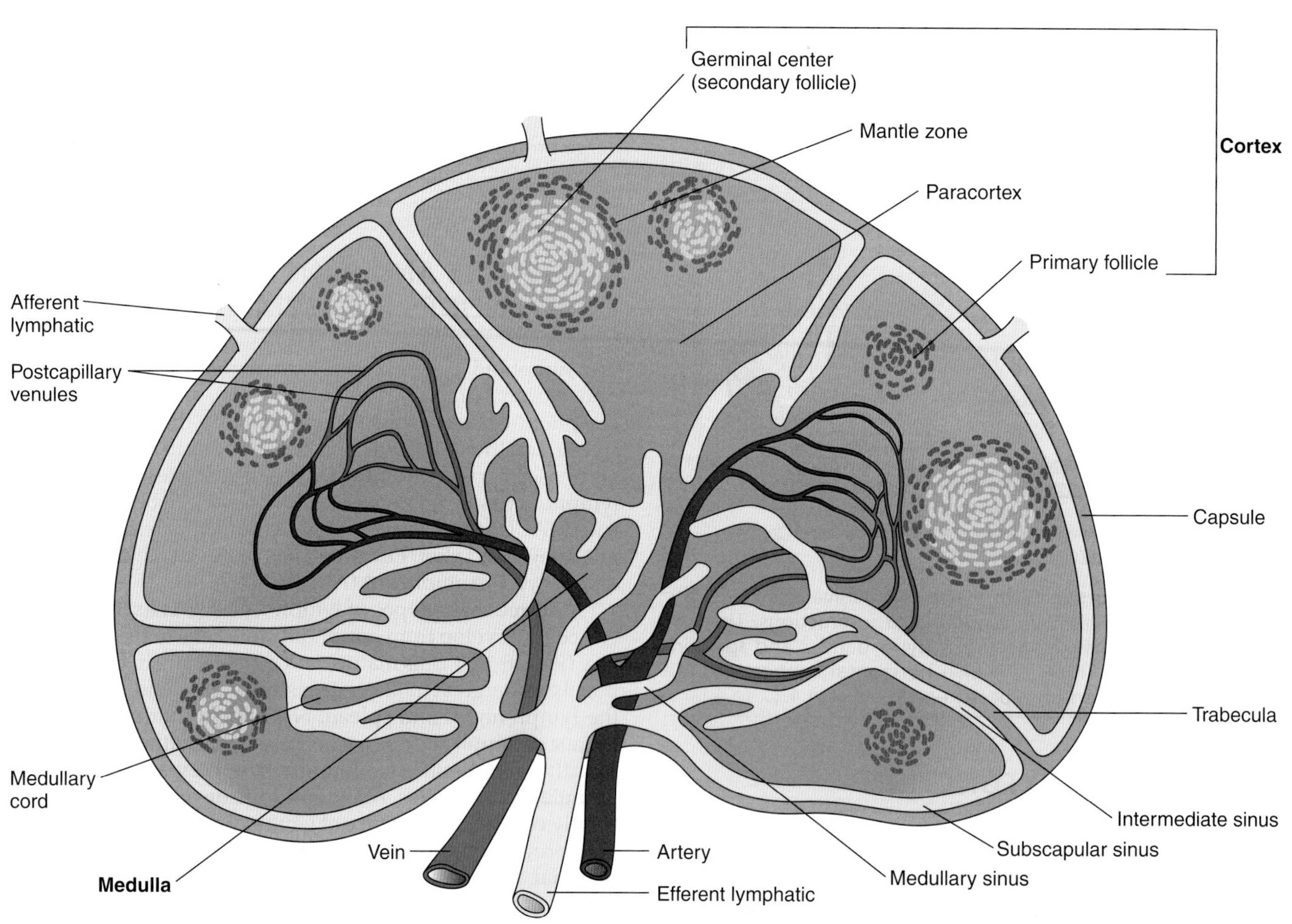

FIGURE 18-4. Structure of normal lymph node.

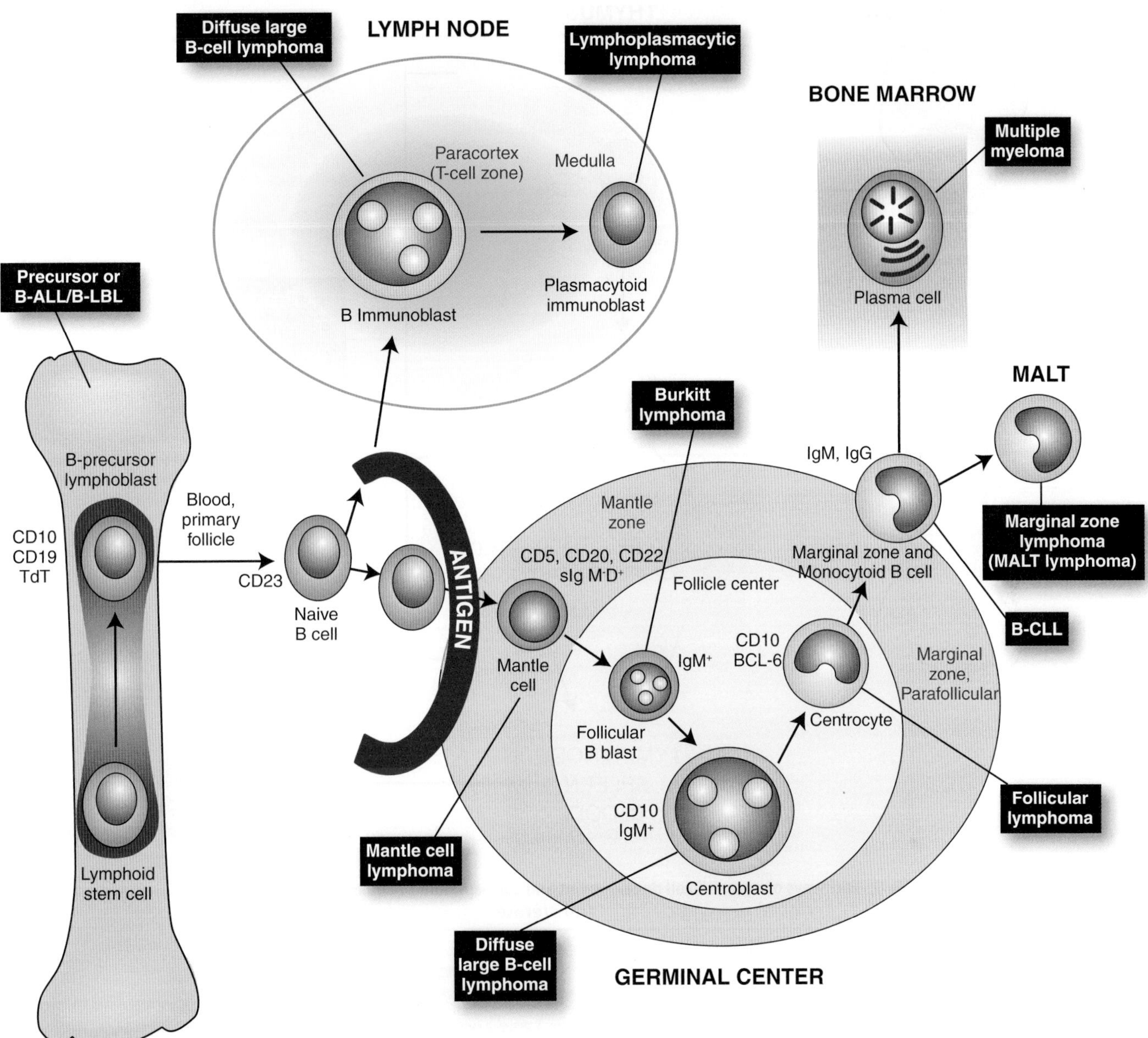

FIGURE 18-5. Pathway of normal B-cell differentiation and corresponding B-cell neoplasms. Following the lymphoid stem cell and precursor stage in the bone marrow, B cells mature into naive B lymphocytes and home to the secondary lymphoid organs (primarily lymph nodes). The germinal center reaction represents an important turntable for immunoglobulin (Ig) variable region gene mutations, Ig heavy-chain switch and differentiation into plasma cells and memory B cells. Cluster designation (CD) markers are shown. B-cell immunoblasts and plasmacytoid immunoblasts reside in the T-cell–rich paracortex and medulla, respectively. Marginal zone B cells home to mucosa-associated lymphoid tissue (MALT) sites and bone marrow. Neoplastic transformation occurs at all phases of B-cell differentiation. ALL/LBL, acute lymphoblastic leukemia/lymphoma; B-CLL, B-cell chronic lymphocytic leukemia; TdT, terminal deoxynucleotidyl transferase.

generates a diverse population of T cells, each of which can recognize a single antigen. T cells that cannot bind a foreign antigen with high affinity and T cells that recognize self-antigens are eliminated via apoptosis. Once mature and educated, T cells leave the thymus to reside in lymph nodes, spleen, and peripheral blood, where they become **post-thymic T cells**.

Natural killer (NK) cells, a small subset of lymphocytes lacking the usual T- or B-cell antigens, are cytotoxic effectors that do not require antigen recognition to initiate their killing function. They are large lymphocytes with granular cytoplasm (**large granular lymphocytes**). They differ from mature T cells in their lack of surface CD3 and possess other surface antigens, such as CD16 and CD56.

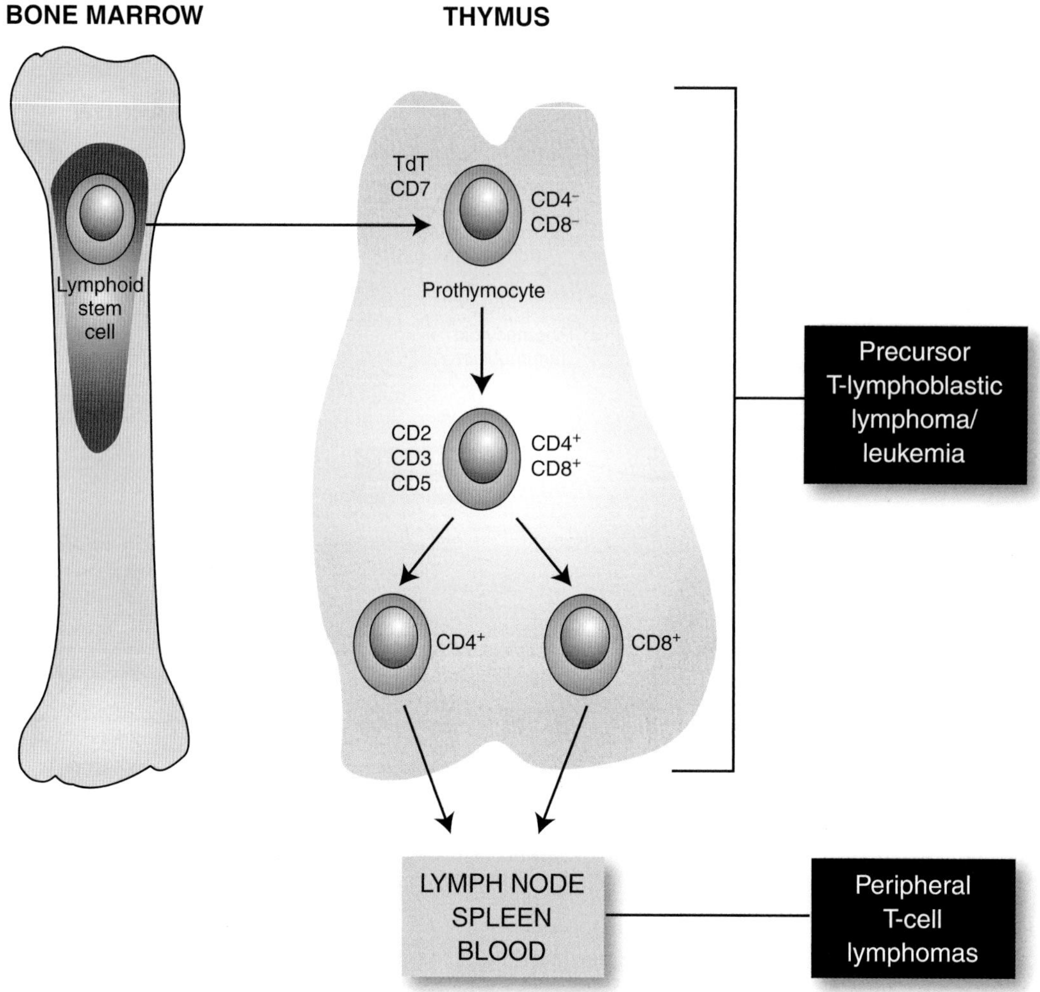

FIGURE 18-6. Pathways of normal T-cell development and corresponding T-cell neoplasms. CD, cluster designation; TdT, terminal deoxynucleotidyl transferase.

ANEMIA

Anemia is defined as a reduced circulating erythrocyte mass and is diagnosed as low hemoglobin, hematocrit (Hct, or RBC count. The low number of circulating erythrocytes in anemia results in decreased oxygen transport by the blood and ultimately tissue hypoxia. Anemias are divided into three groups based on cell size: **microcytic** (decreased mean corpuscular volume [MCV]), (2) **normocytic**, and (3) **macrocytic** (increased MCV) (Table 18-3). Abnormally shaped RBCs (**poikilocytes**) are seen on blood smears in many anemias (Fig. 18-7). Anemias can arise from four different mechanisms (Table 18-4):

- Acute blood loss
- Decreased production of red cells by the bone marrow because of stem cell or progenitor cell defects
- Ineffective hematopoiesis with reduced release of RBCs from bone marrow
- Increased RBC destruction outside the marrow, either intrinsic to the RBCs or the result of an external cause. In anemias with increased RBC destruction, the level of circulating reticulocytes is elevated (**reticulocytosis**) as a response to hypoxia.

Table 18-3

Morphologic Classification of Anemia

Macrocytic
Nutritional deficiency
Alcohol use
Liver disease
Microcytic
Iron deficiency
Thalassemias
Sideroblastic
Normocytic
Anemia of chronic disease/inflammation
Anemia of renal disease
Acute blood loss
Hypothyroidism
Reticulocytosis
Primary bone marrow disease

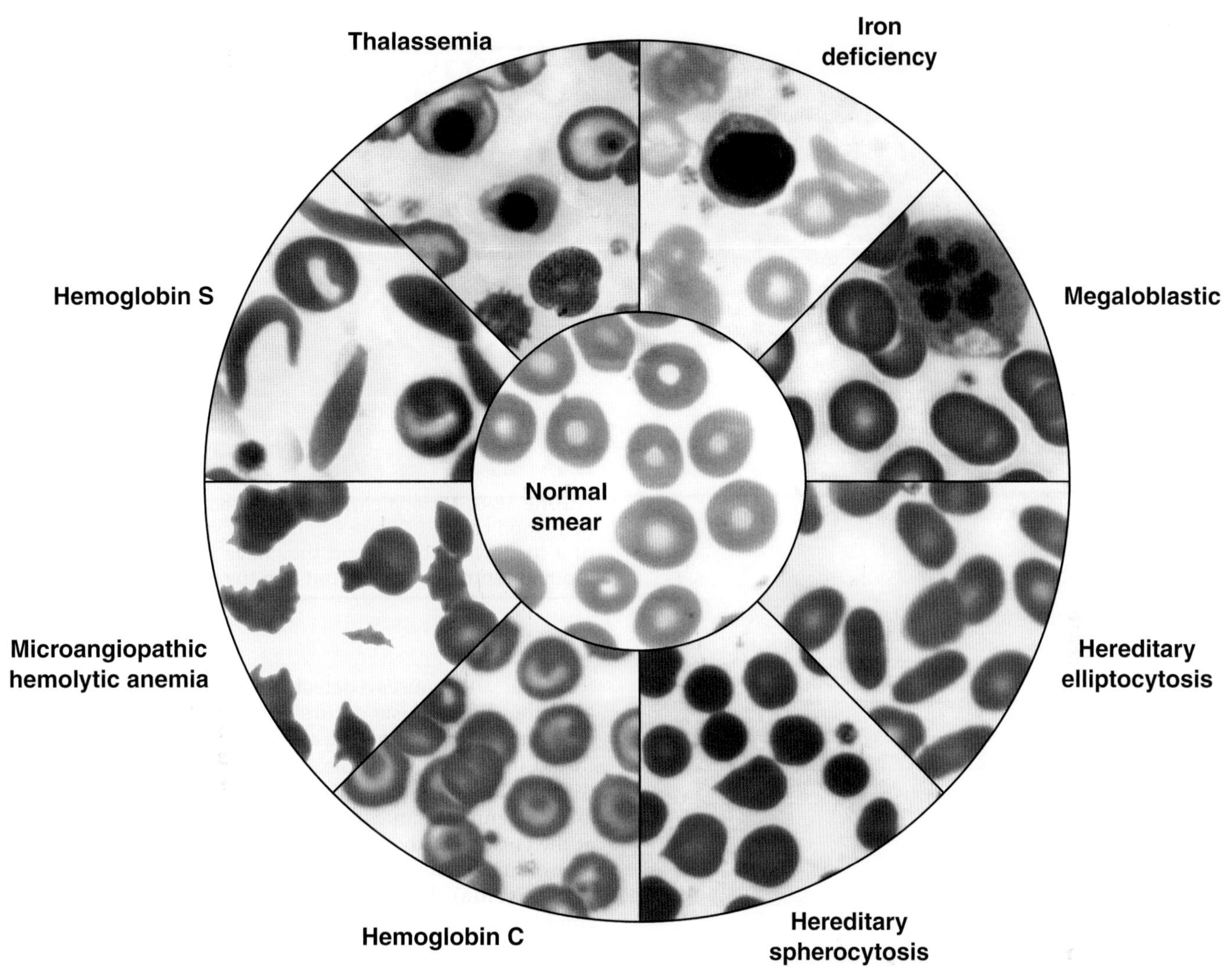

FIGURE 18-7. Abnormal red blood cell morphologies associated with various types of anemia. The morphology of normal erythrocytes is shown in the center. **Clockwise from 12:00: A. Iron deficiency (disturbance in hemoglobin synthesis; lack of iron):** Hypochromic, microcytic erythrocytes. A small lymphocyte is present for comparison. **B. Megaloblastic anemia (disturbance in DNA synthesis, most often caused by deficiency of vitamin B_{12} or folic acid):** Oval macrocytes, some irregularly shaped cells, and hypersegmented neutrophils. **C. Hereditary elliptocytosis (membrane defect):** Elliptocytes. **D. Hereditary spherocytosis (membrane defect):** Spherocytes lacking central pallor. **E. Hemoglobin C disease (abnormal globin chain):** Target cells. **F. Microangiopathic hemolysis (mechanical damage to erythrocytes;** disseminated intravascular coagulation [DIC], thrombocytic thrombocytopenic purpura [TTP], heart valve prosthesis sequela): Schistocytes/fragments. **G. Sickle cell (hemoglobin S) disease (abnormal globin chain):** Sickle cells. **H. Thalassemia (disturbance in hemoglobin synthesis):** Hypochromic, microcytic erythrocytes; poikilocytosis; basophilic stippling; target cells, nucleated red blood cells.

Anemia Secondary to Acute Blood Loss

Acute anemia reflects blood loss from the intravascular compartment. Initial signs of acute blood loss reflect volume depletion and decreased tissue perfusion. Because whole blood is lost, the severity of the anemia may not be appreciated at first. Within 24 to 48 hours after significant hemorrhage, fluid is mobilized from extravascular locations into the intravascular space to restore overall blood volume. This is the time when the extent of the anemia becomes apparent because red cell replacement is not as rapid as that of fluid. If the underlying bleeding is stopped, EPO-driven erythroid hyperplasia in the bone marrow will gradually correct the anemia. The blood smear shows no specific abnormalities, although polychromasia occurs during the recovery phase.

Anemia Secondary to Decreased Red Blood Cell Production

Some disorders in which RBC production is decreased are inherited or acquired diseases of hematopoietic stem cell or of their committed derivatives such as iron-deficiency anemia.

Table 18-4

Pathophysiologic Classification of Anemia

Acute Blood Loss
Decreased Production
Stem Cell and Progenitor Cell Defects
Iron deficiency
Anemia of chronic disease
Aplastic anemia
Pure red cell aplasia
Paroxysmal nocturnal hemoglobinuria
Leukemia
Myelodysplastic syndromes
Marrow infiltration
Lead poisoning
Anemia of renal disease
Ineffective Hematopoiesis
Megaloblastic anemia
Myelodysplastic syndromes
Thalassemia
Increased Destruction
Intracorpuscular
Membrane defect
Enzyme defect
Hemoglobinopathies
Extracorpuscular
Immunologic
Autoimmune
Alloimmune
Nonimmunologic
Mechanical
Hypersplenism
Infectious
Chemical

Iron-Deficiency Anemia

Iron deficiency interferes with normal heme (hemoglobin) synthesis and leads to impaired erythropoiesis and anemia. It is the most common cause of anemia worldwide. Iron deficiency is associated with a microcytic, hypochromic anemia (Fig. 18-8). Many underlying conditions cause iron deficiency. In infants and children, dietary iron may be insufficient for growth and development. Iron need also increases during **pregnancy** and **lactation**. In adults, iron deficiency typically results from **chronic blood loss** or, less often, **intravascular hemolysis**. In reproductive-aged women, **gynecologic blood loss** (menstruation, parturition, and vaginal bleeding) is most common. In postmenopausal women and men, unexplained iron deficiency should prompt a search for gastrointestinal **tumors** or **vascular lesions** because these are the most common sites of chronic blood loss.

Variation in RBC size (**anisocytosis**) and shape (**poikilocytosis**) results in increased variability in blood cell width.

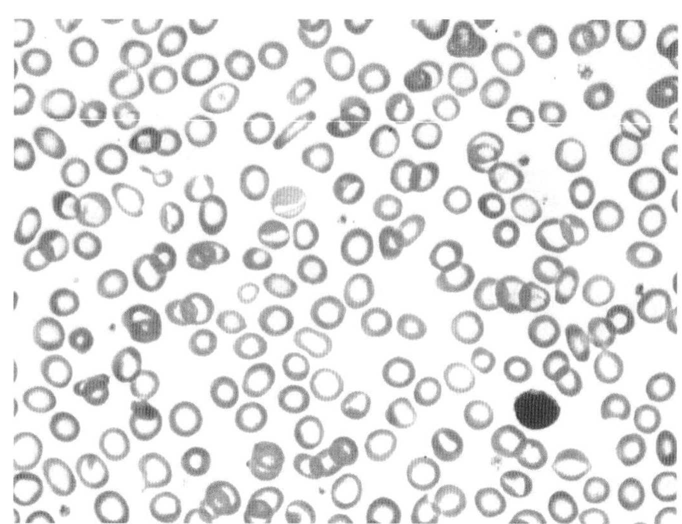

FIGURE 18-8. Microcytic hypochromic anemia caused by iron deficiency. Red blood cells (RBCs) are significantly smaller than the nucleus of a small lymphocyte, and they have increased central pallor (normal central pallor is about one third of the RBC diameter).

Iron deficiency causes a defect in RBC production, so marrow erythroid hyperplasia occurs but blood reticulocytosis does not. Prussian blue staining shows that iron storage and erythroid iron are absent. The symptoms of iron deficiency are those of anemia in general. With advanced disease, a smooth and glistening tongue (**atrophic glossitis**) and inflammation at the corners of the mouth (**angular cheilitis or stomatitis**) may occur, as may a spoon-shaped deformity of the fingernails (**koilonychia**). Treatment requires correcting the source of chronic blood loss and oral or parenteral iron supplementation.

Anemia of Chronic Disease

A mild-to-moderate anemia may occur in chronic inflammatory and malignant diseases.

Red cells are often normocytic and normochromic but can be microcytic. Reticulocyte counts are not appropriately increased for the degree of anemia. Chronic disease causes ineffective use of iron from macrophage stores in bone marrow, resulting in a functional iron deficiency, even though iron stores may be normal or even increased. Other factors that may contribute to anemia are shorter RBC life span, blunted renal EPO response to tissue hypoxia, and poor bone marrow response to EPO. Inflammatory cytokines (lactoferrin, IL-1, TNF-α, and interferon) may inhibit iron mobilization.

Anemia of Renal Disease

Anemia associated with chronic renal disease is normocytic and normochromic, the severity being proportional to the extent of renal insufficiency. Erythrocytes with scalloped cell membranes may sometimes be seen (**Burr cells**). If the renal insufficiency is due to malignant hypertension, red cells may be fragmented and form schistocytes. In some patients with chronic renal diseases, decreased renal production of EPO leads to anemia. A "uremic toxin," which suppresses erythroid precursors, and a minor hemolytic component may contribute to the anemia of chronic renal disease. Administration of recombinant EPO is the treatment of choice.

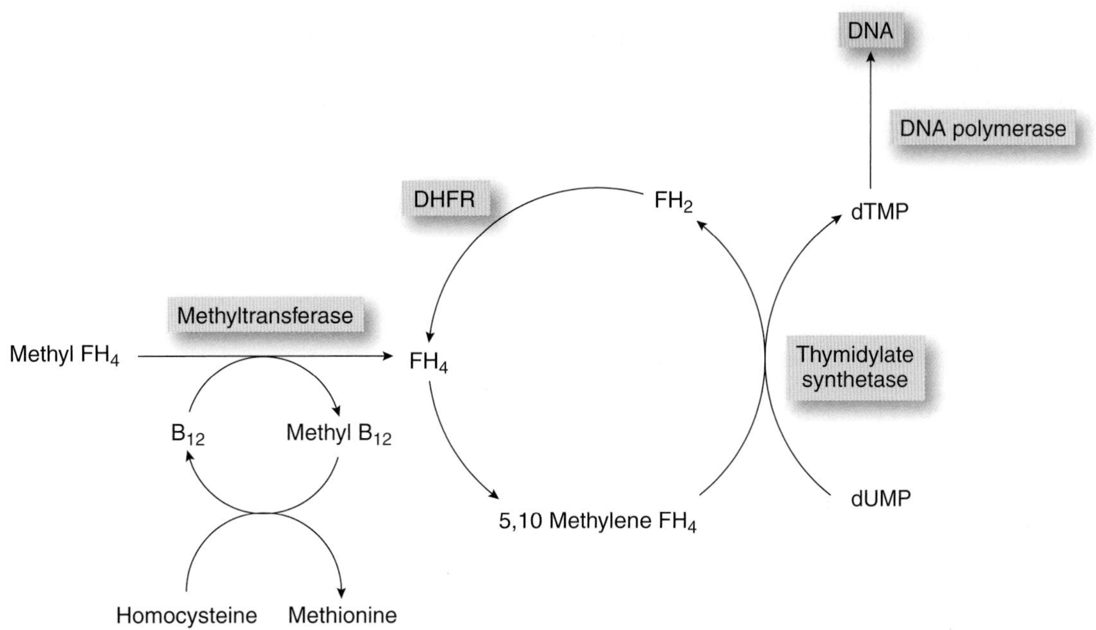

FIGURE 18-9. Relationship of folic acid to vitamin B_{12}. A 1-carbon transfer mediated by folic acid methylates dUMP to dTMP, which is then used for the synthesis of DNA. To enter this cycle, folate (methyl FH_4) is demethylated to FH_4, vitamin B_{12} acting as the cofactor. Thus, both vitamin B_{12} and folic acid deficiencies lead to impaired DNA synthesis and megaloblastic anemia. DHFR, dihydrofolate reductase; dTMP, deoxythymidine monophosphate; dUMP, deoxyuridine monophosphate; FH_2, dihydrofolate; FH_4, tetrahydrofolate.

Anemia Associated With Marrow Infiltration (Myelophthisic Anemia)

Myelophthisic anemia is a hypoproliferative, moderate-to-severe, normocytic anemia associated with marrow infiltration, which features anisopoikilocytosis and teardrop cells. Circulating immature granulocytes and nucleated erythrocytes (**leukoerythroblastosis**) are common. Any infiltrative process (e.g., myelofibrosis, hematologic malignancies, metastatic carcinoma, and granulomatous disease) may replace normal hematopoietic elements and cause anemia (and often leukopenia and thrombocytopenia). In an attempt to maintain blood cell production, extramedullary hematopoiesis may develop, mostly in the spleen and liver.

Anemia Secondary to Ineffective Red Cell Production

Various anemias reflect abnormal erythrocyte production secondary to ineffective hematopoiesis. Sufficient erythroid precursors are formed in the bone marrow, but erythrocytes do not enter the circulation.

Megaloblastic Anemias

Megaloblastic anemias are caused by impaired DNA synthesis, usually because of vitamin B_{12} or folic acid deficiency. Folate and B_{12} (cyanocobalamin) are critical for normal DNA synthesis (for biochemical details, see Fig. 18-9). All proliferating cell types, including myeloid precursors, and cervical and gastrointestinal mucosal cells are affected. In addition to vitamin deficiency, chemotherapeutic agents (methotrexate and hydroxyurea) or antiretroviral drugs (5-azacytidine), and, rarely, inherited defects in purine or pyrimidine metabolism may be responsible. The demand for folic acid is increased in pregnancy, lactation, periods of rapid growth, and chronic hemolytic disease. During these times, folate deficiency may occur unless folate supplementation is provided. Primary intestinal diseases (inflammatory bowel disease and sprue) may also interfere with folic acid absorption.

The hematologic manifestations of both folic acid and vitamin B_{12} deficiency are identical. With impaired DNA synthesis, nuclear development is delayed, but the cytoplasm matures normally. This leads to **nuclear to cytoplasmic asynchrony** and results in the formation of large, nucleated, erythrocyte precursors (**megaloblasts**). Because these cells do not mature enough to be released into the blood, they undergo intramedullary destruction. Released erythrocytes are macrocytic (Fig. 18-10). The myeloid series shows similar dyssynchrony,

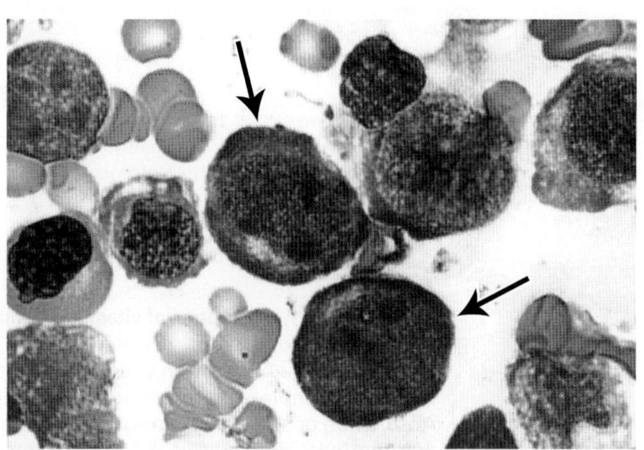

FIGURE 18-10. Megaloblastic anemia. A bone marrow aspirate from a patient with vitamin B_{12} deficiency (pernicious anemia) showing prominent megaloblastic erythroid precursors (*arrows*).

with giant bands and metamyelocytes, and hypersegmented nuclei in mature granulocytes. The megakaryocytes may also be large. The magnitude of the anemia varies but may be severe. Erythrocytes are macrocytic, and many are oval (oval macrocytes). Anisopoikilocytosis is usually prominent, sometimes with teardrop cells. Circulating neutrophils often show nuclear hypersegmentation (>5 lobes). Reticulocytes are not increased.

Vitamin B_{12} cannot be synthesized by humans and must come from diet. It occurs in a variety of animal food sources and is produced by intestinal microorganisms. Proper vitamin B_{12} absorption requires intrinsic factor, which is produced in the stomach (see Chapter 11) and protects vitamin B_{12} from degradation by intestinal enzymes (Fig. 18-11).

Inadequate dietary intake of vitamin B_{12} is rare and usually occurs only in strict vegetarians (vegans). Most

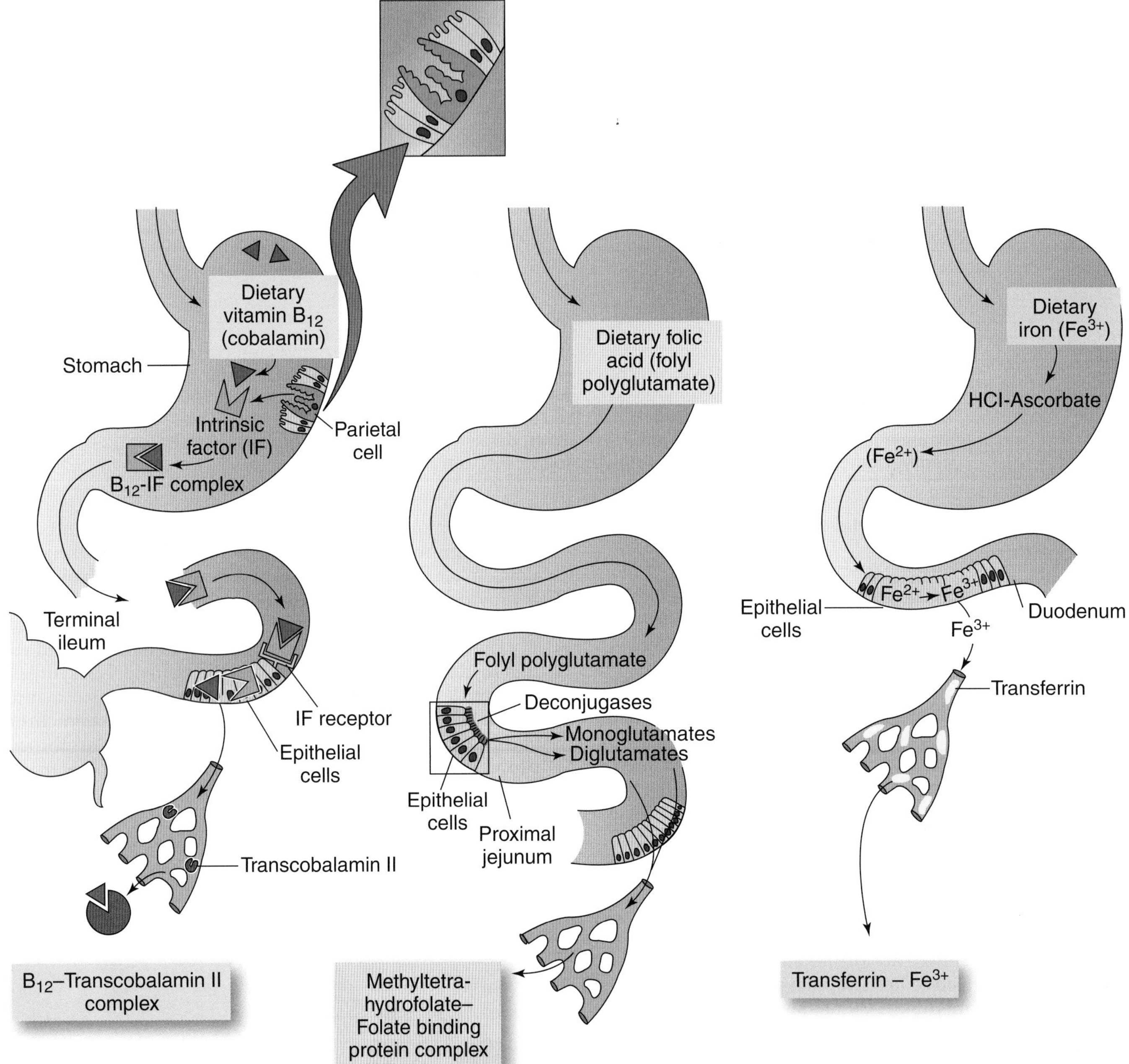

FIGURE 18-11. Absorption of vitamin B_{12}, folic acid, and iron. Absorption of vitamin B_{12} requires initial complexing with intrinsic factor (IF), which is produced by the parietal cells of the gastric mucosa. Absorption then occurs in the terminal ileum, where there are receptors for the IF–B_{12} complex. Dietary folic acid is conjugated by conjugase enzymes to polyglutamate. Absorption occurs in the jejunum following deconjugation in the intestinal lumen. Reduction and methylation result in the generation of methyl tetrahydrofolate, which is then transported by folate-binding protein. Dietary ferric iron (Fe^{3+}) is reduced to ferrous iron (Fe^{2+}) in the stomach and absorbed principally in the duodenum. Iron is transported by transferrin in the circulation. HCl, hydrochloric acid.

often, a lack of intrinsic factor impairs the absorption of the vitamin.

Pernicious anemia, an autoimmune disorder in which patients develop antibodies against parietal cells and intrinsic factor, leads to intrinsic factor deficiency. Antiparietal cell antibodies also cause atrophic gastritis with achlorhydria. Primary intestinal disorders (inflammatory bowel disease) or previous intestinal surgery (ileal bypass) can also impair vitamin B_{12} absorption.

The clinical presentation of megaloblastic anemia is similar, whether caused by a deficiency of B_{12} or folate. In general, the latter develops more rapidly (months) than the former (years). The most important difference clinically is that B_{12} (but not folate) deficiency is complicated by neurologic symptoms, owing to demyelination of posterior and lateral column in the spinal cord (subacute combined degeneration). This may cause sensory and motor deficiencies (see Chapter 24), which unless treated quickly may be irreversible.

Thalassemia

Thalassemias are congenital anemias caused by reduced or absent globin chain synthesis. The globin chain affected controls the type of disease; β-thalassemia (defective β-chain production), α-thalassemia (defective α-chain production), and β−δ-thalassemia. However, a minority of thalassemia cases have structural hemoglobin variants yielding unstable globins. Because α- and β-chains normally pair to form hemoglobin tetramers, the lack of one type of chain leads to unpaired normal globin chains in thalassemic erythrocytes. In β-thalassemia, the excess normal α-chains form an unstable structure that precipitates at the cell membrane. Because this effect makes the RBCs very fragile, they are destroyed within the bone marrow. In α-thalassemia, β-chains are in excess, resulting in hemoglobin with only β-chains. In intrauterine life, the excess of γ-chains yields a hemoglobin with only γ-chains. In both cases, there is excessive RBC destruction.

Thalassemia is most common in the Mediterranean area, especially Italy, Greece, and other areas where malaria has been endemic. Heterozygosity for thalassemia may help protect against malaria, thereby increasing the reproductive potential of heterozygotes.

Normal hemoglobin contains four globin chains: two α-chains and two non–α-chains. There are three normal hemoglobin variants, based on the nature of the non–α-chains (Fig. 18-12). Adult hemoglobin is 95% to 98% HgbA ($\alpha_2\beta_2$), plus small amounts of HgbF ($\alpha_2\gamma_2$) and $HgbA_2$ ($\alpha_2\delta_2$). The most important different types of hemoglobin and the globin chains that contribute to each are presented in Table 18-5.

β-Thalassemia

Homozygous β-thalassemia (**Cooley anemia**) is characterized by moderate-to-severe, microcytic and hypochromic anemia (Fig. 18-13). The disorder is heterogenous and most often caused by point mutations in the β-globin gene's promoter region, a splice site or other coding regions. An inappropriate stop codon may also cause Cooley anemia. Occasionally, a mutation may also affect the adjacent δ-globin gene, leading to a β−δ-thalassemia. In the β° type, most hemoglobin is fetal hemoglobin, although increased (5%–8%) $HgbA_2$ is also present. In the β_1 type, some HgbA may be present (depending on the nature of the underlying defect), and $HgbA_2$ is mildly increased. A modest increase in $HgbA_2$ is characteristic of all forms of β-thalassemia because δ-globin genes are upregulated.

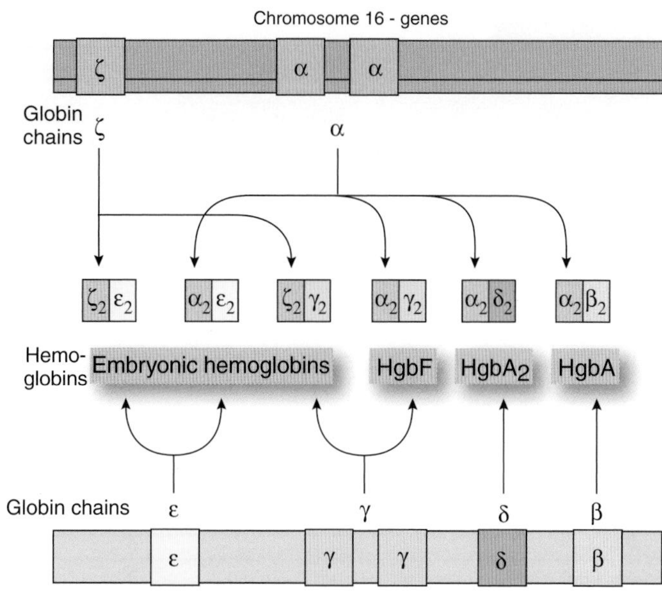

FIGURE 18-12. Hemoglobin (Hb) assembly scheme using globin chains coded on chromosomes 11 and 16.

β-Thalassemia is characterized by a marked excess of α-chains, which form unstable tetramers (α_4) that precipitate in the cytoplasm of developing erythroid precursors.

Blood smears show microcytosis, hypochromia, and striking anisopoikilocytosis (uneven size and shape). Target cells, basophilic stippling, and circulating normoblasts (especially after splenectomy) are common. The increased oxygen affinity of HgbF, plus the underlying anemia, impairs oxygen delivery and elicits increased EPO, which results in marked bone marrow erythroid hyperplasia. The marrow space is expanded, causing facial and cranial bone deformities. Extramedullary hematopoiesis contributes to hepatosplenomegaly and may be reflected in soft tissue masses. Excess erythropoiesis stimulates iron absorption, which together with repeated transfusions, results in iron overload. Excess iron deposition in tissues results in excess morbidity and mortality in thalassemic patients and often requires aggressive chelation therapy.

Heterozygous β-thalassemia (heterozygous carrier of β-thalassemia) is associated with microcytosis and hypochromia. Anemia is generally mild or absent. Most patients are asymptomatic, but iron absorption is increased.

α-Thalassemia

α-Thalassemias are most often caused by gene deletions in one or more of the four α-globin genes. The genetics of the several α-thalassemias are illustrated in Figure 18-14. α-Thalassemia is associated with excess β- or γ-chains, which can form the tetrameric HgbH (β_4) and Hgb Bart (γ_4). Hemoglobins H and Bart are both unstable and precipitate in the cytoplasm, forming Heinz bodies, but to a lesser degree than α_4 tetramers.

The types of α-thalassemia depend on the number of genes affected:

- **Silent carrier α-thalassemia** (one gene affected) is difficult to diagnose because patients' only hematologic abnormality is small amounts of Hgb Bart, detectable only in infancy. There is no anemia, and patients are asymptomatic.

Table 18-5

Major Forms of Hemoglobin and Their Chain Composition

	Contribution of Globin Chains					
Type of Hemoglobin	α	β	γ	δ	ζ	**Explanation**
A	2	2				Principal normal hemoglobin (>95% of total) in postnatal life.
A_2	2			2		Usually <3% of total hemoglobin but may be slightly increased in β-thalassemia.
F	2		2			Normal hemoglobin for most of intrauterine life. Production usually ends by early infancy; hemoglobin F is largely undetectable after 6 months of age. Persists in β-thalassemia.
H		4				Mainly seen in α-thalassemia, where deficiency of α-chains leads to hemoglobins composed of β-chain tetramers. Responsible for formation of Heinz bodies.
Bart's			4			Seen in babies with α-thalassemia. Heinz bodies seen.
Portland			2		2	Hemoglobin present very early in fetal life. May persist in very severe α-thalassemia.

- **α-Thalassemia trait** (two genes affected) is associated with a mild microcytic anemia. $HgbA_2$ is not increased, allowing a distinction between α- and β-thalassemia traits. Up to 5% Hgb Bart can be seen during infancy. Two different genotypes are possible in heterozygous α-thalassemia. There may be a single gene deleted from each chromosome 16 or, alternatively, both genes may be deleted from the same chromosome 16. Clinically, both genotypes present similarly, but homozygous α-thalassemia (see below) can only develop if both genes are deleted from the same chromosome.
- **Hemoglobin H disease** (three genes affected) is associated with moderate microcytic anemia. Increased Hgb Bart (up to 25% in infancy) and variable levels of HgbH are seen. Precipitated HgbH (Heinz bodies) also appears on supravital staining of blood smears.

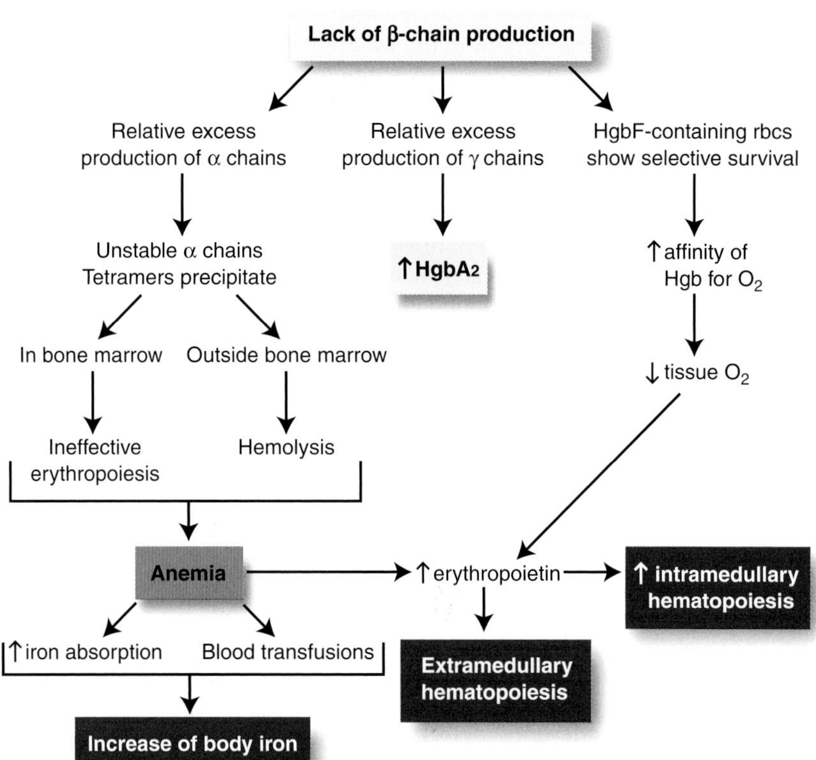

FIGURE 18-13. Pathogenesis of disease manifestations in β-thalassemia.

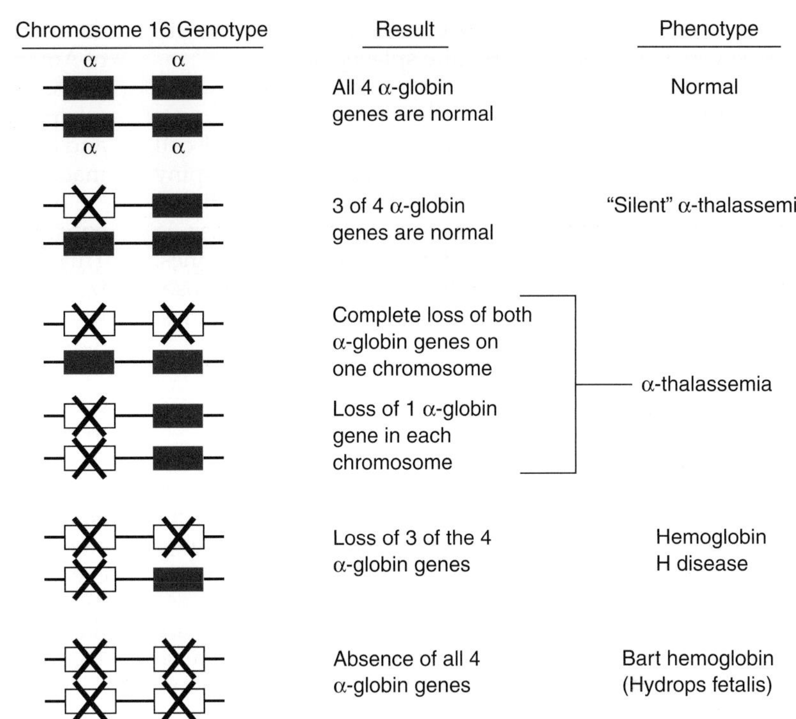

FIGURE 18-14. Genetics of α-globin deficiencies and their manifestations.

- **Homozygous α-thalassemia** (all four genes affected), also called α-hydrops fetalis, is incompatible with life. Affected infants die in utero or shortly after birth with severe anemia, along with marked anisopoikilocytosis and large amounts of Hgb Bart. Severe impairment in tissue oxygen delivery is associated with heart failure and generalized edema. Massive hepatosplenomegaly is caused by extramedullary hematopoiesis.

Anemia Secondary to Increased Red Cell Destruction (Hemolytic Anemia)

Hemolysis (premature elimination of circulating RBCs) causes **hemolytic anemia**. These anemias are classified by the site of red cell destruction. In **extravascular hemolysis**, the monocyte/macrophage system in the spleen and, to a lesser extent, the liver is involved. In **intravascular hemolysis**, RBCs are destroyed while circulating.

Hemolytic anemias are characterized by a compensatory increase in red cell production and release. In the blood, this manifests as red cell polychromasia because of increased reticulocytes. Other laboratory findings commonly associated with hemolysis include increased LDH (particularly isoenzyme 1) and unconjugated (indirect) bilirubin, decreased haptoglobin, free (extracellular) hemoglobin in the blood and urine, increased urobilinogen, and urine hemosiderin.

Erythrocyte Membrane Defects

Erythrocyte membranes are remarkably deformable, which allows red cells to pass unimpaired through the microcirculation and splenic vasculature. Alterations in any part of the red cell membrane can impair RBC plasticity, impacting the "vertical linkages" and rendering erythrocytes susceptible to hemolysis. These membrane defects include hereditary spherocytosis, hereditary elliptocytosis, and acanthocytosis.

Hereditary Spherocytosis

Hereditary spherocytosis (HS) is a diverse group of inherited disorders of the RBC cytoskeleton, in which spectrin or another cytoskeletal component (ankyrin, protein 4.2, and band 3) is deficient. HS is the most common congenital hemolytic anemia in Caucasians and leads to moderate normocytic anemia. Cells undergo a progressive loss of membrane surface area, resulting in **spherocyte** formation. These abnormal red cells are more rigid and fragile and so cannot easily traverse splenic sinusoids. While circulating through the spleen, spherocytes lose additional surface membrane, are trapped, and ultimately succumb to extravascular hemolysis. About 75% of HS cases are inherited as autosomal dominant traits. Most patients have splenomegaly caused by chronic extravascular hemolysis. They may appear jaundiced, and up to 50% develop cholelithiasis, with pigmented (bilirubin) gallstones. Despite chronic hemolysis, transfusion is not usually needed. An exception is a sudden decline in hemoglobin and reticulocytes, which heralds **aplastic crisis** (usually caused by infection with parvovirus B19). Anemia may also become more severe in the so-called **hemolytic crisis** when hemolysis accelerates transiently. Patients with HS can be managed effectively by splenectomy, although spherocytes still persist in the circulation. Splenectomy, however, renders patients more susceptible to certain infections, particularly with *Streptococcus* spp.

Hereditary Elliptocytosis

Hereditary elliptocytosis (HE) is a diverse group of inherited disorders affecting the erythrocyte cytoskeleton. The most commonly described HE variants include defects in self-assembly of spectrin, spectrin–ankyrin binding, protein 4.1, and glycophorin C. Patients with HE usually have only mild normocytic anemia, and many are asymptomatic. HE is characterized by elliptical or oval red blood cells. RBCs have an area of central pallor because there is no loss of the lipid bilayer (as seen in HS). Most forms of HE are autosomal dominant. HE is more common in malaria endemic regions of West Africa. Occasionally, patients with more severe hemolysis may require splenectomy.

Acanthocytosis

Acanthocytosis results from a defect within the red cell membrane lipid bilayer and features irregularly spaced spiny projections of the surface, which may be associated with hemolysis. The most common cause is chronic liver disease, in which increased free cholesterol deposits in cell membranes. Acanthocytes also occur in abetalipoproteinemia, an autosomal recessive disorder with lipid membrane abnormalities. Hemolysis and anemia in acanthocytosis are mild.

Hereditary Nonspherocytic Anemia

Erythrocytes mainly generate energy by glycolysis. Inherited defects of enzymes in the glycolytic pathway can predispose circulating red cells to hemolysis. The most common enzyme defect involves glucose-6-phosphate dehydrogenase (G6PD), which catalyzes conversion of glucose-6-phosphate to 6-phosphogluconate. Deficiencies of other glycolytic enzymes are rare and autosomal recessive. Among these, pyruvate kinase deficiency is the most common. Clinically, these defects cause variable degrees of anemia and are classified as **hereditary nonspherocytic anemias**.

Glucose-6-Phosphate Dehydrogenase Deficiency

Glucose-6-phosphate dehydrogenase deficiency is an X-linked disease in which RBCs are abnormally sensitive to oxidative stress, which triggers hemolytic anemia. The various G6PD mutations appear to protect somewhat against malaria. Because G6PD helps to recycle reduced glutathione, red cells deficient in this enzyme are susceptible to oxidative stress resulting from infections, drugs, or fava bean ingestion (favism). Hemoglobin oxidation generates methemoglobin, in which Fe^{2+} ions are converted to ferric (Fe^{3+}). Methemoglobin cannot transport oxygen, is unstable, and precipitates in the cytoplasm as Heinz bodies. These precipitates increase cell rigidity and lead to hemolysis.

Full expression of G6PD deficiency is seen only in males; females are asymptomatic carriers. The A variant of G6PD seen in 10% to 15% of American blacks is associated with 10% of normal enzyme activity because of instability of the molecule. In affected patients, exposure to oxidant drugs, such as the antimalarial primaquine, may trigger hemolysis. In the Mediterranean type of G6PD mutation, enzyme activity is entirely absent. Thus, exposure to oxidant stress sets off more sustained and severe hemolysis. Potentially, lethal hemolysis may follow ingestion of fava beans (**favism**) in susceptible patients.

In quiescent periods, erythrocytes in G6PD deficiency appear normal. But, in a hemolytic episode precipitated by oxidative stress, passage through the spleen may remove part of red blood cell membranes, to form the so-called **bite cells**.

Hemoglobinopathies

Most clinically relevant hemoglobinopathies are caused by point mutations in the β-globin chain gene.

Sickle Cell Disease

In sickle cell disease, an abnormal hemoglobin, HgbS, causes RBCs to sickle upon deoxygenation. HgbS is most common in people of African ancestry; in some regions of Africa, up to 40% of the population is heterozygous for HgbS. Ten percent of American blacks are heterozygous, and 1 in 650 is homozygous. Heterozygosity for HgbS may partially protect against falciparum malaria. Infected erythrocytes selectively sickle and are removed from the circulation by splenic and hepatic macrophages, effectively destroying the parasite.

A point mutation in the gene for the β-globin chain gene substitutes valine for glutamic acid at amino acid residue six. This single change makes an unstable molecule that polymerizes upon deoxygenation. Polymerization of HgbS transforms the cytoplasm into a rigid filamentous gel and produces less deformable sickled erythrocytes.

The inflexibility of sickled erythrocytes obstructs the microcirculation, leading to tissue hypoxia and ischemic injury in many organs. It also renders the cells susceptible to destruction (hemolysis) during passage through the spleen. Thus, the two primary manifestations of sickle cell disease are recurrent ischemic events and chronic extravascular hemolytic anemia. At first, reoxygenation can reverse the sickling, but after several cycles of sickling and unsickling, the process becomes irreversible. Sickled erythrocytes also have changes in their membrane phospholipids and so adhere more strongly to endothelial cells. This effect further impairs capillary blood flow.

Homozygous patients (HgbSS) have severe normocytic or macrocytic anemia. The macrocytosis reflects increased numbers of reticulocytes, owing to chronic hemolysis. Blood smears show marked anisopoikilocytosis and polychromasia. There are classic sickle cells and target cells, as well as other abnormally shaped erythrocytes (Fig. 18-15). Howell–Jolly bodies, which represent nuclear remnants, are evident in most patients beyond childhood.

People homozygous for HgbS show the full clinical picture of sickle cell disease. Heterozygotes for HgbS (sickle trait), however, do not develop red cell sickling because their HgbA prevents HgbS polymerization. HgbF also interferes with HgbS polymerization; patients who are homozygous for HgbS and have increased HgbF have a milder form of disease. HgbS accounts for 80% to 95% of the total hemoglobin, and HgbA is absent. HgbF and $HgbA_2$ comprise the remaining hemoglobin.

Although patients with SS suffer from lifelong hemolysis, adaptation occurs over time and may not require regular

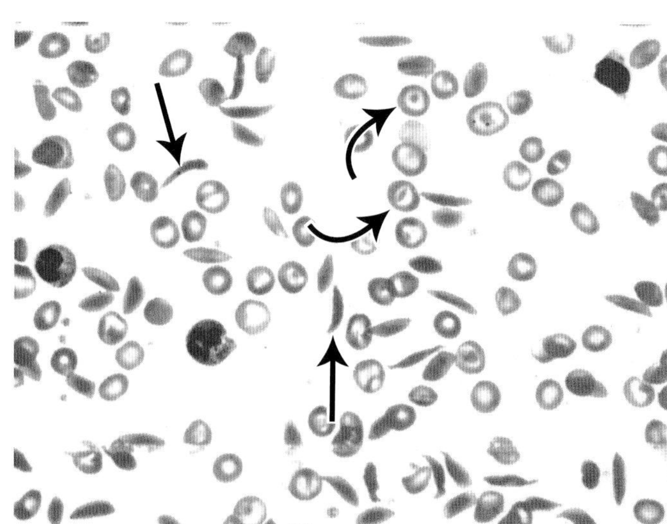

FIGURE 18-15. Sickle cell anemia. Sickled cells (*straight arrows*) and target cells (*curved arrows*) are evident in the blood smear.

transfusions. Instead, the clinical picture is dominated by sequelae of repeated **vaso-occlusive disease.** In an attempt to minimize these complications by decreasing the amount of HgbS in circulation, chronic exchange transfusions may be necessary. Sickle cell anemia is a systemic disorder and eventually impairs the functions of most organ systems and tissues (Fig. 18-16).

Patients with sickle cell disease develop episodic crises of pain in the chest, abdomen, and bone as a result of capillary occlusion, ischemia, and hypoxic cell injury. The painful crises can be triggered by various stimuli (e.g., underlying infection, acidosis, or dehydration). **Aplastic crisis,** associated with rapidly falling hemoglobin levels and no reticulocyte response, occurs when the bone marrow fails to compensate for the high level of red cell loss. Parvovirus B19 (and occasionally other viral and bacterial infections) is a frequent trigger. In **sequestration crisis,** sudden pooling of erythrocytes, especially in the spleen, decreases circulating blood volume and lowers hemoglobin levels. The etiology is unclear, but it occurs most often in young children who still have functioning spleens. This complication may be followed by hypovolemic shock and is the most common cause of death early in life.

Patients with sickle cell disease also can have systemic issues. Chronic demand for increased cardiac output may lead to **cardiomegaly and congestive heart failure.** In addition, obstruction of coronary microcirculation may cause myocardial ischemia. Up to one third of patients with sickle cell anemia suffer a sometimes-fatal **acute chest syndrome** and rapidly **lose respiratory function,** with pulmonary infiltrates on chest radiography. **Splenomegaly** often occurs in childhood, and repeated splenic infarction gives rise to functional autosplenectomy by adulthood. The asplenic state renders the patient susceptible to infections with encapsulated bacteria, especially pneumococcus. Patients with sickle cell anemia suffer **neurologic complications** related to vascular obstruction, including transient ischemic attacks, strokes, and

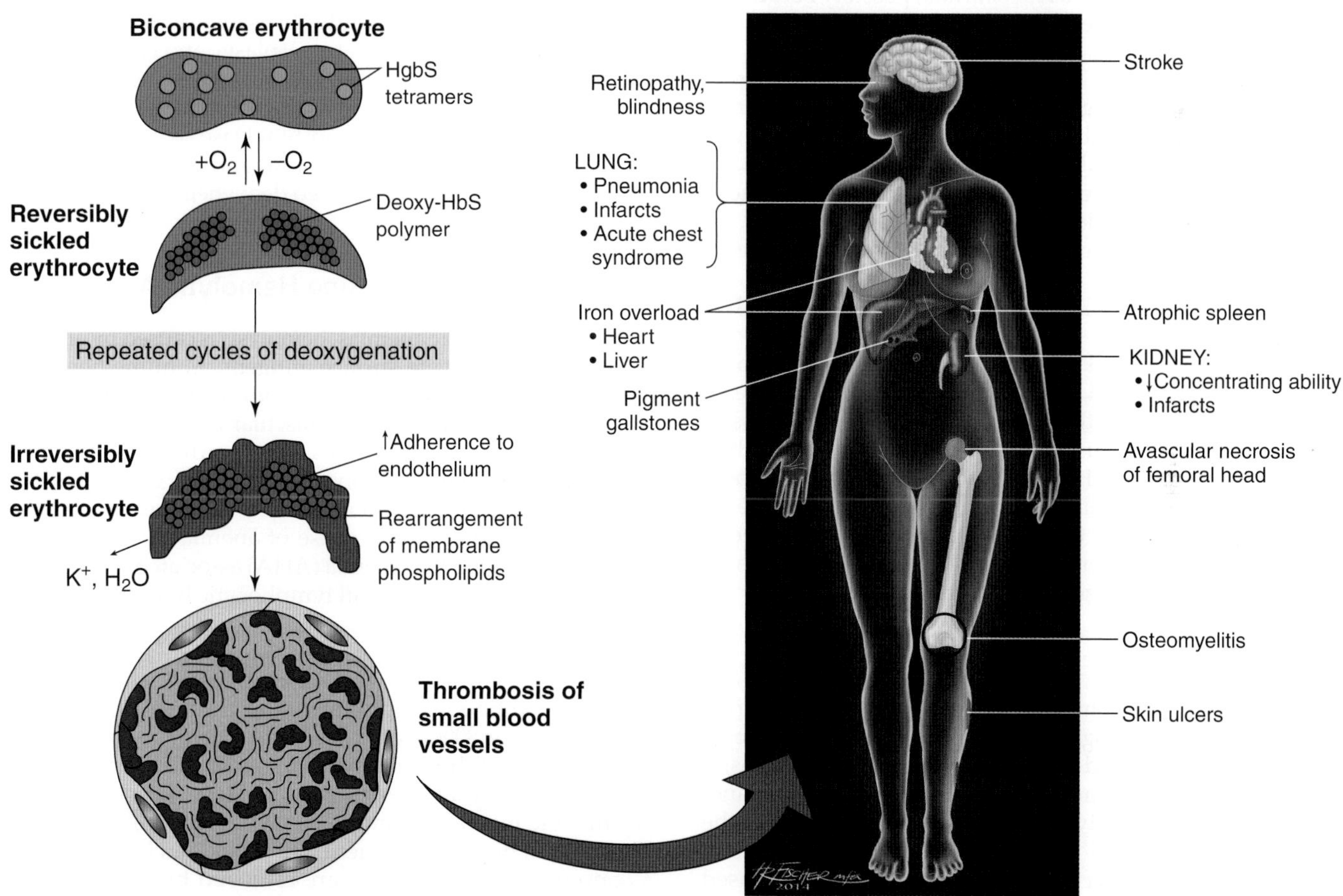

FIGURE 18-16. Pathogenesis of the vascular complications of sickle cell anemia. Substitution of valine for glutamic acid leads to an alteration in the surface charge of the hemoglobin molecule. Upon deoxygenation ($-O_2$), sickle hemoglobin (HbS) tetramers aggregate to form poorly soluble polymers. The erythrocytes change shape from a biconcave disk to a sickle form with the polymerization of HbS. This process is initially reversible upon reoxygenation ($+O_2$), but with repeated cycles of deoxygenation and reoxygenation, the erythrocytes become irreversibly sickled. Irreversibly sickled cells display a rearrangement of phospholipids between the outer and inner monolayers of the cell membrane, in particular an increase in aminophospholipids in the outer leaflet. Potassium (K^+) and water (H_2O) are lost from the cells. The erythrocytes are no longer deformable and are more adherent to endothelial cells, properties that predispose to thrombosis in small blood vessels. The resulting vascular occlusions lead to widespread ischemic complications.

cerebral hemorrhages. Occlusion of retinal microvasculature may lead to retinal hemorrhage and detachment, proliferative retinopathy, and blindness. The hypoxic, acidotic, and hypertonic environment in the renal medulla often produces sickling in that location. This complication impairs the ability to form concentrated urine and causes renal infarcts and papillary necrosis. Men may develop priapism, which, if not treated promptly, results in permanent erectile dysfunction. As in any form of chronic hemolytic anemia, patients with sickle cell anemia have **increased levels of unconjugated (indirect) bilirubin**, which can predispose to pigmented bilirubin gallstones. Hepatomegaly and increased hepatic iron deposition are also seen. **Cutaneous ulcers** over the lower extremities, especially near the ankles, are common and reflect obstruction of dermal capillaries. Children may develop "hand–foot syndrome," with self-limited swelling of the hands and feet because of underlying bone infarcts. Avascular necrosis of the femoral head requires corrective hip surgery. Sickle cell disease is also associated with an increased incidence of osteomyelitis, particularly with *Salmonella typhimurium*, possibly because of the underlying impairment in splenic function.

Sickle Cell Trait

Heterozygosity for the HgbS mutation is called sickle cell trait. In such patients, the HgbA in their red cells prevents HgbS polymerization. As a result, their erythrocytes do not normally sickle except under extreme conditions (e.g., high altitudes and deep-sea diving). Heterozygotes are asymptomatic, do not develop hemolytic anemia, and live normal life spans.

Double Heterozygosity for Hemoglobin S and Other Hemoglobinopathies

Some patients with a sickling disorder are actually heterozygous for both HgbS and other abnormal hemoglobins (e.g., HgbC or HgbD) or for thalassemia. Double heterozygosity for HgbS and HgbC causes a milder sickle phenotype than does homozygosity for HgbS. These patients have episodic skeletal or abdominal pain. However, they commonly develop a retinopathy that tends to be severe. They are also prone to undergo necrosis of the femoral heads. These features probably reflect the high blood viscosity conferred by HgbSC.

Hemoglobin C Disease

HgbC disease results from homozygous inheritance of a structurally abnormal hemoglobin, which increases erythrocyte rigidity and causes mild chronic hemolysis. Homozygosity for HgbC disease is characterized a mild normocytic anemia. In HgbC disease, lysine replaces glutamic acid at the sixth amino acid of β-globin. Because HgbC precipitates in erythrocyte cytoplasm, cellular dehydration and decreased deformability occur. When passing through the spleen, the abnormal red cells are removed from the circulation, resulting in mild anemia and splenomegaly. The reduced oxygen affinity of HgbC increases tissue oxygen delivery, an effect that mitigates the severity of disease. HgbC is mostly found in the same populations as HgbS, although it is less common.

Hemoglobin E Disease

HgbE disease is a result of homozygosity for a structurally abnormal hemoglobin. In this condition, a thalassemia-like defect is associated with mild chronic hemolysis. Patients homozygous for HgbE (EE) have a mild microcytic anemia. In haemoglobin E, lysine substitutes for glutamic acid at position 26 of the β-globin chain. This is at a splice site in the gene, so the mutation results in a structurally abnormal molecule, decreased gene transcription, and unstable β-globin messenger RNA (mRNA). The last allows diminished synthesis of HgbE, creating a situation like that seen in thalassemia. HgbE is relatively unstable and may precipitate in the cell and lead to hemolysis.

Other Hemoglobinopathies

Several hundred additional hemoglobin variants result from mutations in α- or β-globin genes. These mutations may produce structural or functional derangement of the hemoglobin molecule. Some mutations alter hemoglobin tertiary structure, and by destabilizing, it causes it to precipitate in the cytoplasm. As a group, these are **unstable hemoglobins** and are often named after the place where they were first discovered (e.g., hemoglobin Köln). Patients may suffer jaundice and splenomegaly.

Other hemoglobin mutations result in **abnormal oxygen affinity**. **Increased oxygen affinity** decreases tissue oxygen delivery. Hypoxia subsequently elicits increased EPO production, bone marrow erythroid hyperplasia, and erythrocytosis. Patients are mostly asymptomatic, but some may have symptoms related to hyperviscosity. Abnormal hemoglobins with **decreased oxygen affinity** readily release oxygen in tissues. In such patients, EPO levels are low, and most patients have mild anemia. Because of increased deoxyhemoglobin, patients may appear cyanotic.

Immune and Autoimmune Hemolytic Anemias

In immune hemolytic anemias, hemolysis is caused by antibodies against erythrocyte surface antigens. Immune hemolytic anemia can reflect autoantibodies or alloantibodies, and the site of hemolysis may be extravascular or intravascular. Autoantibodies can be classified as either warm or cold antibodies. In immune hemolytic anemias, the red cells themselves are intrinsically normal but are targets for immune-mediated attack. The most common cause of anemia in the elderly is autoimmune hemolytic anemia (AHA) associated with chronic lymphocytic leukemia/small lymphocytic lymphoma.

Warm Antibody Autoimmune Hemolytic Anemia

Warm autoantibodies optimally bind their antigens at 37°C and account for 80% of cases of AIHA. Warm antibody AIHA is associated with normocytic or, occasionally, macrocytic anemia. The antibodies are usually IgG directed against erythrocyte membrane antigens, such as **Rh group proteins**. They do not bind complement, but "coat" red blood cells. As a consequence, these RBCs are removed by macrophages, mainly in the spleen (extravascular hemolysis). Warm antibody AIHA affects women more than men, and half of the cases are idiopathic. In the remaining instances, the antibody reflects an underlying condition (e.g., infection, collagen vascular disease, lymphoproliferative disorders, and drug reactions).

Drug-Induced Warm Antibodies

Drugs induce antibodies by several different mechanisms. When **hapten** mediated, a drug such as penicillin attaches to the RBC surface. With this modification, the red cell–drug complex elicits antibodies, some of which react with the erythrocyte itself. In the case of **immune complex** mediation, a drug (like quinidine) may react with a specific circulating antibody to form immune complexes, which then bind to red cell membranes. Alternatively, a drug (e.g., α-methyldopa) may elicit **autoantibodies** that cross-react with red cell membrane components. When hapten and immune complex mechanisms are responsible, the drug is required for hemolysis, whereas in the case of autoantibodies, hemolysis occurs in the absence of the initiating drug. Refractory cases may require splenectomy or transfusions.

Cold Antibody (Cold Agglutinin) Autoimmune Hemolytic Anemia

Some 20% of cases of AIHA are caused by cold IgM or, occasionally, IgG antibodies, which occur as cold agglutinins or hemolysins. These are activated when blood cools to room temperature, most commonly with cold reactive IgM antibodies. Significant hemolysis is uncommon with cold agglutinins, and patients are more likely to develop peripheral vascular symptoms (Raynaud phenomenon; see Chapter 8), owing to red cell agglutination with cold exposure. Cold antibodies may fix and then activate complement to a variable extent.

Cold agglutinins may be idiopathic or may be due to an underlying condition, mostly infections with Epstein–Barr virus or *Mycoplasma* or lymphoproliferative disorders. Cold agglutinins are mostly IgM directed against I/i antigens on red cells.

Intravascular hemolysis resulting in hemoglobinemia and hemoglobinuria occurs with activation of the complement membrane attack complex. Alternatively, complement may only be activated through C3. In that case, complement-coated red cells are removed in the liver because Kupffer cells have more complement receptors than do splenic macrophages.

Cold Hemolysin Disease (Paroxysmal Cold Hemoglobinuria)

Cold hemolysins (**Donath–Landsteiner antibodies**) as opposed to cold agglutinins are usually biphasic IgGs directed against P antigens on red cells and rarely cause AIHA. The antibody binds to erythrocytes at low temperatures and fixes complement, but intravascular hemolysis does not occur at these temperatures. Because the antibody is IgG, red cells do not agglutinate. Upon warming to 37°C, the cold hemolysin remains attached, complement is activated, and intravascular hemolysis occurs. Patients may develop severe anemia and hemoglobinuria as a result of intravascular hemolysis. The clinical syndrome caused by cold hemolysins is **paroxysmal cold hemoglobinuria**, which often follows viral illness. Immunosuppressive therapy and splenectomy are usually ineffective. Cold avoidance and supportive therapy, such as RBC transfusions, are required.

Alloimmune Antibody

Hemolytic transfusion reaction and hemolytic disease in the newborn are examples of **alloimmune hemolytic anemia**, in which alloantibodies (antibodies formed in response to human nonself antigens) cause destruction of red cells. An **immediate hemolytic transfusion** reaction occurs when a patient with preformed alloantibodies receives grossly incompatible blood, usually because of a clerical error. Massive hemolysis of the transfused blood may cause severe complications, including hypotension, renal failure, and death.

Delayed hemolytic transfusion reactions usually involve antibodies to minor red cell antigens. After a first exposure to such antigens, antibody levels rise, but then may fall to become undetectable by routine pretransfusion screening. Subsequent re-exposure to the offending antigen elicits an anamnestic antibody response; hemolysis occurs several days later. Delayed hemolytic transfusion reactions are usually less severe than immediate reactions and may be clinically undetectable.

Hemolytic disease of the newborn (HDN) reflects incompatibility of blood types between a mother and her developing fetus; the mother lacks an antigen present on fetal red blood cells. Maternal IgG alloantibodies can cross the placenta and cause hemolysis of fetal erythrocytes. Erythroblasts (immature RBCs) are released from the fetal bone marrow in an effort to compensate for the RBC loss. HDN antibodies are mostly directed against ABO or Rh antigens (see Chapter 5).

Anemia Secondary to Nonimmune Causes

Mechanical Red Cell Fragmentation Syndromes (Microangiopathic Hemolytic Anemias)

In red cell fragmentation syndromes, intrinsically, normal erythrocytes undergo intravascular hemolysis when they are damaged mechanically as they circulate in the blood resulting in microangiopathic hemolyic anemia (MAHA). In **thrombotic microangiopathic** hemolytic anemia, red cells are fragmented mechanically either by (1) contact with an artificial surface (e.g., prosthetic heart valve and synthetic vascular graft) or (2) by collision with microthromboses accompanied by fibrin deposition and platelet aggregation. Classic examples of microangiopathic hemolysis include **disseminated intravascular coagulation** (DIC), **thrombotic thrombocytopenic purpura** (TTP), and hemolytic–uremic syndrome (HUS) (see section on "Coagulopathies"). Laboratory findings in microangiopathic hemolytic anemia include a mild-to-moderate microcytic or normochromic anemia with appropriate reticulocyte response. Altered blood flow, as occurs in malignant hypertension or vasculitis, may also lead to mechanical fragmentation of erythrocytes. Long-distance running or walking ("march hemoglobinuria") or prolonged vigorous exercise can cause repetitive trauma to red cells and lead to hemolysis.

Hypersplenism

A mild hemolytic anemia may develop in patients with hypersplenism and congestive splenomegaly. Splenomegaly causes pooling of blood and delayed transit of blood cells through the splenic circulation. Prolonged exposure of red cells to splenic macrophages may give rise to their premature destruction. The anemia of hypersplenism shows no specific morphologic features. Leukopenia and thrombocytopenia are common and are caused by sequestration of these elements in the enlarged spleen, not destruction. The bone marrow shows compensatory hyperplasia of all cell lines.

Anemia Secondary to Nonmalignant Stem Cell Disorders

Aplastic Anemia

Aplastic anemia is a disorder of pluripotential hematopoietic stem cells that leads to bone marrow failure. The marrow is hypocellular, and all blood cell lineages are decreased (pancytopenia).

The disease generally results from an insult to the bone marrow, such as a predictable, dose-dependent, toxic injury (e.g., certain chemotherapeutic drugs, chemicals, and ionizing radiation). Marrow damage can also follow an idiosyncratic, dose-independent, immunologic injury, as occurs with idiopathic cases or after certain drug or viral exposures. The most common inherited type of aplastic anemia is Fanconi anemia. Depending on its cause, stem cell injury may or may not be reversible (Table 18-6).

The bone marrow in aplastic anemia shows variably reduced cellularity, depending on the clinical stage of the disease. Myeloid, erythroid, and megakaryocytic lineages are decreased, with a relative increase in marrow lymphocytes and plasma cells. As marrow cellularity declines, there is a corresponding increase in fat (Fig. 18-17). Anemia, leukopenia (mainly granulocytopenia), and thrombocytopenia characterize aplastic anemia. Despite elevated EPO levels, reticulocytosis is absent, a finding that underscores the underlying stem cell defect.

Patients with aplastic anemia show signs and symptoms due to pancytopenia (i.e., weakness, fatigue, infection, and bleeding). Immunosuppressive therapy often leads to transient remissions. Bone marrow or stem cell transplantation may be curative.

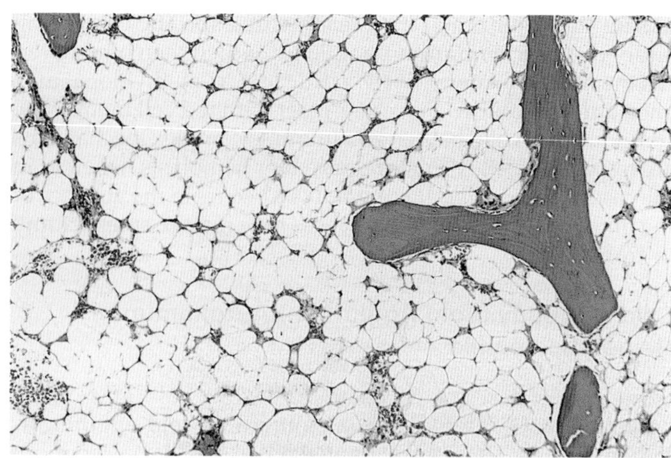

FIGURE 18-17. Aplastic anemia. The bone marrow consists largely of fat cells and lacks normal hematopoietic activity.

Fanconi Anemia

Fanconi anemia (FA) is the most common hereditary bone marrow failure syndrome. The disorder may be obvious at birth or shortly afterward because patients often have abnormalities of their thumbs and radii, as well as cutaneous, renal, and other malformations. The incidence of Fanconi anemia is less than 1 per 100,000 live births.

The underlying defect in Fanconi anemia is in DNA repair, in particular repair of cross-links between DNA strands, such as may occur during DNA duplication. A total of 15 associated genes are labeled *FANC* (for Fanconi complementation group). Different members of the Fanconi gene family mediate key functions in this pathway and interact with other DNA damage/repair genes, such as *ATM*, *ATR*, and *BRCA1*.

Table 18-6

Etiology of Aplastic Anemia

Etiology of Aplastic Anemia
Idiopathic (two thirds of cases)
Ionizing radiation
Drugs
Chemotherapeutic agents
Chloramphenicol
Anticonvulsants
Nonsteroidal anti-inflammatory agents
Gold
Chemicals
Benzene
Viruses
Hepatitis C virus
Epstein–Barr virus
HIV
Parvovirus B19
Hereditary
Fanconi anemia

Aplastic anemia associated with Fanconi anemia usually occurs in the first decade of life and may be the initial symptom. Fanconi patients do not respond to immunosuppressive treatments used for people with idiopathic aplastic anemia. Androgens may be useful in treating bone marrow failure due to FA, but HSC transplantation is the treatment of choice. Unfortunately, the sensitivity of these patients to DNA damaging agents complicates pretransplant conditioning.

Long-term complications of Fanconi anemia in patients who survive hematopoietic failure events include development of myelodysplastic syndromes and acute myeloid leukemia (see below) during their teenage years or as young adults. As well, because the DNA repair defect affects all cells, FA patients are likely to develop epithelial tumors later in life.

Pure Red Cell Aplasia

Pure red cell aplasia (PRCA) is selective marrow suppression of committed erythroid precursors. White blood cells and platelets are unaffected. PRCA most often results from immune suppression of red cell production. Acute acquired PRCA may be caused by viral infection (parvovirus B19). Chronic and relapsing acquired PRCA may be idiopathic or result from thymic lesions (e.g., thymoma and thymic hyperplasia).

Diamond–Blackfan syndrome is a PRCA caused by de novo or inherited mutations in one of many ribosomal proteins. It manifests within the first 2 years of life with anemia, with or without physical abnormalities, including cleft lip or palate, micrognathia, limb abnormalities, and short stature. Anemia is caused by defective erythroid precursors that show a diminished response to EPO and decreased erythroid burst- and colony-forming capacities. Patients with PRCA develop moderate-to-severe anemia, which is often macrocytic. Despite increased EPO, there is no accompanying reticulocytosis. Diamond–Blackfan syndrome is usually life-threatening, owing to severe anemia and the gradual impact of iron overload. Some patients respond to glucocorticoids.

Paroxysmal Nocturnal Hemoglobinuria

Paroxysmal nocturnal hemoglobinuria (PNH) is an acquired clonal stem cell disorder characterized by episodic intravascular hemolytic anemia because of increased RBC sensitivity to complement-mediated lysis. The underlying defect in PNH involves somatic mutation of the *phosphatidylinositol glycan-class A* (*PIG-A*) gene, on the short arm of the X chromosome (Xp22.1) in HSCs. This mutation disrupts synthesis of GPI, which normally anchors many proteins to RBC membranes. This abnormality results in loss of **decay acceleration factor** (CD55) and, more importantly, **membrane inhibitor of reactive lysis** (CD59) from their surfaces. The loss of these proteins makes red blood cells more susceptible to lysis by complement. Leukocytes and platelets derived from the abnormal stem cells also demonstrate the defect.

PNH may develop as a primary disorder or evolve from preexisting aplastic anemia. Because the defect is clonal, it may progress to **myelodysplasia** or overt **acute leukemia** (see below).

During hemolytic episodes, patients develop varyingly severe normocytic or macrocytic anemia, with an appropriate reticulocyte response. Patients may have intermittent intravascular hemolysis, although only a minority have it at night. Because the hemolysis is intravascular, hemoglobinuria is present, and iron deficiency may develop over time from recurrent iron loss in the urine. Leukopenia and thrombocytopenia are frequent, and sensitivity to complement may result in inappropriate platelet activation, resulting in venous and arterial thrombosis, notably Budd–Chiari syndrome. Thrombocytopenia may lead to bleeding. Bone marrow transplantation when available is curative. Use of a monoclonal antibody (eculizumab) directed against a complement receptor protein alleviates the symptoms of PNH. However, therapy must continue for the life of the patient.

POLYCYTHEMIA

Polycythemia (erythrocytosis) is an increase in RBC mass, which is defined arbitrarily as a hematocrit (Hct) greater than 54% in men and greater than 47% in women. Blood viscosity increases exponentially at Hcts over 50%, and cardiac function and peripheral blood flow may be impaired. If the Hct exceeds 60%, blood flow may be so compromised as to cause tissue hypoxia.

Polycythemia can be further divided on the basis of overall red cell mass into relative and absolute categories.

- **Relative polycythemia** occurs in dehydration. Plasma volume is decreased, but red cell mass is normal. Hence, it is not a true increase in red cell mass, but rather a reflection of altered total blood volume.
- **Absolute polycythemia** is a true increase in red cell mass. It can be primary or secondary.
- **Primary polycythemia,** or **polycythemia vera (PV)**, is an autonomous, EPO-independent, proliferation of erythroid cells caused by a clonal HSC disorder. PV is a chronic myeloproliferative disorder (see below).
- **Secondary polycythemia** arises from EPO stimulation of erythropoiesis, usually to compensate for general tissue hypoxia. Tissue hypoxia may arise from chronic lung disease, cigarette smoking, residence at high altitudes, a right-to-left cardiac shunt, or an abnormal hemoglobin with high oxygen affinity.

BENIGN DISORDERS OF THE LYMPHOID SYSTEM

Benign Lymphocytosis

Benign lymphocytosis is characterized by a transient increase in the number of circulating lymphocytes. The upper limits of normal are 4,000/μL in adults, 7,000/μL in children, and 9,000/μL in infants. Lymphocytes in benign lymphocytosis usually appear reactive and are morphologically heterogeneous, although atypical lymphocytes may also be seen (Figs. 18-18 and 18-19). Infectious mononucleosis due to EBV infection is the most common cause of reactive lymphocytosis, but other viral infections can produce similar syndromes (e.g., CMV). Persistent absolute lymphocytosis, greater than 4,000/μL, particularly in adults, raises suspicion for a lymphoproliferative disorder and deserves further evaluation.

Bone Marrow Plasmacytosis

It is uncommon to find plasma cells in the blood. When seen, they are usually part of the spectrum of lymphoid cells in infectious mononucleosis–like syndromes caused by viruses other than EBV. The presence of circulating plasma cells in the blood of an adult raises suspicion for a plasma cell neoplasm.

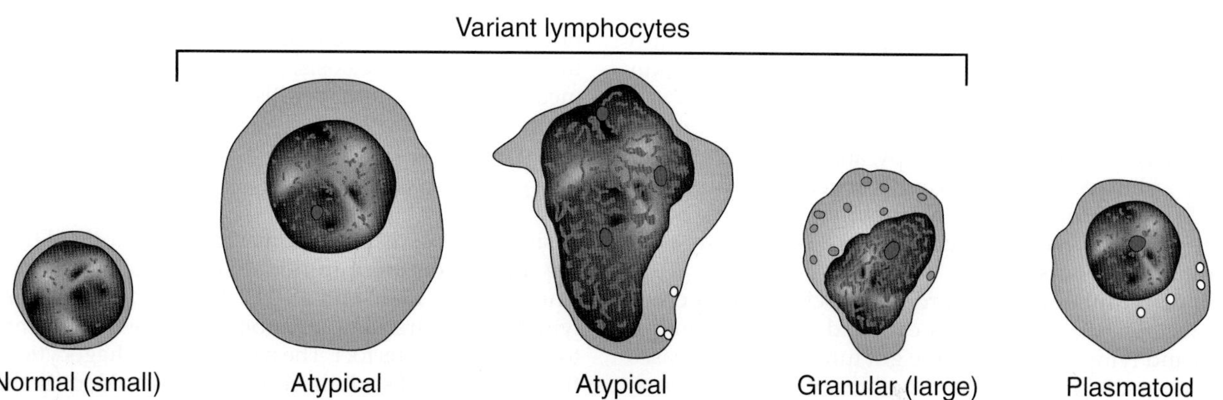

FIGURE 18-18. Lymphocyte morphology. The term "variant lymphocytes" covers atypical lymphocytes and large granular lymphocytes. **Atypical lymphocytes** are large and exhibit deep blue to pale gray cytoplasm; they are seen in benign reactive processes. **Large granular lymphocytes** are medium to large lymphoid cells with some pink cytoplasmic granules. They are suppressor T lymphocytes, some with natural killer function, and may be increased in benign or malignant disorders. **Plasmacytoid lymphocytes** have abundant blue cytoplasm and are seen in some reactive disorders.

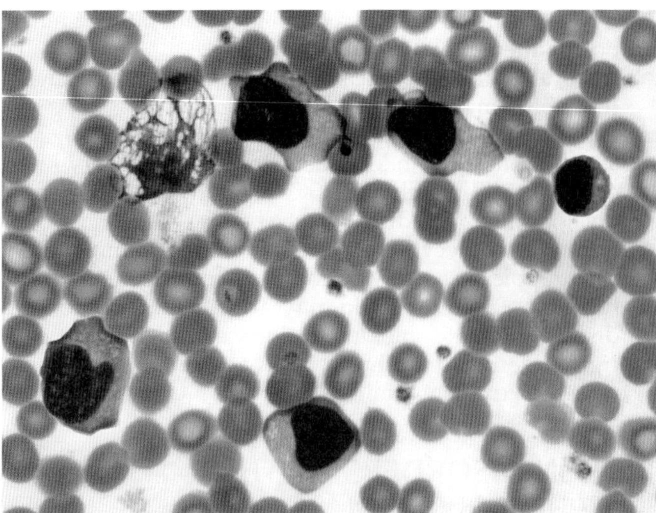

FIGURE 18-19. Infectious mononucleosis. An absolute lymphocytosis caused by a heterogeneous population of small and larger lymphoid cells, including atypical lymphocytes, is characteristic of this Ebstein–Barr virus–driven disorder.

Plasma cells normally account for less than 3% of hematopoietic cells in the bone marrow. In children and young adults, plasmacytosis is caused by reactive conditions, such as chronic infections or systemic inflammatory disorders. Autoimmune diseases are a particularly common cause of bone marrow plasmacytosis, especially in women. Bone marrow plasmacytosis greater than 10% is typically associated with a plasma cell neoplasm, that is, plasma cell myeloma (see below).

Lymphocytopenia

Peripheral blood lymphocytopenia is defined as a blood lymphocyte count less than 1,500/µL in adults or less than 3,000/µL in children. Because the predominant lymphocytes in the blood are T-helper ($CD4^+$) cells, lymphocytopenia generally means decreased $CD4^+$ T cells. There are several mechanisms by which lymphocytopenia occurs:

- **Decreased lymphocyte production:** Several congenital and acquired immunodeficiency syndromes feature reduced generation of lymphocytes. Impaired T-cell production also occurs with some lymphomas, such as classic Hodgkin lymphoma, particularly in advanced stages.
- **Increased lymphocyte destruction:** Certain therapies, such as irradiation, chemotherapy, and administration of antilymphocyte globulin, adrenocorticotropic hormone (ACTH) or corticosteroids, destroy lymphocytes. Some viral infections, particularly HIV, cause T-cell death, with resultant lymphopenia.
- **Loss of lymphocytes:** Disorders associated with damage to intestinal lymphatics can lead to loss of lymph fluid and lymphocytes into the gut lumen. Such diseases include protein-losing enteropathies, Whipple disease, and conditions of increased central venous pressure (e.g., right-sided heart failure and chronic constrictive pericarditis). Immunologic damage to lymphocytes may occur in collagen vascular diseases, such as systemic lupus erythematosus.

Reactive Lymphoid Hyperplasia

Lymph nodes may undergo hyperplasia of all cellular components, or any combination of B cells, T cells, and macrophages, in response to a variety of infectious, inflammatory, and neoplastic disorders (Fig. 18-20).

Acute suppurative and necrotizing lymphadenitis occurs in lymph nodes that drain sites of acute bacterial or fungal infections. Such nodes enlarge rapidly because of edema and hyperemia and are usually tender because the capsule becomes distended. Lymph node sinuses and stroma are infiltrated by neutrophils and variable numbers of bland macrophages. Well- or poorly defined granulomas are common, and necrosis can be focal and geographic or extensive. The location of the nodes involved in reactive lymphadenopathy often provides a clue to its cause in proximate or draining tissue. Generalized lymphadenopathy may occur in systemic infections, hyperthyroidism, drug hypersensitivity reactions, and autoimmune diseases.

Follicular Hyperplasia

Hyperplasia of secondary follicles (germinal centers) and plasmacytosis of medullary cords indicate B-cell immunoreactivity. In **nonspecific reactive follicular hyperplasia**, prominent hyperplastic follicles occur mainly in the cortices of the lymph node (Fig. 18-20). Follicles are round or irregularly shaped and may be fused or confluent. The activated B cells in these follicles range from small cells with irregular, cleaved nuclei to large immunoblasts A well-defined mantle of normal small B cells surrounds the follicles, sharply separating them from interfollicular regions.

The cause of nonspecific reactive follicular hyperplasia is often unknown, although a virus, drug, or inflammatory process is often likely. The clinical course involves rapid and complete resolution of lymphadenopathy after the inciting stimulus disappears.

Interfollicular Hyperplasia

Interfollicular or diffuse hyperplasia of the deep cortex or paracortex is characteristic of T-lymphocyte immunoreactivity.

Nonspecific reactive interfollicular hyperplasia (Fig. 18-20) is most commonly caused by viral infections or immunologic reactions. Although the precise cause is often unknown, the condition usually resolves promptly. Interfollicular lymph node hyperplasia is common in viral diseases, including infectious mononucleosis, varicella-herpes zoster infection, measles, CMV lymphadenitis, and often occurs in systemic lupus erythematosis.

Sinus Histiocytosis

In sinus histiocytosis, tissue macrophages derived from blood are more prominent in nodal subcapsular and trabecular sinuses (Figs. 18-20 and 18-21). The condition is common in lymph nodes draining carcinomas and, less often, inflammatory and infectious foci. The nature of the phagocytic debris in the cytoplasm of such macrophages helps identify the origin of the process. For example, anthracotic pigment accumulates in macrophages in mediastinal lymph nodes showing sinus histocytosis. Macrophages containing erythrocytes and hemosiderin pigment characterize autoimmune hemolytic anemias and sites draining hemorrhages.

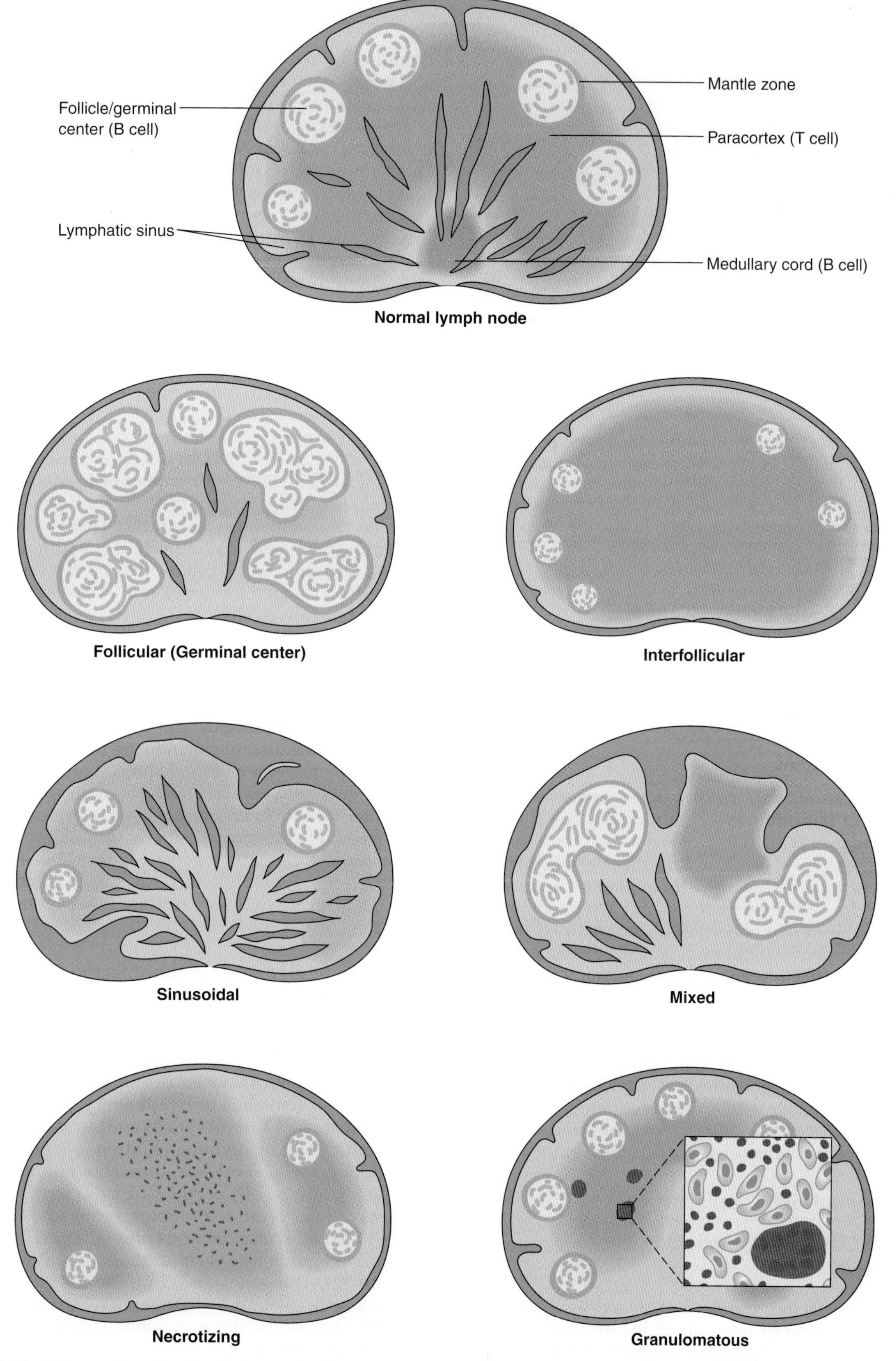

FIGURE 18-20. Patterns of reactive lymphadenopathy. The major patterns of reactive hyperplasia are contrasted with the architecture of a normal lymph node. **Follicular hyperplasia**, with an increased number of enlarged and irregularly shaped follicles, is characteristic of B-cell immunoreactivity. **Interfollicular hyperplasia** with expansion of the paracortex is typical of T-cell immunoreactivity. The **sinusoidal pattern** is typified by expansion of sinuses by bland macrophages. This pattern is seen in reactive proliferations of the mononuclear–phagocyte system. A **mixed pattern** of follicular, interfollicular, and sinusoidal hyperplasia is common in a variety of complex immune reactions. In **necrotizing lymphadenitis**, variable zones of necrosis are found within the lymph nodes, with or without the presence of neutrophils. Cohesive clusters of macrophages and occasional multinucleated giant cells are characteristic of the **granulomatous inflammation pattern**.

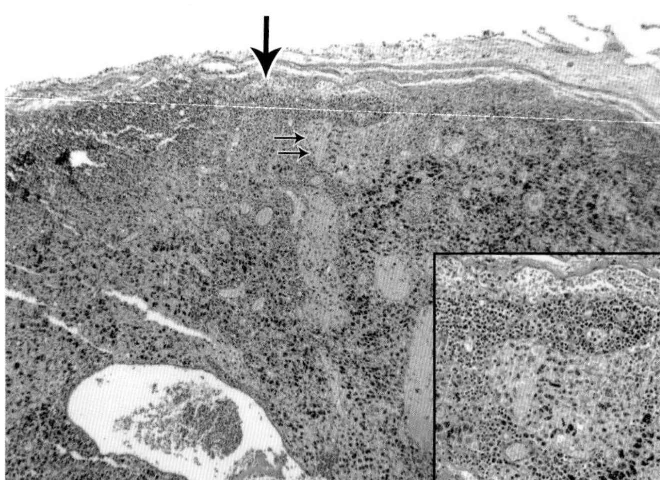

FIGURE 18-21. Sinus histiocytosis. In this hilar lymph node, macrophages are prominent in the subcapsular sinus (*single arrow*) and also in draining sinuses (*double arrows*). (*Inset*) A higher power view demonstrates the large, pink macrophages both at the bottom of the subcapsular sinus and in the draining sinus.

LEUKEMIA AND LYMPHOMA

Three sets of descriptive words help in understanding neoplasms of the bone marrow:

- Lymphoid versus myeloid
- Leukemia versus lymphoma
- Acute versus chronic

The separation of bone marrow–derived neoplasms into **leukemias** and **lymphomas** is arbitrary and based on the location of the neoplastic cells. Leukemias are characterized by circulating neoplastic cells and bone marrow involvement. In lymphomas the neoplastic cells are most often restricted to the lymph nodes and other predominantly lymphoid tissues. For example, chronic lymphocytic leukemia (CLL) and small lymphocytic lymphoma (SLL) are essentially the same disease differing primarily in the location of the neoplastic lymphocytes. In acute leukemias, large, primitive precursor cells with a high nuclear to cytoplasmic ratio (blasts) are prominent, whereas in the chronic leukemias, blasts are uncommon. Seventy percent of acute leukemias originate from the cells of the myeloid lineage (myeloid or myelogenous leukemias); 30% drive from the lymphoid lineage. As the terms imply, acute leukemias tend to have a sudden onset of disease, but chronic leukemias are often indolent and may not be associated with significant symptoms.

Common Lymphoid Neoplasms

Precursor B-Cell Acute Lymphoblastic Leukemia/Lymphoma

The malignant cells in precursor B-ALL and B-cell lymphoblastic lymphoma (B-LBL) are immature (precursor) cells, or **lymphoblasts.** If the B-lymphoblast proliferation involves the bone marrow and peripheral blood, it is termed **acute lymphoblastic leukemia**. However, if it mainly involves extramedullary tissues (e.g., lymph nodes), it is called **lymphoblastic lymphoma**.

Precursor B-ALL is the most common childhood leukemia. Although the disease can present at any age, 75% of cases occur in children younger than age 6. Several environmental and genetic factors have been incriminated in the genesis of ALL, including Down syndrome, Bloom syndrome, ataxia-telangiectasia, neurofibromatosis type I, and in utero exposure to ionizing radiation. Most cases of precursor B-ALL are leukemic rather than lymphomatous at presentation, in contrast to its T-cell counterpart.

Chromosomal abnormalities are present in most cases of precursor B-ALL, including both numerical and structural abnormalities (Table 18-7). Translocations are common (Table 18-7) and include those involving chromosomes 9 and 22 (*BCR/ABL* fusion; Philadelphia chromosome), which tends to generate a smaller protein in childhood B-ALL than in adult B-ALL and chronic myeloid leukemia (CML).

Lymphoblasts are small- to medium-sized cells, with high nucleus to cytoplasm ratios, fine chromatin, inconspicuous nucleoli, and agranular cytoplasm (Fig. 18-22). Lymphoblasts typically comprise 20% or more of bone marrow cellularity and variable numbers of blast cells circulate in the blood. All cases show evidence of B-lymphoblast differentiation, but immunophenotypic patterns in precursor B-ALLs are variable and reflect different stages of early B-cell maturation (Fig. 18-5). The earliest antigens that indicate B-cell differentiation are CD10, CD19, and TdT. B-cell neoplasms that express surface Ig are not considered precursor neoplasms because such is a feature of mature B cells.

The leukemic cells of precursor B-ALL proliferate in the bone marrow and displace the normal marrow elements, resulting in anemia, thrombocytopenia, neutropenia, bone pain, and arthralgias. The last may be the earliest presenting symptoms in children. Organomegaly and CNS involvement are common because the disease disseminates from the bone marrow.

The prognosis for childhood precursor B-ALL after treatment is generally excellent, with complete remission rates of greater than 90%. Poor prognostic indicators include age younger than 1 year or older than 12 years, older adult onset, or the presence of certain cytogenetic abnormalities (e.g., t(9;22), t(1;19), t(4;11), hypodiploidy). All translocations involving the *MLL* gene at 11q23 are associated with a poor prognosis regardless of age.

Precursor T-Cell Acute Lymphoblastic Leukemia/Lymphoma

Precursor T-cell acute lymphoblastic leukemia (T-ALL) and T-cell lymphoblastic lymphoma (T-LBL) are immature T-cell neoplasms. As with precursor B-ALL, the decision whether to call the tumor **leukemia** or **lymphoma** is arbitrary.

Precursor T-ALL occurs at any age but affects adolescents more commonly than young children, accounting for 15% of childhood ALL. T-ALL is more common in males than females. In adults, 25% of ALLs are precursor T-cell variety. Compared to its B-cell counterpart, precursor T-ALL is more likely to have a lymphomatous presentation. The morphology of T lymphoblasts is similar to that of B lymphoblasts (Fig. 18-22). The genes encoding the four T-cell receptor chains (α-, β-, γ-, and δ-chains) often participate in chromosomal translocations with genes encoding transcription factors (Table 18-7).

The immunophenotype in T-ALL reflects normal T-cell differentiation and maturation in the bone marrow and thymus (Fig. 18-6). The earliest T-cell antigen is CD7, followed by CD2 and CD5. During thymic differentiation, T cells become positive for CD1a and cytoplasmic CD3, CD4, and CD8. Like precursor B-ALL, lymphoblasts in most cases of T-ALL express TdT.

Table 18-7

Common Genetic Abnormalities Associated With Proliferations of Lymphoid Cells

Disease	Associated Genetic/Chromosomal Abnormality	Importance
B-lymphoblastic leukemia/ lymphoma	t(9;22) translocations involving *MLL* at 11q23	Children often make p190 bcr/abl, whereas adults make p210 bcr/abl from t(9;22)
	Hyperdiploidy	Better prognosis
	Hypodiploidy	Worse prognosis
T-lymphoblastic leukemia/ lymphoma	*TCR* genes translocate to sites involving *MYC, TAL1, RBTN1, RBTN2, HOX11*	Disturbed transcriptional regulation results
B-cell chronic lymphocytic leukemia/ small lymphocytic lymphomas	del 13q12-14; frequent *IgVH* gene rearrangements	
	del 11q; trisomy 12; del 17p	17p locus encodes p53; these changes imply worse prognosis
Follicular lymphoma	t(14;18)(q32;q21)	Characteristic, leads to overexpression of Bcl-2
	Inactivation of p53; activation of *MYC*	Transformation to more aggressive phenotype
Mantle cell lymphoma	t(11;14)(q13;q32)	Primary genetic event, upregulates cyclin D1
	Mutation at 11q22-23	Inactivates *ATM*
Marginal zone lymphoma	t(11;18); t(1;14)	No longer responds to antibiotic treatment alone
	Mutations of IgV region genes; trisomy 3	
Diffuse large B-cell lymphoma	Rearrangements involving 3q27	3q27 carries *BCL6* locus
	t(14;18) rearrangements involving *MYC*	Tend to portend worse prognosis
Burkitt lymphoma	Rearrangements involving *MYC:* t(8;14) or t(2:8) or t(8;22)	Characteristic rearrangement
Plasma cell myeloma	Clonal rearrangements involving Ig H and L genes	
	Abnormalities of chromosome number	Poor prognosis
	IgH translocations with *cyclin D1, C-MAF, FGFR3, cyclin D3, MAFB*; monosomy or partial deletion of chromosome 13	
	t(4;14); t(14;16); t(14;20); del 17p	Poorer prognosis
Anaplastic large cell lymphoma	t(2;5) (involving anaplastic lymphoma kinase and *NPM* genes)	Tends to occur in younger patients, upregulates *ALK*, better prognosis

H, heavy; Ig, immunoglobulin; L, light; TCR, T-cell receptor.

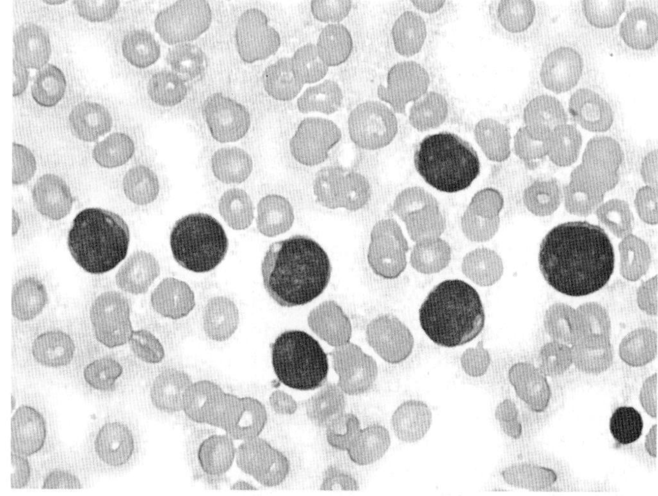

FIGURE 18-22. Acute lymphoblastic leukemia. The lymphoblasts in peripheral blood have irregular and indented nuclei with fine nuclear chromatin, visible nucleoli, and variable amounts of agranular cytoplasm.

The blood and bone marrow are almost always involved in precursor T-ALL. Presenting white blood cell counts are usually high, and a mediastinal mass or other tissue mass (lymphoma) is often present. Lymphadenopathy and organomegaly are common, as are pleural effusions. **Mediastinal adenopathy** occurs particularly often in adolescent males. In general, precursor T-ALL has a worse prognosis than precursor B-ALL in children, but it has a slightly better outcome than B-ALL in adults.

B-Cell Chronic Lymphocytic Leukemia/Small Lymphocytic Lymphoma

B-cell CLL, the most common form of leukemia in adults in the Western world, is a mature CD5$^+$ B-cell tumor. It is characterized by a monomorphic population of small lymphocytes with round to slightly irregular nuclear contours mixed with less abundant larger cells that have round nuclei and single basophilic nucleoli (Fig. 18-23). B-cell CLL/SLL may involve the blood, bone marrow, lymph nodes, or extranodal sites. When the disease only affects the blood and bone marrow (leukemia), the term **CLL** is preferred; uncommonly, when lymphadenopathy or solid tumor masses predominate, **SLL** is

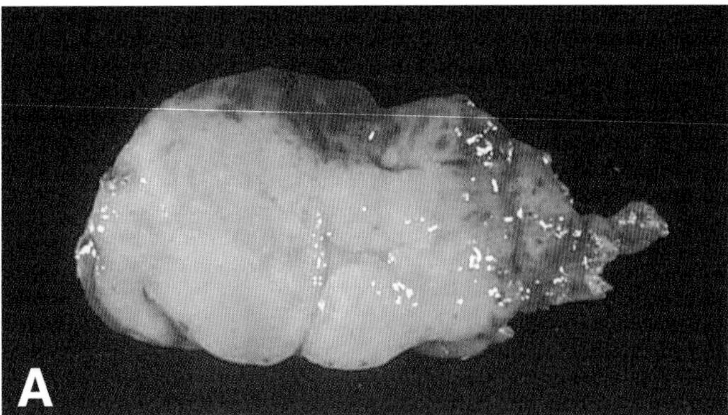

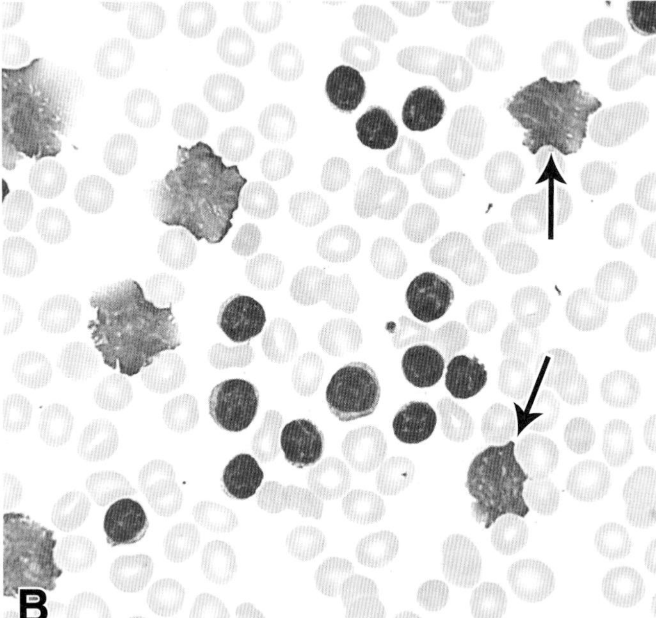

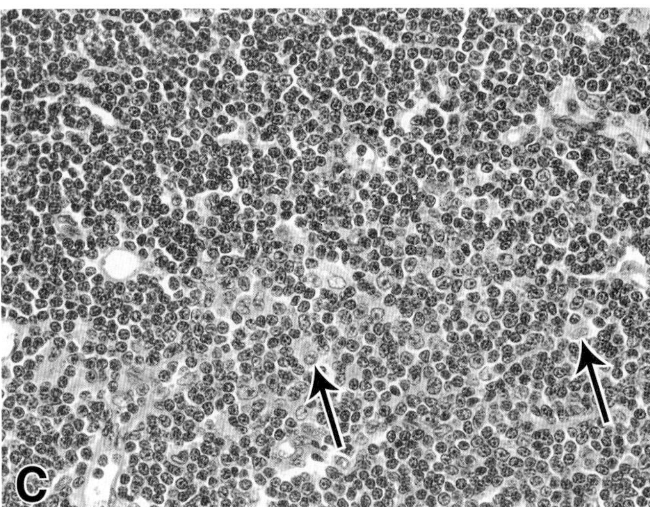

FIGURE 18-23. B-cell small lymphocytic lymphoma/chronic lymphocytic leukemia. A. Gross image of a bisected, enlarged lymph node showing the characteristic uniform, glistening, fish-flesh appearance seen in tissues involved by lymphoma. **B.** A smear of peripheral blood exhibiting numerous small- to medium-sized lymphocytes with clumped nuclear chromatin. Scattered smudge cells (osmotically fragile cells) are present (*arrows*). **C.** On microscopic examination, the nodal architecture is replaced by a diffuse proliferation of small lymphocytes admixed with a low number of larger cells known as paraimmunoblasts (*arrows*) found in scattered proliferation centers.

used. Because these two presentations are otherwise indistinguishable, the term "B-cell CLL/SLL" is sometimes employed. This malignancy generally follows an indolent clinical course and is more frequent in men than in women.

Most B-cell CLL/SLL tumors have cytogenetic abnormalities, the most common of which are shown in Table 18-7. In tissue, the vaguely nodular pattern of B-cell CLL/SLL (with noticeably light and darker staining areas) is most apparent at low magnification (Fig. 18-23C). B-cell CLL/SLL infiltrates the splenic white and red pulp and portal areas of the liver. Bone marrow involvement ranges from complete effacement of the marrow space to patchy interstitial or nonparatrabecular infiltrates of varying degree. The immunophenotype of B-cell CLL/SLL is distinct. The neoplastic cells express pan B-cell antigens, including CD19, CD20, CD22, and CD79, as well as CD5, CD23, and surface Ig light chain.

Most patients with B-cell CLL/SLL are asymptomatic and are diagnosed incidentally. Often the first hint of the disease is an abnormal complete blood count showing absolute lymphocytosis. The total lymphocyte count is variable, but an absolute monoclonal B-cell count of at least 5,000 cells/μL is needed to establish a diagnosis of CLL in the blood.

Immune deficiencies, mainly of B cells but also of T cells, are common. Hypogammaglobulinemia occurs in 50% to 75% of cases at some point during the disease; the degree of hypogammaglobulinemia generally correlates with disease stage and is responsible for infectious complications. Patients with B-CLL also have increased peripheral blood T cells (>3,000/μL). The T cells, though increased in number, often show impaired delayed-type hypersensitivity reactivity, which may contribute to the increased risk of infection. The most common complicating infections are bacterial, then viral and fungal. Asymptomatic patients with B-CLL/SLL who have stable lymphocyte counts may not need treatment. Multiagent chemotherapy or treatment with humanized monoclonal antibodies (e.g., Rituxaimab) is used in patients with high-stage or aggressive disease, but the condition generally remains incurable.

Transformation to prolymphocytic leukemia occurs in 15% to 30% of cases and is the most common form of progression. This type of transformation is heralded by worsening cytopenias, increasing splenomegaly, and relentless increases in prolymphocytes in the blood or paraimmunoblasts in lymph nodes or other tissues. Transformation to diffuse large B-cell lymphoma (**Richter syndrome)** occurs in 10% of cases. This form of progression is marked by the appearance of a rapidly enlarging mass, worsening of systemic symptoms, and a high lactate dehydrogenase level in the serum. Most patients who undergo prolymphocytic or Richter transformation survive less than 1 year.

Mature B-Cell Lymphomas

Mature B-cell malignancies, which make up more than 90% of lymphoid neoplasms worldwide, are clonal proliferations of differentiated B cells. As B cells progress through the steps of differentiation and maturation, from naive B lymphocytes to plasma cells, lymphomas may arise at any point along the way (Fig. 18-5). SLL (more commonly seen in its leukemic form as CLL) has been discussed above under common lymphoid neoplasms.

The frequency of the specific types of B-cell lymphoma varies in different parts of the world. For example, Burkitt lymphoma is endemic in equatorial Africa (where it is the most common childhood malignancy), but it accounts for only 1% to 2% of lymphomas in industrialized nations. Similarly, follicular lymphoma occurs more frequently in the United States and western Europe, compared to South America, eastern Europe, and Asia. Worldwide, the most common lymphomas are follicular lymphoma (29%) and diffuse large cell lymphoma (37%), exclusive of Hodgkin lymphoma (see below) and plasma cell myeloma (multiple myeloma see below) (Table 18-8).

Most mature B-cell lymphomas occur in the sixth and seventh decades of life.

Other than Burkitt lymphoma and diffuse large B-cell lymphoma , they are distinctly uncommon in children.

Risk factors for the development of B-cell lymphoma have been reported to include (1) abnormalities of the immune system, AIDS, iatrogenic immunosuppression, and autoimmune diseases; (2) certain infectious agents (e.g., EBV, hepatitis C, *Helicobacter pylori*, and *Chlamydia*); (3) environmental exposures (e.g., herbicides and pesticides); and (4) genetic polymorphisms in a number of immunoregulatory genes (Table 18-9).

Lymphomas are classified according to their respective normal lymphocyte counterparts (Fig. 18-5). After the precursor stage, B cells undergo Ig *VDJ* gene rearrangements and mature to surface IgM- and IgD-positive naive B cells, which often express CD5. These cells give rise to **mantle cell lymphoma**. Large activated B cells (**centroblasts**) home to germinal centers, where they mature into smaller cells with cleaved nuclei (**centrocytes**). Centroblasts and centrocytes express the germinal center cell markers BCL-6 and CD10 and lack the expression of Bcl-2 antiapoptotic protein. **Follicular lymphomas** derive from germinal center B cells and contain a mixture of centroblasts and centrocytes that overexpress Bcl-2, which gives them a survival advantage. **Burkitt lymphoma** and diffuse large **B-cell** germinal center–type lymphomas also come from germinal center lymphocytes.

Late-stage memory B cells reside in marginal zones, the outermost compartment of lymphoid follicles. **Marginal zone lymphomas** include **splenic marginal zone lymphoma, nodal marginal zone lymphoma,** and **MALT lymphoma**. The last, particularly, involves extranodal sites such as the stomach and other mucosal tissues. Ultimately, some B cells differentiate into plasma cells. These are the only B cells to secrete antibodies, although they lack detectable cell surface Ig. Plasma cells home to the bone marrow, where they may give rise to **multiple myeloma**.

Usually mature B-cell lymphomas contain small lymphocytes and follow an indolent clinical course, whereas other B lymphomas, composed mostly of large cells, follow an aggressive course that is rapidly fatal if untreated. Ironically, although indolent lymphomas follow a prolonged clinical course, they are usually incurable using standard therapy. By contrast, aggressive lymphomas progress rapidly, but many are curable with conventional therapies. Unfortunately, not all lymphomas fall unequivocally into either category.

The following discussion of B-cell lymphomas follows the B-cell development paradigms outlined in Figure 18-5 and concentrates on the more common entities (Table 18-8).

Table 18-8

Frequency of B- and T-/NK-Cell Lymphomas

Diagnosis	% of Total Cases
Diffuse large B-cell lymphoma	30.6
Follicular lymphoma	22.1
MALT lymphoma	7.6
Mature T-cell lymphomas (except ALCL)	7.6
Chronic lymphocytic leukemia/small lymphocytic lymphoma	6.7
Mantle cell lymphoma	6.0
Mediastinal large B-cell lymphoma	2.4
Anaplastic large cell lymphoma (ALCL)	2.4
Burkitt lymphoma	2.5
Nodal marginal zone lymphoma	1.8
Precursor T-cell lymphoblastic lymphoma	1.7
Lymphoplasmacytic lymphoma	1.2
Other types	7.4

MALT, mucosa-associated lymphoid tissue; NK, natural killer.

Table 18-9

Disorders With Increased Risk of Secondary Malignant Lymphoma

Sjögren syndrome
Hashimoto thyroiditis
Renal and cardiac transplant recipients
AIDS
EBV infection
HHV-8 infection
Helicobacter pylori–positive gastritis
Hepatitis C
Congenital immune deficiency syndromes
Chédiak–Higashi
Wiskott–Aldrich
Ataxia-telangiectasia
IgA deficiency
Severe combined immune deficiency
α Heavy-chain disease
Celiac disease
Hodgkin lymphoma (post-treatment)

EBV, Epstein–Barr virus; HHV, human herpesvirus; Ig, immunoglobulin.

Diffuse Large B-Cell Lymphoma

DLBCLs are a heterogeneous group of aggressive—but potentially curable—B-cell tumors. Their heterogeneity is evident at the morphologic, immunophenotypic, genetic, and clinical levels. While some cases of DLBCL arise de novo, others represent transformation or progression from a more indolent type of lymphoma. Although DLBCL most often involves lymph nodes, it commonly presents at extranodal sites, especially the GI tract. DLBCLs are the most common B-cell lymphoma worldwide. They occur at all ages but are most prevalent between the ages of 60 and 70 and are slightly more common in men than in women.

Cases of DLCBL are associated with viral infections, such as EBV, HIV, or (rarely) HHV-8 or chromosomal rearrangements

(Table 18-7). The latter may involve genes that directly or indirectly impair apoptosis and substantially influence prognosis. Some translocations overlap with characteristic follicular lymphoma rearrangements.

The immunophenotype of the malignant cells of DLBCL varies. Often, but not always, the cells express pan B-cell antigens, such as CD19 and CD20. If these are absent, additional markers of B-cell differentiation, such as CD22, CD79a, and PAX-5, may be useful to distinguish DLBCL from other morphologically similar neoplasms. DLBCL cells may or may not express CD10 and BCL-6, markers of germinal center cell differentiation. Sometimes, they express CD5. Surface Ig light-chain restriction occurs most of the time. All cases are negative for TdT and cyclin D1, distinguishing DLBCLs from B-cell lymphoblastic lymphoma (TdT positive) and mantle cell lymphoma (cyclin D1), respectively. DLBCLs show diffuse proliferation of large neoplastic B cells (Fig. 18-24). The large lymphoma cells are comparable in size to the nucleus of a macrophage or roughly twice the size of a normal lymphocyte.

Patients with DLBCL most often present with a rapidly growing tumor in nodal and/or extranodal sites. One or more sites may be involved, but half of patients have limited disease (stage I or II) at presentation. Bone marrow involvement may occur but is usually a late event in this disease. Tumor cells rarely appear in the peripheral blood. Symptoms reflect the site(s) of involvement.

DLBCL is an aggressive neoplasm and is rapidly fatal if left untreated. However, it is sensitive to chemotherapeutic agents that target rapidly dividing cells. Complete remissions are achieved in 60% to 80% of patients. The ultimate outcome depends on tumor stage; patients with limited disease at diagnosis do better compared to those with widespread (high-stage) disease.

Follicular Lymphoma

FL is a mature B-cell lymphoma of follicle center B cells (germinal center cells) and is the second most common lymphoma worldwide. However, it is the most common non-Hodgkin lymphoma in the United States, constituting 20% of all adult lymphomas. FL is mainly a disease of adults, with a peak incidence in the sixth decade. It only rarely occurs in people under age 20 and is more common in women than men. Its behavior varies from indolent to aggressive, depending on tumor grade.

The t(14:18) translocation is the characteristic genomic abnormality in FL and occurs in up to 90% of cases (Table 18-7). This chromosomal aberration places expression of the antiapoptotic protein Bcl-2 under control of the IgH promoter. As a result of Bcl-2, an inhibitor of apoptosis is overexpressed and provides a survival advantage to the lymphoma cells.

FLs express pan B-cell antigens, including CD19, CD20, CD22, CD79a, PAX-5, and cell surface Ig. In most cases, the last contains only one type of light chain (κ or λ). In addition, FLs express the germinal center cell markers CD10 and Bcl-6, as would be expected given that they originate from follicle centers. Unlike mantle cell lymphoma and B-cell CLL/SLL, FLs do not express CD5.

Lymph nodes (or other tissues) involved by follicular lymphoma have a distinctly nodular (follicular) pattern or a combination of nodular and diffuse architectural patterns (Fig. 18-25). The neoplastic follicles are present in high density and are often in a back-to-back arrangement, with little intervening paracortex. The neoplastic follicle centers (germinal centers) contain a mixture of small and large cells with irregular nuclear contours (centrocytes/cleaved cells) and scattered centroblasts. The latter have round nuclear contours and multiple nucleoli attached to the nuclear membrane. High-grade disease presents with an increased density of centroblasts. The bone marrow is involved in 40% to 60% of cases, in a characteristic paratrabecular pattern. Circulating FL cells are present in the blood in 10% of cases; they show prominent nuclear irregularity and deep nuclear clefts.

Most patients with FL present with generalized adenopathy. Over 80% have high-stage disease at the time of initial diagnosis. The lymphadenopathy is painless and may have followed a waxing and waning course before the patient seeks medical attention. Some patients will report having fevers, fatigue, and night sweats (B symptoms).

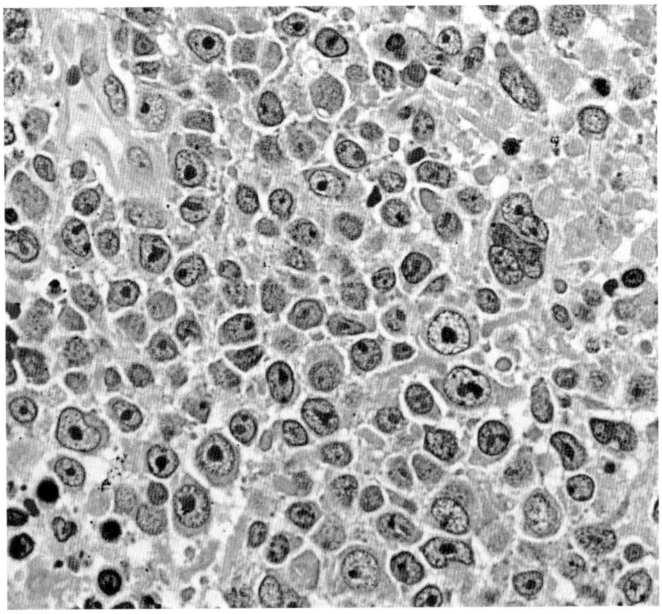

FIGURE 18-24. Diffuse large B-cell lymphoma. Sheets of large lymphoma cells with prominent nucleoli are present.

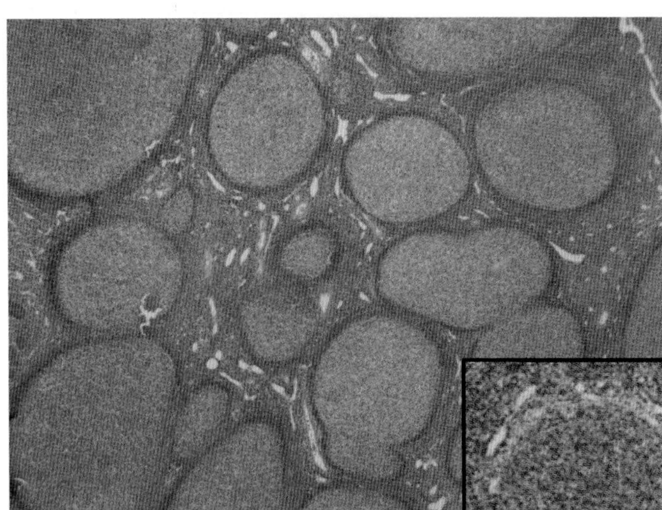

FIGURE 18-25. Follicular lymphoma. The normal lymph node architecture is replaced by malignant lymphoid follicles in a back-to-back pattern. (*Inset*) Malignant lymphoid follicle germinal centers can be distinguished from normal/reactive germinal centers using immunohistochemistry for Bcl-2.

Because most cases of FL follow an indolent clinical course, and the disease is usually incurable, treatment is not always needed at diagnosis. Overall median survival is 7 to 9 years, which does not improve dramatically with high-dose chemotherapy.

Marginal Zone Lymphoma (Mucosa-associated Lymphoid Tissue Lymphoma)

Marginal zone lymphomas comprise a heterogeneous group of mature B-cell tumors that arise in lymph nodes, spleen, and, importantly, in extranodal tissues. The lymphoma cells are thought to arise from the marginal zone of the lymphoid follicle, which contains memory B cells that have gone through the germinal center reaction (postgerminal center). Regardless of the primary site of involvement, all marginal zone lymphomas share similar morphologic and immunophenotypic features. **MALT lymphomas**, or **MALTomas**, are extranodal marginal zone lymphomas arising in the **m**ucosa-**a**ssociated **l**ymphoid **t**issues. They account for 5% to 10% of B-cell lymphomas and are the most common type of gastric lymphoma. Most cases occur in adults with a median age of 60; they are rare in children and young adults.

MALT lymphomas are monoclonal B-cell tumors that arise in the setting of chronic inflammation, most often due to autoimmunity or infection. What begins as a benign polyclonal reaction acquires mutations or chromosomal lesions in B cells. The prototypical infection-driven MALToma is gastric lymphoma associated with *H. pylori* gastritis (see Chapter 11). In their earliest phases of development and prior to acquiring chromosomal translocations (Table 18-7), such lymphomas may regress with antibiotic therapy to eradicate *H. pylori*. Dissemination to distant sites or transformation to diffuse large B-cell lymphomas occurs as additional genetic lesions accrue.

MALTomas have no specific immunophenotype. Most tumor cells express IgM and show light-chain restriction. They express B-cell–associated antigens and are negative for CD5, CD23, and cyclin D1, which distinguishes them from B-CLL/SLL and mantle cell lymphoma. Unlike FL, MALTomas do not express CD10.

Most MALT lymphomas involve the stomach or other mucosal sites, including the respiratory tract. They may also occur in the salivary glands, ocular adnexa, skin, thyroid, and breast. These tumors may remain localized for prolonged periods and tend to follow an indolent clinical course.

Mantle Cell Lymphoma

MCL is a mature CD5$^+$ B-cell tumor that presents a picture of monotonous small- to medium-sized lymphocytes with irregular nuclear contours. They resemble the normal lymphocytes of the mantle zone around germinal centers. MCL accounts for less than 10% of B-cell lymphomas.

The reciprocal chromosomal translocation t(11;14) is considered the primary genetic event in 80% to 90% of all cases of MCL (Table 18-7). The lesion causes overexpression of cyclin D1, which drives cell cycle progression at the G_1 to S phases transition by binding to Cdk4/6 (see Chapter 4). Several other oncogenic changes may occur in MCL and are listed in Table 18-7. MCL expresses the B-cell markers CD19 and CD20 and shows surface light-chain restriction. As noted the lymphoma cells are also positive for CD5, but they are negative for CD10 and CD23. Importantly, MCL cells are positive for cyclin D1 (Fig. 18-26B).

Lymph nodes with MCL show a diffuse to vaguely nodular lymphoid infiltrate composed of small to medium-sized B cells with irregular nuclear contours. In some cases, MCL lymphocytes are round and resemble the cells of B-cell CLL/SLL. Characteristic features in typical cases of MCL are the striking monotony of the lymphoma cells with respect to size and shape (Fig. 18-26A) and the presence of scattered epithelioid histiocytes and hyalinized small blood vessels.

There are two major variants of MCL: one with a more nodular-appearing pattern in which the lymphoma cells surround the germinal centers (**mantle zone pattern**), and another where the cells are larger and resemble lymphoblasts (**blastic/blastoid variant**). The latter is the more aggressive type. MCL is mainly a nodal-based disease, but it involves many different tissues and organs, particularly the spleen, bone marrow, and GI tract. Multifocal mucosal involvement of the gut (mostly small intestine and colon) may produce a pattern known as **lymphomatous polyposis**.

Most patients with MCL present with high-stage disease. About one third have peripheral blood involvement at diagnosis. Despite its small cell morphology, MCL is clinically aggressive and is considered incurable by standard chemotherapy. The median survival is 5 years for the typical type of MCL and 3 years for the blastic/blastoid variant.

Burkitt Lymphoma

BL is one of the most rapidly growing malignancies known and is defined by a chromosomal translocation that activates the *MYC* oncogene (see Chapter 4). BL often presents at extranodal sites, contains a monomorphic population of medium-sized cells, and tends to show involvement of the blood or bone marrow. The MYC translocation is highly characteristic, but is not specific to BL, and a combination of other diagnostic features is required to confirm the diagnosis.

BL occurs in three distinct variants, each with different clinical presentations, morphology, and pathogenesis. In equatorial Africa and Papua-New Guinea, **endemic BL** is the most common childhood malignancy, with a peak incidence in 4- to 7-year-olds. The malignancy commonly involves the jaw, other facial bones, and the abdominal viscera. **Sporadic BL** occurs worldwide and mainly affects children and young adults. In the Western world, sporadic BL is uncommon (1% to 2% of lymphomas overall), but accounts for 30% to 50% of childhood lymphomas. The median age for adult patients is 30 years. Unlike endemic BL, sporadic BL often presents as an abdominal mass involving the ileocecum. **Immunodeficiency-associated BL** mainly occurs in HIV-infected people and may be the initial manifestation of AIDS.

All cases of BL are associated with translocations that upregulate the expression of the *c-MYC* oncogene on chromosome 8, either by placing it under the control of IgH [t(8;14)] or IgL [t(2;8 for κ) or t(8;22 for λ)] promoters (Table 18-7). In endemic cases, the breakpoint on chromosome 14 occurs in the heavy-chain–joining region, as seen in early B cells. In sporadic BL, the translocation occurs in the Ig switch region, which is more characteristic of mature B lymphocytes. EBV infection is present in virtually all cases of endemic BL but is responsible for less than 30% of sporadic and immunodeficiency-related cases. Many patients experience prodromal polyclonal B-cell activation caused by bacterial, viral, or parasitic infections (e.g., malaria). BL cells express surface IgM and Ig light chain and are positive for common B-cell antigens (CD19, CD20, and CD22). They also express CD10 and BCL-6, which suggests that they originate from germinal centers. BL cells do not express TdT, a feature that helps to distinguish these tumors from precursor B-cell acute lymphoblastic leukemia/lymphoma.

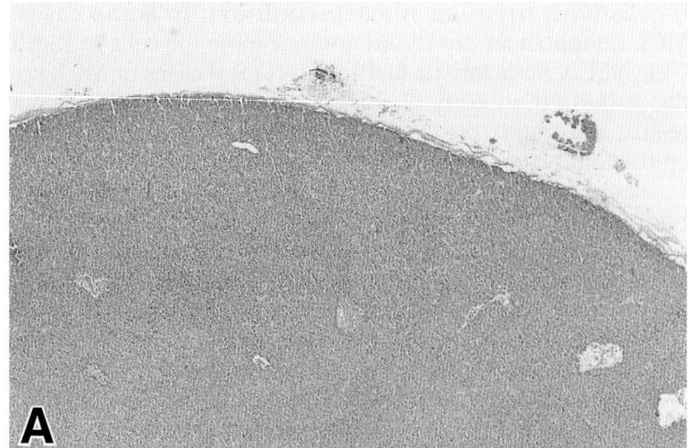

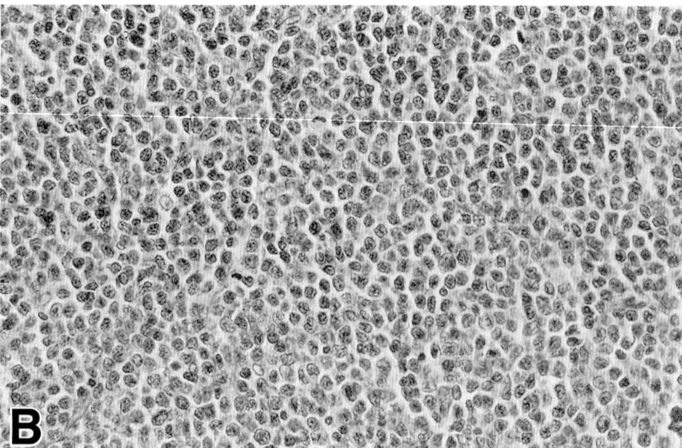

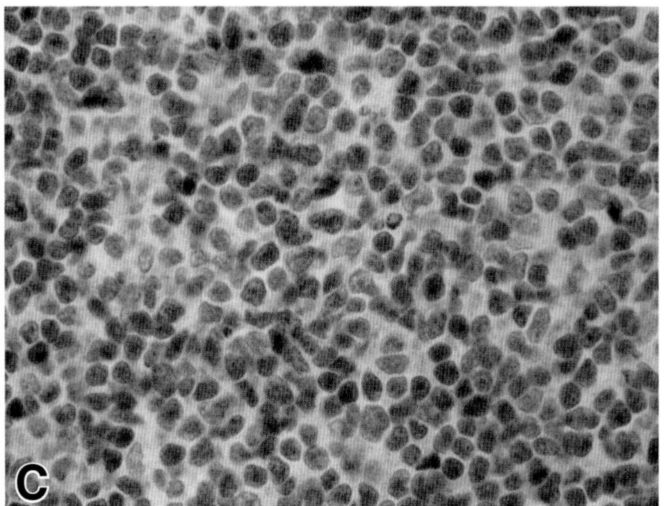

FIGURE 18-26. Mantle cell lymphoma (MCL). A. Lymph node architecture is completely effaced by a small lymphocytic infiltrate. **B.** At closer examination, the population of lymphocytes consists of monotonous, small cells with irregular nuclei. Unlike small lymphocytic lymphomas, MCL has very few admixed larger cells. **C.** A nuclear stain for Bcl-1 (cyclin D1) is positive. This finding correlates with the presence of t(11;14), the typical translocation in MCL.

BL typically produces extranodal tumors rather than lymphadenopathy. All variants of this lymphoma have a high risk for CNS involvement. The classic presentation for endemic BL is a destructive tumor in the jaws or other facial bones (Fig. 18-27A). Patients with sporadic BL typically present with abdominal masses. All types may involve ovaries, kidneys, and breast. Patients with sizable bulky tumors sometimes present with Burkitt leukemia and extensive bone marrow involvement. Involved nodes demonstrate a characteristics "starry-sky" appearance with lighter staining macrophage "stars" scattered among the deeply basopholic BL cell "sky" (Fig. 18-27B and C).

All variants of BL are highly aggressive, and most patients have bulky extranodal tumors, high tumor burdens, and disseminated disease at presentation. Because of its high proliferative rate, BL responds to intensive chemotherapy. Thus, up to 90% of people with early-stage disease and 60% to 80% of those with high-stage disease may be cured. Children and young adults with BL tend to fare better than adults. As a result of rapid tumor cell death during treatment, tumor lysis syndrome, a potentially lethal complication, can occur.

Plasma Cell Neoplasia

Plasma cell neoplasms result from clonal expansion of plasma cells, that is, terminally differentiated B lymphocytes that can produce a monoclonal paraprotein (**monoclonal gammopathy**). The major plasma cell neoplasms **include monoclonal gammopathy of undetermined significance (MGUS)** and **plasma cell myeloma** (multiple myeloma). These maladies almost exclusively affect adults. Risk factors include a genetic predisposition, exposure to ionizing radiation, and chronic antigen stimulation. Further discussion will be limited to MGUS and plasma cell myeloma.

Monoclonal Gammopathy of Undetermined Significance

MGUS occurs in about 3% of people older than age 50 and in more than 5% of those older than 70. Criteria for diagnosing MGUS include (1) monoclonal paraproteinemia of less than 3.0 g/dL; (2) less than 10% plasma cells in the bone marrow; (3) lack of end-organ damage (CRAB: hyper*c*alcemia, *r*enal insufficiency, *a*nemia, *b*one lesions); and (4) exclusion of other B-cell neoplasms or diseases known to produce a monoclonal paraprotein (M-protein).

IgM MGUS is most often associated with a clone of Ig-secreting B cells and can progress to a small B-cell lymphoma. Non-IgM MGUS is most often associated with clonal plasma cells, which becomes overt plasma cell neoplasia (multiple myeloma) in about 1% of affected patients per year.

Plasma Cell Myeloma (Multiple Myeloma)

PCM is a malignancy of plasma cells, in which the serum or urine or both contains an M-protein. The disease is primarily based in the bone marrow and tends to be multifocal. PCM

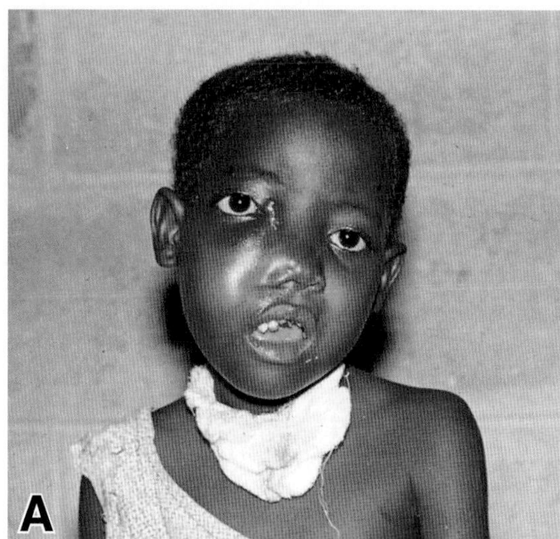

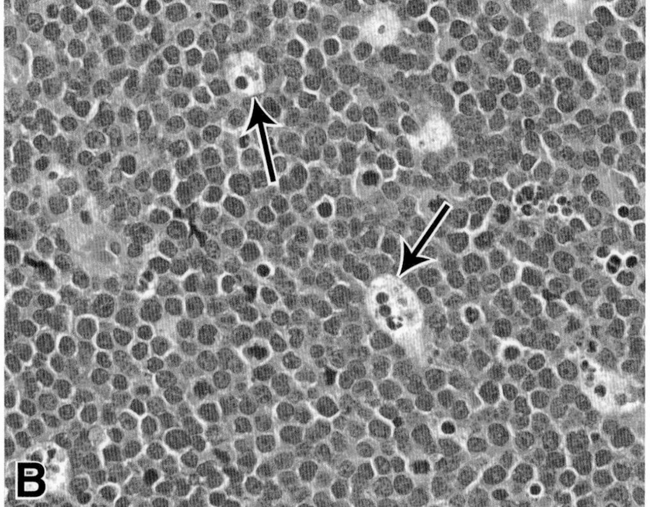

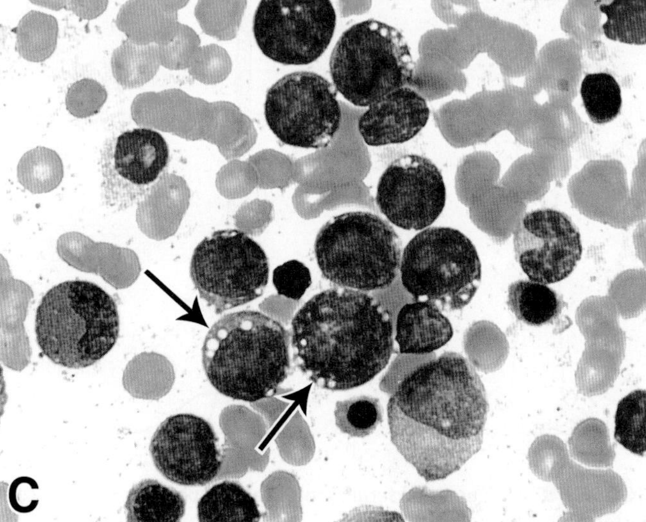

FIGURE 18-27. Burkitt lymphoma. A. A tumor of the jaw distorts the child's face. **B.** Lymph node is effaced by neoplastic lymphocytes with several starry-sky macrophages (*arrows*). **C.** Bone marrow aspirate smear showing typical cytologic features of Burkitt lymphoma. Note the deeply basophilic cytoplasm and lipid vacuoles (*arrows*).

varies from asymptomatic and indolent to highly aggressive with leukemic involvement.

PCM accounts for 10% of hematologic malignancies, with 22,000 cases reported annually in the United States. Its overall incidence is about 6 cases per 100,000 people. Men are more affected than women, and the disease is twice as common in blacks as in whites. The incidence of PCM increases with age; the median age at diagnosis is 69 years, and it is extremely rare in adults under age 30. People who have a first-degree relative with PCM have a fourfold greater risk of developing the disease.

Plasma cell myeloma produces multifocal destructive bone lesions with a lytic or "punched-out" radiographic appearance throughout the skeleton. The vertebral column, ribs, skull, pelvis, femurs, clavicles, and scapulae are most commonly affected. Plasma cells focally fill the medullary cavity, erode cancellous bone, and eventually destroy the bony cortex, causing pathologic fractures. The affected bone contains gelatinous red-brown soft tissue masses that are sharply demarcated from the surrounding normal tissue (Fig. 18-28). If the tumors breach the bony cortex, they may spread beyond the medullary cavity into surrounding soft tissues.

All cases of PCM demonstrate rearrangement of the Ig L- and H-chain genes. The pattern of somatic hypermutation in the variable regions of Ig heavy chains is consistent with the postgerminal center origin of the neoplastic cells. Both numerical and structural chromosomal abnormalities occur in PCM. The IgH gene frequently participates in translocations, which involve diverse oncogenes (Table 18-7). Loss or partial loss of one chromosome 13 occurs in 50% of cases and is thought to be an early genetic event in plasma cell neoplasia.

The bone marrow in PCM shows interstitial clusters, distinct nodules, or confluent sheets of plasma cells; variable amounts of normal bone marrow are often present. PCM is likely if plasma cell infiltrates involve over 30% of the marrow volume or if there are large confluent masses of plasma cells without admixed normal hematopoietic cells.

Plasma cells in PCM usually express the B-cell marker CD79a, plasma cell markers CD38 and CD138, and monotypic *cytoplasmic* Ig. Unlike normal plasma cells, myeloma cells usually lack CD19, and unlike mature B cells, they usually do not express CD20. Myeloma plasma cells may resemble normal plasma cells (Fig. 18-29A), or they may show immature,

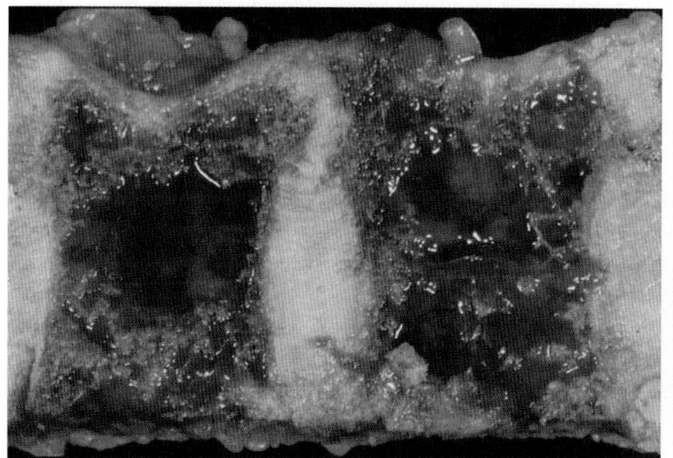

FIGURE 18-28. Plasma cell myeloma. Multiple lytic bone lesions are present in the vertebra. Bones such as this are prone to pathologic fracture.

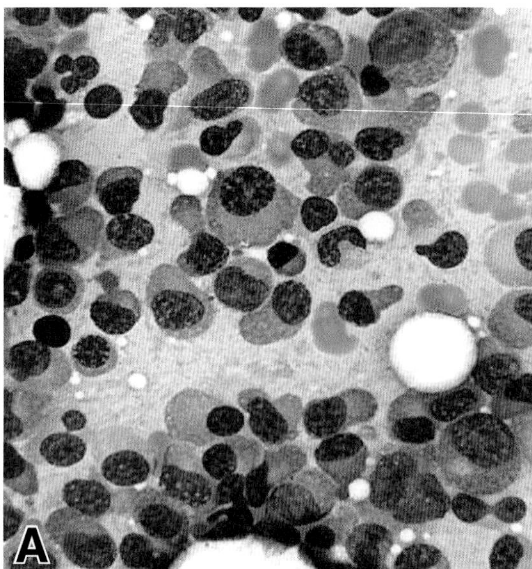

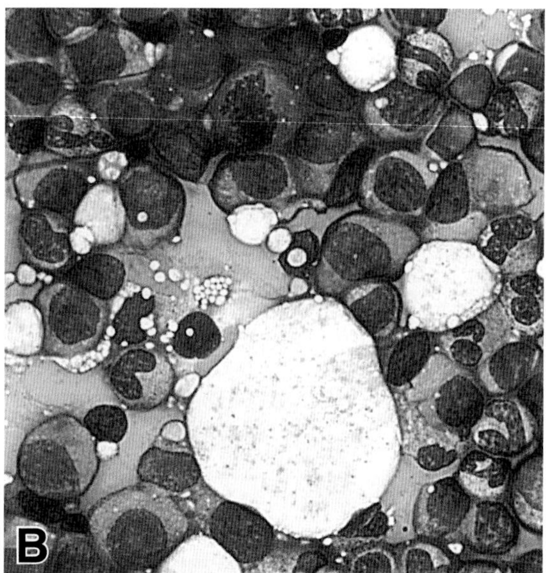

FIGURE 18-29. Plasma cell myeloma (PCM). Neoplastic plasma cells can show variable cytologic features ranging from normal-appearing cells (**A**) to cells resembling blasts (**B**). Total number, clonality, and clinicopathologic findings help distinguish PCM from other plasma cell proliferations.

plasmablastic, or pleomorphic features (Fig. 18-29B). Cytoplasmic and nuclear inclusions, representing accumulated or partially degraded Ig, are occasionally present.

Erythrocyte rouleaux in peripheral blood smears occur when high levels of M-protein cause red blood cells to stick together end on end, like a stack of coins. In a minority of cases, plasma cells may circulate in the blood. Marked peripheral blood plasmacytosis establishes a diagnosis of plasma cell leukemia. Renal disease occurs in more than 50% of cases (see Chapter 14).

In most instances, the heavy chain in the monoclonal paraprotein is IgG or IgA. Rarely, it is IgD or IgE. Immunoglobulins produced in 85% of cases are whole antibody molecules, and the remainder are exclusively light chains (**light-chain disease**). In some cases, there is no detectable serum or urine paraprotein (nonsecreting myelomas). Laboratory assessment for monoclonal gammopathy entails serum (or urine) protein electrophoresis and immunoanalysis to detect a monoclonal restricted protein (spike) (Fig. 18-30).

Symptomatic myeloma is characterized by end-organ damage (CRAB: hypercalcemia, renal insufficiency, anemia, bone lesions). Radiography reveals lytic bone lesions often associated with bone pain and hypercalcemia. Calcium released from injured or resorbed bone may precipitate in the kidneys (nephrocalcinosis) and impair renal function.

Monoclonal light-chain proteinuria can damage renal tubular epithelium and lead to kidney failure. M-proteins can suppress normal antibody responses and so predispose to infectious complications. Anemia develops in 70% of patients, both because the neoplastic plasma cells displace normal bone marrow and because renal injury limits erythropoietin production. Additional findings and complications associated with PCM include amyloidosis, hyperviscosity syndrome, coagulation abnormalities, humoral immune deficiency, and treatment-related myeloid malignancies (e.g., myelodysplasia and acute myeloid leukemia). The serum or urine or both have detectable M-proteins in 97% of patients (see above), the isotype of which predicts disease progression. Uncommon IgD- and IgE-secreting myelomas and light-chain disease are the most aggressive.

Plasma cell myeloma remains an incurable disease; however, targeted therapies such as bortezomib, a proteasome inhibitor, portend increasingly better prognoses. Median survival is 3.75 years but is highly variable, ranging from less than 6 months to more than 10 years.

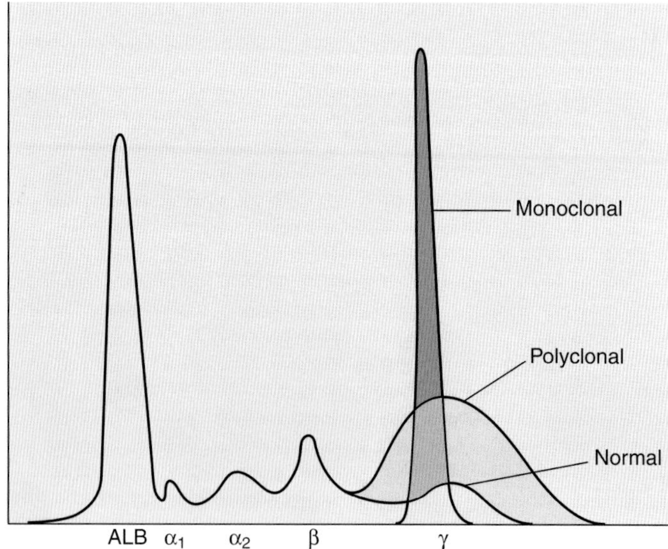

FIGURE 18-30. Abnormal serum protein electrophoretic patterns contrasted with a normal pattern. Polyclonal hypergammaglobulinemia, characteristic of benign reactive processes, shows a broad-based increase in immunoglobulins as a result of immunoglobulin secretion by myriad reactive plasma cells. Monoclonal gammopathy of unknown significance or plasma cell neoplasia shows a narrow peak, or spike, as a result of the homogeneity of the immunoglobulin molecules secreted by a single clone of aberrant plasma cells. ALB, albumin.

Peripheral T-Cell and Natural Killer Cell Lymphomas

These neoplasms are a heterogeneous group of mature lymphoid tumors that arise in lymphoid tissues outside the thymus, such as lymph nodes, spleen, gut, and skin (Fig. 18-6). They occur rarely compared to B-cell lymphomas, accounting for 12% of non-Hodgkin lymphomas, and generally have a poorer prognosis.

They are more common in Asia than in the Western world. Major risk factors for T-cell neoplasia include the prevalence of human T-cell leukemia virus type 1 (HTLV-1) and EBV, plus genetic predispositions to those viruses. HTLV-1 is endemic in southwestern Japan where 8% to 10% of the population is seropositive, and the lifetime risk for adult T-cell leukemia/lymphoma (ATLL) is 5%. EBV-associated T-cell lymphomas are more common in Asians than in other racial groups.

Mature T-cell lymphomas express surface CD3, as well as a variable number of other pan T-cell antigens, such as CD2, CD5, and CD7; CD4 or CD8; and either $\alpha-\beta$ or $\gamma-\delta$ T-cell receptor subunits. Most peripheral T-cell lymphomas are of the a−b type. $\gamma-\delta$ T cells comprise less than 5% of the T-cell repertoire and congregate at epithelial surfaces and in the splenic red pulp; they do not express CD4, CD5, or CD8. Unlike immature T-cell neoplasms (such as T-cell lymphoblastic lymphoma), mature T-cell neoplasms lack TdT.

Peripheral T-cell neoplasms show variable morphologic features. Involved lymph nodes and other tissues are usually diffusely effaced by a heterogeneous population of malignant lymphoid cells. These vary from small to large and from relatively bland to overtly anaplastic in appearance. Eosinophils and benign macrophages often comingle with the neoplastic T cells, probably recruited to the site of involvement by cytokines secreted by the lymphoma cells. Some of these tumors show prominent vascularity.

Some mature T-cell lymphomas have a **cytotoxic** phenotype and are positive for the granule-associated proteins perforin, granzyme B, and T-cell intracellular antigen.

NK-cell lymphomas lack surface CD3, but they do express the CD3 ε-subunit, which is intracellular. They also express other T-cell–associated markers, including, CD2, CD7, CD8, CD16, and CD56.

Peripheral T-cell and NK-cell tumors are grouped clinically into leukemic, nodal, extranodal, and cutaneous forms. They are usually widely disseminated at presentation (high stage) and hence are generally more aggressive than are B-cell neoplasms. Systemic manifestations, such as fever, pruritus, eosinophilia, fever, and weight loss, are common. T- and NK-cell lymphomas are treated with multiagent chemotherapy, but most respond poorly. Overall, 5-year survival is 20% to 30%.

Adult T-Cell Leukemia/Lymphoma

ATLL, caused by the human retrovirus **HTLV-1**, has a long latency period. The normal counterparts of ATLL cells are mature, activated, CD4$^+$ T cells. Exposure to HTLV-1 occurs early in life in people who live in endemic regions. The virus may be transmitted in breast milk and via blood and blood products. Even though exposure occurs early in life, ATLL only occurs in adults, with a mean age of 58. Viral infection alone is not sufficient for neoplastic transformation, and other genetic lesions are required to progress from lymphocyte infection to malignancy.

The neoplastic lymphoid cells vary widely in appearance (Fig. 18-31). They commonly have prominent nuclear convolutions and lobations, sometimes likened to flowers (flower cells). They express T-cell–associated antigens, including CD2, CD3, and CD5, but usually lack CD7. Nearly all cases strongly express CD25, and most express CD4. Tumor cells show clonal T-cell receptor gene rearrangements and have clonally integrated HTLV-1. A viral protein, p40 (Tax), directs transcriptional activation of several genes in infected lymphocytes

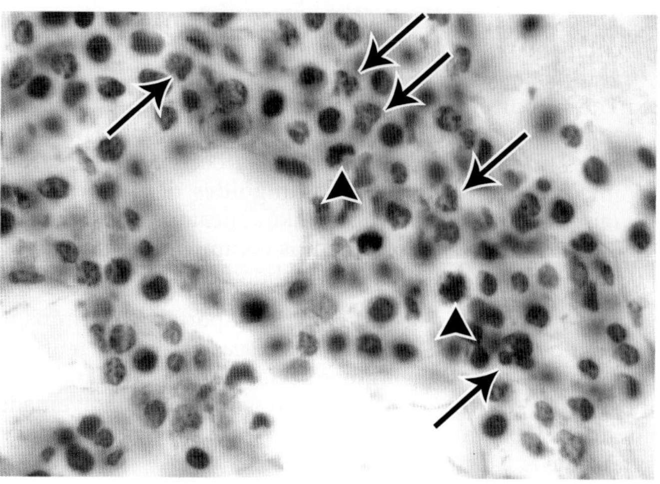

FIGURE 18-31. Adult T-cell leukemia/lymphoma. This disease is characterized by proliferation of malignant T lymphocytes (here, in the bone marrow) with extremely irregular, knobby nuclei (*arrows*). The mitotic rate among the malignant cells is characteristically high (*arrowheads*).

ATLL is a systemic disease and is usually widespread at presentation often involving lymph nodes, spleen, bone marrow, peripheral blood, and skin (the most common extralymphatic site). Hypercalcemia, with or without lytic bone lesions, and peripheral leukocytosis are typical. Acute ATLL has a poor prognosis, and most patients survive less than 1 year, despite aggressive systemic chemotherapy. Death frequently occurs from infectious complications, such as those seen in HIV-infected patients. Chronic and smoldering forms of the disease have a somewhat better prognosis.

Mycosis Fungoides and Sézary Syndrome

MF is the most common form of primary cutaneous T-cell lymphoma. It is characterized by infiltration of the epidermis by malignant CD4$^+$ (helper-type) T cells with marked nuclear folding. Sézary syndrome is a variant of MF, defined by a triad of erythroderma, generalized lymphadenopathy, and circulating lymphoma cells in the blood (Sézary cells).

The MF cells have a T-helper cell immunophenotype and generally express CD2, CD3, CD5, CD4, and T-cell receptor (TCR)- α, β. As in other mature T-cell lymphomas, CD7, the pan T-cell antigen, is absent. Clonal T-cell receptor gene rearrangements are common, which helps to distinguish subtle cases of MF from inflammatory dermatoses.

MF is an indolent lymphoma that progresses slowly over years (and sometimes decades) from patches to plaques to mass lesions.

- The **premycotic or eczematous stage** lasts years and is difficult to distinguish from many benign chronic dermatoses. Skin biopsies show nonspecific perivascular and periadnexal lymphocytic infiltration, with accompanying eosinophils and plasma cells.

- The **plaque stage** follows, with well-demarcated, raised cutaneous plaques. It is usually possible to diagnose MF at this stage.
- The **tumor stage is characterized by** raised cutaneous tumors, mostly on the face and in body folds. These tumors frequently ulcerate and may become secondarily infected. The name, **mycosis fungoides**, derives from the raised, fungating, mushroom-like appearance of the tumor. Extracutaneous involvement is common, particularly of the lymph nodes, spleen, liver, bone marrow, and lungs.

The extent of disease is the most important determinant of prognosis. Patients with limited disease generally have an excellent prognosis; their life expectancies are comparable to those of the general population. Extracutaneous involvement augurs a poor prognosis, and the 5-year survival in Sézary syndrome is 10% to 20%.

Anaplastic Large Cell Lymphoma

ALCL is a mature T-cell tumor that features large pleomorphic cells that express the CD30 lymphoid activation marker. These lymphomas often involve both nodal and extranodal sites (frequently skin). This disease has a bimodal age distribution, in which one peak occurs in young people and a second in older people.

Some cases of ALCL show translocations involving the *ALK* gene (Table 18-7) and have a relatively good prognosis. ALK-negative ALCL tends to be more aggressive. And the prognosis is like that of unspecified types of peripheral T-cell lymphoma.

The histology of ALCL is variable, but all cases have a population of cells with irregularly shaped nuclei (often horseshoe or kidney shaped) and abundant cytoplasm, which often has a distinct eosinophilic area near the nucleus (Fig. 18-32). These cells, which are usually large, are diagnostic **hallmark cells** and, as noted, express CD30. ALCL cells also express several pan T-cell antigens and cytotoxic T-cell antigens (TIA-1, granzyme B), but most cases are negative for CD3. Over 90% of cases have T-cell receptor rearrangements, even if the tumor cells do not express T-cell antigens.

Most patients with ALCL have advanced disease at presentation. Peripheral and central lymphadenopathy are common, as are extranodal and bone marrow involvement. Patients often have B symptoms, especially fever. The overall 5-year survival of ALK-positive ALCL is 80%. This drops to 48% for patients in the case of ALK-negative tumors.

Angioimmunoblastic T-Cell Lymphoma

AITL is an aggressive peripheral (mature) T-cell lymphoma of adults and the elderly. Patients present with generalized adenopathy and symptoms consistent with a systemic disease process. Neoplastic T-cell infiltrates expand the paracortical regions of lymph nodes and are associated with a striking proliferation of high endothelial venules. EBV is present in nearly all cases, but the virus infects only B cells, not the neoplastic T cells.

Neoplastic T cells express most pan T-cell antigens (CD2, CD3, CD5, and CD7), plus CD4 in most cases. They also usually show a phenotype of follicular T-helper cells with expression of CD10, CXCL13, and PD-1. Clonal rearrangement of the T-cell receptor occurs in most cases of AITL.

At the outset, most patients with AITL have high-stage disease, generalized lymphadenopathy, hepatosplenomegaly, bone marrow involvement, hypergammaglobulinemia, and body cavity effusions. A pruritic skin rash is also common. The tumor renders people with AITL immunodeficient, and the high incidence of EBV-positive B cells in these patients reflects their altered immune function. This is an aggressive lymphoma, with a median survival of less than 3 years. Patients often die from infectious complications, and some patients develop a concomitant large B-cell lymphoma.

Hodgkin Lymphomas

There are two types of HL: **classic Hodgkin lymphoma** and **nodular lymphocyte-predominant Hodgkin lymphoma**. Unlike the non-Hodgkin tumors discussed above, classic HL arises in a single lymph node or lymph node chain and spreads in

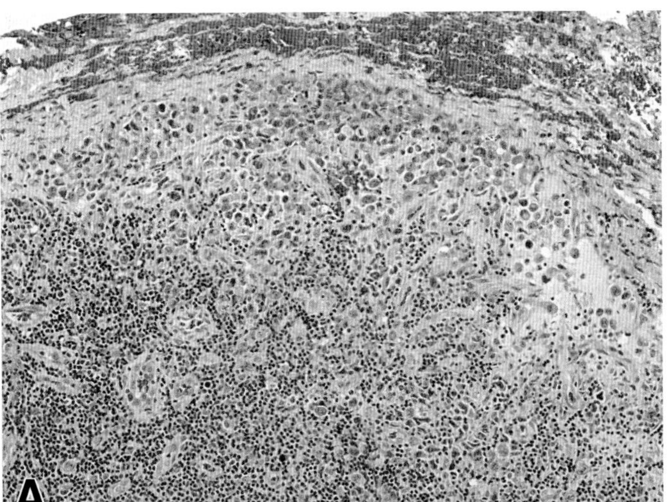

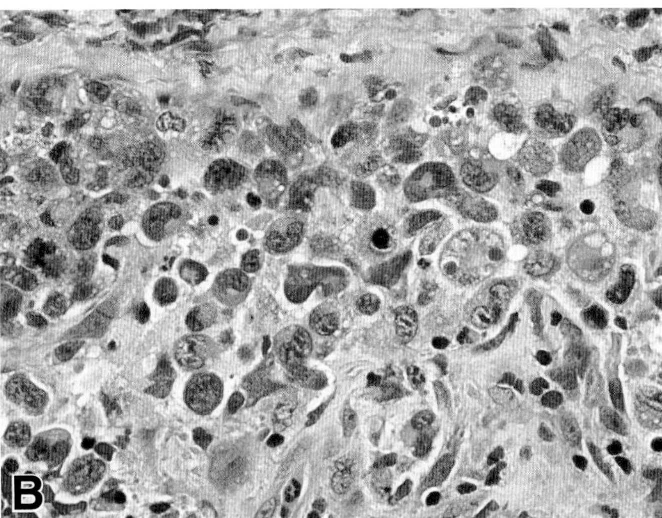

FIGURE 18-32. Anaplastic large cell lymphoma (ALCL). Partially effaced lymph node with accumulation of malignant cells in the subcapsular sinus. This common ALCL pattern may be confused with metastatic carcinoma. (*Inset*) The intrasinusoidal lymphoma cells are large and pleomorphic. Cells with kidney-shaped nuclei and an eosinophilic zone near the nucleus are known as hallmark cells and are seen in all variants of ALCL.

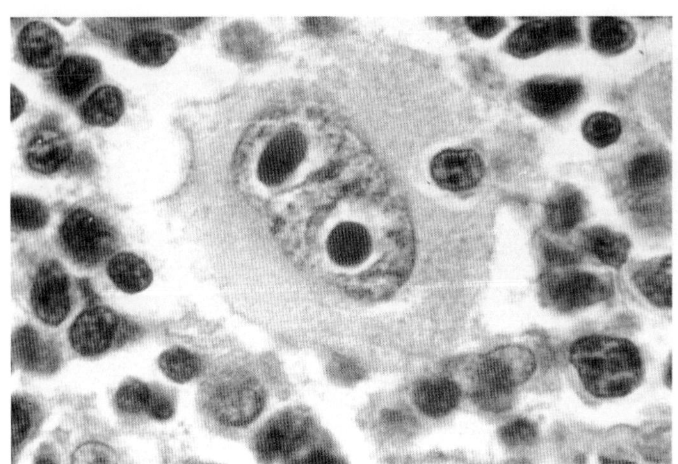

FIGURE 18-33. Classic Reed–Sternberg cell. Mirror-image nuclei contain large eosinophilic nucleoli.

a contiguous manner. It occurs mostly in younger people and has relatively few neoplastic cells, amid a prominent mixed inflammatory cell background. In the majority of cases, the neoplastic cells in HL, namely, the Reed–Sternberg (RS) cells are derivatives of germinal center B cells (Fig. 18-33). RS cells are often less than 1% of the total cell content of affected tissues.

HL is the most common malignancy of Americans between the ages of 10 and 30.

Young adults who have had EBV infectious mononucleosis have a threefold higher risk of developing HL, and the EBV genome is frequently identified in RS cells, suggesting an infectious etiology.

Genetic factors may play a role in HL. Siblings of HL patients have a sevenfold increased risk of the disease, which rises to 100-fold if they are monozygotic twins.

Immune status also seems to be a factor, at least in some cases. HL occurs more often in people with altered immunity or with autoimmune diseases, such as rheumatoid arthritis. HL accounts for 7% of the malignancies seen in people with ataxia-telangiectasia, who develop cancer 100 times more often than the general population.

Classic Hodgkin Lymphoma

This lymphoma (formerly called Hodgkin disease) is a B-cell neoplasm composed of multinucleated RS cells (and a variant mononuclear type termed "Hodgkin cells") (Fig. 18-33) in a reactive inflammatory cell milieu, consisting of small lymphocytes (mostly T cells), plasma cells, bland macrophages, and eosinophils. RS cells are typically scattered and comprise only a small fraction of the total cells in involved lymph nodes. Classic HL, which constitutes 95% of all HLs, is divided into four histologic subtypes, largely based on the nature of the associated inflammatory and fibroblastic background and the appearance of the RS cells. These varieties are (1) **nodular sclerosis,** (2) **mixed cellularity,** (3) **lymphocyte rich**, and (4) **lymphocyte depleted**. RS cells in all subtypes share similar immunophenotypes and genetic alterations.

Lymph nodes involved in classic HL show architectural effacement by a number of RS cells in a mixed inflammatory cell background with variable amounts of fibrosis (sclerosis) (Fig. 18-34). Prototypical RS cells are large with at least two nuclear lobes or nuclei and abundant light blue cytoplasm (Fig. 18-34). The nuclei have irregular nuclear contours, prominent eosinophilic nucleoli, and a perinuclear halo, giving the cells the appearance of "owl's eyes" or viral inclusions. RS cells may undergo apoptosis, resulting in mummified-appearing cells with condensed cytoplasm and pyknotic nuclei. RS cells may hide amid the dense reactive background and typically account for 1% to 3% of the cells in involved tissues.

In nearly all cases, RS cells express the lymphoid activation marker CD30 (Fig. 18-35). They also express the macrophage/monocyte marker, CD15, in 85% of cases. Unlike B-cell non-Hodgkin lymphomas, RS cells do not typically express B-cell antigens such as CD20 and CD79a, nor do they demonstrate CD45 (leukocyte common antigen). However, a clonal Ig gene rearrangement occurs in more than 98% of RS cells.

HL usually presents as nontender peripheral adenopathy in a single lymph node or group of nodes. Cervical and mediastinal nodes are involved in over half of cases. The anterior mediastinum is frequently involved, especially in the nodular sclerosis type. Less commonly, axillary, inguinal, and retroperitoneal lymph nodes are affected. HL spreads predictably between contiguous lymph node groups via efferent lymphatics. As the disease progresses, spread becomes less predictable because of vascular invasion and hematogenous dissemination (Fig. 18-36).

Constitutional B-type symptoms are present in 40% of HL patients. These include low-grade fever, which may be cyclical (Pel–Ebstein fever); night sweats; and weight loss. Pruritus may occur as the disease progresses. For unknown reasons, drinking alcoholic beverages induces pain at involved sites in 10% of patients.

Patients with HL often have deficient T-lymphocyte function, which worsens as the illness progresses. Absolute lymphocytopenia (<1,500 cells/μL) is present in half of the cases, most often those with advanced HL. Humoral immunity is usually intact until late in the course of the disease.

HL prognosis depends mainly on the patient's age and anatomic extent (stage) of the disease. Good prognostic factors include (1) younger age, (2) lower clinical stage (localized disease), and (3) the absence of B signs and symptoms. The comprehensive Ann Arbor Staging System (Table 18-10) relies on clinical evaluation and radiographic and pathologic findings (including bone marrow biopsy) to assign stage.

Complications of HL include compromise of vital organs by enlarging tumor and secondary infections, the latter owing to both primary defects in delayed-type hypersensitivity and immunosuppressive effects of therapy. Development of second malignancies after therapy is of special concern, and eventually affects over 15% of patients. Acute myeloid leukemia develops in 5% of patients; aggressive large cell lymphomas occur somewhat less often.

RS cells produce cytokines that elicit characteristic tissue effects seen in the disease subtypes. The combined effects of IL-5 and eotaxin attract eosinophils, and IL-6 recruits plasma cells. TGF-β activates fibroblasts and may account for nodular fibrosis. Other growth factors and cytokines made by RS cells include IL-2, IL-7, IL-9, IL-10, and IL-13.

Nodular Sclerosis Hodgkin Lymphoma

Nodular sclerosis Hodgkin lymphoma is characterized by a fibrous capsular thickening of involved lymph nodes, with bands of fibrosis extending from the capsule into the nodal cortex and forming nodules (Fig. 18-34A). **Lacunar cells** are helpful in diagnosis but result from a retraction artifact in formaldehyde-fixed tissue

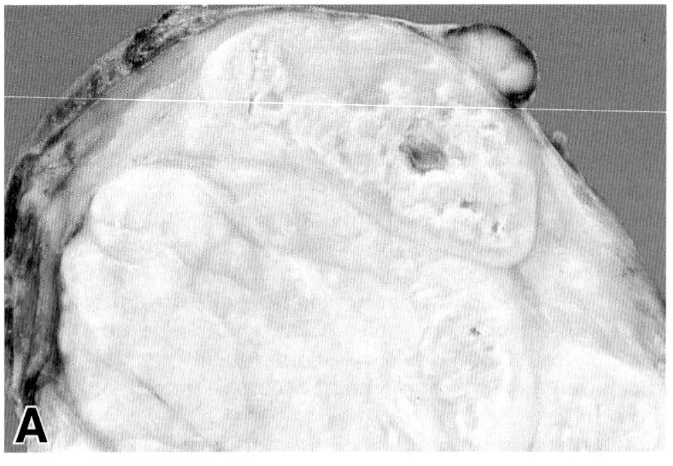

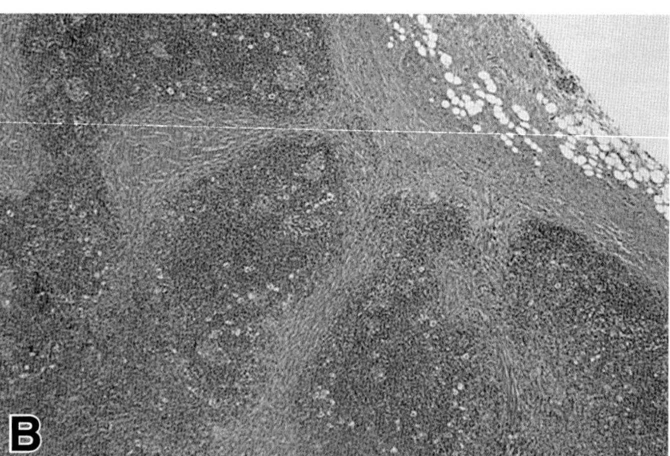

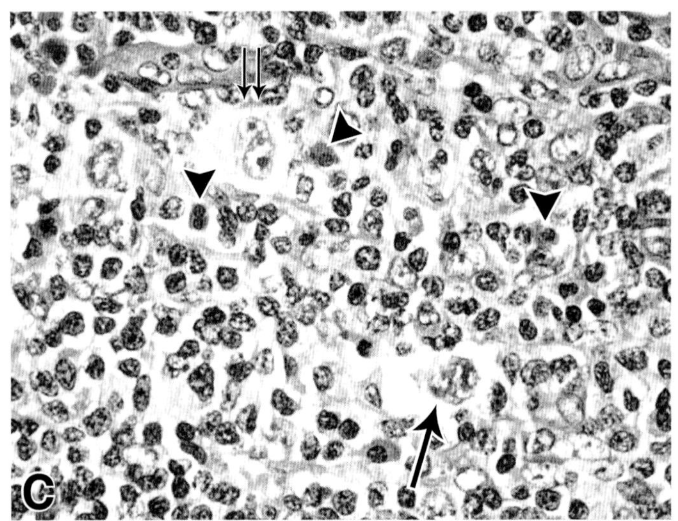

FIGURE 18-34. Nodular sclerosis Hodgkin lymphoma (NSHL). A. Gross photograph showing an enlarged lymph node with a thickened capsule and broad bands of fibrosis dividing the parenchyma into distinct nodules. Several foci of necrosis are evident (red-brown discolorations). **B.** A low-power photomicrograph demonstrating broad bands of fibrosis. There is a dense inflammatory background. Reed–Sternberg cells are rare. **C.** A photomicrograph of NSHL showing a mixed inflammatory background with eosinophils (*arrowheads*), Reed–Sternberg cells (*double arrows*), and lacunar cells (*arrow*).

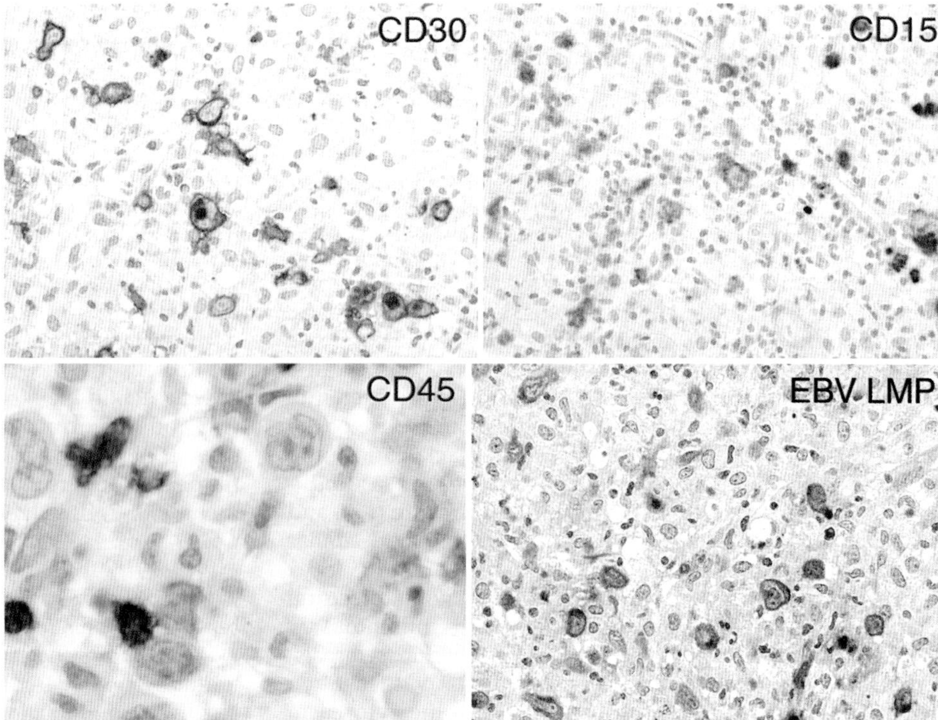

FIGURE 18-35. Reed–Sternberg and Hodgkin cells. The Hodgkin/Reed–Sternberg (HRS) cells are uniformly positive for CD30, CD15, and Epstein–Barr virus latent membrane protein antigen (EBV LMP) (immunohistochemistry; red chromogen). Common leukocyte antigen CD45 is not expressed on HRS cells.

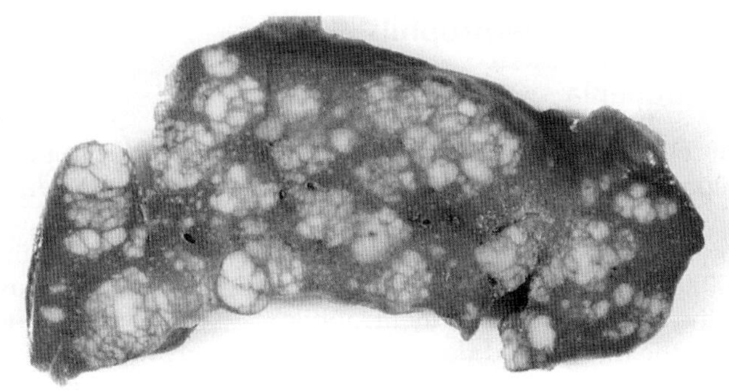

FIGURE 18-36. Hodgkin lymphoma involving the spleen. Multiple masses replace the normal splenic parenchyma. Laparotomy and splenectomy are no longer routinely performed for diagnostic and staging purposes.

(Fig. 18-34C). The nodules contain the mixed inflammatory cell population described above and variable numbers of classic RS and lacunar cells. The nodular sclerosis subtype accounts for 70% of cases of classic HL and most often affects 15- to 30-year-olds. Over 80% of patients have mediastinal involvement, with bulky disease in over half of these. B symptoms (Table 18-10) occur in up to 40% of patients. The frequency of bone marrow involvement and association with EBV is low. The illness has a better prognosis than the other subtypes.

Table 18-10

Ann Arbor Staging System for Hodgkin Disease

Stage I A or B[a]	I I_E	Involvement of a single lymph node region or A single extralymphatic organ or site
Stage II A or B	II II_E	Involvement of two or more lymph node regions on the same side of the diaphragm or With localized contiguous involvement of an extralymphatic organ site
Stage III A or B	III III_E III_S III_{ES}	Involvement of lymph node regions on both sides of the diaphragm or With localized contiguous involvement of an extralymphatic organ or site or With involvement of spleen or Both extralymphatic organ or site and spleen involvement
Stage IV A or B	IV	Diffuse or disseminated involvement of one or more extralymphatic organs with or without associated lymph node involvement

[a]A, asymptomatic; B, presence of constitutional symptoms (fever, night sweats, and weight loss exceeding 10% of baseline body weight in preceding 6 months).

Mixed Cellularity Hodgkin Lymphoma

In mixed cellularity HL, RS cells are present amid a mixed inflammatory background of eosinophils, neutrophils, macrophages, and plasma cells (Fig. 18-37), but the nodular fibrosis is absent. Mixed cellularity represents one fourth of classic HL. *It is the most frequent subtype in HIV-1–infected patients and shows the highest association with EBV.* The malignancy is most common in the fourth and fifth decades. Cervical lymph nodes are the most common initial site of involvement; unlike nodular sclerosis HL, mediastinal involvement is uncommon in mixed cellularity HL. The prognosis for patients with this subtype is similar to that for patients with nodular sclerosis HL.

Lymphocyte-Rich Hodgkin Lymphoma

In lymphocyte-rich HL, classic RS cells are surrounded by a nodular (or rarely diffuse) lymphoid infiltrate of small B cells. Hallmarks of other forms of classic HL—eosinophils, neutrophils, and sclerosis—are absent. This subtype accounts for only 5% of classic HL and tends to occur in older people. Patients generally present with low-stage disease, without B symptoms. Overall survival for lymphocyte-rich HL is better than for all other subtypes of classic HL and is similar to that seen in nodular lymphocyte-predominant HL (see below).

Lymphocyte-Depleted Hodgkin Lymphoma

Lymphocyte-depleted HL is the least common subtype of classic HL, affecting less than 1% of HL patients. In this subtype, RS cells predominate; background lymphocytes are largely absent (Fig. 18-38). Typical patients with lymphocyte-depleted HL are 30- to 40-year-old men. This subtype is also often associated with concomitant HIV infection. Involvement of retroperitoneal lymph nodes and infiltration of abdominal organs and bone marrow, which is rare in other subtypes, is not uncommon in this subtype. Patients with associated HIV infection fare worse, but in others, the disease course and outcome are like those in the other subtypes.

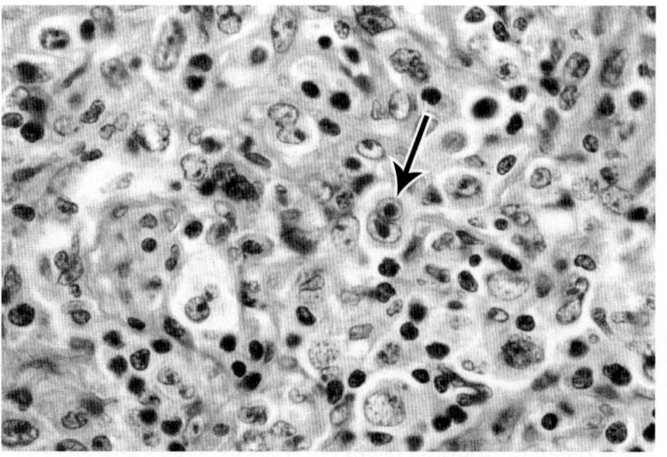

FIGURE 18-37. Mixed cellularity Hodgkin lymphoma. A photomicrograph of a lymph node showing classic, binucleated, and mononuclear Reed–Sternberg cells (*arrow*) in a mixed inflammatory background that includes many small lymphocytes (T cells). Note the absence of fibrotic bands, which helps distinguish this subtype from nodular sclerosis Hodgkin lymphoma.

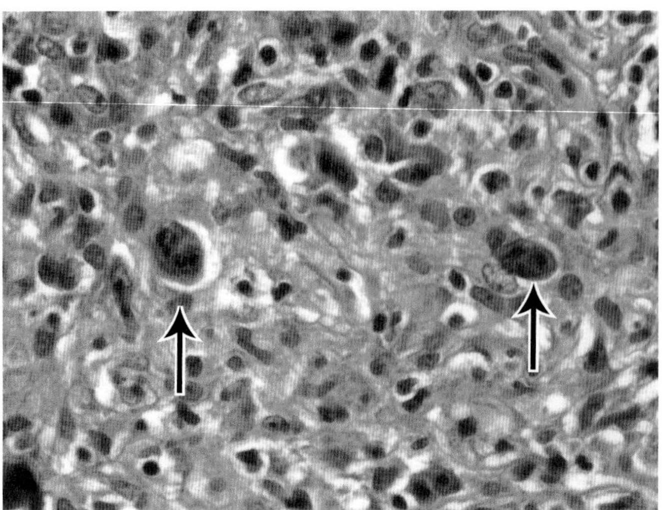

FIGURE 18-38. Lymphocyte-depleted Hodgkin lymphoma. Two Hodgkin/Reed–Sternberg cells are seen (*arrows*). The number of reactive lymphocytes in the fibrotic background is markedly reduced. The differential diagnosis in cases like this includes large cell lymphoma.

Nodular Lymphocyte-Predominant Hodgkin Lymphoma

Nodular lymphocyte-predominant HL is different from classic HL discussed above. Although classified as HL, its immunomorphologic, clinical, and pathologic features resemble indolent, B-cell non-Hodgkin lymphomas. In this subtype, the characteristic cells are called **L&H cells** (for lymphocyte and histiocytic cells), or "popcorn" cells, because of their characteristic appearance. As in classic HL, these neoplastic cells are infrequent in tissues with nodular lymphocyte-predominant HL.

This variety is also a tumor of germinal center B-cell origin. Unlike classic HL, lymphoma cells express specific B-cell lineage antigens (CD20, CD79a, and surface Ig) and are negative for CD15 and CD30. Clonal Ig gene rearrangement occurs in almost all cases. Rearranged heavy-chain genes show a high degree of somatic hypermutation in the variable region, indicating that they most likely derive from germinal center B cells.

Nodular lymphocyte-predominant HL represents about 5% of HL. It mainly affects men aged 30 to 50 years. However, it also occurs in younger people, including children. It is typically localized at the time of diagnosis (i.e., stage I). Cervical, axillary, or inguinal lymph nodes are common sites of disease. Unlike classic HL, mediastinal, splenic, and bone marrow involvement is rare. Visceral involvement is also uncommon. This form of HL tends to skip anatomic lymph node regions (i.e., noncontiguous spread). Only 20% of cases present with B signs and symptoms. These tumors follow an indolent clinical course and are rarely fatal. The 10-year survival for patients with low-stage disease is greater than 80%. Complications include recurrences, which are common; progression to diffuse large B-cell lymphoma occurs in 3% to 5% of cases.

NONMALIGNANT DISORDERS OF MYELOID BLOOD CELLS

Chapters 2 and 3 discuss white blood cell structure and function.

Disorders of Neutrophils

Neutropenia

The clinical consequences of neutropenia (granulocytopenia) depend entirely on its extent. In mild cases, absolute neutrophil counts (ANCs) are 1,000 to 1,500/µL, which is adequate for host defense. In severe cases with ANCs that are less than 500/µL, the risk of serious infection is high. **Agranulocytosis** is the virtual absence of neutrophils, caused by depletion of both the marginated pool and the bone marrow reserve.

Neutropenia reflects either decreased production or increased destruction of neutrophils (Table 18-11). Most cases are asymptomatic and unexplained, to which the term **chronic benign neutropenia** is applied.

DECREASED NEUTROPHIL PRODUCTION: Radiation or chemotherapeutic drugs suppress normal hematopoiesis and so interfere with the generation of neutrophils. Certain drugs, such as phenothiazines, phenylbutazone, antithyroid drugs, and indomethacin, can cause marrow suppression. Viral infection and alcohol intake may also suppress myelopoiesis. Decreased granulocyte production can also result from constitutional genetic alterations in several rare hereditary disorders. Autosomal dominant mutations in the neutrophil elastase gene (*ELANE*) cause the most common form of severe congenital agranulocytosis (Kostmann disease). Autosomal recessive mutations in *HAX*, a gene regulating apoptosis, also result in this condition.

INCREASED PERIPHERAL DESTRUCTION OF GRANULOCYTES: Accelerated elimination of granulocytes is caused by increases in the following:

- Consumption of neutrophils in overwhelming infections
- Sequestration in hypersplenism
- Destruction by antibodies

Table 18-11

Principal Causes of Neutropenia

Principal Causes of Neutropenia
Decreased Production
Irradiation
Drug induced (long and short term)
Viral infections
Congenital
Cyclic
Ineffective Production
Megaloblastic anemia
Myelodysplastic syndromes
Increased Destruction
Isoimmune neonatal
Autoimmune
Idiopathic
Drug induced
Felty syndrome
Systemic lupus erythematosus
Dialysis (induced by complement activation)
Splenic sequestration
Increased margination

Many **drugs** can lead to immune-mediated neutrophil destruction, especially sulfonamides, phenylbutazone, and indomethacin. The toxic effect results from attachment of circulating antigen–antibody complexes to granulocyte surfaces, with subsequent complement-mediated injury.

Neutropenia is common in AIDS patients and is multifactorial. Virus-induced depression of neutrophil production is aggravated by infectious consumption of neutrophils and often by antiretroviral drugs (e.g., zidovudine).

Neutrophilia

Neutrophilia has many causes (Table 18-12) and reflects (1) **increased mobilization** of neutrophils from bone marrow storage, (2) **enhanced release** from the peripheral blood marginal pool, or (3) **stimulation of marrow granulopoiesis**. Increased mobilization of neutrophils from the marrow pool or from peripheral marginal pools occurs in settings of acute trauma or infections. Mild neutrophilia is seen in 20% of women in the third trimester of pregnancy, but the mechanism is poorly defined.

LEUKEMOID REACTION: In acute infections and occasionally in times of severe hemorrhage or acute hemolysis, white blood cell (WBC) counts may be so high as to be mistaken for leukemia, especially chronic myeloid leukemia (CML). Such nonneoplastic increases in leukocyte counts are **leukemoid reactions**. Clues to the benign (or reactive) nature of a leukemoid reaction include the following: (1) the cells in the peripheral blood are usually segmented neutrophils, with few neutrophilic myeloid precursors; (2) leukocyte alkaline phosphatase activity is high in leukemoid reactions but low in CML; (3) WBC counts are usually under 50,000/μL; and (4) reactive neutrophils often contain large blue cytoplasmic inclusions (**Döhle bodies**) or prominent blue-black granulation of the cytoplasm (**toxic granulation**).

Table 18-12

Principal Causes of Neutrophilia
Infections
Primarily bacterial
Immunologic/Inflammatory
Rheumatoid arthritis
Rheumatic fever
Vasculitis
Neoplasia
Hemorrhage
Drugs
Glucocorticoids
Colony-stimulating factors
Lithium
Hereditary
CD18 deficiency
Metabolic
Acidosis
Uremia
Gout
Thyroid storm
Tissue Necrosis
Infarction
Trauma
Burns

Disorders of Other White Blood Cell Series

Eosinophilia

Eosinophils differentiate in the bone marrow under the influence of eosinophil growth factors (e.g., IL-5). Eosinophils respond to chemotactic substances made by mast cells or are induced by persistent antigen–antibody complexes, such as occur in chronic parasitic, dermatologic, and allergic conditions. The main causes of eosinophilia are listed in Table 18-13.

In **idiopathic hypereosinophilic syndrome**, circulating eosinophils exceed 1,500/μL for more than 6 months without evident underlying disease. Eosinophil counts in this condition may reach 50,000 to 100,000/μL.

Hypereosinophilia may accompany mast cell disease (see below), tumors like Hodgkin or non-Hodgkin lymphoma or myeloproliferative disorders (see below).

Regardless of the cause, the accumulation of eosinophils in tissues often leads to necrosis, particularly in the myocardium, where it produces endomyocardial disease.

The prognosis of untreated idiopathic hypereosinophilic syndrome is grave: only 10% of untreated patients survive 3 years. With aggressive corticosteroid therapy, 70% live over 5 years, even with cardiac involvement.

Basophilia

The basophil is the least abundant of all leukocytes. Basophilia occurs most often in immediate-type hypersensitivity reactions and together with chronic myeloproliferative neoplasms. The major causes of basophilia are listed in Table 18-14.

Monocytosis

Monocytosis is defined as a peripheral blood monocyte count above 800/μL. The main causes include hematologic malignancies, immunologic and inflammatory conditions, infectious diseases, and solid cancers. Hematologic causes

Table 18-13

Principal Causes of Eosinophilia
Allergic Disorders
Skin Diseases
Parasitic (Helminth) Infestations
Malignant Neoplasms
Hematopoietic
Solid tumors
Collagen Vascular Disorders
Miscellaneous
Hypereosinophilic syndromes
Eosinophilia–myalgia syndrome
Interleukin-2 therapy

Table 18-14

Principal Causes of Basophilia

Allergic (Drug, Food)
Inflammation
Juvenile rheumatoid arthritis
Ulcerative colitis
Infection
Viral (chickenpox, influenza)
Tuberculosis
Neoplasia
Myeloproliferative syndromes
Basophilic leukemia
Carcinoma
Endocrine
Diabetes mellitus
Myxedema
Estrogen administration

account for at least half of peripheral blood monocytoses. For example, monocytes may constitute a component of myeloproliferative or myelodysplastic syndromes such as chronic myelomonocytic leukemia (see below) and also Hodgkin or non–Hodgkin lymphoma. In such cases, monocytes may be either morphologically normal or immature and dysplastic.

Proliferative Disorders of Mast Cells

Mast cell disorders are diverse and include many benign and malignant diseases. Reactive conditions of mast cells are important to recognize and differentiate from malignant syndromes. Mast cells derive from precursor cells in the bone marrow and are found in the connective tissues, usually in close proximity to blood vessels (see Chapter 2). Mast cell proliferative diseases feature the release of mediators, such as histamine, heparin, and other factors. Clinical symptoms include flushing, pruritus, and hives. Secretion of heparin also causes bleeding from the nasopharynx or GI tract.

Reactive mast cell hyperplasia is a nonmalignant process that occurs in immediate- and delayed-type hypersensitivity reactions and in lymph nodes that drain the sites of malignant tumors. It is also observed in the bone marrow of women with postmenopausal osteoporosis, myelodysplastic syndromes, and after chemotherapy for leukemia.

MYELOID CELL MALIGNANCIES

Malignant proliferations of myeloid cells are derived from bone marrow cells and manifest as as acute myeloid leukemias, myelodysplastic syndromes or myeloproliferative neoplasms including chronic myeloid leukemia.

Myeloproliferative neoplasms (MPNs) are clonal hematopoietic, stem cell disorders with unregulated, increased proliferation of one or more myeloid lineages (granulocytes, erythrocytes, megakaryocytes, or mast cells; Table 18-15).

MPNs typically affect adults aged 40 to 80 years. They are relatively uncommon, with a yearly incidence of 6 to 10 cases per 100,000. Radiation and benzene exposure are implicated in a few historical cases, but the etiology is largely unknown. There is also evidence of inherited predisposition to develop MPNs. Characteristic features of all subtypes include bone marrow hypercellularity and increased numbers of red cells, granulocytes, and platelets. Bone marrow fibrosis of different degrees and splenomegaly often accompany MPNs. Specific oncogene mutations and/or translocations are diagnostic of certain myeloproliferative neoplasms (Table 18-16 and see below).

Myeloproliferative Neoplasms

Chronic Myelogenous Leukemia

CML is derived from abnormal, pluripotent bone marrow stem cells and results in prominent neutrophilic leukocytosis over the full range of myeloid maturation. The **Philadelphia chromosome**, or demonstration of the ***BCR/ABL* fusion gene**, is required to establish the diagnosis.

CML is the most common MPN and accounts for 15% to 20% of all cases of leukemia. The leukemic cells can differentiate along myeloid or, in some cases, lymphoid pathways; however, most cases show mainly granulocytic differentiation. Some 95% of patients demonstrate a reciprocal balanced translocation involving exchange of genetic material between chromosomes 9 and 22, resulting in a Philadelphia chromosome [t(9;22)(q34;q11)] (Table 18-16 and Fig. 18-39A). The *BCR* (*b*reakpoint *c*luster *r*egion) gene on chromosome 22 is fused to the *ABL* gene on chromosome 9 to form a *BCR/ABL* fusion gene, which is a constitutively active tyrosine kinase and is central to the pathogenesis of the neoplasm. This activated tyrosine kinase promotes downstream signaling pathways that trigger cell proliferation, differentiation, and survival.

Most cases of CML display a 210-kd fusion protein (p210). Much less commonly, the *BCR/ABL* fusion gene results from a breakage in the minor breakpoint cluster regions, yielding alternative fusion proteins such as p190. The event is more often seen in Philadelphia chromosome–positive acute lymphoblastic leukemia, occurring outside the setting of CML. Additional chromosomal abnormalities (e.g., second Philadelphia chromosome, trisomy 8) usually herald disease progression to clinically more aggressive phases.

CML may present in **chronic, accelerated,** or **blast phase**.

- **CML, chronic phase:** These patients have leukocytosis, consisting of neutrophils in all stages of maturation with a peak of myelocytes and mature neutrophils. By definition, blasts make up less than 10% of circulating or bone marrow leukocytes. Basophilia and eosinophilia are common. Platelets are normal or increased and may exceed $10^6/\mu L$. Bone marrow biopsies show hypercellularity, usually with total effacement of the marrow space by mostly myeloid cells and their precursors (Fig. 18-40).
- **CML, accelerated phase:** This condition represents disease progression from the chronic phase and is defined by one of the following criteria: (1) persistent or increasing WBC count, (2) persistent or increasing splenomegaly, (3) persistent thrombocytopenia or thrombocytosis, (4) additional chromosomal abnormalities, (5) 20% or more blood basophils, and (6) 10% to20% blasts in the blood or bone marrow.
- **CML, blast phase:** Blast phase represents the evolution to acute leukemia and features (1) 20% or more blasts in the blood or bone marrow, (2) extramedullary proliferation of blasts (skin, lymph nodes, spleen, bone, and brain), and (3) clusters of blasts in the bone marrow. Blast phase heralds

Table 18-15

Myeloproliferative Neoplasms

	Chronic Myelogenous Leukemia, BCR-ABL1 Positive	Polycythemia Vera	Primary Myelofibrosis	Essential Thrombocythemia
Clinical Features				
Peak age range (years)	25–60	40–60	50–70	50–70
Splenomegaly	90%	75%	100%	30% (slight)
Hepatomegaly	50%	40%	80%	40% (slight)
Acute leukemic conversion	80%	5%–10%	5%–10%	2%–5%
Median survival (years)	3–4	13	5	>10
Bone Marrow				
Histopathology	Panhyperplasia (predominantly granulocytic)	Panhyperplasia (predominantly erythroid)	Panhyperplasia with fibrosis	Large megakaryocytes in clusters
M:E ratio	10:1 to 50:1	≤2:1	2:1 to 5:1	2:1 to 5:1
Fibrosis	<10%	15%–20%	90%–100%	<5%
Laboratory Findings				
Hemoglobin	Mild anemia	>20 g/dL	Mild anemia	Mild anemia
RBC morphology	Slight anisokilocytosis and poikilocytosis	Slight anisokilocytosis and poikilocytosis	Immature erythrocytes and marked anisokilocytosis and poikilocytosis	Hypochromic microcytes
Granulocytes	Moderate to markedly increased with spectrum of maturation	Normal to mildly increased; may show a few immature forms	Normal to moderately increased; some immature WBCs	Normal to slightly increased
Platelets	Normal to moderately increased	Normal to moderately increased	Increased to decreased	Markedly increased with abnormal forms
Genetics	Philadelphia chromosome: *BCR/ABL* gene rearrangement	JAK2 activating mutation	JAK2 activating mutation	JAK2 activating mutation

Other myeloproliferative neoplasms include chronic neutrophilic leukemia, chronic eosinophilic leukemia, mastocytosis, and myeloproliferative neoplasm, unclassifiable.
M:E ratio, ratio of myeloid and erythroid; RBC, red blood cell; WBC, white blood cell.

a poor prognosis. In 70% of blast crises, the leukemic blasts show myeloid morphology and immunophenotype; in 30%, they are lymphoblasts, usually of the B-cell precursor lymphoblast immunophenotype (expressing CD10, CD19, CD34, and TdT). In 80% of cases, transformation to accelerated phase or blast crisis entails additional cytogenetic alterations (Table 18-16).

The peak incidence of CML is in the fifth and sixth decades, with a slight male predominance. Patients with CML report fatigue, anorexia, weight loss, and vague abdominal discomfort caused by hepatosplenomegaly. Blood findings include mild-to-moderate anemia, leukocytosis, and absolute basophilia. Peripheral granulocytes are markedly increased, with a full maturation range, including increases in myelocytes and segmented neutrophils. Clinical deterioration often heralds the onset of the blast phase.

CML is a model of targeted drug therapy in human malignancies. The drug imatinib, a tyrosine kinase inhibitor, blocks the ATP-binding site on the *BCR/ABL* tyrosine kinase, thereby inactivating it. Survival of 70% to 90% is typical with imatinib treatment. However, increasingly, subclones with point mutations within the ATP-binding pocket emerge and demonstrate resistance to the drug. Second-generation tyrosine kinase inhibitors and allogeneic bone marrow transplantation have greatly improved the outcome in CML patients.

Polycythemia Vera

PV is a myeloproliferative neoplasm that arises from a clonal HSC and is characterized by autonomous production of RBCs, not responsive to EPO. It is a clonal proliferation not only of erythroid elements but also of megakaryocytes and granulocytes in the bone marrow. Proliferation of the neoplastic clone occurs mainly in the bone marrow but may involve extramedullary sites, such as the spleen, lymph nodes, and liver (**myeloid metaplasia**). Autonomous (EPO-independent) proliferation of these PV cells gives them a proliferative advantage. The increased RBC mass suppresses EPO secretion and thus the proliferation of normal RBC progenitors. Serum EPO levels in PV are normal or low, whereas in secondary (functional) erythrocytosis, EPO is increased.

To distinguish PV from secondary benign polycythemias and other MPNs diagnosis requires that both major criteria

Table 18-16

Common Genetic Abnormalities Associated With Myeloid Proliferations

Disease	Associated Genetic/ Chromosomal Abnormality	Importance
Paroxysmal nocturnal hemoglobinuria (PNH)	PIG-A mutations	Characteristic of PNH
Chronic myeloid leukemia (CML)	t(9;22)(q34;q11) (Philadelphia chromosome)	Largely defines CML
	Trisomy 8; trisomy 19; isochromosome 17q; second Philadelphia chromosome	Occur in some cases in blast phase of CML
Polycythemia vera	Trisomy 8 or 9; del 20q; del 13q; del 9p	Associated in some cases
	JAK2 V617F	Seen in 95% of polycythemia vera cases
Primary myelofibrosis (PMF)	del(13)(q12–22)	Associated in some cases
	der(6)t(1;6)(q21–23;p21.3)	Strongly associated in some cases
	JAK2 V617F	Seen in 50% of PMF
Essential thrombocythemia (ET)	del 20q; trisomy 8	Diagnostically helpful if present
	JAK2 V617F	Seen in 40% of ET cases
	MPL mutations	Seen in rare cases of ET
Myelodysplastic syndromes	5q–	Suggests favorable prognosis
	7q–	Suggests unfavorable prognosis
Acute myelogenous leukemia (AML)	t(8;21)(q22;q22); inv(16)(p13;q22); t(16;16)(p13.1;q22); t(9;11)(p22;q23); t(6;9)(p3;q34); inv(3)(q21;q26.2)	Seen in some cases of AML with recurring chromosomal abnormalities
Acute promyelocytic leukemia (APL)	t(15;17)(q22;q12)	Defines APL
Acute monocytic leukemia (AMoL)	del(11q); t(9;11); t(11;19)	Seen in some cases of AMoL
Acute myelomonocytic leukemia (AMML)	inv(16)(p13;q22); del(16q)	Seen in some cases of AMML
Acute megakaryoblastic leukemia	t(1:22)(p13;q13)	Seen in some cases, particularly in children
Myeloid sarcoma	Translocations involving (11q23), NPM mutations	Seen in some cases, not unique to myeloid sarcomas

PIG-A, phosphatidylinositol glycan class A gene; MPL, gene for thrombopoietin receptor; NPM, nucleophosmin gene

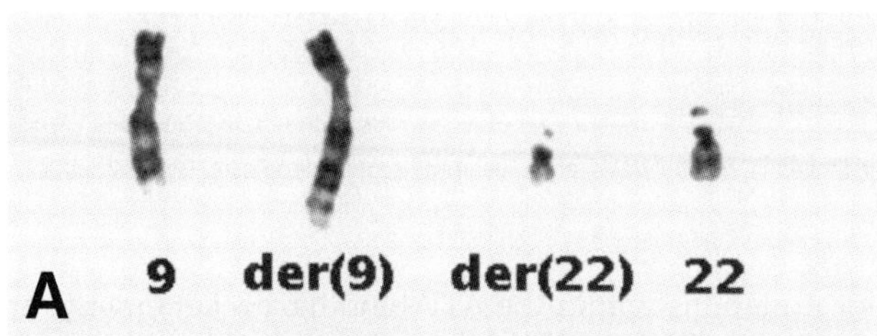

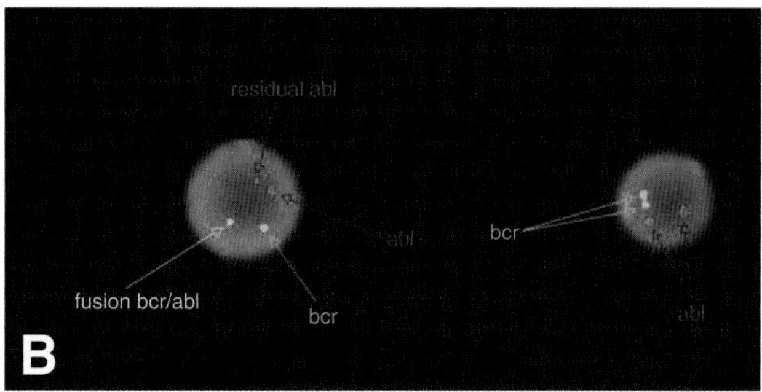

FIGURE 18-39. Chronic myelogenous leukemia. A. The Philadelphia chromosome der(22) is shown. **B.** Fluorescence in situ hybridization in a patient with t(9;22) (Philadelphia chromosome)-positive chronic myeloid leukemia. *Right image.* A normal cell contains two separate bcr (chromosome 22) and abl (chromosome 9) genes. *Left image.* A leukemic cell with a fusion bcr/abl signal; residual abl signal; and two normal abl and bcr signals derived from normal chromosomes 9 and 22, respectively.

and one minor criterion, or the first major criterion and two minor criteria, be present. Major criteria include (1) increased RBC mass or Hgb greater than 18.5 g/dL in men or 16.5 g/dL in women and (2) a Janus kinase 2 (JAK2) mutation. Minor criteria include (1) no elevation of EPO; (2) hypercellular marrow with panmyelosis, which includes erythroid, granulocytic, and megakaryocytic hyperplasia; and (3) erythroid colony formation in vitro without growth factor stimulation (endogenous production).

Over 95% of patients with PV have a somatic mutation in JAK2 (V617F). This gain-of-function mutation, occurring in the HSC and found in all myeloid lineages, makes daughter hematopoietic cells hypersensitive to growth factors and cytokines, including EPO. This JAK2 mutation is not specific for PV; it occurs in other a myeloproliferative neoplasms. Abnormal cytogenetic karyotypes occur in 20% of patients with PV (Table 18-16).

The bone marrow in PV is hypercellular, and all elements—erythroid, granulocytic, megakaryocytic—are hyperplastic (Table 18-15). Panmyelosis is characteristic, but morphologic findings and clinical course vary, depending on the stage of disease. Ultimately, a postpolycythemic, "spent phase" occurs, in which erythropoiesis decreases and the marrow becomes replaced by fibrosis.

The spleen is typically enlarged, with prominent accumulation of erythrocytes in the red pulp cords and sinuses.

Blood hemoglobin concentrations may exceed 20 g/dL, and the Hct surpasses 60% (Table 18-16 summarizes laboratory findings). Anemia characterizes the later, spent phase of

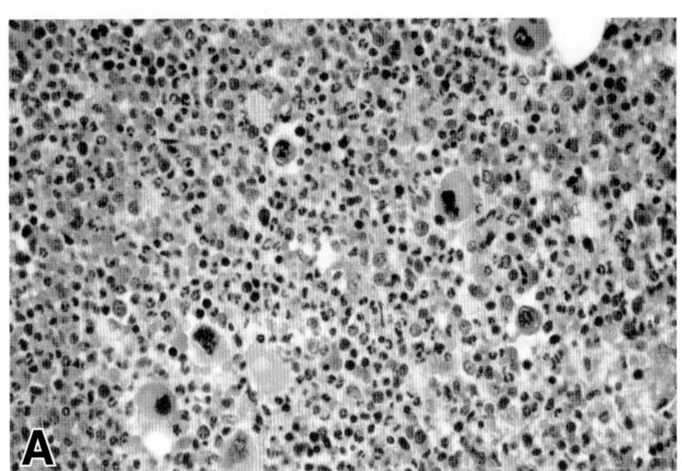

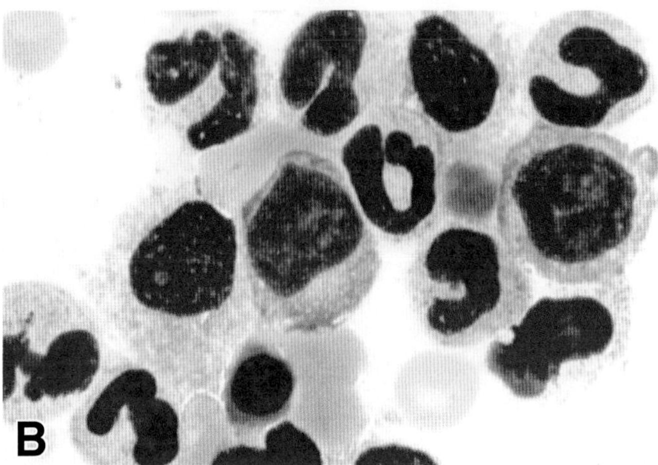

FIGURE 18-40. Chronic myeloid leukemia. A. The bone marrow is conspicuously hypercellular because of an increase in granulocyte precursors, mature granulocytes, and megakaryocytes. **B.** A smear of the bone marrow aspirate from the same patient revealing numerous granulocytes at various stages of development.

PV. Hyperuricemia and secondary gout may occur and are as a result of rapid cell turnover. Peripheral blood smears in the polycythemic phase show crowding of usual RBCs. Hypochromia and microcytosis may occur because iron-deficiency anemia is common in PV.

The mean age at diagnosis of PV is 60 years. The onset tends to be insidious, and symptoms are generally nonspecific, typically relating to the increased erythrocyte mass. Plethora and splenomegaly are early findings. Headache, dizziness, and visual problems reflect hypertension or vascular disturbances in the brain and retina. Angina pectoris, from slowing of coronary blood flow, and intermittent claudication caused by sluggish peripheral blood flow in the lower extremities may be complaints. Major thrombotic complications, including stroke, myocardial infarction, and deep vein thrombosis, occur in 20% of cases. Acute myeloid leukemia (AML) or myelodysplasia occurs in up to 15% of cases. Disease progression is often the result of karyotypic evolution and acquisition of complex chromosomal abnormalities. Median survival with PV is 13 years. Specific causes of death related to the disease itself include thrombosis, hemorrhage, AML, and the spent phase. Repeated phlebotomy or chemotherapy with urea to reduce erythrocyte mass is effective management in most cases. Ruxolitinib, a JAK2 inhibitor has been licensed for use in PV.

Primary Myelofibrosis

PMF is a clonal myeloproliferative neoplasm in which prominent megakaryopoiesis and granulopoiesis accompany marrow fibrosis. Extramedullary hematopoiesis is present in fully developed disease.

As in other MPNs, exposures to benzene or radiation have historically been implicated in the development of primary myelofibrosis. The neoplastic megakaryocytes in PMF produce PDGF and TGF-β, both of which are powerful fibroblast mitogens. Ultimately, although fibroblasts are not part of the clonal stem cell disorder, their stimulation by those cytokines causes the entire marrow space to be replaced by connective tissue. In the fibrotic phase, clonal stem cells enter the circulation to cause extramedullary hematopoiesis at multiple sites, especially the spleen. Half of patients with PMF have the JAK2 V617F mutation, which is important in the pathogenesis of the disease. A minority of cases have mutations of *MPL,* which encodes the thrombopoietin receptor. Some chromosomal abnormalities suggest, but do not prove a diagnosis of PMF (Table 18-16).

PMF evolves through two stages, namely, an early prefibrotic stage and a fibrotic stage. The **prefibrotic stage** usually presents with unexplained thrombocytosis. The hypercellular bone marrow has minimal fibrosis and prominent neutrophilic and megakaryocytic proliferation. The megakaryocytes are densely clustered and atypically lobated, with a high nuclear to cytoplasmic ratio. In the **fibrotic stage**, the blood shows leukopenia or marked leukocytosis; in the latter instance, with myeloid precursors and nucleated RBCs (leukoerythroblastosis) are usually evident. The red cells exhibit poikilocytosis and teardrop forms (Fig. 18-41A). Bone marrow cellularity gradually decreases, and foci of hematopoiesis containing mostly atypical megakaryocytes alternate with hypocellular or acellular regions and fibrosis (Fig. 18-41B). Extramedullary hematopoiesis leads to splenomegaly, hepatomegaly, and lymphadenopathy.

The peak incidence of PMF is in the seventh decade. One quarter are asymptomatic at diagnosis, the disease being detected by splenomegaly on physical examination, by identifying teardrop red cells, or by finding thrombocytosis. Early clinical symptoms are nonspecific and include fatigue, low-grade fever, night sweats, and weight loss. Platelet function may be impaired and associated with either increased platelet aggregation and thrombosis or decreased platelet aggregation with a bleeding diathesis. Transformation to AML occurs in 5% to 30% of cases (Table 18-16). The Jak2 inhibitor ruxolitinib is useful in those patients who demonstrate mutations in the gene.

Essential Thrombocythemia

ET is an uncommon MPN in which megakaryocytes proliferate without restraint. The disorder is thought to derive from neoplastic transformation of a single HSC with principal, but not exclusive, commitment to megakaryocytic lineage. Blood platelet counts remain increased (>450,000/μL), and recurrent episodes of thrombosis and hemorrhage are common. The disease affects middle-aged people, both genders equally (Table 18-16).

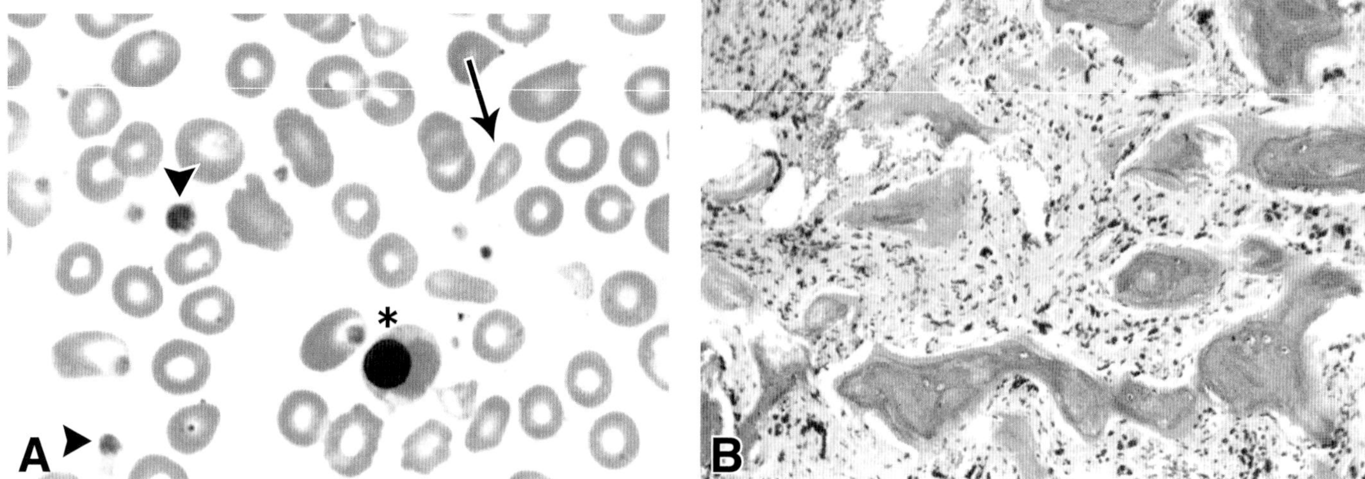

FIGURE 18-41. Chronic idiopathic myelofibrosis. A. Peripheral smear showing anisocytosis (red blood cells of different size), poikilocytosis with teardrop forms (*arrow*), and nucleated erythrocytes (*asterisk*). Large to giant platelets are also present (*arrow head*). **B.** A section of bone marrow showing collagenous fibrosis, osteosclerosis, and numerous abnormal megakaryocytes.

ET features a marked proliferation of megakaryocytes, with up to a 15-fold or greater increase in platelet production and consequent marked thrombocytosis (sometimes $>10^6/\mu L$). About 40% to 50% have a *JAK2* V617F mutation or other functionally similar abnormality. One to two percent of cases have an *MPL* gene mutation. Chromosomal abnormalities, which occur in 5% to 10% of cases, include deletion 20q and trisomy 8.

To diagnose ET, other chronic MPNs and reactive thrombocytosis must be excluded. In this context, abnormalities of platelet function are common in primary thrombocythemia. Recurrent episodes of thrombosis in arteries or veins are attributed to severe thrombocytosis, and hemorrhage reflects defective platelet function. Thromboses in the spleen, with subsequent infarction, may cause splenic atrophy. The bone marrow is normocellular or moderately hypercellular, with fewer fat cells. Increased numbers of large, hyperlobulated, "stag-horn–shaped" megakaryocytes form cohesive clusters or sheets in the marrow. Marrow fibrosis sometimes slightly increased.

The clinical course of ET is indolent, with median survival exceeding 10 to 15 years. In untreated cases, thrombosis of large arteries and veins is common, especially in the legs, heart, intestine, and kidneys. Hemorrhage is less common, usually from mucosal surfaces, and is mild, not life-threatening. AML supervenes in up to 5% of cases. The disease is treated with platelet pheresis and myelosuppressive chemotherapy.

Mastocytosis

Mastocytosis is a clonal hematopoietic disorder in which neoplastic mast cells accumulate in a number of tissues, mainly skin and bone marrow. Systemic neoplastic mast cell disorders are considered to be in the category of MPN. Cutaneous and systemic subtypes occur.

CUTANEOUS MASTOCYTOSIS: This disorder can present as either single or multiple lesions. The most common type is **urticaria pigmentosa**. This condition presents as multiple, symmetrically distributed, tan-brown, cutaneous macules or papules, most commonly in infants and young children. The skin of the trunk is mostly affected, but any skin site may be involved. There is a disseminated perivascular and periadnexal dermal infiltrate of spindle-shaped mast cells. Spontaneous resolution usually occurs at puberty, and systemic involvement does not happen.

SYSTEMIC MASTOCYTOSIS: This disorder is a rare MPN, with mast cell infiltration of many organs, including the bone marrow, skin, lymph nodes, spleen, liver, bones, and GI tract. Systemic mastocytosis has diverse manifestations, including (1) an indolent form; (2) a subtype associated with clonal hematologic, non–mast cell lineage disease; (3) an aggressive form; and (4) a leukemic form (mast cell leukemia). In most cases, there is an activating mutation in the tyrosine kinase domain (D816V) of *c-kit* proto-oncogene, underscoring the neoplastic nature of this disorder.

In mast cell leukemia, the bone marrow and peripheral blood show a significant increase in atypical mast cells ($\geq$20% in the marrow) and depletion of fat and normal hematopoietic elements in the marrow. The circulating cells often exhibit cytologic atypia, including hypogranulation or nuclear irregularity, or less differentiated forms with blastlike morphology. Lymph nodes are rarely involved and initially show perifollicular, paracortical, and perivascular infiltration by mast cells (Fig. 18-42). The spleen shows nodular aggregates of mast cells, with accompanying dense fibrosis in both red and white pulp. In the liver, portal triads are involved first. Involvement of the bone marrow may be peritrabecular, perivascular, or diffuse, and there is often accompanying fibrosis and eosinophilia.

Adults with systemic mastocytosis are most commonly affected in the sixth and seventh decades. Symptoms reflect the overproduction of a number of mediators normally made by mast cells and basophils, including histamine, prostaglandin D_2, and thromboxane B_2. Most patients experience gastrointestinal pain and diarrhea. Anaphylactic episodes—with pruritus, flushing, hypotension, and asthmatic symptoms—are common. Extensive mast cell infiltration of the bone marrow leads to secondary anemia, neutropenia, and thrombocytopenia. Prognosis is variable, depending on the subtype. The indolent form of systemic mastocytosis has a chronic course, and half of the patients survive 5 years or more. Partial relief is obtained with H_1- and H_2-receptor antagonists. There is no effective therapy for the underlying disease process.

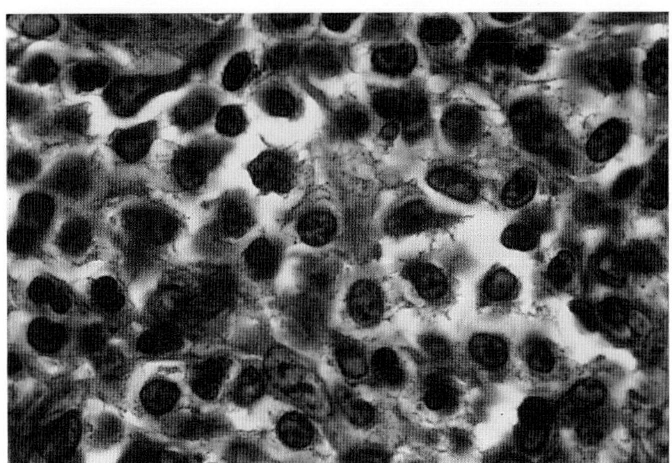

FIGURE 18-42. Mastocytosis. A section of lymph node showing effacement of the normal architecture by sheets of mast cells. The centrally situated nuclei are round to elongated, and occasionally indented. The cytoplasm is pale pink and finely granular.

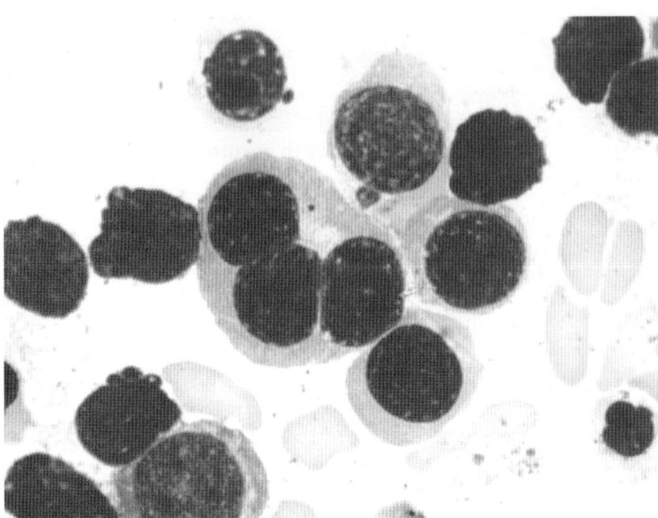

FIGURE 18-43. Myelodysplastic syndrome. Dysplastic, multinucleated, megaloblastoid erythroid precursors are shown.

Myelodysplastic Syndrome

In MDS, peripheral blood cytopenias accompany a hypercellular marrow with ineffective hematopoiesis and increased apoptosis. The disease features dysplastic morphologies in one or more hematopoietic lineages and an increased risk of transformation to AML. There is a discrepancy between the paucity of peripheral blood elements and the hypercellularity in the bone marrow.

There are several subtypes of MDS, depending on whether dysplasia involves one or more cell lineages and the percentage of blasts in the blood or bone marrow. All subtypes show refractory anemia or other cytopenia. Erythrocytosis, leukocytosis, and thrombocytosis do not occur in MDS, unlike the MPNs (see above). In MDS, unlike acute leukemias, there are less than 20% blasts in the blood or bone marrow. Progression of MDS to AML (i.e., progression from ineffective hematopoiesis to a proliferative state) occurs in 30% to 40% of cases, which usually have genetic instability. This progression coincides with an increase in genetic abnormalities.

MDS may be either primary (de novo) or secondary (therapy related). Patients with secondary MDS have usually received radiation or chemotherapy (particularly alkylating agents or topoisomerase II inhibitors). Other risk factors include benzene exposure (historically), cigarette smoking, and congenital disorders, such as Fanconi anemia or Kostmann syndrome.

Subclassification of MDS is based on whether one or more of the hematopoietic lineages shows **dysplasia**, and on the percentage of myeloblasts. Dysplasia is most often seen in erythroid precursors, which exhibit megaloblastoid changes, multinucleation, nuclear budding, bridging between nuclei, and karyorrhexis (Fig. 18-43). Careful elucidation of the blast percentage is important in assigning an MDS subcategory and predicting the likely clinical course of the disease.

Cytogenetic and molecular studies are essential to diagnosing, treating, and assessing prognosis of MDS (Table 18-16).

The disease usually occurs in older patients, with a median age of 70. In general, MDSs present with symptoms related to peripheral blood cytopenias, including weakness, anemia, recurrent infections in neutropenia, and bleeding with thrombocytopenia. Up to 40% of patients with MDS progress to AML. Some low-grade MDS subsets have more stable clinical courses and do not progress to AML.

Acute Myeloid Leukemia

A diagnosis of AML requires 20% or more myeloblasts in the blood or bone marrow. These criteria are relaxed in cases of several AML types with specific cytogenetic abnormalities (Table 18-16). For example, AML with t(15;17)(q22;q12) is acute promyelocytic leukemia (APL) and is defined as AML regardless of blast cell count. If less than 20% blasts are present in AML without recurrent cytogenetic abnormalities, the disease should be classified in the MDS or MPN categories. There are six distinct types of AML (Table 18-17):

- AML with recurrent genetic abnormalities
- AML with myelodysplasia-related changes
- Therapy-related myeloid neoplasms
- AML, not otherwise specified
- Myeloid sarcoma
- Myeloid proliferations related to Down syndrome

Most cases of AML are of unknown etiology. Some cases are attributed to prior radiation, cytotoxic chemotherapy, or (historically) benzene exposure. AML increased after the detonation of atomic bombs in Hiroshima and Nagasaki. Cigarette smoking doubles the risk for AML.

Immunophenotyping by flow cytometry, cytogenetic studies, and molecular analysis are essential for correct classification of AML. Myeloid antigens frequently expressed include CD13, CD15, CD33, and CD117 (*c-kit*), in addition to the progenitor cell marker CD34. AML with megakaryoblastic differentiation may show the platelet/megakaryocyte markers CD41 and CD61 (platelet Gp IIb/IIIa complex).

Most cases of AML occur in adults, with a median age of 67 at onset. The major problems associated with AML reflect progressive accumulation in the marrow of immature myeloid cells that cannot differentiate and mature further. Although leukemic myeloblasts divide more slowly than do normal hematopoietic precursor cells, they also undergo spontaneous

Table 18-17

WHO Classification of Acute Myeloid Leukemia

Acute Myeloid Leukemia (AML) With Recurrent Genetic Abnormalities
AML with t(8;21)(q22;q22); RUNX1-RUNX1T1
AML with abnormal bone marrow eosinophils inv(16)(p13q22) or t(16;16)(p13;q22); CBFβ/MYH11
Acute promyelocytic leukemia [AML with t(15;17)(q22;q12)(PML/RARα] and variants **(M3)**
AML with (9;11)(p22;q23); MLLT3-MLL
AML with t(6;9)(p23:q34); DEK-NUP214
AML with inv(3)(q21q24.2) or t(3;3)(q21;126.2); RPN1-EVI1
AML (megakaryoblastic) with t(1;22)(p13;q13); RBM15-MKL1
AML with gene mutations (NPM1, CEBPA, FLT3, etc.)
Acute Myeloid Leukemia With Myelodysplasia-Related Changes
Following a myelodysplastic syndrome or myelodysplastic syndrome/myeloproliferative disorder
Without antecedent myelodysplastic syndrome
Therapy-Related Myeloid Neoplasms
Alkylating agent related
Topoisomerase type II inhibitor related (some may be lymphoid)
Other types
Acute Myeloid Leukemia Not Otherwise Categorized
AML minimally differentiated **(M0)**
AML without maturation **(M1)**
AML with maturation **(M2)**
Acute myelomonocytic leukemia **(M4)**
Acute monoblastic and monocytic leukemia **(M5)**
Acute erythroid leukemia **(M6)**
Acute megakaryoblastic leukemia **(M7)**
Acute basophilic leukemia
Acute panmyelosis with myelofibrosis
Myeloid Sarcoma
Myeloid Proliferations Related to Down Syndrome

PML, promyelocytic leukemia; RAR, retinoic acid receptor; WHO, World Health Organization.

cell death less often than normal cells. Thus, the expanded pool of abnormal leukemic blasts overwhelms the marrow and suppresses normal hematopoiesis.

The major clinical problems in AML are leukopenia, thrombocytopenia, and anemia. Infections, especially with opportunistic organisms (e.g., fungi), are common, as are cutaneous bleeding (petechiae and ecchymoses) and serosal hemorrhages over viscera. Untreated AML has a dismal prognosis. Chemotherapy leads to remission in over half of patients, but relapses are common, and overall 5-year survival is under 30%. Bone marrow transplantation is a common mode of treatment.

HISTIOCYTIC DISORDERS

Hemophagocytic Disorders

All hematophagocytic disorders have in common an immunologic defect that results in immune dysregulation. Consequent increases in certain cytokines result in inadequately regulated T-cell and macrophage activation and lead to uncontrolled activation of $CD8^+$ T cells. Proinflammatory cytokines, such as TNF-α, IL-6, and interferon-γ, are increased.

Hemophagocytic syndromes may be genetic or acquired. The diagnosis requires a combination of clinical and pathologic criteria: (1) fever over 38.5°C, (2) splenomegaly, (3) anemia, (4) thrombocytopenia, (5) hypertriglyceridemia, and (6) hypofibrinogenemia. These criteria are accompanied by hemophagocytosis in bone marrow, spleen, and lymph nodes. In these organs, one finds macrophages engulfing normal hematopoietic cells (Fig. 18-44).

Inherited hemophagocytic syndromes commonly involve mutations of the perforin *PFR1* gene and typically present in children.

Acquired hemophagocytic syndromes occur in several settings. These include viral infections (primary infections with EBV, CMV, HIV, and parvovirus), malaria, *Escherichia coli*, and histoplasmosis. Hematologic malignancies such as T-cell and NK-cell lymphomas may underlie reactive hemophagocytic diseases. Autoimmune diseases (juvenile rheumatoid arthritis and systemic lupus erythematous) are also occasionally implicated.

Langerhans Cell Histiocytosis

LCH represents a spectrum of uncommon Langerhans cell proliferations. Langerhans cells are mononuclear phagocytes derived from precursor cells in the bone marrow. They are present in the epidermis, lymph nodes, spleen, thymus, and mucosal tissues, and their role is to ingest, process, and present antigens to T cells. Disorders arising from these cells range from asymptomatic involvement at a single site, such as bone or lymph nodes, to aggressive systemic multiorgan disease.

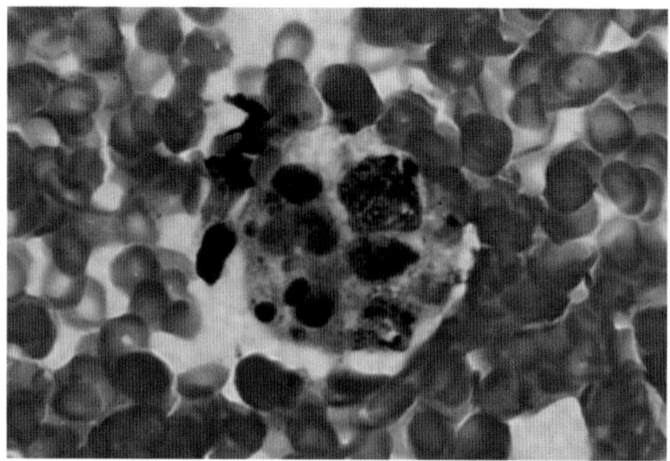

FIGURE 18-44. Hemophagocytic syndrome. This disorder is characterized morphologically by phagocytosis of hematopoietic cells by tissue macrophages. Shown here is a macrophage engulfing bone marrow cells.

The etiology and pathogenesis of LCHs are unknown. Langerhans cells in all forms of LCH are clonal, which strongly suggests that these are neoplastic diseases. LCHs mostly affect infants, children, and young adults. The extent of disease and rate of progression correlate inversely with age at presentation. There were once eponyms attached to various presentations of LCH, but these terms are now used infrequently.

The least aggressive form of LCH is called **eosinophilic granuloma.** It is a localized, usually self-limited, disorder, usually involving one bone or, less often, lymph nodes, skin, and lungs. This form of LCH affects older children (5 to 10 years old) and young adults (under 30), mostly males. Eosinophilic granuloma represents 75% of LCH cases.

In some instances, these lesions present as a multifocal, typically indolent disorder, localized to one organ system, largely bone. Children ages 2 to 5 generally present with multiple bony lesions that may be associated with soft tissue masses. This was once called **Hand–Schüller–Christian disease**.

The rarest of all forms of LCH (<10% of cases) is an acute, disseminated variant that usually occurs in infants and children under age 2. Skin lesions, hepatosplenomegaly, lymphadenopathy, and bone lesions, along with pancytopenia, are typical. In older literature, this was **Letterer–Siwe** disease.

LCHs share common histopathologies (Fig. 18-45). The cells accumulate in an environment with eosinophils, histiocytes, and small lymphocytes. Langerhans cells are large (15–25 μm), with grooved nuclei, delicate vesicular chromatin, and small nucleoli. These cells contain distinctive rod-shaped or tubular cytoplasmic inclusions with dense cores and a double outer sheath, called Birbeck granules. One end of these granules is bulbous, in which case they resemble tennis rackets. Cell markers are identical to those of epidermal Langerhans cells and include S-100 protein and CD1a.

Clinical manifestations of LCH reflect the sites involved. Skin involvement, mainly in the Letterer–Siwe variant, resembles seborrheic or eczematoid dermatitis, and is most prominent on the scalp, face, and trunk. Otitis media is common. Patients show painless localized or generalized lymphadenopathy and hepatosplenomegaly. Lytic lesions of bone cause pain or tenderness to palpation. Proptosis (protrusion of the eyeball) may reflect infiltration of the orbit. Diabetes insipidus occurs if the hypothalamic–pituitary axis is affected. However, the classic triad of Hand–Schüller–Christian disease, namely, diabetes insipidus, proptosis, and defects in membranous bones, occurs in only 15% of cases.

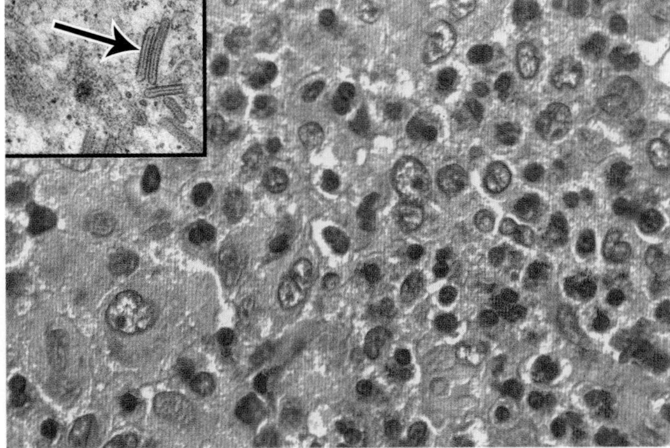

FIGURE 18-45. Eosinophilic granuloma. A section of an affected rib showing proliferated Langerhans cells and numerous eosinophils. (*Inset*) Electron micrograph showing a Birbeck granule (*arrow*) in Langerhans histiocytosis.

The prognosis in LCH depends mainly on age at presentation, extent of disease, and rate of progression.

SPLEEN

The spleen is a lymphoid organ that plays a major role in blood filtration, removing abnormal or senescent cells, immune complexes, and opsonized bacteria. A normal spleen weighs 100 to 170 g and is not palpable on physical examination. The spleen's supporting structure includes a fibrous capsule, radiating fibrous trabeculae, and a delicate stromal framework of reticulum fibers (Fig. 18-46). The splenic artery enters at the hilum and branches into trabecular arteries, following the course of the fibrous trabeculae. The organ is subdivided into areas of red and white (lymphoid) pulp. This division is useful because most diseases affect either one or the other.

Disorders of the Spleen

- **Hypersplenism** is a functional disorder, which features anemia, leukopenia, thrombocytopenia, and compensatory bone marrow hyperplasia.
- **Hyposplenism** occurs when normal splenic functions are impaired by disease or are absent after splenectomy. The spleen's normal filtering function is absent, which increases risk of severe bacteremia and causes mild leukocytosis and thrombocytosis.
- **Asplenia**, congenital absence of the spleen, occurs once in 40,000 births and often accompanies other congenital anomalies.
- **Accessory spleens** are common congenital anomalies and occur in one sixth of pediatric splenectomies.
- **Reactive splenomegaly** is common in many unrelated benign and malignant diseases (Table 18-18).
- **Congestive splenomegaly** occurs most often in patients with portal hypertension due to cirrhosis, thrombosis of the portal or splenic veins, or right-sided heart failure. Splenic congestion also complicates hereditary hemolytic anemias and hemoglobinopathies.
- **Infiltrative splenomegaly** may be the result of extramedullary hematopoiesis or the infiltration of neoplastic cells.
- **Primary malignant tumors of the spleen** are rare, the most common being hemangiosarcoma, a highly malignant neoplasms of vascular endothelial cells.

THYMUS

The thymus elaborates many factors (thymic hormones) that play key roles in maturation of the immune system and development of immune tolerance. Hence, thymic agenesis and developmental dysplasia are associated with immunodeficiency states and are discussed in Chapter 3.

Thymoma

Thymomas are neoplasms of thymic epithelial cells. They almost always occur in adult life, and most (80%) are benign. Type I malignant thymoma is the most common cancer of the

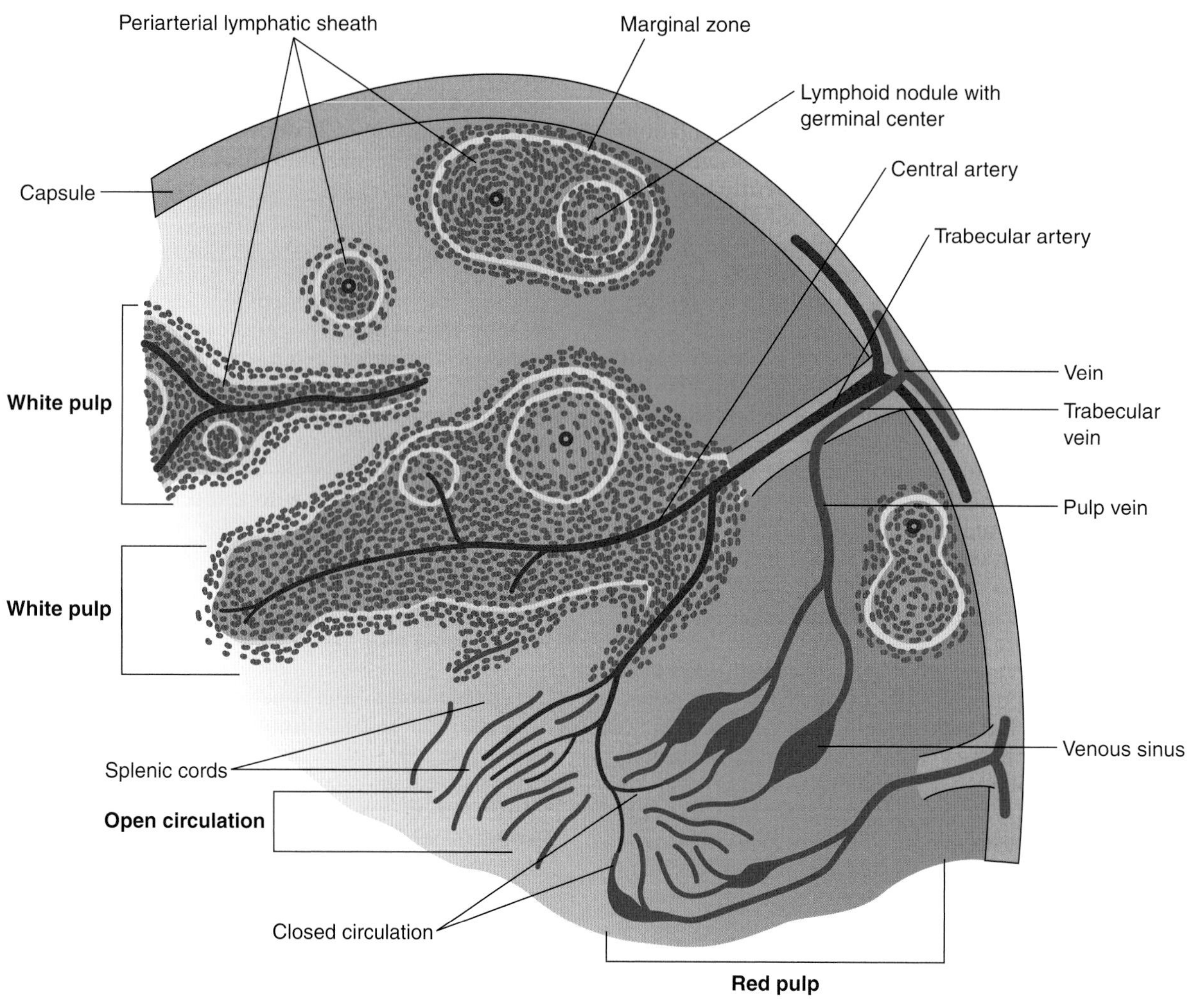

FIGURE 18-46. **Structure of the normal spleen.**

thymus and is virtually indistinguishable histologically from encapsulated, benign thymomas.

Most thymomas are in the anterosuperior mediastinum, although a few may occur at other sites where thymic tissue is present, such as the neck, middle and posterior mediastinum, and pulmonary hilus. Benign thymomas are irregularly shaped masses that vary from a few centimeters to 15 cm or more. They are encapsulated, firm, and gray to yellow tumors that are divided into lobules by fibrous septa (Fig. 18-47).

Thymomas contain a mixture of neoplastic epithelial cells and nontumorous lymphocytes (Fig. 18-48). The proportions of these elements vary from case to case and even among different lobules. The epithelial cells are plump or spindle shaped, with vesicular nuclei. In cases in which epithelial cells predominate, they may show organoid differentiation, including perivascular spaces with lymphocytes and macrophages, tumor cell rosettes, and whorls, suggesting abortive Hassall corpuscles.

MYASTHENIA GRAVIS: Thymic epithelial and myoid cells contain nicotinic acetylcholine receptor protein, which may stimulate the development of antibodies against that receptor and result in myasthenia gravis (see Chapter 23). Fifteen percent of patients with myasthenia gravis have thymomas. Conversely, one third to one half of patients with thymomas develop myasthenia gravis. When thymoma is associated with myasthenic symptoms, the epithelial cells are plump, rather than spindly.

OTHER ASSOCIATED DISEASES: Over 10% of patients with thymoma have hypogammaglobulinemia, and 5% exhibit erythroid hypoplasia. In these patients, unlike those with myasthenia gravis, the epithelial component of the thymoma is spindle shaped. Other associated diseases include myocarditis, dermatomyositis, rheumatoid arthritis, lupus erythematosus, scleroderma, and Sjögren syndrome. Certain malignant tumors may also occur with thymoma, including T-cell leukemia/lymphoma and multiple myeloma.

Germ Cell Tumors

Thymic germ cell tumors account for 20% of mediastinal tumors and may arise from cells left behind when germ cells migrate during embryogenesis. The histologic appearance of mediastinal germ cell tumors are like those in the gonads (see Chapters 15 and 16).

Table 18-18

Principal Causes of Splenomegaly
Infections
Acute
Subacute
Chronic
Immunologic Inflammatory Disorders
Felty syndrome
Lupus erythematosus
Sarcoidosis
Amyloidosis
Thyroiditis
Hemolytic Anemias
Immune Thrombocytopenia
Splenic Vein Hypertension
Cirrhosis
Splenic or portal vein thrombosis or stenosis
Right-sided cardiac failure
Primary or Metastatic Neoplasm
Leukemia
Lymphoma
Hodgkin disease
Myeloproliferative syndromes
Sarcoma
Carcinoma
Storage Diseases
Gaucher
Niemann–Pick
Mucopolysaccharidoses

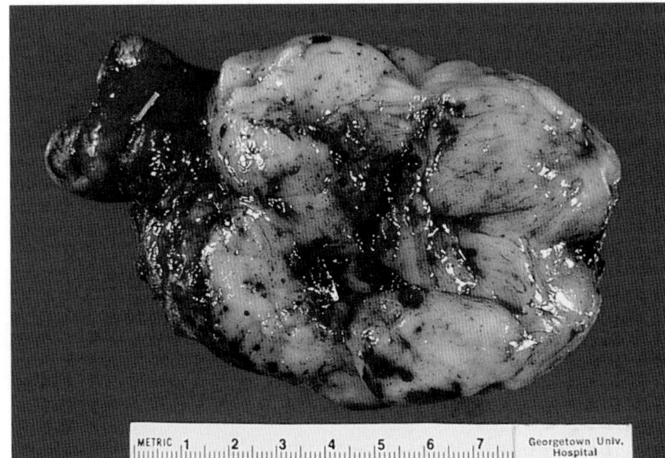

FIGURE 18-47. Thymoma. The tumor in cross section is whitish and has a bulging surface with areas of hemorrhage. Note the attached portion of normal thymus.

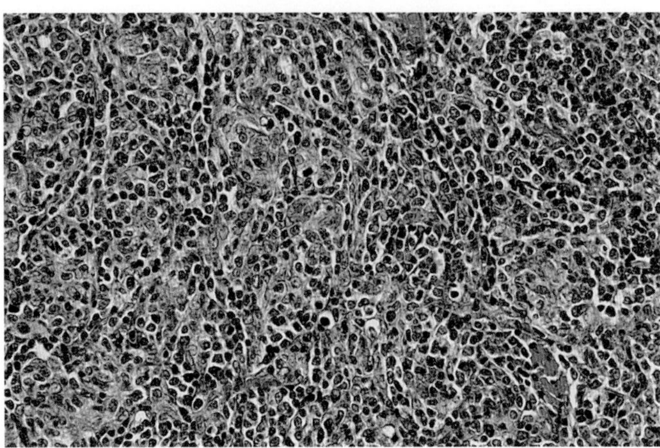

FIGURE 18-48. Microscopic features of thymomas. The tumor consists of a mixture of neoplastic epithelial cells and nontumorous lymphocytes.

HEMOSTASIS AND THROMBOSIS

Hemostasis is a controlled physiologic process that arrests hemorrhage by forming a blood clot. Normal hemostasis requires that platelets, endothelial cells, coagulation factors, endogenous anticoagulants, and thrombolytics exist in a resting nonthrombotic state. However, the system can respond instantly to vascular damage and form a clot. Local vasoconstriction and tissue swelling occur in response to injury. Platelets adhere, aggregate, and activate at the site of endothelial injury to form a platelet aggregate. Fibrin, the end product of coagulation cascade activation, stabilizes the platelet aggregate to form a blood clot (so termed when outside the circulation) or thrombus (when within the circulation), containing platelets, fibrin, leukocytes, and red blood cells. Thrombosis refers to the pathologic formation of a thrombus, a process that is discussed in Chapter 8.

Hemostasis can be best understood as a series of interlocking processes that begin with disruption of the endothelial barrier to expose a procoagulant (thrombogenic) subendothelial surface. Platelets then adhere to the exposed surface and are activated to release agonists promoting platelet aggregation. This platelet-dependent phase is termed **primary hemostasis**. Exposure of the subendothelium also initiates the coagulation cascade, which is dependent on humoral plasma proteins, a process termed **secondary hemostasis** (Fig. 18-49). The result is the production of fibrin, a critical and stabilizing component of the thrombus. Defects in either primary or secondary hemostasis result in a hemostatic disorder (**bleeding diathesis**).

Primary Hemostasis

Platelets are small discoid cells, 2 to 3 μm in diameter (Fig. 18-50), with a life span of about 10 days. They contain mitochondria, glycogen particles, dense granules, and α-granules. Dense granules contain ADP, a potent aggregating molecule, adenosine ATP, calcium, histamine, serotonin, and epinephrine. α-Granules express the adhesive protein P-selectin on their membranes and contain fibrinogen, von Willebrand factor (vWF), fibronectin, and thrombospondin. The α-granules are also characterized by the chemokines platelet factor 4, neutrophil-activating peptide 2, PDGF, and TGF-α.

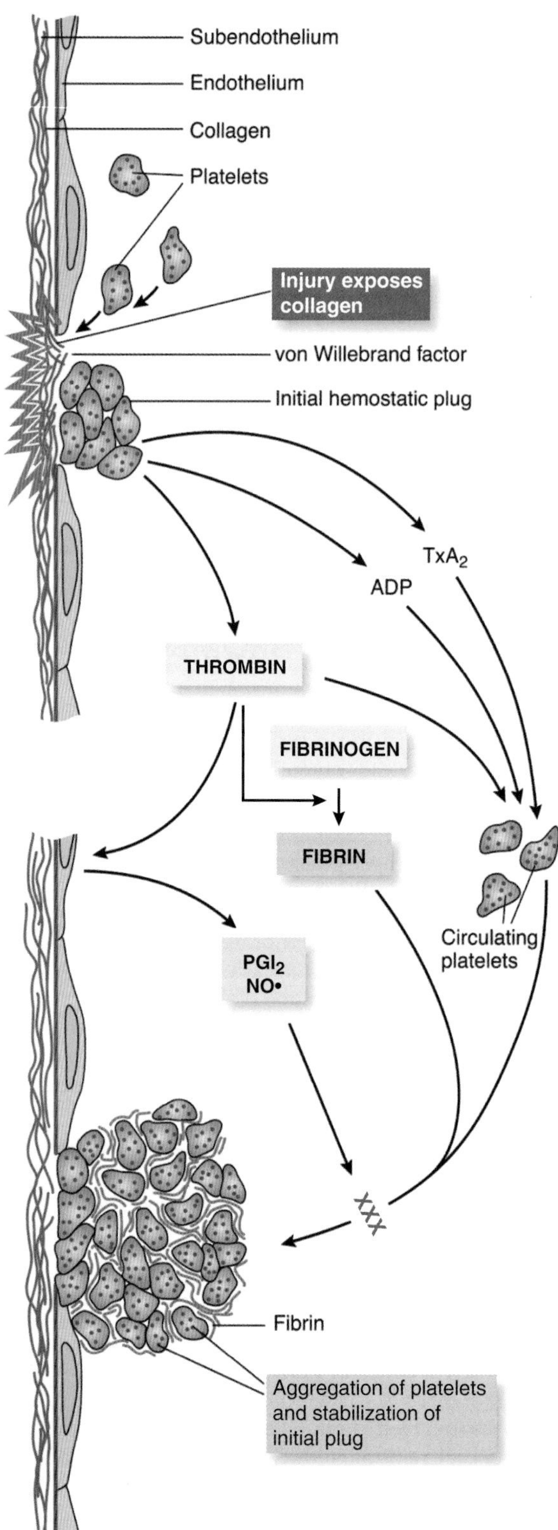

FIGURE 18-49. The role of platelets in thrombosis. Following vessel wall injury and alteration in flow, platelets adhere and then aggregate. Adenosine diphosphate (ADP) and thromboxane A_2 (TxA_2) are released and, along with locally generated thrombin, recruit additional platelets, causing the mass to enlarge. The growing platelet thrombus is stabilized by fibrin. Other elements, including leukocytes and red blood cells, are also incorporated into the thrombus. The release of prostacyclin (PGI_2) and nitric oxide (NO•) by endothelial cells regulates the process by inhibiting platelet aggregation.

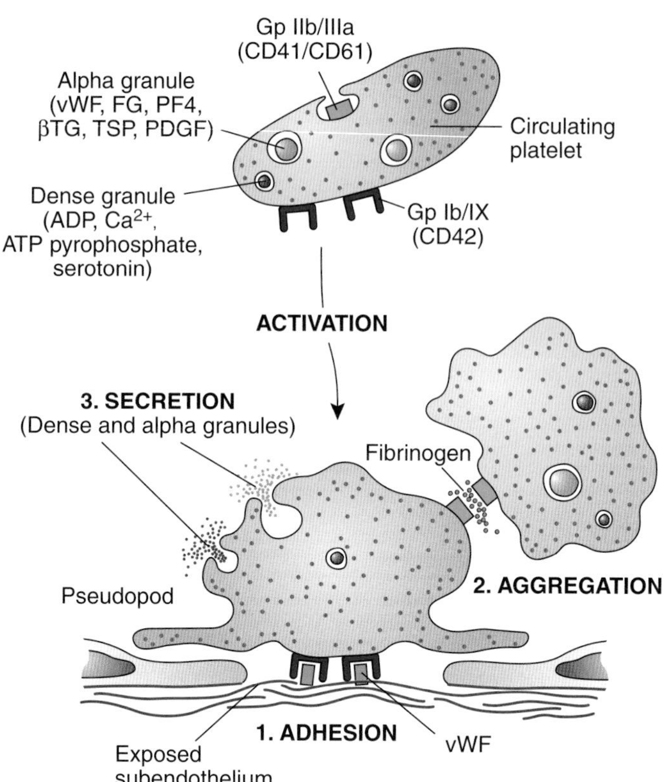

FIGURE 18-50. Platelet activation involves three overlapping mechanisms. (*1*) Adhesion to the exposed subendothelium is mediated by the binding of von Willebrand factor (vWF) to glycoprotein (Gp) Ib/IX (CD42) and is the initiation signal for activation. (*2*) Exposure of Gp IIb/IIIa (CD41/61) to the fibrinogen (FG) receptor on the platelet surface allows for platelet aggregation. (*3*) At the same time, platelets secrete their granule contents, which facilitates further activation. α-Granules contain vWF, fibrinogen, platelet factor 4 (PF4), thromboglobulin (TG), thrombospondin (TSP), and platelet-derived growth factor (PDGF). ADP, adenosine diphosphate; ATP, adenosine triphosphate; Ca^{2+}, calcium ion; CD, cluster designation.

Platelet Adhesion

Normally, circulating platelets do not adhere to each other or to the endothelial surface of the vessel wall. The endothelial cells synthesize anticoagulant factors, which inhibit primary hemostasis. These include **PGI_2**, which inhibits platelet aggregation, and endothelial NO•, which strongly inhibits aggregation and adhesion. Endothelial cells metabolize ADP, a promoter of thrombogenesis, into antithrombogenic metabolites. In addition, the endothelium inhibits secondary hemostasis, the activation of the coagulation cascade, by being coated with heparan sulfate. This molecule binds a number of clotting factors, including the antiprotease β_2-macroglobulin. Endothelial heparan sulfate activates the antiprotease antithrombin III, which inactivates coagulation factors, IIa, IXa, and Xa. Endothelium-derived modulators of coagulation are listed in Table 18-19.

When vascular endothelium is disrupted, platelet contact with the extracellular matrix, particularly type I collagen, initiates a sequence of steps of platelet activation (Fig. 18-50):

1. **Platelets adhere** to subendothelial matrix proteins with specific platelet surface glycoproteins (GPs). Major adhesive ligands include collagen via the Gp Ia/IIa ($\alpha_2\beta_1$ integrin) and Gp VI receptors, and vWF via the Gp Ib/IX receptor.
2. **Shape change**, from discoid to spherical to stellate, follows initial adhesion.

Table 18-19

Regulation of Coagulation at the Endothelial Cell Surface

Downregulation
1. Thrombin inactivators
a. Antithrombin III
b. Thrombomodulin
2. Activated protein C pathway
a. Synthesis and expression of thrombomodulin
b. Synthesis and expression of protein S
c. Thrombomodulin-mediated activation of protein C
d. Inactivation of factor V_a and factor VIII_a by APC–protein S complex
3. Tissue factor pathway inhibition
4. Fibrinolysis
a. Synthesis of tissue plasminogen activator, urokinase plasminogen activator, and plasminogen activator inhibitor-1
b. Conversion of Glu-plasminogen to Lys-plasminogen
c. APC-mediated potentiation
5. Synthesis of unsaturated fatty acid metabolites
a. Lipoxygenase metabolites—13-HODE
b. Cyclooxygenase metabolites—PGI_2 and PGE_2
Procoagulant Pathways
1. Synthesis and expression of:
a. Tissue factor (thromboplastin)
b. Factor V
c. Platelet-activating factor
2. Binding of clotting factors IX/IX_a, X (prothrombinase complex)
3. Downregulation of APC pathway
4. Increased synthesis of plasminogen activator inhibitor
5. Synthesis of 15-HPETE

APC, adenomatous polyposis coli; 13-HODE, 13-hydroxy-octadeca-dienoic acid; 15-HPETE, 15-hydroperoxyeicosatetraenoic acid; PGE_2, prostaglandin E_2; PGI_2, prostacyclin.

3. **Secretion of platelet granule contents from both the dense granules and α-granules** results in the release of ADP, epinephrine, calcium, vWF, and PDGF.
4. **Thromboxane A_2** is generated by platelet cyclooxygenase 1.
5. **Membrane changes** expose platelet P-selectin and procoagulant anionic phospholipids, such as phosphatidylserine.
6. **Aggregation of platelets** occurs by fibrinogen receptor Gp IIb/IIIa cross-linking.

Each of these functional steps has specific consequences. Initial adhesion signals platelet activation. Secreted granule contents and thromboxane A_2 provide positive feedback to activate additional platelets via their surface receptors. The stellate shape projects the procoagulant membrane surface and activated Gp IIb/IIIa/fibrinogen to the site of interaction with coagulation factors and other platelets. Thus, the surface of activated platelets is an optimal environment for propagating the assembly of the coagulation–factor complex, including the thrombin-generating prothrombinase complex of secondary hemostasis. The resulting thrombin simulates further release of platelet granules and subsequent recruitment of new platelets. Finally, P-selectin participates in binding leukocytes and localizing them to participate in healing, together with substances secreted by platelets, such as PDGF. As a result of these steps, activated platelets form a strong primary plug and then an aggregate within a platelet–fibrin meshwork, which stops bleeding and begins healing.

Secondary Hemostasis

Activation of platelets and coagulation factors is highly constrained in space and time, to prevent thrombi from spreading through the circulation. Platelets and leukocytes circulate in an inactive state. Similarly, coagulation factors are present as inactive zymogen forms. The localization of coagulation–factor complexes to the phospholipid surface of blood cells, especially platelets, accelerates activation of coagulation factors and avoids the many anticoagulant factors in plasma.

Activation of the coagulation cascade by damaged tissue exposes tissue factor and culminates in the conversion of prothrombin (factor II) to thrombin (factor IIa) and generation of fibrin from fibrinogen (Fig. 18-51).

There are three essential procoagulant complexes (Fig. 18-51). Generally, each active enzyme in the cascade is assisted by a nonenzymatic cofactor (tissue factor [TF], F.V, and F. VIII) and localized to a phospholipid surface (PL).

PROCOAGULANT PATHWAYS:

1. **Initiating complex:** Coagulation begins with the release of **tissue factor (TF)** from subendothelial cells, activated monocytes, or endothelial cells. TF then combines with **factor VIIa** to continue the process. The TF/VIIa/PL complex activates factors X to Xa. However, this activation is then rapidly shut off by **TF pathway inhibitor (TFPI)**. The TF/VIIa/PL complex also activates a small amount of factor IX to IXa.
2. **Xase complex:** The **IXa/VIIIa/PL complex** also activates factors X to Xa with ongoing activation of factor IX by XIa.
3. **Prothrombinase complex:** Factor Xa, together with its cofactor Va (Xa/Va complex), cleaves factor II (prothrombin) to factor IIa (thrombin).

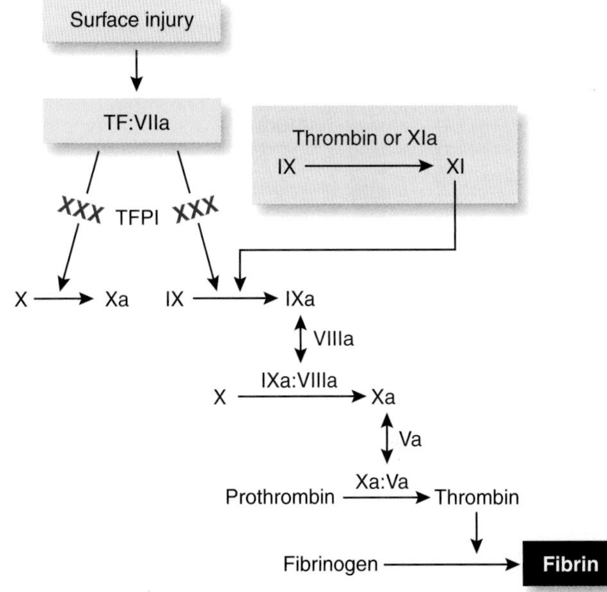

FIGURE 18-51. Coagulation cascade. The coagulation cascade is initiated by endothelial injury, which releases tissue factor (TF). The latter combines with activated factor VII (VIIa) to form a complex that activates small amounts of X to Xa and IX to IXa. The complex of IXa with VIIIa further activates X. The complex of Xa with Va then catalyzes the conversion of prothrombin to thrombin, after which fibrin is formed from fibrinogen. TFPI, tissue factor pathway inhibitor.

In addition to the formation of fibrin from fibrinogen thrombin has several other roles, which include (1) accelerating the Xase complexes by activating cofactors VIII and V; (2) activating factor XIII to promote the formation of cross-linked fibrin strands, which serve to stabilize the clot; (3) producing fibrinolytic molecules; (4) regulating growth factors and leukocyte adhesion molecules; and (5) mediating the protein C anticoagulant pathway (see below).

ANTICOAGULANT PATHWAYS: An anticoagulant complex (thrombin–thrombomodulin) activates protein C (Fig. 18-52). The **protein C$_{ase}$ complex** contains thrombin and thrombomodulin in endothelial cell plasma membranes. Endothelial protein C receptor also participates in forming this cell surface complex. Activated protein C, with its cofactor protein S, inactivates the key cofactors VIIIa and Va, thereby limiting further generation of Xa and IIa.

Antithrombin III, as previously mentioned, inhibits thrombin activity. Antithrombin III also inhibits activated factors IXa, Xa, Xia, and XIIa. In vivo, this effect is accentuated by heparan sulfate proteoglycans and, most dramatically, by therapeutic administration of heparin AT (Fig. 15-52).

Thrombolysis (Fibrinolysis)

A thrombus may undergo several fates, including (1) lysis, (2) growth and propagation, (3) embolization, and (4) organization and canalization. The combination of aggregated platelets and clotted blood is made unstable by activation of the fibrinolytic enzyme plasmin (Fig. 18-53). During clot formation, plasminogen is bound to fibrin and is an integral part of the forming the platelet mass. However, in larger thrombi, circulating plasminogen may also be converted to plasmin by products of the coagulation cascade. Endothelial cells synthesize plasminogen activator, which binds to fibrin and activates plasmin. In turn, by digesting fibrin strands into smaller fragments, plasmin lyses clots and disrupts the thrombus. These smaller fragments inhibit thrombin and fibrin formation. Endothelial cells also (1) synthesize plasminogen activator inhibitor-1 (PAI-1), (2) antiplasmin and thrombin-activatable fibrinolysis inhibitor (TAFI) and (3) α_2-antiplasmin. Thus, a regional fibrinolytic state reflects the balance between plasminogen and plasmin activation and inhibition.

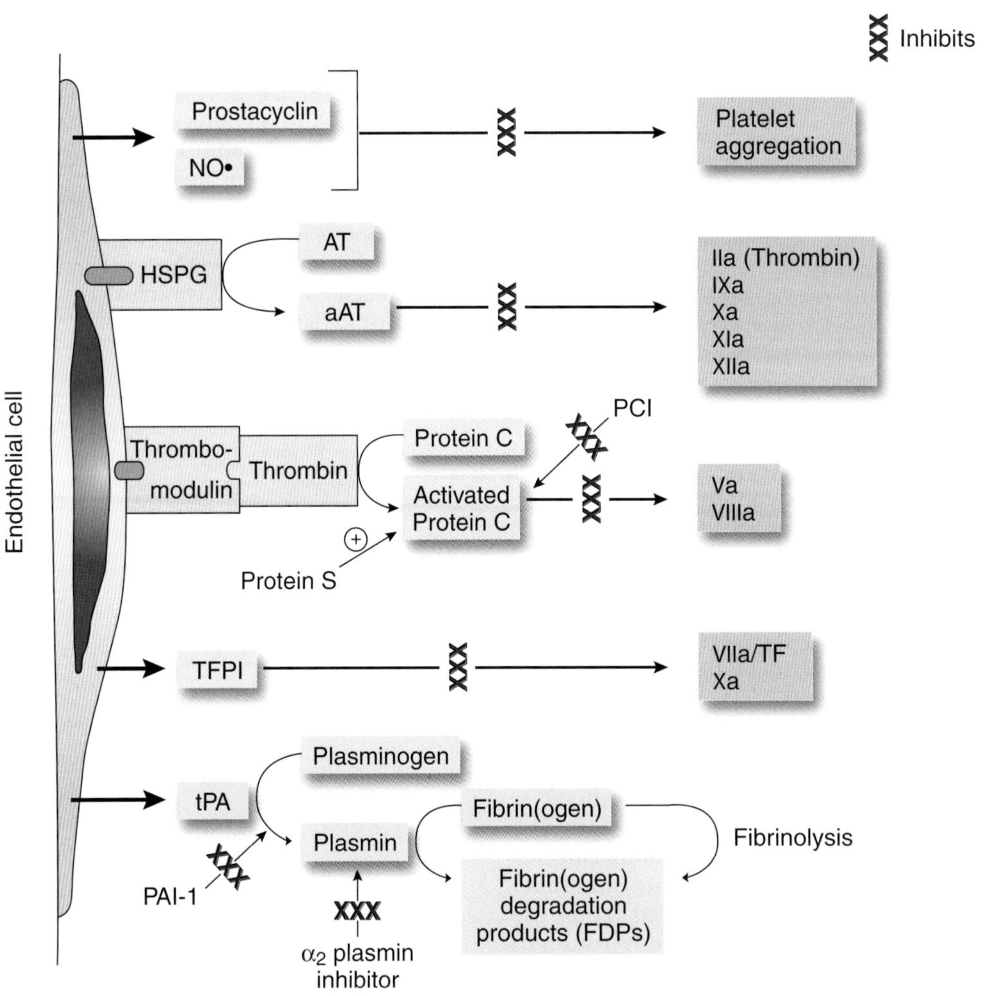

FIGURE 18-52. The role of endothelium in anticoagulation, platelet inhibition, and thrombolysis. The endothelial cell plays a central role in the inhibition of various components of the clotting mechanism. Heparan sulfate proteoglycan potentiates the activation of antithrombin (AT) 15-fold. Thrombomodulin stimulates the activation of protein C by thrombin 30-fold. *HSPG* = heparan sulfate proteoglycan; NO•, nitric oxide; PAI-I, plasminogen activator inhibitor-I; PCI, protein C inhibitor; tPA, tissue plasminogen activator. TFPI, tissue factor pathway inhibitor.

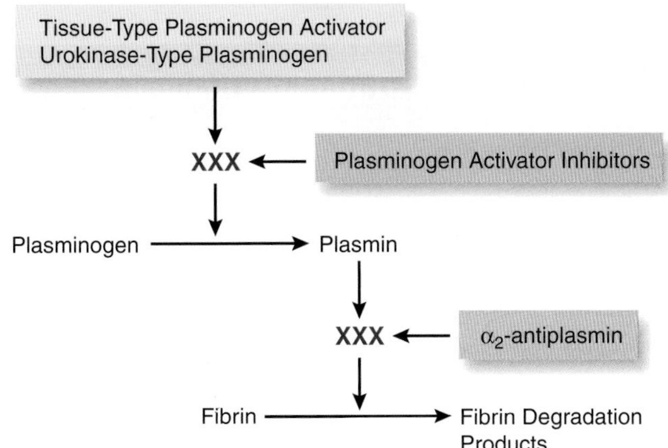

FIGURE 18-53. **Mechanisms of fibrinolysis.** Plasmin formed from plasminogen lyses fibrin. The conversion of plasminogen to plasmin and the activity of plasmin itself are suppressed by specific inhibitors.

Thrombi may undergo organization and become incorporated into vessel walls. The fibrin meshwork contracts to reduce the size of the thrombus. Arterial smooth muscle cells or venous fibroblasts migrate into the thrombus meshwork of cross-linked fibrin and produce extracellular matrix. Proteolytic enzymes and their inhibitors, which are secreted by smooth muscle cells and macrophages, remodel the thrombus, digest the fibrin, and form a fibrous structure. New blood vessels are formed by angiogenic factors present in the thrombus, a process called **canalization.** However, blood flow through canalized thrombi is usually limited.

Thrombolysis coincides with the start of wound repair (see Chapter 2), which involves (1) fibroblasts and endothelial cells migrating and proliferating, (2) secretion of new extracellular matrix, and (3) restoration of blood vessel patency. Angiogenesis (i.e., new blood vessels budding from existing ones) occurs in the setting of tissue ischemia or damage. Many products of coagulation and fibrinolysis are potent angiogenic agents.

HEMOSTATIC DISORDERS

Defects in hemostasis occur when the balance of procoagulant and anticoagulant activities tilts toward one or the other. Clinical manifestations of hemorrhage associated with disorders of each component of the hemostatic system are distinctive (Table 18-20). Platelet abnormalities result in both **petechiae** and purpuric hemorrhages in the skin and mucous membranes. Deficiencies of coagulation factors lead to hemorrhage into muscles, viscera, and joint spaces. Disorders of the blood vessels usually cause **purpura (bruises)**.

Dysfunction of Vascular or Extravascular Tissues

Dysfunction of the extravascular or vascular tissues may cause hemorrhages, ranging from cosmetic blemishes to life-threatening blood loss.

Extravascular Dysfunction

SENILE PURPURA: The most common disorder in extravascular dysfunction, senile purpura, is age-related atrophy of supporting connective tissues. Senile purpura is associated with superficial, sharply demarcated, persistent purpuric spots on the forearms and other sun-exposed areas.

Table 18-20

Principal Causes of Bleeding
Vascular Disorders
Senile purpura
Purpura simplex
Glucocorticoid excess
Dysproteinemias
Allergic (Henoch–Schönlein) purpura
Hereditary hemorrhagic telangiectasia
Platelet Abnormalities
Thrombocytopenia (see Table 18-21)
Qualitative disorders
Inherited
Glycoprotein IIb/IIIa deficiency (Glanzmann thrombasthenia)
Glycoprotein Ib/IX/V deficiency (Bernard–Soulier syndrome)
Storage pool diseases (α and δ)
Abnormal arachidonic acid metabolism
Acquired
Uremia
Drugs
Cardiopulmonary bypass
Myeloproliferative disorders
Liver disease
Coagulation Factor Deficiencies
Inherited
von Willebrand disease
Hemophilia A
Hemophilia B
Acquired
Vitamin K deficiency/antagonism
Liver disease
Disseminated intravascular coagulation

SCURVY: Vitamin C deficiency (scurvy) impairs collagen synthesis and leads to purpura. Perifollicular hemorrhages are characteristic.

Vascular Dysfunction

Hereditary Hemorrhagic Telangiectasia (Rendu–Osler–Weber Syndrome)

Hereditary hemorrhagic telangiectasia (HHT) is an uncommon, autosomal dominant disorder of blood vessel walls (venules and capillaries) in which arteriovenous malformations (AVMs) and telangiectasia (dilated, tortuous small blood vessels) form in solid organs, mucous membranes, and dermis. The underlying defect is dilation and thinning of vessel walls owing to inadequate elastic tissue and smooth muscle. The disorder is caused by mutations in TGF-β family members, endoglin (*ENG*), or an activin receptor–like kinase 1 (*ALK1*). Initially, telangiectasias are punctate reddish spots on the lips and nose, which can remain as such or progress to arteriovenous malformations or aneurysmal dilations throughout the body. Patients with HHT have recurrent hemorrhages.

Allergic Purpura (Henoch–Schönlein Purpura)

Allergic purpura is a vascular disease that results from immunologic damage to blood vessel walls (also see Chapter 14). In children, it often follows viral infections and is self-limited. In adults, allergic pupura often reflects exposure to a variety of drugs and may be chronic. The disease is characterized by **leukocytoclastic vasculitis**, characterized by perivascular infiltration of neutrophils and eosinophils, fibrinoid necrosis of vessel walls, and platelet plugs in vascular lumens. IgA and complement complexes circulate in the blood and often deposit in vessel walls.

PLATELET DISORDERS

Patients with ailments related to platelets may have histories of (1) easy bruising; (2) mucocutaneous bleeding, including gingival bleeding, epistaxis, and menorrhagia; or (3) life-threatening hemorrhages into the gastrointestinal tract, genitourinary tract, and brain. Platelet disorders may reflect decreased production, increased destruction, or impaired function.

Thrombocytopenia

Thrombocytopenia, defined as platelet counts under 150,000/mL, results from either decreased production or increased destruction. Manifestations of thrombocytopenia include spontaneous bleeding, prolonged bleeding time (a clinical test providing a standardized measure of the response to superficial skin wounds), and normal prothrombin time (PT) and partial thromboplastin time (PTT), Both PT and PTT measure the activity of components of secondary (humoral) coagulation. The lower the platelet count, the greater the risk of bleeding. Patients with less than 10,000 platelets/μL are at greatest risk of spontaneous hemorrhage (Table 18-21).

Decreased platelet production can result from defects in megakaryocytopoiesis, including diseases that affect the marrow generally, abnormalities that selectively impair platelet production, or conditions that lead to ineffective megakaryocytopoiesis (see above). Marrow infiltration with malignant cells or bone marrow failure (e.g., in patients with aplastic anemia or who received radiotherapy or chemotherapy) may cause pancytopenia, including thrombocytopenia. Certain viral infections, such as CMV and HIV, and certain drugs impair platelet production. (HIV may also increase platelet destruction; see below.) Megaloblastic anemia and myelodysplasia may cause thrombocytopenia owing to ineffective megakaryopoiesis.

May–Hegglin anomaly is a congenital form of thrombocytopenia that entails decreased platelet production. It is the most common of a family of inherited thrombocytopenias called myosin heavy-chain 9 (MYH9)-related platelet disorders.

Increased platelet destruction can result from immune-mediated damage, with consequent removal of circulating platelets, as in idiopathic (immune) thrombocytopenic purpura and drug-induced thrombocytopenia. Excessive platelet destruction also occurs in nonimmunologic conditions, such as intravascular platelet aggregation (e.g., in TTP).

Abnormal platelet distribution, or pooling, is seen in disorders of the spleen and hypothermia.

Table 18-21

Principal Causes of Thrombocytopenia

Principal Causes of Thrombocytopenia
Decreased Production
Aplastic anemia
Bone marrow infiltration (neoplastic, fibrosis)
Bone marrow suppression by drugs or radiation
Ineffective Production
Megaloblastic anemia
Myelodysplasias
Increased Destruction
Immunologic (idiopathic, HIV, drugs, alloimmune, post-transfusion purpura, neonatal)
Nonimmunologic (DIC, TTP, HUS, vascular malformations, drugs)
Increased Sequestration
Splenomegaly
Dilutional
Blood and plasma transfusions

DIC, disseminated intravascular coagulation; HUS, hemolytic–uremic syndrome; TTP, thrombocytic thrombocytopenic purpura.

Diseases Associated With Thrombocytopenia

Idiopathic (Immune) Thrombocytopenic Purpura

Idiopathic (immune) thrombocytopenic purpura (ITP) is a syndrome in which antibodies against platelet or megakaryocytic antigens cause thrombocytopenia. ITP occurs in two forms: (1) an acute, self-limited, hemorrhagic syndrome in children and (2) a chronic bleeding disorder in adolescents and adults. The autoantibodies often recognize the platelet membrane glycoproteins, Gp IIb/IIIa or Ib/IX, which are involved in platelet adhesion and clot formation (see above). Similar to autoimmune hemolytic anemia, ITP reflects antibody-mediated destruction of platelets or their precursors. In most cases, these are IgGs, although IgM antiplatelet antibodies also occur.

Acute ITP typically appears in children of either sex after a viral illness and is likely caused by virus-induced changes in platelet antigens that elicit autoantibodies. Complement bound at the surface lyses platelets in the blood or mediates their phagocytosis and destruction by splenic and hepatic macrophages.

Chronic ITP occurs mainly in adults (male to female ratio = 1:2.6) and may be associated with autoimmune or lymphoproliferative diseases. It is also common in people infected with HIV. The degree of thrombocytopenia in ITP reflects the balance between levels of antiplatelet antibodies and the extent to which platelet production in the marrow is impaired by antibody binding to megakaryocytes. In acute ITP, the platelet count is typically less than 20,000/μL. In chronic adult ITP, platelet counts vary from a few thousand to 100,000/μL. The bone marrow shows compensatory increases in megakaryocytes. Platelets carry detectable IgG in more than 80% of patients with chronic ITP; in half of these, platelet-associated C3 is also detectable.

Peripheral blood smears show many large platelets, owing to accelerated release of young platelets by bone marrow actively engaged in platelet production. The bone marrow thus shows compensatory increases in megakaryocytes (Fig. 18-54).

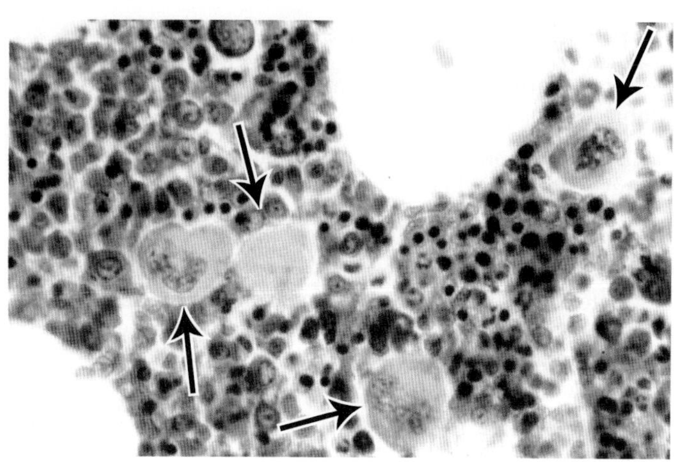

FIGURE 18-54. Idiopathic thrombocytopenic purpura. A section of the bone marrow revealing increased megakaryocytes (*arrows*).

Drug-Induced Autoimmune Thrombocytopenia

Many drugs cause immune-mediated platelet destruction: quinine, quinidine, heparin, sulfonamides, gold salts, antibiotics, sedatives, tranquilizers, and anticonvulsants. The drugs often complex with a platelet-related protein to make a neoepitope that elicits antibody production. Chemotherapeutic agents, ethanol, and thiazides cause thrombocytopenia by directly suppressing platelet production.

Heparin-induced thrombocytopenia (HIT) is a distinct type of drug-induced thrombocytopenia in which heparin paradoxically activates platelet aggregation. Some 25% of patients with HIT demonstrate **type I disease**, which is mild and transient, involving aggregation of platelets by nonimmune mechanisms.

Type II HIT occurs in 1% to 3% of patients treated with unfractionated heparin and is immunologically mediated. It is caused by acquired IgG antibodies against platelet factor 4–heparin complexes. Patients develop severe consumptive thrombocytopenia, platelet activation, and thus a hypercoagulable state. Patients with HIT are predisposed to arterial and venous thromboembolic events, which may be lethal. A low–molecular-weight version of heparin has a lower risk of HIT.

Pregnancy-Associated Thrombocytopenia

Minimal thrombocytopenia often occurs during the third trimester of pregnancy, owing to dilution of platelets. Because platelet counts are usually above 100,000/μL, no special management is needed. Conversely, preeclampsia/eclampsia syndromes can result in maternal thrombocytopenia. A condition related to preeclampsia is called **HELLP** (*h*emolysis, *e*levated *l*iver enzyme tests and *l*ow *p*latelets; see Chapter 16).

Neonatal and Inherited Thrombocytopenia

Neonatal thrombocytopenia is either **inherited** or **acquired**. **Inherited causes** associated with increased platelet destruction include **Fanconi anemia** (see above) and **Wiskott–Aldrich syndrome** (WAS). The latter is an X-linked recessive disorder caused by a defect in the Wiskott–Aldrich syndrome protein (*WASP*) gene. Affected boys have small platelets, eczema, and immunodeficiency. A variant of WAS is **X-linked thrombocytopenia**, displaying mutations in the same gene, but which only involves thrombocytopenia. Thrombocytopenia can also be seen in infants with trisomy 13, 18, or 21.

Neonatal alloimmune thrombocytopenia (NAIT) is caused by increased destruction of platelets. The pregnant mother lacks platelet-specific antigens (HPA-1) present in the fetus and becomes alloimmunized. The fetus or neonate, but not the mother, exhibits thrombocytopenia, which predisposes to intracranial hemorrhage.

Post-Transfusion Purpura

This complication of blood transfusion typically develops in women who are HPA-1 negative and who were sensitized to HPA-1 as a result of previous pregnancies. It may also occur in HPA-1 negative men who have had previous blood transfusions. Any HPA-1–positive platelets infused thereafter are destroyed by those antibodies. Curiously, the patient's own HPA-1–negative platelets are also destroyed.

Thrombotic Thrombocytopenic Purpura

Thrombotic microangiopathies (TMAs) comprise a heterogeneous group of syndromes that all cause thrombocytopenia, microangiopathic hemolytic anemia, neurologic symptoms, fever, and renal impairment. TMAs include TTP and hemolytic uremic syndrome (see below). Their pathology reflects widespread platelet aggregation and deposition of hyaline thrombi in the microcirculation. In TTP, platelet cross-linking by inappropriate vWF multimers from injured endothelial cells reflects altered cleavage of vWF.

In TTP, ADAMTS13, the cleaving agent of vWF, is deficient, causing ultralarge vWF multimers to accumulate and bind platelets. Thrombi form in the microvasculature, depleting platelets and causing thrombocytopenia. ADAMTS13 is genetically absent or defective in familial TTP and is inactivated by autoantibodies in idiopathic TTP.

TTP may also complicate systemic diseases, such as autoimmune collagen vascular disorders (systemic lupus erythematosus, rheumatoid arthritis, and Sjögren syndrome), drug-induced hypersensitivity reactions, and malignant hypertension.

TTP may occur at any age but is most common in women in the fourth and fifth decades. It may be chronic and recurrent for years or, more frequently, occur as an acute, fulminant disease that is potentially fatal. Most patients present with neurologic symptoms, including seizures, focal weakness, aphasia, and alterations in consciousness.

Hemolytic–Uremic Syndrome

HUS is a thrombotic microangiopathy that resembles TTP, but its pathogenesis is entirely different. HUS is characterized by thrombocytopenia, microangiopathic hemolysis, and acute renal failure. Classic HUS occurs in children, usually after an acute gastroenteritis caused by *E. coli* strain O157:H7 or *Shigella dysenteriae*. Production of a bacterial toxin damages vascular endothelium and activates platelets. Fibrinogen then binds activated platelet Gp IIb/IIIa complex, after which platelets aggregate. In HUS, aggregated platelet thrombi are primarily in the renal microvasculature. Kidney failure, rather than neurologic abnormalities, is the main clinical feature (see Chapter 14).

Splenic Sequestration of Platelets

Many patients with splenomegaly, irrespective of the cause, show **hypersplenism**, a syndrome that includes sequestration of platelets in the spleen. One third of platelets are normally stored temporarily in the spleen, but in massive splenomegaly, up to 90% of the total platelet pool may be sequestered in that organ. Interestingly, the platelet life span is normal, or only slightly reduced. Thrombocytopenia associated with hypersplenism is rarely severe and by itself does not produce a hemorrhagic diathesis.

Hereditary Disorders of Platelets

Bernard–Soulier Syndrome (Giant Platelet Syndrome)

Bernard–Soulier syndrome is an uncommon, autosomal recessive disorder in which platelets have a quantitative or qualitative defect in the membrane glycoprotein complex (Gp Ib/IX [CD42]), which serves as a receptor for vWF. The complex helps mediate platelet adhesion to vWF in injured subendothelial tissues. In Bernard–Soulier syndrome, platelets vary widely in size and shape, and the diagnosis is suggested by the combination of thrombocytopenia and giant platelets on a blood smear.

Children demonstrate abnormal platelet function, such as ecchymoses, epistaxis, and gingival bleeding, which progresses to traumatic hemorrhage, gastrointestinal bleeding, and menorrhagia in adults. Patients may have a mild or, in some cases, a more severe, hemorrhagic disease, which may be fatal.

Glanzmann Thrombasthenia

Glanzmann thrombasthenia is an autosomal recessive defect in platelet aggregation caused by a quantitative or qualitative abnormality in the glycoprotein complex IIb/IIIa (CD41/61). In normal platelets, this complex is activated during platelet adhesion acting as a receptor for fibrinogen and vWF to mediate platelet aggregation and generate a solid plug. The IIb/IIIa complex is also linked to the platelet cytoskeleton and transmits the force of contraction to adherent fibrin, which promotes clot retraction. In Glanzmann thrombasthenia, impairment of aggregation and clot retraction hampers hemostasis and causes bleeding, despite a normal platelet count.

The disease becomes clinically apparent shortly after birth with mucocutaneous or gingival hemorrhage, epistaxis, or bleeding after circumcision. Later, patients may suffer unexpected hemorrhage after trauma or surgery. The severity of disease varies, and only a few patients experience life-threatening hemorrhage.

α-Storage Pool Disease (Gray Platelet Syndrome)

α-Storage pool disease is a rare inherited disease in which platelets lack morphologically recognizable α-granules. Thrombocytopenia is common; platelets are large and pale. The bleeding diathesis tends to be mild.

α-Storage Pool Disease

This heterogeneous illness affects the dense granules of platelets. It is sometimes associated with other multisystem hereditary disorders, including Chédiak–Higashi syndrome and Hermansky–Pudlak syndrome (both of which include oculocutaneous albinism). Bleeding manifestations are mild to moderate.

Acquired Qualitative Platelet Disorders

Several acquired disorders may impair platelet function (Table 18-21).

- **Drugs:** Various drugs can limit platelet activity. Aspirin irreversibly acetylates cyclooxygenase, primarily COX-1, by blocking production of platelet thromboxane A_2, which is important for platelet aggregation. Platelets cannot synthesize cyclooxygenase so the aspirin effect lasts for the life span of platelets (7–10 days). Nonsteroidal analgesics, such as indomethacin or ibuprofen, impair platelet function because their inhibition of cyclooxygenase is reversible and their effect on platelets is short. Antibiotics, particularly β-lactams (penicillin and cephalosporins), can cause platelet dysfunction.
- **Renal failure:** Qualitative platelet defects that lead to prolonged bleeding times and a tendency toward hemorrhage may complicate kidney disease. These platelet abnormalities are aggravated by uremic anemia.
- **Hematologic malignancies:** Platelet dysfunction in chronic myeloproliferative neoplasms and myelodysplastic syndromes reflects intrinsic platelet defects. In paraproteinemias platelets are coated with the plasma paraprotein, thereby impairing their function.

Thrombocytosis

Thrombocytosis (increase in platelets) can occur in association with (1) iron-deficiency anemia, especially in children; (2) splenectomy; (3) cancer; and (4) chronic inflammatory disorders. Such increases may be reactive or clonal. Reactive thrombocytosis is rarely symptomatic, but it may trigger thrombotic episodes, especially in patients bedridden after splenectomy. Myeloproliferative neoplasms, such as polycythemia vera and essential thrombocythemia, entail malignant proliferations of megakaryocytes. The resulting increases in circulating platelets often lead to episodic thrombosis or bleeding.

COAGULOPATHIES

Quantitative and qualitative disorders of all of the coagulation factors may be **inherited** or **acquired**. They result from deficiency or dysfunction of a protein factor, producing inadequate hemostasis and concomitant bleeding. Only hereditary deficiencies of factor VIII (hemophilia A), factor IX (hemophilia B), and vWF (von Willebrand factor) are common.

Hemophilia A (Factor VIII Deficiency)

Hemophilia A is the most common X-linked, inherited, bleeding disorder (1 per 5,000–10,000 males). Causative mutations in the factor VIII gene on the long arm of the X chromosome (Xq28) include deletions, inversions, point mutations, and insertions. Because the factor VIII gene is X-linked, women are most often asymptomatic carriers, males express the disease.

Patients with hemophilia A exhibit variable bleeding tendencies, the severity paralleling factor VIII activity in the blood. Half of patients have virtually no factor VIII activity and often suffer spontaneous bleeding. One fifth have factor VIII activity levels from 5% to 40% of normal and bleed only after significant trauma or surgery.

The most frequent complication of hemophilia A is a degenerative joint disease caused by repeated bleeding into many joints. Although uncommon today, bleeding into the brain was formerly the most frequent cause of death.

Screening blood donors for HIV, treating purified factor VIII to inactivate HIV, and, now, the use of human recombinant factor VIII have eliminated the prior risks of hepatitis and AIDS associated with replacement therapy. Screening to detect female carriers and prenatal diagnosis using DNA markers are highly accurate.

Hemophilia B (Factor IX Deficiency)

Hemophilia B is an X-linked inherited disorder caused by factor IX deficiency. It is one fourth as common as hemophilia A (1 in 20,000 male births) and accounts for 15% of cases of hemophilia. Factor IX is a vitamin K–dependent protein made in the liver. Many different mutations, from single base substitutions to gross deletions, may cause hemophilia B. Bleeding manifestations in hemophilia B are similar to those of hemophilia A. Treatment relies on infusion of purified or recombinant factor IX.

von Willebrand Disease

vWD is a heterogeneous complex of hereditary bleeding disorders related to deficiency or abnormality of von Willebrand disease. A simplified classification (see below) recognizes three major categories. vWD is probably the most common inherited coagulopathy (1%–2% of the population).

vWF is an adhesive molecule made by endothelial cells and megakaryocytes. It is secreted as a monomer, which polymerizes to form multimers, with molecular weights in the millions. vWF is stored in cytoplasmic Weibel–Palade bodies of endothelial cells, from which it is released into subendothelial tissues and plasma after an endothelial insult, thereby triggering platelet adherence and sealing the injury (Fig. 18-55). vWF also binds Gp IIb/IIIa (CD41/CD61) to promote platelet aggregation. In plasma, it binds and protects factor VIII; in its absence, factor VIII activity is always impaired.

vWD is an autosomal disease, affecting men and women. The *vWF* gene on chromosome 12 is large and complex. Three types of the disease are recognized, each of which is heterogeneous:

- **Type I vWD:** These variants constitute 75% of cases of vWD and are inherited as autosomal dominant traits with variable penetrance. Type I vWD is a **quantitative deficiency in vWF**, in which levels of **all** multimers are reduced, although their relative concentrations remain unchanged. Factor VIII levels are also reduced roughly in proportion to the levels of vWF.
- **Type II vWD: Qualitative defects in vWF** characterize type II variants, which account for 20% of vWD. In type II disease, interactions of vWF and the blood vessel wall are defective. The plasma activities of both vWF and factor VIII are low. In type IIa, higher molecular-weight multimers are **absent** from platelets and plasma. Type IIb, an **abnormal** vWF, features increased affinity for platelets and may cause thrombocytopenia.
- **Type III vWD:** This severe form of vWD is least common. Both vWF alleles produce little or no protein, and hence this

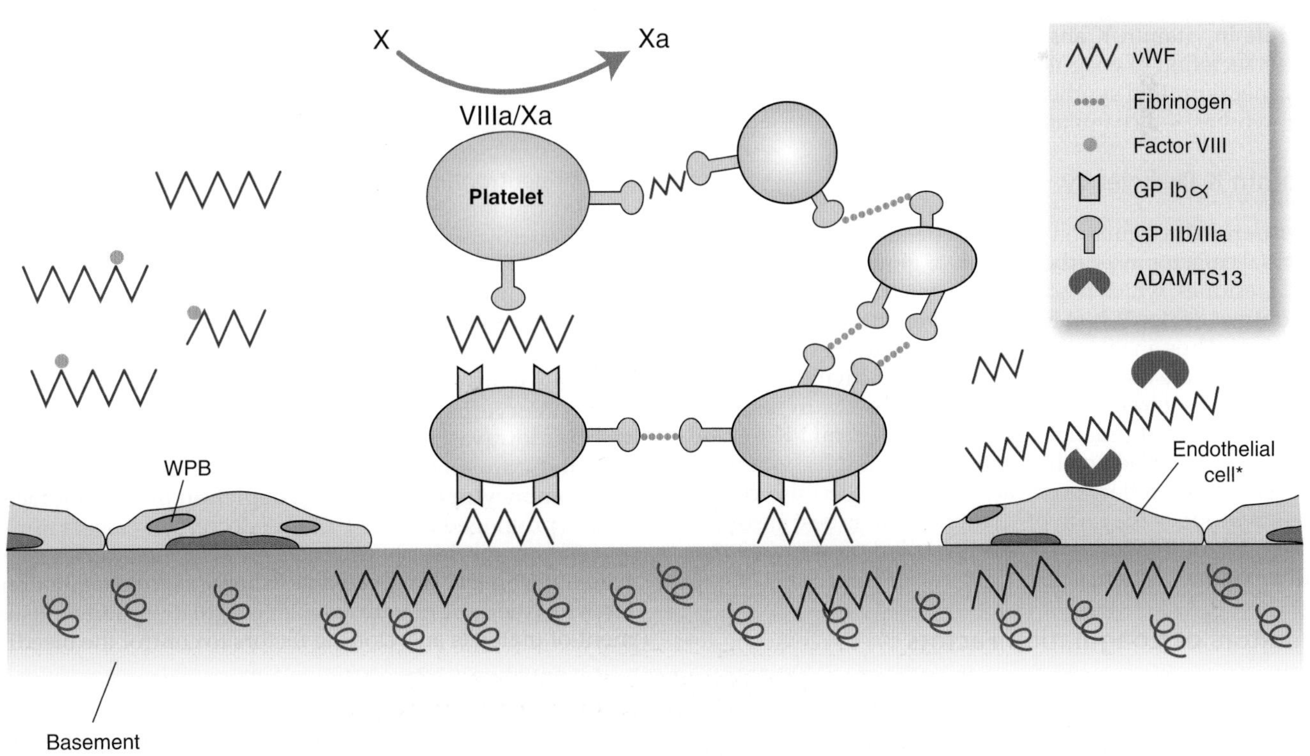

FIGURE 18-55. von Willebrand factor (vWF). vWF is stored in Weibel–Palade bodies (WPBs) of endothelial cells and is secreted from activated endothelial cells (*asterisk*) into the subendothelial space. vWF is also secreted from platelet α-granules. After endothelial injury, vWF binds to platelet glycoprotein (Gp) receptors Gp Ibα and promotes platelet adherence and protects factor VIII. Released vWF stabilizes platelet adhesion to the damaged vessel wall and promotes platelet–fibrin interactions. vWF also binds Gp IIB/IIA on the activated platelet surface to promote platelet aggregation. ADAMTS13 is the protease that cleaves ultralarge multimers of vWF.

disorder appears to be recessive. However, some patients are compound heterozygotes, with different mutations in the two vWF alleles. vWF activity is absent, and plasma factor VIII levels are less than 10% of normal.

Except for type III, most cases of vWD entail only a mild bleeding diathesis.

In contrast to hemophilia-related bleeding, patients with vWD show mucocutaneous bleeding, such as easy bruising and epistaxis, GI bleeding, and (in women) menorrhagia. However, patients with type III vWD may have life-threatening hemorrhage from the gut. Hemarthroses, like those in hemophilia, are occasionally encountered.

All forms of vWD respond well to vWF concentrates or cryoprecipitate. A vasopressin analog desmopressin (DDAVP) is the treatment of choice in types I and IIa because it increases the release of preformed vWF from endothelial storage pools.

Other Coagulation Factor Deficiencies

Deficiencies of all coagulation factor proteins, including factors VII, X, V, XI, and II (prothrombin) and fibrinogen, have been reported in humans. As expected, the severity of bleeding usually correlates with the level of functional protein activity. Deficiency of fibrinogen causes bleeding. By contrast, dysfibrinogenemia (functionally abnormal fibrinogen) more often promotes thrombosis.

Role of Liver in Coagulation

Many coagulation factors are produced by hepatocytes (e.g., factors II, V, VII, IX, and X). Factor VIII is made in part in liver sinusoidal endothelial cells (not hepatocytes) and also in monocyte/macrophages. In addition, the liver plays a key role in vitamin K absorption. Severe liver disease may impair secretion of coagulation factors as a manifestation of the general protein synthetic defect. In this case, levels of all liver-synthesized coagulation factors are low.

Vitamin K Deficiency

Liver-derived coagulation factors depend on vitamin K as an essential cofactor in γ-carboxylation of glutamic acid residues to Gla residues, which renders the secreted protein functional. By contrast, factor V is made in the liver but does not require vitamin K. Thus, in vitamin K deficiency, activities of factors II, VII, IX, and X are low, but factors V and VIII activity are normal.

Levels of vitamin K are physiologically low in neonates, and it is standard practice to administer vitamin K to newborns to prevent hemorrhagic disease. In adults, vitamin K deficiency may reflect poor dietary intake. Because colonic bacteria produce the form of vitamin K that is best absorbed, prolonged antibiotic intake or large colonic resections may lead to vitamin K deficiency.

Inhibitors of Coagulation Factors

Acquired inhibitors of coagulation factors, **circulating anticoagulants**, are usually IgG autoantibodies. Most are directed against factor VIII, but rarely antibodies to any of the other coagulation factors can be present. In hereditary coagulation disorders, especially hemophilia, circulating anticoagulants arise because of replacement therapy. Anticoagulants also develop in some patients with autoimmune disorders (e.g., systemic lupus erythematosus and rheumatoid arthritis), presumably owing to abnormal immune regulation. Finally, acquired anticoagulants occasionally appear in apparently normal people. Acquired anticoagulants may be asymptomatic laboratory findings, or they may cause life-threatening hemorrhage.

DISSEMINATED INTRAVASCULAR COAGULATION

DIC refers to widespread intravascular activation of coagulation, which generates thrombin and microvascular fibrin thrombi and triggers fibrinolysis. Platelets and clotting factors are consumed so patients also tend to hemorrhage. DIC is a serious and often fatal. It may follow massive trauma, burns, sepsis, and obstetric emergencies. It is also associated with metastatic cancer, hematopoietic malignancies, cardiovascular and liver disease, and many other conditions.

DIC begins with activation of clotting cascades within the vascular compartment by tissue injury or endothelial damage or both. Subsequent generation of substantial amounts of thrombin (Fig. 18-56), combined with the failure of natural inhibitory mechanisms to neutralize thrombin, triggers DIC. This situation promotes consumption of clotting factors, platelets, and fibrinogen and a consequent hemorrhagic diathesis.

DIC is triggered when procoagulant TF is released into the circulation after many kinds of injury. **Bacterial endotoxin** also stimulates macrophages to release TF (see Chapter 2). **Certain tumor cells** cause DIC by releasing TF or TF-like substances. With activation of the clotting cascade, intravascular fibrin microthrombi deposit in the smallest blood vessels. Stimulation of the fibrinolytic system by fibrin generates fibrin split products, which possess anticoagulant properties and contribute to the bleeding diathesis. **Endothelial injury** often plays an important role in the development of DIC. The anticoagulant properties of the endothelium (Fig. 18-52) are impaired by diverse injuries, including (1) TNF in Gram-negative sepsis; (2) other inflammatory mediators, such as activated complement, IL-1, or neutrophil proteases; (3) viral or rickettsial infections; and (4) trauma (e.g., burns). Thus, platelet aggregates form in the microvasculature. Arterioles, capillaries, and venules throughout the body are occluded by **microthrombi** made of fibrin and platelets. Microvascular obstruction is associated with widespread **ischemic changes**, particularly in the brain, kidneys, skin, lungs, and GI tract. These organs are also sites of bleeding, which, in the case of the brain and gut, may be fatal.

Erythrocyte fragments (**schistocytes**) form in passing through webs of intravascular fibrin, resulting in **microangiopathic hemolytic anemia**. Consumption of activated platelets leads to **thrombocytopenia**, whereas **depletion of clotting factors** causes prolonged PT and PTT and decreased plasma fibrinogen. Plasma fibrin split products prolong the thrombin time. Patients with DIC are treated with heparin anticoagulation to interrupt the cycle of intravascular coagulation, and replenishment of platelets and clotting factors to control the bleeding.

HYPERCOAGULABILITY

Hypercoagulability refers to an increased tendency to form thrombi, compared to normal.

Disorders that enhance thrombosis are also covered in Chapter 8. Hypercoagulable states are either inherited or acquired (Table 18-22).

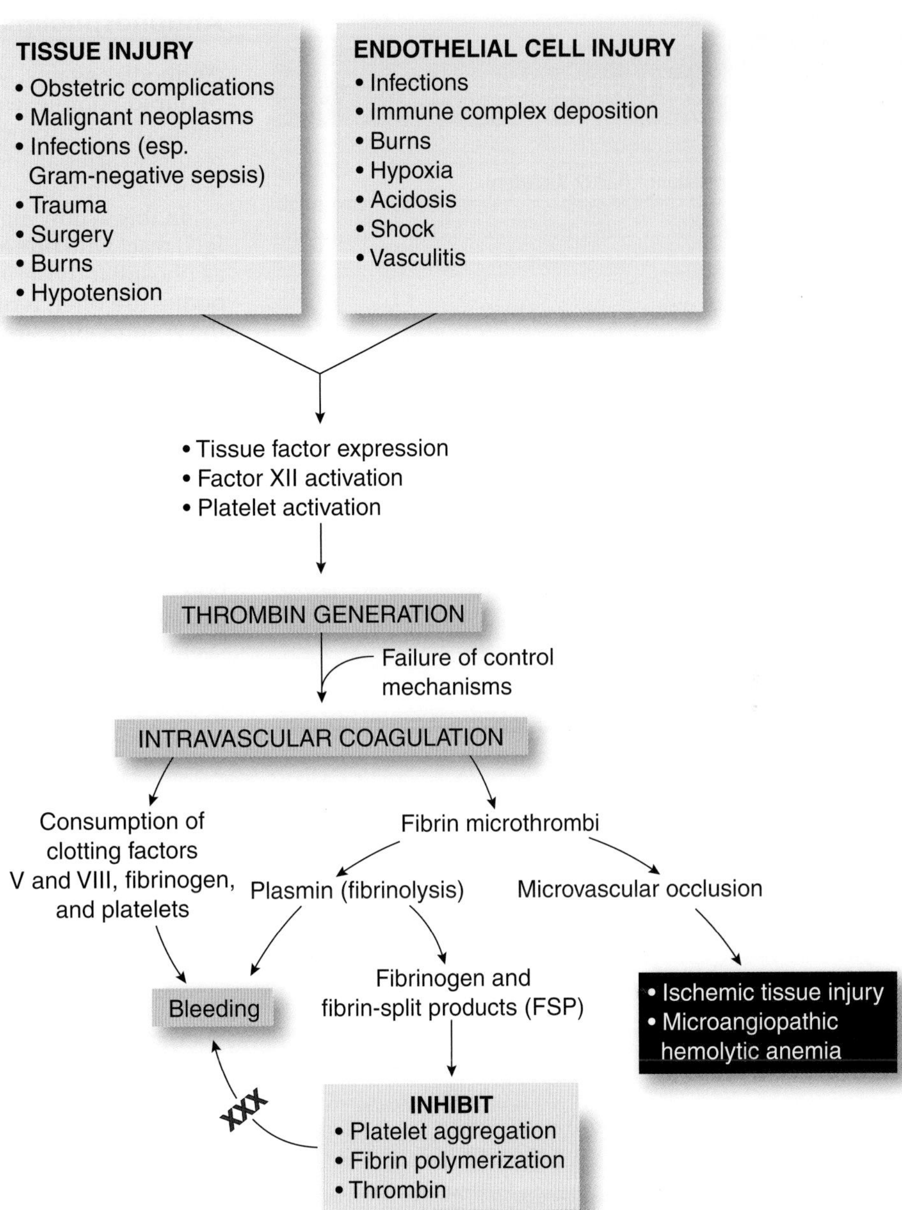

FIGURE 18-56. The pathophysiology of disseminated intravascular coagulation (DIC). The DIC syndrome is precipitated by tissue injury, endothelial cell injury, or a combination of the two. These injuries trigger increased expression of tissue factor on cell surfaces and activation of clotting factors (including XII and V) and platelets. With the failure of normal control mechanisms, generation of thrombin leads to intravascular coagulation.

Inherited Hypercoagulability

Inherited hypercoagulability reflects alterations in the natural anticoagulant pathways. A hereditary tendency to clot excessively, regardless of its origin, is **thrombophilia**.

- **Activated protein C (APC) resistance—factor V Leiden:** A point mutation in the *factor V* gene (factor V Leiden) renders it resistant to inhibition by APC. Resistance to APC action is the most common genetic hypercoagulability disorder and accounts for some 65% of patients with venous thrombosis. The factor V Leiden mutation occurs worldwide, but more so in whites (up to 5% of the general population) and much less so in Africans (near 0%). Compared with nonaffected individuals, heterozygotes for factor V Leiden have a sevenfold increased risk for deep venous thrombosis. In homozygotes, the increased risk is 80-fold.
- **Antithrombin (ATIII) deficiency:** This autosomal dominant disorder, which has incomplete penetrance, occurs in 0.2% to 0.4% of the general population and can result in either a quantitative or a qualitative effect on ATIII. The risk of a thrombotic event (usually venous) is 20% to 80% in different families.
- **Protein C and protein S deficiencies:** Homozygous protein C deficiency causes life-threatening neonatal thrombosis with **purpura fulminans**. Up to 0.5% of the general population has heterozygous protein C deficiency, but many of them are symptom free. Clinically, deficiencies of proteins C and S resemble ATIII deficiency.
- **Other causes of hypercoagulability:** A genetic variant (G20210A) in the 3′-untranslated region of prothrombin mRNA is associated with thrombosis. The mechanism is unclear but may involve excessively high prothrombin levels in people with this variant. Unusually, high levels of fibrinogen and factors VII and VIII are associated with thrombosis. Again, how the elevated levels occur remains to be elucidated. Some dysfibrinogenemias are also associated with thrombosis.

Table 18-22

Principal Causes of Hypercoagulability

Inherited
Activated protein C resistance (factor V Leiden)
Antithrombin deficiency
Protein C deficiency
Protein S deficiency
Dysfibrinogenemias
Acquired
Lupus inhibitor
Malignancy
Nephrotic syndrome
Therapy
Factor concentrates
Heparin
Oral contraceptives
Hyperlipidemia
Thrombotic thrombocytopenic purpura

Antiphospholipid Antibody Syndrome

Antibodies against several negatively charged protein/phospholipid complexes are associated with anti-phospholipid antibody syndrome. This is an autoimmune disorder that results in arterial and venous thrombosis, spontaneous abortions, and immune-mediated thrombocytopenia or anemia.

In this syndrome, antibodies (mainly, but not exclusively, IgG) react with proteins that bind anionic phospholipids, such as phosphatidylserine or cardiolipin. Collectively, such antibodies are often termed **lupus anticoagulants** (a misnomer: these antibodies are not restricted to patients with systemic lupus erythematosus and cause increased coagulability). Such antibodies occur in patients with systemic lupus erythematosus, other autoimmune conditions, or in otherwise previously asymptomatic people. Because they inhibit phospholipids, lupus anticoagulants prolong PTT in vitro, but these patients actually tend to be prone to hypercoagulability.

Anti-phospholipid antibody syndrome is the leading acquired hematologic cause of thrombosis. Resulting thromboses may occur via several possible mechanisms, including platelet activation, endothelial cell activation, and altered coagulation factor assembly on membranes. Thrombosis in the uteroplacental vasculature is the likely mechanism in recurrent fetal loss.

19 Endocrine System, Diabetes, and Nutritional Diseases

Maria J. Merino ▪ David S. Klimstra ▪ Edward B. Stelow ▪ David S. Strayer ▪ Emanuel Rubin ▪ Kevin Jon Williams ▪ Elias S. Siraj

LEARNING OBJECTIVES

- Describe the anatomic structure and embryologic origin of the components of the pituitary gland.
- List the names and functions of the hormone-producing cells of the anterior pituitary.
- Describe the function of the hypothalamus and neurohypophysis in hormone production.
- Describe the pathophysiology of common causes of hypopituitarism.
- What mutations are responsible for isolated growth hormone deficiencies and for panhypopituitarism?
- Distinguish between Laron syndrome, isolated growth hormone deficiency, and Kallmann syndrome.
- Discuss functional adenomas of the anterior pituitary and their clinical effect.
- Discuss the pathophysiology that results in central and nephrogenic diabetes insipidus and the syndrome of inappropriate antidiuretic hormone (SIADH) secretion.
- Differentiate between toxic and nontoxic goiter in terms of pathologic and clinical features.
- What are the common causes and clinical manifestations of hypothyroidism?
- Define the term "cretinism" and discuss its etiology.
- Discuss the pathophysiology of Graves disease.
- Discuss the pathophysiology of toxic multinodular goiter.
- Discuss the pathophysiology of chronic autoimmune thyroiditis.
- Distinguish between subacute, silent, and Riedel thyroiditis.
- Discuss the pathophysiology of benign follicular adenomas. How are they distinguished from malignant thyroid tumors?
- Distinguish between papillary and follicular thyroid cancer in terms of etiology, histopathology, and clinical features.
- Distinguish medullary thyroid cancer from other common forms of thyroid cancer in terms of molecular pathogenesis, cell of origin, histopathology, and diagnostic and clinical features.
- Discuss the products and physiologic function of the parathyroid gland.
- What are the causes and clinical features of primary hyperparathyroidism?
- Distinguish between primary, secondary, and tertiary hypoparathyroidism.
- Describe the histologic components of the cortex and medulla of the adrenal gland. What hormonal products are produced by each region?
- What are the pathophysiologic and clinical features of congenital adrenal hyperplasia?
- What are the most common etiologies for primary chronic adrenal insufficiency (Addison disease)? Discuss the pathologic and clinical features of the disorder.
- What are mechanisms for acute adrenal insufficiency?
- Distinguish between Cushing disease and Cushing syndrome.
- Distinguish between ACTH-dependent and independent mechanisms of adrenal hyperfunction, providing examples of each.
- Distinguish between pheochromocytomas and paragangliomas. What are the histopathology and clinical consequences of each?
- Distinguish between the types of MEN in terms of molecular etiology, pathology, and clinical consequences.
- Compare neuroblastoma and ganglioneuromas.
- What are the cellular components and endocrine products of the islets of Langerhans?
- Define the term PanNET and discuss the etiology and histopathology. What are the clinical consequences of such tumors?
- What are the major glucose-related and glucose-unrelated physiologic roles of insulin?
- Contrast type 1 and type 2 diabetes mellitus in terms of epidemiology, etiology, histopathology, and clinical consequences.
- Compare the metabolic syndrome to diabetes in terms of risk factors.
- What are major mechanisms postulated to result in insulin resistance for glucose?
- What are the roles of insulin resistance and beta-cell dysfunction in the clinical progression of diabetes?
- List the major clinical complications of diabetes.

- Distinguish between microvascular and macrovascular complications of diabetes. What are potential mechanisms for such complications?
- Outline the mechanisms that modulate central weight control.
- List endogenous factors that regulate hunger and satiety. What is their site of synthesis and mode of action?
- How is body mass and obesity defined clinically?
- What are heritable causes of obesity?
- Differentiate between marasmus and kwashiorkor.
- Be able to list essential vitamins, their biochemical mode of action, and the clinical consequences of deficiency and excess.

ENDOCRINE SYSTEM

The main function of the endocrine system is communication. Although the nervous and endocrine systems use some of the same soluble mediators and sometimes overlap functionally, the endocrine system is unique in its ability to communicate at a distance using soluble mediators termed hormones. *To qualify as a hormone, a chemical messenger must bind a receptor on the surface or in the interior of a cell.* Hormones act either on the final effector target or on other glands that in turn produce other hormones. For instance, thyroid-stimulating hormone (TSH) is released by the pituitary and promotes thyroid hormone secretion by the thyroid gland. Thyroid hormone, then, directly affects many types of peripheral cells. Diseases of the endocrine system may entail too little or too much hormone secretion. Target tissue insensitivity may simulate the clinical picture of hormone underproduction.

The endocrine system includes the pituitary gland, the hypothalamus, the parathyroid, adrenal glands, and the endocrine pancreas.

PITUITARY GLAND

The pituitary gland, or the hypophysis, is a small gland that weighs 0.5 g and measures 1.3 × 0.9 × 0.5 cm. It sits at the base of the brain in a bony cavity called the sella turcica, within the sphenoid bone.

Anatomically, the pituitary gland is composed of two lobes. The anterior lobe, or **adenohypophysis**, arises from the ectoderm, comprises 80% of the gland, and is populated by epithelial cells. The posterior lobe, or **neurohypophysis**, originates from neuroectoderm as a prolongation of the hypothalamus (Fig. 19-1). The pituitary gland is near the optic chiasm and cranial nerves III, IV, V, and VI; thus, pituitary enlargement may impair vision or cause palsies by impinging on various cranial nerves.

The cells of the anterior pituitary are arranged in cords or nests in a highly vascular stroma. The hormone-producing cells in the anterior pituitary are as follows:

- **Corticotrophs:** These basophilic cells secrete **proopiomelanocortin (POMC)** and its derivatives, including **adrenocorticotropic hormone (ACTH, corticotropin)**, which controls adrenal secretion of **corticosteroids, melanocyte-stimulating hormone (MSH), lipotropic hormone (LPH),** and **endorphins**.
- **Lactotrophs:** These acidophilic cells secrete **prolactin**, which is essential for lactation and other metabolic activities.
- **Somatotrophs:** These acidophilic cells produce and secrete growth hormone and constitute half of the hormone-producing cells of the adenohypophysis.
- **Thyrotrophs:** TSH is produced by pale basophilic or amphophilic cells, which constitute only 5% of the cells of the anterior lobe.
- **Gonadotrophs: Follicle-stimulating hormone (FSH)** and **luteinizing hormone (LH)** are secreted by the same basophilic cell. FSH stimulates Graafian follicle formation in the ovary. LH induces ovulation and the formation of corpora lutea.

Axons and unmyelinated nerve fibers from the hypothalamus proceed along the pituitary stalk to the neurohypophysis and supply the posterior lobe. These nerves regulate secretion of **arginine vasopressin (antidiuretic hormone [ADH])** and **oxytocin**. These hormones are made in the hypothalamus, stored in the posterior lobe, and later released into the systemic circulation via a rich network of capillaries, which surround the axon terminals.

The posterior lobe **pituicytes** are modified glial cells with no secretory function; they facilitate hormone release into the vasculature. ADH promotes water resorption from distal renal tubules. Oxytocin stimulates contraction of the pregnant uterus at term and also of cells around lactiferous ducts in the breasts.

Hypopituitarism

Hypopituitarism is a rare disorder in which the pituitary secretes insufficient amounts of one or a few pituitary hormones. Occasionally **panhypopituitarism** occurs, in which the gland fails totally. The effects of hypopituitarism vary with the extent of the loss, specific hormones involved, and age of the patient. In general, symptoms relate to deficient function of the thyroid and adrenal glands and the reproductive system. In children, growth retardation and delayed puberty also occur.

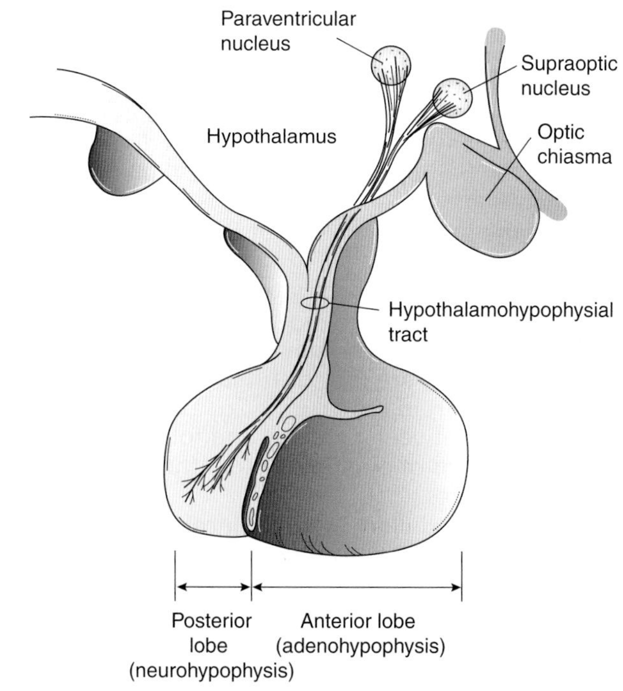

FIGURE 19-1. The pituitary gland.

Pituitary Tumors

Over half of hypopituitarism in adults is caused by pituitary tumors, usually adenomas. The tumor itself may be functional, but symptoms of hypopituitarism often result because the tumor compresses adjacent pituitary tissue.

Sheehan Syndrome

In this condition, ischemic necrosis of the pituitary causes panhypopituitarism. It is often caused by severe hypotension from postpartum hemorrhage or, rarely, without massive bleeding or after normal delivery. The pituitary is particularly vulnerable during pregnancy because of reduced blood flow associated with its enlargement at this time. The result of the damage to the gland is permanent underproduction of essential pituitary hormones (hypopituitarism). Agalactia, amenorrhea, hypothyroidism, and adrenocortical insufficiency are important consequences (Fig. 19-2). Treatment of Sheehan syndrome is hormone replacement therapy. This syndrome has become rare in developed countries.

Pituitary Apoplexy

Hemorrhage or infarction can occur in a normal pituitary, but at least half of cases arise in association with nonsecreting inactive adenomas. On occasion, pituitary apoplexy leads to hypopituitarism. The initial symptoms include headaches and associated visual problems.

Iatrogenic Hypopituitarism

Damage to the hypothalamic–pituitary axis by radiation or neurosurgical procedures may cause neuroendocrine abnormalities, including hypopituitarism.

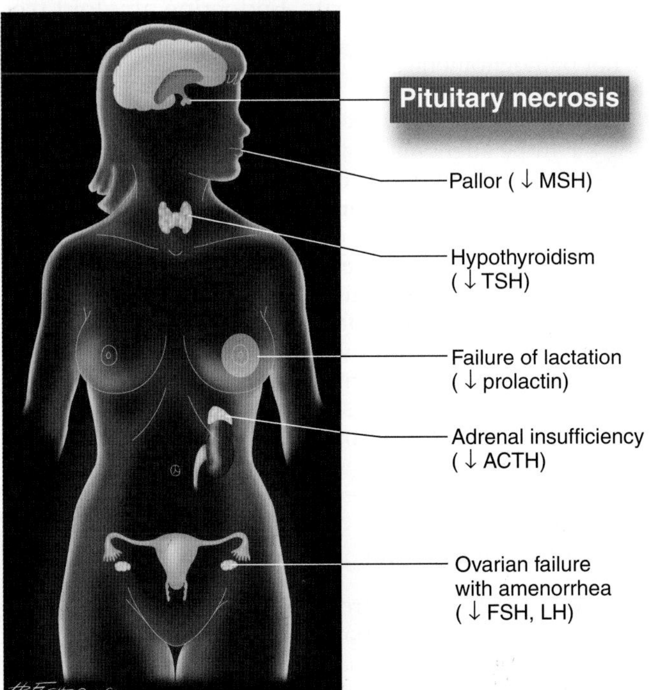

FIGURE 19-2. Major clinical manifestations of panhypopituitarism. ACTH, adrenocorticotropic hormone; FSH, follicle-stimulating hormone; LH, luteinizing hormone; MSH, melanocyte-stimulating hormone; TSH, thyroid-stimulating hormone.

Trauma

Traumatic brain injury entails significant risk to the pituitary gland, with potential development of diabetes insipidus, hypopituitarism, and other endocrinopathies.

Infiltrative Diseases

Bacterial and viral infections may give rise to inflammation, which can damage the gland. Langerhans cell histiocytosis (see Chapter 18) and hemochromatosis (see Chapter 12) also may result in hypopituitarism.

Genetic Abnormalities of Pituitary Development

Congenital growth hormone deficiency may be sporadic or familial. The condition may occur as an **isolated growth hormone deficiency (IGHD)** or emerge together with other pituitary hormone deficiencies. Familial IGHD is recessive, dominant, or sex linked. It can result from mutations in the genes for **human growth hormone** (*GH1*) or growth hormone–releasing hormone (*GHRH*) receptor, or occasionally in the Bruton tyrosine kinase (*BTK*) gene. The most severe form of the disease (type IA) results from a total lack of growth hormone. Recombinant GH is the treatment of choice for children with this disorder.

Several mutations target transcription factors during embryogenesis and result in panhypopituitarism. Among them are the following:

- **Pit-1:** Pit-1 is a POU homeodomain transcription factor encoded by the *POU1F1* gene, which is important for pituitary development. Mutations in this gene cause combined pituitary hormone deficiency (CPHD) with low levels or absence of GH, prolactin (PRL), and TSH.
- **PROP1 (5q):** Prop 1 is a pituitary-specific transcription factor. Mutations inactivate LH, FSH, GH, PRL, and TSH. This trait is inherited as an autosomal recessive condition.
- **LX3/LX4:** These genes belong to the LIM family of homeobox genes that are expressed early in the Rathke pouch. Its mutations are associated with deficiencies in GH, TSH, LH, FSH, and PRL. Rarely, mutation of the *LX4* gene may present as deficiency of GH, TSH, and ACTH.

Growth Hormone Insensitivity (Laron Syndrome)

Laron dwarfism is a rare, autosomal recessive disorder characterized by short stature as a result of extreme resistance to GH because of abnormalities in the growth hormone receptor (GHR). These pituitary dwarfs tend to be obese and have high serum GH levels, but low concentrations of insulin-like growth factor I (IGF-I). Laron syndrome occurs mainly in people of Mediterranean origin, such as Sephardic Jews. The same mutation is responsible for dwarfism in African pygmies. Because GH exerts its effects by promoting IGF-I secretion, the latter is effective replacement therapy for Laron syndrome, mimicking most effects ascribed to GH itself.

Isolated Gonadotropin Deficiency (Kallmann Syndrome)

Kallmann syndrome is characterized by hypogonadotropic hypogonadism (owing to gonadotropin-releasing hormone [GnRH] deficiency) and anosmia (absent sense of smell). Cleft lip/palate and other anomalies may also be present. Kallmann syndrome is usually diagnosed at puberty because of a delay in the appearance of secondary sex characteristics. It occurs three to five times more often in males (1:30,000) than in females. Mutations in at least 20 genes are associated with Kallman syndrome, some of which are X-linked, whereas others are autosomal dominant or recessive.

Empty Sella Syndrome

This is primarily a radiologic term for an enlarged sella containing a thin, flattened pituitary at the base. It is due to a congenitally defective or absent diaphragma sellae, which permits transmission of cerebrospinal fluid pressure into the sella. The syndrome can also result from pituitary gland regression after an injury, surgery, or radiation therapy. Empty sella syndrome can cause varying degrees of pituitary dysfunction and endocrine abnormalities.

Pituitary Adenomas

Pituitary adenomas are benign tumors of the anterior lobe of the pituitary. They often cause excess secretion of one or more pituitary hormones and corresponding endocrine hyperfunction (Table 19-1). The tumors are most common in adults and rare in children. **PRL-producing adenomas** are the most frequent hormone-secreting tumors of adults and children. **Gonadotrope adenomas** are more common in the elderly. Small, apparently **nonfunctioning pituitary adenomas** are found incidentally in as many as a quarter of adult autopsies.

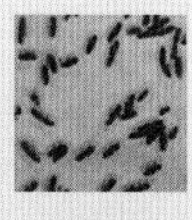
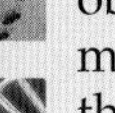

ETIOLOGIC FACTORS AND MOLECULAR PATHOGENESIS: The etiology of pituitary adenomas is obscure, but it is clear that hormonal, environmental, and genetic factors are involved. Rarely, they occur in the context of multiple endocrine neoplasia (MEN) type 1, a hereditary syndrome in which patients develop pituitary adenomas, parathyroid hyperplasia or adenoma, and islet cell adenomas of the pancreas (see below). They are also associated with Carney complex, an uncommon syndrome associated with multiple endocrine tumors.

Acquired mutations in the stimulatory subunit of the G_s protein that activates adenylyl cyclase have been reported in 40% of growth hormone–secreting pituitary adenomas. More specifically, elevation of intracellular cAMP levels is thought to stimulate hypersecretion of GH and cell proliferation.

Table 19-1
Frequency of Adenomas of the Anterior Pituitary

Cell Type	Hormone	Frequency (%)
Lactotrope	Prolactin	26
Null cell	None	17
Corticotrope	ACTH (corticotropin)	15
Somatotrope	Growth hormone	14
Plurihormonal	Multiple	13
Gonadotrope	FSH, LH	8
Oncocytoma	None	6
Thyrotrope	TSH	1

ACTH, adrenocorticotropic hormone; FSH, follicle-stimulating hormone; LH, luteinizing hormone; TSH, thyroid-stimulating hormone.

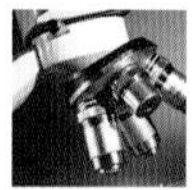

PATHOLOGY: Because the routine staining properties of the tumor cells do not correlate with the type of hormone secreted, pituitary adenomas are now classified by the hormone(s) they produce.

Pituitary adenomas range from small lesions that do not enlarge the gland to expansive tumors that erode the sella turcica and impinge on adjacent cranial structures. In general, adenomas smaller than 10 mm are called microadenomas; larger tumors are macroadenomas. Microadenomas are not symptomatic until they secrete hormones. Macroadenomas tend to cause local compression by virtue of their size and systemic manifestations owing to overproduction of hormones.

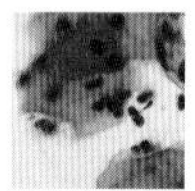

CLINICAL FEATURES: They may compress the optic chiasm, causing severe headaches, bitemporal hemianopsia, and loss of central vision. Oculomotor palsies occur when a tumor invades the cavernous sinuses. Large adenomas may penetrate the hypothalamus, interfere with normal hypothalamic input to the pituitary, and lead to loss of temperature regulation, hyperphagia, and hormonal syndromes.

Lactotrope Adenomas

Lactotrope adenomas are the most common pituitary adenomas, comprising a quarter of the gland's benign tumors. Although the true incidence of such adenomas is similar in both sexes they are most often symptomatic in young women. Lactotrope adenomas mostly occur in the lateral or posterior parts of the pituitary gland.

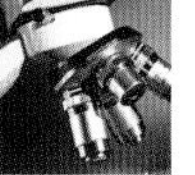

PATHOLOGY: These adenomas tend to contain spheroid nuclei with prominent nucleoli. They are sparsely granulated and may show diffuse or papillary growth patterns. Endocrine amyloid (see Chapter 7) and psammoma bodies (calcospherites) occur but are not pathognomonic.

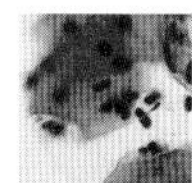

CLINICAL FEATURES: In women, functional lactotrope adenomas lead to amenorrhea, galactorrhea, and infertility. The consistently elevated blood PRL levels inhibit the surge of pituitary LH necessary for ovulation. Men tend to suffer from decreased libido and impotence. Functional lactotrope microadenomas are successfully treated with dopamine agonists (bromocriptine, cabergoline) to inhibit PRL secretion, but macroadenomas may require surgery or radiation therapy. Excess PRL secretion may be caused by factors other than pituitary adenomas, including pregnancy, lactation, administration of certain drugs, or pressure on the hypothalamus by other tumors. Radiologically, they are mostly microadenomas and are frequently part of MEN1. The prognosis of these patients is good.

Somatotrope Adenomas

Dramatic changes result from excess GH secretion. Most tumors are macroadenomas and cause mass effects and tumor-induced adenohypophyseal hypofunction. The majority of GH-producing adenomas are sporadic, but some arise as part of MEN1 and Carney syndrome.

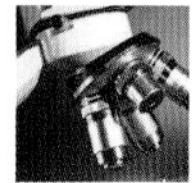

PATHOLOGY: Of patients with acromegaly, 75% have a somatotrope macroadenoma within the gland. Most of the rest have microadenomas. GH-producing

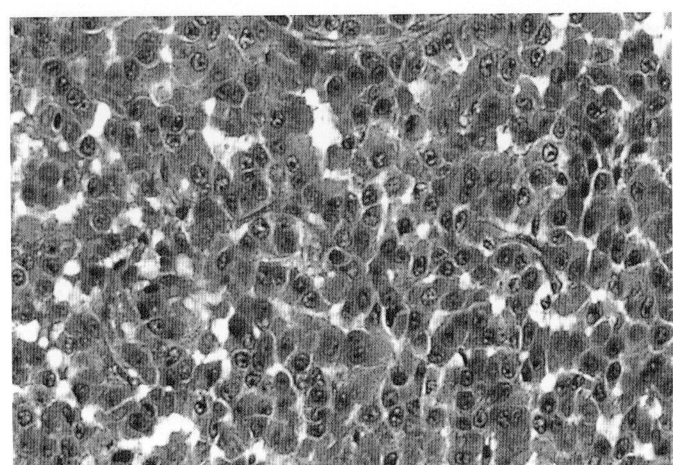

FIGURE 19-3. Pituitary somatotrope adenoma from a man with acromegaly. The tumor cells are arranged in thin cords and ribbons.

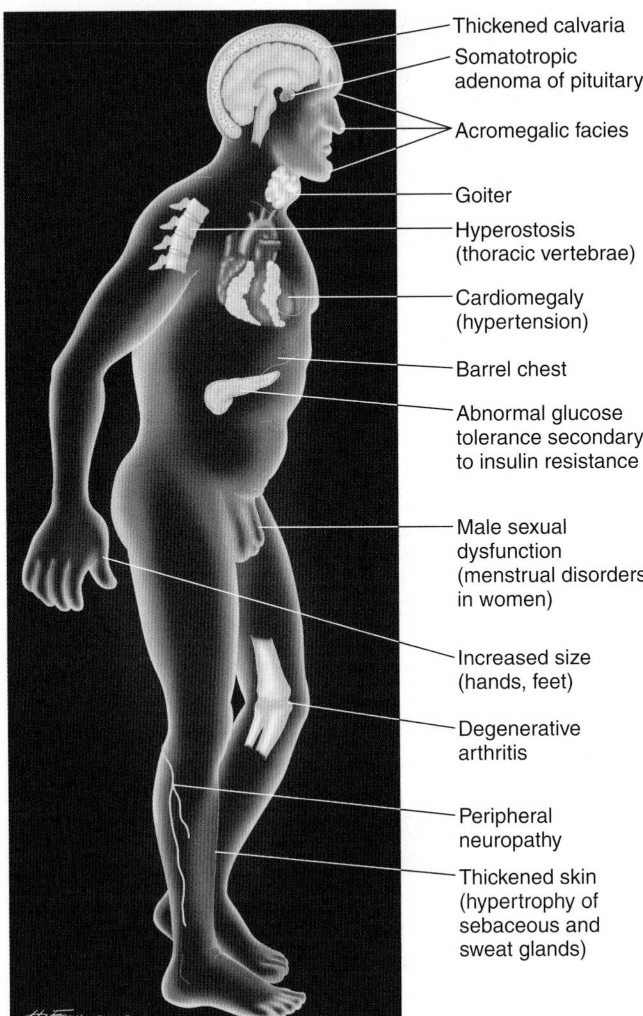

FIGURE 19-4. Clinical manifestations of acromegaly.

tumors include both densely granulated acidophilic and sparsely granulated chromophobic (weakly staining) somatotrope adenomas (Fig. 19-3). The latter variant tends to grow faster and to invade. It also shows cellular and nuclear pleomorphism. Mammosomatotrope adenomas are monomorphous with a single cell type expressing both GH and PRL.

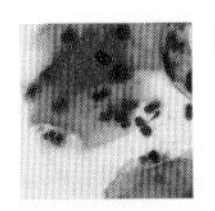

CLINICAL FEATURES: A somatotrope adenoma that arises before the epiphyses close in a child or adolescent causes **gigantism**. After the long bone epiphyses have fused and adult height has been attained, the same tumor produces **acromegaly**. The condition is uncommon, with an annual incidence of three cases per million. Over many years, patients with acromegaly gradually develop coarse facial features (Fig. 19-4), with overgrowth of the mandible (prognathism) and maxilla, increased space between the upper incisor teeth, and a thickened nose. Their hands, feet, and heads often become enlarged. Cardiovascular, cerebrovascular, and respiratory complications may be fatal.

Treatment for somatotrope adenomas is usually transsphenoidal hypophysectomy, after which circulating GH levels may decline to normal levels within hours. Radiation therapy is an alternative if surgery is contraindicated. A long-acting analog of somatostatin, an antagonist of GH, is a useful therapeutic adjunct. Most of these tumors are associated with a good prognosis.

Corticotrope Adenomas

ACTH excess induces adrenal cortical hypersecretion, causing **Cushing disease** (see below). In most cases, these tumors are microadenomas that are intensely basophilic and PAS positive. Immunohistochemistry shows ACTH and related peptides, such as endorphins and lipotropin. A few functional corticotrope adenomas are chromophobic and more aggressive than their basophilic counterparts and may demonstrate pleomorphic features and apoptosis. **Crooke adenomas** represent ACTH-producing tumors with massive hyaline deposition.

The prognosis of these patients depends on the severity of the symptoms.

Gonadotrope Adenomas

Most of these tumors are hormonally inactive macroadenomas, which are detected either incidentally or because of local compressive effects secondary to suprasellar extension. Clinical presentations include headache, visual disturbance, and hypopituitarism.

In general, gonadotrope adenomas are chromophobic and PAS negative and grow in a diffuse pattern. They proliferate slowly. Tumor cells are strongly immunopositive for FSH, LH, or both. Treatment is surgical resection. The prognosis depends on the results of the surgery.

Thyrotrope Adenomas

These are the rarest of pituitary adenomas. They come to medical attention when there are symptoms of hyperthyroidism, goiter, or a pituitary mass lesion. Circulating TSH and thyroid hormone levels are usually elevated, a situation that is unique to this tumor. Thyrotrope adenomas are predominantly macroadenomas and can be invasive and fibrotic. They are chromophobic, with polyhedral or columnar cells that form collars around blood vessels. They stain for α- and β-TSH and tend to have high proliferative indices.

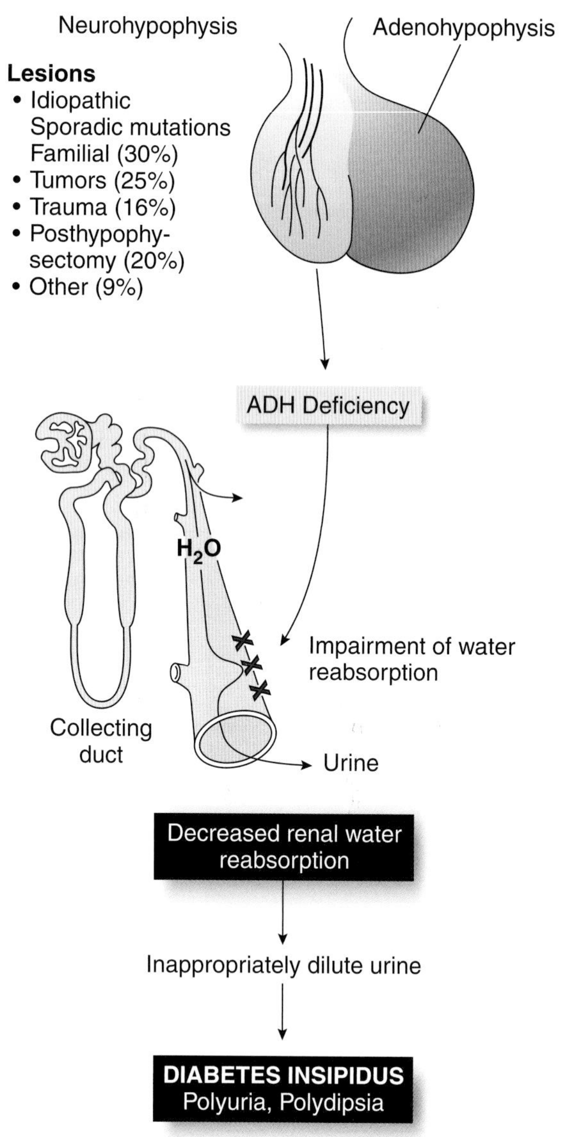

FIGURE 19-5. Mechanism of diabetes insipidus. ADH, antidiuretic hormone.

Patients with long-standing hypothyroidism may develop hyperplasia of pituitary thyrotropes (thyroid deficiency cells), presumably owing to inadequate feedback inhibition by thyroid hormone.

Nonfunctional Pituitary Adenomas

One quarter of pituitary tumors removed surgically do not secrete excess hormones. They are slowly growing macroadenomas that occur in older people and come to medical attention because of their mass effect.

Null cell adenomas are usually chromophobic and arise in the adenohypophysis, are PAS negative, and grow in a pseudopapillary pattern. The tumor cells are negative or sparsely positive for all anterior pituitary hormones. They are typically immunopositive for chromogranin A and synaptophysin.

Pituitary Carcinomas

It is not possible to distinguish between pituitary adenomas and carcinomas on morphologic grounds. Pituitary carcinomas spread to cerebrospinal or extracranial sites. When functional, they primarily secrete PRL or ACTH.

Imaging reveals a tumor extending beyond the sella turcica. The tumors are very rare and their prognosis is poor.

Posterior Pituitary

Central diabetes insipidus (Fig. 19-5) is the only significant disease associated with the posterior pituitary. Affected patients cannot concentrate urine and so have chronic water diuresis (polyuria), thirst, and polydipsia because they lack sufficient ADH (vasopressin). ADH is secreted by the posterior pituitary under the influence of the hypothalamus. One third of cases of central diabetes insipidus are of unknown etiology or can be attributed to sporadic or familial mutations in the vasopressin-neurophysin II gene. Mutations or deletions in the vasopressin V2 receptor and the vasopressin-sensitive aquaporin-2 water channel genes may cause **nephrogenic diabetes insipidus**.

One fourth of cases of central diabetes insipidus are associated with brain tumors, particularly **craniopharyngiomas** (Fig. 19-6; see Chapter 24). These tumors arise above the sella turcica from remnants of the Rathke pouch and invade and compress adjacent tissues. Trauma and hypophysectomy for anterior pituitary tumors account for most of the remaining cases of diabetes insipidus. Polyuria is often controlled using desmopressin, a synthetic vasopressin analog. Inappropriate ADH secretion (SIADH) may be caused by paraneoplastic secretion of ADH by tumors (see below).

HYPOTHALAMIC–PITUITARY AXIS

The hypothalamus, pituitary stalk, and pituitary gland constitute an anatomically and functionally integrated "neuroendocrine system." Hypothalamic neurons secrete factors that stimulate the anterior pituitary (Table 19-2). Secretion of these hypothalamic factors is, in turn, antagonized by hormones made in peripheral target organs, thereby completing a feedback loop. There are also specific hypothalamic inhibitory hormones. For example, dopamine inhibits pituitary secretion of PRL.

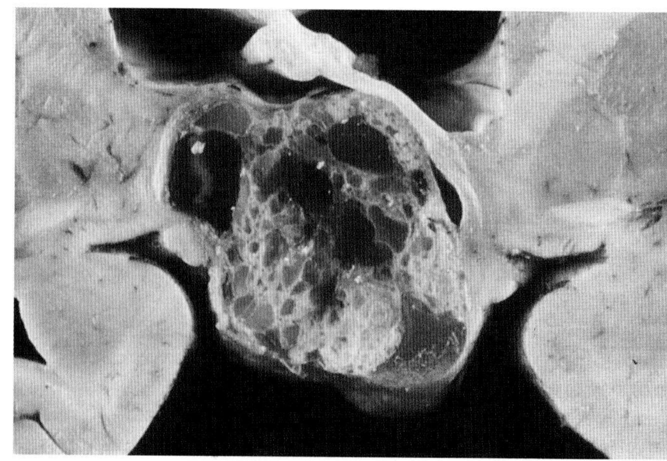

FIGURE 19-6. Craniopharyngioma. Coronal section of the brain shows a large, cystic tumor mass replacing the midline structures in the region of the hypothalamus.

Table 19-2

Hormones of the Hypothalamic–Pituitary–Target Gland Axis

Hypothalamus	Pituitary	Target Gland	Peripheral Inhibitory Hormone
CRH	ACTH	Adrenal	Corticosteroids
TRH	TSH	Thyroid	T_3, T_4
GHRH	Growth hormone	Varied	IGF-I
Somatostatin	Growth hormone	Varied	IGF-I
LHRH	LH	Gonads	Estradiol, testosterone
	FSH	Gonads	Inhibin, estradiol, testosterone
Dopamine	Prolactin	Breast	Unknown

ACTH, adrenocorticotropic hormone; CRH, corticotropin (ACTH)-releasing hormone; FSH, follicle-stimulating hormone; GHRH, growth hormone–releasing hormone; IGF-I, insulin-like growth factor I; LH, luteinizing hormone; LHRH, luteinizing hormone–releasing hormone; T_3, triiodothyronine; T_4, tetraiodothyronine (thyroxine); TRH, thyrotropin-releasing hormone; TSH, thyroid-stimulating hormone.

THYROID GLAND

The thyroid is one of the largest endocrine organs. The adult thyroid has two lobes connected by an isthmus and is below the thyroid cartilage anterior to the trachea. Follicles average 200 μm in diameter and are formed by a single row of cuboidal epithelial cells surrounded by a delicate basement membrane. Follicles become filled by an eosinophilic, proteinaceous **colloid**, which represents secreted thyroglobulin, from which active thyroid hormones are released.

In addition to follicular epithelial cells, the thyroid also contains **parafollicular,** or **C cells,** in the lateral aspects of both thyroid lobes. These cells probably derive from the neural crest and are more prominent in children. They produce **calcitonin,** a calcium-lowering hormone, and can also secrete smaller amounts of other peptides, such as serotonin and somatostatin. C cells are difficult to identify using routine stains but are readily seen by immunostaining for calcitonin or neuroendocrine markers including chromogranin and synaptophysin.

Thyroid Function

The main function of the **follicular cells** in the thyroid gland is to make the thyroid hormones **triiodothyronine** (T_3) and tetraiodothyronine (**thyroxine,** T_4). T_4 is principally a prohormone; the major effector of thyroid function is T_3. These molecules are formed by iodination of tyrosines in thyroglobulin by the follicular cells. Iodinated thyroglobulin is then secreted into the follicular lumen. Alone among endocrine glands, the thyroid can store a large amount of preformed hormone.

On demand, follicular cells reabsorb thyroglobulin, liberate T_4 and T_3 by proteolytic cleavage, and release them into the blood. Most secreted hormone is T_4, which is deiodinated in peripheral tissues to its more active form, T_3. Thyroid hormones in the blood are both free and bound to thyronine-binding thyronine-binding globulin (TBG). Peripheral cells take up only free hormone, which binds to nuclear receptors and initiates specific protein synthesis.

Thyroid hormone affects almost all organs. It stimulates basal metabolic rate and metabolism of carbohydrates, lipids, and proteins. It increases body heat and hepatic glucose production by increasing gluconeogenesis and glycogenolysis. The hormone promotes the synthesis of many structural proteins, enzymes, and other hormones. Glucose use, fatty acid synthesis in the liver, and adipose tissue lipolysis all increase. In general, thyroid hormone upregulates overall metabolic activities, both anabolic and catabolic.

Thyroid structure and function is mainly governed by pituitary TSH. In turn, thyroid hormone suppresses TSH secretion, to complete a feedback loop. Normal thyroid hormone production requires an adequate dietary supply of iodine.

Congenital Anomalies

Thyroid Agenesis

Complete absence of thyroid tissue (athyrosis) is a rare congenital abnormality, usually not discovered until several weeks after birth because maternal thyroid hormone supplies the fetus through the placenta.

Ectopic Thyroid

Thyroid tissue may be found outside the thyroid gland in several locations, as a result of abnormal migration during development. Such ectopic thyroid tissues are functionally normal and can produce thyroid hormone. Malignant tumors may develop in such tissue.

Lingual Thyroid

If the thyroid fails to descend during embryogenesis, it stays at its origin as a nodule at the base of the tongue, which resembles normal thyroid histologically. Lingual thyroid happens more often in females and usually is detected because of difficulty in swallowing, speaking, or breathing. Removal may lead to total hypothyroidism. These tissues resemble normal thyroid histologocally.

Thyroglossal Duct Cyst

Failure of the thyroglossal duct to involute completely can result in a cystic, fluid-filled remnant anywhere along the duct's route. This condition affects patients in all age groups. It presents as cystic masses of variable size (1 to 4 cm), often in the middle of the neck and attached to the hyoid bone or soft tissues. The cysts can be lined by squamous or respiratory-type epithelium and contain variable amounts of thyroid tissue. Malignancies can develop in these cysts, usually papillary carcinomas. Surgical excision is curative.

Nontoxic Goiter

Goiter is defined as thyroid gland enlargement, either nodular or diffuse, which is classified according to its function.

Nontoxic goiter, also called simple, colloid, or multinodular goiter or nodular hyperplasia, is thyroid enlargement without functional, inflammatory, or neoplastic changes. Thus, patients with nontoxic goiter are euthyroid and do not have thyroiditis (see below). The disease is far more common in women than in men (8:1). Nontoxic goiter results from a deficiency in thyroid hormone synthesis leading to increased production of TSH. As a result of this increase, thyroid gland hyperplasia occurs so as to normalize thyroid hormone production. Nontoxic goiters range from double the size of a normal gland (40 g) to a massive thyroid weighing hundreds of grams (Fig. 19-7).

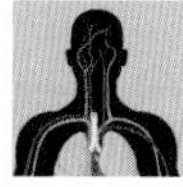

PATHOPHYSIOLOGY: The cause of the decrease in thyroid hormone production may be unknown. However, in some endemic cases decreased hormone production is caused by low iodine content in the diet or drinking water. Goiters can develop in patients receiving a variety of medications, such as sulfonamides or after an excess of iodine intake.

Simple nodular thyroid enlargement tends to be familial, suggesting a genetic factor in the disorder. Indeed, mutations in the thyroglobulin gene occur in a number of families who have simple goiter.

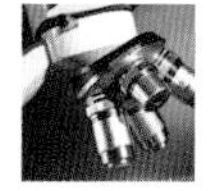

PATHOLOGY: **Diffuse nontoxic goiter** characterizes the early stages of the disease. The gland is diffusely enlarged, with hypertrophy and hyperplasia of follicular epithelial cells. On occasion, the epithelium is papillary. At this stage, follicles contain decreased colloid.

Multinodular nontoxic goiter reflects more chronic disease. These nodules vary considerably in size and shape. Some are distended with colloid, whereas others are collapsed. Large colloid-containing follicles sometimes fuse to form even larger "colloid cysts." Lining epithelial cells are flat to cuboidal and are occasionally arrayed as papillae that project into the follicular lumen. Hemorrhage and chronic inflammation are common (Fig. 19-7C).

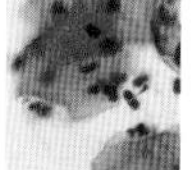

CLINICAL FEATURES: Patients with nontoxic goiter are typically asymptomatic and come to medical attention because of a mass in the neck. Large goiters may compress structures in the neck and cause dysphagia (esophagus), inspiratory stridor (trachea), venous congestion of the head and face (neck veins), or hoarseness (recurrent laryngeal nerve). Patients tend to be euthyroid and blood T_4, T_3, and (usually) TSH are normal.

Nontoxic goiters are most commonly treated with thyroid hormone to reduce TSH levels and, thus, the stimulus to thyroid growth. ***Many patients with nontoxic goiter eventually develop hyperthyroidism, in which case the term "toxic multinodular goiter" is applied (see below).***

Hypothyroidism

Hypothyroidism is the clinical manifestations of thyroid hormone deficiency. It can be the consequence of three general processes:

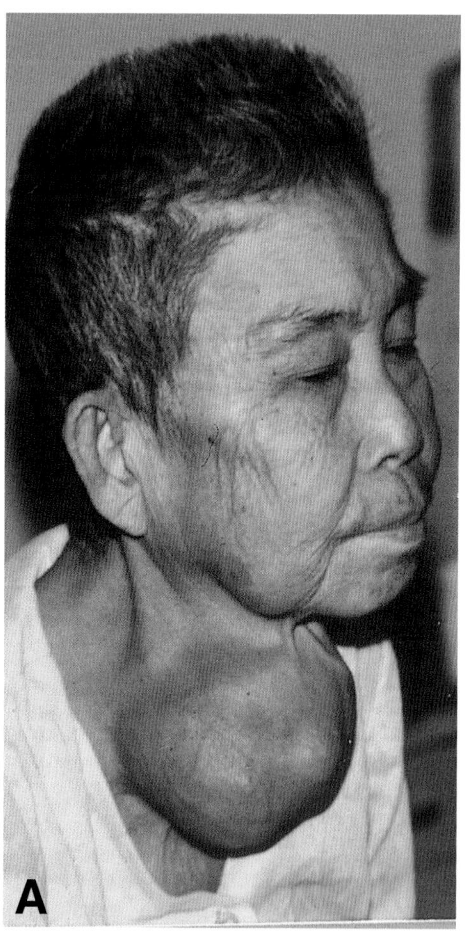

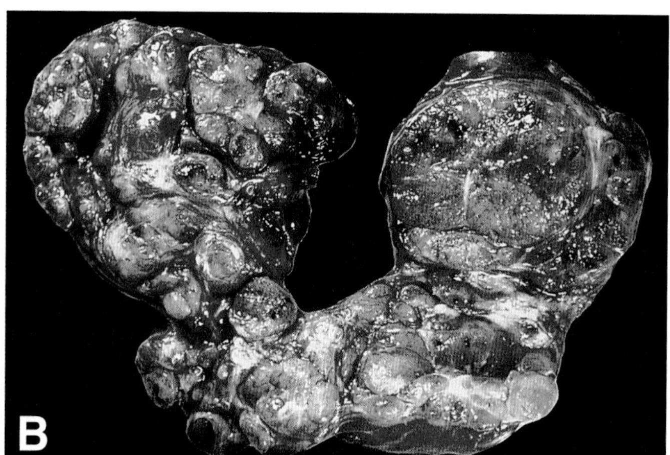

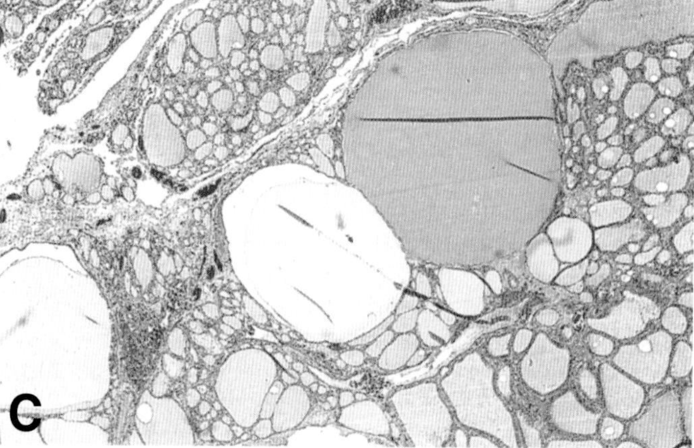

FIGURE 19-7. Nontoxic goiter. A. In a middle-aged woman with nontoxic goiter, the thyroid has enlarged to produce a conspicuous neck mass. **B.** Coronal section of the enlarged thyroid gland shows numerous irregular nodules, some with cystic and old hemorrhage. **C.** Microscopic view of one of the macroscopic nodules shows marked variation in the size of the follicles.

- **Defective thyroid hormone synthesis**, with compensatory goitrogenesis (goitrous hypothyroidism)
- **Inadequate thyroid parenchyma function**, usually because of thyroiditis, surgical resection of the gland, or therapeutic radioiodine administration
- **Inadequate secretion of TSH** by the pituitary or of **thyroid-releasing hormone (TRH) by the hypothalamus**

Other causes include pregnancy (postpartum thyroiditis), congenital conditions, and certain medications such as lithium.

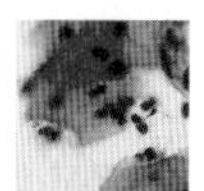

CLINICAL FEATURES: Symptoms of hypothyroidism, which develop insidiously, reflect decreased circulating thyroid hormone. Often the first manifestations are tiredness, lethargy, sensitivity to cold, and inability to concentrate. Many organ systems are affected (Fig. 19-8). Hypothyroidism is treated effectively with thyroid hormone.

Skin

Cutaneous signs are almost universal in patients with clinical hypothyroidism. Proteoglycans accumulate in the extracellular matrix and bind water, resulting in a peculiar form of edema called **myxedema.**

Nervous System

Hypothyroidism in pregnancy has grave neurologic consequences for the fetus, expressed after birth as cretinism (see below). Hypothyroid adults are lethargic and somnolent and show memory loss and slowed mental processes. Psychiatric symptoms are common and severe agitation, **myxedema madness**, may develop.

Heart

In early hypothyroidism, heart rate and stroke volume are reduced, resulting in decreased cardiac output. In untreated hypothyroidism, so-called **myxedema heart** develops, with cardiac dilation and pericardial effusion. Such hearts are flabby and show interstitial edema and myocyte swelling. Coronary atherosclerosis is common.

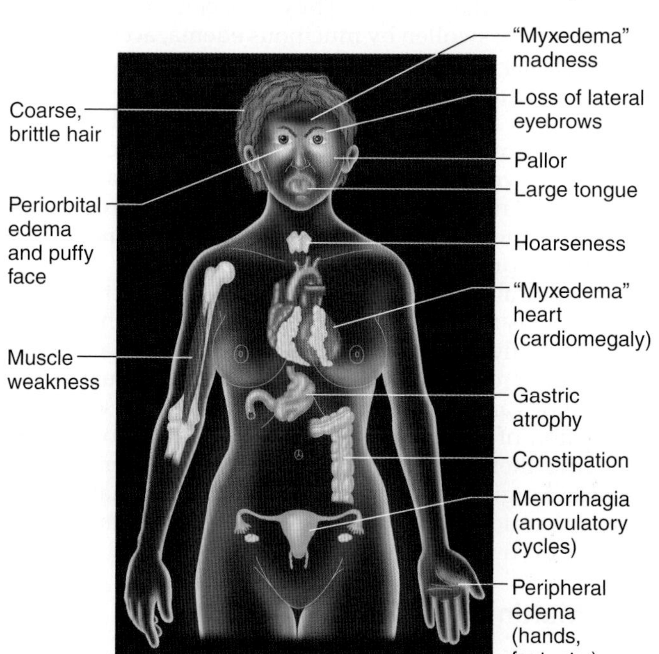

FIGURE 19-8. Dominant clinical manifestations of hypothyroidism.

Gastrointestinal Tract

Constipation, owing to decreased peristalsis, is common and may be severe enough to result in fecal impaction (**myxedema megacolon**).

Reproductive System

Women with hypothyroidism suffer ovulatory failure, progesterone deficiency, and irregular and excessive menstrual bleeding. In men, erectile dysfunction and oligospermia are common.

Hypothyroidism can reflect a variety of causes including the following:

- **Autoimmunity:** Autoimmune hypothyroidism results from circulating antibodies to thyroid antigens, which eventuate in end-stage autoimmune thyroiditis (see below). Antibodies may also block TSH or TSH receptor and prevent thyroid activation.
- **Goitrous hypothyroidism:** Iodine deficiency, antithyroid agents (drugs such as lithium or dietary goitrogens including cassava), long-term iodide intake, and hereditary defects in thyroid hormone synthesis all may result in thyroid enlargement and glandular hypofunction. **Endemic goiter** is goitrous hypothyroidism because of dietary iodine deficiency in areas with a high prevalence of the disease.
- **Congenital hypothyroidism (cretinism):** The condition may result from endemic iodine deficiency, developmental defects of the thyroid (**thyroid dysgenesis**), or inherited defects. The last include mutations in genes for TRH and its receptor, TSH and its receptor, sodium–iodide symporter, thyroglobulin, and thyroid oxidase. Hypothyroid cretinism arises from iodine deficiency in late fetal life and in the neonatal period. The clinical course in these children is similar to that of other forms of congenital hypothyroidism. Affected infants are apathetic and sluggish, with large abdomens often showing umbilical hernias. Body temperatures are often below 35°C (95°F), and the skin is pale and cold. Refractory anemia and dilated hearts are common. By 6 months, mental retardation, stunted growth (because of defective osseous maturation), and characteristic facies are evident. Levels of serum T_4 and T_3 are low and those of TSH levels are high (unless the problem involves defective TSH secretion).

Hyperthyroidism

Hyperthyroidism is the clinical syndrome of excessive circulating thyroid hormone. In general, signs and symptoms of hyperthyroidism reflect a hypermetabolic state of target tissues. Prolonged hypersecretion of thyroid hormone can result from abnormal thyroid stimulator (Graves disease), intrinsic thyroid disease (toxic multinodular goiter or functional adenoma), and, rarely, excess TSH production by a pituitary adenoma.

Graves Disease

Also known as diffuse toxic goiter, Graves disease is an autoimmune disorder characterized by diffuse goiter, hyperthyroidism, exophthalmos (Fig. 19-9), tachycardia, weight loss, and dermopathy. It is the most prevalent autoimmune disease in

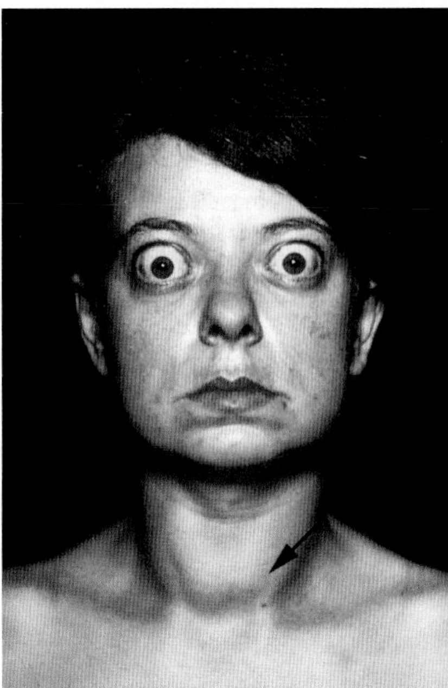

FIGURE 19-9. Graves disease. A young woman with hyperthyroidism displays a mass in the neck and exophthalmos. Sandoz Pharmaceutical Corporation.

the United States, affecting 0.5% to 1% of the population under age 40. Graves disease can also affect children.

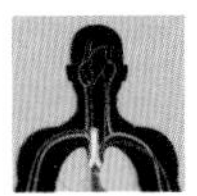

PATHOPHYSIOLOGY: The cause of Graves disease is not fully understood and seems to involve an interplay between immune mechanisms, heredity, sex, and possibly emotional factors. Like other autoimmune diseases, Graves disease is far more common (7- to 10-fold) in women than in men. It tends to arise during periods of hormonal imbalance, including puberty, pregnancy, and menopause.

Immune mechanisms: Patients have IgG antibodies that bind to specific domains of the plasma membrane TSH receptor (Fig. 19-10). These antibodies act as agonists, that is, they stimulate the TSH receptor and activate adenylyl cyclase, thereby increasing thyroid hormone secretion. Under such continued stimulation, the thyroid becomes diffusely hyperplastic and highly vascular.

Graves autoantibodies are heterogeneous; some antibodies seem to be cytotoxic and may cause thyroid failure that often follows long-standing Graves disease.

Genetic factors: The strongest risk factor for Graves disease is a positive family history. No single gene is responsible. The concordance rate in monozygotic twins is only 30% to 50%. Thus, both genetic and environmental factors are probably involved.

HLA class II molecules exposed on thyrocytes (e.g., HLA-DR3, HLA-DQA1) have been established as susceptibility loci. Graves disease is also associated with polymorphism of cytotoxic T-lymphocyte antigen-4 (CTLA-4), which indicates the importance of autoreactive T cells. Patients with Graves disease and their relatives have a much higher incidence of other autoimmune diseases (e.g., pernicious anemia and Hashimoto thyroiditis).

Smoking: Smoking increases the risk of Graves disease, and particularly the severity of the eye disease in patients who develop ophthalmopathy.

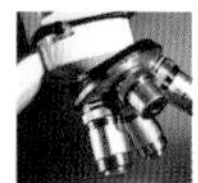

PATHOLOGY: The thyroid is symmetrically enlarged, usually 35 to 100 g. The cut surfaces are firm and dark red. There is diffuse follicular hyperplasia and increased vascularity. Thyroid epithelial cells are tall and columnar and array themselves on papillae that project into the lumens of the follicles. Thyroid colloid tends to be depleted and appears pale, scalloped, or "moth-eaten" where it abuts the epithelial cells. Scattered B and T lymphocytes and plasma cells infiltrate the interstitial tissue. B cells may form germinal follicles but T cells predominate. Hyperplastic follicles may occur outside the gland's capsule and in adjacent muscle.

Therapy with antithyroid medication (e.g., methimazole or propylthiouracil) commonly results in increased thyroid hyperplasia and complete lack of colloid.

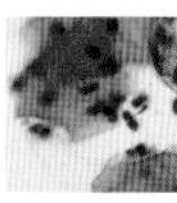

CLINICAL FEATURES: Patients with Graves disease note the gradual onset of nonspecific symptoms, such as nervousness, emotional lability, tremor, weakness, and weight loss (Fig. 19-11). They tolerate heat poorly, tend to sweat profusely, and may report palpitations. Excess thyroid hormone reduces systemic vascular resistance, enhances cardiac contractility, and increases the heart rate. In patients with preexisting heart disease, congestive heart failure may ensue. Women develop oligomenorrhea, which may progress to amenorrhea.

Patients have symmetrically enlarged thyroids, often with an audible bruit and a palpable thrill. Proptosis and retraction of the eyelids expose the sclera above the superior margin of the limbus. The skin is warm and moist. Some patients show **Graves dermopathy**, a peculiar pretibial edema caused by the accumulation of fluid and glycosaminoglycans. The diagnosis is confirmed by increased thyroid radioactive iodine uptake and elevated levels of serum T_4 and T_3. Serum TSH is very low.

Ophthalmopathy: Exophthalmos (protrusion of eyeballs) is a common feature of Graves disease (Fig. 19-9), but its occurrence and severity correlate poorly with levels of thyroid hormone. The condition is caused by enlargement of orbital extraocular muscles. These muscles themselves are normal but are swollen by mucinous edema, accumulation of fibroblasts, and lymphocyte infiltration. The increased orbital contents displace the eye forward. T lymphocytes sensitized to antigens shared by thyroid follicular cells and orbital fibroblasts (possibly TSH receptor) accumulate around the eye, where they secrete cytokines that activate fibroblasts. Antibodies that stimulate orbital fibroblasts to proliferate and produce collagen and glycosaminoglycans may also be produced.

The clinical course of Graves disease is characterized by exacerbations and remissions. Untreated, hyperthyroidism may eventually lead to progressive thyroid failure and hypothyroidism. Treatment depends on many individual factors and includes antithyroid medication such as thioisocyanate, destruction of thyroid tissue with radioactive iodine and adjunctive therapy with corticosteroids and adrenergic antagonists. Surgical ablation is uncommon. Unfortunately, even if hyperthyroidism is relieved, exophthalmos often persists and may even worsen.

Toxic Multinodular Goiter

Many patients over the age of 50 with nontoxic multinodular goiter eventually develop a toxic form of the disease. Toxic goiter is more common in women (10:1).

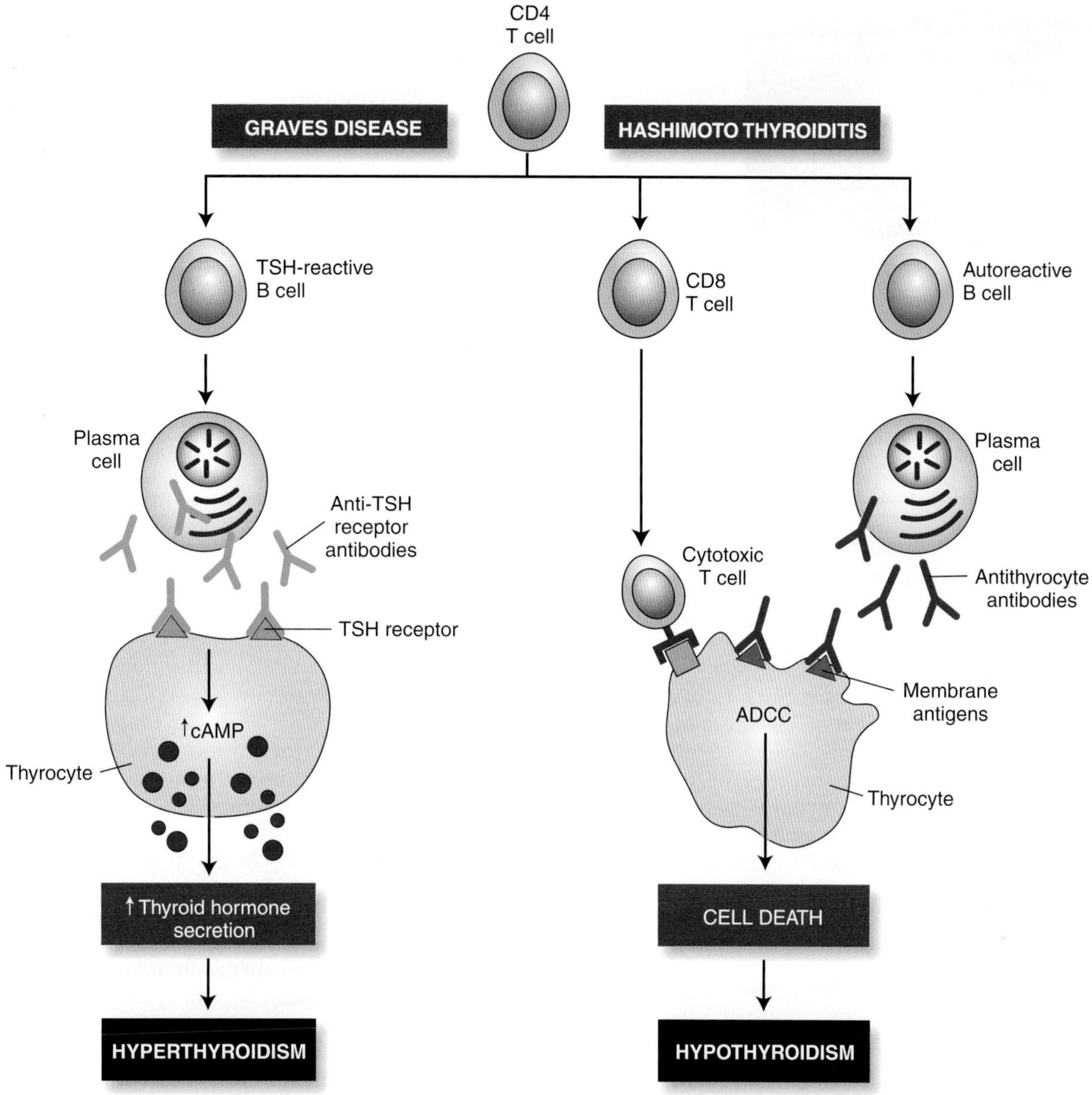

FIGURE 19-10. Immune mechanisms of Graves disease and Hashimoto thyroiditis. $CD4^+$ T cells stimulate antibody production by autoreactive B cells. Anti–thyroid-stimulating hormone (TSH) receptor antibodies stimulate thyroid hormone synthesis in Graves disease. Antibodies induce thyrocyte cell death in Hashimoto thyroiditis by complement-dependent cytotoxicity and antibody-dependent cell-mediated cytotoxicity (ADCC). Thyrocyte death also results from attack by $CD8^+$ (cytotoxic) T cells. cAMP, cyclic adenosine 3′,5′-monophosphate; CD, cluster differentiation.

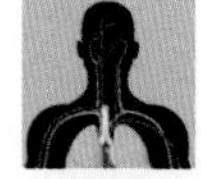

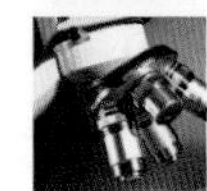

PATHOPHYSIOLOGY AND PATHOLOGY: There are two patterns by which nontoxic multinodular goiter assumes functional autonomy and progresses to a toxic condition. (1) In some patients, iodine uptake is diffuse and not affected by administration of thyroid hormone. The thyroid shows groups of small hyperplastic follicles mixed with other nodules of varying size that appear to be inactive. (2) In other patients, iodine accumulates focally in one or more nodules. These hyperfunctional nodules suppress the rest of the gland. Exogenous thyroid hormone produces no further suppression of iodine uptake. The functional nodules show large hyperplastic follicles resembling adenomas and are clearly distinct from the inactive areas.

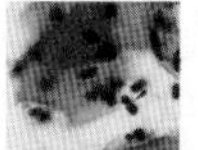

CLINICAL FEATURES: Patients with toxic multinodular goiter tend to have less severe symptoms of hyperthyroidism than those with Graves disease, and they do not develop exophthalmos. Cardiac complications, including atrial fibrillation and congestive heart failure, may dominate the clinical presentation. Serum T_4 and T_3 levels are only minimally high, and radiolabeled iodine uptake is normal or only slightly elevated. Radiolabeled iodine after a course of antithyroid therapy is the most common therapy.

Toxic Adenoma

Toxic adenoma refers to a solitary, hyperfunctioning, benign follicular tumor in an otherwise normal thyroid. It is an

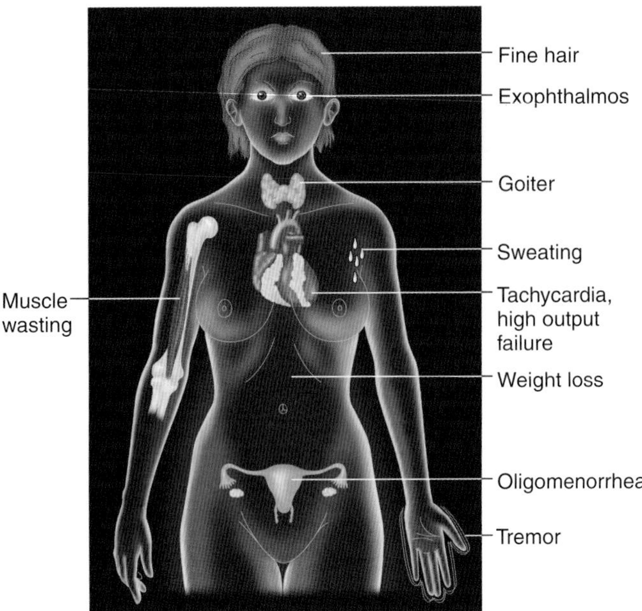

FIGURE 19-11. Major clinical manifestations of Graves disease.

uncommon cause of hyperthyroidism. Such tumors display autonomous function independent of TSH and are not suppressed by exogenous thyroid hormone. A toxic adenoma eventually suppresses the rest of the thyroid, which then atrophies. Many toxic adenomas have a variety of somatic activating mutations of the TSH receptor gene, leading to constitutive upregulation of the cAMP cascade and less commonly the inositol phosphate–diacylglycerol system.

THYROIDITIS

Thyroiditis refers to a heterogeneous group of inflammatory disorders of the thyroid gland, including those caused by autoimmune mechanisms and infectious agents.

Acute Thyroiditis as a Result of Bacterial or Fungal Infections

The disease usually develops during a systemic infection that reaches the thyroid by hematogenous spread. It occurs in patients of all ages, but children, the elderly, or immunocompromised persons are most commonly affected.

Symptoms begin with fever, chills, malaise, and a painful, swollen neck. Infection may involve one lobe or the entire gland. There is diffuse acute and chronic inflammation with focal microabscess formation. Rarely, the infection spreads into the trachea, mediastinum, and esophagus. The prognosis is excellent when the infection is promptly treated with antibiotics.

The most common causative organisms are streptococcus, staphylococcus, and pneumococcus. Other causes include fungi and cytomegalovirus (CMV), and rarely tuberculosis thyroiditis is rare but can occur in immunosuppressed patients.

Chronic Autoimmune Thyroiditis (Hashimoto Thyroiditis)

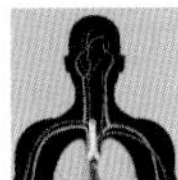

PATHOPHYSIOLOGY: Hashimoto thyroiditis (HT) is usually part of the spectrum of autoimmune diseases. It can affect several family members who often also suffer other autoimmune conditions such as lupus, Graves disease, arteritis, and scleroderma (see Chapter 3).

Immune Mechanisms

Unlike the case in Graves disease, the pathogenesis of HT involves cellular and humoral autoimmunity, as detailed in Figure 19-10. Viral or bacterial infection appears to initiate the activation of CD4 (helper) T cells sensitized to thyroid antigens. Subsequently autoreactive cytotoxic ($CD8^+$) T cells attack thyrocytes. Lymphocyte-produced interferon-γ causes thyrocytes to express MHC class II molecules, thereby expanding the autoreactive T-cell population. These effects account for the striking accumulation of lymphocytes in the glands of patients with autoimmune thyroiditis. Autoreactive B cells are also recruited and produce antibodies against thyroid antigens, including microsomal peroxidase (95%), thyroglobulin (60%), and the TSH receptor.

Half of all first-degree relatives of patients with HT display antithyroid antibodies. Moreover, both Graves disease and chronic autoimmune thyroiditis are described in these family members. A familial tendency for HT is further suggested by the higher prevalence of other autoimmune diseases in patients and their relatives, including MEN syndrome type 2, type 1 diabetes, pernicious anemia, Addison disease, and myasthenia gravis. HT is most common where **iodine intake** is greatest, for example, Japan and the United States. In iodine-deficient areas, iodine supplementation significantly increases the prevalence of chronic inflammation of the thyroid and the presence of thyroid autoantibodies.

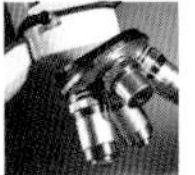

PATHOLOGY: The gland in patients with HT is diffusely enlarged and firm, weighing 60 to 200 g. The cut surface is pale tan and fleshy with a vaguely nodular pattern (Fig. 19-12). The capsule is intact and perithyroid tissues are not involved. The thyroid shows a conspicuous infiltrate of lymphocytes and plasma cells, with destruction and atrophy of follicles. Oncocytic cells (i.e., showing granular pink staining of cytoplasm related to a high concentration of mitochondria) (**Hürthle** or **Askanazy cells**) are conspicuous. Lymphoid follicles, often with germinal centers, are present. Interstitial fibrosis is variable and is prominent in 10% of cases (fibrous variant). The thyroid eventually undergoes atrophy in some patients, who are left with a small, fibrotic gland infiltrated by lymphocytes. Thyroid lymphoma is a rare complication of HT.

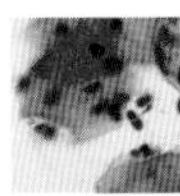

CLINICAL FEATURES: HT mainly affects women between 30 and 50 years of age. Patients often present with nonspecific symptoms such as fatigue, depression, and fibromyalgia. Clinically they show diffuse thyroid enlargement and either mild hyperthyroidism or hypothyroidism. Most patients note the gradual onset of a goiter, although sometimes the gland enlarges rapidly. Eventually, one third to one half of patients progress to an overt hypothyroid state, the risk of which is much greater among men than women. The diagnosis of HT is made by identifying circulating antithyroid antibodies. Such patients show low levels of T_4, elevated serum thyrotropin, and elevated TSH. HT frequently coexists with papillary cancer of the thyroid.

Many patients need no therapy. Thyroid hormone is given to treat hypothyroidism and decrease the size of the gland. Surgery is reserved for patients who do not respond to suppressive hormone therapy or who complain of troublesome pressure symptoms.

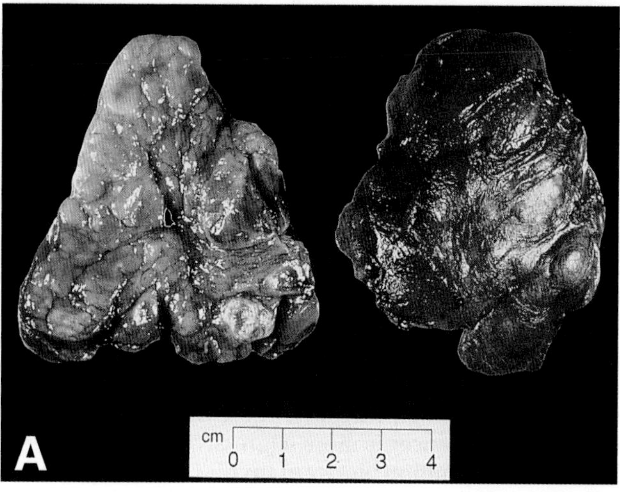

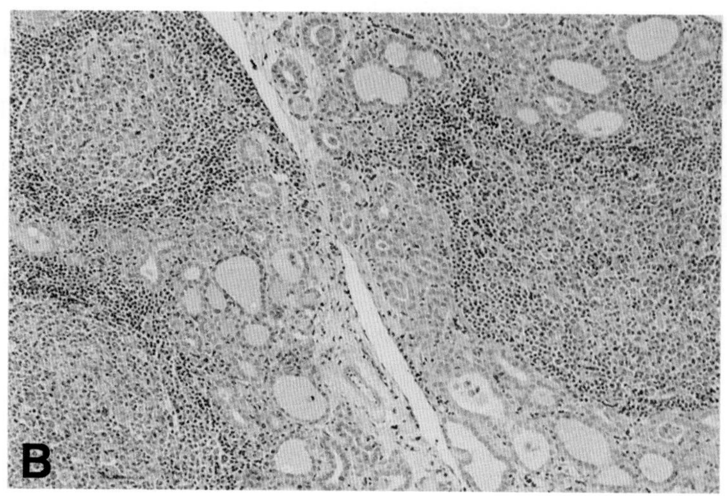

FIGURE 19-12. Chronic autoimmune (Hashimoto) thyroiditis. The thyroid gland is symmetrically enlarged and coarsely nodular. **A.** A coronal section of the right lobe shows irregular nodules and an intact capsule. **B.** A microscopic section of the thyroid reveals a conspicuous chronic inflammatory infiltrate and many atrophic thyroid follicles. The inflammatory cells form prominent lymphoid follicles with germinal centers.

Subacute Thyroiditis (de Quervain, Granulomatous, or Giant Cell Thyroiditis)

Subacute thyroiditis, also known as granulomatous, de Quervain, or nonsuppurative thyroiditis, is an uncommon, self-limited disorder characterized by granulomatous inflammation. It typically occurs after upper respiratory viral infections, such as with influenza virus, adenovirus, echovirus, or coxsackievirus. Mumps virus has also been incriminated in some cases. de Quervain thyroiditis principally affects women 30 to 50 years old.

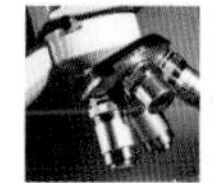

PATHOLOGY: The thyroid is enlarged to 40 to 60 g. Its cut surface is firm and pale. Acute inflammation, often with microabscesses, is followed by a patchy infiltrate of lymphocytes, plasma cells, and macrophages throughout the thyroid. Destruction of follicles releases colloid, which elicits a conspicuous granulomatous reaction (Fig. 19-13). Abundant foreign body–type multinucleated giant cells, often containing colloid, are present. Fibrosis may follow resolution of the inflammatory reaction, but normal thyroid architecture is usually restored.

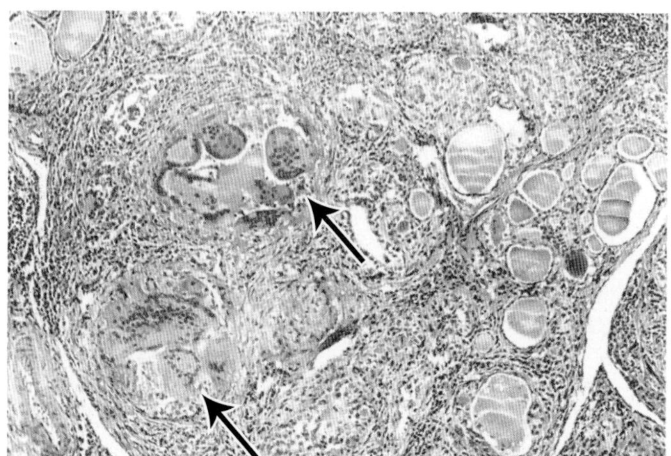

FIGURE 19-13. Subacute thyroiditis. The release of colloid into the interstitial tissue has elicited a prominent granulomatous reaction, with numerous foreign body giant cells (*arrows*).

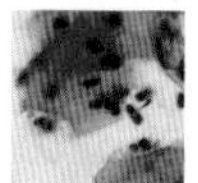

CLINICAL FEATURES: Patients with subacute thyroiditis typically notice pain in the anterior neck, sometimes with fever, malaise, fatigue, and pain in the neck or radiating to the jaw. Other patients follow a mild course with only minimal symptoms. Subacute thyroiditis generally resolves within a few months without any clinical sequelae. Release of preformed thyroid hormone by destruction of the follicles often raises serum T_4 and T_3, which may be high enough to cause transient clinical hyperthyroidism. The consequent suppression of TSH leads to decreased radiolabeled iodine uptake. This phase is followed by decreased serum T_4 and T_3 levels, but as inflammation resolves, a euthyroid state returns. There may be low levels of antithyroid antibodies.

Silent Thyroiditis

In silent thyroiditis, also called **painless subacute thyroiditis** or **lymphocytic thyroiditis**, patients experience painless thyroid enlargement, self-limited hyperthyroidism, and destruction of gland parenchyma, with lymphocytic infiltration. Thus, it resembles subacute thyroiditis clinically but is closer to HT pathologically. Silent thyroiditis differs from the latter by the lack of antithyroid antibodies or other evidence of autoimmune thyroiditis. Silent thyroiditis mainly affects women, often in the postpartum period, causing hyperthyroidism that usually persists for 2 to 4 months. Treatment is symptomatic, and most patients become euthyroid.

Riedel Thyroiditis

The "thyroiditis" in Riedel thyroiditis is something of a misnomer, as this rare disease also involves extrathyroidal soft tissues of the neck. Often progressive fibrosis occurs in other locations, including the retroperitoneum, mediastinum, and orbit. Riedel thyroiditis is mainly a disease of middle age. The female-to-male ratio is 3:1. The condition is considered to be a manifestation of IgG4-related systemic disease.

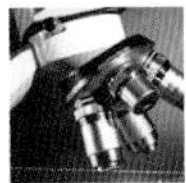

PATHOLOGY: Part or all of the thyroid is stony hard and "woody." The process is usually asymmetric and often affects only one lobe. The fibrous infiltrate extends into the thyroid gland and other tissues of the neck, including skeletal muscle and nerves. It may also surround and infiltrate lymph nodes and parathyroid glands. Dense, hyalinized fibrous tissue and chronic inflammation are present throughout involved portions of the thyroid. Eosinophils may also be present. Follicles are normal in unaffected parts of the gland.

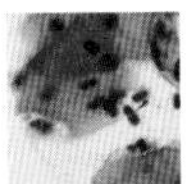

CLINICAL FEATURES: Patients with Riedel thyroiditis notice the gradual onset of painless goiter and present with a hard thyroid mass. They may also have fibrosing lesions at other sites, such as the retroperitoneum, mediastinum, and retro-orbital tissues. Symptoms may be due to compression of neck organs: the trachea (stridor), esophagus (dysphagia), and recurrent laryngeal nerve (hoarseness). Treatment is primarily surgical to relieve symptomatic compression of local structures.

FOLLICULAR ADENOMA OF THE THYROID

Follicular adenomas are benign neoplasms with follicular differentiation. They are the most common thyroid tumors and typically present in euthyroid people as solitary "cold" nodules (no uptake of radioiodine). Follicular adenomas occur frequently in iodine-deficient areas. They can also arise in irradiated glands and as part of Cowden syndrome (see Chapter 4). Adenomas are solitary encapsulated neoplasms in which cells are arranged in follicles that resemble normal adult thyroid tissue or mimic stages in the gland's embryonic development. Multiple adenomas are uncommon. Follicular adenomas are most common in the fourth and fifth decades, with a female-to-male ratio of 7:1. The clonal origin of follicular adenomas has been established.

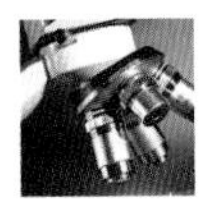

PATHOLOGY: Follicular adenomas are solitary, circumscribed, 1 to 3 cm nodules that protrude from the surface of the thyroid. They are completely enclosed by a thin fibrous capsule. The tumor cut surface is soft and paler than the surrounding gland. Hemorrhage, fibrosis, and cystic change are common.

These benign lesions should be differentiated from follicular carcinomas, which usually have thicker capsules. Careful evaluation of the capsule for capsular or vascular invasion is mandatory to make this distinction. *Malignancies can develop in association with or within benign nodules.* Surgical lobectomy to remove the lesion is curative.

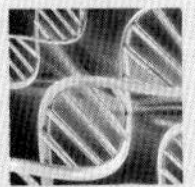

MOLECULAR PATHOGENESIS: Adenomas are clonal in over 60% of cases. Other molecular alterations include trisomy 7, translocations in 19q13, deletions in chromosomes 3p, 10, and 13, and sometimes mutations in the RAS oncogene.

Papillary Hyperplastic Nodules

Papillary hyperplastic nodules occur mainly in children and young women. They are solitary, well circumscribed, and well encapsulated and contain papillae of different sizes. The papillae are lined by cuboidal cells with characteristic follicular nuclei (i.e., dense with dispersed chromatin). The center of nodules is often cystic and can contain colloid-like material. These lesions are often misdiagnosed as papillary cancer.

Thyroid Cancer

In the United States, some 57,000 new cases of thyroid cancer are diagnosed each year. Mortality from thyroid cancer exceeds that from malignant tumors of all other endocrine organs.

Thyroid nodules occur in up to 10% of the population, but thyroid cancers represent only 1% of all cancers. A single nodule has 12% probability of being malignant, and those odds decrease significantly to 3% if a nodule is palpable.

Most cases of thyroid carcinoma occur between the third and seventh decades, but they do not spare children. These tumors occur in women threefold more often than in men. However, thyroid cancer is more aggressive in older males.

Fine-needle aspiration biopsy of thyroid nodules provides a diagnosis in most cases. Prognosis is a function of the tumor morphology, and the clinical course ranges from virtually benign to rapidly fatal. Fortunately, the latter is uncommon.

Thyroid radioscintigraphy is helpful, because hyperfunctioning nodules are usually benign. "Cold" or nonfunctioning nodules, although more often malignant, may also be benign.

Papillary Thyroid Carcinoma

PTC accounts for up to 90% of sporadic thyroid cancers in the United States. It occurs most often between the ages of 20 and 50, with a female-to-male ratio of 3:1. However, it may arise at any age, even in children and young adolescents in whom it is the most common type.

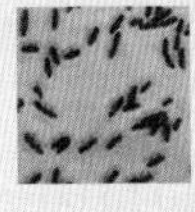
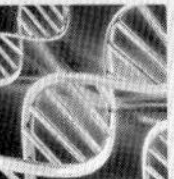

ETIOLOGIC FACTORS AND MOLECULAR PATHOGENESIS: The etiology of PTC is uncertain, but there are several potentially important connections.

- **Iodine excess:** In endemic goiter regions, addition of iodine to the diet increased the proportion of thyroid cancers showing papillary, as compared with follicular, morphology.
- **Radiation:** External radiation to the neck of children and adults increases the incidence of later PTC. Children living in contaminated areas surrounding the Chernobyl nuclear disaster had an almost 100-fold higher rate of PTC, especially if they were under 15 at the time of the incident. The younger the children, the higher the risk, because younger children have a higher uptake of radioactive iodine. Radiation leads to mutations and translocations including RET rearrangements important in the etiology of this cancer.
- **Genetic factors:** First-degree relatives of PTC patients have a 4- to 10-fold greater risk for PTC than does the general population. PTC also occurs in association with familial polyposis syndrome (*APC* gene; see Chapter 4).
- ***RET* mutations:** Somatic rearrangements of *RET* proto-oncogene on chromosome 10 (10q11.2) are common in PTC. These rearrangements cause the tyrosine kinase domain of *RET* to fuse to various other genes, creating *RET/PTC* fusion oncogenes.
- ***BRAF* and RAS mutations:** Point mutations of the *BRAF* gene are present in up to 70% of papillary thyroid cancers. This mutation is linked to specific characteristics

of PTC that predict tumor behavior and progression. *RAS* proto-oncogene mutations are present in 10% of PTCs and may be increasing.

PATHOLOGY: PTCs vary from common microscopic lesions to tumors larger than a normal gland. Papillary cancers may occur in either lobe or the isthmus. They are firm, solid, and white-yellowish, with irregular and infiltrative borders. Lesions may be multiple and are occasionally encapsulated (Fig. 19-14A).

Branching papillae contain a central fibrovascular core and a single or stratified lining of cuboidal to columnar cells (Fig. 19-14B). There are usually irregularly shaped or tubular neoplastic follicles, but relative proportions of papillary and follicular elements vary greatly. Nuclear atypia is an important diagnostic feature and includes clear (**ground-glass** or **Orphan Annie**) nuclei, eosinophilic pseudoinclusions (which are invaginations of cytoplasm into the nucleus) and nuclear grooves. Many papillary cancers show dense fibrosis and psammoma bodies (calcospherites), the latter being virtually diagnostic. The stroma may be infiltrated by lymphocytes and Langerhans cells. Vascular invasion is uncommon.

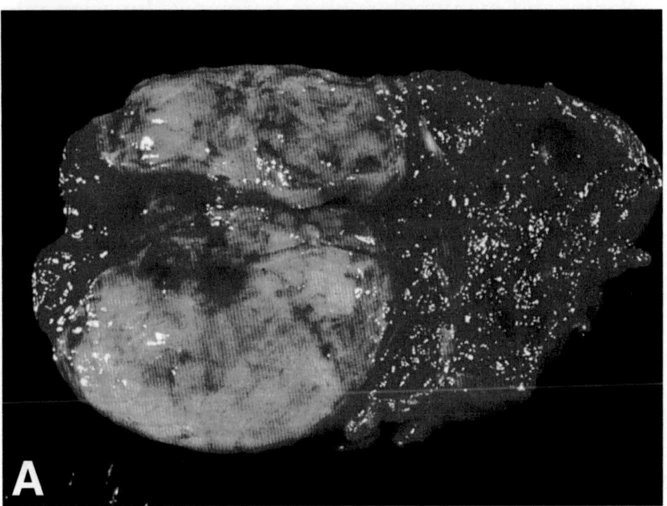

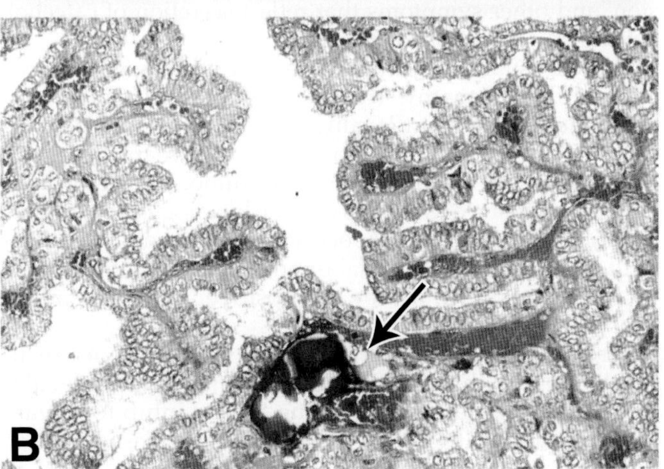

FIGURE 19-14. Papillary carcinoma of the thyroid. A. The cut surface of a surgically resected thyroid displays a circumscribed pale tan mass with foci of cystic change. **B.** Branching papillae are lined by neoplastic columnar epithelium with clear nuclei. A calcospherite, or psammoma body, is evident.

Several morphologic types of papillary carcinoma are known, some associated with good prognosis such as **microcarcinoma** (≤1 cm), not requiring further treatment. The **diffuse sclerosis, tall cell,** and **columnar** variants have worse prognoses.

PTC typically invades lymphatics and spreads to regional cervical lymph nodes. Lymph node metastases vary from tiny foci in otherwise normal lymph nodes to large masses that dwarf the primary lesion. Direct extension of PTC into soft tissues of the neck occurs in one fourth of cases. Hematogenous metastases are less common than in other types of thyroid cancer, but they do happen occasionally, mostly to the lungs.

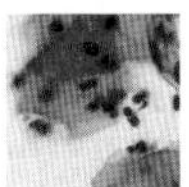

CLINICAL FEATURES: PTC generally presents as (1) a painless, palpable nodule in an otherwise normal gland; (2) a nodule with enlarged cervical lymph nodes; or (3) cervical lymphadenopathy without a palpable thyroid nodule. In general, the prognosis of PTC is excellent, and life expectancy for patients differs little from that of the general population.

The presence of metastases to cervical nodes at the time of surgery does not change the prognosis, as less than 10% of such patients die of the tumor. In fatal cases of PTC, death is caused principally by metastases to the lungs or brain or by obstruction of the trachea or esophagus.

Therapies include surgery (lobectomy or total thyroidectomy), with or without neck dissection, followed by administration of radioiodine.

Follicular Thyroid Carcinoma

FTC is a purely follicular malignant tumor with no papillary or other elements. It comprises 15% to 20% of thyroid tumors. Most patients are older than 40 and female (3:1). FTC is extremely rare in children. However, in areas where salt is iodized, FTC is uncommon, representing as few as 5% of thyroid cancers.

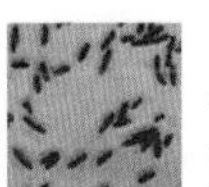

ETIOLOGIC FACTORS: The incidence of follicular carcinoma is higher in endemic goiter areas among people who do not receive iodine supplements. Irradiation to the gland may precede FTC in some cases. Genetically, follicular tumors may occur in patients with Cowden and other syndromes (see Chapter 4).

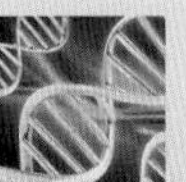

MOLECULAR PATHOGENESIS: Molecular changes associated with follicular thyroid carcinoma include point mutations in oncogenes of the *RAS* family (*NRAS, KRAS, HRAS*), which occur in 20% to 45% of the tumors, and *PAX8/PPARγ* (paired box 8/peroxisome proliferator–activated receptor γ) rearrangement, with a t(2;3)(q13;p25) translocation. Such mutations affect 20% to 40% of patients. Mutations of *TP53* tumor suppressor and *PTEN* do occur and may play a role in tumor progression.

Follicular tumors with oncocytic morphology have chromosomal changes and abnormalities in mitochondrial DNA, similar to other thyroid tumors with oncocytic features.

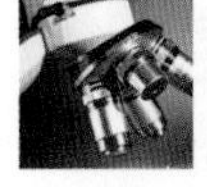

PATHOLOGY: Follicular cancers vary in size, are yellow-tan, and have thick white fibrous capsules. Areas of hemorrhage and necrosis and foci of cystic degeneration are common. FTCs are subdivided into minimally invasive and widely invasive variants.

Minimally invasive FTCs are well-defined, encapsulated tumors. They are soft and pale tan to pink, and bulge from within their capsules. Most resemble follicular adenomas but mitoses are common. Hemorrhagic necrosis may occur in their centers. Unlike adenomas, minimally invasive FTCs extend into, but not entirely through, the capsule or show areas of vascular invasion.

Invasive FTC usually presents few diagnostic problems, because it extends through its capsule or shows vascular invasion (Fig. 19-15), often within or adjacent to the capsule. The tumor may also extend into surrounding soft tissues.

Oncocytic (Hürthle cell) carcinomas are tumors of follicular derivation composed mainly (>75%) of oncocytes. The criteria for malignancy are the same as for follicular cancer: capsular and vascular invasion. These tumors account for 5% of thyroid malignancies and tend to behave more aggressively than usual follicular cancer.

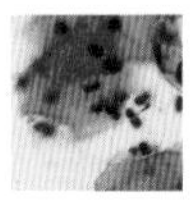

CLINICAL FEATURES: FTC differs from PTC in that its metastases are blood-borne, not lymphatic, and go mainly to the lung and bones of the shoulder, pelvic girdle, sternum, and skull. Most follicular cancers present as solitary palpable nodules or enlarged thyroids. However, in some cases, the presenting sign is a pathologic fracture through a bony metastasis or a pulmonary lesion. Both primary tumors and metastases take up radiolabeled iodine and ^{131}I may be used therapeutically. Minimally invasive follicular tumors have a cure rate of at least 95%, compared with a survival of about 50% for the widely invasive form. FTC is treated with unilateral lobectomy. Metastases can be treated with radioiodine.

Medullary Thyroid Carcinoma

MTC constitutes about 5% of thyroid cancers. The tumor cells derive from the parafollicular (C) cells, which secrete multiple hormones, including calcitonin, serotonin, ACTH, and somatostatin.

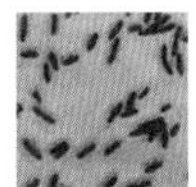

ETIOLOGIC FACTORS: The tumor occurs in sporadic and familial forms, the latter accounting for **25%** of cases. Patients with familial forms of medullary carcinoma often have autosomal dominant MEN type 2B or 2A. There are no known etiologic factors.

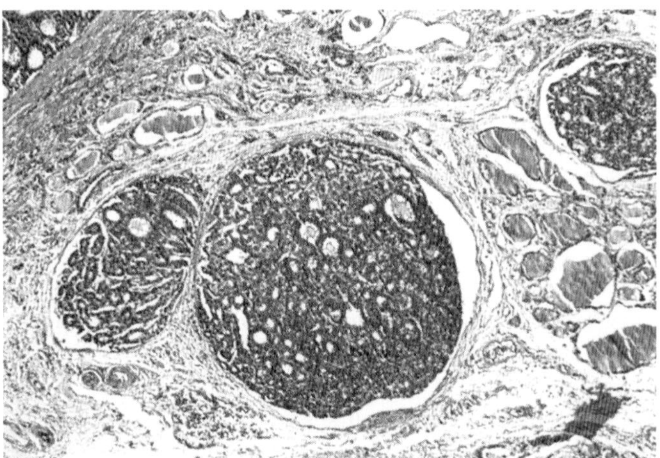

FIGURE 19-15. Follicular carcinoma of the thyroid. A microfollicular tumor has invaded veins in the thyroid parenchyma.

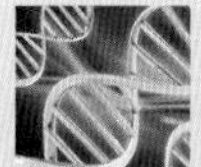

MOLECULAR PATHOGENESIS: Somatic mutations in *RET* proto-oncogene on chromosome 10 are present in 25% to 70% of sporadic MTCs. Most of these are in the tyrosine kinase domain of Ret protein and portend a poorer prognosis than do tumors without *RET* mutations. *RET* is discussed more fully in the section on MEN syndromes (see below).

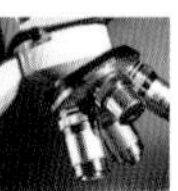

PATHOLOGY: MTC tends to arise in the superior portion of the thyroid, which is the region richest in C cells. In the setting of MEN type 2, tumors are often multicentric and bilateral. MTCs are not encapsulated but are usually circumscribed. The cut surfaces are firm and grayish white. Characteristically, these tumors are solid, with polygonal granular cells separated by a highly vascular stroma (Fig. 19-16). However, the architectural patterns and appearances of the cells are highly variable. *A conspicuous feature is stromal amyloid, representing deposition of procalcitonin.* Nests of tumor cells are embedded in a hyalinized collagenous framework. Focal calcification is often present and may be extensive enough to be detected radiologically. Besides amyloid, medullary carcinoma may contain mucin, melanin, and many polypeptide hormones. Invasion into adjacent tissues is common.

Almost all MTCs express carcinoembryonic antigen (CEA). Many are also positive for ACTH, serotonin, substance P, glucagon, insulin, and human chorionic gonadotropin (hCG).

MTCs extend by direct invasion into soft tissues. They metastasize to regional lymph nodes and to lung, liver, and bone. Sometimes, the initial presentation may be as metastatic disease. Metastases resemble primary tumors and also contain amyloid.

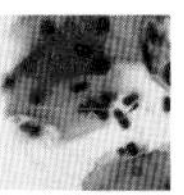

CLINICAL FEATURES: Patients with MTC often suffer symptoms related to endocrine secretion, including carcinoid syndrome (serotonin) and Cushing syndrome (ACTH). Watery diarrhea in a third of patients is caused by secretion of vasoactive intestinal peptide (VIP), prostaglandins, and several kinins. In cases of familial MTC, patients may have hyperparathyroidism, episodic hypertension, and other symptoms that reflect secretion of catecholamines by pheochromocytoma.

MTCs usually present as firm thyroid masses or cervical lymphadenopathy. Treatment is total thyroidectomy, but tumors often recur locally. Overall survival of patients with MTC is 86% at 5 years and 65% at 10 years. Prognosis depends on age (women do better), tumor size, and stage. Other prognostic parameters include histologic type, mitotic count, necrosis, and amount of calcitonin present. All patients with MTC (whether familial or sporadic) should be tested for *RET* mutations; if they are positive, family members should also be tested.

Treatment is total thyroidectomy, but tumors recur locally in one third of patients. Several new molecular targeted therapies with tyrosine kinase inhibitors (vandetanib, cabozantinib) have resulted in increased median progression-free survival.

Anaplastic Thyroid Carcinoma

Anaplastic thyroid cancer is a highly malignant tumor that mostly afflicts women (female-to-male ratio, 4:1) over age 60.

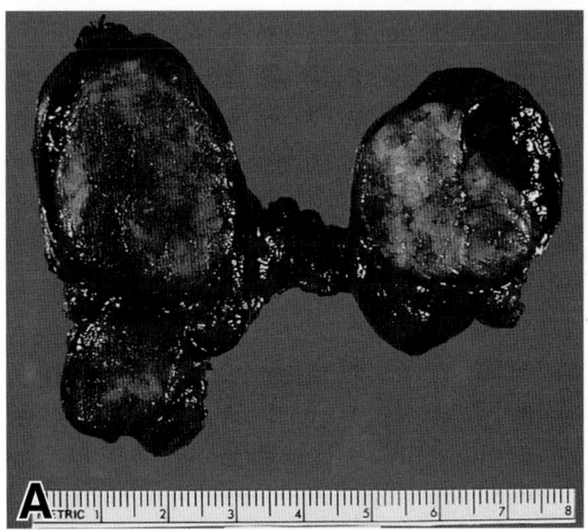

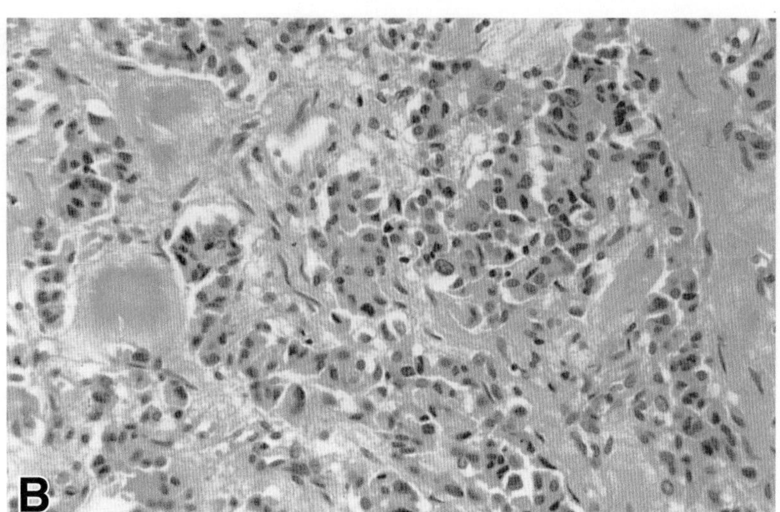

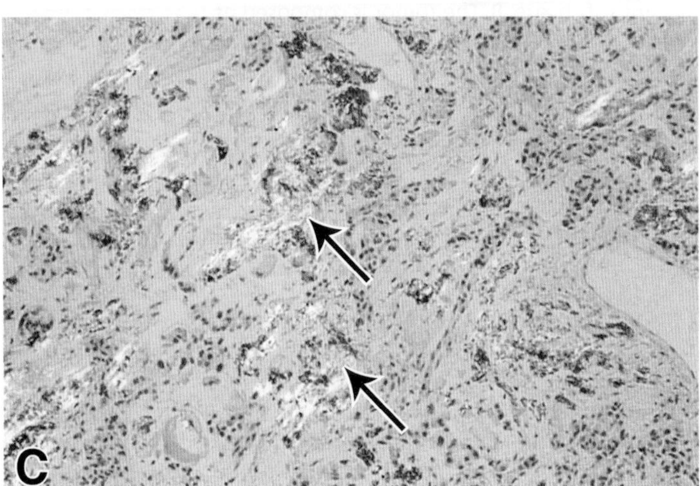

FIGURE 19-16. Medullary thyroid carcinoma. A. Coronal section of a total thyroid resection shows bilateral involvement by a firm, pale tumor. **B.** The tumor features nests of polygonal cells embedded in a collagenous framework. The connective tissue septa contain eosinophilic amyloid. **C.** A section stained with Congo red and viewed under polarized light demonstrates the pale green birefringence (*arrows*) of amyloid.

This tumor constitutes 10% of thyroid cancers. At least half of patients suffer from long-standing goiter. Many patients with anaplastic carcinoma also have histories of lower-grade thyroid cancers. Thus, the anaplastic variant probably often represents transformation of a benign or low-grade thyroid neoplasm into a more poorly differentiated, more aggressive cancer. External radiation appears to increase the risk of such an event.

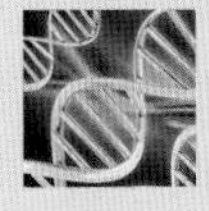

MOLECULAR PATHOGENESIS: Anaplastic carcinomas have more chromosomal imbalances than do other thyroid tumors. Mutations in *TP53* are common in anaplastic cancers.

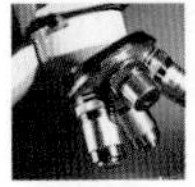

PATHOLOGY: Anaplastic carcinoma of the thyroid presents as large poorly circumscribed masses in the gland, frequently extending into the soft tissues of the neck. The cut surface is hard and grayish white. The most common histologic pattern is a sarcoma-like proliferation of bizarre spindle and giant cells, with polyploid nuclei, many mitoses, necrosis, and stromal fibrosis (Fig. 19-17). Other patterns include epithelial and giant cell differentiation. The tumor tends to invade veins and arteries, often occluding them and producing foci of infarction and necrosis within the tumor.

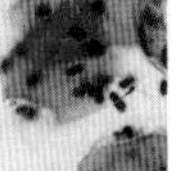

CLINICAL FEATURES: Anaplastic carcinomas compress and destroy local structures. Accordingly, the tumor presents as a rapidly enlarging neck mass, with symptoms such as dysphagia, hoarseness, dyspnea, and enlargement of cervical nodes. The prognosis is dismal, and widespread metastases are common. Less than 10% of patients survive 5 years. Treatment with radiation and chemotherapy has had little success.

PARATHYROID GLANDS

Most people have four parathyroid glands, but numbers vary from 1 to 12. Normally, they are on the posterior thyroid surface, but they occasionally occur intrathyroidally or in ectopic locations such as mediastinum, pericardium, or near the recurrent laryngeal nerve.

They are the size and color of a grain of saffron-cooked rice. All glands combined weigh about 130 mg. Individual gland weights vary considerably, but anything over 50 mg probably represents enlargement. They measure 4 to 6 mm in length. About three fourths of the cells are chief and oxyphil cells, the remainder being fat cells scattered throughout the parenchyma.

Chief cells secrete parathyroid hormone (PTH) and PTH-related protein. They are polyhedral cells with pale,

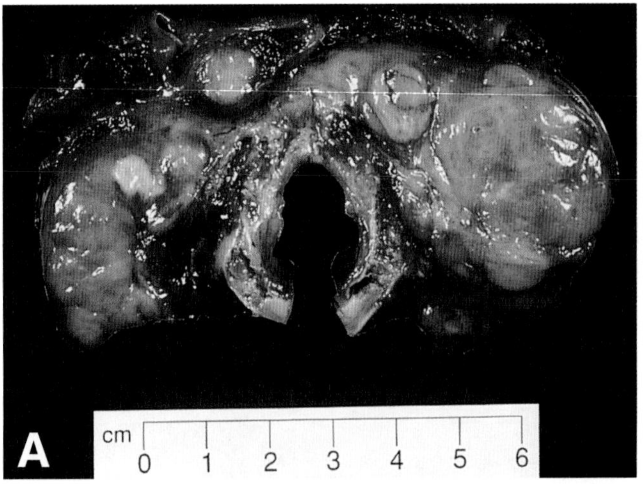

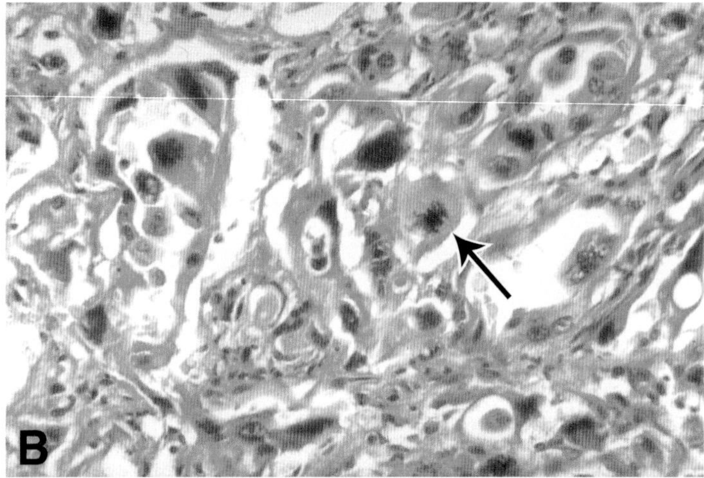

FIGURE 19-17. Anaplastic carcinoma of the thyroid. A. The tumor in transverse section partially surrounds the trachea and extends into the adjacent soft tissue. **B.** The tumor is composed of bizarre spindle and giant cells with polyploid nuclei and prominent mitotic activity (*arrow*).

eosinophilic-to-amphophilic cytoplasm that contains glycogen and fat droplets. These cells stain positively for cytokeratins, chromogranin A, and synaptophysin. Chief cells are the most sensitive to calcium concentrations. **Clear cells** are chief cells whose cytoplasm is packed with glycogen. **Oxyphil cells** appear after puberty, are larger than chief cells, and have deeply eosinophilic cytoplasm, owing to many mitochondria. They have no secretory granules and do not secrete PTH.

The parathyroids respond to blood levels of ionized calcium and magnesium. In turn, PTH controls plasma calcium. Magnesium, a cation closely related to calcium, acts as a brake on PTH secretion. Other PTH functions also include regulation of renal phosphate excretion, increased tubular and intestinal reabsorption of calcium, and bone resorption.

Hypoparathyroidism

Hypoparathyroidism results from decreased secretion of PTH or end-organ insensitivity to it (pseudohypoparathyroidism), whether congenital or acquired. It is clinically characterized by hypocalcemia and hyperphosphatemia.

The symptoms of hypoparathyroidism relate to hypocalcemia. Increased neuromuscular excitability may cause mild tingling in the hands and feet, severe muscle cramps, tetany, laryngeal stridor, and convulsions. Neuropsychiatric manifestations include depression, paranoia, and psychoses. High cerebrospinal fluid pressure and papilledema may mimic a brain tumor. Patients with all forms of hypoparathyroidism are successfully treated with vitamin D and calcium supplementation. Of patients undergoing surgery for primary hyperparathyroidism, 1% develop irreversible hypoparathyroidism.

Familial hypoparathyroidism is a rare disease that can be inherited as autosomal dominant, X-linked recessive, or autosomal recessive. It may also be part of a polyglandular syndrome that includes adrenal insufficiency and mucocutaneous candidiasis (see below). Hypoparathyroidism can occur with other congenital abnormalities as in DiGeorge syndrome (see Chapter 3), in which there is agenesis of the parathyroid glands. **Familial isolated hypoparathyroidism** is rare and has variable inheritance patterns, reflecting deficient PTH secretion. Mutations in *GCM2* exon 3 may be responsible for some cases of congenital hypoparathyroidism. **Idiopathic hypoparathyroidism** is a heterogeneous group of rare disorders, sporadic and familial, that share deficient secretion of PTH.

Pseudohypoparathyroidism

PHP reflects hereditary conditions and is characterized by hypocalcemia, hyperphosphatemia, increased serum concentration of PTH, and lack of response to the hormone. **Albright hereditary osteodystrophy** reflects mutation of the *GNAS1* gene on chromosome 20q, which codes for the G_S protein that couples the hormone receptor to adenylyl cyclase. This mutation impairs the renal tubular epithelium's response to PTH, causing inadequate calcium resorption from glomerular filtrate. Patients are also often resistant to other cAMP-coupled hormones, including TSH, glucagon, FSH, and LH. A characteristic phenotype includes short stature, obesity, mental retardation, subcutaneous calcification, and a number of congenital anomalies of bone, particularly abnormally short metacarpals and metatarsals. Some patients with pseudohypoparathyroidism have normal G_S activity and a normal phenotype. The basis for their resistance to PTH is unclear.

Primary Hyperparathyroidism

Excessive PTH Secretion

In primary hyperparathyroidism, PTH production persists without intestinal or renal stimulation of the parathyroid glands. This condition is rare, with an incidence of 1 in 1,000, and is most common in women in the fifth decade. Patients may be asymptomatic or present with hypercalcemia, hypophosphatemia, nephrolithiasis, and bone disease.

Hyperparathyroidism may be due to a parathyroid adenoma (80% to 90%), hyperplasia involving all parathyroids (10% to 15%), or (rarely) parathyroid carcinoma (1% to 5%). Primary hyperparathyroidism can be sporadic or part of familial syndromes such as MEN1 or MEN2A.

Parathyroid Adenomas

Solitary parathyroid adenomas cause 85% of cases of primary hyperparathyroidism.

These tumors are monoclonal proliferations that arise sporadically or (20%) in the context of MEN1 (see below). Loss of heterozygosity at the MEN1 locus occurs in 20% to 40% of adenomas with somatic mutations.

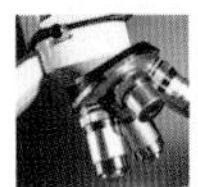

PATHOLOGY: Parathyroid adenomas are circumscribed, red-brown, 1 to 3 cm solitary masses, weighing 0.05 to 200 g. Hemorrhagic areas are common, and cystic changes are occasionally noted. Adenomas show sheets of neoplastic chief cells in a rich capillary network. A rim of normal parathyroid tissue is usually evident outside the capsule and distinguishes adenomas from parathyroid hyperplasias. Adenoma cells mostly resemble normal chief cells. Immunostaining for PTH documents the tumor's activity. Surgical removal of the tumor relieves the symptoms of hyperparathyroidism. Most parathyroid adenomas only involve one or rarely two glands.

Primary parathyroid hyperplasia causes 15% of hyperparathyroidism. About 75% of parathyroid hyperplasias occur in women. Of these, 20% involve familial hyperparathyroidism or MEN syndromes (MEN types 1, 2A). Factors associated with sporadic primary hyperparathyroidism include external radiation and lithium ingestion.

All four parathyroid glands are enlarged, with the normal glandular adipose tissue replaced by hyperplastic chief cells arranged in sheets or trabecular or follicular patterns (Fig. 19-18). Scattered oxyphil cells are common, and small foci of adipose tissue may remain.

Parathyroid Carcinoma

Parathyroid carcinomas are rare and afflict both sexes, mainly between the ages of 30 and 60. They are usually functioning tumors, and most patients present with symptoms of hyperparathyroidism. Hypercalcemia in these patients is often severe, with serum calcium in excess of 14 mg/dL. The etiology of these tumors is not known. Neck radiation and hereditary syndromes with histories of parathyroid adenomas are risk factors. Factors that increase risk include hyperparathyroidism–jaw tumor syndrome and familial isolated hyperparathyroidism.

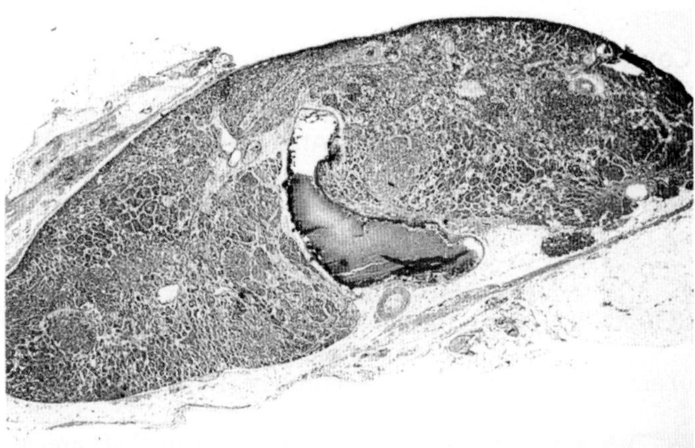

FIGURE 19-18. Primary parathyroid hyperplasia. The normal adipose tissue of the gland has been replaced by sheets and trabeculae of hyperplastic chief cells.

Parathyroid carcinomas tend to be larger than adenomas and appear as lobulated, firm, tannish, unencapsulated masses. They often adhere to surrounding soft tissues. Most carcinomas show trabecular cell arrangements, with significant mitotic activity and thick fibrous bands. Tumors occasionally invade capsules or blood vessels.

Treatment of PTH carcinoma includes surgery and, when invasive disease or metastases are present, chemotherapy and radiation therapy. After surgical removal, local recurrence is common. About one third of patients develop metastases to regional lymph nodes, lungs, liver, and bone. Death is most often due to hyperparathyroidism rather than carcinomatosis. Ten-year survival is 50%.

Clinical Features of Hyperparathyroidism

Some patients with hyperparathyroidism have asymptomatic hypercalcemia, detected on routine blood analysis. Others show florid systemic, renal, and skeletal disease (Fig. 19-19). The systemic symptoms of hyperparathyroidism are often expressed by the following mnemonic: **stones** (renal stones, nephrocalcinosis, polyuria, and polydipsia), **bones** (**osteitis fibrosa cystica** [see Chapter 22]), **groans** (peptic ulcer disease and other GI symptoms), and **moans** (psychiatric changes, depression, and emotional lability).

Secondary Hyperparathyroidism

Secondary parathyroid hyperplasia occurs mainly in patients with chronic renal failure, but also in association with vitamin D deficiency, intestinal malabsorption, Fanconi syndrome, and renal tubular acidosis (Fig. 19-20). Chronic hypocalcemia secondary to renal retention of phosphate, inadequate $1,25(OH)_2D$ production by diseased kidneys, and skeletal resistance to PTH all cause compensatory PTH hypersecretion.

The condition results in hyperplasia of all parathyroids and excess levels of PTH, which produces the main clinical manifestations.

Tertiary hyperparathyroidism refers to autonomous parathyroid hyperplasia following long-standing secondary hyperplasia because of renal failure. In such cases, parathyroid

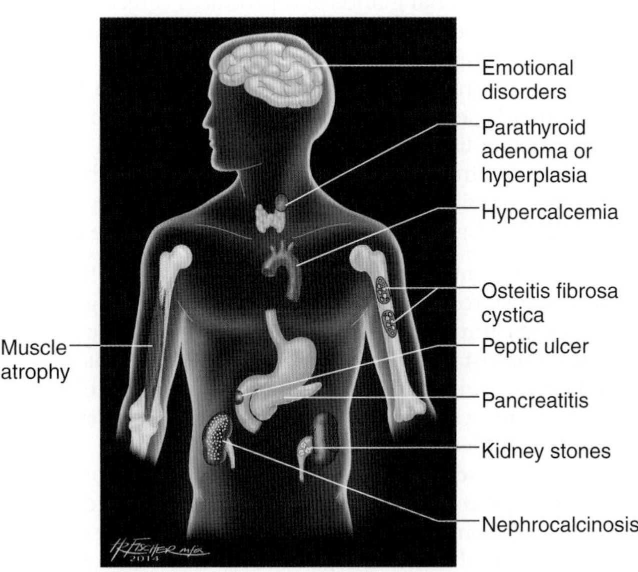

FIGURE 19-19. Major clinical features of hyperparathyroidism.

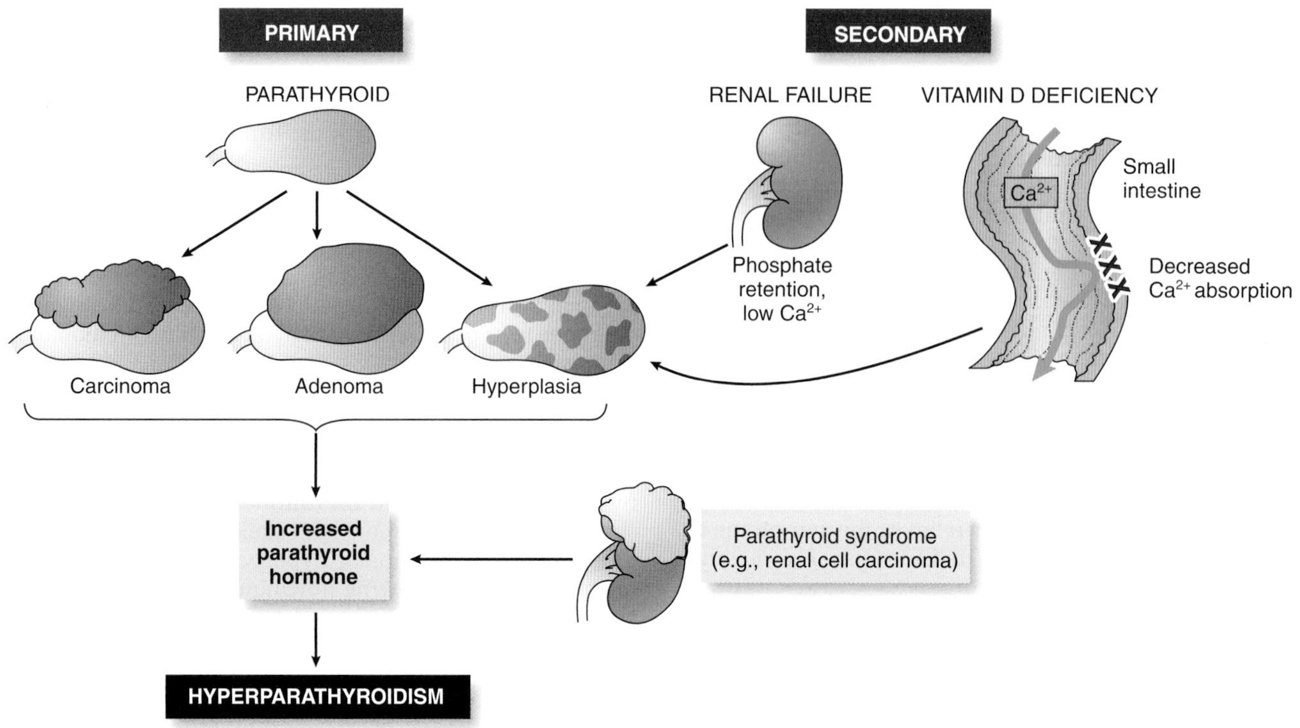

FIGURE 19-20. Major pathogenetic pathways leading to clinical primary and secondary hyperparathyroidism. Ca^{2+}, calcium ion.

hyperplasia does not regress after renal transplantation, and parathyroidectomy is required.

ADRENAL CORTEX

Each adrenal gland contains two independent endocrine organs: the cortex and the medulla. They are distinct anatomically, functionally, and embryologically. The cortex arises from celomic mesenchymal cells near the urogenital ridge and secretes steroid hormones such as aldosterone, cortisol, and testosterone. The medulla arises from neuroectoderm invading fetal adrenal glands and produces catecholamines.

Adult adrenal glands are pyramidal organs above each kidney, found anteriorly in the retroperitoneum. Each gland is 4 to 6 cm in greatest dimension and weighs **4 to 6** g. The adrenal glands secrete steroid hormones or corticosteroids, regulate metabolism and immune system function, and aid in response to stress. Grossly, and on cut section, the cortex has a characteristic yellow color because of lipid deposits. The medulla is paler gray-tan. The cortex contains three zones:

- The **zona glomerulosa** is the outermost layer. In that location, aldosterone production is stimulated by angiotensin and potassium and inhibited by atrial natriuretic peptide and somatostatin. The zona glomerulosa forms 15% of the cortex, with indistinct spherical nests of cells with dark-staining nuclei and moderate numbers of cytoplasmic fat droplets.
- The **zona fasciculata** constitutes 75% of the cortex and produces glucocorticoids, such as cortisol. It is not distinctly separated from the zona glomerulosa. This zone contains radial cords of larger cells, each with a small nucleus and a large, foamy, clear cytoplasm, representing stored lipid.
- The **zona reticularis** secretes androgens and is the innermost layer, adjacent to the medulla. Irregular anastomosing cords are composed of compact smaller cells with a lipid-poor, slightly granular, eosinophilic cytoplasm and bland nuclei.

The medulla is in the center of the gland, surrounded by cortex. It secretes epinephrine (adrenalin) and norepinephrine.

Ectopic adrenal tissue can occur in many places outside the gland because the cells migrate alongside the gonads. Common locations include the retroperitoneum, broad ligament near the ovary and near the epididymis, the kidney, and the liver. Ectopic adrenal tissue contains only cortex, not medulla.

Congenital Adrenal Hypoplasia

This condition is quite rare and may accompany renal agenesis. It is X-linked and caused by mutations in the *DAX-1* gene at Xp21.

Congenital Adrenal Hyperplasia

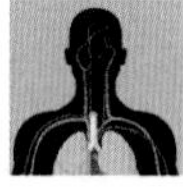

PATHOPHYSIOLOGY AND ETIOLOGIC FACTORS: CAH results from several autosomal recessive enzyme defects in the biosynthesis of cortisol from cholesterol. Deficiencies vary from mild to complete lack of cortisol. In general, impaired corticosteroid synthesis leads to unopposed action of ACTH and therefore adrenal hyperplasia. CAH occurs equally in males and females and is the most common cause of ambiguous genitalia in newborn girls (Fig. 19-21A).

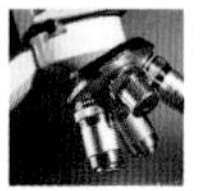

PATHOLOGY: The adrenal glands in CAH are enlarged, weighing as much as 30 g (Fig. 19-21B). Their cut surfaces are soft, tan to brown and either diffusely enlarged or nodular. The cortex is widened between the medulla and zona glomerulosa. The hyperplastic zone is filled by compact, granular, eosinophilic cells. In most cases,

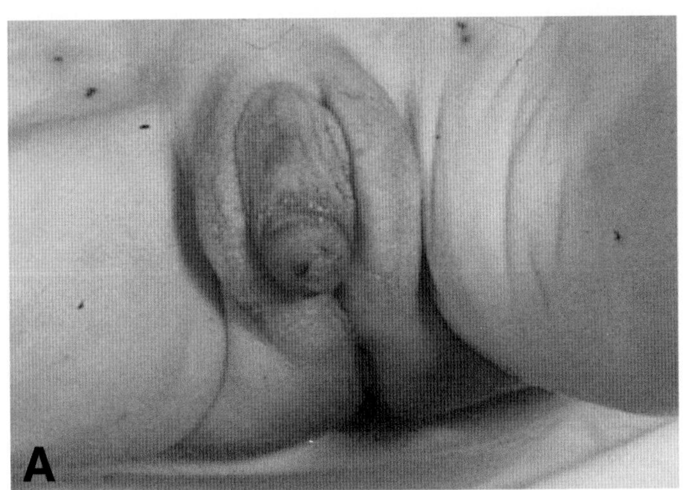

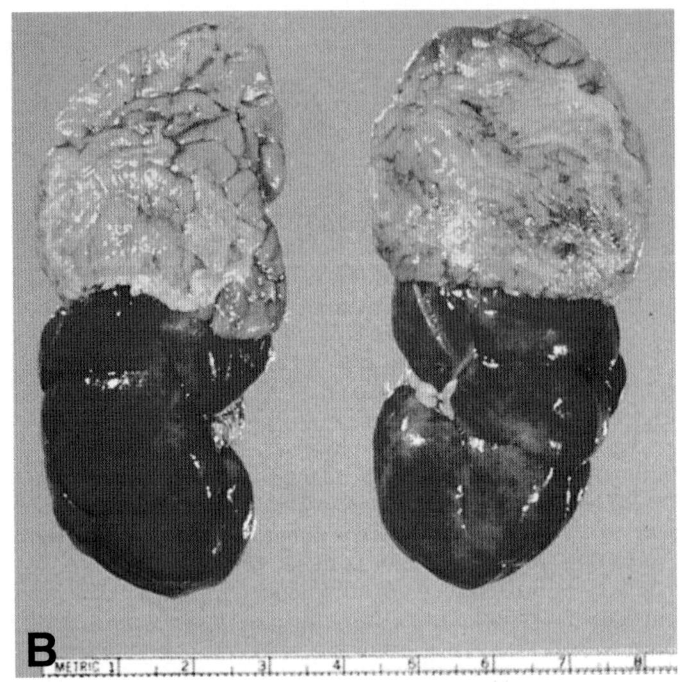

FIGURE 19-21. Congenital adrenal hyperplasia. A. A female infant is markedly virilized with hypertrophy of the clitoris and partial fusion of labioscrotal folds. **B.** A 7-week-old male infant died of severe salt-wasting congenital adrenal hyperplasia. At autopsy, both adrenal glands were markedly enlarged.

the zona glomerulosa is also hyperplastic, but not to the extent of the other zones, especially the zona fasciculata.

21-Hydroxylase ($P450_{C21}$) Deficiency

This enzyme defect is responsible for 90% of cases of CAH. The gene for $P450_{C21}$ (CYP21) is linked to the *MHC* locus on the short arm of chromosome 6 (6p21.3) and is closely associated with *HLA-B* and *C4A* and *C4B* complement genes. The incidence of CAH varies from 1 in 10,000 among whites to 1 in 500 in Alaskan Eskimos.

$P450_{C21}$ is a microsomal enzyme that converts 17-hydroxyprogesterone to 11-deoxycortisol. A deficiency in this enzymatic activity limits cortisol biosynthesis. Accumulated precursors are instead converted to androgens.

Classic CAH, the more severe form of the disease, is usually detected in infancy. It also occurs as a less severe, late-onset (nonclassic) variant.

- **Simple virilizing CAH** occurs when residual enzyme activity is at least 2%. Female infants show pseudohermaphroditism, whereas males have no abnormalities of the sexual organs. Conversion of cortisol precursors into adrenal androgens is amplified by the ACTH-dependent increase in the size of the gland. Female newborns exposed to a large excess of adrenal androgens in utero may be born with fused labia, an enlarged clitoris, and a urogenital sinus that may be mistaken for a penile urethra (Fig. 19-21A). As a result, the infant may be mislabeled as male. Normal appearing infant girls may, with time, develop a syndrome of androgen excess, with clitoral enlargement and pubic hair. Infant boys may exhibit sexual precocity. Eventually, the high levels of adrenal androgens lead to premature closure of epiphyses and short stature. Adult women with CAH tend to be infertile because elevated levels of androgens and progestogens disturb the menstrual cycle and inhibit ovulation. Men with CAH may be fertile, but some have azoospermia.
- **Salt-wasting CAH** results from mutations that completely inactivate the 21-hydroxylase. As a result, aldosterone synthesis is impaired and leads to hypoaldosteronism, which develops in the first few weeks of life in two thirds of cases. Hyponatremia, hyperkalemia, dehydration, hypotension, and increased renin secretion are typical. These effects may be rapidly fatal if not treated.
- **Late-onset CAH produces** no abnormalities at birth but results in virilizing symptoms at puberty. In young women, late-onset CAH may closely resemble polycystic ovary syndrome (see Chapter 16). Most young men with the disorder are asymptomatic.

11β-Hydroxylase Deficiency

This deficiency is uncommon in the general population, but among Jews of Iranian or Moroccan ancestry in Israel, it is the most common cause of CAH. This disorder is inherited as an autosomal recessive trait. In addition to the androgenic complications of CAH, high levels of 11-deoxycortisol, which is a weak mineralocorticoid, often cause sodium retention and accompanying hypertension.

Adrenal Cortical Insufficiency

Deficient production of adrenal cortical hormones can result from (1) adrenal gland destruction, (2) pituitary or hypothalamic dysfunction with decreased ACTH production, or (3) chronic corticosteroid therapy.

Primary Chronic Adrenal Insufficiency (Addison Disease)

Addison disease is a fatal wasting disorder caused by failure of the adrenal glands to produce glucocorticoids, mineralocorticoids, and androgens. It causes weakness, weight loss, muscle pain, gastrointestinal symptoms, hypotension, electrolyte imbalance, and hyperpigmentation. In Western societies, autoimmunity is responsible for 75% of cases, but tuberculosis of the adrenal glands is a common cause worldwide. Metastatic carcinoma, amyloidosis, hemorrhage, sarcoidosis, fungal infection, and adrenoleukodystrophy (see Chapter 24) may also result in Addison disease. Rarely, adrenal insufficiency is due to congenital adrenal hypoplasia or familial glucocorticoid deficiency (defective ACTH receptor).

Autoimmune adrenalitis may be an isolated disorder or a part of two different polyglandular autoimmune syndromes.

IMMUNE MECHANISMS: Antiadrenal antibodies that react with tissue from all three zones of the adrenal cortex are present in two thirds of patients with Addison disease. The major autoantigens are adrenal steroidogenic enzymes, particularly $P450_{C21}$. In Addison disease, autoantibodies do occur, but cell-mediated immunity is probably predominant.

POLYENDOCRINE SYNDROMES: Half of patients with autoimmune adrenal insufficiency suffer from other autoimmune endocrine diseases. These are grouped into two polyendocrine syndromes.

Type I polyendocrine autoimmune syndrome (candidiasis–hypoparathyroidism–Addison disease syndrome) is a rare, autosomal recessive condition seen in older children and adolescents. In addition to adrenal insufficiency, most (60%) patients also have hypoparathyroidism and chronic mucocutaneous candidiasis. Insulin-dependent diabetes (type 1) is common. Premature ovarian failure, hypothyroidism, infertility, malabsorption syndromes, pernicious anemia, chronic hepatitis, alopecia totalis, and vitiligo are also frequent. The gene associated with the disorder is *AIRE* (autoimmune regulator; see Chapter 3), which is important in the generation of immune tolerance.

Type II polyendocrine autoimmune syndrome (Schmidt syndrome) is more common than type I and always includes adrenal insufficiency. Women are affected twice as often as men. The disorder usually presents in young adults, ages 20 to 40. Half of cases are familial, but several modes of inheritance are known. Hashimoto thyroiditis and occasionally Graves disease occur in over two thirds of cases. Type I diabetes and premature ovarian failure are common. Rarely, other autoimmune diseases are present. This condition is considered as a polygenic disorder linked to HLA-DR3.

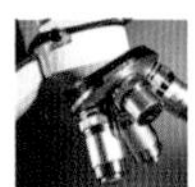

PATHOLOGY: Over 90% of the adrenal gland must be destroyed in order for chronic adrenal insufficiency to be symptomatic. Autoimmune adrenalitis leads to pale, irregular, shrunken glands, weighing 2 to 3 g or less. The medulla is intact but surrounded by fibrous tissue with small islands of atrophic cortical cells (Fig. 19-22). Depending on the stage of the disease, variably intense lymphoid infiltrates, mainly T cells, are seen.

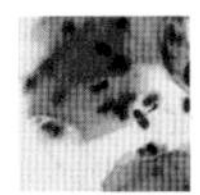

CLINICAL FEATURES: Typically, the first symptom is insidious onset of weakness, which may become so profound that a patient is bedridden. Anorexia and weight loss are always present. A diffuse, tan pigmentation usually develops on the skin, and dark patches may appear on the mucous membranes. This hyperpigmentation is related to stimulation of skin melanocytes by pituitary POMC. Hypotension, with blood pressures around 80/50 mm Hg, is the rule. A variety of GI symptoms, including vomiting, diarrhea, and abdominal pain, affect most patients and may be the presenting complaint. Patients with Addison disease often show marked personality changes and even organic brain syndromes.

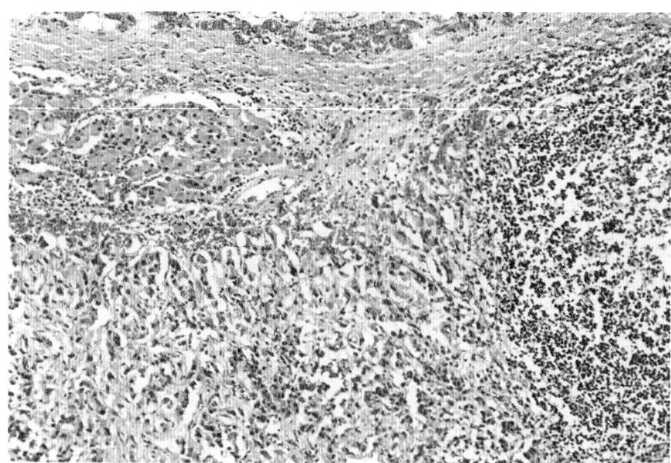

FIGURE 19-22. Autoimmune adrenalitis. A section of the adrenal gland from a patient with Addison disease shows chronic inflammation and fibrosis in the cortex, an island of residual atrophic cortical cells and an intact medulla.

Deficient mineralocorticoid secretion, together with other metabolic derangements, gives rise to low serum sodium and high potassium levels. The absence of glucocorticoids leads to lymphocytosis and mild eosinophilia. With glucocorticoid and mineralocorticoid replacement, patients live normal lives.

Acute Adrenal Insufficiency

Acute adrenal insufficiency, or adrenal crisis, is characterized by sudden loss of adrenal cortical function. Symptoms relate more to mineralocorticoid deficiency than to inadequate glucocorticoids. Adrenal crisis occurs in three settings:

- Abrupt withdrawal of corticosteroid therapy in patients with adrenal atrophy because of long-term steroid administration. This is the most common cause of acute adrenal insufficiency.
- Stress of infection or surgery may precipitate a sudden, devastating worsening of chronic adrenal insufficiency.
- ***Waterhouse–Friderichsen syndrome*** *refers to acute, bilateral, hemorrhagic infarction of the adrenal cortex, most often secondary to meningococcus or* Pseudomonas *septicemia.* Acute adrenal insufficiency due to adrenal hemorrhage is also seen in newborns subjected to birth trauma.

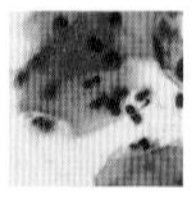

CLINICAL FEATURES: The initial manifestations of adrenal crisis are usually hypotension and shock. Nonspecific symptoms commonly include weakness, vomiting, abdominal pain, and lethargy, which may progress to coma. Typically, in Waterhouse–Friderichsen syndrome, a young person suddenly develops hypotension and shock, abdominal or back pain, fever, and purpura. Adrenal crisis is almost always fatal unless diagnosed quickly and aggressive therapy with corticosteroids and supportive measures is instituted.

Secondary Adrenal Insufficiency

Destruction of the pituitary and consequent panhypopituitarism (see earlier) result in secondary adrenal insufficiency. Causes include pituitary tumors, craniopharyngioma, empty sella syndrome, and pituitary infarction. Trauma, surgery, and radiation therapy may also cause a loss of pituitary function. Isolated ACTH deficiency is often associated with autoimmune endocrinopathies.

Adrenal Hyperfunction (Cushing or Conn Syndrome)

Excess corticosteroid secretion occurs in adrenal hyperplasia or neoplasia (Fig. 19-23). Such hyperfunction takes one of two forms: **hypercortisolism** (Cushing syndrome) or **hyperaldosteronism** (Conn syndrome), for the two major classes of adrenal steroids.

The combination of pituitary hyperfunction and chronic glucocorticoid excess is called **Cushing disease**. Hypercortisolism from any cause is now called **Cushing syndrome**; the term **Cushing disease** is reserved for excessive ACTH secretion by pituitary corticotrope tumors.

The most common cause of Cushing syndrome in the United States is chronic corticosteroid administration to treat immune and inflammatory disorders. The second most common cause is paraneoplastic syndromes associated with nonpituitary cancers that inappropriately produce ACTH (see below). Cushing disease is fivefold more common than Cushing syndrome associated with adrenal tumors.

ACTH-Dependent Adrenal Hyperfunction

Pathophysiology

Women, usually ages 25 to 45, are five times more likely than men to develop Cushing disease. Excessive ACTH secretion

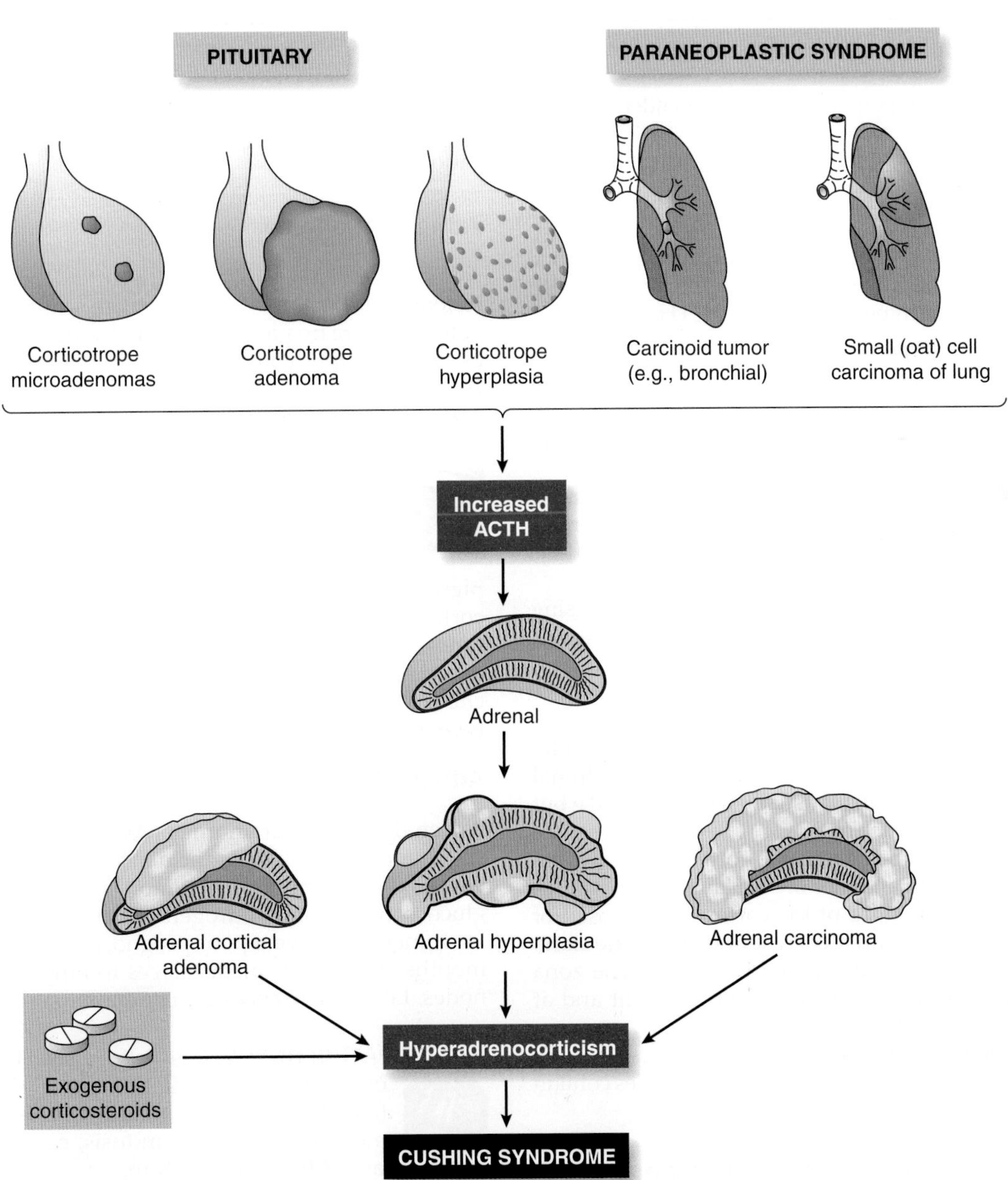

FIGURE 19-23. The pathogenetic pathways of Cushing syndrome. The ACTH-dependent pathway is called Cushing disease. ACTH, adrenocorticotropic hormone (corticotropin).

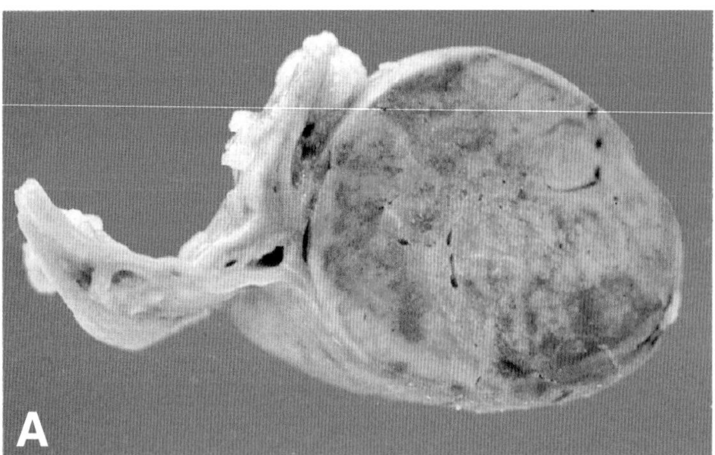

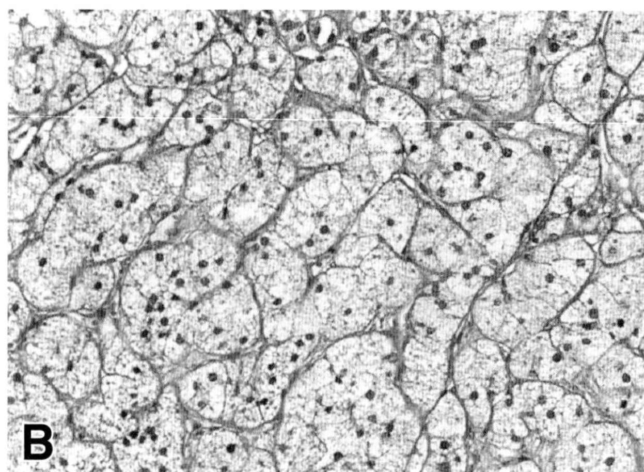

FIGURE 19-24. Adrenal adenoma. A. The cut surface of an adrenal tumor removed from a patient with Cushing syndrome is a mottled yellow with a rim of compressed normal adrenal tissue. **B.** A microscopic view reveals nests of clear, lipid-laden cells.

leads to adrenal cortical hyperplasia. ACTH-dependent adrenal hyperfunction results from the following:

- Ectopic ACTH production by a nonpituitary tumor
- Primary hypersecretion of ACTH by the pituitary (Cushing disease)
- Inappropriate secretion of corticotropin-releasing hormone (CRH) by tumors arising outside the hypothalamus, with secondary pituitary hypersecretion of ACTH

ECTOPIC PRODUCTION OF ACTH: Inappropriate CRH secretion by a malignant tumor accounts for most cases of ACTH-dependent hyperadrenalism. Cancers of the lung, particularly small cell carcinoma, are responsible for over half of the cases of ectopic ACTH syndrome.

PRIMARY HYPERSECRETION OF ACTH: Cushing disease usually results from pituitary corticotrope microadenomas, although it may be due to a macroadenoma or, rarely, diffuse corticotrope hyperplasia.

ECTOPIC CRH PRODUCTION: Ectopic ACTH-releasing enzyme (CRH) syndrome is like ectopic ACTH syndrome, except that the tumor secretes CRH. In turn, CRH stimulates pituitary ACTH secretion, leading to adrenal hyperplasia.

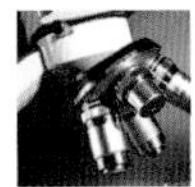

PATHOLOGY: Cushing disease is characterized by bilateral, diffuse (75%), or nodular (25%) adrenal hyperplasia. Each gland usually weighs 8 to 10 g but may weigh as much as 20 g.

In **diffuse adrenal hyperplasia**, the cortex is grossly visible and broadened, with an inner brown layer and a yellow, lipid-rich cap. The inner third of the cortex is composed of a compact cell layer. The area corresponding to the zona fasciculata has large clear cells packed with lipid. The zona glomerulosa varies: it may sometimes be prominent and at other times be difficult to identify.

Nodular adrenal hyperplasia is limited to grossly visible nodules up to 2.5 cm in diameter. Hyperplastic nodules contain large, lipid-laden, clear cells.

ACTH-Independent Adrenal Hyperfunction

In adults, the incidence of adrenal carcinoma peaks at age 40, and that of adenoma a decade later. In children, adrenal carcinomas account for half of cases of Cushing syndrome; 15% are caused by adenoma. At all ages, the female-to-male ratio is 4:1.

Adrenal Adenoma

Adrenal adenomas derive from the cortex. The incidence of these lesions is unknown because they are so often asymptomatic. Adenomas are frequently identified as part of syndromes such as MEN1, Carney complex, and McCune–Albright syndrome. Adenomas can produce hormones, the most common being cortisol and aldosterone.

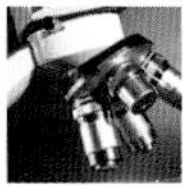

PATHOLOGY: A typical adenoma is 1 to 4 cm, encapsulated, firm, yellow, and slightly lobulated (Fig. 19-24). Cut surfaces are mottled yellow and brown, and occasionally black, owing to lipofuscin pigment deposition. A thin rim of compressed normal adrenal cortex surrounds the tumor. Necrosis and calcifications are rare. Adenomas show clear, lipid-laden (fasciculata type) cells arranged in sheets or nests. They are often interspersed with clusters of compact, lipid-depleted, eosinophilic (reticularis type) cells.

Adrenal Cortical Carcinoma

Adrenal cortical carcinomas (ACCs) are rare and aggressive tumors that have an incidence of 1 case per million per year. Sixty percent of these tumors are functional and secrete glucocorticoids and androgens. They occur more commonly in women and have a poor prognosis. Median survival is 30 months. The tumor metastasizes to lung, liver, and lymph nodes. Local recurrences are common.

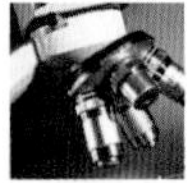

PATHOLOGY: ACC is distinguished from an adenoma by the presence of mitotic figures (>5/50 high-power fields), clear cell cytoplasm, necrosis, nuclear pleomorphism, atypical mitosis, capsular or vascular invasion, and diffuse architecture.

Most adrenal cortical carcinomas cannot be resected completely, and micrometastases in other organs are almost always already present. Metastases to lung, liver, and bone are common. The

5-year survival for patients with ACC limited to the adrenal gland is better (65%) than for patients with distant metastases (18%).

IATROGENIC CUSHING SYNDROME

The synthetic hormones ordinarily used (e.g., dexamethasone, prednisone) have only glucocorticoid activity and little or no mineralocorticoid or androgen effect. Thus, hypertension and hirsutism, features common in Cushing syndrome because of adrenal hyperplasia or neoplasia, are usually absent in this iatrogenic disorder.

Clinical Features of Cushing Syndrome

The manifestations of Cushing syndrome are illustrated in Figures 19-25 and 19-26. They depend on the degree and duration of excessive corticosteroid levels, as well as on levels of adrenal androgens and mineralocorticoids. Most (70%) patients are females, and fewer than 20% of cases occur before puberty.

In all forms of Cushing syndrome, glucocorticoid levels are increased. The dexamethasone suppression test distinguishes ACTH-dependent and ACTH-independent forms of Cushing syndrome. Dexamethasone suppresses pituitary ACTH secretion, and hence hypercortisolism, but it is without effect on adrenal tumors.

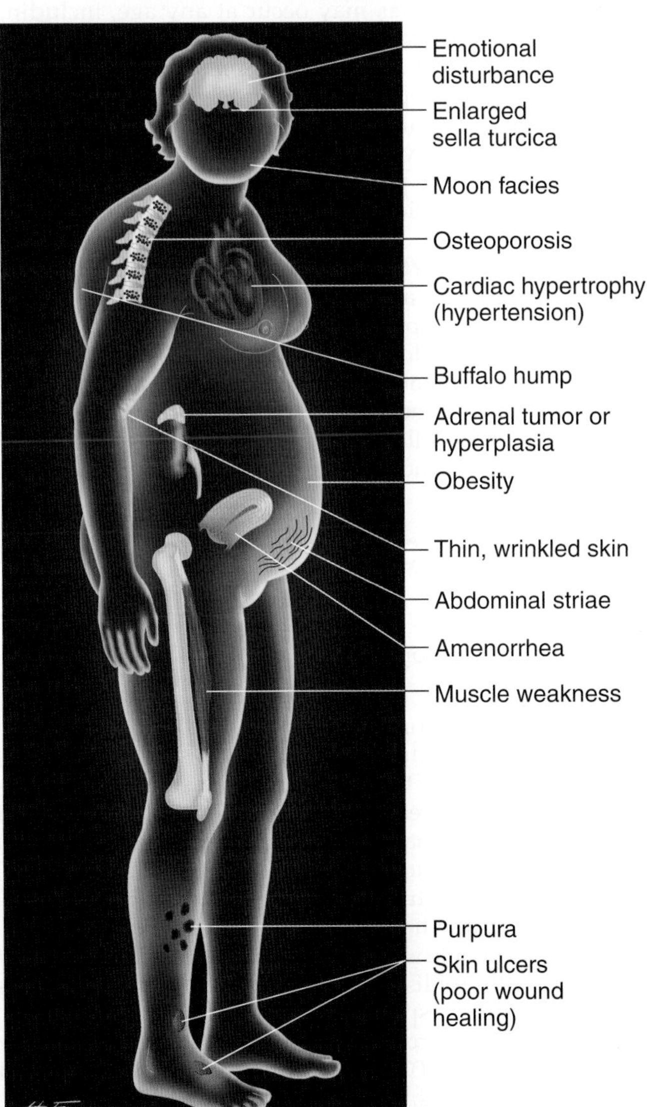

FIGURE 19-25. Major clinical manifestations of Cushing syndrome.

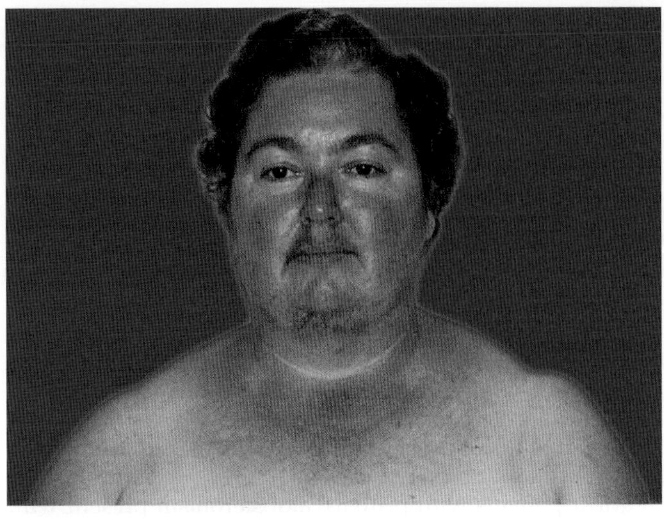

FIGURE 19-26. Cushing syndrome. A woman who had a pituitary adenoma that produced adrenocorticotropic hormone exhibits a moon face, buffalo hump, increased facial hair, and thinning of the scalp hair.

Primary Aldosteronism (Conn Syndrome)

Excess secretion of aldosterone occurs with adrenal adenomas or hyperplasia. Such overproduction causes potassium to be lost and sodium to be retained in the urine.

Aldosterone-secreting adenomas are more common in women than in men (3:1) and usually occur between the ages of 30 and 50.

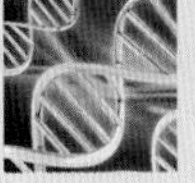

MOLECULAR PATHOGENESIS: Most (75%) primary aldosteronism is due to solitary adrenal adenomas (aldosteronoma). In one fourth of cases, adrenal hyperplasia is responsible. The rest reflect bilateral hyperplasia of the zona glomerulosa. Only a few cases of primary aldosteronism are caused by adrenal carcinomas.

There are three types of familial hyperaldosteronism:

- **Type I (glucocorticoid suppressible)** is an autosomal dominant disease resulting from the abnormal fusion of two genes on chromosome 8: the ACTH-responsive regulators of the 11β-hydroxylase (*CYP11B1*) and the aldosterone synthase gene (*CYP11B2*). The result is a hybrid constitutively active gene in the zona fasciculata which results in bilateral hyperplasia of the zone. By suppressing ACTH release, glucocorticoids prevent type I disease, which also responds to glucocorticoids.
- **Type II familial hyperaldosteronism** is most often the result of adrenal cortical adenomas, which do not turn off with glucocorticoid administration. In type II, hypertension usually appears in early adulthood.
- **Type III hyperaldosteronism** is characterized by marked adrenal enlargement. Patients suffer childhood onset of

severe hypertension that eventually damages the heart and kidneys.

Aldosterone hypersecretion enhances renal tubular sodium reabsorption, thereby increasing body sodium. Hypertension results not only from retention of sodium and consequent volume expansion, but also from increased peripheral vascular resistance. Hypokalemia reflects aldosterone-induced loss of potassium in the distal renal tubule.

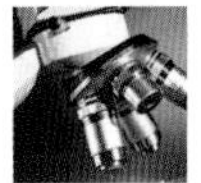

PATHOLOGY: The dominant cells in most aldosterone-secreting adenomas are clear and lipid-rich, similar to those in the zona fasciculata. They are arranged in cords or alveoli and demonstrate little nuclear pleomorphism. In contrast to cortisol-producing adenomas, the nontumorous cortex in cases of hyperaldosteronism is not atrophic, because aldosterone does not inhibit ACTH secretion by the pituitary.

Most patients with primary aldosteronism present with asymptomatic diastolic hypertension. Skeletal muscle weakness and fatigue are caused by potassium depletion. Polyuria and polydipsia result from impaired renal concentrating capacity, probably a result of hypokalemia. Metabolic alkalosis and an alkaline urine are common.

Bilateral adrenal hyperplasia in Conn syndrome is treated medically with aldosterone antagonists, and sometimes with dexamethasone in the case of glucocorticoid-suppressible hyperaldosteronism.

ADRENAL MEDULLA AND PARAGANGLIA

The adrenal medulla is entirely surrounded by the adrenal cortex and accounts for 10% of the gland's weight. It consists of neuroendocrine cells, or **chromaffin cells** (Fig. 19-27). These cells are also present at sites in the extra-adrenal sympathetic nervous system, such as the preaortic sympathetic plexuses and paravertebral sympathetic chain.

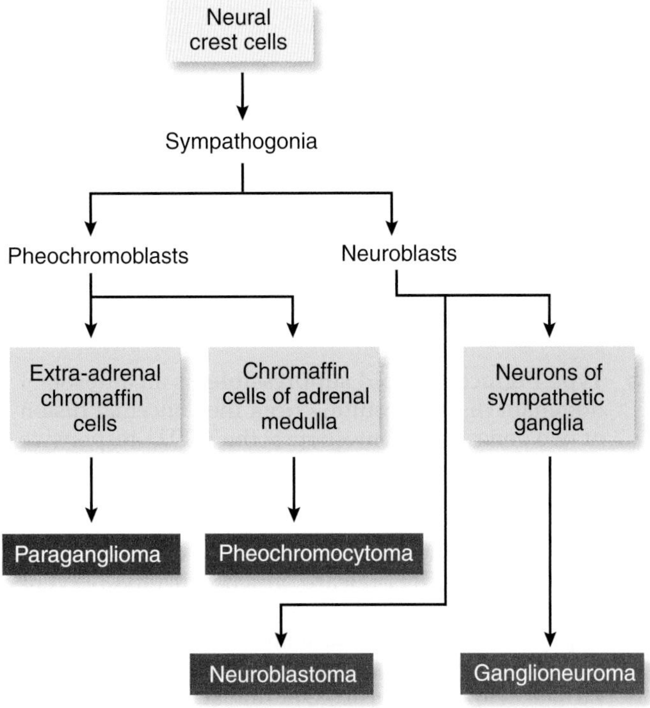

FIGURE 19-27. Histogenesis of tumors of the adrenal medulla and extra-adrenal sympathetic nervous system.

Chromaffin cells appear as nests of small polyhedral cells with pale amphophilic cytoplasm and vesicular nuclei. The cells of the adrenal medulla have many electron-dense, 100 to 300 nm chromaffin (catecholamine-containing) granules, resembling those of sympathetic nerve endings. Epinephrine accounts for 85% of the content of these granules, with the remainder being norepinephrine and other noncatecholamine hormones. Interspersed among the chromaffin cells are postganglionic neurons and small autonomic nerve fibers. Stored catecholamines are secreted on sympathetic stimulation as a response to stress (exercise, cold, fasting, trauma) or emotional excitation accompanying fear and anger.

Pheochromocytoma

Pheochromocytomas are rare catecholamine-secreting tumors of chromaffin cells of the adrenal medulla and elsewhere. They may arise in extra-adrenal sites, in which case they are called **paragangliomas**.

Pheochromocytomas may occur at any age, including infancy, but are uncommon after age 60. Many are unexpected findings at autopsy. The presenting symptoms reflect sustained or episodic hypertension, in addition to include headaches, pallor, anxiety, and cardiac arrhythmias. If detected early, they are amenable to surgical resection, but if left untreated, patients can die of complications of prolonged hypertension.

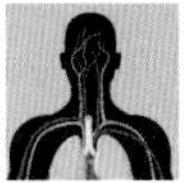

PATHOPHYSIOLOGY: Pheochromocytomas are mostly sporadic. A minority are inherited, either alone or as part of hereditary syndromes, such as multiple endocrine neoplasia (MEN) types 2A or 2B, **paraganglioma–pheochromocytoma syndrome**, von Hippel–Lindau disease, neurofibromatosis type 1, or McCune–Albright syndrome. Bilateral tumors strongly suggest familial disease. Sporadic tumors are unilateral in 80% of cases.

MULTIPLE ENDOCRINE NEOPLASIA (MEN) SYNDROMES

The features of autosomal dominant MEN syndromes are as follows (Fig. 19-28):

- **MEN type 1 (Wermer Syndrome)** includes (1) pituitary adenoma, (2) parathyroid hyperplasia or adenoma, and (3) islet cell tumors of the pancreas (e.g., insulinomas, gastrinomas). The pancreatic tumors tend to be multicentric and more malignant than in sporadic cases. Most (two thirds) patients have adenomas of two or more endocrine organs, and 20% develop tumors of three or more. Carcinoid, adrenocortical, and lipoid tumors may also occur in MEN1. Almost all people with MEN type 1 (>95%) have primary hyperparathyroidism. Mutation of the *MEN1* tumor suppressor gene is responsible for the disorder.
- **MEN type 2 syndromes** almost always include medullary thyroid cancer (MTC), and pheochromocytoma is included in half of the cases.
- ***MEN2A (Sipple syndrome):*** Most (95%) MEN2 patients are classified as type 2A. In addition to MTC and pheochromocytoma, one third of patients show hyperparathyroidism

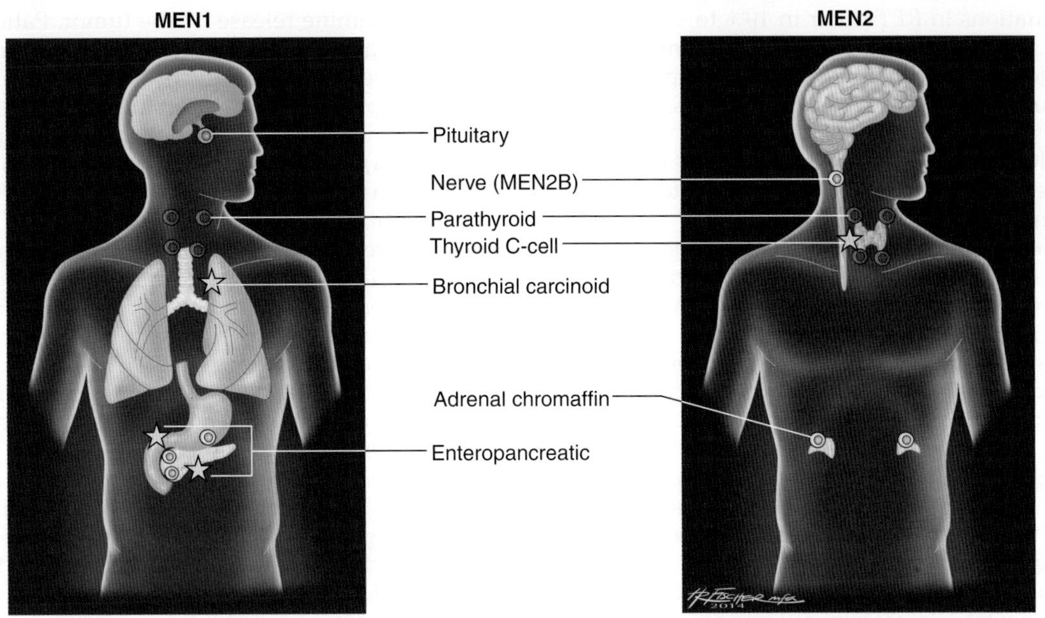

FIGURE 19-28. Multiple endocrine neoplasia (MEN) syndromes. The locations of the most common endocrine tumors in hereditary MEN syndrome types 1 and 2 are shown.

because of parathyroid hyperplasia or adenomas. Several neural crest tumors may occur in MEN type 2A, including gliomas, glioblastomas, and meningiomas. Hirschsprung disease is also associated with MEN type 2A.

- *MEN2B:* This disorder resembles MEN2A, but it develops about 10 years earlier and rarely includes parathyroid disease. The **mucosal neuroma syndrome** (ganglioneuromas of the conjunctiva, oral cavity, larynx, and gut) is a feature of MEN2B. Mucosal neuromas are always present, but only half of patients express the full phenotype. Many patients have a habitus resembling that of Marfan syndrome.

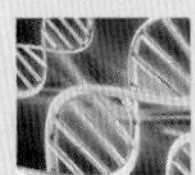

MOLECULAR PATHOGENESIS: The ***RET* proto-oncogene** on chromosome 10q11.2 is responsible for MEN2 syndromes. Several germline, missense, and activating mutations in the cysteine-rich extracellular domain of RET occur in 95% of families with MEN2A and in 85% of those with familial thyroid carcinomas (Fig. 19-29). The most common mutation (codon 634) constitutively activates the receptor by promoting its dimerization, which recapitulates the result of ligand binding. A different activating mutation in *RET* at codon 918 of the tyrosine kinase domain of *RET* is present in 95% of patients with MEN2B.

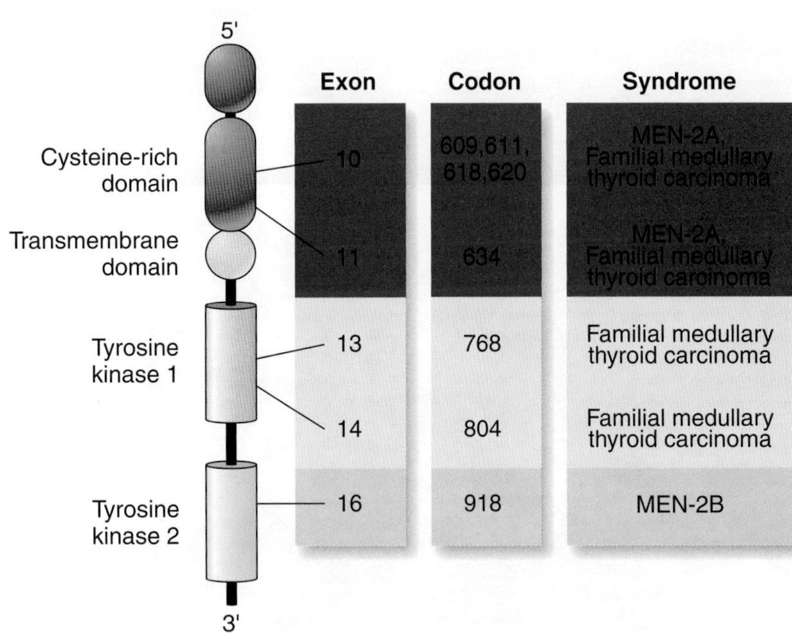

FIGURE 19-29. Representative RET proto-oncogene mutations in multiple endocrine neoplasia type 2 (MEN2).

Somatic mutations in *RET* occur in 10% to 20% of cases of sporadic pheochromocytomas. In addition, some sporadic pheochromocytomas have mutations in the von Hippel-Lindau (*VHL*) and neurofibromatosis type 1 (*NF1*) genes.

PATHOLOGY: MEN tumors vary from 1 cm to large masses of more than 2 kg. Most are 5 to 6 cm and weigh 80 to 100 g.

Pheochromocytomas tend to be encapsulated, spongy, and reddish, with prominent central scars, hemorrhage, and foci of cystic degeneration (Fig. 19-30A). Typically, circumscribed nests (**zellballen**) of polyhedral to fusiform neoplastic cells contain granular, amphophilic or basophilic cytoplasm, and vesicular nuclei. Eosinophilic cytoplasmic globules are common. Cellular pleomorphism may be prominent, including multinucleated tumor giant cells (Fig. 19-30B). Tumors are highly vascular, with many capillaries.

Immunostains attest to the neuroendocrine nature of the tumor and show neuron-specific enolase, chromogranin (Fig. 19-30C), and synaptophysin.

Up to 10% of adrenal pheochromocytomas are malignant, especially among extra-adrenal tumors. Only a tumor's behavior (i.e., metastases), and not its histology, defines malignancy. Both benign and malignant pheochromocytomas show mitoses, cellular pleomorphism, capsular or vascular invasion, and necrosis. The tumors spread most often to regional lymph nodes, bone, lung, and liver.

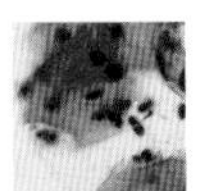

CLINICAL FEATURES: With few exceptions, the clinical features of pheochromocytomas are caused by catecholamine release by the tumor. Patients may come to medical attention because of (1) asymptomatic hypertension discovered on routine physical examination; (2) symptomatic hypertension resistant to antihypertensive therapy; (3) malignant hypertension (e.g., encephalopathy, papilledema, proteinuria); (4) myocardial infarction or aortic dissection; or (5) paroxysms of convulsions, anxiety, or hyperventilation.

There are other consequences of high catecholamine levels. Orthostatic hypotension results from decreased plasma volume and poor postural tone. Increased basal metabolism, sweating, heat intolerance, and weight loss may mimic hyperthyroidism. Angina and myocardial infarction occur in the absence of coronary artery disease. The cardiac complications reflect myocardial necrosis caused by elevated catecholamine levels ***(catecholamine cardiomyopathy).***

Increased urinary levels of catecholamine metabolites, particularly vanillylmandelic acid (VMA), metanephrine, and unconjugated catecholamines, help to confirm that a patient has a pheochromocytoma. Treatment for the tumor is surgical removal. β-Adrenergic blocking agents may help control hypertensive crises, and β-adrenergic receptor antagonists are helpful adjuncts.

Paraganglioma

Paragangliomas, namely pheochromocytomas arising at extra-adrenal sites, may occur in any location, including the retroperitoneum, neck, and bladder. They are frequently familial and inherited as autosomal dominant traits. Germline

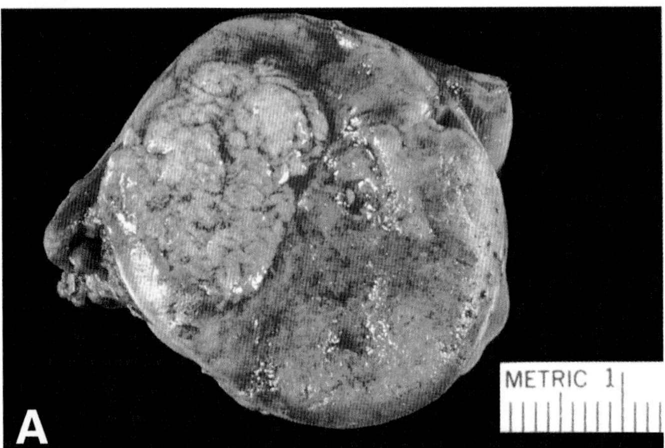

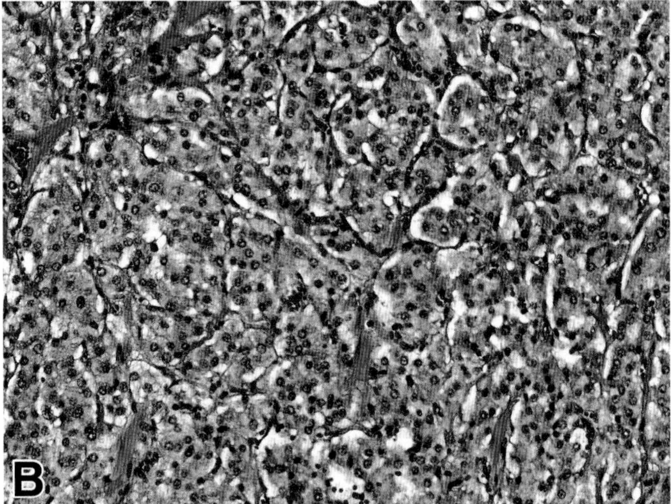

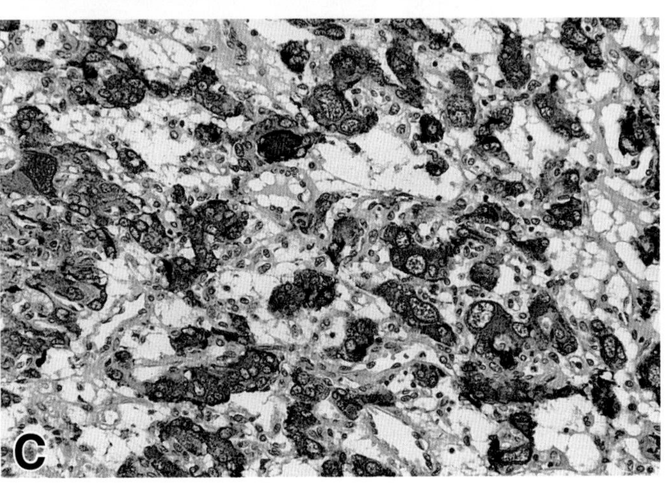

FIGURE 19-30. Pheochromocytoma. A. The cut surface of an adrenal tumor from a patient with episodic hypertension is reddish brown with a prominent area of fibrosis. Foci of hemorrhage and cystic degeneration are evident. **B.** A photomicrograph of the tumor shows polyhedral tumor cells with ample finely granular cytoplasm. Note the enlarged hyperchromatic nuclei. Courtesy of John Woosley, MD, PhD. **C.** Many of the tumor cells show positive immunohistochemical staining for chromogranin A, a marker of neuroendocrine differentiation.

mutations in *SDHB, SDHC, SDHD,* and *SDHAF2* genes are involved in the structure and function of succinate dehydrogenase. For unknown reasons, the inheritance of some subtypes of paragangliomas is paternal.

***Carotid body tumors** are prototypical paragangliomas.* They arise at the carotid bifurcation and form palpable masses in the neck. Interestingly, carotid body tumors are 10-fold more common in people living at high altitude than in those at sea level, suggesting that these tumors reflect hyperplastic responses to prolonged carotid body sensing of hypoxia.

Neuroblastoma

Neuroblastomas are malignant embryonal tumors of neural crest origin that arise in the adrenal medulla, paravertebral sympathetic ganglia, and sympathetic paraganglia and are composed of neoplastic neuroblasts, an intermediate stage in the development of sympathetic ganglion neurons (Fig. 19-27). These tumors are the most common solid extracranial neoplasms of childhood, accounting for up to 10% of childhood cancers and 15% of cancer deaths in children. The overall incidence peaks in the first 3 years and half of cancers diagnosed in the first month of life.

Adolescents or adults may rarely develop them. Although neuroblastomas are sporadic, a few instances are familial. Those genetically predisposed to this disease usually have multifocal tumors at an early age and follow autosomal dominant inheritance. These tumors may occur with neurofibromatosis type 1, Beckwith–Wiedemann syndrome, and Hirschsprung disease. Germline mutations in *PHOX2b* or *ALK* genes may be responsible for familial cases.

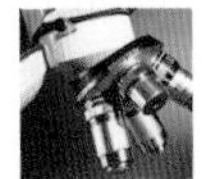

PATHOLOGY: Neuroblastomas can arise at any site that contains neural crest–derived cells (i.e., from the posterior cranial fossa to the coccyx). One third of the tumors are in the adrenal, another one third elsewhere in the abdomen, and 20% in the posterior mediastinum.

The tumors vary from minute, barely discernible nodules to tumors readily palpable through the abdominal wall. They are round, irregularly lobulated masses that may weigh 50 to 150 g or more (Fig. 19-31A). The cut surface is soft, friable, and variegated maroon in color. Necrosis, hemorrhage, calcification, and cystic changes are common.

Neuroblastomas contain dense sheets of small, round to fusiform cells with scant cytoplasm and hyperchromatic nuclei, resembling lymphocytes. Mitoses are frequent. Characteristic Homer Wright rosettes are defined by a rim of dark tumor cells in a circumferential arrangement around a central pale fibrillar core (Fig. 19-31B).

Neuroblastomas readily infiltrate surrounding structures and metastasize to regional lymph nodes, liver, lungs, bones, and other sites. The tumors may differentiate into ganglioneuromas (see below).

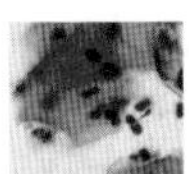

CLINICAL FEATURES: Clinical presentations are highly variable, reflecting the many sites where the primary tumors may develop and metastasize. The first sign is often an enlarging abdomen in a young child. Respiratory distress accompanies large masses in the thorax, and tumors in the pelvis may obstruct the bowel or ureters. Spinal cord compression may lead to gait disturbance and sphincter dysfunction. Tumor secretion of vasoactive intestinal peptide (VIP) may cause diarrhea. Some patients show paraneoplastic opsoclonus-myoclonus syndrome.

Urinary catecholamines and their metabolites are almost invariably elevated, particularly **norepinephrine, VMA, homovanillic acid (HVA)**, and **dopamine**.

Localized neuroblastomas are treated by surgical resection alone. Patients with disseminated tumors receive chemotherapy and sometimes irradiation.

Ganglioneuroma

Ganglioneuromas, like neuroblastomas, are tumors of neural crest origin. They occur in older children and young adults.

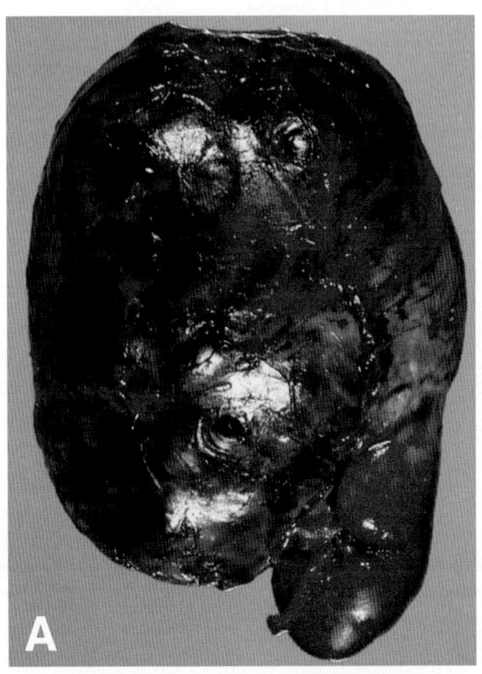

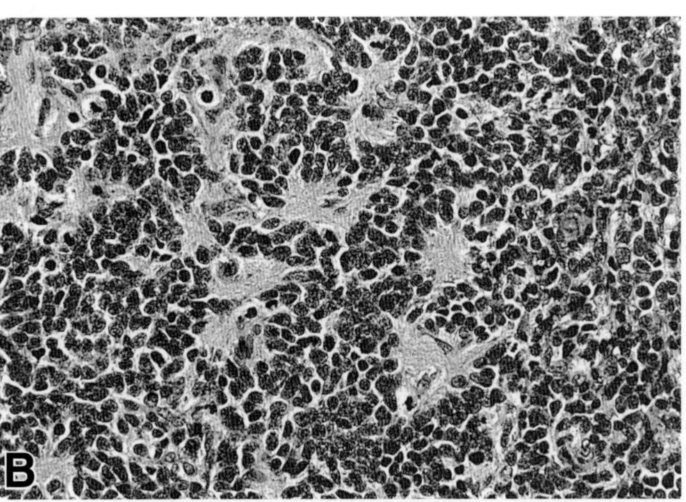

FIGURE 19-31. Neuroblastoma. A. A large, lobulated, hemorrhagic, and cystic tumor, adherent to the upper pole of the kidney, was removed from a child who presented with an abdominal mass. **B.** A photomicrograph illustrates the characteristic rosettes, formed by small, regular, dark tumor cells arranged around a central, pale fibrillar core.

Ganglioneuromas are benign and arise in sympathetic ganglia, typically in the posterior mediastinum. Up to 30% of these tumors develop in the adrenal medulla. In keeping with their degree of differentiation, ganglioneuromas do not manifest chromosomal abnormalities characteristic of neuroblastomas.

Ganglioneuromas are well encapsulated, with myxoid, glistening cut surfaces. They show well-differentiated, mature ganglion cells associated with spindle cells in a loose, abundant fibrillar stroma (Fig. 19-32). The fibrils represent neurites extending from tumor cell bodies. Various intracellular neuroendocrine markers may be demonstrated.

PINEAL GLAND

The pineal gland resembles a 5- to 7-mm minute pine cone. It is below the posterior edge of the corpus callosum, suspended from the roof of the third ventricle over the superior colliculi. The pineal has a lobulated architecture, compartmentalized by fibrovascular septa, with cords and clusters of large epithelial-like cells, termed **pinealocytes**. These have modified photosensory and neuroendocrine functions. Astrocytes make up 10% of pineal gland cellularity.

The pineal gland produces several neurotransmitters, of which **melatonin** is among the most abundant. Because melatonin levels are distinctly higher at night than during waking hours, it may act as a sleep inducer.

Serotonin and several other substances are also produced by the pineal. The most significant of these is arginine vasotocin, a hormone that has important antigonadotropic activity. Melatonin may be a releasing factor for arginine vasotocin.

Beginning at puberty, calcifications (corpora arenacea or "brain sand") develop in the pineal gland. These mineralized concretions accumulate increasingly with age and are accompanied by cystic degeneration and gliosis of no known clinical significance.

Pineal Neoplasms

Tumors of the pineal gland are rare and represent less than 1% of brain tumors. Pineal tumors include neoplasms (1) originating from the pineal parenchyma, presumably from pinealocytes; (2) in the pineal gland region (**astrocytomas**) but derived from cells other than pinealocytes; (3) germ cell tumors derived from misplaced germ cells, and, rarely, (4) metastasis from other sites. Germ cell tumors are the most common pineal neoplasms and are indistinguishable from their gonadal counterpart.

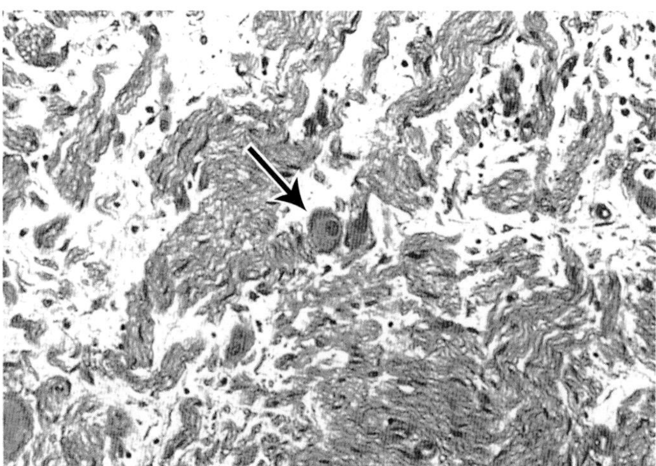

FIGURE 19-32. Ganglioneuroma. A photomicrograph shows mature ganglion cells (*arrow*) interspersed among wavy spindle cells embedded in a myxoid matrix.

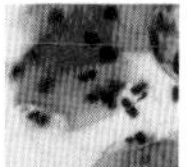

CLINICAL FEATURES: Regardless of histologic type, pineal gland tumors present with signs and symptoms related to their impact on surrounding structures, including headaches and visual and behavioral disturbances. In children, these tumors may precipitate precocious puberty, especially in boys. The prognosis of malignant pinealocyte tumors, pinealoblastomas, is poor. However, even benign pineal tumors and nonneoplastic pineal cysts carry guarded prognoses and pose a great threat to life, because they are difficult to excise surgically.

ENDOCRINE PANCREAS

The islets of Langerhans form the endocrine pancreas. These structures are irregularly scattered throughout the pancreas and consist of richly vascularized aggregates of endocrine cells arranged in spherical clusters (compact islets) or irregular trabeculae (diffuse islets). Four major distinct cell types are present in the islets, and each cell produces only one specific peptide hormone (Table 19-3).

- **Alpha cells** synthesize glucagon and are found at the periphery of islet lobules. They comprise 15% to 20% of the total islet cell population. Glucagon induces glycogenolysis and gluconeogenesis in the liver, thereby raising blood glucose levels. Its secretion is stimulated by hypoglycemia and by ingestion of a low-carbohydrate, high-protein meal.

Table 19-3

Secretory Products of Islet Cells and Their Physiologic Actions

Cell	Secretory Product	Physiologic Actions
Alpha	Glucagon	Catabolic; stimulates glycogenolysis and gluconeogenesis; raises blood glucose
Beta	Insulin	Anabolic; stimulates glycogenesis, lipogenesis, and protein synthesis; lowers blood glucose
Delta	Somatostatin	Inhibits secretion of alpha, beta, D_1, and acinar cells
D_1	Vasoactive intestinal polypeptide	Same as glucagon; also regulates tone and motility of the GI tract and activates cAMP of intestinal epithelium
PP	Human pancreatic polypeptide	Stimulates gastric enzyme secretion; inhibits intestinal motility and bile secretion

cAMP, cyclic adenosine 3′,5′-monophosphate; GI, gastrointestinal; PP, pancreatic polypeptide.

By virtue of these responses, glucagon, together with insulin, serves to maintain glucose homeostasis.

- **Beta cells** constitute 60% to 70% of islet cells and produce insulin. They are found toward the centers of islets. Insulin secretion is activated when glucose binds to receptors on the beta-cell surface.
- **Delta cells** secrete somatostatin. They are few in number (5% to 10%) and, like alpha cells, tend to be at the periphery of islets. Pancreatic somatostatin inhibits the pituitary release of growth hormone; secretion by pancreatic alpha, beta, and acinar cells; and activities of certain hormone-secreting cells in the gastrointestinal tract. These hormonal interactions suggest that somatostatin plays a regulatory role in glucose homeostasis.
- **Pancreatic polypeptide-secreting cells** are primarily in the diffuse islets within the head of the pancreas. They synthesize a polypeptide that appears to have diverse functions, including stimulation of enzyme secretion by the gastric mucosa, inhibition of smooth muscle contraction in the intestine and gallbladder, production of gastric acid, and secretion by the exocrine pancreas and biliary system.

Pancreatic Neuroendocrine Tumors

Well-differentiated pancreatic neuroendocrine tumors amount to about 5% of pancreatic neoplasms. PanNETs resemble normal islet cells and other well-differentiated endocrine (or neuroendocrine) tumors of the body, such as carcinoid tumors. Previously called "islet cell tumors," PanNETs may secrete hormones that cause dramatic paraneoplastic syndromes, or they may not function at all. Functioning varieties include insulinoma, glucagonoma, somatostatinoma, gastrinoma, VIPoma, and other rare types.

PanNETs show a range of clinical aggressiveness. If small, they can be cured by surgical resection, but larger tumors may develop incurable metastases. Predicting their likely clinical behavior is difficult, but features such as large size, high proliferative activity, and more extensive invasion increase the chance of recurrence. Even in the presence of distant metastases, PanNETs often grow slowly, and patients can survive for years. Although most tumors are nonfunctional, those that do function result in hormonal syndromes, which are often debilitating. Functioning insulinomas are most common. ***The distinctive paraneoplastic syndromes of the more common functioning types are shown in*** **Figure 19-33.**

PanNETs occur at any age but are most common between the age of 40 and 60, affecting men and women equally.

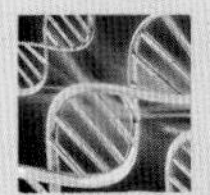

MOLECULAR PATHOGENESIS: PanNETs are a component of multiple endocrine neoplasia syndrome type 1 (MEN1) (see earlier). Patients with von Hippel-Lindau (VHL) syndrome also develop nonfunctioning PanNETs, which may be histologically distinguished by their clear cytoplasm. The genes involved in MEN1 and VHL syndromes (*MEN1* and *VHL* tumor suppressors, respectively) show biallelic inactivation in hereditary PanNETs.

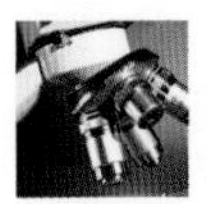

PATHOLOGY: Functioning and nonfunctioning PanNETs appear similar. They are usually solitary, circumscribed masses of pink to tan, soft tissue. Larger tumors are multinodular and have areas of hemorrhage. Cystic degeneration can occur, and some cases are firm and fibrotic. They have uniform cells, arranged in so-called organoid patterns, including nests, ribbons, glands, and festoons (Fig. 19-34). Nuclei are uniform and the chromatin is coarsely stippled. The proliferative rate is low; by definition, there should be fewer than 20 mitotic figures in 10 high-power microscopic fields, and under 20% of nuclei should be positive for the proliferation marker Ki67. Low- and intermediate-grade groups of PanNETs can be further defined based on these measures of proliferation, and the grade correlates well with prognosis. Sometimes the stroma contains amyloid, or it may be sclerotic.

Paraneoplastic Syndromes

- **Insulinomas,** the most common functioning PanNETs, secrete sufficient insulin to cause hypoglycemia. Insulin secretion by the tumor cells is not regulated by blood glucose levels, so the tumors secrete insulin continuously. Although these neoplasms are usually small (75% are <2 cm), the symptoms may be profound and include both the direct effects of hypoglycemia on the CNS and the secondary effects of the resulting catecholamine response. Insulinomas tend to have a benign clinical course, perhaps because they are usually very small when detected. Surgical removal, even by enucleation, is usually curative.
- **Glucagonomas** are associated with a syndrome of (1) mild diabetes; (2) a necrotizing, migratory, erythematous rash; (3) anemia; (4) diarrhea; and (5) deep vein thromboses. Psychiatric disturbances also occur. Glucagonomas constitute up to 13% of functioning PanNETs and occur between the ages of 40 and 70, with a slight female predominance.
- **Somatostatinomas** are rare and produce a syndrome of mild diabetes, gallstones, steatorrhea, hypochlorhydria, anemia, and weight loss. Symptoms are due to the inhibitory actions of somatostatin on other cells of the pancreatic islets and on neuroendocrine cells of the gastrointestinal tract. Consequently, blood levels of insulin and glucagon are low.
- **Pancreatic gastrinoma** is a functioning PanNET composed of so-called G cells, which produce gastrin, a potent hormonal stimulus for gastric acid secretion. The location of this tumor in the pancreas is curious because gastrin-producing cells do not normally occur in the islets. Pancreatic gastrinoma causes Zollinger–Ellison syndrome, a disorder showing (1) intractable gastric hypersecretion, (2) severe peptic ulceration of the duodenum and jejunum, and (3) high blood gastrin levels. Pancreatic gastrinomas are aggressive, although those arising in the duodenum usually remain localized, even when lymph node metastases are present.
- **VIPomas** are functioning PanNETs that produce **vasoactive intestinal polypeptide** (VIP). Like gastrin, VIP is not normally found in nonneoplastic islet cells but rather is made in ganglion cells and nerve fibers of the pancreas, gut, and brain. VIP induces glycogenolysis and hyperglycemia and regulates ion and water secretion by the gastrointestinal epithelium. VIPomas induce Verner–Morrison syndrome, which is characterized by explosive and profuse watery diarrhea, hypokalemia, and achlorhydria. VIPomas are rare (3% to 8% of all PanNETs and 10% of functioning PanNETs) and are usually large and solitary.
- PanNETs may rarely secrete **other hormones not ordinarily produced by the pancreas** (**ectopic hormones**), including ACTH, parathyroid hormone, calcitonin, and vasopressin.

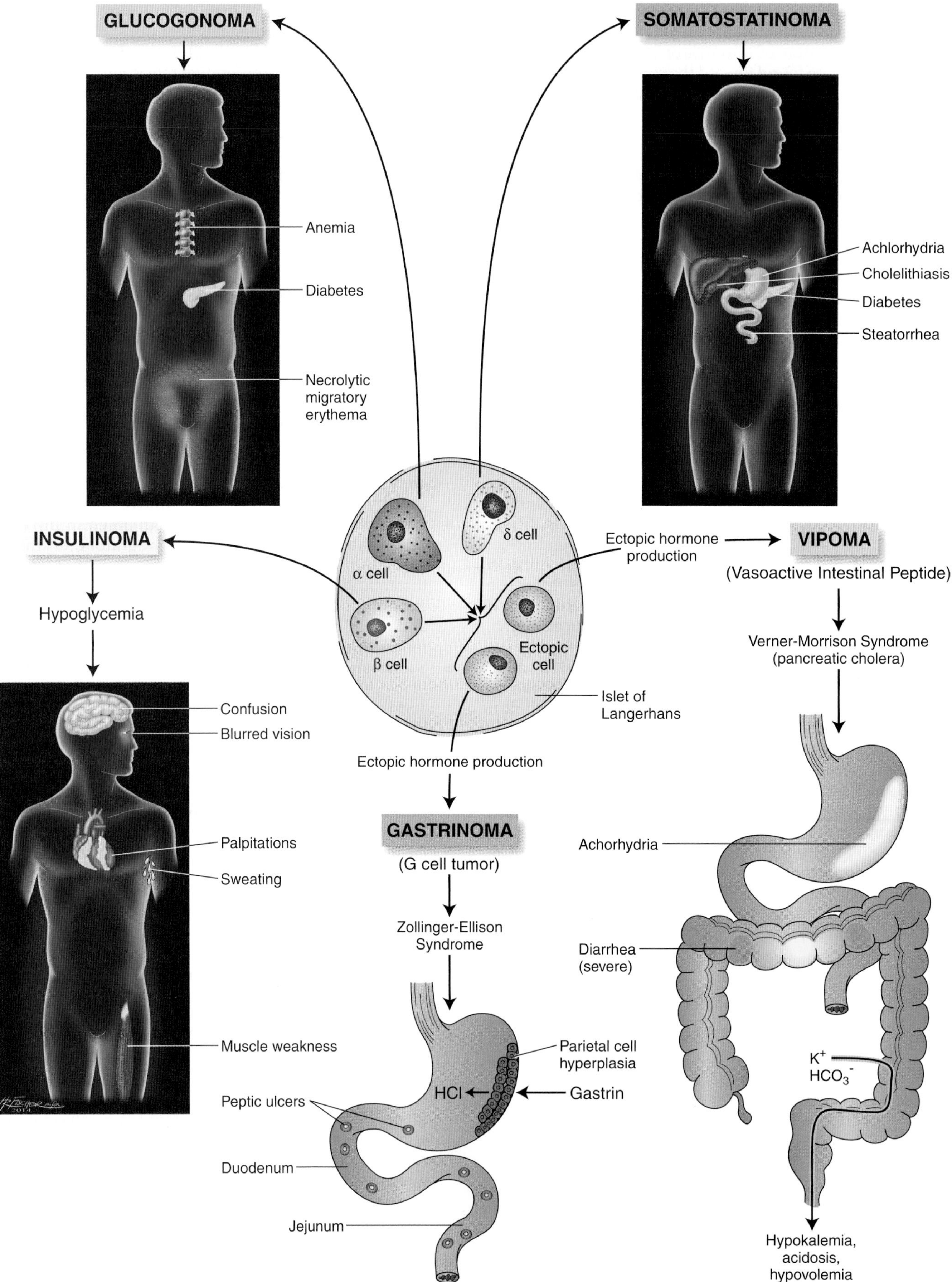

FIGURE 19-33. Syndromes associated with well-differentiated pancreatic neuroendocrine tumors.

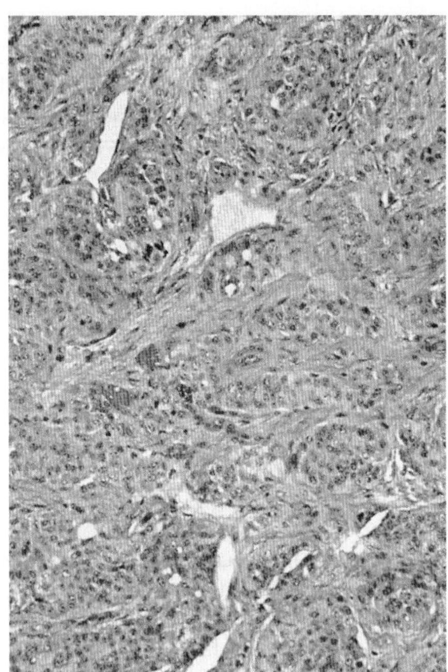

FIGURE 19-34. Insulinoma. Nests of tumor cells are surrounded by numerous capillaries.

DIABETES MELLITUS

Two major forms of diabetes are recognized and are distinguished by different underlying etiologies. **Type 1 diabetes mellitus (T1DM)**, formerly known as **insulin-dependent diabetes mellitus (IDDM)** or **juvenile-onset diabetes**, is caused by the autoimmune destruction of insulin-producing beta cells in the islets of Langerhans. It affects fewer than 10% of all patients with diabetes. By contrast, **type 2 diabetes mellitus (T2DM),** formerly known as **non–insulin-dependent diabetes mellitus (NIDDM)** or **maturity-onset diabetes**, is often associated with obesity. It results from a complex interrelationship between insulin resistance of target tissues and an oversecretion of insulin by the pancreas. The balance between oversecretion and resistance may, or may not, be sufficient to control plasma glucose concentrations. Table 19-4 compares the key features of type 1 and type 2 diabetes.

Gestational diabetes develops in some pregnant women, owing to resistance to the glucose-lowering actions of insulin in pregnancy, combined with a beta-cell defect in the pancreas. It almost always abates after delivery (see below). Diabetes can also occur in other endocrine conditions or drug therapy, especially in Cushing syndrome or during treatment with glucocorticoids.

Table 19-4

Comparison of Type 1 and Type 2 Diabetes Mellitus

	Type 1 Diabetes	Type 2 Diabetes
Age at onset	Usually before 20	Usually after 30
Type of onset	Abrupt; symptomatic (polyuria, polydipsia, dehydration); often severe with ketoacidosis	Gradual; usually subtle; often asymptomatic
Usual body weight	Normal; recent weight loss is common	Overweight
Family history	<20%	>60%
Monozygotic twins	50% concordant	90% concordant
HLA associations	+	No
Antibodies to islet cell antigens (insulin, GAD-65, IA-2)	+	No
Islet lesions	Early—inflammation Late—atrophy and fibrosis	Late—fibrosis, amyloid
β-cell mass	Markedly reduced	Normal or slightly reduced
Circulating insulin levels	Markedly reduced or absent	Elevated (early)
Insulin resistance for glucose (i.e., selective resistance to the glucose-lowering actions of insulin)	Normal sensitivity to glucose-lowering actions of insulin	Significant insulin resistance for glucose, but with continued insulin responsiveness of other pathways
Clinical management	Administration of exogenous insulin absolutely required	Exogenous insulin usually not needed initially; insulin supplementation may be needed at later stages; weight loss typically improves the condition

GAD, glutamic acid decarboxylase; HLA, human leukocyte antigen; IA-2, islet cell antigen-512.

Diagnostic Criteria

The American Diabetes Association suggests any of four criteria to diagnose diabetes (Table 19-5). One of the four criteria have to be present for the diagnosis. In addition, three categories of increased risk for diabetes are defined (Table 19-6). Some of those are commonly referred to as "prediabetes," but the term should be used with caution, because only half of those patients will ultimately develop diabetes. These criteria are based on abnormal threshold levels for glucose or hemoglobin A_{1c}, which are closely associated with the chronic complications of this disorder. In particular, hyperglycemia causes the microvascular changes of diabetic retinopathy and renal glomerular damage. In a younger patient with an abrupt onset of hyperglycemia and elevated plasma ketones or frank ketoacidosis, T1DM arises from absolute insulin deficiency. By contrast, T2DM typically develops gradually over years before it is recognized, most often in an overweight, middle-aged person with a genetic predisposition.

Table 19-5

Criteria for the Diagnosis of Diabetes

1. HbA_{1c}[a] ≥6.5%
   OR
2. FPG ≥126 mg/dL (7.0 mmol/L). Fasting is defined as no caloric intake for at least 8 hours
   OR
3. 2-h plasma glucose ≥200 mg/dL (11.1 mmol/L) during an OGTT
   OR
4. In a patient with classic symptoms of hyperglycemia or hyperglycemic crisis, a random plasma glucose ≥200 mg/dL (11.1 mmol/L)

FPG, fasting plasma glucose; HbA_{1c}, hemoglobin A_{1c}; OGTT, oral glucose tolerance test.

[a]In the absence of unequivocal hyperglycemia, criteria 1 to 3 should be confirmed by repeat testing.

Modified with permission from the American Diabetes Association. *Diabetes Care.* Vol. 36; 2013. © 2013 American Diabetes Association.

Role of Insulin

The **insulin receptor** is a tetrameric glycoprotein; two extracellular α-subunits bind insulin and two transmembrane β-subunits demonstrate insulin-stimulated tyrosine kinase activity. Activation of the receptor kinase leads to tyrosine phosphorylation of several adaptor proteins (insulin receptor substrates [IRS]). These, in turn, activate downstream kinases. As a result, lipid and protein substrates are phosphorylated, giving rise to translocation of glucose transport proteins from the interior of the cell to the plasma membrane. This effect facilitates glucose entry, particularly into skeletal muscle and, to a lesser extent, adipocytes (Fig. 19-35).

Insulin has several additional functions unrelated to importing glucose:

- Suppression of hepatic glycogenolysis and gluconeogenesis, thus inhibiting hepatic glucose production in the postprandial state.
- Induction of hepatic fatty acid and triglyceride biosynthesis (de novo lipogenesis) to export and store calories in a compact, osmotically inactive form.
- Activation of endothelial nitric oxide synthase (eNOS) to produce nitric oxide (NO), a vasodilator that increases blood flow and hence glucose availability to skeletal muscle.
- Activation of extracellular signal-regulated kinase (ERK), a mitogen-activated protein (MAP) kinase. This kinase drives protein synthesis and cell division and increases endothelial production of endothelin-1, a vasoconstrictor that may modulate eNOS-mediated vasodilation.

Table 19-6

Categories of Increased Risk for Diabetes (Prediabetes)[a]

FPG 100 mg/dL (5.6 mmol/L) to 125 mg/dL (6.9 mmol/L) (IFG)
2-h PG in the 75-g OGTT 140 mg/dL (7.8 mmol/L) to 199 mg/dL (11.0 mmol/L) (IGT)
HbA_{1c} 5.7%–6.4%

FPG, fasting plasma glucose; HbA_{1c}, hemoglobin A_{1c}; IFG, impaired fasting glucose; IGT, impaired glucose tolerance; OGTT, oral glucose tolerance test; PG, plasma glucose.

[a]For all three tests, risk is continuous, extending below the lower limit of the range and becoming disproportionately greater at the higher ends of the range.

Modified with permission from the American Diabetes Association. *Diabetes Care.* Vol. 36; 2013. © 2013 American Diabetes Association.

Type 1 Diabetes Mellitus

T1DM is a lifelong disorder of glucose homeostasis that results from autoimmune destruction of beta cells in the islets of Langerhans. Triggers for this autoimmune reaction remain unknown (see below). Because T1DM reflects insulin deficiency, rather than complex defects in insulin action, these patients can be made almost metabolically normal by closely controlling the amounts, timing, and preparations of exogenous insulin.

T1DM is characterized by few, if any, functional beta cells and extremely limited or nonexistent insulin secretion. Without insulin, the body switches energy use to a pattern that resembles starvation, regardless of the availability of food. Thus, adipose stores, rather than exogenous glucose, are preferentially metabolized for energy. Oxidation of fat overproduces **ketone bodies** (acetoacetic acid and β-hydroxybutyric acid), which are released into the blood from the liver and lead to metabolic ketoacidosis. Hyperglycemia results from unsuppressed hepatic glucose output and reduced glucose uptake into skeletal muscle and adipose tissue. Blood glucose levels exceed the kidneys' ability to resorb it, leading to glycosuria. This effect, in turn, causes osmotic diuresis, which can give rise to dehydration from accompanying loss of body water. If uncorrected, progressive acidosis and dehydration cause coma and death. Only when 80% or more of insulin-secreting cells are eliminated, and insulin deprivation is severe, is T1DM with hyperglycemia or ketoacidosis clinically evident.

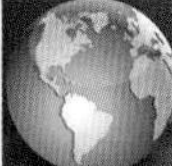

EPIDEMIOLOGY: It is estimated that more than 1 million Americans suffer from T1DM. Most develop this disease within the first two decades of life, but more and more cases are being recognized in older people. In some older patients, autoimmune beta-cell destruction may develop slowly over many years. The name **latent autoimmune diabetes in adults (LADA)** is commonly applied to those patients.

T1DM is most common among northern Europeans and their descendants and occurs less often in other ethnic groups. For example, T1DM develops in Finland 20 to 40 times more than in Japan. Although it can develop at any age, the peak age of onset coincides with puberty. In many geographical areas, an increased incidence in late fall and early winter suggests seasonal infections as autoimmune triggers (see below).

AUTOIMMUNITY: The concept of an autoimmune pathogenesis for T1DM is suggested by the observation that pancreatic islets from patients who die shortly after the onset of the disease show mononuclear infiltrates, or **insulitis**, in their pancreatic islets (Fig. 19-36). $CD8^+$ T lymphocytes predominate among these inflammatory cells. The infiltrating cells also elaborate proinflammatory cytokines, for example, IL-1, IL-6, interferon-α, and nitric oxide, which may further contribute to beta-cell injury.

Most newly diagnosed children with T1DM have circulating antibodies against components of the beta cells, including insulin. However, these antibodies are now regarded as responses to beta-cell antigens released during destruction of beta cells by cell-mediated immune mechanisms, rather than the cause of beta-cell depletion.

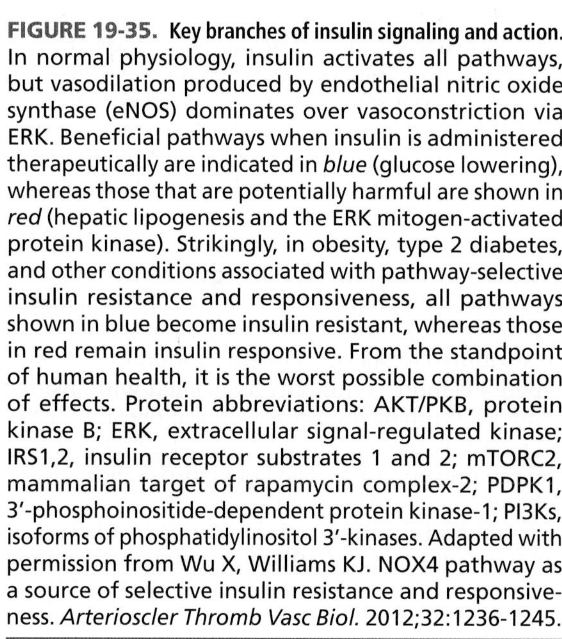

FIGURE 19-35. Key branches of insulin signaling and action. In normal physiology, insulin activates all pathways, but vasodilation produced by endothelial nitric oxide synthase (eNOS) dominates over vasoconstriction via ERK. Beneficial pathways when insulin is administered therapeutically are indicated in *blue* (glucose lowering), whereas those that are potentially harmful are shown in *red* (hepatic lipogenesis and the ERK mitogen-activated protein kinase). Strikingly, in obesity, type 2 diabetes, and other conditions associated with pathway-selective insulin resistance and responsiveness, all pathways shown in blue become insulin resistant, whereas those in red remain insulin responsive. From the standpoint of human health, it is the worst possible combination of effects. Protein abbreviations: AKT/PKB, protein kinase B; ERK, extracellular signal-regulated kinase; IRS1,2, insulin receptor substrates 1 and 2; mTORC2, mammalian target of rapamycin complex-2; PDPK1, 3′-phosphoinositide-dependent protein kinase-1; PI3Ks, isoforms of phosphatidylinositol 3′-kinases. Adapted with permission from Wu X, Williams KJ. NOX4 pathway as a source of selective insulin resistance and responsiveness. *Arterioscler Thromb Vasc Biol.* 2012;32:1236-1245.

Ten percent of patients with T1DM develop at least one other organ-specific autoimmune disease, including Hashimoto thyroiditis, Graves disease, myasthenia gravis, Addison disease, and pernicious anemia.

Evidence for the role of genetic factors in the pathogenesis of T1DM include the following:

- Relatives of people with T1DM have an increased risk for development of this disorder. An identical twin of a T1DM patient has a 30% to 50% risk of developing T1DM.
- T1DM is strongly linked to HLA class II molecules—DR and DQ. Although only 45% of the population in the United States express DR3 or DR4, 95% of those who develop T1DM express these haplotypes.
- Many other independent chromosomal regions (several of them non-HLA) are also associated with susceptibility to T1DM, but their contributions to the overall incidence of T1DM are small.

ENVIRONMENTAL FACTORS: Evidence for the role of environmental factors in the pathogenesis of T1DM includes the following:

- Only one third to one half of monozygotic twins of T1DM patients develop T1DM.
- About 80% to 90% of patients with T1DM have no family history of the disease.
- There are seasonal differences in the incidence of T1DM.

Viruses have been implicated in at least some cases. Thus, T1DM occasionally develops after infection with coxsackie B virus and, less often, mumps virus.

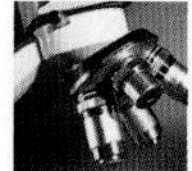

PATHOLOGY: The most characteristic early lesion in the pancreas of T1DM is a chiefly lymphocytic infiltrate in the islets (insulitis), sometimes with scattered macrophages and neutrophils (Fig. 19-36). As the disease becomes chronic, islet beta cells

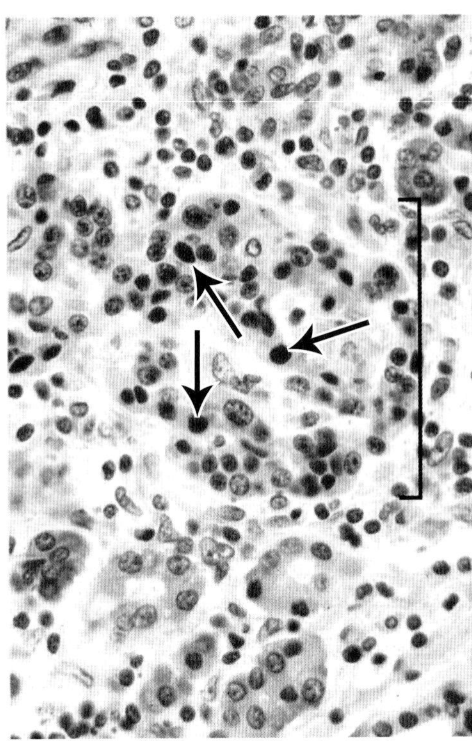

FIGURE 19-36. Insulitis in type 1 diabetes mellitus. A lymphocytic inflammatory infiltrate (*arrows*) is seen in and around the islet (*left of bracket*).

become progressively depleted; eventually insulin-producing cells are no longer discernible. Loss of beta cells results in variably sized islets, many of which appear as ribbon-like cords that may be difficult to distinguish from surrounding acinar tissue. Islet fibrosis is uncommon. However, chronic T1DM often shows diffuse interlobular and interacinar fibrosis, accompanied by atrophy of the acinar cells. Unlike T2DM (see later) amyloid is not seen in pancreatic islets in T1DM.

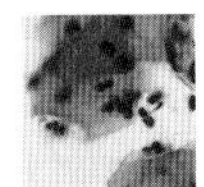

CLINICAL FEATURES: The clinical picture of T1DM reflects a lack of insulin and its unique role in energy metabolism. The disease classically presents with acute metabolic decompensation, characterized by hyperglycemia and ketoacidosis. Depending on the degree of absolute insulin deficiency, severe ketoacidosis may be preceded by weeks to months of increased urine output (**polyuria**) and increased thirst (**polydipsia**). Weight loss in spite of increased appetite (**polyphagia**) results from unregulated catabolism of body stores of fat, protein, and carbohydrate.

Type 2 Diabetes Mellitus

T2DM is characterized by a combination of reduced tissue sensitivity to the effects of insulin and oversecretion of insulin from the pancreas. This combination eventuates in an inadequate control of plasma glucose concentrations.

T2DM usually develops in adults, mostly in obese people and in the elderly. However, the disease has been appearing increasingly in younger adults and adolescents, as severe obesity and lack of exercise become more common in this age group. Patients with T2DM exhibit hyperinsulinemia, but these excessive insulin concentrations fail to control blood sugar levels. When T2DM patients require administration of exogenous insulin, their total daily doses are much higher than those in lean T1DM (insulin-deficient) patients.

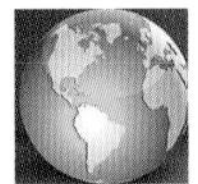

EPIDEMIOLOGY: About 10% of the U.S. population has diabetes and over 25% are prediabetic. The prevalence differs among ethnic groups, being higher in American Indians, blacks, and Hispanics, compared to Asians and non-Hispanic whites.

Diabetes is the leading cause of kidney failure, nontraumatic lower limb amputations, and new cases of blindness among American adults. It is also a major factor in heart disease and stroke and is the seventh leading cause of death.

Risk Factors

T2DM is a two-hit disease. The first "hit" is resistance to the glucose-lowering actions of insulin in its target tissues (liver, skeletal muscle, adipose tissue). This defect alone provokes an increased pancreatic output of insulin and may later be followed by moderate defects in glucose handling, indicative of prediabetes. The second "hit" occurs when increased insulin output no longer compensates for the increased demand for insulin to control blood sugar levels. Pancreatic islets often show degenerative changes in these patients. Progression to overt diabetes occurs most commonly in patients with both of these "hits" (Fig. 19-37).

Several risk factors are clearly associated with T2DM. The most important ones are **obesity, overnutrition, and low levels of physical activity**. The risk of T2DM increases linearly with body mass index (BMI), and more than 80% of cases can be attributed to obesity. Visceral–abdominal obesity ("apple shaped") is more commonly associated with insulin resistance and T2DM than is gluteal–femoral obesity ("pear shaped") (Fig. 19-38). Accordingly, weight loss lowers the risk of T2DM and can prevent progression of high-risk individuals to frank diabetes.

Multifactorial and multigenic inheritance is a key contributor to the development of T2DM. Several observations demonstrate genetic influences in the development of T2DM:

- More than one third of patients with T2DM have at least one parent with the disease.
- Among monozygotic twins, concordance for T2DM approaches 100%.
- The prevalence of T2DM among different ethnic groups who are living in similar environments is highly variable.
- First-degree relatives of patients with T2DM have a significantly higher lifetime risk of the disease compared with those without a family history.

Despite the high familial prevalence of the disease, inheritance is complex and involves multiple interacting susceptibility genes. Monogenic causes of T2DM represent only a small fraction of cases, and common inherited polymorphisms contribute only small degrees of risk for, or protection from, T2DM.

A rare autosomal dominant form of inherited diabetes, known as **maturity-onset diabetes of the young (MODY)**, is associated with gene defects that affect beta-cell function, including the gene for glucokinase, a key sensor for glucose metabolism within the beta cell. Several mutations in genes that control beta-cell development and function have been described. Mutations in these genes, however, do not account for typical T2DM.

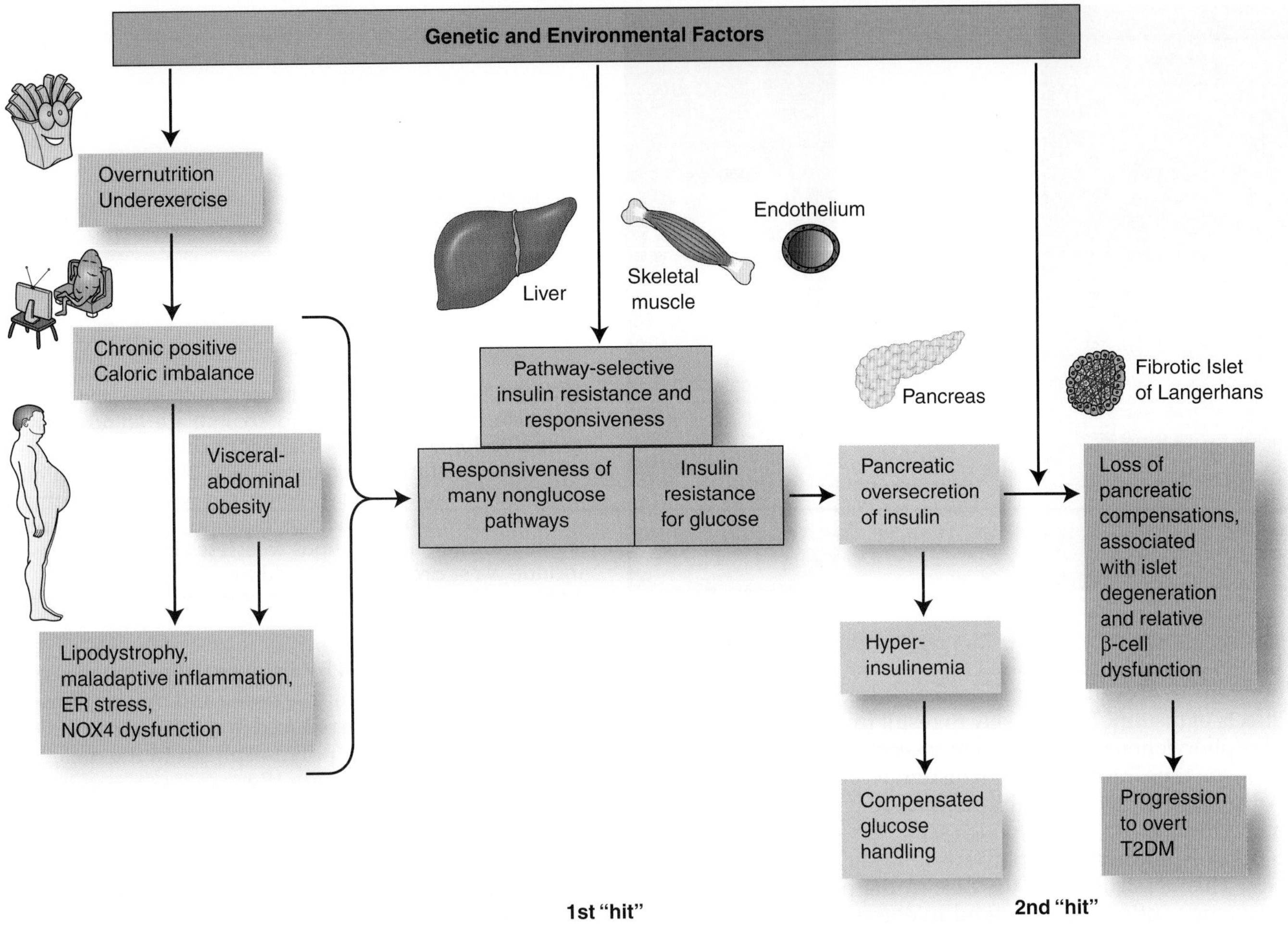

Genetic and Environmental Factors

Overnutrition
Underexercise

Chronic positive
Caloric imbalance

Visceral-
abdominal
obesity

Lipodystrophy,
maladaptive inflammation,
ER stress,
NOX4 dysfunction

Liver

Skeletal
muscle

Endothelium

Pathway-selective
insulin resistance and
responsiveness

Responsiveness of
many nonglucose
pathways

Insulin
resistance
for glucose

Pancreas

Pancreatic
oversecretion
of insulin

Hyper-
insulinemia

Compensated
glucose
handling

Fibrotic Islet
of Langerhans

Loss of
pancreatic
compensations,
associated
with islet
degeneration
and relative
β-cell
dysfunction

Progression
to overt
T2DM

1st "hit"

2nd "hit"

FIGURE 19-37. Pathogenesis of obesity-related type 2 diabetes mellitus (T2DM). The expanded visceral fat mass in upper body obesity elaborates several factors that may contribute to insulin resistance for glucose. These include an increase in circulating free (nonesterified) fatty acids and other cytokines and proteins that inhibit insulin action, as well as a decrease in factors that enhance insulin signaling, such as adiponectin. These changes result in impairments to insulin action in liver and skeletal muscle at the level of the insulin receptor and at postreceptor signaling sites, resulting in a failure of insulin to suppress hepatic glucose production and to promote glucose uptake into muscle. The resulting hyperglycemia is normally countered by increased insulin secretion by pancreatic beta cells. Continuing responsiveness of pathways downstream of the insulin receptor that are unrelated to glucose control, such as lipogenesis in the liver and activation of the extracellular signal-regulated kinase mitogen-activated protein kinase, may contribute to fatty liver, dyslipoproteinemia, and hypertension. In many individuals, the combination of resistance to the glucose-lowering actions of insulin and a genetically determined impairment of the beta-cell response to hyperglycemia eventually results in hyperglycemia, and T2DM ensues. ER, endoplasmic reticulum.

Insulin Resistance

After a carbohydrate-rich meal, the gut absorbs glucose. The consequent increases in blood glucose stimulates insulin secretion by pancreatic beta cells. In turn, insulin increases glucose uptake by skeletal muscle and adipose tissue (Fig. 19-39). Insulin also suppresses hepatic glucose production by (1) inhibiting glycogenolysis and gluconeogenesis, (2) enhancing glycogen synthesis, (3) blocking the effects of glucagon on the liver, and (4) antagonizing glucagon release from the pancreas.

All of these effects of insulin are impaired in T2DM. Insulin resistance (for glucose) (IRg) increases hepatic glucose output and reduces glucose uptake by peripheral tissues, primarily muscles and adipose tissue.

By itself, insulin resistance rarely causes T2DM because increased insulin secretion (hyperinsulinism) by beta cells compensates for these defects and prevents blood glucose levels from rising. In many obese and prediabetic patients, subclinical beta-cell dysfunction exists before overt diabetes. Only when the pancreas can no longer keep step with this high demand do blood glucose levels start to increase.

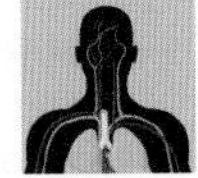

PATHOPHYSIOLOGY OF IRg: There are currently several suggested mechanisms to explain IRg. Although no one hypothesis satisfactorily accounts for IRg, the clear role of obesity in furthering T2DM strongly suggests the involvement of adipose tissue.

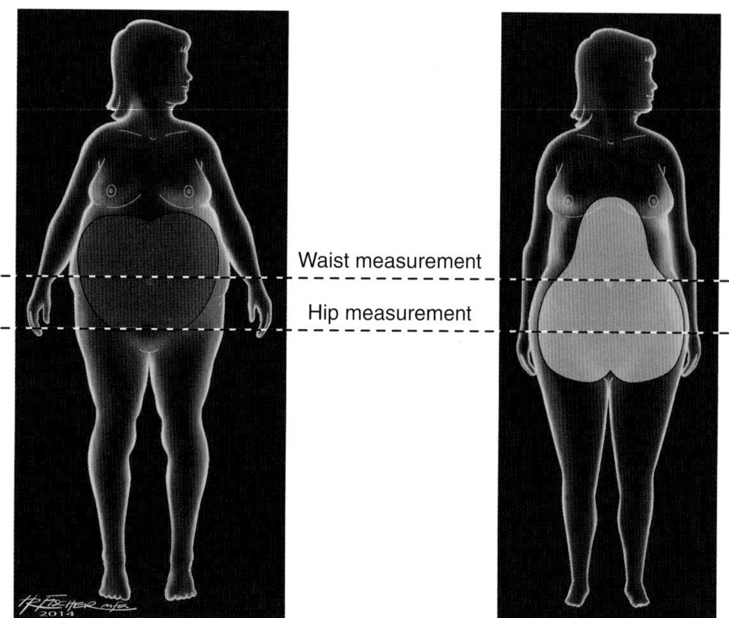

FIGURE 19-38. Regional adipose distribution and cardiometabolic risk. Individuals who accumulate adipose tissue in the abdomen ("apple shaped") exhibit increased risk of insulin resistance for glucose, type 2 diabetes mellitus, and cardiovascular disease, compared with those with fat accumulations around the hips, buttocks, and thighs ("pear shaped"). Standard methods to assess abdominal obesity include waist circumference and the waist:hip ratio.

- **Lipotoxicity:** High circulating levels of free fatty acids that occur in obesity can impair skeletal muscle sensitivity to the effects of insulin. This is likely to result from inhibition of phosphorylation of insulin receptor substrate (IRS) adaptor proteins thus interfering with insulin receptor signaling.
- **Adipokine secretion:** Adipose tissue may be considered an endocrine-like organ, which secretes a variety of proteins (**adipokines**) that play a role in the generation of IRg. This is particularly the case in the presence of the low-grade inflammation found in obese adipose tissue. Among the adipokines most likely to play a role in IRg are the following:
  - **Adiponectin secreted by adipose tissue** enhances the effects of insulin in adipose tissue and muscle. Plasma levels of adipokine are reduced in obesity and in T2DM. In addition, a genetic polymorphism in the molecule is strongly associated with IRg.
  - **TNF-α** levels are increased in visceral–abdominal obesity. This cytokine also induces IRg in experimental animals and cultured cells. However, in early stages of human overnutrition syndromes, TNF-α and other cytokines are not elevated; yet, these people already display IRg.
  - **Retinol binding protein 4 (RBP4)** is an adipokine that is increased in persons with metabolic syndrome (see below)

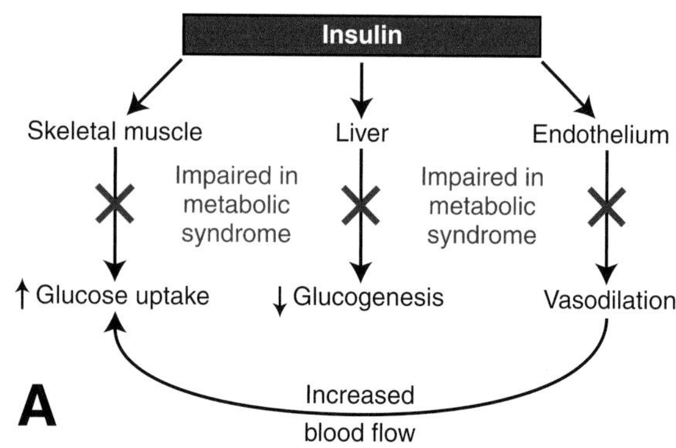

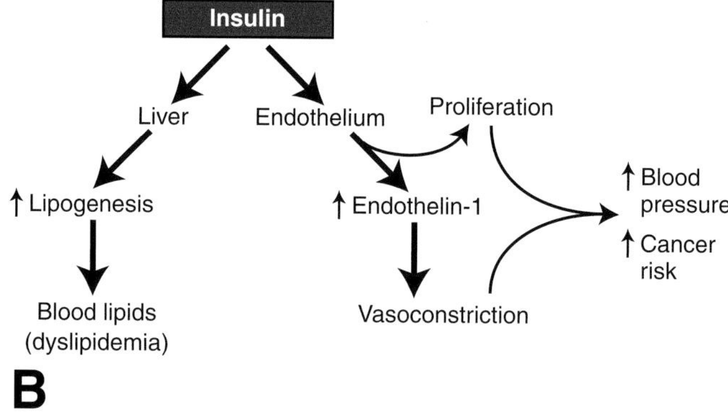

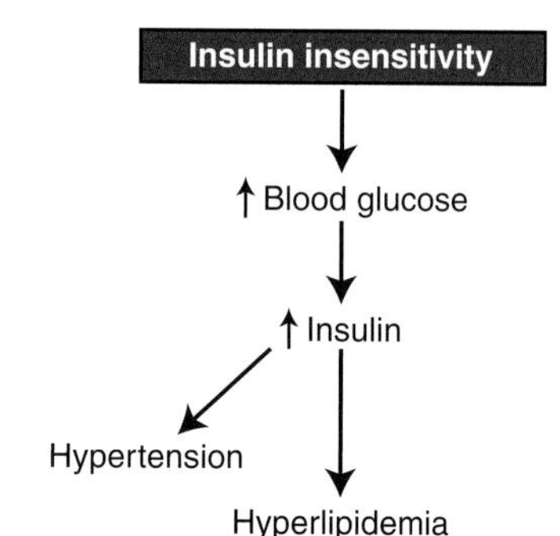

FIGURE 19-39. Mechanisms of insulin action that are impaired and that are intact in metabolic syndrome. A. Insulin activities that are impaired in metabolic syndrome. **B.** Insulin functions that remain intact in metabolic syndrome. **C.** Summary of insulin resistance for glucose and its consequences.

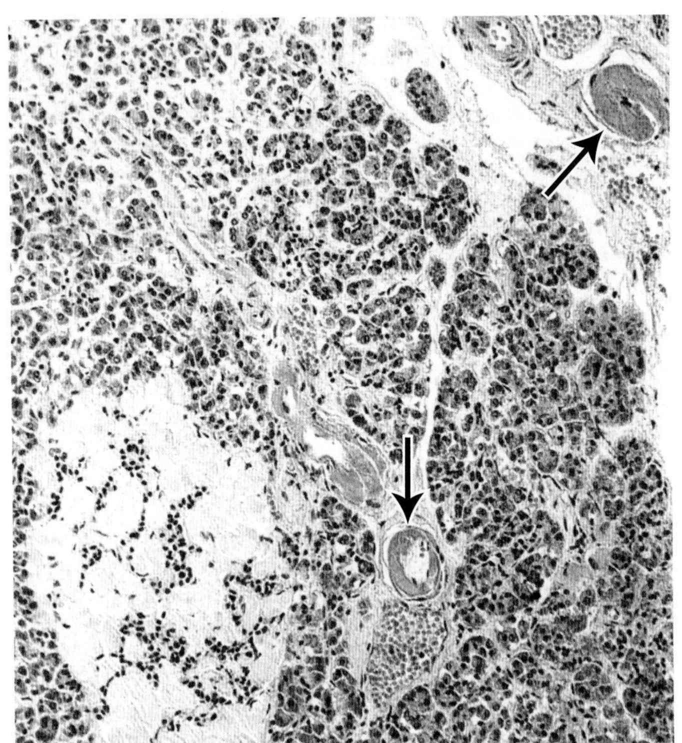

FIGURE 19-40. Amyloid deposition (hyalinization) of an islet in the pancreas of a patient with type 2 diabetes mellitus (*lower left*). Blood vessels adjacent to the islet show the advanced hyaline arteriolosclerosis (*arrows*) characteristic of diabetes.

and IRg. Unlike other adipokines, serum levels of RBP4 appear to be independent of obesity per se and hence may be an independent risk factor for T2DM-associated cardiovascular risk.

- **Endoplasmic reticulum (ER) stress:** Chemical induction of ER stress in cultured cells impairs insulin signaling, and relief of ER stress in obese animals improves their glucose handling. Evidence for this pathway in obese humans, however, has been mixed.

Beta-Cell Dysfunction

In T2DM an impairment in the first phase of insulin secretion following glucose stimulation precedes glucose intolerance. Later, in the second phase of the disease, the release of newly synthesized insulin is faulty. This effect can be reversed, at least in some patients, by restoring good control of glycemia. This partially reversible reduction in insulin secretion results from a paradoxical inhibitory effect of glucose upon insulin release, which may be seen at high blood glucose levels ("glucose toxicity").

Impaired first-phase insulin secretion can serve as a marker of risk for T2DM in family members and may be seen in patients with prior gestational diabetes. Over a long time, insulin secretion in T2DM gradually declines, together with beta-cell mass.

PATHOLOGY: Lesions may be found in the islets of Langerhans of many, but not all, patients with T2DM. Unlike T1DM (see above), the number of beta cells is not consistently reduced in T2DM, and no morphologic lesions of these cells have been found by light or electron microscopy.

In some islets, fibrous tissue accumulates, sometimes to the extent that islets are obliterated. Islet amyloid is often present (Fig. 19-40), particularly in patients older than 60 years. This type of amyloid is composed of a polypeptide molecule known as **amylin**, which is secreted with insulin by the beta cell. Importantly, some 20% of aged nondiabetics also have amyloid in the pancreatic islets, a finding that has been attributed to the aging process itself.

Metabolic Syndrome

Imbalanced insulin action in target tissues and compensatory hyperinsulinemia are closely tied to a diverse set of cardiovascular risk factors that are prevalent in obese, sedentary people and patients with diabetes. These risk factors, together called the **metabolic syndrome**, include (1) abdominal adiposity with increased waist circumference, (2) mild hypertension (perhaps related to failure of endothelium-dependent vascular relaxation), (3) elevated plasma glucose levels, and (4) dyslipoproteinemia with elevated plasma triglycerides and low plasma high-density lipoprotein (HDL) cholesterol (Table 19-7). Some consider metabolic syndrome as a precursor to T2DM.

Therapeutic Implications

Early in T2DM, IRg and hyperinsulinemia predominate. Both can improve dramatically with even modest weight loss and exercise. In addition, insulin sensitizers are useful in those patients. Metformin is considered an "insulin sensitizer" because it improves glucose uptake by muscle and inhibits hepatic glucose production, although its mechanism of action at a molecular level remains problematic.

Later in the course of diabetes, as beta-cell dysfunction sets in, insulin sensitizers alone cannot control T2DM. Other agents, and ultimately exogenous insulin, are needed.

Table 19-7

Frequently Observed Concomitants of the Metabolic Syndrome

Clinical Signs
Central (upper body) obesity with increased waist circumference
Acanthosis nigricans (hypertrophic, hyperpigmented skin changes)
Laboratory Abnormalities
Elevated fasting and/or postprandial glucose
Insulin resistance for glucose, with hyperinsulinemia, but continued responsiveness—and hence overactivity—of other pathways downstream of the insulin receptor
Dyslipidemia characterized by increased triglycerides and low high-density lipoprotein cholesterol
Hypercoagulability and abnormal thrombolysis
Hyperuricemia
Endothelial and vascular smooth muscle dysfunction
Albuminuria
Comorbid Illnesses
Hypertension
Atherosclerosis
Hyperandrogenism with polycystic ovary syndrome

Complications of Diabetes

The severity and chronicity of hyperglycemia in both T1DM and T2DM are the major pathogenetic factors that lead to the "microvascular" complications of diabetes. These include retinopathy, nephropathy, and neuropathy. Thus, control of blood glucose remains the major means by which the development of microvascular diabetic complications can be minimized. It has been more difficult to demonstrate that glucose control can prevent "macrovascular" (large-vessel) complications, meaning atherosclerosis and its sequelae (coronary artery disease, peripheral vascular disease, and cerebrovascular disease). These macrovascular complications are especially common in patients with T2DM, in part because the patients tend to be older and frequently harbor additional cardiovascular risk factors, particularly dyslipoproteinemia, hypertension, and hypercoagulability.

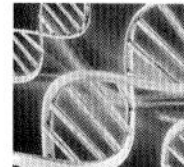

PATHOGENESIS: Several biochemical mechanisms have been proposed to account for the development of complications in diabetes.

- **Cardiovascular risk factors:** In T2DM, the harmful pattern of pathway-selective insulin resistance and responsiveness promotes the following: (1) fatty liver, (2) overproduction of triglyceride-rich apoB lipoproteins, (3) impaired hepatic removal of atherogenic postprandial lipoproteins from the circulation, (4) vasoconstriction, (5) overexpression of tissue factor, and (6) possibly salt retention. Benefits have been shown from lipid-lowering agents (statins); treatment of hypertension, particularly with angiotensin-converting enzyme (ACE) inhibitors; and low daily doses of aspirin to inhibit platelet function. In T1DM, significant hypertriglyceridemia can develop in the context of poor glycemic control, but this effect usually corrects quickly once insulin is administered.
- **Protein glycation:** Glucose covalently attaches to an assortment of proteins roughly in proportion to the severity of hyperglycemia. A specific fraction of glycated hemoglobin in circulating red blood cells, namely hemoglobin A_{1c}, is used routinely to monitor the overall degree of hyperglycemia during the preceding 6 to 8 weeks. Because glycation of hemoglobin is irreversible, hemoglobin A_{1c} levels serve as a marker for glycemic control. With time, the initial glycation products form stable **advanced glycosylation end-products (AGEs)**, which consist of glucose derivatives bound covalently to protein amino groups. AGE formation permanently alters protein structure and leads to cross-linking of nearby proteins, possibly contributing to the characteristic thickening of vascular basement membranes in diabetes. Nevertheless, the role of AGEs in diabetic microvascular disease remains uncertain.

Atherosclerosis

Atherosclerotic heart disease and ischemic strokes account for over half of all deaths among adults with diabetes. The extent and severity of atherosclerotic lesions in medium-sized and large arteries are increased in patients with long-standing diabetes. Diabetes eliminates the usual protective effect of being female, and coronary artery disease develops at a younger age than in nondiabetic people. Moreover, mortality from myocardial infarction is higher in diabetics than in nondiabetics. Patients with T2DM often have multiple risk factors of the metabolic syndrome that contribute to atherogenesis.

Atherosclerotic peripheral vascular disease, particularly of the lower extremities, commonly complicates diabetes. Vascular insufficiency may cause ulcers and gangrene of the toes and feet, ultimately necessitating amputation. ***Diabetes accounts for more than 60% of nontraumatic limb amputations in the United States.***

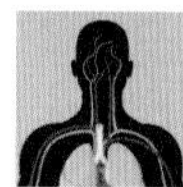

PATHOPHYSIOLOGY: How diabetes promotes atherosclerosis is uncertain. There are at least three general schools of thought:

1. **Direct effects of diabetes or hyperglycemia on the arterial wall.** As noted earlier, however, none of the clinical therapies based on this idea reduces this type of complication of T2DM.
2. **Side effects of diabetic therapy,** such as high insulin concentrations associated with certain forms of treatment.
3. **Exacerbation of general risk factors for** atherosclerosis (e.g., hypertension, dyslipoproteinemia, hypercoagulability). Dyslipoproteinemia in T2DM is partly due to hepatic and intestinal overproduction of triglyceride-rich apoB lipoproteins. A defect in lipoprotein lipase impairs clearance of chylomicrons and causes postprandial hypertriglyceridemia. In addition, the liver's uptake of atherogenic postprandial remnant lipoprotein particles is impaired. The most successful strategies to reduce cardiovascular events in T2DM involve management of these risk factors (e.g., administration of statins, antihypertensive agents, and low-dose aspirin).

Microvascular Disease

Arteriolosclerosis and capillary basement membrane thickening are characteristic vascular changes in diabetes (see Chapter 14). The frequent occurrence of hypertension contributes to the development of the arteriolar lesions. Deposition of basement membrane proteins, which may also become glycated, increases in diabetes. Platelet aggregation in smaller blood vessels and impaired fibrinolysis may also contribute to diabetic microvascular disease.

The effects of microvascular disease on tissue perfusion and wound healing are profound. Blood flow to the heart, already compromised by large-vessel disease (coronary atherosclerosis), is reduced. Chronic ulcers due to trauma and infection of the feet heal poorly in diabetic patients, in part because of microvascular disease. The major complications of diabetic microvascular disease involve the kidney and the retina (Fig. 19-41).

Nephropathy

Diabetes is the leading cause of renal failure in the United States, accounting for almost half of new cases. One third of patients with T1DM ultimately develop renal failure, as do up to 20% of patients with T2DM. Some patients with T1DM may die from uremia, but most of those who develop nephropathy die of cardiovascular disease. The latter is 40 times more common in T1DM patients who have end-stage renal disease. The prevalence of diabetic nephropathy increases with the severity and duration of hyperglycemia. Kidney disease due to diabetes is the most common reason for renal transplantation in adults (Fig. 19-42) (see Chapter 14).

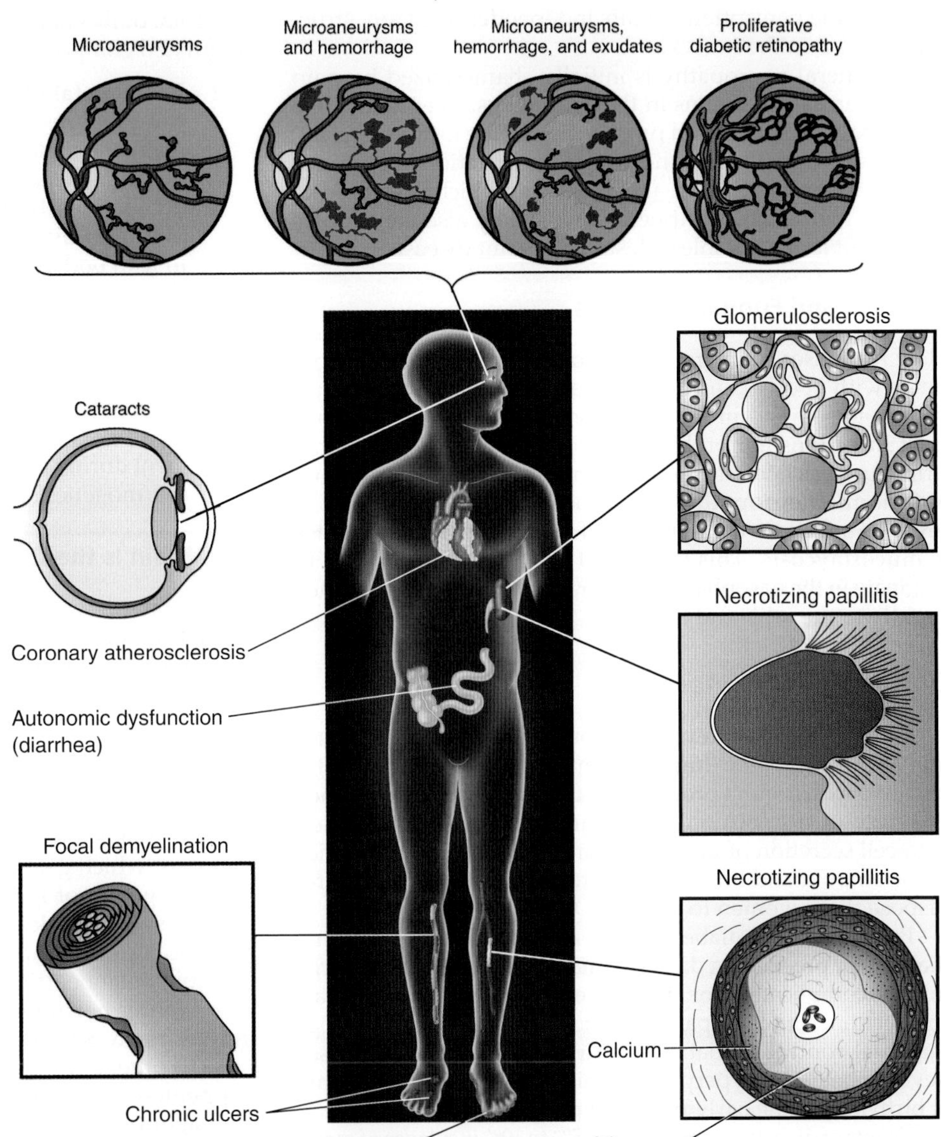

FIGURE 19-41. Secondary complications of diabetes. The effects of diabetes on a number of vital organs result in complications that may be incapacitating (cerebral and peripheral vascular disease), painful (neuropathy), or life-threatening (coronary artery disease, pyelonephritis with necrotizing papillitis).

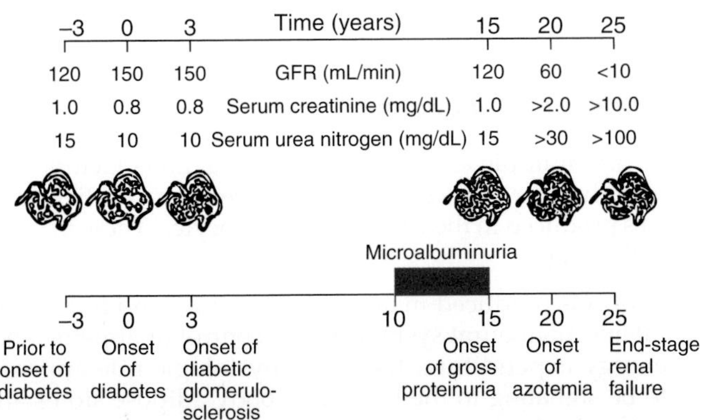

FIGURE 19-42. Natural history of diabetic nephropathy. Initially, renal hypertrophy and hyperfiltration lead to an increase in the glomerular filtration rate (GFR). Once the decline in renal function begins, on average at least 10 years after the onset of diabetes, leakage of a small amount of serum albumin into the urine (microalbuminuria) is the first abnormality that is easily and reliably measured. The elevation in serum creatinine and gross proteinuria occur much later. Courtesy of the American Diabetes Association.

Retinopathy

Diabetic retinopathy is the leading cause of blindness in the Unites States in adults under age 74. The risk is higher in T1DM than in T2DM. In fact, 10% of patients with T1DM of 30 years' duration become legally blind. Nevertheless, as there are many more patients with T2DM, they are the most numerous patients with diabetic retinopathy. Retinopathy is the most devastating ophthalmic complication of diabetes, although glaucoma, cataracts, and corneal disease are also increased. Like nephropathy, the prevalence of diabetic retinopathy reflects the duration and degree of glycemic control.

Neuropathy

Peripheral sensory impairment and autonomic nerve dysfunction are among the most common and distressing complications of diabetes. Changes in the nerves are complex, with abnormalities in axons, the myelin sheath, and Schwann cells. Microvascular pathology involving the small blood vessels of nerves contributes to diabetic neuropathy. Hyperglycemia increases the perception of pain, independently of any structural lesions in the nerves.

Peripheral neuropathy is initially characterized by pain and abnormal sensations in the extremities. Eventually, fine touch, pain detection, and proprioception are lost. As a result, patients with diabetes tend to ignore irritation and minor trauma to the feet, joints, and legs, after which they tend to develop foot ulcers. Peripheral neuropathy also contributes to Charcot joint, a painless destructive joint disease.

Bacterial and Fungal Infections

Host responses to microbial pathogens are abnormal in patients with poorly controlled diabetes. Leukocyte function is compromised and immune responses are blunted. **Urinary tract infections** are problematic because glucose makes the urine an enriched culture medium. Urinary retention from autonomic neuropathy may exacerbate this tendency. A dreaded infectious complication of poorly controlled diabetes is **mucormycosis**. This often-fatal fungal infection tends to originate in the nasopharynx or paranasal sinuses and spreads rapidly to the orbit and brain.

Gestational Diabetes

Gestational diabetes develops in only a few percent of seemingly healthy women during pregnancy. It may continue after parturition in a small proportion of these patients. Pregnancy is a state of IRg, but only pregnant women with impaired beta-cell secretion of insulin become diabetic. Abnormalities in the amount and timing of pancreatic insulin secretion predispose these women to overt T2DM later in life.

Poor control of diabetes in pregnancy (either gestational diabetes or preexisting diabetes) may lead to the birth of large infants, complicate labor and delivery, and necessitate a cesarean section. The fetal pancreas tries to compensate for poor maternal control of diabetes during gestation. Such fetuses develop beta-cell hyperplasia, which leads to hypoglycemia at birth and in the early postnatal period.

Infants of diabetic mothers have a 5% to 10% incidence of major developmental abnormalities, including anomalies of the heart and great vessels and neural tube defects, such as anencephaly and spina bifida. The frequency of these lesions is a function of the control of maternal diabetes during early gestation.

NUTRITIONAL DISEASES

In industrialized countries obesity, rather than starvation, is the overwhelming cause of nutritional disease. Metabolic syndrome and subsequent T2DM may be classified as nutritional diseases because of their strong association with obesity. Nevertheless, starvation, particularly in children, and vitamin deficiencies remain common problems in the nonindustrialized world.

Obesity

Energy Intake and Expenditure

Weight increases when energy intake exceeds expenditure; you are what you eat, minus what you burn. The normal human gastrointestinal (GI) tract absorbs essentially all simple fuels that enter it.

Total daily energy expenditure (TDEE) consists of several regulated components:

1. **Basal metabolic rate:** BMR is the energy expended at complete rest, in the postabsorptive state. It includes maintenance levels of breathing, circulation of blood, and essential metabolic functions. For people with sedentary occupations, BMR accounts for ~60% of TDEE. Over 75% of interindividual variation in BMR reflects differences in lean body mass.
2. **Calories spent to digest, absorb, and store ingested calories** (6% to 12% of TDEE).
3. **Energetic costs of emotion, medication, and adaptive thermogenesis** (e.g., changes in temperature, exposure to infectious agents).
4. **Activity thermogenesis** generated by physical movement during purposeful exercise and nonexercise activity thermogenesis.

The Brain Is the Central Controller of Body Weight

The brain receives hormonal and neuronal signals about food deficits or surpluses and the rate of fuel utilization. To maintain homeostasis, it then coordinates responses, modulating behavior and the endocrine and autonomic nervous systems to adjust energy balance.

The **hypothalamus** is the main processor of signals from the periphery and is crucial to managing energy balance. Although many hypothalamic nuclei regulate metabolism, the arcuate nucleus plays a central role via two distinct populations of neurons, which generate opposing actions on food intake.

One group of neurones makes **anorexigenic** (appetite-suppressing) peptides, including proopiomelanocortin (POMC) and cocaine- and amphetamine-regulated transcripts (CARTs). proopiomelanocortin (POMC) is cleaved into α-melanocyte–stimulating hormone (α-MSH), which binds melanocortin receptors MC3R and MC4R to decrease appetite.

The other population of neurons produces two **orexigenic** (appetite-stimulating) neuropeptides: **neuropeptide Y** (NPY) and **agouti-related protein** (AgRP). NPY is among the most abundant neuropeptides in the mammalian brain and strongly stimulates feeding. AgRP antagonizes melanocortin receptors, thereby blocking α-MSH anorexigenic effects and stimulating food intake.

Regulation of Hunger and Satiety

There are multiple endogenous and exogenous factors that regulate hunger and satiety. Several are hormone-like substances produced in the GI tract and adipocytes. These include the following:

- **Leptin** is produced mainly by adipocytes and links neural and nonneural systems in the control of appetite and energy expenditure. Its chief physiologic role appears to be signaling to the brain that body adipose stores are sufficient. Low-serum leptin levels increase appetite and decrease energy expenditure. Mutations in the leptin and leptin receptor genes are rarely associated with obesity.
- **Endocannabinoids** are endogenous lipids that bind to cannabinoid receptors in hypothalamic nuclei that are involved in the control of energy balance and weight. They are also present in adipose tissue and the GI tract. Activated CB1 receptor stimulates food intake and may play a role in the development and maintenance of obesity.

- **The GI tract** contains a diverse group of mechanoreceptors and chemosensitive receptors. These molecules relay information via vagal afferent fibers that terminate in the nucleus tractus solitarii in the brainstem. Several hormones produced by the GI tract signal the CNS to regulate energy intake. These include the following:
  - **Glucagon-like peptide 1** (GLP-1) is derived from proglucagon in the mucosa of the distal ileum and colon. GLP-1 (1) decreases food intake, (2) slows gastric emptying, (3) generates a feeling of satiety, (4) augments postprandial glucose-stimulated insulin secretion, and (5) decreases secretion of glucagon, a hormone that opposes insulin action. Long-acting GLP-1 analogs (exenatide and liraglutide) are used to treat type 2 diabetes mellitus and to induce weight reduction.
  - **Ghrelin** is a hormone that stimulates the sensation of hunger. It is produced primarily by endocrine cells in the stomach and, to a lesser extent, in the duodenum, ileum, and colon. Ghrelin stimulates orexigenic NPY neurons in the arcuate nucleus of the hypothalamus. Serum ghrelin increases after diet-induced weight loss, an effect that may contribute to poor long-term results of clinical weight loss programs.
  - **Cholecystokinin (CCK)** is made mainly in the duodenal and jejunal mucosa, particularly after fat and protein intake. CCK stimulates the release of enzymes from the pancreas and gallbladder to aid digestion, slow gastric emptying, and reduce food intake.
  - **Peptide YY** (PYY) and the related **pancreatic polypeptide** are secreted mostly in the ileum and colon and pancreas respectively. They are released in response to food intake and decrease appetite and total caloric intake.
- **Gut flora** may affect body weight. Distal gut flora from obese people contain microbes that are different from the flora of lean individuals. Gut bacteria from obese individuals may extract calories from complex components of the diet more efficiently than do microbiota from their lean counterparts. Regulatory effects on the host from variations in gut flora are likely to be important but are poorly understood.

Body Mass Index and Obesity

The standard most often used to define obesity is body mass index (BMI)

$$\text{BMI} = [\text{weight (kg)}]/[\text{height (m)}]^2$$

Although BMI is an excellent indicator of obesity, it does not formally distinguish between fat mass and lean mass. Most health organizations define overweight as a BMI between 25 and 30 kg/m^2. A BMI over 30 defines obesity, 30 to 35 class I obesity, 35 to 40 class II obesity, and a BMI exceeding 40 extreme (class III) obesity. A high BMI correlates with excess morbidity, largely owing to metabolic abnormalities such as dyslipoproteinemia, hypertension, impaired regulation of plasma glucose concentrations, hypercoagulability, and T2DM. A BMI above 35 (class II and class III obesity) is consistently associated with excess all-cause mortality, but BMIs of 25 to 30 (overweight) or 30 to 35 (class I obesity) are not.

As noted above, regional body fat distribution also determines health risks associated with obesity. Fat depots in various parts of the body play different roles, including (1) energy metabolism, (2) secretion of circulating proteins and metabolites into the bloodstream, and (3) physical cushioning and protection of internal organs. Compared with gluteal–femoral obesity (lower-body obesity or "pear shaped"; Fig. 19-38), visceral–abdominal obesity (central adiposity or "apple shaped") carries a greater risk of dyslipoproteinemia, hypertension, heart disease, diabetes, and some forms of cancer.

BMI does not account for fat distribution, so abdominal obesity is better assessed by measuring waist circumference or the waist:hip ratio. Waist circumference above 102 cm (40 inches) and waist:hip ratio over 0.9 in men are associated with adverse outcomes. The same holds true for women with a waist circumference more than 88 cm (35 inches) or waist:hip ratio larger than 0.85. Thus, the amounts of visceral fat and modifiable cardiovascular risk factors provide better guides to therapy than does BMI.

Studies of Heritable Causes of Obesity

Most persons who live in developed countries are exposed to a calorie-rich, sedentary environment; yet BMIs vary considerably, from extremely thin to morbidly obese. An inherited propensity toward obesity is clear, based on comparisons of BMIs (1) between monozygotic and dizygotic twins, (2) between genetically full or half-siblings raised apart after adoption in infancy, and (3) in multigenerational kindreds. These reports yield estimates of heritability for obesity ranging from 20% to 80%. Notably, a study of twin children found that BMI and waist circumference each showed 77% heritability. Moreover, behaviors linked to obesity all have substantial inherited components.

Many genetic studies have identified specific gene variants that, altogether, contribute only slightly to the population-wide development of obesity:

- **Leptin gene and receptor mutations** have both been linked to rare monogenic syndromes of severe obesity in humans. Homozygotes present with hyperphagia and severe, early-onset obesity. In the case of leptin gene mutations, replacement therapy with injections of recombinant leptin is effective.
- **Melanocortin 4 receptor gene (*MC4R*) mutations**, both dominant and recessive, are the leading cause of severe, monogenic, childhood-onset obesity, accounting for 5% of such cases. Patients tend to have no phenotype other than overeating, obesity, and the well-known cardiometabolic sequelae of obesity.
- **Genome-wide association studies** have identified several genes that encode brain/hypothalamic proteins and are associated with variations in BMI. However, all specific gene polymorphisms identified to date account for less than 1% of the genetic basis for obesity.

Body weight control mechanisms are believed to have evolved to protect from weight loss in times of scarcity, not obesity in times of plenty. Striking examples of environmental influence on genetic predisposition include the Pima Native Americans in Arizona. Pimas are now largely sedentary and eat a diet in which 50% of energy derives from fat, unlike their traditional low-fat diets. They have experienced huge increases in obesity and diabetes. By contrast, the genetically related Pimas in the Sierra Madre Mountains of Northern Mexico are more physically active, maintain more traditional low-fat diets, and have much lower rates of obesity and type 2 diabetes.

Diabetes risk among the Pima community varies inversely with the extent of European ancestry in each. This is consistent with the threefold difference in disease prevalence between the two parental populations (i.e., Pima and European).

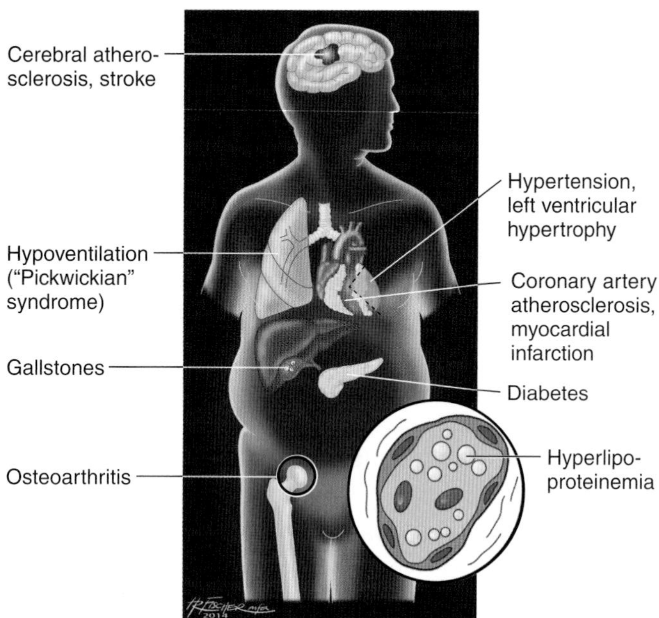

FIGURE 19-43. Medical complications of obesity.

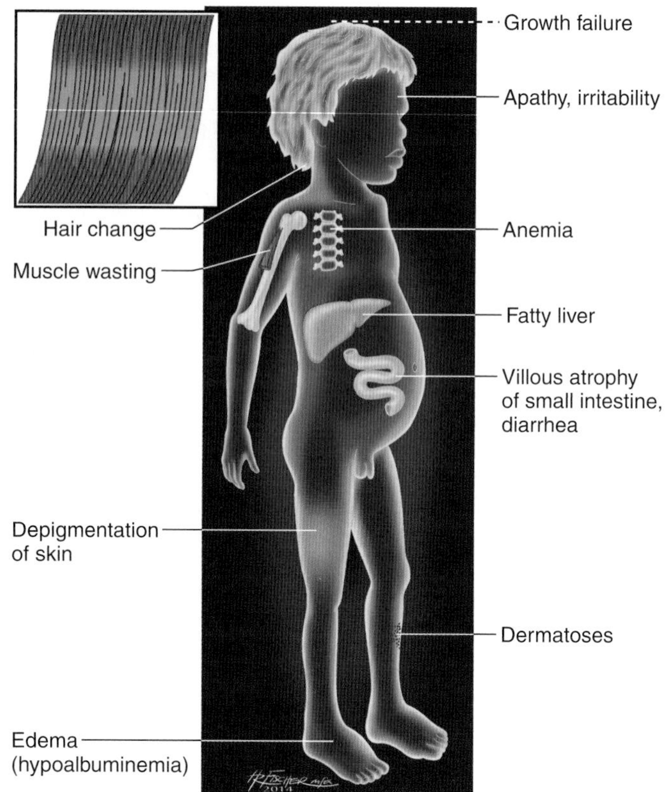

FIGURE 19-44. Complications of kwashiorkor.

Complications of Obesity

Obesity and central adiposity are associated with increased morbidity and, for class II and III obesity, increased mortality as well (Fig. 19-43). Fat cells undergo both hyperplasia and hypertrophy. The excess from the imbalance between energy intake and energy expenditure is stored in adipocytes, which enlarge, increase in number, or both. An extremely obese adult can have four times as many adipocytes as a lean person, each cell containing twice as much lipid. Given the close association between T2DM, obesity, and the metabolic syndrome, clinical complications of these conditions are discussed earlier and in Chapters 8 and 10.

Starvation

Marasmus refers to a deficiency of calories from all sources. **Kwashiorkor** is a form of malnutrition in children caused by a diet deficient in protein alone.

Marasmus

Global starvation in children (i.e., a deficiency of all elements of the diet) produces marasmus. Pathologic changes are similar to those in starving adults and include decreased body weight, diminished subcutaneous fat, a protuberant abdomen, muscle wasting, and a wrinkled face. Wasting and increased lipofuscin pigment are seen in most visceral organs, especially the heart and the liver. Pulse, blood pressure, and temperature are low and diarrhea is common. Because immune responses are impaired, the child suffers from numerous infections. An important consequence of marasmus is **growth failure**. If these children are not provided with adequate food in childhood, they do not reach their full potential stature as adults. Severe marasmus accompanied by iron deficiency anemia in early childhood, when brain development is under way, may result in permanent intellectual deficits.

Kwashiorkor

Kwashiorkor (Fig. 19-44) results from a **deficiency of protein** in diets relatively high in carbohydrates. Like marasmus, it usually occurs after an infant is weaned, when a protein-poor diet, consisting principally of staple carbohydrates, replaces mother's milk. There is generalized growth failure and muscle wasting, as in marasmus, but subcutaneous fat is normal because caloric intake is adequate. Extreme apathy is notable, in contrast to children with marasmus, who may be alert. Also, in contrast to marasmus, severe edema, hepatomegaly, depigmentation of the skin, and dermatoses are usual. "Flaky paint" lesions of the skin on the face, extremities, and perineum are dry and hyperkeratotic. Hair becomes a sandy or reddish color; a characteristic linear depigmentation of the hair ("flag sign") provides evidence of particularly severe periods of protein deficiency. The abdomen is distended because of flaccid abdominal muscles, hepatomegaly, and ascites as a result of hypoalbuminemia. Along with general atrophy of the viscera, villous atrophy of the intestine may interfere with nutrient absorption. Diarrhea is common. Anemia is the rule, but it is not generally life-threatening. The nonspecific effects on growth, pulse, temperature, and the immune system are similar to those in marasmus.

Vitamin Deficiency and Toxicity

Vitamins are organic catalysts that are essential for normal metabolism and available only from dietary sources. Vitamin deficiencies are uncommon in all but the most disadvantaged populations in industrialized countries.

Vitamin A

Vitamin A is a fat-soluble substance that is important for skeletal maturation and maintenance of specialized epithelial linings and cell membrane structure. In addition, it is an important constituent of the photosensitive pigments in the retina. Also, vitamin A appears to be important in immune function and nonimmune defense mechanisms. Vitamin A occurs naturally as **retinoids** or as a precursor, **β-carotene**. The source of the precursor—carotene—is in plants, principally leafy, green vegetables. Fish livers are a particularly rich source of vitamin A itself (retinoids).

Vitamin A deficiency is associated with poor resistance to infection. Administration of vitamin A to deficient people reduces overall mortality. In addition, in underdeveloped countries, vitamin A supplementation to pregnant women and their children has reduced infant mortality.

β-Carotene is modified in the intestinal mucosa to retinoids, which are absorbed with chylomicrons. It is stored in the liver, where 90% of the body's vitamin A is located. At times when fat absorption is impaired (e.g., diarrhea), vitamin A absorption decreases.

Although vitamin A deficiency is uncommon in developed countries, it is a significant health problem in poorer regions of the world, including much of Africa, China, and Southeast Asia.

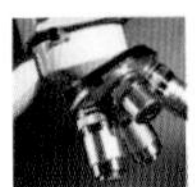

PATHOLOGY: *Deficiency of vitamin A results principally in squamous metaplasia, especially in glandular epithelium* (Fig. 19-45). As a result, persons with this vitamin deficiency may suffer numerous disorders. These include bronchopneumonia, xerophthalmia (dryness of cornea and conjunctiva), corneal ulceration, and blindness.

The earliest sign of vitamin A deficiency is often diminished vision in dim light. Vitamin A is a necessary component in retinal rod pigment and is active in light transduction. Because vitamin A aldehyde, termed retinal, is constantly degraded in generating the light signal, a continuous supply of vitamin A is necessary for night vision.

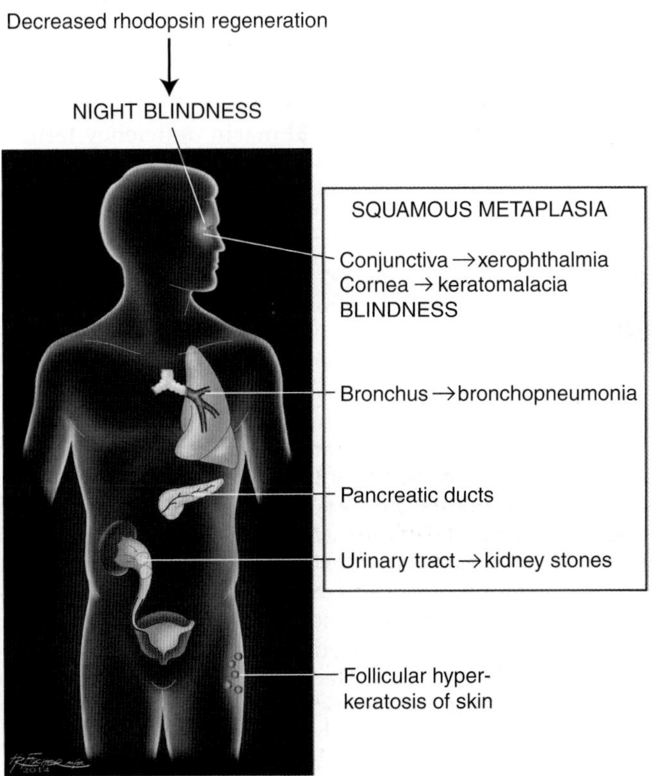

FIGURE 19-45. Complications of vitamin A deficiency.

Vitamin A toxicity

Vitamin A poisoning is usually caused by overenthusiastic administration of vitamin supplements to children. Enlargement of the liver and spleen is common; microscopically, these organs show lipid-laden macrophages. In the liver, vitamin A is also present in hepatocytes, and prolonged hypervitaminosis A has been incriminated in rare cases of cirrhosis. Bone pain and neurologic symptoms, such as hyperexcitability and headache, may be the presenting symptoms. Excessive carotene intake is benign and simply stains the skin yellow, which may be mistaken for jaundice.

Vitamin B Complex

Vitamins in the B group of water-soluble vitamins are numbered 1 through 12, but only eight are distinct vitamins (Table 19-8). Deficiencies of thiamine, riboflavin, and niacin are unusual in industrialized countries because bread and cereals are fortified with these vitamins.

Thiamine (B_1)

Thiamine is an essential cofactor in the activity of several enzymes crucial to energy metabolism, mainly in the tricarboxylic acid (Krebs) cycle. In Western countries, the disease occurs in alcoholics, people with poor overall nutrition, and food faddists. ***The cardinal symptoms of thiamine deficiency are polyneuropathy, edema, and cardiac failure*** (Fig. 19-46). The deficiency syndrome is classically divided into **dry beriberi**, with symptoms referable to the neuromuscular system, and **wet beriberi**, in which manifestations of cardiac failure predominate.

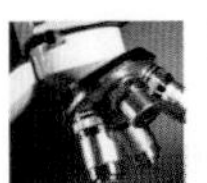

PATHOLOGY: A characteristic alteration in thiamine deficiency is myelin sheath degeneration, which often begins in the sciatic nerve and then involves other peripheral nerves and sometimes the spinal cord itself. In advanced cases, axon fragmentation may be seen. Thiamine deficiency in chronic alcoholics may be manifested by CNS involvement, in the form of **Wernicke syndrome**, in which progressive **dementia, ataxia, and ophthalmoplegia** (paralysis of the extraocular muscles) are prominent. The most striking lesions in Wernicke encephalopathy are found in the mammillary bodies and surrounding areas that abut on the third ventricle (see Chapter 24).

The changes in the heart are also nonspecific. Grossly, the heart is flabby, dilated, and increased in weight. The process

Table 19-8

B Vitamins

Vitamin	Biochemical Name
B_1	Thiamine
B_2	Riboflavin
B_3	Niacin
B_5	Pantothenic acid
B_6	Pyridoxine
B_7	Biotin
B_9	Folic acid
B_{12}	Cyanocobalamin

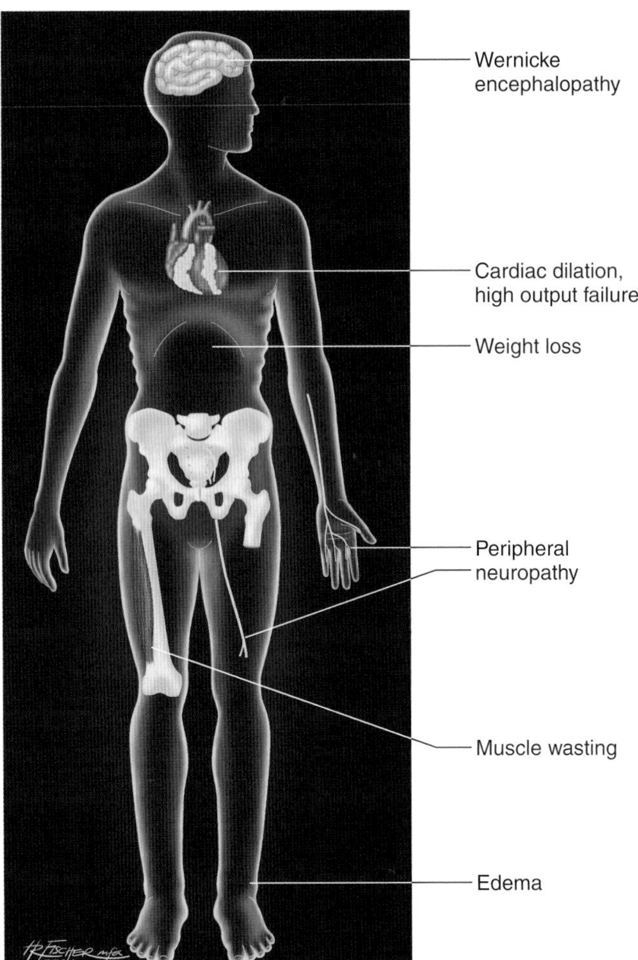

FIGURE 19-46. Complications of thiamine deficiency (beriberi).

may affect either the right or the left side of the heart or both. The microscopic changes are nondescript and include edema, inconsistent fiber hypertrophy, and occasional foci of fiber degeneration.

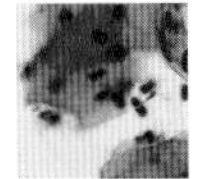

CLINICAL FEATURES: Patients with dry beriberi present with paresthesias, depressed reflexes, and weakness and muscle atrophy in the extremities. Wet beriberi is characterized by generalized edema, a reflection of severe high-output congestive failure secondary to extreme vasodilation.

Riboflavin (B_2)

Riboflavin is a vitamin derived from many plant and animal sources. It is important for the synthesis of flavin nucleotides, which are important in electron transport and other reactions in which energy transfer is crucial. Riboflavin is converted within the body to flavin mononucleotides and dinucleotides. Clinical symptoms of riboflavin deficiency are uncommon; they are usually seen only in debilitated patients with a variety of diseases and in poorly nourished alcoholics.

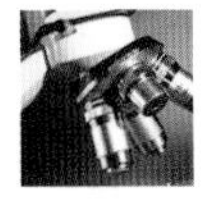 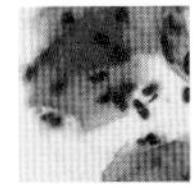

PATHOLOGY AND CLINICAL FEATURES: Riboflavin deficiency is usually seen in conjunction with deficiencies of other water-soluble vitamins. It is manifested principally by lesions of the facial skin and corneal epithelium. **Cheilosis**, a term used for fissures in the skin at the angles of the mouth, is a characteristic feature (Fig. 19-47). These cracks in the skin may be painful and often become infected.

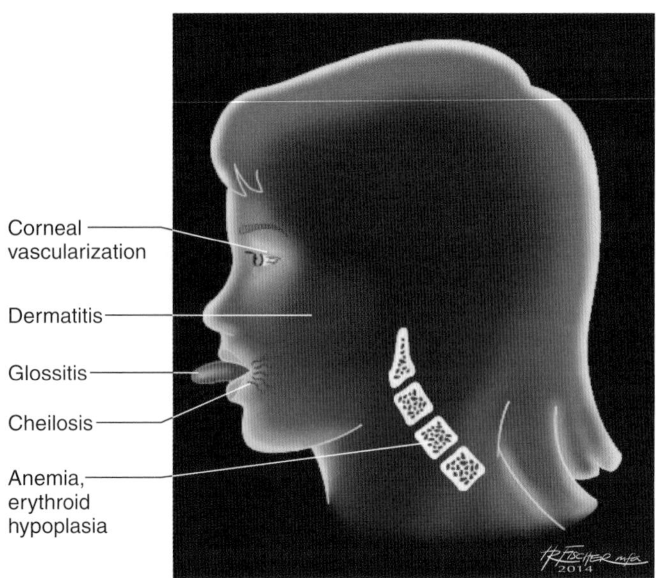

FIGURE 19-47. Complications of riboflavin deficiency.

Niacin (B_3)

Niacin (nicotinic acid) is derived from dietary sources or biosynthesized from tryptophan. In the body, nicotinic acid is converted to nicotinamide, which plays a major role in the formation of NAD. This compound and its phosphorylated derivative, NADP, are important in intermediary metabolism and an extensive variety of oxidation–reduction reactions. Animal protein, as found in meat, eggs, and milk, is high in tryptophan and is therefore a good source of endogenously synthesized niacin. Niacin itself is available in many types of grain. Clinical niacin deficiency termed pellagra is uncommon today and is seen principally in patients who have been weakened by other diseases and in malnourished alcoholics.

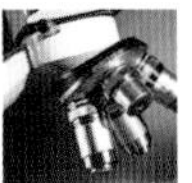

PATHOLOGY: Pellagra is characterized by the three "Ds" of niacin deficiency: **dermatitis, diarrhea,** and **dementia** (Fig. 19-48). Areas exposed to light, such as the face and the hands, and those subjected to pressure, for instance, the knees and the elbows, exhibit a rough, scaly dermatitis. The involvement of the hands leads to so-called glove dermatitis. Similar lesions are found in the mucous membranes of the mouth and vagina. In the mouth, inflammation and edema give rise to a large, red tongue, which in the chronic stage is fissured and is likened to raw meat. Chronic, watery diarrhea is typical for the disease, presumably a result of mucosal atrophy and ulceration in the entire gastrointestinal tract, particularly in the colon. Dementia, characterized by aberrant ideation bordering on psychosis, is represented in the brain by degeneration of ganglion cells in the cortex.

Pyridoxine (B_6)

Vitamin B_6 activity is found in three related, naturally occurring compounds: pyridoxine, pyridoxal, and pyridoxamine

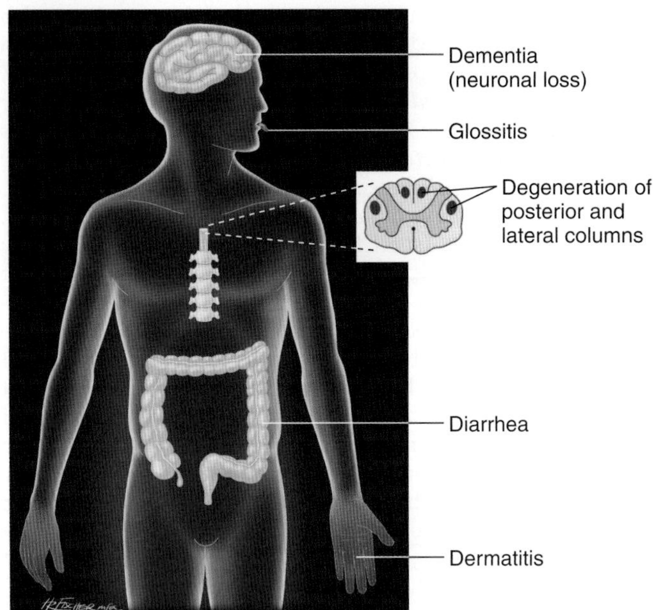

FIGURE 19-48. Complications of niacin deficiency (pellagra).

collectively termed pyridoxine. These compounds are widely distributed in vegetable and animal foods. Vitamin B_6 functions as a coenzyme in numerous metabolic pathways, including those related to amino acids, lipids, methylation, decarboxylation, gluconeogenesis, and heme and neurotransmitter synthesis. Some studies also suggest a role for vitamin B_6 in maintaining normal B- and T-cell immune function.

Pyridoxine deficiency is rarely caused by an inadequate diet. Of particular concern is the deficiency of pyridoxine that follows prolonged medication with a number of drugs, particularly isoniazid, cycloserine, and penicillamine. A deficiency state is also occasionally reported in alcoholics.

There are no clinical manifestations of pyridoxine deficiency that can be considered characteristic or pathognomonic. The usual dermatologic complications of other B-vitamin deficiencies occur with pyridoxine deficiency. ***The primary expression of the disease is in the CNS, a feature consistent with the role of this vitamin in the formation of pyridoxal-dependent decarboxylase of the neurotransmitter GABA.*** In infants and children, diarrhea, anemia, and seizures have occurred.

Biotin (B_7)

Most biotin is found in meats and cereals, where it is largely bound to protein. Biotin is an obligatory cofactor for five carboxylases that participate in intermediary metabolism, including the Krebs cycle.

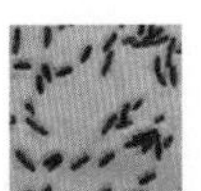

ETIOLOGIC FACTORS: Biotin deficiency is reported in people who consume large amounts of raw eggs that contain the biotin binding compound avidin. It also occurs in those with prolonged malabsorption syndrome and in children with severe protein-calorie malnutrition. Chronic administration of anticonvulsant drugs can also lead to biotin depletion.

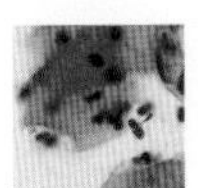

CLINICAL FEATURES: Symptoms of biotin deficiency include seborrheic and eczematous skin rash. In adults, neurologic symptoms are evidenced by lethargy, hallucinations, and paresthesias. In infants, hypotonia and developmental delay have been reported.

Folic Acid (B_9)

Folic acid is a heterocyclic derivative of glutamic acid and serves as a methyl group donor, especially in nucleotide synthesis. Folate, together with vitamin B_{12} (see later), is a key cofactor in methylation reactions. One of the key reactions in question is the conversion of homocysteine to methionine, which is needed to generate S-adenosyl methionine (SAM). SAM is a key methyl donor in the synthesis of neurotransmitters (norepinephrine to epinephrine), phospholipids (phosphatidylethanolamine to phosphatidylcholine), methylated nucleotides, and histones. Folate and vitamin B_{12} are also critical in the generation of purine nucleotides and in the conversion of uracil to thymidine. The latter reaction is important for understanding the consequences of folate deficiency in causing megaloblastic anemia (see Chapter 18).

Folate is present in almost all foods, including meat, dairy products, seafood, cereals, and vegetables. Deficiency is thus usually a consequence of a generally poor diet, as is seen in some alcoholics, rather than a diet deficient in any single constituent. Malabsorption syndromes may also result in folate deficiency. Because the settings in which folate deficiency occurs affect many nutrients, isolated folate deficiency is rare.

Importantly, folate supplements given during early pregnancy have been shown to decrease the incidence of fetal neural tube defects. Because neural tube formation occurs before many women know they are pregnant, fortification of cereal and grain products with folic acid is mandated in the United States.

Cyanocobalamin (B_{12})

Deficiency of vitamin B_{12} is characteristic of pernicious anemia and results from the lack of secretion of intrinsic factor in the stomach (see Chapter 11), which is necessary for absorption of the vitamin in the ileum.

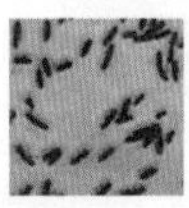

ETIOLOGIC FACTORS: Because vitamin B_{12} is found in almost all animal protein, including meat, milk, and eggs, dietary deficiency is seen only in rare cases of extreme vegetarianism and then only after many years of a restricted diet. Parasitization of the small intestine by the fish tapeworm *Diphyllobothrium latum* (from undercooked fish) may lead to vitamin B_{12} deficiency because the parasite absorbs the vitamin in the gut lumen.

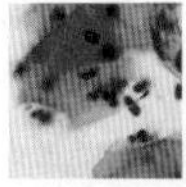

CLINICAL FEATURES: Deficiency of vitamin B_{12} is associated with megaloblastic anemia. In addition, pernicious anemia is complicated by a neurologic condition termed subacute combined degeneration of the spinal cord. A comprehensive discussion of vitamin B_{12} deficiency is found in Chapter 18.

Vitamin C (Ascorbic Acid)

The effects of vitamin C deficiency, namely **scurvy**, have been known for millennia. Ascorbic acid is a water-soluble vitamin that is a powerful biologic reducing agent. It is involved in many oxidation/reduction reactions and in proton transfer. The vitamin is important for chondroitin sulfate synthesis and for proline hydroxylation to form hydroxyproline of collagen. Ascorbic acid serves many other important functions: it prevents oxidation of tetrahydrofolate and augments absorption of iron from the gut. Without vitamin C, biosynthesis of certain neurotransmitters is impaired, leading to, for example, a reduction in dopamine β-hydroxylase activity. Wound healing and immune functions are also impaired in deficiency of ascorbic acid. The best dietary sources of vitamin C are citrus fruits, green vegetables, and tomatoes.

Scurvy is today uncommon in the Western world, but is often noted in nonindustrialized countries, where other forms of malnutrition are prevalent. In industrialized countries, scurvy is now a disease of people afflicted with chronic diseases who do not eat well, the aged, and malnourished alcoholics.

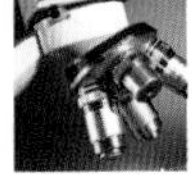

PATHOLOGY: *Most of the events associated with vitamin C deficiency are caused by formation of abnormal collagen that lacks tensile strength* (Fig. 19-49). Within 1 to 3 months, subperiosteal hemorrhages produce pain in bones and joints. Petechial hemorrhages, ecchymoses, and purpura are common, particularly after mild trauma or at pressure points. Perifollicular hemorrhages in the skin are particularly typical of scurvy. In advanced cases, swollen, bleeding gums are a classic finding. Alveolar bone resorption results in loss of teeth. Wound healing is poor, and dehiscence of previously healed wounds occurs. Anemia may result from prolonged bleeding, impaired iron absorption, or associated folic acid deficiency.

Vitamin D

Vitamin D is a fat-soluble steroid hormone found in two forms: vitamin D_3 (cholecalciferol) and vitamin D_2 (ergocalciferol), both of which have equal biologic potency in humans. Vitamin D_3 is produced in the skin and vitamin D_2 is derived from plant ergosterol. The vitamin is absorbed in the jejunum along with fats and is transported in the blood bound to an α-globulin (vitamin D–binding protein). ***To achieve biologic potency, vitamin D must be hydroxylated to active metabolites in the liver and kidney. The active form of the vitamin promotes calcium and phosphate absorption from the small intestine and may directly influence mineralization of bone.***

In children, vitamin D deficiency causes ***rickets****; in adults,* ***osteomalacia*** *occurs* (see Chapter 22). Vitamin D deficiency results from (1) insufficient dietary vitamin D, (2) inadequate production of vitamin D in the skin because of limited sunlight exposure, (3) poor absorption of vitamin D from the diet (as in the fat malabsorption syndromes), or (4) impaired conversion of vitamin D to its bioactive metabolites. The last occurs in liver disease and chronic renal failure. Addition of vitamin D to milk and many processed foods, administration of vitamin preparations to young children, and generally improved levels of nutrition have made rickets a curiosity in industrialized countries.

Hypervitaminosis D

The most common cause of excess vitamin D is the inordinate consumption of vitamin preparations. Deficient conversion of vitamin D to biologically active metabolites is occasionally seen in granulomatous diseases such as sarcoidosis. In cases of calcium

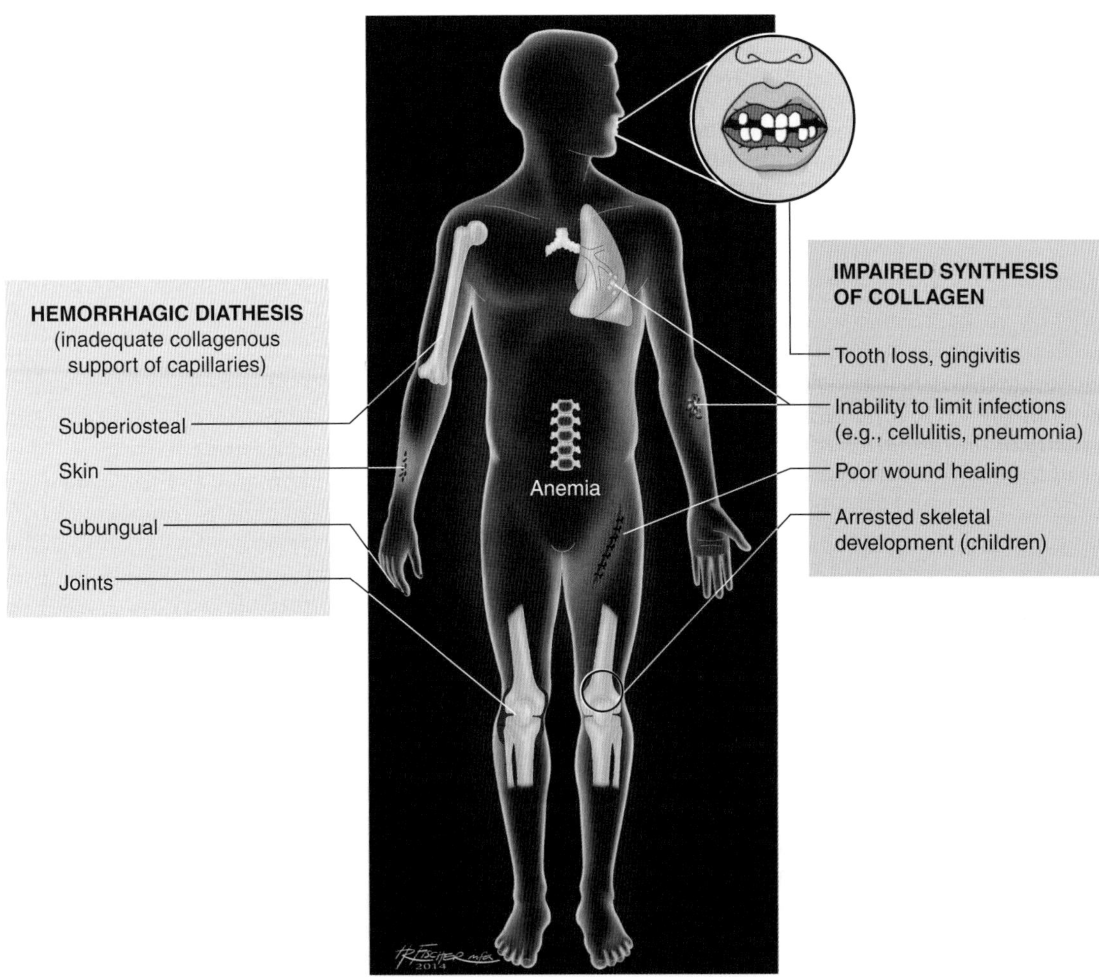

FIGURE 19-49. Complications of vitamin C deficiency (scurvy).

malabsorption, when the underlying disease is corrected, the sensitivity of target tissues to vitamin D is increased. The initial response to excess vitamin D is **hypercalcemia**, which results in nonspecific symptoms, such as weakness and headaches. Increased renal calcium excretion results in **nephrolithiasis** or **nephrocalcinosis. Ectopic calcification** in other organs, such as blood vessels, heart, and lungs, may occur.

Vitamin E

Vitamin E is an antioxidant that (experimentally) protects membrane phospholipids against lipid peroxidation by free radicals formed by cellular metabolism. The activity of this fat-soluble vitamin is found in a number of dietary constituents, principally in α-tocopherol. Corn and soy beans are particularly rich in vitamin E.

Dietary deficiency of vitamin E can occur in children as a result of mutations in the α-tocopherol transfer protein and in adults with various malabsorption syndromes. The deficiency may present clinically as spinocerebellar ataxia, skeletal myopathy, and pigmented retinopathy.

Vitamin K

Vitamin K, a fat-soluble compound, occurs in two forms: vitamin K_1 from plants and vitamin K_2 that is principally synthesized by the normal intestinal bacteria. Green leafy vegetables are rich in vitamin K, and liver and dairy products contain smaller amounts.

Dietary deficiency is very uncommon in the United States; most cases are associated with other disorders. Vitamin K deficiency is common in severe fat malabsorption, as seen in sprue and biliary tract obstruction. Destruction of intestinal flora by antibiotics may also result in vitamin K deficiency. Newborn infants may exhibit vitamin K deficiency because the vitamin is not transported well across the placenta, and the sterile gut of the newborn does not have bacteria to produce it. Vitamin K confers calcium-binding properties to certain proteins and is important for the activity of four clotting factors: prothrombin, factor VII, factor IX, and factor X. *Deficiency of vitamin K can be serious, because it can lead to catastrophic bleeding.* Parenteral vitamin K therapy is rapidly effective (see Chapter 18).

Essential Trace Minerals

Essential trace minerals include iron, copper, iodine, zinc, cobalt, selenium, manganese, nickel, chromium, tin, molybdenum, vanadium, silicon, and fluorine. Dietary deficiencies of these minerals are clinically important in the case of iron and iodine. These are discussed earlier and in Chapter 18.

20 The Skin

Ronnie M. Abraham ▪ Emily Y. Chu ▪ David E. Elder

LEARNING OBJECTIVES

- Describe the histologic layers of the epidermis and dermis.
- What are two distinguishing structural products of keratinocytes?
- Describe the origin, function, and histology of the following cells: melanocytes, Langerhans cells, and Merkel cells.
- Describe the structure and function of the basement membrane zone of the skin.
- Describe the structure of hair follicles and outline the process of hair growth.
- Distinguish between androgenetic alopecia and alopecia areata.
- What are the potential molecular mechanisms responsible for ichthyoses?
- What is the characteristic ratio between the stratum corneum and the nucleated epidermal layers in ichthyoses versus chronically irritated skin, as found in lichen simplex chronicus?
- Delineate the factors implicated in the molecular pathogenesis of psoriasis.
- Describe the histopathology and clinical consequences of psoriasis.
- Define the terms "hyperkeratosis" and "parakeratosis."
- Describe the molecular pathogenesis, histopathology, and clinical consequences of pemphigus vulgaris.
- Distinguish between the following blistering diseases of the dermal–epidermal interface in terms of molecular mechanism, histopathology, and clinical consequences: epidermolysis simplex, junctional epidermolysis bullosa, bullous pemphigoid, dermatitis herpetiformis, and erythema multiforme.
- Distinguish between the histopathology and clinical consequences of chronic cutaneous (discoid) lupus erythematosus and acute systemic disease.
- Explain the term "lichenoid inflammation" of the skin. What role does it play in the pathogenesis of lichen planus?
- How does the histopathology of cutaneous necrotizing vasculitis account for the disease's presentation as palpable purpura?
- Describe the mechanism of delayed hypersensitivity. Use contact dermatitis relating to *Rhus* as an example.
- Describe the etiology and pathogenesis of erythema nodosum. What is a common clinical presentation of the disease?
- Differentiate between septal and lobular panniculitis.
- Describe the etiologic factors and pathogenesis of acne vulgaris.
- Define the term "dermatophyte" and list several common dermatophytic infections.
- Describe the appearance, etiology, and molecular pathogenesis of melanocytic nevi.
- What histopathologic features differentiate dysplastic from simple melanocytic nevi?
- Describe the growth pattern of superficial spreading melanoma. What are the molecular changes associated with the disease?
- What are the clinical consequences of superficial spreading melanoma in the radial growth phase?
- Define the "ABCDE" rule.
- What are the characteristic histopathologic features of the vertical growth phase of melanoma?
- Differentiate between nodular melanoma, lentigo maligna melanoma, and acral lentiginous melanoma in terms of histopathology and clinical signs.
- What are important factors considered in staging and defining the prognosis of melanoma?
- What is Breslow thickness?
- Describe the etiology and histopathology of verruca vulgaris.
- Differentiate between the following keratotic conditions: seborrheic keratosis, actinic keratosis, and keratoacanthoma.
- Describe the etiology, molecular pathogenesis, histopathology, and clinical consequences of basal cell carcinoma and squamous cell carcinoma of the skin.
- What is the pathologic appearance and clinical consequences of Merkel cell carcinoma?
- List common adnexal tumors and their likely cell of origin.
- Describe the etiology and histopathology of mycosis fungoides.
- Describe the etiology and histopathology of Kaposi sarcoma.
- What is the appearance and clinical significance of acanthosis nigricans?

HISTOLOGY OF THE SKIN

KERATINOCYTES: The epidermis is a multilayered sheet of keratin-producing cells. It forms undulating folds at the interface with the dermis, called **dermal papillae.** A progressive change in morphology occurs from (1) the replicating columnar cells of the basal layer (**stratum basalis**), (2) through the spinous (**stratum spinosum**) and the granular layers (**stratum granulosum**), to (3) the nonviable flattened cells of the cornified layer (**stratum corneum**) (Figs. 20-1 and 20-2). The basal cells harbor most of the mitotic activity of the epidermis. As keratinocytes approach the surface, they lose their nuclei and form flattened plates of dead cells on the outer boundary of the skin (the cornified or keratin layer). Keratinocytes synthesize sulfur-poor, filamentous **tonofibrils**, which are composed of varying blends of acidic and basic intermediate keratin filaments; they result in over 30 different keratins that are responsible for structures, such as the stratum corneum, hair, and nails. Bundles of tonofibrils converge on, and terminate at, the plasma membrane in attachment plates, called **desmosomes**.

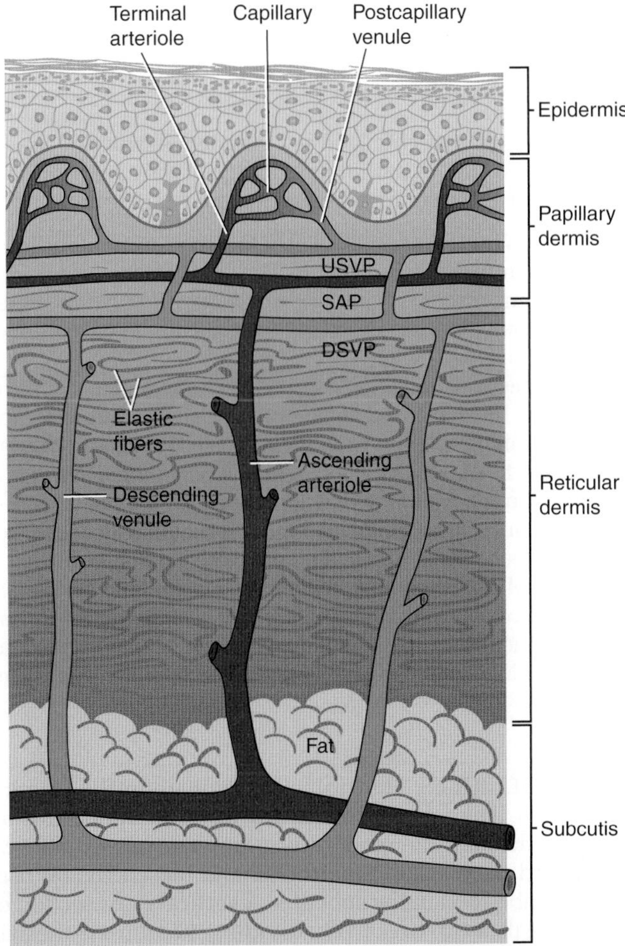

FIGURE 20-1. The dermis and its vasculature. The dermis is divided into two distinct anatomic regions. The papillary dermis with its vascular plexus and the epidermis usually react together in diseases that are primarily limited to the skin. The reticular dermis and the subcutis are altered in association with systemic diseases that manifest in the skin. DSVP, deep superficial venular plexus; SAP, superficial arterial plexus; USVP, upper superficial venular plexus.

Keratinocytes are also distinguished by two other structural products: "**keratohyaline granules**" and **"Odland bodies."** Keratohyaline granules are the defining feature of the granular layer and are composed of a histidine-rich, electron-dense, basophilic protein—profilaggrin—which is associated with intermediate filaments. Odland bodies (keratinosomes or lamellar bodies) are the only structurally distinctive, epidermal secretory product (Fig. 20-3). They form in the outer spinous and granular layers and discharge their contents into intercellular spaces, appearing there as lamellar masses parallel to the surface of the skin. Odland bodies and the discharged lamellated products are most obvious in the outer granular layer and are related to epidermal barrier function.

The epidermis harbors immigrant cells of neuroectodermal and mesenchymal origin, which do not synthesize keratin but have their own highly distinctive organelles. Their numbers vary among the several different levels of the epidermis. Two of these cells, **melanocytes** and **Langerhans cells**, are dendritic. The third, the **Merkel cell**, is associated with a terminal neuronal axon (Fig. 20-2).

*MELANOCYTES: **Melanocytes are dendritic cells of neural crest origin that largely determine skin color.*** They lie in the basal layer of the epidermis, separated from the dermis by the epidermal basement membrane zone. A single melanocyte may supply dendrites to over 30 keratinocytes.

The **melanosome** is a cytoplasmic membrane–bound complex in which melanin is synthesized. When melanin synthesis is active, melanosomes contain filaments in parallel arrays along the long axis of the organelle. As they mature, the orderly internal structure of melanosomes is progressively obliterated, and they become electron-opaque granules. These structures are transferred to keratinocytes, where they form a supranuclear cap, protecting the nuclear material from ultraviolet light.

Skin color is largely based on the number, size, and packaging of melanosomes in keratinocytes. In hair and epidermal keratinocytes, melanins are packaged and absorb and reflect visible light, thereby forming the integumentary colors.

LANGERHANS CELLS: These cells arrive in embryonic skin in the last month of the first trimester, following the melanocytes by a month. These HLA-DR–positive cells allow skin to recognize and process antigens, and so become a part of the immune system. Langerhans cells are uncommon in the dermis but are distributed throughout the nucleated layers of the epidermis, where they constitute about 4% of the cells. They are difficult to see by routine light microscopy. In electron micrographs, their cytoplasm contains a moderate number of specialized organelles, termed **Birbeck granules.** In two dimensions, these structures appear to be racquet shaped, but three-dimensional reconstruction shows them to be cup shaped. These unique organelles are derived from the plasma membrane and probably participate in antigen presentation by Langerhans cells (antigenic material being internalized into Birbeck granules). Langerhans cells express MHC-I, MHC-II, and receptors for Fc IgG and Fc IgE.

MERKEL CELLS: Although sometimes classified as "immigrant" cells, Merkel cells may be specialized basal keratinocytes. They form desmosomes with keratinocytes and express keratins similarly to the latter. Merkel cells do not appear in all areas of the epidermis but are seen in special regions, such as the lips, oral cavity, external root sheaths of hair follicles, and palmar skin of the digits. They have a distinctive organelle, a membrane-bound, dense-core granule, 100 nm or wider.

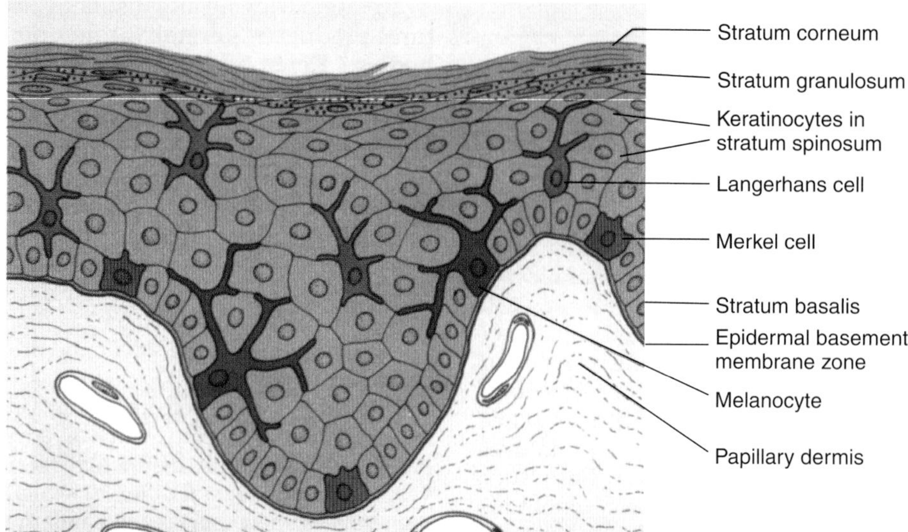

FIGURE 20-2. Normal epidermis and the epidermal immigrant cells. Keratinocytes form the multilayered epidermis, protecting against water loss and bacterial invasion. Melanocytes provide color as well as protection against ultraviolet radiation. Langerhans cells are among the cells responsible for the skin's function as an immunologic organ. Merkel cells may represent one of the enablers of tactile function of the skin.

The basal aspect of the cell is apposed to a small nerve plate that connects to a myelinated axon by a short, nonmyelinated axon. This complex structure may be a tactile mechanoreceptor.

BASEMENT MEMBRANE: The basement membrane zone (BMZ) is an interface between the dermis and epidermis and is as diverse in function as it is complex in structure (Fig. 20-4). It mediates dermal–epidermal adherence and probably acts as a selective macromolecular filter as well. It is also a site of immunoglobulin and complement deposition in certain cutaneous diseases. Most structures of the BMZ are elaborated by epidermal cells. The basal lamina is the primary organizational feature of the BMZ and is responsible for epithelial cell polarity as well as some keratin gene expression. The basal lamina is divided into a **lamina lucida**, an electron-lucent layer containing adherence proteins, and a **lamina densa**, composed principally of type IV collagen.

The **dermis** is a complex organization of connective tissue deep to the BMZ, containing mostly collagen, which is embedded in a ground substance rich in hyaluronic acid. The dermis has two zones:

- *PAPILLARY DERMIS:* The papillary dermis is a narrow zone immediately below the BMZ of the epidermis. It has a pale pink eosinophilic appearance and has little organization when viewed with the light microscope (Figs. 20-1 and 20-2). Delicate collagen fibrils are the most apparent structures. This fine connective tissue extends into the dermal papillae and also functions as a sheath about blood vessels, nerves, and adnexal structures. This entire network of periadnexal collagen is known as the **adventitial dermis**. The papillary dermis is generally altered in epidermal diseases and disorders affecting the superficial vascular bed. The epidermis, papillary dermis, and superficial vascular bed react jointly and influence each other in complex ways.
- *RETICULAR DERMIS:* The reticular *dermis* is deep to the papillary dermis and contains most of the dermal collagen, which is organized into coarse bundles and is associated with elastic fibers (Fig. 20-1). The reticular dermis and subcutis (also recognized as a cutaneous structure) are less common sites of pathologic change. If they are diseased, it is often as a manifestation of a systemic disorder.

CUTANEOUS VASCULATURE: Circulating blood in the skin has a number of functions. The skin, via its vascular network, is important in temperature regulation. Many aspects of cutaneous inflammation involve the superficial cutaneous vasculature (Fig. 20-1).

Cutaneous lymphatic vessels form a random network, starting as lymphatic capillaries near the epidermis. A superficial lymphatic plexus then sends forth lymphatic channels that drain to regional lymph nodes. Lymphatic channels are involved in the drainage of tissue fluids and metastasis of cutaneous cancers, especially malignant melanoma. Cutaneous lymphatics have, at best, an incomplete basal lamina.

Mast cells are derived from the bone marrow and are normally present around dermal venules. They release vasoactive and chemotactic substances, mediate all types of inflammation, and proliferate in a spectrum of diseases, called **urticaria pigmentosa**.

Hair

HAIR FOLLICLES: Hair follicles originate in the primitive epidermis. They grow downward through the dermis and upward through the epidermis. Growing hairs of the scalp and beard have bulbs of epithelial and mesenchymal tissue firmly embedded in the subcutis. A vertical cross section of a bulb reveals a cap of actively dividing, keratin-synthesizing cells. These cells become arrayed in layers that join at the top of the bulb to form the cylindrical hair shaft. The differentiating hairs form the roof of the epithelial bulb and interact with an island of melanocytes that contribute melanin to the passing keratinocytes. **This process results in hair color.** The colored keratinocytes lose their nuclei as they form the final product, the cylindrical hair shaft. Curly hair is formed from angulated bulbs; straight hair develops from round bulbs.

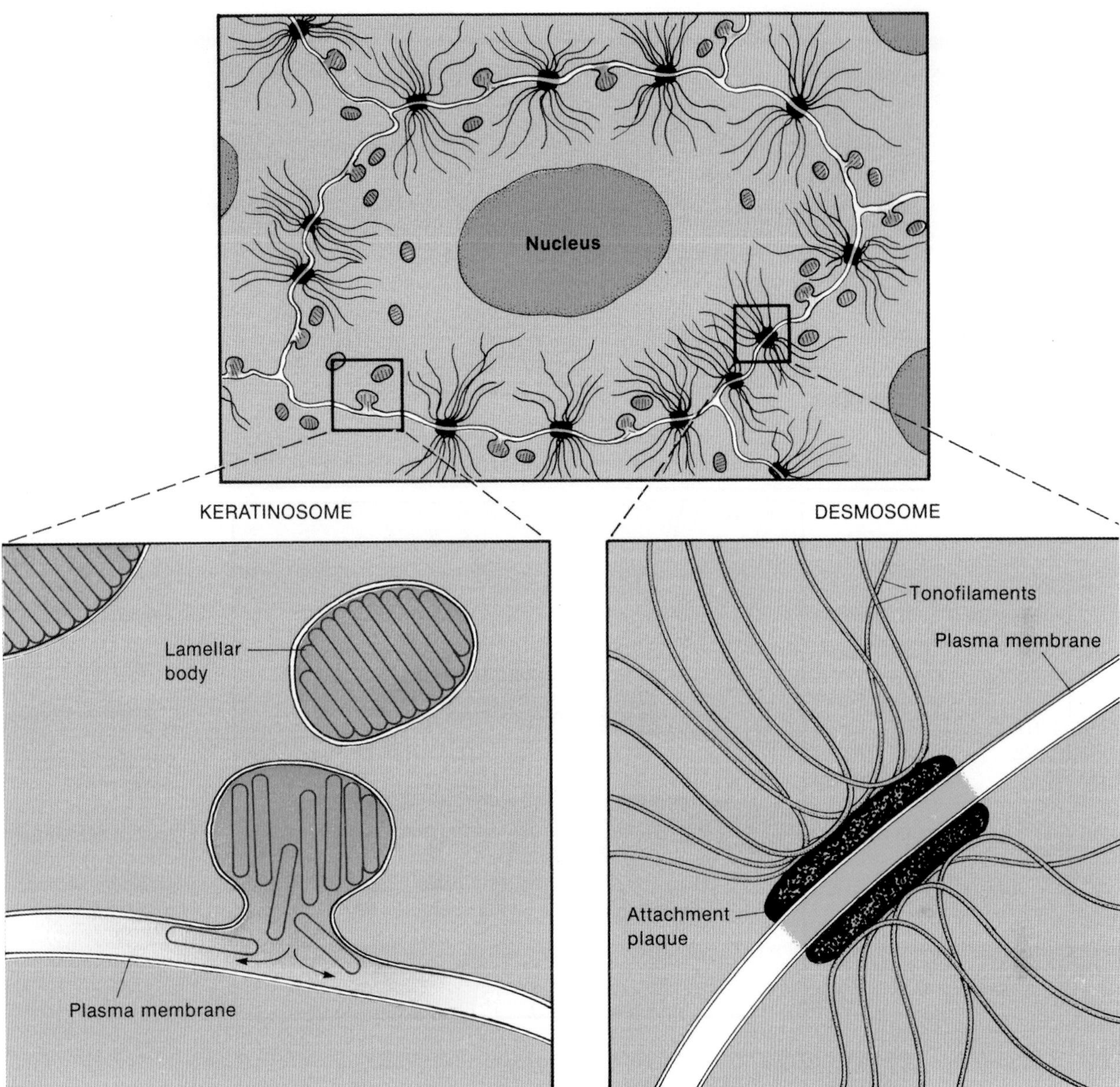

FIGURE 20-3. The keratinocyte, keratinosome, and desmosome. The keratinocyte cytoplasm is dominated by delicate keratin fibrils, the tonofilaments. These are part of the cytoskeleton of the cell and loop within the attachment plaque of the desmosome. The lamellar body of the keratinocyte extrudes its contents into the intercellular space. This material probably has a role in cellular cohesion.

THE HAIR CYCLE: Hair grows in a cyclical manner. At any given time, 90% of hairs are normally in the actively growing, or **anagen**, phase. These hairs are interspersed with others that show no evidence of active growth, termed **telogen** hairs. Hairs in the process of ceasing growth, namely, **catagen** hairs, still have hair shafts. Catagen hairs end in the lower reticular dermis as slightly widened clublike structures, each surrounded by a rim of nucleated keratinocytes. Hair bulbs are no longer evident, and the lamina densa around the catagen hair is strikingly thickened.

VELLUS HAIRS: These fine hairs may play a role in touch perception in many mammals, but in humans, they have no function.

SEBACEOUS FOLLICLES: These structures develop with puberty and are the sites of **acne**. Sebaceous follicles have a minute vellus hair at the base. The central face has large sebaceous glands that dwarf the vellus hairs and fill the follicular canal with sebum.

Alopecia

Alopecia, commonly known as baldness, is loss of hair. **Androgenetic alopecia,** or **common alopecia**, affects both men and women and results from a complex and poorly understood interaction of heritable and hormonal factors. Men castrated before puberty retain scalp hair and fail to grow a beard. On the other hand, administering testosterone to such castrated men results in growth of a beard and male-pattern baldness. Loss of scalp hair leads to replacement of large terminal hair follicles by tiny "vellus" hair follicles, the source of the delicate "fuzz" on the cheeks of women and the upper cheeks of men.

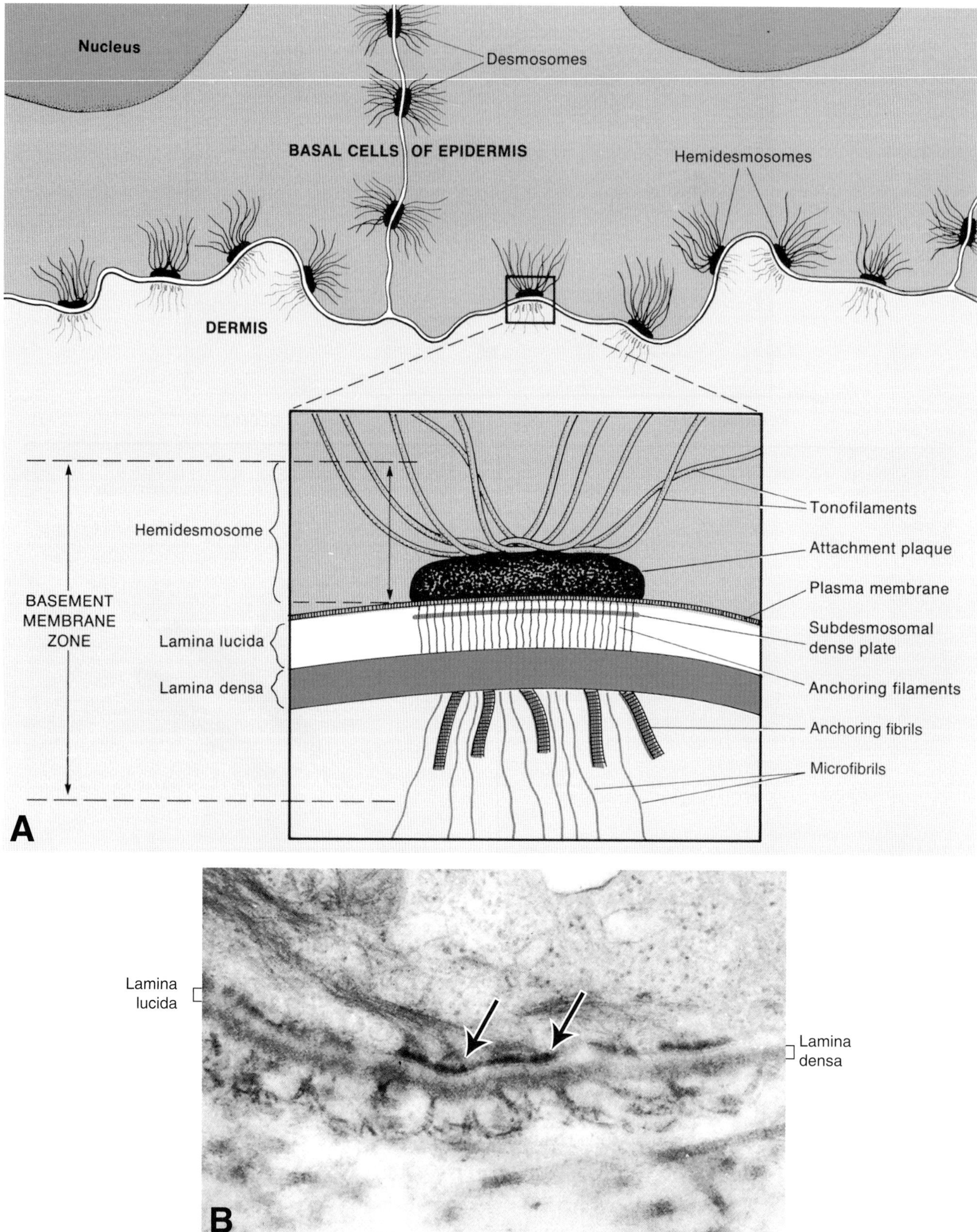

FIGURE 20-4. The dermal–epidermal interface and the basement membrane zone. A. This epithelial–mesenchymal interface is the site of the basement membrane zone, a complex structure that is mostly synthesized by the basal cells of the epidermis. Each of its complex structures is a site of change in specific disease, from tonofilaments and attachment plaques of basal cells to anchoring fibrils and microfibrils. **B.** An electron micrograph showing the hemidesmosomal attachment plaques with their inserting tonofilaments (*arrow*). The subdesmosomal dense plates, the lamina lucida, the lamina densa, and the subjacent anchoring fibrils are well demonstrated.

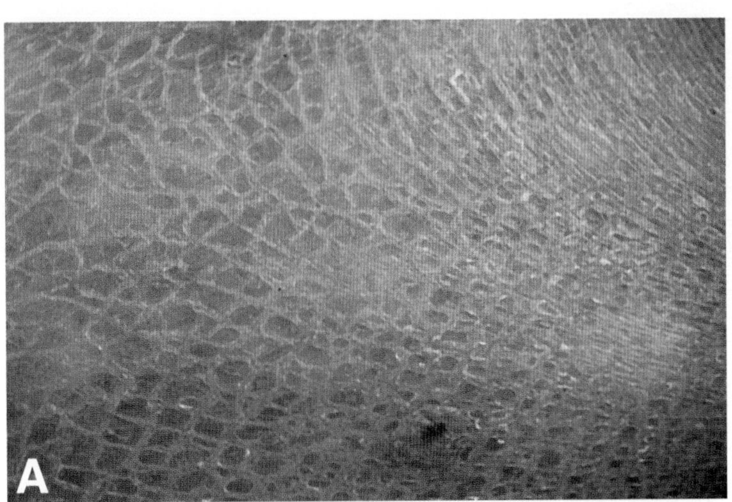
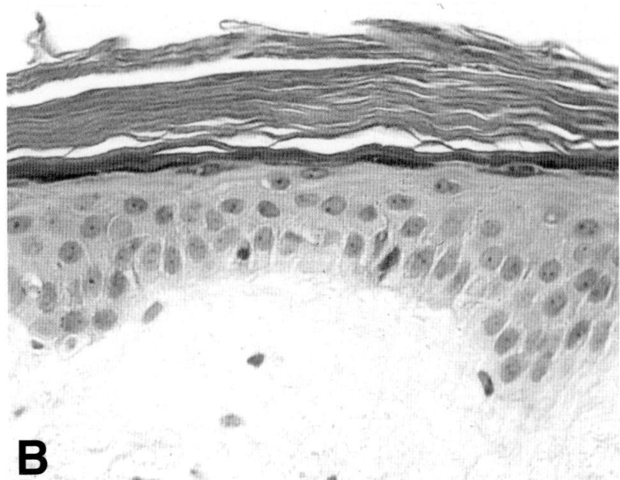

FIGURE 20-5. Ichthyosis vulgaris. A. Noninflammatory fishlike scales are evident on the thigh of a patient with a strong family history of ichthyosis vulgaris. **B.** There is disproportionate thickening of the stratum corneum relative to the normal thickness of the nucleated epidermal layer. The stratum granulosum is thin and focally absent. 20-5A From Elder AD, Elenitsas R, Johnson BL, et al. *Synopsis and Atlas of Lever's Histopathology of the Skin*. Philadelphia, PA: Lippincott Williams & Wilkins; 1999.

Actively growing hair is a site of mitosis. Many systemic diseases inhibit hair mitosis and give rise to alopecia. If the condition passes, mitotic activity is renewed and hair regrows. If a patient is treated with potent antimitotic drugs (e.g., chemotherapy), hair follicles stop growing, the hair is lost, and a telogen follicle follows. When therapy stops, hair cycling resumes. Almost any kind of follicular inflammation can trigger the telogen phase. The synchronous onset of telogen hairs in multiple follicles may result in rapid hair loss, called "telogen effluvium."

Alopecia areata is a circumscribed area of hair loss, usually on the scalp, although other body areas may be involved. Brisk lymphocytic infiltrates around the hair bulb result in formation of telogen hairs and hair loss. This pattern and its association with the inheritance of HLA class II alleles (especially HLA-DQ3) suggest an autoimmune etiology. Generally, scarring does not occur, and hair may regrow normally after varying time periods. **Alopecia totalis** is an autoimmune disease that causes loss of all body hair. Aside from cosmetic problems, it is harmless.

DISEASES OF THE EPIDERMIS

Ichthyoses

Ichthyosiform dermatoses, many of which are heritable, are diverse diseases characterized by thickening of the stratum corneum. The term **ichthyosis** reflects the similarity of the diseased skin to coarse, fishlike scales (Fig. 20-5). Several rare ichthyoses are associated with other abnormalities, such as abnormal lipid metabolism, neurologic or bone diseases, and cancer.

MOLECULAR PATHOGENESIS: Three general defects are involved in the excessive epidermal cornification of ichthyoses:

- **Increased cohesiveness** of the cells of the stratum corneum, possibly reflecting altered lipid metabolism
- **Abnormal keratinization**, manifested as impaired tonofilament formation, keratohyaline synthesis, and excessive cornification
- **Increased basal cell proliferation**, associated with a decrease in transit time of keratinocytes across the epidermis

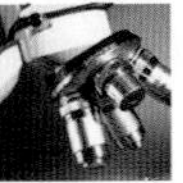

PATHOLOGY: In all ichthyoses, the stratum corneum is *disproportionately* thick compared to the nucleated epidermal layers. By contrast, other diseases characterized by thickening of the nucleated epidermal layers exhibit a *proportional* hyperkeratosis. For example, chronic scratching or rubbing of normal skin causes a thickened epidermis, hyperkeratosis, and dermal fibrosis, a condition known as **lichen simplex chronicus**. In this entity, the nucleated epidermis and stratum corneum may each be threefold thicker than normal. By contrast, in ichthyosis, although the stratum corneum may be five times thicker than normal, it overlies a disproportionately thin nucleated epidermis. There are a number of different icthyotic conditions:

- **Ichthyosis vulgaris** is the prototype of disproportionate corneal thickening and is the most common of the ichthyoses. The condition is an autosomal dominant disorder of keratinization, characterized by hyperkeratosis and reduced or absent epidermal keratohyaline granules (Fig. 20-6). Scaly skin results from increased cohesiveness of the stratum corneum. The attenuated stratum granulosum is a single layer with small, defective keratohyaline granules, and often appears absent. The stratum corneum differs from normal only in amount. The granular layer is greatly diminished and is often absent. ***Decreased or absent synthesis of* profilaggrin*, a keratin filament "glue," is responsible for these defects.*** The condition begins in early childhood. Small white scales occur on the extensor surfaces of extremities and on the trunk and face. The disease is lifelong, but with topical treatment, most patients can be maintained free of scales.

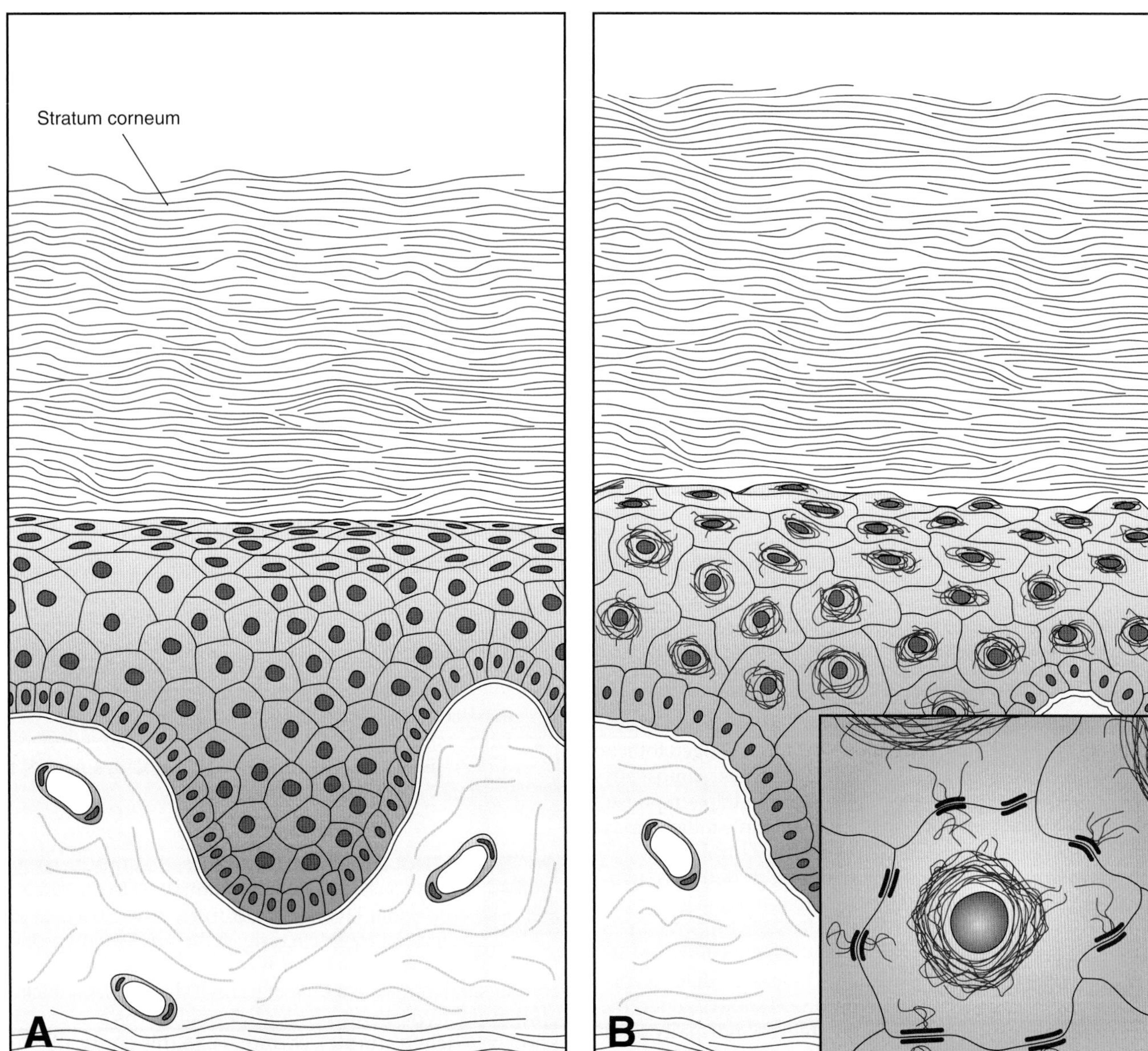

FIGURE 20-6. **Icthyoses. A. Ichthyosis vulgaris. B. Epidermolytic hyperkeratosis.** Both diseases are characterized by thickening of the stratum corneum relative to the nucleated layers. Epidermolytic hyperkeratosis is characterized by abnormal keratin synthesis, manifested by whorled keratin filaments about the nucleus (*inset*).

- **X-linked icthyosis** is a heritable epidermal disorder that, in recessive form, is characterized by delayed dissolution of desmosomal disks in the stratum corneum, owing to a deficiency of steroid sulfatase. Failure of steroid sulfatase action on cholesterol sulfate leads to persistent cohesion of the stratum corneum, but unlike icthyosis vulgaris, the granular layer is preserved.
- **Epidermolytic hyperkeratosis** is a congenital, autosomal dominant ichthyosis, which features generalized erythroderma, ichthyosiform skin, and blistering. It is thus also known as "bullous congenital ichthyosiform erythroderma." This disease results from mutations in the K1 or K10 keratin genes, which encode the keratins in the suprabasal epidermis. These abnormalities result (1) in faulty assembly of keratin tonofilaments, (2) impair their insertion into desmosomes, and (3) give rise to epidermal "lysis" and a tendency to form vesicles. Suprabasal keratinocytes contain thick, eosinophilic tonofilaments that whorl around the nucleus in a concentric manner (Figs. 20-6 and 20-7). The cytoplasm has a clear zone (vacuolization) around the perinuclear tonofilaments, but these filaments again condense at the outer margins of the cell. The stratum corneum is disproportionately thickened (Fig. 20-6). Epidermolytic hyperkeratosis manifests with generalized or localized blistering at or shortly after birth. Lesions tend to appear dark and even verrucous. Other than cosmetic disfigurement, the major problem is secondary bacterial infection.
- **Lamellar icthyosis** is an autosomal recessive congenital disorder of cornification, which is characterized by severe and generalized ichthyosis. Typically, increased cohesiveness of the stratum corneum is accompanied by numerous keratinosomes and an abnormally large amount of intercellular substance. The disease is genetically heterogeneous

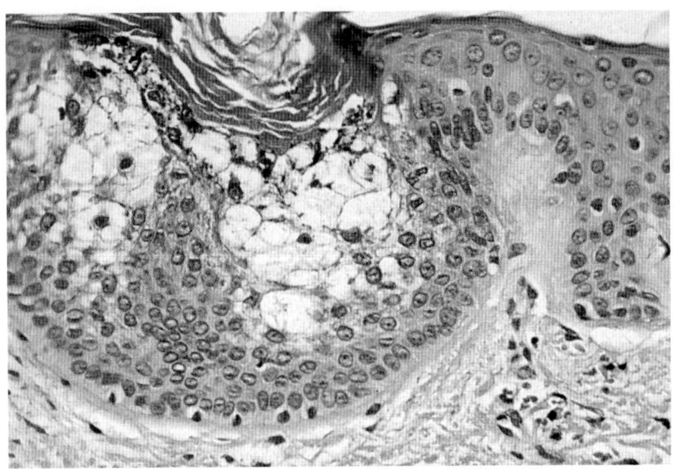

FIGURE 20-7. Epidermolytic hyperkeratosis. The keratinocytes of the stratum spinosum have clumped tonofilaments. As a result, their cytoplasm is relatively clear. In the outer stratum spinosum, the clumped fibrils are further compacted and whorl about the nuclei, resulting in dark cytoplasm condensed about the nuclei. These cells separate from each other to produce epidermolysis. A normal portion of epidermis is seen on the *right*.

but is often caused by mutations in the gene encoding transglutaminase 1 (*TGM1*; chromosome 14q11), resulting in defective lamellar body (Odland body) secretion.

- **Darier disease**, also called **keratosis follicularis**, and the similar **Hailey–Hailey disease**, are autosomal dominant conditions characterized by multifocal keratoses. The diseases are linked to defects in the intercellular matrix caused by mutations in the genes for two calcium pumps of the endoplasmic reticulum (*ATP2A2* on chromosome 12q23-24 and the *ATP2C1* gene on chromosome 3, respectively). The warty papule of Darier disease (and similarly Hailey–Hailey disease) has a suprabasal cleft. Above and to the side of the cleft, dyskeratotic keratinocytes with eosinophilic cytoplasm contain keratin fibrils that whorl about the nucleus (Fig. 20-8). The conditions first appear late in childhood or in adolescence as skin-colored papules that later become crusted. Affected areas have many warty elevations, 2 to 4 mm in diameter, largely on the chest, nasolabial folds, back, scalp, forehead, ears, and groin.

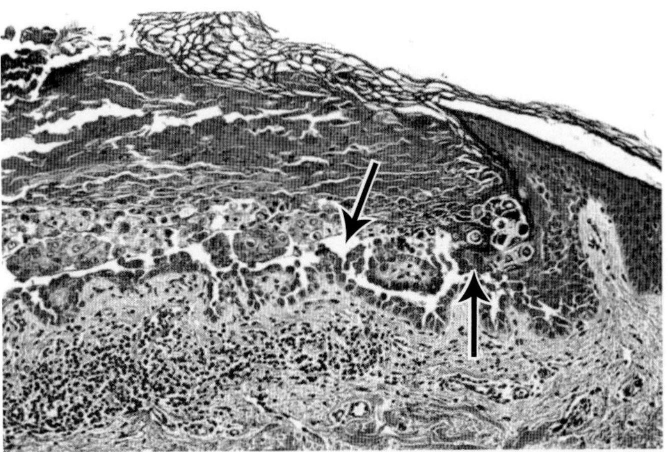

FIGURE 20-8. Darier disease. Virtually the entire epidermis exhibits focal acantholytic dyskeratosis. A small portion of normal epidermis is present (*right*). In the lesion, there is a suprabasal cleft (*arrows*) with a few dyshesive (acantholytic) keratinocytes surmounted by hyperkeratosis and parakeratosis. The cleft is not a vesicle because true vesicles contain inflammatory cells and tissue fluid. Dyskeratosis is present above the cleft.

Psoriasis

Psoriasis is a chronic, frequently familial disorder that features large, erythematous, scaly plaques, commonly on extensor cutaneous surfaces. It affects 1% to 2% of the population worldwide. Psoriasis may arise at any age but shows a peak in late adolescence. Interestingly, the condition is not seen among Native Americans and is infrequent among Asians (Fig. 20-9).

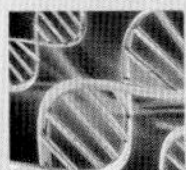

MOLECULAR PATHOGENESIS: The pathogenesis of psoriasis is multifactorial, with genetic, immunologic, and environmental factors contributing to the development of psoriatic lesions.

GENETIC FACTORS: Psoriasis unquestionably has a genetic component, although only one third of patients with psoriasis have a family history of the disease. (1) There is an increased incidence among relatives and offspring of patients with psoriasis; the more severe the illness, the greater is the likelihood of a familial background; (2) There is a 65% concordance for psoriasis in monozygotic twins; and (3) an increased prevalence is noted with certain HLA haplotypes, particularly HLA-Cw6. People with HLA-Cw6 are 10 to 15 times more likely to develop psoriasis than the general population. A 300-kb segment in the MHC-I region of chromosome 6p21, PSORS1, is believed to be a major genetic determinant of susceptibility.

IMMUNOLOGIC FACTORS: T lymphocytes are crucial to the pathogenesis of psoriatic lesions. T_H1 and T_H17 cells appear to drive the inflammatory response and subsequent dermatosis. These subsets of T cells, $CD8^+$ T cells and antigen-presenting dendritic cells, secrete pro-inflammatory cytokines, as well as keratinocyte growth factors. The combination of these cytokines and epidermal growth factors likely causes the constellation of changes seen in psoriasis. For these reasons, therapeutics targeting cytokines, such as TNF-α inhibitors, and those targeting IL-12, IL-17, and IL-23, are currently being used.

ENVIRONMENTAL FACTORS: Stimuli such as physical injury ("Köbner phenomenon"), infection, certain drugs, and photosensitivity may produce psoriatic lesions in apparently normal skin. Chronic irritation of normal skin, as in repeated rubbing, produces a tough, scaly, cutaneous plaque that is clinically and histologically psoriasiform. However, the lesion disappears when the trauma ceases. In psoriatic patients, even less trauma generates psoriatic plaques that may persist for years after an initial injury.

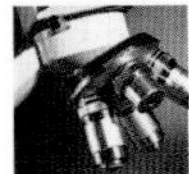

PATHOLOGY: The most distinctive pathologic change is at the edges of chronic psoriatic plaques. The epidermis is thickened, with **hyperkeratosis** and focal or diffuse **parakeratosis** (persistence of nuclei in cells of the stratum corneum, which occurs with increased epidermal turnover). In the latter case, the granular layer is diminished or absent. The nucleated layers of the epidermis are thickened several-fold in the rete pegs and are frequently thinner over dermal papillae (Fig. 20-9B). In turn, the papillae are elongated and appear as sections of cones, with their apices toward the

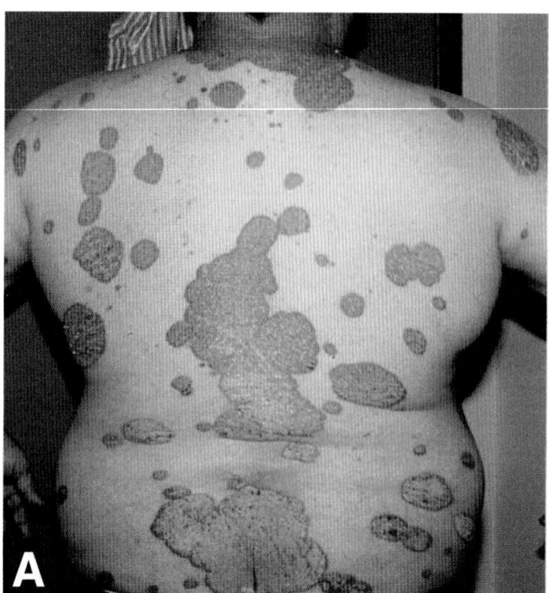

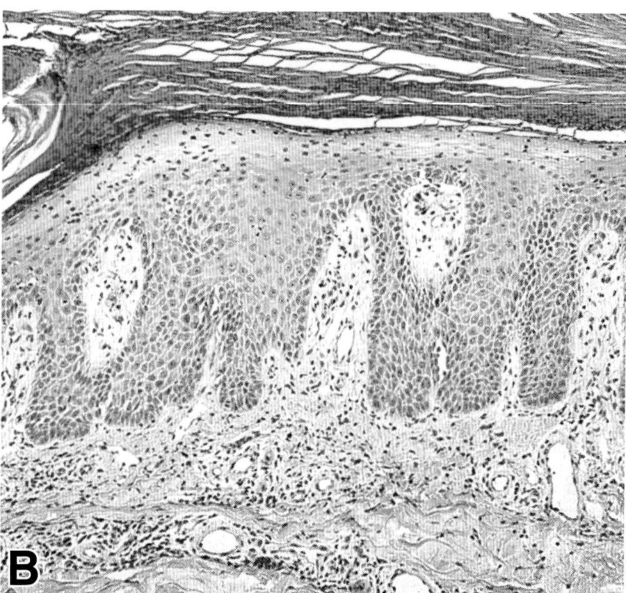

FIGURE 20-9. Psoriasis. This disorder is the prototype of psoriasiform epidermal hyperplasia. **A.** A patient with psoriasis shows large, confluent, sharply demarcated, erythematous plaques on the trunk. **B.** Microscopic examination of a lesion demonstrating that the rete ridges are uniformly elongated, as are the dermal papillae, giving an interlocking pattern of alternately reversed "clubs." The dermal papillae are edematous and reside beneath a thinned epidermis (suprapapillary thinning). There is striking parakeratosis, which is the scale observed clinically.

dermis. In chronic lesions, dermal papillae may appear as bulbous "clubs" with short handles (Figs. 20-9 and 20-10). The rete ridges of the epidermis have a profile reciprocal to that of the dermal papillae, resulting in interlocked dermal and epidermal "clubs" with alternately reversed polarity. Capillaries of dermal papillae are dilated and tortuous (Fig. 20-10). In very early lesions, changes may be limited to capillary dilation, with a few neutrophils "squirting" into the epidermis. Epidermal hyperplasia and hyperkeratosis occur mainly in chronic lesions.

The capillaries are venule like; neutrophils may emerge at their tips and migrate into the epidermis above the apices of the papillae. Neutrophils are sometimes localized in the epidermal spinous layer or in small microabscesses (of Munro) in the stratum corneum and may be associated with limited areas of parakeratosis (Fig. 20-11). The dermis below the papillae contains variable mononuclear inflammation, mostly lymphocytes, around the superficial vascular plexus. The inflammatory process does not extend into the subjacent reticular dermis.

The psoriasiform histologic appearance is common in cutaneous pathology and may also be seen in seborrheic dermatitis, reaction to chronic trauma (lichen simplex chronicus), subacute and chronic spongiotic dermatitis (eczema), and cutaneous T-cell lymphoma (mycosis fungoides).

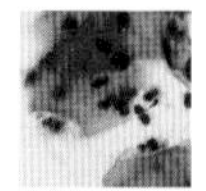

CLINICAL FEATURES: The initial presentation of psoriasis is variable, and disease activity is intermittent. Its severity varies from annoying scaly lesions over the elbows to a serious debilitating disorder that involves most of the skin and is often associated with arthritis. A single lesion of psoriasis may be a small focus of scaly erythema or an enormous confluent plaque covering much of the trunk (Fig. 20-9A). A typical plaque is 4 to 5 cm, sharply demarcated at its margin, and covered by a surface of silvery scales. If the scales are detached, pinpoint foci of bleeding from the dilated capillaries in the dermal papillae dot the underlying glossy erythematous surface ("Auspitz sign").

Seronegative arthritis develops in 7% of patients with psoriasis. The tendency to arthropathy is linked to several HLA haplotypes, particularly HLA-B27. Psoriatic arthritis closely resembles its rheumatoid counterpart, but it is usually milder and may cause little disability.

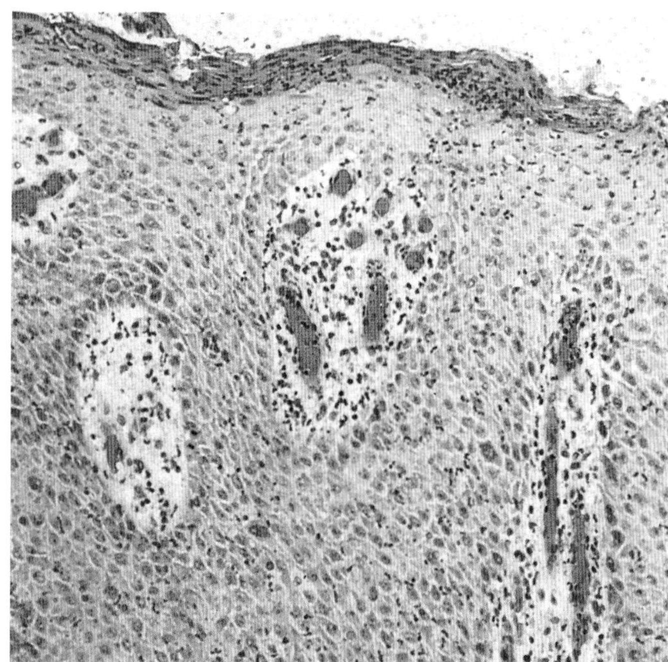

FIGURE 20-10. Psoriasis. The clubbed papillae contain tortuous dilated venules. The prominent venules are part of the venulization of capillaries, which may be of histogenetic importance in psoriasis. The papilla to the *right* has one cross section of its superficial capillary venule loop, which is normal. The papilla in the *center* shows numerous cross sections of its venule, indicating striking tortuosity.

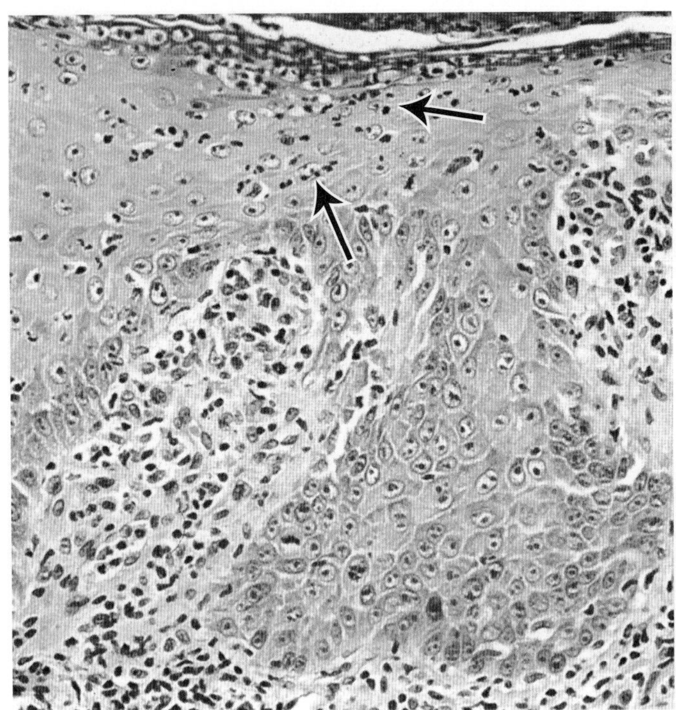

FIGURE 20-11. Psoriasis. Neutrophils migrate into the epidermis, emerging from the venulized capillaries at the tips of the dermal papillae. They migrate to the upper stratum spinosum and stratum corneum (*arrows*). In some forms of psoriasis, pustules are common clinical lesions.

Psoriasis has long been treated with coal tar or wood tar derivatives and anthralin, a strong reducing agent. Topical and systemic corticosteroids have also been used. Severe, generalized psoriasis justifies systemic treatment with methotrexate. Phototherapy ("PUVA") after administration of psoralens, a UV-absorbing compound that binds to DNA, is often effective. Synthetic vitamin A and vitamin D derivatives have also been used. Treatments that target immunologic and inflammatory mediators, such as anticytokine monoclonal antibodies, are also employed.

Pemphigus Vulgaris

Dyshesive disorders are cutaneous diseases in which blisters form because of diminished cohesiveness between epidermal keratinocytes. PV, the prototype of dyshesive diseases, is a chronic, blistering skin disorder, which is most common in people 40 to 60 years old but is seen at all ages, including children. Although all races are susceptible, persons of Jewish or Mediterranean heritage are at greatest risk.

MOLECULAR PATHOGENESIS: PV is an autoimmune disease. Patients have circulating IgG against an epidermal surface protein, **desmoglein 3**. Immune complex formation results in dyshesion, which is augmented by the release of plasminogen activator and, hence, activation of plasmin. This proteolytic enzyme acts on the intercellular substance and may be the dominant factor in dyshesion. Internalization of antigen–antibody complexes, disappearance of attachment plaques, and retraction of perinuclear tonofilaments may all act in concert with proteinases to cause dyshesion and vesiculation. Blisters in PV are intraepidermal, whereas other blistering disorders that affect the basement membrane zone (discussed below), subepidermal blisters are formed.

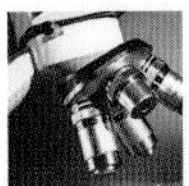

PATHOLOGY: Suprabasal dyshesion results in a blister with an intact basal layer as a floor and the remaining epidermis as a roof (Fig. 20-12). Desmoglein 3 is concentrated in the lower epidermis, explaining the location of the blister. The blister contains lymphocytes, macrophages, eosinophils, and neutrophils. Distinctive, rounded keratinocytes (acantholytic cells) are shed into the vesicle during dyshesion. Basal cells remain adherent to the basal lamina and form a layer of "tombstone cells." Dyshesion may extend along dermal adnexa. The subjacent areas contains lymphocytes, macrophages, eosinophils, and neutrophils, predominantly around the capillary venular bed.

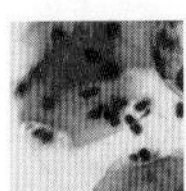

CLINICAL FEATURES: The characteristic lesion of PV is a large, easily ruptured blister that leaves extensive denuded or crusted areas. They are most common on the scalp and mucous membranes and in periumbilical and intertriginous areas. Without corticosteroid treatment, much of the skin surface may become denuded. PV is progressive and usually fatal. Immunosuppression is also useful for maintenance therapy. With appropriate treatment, the 10-year mortality rate for PV is less than 10%.

DISEASES OF THE DERMAL–EPIDERMAL INTERFACE

Epidermolysis Bullosa

EB is a heterogeneous group of disorders of hereditary nature that have a tendency to form blisters at sites of minor trauma. The clinical spectrum ranges from a minor annoyance to a widespread, life-threatening blistering disease. ***These blisters are almost always present at birth or shortly thereafter.*** The classification of EB is based on a combination of clinical features and the site of blister formation in the BMZ. The different mechanisms of blister formation underlie each of the four major categories of EB (Fig. 20-13).

- **Epidermolytic epidermolysis bullosa (EB simplex)** is a group of autosomal dominant and autosomal recessive skin diseases in which blisters form. EB simplex is caused by disruption of basal keratinocytes as a result of mutations of genes encoding cytokeratin intermediate filaments 5 and 14, which provide mechanical stability to the epidermis. Initially, small, subnuclear, cytoplasmic vacuoles develop, enlarge, coalesce, and eventually result in cell lysis and intraepidermal vesicle formation. The roof of the vesicle is an almost intact epidermis with a fragmented basal layer. The vesicle floor shows bits of basal cell cytoplasm attached to the lamina densa, which appears as a well-preserved pink line. Inflammatory cells are sparse. Blisters develop after minor trauma, such as merely rubbing the skin, but heal without scarring (thus the term "simplex"). Epidermolytic EB is cosmetically disturbing and sometimes debilitating but is not life-threatening.
- **Junctional epidermolysis bullosa** refers to a group of both benign and severe, autosomal recessive skin diseases, in which blisters form within the lamina lucida. The benign form

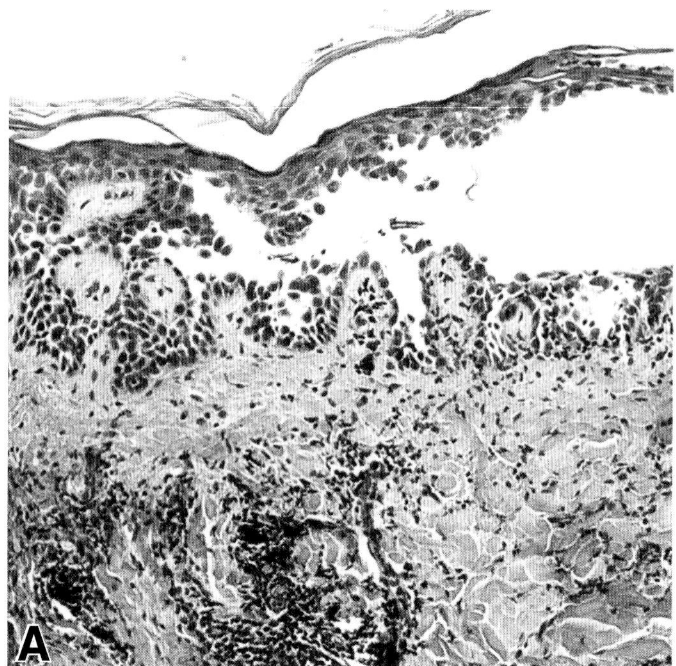

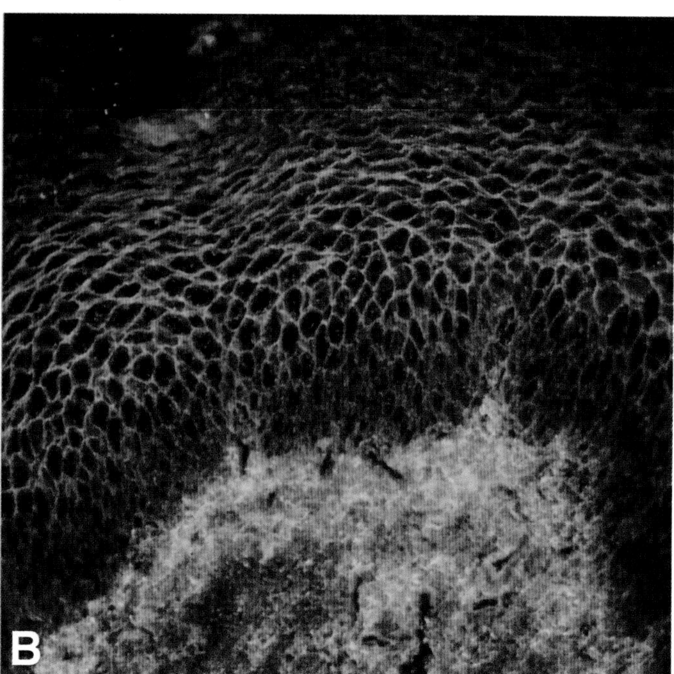

FIGURE 20-12. Pemphigus vulgaris. A. Suprabasal dyshesion leads to an intraepidermal blister containing acantholytic keratinocytes. The basal keratinocytes are slightly separated from each other and totally separated from the stratum spinosum. The basal keratinocytes are firmly attached to the epidermal basement membrane zone. **B.** Direct immunofluorescence examination of perilesional skin reveals antibodies, usually of the immunoglobulin G (IgG) type, deposited in the intercellular substance of the epidermis, yielding a lacelike pattern outlining the keratinocytes.

reflects mutations in the gene for type XVII collagen. In the severe type, mutations in the genes for certain isoforms of laminin and integrins occur. An intact epidermis forms the roof of the vesicle in junctional EB. Plasma membranes of basal keratinocytes are unchanged. The vesicle floor is an intact lamina densa, as in epidermolytic EB, but there are no attached fragments of basal cell cytoplasm. Benign disease has no effect on life span, whereas the severe variety may be fatal within the first 2 years of life.

- **Dystrophic EB** or **dermolytic EB** comprises a group of autosomal dominant and more severe autosomal recessive diseases. As a result of defects in anchoring fibrils related to mutations in the gene for collagen type VII, blisters are immediately deep to the lamina densa. These fibrils are abnormally arranged and reduced in number in apparently normal skin of affected newborns. Normally anchoring fibrils attach the epidermis to the underlying dermis. Hence, disruption results in subepidermal bullae arising in the sublamina densa zone. The vesicle roof is normal epidermis with an attached, intact lamina lucida and lamina densa. The base of the vesicle is the outer part of the papillary dermis. Healed blisters show atrophic ("dystrophic") scarring. Nails and teeth may also be involved.

Bullous Pemphigoid

BP is a common, autoimmune, blistering disease, which has clinical similarities to PV (hence the term "pemphigoid"), but which lacks acantholysis. The disease is most common in the later decades of life and affects all races and both sexes.

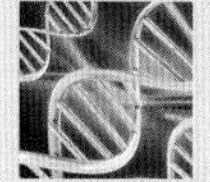

MOLECULAR PATHOGENESIS: Like PV, BP is an autoimmune disease, but in BP, complement-fixing IgG antibodies are directed against the basement membrane proteins BPAG1 and BPAG2. The antigen–antibody complexes injure the basal cell plasma membrane via the C5b–C9 membrane attack complex (see Chapter 3), which interferes with the elaboration of adherence factors by basal keratinocytes. Anaphylatoxins C3a and C5a trigger mast cell degranulation and the release of factors chemotactic for eosinophils, neutrophils, and lymphocytes. Levels of IL-5 and eotaxin play significant roles in recruitment and function of eosinophils. The granules of these inflammatory cells contain tissue-damaging substances, including eosinophil peroxidase and major basic protein. These molecules, together with neutrophil and mast cell proteases, cause dermal–epidermal separation within the lamina lucida.

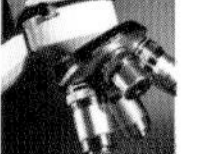

PATHOLOGY: The blisters of BP are subepidermal; the roof is intact epidermis, and the base is the lamina densa of the BMZ (Fig. 20-14). The blisters contain many eosinophils, plus fibrin, lymphocytes, and neutrophils. With the onset of erythema, eosinophils appear in the upper dermis and may be arrayed along the epidermal BMZ. Immunofluorescence shows linear deposition of C3 and IgG at the epidermal BMZ and the presence of serum antibodies against BPAG1 and BPAG2.

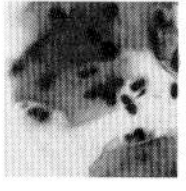

CLINICAL FEATURES: The blisters of BP are large and tense and may appear on normal-appearing skin or on an erythematous base (Fig. 20-14). The medial thighs and flexor aspects of the forearms are

EPIDERMOLYTIC EB

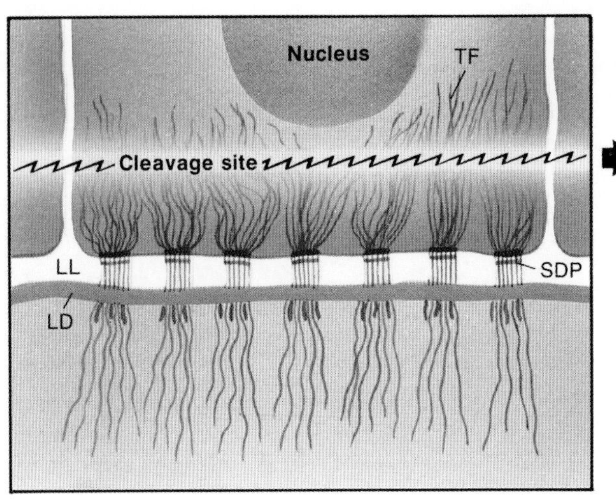

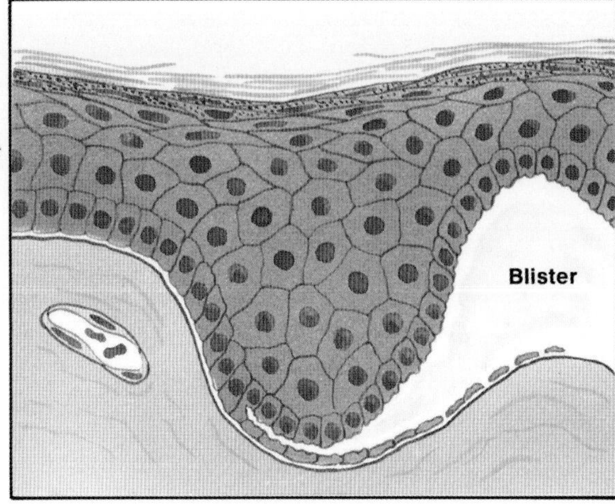

JUNCTIONAL EB

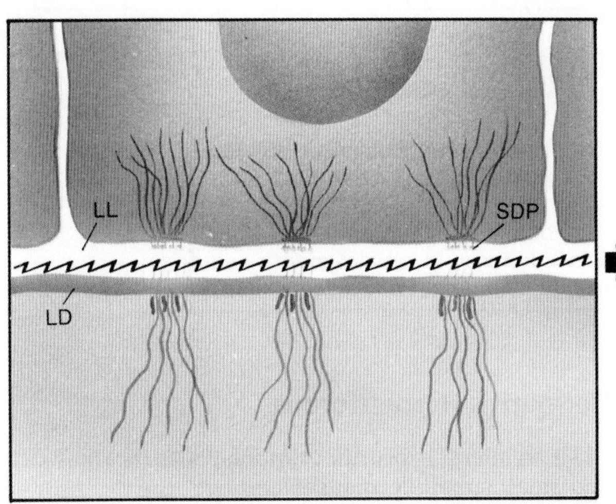

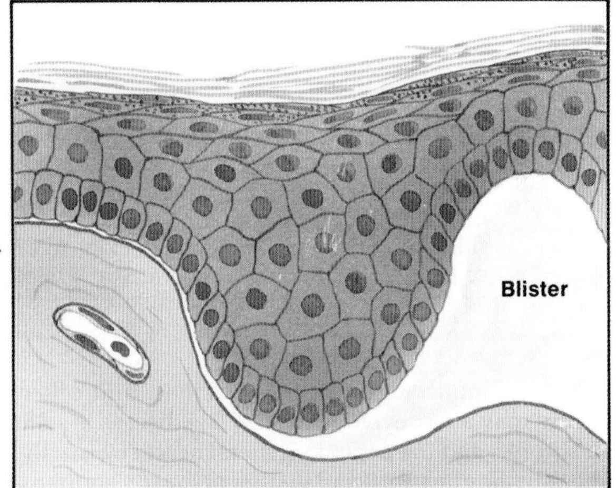

DERMOLYTIC EB

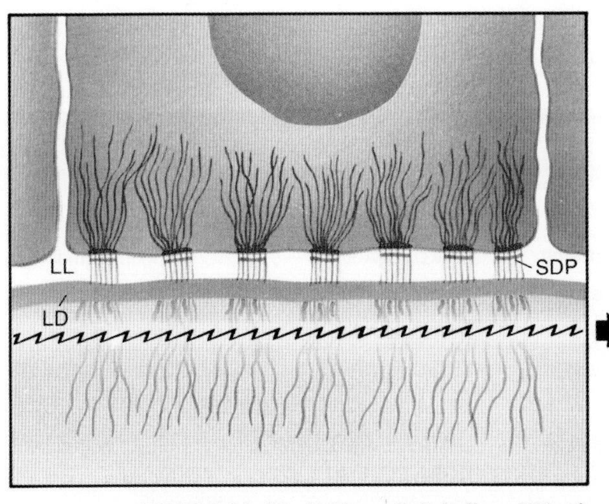

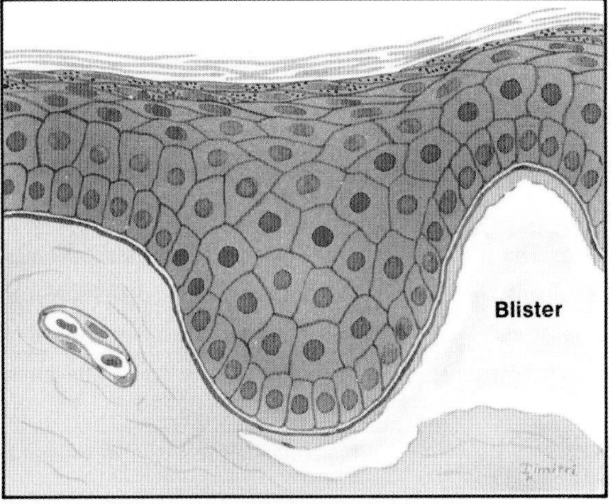

FIGURE 20-13. Epidermolysis bullosa (EB). Three distinct mechanisms of blister formation are shown. Electron microscopic images are diagrammed on the *left*; light microscopic images are on the *right*. **Epidermolytic EB** is caused by disintegration of the lowermost regions of the epidermal basal cells. The bottom portions of the basal cells cleave, and the remainder of the epidermis lifts away. Small fragments of basal cells remain attached to the basement membrane zone. **Junctional EB** is characterized by cleavage in the lamina lucida. **Dermolytic EB** is associated with rudimentary and fragmented anchoring fibrils. The entire basement membrane zone and epidermis split away from the dermis in relationship to these flawed anchoring fibrils. LD, lamina densa; LL, lamina lucida; SDP, subdesmosomal dense plate; TF, tonofilaments .

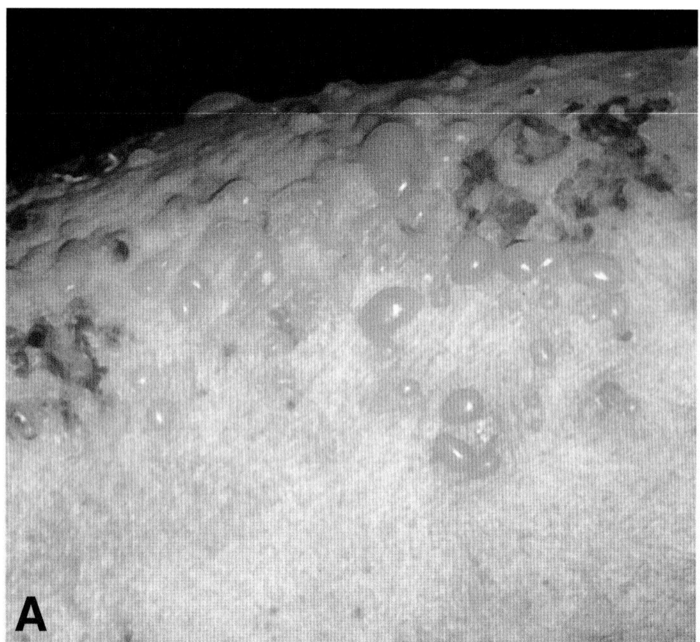

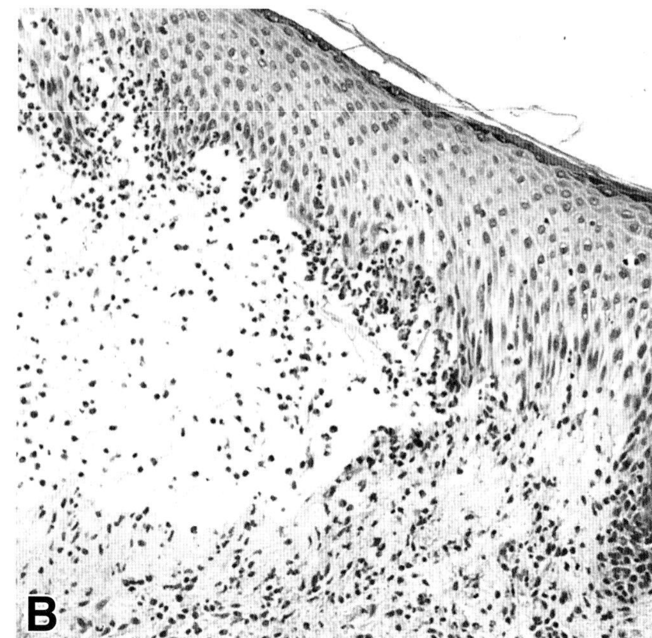

FIGURE 20-14. Bullous pemphigoid. A. The skin showing multiple tense bullae on an erythematous base and erosions, distributed primarily on the medial thighs and trunk. **B.** A subepidermal blister has an edematous papillary dermis as its base. The roof of the blister consists of the intact, entire epidermis, including the stratum basalis. Inflammatory cells, fibrin, and fluid fill the blister. 20-14A From Elder AD, Elenitsas R, Johnson BL, et al. *Synopsis and Atlas of Lever's Histopathology of the Skin*. Philadelphia, PA: Lippincott Williams & Wilkins; 1999.

commonly affected, although the groin, axillae, and other cutaneous sites may also develop blisters. The disease is self-limited but chronic, and the patient's general health is usually unaffected. Systemic glucocorticoid treatment greatly shortens the course of the disease.

Table 20-1 summarizes the molecular pathogenesis immunobullous and acantholytic disorders.

Dermatitis Herpetiformis

DH is an intensely pruritic eruption with urticaria-like plaques and small subepidermal vesicles over the extensor surfaces of the body.

Table 20-1

Pathogenesis of Immunobullous and Acantholytic Disorders

Condition	Pathogenetic Mechanism	Gene Target	Result
Bullous pemphigoid	Autoantibody against basal cell hemidesmosome	BPAG1, BPAG2	Subepidermal blister
Pemphigus vulgaris	Autoantibody against desmosomal proteins	Desmoglein 1, 3	Intraepidermal blister
Pemphigus foliaceous	Autoantibody against desmosomal proteins	Desmoglein 1	Intraepidermal blister
Epidermolysis bullosa (EB) simplex	Molecular defect in cytokeratin intermediate filaments	KRT5 KRT14	Intraepidermal blister
Junctional EB	Molecular defect in laminin, integrins, collagen	LAMA3, LAMB3, LAMC2, ITGB4, COL17A1	Blister within lamina densa
Dermolytic EB	Molecular defect in anchoring fibrils	COL7A1	Blister below lamina densa
Kindler syndrome	Molecular defect in basal keratinocyte adhesion	KIND1	Blistering, photosensitivity
Darier disease	Molecular defect in keratinocyte adhesion	ATP2A2	Acantholysis, dyskeratosis
Hailey–Hailey disease	Molecular defect in keratinocyte adhesion	ATP2C1	Acantholysis, dyskeratosis

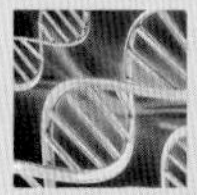

MOLECULAR PATHOGENESIS: DH accompanies gluten sensitivity in patients with HLA-B8, HLA-DR3, and HLA-DQw2 haplotypes. Although gluten-sensitive enteropathy may be subclinical, most patients will show features of celiac disease on small intestinal biopsy (see Chapter 11). DH cutaneous lesions reflect granular deposits of IgA, mainly at the tips of dermal papillae (Fig. 20-15). Such IgA immune complexes are more prominent in perilesional skin than in normal-appearing skin. These complexes do not activate complement efficiently (alternate pathway), and few neutrophils are attracted to the site. However, those neutrophils that do accumulate elaborate leukotrienes, which attract more neutrophils. The neutrophils release lysosomal enzymes that degrade laminin and type IV collagen, cleaving the epidermis from the dermis and eventually causing blisters.

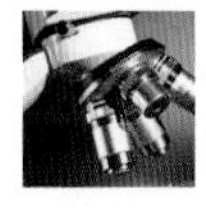

PATHOLOGY: There are two related mechanisms of dermal–epidermal separation. One is associated with the sheetlike spread of a layer or two of neutrophils at the dermal–epidermal interface. In this case, the entire epidermis detaches from the papillary dermis (Fig. 20-16B). The vesicle roof contains the epidermis; the floor is composed of the lamina densa and the papillary dermis. Unlike bullous pemphigoid, eosinophils are uncommon early in the course of DH. In the second route of vesicle formation, many neutrophils accumulate rapidly in the tips of the dermal papillae. Release of their lysosomal enzymes into the superficial portion of the dermal papillae (1) uncouples the epidermis from the dermis at the tips of dermal papillae, (2) disrupts the BMZ in the lamina lucida and superficial part of the papillae, and (3) tears the epidermis across the adjacent rete ridges. The roofs of resulting vesicles have alternating tears across their epidermal covering, and their floors show residual epidermal pegs that alternate with the basal half of dermal papillae. In both cases, granular IgA is deposited at the dermoepidermal junction (Fig. 20-16C).

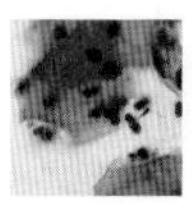

CLINICAL FEATURES: The lesions of DH are especially prominent over the elbows, knees, and buttocks (Fig. 20-16A). These intensely pruritic vesicles appear similar to those of herpes simplex infections (hence "herpetiformis") and are almost invariably rubbed until broken. Thus, patients may present with only crusted lesions and no intact vesicles. DH is of varying severity and characterized by remissions, but it is disturbingly chronic. Healing lesions often leave scars. Besides a gluten-free diet, dapsone or sulfapyridine may control the signs and symptoms of DH. An increased risk for lymphoproliferative disorders and systemic lupus erythematosus has been reported.

Erythema Multiforme

EM is an acute, self-limited disorder that varies from a few annular (ringlike) and targetoid erythematous macules and blisters (EM minor) to a life-threatening, widespread ulceration of the skin and mucous membranes (EM major; Stevens–Johnson syndrome). ***It is usually a reaction to a drug or an infectious agent, in particular, herpes simplex virus infection.***

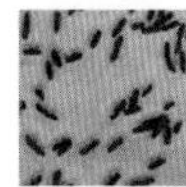

ETIOLOGIC FACTORS: A long list of agents may provoke EM, including herpesvirus, *Mycoplasma*, and sulfonamides, but precipitating factors are identified in only half of cases. In postherpetic EM, viral antigens, IgM, and C3 deposit in a perivascular location and at the epidermal BMZ. The combination of infiltrating lymphocytes and antigen–antibody complexes within the lesions suggests that humoral and cellular hypersensitivity are both involved.

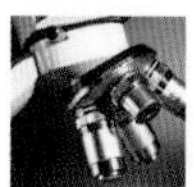

PATHOLOGY: The dermis in EM shows a sparse lymphocytic infiltrate about the superficial vascular bed and at the dermal–epidermal interface. The characteristic morphologic feature in the epidermis is apoptotic ("dyskeratotic") keratinocytes, with pyknotic nuclei and eosinophilic cytoplasm. Apoptosis may be extensive and associated with a subepidermal vesicle, whose roof is an almost completely necrotic epidermis. Because of the acute onset of the disease, in most cases, there is little or no change in the stratum corneum. The dermis shows a perivascular lymphocytic infiltrate, without eosinophils.

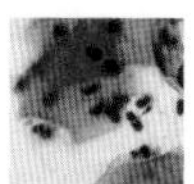

CLINICAL FEATURES: The characteristic "target" or "iris" lesions of EM have a central, dark red zone, occasionally with a blister, surrounded by a paler area (Fig. 20-17). In turn, the latter is encompassed by a peripheral red rim. Urticarial plaques are common. The presence of vesicles and bullae usually predicts a more severe course. EM is a common condition, with a peak incidence in the second and third decades of life. It is occasionally encountered in association with other presumably immunologic cutaneous disorders, including erythema nodosum, toxic epidermal necrolysis, and necrotizing vasculitis. **Stevens–Johnson syndrome** and **toxic epidermal necrolysis** (TEN) refer to unusually severe forms of EM that involve mucosal surfaces and internal organs and are often fatal.

Systemic Lupus Erythematosus

Cutaneous involvement in SLE (see Chapter 3) may be severe and cosmetically devastating but is not life-threatening. However, the nature and pattern of immune reactants in the skin are an excellent guide to the likelihood of systemic disease.

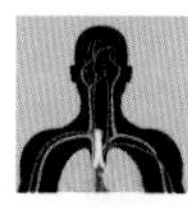

PATHOPHYSIOLOGY: Immune complexes are present in both lesional and normal-appearing skin in SLE. Deposition of immune reactants along the epidermal BMZ of normal-appearing skin is important in making the diagnosis. Epidermal injury seems to be initiated by exogenous agents such as UV light, and perpetuated by cell-mediated immune reactions, similar to those in graft-versus-host disease. The manifestations of epidermal injury include (1) vacuolization of basal keratinocytes, (2) hyperkeratosis, (3) diminished epidermal thickness, (4) release of DNA and other nuclear and cytoplasmic antigens to the circulation, and (5) deposition of DNA and other antigens in the epidermal BMZ (lamina densa and immediately subjacent dermis). Thus, epidermal injury, local immune complex formation, deposition of circulating immune complexes, and lymphocyte-induced cellular injury all seem to act in concert.

The various forms of cutaneous lupus are classified according to their chronicity, but considerable overlap in features is possible. There is an inverse relationship between the prominence of skin lesions and the extent of systemic disease.

CHRONIC CUTANEOUS (DISCOID) LUPUS ERYTHEMATOSUS: This form of lupus is usually limited to the skin. It generally affects skin above the neck, on the face (especially

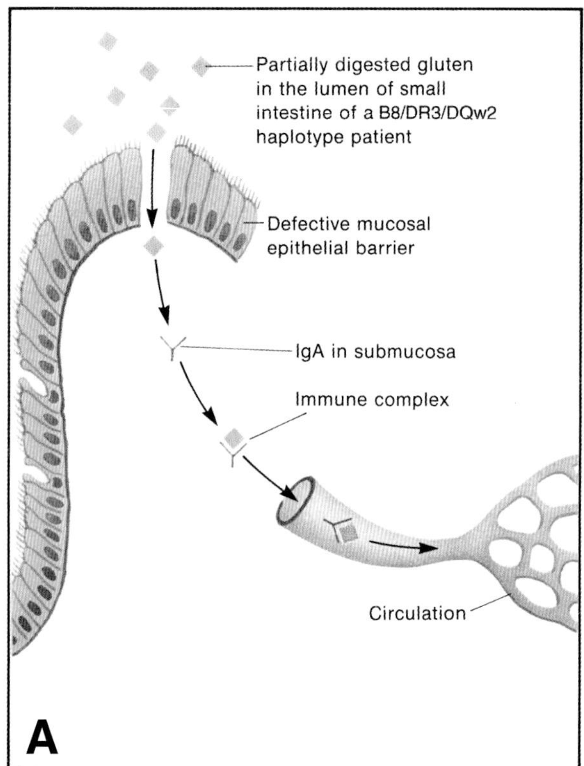

1. Formation of immune complexes in submucosa of small intestine. Passage of immune complexes into **the circulation.**

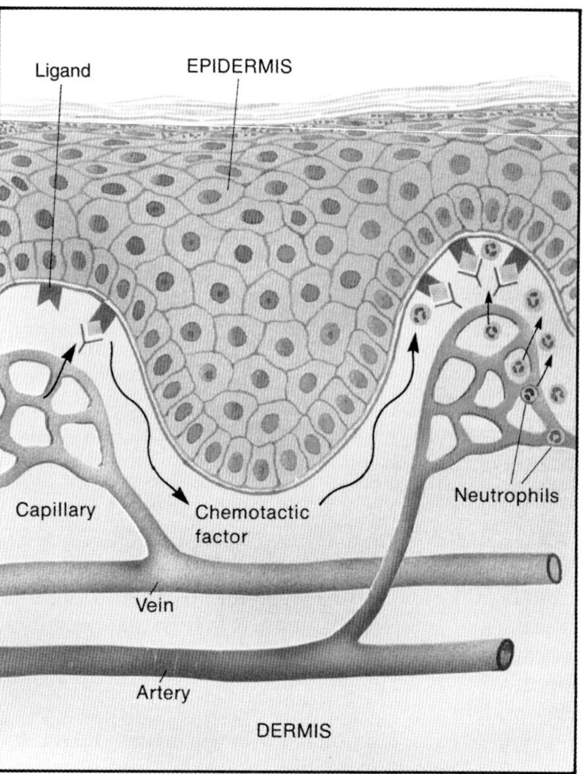

2. Ligand–immune complex union releases neutrophil chemotactic factor. Neutrophils migrate to the tips of the papillae.

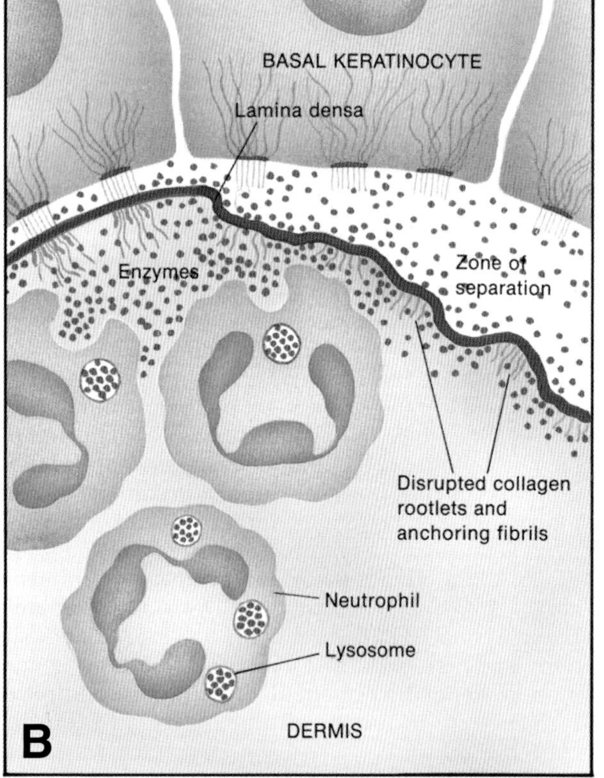

3. Dissolution of basal rootlets and anchoring fibrils by enzymes released by neutrophils. Early dermo-epidermal separation.

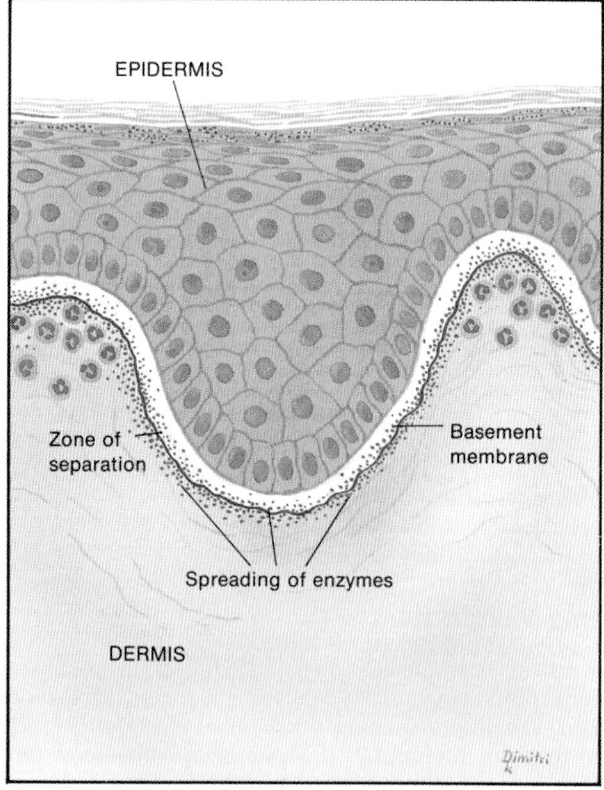

4. Concentration of neutrophils at the tips of the papillae. Spreading of enzymes along basement membrane. Lifting away of lamina densa.

FIGURE 20-15. Dermatitis herpetiformis. A. Immune mechanisms. **B.** Mechanisms of blister formation. Proposed pathogenesis for cutaneous lesions. The disease is initiated in the small intestine and is likely expressed in the skin because of the presence of a ligand immediately deep to the lamina densa. IgA, immunoglobulin A.

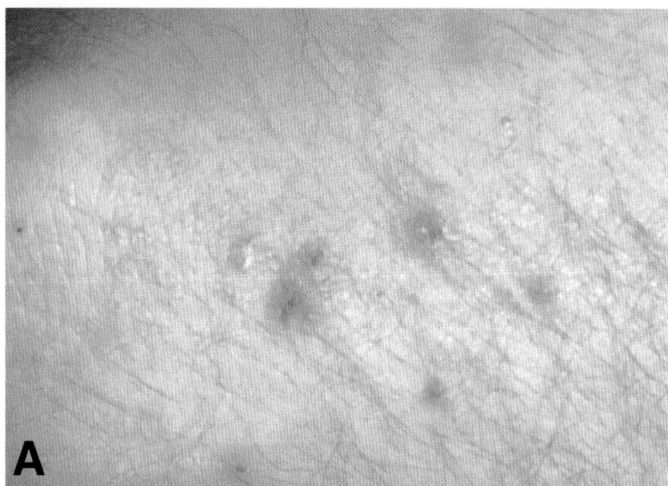

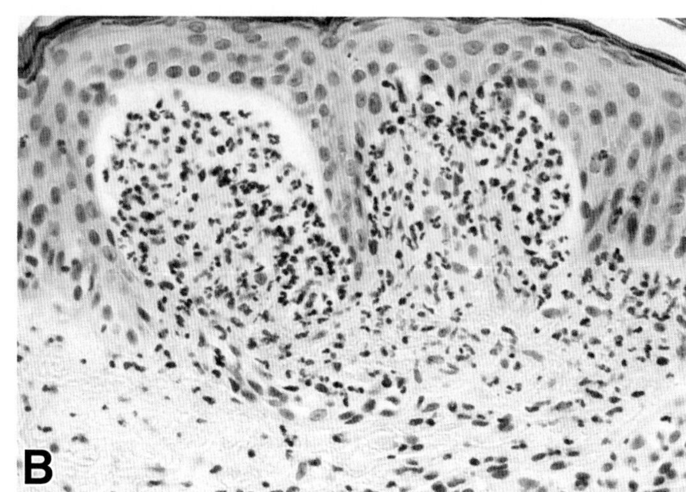

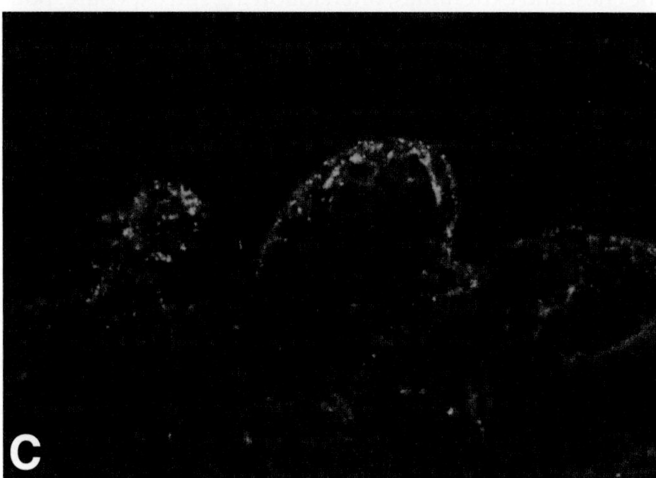

FIGURE 20-16. Dermatitis herpetiformis. A. Pruritic, symmetric, grouped vesicles on an erythematous base are seen on the elbows and knees. **B.** Dermal papillary abscesses of neutrophils with vesicle formation at the dermal–epidermal junction are characteristic. **C.** Direct immunofluorescence revealing immunoglobulin A deposited in dermal papillae in association with (but not necessarily directly upon) anchoring fibrils and elastic tissue fibers. This is the site of neutrophil infiltration and subepidermal vesicle formation. 20-16A From Elder AD, Elenitsas R, Johnson BL, et al. *Synopsis and Atlas of Lever's Histopathology of the Skin*. Philadelphia, PA: Lippincott Williams & Wilkins; 1999.

the malar area), scalp, and ears. Lesions begin as slightly elevated violaceous papules with a rough scale of keratin. They enlarge to assume a disc shape, with a hyperkeratotic margin and a depigmented center. The cutaneous lesions may culminate in disfiguring scars. Elevated circulating antinuclear antibody (ANA) levels are uncommon (less than 10% of patients).

FIGURE 20-17. Erythema multiforme. Steroid-responsive "target" papules, characterized by central bullae with surrounding erythema, appeared after antibiotic therapy. From Elder AD, Elenitsas R, Johnson BL, et al. *Synopsis and Atlas of Lever's Histopathology of the Skin*. Philadelphia, PA: Lippincott Williams & Wilkins; 1999.

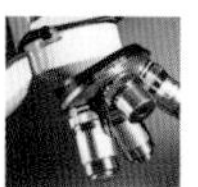

PATHOLOGY: In discoid lupus, nucleated epidermal layers are modestly thickened or somewhat thin. Hyperkeratosis, without prominent parakeratosis, and plugging of hair follicles are prominent. The rete-papillae pattern of the dermal–epidermal interface is partially effaced. Basal keratinocytes are vacuolated, and eosinophilic apoptotic bodies are noted. The lamina densa is greatly thickened and reduplicated. These changes all suggest that injury to basal keratinocytes is an essential pathogenetic characteristic of discoid lupus (Figs. 20-18 and 20-19).

The basal keratinocytes and BMZ contain a diffuse lymphocytic infiltrate that penetrates the basal layer focally. Deeper in the dermis, dense patches of helper and cytotoxic/suppressor T lymphocytes, often with plasma cells, are commonly found around skin appendages. Immune complexes are mainly deep to the lamina densa but also occur as granular deposits on the lamina densa and within the lamina lucida.

SUBACUTE CUTANEOUS LUPUS ERYTHEMATOSUS: This disorder primarily afflicts young and middle-aged white women. Unlike discoid lupus, subacute cutaneous lupus may also involve the musculoskeletal system and kidneys. Initially, scaly erythematous papules develop and then enlarge into psoriasiform or annular lesions, which may

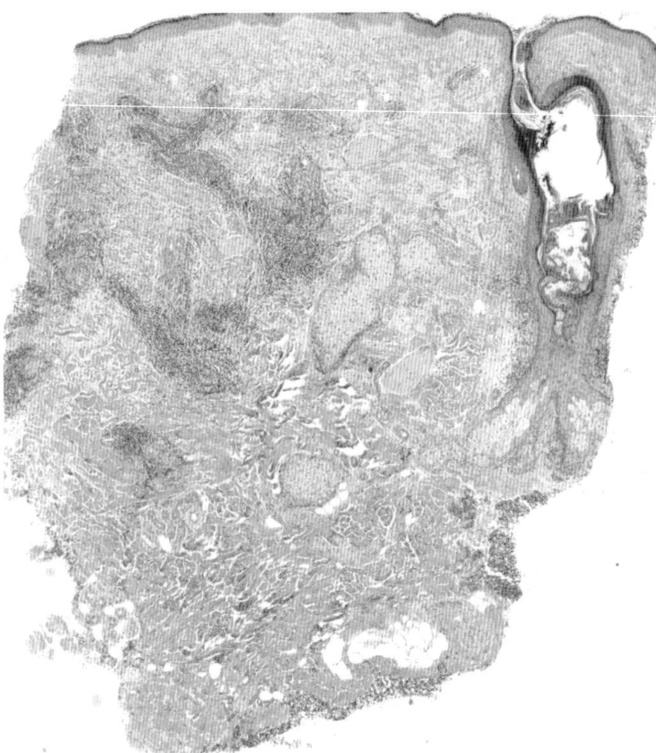

FIGURE 20-18. Lupus erythematosus. Perivascular and periappendageal lymphocytic inflammation is present in the superficial and deep dermis. A hair follicle plugged with keratin is present near the right edge.

fuse. Skin changes occur in the upper chest, upper back, and extensor surfaces of the arms, suggesting that light exposure plays a role in the pathogenesis of the disorder. Significant scarring does not occur. About 70% of patients have circulating anti-Ro (SS-A) antibodies. ANA levels are elevated in 70%.

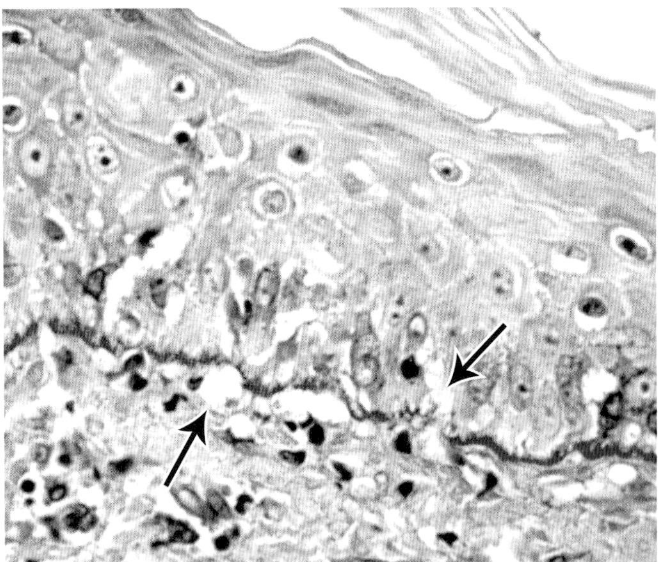

FIGURE 20-19. Lupus erythematosus. Basal cell necrosis with resultant basal keratinocytic migration and synthesis of new basement membrane zone leads to thickening of the epidermal basement membrane zone (BMZ), as evident in this periodic acid–Schiff stain. Notice the vacuoles (*arrows*) on either side of the BMZ, an indicator of cellular injury.

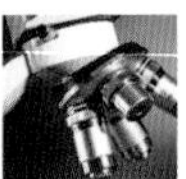

PATHOLOGY: Subacute cutaneous lupus features edema of the papillary dermis, thickening of the lamina densa, and prominent vacuolar degeneration of basilar keratinocytes. Although there is some lymphocytic infiltration of the BMZ, deeper patches of lymphocytes are not observed.

ACUTE SYSTEMIC LUPUS ERYTHEMATOSUS: Over 80% of patients with SLE have acute skin disease during their illness, in association with disease of the kidneys and joints. The rash is often the first manifestation of the disease and may precede the onset of systemic symptoms by a few months. The typical "butterfly" rash of SLE is a delicate erythema of the malar area of the face, which may pass in a few hours or a few days. Many patients have a maculopapular eruption of the chest and extremities, often following sun exposure. Both rashes heal without scarring. Lesions indistinguishable from discoid lupus may occur. ANA levels are elevated in more than 90% of patients.

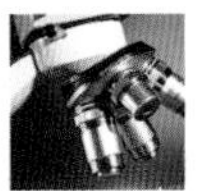

PATHOLOGY: The earliest malar blush of acute cutaneous lupus may show only edema of the papillary dermis. More often, changes are like those in the subacute form of lupus. The histopathologic picture of lupus can be indistinguishable from other connective tissue diseases, such as dermatomyositis.

Lichen Planus

"Lichenoid" tissue reactions are so named because the clinical lesions resemble certain lichens that form scaly growths on rocks or tree trunks. Lichenoid infiltrates are characterized by a bandlike congregation of lymphocytes that obscures the dermal–epidermal junction. LP is the prototypic disorder of this group, which includes entities such as lichenoid drug eruptions.

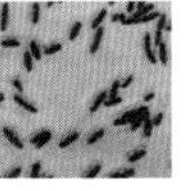

ETIOLOGIC FACTORS: The etiology of LP is unknown. It is occasionally familial and may also accompany autoimmune disorders, such as SLE and myasthenia gravis. LP is more common in patients with ulcerative colitis. Some drugs—gold, chlorothiazide, chloroquine—may induce lichenoid reactions. External agents such as photographic chemicals may also evoke a lichenoid response. LP sometimes coexist with hepatitis C.

The presence of apoptotic bodies and reduced epidermal cell turnover suggests that the lesions of LP result from basal layer cell destruction, creating reduced and subsequent reactive epidermal proliferation. Evidence suggests that LP is a delayed type of hypersensitivity reaction initiated and amplified by cytokines, such as IFN-γ and IL-6, which are produced both by infiltrating lymphocytes and by stimulated keratinocytes.

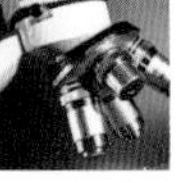

PATHOLOGY: The epidermis in LP features compact hyperkeratosis with little or no parakeratosis. The absence of the latter correlates with reduced epidermal turnover associated with damage to basal keratinocytes. The stratum granulosum is thickened, frequently in a distinctive, focal, wedge-shaped pattern, with the base of the wedge abutting the stratum corneum. The stratum spinosum is variably thickened.

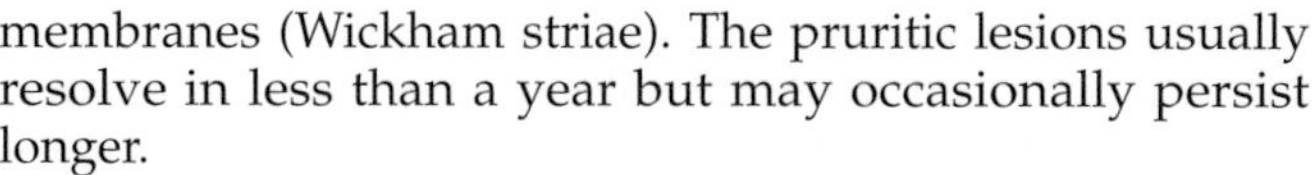

The distinctive pathology of LP is at the dermal–epidermal interface. The basal row of cuboidal cells is replaced by flattened or polygonal keratinocytes. The undulating interface between the dermal papillae and the rounded profiles of the rete ridges is obscured by a dense infiltrate of helper/inducer lymphocytes and macrophages, many of the latter containing melanin pigment (**melanophages**) (Fig. 20-20). Sharply pointed ("saw-toothed") rete ridges of keratinocytes project into the inflammatory infiltrate.

Commonly admixed with the infiltrate (in the epidermis or dermis) are globular, fibrillary, eosinophilic bodies, 15 to 20 µm (Fig. 20-20), which represent apoptotic keratinocytes. These structures are variably called *apoptotic, colloid, Civatte,* or *fibrillary bodies.* The fibrils within the apoptotic bodies are keratin filaments. Epidermal Langerhans cells are increased early in LP.

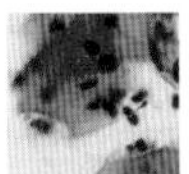

CLINICAL FEATURES: LP is a chronic eruption with violaceous, flat-topped papules, usually on the flexor surfaces of the wrists (Fig. 20-20A). White patches or streaks may also be present on oral mucous membranes (Wickham striae). The pruritic lesions usually resolve in less than a year but may occasionally persist longer.

INFLAMMATORY DISEASES OF THE SUPERFICIAL AND DEEP VASCULAR BED

Urticaria and Angioedema

These reactions are initiated by degranulation of mast cells sensitized to a specific antigen. **Urticaria** ("hives") are raised, pale, pruritic papules and plaques that appear and disappear within a few hours. The lesions represent edema of the superficial dermis. **Angioedema** is a condition in which the edema involves the deeper dermis or subcutis, resulting in an egglike swelling. Both entities have a rapid onset and range in severity from simply annoying lesions to life-threatening anaphylactic reactions. The mainstays of treatment are avoiding the offending agent and prompt administration of antihistamines.

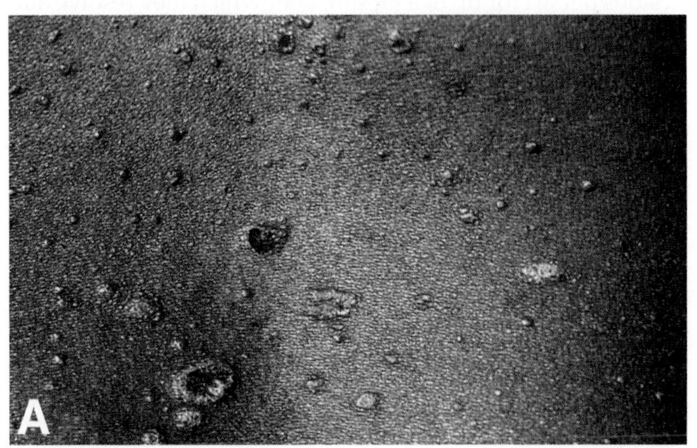

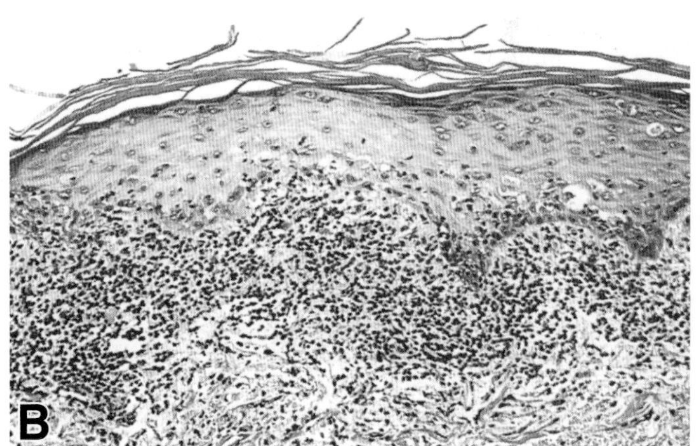

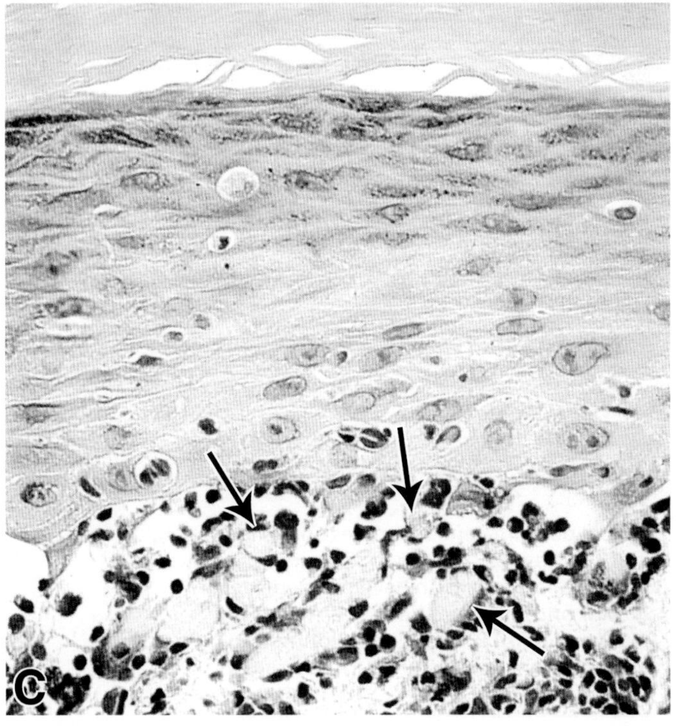

FIGURE 20-20. Lichen planus. A. The skin displaying multiple flat-topped violaceous polygonal papules. **B.** A cell-rich, band-like, lymphocytic infiltrate disrupting the stratum basalis. Unlike lupus erythematosus, there is usually epidermal hyperplasia, hyperkeratosis, and wedgelike hypergranulosis. **C.** Hypergranulosis and loss of rete ridges are noted. The site of pathologic injury is at the dermal–epidermal junction where there is a striking infiltrate of lymphocytes, many of which surround apoptotic keratinocytes (*arrows*). 20-20A From Elder AD, Elenitsas R, Johnson BL, et al. *Synopsis and Atlas of Lever's Histopathology of the Skin*. Philadelphia, PA: Lippincott Williams & Wilkins; 1999: p. 2, clin.

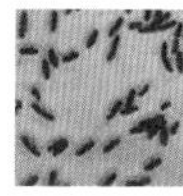

ETIOLOGIC FACTORS: Most cases of urticaria are IgE dependent and reflect exaggerated venule permeability owing to mast cell degranulation. An almost endless list of materials may react with IgE antibodies on the surface of the mast cell. Urticaria may occur in both atopic and nonatopic people. Atopic patients have intensely pruritic skin eruptions, a family history of similar eruptions, and a personal or family history of allergies. They commonly have elevated circulating IgE (see Chapter 3).

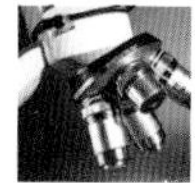

PATHOLOGY: In urticaria, collagen fibers and fibrils are splayed apart by excess fluid. Lymphatic vessels are dilated; venules show margination of neutrophils and eosinophils. Vessels are cuffed by a few lymphocytes. In persistent urticaria, lymphocytes and eosinophils are increased, but neutrophils are sparse.

Cutaneous Necrotizing Vasculitis

CNV presents as **"palpable purpura"** and has also been called **allergic cutaneous vasculitis, leukocytoclastic vasculitis,** and **hypersensitivity angiitis** (see also Vasculitis in Chapter 8).

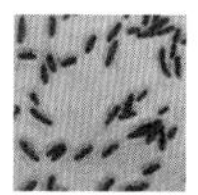

ETIOLOGIC FACTORS: In CNV, circulating immune complexes deposit in vessel walls at sites of injuries, at branch points where turbulence is increased, or where venous circulation is slowed, as in the lower extremities. Elaborated C5a complement component attracts neutrophils, which degranulate and release lysosomal enzymes, causing endothelial damage and fibrin deposition.

CNV is primary, that is, without a known precipitating event, in half of the cases. The disorder may also be associated with a specific infectious agent (e.g., hepatitis B or C). It may also be a secondary process in a variety of chronic diseases, such as rheumatoid arthritis, SLE, and ulcerative colitis. CNV may also be linked to (1) underlying malignancies such as lymphoma, (2) a drug or some other allergy, or (3) a postinfectious process, such as Henoch–Schönlein purpura.

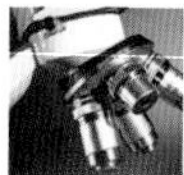

PATHOLOGY: Lesions of CNV show vessel walls obliterated by a neutrophilic infiltrate. Endothelial cells are difficult to visualize, and vessel damage is manifested by fibrin deposition and erythrocyte extravasation (Fig. 20-21). Many of the neutrophils are also damaged, resulting in dustlike nuclear remnants, a process known as "leukocytoclasia." The collagen fibers between affected vessels are separated by neutrophils, eosinophils, and leukocytoclastic cellular remnants, as well as the extravasated erythrocytes that account for the characteristic palpable purpura.

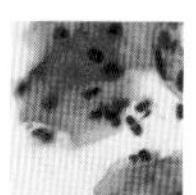

CLINICAL FEATURES: CNV is distinguished by 2- to 4-mm red, palpable lesions that do not blanch under pressure ("palpable purpura") (Fig. 20-21). Multiple lesions characteristically appear in crops on the legs or at sites of pressure. Lesions may be confined to the skin in an otherwise healthy person or may involve small blood vessels in the joints, gastrointestinal tract, or kidneys. Individual lesions persist for up to a month, after which they resolve and leave hyperpigmentation or atrophic scars. Despite removal of the offending agent, episodes of CNV may recur.

Allergic Contact Dermatitis

Members of the *Rhus* genus of plants are common sensitizing agents, so that 90% of the population of the United States is sensitive to the common offenders: *Rhus radicans* (poison ivy), *Rhus diversiloba* (poison oak), and *Rhus vernix* (poison sumac).

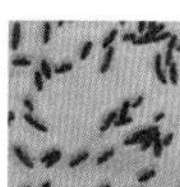

ETIOLOGIC FACTORS: The offending plant contains low–molecular-weight **haptens** (see Chapter 3), in particular, oleoresins. They are active in

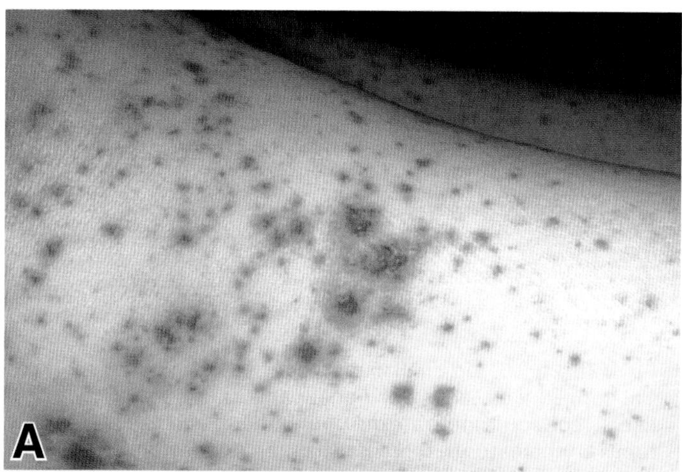

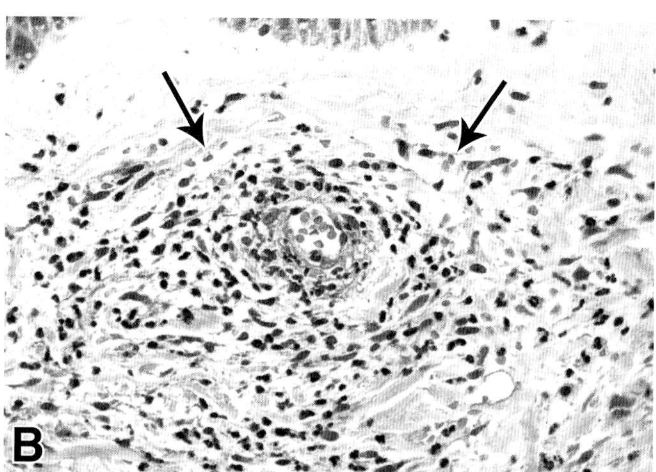

FIGURE 20-21. Cutaneous necrotizing vasculitis. A. Palpable purpuric tender papules on the legs of a 25-year-old woman. The condition resolved after therapy for streptococcal pharyngitis. **B.** The vessel is surrounded by pink fibrin and neutrophils, many of which have disintegrated (leukocytoclasis). Extravasated red blood cells (*arrows*) and inflammation give the classic clinical appearance of "palpable purpura." 20-21A From Elder AD, Elenitsas R, Johnson BL, et al. *Synopsis and Atlas of Lever's Histopathology of the Skin*. Philadelphia, PA: Lippincott Williams & Wilkins; 1999.

sensitization only when they combine with a carrier protein (see Chapter 3). This likely happens at the cell membrane of the Langerhans cell in the **sensitization phase**, a process that has been studied as a prototype of antigenic sensitization in delayed-type hypersensitivity. Formation of a **hapten–carrier complex** requires about 1 hour, after which it is processed as an antigen by Langerhans cells. These cells carry the antigen through the lymphatics to regional lymph nodes and present it to $CD4^+$ T cells. After 5 to 7 days, some of these T lymphocytes recognize the antigen, become activated, multiply, and circulate in the blood as memory cells. Some migrate to the skin, ready to react with the antigen if they encounter it again. IL-1, made by Langerhans cells, supports proliferation of $CD4^+$ T_H1 cells, the effectors of delayed hypersensitivity.

In the **elicitation phase**, specifically sensitized T lymphocytes in the circulation enter the skin. At the site of antigen challenge, Langerhans cells, endothelial cells, perivascular dendritic cells, and monocytes process the antigen and present it to the specifically sensitized T cells, which then migrate into the epidermis. Cytokine production causes accumulation of more T cells and macrophages, which are responsible for epidermal cell injury.

PATHOLOGY: Allergic contact dermatitis is a type of **spongiotic dermatitis**. In the 24 hours after reexposure to the offending plant (elicitation phase), lymphocytes and macrophages congregate about superficial venules and extend into the epidermis. Epidermal keratinocytes are partially separated by the edema fluid, creating a spongelike appearance (**spongiosis**) (Fig. 20-22). The stratum corneum contains coagulated eosinophilic fluid and plasma proteins. Later, many mononuclear inflammatory cells and eosinophils accumulate. Vesicles containing lymphocytes and macrophages are present, and abundant eosinophilic coagulated fluid accrues in the stratum corneum.

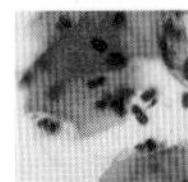

CLINICAL FEATURES: At first contact with poison ivy, for example, there is no immediate reaction. Five to 7 days after a re-exposure, the site of contact becomes intensely pruritic. Then, erythema and small vesicles rapidly develop (Fig. 20-22). Over the next few days, the area enlarges, becomes fiery red, develops vesicles and exudes a large amount of clear proteinaceous fluid. Pruritus is intense. The entire process lasts about 3 weeks. Exudation gradually subsides, and the area is covered by an irregular crust that eventually falls off. Pruritus diminishes and healing occurs without scarring.

When a sensitized patient again comes into contact with poison ivy, the process is faster. Lesions appear within 1 to 2 days, spread rapidly, and produce the same clinical appearance. However, the reaction is usually more intense. Lesions again clear in about 3 weeks. Allergic contact dermatitis responds to topical or systemic corticosteroids.

Sarcoidosis

Cutaneous manifestations of sarcoidosis are asymptomatic papules, plaques, and nodules in the dermis and subcutis. Some dermal plaques are annular, and those that involve the subcutis appear as irregular nodules. In severe cases, cutaneous lesions are so prominent that they simulate a diffusely infiltrative neoplasm (see Chapter 10).

SCLERODERMA

Scleroderma displays variable structural and functional involvement of internal organs as well as the skin. **Morphea** is similar to scleroderma but involves only patchy, circumscribed areas of the skin. The pathogenesis and systemic manifestations of scleroderma are discussed elsewhere (see Chapter 3).

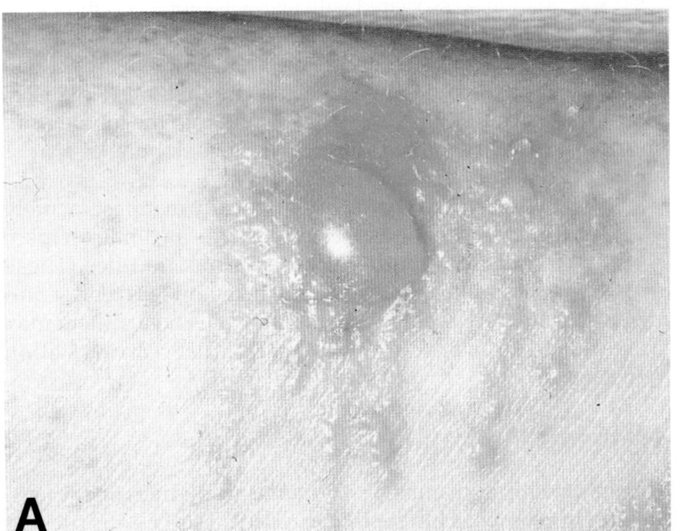

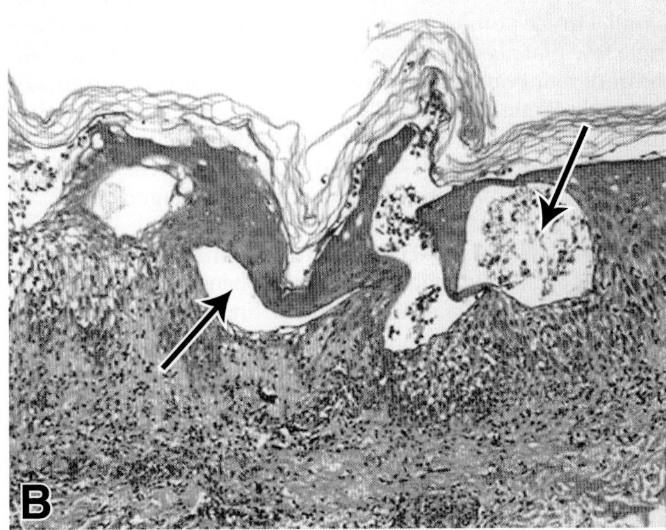

FIGURE 20-22. Allergic contact dermatitis. A. Vesicles and bullae developed on the volar forearm after application of perfume. **B.** Epidermal spongiosis and spongiotic vesicles (*arrows*) are present in this biopsy of "poison ivy." Infiltrating lymphocytes are apparent in the epidermis, where they effect the cell-mediated delayed hypersensitivity reaction. 20-22A From Elder AD, Elenitsas R, Johnson BL, et al. *Synopsis and Atlas of Lever's Histopathology of the Skin*. Philadelphia, PA: Lippincott Williams & Wilkins; 1999.

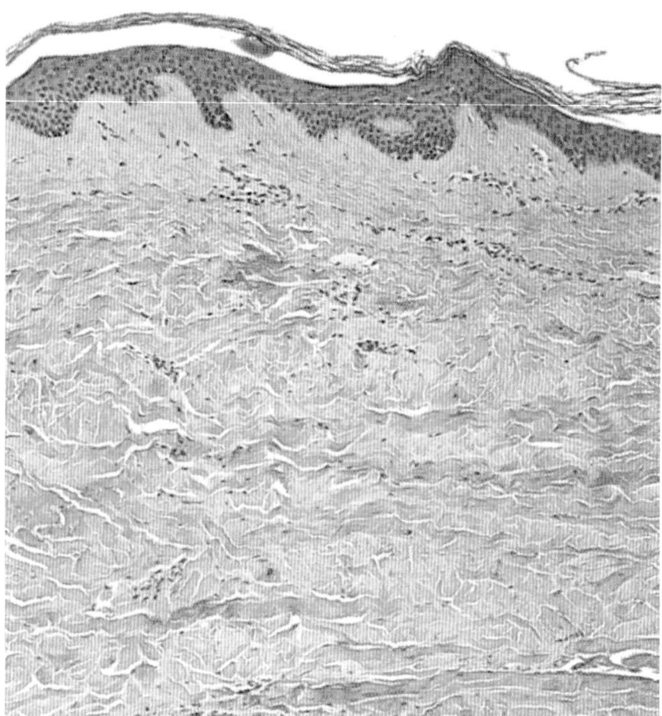

FIGURE 20-23. Scleroderma. The dermis is characterized by large, reticular collagen bundles that are oriented parallel to the epidermis. The large size and loss of basket-weave pattern of these collagen bundles are abnormal. No appendages are apparent because these structures have been destroyed.

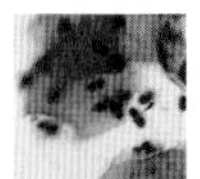

PATHOLOGY: The initial cutaneous lesions of scleroderma are in the lower reticular dermis, but eventually, the entire reticular dermis and even the papillary dermis are involved. There is diminished space among collagen bundles in the reticular dermis and a tendency for the collagen bundles to be enlarged, hypocellular, and parallel to each other. A patchy lymphocytic infiltrate containing a few plasma cells is common and may also be present in the underlying subcutaneous tissue. Sweat ducts are entrapped in the thickened fibrous tissue, and the fat that is usually around them is lost. Hair follicles are completely obliterated (Fig. 20-23). In late stages of the disease, large areas of subcutaneous fat are replaced by newly formed collagen.

CLINICAL FEATURES: Patients with early scleroderma usually present with Raynaud phenomenon or nonpitting edema of the hands or fingers. Affected areas become hard and tense. The skin of the face becomes mask like and expressionless, and the skin around the mouth exhibits radial furrows. In late stages of the disease, the skin over large parts of the body is thickened, densely fibrotic, and fixed to the underlying tissue. Prognosis is related to the extent of disease in visceral organs, particularly the lung and kidney.

INFLAMMATORY DISORDERS OF THE PANNICULUS

Panniculitis denotes a diverse group of diseases characterized by inflammation, mainly in the subcutis (panniculus). The disorders gathered under the umbrella of panniculitis are classified according to the location of the inflammation. **Septal panniculitis** is an inflammation in connective tissue septa, whereas **lobular panniculitis** entails involvement of fat lobules. These two entities may occur with or without accompanying vasculitis.

Erythema Nodosum

EN is a cutaneous disorder that manifests as nonsuppurative, self-limited, tender nodules over extensor surfaces of the legs. It has a peak incidence in the third decade of life and is three times more common in women than in men.

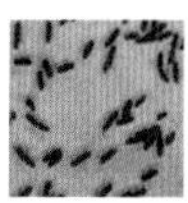

ETIOLOGIC FACTORS: EN is triggered by a variety of agents, such as drugs and microorganisms, and accompanies a number of benign and malignant systemic diseases. Common infections complicated by EN include streptococcal diseases (especially in children), tuberculosis, and *Yersinia* infection. In endemic areas, deep fungal infections (blastomycosis, histoplasmosis, and coccidioidomycosis) are common causes. EN also frequently occurs after acute respiratory tract infections, which are likely viral. The agents most commonly implicated in drug-induced EN are sulfonamides and oral contraceptives. Finally, people with Crohn disease and ulcerative colitis may develop EN.

EN most likely represents an immunologic response to foreign antigens. For example, patients with tuberculosis or coccidioidomycosis do not develop EN until skin tests for reactions to antigens of those infectious agents become positive. The early acute inflammation suggests that EN may be a response to complement activation, with resulting neutrophil chemotaxis. Subsequent chronic inflammation, foreign-body giant cells, and fibrosis are caused by adipose tissue necrosis at the interface of septa and lobules.

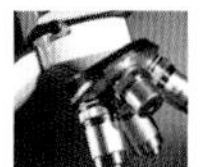

PATHOLOGY: Early EN lesions are in the fibrous septa of the subcutaneous tissue, where neutrophilic inflammation is associated with extravasation of erythrocytes. In chronic lesions, the septa are widened, with focal collections of giant cell macrophages around small areas of altered collagen and an ill-defined lymphocytic infiltrate (Fig. 20-24). Giant cells and inflammatory cells extend into the lobule from the interface between the septum and the fat lobule.

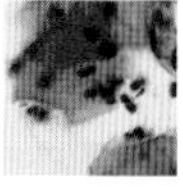

CLINICAL FEATURES: EN typically manifests acutely on the anterior aspects of the legs as dome-shaped, exquisitely tender, erythematous nodules. These lesions eventually become firm and less tender and disappear in 3 to 6 weeks. As some nodules heal, others may arise, but all lesions resolve without residual scarring within 6 weeks.

Erythema Induratum

EI refers to chronic recurrent subcutaneous nodules on the legs, mostly in women. *Mycobacterium tuberculosis* DNA is present in most biopsies, suggesting the condition is a hypersensitivity reaction to the organism.

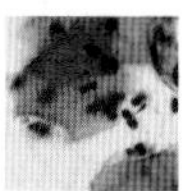

CLINICAL FEATURES: Patients with EI present with recurrent, tender, erythematous, subcutaneous nodules on the legs, particularly the calves (as opposed to the shins, which are the usual location of EN).

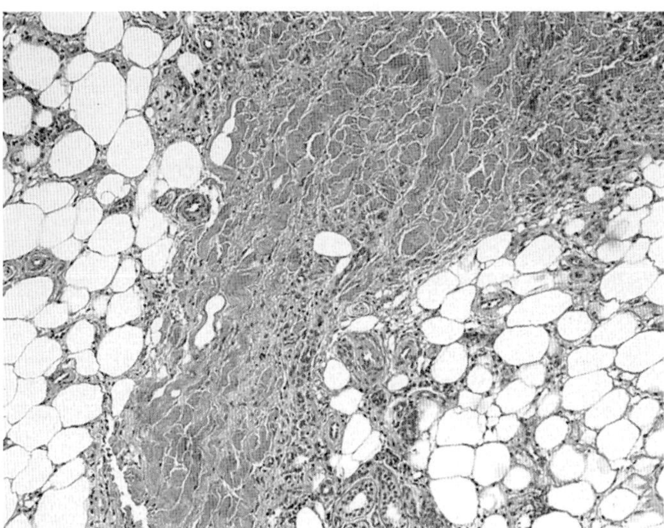

FIGURE 20-24. Erythema nodosum. The reticular dermis is present in the *upper right.* Within the panniculus is a widened septum (*extending through the middle of the field*). Lymphocytes and macrophages are present at its interface with the adipose tissue lobules. The vessels palisading along the interface of the septum are infiltrated by lymphocytes.

Lesions tend to ulcerate and heal with an atrophic scar. The course may last many years. Systemic steroids are usually necessary to control the disease.

Acne Vulgaris

Acne vulgaris is a self-limited, inflammatory disorder of sebaceous follicles that typically afflicts adolescents, results in intermittent formation of discrete papular or pustular lesions and may lead to scarring. In some cases, acne extends to the third decade.

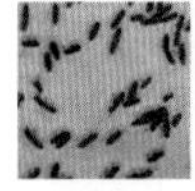

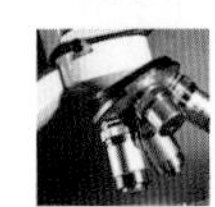

ETIOLOGIC FACTORS AND PATHOLOGY: The development of acne is related to (1) excessive hormonally induced production of sebum, (2) abnormal cornification of portions of the follicular epithelium, (3) a response to the anaerobic diphtheroid *Propionibacterium acnes*, and (4) follicle rupture and subsequent inflammation. The sebaceous follicle contains a vellus hair and prominent sebaceous glands. Changes in hormonal status at puberty generate sebum production in the follicle and altered cornification in the neck of the sebaceous follicle (infundibulum). These effects lead to dilation of the follicular canal. Continuing excessive sebum production is associated with desquamation of squamous cells and accretion of keratinous debris, providing a rich environment for *P. acnes* proliferation. These combined changes produce a distended, plugged follicle termed a **comedone**. Neutrophils attracted to the area by chemotactic factors released by *P. acnes* form a follicular abscess (**pustule**). They also attack the follicle wall, thereby permitting escape of sebum, keratin, and bacteria into perifollicular tissue, where they stimulate further acute inflammation and a perifollicular abscess (Fig. 20-25). The development of allergy to *P. acnes* intensifies the inflammatory response. Fully evolved lesions show intense neutrophilic inflammation surrounding a ruptured sebaceous follicle. In addition, abundant macrophages, lymphocytes, and foreign-body giant cells accumulate in response to rupture of the sebaceous follicle.

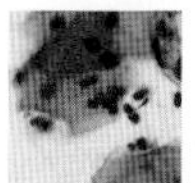

CLINICAL FEATURES: Acne vulgaris features a variety of skin lesions in different stages of development, including comedones, papules, pustules, nodules, cysts, and pitted scars. Comedones, the primary noninflammatory lesions of acne, are either open (**blackheads**) or closed (**whiteheads**). More advanced inflammatory lesions vary from small, erythematous papules to large, tender, purulent nodules, and cysts.

Acne vulgaris is treated with topical cleansing and keratolytic and antibacterial agents. Severe cases are managed with topical vitamin A, systemic antibiotics, or synthetic oral retinoids (isotretinoin).

INFECTIONS AND INFESTATIONS

The skin is under constant assault from countless marauders and is an effective but imperfect barrier against them; bacteria, fungi, viruses, parasites, and insects sometimes penetrate this first line of defense.

Impetigo

Superficial bacterial infections of the skin, known as **impetigo**, occur mostly in children, who are often infected through minor breaks in the skin (see also Chapter 6). Adults tend to contract impetigo after an underlying disease process compromises the barrier function of the skin. Honey-colored crusted erosions or ulcers, often with central healing, occur most commonly on exposed areas, such as the face, hands, and extremities. A combination of topical and systemic antimicrobial agents against staphylococci or streptococci is the mainstay of therapy.

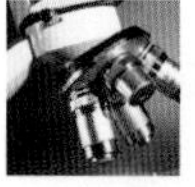

PATHOLOGY: Neutrophils accumulate beneath the stratum corneum, and bacteria may be visualized with special stains. Vesicles or bullae form and eventually rupture, allowing a thin, seropurulent discharge to appear. This discharge dries and forms the characteristic layers of exudate containing neutrophils and cell debris. Reactive epidermal changes (spongiosis, elongation of rete ridges) and superficial dermal inflammation are usually present.

Dermatophytic (Superficial Fungal) Infections

Dermatophytes are fungi that can infect nonviable keratinized epithelium, including stratum corneum, nails, and hair. They synthesize keratinases that digest keratin, thereby providing themselves with sustenance. Superficial fungal infections are often caused by a change in the skin microenvironment, allowing overgrowth of transient or resident flora. For example, use of immunosuppressive agents, such as topical or systemic glucocorticoids, may impair cell-mediated immune responses that normally eliminate dermatophytes. Excessive sweating or occlusion of a body part may provide an environment that "tips the balance" between fungal proliferation and elimination in favor of proliferation.

Of the 10 or so dermatophyte species that often cause human cutaneous infection, *Trichophyton rubrum* is the most common. A superficial dermatophyte infection is called a **dermatophytosis,**

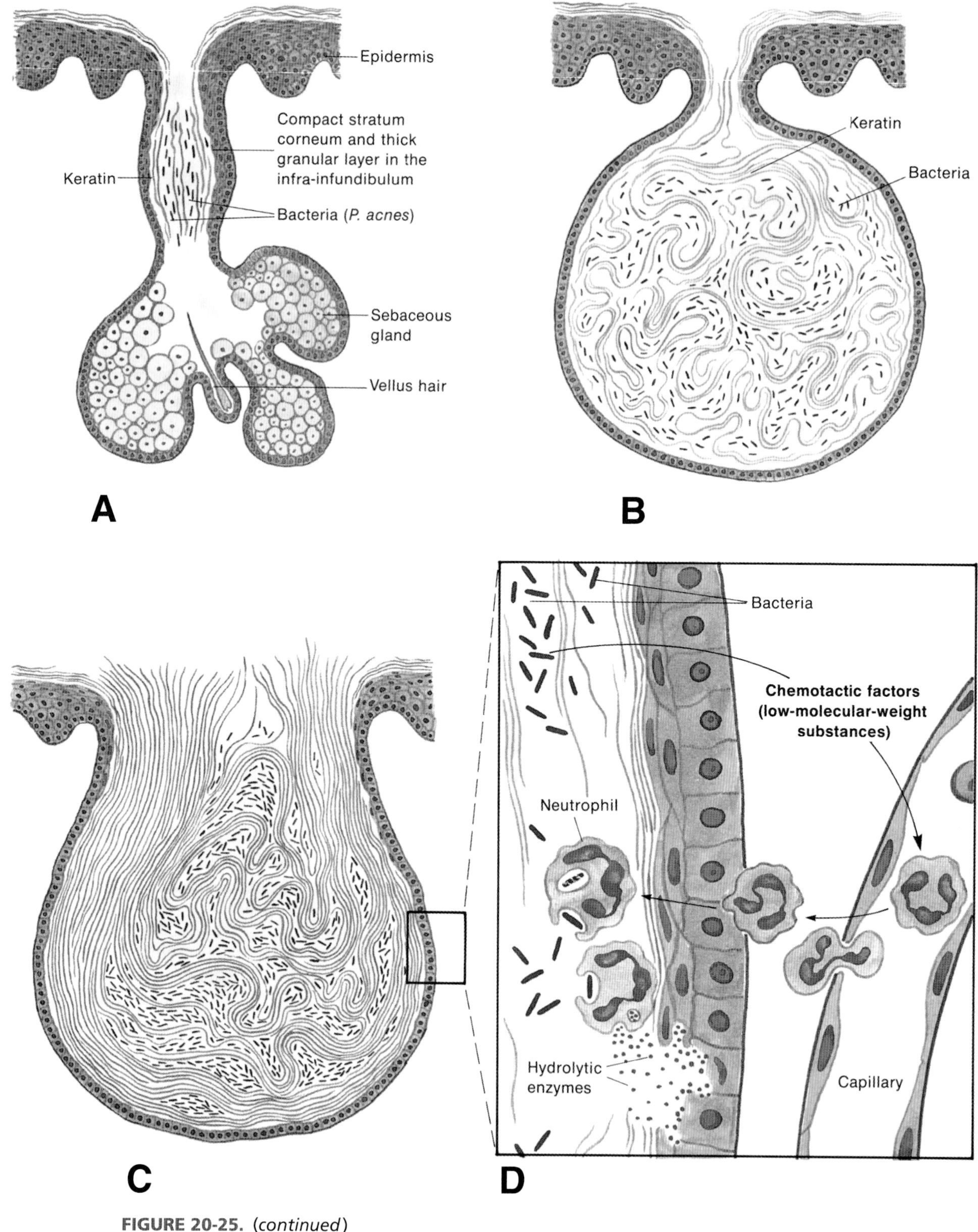

FIGURE 20-25. *(continued)*

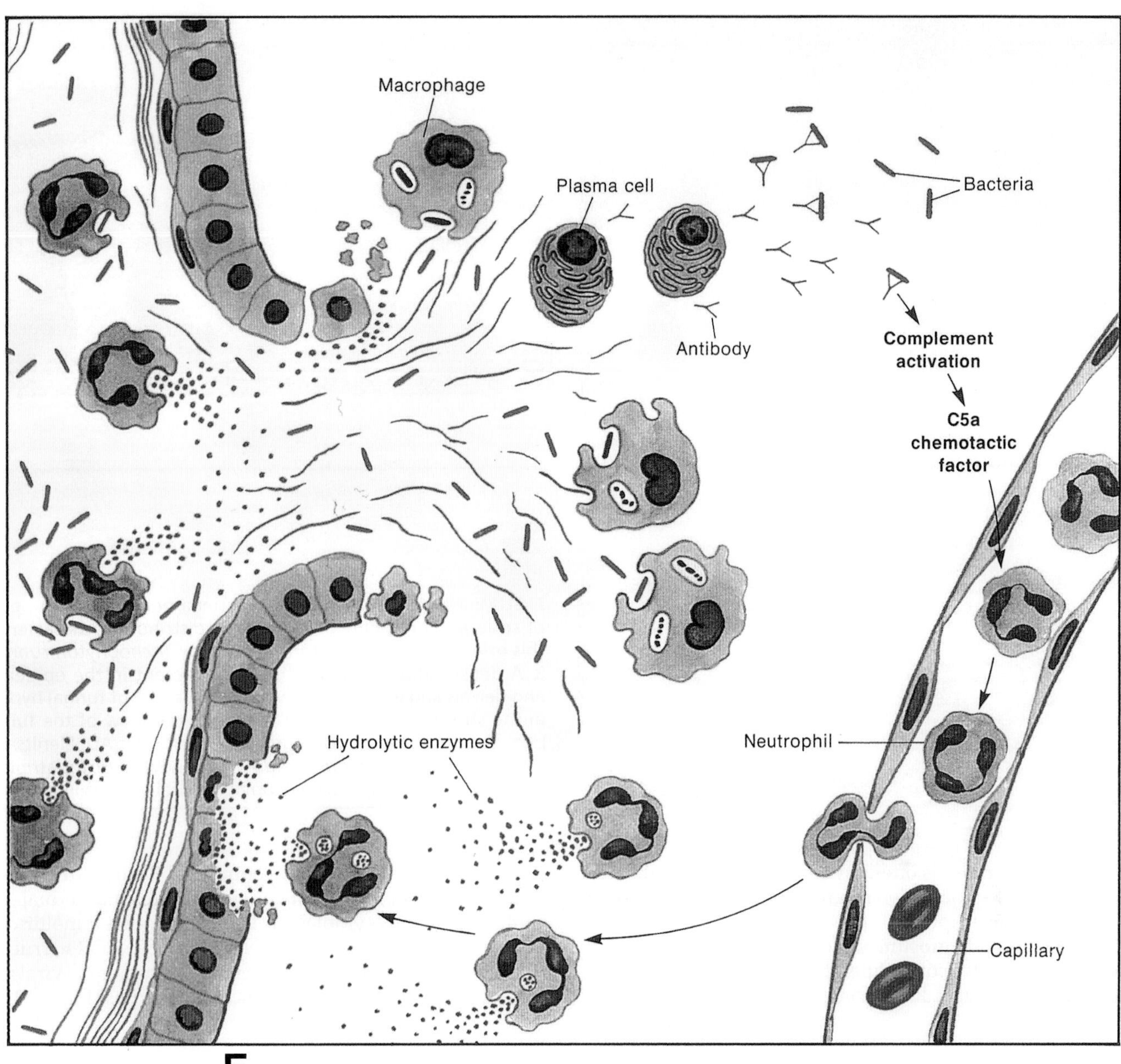

FIGURE 20-25. Acne vulgaris. The pathogenesis of follicular distention, rupture, and inflammation is depicted. Acne is a disease of the follicular canal of a sebaceous follicle. A compact stratum corneum and a thickened granular layer in the infrainfundibulum are the beginning of the formation of a comedone. Microcomedones **(A)** and closed **(B)** and open **(C)** comedones form. Excessive sebum secretion occurs, and the bacterium *Propionibacterium acnes* proliferates. The organism produces chemotactic factors, leading to neutrophil migration into the intact comedone. Neutrophilic enzymes are released, and the comedone ruptures, inducing a cycle of chemotaxis and intense neutrophilic inflammation **(D, E)**.

tinea, or **ringworm.** The tineas have distinctive clinical features depending on the site of infection. They are divided as follows: (1) **tinea capitis** (scalp; "ringworm"), (2) **tinea barbae** (beard), (3) **tinea faciei** (face), (4) **tinea corporis** (trunk, legs, arms, or neck, excluding the feet, hands, and groin), (5) **tinea manus** (hands), (6) **tinea pedis** (feet; "athlete's foot"; Fig. 20-26A), (7) **tinea cruris** (groin, pubic area, and thigh; "jock itch"), and (8) **tinea unguium** (nails; "onychomycosis") (see also Chapter 6).

Viral Skin Infections

Some viruses (see Chapters 6 and 16), such as the poxvirus **molluscum contagiosum** or **human papillomaviruses** (HPVs), cause transient benign epithelial proliferations that resolve spontaneously. Others (e.g., measles or *parvovirus* [**erythema infectiosum**]) produce febrile illnesses with self-limited cutaneous eruptions (**exanthems**). Primary infection by most

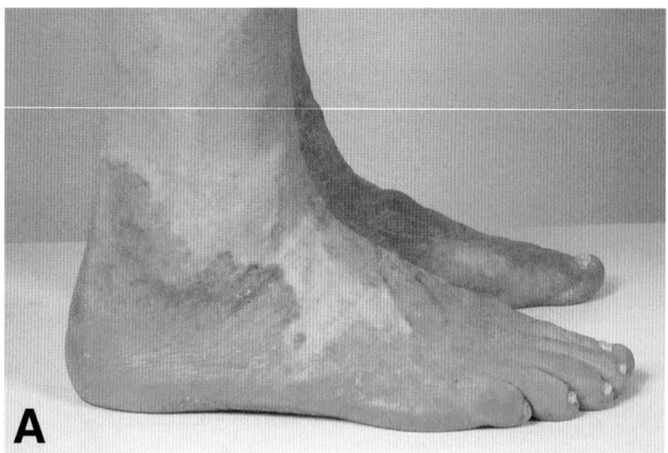

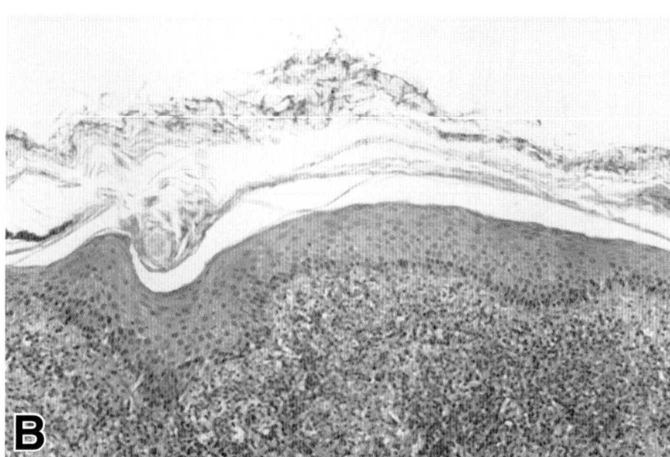

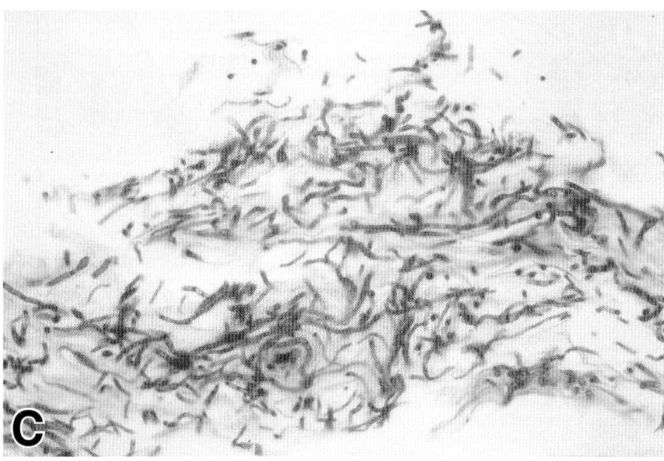

FIGURE 20-26. Dermatophytosis. A. Tinea pedis. A leading edge of scale and erythema in a moccasin distribution characterizes this infection, most commonly caused by *Trichophyton rubrum*. **B.** A dense inflammatory infiltrate is present in the epidermis and dermis and is associated with the presence of fungal hyphae in the stratum corneum. **C.** A higher power view of the fungal hyphae in the stratum corneum. 26A From Elder AD, Elenitsas R, Johnson BL, et al. *Synopsis and Atlas of Lever's Histopathology of the Skin*. Philadelphia, PA: Lippincott Williams & Wilkins; 1999.

human herpesviruses is often asymptomatic but results in a state of latent infection. Upon reactivation, the virus causes a painful, vesicular eruption.

Molluscum contagiosum is a common infection among children and sexually active adults. It is self-limited and is easily spread by direct contact. Firm, dome-shaped, smooth-surfaced papules with a characteristic central umbilication are usually found on the face, trunk, and anogenital area. Epidermal cells contain large intracytoplasmic inclusion bodies ("molluscum bodies") within cup-shaped areas that also exhibit verrucous (papillomatous) epidermal hyperplasia. Numerous viral particles are present within these inclusion bodies (Fig. 20-27).

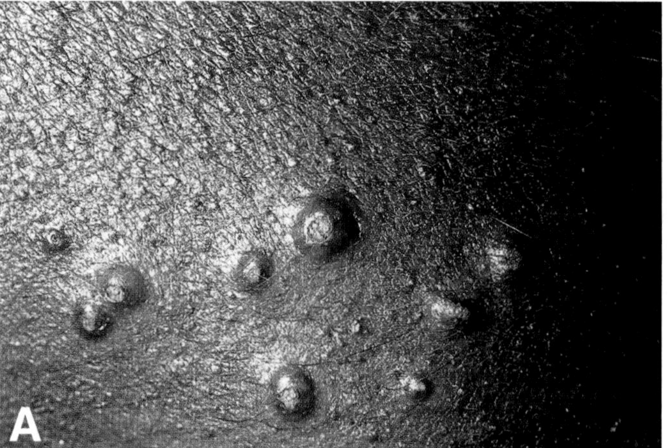

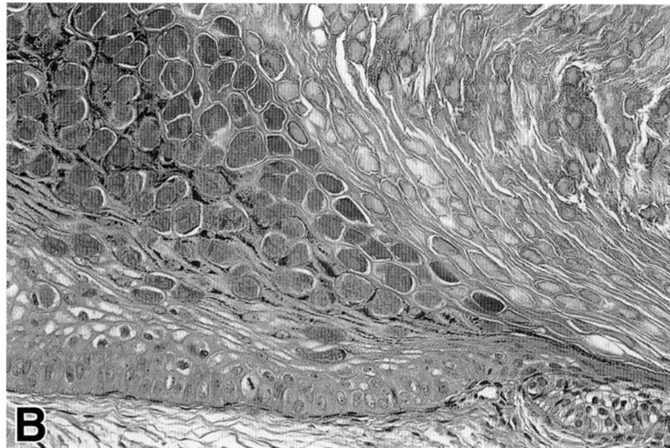

FIGURE 20-27. Molluscum contagiosum. A. Multiple umbilicated papules in an HIV-positive patient. **B.** The keratinocytes that are infected with this poxvirus show large eosinophilic cytoplasmic inclusions called "molluscum bodies." From Elder AD, Elenitsas R, Johnson BL, et al. *Synopsis and Atlas of Lever's Histopathology of the Skin*. Philadelphia, PA: Lippincott Williams & Wilkins; 1999.

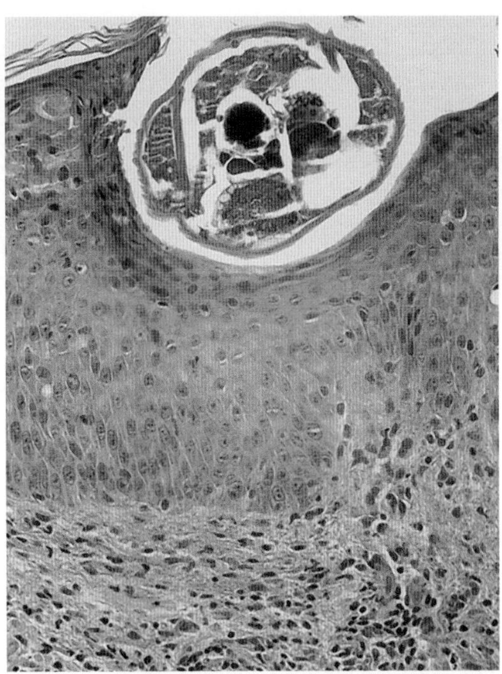

FIGURE 20-28. Scabetic nodule. A scabies mite is present in the stratum corneum. From Elder AD, Elenitsas R, Johnson BL, et al. *Synopsis and Atlas of Lever's Histopathology of the Skin*. Philadelphia, PA: Lippincott Williams & Wilkins; 1999.

Arthropod Infestations

Mites and lice, other insects, and spiders cause local lesions that are often very pruritic.

- ***Scabies*** is a severely pruritic, eczematous dermatitis caused by the mite *Sarcoptes scabiei*. The female mite burrows beneath the stratum corneum on the fingers, wrists, trunk, and genital skin (Fig. 20-28). Intense lymphocytic and eosinophilic dermatitis is induced as a hypersensitivity reaction to the mite and its eggs and feces.
- ***Pediculosis***, another pruritic dermatosis, may be caused by a variety of human lice. Eggs ("nits") of the lice tend to be attached to hair shafts.
- **Biting insects** produce lesions that vary from small, pruritic papules to large, weeping nodules. The reaction varies with the arthropod species and host immune response. For example, tick bites are usually large, with a striking lymphocytic and eosinophilic infiltrate. Lymphoid follicles may also form. Flea bites are mostly urticarial, with a scant neutrophilic infiltrate. The venoms injected by arthropods, such as the brown recluse spider, may give rise to severe local tissue necrosis.

PRIMARY NEOPLASMS OF THE SKIN

Benign Tumors of Melanocytes

Congenital Melanocytic Nevus

About 1% of white children are born with some form of pigmented skin lesion, sometimes as inconspicuous as a small patch of pale tan hyperpigmentation. Much more rarely, the trunk or an extremity is covered by a large pigmented patch or plaque that is cosmetically deforming ("giant hairy" or "garment" nevus). Such areas display a striking increase in intraepidermal and dermal melanocytes, which may extend deep into the subcutaneous tissue. Malignant melanomas may, at times, develop during childhood in these large congenital melanocytic nevi. Attempts are sometimes made to remove these conspicuous lesions, but their size may make surgical removal problematic.

Spitz Nevus/Tumor

Spitz tumors (also known as spindle and epithelioid cell nevi) occur in children or adolescents and, less often, in adults. They are elevated, spheroid, pink, smooth nodules, usually on the head or neck. Spitz tumors grow rapidly, reaching 3 to 5 mm in 6 months or less. The lesions are composed of large spindle or epithelioid melanocytes in the epidermis and dermis (Fig. 20-29). The cells are so atypical that an incorrect diagnosis of melanoma may be made, even though melanoma is rare in childhood. Most Spitz tumors are benign and are called Spitz nevi. A few have metastasized, although usually not beyond regional nodes. Therefore, the prognosis is to some extent uncertain, especially in adults. Most Spitz tumors have fusion gene rearrangements that form constitutively activated chimeric oncogenes, rather than the point mutations that are the rule in melanomas (see below).

Blue Nevus

Blue nevi appear in childhood or late adolescence as dark blue, gray, or black, firm, papules or nodules on the dorsal hands or feet or on the buttocks, scalp, or face. Their clinical appearance may prompt an excisional biopsy to rule out nodular melanoma. Melanin-containing melanocytes with long, thin dendrites are present in the superficial to mid-dermis, where they are often admixed with numerous melanin-containing macrophages (Fig. 20-30). There are also rare examples of "malignant blue nevi."

Freckle and Lentigo

Freckles, or **ephelides**, are small, brown macules that occur on sun-exposed skin, especially in people with fair skin. They show hyperpigmentation of basal keratinocytes without a concomitant increase in the number of melanocytes. The pigmentation of a freckle deepens with exposure to sunlight and fades when light exposure ceases. A **lentigo** is a discrete, brown macule that appears at any age and on any part of the body. A **solar lentigo**, or "liver spot," appears at an older age after long-term sun exposure. Unlike ephelides, the pigmentation of a lentigo does not depend on sun exposure. Lentigines display elongated rete ridges, increased melanin pigment in both basal keratinocytes and melanocytes, and increased melanocytes. Larger lesions may need to be biopsied to rule out lentigo maligna melanoma.

Lentigines, often called freckles by the public and by clinicians, are strong risk factors for melanoma, acting synergistically with nevi, dysplastic nevi, and other risk factors. Their prevalence is strongly related to polymorphisms of the melanocortin receptor gene (*MC1R*, which has been named the "freckle gene").

Verrucae

Verrucae are elevated, circumscribed cutaneous tumors, which often appear papillary. ***HPV infection is the cause of verrucae*** (see Chapter 16).

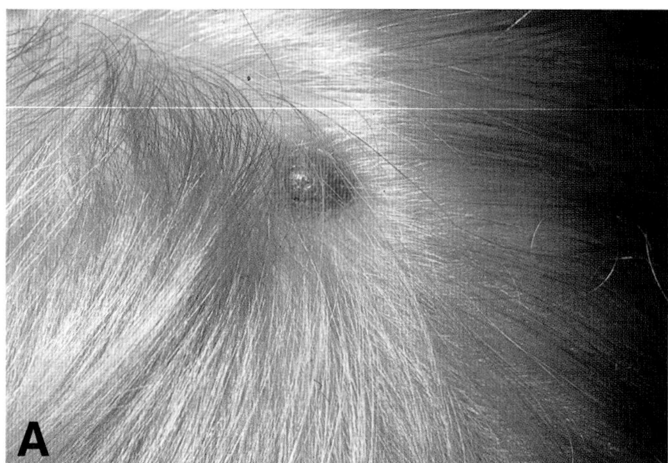
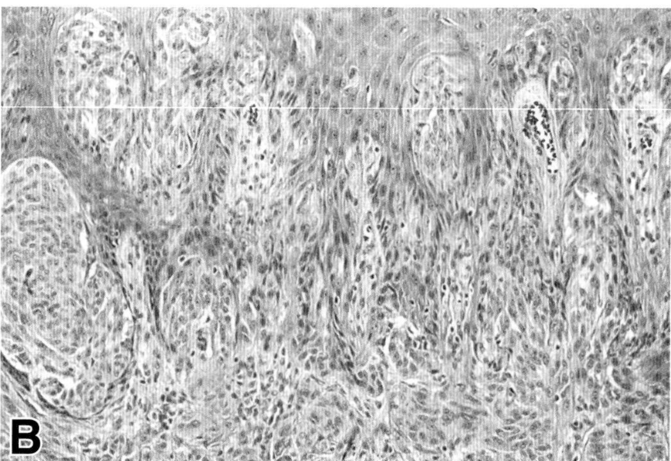

FIGURE 20-29. Spindle and epithelioid cell (Spitz) nevus. A. A symmetric pink nodule appeared suddenly in a child but then remained stable for several weeks until it was excised. **B.** Spitz tumors are composed of large melanocytes with prominent nuclei. Within a hyperplastic epidermis, the melanocytes are present in large nests. Even though the cells are large and, at first glance, suggest melanoma, they are much more uniform than the cells of most malignant melanomas. 20-29A From Elder AD, Elenitsas R, Johnson BL, et al. *Synopsis and Atlas of Lever's Histopathology of the Skin*. Philadelphia, PA: Lippincott Williams & Wilkins; 1999.

PATHOLOGY:

- **Verruca vulgaris**, or the **common wart**, is an elevated papule with a verrucous (papillomatous) surface. Such lesions may be single or multiple and occur most commonly on the dorsal surfaces of the hands or on the face. Verruca vulgaris displays hyperkeratosis and papillary epidermal hyperplasia (Fig. 20-31). **Koilocytes** (i.e., enlarged keratinocytes with a pyknotic nucleus surrounded by a halo-like cleared area) are seen within the upper epidermis. Viral inclusions are difficult to identify (Fig. 20-32). HPV, especially serotypes 2 and 4, is commonly found in verruca vulgaris. There is no malignant potential.
- **Plantar warts** are benign, frequently painful, hyperkeratotic nodules on the soles of the feet. Occasionally, similar lesions appear on the palms of the hands (**palmar warts**). Plantar warts are endophytic or exophytic, papillary, squamous epithelial proliferations. The cells contain abundant cytoplasmic inclusions that resemble the darker-staining keratohyaline granules. The nuclei of keratinocytes near the base of these warts also contain pink nuclear inclusions. HPV type 1 is the etiologic agent.

Melanocytic Nevi

Melanocytic nevi (moles) are localized benign neoplastic proliferations of melanocytes within the epidermis or dermis.

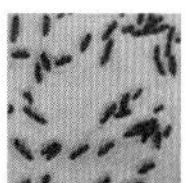

ETIOLOGIC FACTORS: Most people, regardless of skin color, eventually develop 10 to 50 nevi on their skin. The total number depends on light exposure

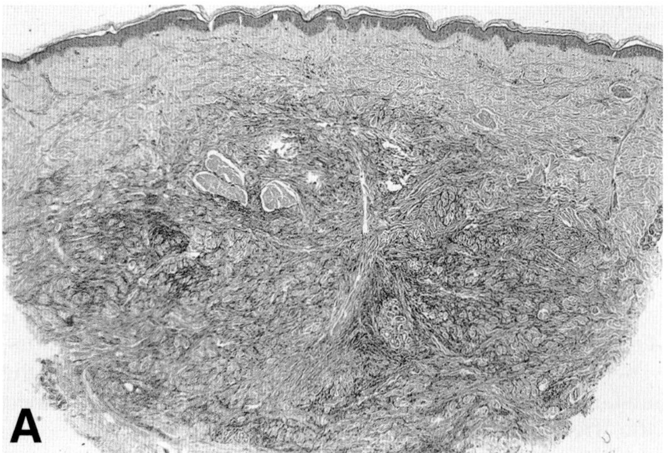
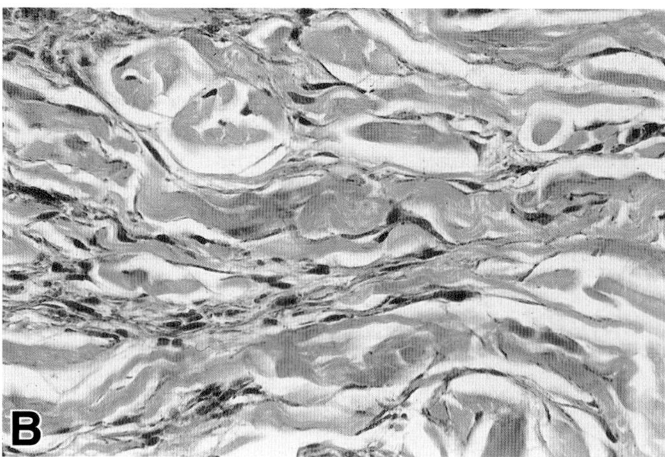

FIGURE 20-30. Blue nevus. A. Within the dermis, there is a poorly defined but symmetric spindle cell proliferation that is dark brown. **B.** The lesion is composed of elongated cells with heavily pigmented dendrites and small bland nuclei. From Elder AD, Elenitsas R, Johnson BL, et al. *Synopsis and Atlas of Lever's Histopathology of the Skin*. Philadelphia, PA: Lippincott Williams & Wilkins; 1999.

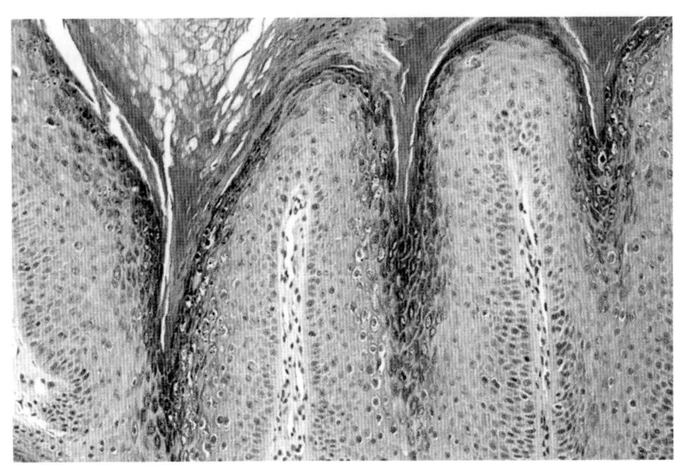

FIGURE 20-31. **Verruca vulgaris.** Verruca vulgaris is the prototype of papillary epidermal hyperplasia. Squamous epithelial-lined fronds have fibrovascular cores. The blood vessels within the cores extend close to the surface of verrucae, making them susceptible to traumatic hemorrhage and the resultant black "seeds" that patients observe.

and innate susceptibility. Nevi are important mainly in relation to melanoma because they serve as markers for an increased risk of developing melanoma. Even though 30% of melanomas arise in relation to a nevus, nevi are much more common than melanomas, and most are stable or undergo senescence over time. Thus, wholesale excision of nevi is not effective as a means of preventing melanoma.

Black skin can develop nevi, but less commonly. Those nevi that develop in the skin of darkly pigmented people are usually not associated with an increased risk of melanoma. However, the risk of melanoma from nevi on the palms of the hands, the soles of the feet, or the genital skin is the same in all races. Nevi, like melanomas, do not ordinarily develop in areas protected from light by at least two layers of clothing, such as the buttocks. There is an unequivocal causal relationship between exposure to ultraviolet light and melanocytic nevi (and malignant melanoma), but the relationship is complex.

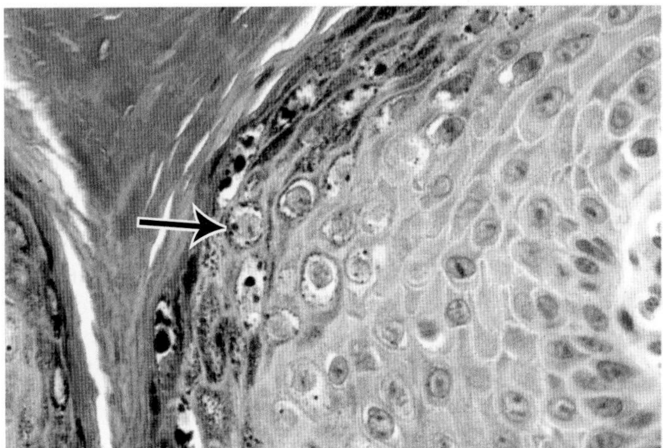

FIGURE 20-32. **Verruca vulgaris.** Characteristic cytopathic changes occur in the outer portion of the stratum spinosum and stratum granulosum, in which there is perinuclear vacuolization and prominent keratohyaline granules, with homogeneous blue inclusions (*arrow*).

Some people with fair skin form relatively few nevi, whereas those with dark skin occasionally develop numerous nevi. The ability to form nevi is partly under genetic control and has been correlated with polymorphic variants of the melanocortin receptor and with subsequent variation in the ratio of pheomelanin and eumelanin. These are the pigments associated with red and brown hair, respectively, and also with susceptibility to burning and tanning. There are at least two distinguishable profiles of persons at risk for melanoma. One group prototypically has skin that may burn but can tan and has an increased number of nevi. The other group consists of red-haired, blue-eyed people with milk-white skin, who are exquisitely sensitive to light and do not tan well. However, they form freckles and do not develop a significant number of nevi.

MOLECULAR PATHOGENESIS: A majority of nevi have an activating mutation of the oncogene *BRAF*, which can lead to growth stimulation through the MAPK pathway. However, after an initial period of growth, nevi are stable lesions that may regress or senesce. Such senescence is mediated by increased activity of p16, which is encoded by the gene *CDKN2A* on chromosome 9p21 and is an inhibitor of CDK4. The p16 protein suppresses cell proliferation and promotes end-stage differentiation of the nevus cells (see Chapter 4).

Epidemiologic studies have shown that melanocytic nevi are strong risk markers for the development of melanomas. Someone with 100 or more nevi that are 2 to 5 mm has a threefold greater risk of developing melanoma than a person with fewer than 25 similar nevi. Patients with clinically atypical-appearing nevi or histologically proven dysplastic nevi are at even greater risk for melanoma. Only 10 or more clinically atypical or dysplastic nevi are sufficient to be associated with a 12-fold increased risk for melanoma. Because nevi are very common and melanomas are not, the risk of progression of any one nevus is small.

Melanocytic nevi begin to appear between the first and second years of life and continue to emerge for the first two decades of life. A nevus first appears as a small tan dot no bigger than 1 to 2 mm. During the next 3 to 4 years, the dot enlarges to become a uniform tan to brown circular or oval area. When it reaches 4 to 5 mm in diameter, it is flat or slightly elevated, stops enlarging peripherally, and is sharply demarcated from surrounding normal skin. Over the next 10 years, the lesion elevates, and its color pales to the point of becoming a tan taglike protrusion. For the next decade or two, it gradually flattens, and the skin may approximate a normal appearance. In most people, the number of nevi gradually decreases over time. Notably, many melanoma patients tend to retain increased numbers of nevi, including atypical ones, in the later decades of life.

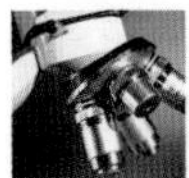

PATHOLOGY: At the inception of a melanocytic nevus, melanocytes are increased in the basal epidermis, with subsequent hyperpigmentation. They eventually form nests, frequently at tips of rete ridges, and then migrate into the dermis where they appear as small clusters. As the lesion becomes elevated, the dermal nevus cells begin to differentiate, an evolution that gradually encompasses the entire dermal component. The nevus may progress or eventually flatten and possibly even disappear. The histologic classification of melanocytic nevi reflects their evolution:

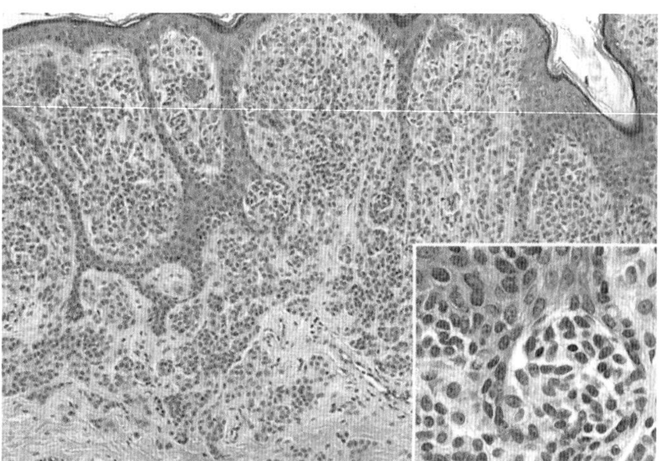

FIGURE 20-33. **Compound melanocytic nevus.** Melanocytes are present as nests within the epidermis and dermis. An intraepidermal nest of melanocytes is surrounded by keratinocytes (*inset*).

- **Junctional nevus:** Melanocytes form nests at the tips of epidermal rete ridges, after which they are termed "nevus cells." They tend to lose their dendritic morphology and retain pigment in their cytoplasm.
- **Compound nevus:** Nests of melanocytes are seen in the epidermis, and some of the cells have migrated into the dermis (Fig. 20-33).
- **Dermal nevus:** Intraepidermal melanocytic growth has ceased, and melanocytes are present only in the dermis (Fig. 20-34). Pigment tends to be lost at this stage.

Dysplastic (Atypical) Nevi

Some common acquired nevi do not follow the pattern of growth, differentiation, and disappearance described above and are termed "dysplastic nevi." These lesions are especially strong risk factors for melanoma. They persist and are often larger than 5 mm. Dysplastic nevi may show foci of aberrant melanocytic growth and become larger and somewhat irregular peripherally (although less so than melanomas). The peripheral area is flat (macular) and extends symmetrically from the parent nevus. Some clinically dysplastic nevi are entirely macular. Not all patients with dysplastic nevi will develop melanomas, and not all melanomas occur in patients with dysplastic nevi. The magnitude of this risk varies with the number of nevi and is especially high in patients with a prior melanoma or a family history of melanoma.

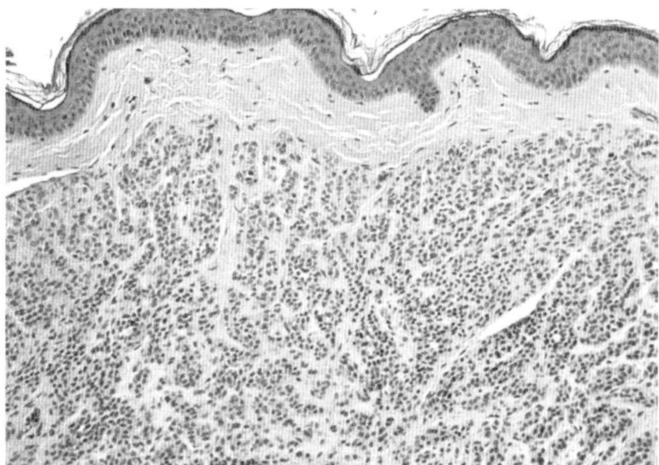

FIGURE 20-34. **Dermal melanocytic nevus.** The melanocytes are entirely confined to the dermis.

Melanocytic Dysplasia

Dysplastic nevi are characterized by junctional proliferation of nevoid to epithelioid melanocytes arranged singly and in nests, with nests predominating. These lesions occur mainly near the dermal–epidermal junction and at the tips and sides of elongated rete ridges. A band of eosinophilic connective tissue ("concentric eosinophilic fibroplasia") is seen around the rete ridges. Horizontal nests of lesional cells extend from some rete to adjacent rete ("bridging"). As these architectural features become more prominent, melanocytes with large atypical nuclei that resemble malignant cells may also appear in the areas of architectural disorder, remaining a minority population and constituting cytologic atypia. **The combination of architectural disorder and cytologic atypia together defines a dysplastic nevus** (Fig. 20-35). Areas of dysplasia may also be associated with a subjacent lymphocytic infiltrate. Although 30% of malignant melanomas have precursor nevi, most of which show melanocytic dysplasia, most dysplastic nevi are stable and never progress to melanoma. In other words, dysplastic nevi are much more common in the population than melanomas. Moderate and severe histologic dysplasia, but not mild dysplasia, is associated with an increased risk of developing melanoma.

Malignant Melanoma

Malignant melanoma (often simply "melanoma") is a neoplasm of melanocytes. Malignant melanoma is a leading cause of cancer mortality in young adults. It is rare in adolescence and exceedingly rare in childhood. Melanomas may progress through two major stages. In the "radial growth phase," the lesion spreads (as viewed clinically) along the radii of an imperfect circle in the skin but remains superficial and thin (the "Breslow thickness"). In the "vertical growth phase," a focal area in the lesion expands to form a tumor mass, with increasing Breslow thickness. Melanomas are dependent, to a greater or lesser extent, on an activated oncogene, *BRAF*, as a driver mutation, which is also mutated in benign nevi. The histopathologic subtypes of melanoma (discussed below) are related to the particular oncogenes involved in their pathogenesis. Loss of p16 (and in some cases other tumor suppressors) is common in melanomas and leads to unrestrained proliferation and the potential for future progression "from bad to worse."

The incidence of malignant melanoma is increasing rapidly. It is estimated that over 1% of children born today will develop malignant melanoma. The prognosis of most melanomas is excellent if lesions are recognized and excised before entering a vertical growth phase. However, a patient is at increased risk of metastatic disease if the tumor exceeds a critical depth in the dermis.

Radial Growth Phase Melanoma

The most common type of melanoma is **superficial spreading melanoma**, which can present in the radial growth phase or vertical growth phase (Fig. 20-36). Excision for histologic examination is the gold standard for the diagnosis of melanoma of any sort.

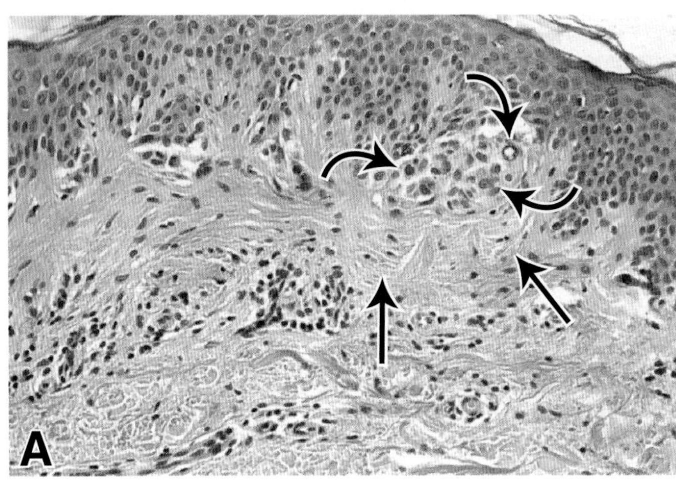

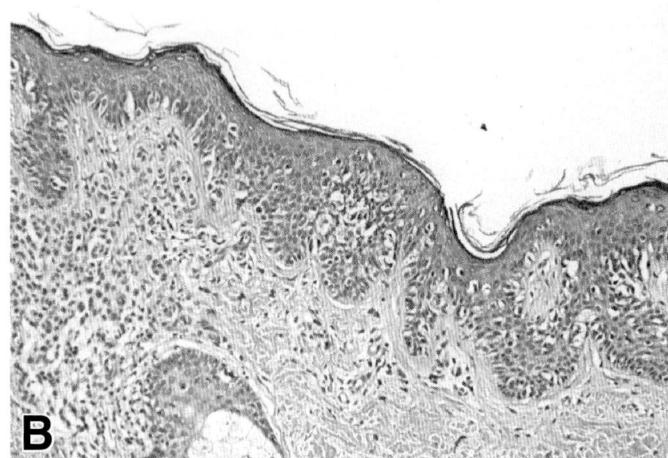

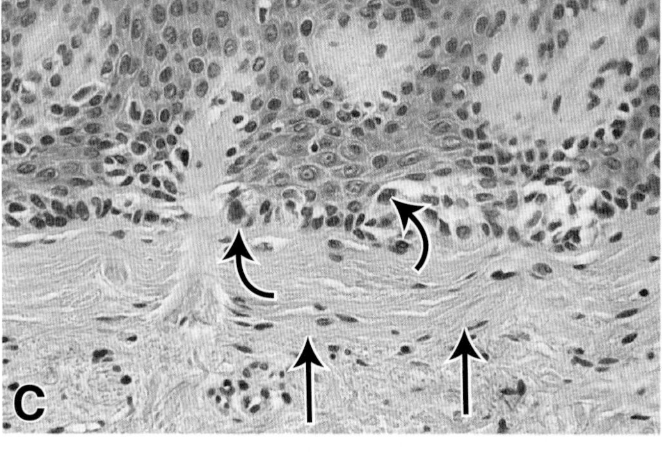

FIGURE 20-35. Dysplastic nevus. A. There is bridging of rete ridges by nests of melanocytes, melanocytes with cytologic atypia (*curved arrows*), lamellar fibroplasia (*straight arrows*), and a scant perivascular lymphocytic infiltrate. **B.** To the *left* is a zone containing typical dermal nevus cells of a compound melanocytic nevus. In the epidermis on the *right* is a proliferation of atypical melanocytes with lamellar fibroplasia. This photomicrograph is taken from the junction of the papular and macular components of this dysplastic nevus. Dysplasia usually develops in the macular portion, which takes up most of the field. **C.** Irregular melanocytic nests resting above lamellar fibroplasia (*straight arrows*) exhibit large epithelioid melanocytes with atypia (*curved arrows*).

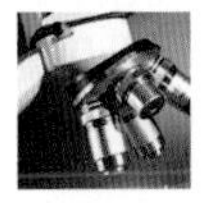

PATHOLOGY: In a superficial spreading melanoma, large, often pigmented epithelioid melanocytes are dispersed in nests and as individual cells through the entire thickness of the epidermis ("pagetoid scatter"). These melanocytes may be limited to the epidermis (**melanoma in situ**) or they may invade into the papillary dermis. In the radial growth phase, no nest has growth preference (larger size) over the other nests (Fig. 20-37), so cells grow evenly in all directions: upward in the epidermis, peripherally in the epidermis, and downward into the dermis (**invasion**). Mitoses are not seen in dermal melanocytes but may be present in the epidermal component. These lesions enlarge at the periphery, hence the term **radial**. A brisk lymphocytic infiltrate typically accompanies melanocytes in the radial growth phase. Such lesions rarely metastasize.

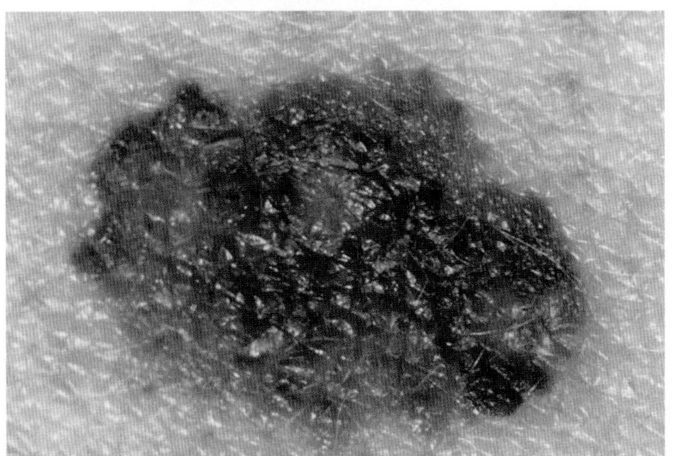

FIGURE 20-36. The clinical appearance of the radial growth phase in malignant melanoma of the superficial spreading type. The larger diameter is 1.8 cm.

MOLECULAR PATHOGENESIS: Melanoma displays several different genetic mutations implicated in its pathogenesis, involving many different molecular pathways. As with nevi, activating *BRAF* mutations are seen in 40% to 50% of melanomas, and *NRAS* mutations are present in 10% to 20%. These kinases both utilize the MAPK pathway, which regulates cell proliferation. Upstream from both NRAS and BRAF is the receptor tyrosine kinase c-Kit, for which mutations account for only 1% of melanomas overall. However, it is the most common mutation seen in acral and mucosal subtypes and often in lentigo maligna melanoma. Downstream from NRAS is the PI3K/AKT pathway, which regulates cell survival and is suppressed by PTEN (see Chapter 4). In this context, PTEN mutations occur in 60% of cases. Mutations in *CDKN2A* are common in sporadic and familial melanomas and account for 30% of cases overall. Because many of the same activating mutations occur in both benign nevi and melanomas, malignancy most likely entails (1) a combination of these mutations, (2) inactivation of senescence genes (like p16), and (3) other still unidentified alterations.

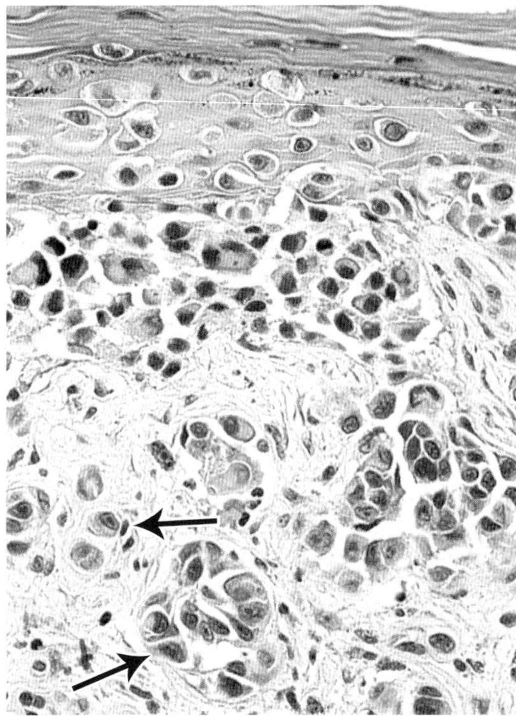

FIGURE 20-37. Malignant melanoma, superficial spreading type, radial growth phase. Melanocytes grow singly within the epidermis at all levels and as large, irregularly sized nests at the dermal–epidermal junction. Tumor cells are present in the papillary dermis (*arrows*), but no nest shows preferential growth over the others.

The increased understanding of melanoma molecular mechanisms in melanoma has spurred the developments of targeted therapies aimed at inhibiting particular genetic pathways, including BRAF inhibitors, with many more in clinical development (Fig. 20-38).

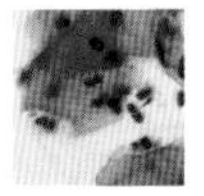

CLINICAL FEATURES: Superficial spreading melanoma (SSM) usually follows a history of intermittent sun exposure and sunburn. Early melanomas in the radial growth phase have slightly elevated and palpable borders. The neoplasm is usually variably and haphazardly pigmented (Fig. 20-38). Alterations in SSM include itching, increase in size, darkening, or bleeding. The "ABCDE rule" is a convenient mnemonic to help recognize changes in nevi that should prompt patients to seek medical attention: **a**symmetry of shape, **b**order irregularity, **c**olor variation, and a **d**iameter more than 6 mm. The letter "E" can stand for "**e**levation" or more importantly "**e**volution."

Vertical Growth Phase Melanoma

After a variable time (usually 1 to 2 years), the character of growth begins to change. Melanocytes exhibit mitotic activity in both the epidermal and dermal components and grow as expanding spheroid nodules in the dermis (Fig. 20-39). The net direction of growth tends to be perpendicular to that of the radial growth phase, hence **vertical** (Figs. 20-39, 20-40, and 20-41).

PATHOLOGY: The vertical growth phase is usually characterized by the following:

- The cellular aggregate that characterizes the vertical growth phase is larger than the clusters of melanocytes that form the epidermal and dermal components of the radial growth phase. Invasion can occur in both the radial growth phase and vertical growth phase, but the dominant direction of tumor growth shifts from the epidermis to

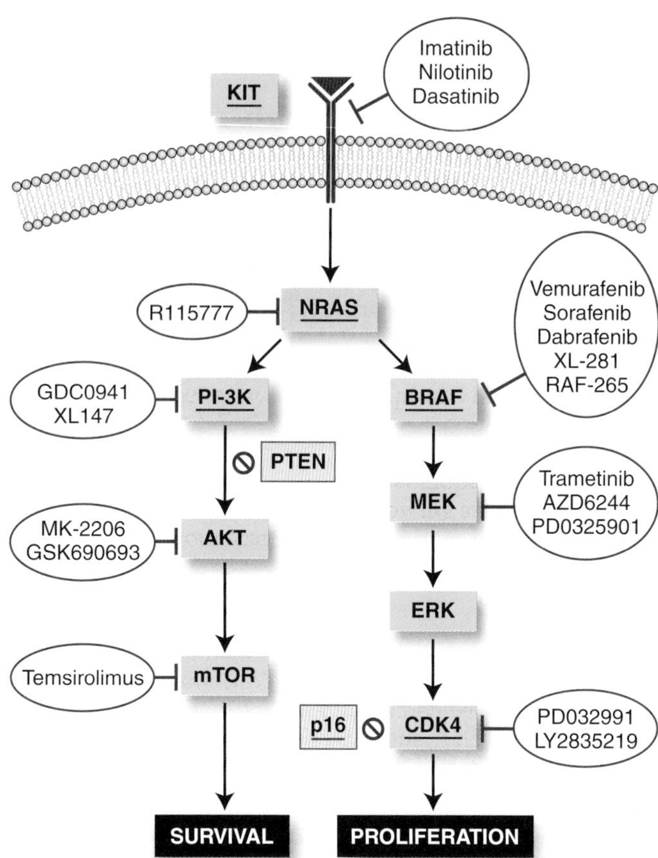

FIGURE 20-38. Simplified melanoma genetic pathway schema. Mitogen-activated protein kinase and phosphatidylinositol-3-kinase/AKT pathways are depicted, which regulate cell proliferation and cell survival, respectively. Red ovals contain examples of targeted therapeutic agents currently in use or in clinical trials. Underlined genes are ones with proven mutations in melanoma.

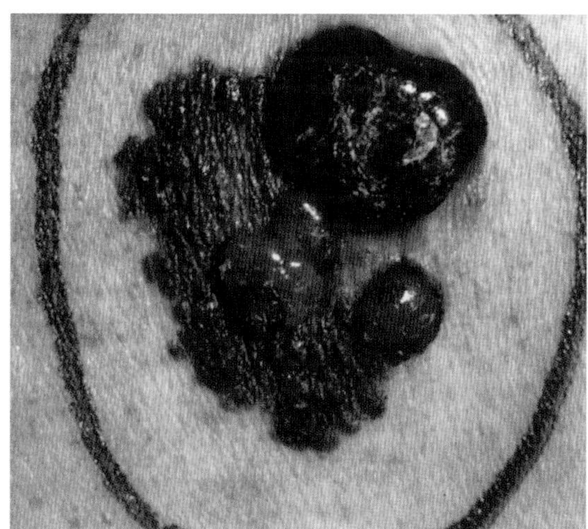

FIGURE 20-39. Malignant melanoma, superficial spreading type, vertical growth phase. Vertical growth is manifested by the distinct spheroid tumor nodule to the *right.* This focus of melanocytes clearly has a growth advantage (larger size of the aggregate) over nests in the adjacent radial growth phase (*left*).

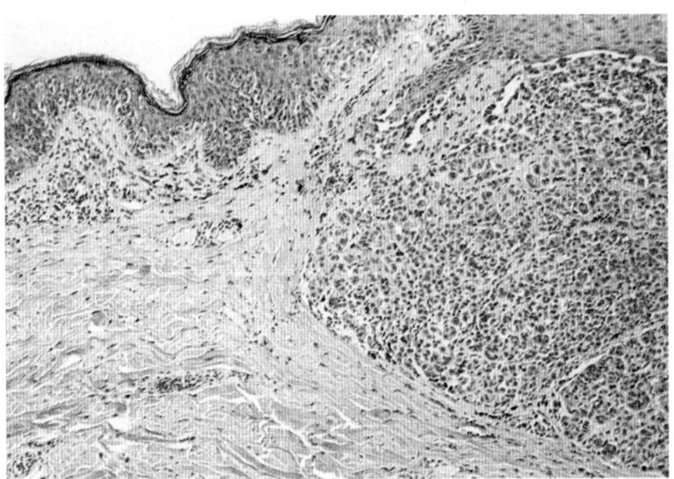

FIGURE 20-40. Malignant melanoma. The superficial spreading type is represented by the relatively flat, dark, brown–black portion of the tumor. Three areas in this lesion are characteristic of the vertical growth phase. All are nodular in configuration; two have a pink coloration, and the largest is a rich, ebony black.

the dermis in the vertical growth phase. This property of expansile growth in the dermis is called *tumorigenicity.*

- Mitotic figures and markers of cell division are common in the vertical growth phase and, along with tumorigenicity, form one of its two defining attributes.
- The melanocytes tend to appear different from those of the radial growth phase. For example, they may contain little or no pigment, whereas the cells in the radial growth phase are melanotic.
- Tumors that involve the reticular dermis are usually considered to be in the vertical growth phase.
- Host response (i.e., lymphocytic inflammation) may be absent or reduced at the base of the vertical growth phase, compared to that in the radial growth phase.

Not all tumors in the vertical growth phase possess the propensity to metastasize. Thus, vertical growth phase melanomas less than 1 mm thick that lack mitoses rarely metastasize. The risk of metastasis can be predicted, albeit imperfectly, through the use of prognostic models (see below).

Nodular Melanoma

Occasionally, a melanoma "bypasses" the stepwise tumor progression described above and manifests all of its malignant characteristics in the initial lesion. Nodular melanoma is an uncommon form of the tumor (10%), which appears as a circumscribed, elevated, spheroidal nodule. It is in the vertical growth phase when initially observed and grows in an expansile manner in the dermis. These lesions lack most of the ABCD criteria. They may be advanced in thickness and thus at high risk of metastasis at the time of diagnosis, despite often being small in diameter, symmetric, and homogeneous in color.

Lentigo Maligna Melanoma

Lentigo maligna melanoma, also known as **Hutchinson melanotic freckle**, is a large, pigmented macule that occurs on sun-damaged skin. It develops almost exclusively in fair-skinned, usually elderly whites, often with a history of being outdoor workers. Thus, it is probably related to chronic ultraviolet light exposure. Lentigo maligna melanoma, like acral and mucosal melanomas (see below), is less likely than superficial spreading melanoma to be associated with mutations of *B-RAF*, while *NRAS* mutations are more common.

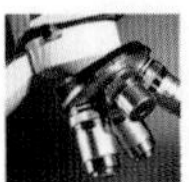

PATHOLOGY: In the radial growth phase, lentigo maligna melanoma is a flat, irregular, brown to black patch that may cover a large part of the face or dorsal hands (Fig. 20-42). The cells of the radial growth phase are predominantly in the basal layer, often forming contiguous rows of atypical single melanocytes, but occasionally forming small nests that hang down into the papillary dermis (Fig. 20-43). The subjacent dermis often shows a modest lymphocytic infiltrate and solar degeneration of the connective tissue.

Acral Lentiginous Melanoma

Acral lentiginous melanoma occurs with about equal frequency in all races. It is thus the most common form of melanoma in dark-skinned people and is generally limited to palms, soles, and subungual regions. Increased copy numbers and often mutations of the cell cycle marker cyclin D are common findings in these lesions. The verticle growth phase is similar to that of lentigo maligna melanoma, but the prognosis is worse than that for the more common cutaneous melanomas.

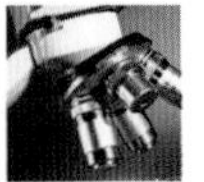

PATHOLOGY: In the radial growth phase, acral lentiginous melanoma forms an irregular, brown to black patch that covers a part of the palm or sole or arises under a nail, usually on a thumb or great toe (Fig. 20-44). Tumor cells are confined mostly to the basal layer of the epidermis and tend to maintain long dendrites (Fig. 20-45). A brisk lichenoid lymphocytic infiltrate is often seen.

Metastatic Melanoma

Metastatic melanoma arises from the melanocytes of the vertical growth phase of any of the various forms of melanoma. Initial metastases usually involve regional lymph nodes, although hematogenous spread to organs is also possible. When the latter occurs, metastases are unusually widespread in comparison with other neoplasms; virtually any organ may be involved. Metastatic melanomas may remain dormant and clinically undetectable for long periods after the excision of a primary melanoma, only to reappear years later.

Staging and Prognosis of Melanoma

The prognosis of a patient with a melanoma is based on the following:

- ***TUMOR THICKNESS:*** Tumor thickness is the strongest prognostic variable for melanomas that are apparently confined to their primary site. The "Breslow thickness" of a melanoma is measured from the most superficial aspect of the stratum granulosum to the point of maximal thickness (Fig. 20-41). Prognosis up to 10 years after removal of the primary lesion may then be estimated.
- ***ULCERATION:*** Ulceration in a primary melanoma is associated with decreased survival.

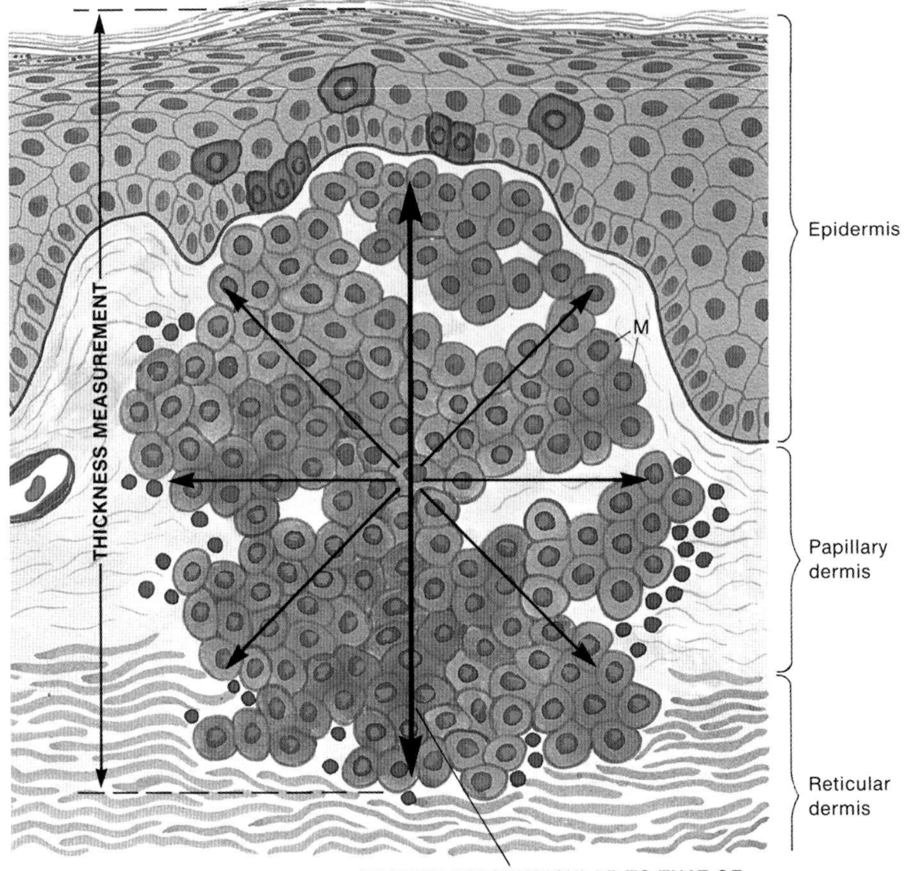

FIGURE 20-41. Malignant melanoma. The evolved vertical growth phase in malignant melanoma of the superficial spreading type is shown, with an indication of how thickness is measured. In this illustration, the vertical growth phase has extended into the reticular dermis. Small nodules of tumor cells that clearly have a growth preference over other tumor cells are a manifestation of the vertical growth phase. Thickness measurements (*arrows*) are taken from the most superficial aspect of the granular layer across the tumor at its thickest point (to its deepest point of invasion).

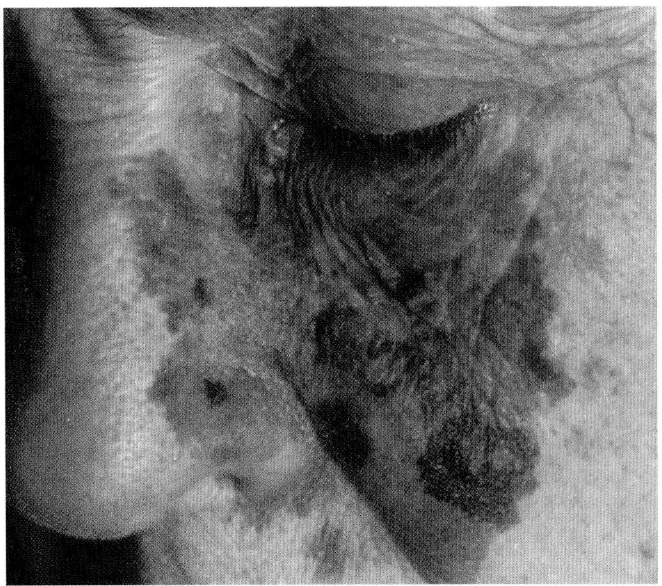

FIGURE 20-42. Malignant melanoma of the lentigo maligna type, radial growth phase.

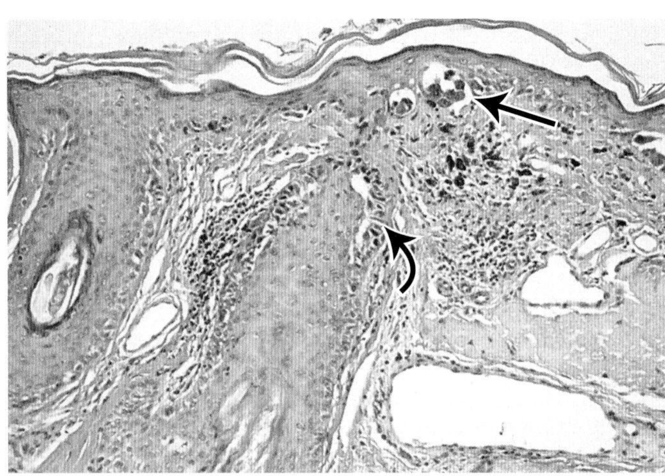

FIGURE 20-43. Lentigo maligna. Atypical melanocytes grow mostly at the dermal–epidermal interface (*straight arrow*), with extension down the external root sheath of follicles (*curved arrow*). Upward growth of melanocytes is much less prominent than in malignant melanoma of the superficial spreading type.

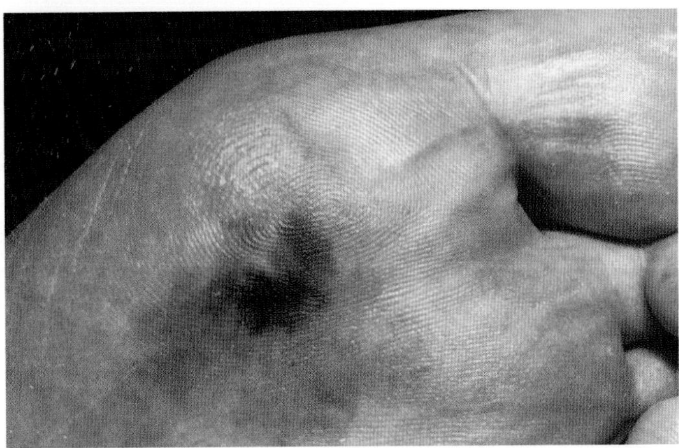

FIGURE 20-44. **Malignant melanoma, acral lentiginous type (radial growth phase).** The clinical appearance of the sole of the foot is depicted.

- *DERMAL MITOTIC RATE:* For tumor cells in the vertical growth phase, the mitotic rate correlates well with survival. Survival becomes progressively worse as the mitotic rate increases.
- *LYMPHOCYTIC INFILTRATE:* Interaction of lymphocytes with tumor cells in the vertical growth phase is an important prognostic indicator. Tumor-infiltrating lymphocytes (TILs) actually penetrate and disrupt the tumor, frequently forming rosettes around tumor cells (Fig. 20-46). The more prevalent the TILs, the better is the prognosis.
- *LOCATION:* Melanomas on the extremities have a better prognosis than those on the head, neck, or trunk (axial). However, melanomas on the sole of the foot or the subungual region have a prognosis similar to, or worse than, axial lesions.
- *SEX:* For every site and thickness, women have better prognoses than men.
- *STAGE:* The stage of the disease is the most important single factor influencing a patient's survival. Lymph node involvement suggests an estimated 40% decrease in 5-year survival, compared with patients with clinically localized tumors. An increasing number of involved lymph nodes is also highly predictive of a poor prognosis.

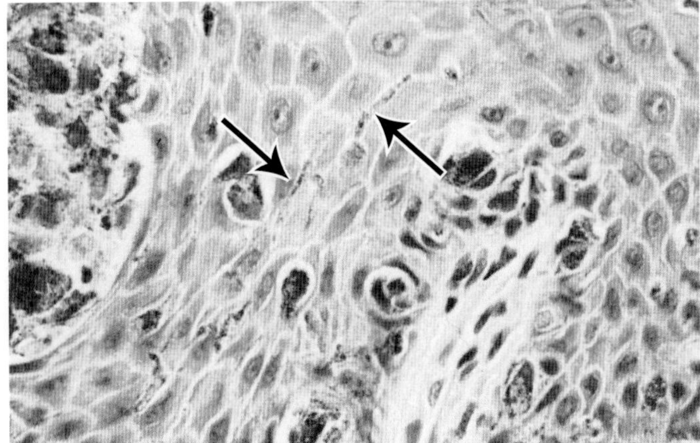

FIGURE 20-45. **Malignant melanoma, acral lentiginous type.** Large melanocytes with prominent dendrites (*arrows*) are present in the basilar region of the epidermis. The tumor cells contain numerous melanosomes, making the perinuclear and dendritic cytoplasms brown.

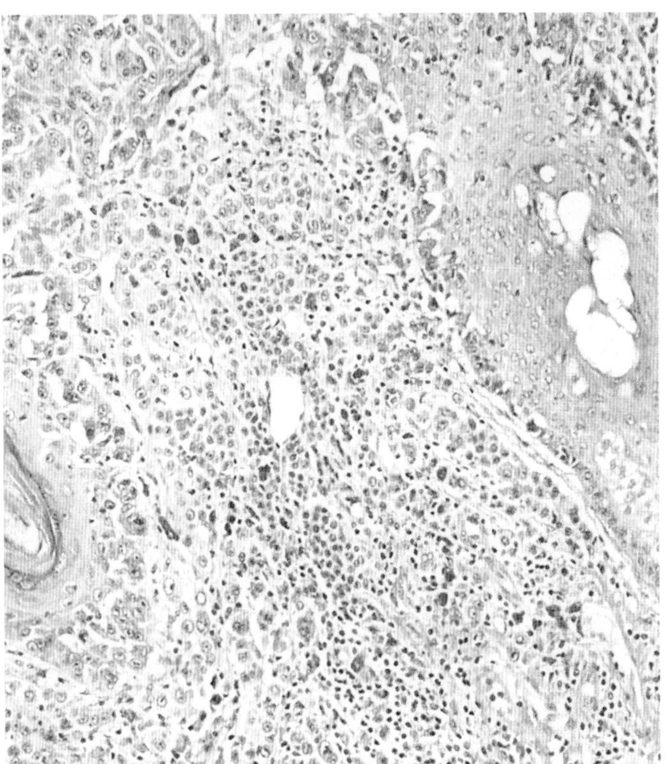

FIGURE 20-46. **Malignant melanoma, vertical growth phase.** The host response consists of lymphocytes infiltrating amid the melanocytes ("tumor-infiltrating lymphocytes").

The tumor–node–metastasis (TNM) system of tumor staging incorporates features of the primary tumor, regional lymph nodes and soft tissues, and distant metastases. It helps define the pathologic stage of disease, which, in turn, reflects the probability of survival. (1) The **T** (primary tumor) attributes of tumor thickness, the presence or absence of ulceration, and mitogenicity are classified histologically after excision of the melanoma. (2) Number of lymph nodes with metastatic tumor is a large part of the **N** (node) classification. (3) The **M (metastasis)** properties incorporate results of evaluation for distant metastases at various anatomic sites.

Current recommendations regarding excision of confirmed melanomas state that (1) a 5-mm margin of uninvolved tissue should be obtained with in situ melanoma, (2) a 1-cm margin with a tumor thickness of 1 mm or less, and (3) a 2-cm margin with a tumor thickness greater than 1 mm. Sentinel lymph node sampling is generally considered with tumor thickness greater than 1 mm or with other risk factors. If metastatic disease ensues, targeted therapeutics, such as BRAF inhibitors, can be employed, and immunomodulatory drugs are also used.

Keratosis

Seborrheic Keratosis

Seborrheic keratoses are scaly, frequently pigmented, elevated papules or plaques with scales that are easily rubbed off. They are common later in life, but their etiology is unknown. Seborrheic keratoses tend to be familial. Clinically and microscopically, they appear "pasted on" and contain broad anastomosing cords of squamous epithelium, forming papillae, and

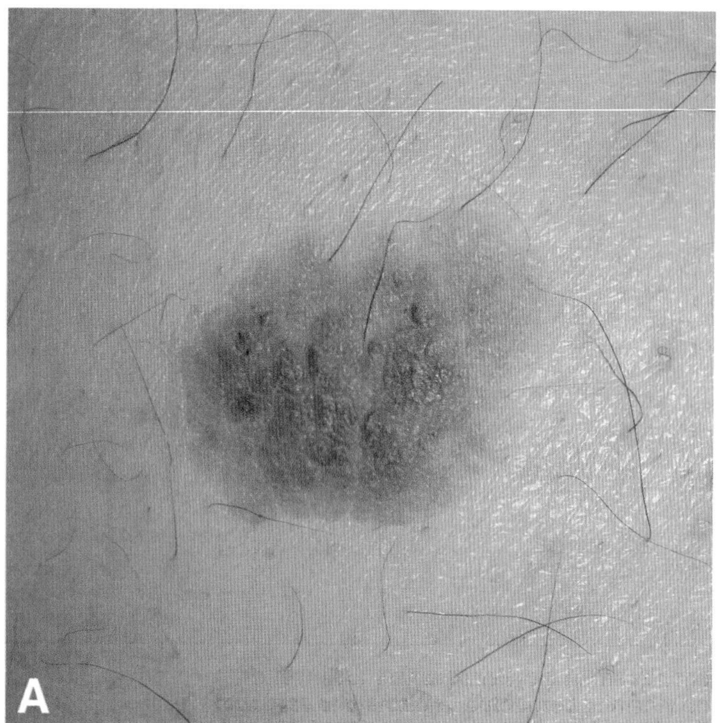

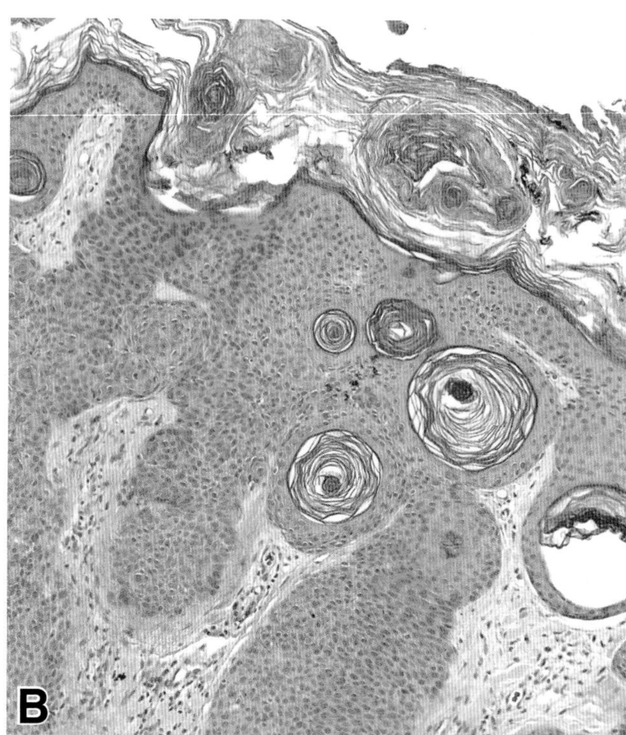

FIGURE 20-47. **Seborrheic keratosis. A.** Sharply defined, "stuck-on" brown lesions are a common presentation. **B.** Broad anastomosing cords of mature stratified squamous epithelium are associated with small keratin cysts.

associated with small cysts of keratin (horn cysts) (Fig. 20-47). Seborrheic keratoses are innocuous but are a cosmetic nuisance. The sudden appearance of many seborrheic keratoses may be associated with internal malignancies ("Leser–Trélat sign"), especially gastric adenocarcinoma.

Actinic Keratosis

Actinic keratoses are keratinocytic neoplasms that develop in sun-damaged skin as circumscribed keratotic patches or plaques, commonly on the backs of the hands or the face. The stratum corneum is no longer loose and basket weaved and is replaced by a dense parakeratotic scale. The basal keratinocytes show significant atypia (Fig. 20-48). Actinic keratoses may evolve into squamous carcinomas in situ and finally into invasive cancers, but most are stable and many regress.

Keratoacanthoma

Keratoacanthomas are rapidly growing keratotic papules on sun-exposed skin that develop over 3 to 6 weeks into craterlike nodules. They reach a maximum size of 2 to 3 cm. Spontaneous regression usually follows within 6 to 12 months, leaving an atrophic scar. Some lesions may cause considerable damage before they regress, and some fail to regress. Keratoacanthomas are considered by some to be self-resolving variants of squamous cell carcinoma.

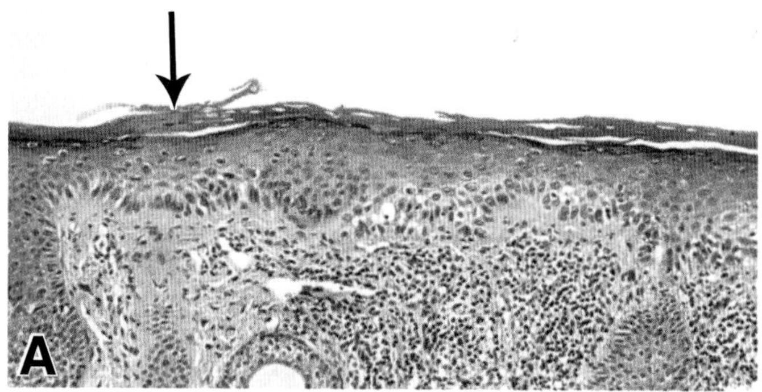

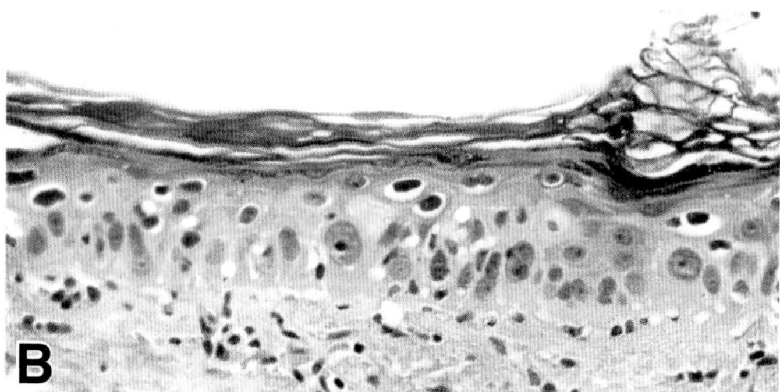

FIGURE 20-48. **Actinic keratosis. A.** A low-power view revealing cytologic atypia within the stratum basalis and lower stratum spinosum with loss of polarity. A lichenoid, bandlike, lymphocytic infiltrate is frequently present. Parakeratosis is present here only in a small focus (*arrow*). **B.** High-power examination of an actinic keratosis revealing striking cytologic atypia of the basal keratinocytes, the hallmark of actinic keratoses.

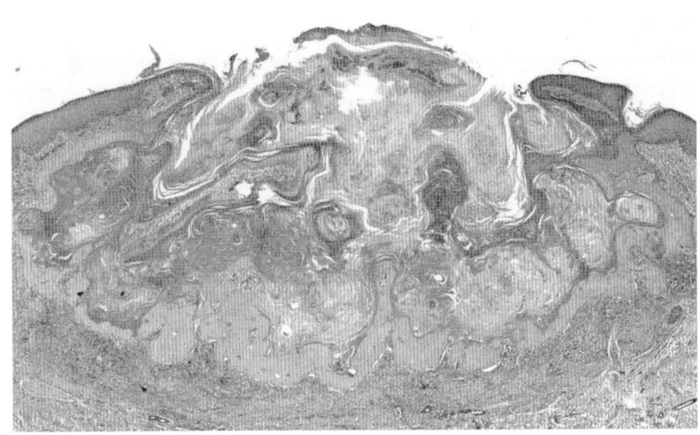

FIGURE 20-49. Keratoacanthoma. A keratin-filled crater (*center*) is lined by glassy proliferating keratinocytes.

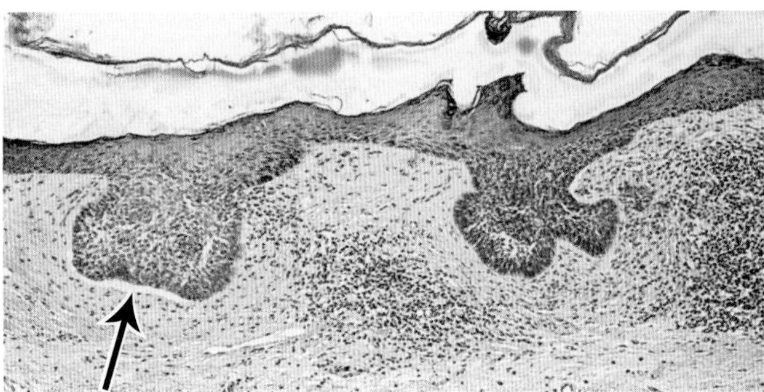

FIGURE 20-50. Basal cell carcinoma, superficial type. Buds of atypical basaloid keratinocytes extend from the overlying epidermis into the papillary dermis. The peripheral keratinocytes mimic the stratum basalis by palisading. The separation artifact (*arrow*) is present because of poorly formed basement membrane components and the hyaluronic acid–rich stroma that contains collagenase.

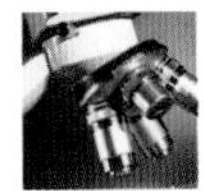

PATHOLOGY: Histologically, keratoacanthomas are endophytic proliferations of keratinocytes. The lesion is cup shaped, with a central, keratin-filled umbilication and overhanging ("buttressing") epidermal edges (Fig. 20-49). At the base of the keratin, keratinocytes are large and have abundant homogeneous, eosinophilic ("glassy") cytoplasm. At the lower aspect of the lesion, irregular tongues of squamous epithelium infiltrate the collagen of the reticular dermis.

Basal Cell Carcinoma

BCC is the most common malignant tumor in people with pale skin. It may be locally aggressive, but metastases are exceedingly rare.

MOLECULAR PATHOGENESIS: ***BCC usually develops on sun-damaged skin of people with fair skin and freckles.*** However, unlike squamous lesions, BCC also arises on areas not exposed to intense sunlight. The tumor is thought to derive from pluripotential cells in the basal layer of the epidermis, more specifically, in the bulge region of the hair follicle.

In several heritable syndromes, BCC originates on skin that has had little light exposure. **Nevoid BCC syndrome** features multiple tumors in the context of a complex multisystem disease. The syndrome also includes pits (dyskeratoses) on the palms and soles, mandibular cysts, hypertelorism, and a predisposition to other neoplasms, including medulloblastoma. The BCCs of this syndrome appear at a young age and may number in the hundreds. Germline mutations in the *PTCH* tumor suppressor gene cause nevoid BCC syndrome. Likewise, somatic mutations in the gene occur in up to 90% of sporadic BCCs and may be targeted in the therapy of advanced lesions.

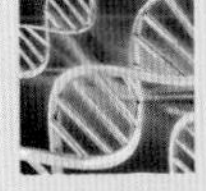

PATHOLOGY: BCCs contain nests of deeply basophilic epithelial cells with narrow rims of cytoplasm that are attached to the epidermis and protrude into the subjacent papillary dermis (Fig. 20-50). At least in early lesions, there is typically a loose mucinous stroma containing fibroblasts and lymphocytes. The central part of each nest contains closely packed keratinocytes that are slightly smaller than normal basal keratinocytes and show occasional apoptosis and mitoses. The periphery of each nest shows an organized layer of polarized, columnar keratinocytes, with the long axis of each cell perpendicular to the surrounding stroma ("peripheral palisading").

CLINICAL FEATURES: Common forms of BCC include the following:

- **Pearly papule** is the prototypic **nodulocystic** type of lesion, so named because it resembles a 2- to 3-mm pearl (Fig. 20-51A). It is covered by tightly stretched epidermis and is laced with small, delicate, branching vessels (telangiectasia).
- **Rodent ulcer** is a small crater in the center of the pearl.
- **Superficial BCC** appears as a scaly, red, sharply demarcated plaque.
- **Morpheaform BCC** is a pale, firm, scarlike tumor that is ill-defined on and especially beneath the skin surface, making it particularly difficult to eradicate (Fig. 20-51B).
- **Pigmented BCC** may grossly resemble malignant melanoma. The pigment comes from reactive melanocytes that populate the tumor.

Treatment of BCC involves various excision or eradication procedures.

Squamous Cell Carcinoma

SCCs are second only to BCCs in skin cancer incidence. SCCs are most common on sun-damaged skin of fair persons with light hair and freckles and often originate in actinic keratoses. They are rare on normal black skin.

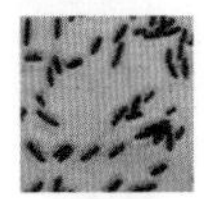

ETIOLOGIC FACTORS: SCCs have multiple causes, UV light being the most common, but also including ionizing radiation, chemical carcinogens, and HPV. SCCs arising in sun-damaged skin rarely metastasize (<2%). They may also arise in chronic scarring processes, such as burn scars ("Marjolin ulcers") and areas of radiation dermatitis. In these settings, they metastasize more often. Over 90% of SCCs, and many actinic keratoses, have mutated *TP53* genes.

20: The Skin

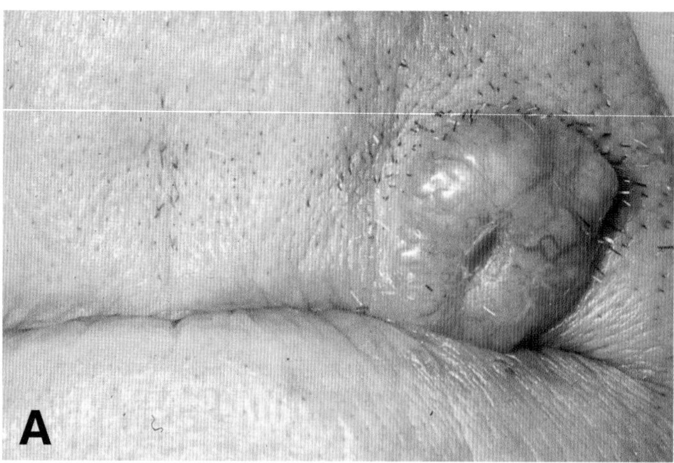
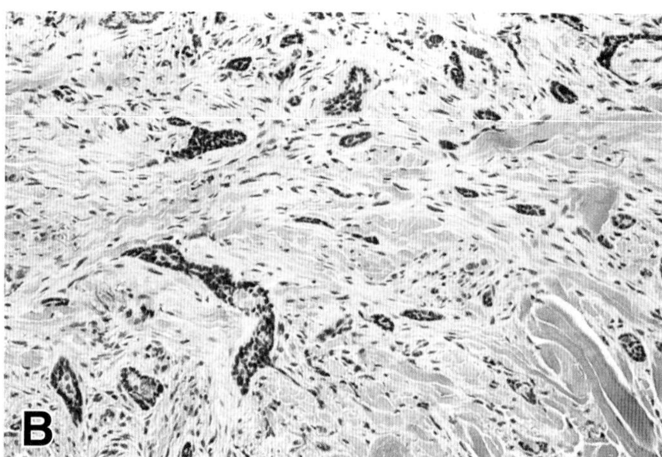

FIGURE 20-51. **Basal cell carcinoma (BCC). A.** Pearly papule: the tumor exhibits typical rolled pearly borders with telangiectases and central ulceration. **B.** Microscopic examination of morpheaform BCC showing a sclerosing and infiltrative lesion. Irregularly branching strands of tumor cells permeate the dermis, with induction of a cellular, fibroblastic, hyaluronic acid–rich stroma. 20-51A From Elder AD, Elenitsas R, Johnson BL, et al. *Synopsis and Atlas of Lever's Histopathology of the Skin*. Philadelphia, PA: Lippincott Williams & Wilkins; 1999.

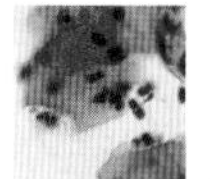

PATHOLOGY: SCC is composed of tumor cells that mimic epidermal stratum spinosum to varying degrees and extend into the subjacent dermis (Fig. 20-52). The edges of many tumors show changes typical of actinic keratosis, namely, a variably thickened epidermis with parakeratosis and significant atypia of basal keratinocytes.

CLINICAL FEATURES: SCCs characteristically arise in chronically sun-exposed areas, such as the backs of the hands, face, lips, and ears (Fig. 20-52A). Early lesions are small, scaly, or ulcerated, erythematous papules, which may be pruritic. They are usually treated by excision, or sometimes by electrosurgery, topical chemotherapy, or radiation therapy.

Merkel Cell Carcinoma

These tumors are typically solitary, dome-shaped, red to violaceous nodules or indurated plaques on the skin of the head and neck in elderly white patients. MCCs are aggressive tumors that are lethal in 25% to 70% of patients within 5 years.

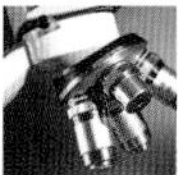

PATHOLOGY: Most MCCs have large nests of undifferentiated cells that resemble small cell carcinoma of the lung (Fig. 20-53). Peripherally, the tumors may show a trabecular pattern. Nuclear chromatin is dense and evenly distributed, cytoplasm is scant, and mitotic figures and nuclear fragments are common. CK 20 is distributed in a "perinuclear dot" cytoplasmic pattern. Tumor cells

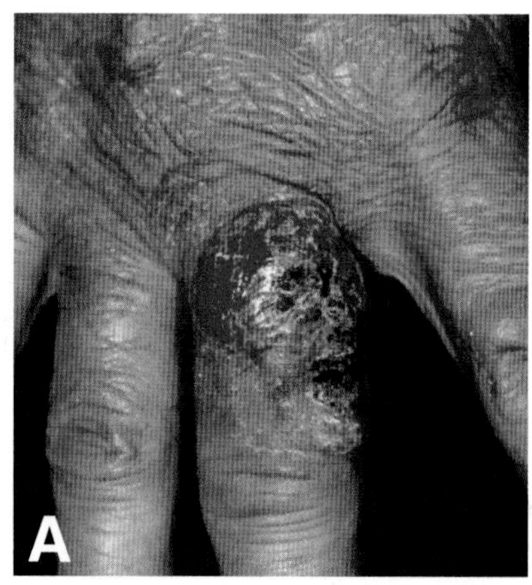
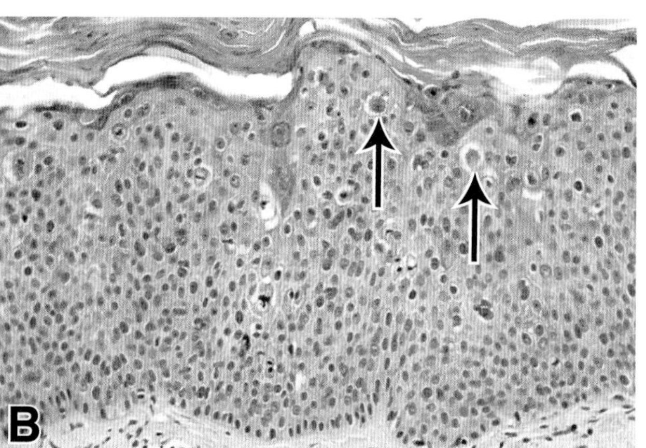

FIGURE 20-52. **Squamous cell carcinoma. A.** An ulcerated, encrusted, and infiltrating lesion is seen on the sun-exposed dorsal aspect of a finger. **B.** A microscopic view of the periphery of the lesion showing squamous cell carcinoma in situ. The entire epidermis is replaced by atypical keratinocytes. Mitoses are apparent, as is apoptosis (*arrows*).

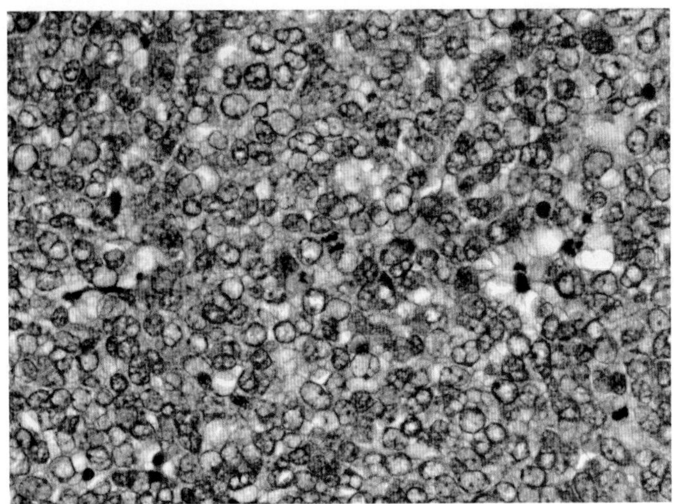

FIGURE 20-53. **Merkel cell carcinoma.** The tumor is composed of solid nests of undifferentiated cells that resemble small cell carcinoma of the lung.

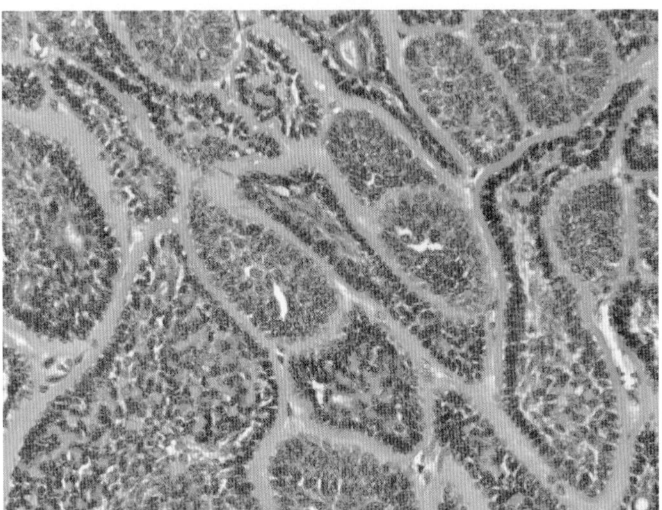

FIGURE 20-54. **Cylindroma.** Sharply circumscribed islands of basophilic epithelial cells reside in a jigsaw puzzle–like array. Dense eosinophilic hyaline sheaths surround each island.

also express neuroendocrine markers, such as chromogranin and synaptophysin.

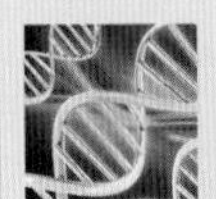

MOLECULAR PATHOGENESIS: The genome of Merkel cell polyoma virus is present in 75% of MCCs and may play a role in tumorigenesis. However, it is a common virus, and the association with MCCs is still speculative. Tumorigenicity is associated with a truncating mutation of the polyoma *Tag* gene.

Adnexal Tumors

Adnexal tumors appear as elevated small skin nodules that often occur in people with family histories of similar tumors. The lesions commonly appear at puberty. Although most are benign, malignant behavior is sometimes observed.

Sebaceous Neoplasms

Sebaceous neoplasms, including sebaceous adenomas, sebaceous epitheliomas (sebaceomas), and sebaceous carcinomas are all tumors of sebaceous gland derivation. Clinically, sebaceous adenomas and epitheliomas are small, slow-growing papules or nodules, commonly on the head and neck. Sebaceous carcinomas, however, often present larger than 1 cm and have a predilection for periocular sites. Histopathologically, **sebaceous adenomas** show a well-circumscribed proliferation of sebaceous lobules, primarily composed of mature sebocytes with some germinative basaloid cells. **Sebaceous epitheliomas** have a preponderance of germinative cells. **Sebaceous carcinomas** show histologic signs of malignancy, such as severe cytologic atypia, high mitotic activity, and infiltrative growth.

Cylindroma

Cylindromas are adnexal neoplasms with features of sweat gland differentiation. They may be solitary or multiple elevated nodules around the scalp. An autosomal dominant, heritable variant features multiple tumors. Occasionally, they become large and cluster about the head ("turban tumors"). Cylindromas show sharply circumscribed nests of deeply basophilic cells surrounded by a hyalinized, thickened BMZ (Fig. 20-54).

Syringoma

Syringomas typically occur about the eyelid and upper cheek as small, elevated, flesh-colored papules. Small ducts resembling intraepidermal portions of eccrine sweat ducts are seen (Fig. 20-55).

Poroma

Poroma is a common, solitary neoplasm histologically similar to seborrheic keratosis but with narrow ductal lumina and occasional cystic spaces. The pattern has been interpreted as eccrine sweat gland differentiation. These tumors are firm, raised lesions, usually less than 2 cm in diameter, that develop on the sole or sides of the foot or on the hands or fingers. Poromas extend from the lower portion of the epidermis into the dermis as broad, anastomosing bands of uniform, cuboidal cells. Occasional malignant lesions with similar differentiation are called **porocarcinomas**.

Trichoepithelioma

Trichoepithelioma is a neoplasm that differentiates toward hair structures. It is usually a solitary lesion, but in "multiple trichoepithelioma syndrome," it occurs as an autosomal dominant trait. Lesions begin to appear at puberty, on the face, scalp, neck, and upper trunk. Trichoepitheliomas resemble basal cell carcinomas but contain many "horn cysts," which are keratinized centers surrounded by basophilic epithelial cells.

Fibrohistiocytic Tumors of the Skin

Dermatofibroma

Dermatofibroma is a common, benign tumor of fibroblast-like cells and macrophages. The former are the neoplastic cells. These tumors occur on the extremities as dome-shaped, firm

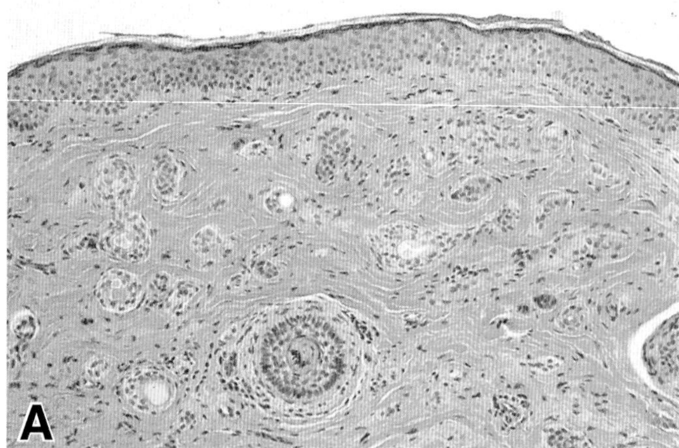

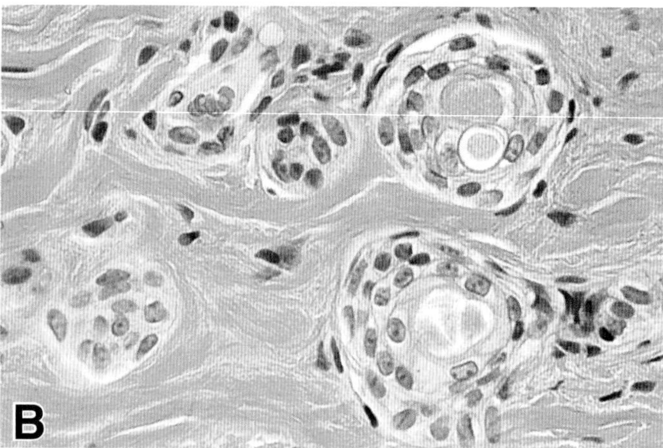

FIGURE 20-55. Syringoma. A. Within the upper dermis is an epithelial proliferation forming ducts, tubules, and solid islands amid a dense fibrous stroma. **B.** The ductal differentiation closely mimics that of the straight dermal eccrine duct, with a central lumen and cuticle formation.

nodules with ill-defined borders, and pink to dark brown pigmentation. They rarely exceed 5 mm. The papillary and reticular dermis are replaced by fibrous tissue that forms ill-defined small cartwheels, with small central vascular spaces (Fig. 20-56). The tumors are not well demarcated and blend into the surrounding dermis. The overlying epidermis is hyperplastic and often hyperpigmented.

Dermatofibrosarcoma Protuberans

DFSP, a tumor with intermediate malignant potential, is a slowly growing nodule or indurated plaque that appears mostly on the trunk of young adults. Local recurrence after attempted complete excision is common, but metastases are rare. The most common histologic pattern is a poorly circumscribed, monotonous population of spindle cells arranged in a dense "storiform" (pinwheel-like) array (Fig. 20-57). The tumor extends into the subcutis along fat septa and interstices, creating an infiltrative, honeycomb-like pattern. Tumor cells display CD34, a marker of endothelial cells and some neural tumor cells, as well as fibroblast-like dendritic cells, the probable cell of origin. Positivity for CD34 may help distinguish this tumor from a dermatofibroma, which does not express this antigen.

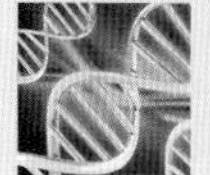

MOLECULAR PATHOGENESIS: More than 90% of DFSPs have a chromosomal translocation t(17;22), which fuses the collagen gene (*COL1A1*) with the *PDGFB* gene. This balanced translocation creates a fusion gene product that causes transcriptional upregulation of the *PDGFB* gene and results in increased growth.

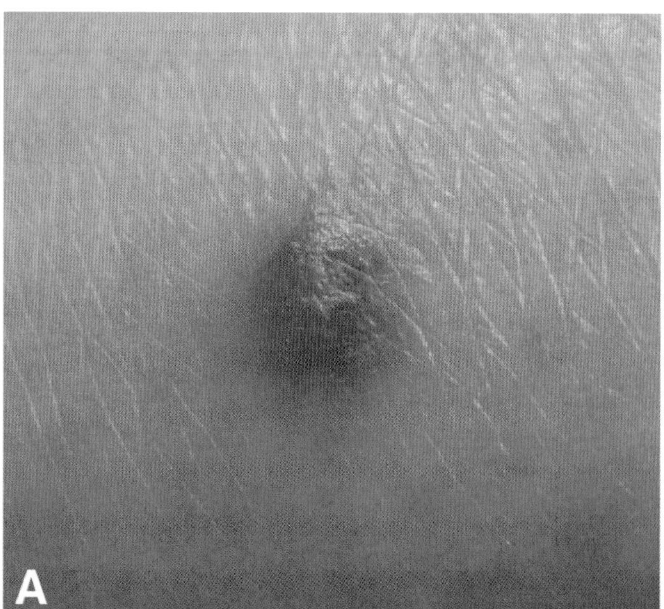

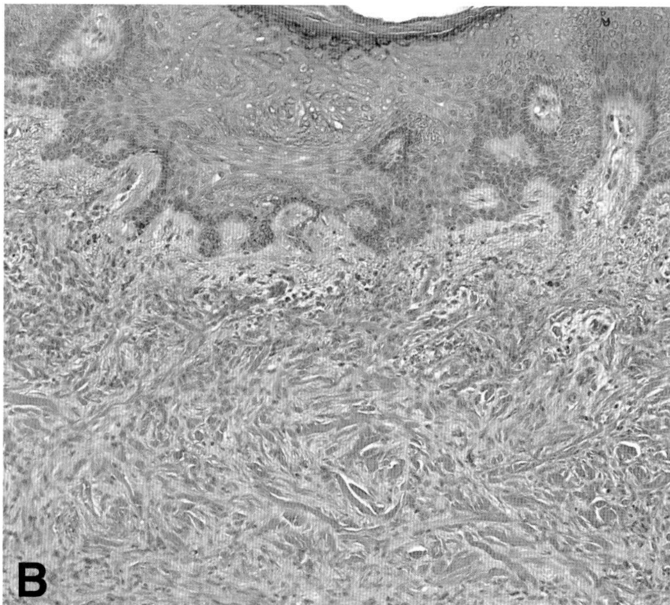

FIGURE 20-56. Dermatofibroma. A. A brown dome-shaped nodule occurring on the lower leg is a common clinical presentation. **B.** Fibrous tissue replaces the dermis and forms poorly defined cartwheels, with overlying epidermal hyperplasia and basaloid proliferation, resembling basal cell carcinoma.

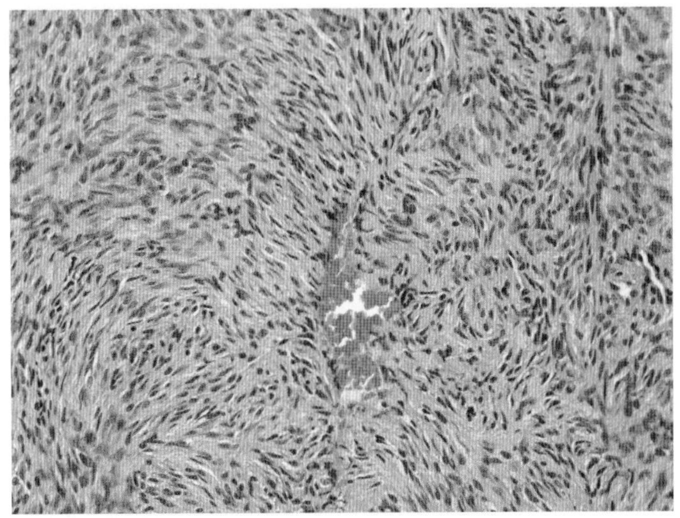

FIGURE 20-57. Dermatofibrosarcoma protuberans. Tumor cells form small cartwheels with central vascular spaces.

Mycosis Fungoides

MF is a variant of cutaneous T-cell lymphoma discussed in detail in Chapter 18.

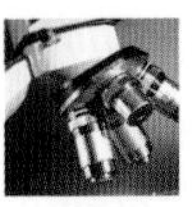

PATHOLOGY: In the early stages of the disease, delicate, erythematous plaques appear, often by the buttocks. These plaques show psoriasiform changes in the epidermis. The early inflammatory cell infiltrates in the dermis are polymorphic and are often not diagnostic of MF.

Skin involvement becomes progressively more prominent and infiltrative (Fig. 20-58). The most important histologic feature of MF is the presence of lymphocytes in the epidermis ("epidermotropism"). In later stages, the dermal infiltrate becomes dense to the point of forming tumor nodules. Increasing numbers of atypical lymphocytes that display hyperchromatic, convoluted ("cerebriform") nuclei are seen in the papillary dermis and epidermis. Circumscribed nests of these atypical lymphocytes ("Pautrier microabscesses") eventually involve the epidermis.

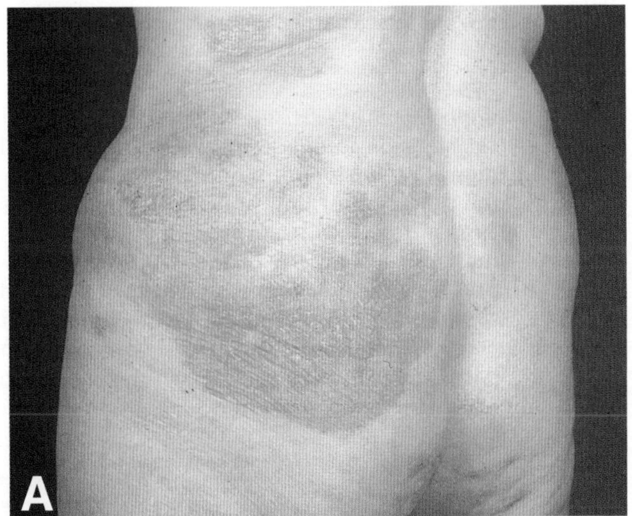

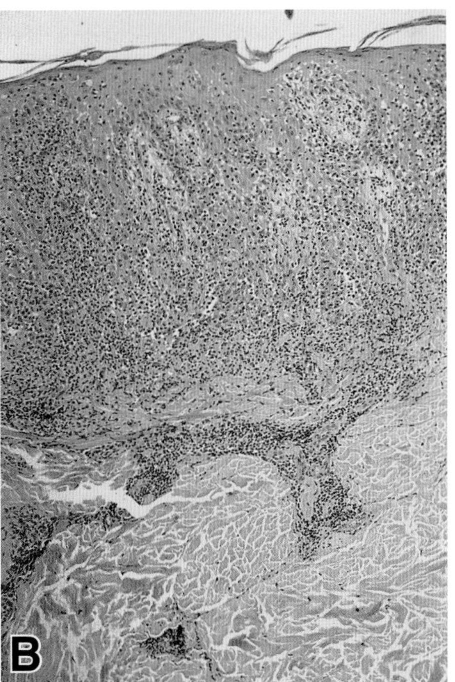

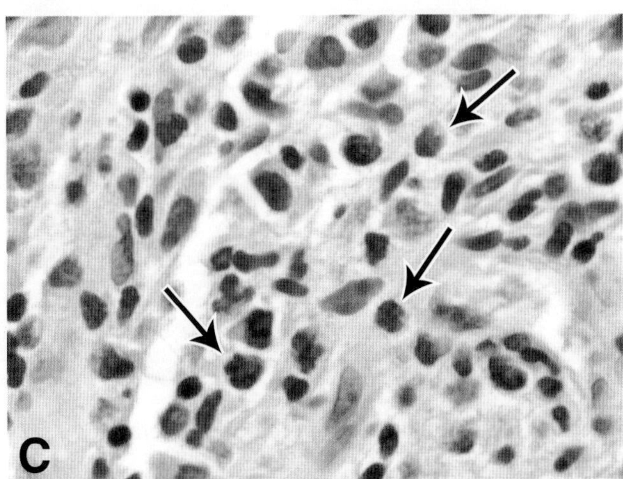

FIGURE 20-58. Mycosis fungoides. A. A 66-year-old woman presented with a 30-year history of erythematous scaly patches and plaques with telangiectases, atrophy, and pigmentation. **B.** An atypical infiltrate of lymphocytes expands the papillary dermis and extends into the epidermis ("epidermotropism"). **C.** Some of the lymphocytes display hyperchromatic and convoluted ("cerebriform") nuclei (*arrows*). 20-58A From Elder AD, Elenitsas R, Johnson BL, et al. *Synopsis and Atlas of Lever's Histopathology of the Skin*. Philadelphia, PA: Lippincott Williams & Wilkins; 1999.

Kaposi Sarcoma

This malignant tumor of endothelial cells of blood vessels was once seen only in older people of Eastern European or Mediterranean descent or in Africans. With the advent of HIV infection, KS is most often seen in patients with AIDS. ***Human herpesvirus 8 (HHV8) is the etiologic agent of KS.***

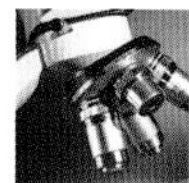

PATHOLOGY: All cases of Kaposi sarcoma evolve through three stages: patch, plaque, and nodule. In the patch stage, a subtle proliferation of irregular vascular channels, lined by a single layer of mildly atypical endothelial cells, radiates from preexisting blood vessels and extends almost imperceptibly into the surrounding reticular dermis. Extravasated red blood cells, hemosiderin deposition, and a sparse inflammatory infiltrate of lymphocytes and plasma cells are common.

In the plaque stage (Fig. 20-59), the entire reticular dermis is involved, with frequent extension into the subcutis and formation of bundles of spindle cells. In the nodule stage (Fig. 20-60), well-circumscribed dermal nodules are composed of anastomosing fascicles of spindle cells surrounding numerous slitlike spaces. Many cases of KS also involve internal organs. In AIDS-related KS, antiretroviral therapy is effective.

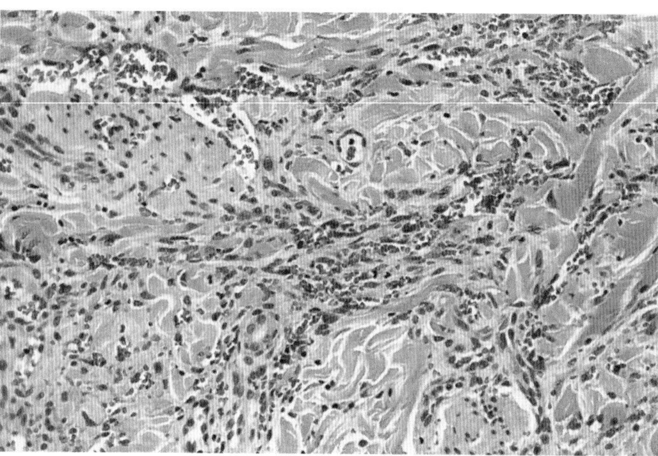

FIGURE 20-59. Kaposi sarcoma, plaque stage. Extending along the vascular arcades and amid reticular dermal collagen is a proliferation of endothelial cells. They form delicate vascular channels filled with red blood cells. Some endothelial cells are not canalized (have not formed lumina).

PARANEOPLASTIC SYNDROMES INVOLVING THE SKIN

Diverse dermatologic manifestations may complicate internal malignancies, often preceding detection of the tumor itself. Pigmented lesions and keratoses are well-recognized paraneoplastic effects.

- **Acanthosis nigricans** is marked by hyperkeratosis and pigmentation of the axilla, neck, flexures, and anogenital region. *It is of particular interest because more than half of patients with acanthosis nigricans have cancer.* The development of the disease may precede, accompany, or follow the detection of the cancer. Over 90% of cases occur in association with gastrointestinal carcinomas, and more than half accompany cancers of the stomach.
- **Sweet syndrome** is a combination of elevated neutrophil count, acute fever, and painful red plaques in the anus, neck, and face. About 20% of cases occur with malignancies, particularly those of the hematopoietic system.

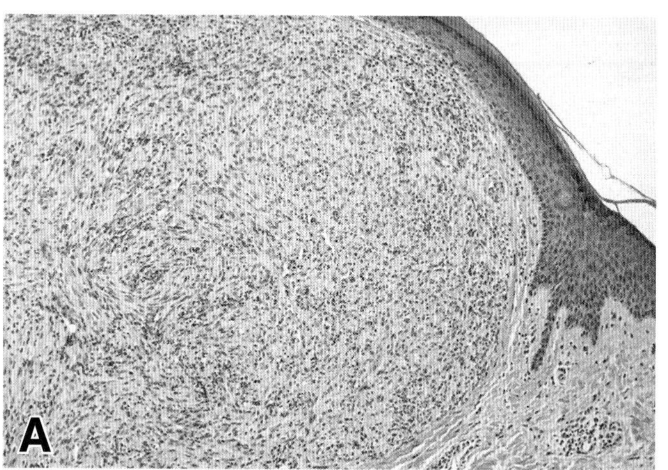

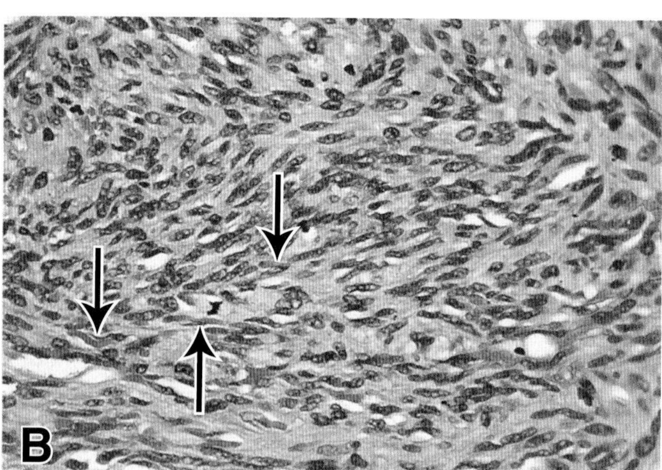

FIGURE 20-60. Kaposi sarcoma, nodule stage. A. A large nodule is composed of proliferating endothelial cells forming fascicles and vascular spaces. **B.** A higher power view showing cytologic atypia of the spindle cells. Red blood cells appear agglutinated (*arrows*). The endothelial cells, in which the agglutinated red blood cells are present, form slitlike spaces.

21 The Head and Neck

Diane L. Carlson

LEARNING OBJECTIVES

- Define the common anatomic location of intraoral ectopic thyroid tissue and the potential complications of therapy.
- Define the following terms related to infections of the oral cavity: cheilitis, gingivitis, glossitis, and stomatitis.
- What are the etiology, pathology, and clinical consequences of Vincent angina?
- What are the etiology, pathology, and clinical consequences of Ludwig angina?
- Both high- and low-risk human papilloma virus infections occur in several of the anatomic divisions of the upper aerodigestive tract. List the pathology and clinical consequences of such infections.
- What is the most common benign tumor of the minor oral salivary gland?
- Describe the pathology of pyogenic intraoral granulomas. Why is the term a misnomer?
- Differentiate between erythroplakia and leukoplakia in terms of potential etiologies, histopathology, and clinical consequences.
- Describe the etiology and molecular pathogenesis of intraoral squamous cell carcinoma.
- Describe the etiology, pathophysiology, and histopathology of dental caries and periodontal disease.
- Describe the histopathology of ameloblastomas.
- List the potential complications of acute and chronic sinusitis.
- Describe the histopathology of inverted Schneiderian papillomas.
- Describe the etiology, histopathology, and clinical consequences of nasal-type angiocentric lymphoma.
- What are the etiologic agents and clinical consequences of peritonsillar abscesses?
- Describe the histopathology of nasopharyngeal angiofibromas. Why are biopsies contraindicated in diagnosing this condition?
- What are the unique epidemiologic features of undifferentiated nonkeratinizing nasopharyngeal carcinoma?
- Differentiate between differentiated and undifferentiated nasopharyngeal carcinoma in terms of etiology and histopathology.
- What are the histopathologic consequences of Sjögren syndrome within salivary glands?
- Describe the distribution, molecular pathogenesis, histopathology, and clinical consequences of pleomorphic salivary gland adenomas.
- Describe the histopathology of Warthin tumors.
- Present an overview of common malignant salivary gland tumors, including their molecular pathology, histopathology, and clinical consequences.
- What are potential complications of acute and chronic otitis media?
- What is the most common benign tumor of the middle ear?

Oral Cavity

The oral cavity extends from the lips to the pharynx (Fig. 21-1).

The mucosa consists of keratinized epithelia of the attached gingiva, hard palate, and the specialized gustatory area of the dorsum of the tongue. It also includes the nonkeratinized mucosal surfaces of the inner lip and inner cheek, the nonattached and movable gingiva that continues into the maxillary and mandibular sulci, ventral tongue, floor of the mouth, soft palate, and tonsillar pillars. The epithelium is three to four times the thickness of the epidermis. Under the epithelium is a lamina propria of fibrous tissue and blood vessels, beneath which is the densely fibrous periosteum of the hard palate or the alveolus of the maxilla and mandible. The term **submucosa** is sometimes loosely applied to the deep connective tissue just above the muscle layer, in which minor salivary glands are often embedded.

Minor salivary glands are scattered throughout the oral cavity as small, unencapsulated lobules within the mucosa and submucosa. There are mucous glands in the lamina propria, particularly in the posterior hard palatal mucosa. The anterior two thirds of the dorsum of the tongue is covered by stratified squamous epithelium that is specialized to form **filiform papillae** (pointed projections of keratin). Between these are **fungiform papillae**, mushroom-shaped mucosal elevations containing taste buds. **Circumvallate papillae** separate the anterior two thirds of the tongue from the posterior one third and contain taste buds at their base. The final group is the **foliate papillae**, in the posterior lateral tongue in a series of

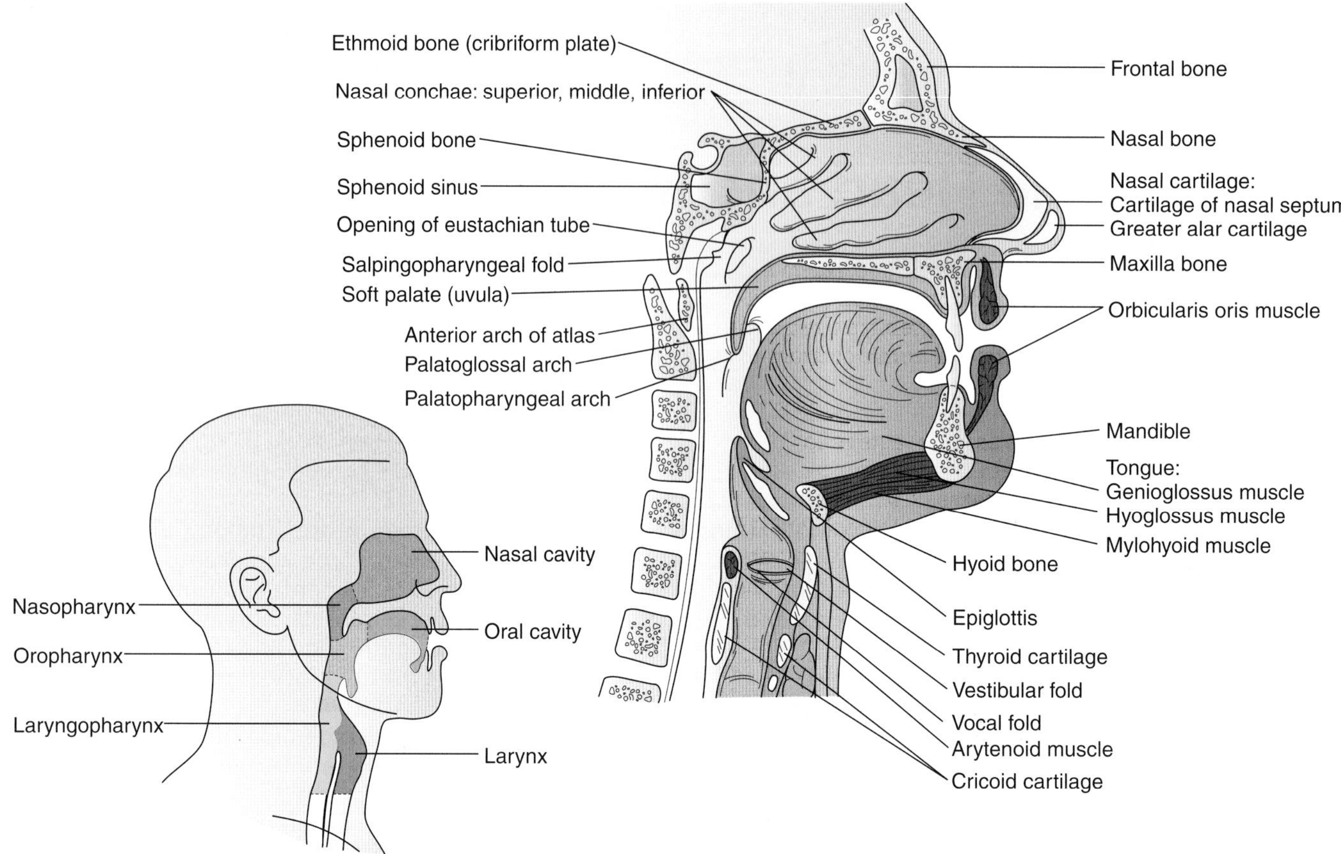

FIGURE 21-1. Structure of the oral cavity, oropharynx, and larynx. Schematic diagram of the oral cavity, palate, oropharynx, and larynx.

ridges. Each taste bud is a barrel-shaped collection of modified epithelial cells that extend vertically from the basal lamina to the epithelial surface, opening via a taste pore.

DEVELOPMENTAL ANOMALIES

FACIAL CLEFTS: If facial structures fail to fuse in the seventh week of embryonic life, facial clefts form. The most common of these is cleft upper lip (**harelip**). It may be unilateral or bilateral and often occurs in association with cleft palate (see Chapter 5).

HAMARTOMAS AND CHORISTOMAS: These lesions are common in the oral cavity. **Fordyce granules** are aggregates of sebaceous glands in the oral cavity (**choristoma**). They occur on the buccal mucosa, lingual surface, and lip in 70% to 95% of adults; rarely, they coalesce to form mass lesions.

Abnormal descent of the thyroid during development may create submucosal foci of **ectopic thyroid** between the tongue and suprasternal notch. The base of the tongue between the foramen cecum and epiglottis is the most common site for ectopic thyroid tissue (**lingual thyroid**). ***Over 75% of patients with lingual thyroid lack a cervical thyroid ("total migration failure"). Thus, surgically removing a lingual thyroid may lead to hypothyroidism and stunted physical growth and mental development*** (**cretinism** see Chapter 19). In fact, 70% of patients with symptomatic lingual thyroid are hypothyroid, and 10% suffer from cretinism. The absence of a normally descended thyroid may also affect development and localization of the parathyroid glands.

Thyroglossal duct cysts result from persistence and cystic dilatation of the thyroglossal duct in the middle of the neck. The anomaly usually occurs above the thyroid isthmus but below the hyoid bone. Patients, mostly under age 40, present clinically with a palpable 4 to 5 cm midline nodule, *which moves up and down upon swallowing.* Surgery is the treatment of choice. Malignancies, commonly papillary thyroid carcinomas, arise in up to 1% of thyroglossal duct cysts.

BRANCHIAL CLEFT CYST: Branchial cleft cysts originate from branchial arch remnants. They occur in the lateral anterior neck or parotid gland, mostly in young adults, and contain thin, watery fluid and mucoid or gelatinous material. These cysts are usually lined by squamous epithelium, with occasional foci of ciliated respiratory or pseudostratified columnar epithelium.

INFECTIONS OF THE ORAL CAVITY

Bacteria and spirochetes are normally present in the oral cavity and are generally harmless. If the mucosa is injured or immunity is impaired, otherwise normal oral flora may become pathogenic.

These terms are used to describe localized inflammation of the oral cavity:

- **Cheilitis** (lips)
- **Gingivitis** (gum)
- **Glossitis** (tongue)
- **Stomatitis** (oral mucosa)

Bacterial and Fungal Infections

SCARLET FEVER: Scarlet fever is mainly a disease of children, caused by several strains of β-hemolytic streptococci (*S. pyogenes*). Damage to vascular endothelium by the erythrogenic toxin results in a rash on the skin and oral mucosa. The tongue acquires a white coating through which the hyperemic fungiform papillae project as small red knobs ("strawberry tongue"). Untreated scarlet fever can lead to glomerulonephritis and heart disease (**acute rheumatic fever**; see Chapter 9).

APHTHOUS STOMATITIS (CANKER SORES): Aphthous stomatitis is a common disease characterized by painful, recurrent, solitary, or multiple, small ulcers of the oral mucosa. Although various etiologies have been suggested, its cause is unknown. The lesion is a shallow ulcer covered by a fibrinopurulent exudate, with underlying mononuclear and polymorphonuclear inflammation. The lesions heal without scarring.

ACUTE NECROTIZING ULCERATIVE GINGIVITIS (VINCENT ANGINA, FUSOSPIROCHETOSIS): Vincent angina is an acute, necrotizing, ulcerative gingivitis caused by infection with two symbiotic organisms, a fusiform bacillus and a spirochete (*Borrelia vincentii*). These organisms are found in the mouths of many healthy people, suggesting the involvement of other factors, particularly decreased resistance to infection owing to inadequate nutrition, immunodeficiency, or poor oral hygiene. Vincent angina is characterized by punched-out erosions of the interdental papillae. The process tends to spread and eventually involves all gingival margins, which become covered by a necrotic pseudomembrane.

LUDWIG ANGINA: Ludwig angina is a rapidly spreading cellulitis originating in the submaxillary or sublingual space but extending to involve both. Several aerobic and anaerobic oral bacteria have been implicated. Ludwig angina is a potentially life-threatening inflammatory process. It is uncommon in developed countries, except in patients with chronic illnesses associated with immunosuppression.

Ludwig angina is most often related to dental extraction or trauma to the floor of the mouth. After extraction of a tooth, hairline fractures may occur in the lingual cortex of the mandible, providing microorganisms ready access to the submaxillary space. Infection may dissect into the parapharyngeal space along fascial planes, and from there into the carotid sheath. A mycotic internal carotid artery aneurysm may result, the erosion of which may cause massive hemorrhage. The inflammation can also dissect into the superior mediastinum to involve the pleural space and pericardium.

DIPHTHERIA: Infection with *Corynebacterium diphtheriae* is characterized by a patchy pseudomembrane, which often begins on the tonsils and pharynx but may also involve the soft palate, gingivam, or buccal mucosa (see Chapter 6).

ACTINOMYCOSIS: Actinomycetes are common denizens of the oral cavity in healthy people. Invasive actinomycosis is most often caused by *Actinomyces bovis,* although *A. israelii* is sometimes seen. The organisms produce chronic granulomatous inflammation and abscesses that drain by fistula formation; suppurative infection contains characteristic yellow "sulfur granules." In cervicofacial actinomycosis, soft tissue infection may extend to adjacent bones, most often to the mandible.

CANDIDIASIS: Also called **thrush** or **moniliasis**, oral candidiasis is caused by *Candida albicans* (see Chapter 6), which is common on the surfaces of the oral cavity, gastrointestinal tract, and vagina. To cause the disease, the fungus must penetrate tissues, albeit superficially. Oral candidiasis is mostly seen in diabetics and people with compromised immune systems. Lesions are white, slightly elevated, soft patches, which consist mainly of fungal hyphae.

Oral Viral Diseases

HERPES SIMPLEX VIRUS TYPE 1: Herpes labialis (cold sores, fever blisters) and herpetic stomatitis are caused by herpes simplex virus (HSV) type 1 and are among the most common viral infections of the lips and oral mucosa in children and young adults. Transmission is via aerosol, and the virus can be recovered from the saliva of infected people. Disease starts with painful inflammation of affected mucosa, followed shortly by formation of vesicles. These result from "ballooning degeneration" of epithelial cells, some of which show intranuclear inclusions (Fig. 21-2). The vesicles rupture to form shallow, painful, 1 to 10 mm ulcers, which heal spontaneously without scarring.

Once HSV enters the body, it remains dormant in the trigeminal ganglion until stresses, such as trauma, allergy, menstruation, pregnancy, exposure to ultraviolet light, or other viral infections, reactivate it. Recurrent oral cavity vesicles almost invariably develop on a mucosa that is tightly bound to periosteum, for example, the hard palate.

HUMAN PAPILLOMA VIRUS–RELATED DISEASES: The HPV family of viruses causes epithelial proliferations, including papillomas (e.g., sinonasal, Schneiderian papillomas, and other papillomas of upper aerodigestive tract sites). "High-risk" HPV, mainly types 16 and 18, as well as 31, 33, and 35, is strongly associated with oropharyngeal squamous cell carcinoma (see below).

EPSTEIN–BARR VIRUS–RELATED DISEASES: Epstein–Barr virus (EBV) is a member of the *Herpesvirus* family that causes oral hairy leukoplakia, various lymphoid diseases (see Chapter 18), and epithelial cancers in the nose and pharynx (see below).

HUMAN HERPES VIRUS 8: This virus is associated with **Kaposi sarcoma**, which occurs most often in the skin (see Chapter 20) but can also involve, among other places, the tongue and oral cavity.

OTHER VIRAL INFECTIONS: Coxsackievirus causes **herpangina**, an acute vesicular oropharyngitis. A brief infection

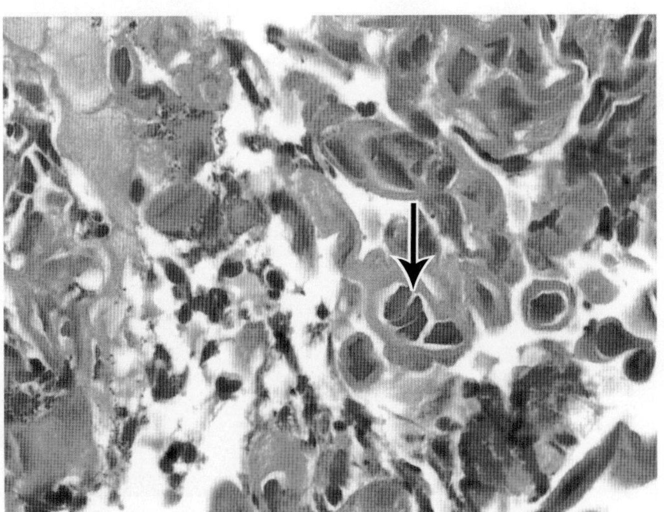

FIGURE 21-2. Herpes simplex virus type 1. A biopsy from a nonhealing ulcer on the tongue demonstrates intranuclear viral inclusions (*arrow*) within squamous cells infected by the virus.

confers lasting immunity. **Cytomegalovirus** (CMV) infection typically presents with surface ulceration. Other viral infections that involve the oral mucosa include measles, rubella, chickenpox, and herpes zoster.

BENIGN TUMORS

Benign tumors found elsewhere in the body (e.g., nevi, fibromas, hemangiomas, lymphangiomas, and squamous papillomas) are seen also in the oral cavity. Trauma may lead to ulceration of the lesions, causing bleeding or infection.

PAPILLOMA: Squamous papillomas are benign, exophytic epithelial tumors with branching fronds of squamous epithelium and fibrovascular cores (Fig. 21-3A). They are the most common benign oral cavity neoplasms and have been associated with HPV types 6 and 11, which are low-risk serotypes *not* associated with malignancy (Fig. 21-3B). They occur mainly in the third to fifth decades. The tongue, palate, buccal mucosa, tonsil, and uvula are most often involved.

BENIGN MINOR SALIVARY GLAND TUMORS: **Pleomorphic adenoma** (benign mixed tumor) is the most common oral salivary gland tumor (see later discussion). Monomorphic adenomas such as myoepithelioma or oncocytoma are less common. Benign mesenchymal tumors that may occur in the oral cavity include hemangiomas, leiomyomas, and lipomas.

LOBULAR CAPILLARY HEMANGIOMA (PYOGENIC GRANULOMA; PREGNANCY TUMOR): Lobular capillary hemangiomas are benign polypoid capillary hemangiomas that occur mainly on the skin, mucous membranes, and, most often, gingiva. The term "pyogenic granuloma" is a misnomer: it is neither infectious nor granulomatous. In the mouth, the lesions are elevated, soft, red, or purple and vary from a few millimeters to a centimeter, with smooth, lobulated, ulcerated surfaces. They show lobules or clusters of submucosal vessels, with central capillaries and smaller ramifying tributaries. In time, the lesions tend to become less vascular and resemble fibromas.

An identical lesion in the gingiva (**pregnancy tumor**) may occur in pregnant women near the end of the third trimester. It may or may not regress after delivery.

PRENEOPLASTIC EPITHELIAL LESIONS

Premalignant lesions of the upper aerodigestive tract include (1) leukoplakia, (2) erythroplakia, or (3) speckled leukoplakia, the terms describing a white, red, or mixed white/red lesion, respectively.

- ***Leukoplakia is an asymptomatic white lesion on the surface of a mucous membrane.*** It affects both sexes equally, mostly after the third decade. Some of these lesions may become squamous cell carcinomas (SCCs). Diverse diseases appear clinically as leukoplakia, including several keratoses and squamous carcinoma in situ. ***Thus, leukoplakia is a descriptive clinical term, not a pathologic diagnosis.*** The causes of leukoplakia include tobacco use, alcoholism, and local irritation. The same factors also appear to be important in the etiology of oral carcinoma.
- ***Erythroplakia is the red equivalent of leukoplakia,*** but occurs less often. Red areas associated with leukoplakic lesions are **speckled leukoplakia (speckled mucosa; erythroleukoplakia)**. Erythroplakia may represent moderate to severe dysplasia or carcinoma. However, not all red erythroplakic lesions indicate dysplasia/carcinoma, because many red oral mucosal lesions are inflammatory.

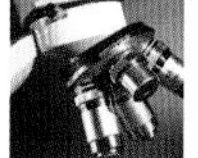

PATHOLOGY: Leukoplakia (Fig. 21-4) occurs mostly on the buccal mucosa, tongue, and floor of the mouth. Plaques may be solitary or multiple small lesions to large patches. Erythroplakia is often associated with ominous histopathologic features, including severe dysplasia, carcinoma in situ, or invasive SCC. In contrast, leukoplakic lesions represent a spectrum of histopathologies, from increased surface keratinization without dysplasia to invasive keratinizing squamous carcinoma. Leukoplakias, unlike erythroplakic lesions, tend to show well-demarcated margins. The risk of malignancy with leukoplakia is 10% to 12%. The same risk in erythroplakia approaches 50%.

Oral hairy leukoplakia demonstrates shaggy parakeratosis and edema, with or without associated inflammation. It occurs mainly in people who are HIV-1 positive, usually

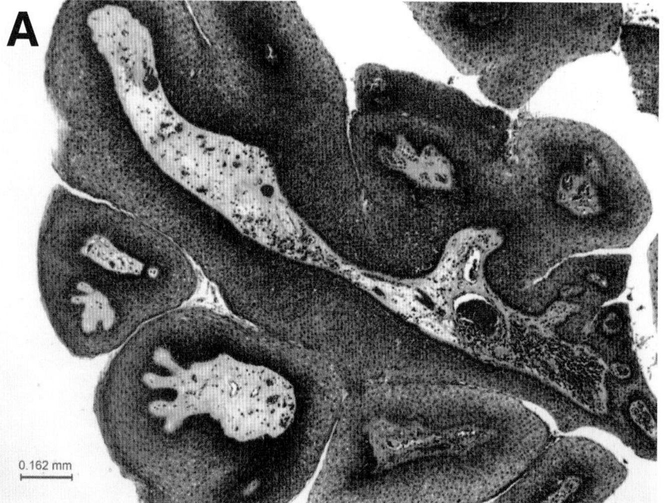

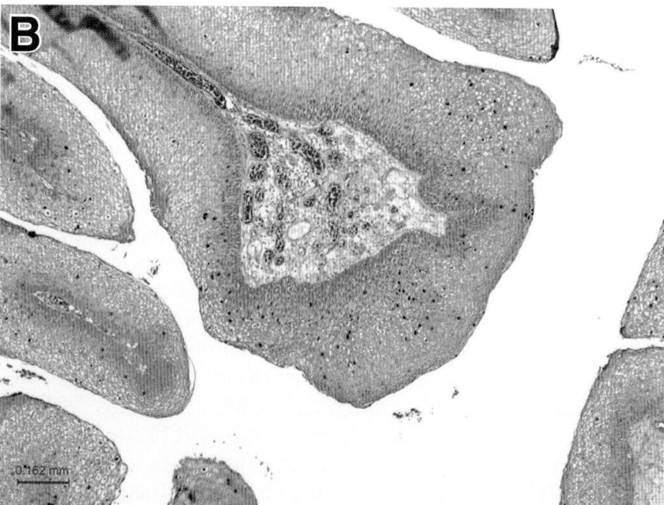

FIGURE 21-3. Squamous Papilloma. A. Histologic appearance. This exophytic frond-like papillary tumor grew off the patient's uvula. **B. In situ hybridization** for low-risk human papillomavirus demonstrates nuclear localization.

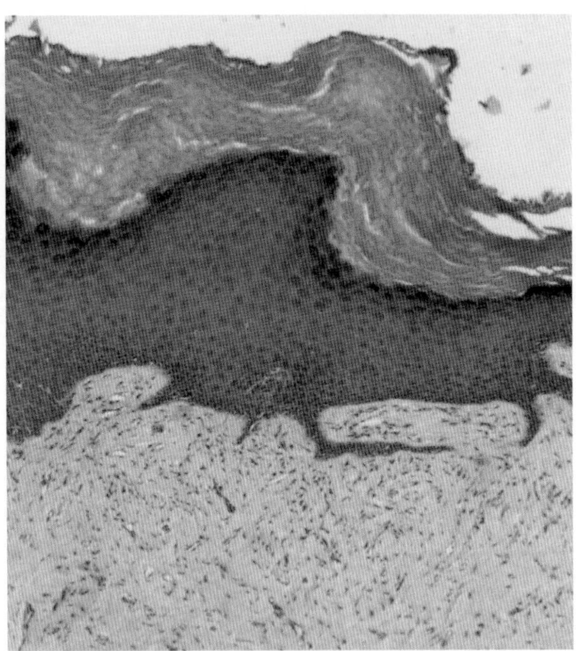

FIGURE 21-4. Leukoplakia. The lesion was seen as a white patch on the buccal mucosa of a heavy smoker. Histologically, epithelial hyperplasia and hyperkeratosis are evident.

with associated candidiasis. The EBV-infected squamous cells are seen just beneath the keratin layer and have dense central eosinophilic inclusions and vacuolated cytoplasm. Oral hairy leukoplakia and candidiasis reflect immune status and together suggest low $CD4^+$ lymphocyte counts and high viral load.

SQUAMOUS CELL CARCINOMA

SCCs are the most common malignant tumors of the oral mucosa and may occur at any site. In the United States, there are over 40,000 cases yearly, most often involving the tongue, followed by the floor of the mouth, alveolar mucosa, palate, and buccal mucosa in that order. The male-to-female ratio is 2:1 for the gums but 10:1 for the lip. The geographic distribution of oral cancer shows wide variation: it is the most common cancer of men in India, where it is associated with betel nut quid (pan) chewing.

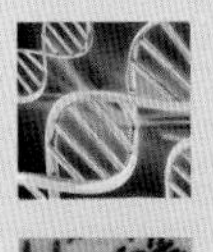

MOLECULAR PATHOGENESIS AND ETIOLOGIC FACTORS: Use of tobacco products, alcoholism, iron deficiency (Plummer–Vinson syndrome), Fanconi anemia, physical and chemical irritants, chewing of betel nuts, ultraviolet light on the lips, and poor oral hygiene (craggy teeth and ill-fitting dentures) predispose a person to oral SCC. Not surprisingly, several of these factors are also connected with leukoplakia. Multiple separate SCCs may be simultaneous (synchronous) or may occur at intervals (metachronous) in the oral mucosa ("field cancerization"). Worldwide, 35% to 50% of head and neck SCCs are associated with high-risk HPV, mostly HPV-16.

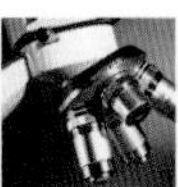

PATHOLOGY: ***Invasive oral cavity SCC resembles the same tumor in other sites. It is generally preceded by carcinoma in situ.*** The tumor ranges from well to poorly differentiated, undifferentiated, and sarcomatoid variants. Well-differentiated, or grade I, tumors are frequently keratinizing (Fig. 21-5). At the other end of the spectrum, tumors may be so poorly differentiated that their origin is difficult to determine.

Oral SCC metastasizes mainly to submandibular, superficial, and deep cervical lymph nodes, and at autopsy 18% of these patients have axillary metastases. More than half of patients who die of head and neck SCC have distant, blood-borne metastases, most often in the lungs, liver, and bones.

Local recurrence is predicted by a tumor's pattern of infiltration: single-cell invasion is less favorable than a broad, "pushing" border. Other prognostic factors include (1) depth of tumor invasion, (2) perineural invasion, and (3) lymphovascular tumor emboli. Negative resection margins are important in local and regional control of the tumor.

Verrucous carcinomas are highly differentiated variants of squamous cell carcinoma that generally occur in the sixth and seventh decades; they are locally destructive but do not usually metastasize. The tumors may arise anywhere in this region. but are most common on the buccal mucosa, gingiva, and larynx. These lesions are usually white, warty to fungating, or exophytic and generally have broad bases (Fig. 21-6A). They are composed of benign-appearing squamous epithelium, with marked surface keratinization and a pushing border of bulbous rete pegs (Fig. 21-6B). Verrucous carcinomas carry a good prognosis if completely removed.

MALIGNANT MINOR SALIVARY GLAND NEOPLASMS

About 50% of intraoral minor salivary gland tumors are malignant. These include mucoepidermoid carcinomas, adenoid cystic carcinomas, and polymorphous low-grade adenocarcinomas (see below). Some tumors that are more common malignancies of major salivary glands occur uncommonly in minor salivary glands (e.g., acinic cell adenocarcinoma), whereas low-grade adenocarcinoma and clear cell carcinoma are more common in the palate than in the major salivary glands.

BENIGN DISEASES OF THE LIPS

The lips are affected by many degenerative, inflammatory, and proliferative processes. Some of these, particularly those expressed in the skin and mucous membranes, are systemic; others reflect localized disease. A **mucocele** is a mucus-filled cystic lesion associated with minor salivary glands that is often caused by trauma.

DENTAL CARIES (TOOTH DECAY)

Caries is the most common chronic disease of the calcified tissues of teeth, affecting both sexes and every age group. Its incidence has plummeted with modern civilization.

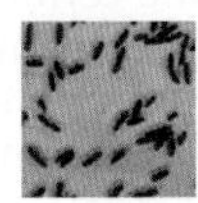

ETIOLOGIC FACTORS: The interactions of several factors cause caries:

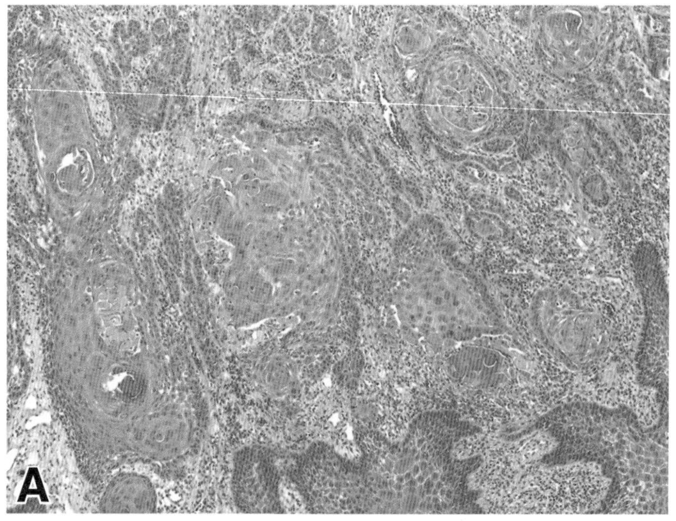

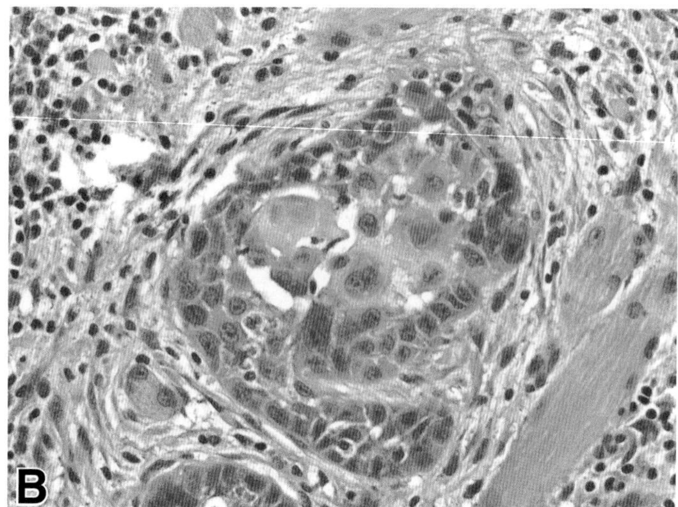

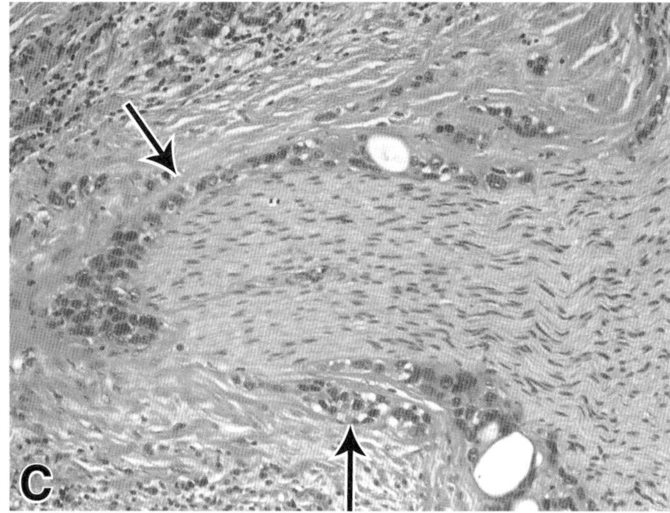

FIGURE 21-5. Squamous cell carcinoma. A. An infiltrative neoplasm is composed of cohesive nests of tumor. **B.** A less differentiated tumor displays cells with pleomorphic nuclei, prominent nucleoli, brightly eosinophilic cytoplasm indicating keratinization and intercellular bridges connecting adjacent cells. **C.** Perineural invasion by squamous cell carcinoma. Tumor surrounds a nerve (*arrows*).

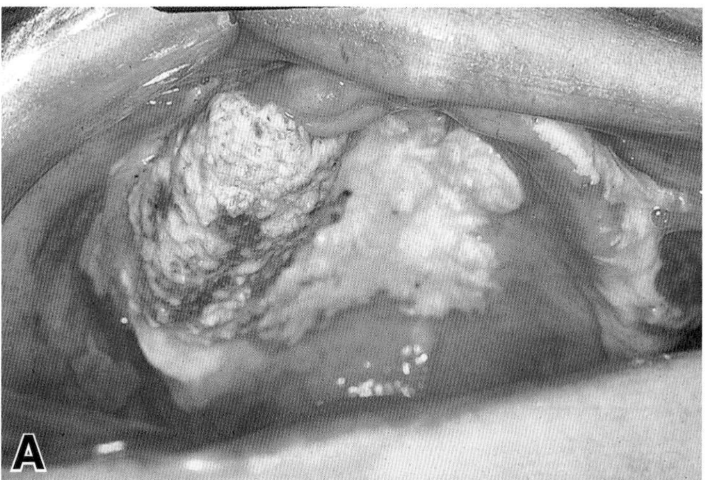

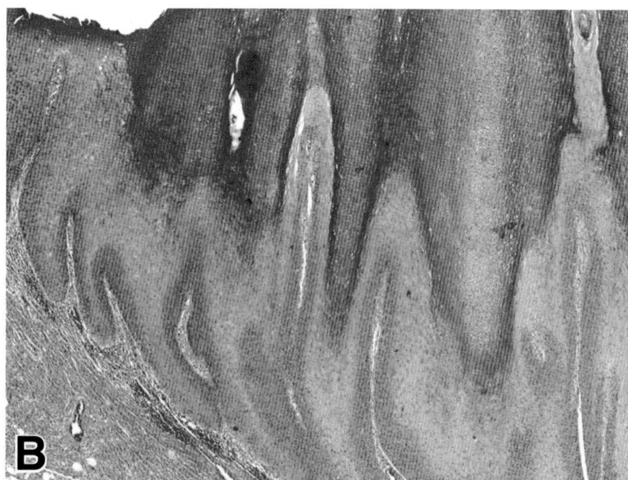

FIGURE 21-6. Verrucous carcinoma. A. The tumor is white with an exophytic appearance involving the alveolar ridge. Note the confluent flat white (leukoplakic) appearance of the palate. **B.** Microscopically, there is prominent surface keratinization ("church-spire" keratosis) composed of bland-appearing uniform squamous cells without dysplasia and broad or bulbous rete pegs with a pushing margin into the submucosa.

BACTERIA: Dental caries is a chronic infectious disease of tooth enamel, dentin, and cementum. Tooth surfaces are colonized by many microorganisms. Unless the surfaces are cleaned thoroughly and frequently, bacterial colonies coalesce into a soft mass known as **dental plaque**.

Carious lesions occur because acids produced from food residues by microorganisms on tooth surfaces leach the minerals in teeth. Responsible agents include streptococci, lactobacilli, and actinomycetes in the oral flora. Indirect evidence points strongly to *Streptococcus mutans* as the primary etiologic agent that initiates caries.

SALIVA: Saliva has a high buffering capacity that helps neutralize microbially produced acids in the mouth. It also contains bacteriostatic factors such as lysozyme, lactoferrin, lactoperoxidases, and secretory immunoglobulins. **Xerostomia** (chronically dry mouth caused by lack of saliva) may be iatrogenic, for example, due to surgery or radiation therapy; it results in rampant caries.

DIETARY FACTORS: One of the most important factors in the pathogenesis of caries is a high-carbohydrate diet. Roughage in raw and unrefined foods necessitates heavy mastication, which cleanses the teeth. By contrast, soft and refined foods tend to stick to the teeth and also require less chewing.

FLUORIDE: Fluoride protects the teeth from caries. It is incorporated into the crystal lattice structure of enamel, where it forms fluoroapatite, which is less acid soluble than is the apatite of enamel. Many communities that fluoridated their drinking water experienced huge reductions in the incidence of dental caries in children.

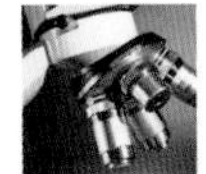

PATHOLOGY: Caries begins with disintegration of enamel prisms after decalcification of the interprismatic substance, events that lead to the accumulation of debris and microorganisms (Fig. 21-7). These changes produce a small pit or fissure in the enamel. When the process reaches the dentinoenamel junction, it spreads laterally and also penetrates the dentin along the dentinal tubules. A substantial cavity then forms in the dentin, producing a flask-shaped lesion with a narrow orifice. Dentin decalcification causes the destroyed dentinal tubules to coalesce. Only when the vascular pulp of the tooth is invaded does an inflammatory reaction (**pulpitis**) appear, accompanied, for the first time, by pain.

PERIODONTAL DISEASE

The gingiva (gum) is the part of the oral mucosa that surrounds the teeth. It ends in a thin edge (free gingiva) that adheres closely to the teeth. A periodontal ligament of collagen fibers holds the teeth in position in the socket (alveolus) of the jawbone. These structures form the periodontium.

Periodontal diseases are acute and chronic disorders of the soft tissues around the teeth, which eventually erode the supporting bone. Chronic periodontal disease typically occurs in adults with poor oral hygiene but may develop even in people with apparently impeccable habits who have strong family histories of periodontal disease. It causes more loss of teeth in adults than does any other disease, including caries.

Periodontal disease occurs when bacteria accumulate under the gingiva in the periodontal pocket. The mass of bacteria adhering to the tooth surface (**dental plaque**) ages, mineralizes, and forms **calculus (tartar)**. Adult periodontitis is mostly associated with *Bacteroides gingivalis, Bacteroides intermedius, Actinomyces* sp., and *Haemophilus* sp.

Inflammation often starts as a marginal gingivitis. Untreated, it progresses to chronic periodontitis, in which the chronic inflammation weakens and destroys the periodontium, causing loosening and eventual loss of teeth.

Hematologic disorders may affect oral tissues. Agranulocytosis may cause necrotizing ulcers anywhere in the oral and pharyngeal mucosa, but especially in the gingiva. Infectious mononucleosis is often complicated by gingivitis and stomatitis, with exudation and ulceration. Acute and chronic

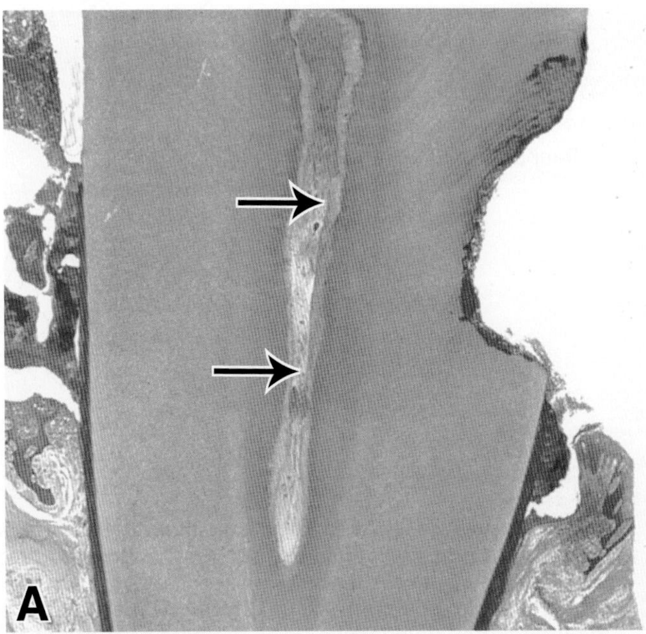

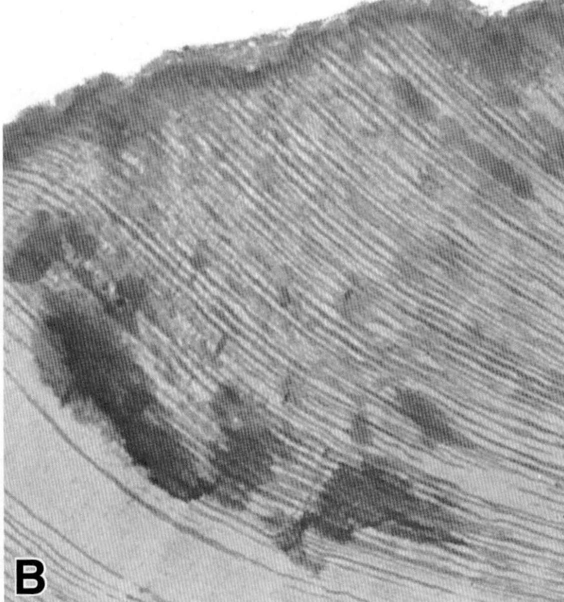

FIGURE 21-7. Dental caries. A. A large cavity close to the gingival margin is illustrated. *Arrows* indicate band of secondary dentin that lines the pulp chamber. This newly formed dentin is opposite the area of tooth destruction and was produced by the stimulated odontoblasts. **B.** Deposits of debris cover the surface. Bacterial colonies (*dark purple*) have extended into dentinal canals.

leukemias of all types are associated with oral lesions. In **acute monocytic leukemia**, 80% of patients have gingivitis, gingival hyperplasia, petechiae, and hemorrhage. Necrosis and ulceration of the gingiva lead to severe superimposed infection, which may cause loss of teeth and alveolar bone. A hemorrhagic diathesis is often reflected in gingival hemorrhage.

Mild scurvy affects the marginal and interdental gingiva, which become swollen and bright red and bleed and ulcerate readily. Hemorrhage into the periodontal membrane causes loosening and loss of teeth.

ODONTOGENIC CYSTS AND TUMORS

- **Odontogenic cysts** may be inflammatory or developmental. Most common are **radicular (apical, periodontal) cysts**, involving tooth apices, usually after infection of the dental pulp.
- **Dentigerous cysts** are associated with the crowns of impacted, embedded, or unerupted teeth, most often involving mandibular and maxillary third molars. They form after the crown has completely developed; fluid accumulates between the crown and overlying enamel epithelium. Dentigerous cysts may be complicated by ameloblastoma or SCC.
- **Ameloblastomas** are tumors of odontogenic epithelia and are the most common odontogenic tumors. They are slow growing and locally invasive, generally follow a benign clinical course, and can be locally destructive. Most arise in the mandibular ramus or molar area, maxilla, or floor of the nasal cavity. The tumors grow slowly as central lesions of bone, showing a characteristic "soap bubble" radiographic appearance. Ameloblastomas resemble the enamel organ in its various stages of differentiation. Thus, tumor cells resemble ameloblasts at the edges of epithelial nests or cords, where columnar cells are oriented perpendicularly to the basement membrane (Fig. 21-8). The prognosis is favorable, but incompletely excised tumors recur. Some may metastasize and yet remain histologically benign (**metastasizing ameloblastoma**).
- **Ameloblastic carcinomas** are frankly malignant, with atypia, necrosis, nuclear pleomorphism, and abundant mitoses. Nuclei of ameloblastomas may show aberrant β-catenin expression. An *APC* gene missense mutation, which plays a role in colon cancer, may also participate in the pathogenesis of odontogenic tumors (see Chapter 11).

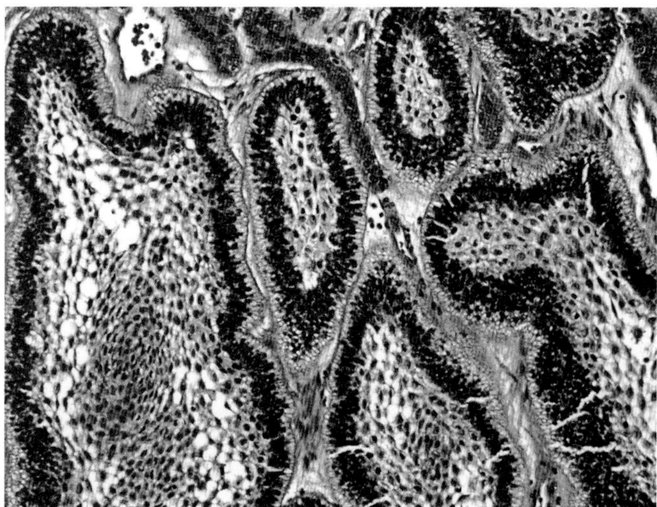

FIGURE 21-8. Ameloblastoma. A common histologic pattern is characterized by islands of odontogenic epithelium with a central stellate reticulum-like area, surrounded by basal cells with a "picket fence" appearance, because of subnuclear vacuoles.

Nasal Cavity and Paranasal Sinuses

ANATOMY: The **nostril apertures** (anterior nares) lead into the **nasal vestibule**, a space lined by skin that contains hairs and sebaceous glands. Beyond the nares, the median septum divides the nasal cavity into two symmetric chambers, called the **nasal fossae**. Each nasal fossa has an **olfactory region**, consisting of the superior nasal concha and the opposed part of the septum, and a **respiratory region**, which is the rest of the cavity. Laterally, the inferior, middle, and superior nasal conchae (**turbinates**) overhang the corresponding nasal passages or meatus.

The paranasal sinuses are paired air spaces that communicate with the nasal cavity. The respiratory portion of the nasal cavity is covered by ciliated, columnar epithelium with interspersed goblet cells.

These anatomic interrelations determine routes of disease spread (Fig. 21-9). Infections can spread to maxillary, ethmoid,

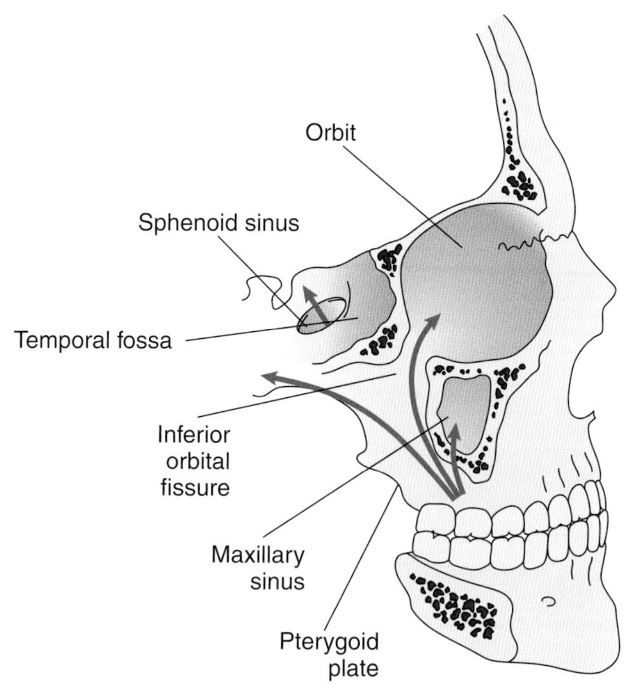

FIGURE 21-9. Pathways of infection to the intracranial cavity. Osseous pathways of infection from the jaws. *Arrows* indicate the direction of spread from the teeth to the maxillary sinus and through the inferior orbital fissure to the orbit. A deeper route is along the lateral pterygoid lamina up to the base of the skull, where, medial to the foramen ovale, a small aperture admits the vein of Vesalius. Through this small vein, the pterygoid plexus communicates with the cavernous sinus.

frontal, and sphenoid sinuses, causing intraorbital and intracranial disease. The vein of Vesalius, medial to the foramen ovale, puts the cavernous sinus at risk.

NONNEOPLASTIC DISEASES OF THE NOSE AND NASAL VESTIBULE

Rosacea is a chronic skin disorder of the cheeks, nose, chin, and central forehead, characterized by telangiectasias, flushing, erythema, papules, pustules, rhinophyma (see below) and ocular manifestations (Fig. 21-10). Bacteria (e.g., *Bacillus oleronius* and *Staphylococcus epidermidis*), as well as Demodex mites, have all been implicated. Inflammation is central to this disease, although the initiating factors and etiology of rosacea remain obscure. Antibiotics, such as tetracycline and metronidazole, are common therapies.

Rhinophyma is a protuberant bulbous mass on the nose caused by marked hyperplasia of sebaceous glands and chronic inflammation of the skin in acne rosacea.

Nosebleed (epistaxis) is most often caused by trauma but has many other causes, including hypertension, diverse hematologic abnormalities, inflammatory conditions, and nasal mucosal tumors. Epistaxis often originates in a triangular area of the anterior nasal septum called "Little area," where the epidermis is thin and arteries anastomose to form the **Kiesselbach plexus**. Many dilated blood vessels, or telangiectasias, are often apparent. Ulcers and perforations, which may be caused by various diseases or by trauma to the septum, occur here (Table 21-1).

NONNEOPLASTIC DISEASES OF THE NASAL CAVITY AND SINUSES

Rhinitis

Rhinitis is inflammation of the mucous membranes of the nasal cavity and sinuses. Its causes range from the common cold to unusual infections such as diphtheria, anthrax, or glanders.

VIRAL RHINITIS: The most common cause of acute rhinitis is viral infection, especially the common cold (**acute coryza**). The virus replicates in epithelial cells, after which degenerating epithelial cells are shed. The mucosa is edematous, engorged, and infiltrated by neutrophils and mononuclear cells. Clinically, mucosal swelling is felt as nasal stuffiness. Abundant mucous secretion and increased vascular permeability lead to **rhinorrhea** (free discharge of a thin, watery mucus).

Secondary infection by normal nasal and pharyngeal flora follow viral rhinitis by a few days. The abundant serous discharge then becomes mucopurulent, after which the surface epithelium is shed. Once inflammation subsides, the epithelium regenerates rapidly.

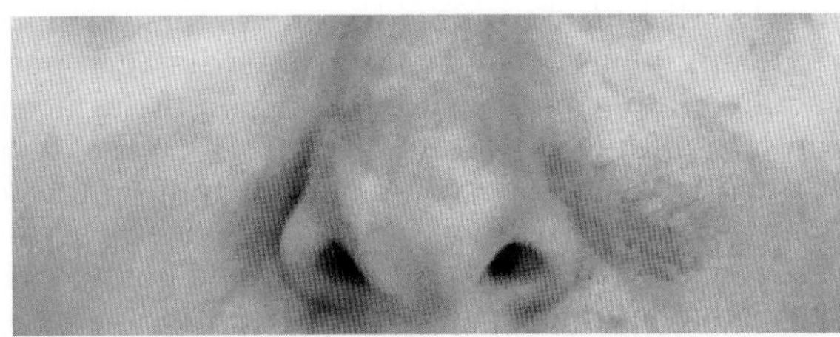

FIGURE 21-10. Rosacea. Typically characterized by erythema over the bridge of the nose and cheeks, as well as pustules and papules.

Table 21-1

Causes of Nasal Septum Perforation

Trauma
Specific infections (tuberculosis, syphilis, leprosy)
Wegener granulomatosis
Lupus erythematosus
Chronic exposure to dust (containing arsenic, chromium, copper, etc.)
Cocaine abuse
Malignant tumors

ALLERGIC RHINITIS (HAY FEVER): Allergens are constantly present in the environment, and sensitivity to any one of them can cause allergic rhinitis. Allergic rhinitis may be acute and seasonal or chronic and perennial (see Chapter 3).

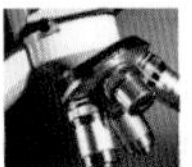

PATHOLOGY: Vasodilation increases vascular permeability to cause edema of the nasal mucosa, especially of the inferior turbinates. Many eosinophils may be seen in the nasal mucosa or secretions. The late phase of mast cell–mediated reactions is associated with persistent mucosal edema and manifests clinically as nasal obstruction.

CHRONIC RHINITIS: Repeated bouts of acute rhinitis may lead to chronic rhinitis. In this condition, the nasal mucosa is thickened by persistent hyperemia, mucous gland hyperplasia, and infiltration with lymphocytes and plasma cells.

Inflammatory Polyps

These structures arise in the nose and sinuses, mostly from the lateral nasal wall or ethmoid recess. They may be unilateral or bilateral, single, or multiple. Symptoms include nasal obstruction, rhinorrhea, and headaches. Multiple etiologies are responsible, including allergy, cystic fibrosis, infections, diabetes mellitus, and aspirin intolerance. These polyps are lined by respiratory epithelium and have mucous glands within a loose mucoid stroma, containing plasma cells, lymphocytes, and eosinophils.

Sinusitis

The disease usually reflects bacterial infections of the paranasal sinuses.

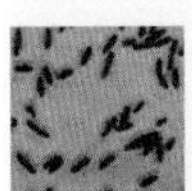

ETIOLOGIC FACTORS: Any condition (inflammation, neoplasm, or presence of foreign body) that interferes with sinus drainage or aeration renders it susceptible to infection. If a sinus ostium is blocked, secretions or exudate accumulate behind the obstruction.

Acute sinusitis is a disorder of less than 3 weeks' duration, caused largely by extension of infection from the nasal mucosa. *H. influenzae* and *Branhamella catarrhalis* are the most common organisms. Maxillary sinusitis may also be caused by odontogenic infections; bacteria from the roots of the first and second molars penetrate the thin bony plate that separates them from the floor of the maxillary sinus. Incomplete resolution of infection or recurrent acute sinusitis may lead to chronic sinusitis, in which the purulent exudate almost always includes anaerobic bacteria.

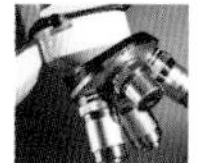

PATHOLOGY: Complications of acute or chronic sinusitis are as follows:

- **Mucocele:** Mucocele is an accumulation of mucous secretions in a nasal sinus. If infected, a mucocele may cause a sinus to fill with mucopurulent exudate, called a **pyocele**. Purulent exudation in a sinus is **empyema** (Fig. 21-11). Mucoceles of anterior ethmoid or frontal sinuses may be large enough to displace the contents of the orbit and occasionally erode into the central nervous system.
- **Osteomyelitis:** Suppurative infection of sinus walls may spread through Volkmann canals to the periosteum, producing periostitis and subperiosteal abscess. Osteomyelitis may also spread rapidly between the outer and inner tables of the skull.
- **Septic thrombophlebitis:** Sinus infections that penetrate the bone may spread to frontal and diploe venous systems. The resulting septic thrombophlebitis may involve the cavernous venous sinus through the superior ophthalmic veins and is a potentially life-threatening condition.
- **Intracranial infections:** Sinusitis may also spread infection to the cranial cavity. Lesions include epidural, subdural, and cerebral abscesses and purulent leptomeningitis. Spread may be via lymphatics and veins and need not involve extensive destruction of bone.

Allergic Fungal Sinusitis

Allergic fungal sinusitis reflects hypersensitivity to fungal antigens, such as allergic bronchopulmonary aspergillosis. The disease occurs at all ages but is most common in children or young adults, especially those who are atopic or immunologically "hypercompetent." Any sinus may be affected, but maxillary and ethmoid sinuses are most often involved.

Fungus balls, or **aspergillomas**, occur in immunologically normal patients, usually with chronic sinusitis and poor drainage. In this setting, fungi proliferate to form a dense mass of hyphae that causes nasal obstruction. Evidence of bone destruction and ocular symptoms may be present.

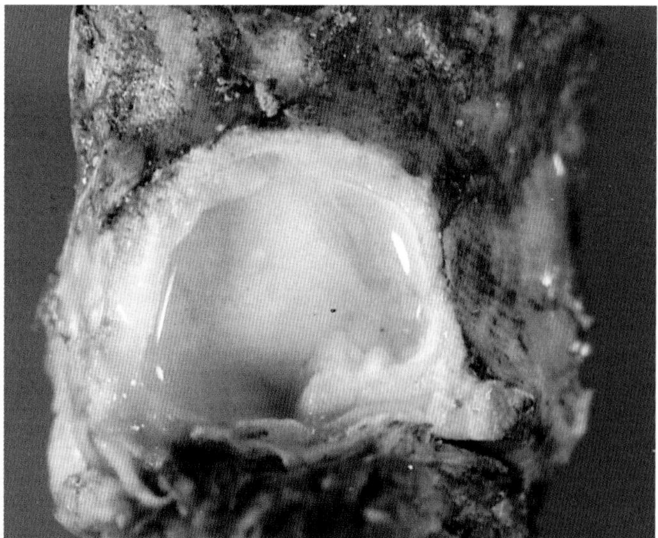

FIGURE 21-11. Empyema of the maxillary sinus (sagittal section). Infection followed chronic obstruction of the orifice caused by adenocarcinoma of the nasal mucosa.

Invasive Fungal Sinusitis

Invasive fungal sinusitis usually affects immunocompromised patients. In the rare **rhinocerebral aspergillosis**, the organisms penetrate venous sinuses and spread to the meninges and brain. Few patients survive.

Mucormycosis is a potentially life-threatening infection, particularly in diabetic and immunosuppressed patients. It typically involves the nasopharynx but can invade the skin, bone, orbit, and brain.

Granulomatosis With Polyangiitis

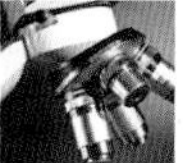

PATHOLOGY: This condition may affect many organs (see Chapters 8 and 14). The sinonasal tract may be the only involved site, or it may be part of a systemic disease. Septal perforation and mucosal ulceration may be followed by slowly progressive destruction of the nose and paranasal sinuses, leading to a saddle nose deformity. Constitutional symptoms, such as fever, malaise, and weight loss, may accompany resulting "runny nose," sinusitis, and nosebleeds. Nasal lesions show ischemic-type necrosis, vasculitis, mixed chronic inflammation, scattered multinucleated giant cells, and microabscesses. Well-formed granulomas are not seen. Elevated serum antineutrophil cytoplasmic antibodies (ANCAs; see Chapter 14) are associated with active disease.

Benign Tumors of the Nasal Cavity and Paranasal Sinuses

SQUAMOUS PAPILLOMA: This is the most common benign tumor of the nasal cavity. It resembles a wart (verruca vulgaris) and almost always occurs in the nasal vestibule.

SCHNEIDERIAN PAPILLOMA: This benign neoplasm arises from the sinonasal (Schneiderian) mucosa and is composed of a squamous or columnar epithelial proliferation with associated mucous cells. There are three morphologically distinct lesions, collectively called Schneiderian papillomas: **inverted, oncocytic** (cylindrical or columnar cell), and **fungiform** (exophytic, septal) papilloma. Schneiderian papillomas represent less than 5% of sinonasal tract tumors.

INVERTED PAPILLOMA: This tumor involves the lateral nasal wall and may spread to the paranasal sinuses. Inverted papillomas occur mainly in middle-aged people. As the name implies, they show inversion of surface epithelium into underlying stroma (Fig. 21-12). HPV types 6 and 11 are often detected but are of uncertain significance. Although benign, these tumors may erode bone by pressure. Surgical resection must extend beyond the boundaries of grossly visible lesions, or they may recur. In 5% of cases, inverted papillomas give rise to SCC. Oncocytic, but not exophytic, papillomas have also been reported to give rise to malignant transformation.

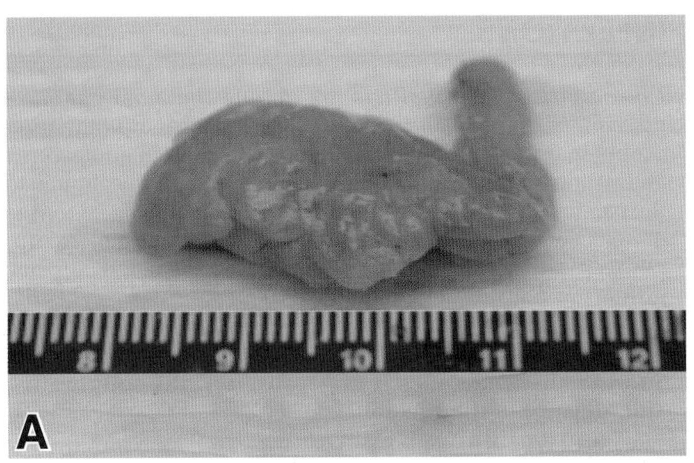

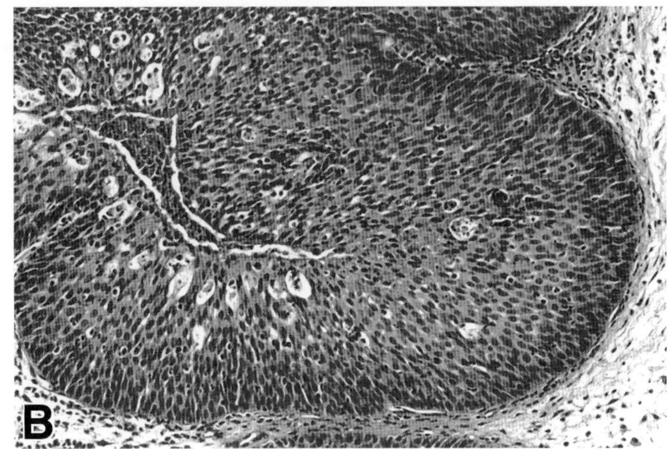

FIGURE 21-12. Sinonasal inverted papilloma. A. Gross photograph of sinonasal inverted papilloma. **B.** Epithelial nests are growing downward (inverted) into the submucosa. They involve uniform cellular proliferation, which displays an inflammatory cell infiltrate and scattered microcysts.

MALIGNANCIES OF THE NASAL CAVITY AND PARANASAL SINUSES

Squamous Cell Carcinoma

Over half of cancers of the nasal cavity and paranasal sinuses arise in the maxillary sinus antrum, one third in the nasal cavity, 10% in the ethmoid sinus, and 1% in sphenoid and frontal sinuses (Fig. 21-13). Most are keratinizing or nonkeratinizing SCCs. Some 15% are adenocarcinoma or undifferentiated carcinoma.

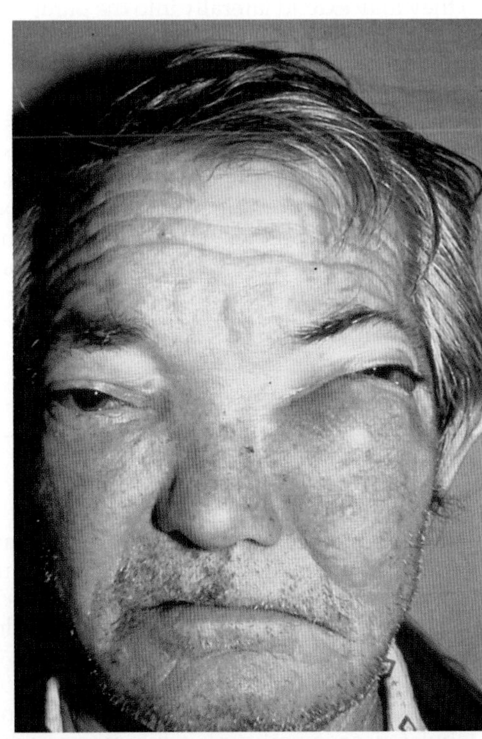

FIGURE 21-13. Squamous cell carcinoma of the maxillary sinus caused an obvious facial deformity, owing to invasion outside the confines of the sinus. Involvement of the orbit and facial nerve is evident. The latter is defined by drooping of the mouth to the side of the facial nerve paralysis.

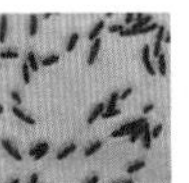

ETIOLOGIC FACTORS: Several industrial chemicals may cause cancer of the nose and sinuses, including nickel, chromium, and aromatic hydrocarbons. Occupational settings reportedly with an increased risk for cancer of the nose and sinuses (but for which a specific chemical agent is not identified) are woodworking in the furniture industry, use of cutting oils, and leather textile industries.

Nickel workers are prone to SCCs, mostly from the middle turbinate, with latencies from 2 to over 30 years. Most other occupational exposures lead mainly to adenocarcinomas and occur mostly in the maxillary and ethmoid sinuses. Because of these occupational risk factors, cancers of the nose and sinuses occur far more often in men and after age 50. These tumors grow relentlessly and invade adjacent structures, but typically do not metastasize. Survival is usually only a few years.

Nasal-Type Angiocentric NK/T-Cell Lymphoma

These tumors, once called **lethal midline granulomas** (also midline malignant reticulosis, and polymorphic reticulosis), are now recognized as malignant lymphomas.

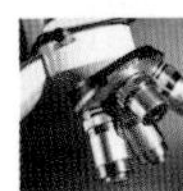

PATHOLOGY: The characteristic lymphoid infiltrate is necrotizing and polymorphic. Similar infiltrates may occur in the upper airways, lungs, and alimentary tract, but any organ can be involved. Tumor cells (1) surround small- to medium-sized blood vessels (angiocentric); (2) infiltrate through their walls (angioinvasion), often occluding vessel lumens like a thrombus; and (3) cause necrosis in adjacent tissues (ischemic type) (Fig. 21-14). ***EBV infection is associated with this type of lymphoma.***

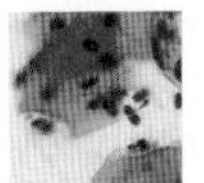

CLINICAL FEATURES: Nasal-type NK/T-cell lymphoma usually begins insidiously as nonspecific rhinitis or sinusitis. Gradually, the nasal mucosa is focally swollen, indurated, and eventually ulcerated. Ulcers are covered by a black crust, under which cartilage

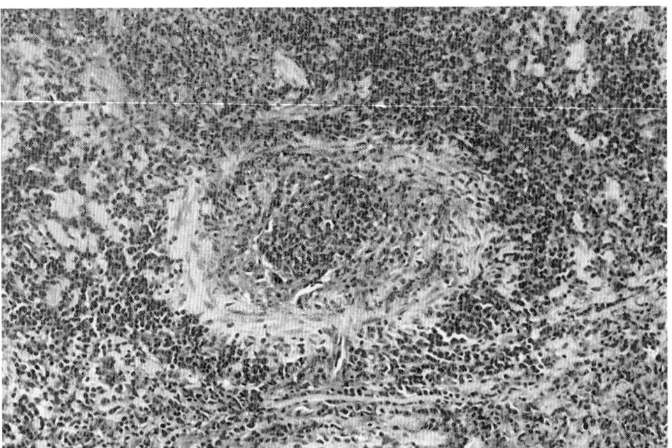

FIGURE 21-14. Angiocentric natural killer /T-cell lymphoma. A malignant cellular infiltrate growing around and into a medium-sized blood vessel with disruption of the external elastic membrane and occlusion of the vessel lumen.

and bone are eroded. The resulting defects of the nasal septum, hard palate, and nasopharynx have serious functional consequences. The skin of the midface is often involved. Half of patients have localized disease, but wide dissemination is common. Death is due to secondary bacterial infection, aspiration pneumonia, or hemorrhage from eroded large blood vessels. These lymphomas are, at least initially, radiosensitive, and remission with cytotoxic agents has also been reported.

Nasopharynx and Oropharynx

ANATOMY: The nasopharynx is continuous anteriorly with the nasal cavities; its roof is formed by the body of the sphenoid bone, and its posterior wall by the cervical vertebrae. Eustachian tube openings are on the lateral walls of the nasopharynx. In newborns, it is covered by pseudostratified, ciliated, columnar epithelium. With advancing age, the nasopharynx is replaced by a stratified squamous epithelium over large areas (80%). The mucosa has many mucous glands and abundant lymphoid tissue.

Waldeyer ring *is a circular band of lymphoid tissue where the oropharynx opens into the respiratory and digestive tracts.* Lymphoid tissue on the superior posterior wall forms the nasopharyngeal tonsils, which, when hyperplastic, are called **adenoids**. The palatine tonsils are lateral where the pharynx connects with the oral cavity. They are covered by stratified squamous epithelium, which lines infoldings (**tonsillar crypts**) into the lymphoid tissue. Crypts normally contain desquamated epithelium, lymphocytes, some neutrophils, and saprophytic organisms, such as bacteria, *Candida*, and actinomycetes. Pathogens (e.g., *Corynebacterium diphtheriae* and meningococcus) may also be seen in the pharynx of healthy people.

Waldeyer ring is well developed in children, and its follicles have germinal centers. In fact, the tonsils represent the largest collections of B lymphocytes in a normal child. Pharyngeal lymphoid tissue diminishes considerably by adulthood. It gradually involutes with age but does not totally disappear.

INFECTIONS

Pharyngitis and tonsillitis are among the most common diseases of the head and neck. Nasopharyngeal inflammation occurs mainly in children but is also common in adolescents and young adults. Viral or bacterial infections may be limited to the palatine tonsils or may also involve nasopharyngeal tonsils or adjacent pharyngeal mucosa, often as part of a general upper respiratory tract infection. Viruses are the usual culprits; influenza, parainfluenza, adenovirus, respiratory syncytial virus, and rhinovirus are spread by droplet or by direct contact.

S. pyogenes **is the most important cause of pharyngitis and tonsillitis, because it may cause serious suppurative and nonsuppurative sequelae.**

Acute tonsillitis is usually caused by *S. pyogenes* (group A β-hemolytic streptococci). In **follicular tonsillitis**, pinpoint exudates are extruded from the crypts.

In **pseudomembranous tonsillitis**, a necrotic mucosa is covered by a coat of exudate.

Recurrent or chronic tonsillitis is not as common as once believed, and enlarged tonsils in children do not necessarily signify chronic tonsillitis. However, repeated infections can cause tonsils and adenoids to enlarge and obstruct air passages. Repeated streptococcal tonsillitis may lead to rheumatic fever or glomerulonephritis in children, who may benefit from tonsillectomy.

Peritonsillar abscesses (quinsy) are collections of pus behind the posterior capsule of the tonsil, usually caused by α- and β-hemolytic streptococci. About one third of patients have histories of tonsillitis. Untreated, such abscesses may be life-threatening because (1) aided by gravity, they may dissect inferiorly to the pyriform sinus to obstruct, or rupture into, the airway; (2) they may extend laterally into the parapharyngeal space (parapharyngeal abscess) and weaken the carotid artery wall; or (3) they may penetrate along the carotid sheath inferiorly into the mediastinum or, superiorly, to the base of the skull or cranial cavity, with disastrous consequences.

Infectious mononucleosis often presents with exudative tonsillitis, pharyngitis, and posterior cervical lymphadenopathy. **Adenoids** represent chronic inflammatory hyperplasia of pharyngeal lymphoid tissue. This condition is often accompanied by chronic tonsillitis or rhinitis, almost always in children. Enlarged adenoids may partly or completely obstruct the eustachian tube, leading to otitis media.

NEOPLASMS

Nasopharyngeal Angiofibroma

These tumors, once called "juvenile nasopharyngeal angiofibromas," are uncommon, highly vascular neoplasms of the nasopharynx. They are histologically benign but locally aggressive. Although these tumors most often arise in adolescent males, they are not restricted to this age group.

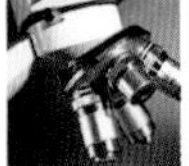

PATHOLOGY: Angiofibromas are multinodular, lobulated, or smooth pink–white masses, which may show surface ulceration and obvious blood vessels (Fig. 21-15A). They typically arise in the submucosa of the **posterolateral nasal wall** and tend to expand into adjacent structures, causing local mass effects. These tumors may grow into fissures and foramina of the skull or destroy

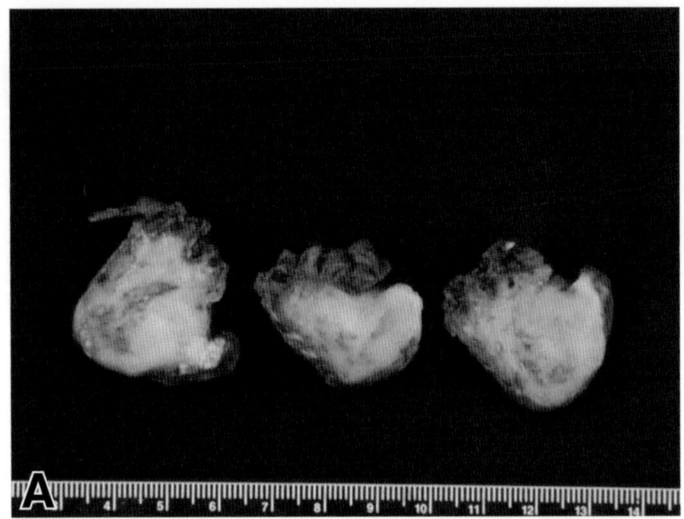

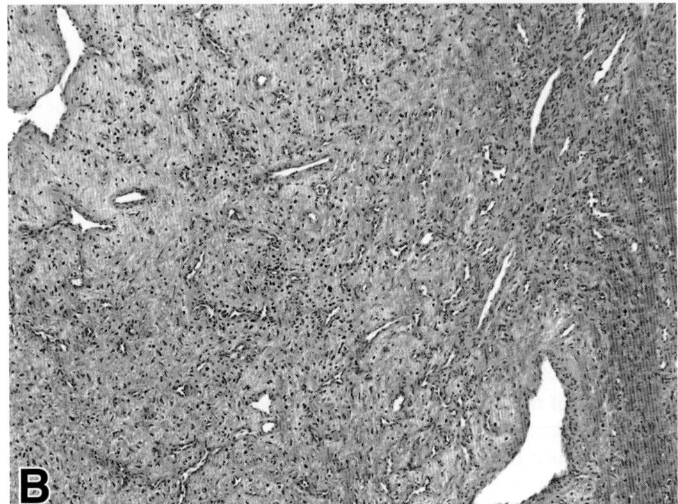

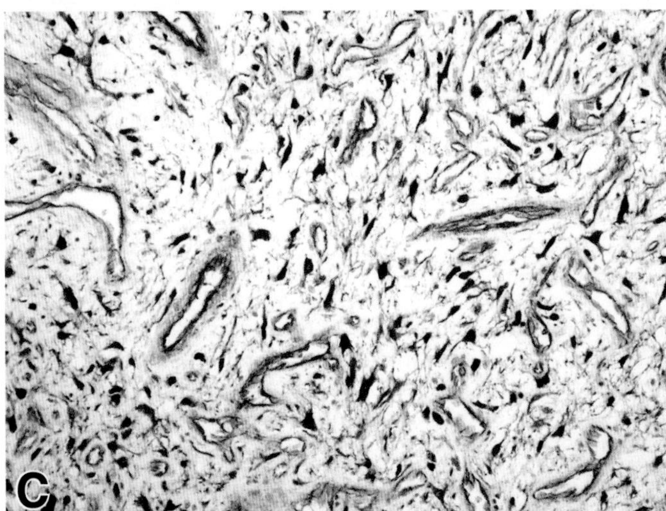

FIGURE 21-15. Nasopharyngeal angiofibroma. A. The cut surface of the tumor appears dense and spongy. **B.** Microscopically, it is composed of slit-like vascular structures in a collagenous stroma. **C.** Immunohistochemistry for β-catenin demonstrates aberrant nuclear labeling.

bone and spread into adjacent structures, such as the nasal cavity, paranasal sinuses, orbit, middle cranial fossa, or pterygomaxillary fossa.

Angiofibromas have vascular and stromal components (Fig. 21-15B). Blood vessels vary in size and shape; the smooth muscle in their walls is not layered, but rather arranged irregularly. Stromal fibroblasts express aberrant nuclear β-catenin (Fig. 21-15C).

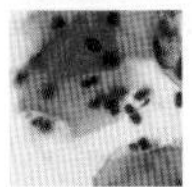

CLINICAL FEATURES: Many angiofibromas regress spontaneously after puberty. They respond to estrogen therapy, and may therefore be hormonally regulated and androgen dependent. Vessel wall defects preclude vasoconstriction, leading to brisk bleeding after trauma. Biopsies may thus be dangerous and are contraindicated. Radiation therapy is also effective. Preoperative embolization is often used to reduce vascularity prior to surgery. There is a familial tendency for these tumors; they occur 25 times more often in patients with familial adenomatous polyposis syndrome.

Oropharyngeal Squamous Cell Carcinoma

In the United States, 80% of oropharyngeal SCCs are associated with high-risk HPV serotypes. These cancers, called HPV-associated head and neck SCCs (HPV-HNSCCs), arise mainly from palatine and lingual tonsils and are nonkeratinizing tumors of the basaloid cell type (Fig. 21-16A). Such tumors may be small and difficult to detect and often present as metastatic cancer in a cervical lymph node.

HPV-associated tumors tend to occur in younger people without the risk factors for HNSCC (i.e., smoking, alcohol) as often seen in older patients. HPV-HNSCCs also are radiosensitive and have a better overall prognosis than do HPV-negative SCCs (Fig. 21-16B and C).

Nasopharyngeal Carcinoma

NPC is divided into keratinizing and nonkeratinizing types. The latter are associated with EBV infection and may be differentiated or undifferentiated.

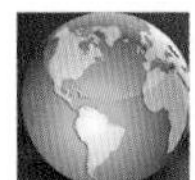

EPIDEMIOLOGY: ***Undifferentiated nonkeratinizing carcinomas are particularly common in southeast Asia and parts of Africa.*** By far the most common cancer of the nasopharynx, NPC is the most common of all cancers in China. In Hong Kong, it represents 18% of all malignancies, compared with 0.25% worldwide. Chinese born in the United States have a 20-fold greater mortality from this tumor than do other ethnicities.

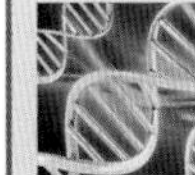

MOLECULAR PATHOGENESIS: Environmental risk factors for NPC have remained elusive. The A2/sin HLA profile is more common in Chinese patients, suggesting a genetic susceptibility. Frequent deletions in several chromosomes, in particular 3p, 9p, and 14q, occur in NPCs.

Some 85% of patients with NPC have antibodies to EBV. The viral genomes are detected in 75% to 100% of nonkeratinizing and undifferentiated types of NPC. EBV is more variable in keratinizing NPCs.

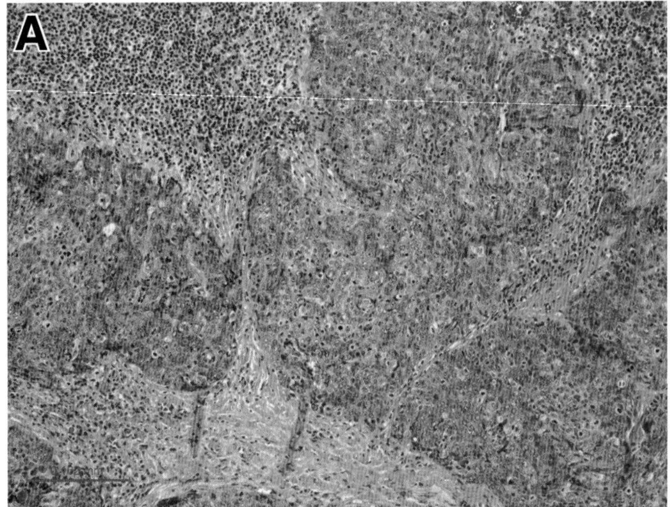

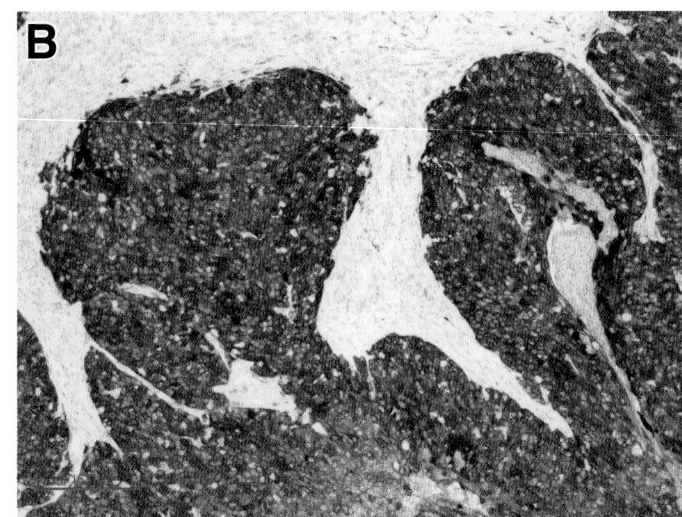

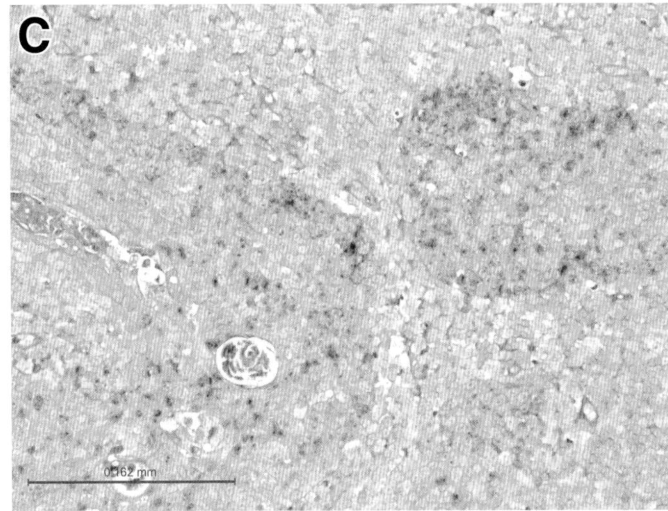

FIGURE 21-16. Human papillomavirus (HPV)–associated squamous cell carcinoma of the tonsil. A. Nests of invasive carcinoma are positive for p16 immunohistochemistry **(B)**. **C.** In situ hybridization for high-risk HPV (including types 16 and 18) demonstrates nuclear localization (blue dots).

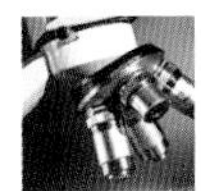

PATHOLOGY: Differentiated nonkeratinizing NPCs have a stratified appearance and distinct cell margins. By contrast, in undifferentiated tumors, clusters of poorly delimited or syncytial cells exhibit large oval nuclei and scant eosinophilic cytoplasm (Fig. 21-17A). Lymphoid infiltrates may be prominent in undifferentiated tumors. Both subtypes express cytokeratin (Fig. 21-17B), but not hematologic or lymphoid markers. In situ hybridization studies usually identify EBV DNA (Fig. 21-17C).

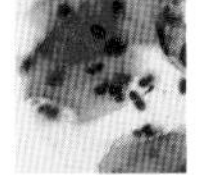

CLINICAL FEATURES: Owing to their location, most NPCs are asymptomatic for a long time, and in half of patients they first present as palpable cervical lymph node metastases. Even then, many patients still have no complaints referable to the nasopharynx. Tumors invade nearby regions, such as the parapharyngeal space, orbit, and cranial cavity, causing neurologic symptoms and hearing disturbances. Invasion of the base of the skull leads to cranial nerve involvement. Tumors in the fossa of Rosenmüller and the lateral wall of the nasopharynx cause symptoms referable to the middle ear. Eustachian tube obstruction is common. The abundant local lymphatic network gives rise to frequent and early metastases to cervical lymph nodes.

Undifferentiated NPC is radiosensitive, and most patients with tumors restricted to the nasopharynx survive 5 years or more. Cranial nerve involvement or metastases to cervical lymph nodes or beyond portend poor survival.

Lymphoma

Lymphomas account for 5% of head and neck cancers. The Waldeyer ring is by far the most common site of origin of lymphoma in this region. These lymphomas are histologically diffuse (90%), and over half are large cell lymphomas. The vast majority are of B-cell origin.

Other Malignancies

Tumors may derive from various components of mucosa or adjacent supportive soft tissues and skeleton. **Embryonal rhabdomyosarcomas** are highly malignant tumors of pharyngeal tissues of young children. They invade contiguous structures and metastasize via the bloodstream and lymphatics. Nasopharyngeal **Kaposi sarcomas** may occur in patients with AIDS, in association with HHV8.

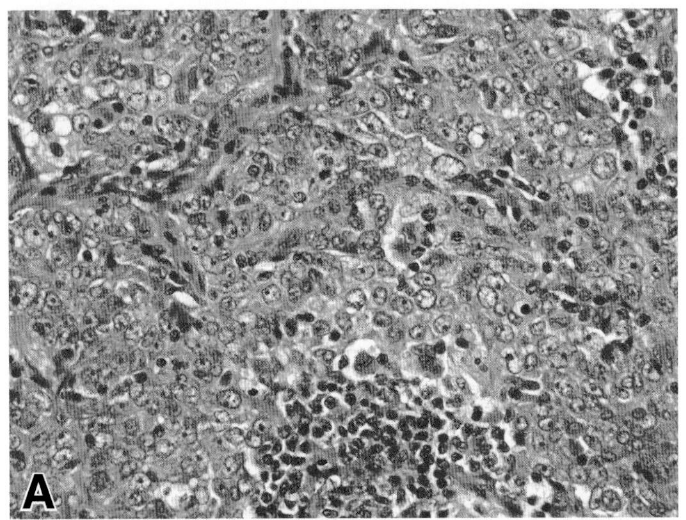

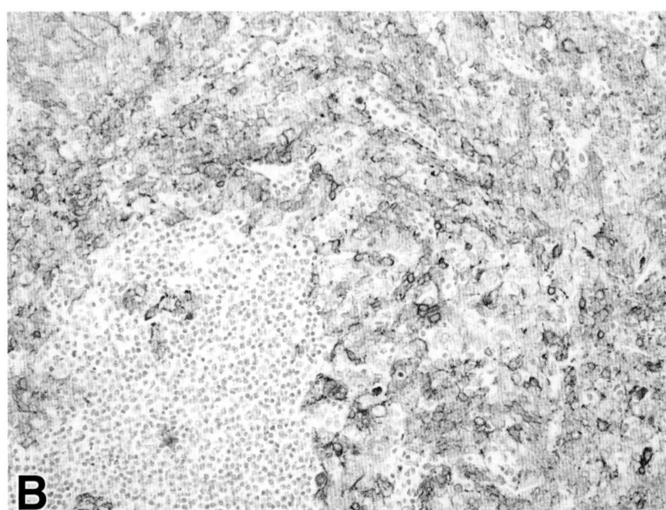

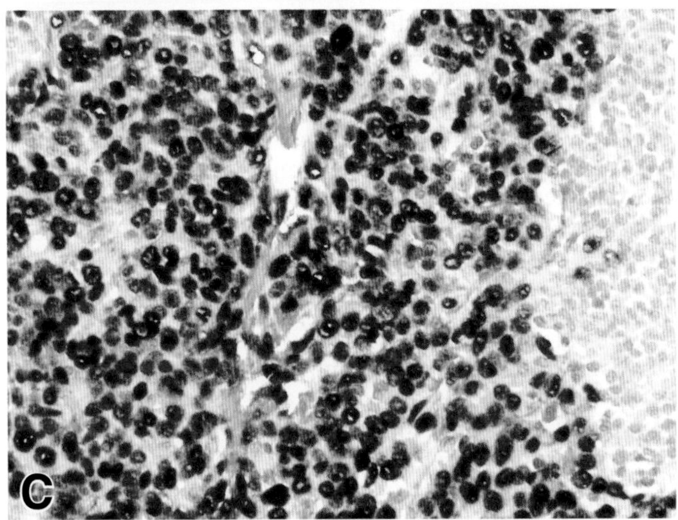

FIGURE 21-17. Nasopharyngeal nonkeratinizing carcinoma, undifferentiated type. A. The cells have large nuclei and prominent eosinophilic nucleoli. **B.** The cells are cytokeratin positive (by immunohistochemistry), indicating an epithelial cell proliferation. **C.** In situ hybridization for Epstein–Barr virus.

Larynx and Hypopharynx

INFECTIONS

EPIGLOTTITIS: Inflammation of the epiglottis is most commonly caused by *H. influenzae* type B. It occurs in infants and young children and may be a life-threatening emergency. ***Swelling of an acutely inflamed epiglottis may obstruct airflow. Inspiratory stridor (loud wheezing on inspiration) and the onset of cyanosis may indicate airway obstruction so severe as to require tracheostomy.***

CROUP: Croup is a laryngotracheobronchitis of young children who have symptoms of inspiratory stridor, cough, and hoarseness, owing to varying degrees of laryngeal obstruction. It is a complication of an upper respiratory infection, with marked laryngeal edema and a "barking cough." This was once a deadly complication of diphtheria. However, today, it is most commonly caused by the parainfluenza viruses.

VOCAL CORD NODULE AND POLYP

Also called *singer's nodules,* these tumors are stromal reactions related to inflammation and/or trauma. They may be seen in all age groups but are most common between the third and sixth decades (Fig. 21-18). Symptoms related to vocal cord

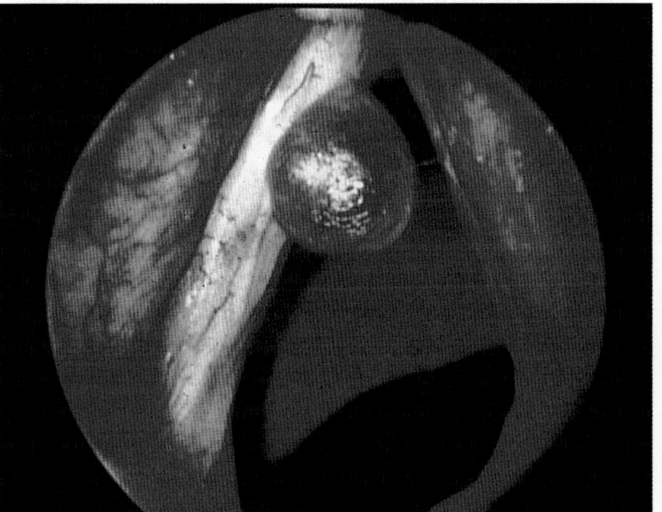

FIGURE 21-18. Vocal cord polyp. A solitary polypoid lesion with a glistening appearance is seen arising from the true vocal cord.

polyps and nodules are similar: hoarseness or voice changes ("cracking" of the voice). Lesions occur after voice abuse, infection (laryngitis), excessive alcohol consumption, smoking or endocrine dysfunction (e.g., hypothyroidism). Histologies vary from a myxoid, edematous, fibroblastic stroma in early stages to a hyalinized, densely fibrotic stroma later.

NEOPLASMS OF THE LARYNX

SQUAMOUS PAPILLOMA AND PAPILLOMATOSIS: These papillomas are solitary or multiple growths of the squamous cells that line the surface of fibrovascular cores. They may be multiple in children or adolescents (**juvenile laryngeal papillomatosis**) and may extend into the trachea and bronchi. HPV, especially serotypes 6 and 11, are the main causes. The condition may result in life-threatening respiratory obstruction and, rarely, evolve into overt SCC, particularly in smokers or after radiation therapy. Surgical excision may not be curative, as the viral infection is often widespread, and these tumors tend to recur over many years. Solitary laryngeal squamous papilloma occurs in adults, mostly men, and is usually cured surgically.

SQUAMOUS CELL CARCINOMA: Almost all laryngeal cancers are SCCs, predominantly in men, most of whom smoke cigarettes. HPV is found in a quarter of cases.

CHONDROSARCOMA: Chondrosarcomas account for 75% of nonepithelial laryngeal malignancies. In the larynx, they grow as exophytic, polypoid masses and can cause airway obstruction. Most patients are men in their 70s. It also occurs in the nasopharynx, mandible, maxilla, and nasal and paranasal sinuses. Patients present with hoarseness, airway obstruction, and dyspnea.

Salivary Glands

The salivary glands, which develop as buds of oral ectoderm, are tubuloalveolar structures that secrete saliva. Major salivary glands are paired organs. Parotid glands secrete serous saliva, and submandibular and sublingual glands make mixed serous and mucous saliva. Minor salivary glands are widespread under the mucosa of the lips, cheeks, palate, and tongue.

XEROSTOMIA: Xerostomia is chronic mouth dryness caused by lack of saliva and has many causes. Diseases that involve major salivary glands and lead to xerostomia include mumps, Sjögren syndrome, sarcoidosis, radiation-induced atrophy, and drug sensitivity (e.g., antihistamines, tricyclic antidepressants, and phenothiazines).

SIALORRHEA: Increased salivary flow is associated with many conditions, including acute inflammation of the oral cavity (e.g., as in aphthous stomatitis), Parkinson disease, rabies, mental retardation, nausea, and pregnancy.

ENLARGEMENT: Unilateral enlargement of major salivary glands is usually caused by cysts, inflammation, or neoplasms. Bilateral enlargement is due to inflammation (mumps, Sjögren syndrome; see below), granulomatous disease (sarcoidosis), or diffuse neoplastic involvement (leukemia or lymphoma).

SIALOLITHIASIS: Calcific stones in salivary gland ducts occur mostly in the submandibular gland. They obstruct ducts and lead to inflammation.

PAROTITIS: Bacteria (usually *S. aureus*) may ascend from the oral cavity when salivary flow is reduced and cause acute suppurative parotitis. It is most often seen in debilitated or postoperative patients. Salivary duct stricture or obstruction by stones may cause acute or chronic parotitis. Stagnant secretions serve as a medium for retrograde bacterial invasion.

Epidemic parotitis (mumps) is an acute viral disease of the parotid glands that spreads via infected saliva. Submandibular and sublingual glands also may be affected. Involved glands have dense lymphocytic and macrophage infiltrates, epithelial degeneration, and necrosis.

SJÖGREN SYNDROME

The disease may be limited to these sites, or it may be associated with a systemic autoimmune disease (see Chapter 3). In the salivary glands, it gives rise to xerostomia. Involvement of the lacrimal glands results in dry eyes (**keratoconjunctivitis sicca**). The pathogenesis and clinical features of Sjögren syndrome are discussed in Chapter 3.

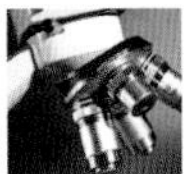

PATHOLOGY: In Sjögren syndrome, parotid glands, and sometimes submandibular glands, are enlarged unilaterally or bilaterally, but their lobulation is preserved. Initial periductal chronic inflammation gradually extends into the acini, until the glands are completely replaced by a sea of polyclonal lymphocytes, immunoblasts, germinal centers, and plasma cells. Proliferating myoepithelial cells surround remnants of damaged ducts and form so-called epimyoepithelial islands (**lymphoepithelial sialadenitis**; Fig. 21-19). Similar changes occur in the lacrimal glands and minor salivary glands. Focal lymphocytic sialadenitis is also present in minor salivary glands. Late in the course of the disease, affected glands become atrophic, with fibrosis and fatty infiltration of the parenchyma. Lymphocytes in Sjögren syndrome may show restricted immunoglobulin types but generally remain localized.

BENIGN SALIVARY GLAND NEOPLASMS

Pleomorphic Adenoma

These neoplasms, also called **mixed tumors**, are benign proliferations with admixed epithelial and stromal elements.

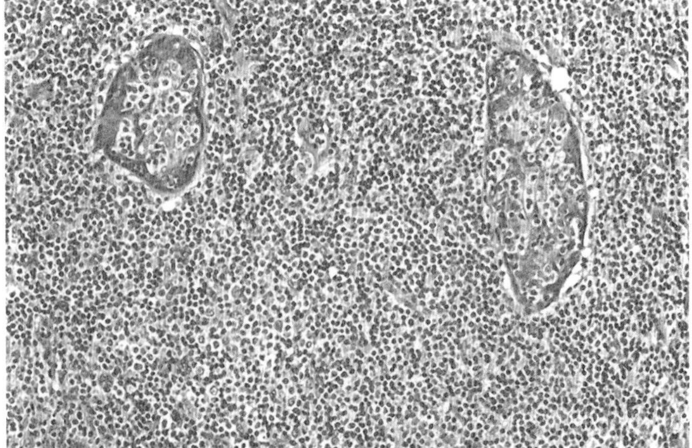

FIGURE 21-19. Sjögren syndrome. There is infiltration of the involved salivary gland by a mixed chronic inflammatory cell infiltrate. Extension of the infiltrate into epithelial (ductal) structures results in metaplasia and characteristic epimyoepithelial islands.

Two thirds of major salivary gland tumors, and about half of those in the minor glands, are pleomorphic adenomas. These tumors occur nine times more often in the parotid than in the submandibular gland and usually arise in the superficial lobe of the former. Middle-aged people and women are most affected.

MOLECULAR PATHOGENESIS: In most of these tumors, PLAG1 (pleomorphic adenoma gene 1), which encodes a zinc finger protein, is activated by reciprocal chromosomal translocations involving 8q12. Carcinomas that develop from pleomorphic adenomas may have 8q12 rearrangements, alterations in 12q13-15, and mutations in *HMGIC* and *MDM2* genes.

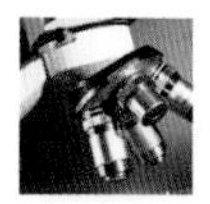

PATHOLOGY: Pleomorphic adenomas are slowly growing, painless, movable, firm masses with smooth surfaces. Those arising deep in the parotid may grow into the parapharyngeal space and appear as swellings of the lateral pharyngeal or tonsillar regions. These tumors show epithelial tissue mingled with myxoid, mucoid, or chondroid areas (Fig. 21-20A). The neoplasm is considered to be of epithelial origin.

The epithelial component consists of myoepithelial and ductal cells. The cells that line the ducts form tubules or small cystic structures and contain clear fluid or eosinophilic, PAS-positive material. Around ductal epithelial cells are smaller myoepithelial cells, which are the main cellular component. These cells form well-defined sheaths, cords, or nests and are often separated by a cellular ground substance that resembles cartilaginous, myxoid, or mucoid material.

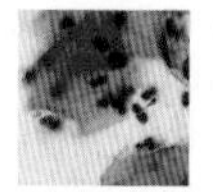

CLINICAL FEATURES: Pleomorphic adenomas have fibrous capsules. As they grow, surrounding fibrous tissue condenses around them. The tumors expand and often protrude focally into adjacent tissues, becoming nodular and occasionally forming "podocytes" (Fig. 21-20B). Recurrences usually represent local regrowth, not malignancy. Definitive surgery may necessitate sacrificing the facial nerve.

On rare occasions, carcinomas may arise in pleomorphic adenomas (**carcinoma ex pleomorphic adenoma**). In such cases, the tumor that was present for many years then begins to grow rapidly or becomes painful. Such carcinomas are most frequently high-grade malignancies set in otherwise benign pleomorphic adenomas.

Monomorphic Adenoma

In monomorphic adenomas, the epithelium is arranged in a regular, usually glandular, pattern with no mesenchymal component.

Warthin Tumor (Papillary Cystadenoma Lymphomatosum)

Warthin tumors are the most common monomorphic adenomas. They are benign parotid gland neoplasms composed of cystic glandular spaces within dense lymphoid tissue. Clearly benign, they are bilateral (15% of cases) or multifocal within one gland. These are the only salivary gland tumors that are more common in men than in women. They generally occur after age 30, and most arise after age 50.

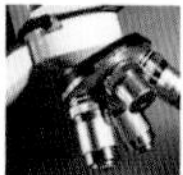

PATHOLOGY: Warthin tumors have glandular spaces that tend to become cystic, with papillary projections. The cysts are lined by eosinophilic epithelial cells (oncocytes), surrounded by dense lymphoid tissue with germinal centers (Fig. 21-21).

The histogenesis of this tumor is uncertain. Lymph nodes are normally found in the parotid gland and its immediate vicinity and usually contain a few ducts or small islands of salivary gland tissue. Warthin tumors may arise from proliferation of these salivary gland inclusions.

MALIGNANT SALIVARY GLAND TUMORS

Salivary gland tumors account for 5% of all head and neck cancers. Most (75%) arise in the parotid glands, 10% in the submandibular glands, and 15% in the minor salivary glands

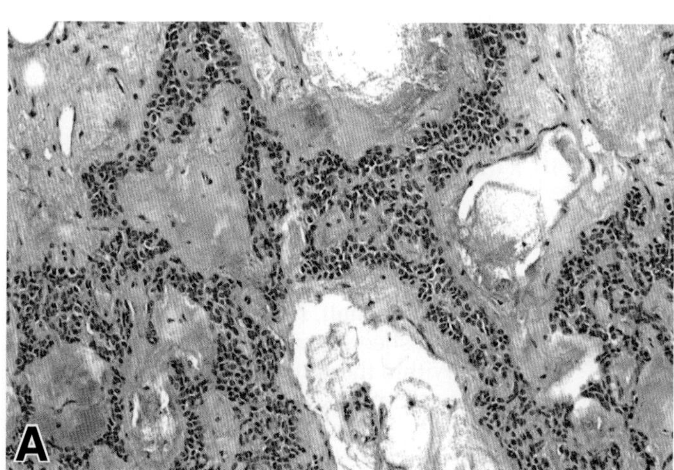

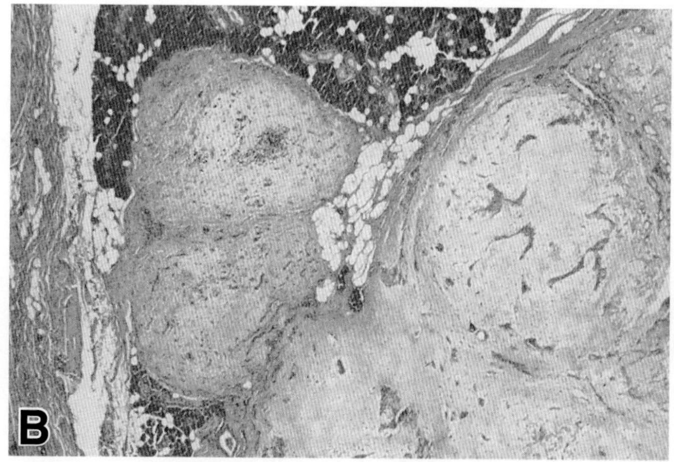

FIGURE 21-20. Pleomorphic adenoma of the parotid gland. A. Cellular components of pleomorphic adenomas include an admixture of glands and myoepithelial cells within a chondromyxoid stroma. **B.** The tumor contains characteristic myxoid and chondroid portions. The tumor is partly encapsulated, but a nodule protruding into the parotid gland lacks a capsule. If such nodules are not included in the resection, the tumor will recur.

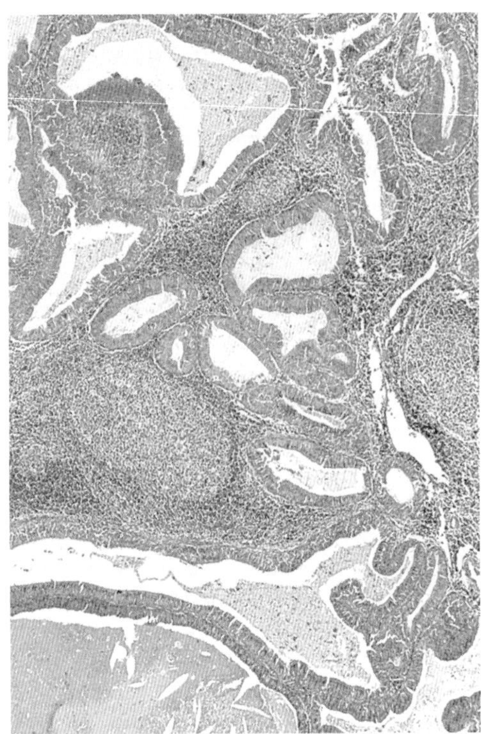

FIGURE 21-21. Warthin tumor. Cystic spaces and duct-like structures are lined by oncocytes. Follicular lymphoid tissue is present.

of the upper aerodigestive tract. Malignancies of the sublingual glands are rare.

Mucoepidermoid Carcinoma

MECs derive from ductal epithelium, which has a great potential for metaplasia. They account for 5% to 10% of major salivary gland tumors and 10% of tumors in minor salivary glands. Over half of MECs in the major glands arise in the parotid. Among minor salivary glands, they develop mostly in the palate. Most MECs present in adult women but may occur in adolescents.

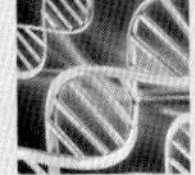

MOLECULAR PATHOGENESIS: Over 60% of MECs are characterized by a t(11;19)(q21-22;p13) translocation. This recombination generates a fusion gene (**MECT1–MAML2** fusion) that disrupts NOTCH signaling (Fig. 21-22).

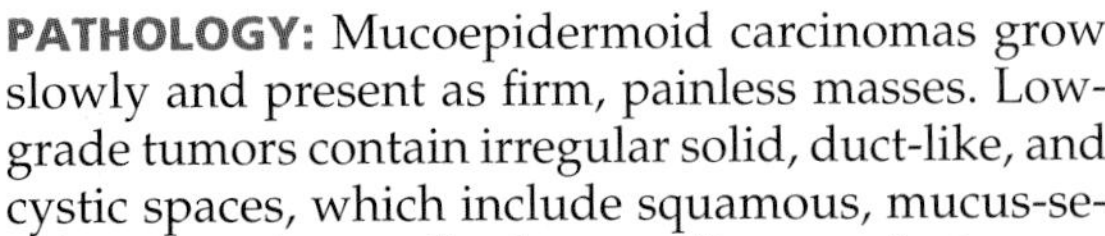

PATHOLOGY: Mucoepidermoid carcinomas grow slowly and present as firm, painless masses. Low-grade tumors contain irregular solid, duct-like, and cystic spaces, which include squamous, mucus-secreting, and intermediate cells. Intermediate-grade tumors tend to grow in more solid patterns, with more epidermoid and intermediate cells and fewer mucus-secreting cells. High-grade MECs are very pleomorphic, with minimal differentiation, save for scattered glandular cells.

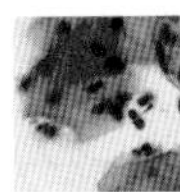

CLINICAL FEATURES: Even low-grade mucoepidermoid carcinomas may metastasize, but over 90% of patients survive 5 years, regardless of the primary

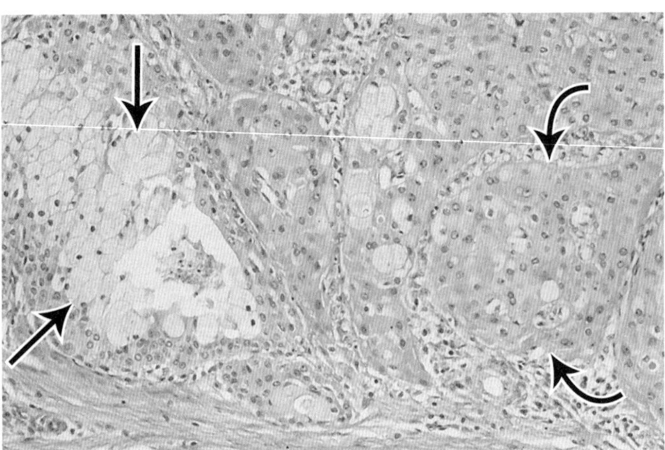

FIGURE 21-22. Mucoepidermoid carcinoma is characterized by an admixture of mucocytes (*straight arrows*), epidermoid cells (*curved arrows*) and intermediate cells. The mucocytes are clustered and have a clear cytoplasm with eccentrically situated nuclei. Epidermoid cells are squamous-like cells but lack keratinization and intercellular bridges. Intermediate cells (best seen at lower left) are smaller than epidermoid cells.

site. Survival with high-grade tumors is much worse (20% to 40%). Treatment is dictated by grade; low-grade tumors are treated surgically, but high-grade ones require both surgery and radiation therapy.

Adenoid Cystic Carcinoma

ACCs tend to grow slowly. One third of these tumors arise in the major salivary glands, and two thirds in the minor ones. They represent 5% of major salivary gland tumors and 20% of those of the minor salivary glands. ACCs may occur not only in the oral cavity but also in the lacrimal glands, nasopharynx, nasal cavity, paranasal sinuses, and lower respiratory tract. They are most common in people 40 to 60 years old.

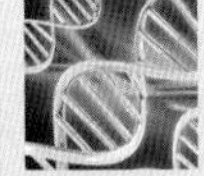

MOLECULAR PATHOGENESIS: ACCs consistently demonstrate t(6;9) translocations and chromosome 6 deletions. The translocation t(6;9)(q22-23;p23-24) results in a novel fusion of the MYB proto-oncogene with NFIB, a transcription factor.

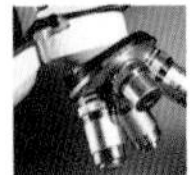

PATHOLOGY: ACCs show variable histology. The tumor cells are small, have scant cytoplasm, and grow in solid sheets or as small groups, strands, or columns. Within these structures, tumor cells interconnect to enclose cystic spaces, resulting in solid, tubular, or cribriform (sieve-like) patterns (Fig. 21-23). Grading ACCs depends on the proportions of tubular and cribriform patterns, with over 30% solid growth defining "high grade." Such high-grade tumors have a 5-year survival rate of about 15%. Tumor cells produce a homogeneous basement membrane material that gives them the characteristic "cylindromatous" appearance.

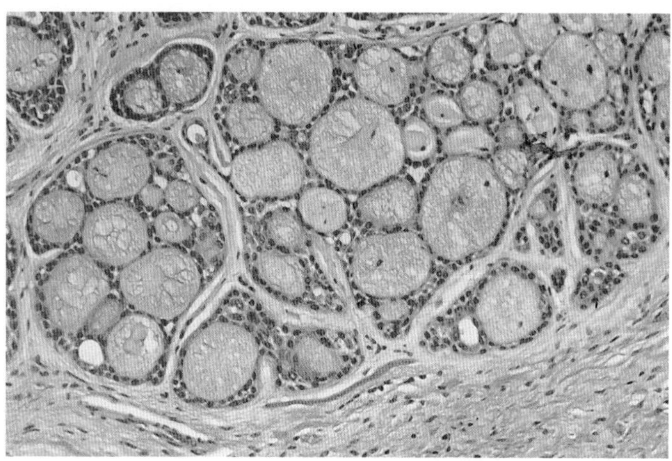

FIGURE 21-23. Adenoid cystic carcinoma showing cribriform growth in which cyst-like spaces are filled with basophilic material. The cyst spaces are really pseudocysts surrounded by myoepithelial cells.

ACCs probably arise from cells that differentiate toward intercalated ducts and myoepithelium. ***They tend to infiltrate perineural spaces and are thus often painful.*** Most do not metastasize for years, but they are often diagnosed late, are difficult to eradicate completely, and have a poor long-term prognosis.

Acinic Cell Adenocarcinoma

These uncommon parotid tumors (10% of salivary gland tumors) arise occasionally in other salivary glands. They occur mainly in young men aged 20 to 30 years. Acinic cell carcinomas are encapsulated, round masses, usually under 3 cm, and may be cystic. They are composed of uniform cells with a small central nucleus and abundant basophilic cytoplasm, similar to the secretory (acinic) cells of normal salivary glands (Fig. 21-24). They may spread to regional lymph nodes. Most (90%) patients survive 5 years with surgery, but one third experience local recurrences. Only half survive for 20 years.

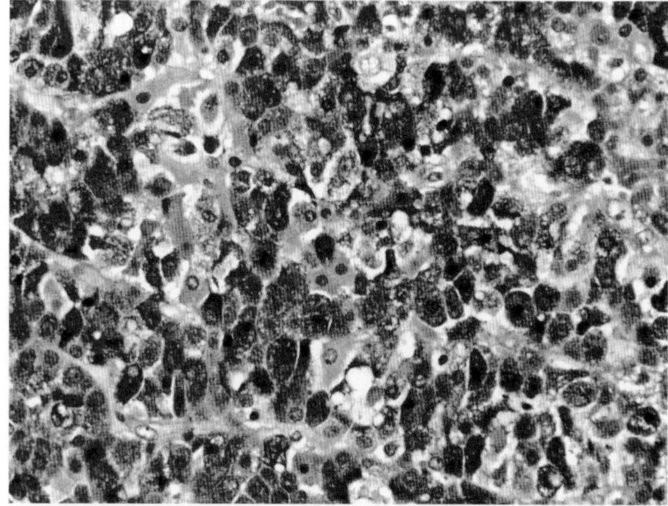

FIGURE 21-24. Acinic cell adenocarcinoma. This tumor demonstrates a solid growth pattern and is composed of basophilic cells with abundant cytoplasm filled with zymogen granules.

The Ear

EXTERNAL EAR

ANATOMY: The outer portion of the external ear includes the auricle or pinna, leading into the external auditory canal. The external auditory canal or meatus extends from the concha medially to the tympanic membrane (eardrum). Its lateral wall is cartilage and connective tissue, and its medial wall is bone. The eardrum sits obliquely at the end of the external auditory canal, separating the external ear and the middle ear.

The outer third of the external auditory canal has ceruminous glands, which produce cerumen. The inner portion of the external auditory canal has no adnexae. The eardrum is airtight. Its outer surface is squamous epithelium, continuous with the skin of the external ear canal. Its inner surface is lined by cuboidal epithelium. Between these two is a middle layer of dense fibrous tissue.

KELOIDS: Keloids are very common on the ear lobes after piercing for earrings or other trauma (see Chapter 2). They are much more common in blacks and Asians than in whites. Keloids can attain considerable size and tend to recur. They are composed of thick, hyalinized bundles of collagen in the deep dermis.

AURAL POLYPS: These benign inflammatory lesions arise in the external ear canal or extrude into the canal from the middle ear. Aural polyps are ulcerated, inflamed granulation tissue, which bleeds readily. Those arising in the middle ear result from chronic otitis media.

NEOPLASMS: Ceruminal gland tumors are unique to this area. Benign tumors include ceruminal gland adenomas and salivary gland-type tumors (e.g., pleomorphic and monomorphic adenomas). Malignant tumors include adenocarcinoma and malignant salivary gland-type tumors (e.g., adenoid cystic and mucoepidermoid carcinomas).

MIDDLE EAR

ANATOMY: The middle ear, or tympanic cavity, is an oblong space in the temporal bone lined by a mucous membrane. Together with the mastoid air sinuses, it forms a closed mucosal compartment, also called the **middle ear cleft**. Most of its lateral wall is the tympanic membrane. Anteriorly, the eustachian tube connects the middle ear to the nasopharynx. This air passage allows air pressure on both sides of the tympanic membrane to equalize. The three auditory ossicles—the malleus, incus, and stapes—are a chain that connects the tympanic membrane with the oval window located at the medial wall of the tympanic cavity. They conduct sound across the middle ear. Free motion of the ossicles, mainly the stapes in the oval window, is more important for hearing than is an intact tympanic membrane. The middle ear opens posteriorly into the mastoid antrum, a honeycomb of small, aerated, bony compartments (air cells) lined by a thin mucous membrane that is continuous with that of the middle ear.

Otitis Media

Otitis media refers to inflammation of the middle ear. It usually results from upper respiratory tract infections that spread from the nasopharynx. Obstruction of the eustachian tube is important in the production of middle ear effusions. When the pharyngeal end of the eustachian tube is swollen, air cannot enter the tube. Air in the middle ear is absorbed through the mucosa, and negative pressure causes transudation of plasma and occasional bleeding. Antibiotics usually cure or suppress the condition.

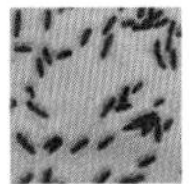

ETIOLOGIC FACTORS: Acute otitis media may be caused by viral or bacterial infection or sterile obstruction of the eustachian tube. Viral otitis media may resolve without suppuration or lead to secondary invasion by pus-forming bacteria. Microorganisms ascend from the nasopharynx and pass through the eustachian tube to the middle ear. Otitis media almost invariably penetrates through the mastoid antrum into the mastoid cells.

ACUTE SEROUS OTITIS MEDIA: Obstruction of the eustachian tube may result from sudden changes in atmospheric pressure (e.g., flying in an aircraft or deep-sea diving). This effect is particularly severe if there is an upper respiratory tract infection, acute allergic reaction or infection at the eustachian tube orifice. Inflammation may also occur without bacterial invasion of the middle ear. Over half of the children in the United States have at least one bout of serous otitis media before their third birthday. Repeated otitis media in early childhood often leads to residual (usually sterile) fluid in the middle ear, which contributes to unsuspected hearing loss.

CHRONIC SEROUS OTITIS MEDIA: The same conditions that cause acute obstruction of the eustachian tube also cause recurrent or chronic middle ear serous effusions. Carcinoma of the nasopharynx may cause chronic serous otitis media in adults and should be suspected in the presence of a unilateral middle ear effusion.

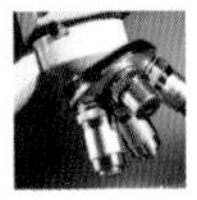

PATHOLOGY: In chronic serous otitis media, mucus-producing (goblet) cell metaplasia may be seen in the mucosal lining of the middle ear. Hemorrhage (e.g., in the mastoid cells) may accompany acute obstruction. Extravasation of blood and degradation of erythrocytes liberate cholesterol. Cholesterol crystals stimulate a foreign body response and granulation tissue, called a **cholesterol granuloma**. If large, these granulomas may destroy tissue in the mastoid or antrum. If they are allowed to persist for many months, the granulation tissue becomes fibrotic, which eventually obliterates middle ear and mastoid.

ACUTE SUPPURATIVE OTITIS MEDIA: One of the most common infections of childhood, acute suppurative otitis media, is caused by pyogenic bacteria that invade the middle ear, usually via the eustachian tube. The most common culprit in all age groups (30% to 40%) is *S. pneumoniae* (pneumococcus). *H. influenzae* is the cause in about 20% of cases, but occurs less often with increasing age. An accumulating purulent exudate in the middle ear may rupture the eardrum, causing a purulent discharge. In most cases, infection is self-limited and heals even without therapy.

ACUTE MASTOIDITIS: Infection of the mastoid bone was once a common complication of acute otitis media before the advent of antibiotics. It is still seen, rarely, if otitis media is not treated adequately. Mastoid air cells are filled with pus, and their thin osseous intercellular walls are destroyed. If the infection spreads to contiguous structures, serious complications may ensue.

CHRONIC SUPPURATIVE OTITIS MEDIA AND MASTOIDITIS: Neglected or recurrent middle ear and mastoid infections give rise to chronic inflammation of the mucosa or destruction of the periosteum of the ossicles (Fig. 21-25). Chronic otitis media occurs much more commonly in people who have had ear disease in early childhood, which may have arrested normal development of air cells in the mastoid.

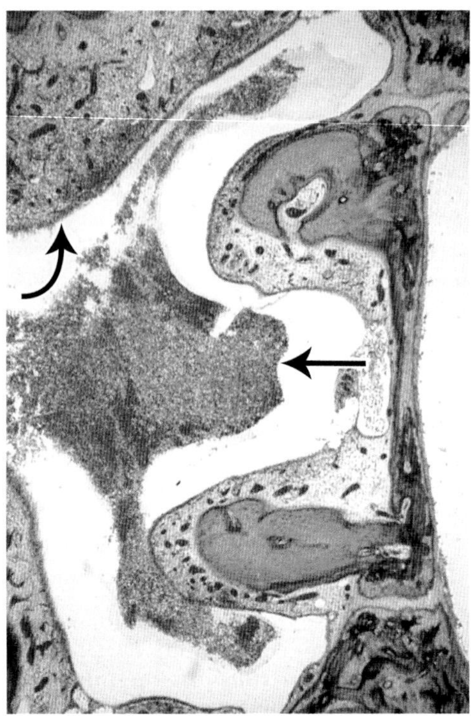

FIGURE 21-25. Chronic suppurative otitis media. A purulent exudate (*straight arrow*) is present in the middle ear cavity. The entire mucosa (*curved arrow*) is thickened by chronic inflammation and granulation tissue. The footplate and the crura of the stapes are at right.

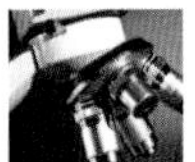

PATHOLOGY: Inflammation tends to be insidious, persistent, and destructive. In chronic otitis media, by definition, the eardrum is always perforated. Painless discharge (**otorrhea**) and variable hearing loss are constant symptoms. Exuberant granulation tissue may form polyps, which can extend through the perforated eardrum into the external ear canal.

A **cholesteatoma** is a mass of accumulated keratin and squamous mucosa produced by growth of squamous epithelium from the external ear canal through a perforated eardrum into the middle ear. In that location, it continues to produce keratin. Cholesteatomas are identical to epidermal inclusion cysts and are surrounded by granulation tissue and fibrosis. The keratin mass often becomes infected and protects bacteria from antibiotics. The main dangers of cholesteatoma arise from bony erosion, which may destroy important contiguous structures (e.g., auditory ossicles, facial nerve, and labyrinth).

COMPLICATIONS OF ACUTE AND CHRONIC OTITIS MEDIA: Antibiotic therapy has, fortunately, made complications of otitis media uncommon. However, suppurative middle ear infections may still cause these serious complications:

- Destruction of the facial nerve
- Deep cervical or subperiosteal abscess, if cortical bone of the mastoid process is eroded

- Petrositis, when infection spreads to the petrous temporal bone through the chain of air cells
- Suppurative labyrinthitis, owing to infection of the internal ear
- Epidural, subdural, or cerebral abscess, when infection extends through the inner table of the mastoid bone
- Meningitis, when infection reaches the meninges
- Sigmoid sinus thrombophlebitis, if infection traverses the dura to the posterior cranial fossa

Jugulotympanic Paraganglioma

Jugulotympanic paragangliomas are the most common benign tumors of the middle ear. They grow slowly but, over years, may destroy the middle ear and extend into the internal ear and cranial cavity. Metastases are rare.

Middle ear paragangliomas resemble those arising elsewhere, with characteristic lobules of cells in richly vascular connective tissue (Fig. 21-26). Paraganglial cells are of neural crest origin and contain varying amounts of catecholamines, mostly epinephrine and norepinephrine.

INTERNAL EAR

ANATOMY: The petrous portion of the temporal bone contains the labyrinth, which shelters the end organs for hearing (**cochlea**) and equilibrium (**vestibular labyrinth**). The complex cavities of the osseous labyrinth contain the **membranous labyrinth**, a series of communicating membranous sacs and ducts. The osseous labyrinth connects to the subarachnoid space via the cochlear aqueduct. It is filled with perilymph, a clear fluid that mingles with cerebrospinal fluid. The membranous labyrinth contains a different fluid, the endolymph, which circulates in a closed system. Because there are no barriers between the cochlear and vestibular labyrinths, injury or disease of the inner ear frequently affects both hearing and equilibrium.

The **cochlea** is coiled upon itself like a snail shell and makes 2-1/2 turns. It has three compartments: two that contain perilymph and a third (the cochlear duct) that contains endolymph. The cochlear duct encompasses the end organ of hearing, **the organ of Corti**, which rests on the basement membrane and is arranged as a spiral, with three rows of outer hair cells and a row of inner hair cells. When hairs of these neuroepithelial cells are bent or distorted by vibration, the mechanical force is converted into electrochemical impulses and interpreted in the temporal cortex as sound. The vestibular part of the membranous labyrinth consists of the utricle, saccule, and semicircular canals, each with specialized neuroepithelium that determines equilibrium.

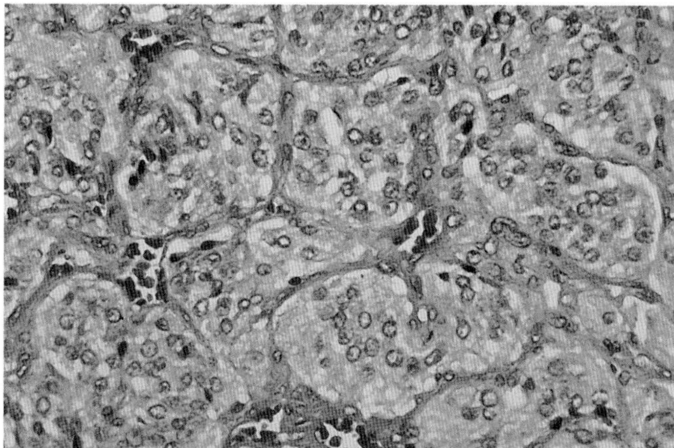

FIGURE 21-26. Jugulotympanic paraganglioma. Tumor cell nests are composed of cells with ill-defined cell borders and prominent eosinophilic cytoplasm (chief cells).

Otosclerosis

Otosclerosis is an autosomal dominant hereditary defect, which is the most common cause of conductive hearing loss in young and middle-aged adults in the United States. This disorder affects 10% of white and 1% of black adult Americans, although 90% of cases are asymptomatic. The female-to-male ratio is 2:1, and both ears are usually affected.

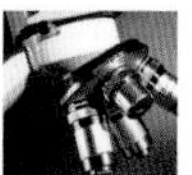

PATHOLOGY: Although any part of the petrous bone may be affected, otosclerotic bone tends to form at particular points. The most frequent (85%) site is immediately anterior to the oval window. The focus of sclerotic bone extends posteriorly and may infiltrate and replace the stapes, progressively immobilizing the footplate of the stapes. The developing bony ankylosis is functionally manifested as a slowly progressive conductive hearing loss.

Otosclerosis begins with resorption of bone and formation of highly cellular fibrous tissue, with wide vascular spaces and osteoclasts. The resorbed bone is later replaced by immature bone, which, with repeated remodeling, becomes mature (Fig. 21-27). Otosclerosis is treated by surgical mobilization of the auditory ossicles.

Ménière Disease

Although several etiologies have been suggested, the cause of **Ménière disease** is uncertain. About 46,000 new cases are

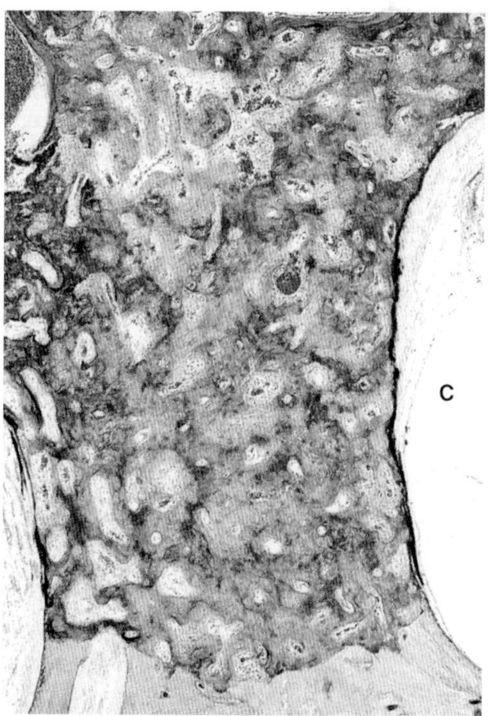

FIGURE 21-27. Otosclerosis. In the lateral wall of the cochlea, the basophilic and more vascular bone is well demarcated. C, organ of Corti.

diagnosed in the United States annually. Viral etiologies, vascular causes, and, possibly, autoimmune mechanisms have all been suggested. Tinnitus is usually unilateral and is most frequent between 40 and 60 years of age. A familial association suggests an underlying genetic predisposition.

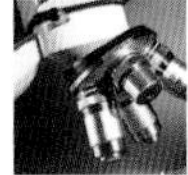

PATHOLOGY: The earliest change is dilation of the cochlear duct and saccule. As the disease (**hydrops**) progresses, the entire endolymphatic system dilates, and the membranous wall may tear (Fig. 21-28). Ruptures can be followed by collapse of the membranous labyrinth, but atrophy of sensory and neural structures is rare. Symptoms occur when endolymphatic hydrops causes rupture, and endolymph escapes into the perilymph.

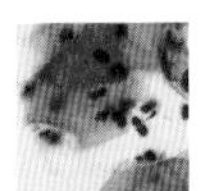

CLINICAL FEATURES: Attacks of vertigo, often with incapacitating nausea and vomiting, last less than 24 hours. Weeks or months go by before another episode. In time, remissions become longer. Hearing loss recovers between attacks but may later become permanent. Ménière disease may improve with a low-salt diet and diuretics.

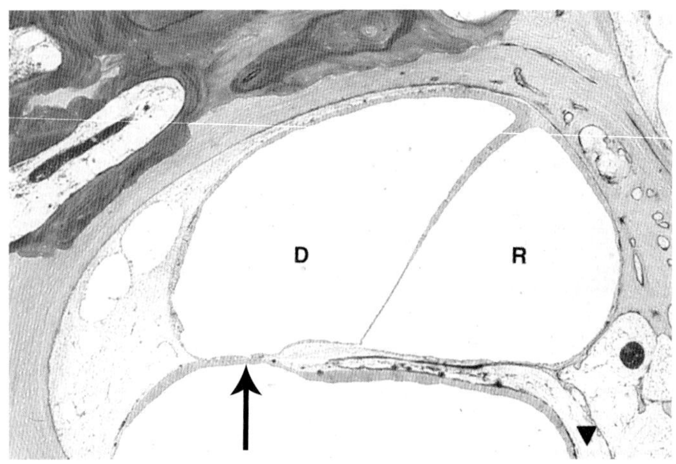

FIGURE 21-28. Ménière disease. The cochlear duct (D) is markedly distended, and the Reissner membrane (R) is pushed back by endolymphatic hydrops. Neither the organ of Corti (*arrow*) nor the spiral ganglion (*arrowhead*) is in its usual location.

Labyrinthine Toxicity

Aminoglycoside antibiotics are the most common ototoxic drugs, producing irreversible damage to vestibular or cochlear sensory cells. Other antibiotics, diuretics, antimalarials, and salicylates may also lead to transient or permanent sensorineural hearing loss. Among antineoplastic drugs, cisplatin causes temporary or permanent hearing loss.

The labyrinth of the developing embryo is very sensitive to some drugs. Maternal use of antimalarials and other drugs may result in congenital deafness.

Viral Labyrinthitis

Viral infections may cause inner ear disorders, particularly deafness. This is mostly caused by viral invasion of the labyrinth. CMV and rubella are the best-known prenatal viral infections that cause congenital deafness via maternal-to-fetal transmission.

Mumps is the most common postnatal viral cause of deafness. It can cause rapid hearing loss, which is unilateral in 80% of cases. By contrast, prenatal infection of the labyrinth with rubella is usually bilateral, with permanent loss of cochlear and vestibular function.

Schwannoma

SCHWANNOMA: Nearly all schwannomas in the internal auditory canal arise from the vestibular nerves. Vestibular schwannomas, which account for about 10% of all intracranial tumors, are slow growing and encapsulated. Larger tumors protrude from the internal auditory meatus into the cerebellopontine angle and may deform the brainstem and adjacent cerebellum. Schwannomas cause slowly progressive vestibular and auditory symptoms. In neurofibromatosis type 2 (NF-2; see Chapters 5 and 24), bilateral vestibular schwannomas, identical to other vestibular schwannomas, occur frequently.

MENINGIOMA: Meningiomas of the cerebellopontine angle originate from the meningothelial cells in the arachnoid villi. The favored sites for these tumors are the sphenoid ridge and petrous pyramid. Meningiomas may extend into the adjacent temporal bone or dural sinuses (see Chapter 24).

22 Bones, Joints, and Soft Tissue

Roberto A. Garcia ▪ Elizabeth G. Dostco ▪ Michael J. Klein ▪ Alan L. Schiller

LEARNING OBJECTIVES

- Define the following terms related to bone structure: growth plate, epiphyseal cartilage plate, epiphysis, metaphysis, diaphysis, endochondral ossification, and intramembranous ossification.
- What are the specific roles of each of the following cells in bone formation, resorption, and remodeling: osteoprogenitor cell, osteoblast, osteocyte, and osteoclast?
- What are the major structural differences between lamellar bone, woven bone, hyaline cartilage, fibrocartilage, and elastic cartilage?
- Outline the process of bone formation and growth during development.
- What are the pathophysiologic mechanisms by which cretinism and achondroplasia result in skeletal disorders?
- Discuss the pathophysiology, gross and microscopic pathology, and clinical consequences of osteopetrosis.
- What molecular defect results in osteogenesis imperfecta? Describe the gross and microscopic pathology and clinical consequences of the disease.
- Outline and describe the major phases of the healing of bone fractures.
- What are the major causes of osteonecrosis?
- Describe the histopathology of myositis ossificans. Is it a reactive or neoplastic process?
- Describe etiologic factors and pathologic progression of osteomyelitis.
- Compare and contrast type 1 and type 2 primary osteoporosis in terms of epidemiology and pathogenesis.
- List the major factors likely to influence bone loss in primary osteoporosis.
- What are the major etiologies of secondary osteoporosis? What endocrinopathies are associated with the condition?
- Compare and contrast osteomalacia and rickets. By what process can disorders of vitamin D metabolism and intestinal malabsorption result in these conditions? Describe the gross and microscopic pathology and clinical consequences of the disorders.
- What disorders of renal phosphate metabolism may result in rickets and osteomalacia?
- What is the molecular pathogenesis of bone disease resulting from primary hyperparathyroidism?
- Define and describe the gross and microscopic appearance of osteitis fibrosa cystica.
- Discuss the pathophysiology, gross and microscopic pathology, and clinical consequences of Paget disease of bone.
- Discuss the pathophysiology, gross and microscopic pathology, and potential clinical consequences of fibrous dysplasia of bone.
- Discuss the etiology, pathophysiology, gross and microscopic pathology, and clinical consequences of osteochondroma.
- Discuss the molecular pathogenesis of giant cell tumor of bone concentrating on the multiple cell populations involved. What is the gross appearance of the tumor and its clinical consequences?
- Describe the molecular pathogenesis of osteosarcoma. What are the etiologic factors and gross, microscopic, and radiographic appearance of the tumor?
- Differentiate between peripheral and central chondrosarcoma in terms of the pathologic appearance and location of lesions.
- Discuss the etiology, pathophysiology, gross and microscopic pathology, and clinical consequences of Ewing sarcoma.
- Describe the histology of the normal synovium and compare it with the synovium during the progression of rheumatoid arthritis.
- What etiologic factors and biochemical abnormalities are associated with osteoarthritis? Compare these with those associated with rheumatoid arthritis.
- Present an overview of the histologic changes associated with the progression of osteoarthritis.
- Describe the process of pannus formation in rheumatoid arthritis. How does this relate to bone loss?
- Describe the histologic appearance and potential clinical correlates of rheumatoid nodules.
- Define the term spondyloarthropathy and list common clinical features with which they are associated.
- Differentiate between ankylosing spondylitis and reactive and enteropathic arthritis in terms of etiology and pathogenesis.

- What are the chronic arthritic conditions included under the classification juvenile arthritis?
- What is the molecular pathogenesis of primary gout and secondary gout?
- Describe the gross and microscopic pathology and clinical consequences associated with gout.
- Differentiate pseudogout from gout in terms of the pathogenesis and clinical consequences of the former.
- What are important general principles relating to soft tissue tumors?
- Discuss the etiology of nodular fasciitis.
- Discuss the pathogenesis of fibromatosis, specifically Dupuytren contractures and Peyronie disease.
- Differentiate between the gross and histopathologic appearance of lipomas and liposarcoma.

Bones

The term **bone** can refer to both an organ and a tissue. The "organ" is composed of bone tissue, cartilage, fat, marrow elements, vessels, nerves, and fibrous tissue. Bone "tissue" is described in microscopic terms and is defined by the relation of its collagen and mineral structure to the bone cells.

ANATOMY

Macroscopically, two types of bone are recognized:

- **Cortical bone** is dense, compact bone, whose outer shell defines its shape. It comprises 80% of the skeleton. Because of its density, its functions are mainly biomechanical.
- **Coarse cancellous bone** (also called **spongy, trabecular,** or **medullary bone**) is located at the ends of long bones within the medullary canal. Cancellous bone has a high surface to volume ratio and contains many more bone cells per unit volume than does cortical bone. **Changes in the rate of bone turnover are manifested principally in cancellous bone.**

All bones contain both cancellous and cortical elements (Fig. 22-1), but their proportions differ. The body or shaft of a long tubular bone, such as the femur, is composed of cortical bone, and its marrow is mainly fat. Toward the ends of the femur, the cortex becomes thin, and coarse cancellous bone becomes the predominant structure. By contrast, the skull is formed by outer and inner tables of compact bone, with only a small amount of cancellous bone within the marrow space, called the **diploë**.

The anatomy of bone is defined in relation to a transverse cartilage plate, which is present in the growing child. This structure is named the **growth plate,** the **epiphyseal cartilage plate,** or **the physis** (Fig. 22-2A to C). The terms **epiphysis, metaphysis,** and **diaphysis** are defined in relation to the growth plate.

- **The epiphysis** is the area of the bone that extends from the subarticular bone plate to the base of the growth plate.
- **The metaphysis** contains coarse cancellous bone and is the region from the side of the growth plate facing away from the joint to the area where the bone develops its fluted or funnel shape.
- **The diaphysis** corresponds to the body or shaft of the bone and is the zone between the two metaphyses in a long tubular bone.

The metaphysis blends into the diaphysis and is the area where coarse cancellous bone dissipates. This area of bone is particularly important in hematogenous infections, tumors, and skeletal malformations.

Two additional terms are essential to an understanding of bone organization:

- **Endochondral ossification** is the process by which bone tissue replaces cartilage.
- **Intramembranous ossification** refers to the mechanism by which bone tissue supplants membranous or fibrous tissue laid down by the periosteum.

All bones are formed by at least some intramembranous ossification. Some bones (e.g., the calvaria of the skull) are forged purely by intramembranous ossification.

The Bone Marrow

The marrow space is enclosed by cortical bone. It is supported by a delicate connective tissue framework that enmeshes marrow cells and blood vessels. Three types of marrow are evident to the naked eye:

- **Red marrow** corresponds to hematopoietic tissue and is found in virtually all bones at birth. In adults, it is confined to the axial skeleton, which includes the skull, vertebrae, sternum, ribs, scapulae, clavicles, pelvis, and proximal humerus and femur.
- **Yellow marrow** is fat tissue and is found in the limb bones. In a normally hematopoietic area, such as a vertebral body, yellow marrow is abnormal at any age.
- **Gray or white marrow** is deficient in hematopoietic elements and is often fibrotic. ***It is always a pathologic tissue in a nongrowing adult bone or in areas distant from the growth plate in a child.***

Periosteum

The periosteum is a fibrous tissue that envelopes the outer surface of the bone and demarcates it from the surrounding soft tissue. If the periosteum is irritated (e.g., infection, trauma, or tumor), it can produce a significant amount of reactive bone that can be seen radiographically.

Bone Matrix

Bone tissue is composed of cells (10% by weight), a mineralized phase (hydroxyapatite crystals, representing 60% of the total tissue), and an organic matrix (30%). ***Thus, except for its cells, bone is a biphasic structure composed of an organic and an inorganic matrix.***

The **mineralized matrix** consists of poorly crystalline hydroxyapatite, $Ca_{10}(PO_4)_6(OH)_2$.

The **organic matrix** consists of 88% type I collagen, 10% other proteins and 1% to 2% lipids, and glycosaminoglycans. ***Thus, type I collagen basically defines the organic matrix.***

Cells of Bone

There are four types of cells in bone tissue, each of which has specific functions related to the formation, resorption, and remodeling of bone.

OSTEOPROGENITOR CELL: The osteoprogenitor cell, which differentiates ultimately into osteoblasts and osteocytes,

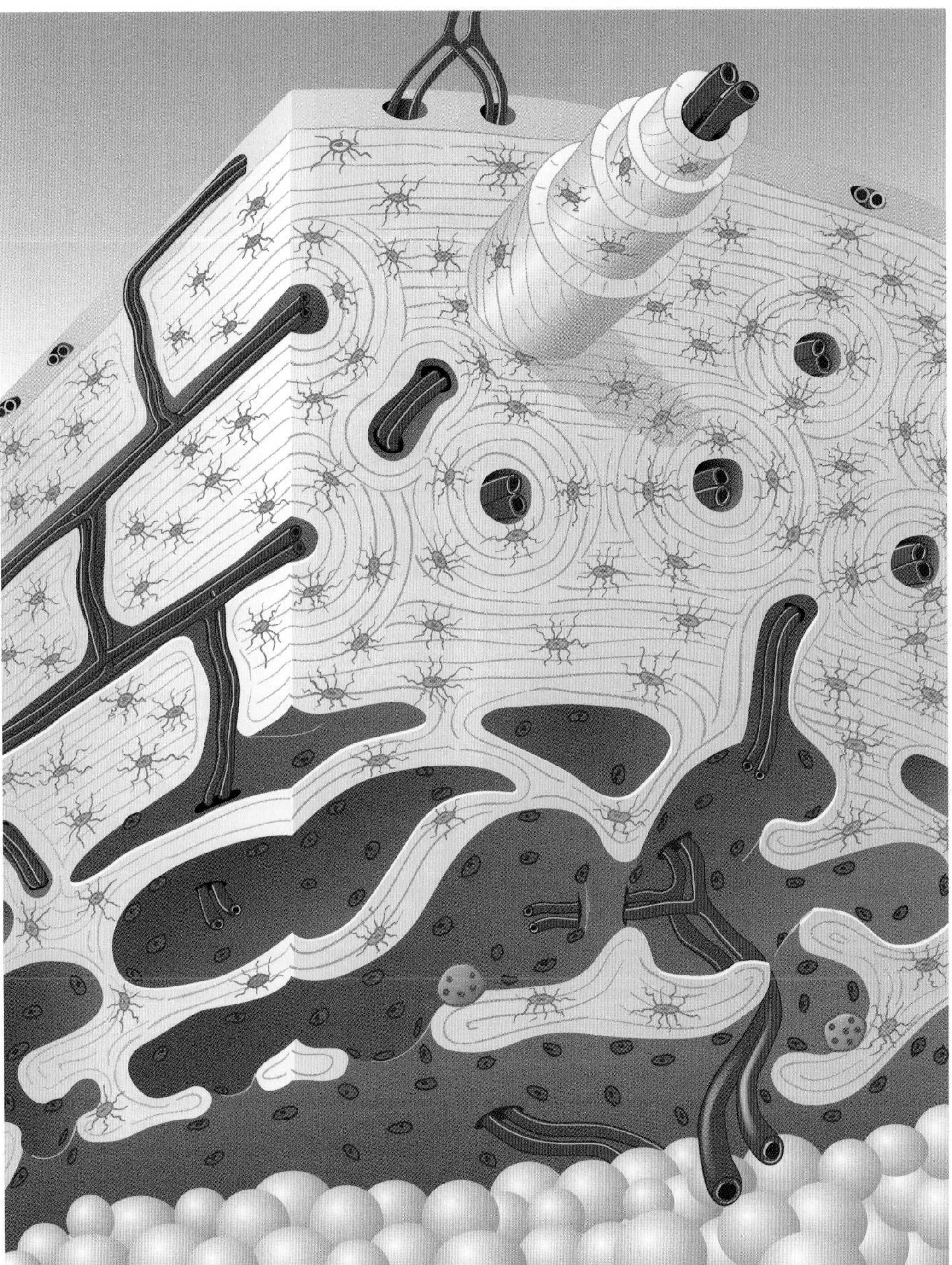

FIGURE 22-1. Anatomy of bone. A schematic representation of cortical and trabecular bone. The longitudinal section (*left*) showing the vasculature entering the periosteum via the periosteal perforating arteries and coursing through the bone perpendicular to the long axis in Volkmann canals. The vessels that proceed longitudinally, or parallel to the long axis, are located in Haversian canals. Each artery is accompanied by a vein. Within the cortex, osteocytes reside in lacunae, and their cell processes extend into the canaliculi. The cross-sectional view (*right*) illustrating the various types of lamellar bone in the cortex. Circumferential lamellar bone is located adjacent to the periosteum and borders the marrow space. Concentric lamellar bone surrounds the central Haversian canals to form an **osteon.** Each layer of the concentric lamellar bone displays a change in the pitch of the collagen fibers, such that each layer has a different arrangement of collagen. The interstitial lamellar bone occupies the space between osteons. The marrow space is filled with fat, and its trabecular bone is contiguous with the cortex. Multinucleated osteoclasts are present, and palisaded osteoblasts surround the bone surfaces. The perforating arteries from the periosteum and the nutrient artery from the marrow space communicate within the cortex via Haversian and Volkmann canals.

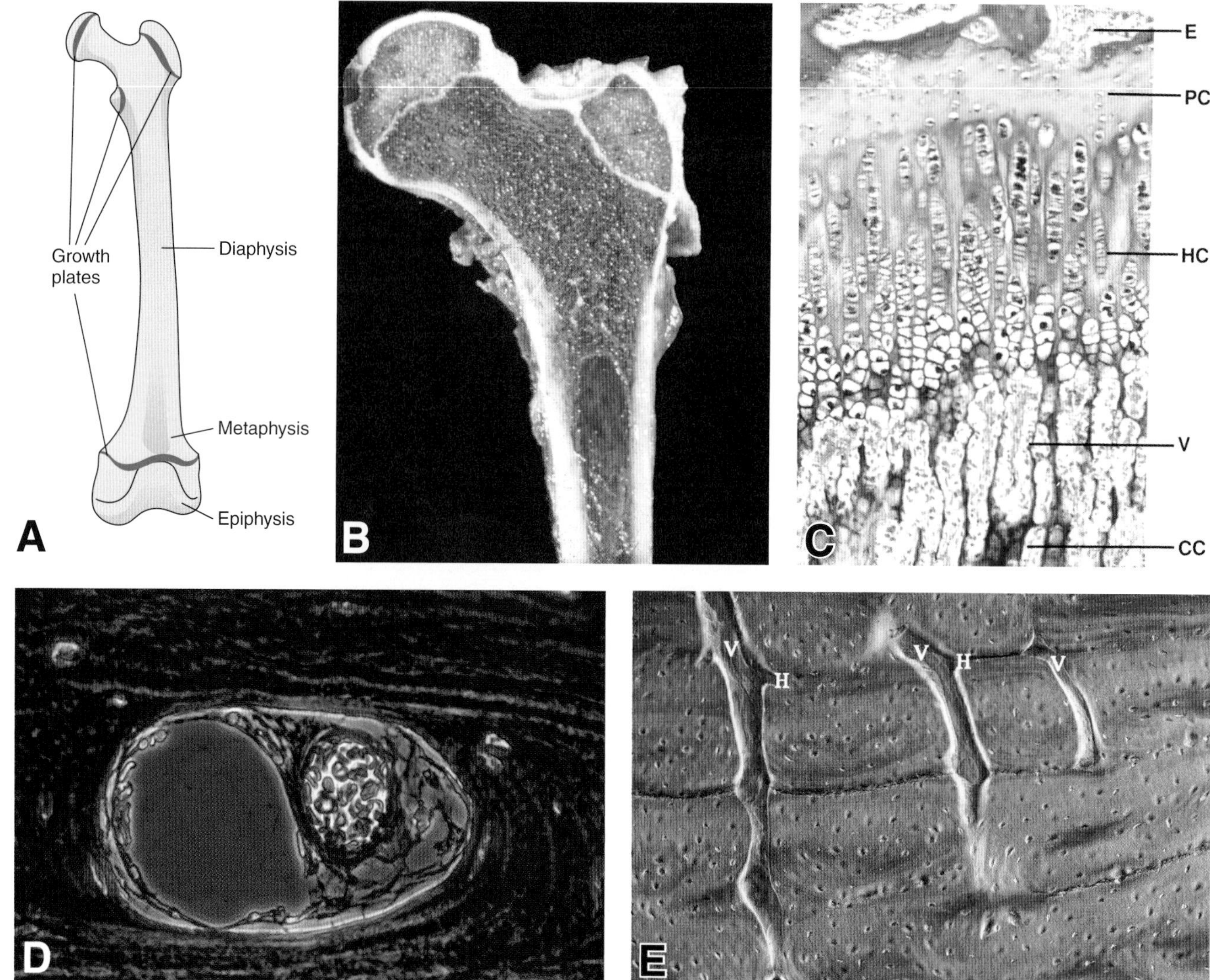

FIGURE 22-2. Anatomy of a long bone. A. Diagram of the femur illustrating the various compartments. **B. Coronal section of the proximal femur** illustrating the various anatomic parts of a long bone. The epiphysis of the femoral head and the apophysis of the greater trochanter are separated from the metaphysis by their respective growth plates. The cortex and the medullary cavity are well visualized. The medullary cavity contains cancellous bone until the metaphysis narrows into the diaphysis (shaft) of the bone, which is almost completely devoid of bone and filled with marrow. **C. A section of the epiphysis** with a zone of proliferating cartilage cells. Beneath this zone, the hypertrophic cartilage cells are arrayed in columns. At the *bottom*, the calcifying matrix is invaded by blood vessels. CC, calcified cartilage; E, epiphysis; HC, hypertrophic cartilage; PC, proliferative cartilage; V, vascular invasion. **D. Haversian canal** containing a venule (thin-walled wider vessel on *left*) and an arteriole (thicker-walled narrow vessel on the *right*). **E. Volkmann canals.** In this photograph, three Volkmann canals are seen running parallel to each other (*V*) and perpendicular to the cortex. The openings of two Haversian canals (*H*) are visible.

is itself derived from a primitive stem cell. The stem cell can develop into adipocytes, myoblasts, fibroblasts, or osteoblasts. Osteoprogenitor cells are found in marrow, periosteum, and all supporting structures within the marrow cavity.

OSTEOBLAST: Osteoblasts are the protein-synthesizing cells that produce and mineralize bone tissue. They are derived from mesenchymal progenitors that also give rise to chondrocytes, myocytes, adipocytes, and fibroblasts. These large cells are arrayed in a line along the bone surface (Fig. 22-3). Underlying the layer of osteoblasts is a thin, eosinophilic zone of organic bone matrix that has not yet been mineralized, called **osteoid**. When an osteoblast is inactive, it flattens on the surface of bone tissue. A number of growth factors are important in regulating bone growth and differentiation, including TGF-β, IGF-I, IGF-2, PDGF, IL-1, FGF, and TNF-α, are produced by osteoblasts. Furthermore, the osteoblast possesses surface receptors for various hormones (e.g., PTH, vitamin D, estrogen, and glucocorticoids), as well as for cytokines and growth factors. ***The osteoblast ultimately controls the activation, maturation, and differentiation of the osteoclast through a paracrine cell signaling mechanism (see below).***

OSTEOCYTE: The osteocyte is an osteoblast that is completely embedded in bone matrix and is isolated in a lacuna (Fig. 22-3B). Osteocytes deposit small quantities of bone around lacunae, but with time, they lose the capacity for protein synthesis. They have small hyperchromatic nuclei and numerous processes that extend through bony canals

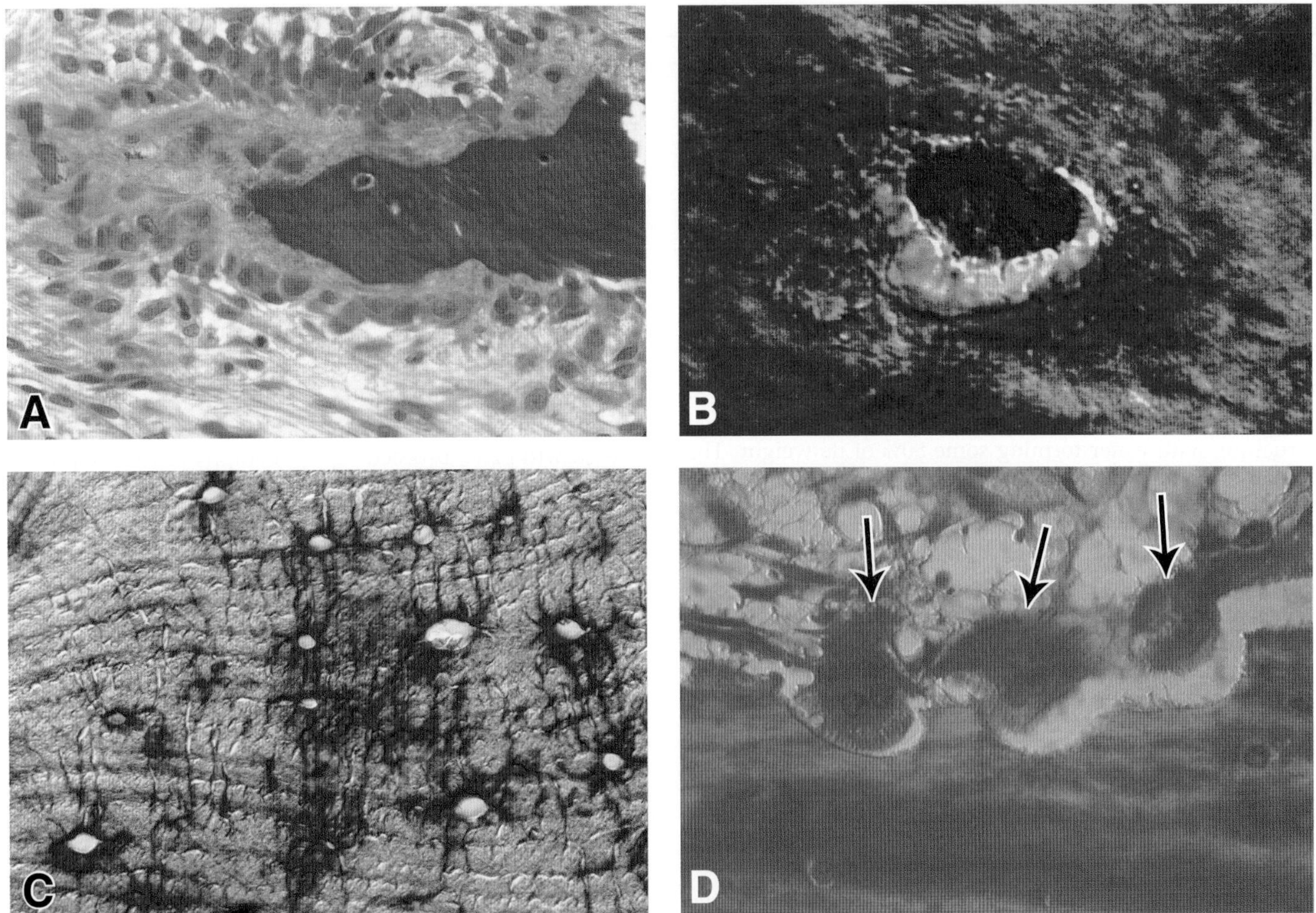

FIGURE 22-3. **The cells of bones. A. A developing bone spicule** demonstrating a prominent layer of plump osteoblasts lining the pink osteoid seam. The dark purple layer beneath the osteoid seam is mineralized bone. **B. Osteocytes.** Osteocytes represent trapped osteoblasts surrounded by bone matrix. The space surrounding the cell is called a **lacuna**. At this power, a few cytoplasmic extensions of the cell can be seen extending into narrow channels in the bone, called **canaliculi. C.** The extensive **intercommunication of osteocyte processes** via their canalicular network in cortical bone is visible in this section. **D. Osteoclasts.** These are multinucleated giant cells (*arrows*) found on bone surfaces within small scalloped reabsorption pits, called **Howship lacunae**.

called **canaliculi**, which communicate with those from other osteocytes and osteoblasts (Fig. 22-3C). ***The osteocytes may be the bone cells that recognize and respond to mechanical forces and are important regulators of bone remodeling.***

OSTEOCLAST: Osteoclasts are the exclusive bone-resorptive cells. They are of hematopoietic origin and are members of the monocyte/macrophage family. Three major factors are required for osteoclastogenesis: (1) TNF-related receptor RANK (receptor activator for nuclear factor-κB [NF-κB]), (2) RANK ligand (RANKL), and (3) macrophage colony-stimulating factor (M-CSF). RANK is expressed by osteoclast precursors. RANKL and M-CSF are produced by osteoblasts and stromal cells.

Osteoclasts are multinucleated cells that contain many lysosomes and are rich in hydrolytic enzymes. They are found in small depressions on bone surfaces called **Howship lacunae** or resorption bays (Fig. 22-3D).

Although the machinery of an osteoclast is superbly suited for bone resorption, it functions only if the matrix is mineralized. ***In fact, any bone that is lined by osteoid or unmineralized cartilage is protected from osteoclastic activity.***

Types of Bone

Bone may be mineralized or unmineralized. Unmineralized bone is called **osteoid**.

Lamellar Bone

Lamellar bone is made slowly and is highly organized. As the stronger bone tissue, it forms the adult skeleton. ***Anything other than lamellar bone in the adult skeleton is abnormal.*** Lamellar bone is defined by (1) a parallel arrangement of type I collagen fibers, (2) few osteocytes in the matrix, and (3) uniform osteocytes in lacunae parallel to the long axis of the collagen fibers.

Woven Bone

Woven bone is identified by (1) an irregular arrangement of type I collagen fibers, hence the term *woven*; (2) numerous osteocytes in the matrix; and (3) variation in osteocyte size and shape. Woven bone is deposited more rapidly than lamellar bone. It is haphazardly arranged and of low tensile strength, serving as a temporary scaffolding for support. It is not surprising that woven bone is found in the developing fetus, in areas surrounding tumors and infections and as part of a healing fracture. ***Its presence in the adult skeleton is always abnormal and indicates that reactive tissue has been produced in response to some stress in the bone.***

Cartilage

Cartilage Matrix

Like bone, cartilage may be viewed as an organic and inorganic biphasic material. The inorganic phase is composed of calcium hydroxyapatite crystals, equivalent to those found in bone matrix. However, the organic matrix is quite different from that of bone. Essentially, cartilage is a hyperhydrated structure, with water forming some 80% of its weight. The remaining 20% is composed principally of two types of macromolecules, type II collagen, and proteoglycans. The water content is extremely important in the function of articular cartilage because it enhances the resilience and lubrication of the joint. Proteoglycans are complex macromolecules composed of a central linear protein core, to which long side arms of polysaccharides, called **glycosaminoglycans**, are attached. The chondroitin sulfates are the most abundant constituents, accounting for 55% to 90% of the cartilage matrix, depending on the age of the tissue. Cartilage may be focally calcified to provide some internal strength in the appropriate areas.

Types of Cartilage

There are three types of cartilage:

- **Hyaline cartilage:** This prototypic cartilage constitutes the articular cartilage of joints; cartilaginous anlage of developing bones; growth plates; costochondral cartilages; cartilages of the trachea, bronchi, and larynx; and nasal cartilages. Hyaline cartilage is the most common cartilage in tumors, in fracture callus, and in areas of relative avascularity.
- **Fibrocartilage:** This tissue is essentially hyaline cartilage that contains numerous type I collagen fibers for tensile and structural strength. It is found in the annulus fibrosus of the intervertebral disk, tendinous and ligamentous insertions, menisci, symphysis pubis, and insertions of joint capsules. Fibrocartilage may also occur in a fracture callus.
- **Elastic cartilage** is found in the epiglottis, in the arytenoid cartilages of the larynx, and in the external ear.

Chondrocytes

Chondrocytes are derived from primitive mesenchymal cells that are similar to the precursors of bone cells. The chondroblast gives rise to the chondrocyte. As in bone, the cell that resorbs calcified cartilage is the osteoclast.

BONE FORMATION AND GROWTH

Bone tissue grows only by appositional growth, defined as deposition of new matrix on a preexisting surface by adjacent surface osteoblasts. By contrast, virtually all other tissues, especially cartilage, increase by interstitial cell proliferation within the matrix as well as by appositional growth.

Bone development in the fetus follows a stereotyped sequence. Most of the skeleton (except the calvaria and clavicles) develops from cartilage anlagen present during fetal development. This cartilage is eventually resorbed and replaced by bone that is formed by **endochondral ossification**. Similar events take place in the cartilaginous ends of the future bone. Resting (reserve) cartilage is stimulated to become columns of proliferating cartilage, which then progress to hypertrophied chondrocytes and, eventually, calcified cartilage forming secondary centers of ossification. As the bony ends expand in the future diaphysis, a zone of cartilage is trapped between the end of the bone and the diaphysis. This cartilage is destined to be the **growth plate** (Fig. 22-4A), which is a layer of modified cartilage between the diaphysis and epiphysis. Its structure is essentially unchanged from early fetal life to skeletal maturity. ***The growth plate controls the longitudinal growth of bones and ultimately determines adult height.*** The chondrocytes of the growth plate are arranged in vertical rows, which, in three dimensions, are really helices. Viewed longitudinally, the growth plate, proceeding from epiphysis to metaphysis, is divided into zones (Figs. 22-2C and 22-4).

The growth plate is normally obliterated at a specific age for each bone.

Closure of the growth plate (Fig. 22-4B) is induced by sex hormones and occurs earlier in girls than in boys. Renewal of chondrocytes slows and ultimately ceases. The entire plate is eventually replaced by bone.

DISORDERS OF THE GROWTH PLATE

Cretinism

Cretinism results from **maternal iodine deficiency** (see Chapter 19) and has profound effects on the skeleton. Thyroid hormone plays a role in regulating chondrocytes, osteoblasts, and osteoclasts through production of cytokines and other factors involved in bone development and growth. Linear growth is severely impaired, resulting in dwarfism, with limbs disproportionately short in relation to the trunk. Delayed closure of the fontanelles of the skull causes an unusually large head. There is a delay in closure of the epiphyses, as well as radiologic stippling of these zones. Shedding of deciduous teeth and eruption of permanent teeth are retarded.

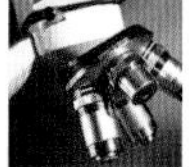

PATHOLOGY: In cretinism, chondrocytes do not follow the orderly endochondral sequence. Endochondral ossification does not proceed appropriately, and transverse bars of bone in the metaphysis seal off the growth plate. The failure of endochondral ossification produces severe dwarfism. The misshapen epiphyses seen on radiography reflect incomplete formation of secondary centers of ossification.

Morquio Syndrome

Many of the mucopolysaccharidoses (see Chapter 5), most notably Morquio syndrome (mucopolysaccharidosis type IV), involve skeletal deformities. These are attributable to the deposition of mucopolysaccharides (glycosaminoglycans) in developing bones.

Achondroplasia

Achondroplasia refers to a syndrome of short-limbed dwarfism and macrocephaly and represents a failure of normal epiphyseal cartilage formation. It is the most common genetic

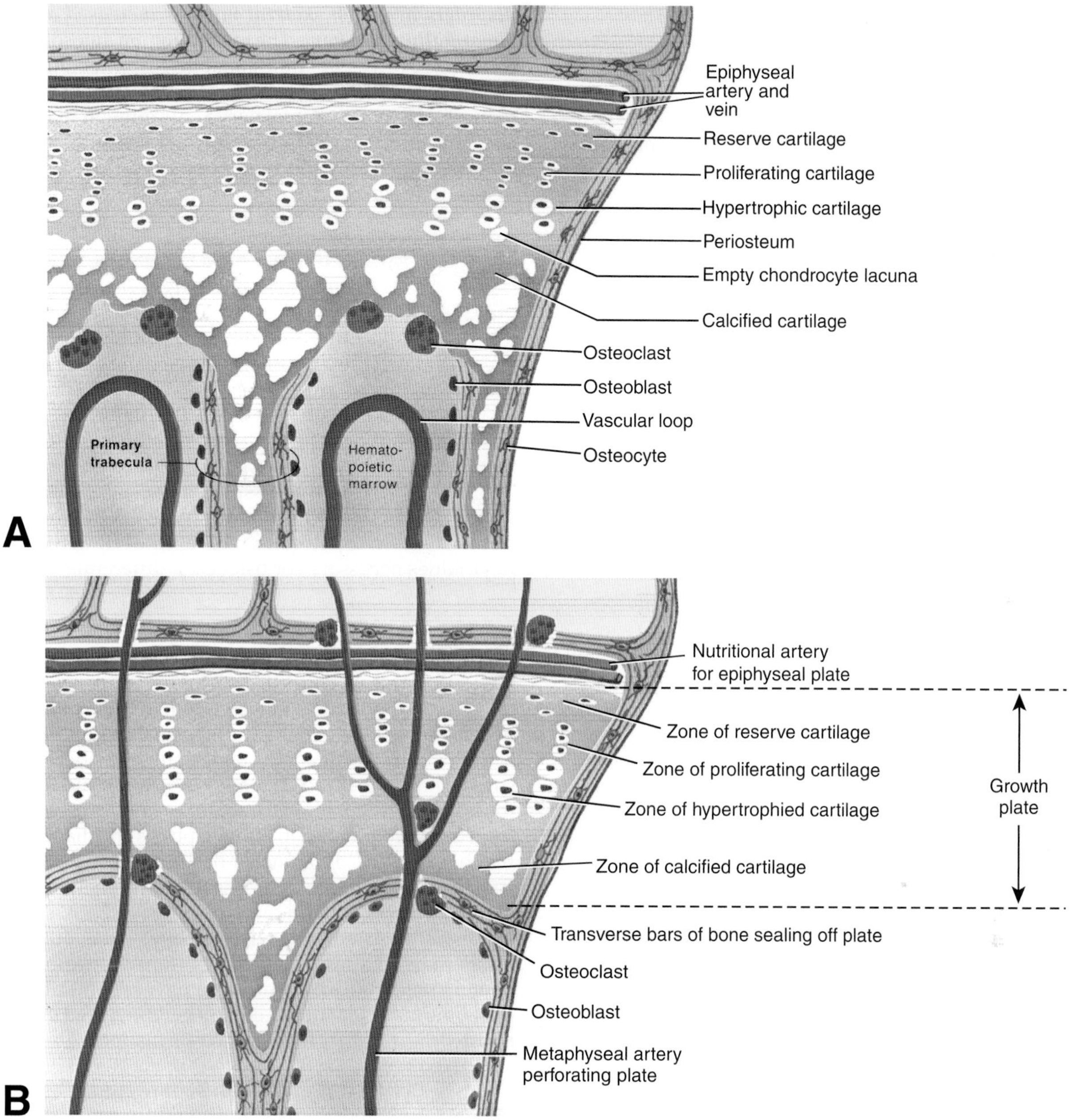

FIGURE 22-4. Anatomy of the epiphyseal growth plate. A. Normal growing epiphyseal plate. The epiphysis is separated from the epiphyseal plate by transverse plates of bone that seal the plate so that it grows only toward the metaphysis. The various zones of cartilage are illustrated. As the calcified cartilage migrates toward the metaphysis, the chondrocytes die, and the lacunae are empty. At the interface of the epiphyseal plate and the metaphysis, osteoclasts bore into the calcified cartilage, accompanied by a capillary loop from the metaphyseal vessels. Osteoblasts follow the osteoclasts and lay down woven bone on the cartilage core, thereby forming the primary spongiosum or primary trabeculae. **B. Normal closure.** The epiphyseal cartilage has ceased to grow, and metaphyseal vessels penetrate the cartilage plate. Transverse bars of bone separate the plate from the metaphysis.

form of dwarfism (1 in 15,000 live births) and is inherited as an autosomal dominant trait. Most cases represent new mutations. Some patients develop severe kyphoscoliosis and its complications.

MOLECULAR PATHOGENESIS: Achondroplasia is caused by an **activating** mutation in the FGF receptor (FGFR3) encoded on chromosome 4p16.3. The mutation constitutively inhibits chondrocyte differentiation and proliferation, an effect that retards growth plate development.

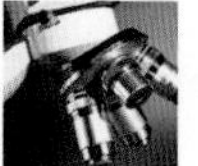

PATHOLOGY: The growth plate in achondroplasia is greatly thinned, and the zone of proliferative cartilage is either absent or extensively attenuated. The zone of provisional calcification, if present, undergoes endochondral ossification, but at a greatly reduced rate. A transverse bar of bone often seals off the growth plate, thereby preventing further bone formation and causing dwarfism. Because intramembranous ossification is undisturbed, the periosteum functions normally, and the bones become very short and thick. For the same reasons, the head of the achondroplastic appears unusually large, compared with the bones formed from the cartilage of the face. The spine is of normal length, but the limbs are abnormally short.

Scurvy

Scurvy refers to the disorder that follows vitamin C deficiency.

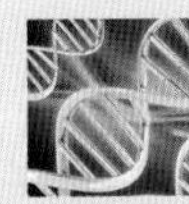

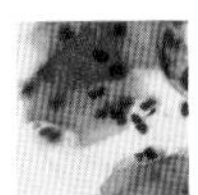

MOLECULAR PATHOGENESIS AND PATHOLOGY: Hydroxyproline and hydroxylysine are important in stabilizing the helical structure of collagen and in cross-linking the tropocollagen fibers into the proper molecular structure of collagen. Vitamin C is a cofactor in hydroxylation of proline and lysine. The skeletal changes of scurvy reflect the inability to produce and normally cross-link collagen. Chondrocytes at the growth plate continue to grow. The zone of calcified cartilage may actually become more prominent because it is more heavily calcified.

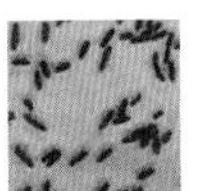

CLINICAL FEATURES: Today, scurvy is a rare disease (see Chapter 19). Wound healing and bone growth are impaired in patients with scurvy. Furthermore, the basement membrane of capillaries is damaged by this condition, and widespread capillary bleeding is common. Subperiosteal bleeding may occur, leading to joint and muscle pain.

Asymmetric Cartilage Growth

Asymmetric cartilage growth, such as occurs in patients with knock knees and bowed legs, develops when one part of the growth plate, either medial or lateral, grows faster than the other. Most cases are hereditary, but mechanical forces near the growth plate, such as trauma, may stimulate one side to grow faster or in an asymmetric manner. Aside from the cosmetic appearance, these conditions may require correction to prevent future incongruity, eventual loss of articular cartilage, and joint destruction.

Scoliosis and Kyphosis

Scoliosis *refers to an abnormal lateral curvature of the spine, usually affecting adolescent girls.* **Kyphosis** *is an abnormal anteroposterior curvature.* When both conditions are present, the term **kyphoscoliosis** is used.

ETIOLOGIC FACTORS: A vertebral body grows in length (height) from the endplates of the vertebrae, which correspond to the growth plates of long tubular bones. As in tubular bones, vertebral bodies increase in width by appositional bone growth from the periosteum. In scoliosis, for unknown reasons, one portion of the endplate grows faster than the other, producing lateral curvature of the spine.

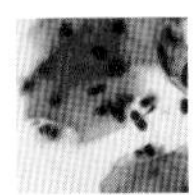

CLINICAL FEATURES: The treatment is appropriate stress on the vertebral body through use of braces or internal fixation to straighten the spine. If kyphoscoliosis is severe, the patient may eventually develop chronic pulmonary disease, cor pulmonale, and joint problems, particularly involving the hip.

BONE MODELING ABNORMALITIES

Osteopetrosis

Osteopetrosis, *also known as* **marble bone disease** *or* **Albers–Schönberg disease,** *is a heterogeneous group of rare inherited disorders in which skeletal mass is increased as a result of abnormally dense bone.* The most common autosomal recessive form is a severe, sometimes fatal disease affecting infants and children. Death of infants with the severe variant is attributable to marked anemia, cranial nerve entrapment, hydrocephalus, and infection. A more benign form, transmitted as an autosomal dominant trait and seen in adulthood or adolescence, is associated with mild anemia or no symptoms at all.

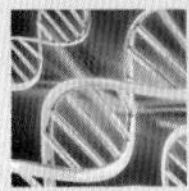

MOLECULAR PATHOGENESIS: ***The sclerotic skeleton of osteopetrosis is the result of failed osteoclastic bone resorption.*** The disease is caused by mutations in genes that govern osteoclast formation or function. The most common mutations cause defects in bone acidification, which is necessary for osteoclastic bone resorption. These include (1) mutations in the *TCIRG1* gene (osteoclast proton pump; autosomal dominant); (2) the *CLCN7* gene (osteoclast chloride channel; autosomal recessive); and (3) the **carbonic anhydrase II** gene, autosomal recessive. Other mutations that cause osteopetrosis involve transcription factors or cytokines necessary for osteoclast differentiation.

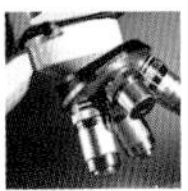

PATHOLOGY: Because osteoclast function is arrested, osteopetrosis is characterized by short, blocklike, radiodense bones (Fig. 22-5A). These bones are extremely radiopaque and weigh two to three times more than normal bone. However, they are weak because their structure is intrinsically disorganized and cannot remodel along lines of stress. The mineralized cartilage is also weak and friable, so that the bones in osteopetrosis fracture easily. Grossly, bones in osteopetrosis are widened in the metaphysis and diaphysis, causing the characteristic "Erlenmeyer flask" deformity (Fig. 22-5A and B). Histologically, the bone tissue is extremely irregular, and almost all areas contain a cartilage core (Fig. 22-5C). The marrow spaces become obliterated. Depending on the mutation, osteoclasts may be absent, present in normal numbers, or even abundant. In the case of normal or increased numbers of osteoclasts, the molecular defect lies in a gene involved in the function of osteoclasts, rather than in their formation.

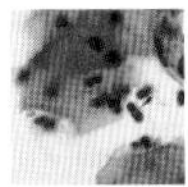

CLINICAL FEATURES: Suppression of hematopoiesis in osteopetrosis is caused by replacement of the marrow by sheets of abnormal osteoclasts or extensive fibrosis, which may be sufficiently severe to lead to severe anemia or pancytopenia. To compensate for loss of marrow hematopoiesis, extramedullary hematopoiesis occurs in the liver, spleen, and lymph nodes. Narrowing of neural foramina causes cranial nerve involvement, and subsequent strangulation of nerves leads to blindness and deafness. Osteopetrosis can be treated by bone marrow transplantation, which gives rise to a new clone of functional osteoclasts.

DELAYED MATURATION OF BONE

Osteogenesis Imperfecta

OI refers to a group of mainly autosomal dominant, heritable disorders of connective tissue caused by mutations in the gene for type I collagen. This disorder affects the skeleton, joints, ears, ligaments, teeth, sclerae, and skin. There are four well-characterized types of OI (see Chapter 5).

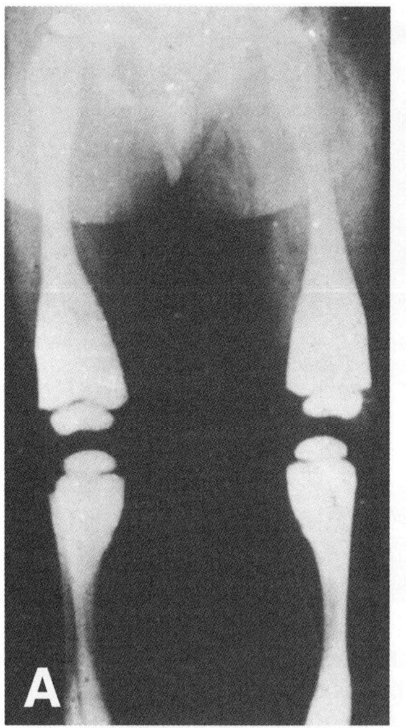

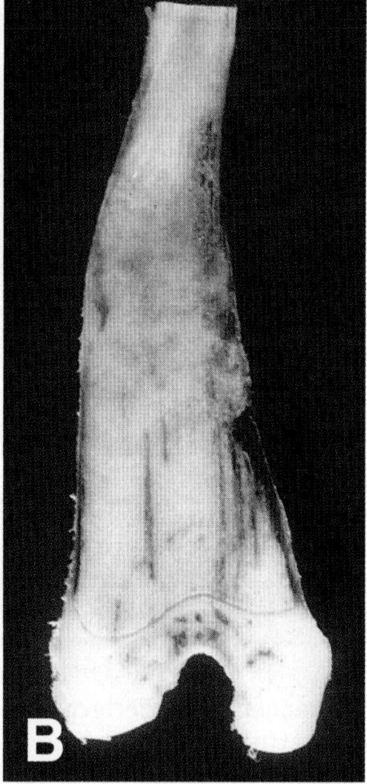

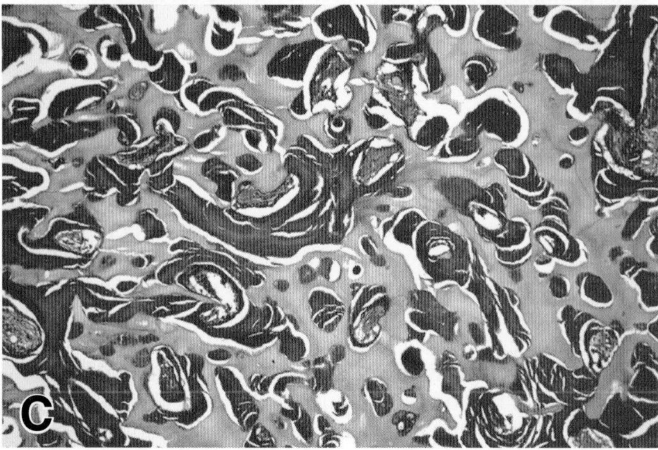

FIGURE 22-5. **Osteopetrosis. A.** A radiograph of a child showing markedly misshapen and dense bones of the lower extremities, characteristic of "marble bone disease." **B.** A gross specimen of the femur showing obliteration of the marrow space by dense bone. **C.** A photomicrograph of the bone of a child with autosomal recessive osteopetrosis demonstrating disorganization of bony trabeculae by retention of primary spongiosa (mixed spicules) and further obliteration of the marrow space by secondary spongiosa. The result is complete disorganization of the trabeculae and absence of marrow.

MOLECULAR PATHOGENESIS: The pathogenesis of OI involves mutations of *COL1A1* and *COL1A2* genes, which encode the α_1- and α_2-chains of type I procollagen, the major structural protein of bone. These genes reside in chromosome 17 (17q21.3–q22) and chromosome 7 (7q21.3–q22), respectively. The resulting phenotype ranges from mild to lethal, depending on (1) which gene is affected, (2) the location in the collagen triple helix at which the substitution occurs, and (3) which amino acid is substituted for glycine.

OI Type 1

Type I disease is the mildest phenotype. It is inherited as an autosomal dominant trait characterized by multiple fractures after birth, blue sclera, and hearing abnormalities. In some patients, abnormalities of the teeth are also conspicuous (dentinogenesis imperfecta).

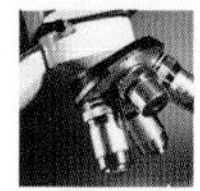

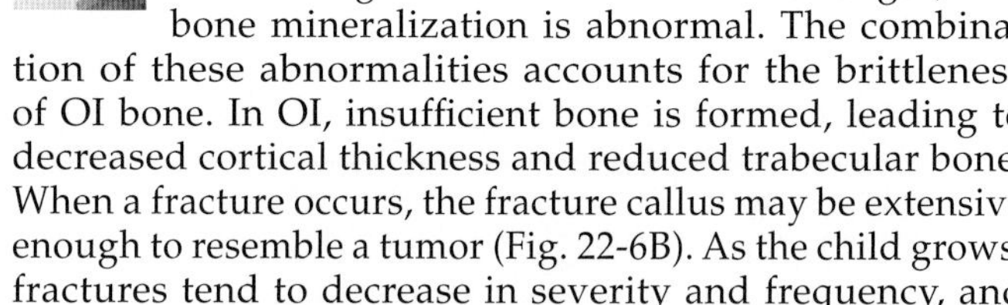

PATHOLOGY AND CLINICAL FEATURES: Initial fractures usually occur after the infant begins to sit and walk. There may be hundreds of fractures a year with minor movement or trauma. On radiologic examination, bones are extremely thin, delicate, and abnormally curved (Fig. 22-6A). Bone collagen has reduced tensile strength, and bone mineralization is abnormal. The combination of these abnormalities accounts for the brittleness of OI bone. In OI, insufficient bone is formed, leading to decreased cortical thickness and reduced trabecular bone. When a fracture occurs, the fracture callus may be extensive enough to resemble a tumor (Fig. 22-6B). As the child grows, fractures tend to decrease in severity and frequency, and stature is generally unaffected.

The sclerae are very thin, with a blue color attributable to the underlying choroid. Progressive hearing loss, which develops to total deafness in adulthood, results from fusion of the auditory ossicles. Joint laxity associated with the condition eventually leads to kyphoscoliosis and flat feet. Because of hypoplasia of the dentine and pulp, the teeth are misshapen and bluish yellow.

OI Type II

OI type II is a lethal, autosomal dominant, perinatal disease. Affected infants are stillborn or die within a few days after birth, in a sense being crushed to death. They are markedly short in stature, with severe limb deformities. Almost all bones sustain fractures during delivery or during uterine contractions in labor.

OI Type III

This progressive, severely deforming disease is characterized by many bone fractures, growth retardation, and severe skeletal deformities. Inheritance is usually autosomal dominant, although (rarely) autosomal recessive forms are reported. Fractures are present at birth, but bones are less fragile than in the type II form. These patients eventually develop severe shortening of their stature because of progressive bone fractures and severe kyphoscoliosis. Although sclerae may be blue at birth, they become white shortly thereafter. Dental abnormalities are common.

OI Type IV

This disease is similar to type I except that sclerae appear normal. The condition is heterogeneous in presentation, and there may or may not be dental disease. In this disorder, abnormal cross-linkages of collagen result in thin, delicate, and weak collagen fibrils. This inappropriate collagen does not allow the bone cortex to mature, so that at birth, the cortex of the bone resembles that of a fetus. Over a period of years, the cortex matures, but this may not occur until adolescence or even later. In any event, the frequency of fractures tends to decrease over a long period. These patients are vigorously

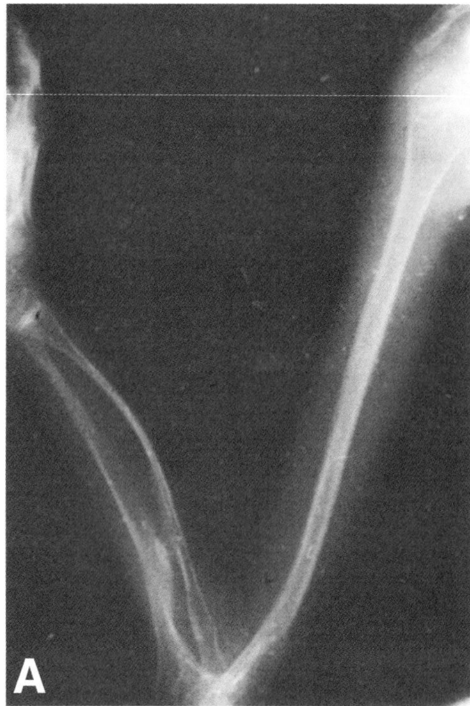

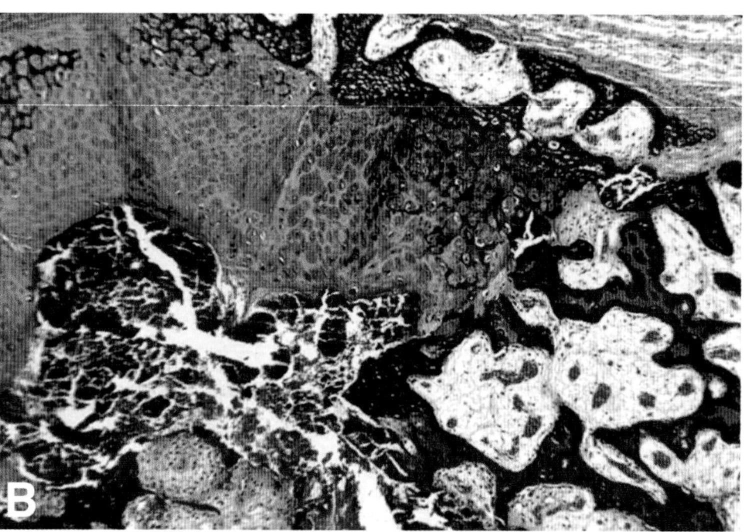

FIGURE 22-6. Osteogenesis imperfecta. A. A radiograph illustrating the markedly thin and attenuated humerus and bones of the forearm. There is a fracture callus in the proximal ulna. **B.** A photomicrograph of the fracture callus with prominent cartilage (*upper left*). The cortex is thin and composed of hypercellular woven bone.

treated with orthopedic devices, including rods inserted into the medullary cavities to prevent the dwarfing effect of multiple fractures.

There is no single treatment for OI. Surgery and orthotics have been the major treatments. However, bisphosphonates (pamidronate) improves types III and IV OI by decreasing the rate of fractures.

FRACTURE

The most common bone lesion is a fracture, which is defined as a discontinuity of the bone. A force perpendicular to the long axis of the bone results in a **transverse fracture**. A force along the long axis of the bone yields a **compression fracture**. Torsional force produces **spiral fractures**, and combined tension and compression shear forces cause angulation and displacement of the fractured ends.

A force powerful enough to fracture a bone also injures adjacent soft tissues. In this situation, there is often (1) extensive muscle necrosis; (2) hemorrhage because of shearing of capillary beds and larger vessels of soft tissues; (3) tearing of tendinous insertions and ligamentous attachments; and (4) nerve damage, caused by stretching or direct tearing of the nerve.

Fracture Healing

The duration of each phase (Fig. 22-7) depends on the patient's age, the site of fracture, the patient's overall health and nutritional status, and the extent of soft tissue injury. Local factors, such as vascular supply and mechanical forces at the site, also play a role in healing. ***In repairing a bone fracture, anything other than formation of bone tissue at the fracture site represents incomplete healing.***

Pathology is presented in detail in Figure 22-7:

- **The inflammatory phase:** (1) The first 1 to 2 days postfracture are characterized by hemorrhage and extensive bone necrosis as a result of disruption of rupture of large blood vessels in the bone. ***Dead bone is characterized by the absence of osteocytes and empty osteocyte lacunae.*** (2) After 2 to 5 days, large clot formation and peripheral neovascularization are observed. (3) By the end of the first week, most of the clot is organized by invasion of blood vessels and early fibrosis. (4) After a week, early woven bone formation corresponding to *the "scar" of bone occurs*. In most fractures, cartilage is also formed and is eventually resorbed by endochondral ossification. Granulation tissue containing bone or cartilage is called a **callus**.
- **The reparative phase:** This period follows the first week after a fracture and may last for months, depending on the degree of movement and the fixation of the fracture. By this time, acute inflammation has dissipated. Pluripotent cells differentiate into fibroblasts and osteoblasts. Repair proceeds from the periphery toward the center of the fracture site and accomplishes two objectives: (1) to organize and resorb the blood clot and, more importantly, (2) to neovascularize construction of the callus, which will eventually bridge the fracture site.
- **The remodeling phase:** Several weeks after a fracture, the ingrowth of callus has sealed the bone ends, and remodeling begins to restore the original cortex. In a child, in whom the growth plates are still open, normal modeling of growing bone overtakes the callus, so that a fracture may not be recognizable in later life.

PRIMARY HEALING: A fracture does not necessarily result in bone displacement and soft tissue injury. In this situation, there is almost no soft tissue reaction and callus formation because the bone remains rigidly fixed or is mechanically held in position. In such cases, the fracture callus grows directly into the fracture site by a process called **primary healing**.

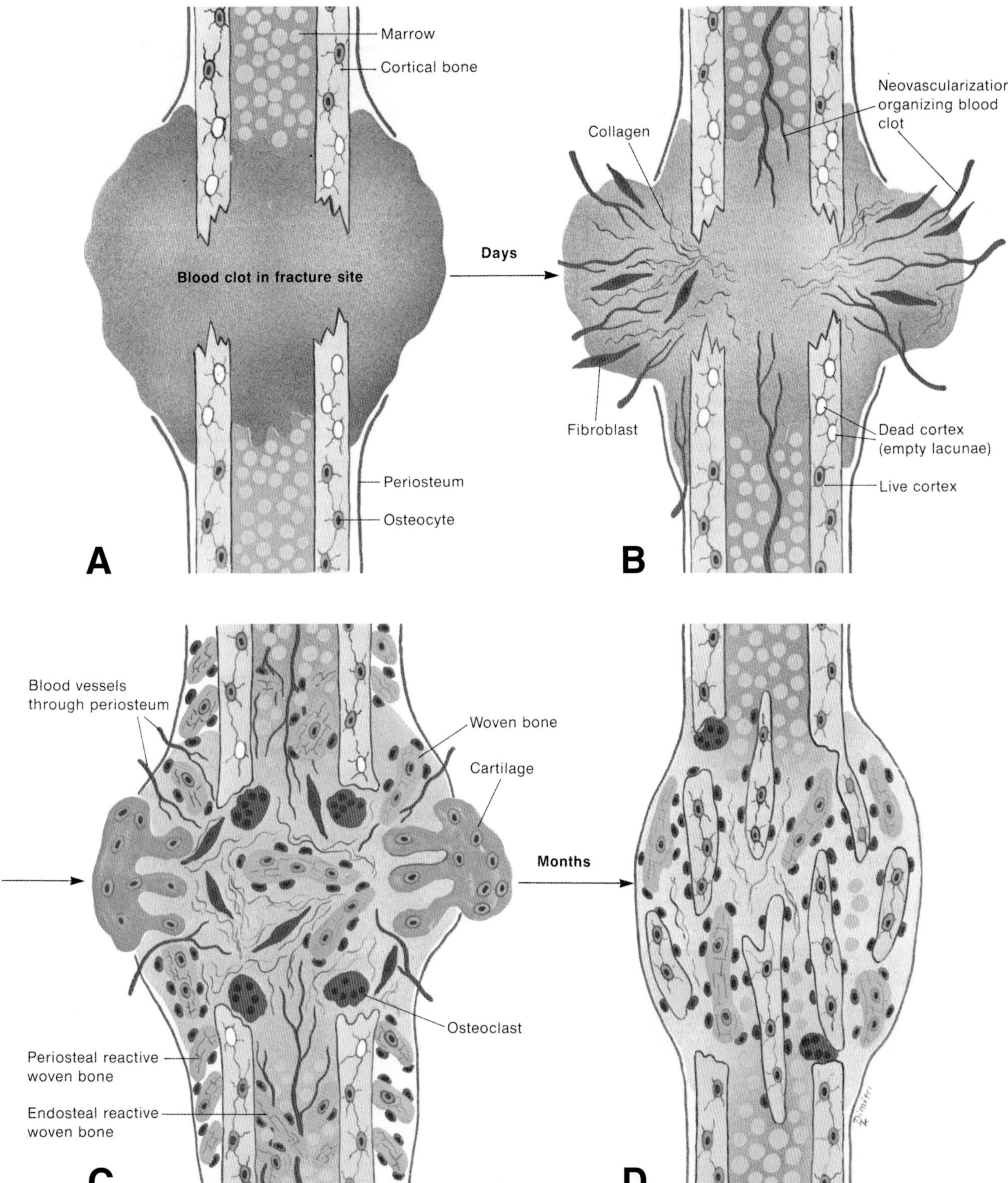

FIGURE 22-7. Healing of a fracture. A. Soon after a fracture is sustained, an extensive blood clot forms in the subperiosteum and soft tissue, as well as in the marrow cavity. The bone at the fracture site is jagged. **B.** The **inflammatory phase** of fracture healing is characterized by neovascularization and beginning organization of the blood clot. Because the osteocytes in the fracture site are dead, the lacunae are empty. The osteocytes of the cortex are necrotic well beyond the fracture site, owing to the traumatic interruption of the perforating arteries from the periosteum. **C.** The **reparative phase** of fracture healing is characterized by the formation of a callus of cartilage and woven bone near the fracture site. The jagged edges of the original cortex have been remodeled and eroded by osteoclasts. The marrow space has been revascularized and contains reactive woven bone, as does the periosteal area. **D.** In the **remodeling phase,** during which the cortex is revitalized, the reactive bone may be lamellar or woven. The new bone is organized along stress lines and mechanical forces. Extensive osteoclastic and osteoblastic cellular activity is maintained.

NONUNION: Failure of a fracture to heal is called **nonunion**. Causes of nonunion include interposition of soft tissues at the fracture site, excessive motion, infection, poor blood supply, and other factors mentioned above.

OSTEONECROSIS (AVASCULAR NECROSIS AND ASEPTIC NECROSIS)

Osteonecrosis refers to the death of bone and marrow in the absence of infection (Fig. 22-8). Causes of osteonecrosis are listed in Table 22-1. Necrotic bone heals differently in the cortex than in the underlying coarse cancellous bone.

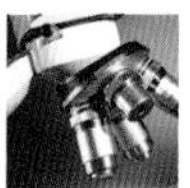

PATHOLOGY: Osteonecrosis is characterized by the death of bone and marrow. The necrotic bone has empty lacunae that lack osteocyte nuclei, and the marrow displays dystrophic calcification (Fig. 22-8B).

Legg–Calvé–Perthes disease refers to osteonecrosis of the femoral head in children; **idiopathic osteonecrosis** occurs in a similar location in adults. In both conditions, collapse of the femoral head may create joint incongruity and eventual severe osteoarthritis. Collapse of the subchondral bone results from several mechanisms:

- Necrotic bone may sustain stress fractures and compaction over a long period.
- The portion peripheral to the necrotic bone may undergo neovascularization. On radiologic examination, there is a lucent area surrounding the necrotic zone.
- The rigid articular cartilage and subchondral bone may actually crack as the subchondral necrotic zone collapses, producing a fracture.

REACTIVE BONE FORMATION

Reactive bone describes intramembranous bone formed in response to stress on bone or soft tissue. Conditions such as tumors, infections, trauma, generalized disorders, or focal disease can stimulate bone formation.

Table 22-1

Causes of Osteonecrosis

Trauma, including fracture and surgery
Emboli, producing focal bone infarction
Systemic diseases, such as polycythemia, lupus erythematosus, Gaucher disease, sickle cell disease, and gout
Radiation, either internal or external
Corticosteroid administration
Specific focal bone necrosis at various sites—for instance, in the head of the femur (Legg–Calvé–Perthes disease) or in the navicular bone (Köhler disease)
Organ transplantation, particularly renal, in patients with persistent hyperparathyroidism
Osteochondritis dissecans, a condition of unknown etiology in which a piece of articular cartilage and subchondral bone breaks off into a joint. It is thought that a focal area of bone necrosis occurs and eventually detaches.
Autografts and allografts
Thrombosis of local vessels secondary to the pressure of adjacent tumors or other space-occupying lesions
Idiopathic factors, as in the high incidence of osteonecrosis of the head and the femur in alcoholics. Necrotic bone heals differently in the cortex and in the underlying coarse cancellous bone.

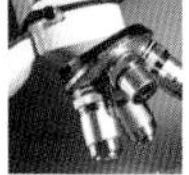

PATHOLOGY: The periosteum may respond with a so-called **sunburst** pattern (Fig. 22-9), as seen with certain tumors, or progressive layering of the periosteum, which yields an **onionskin pattern** of the cortex. The endosteal, that is, the marrow surface, may produce new bone, so that on radiologic studies, the cortex appears to be thickened, and the coarse cancellous bone is denser.

Reactive bone may be either woven or lamellar, depending on the rates of deposition of the reactive bone. Around an indolent infection, as in chronic osteomyelitis, reactive bone may be laid down de novo as lamellar bone from the

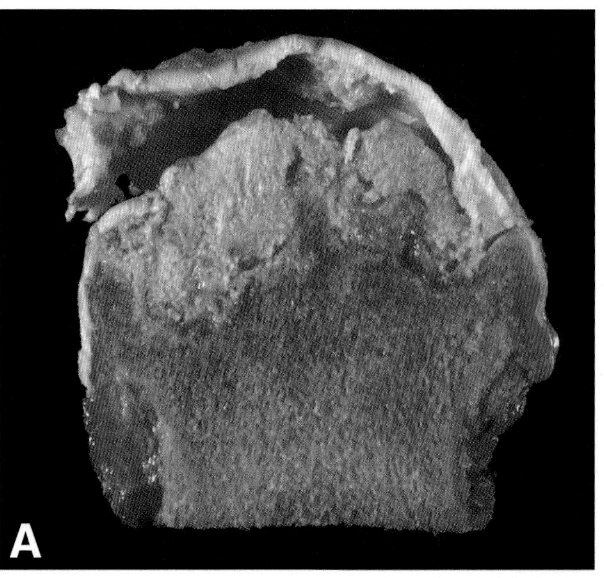

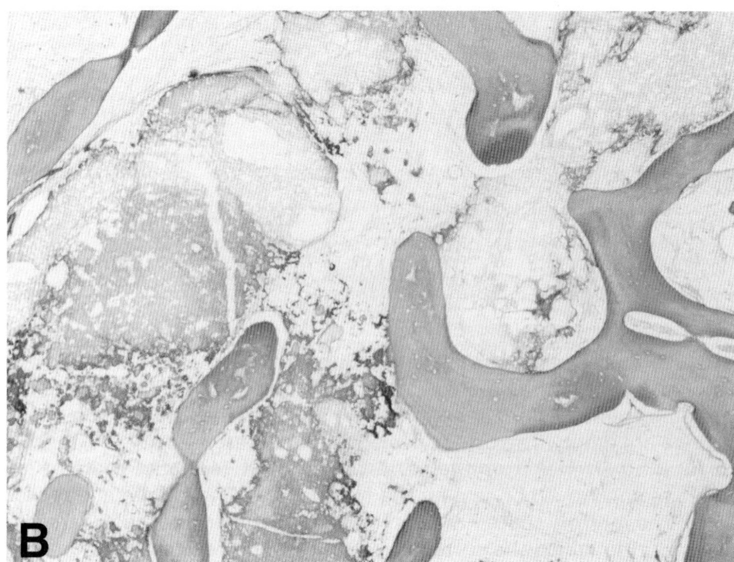

FIGURE 22-8. Osteonecrosis of the head of the femur. A. A coronal section showing a circumscribed area of subchondral infarction with partial detachment of the overlying articular cartilage and subarticular bone. **B.** Microscopically, the necrotic bone is characterized by empty lacunae, and the necrotic marrow shows dystrophic calcification.

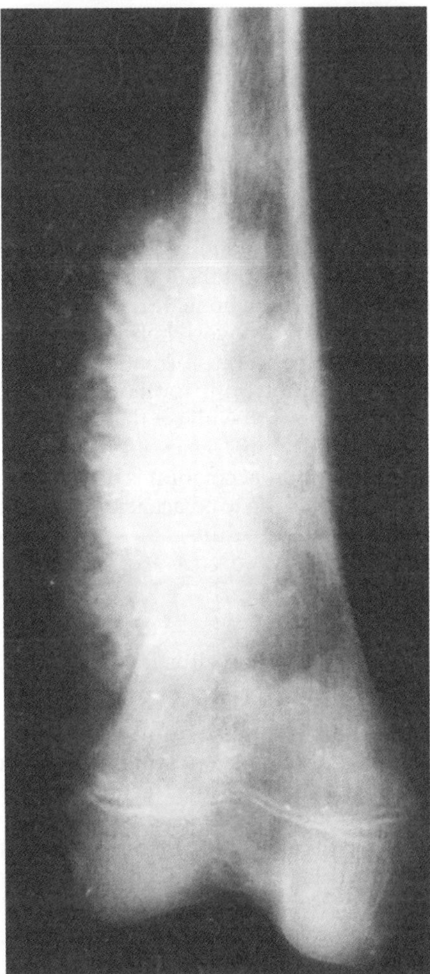

FIGURE 22-9. Reactive bone formation. A radiograph of a resected femur bearing an osteosarcoma showing a sunburst pattern of hyperdense new bone in the distal diaphysis and metaphysis. This radiodensity is because of woven bone produced by the sarcoma and the periosteal reaction of the host bone. The epiphyseal plate is represented as a transverse lucent line that separates the metaphysis from the epiphysis. The radiating radiodense bone extends beyond the periosteum into the soft tissues, obscuring the underlying bone architecture.

periosteum. In this case, the bone has time to respond to the persistent stress. Similarly, a benign tumor may cause a lamellar bone reaction. By contrast, a rapidly enlarging tumor is more likely to promote woven bone. Invariably, reactive bone is of the intramembranous type because it is derived from the periosteum or the endosteal tissue of the marrow.

Heterotopic Ossification

HO is formation of reactive bone (woven or lamellar) in extraskeletal sites, such as the skin, subcutaneous tissue, skeletal muscle, and fibroconnective tissue around joints. HO is not associated with any metabolic disease, and patients have normal serum calcium and phosphorous levels. The disorder occurs in five major clinical settings: genetic, post-traumatic, neurogenic, postsurgical, and as distinctive reactive lesions, such as **myositis ossificans** (see below). A genetic disorder known as **fibrodysplasia ossificans progressiva** is characterized by massive deposits of bone around multiple joints. HO may form in hematomas or skeletal muscle after trauma. Neurogenic HO occurs in muscle and periarticular fibrous tissue at multiple sites in patients with head trauma, spinal cord injury, or prolonged coma. HO can also form in periarticular soft tissue following joint surgery.

Myositis Ossificans

Myositis ossificans is a distinctive form of heterotopic ossification that affects young people and, although it is entirely benign, often mimics a malignant neoplasm. It is a self-limited process and carries an excellent prognosis. Spontaneous regression has been observed. No treatment is required once the diagnosis is established.

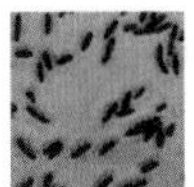

ETIOLOGIC FACTORS: The lesion typically results from blunt trauma to the muscle and soft tissues, usually of the lower limb. However, some cases occur spontaneously. Peripheral neovascularization and fibrosis at the site of damaged tissue, together with associated hemorrhage, lead in a short time to bone spicule formation. Because myositis ossificans often occurs near a bone, such as the femur or tibia, it may be misdiagnosed on radiography as a malignant bone-forming tumor.

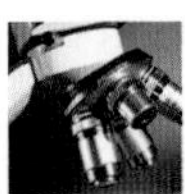

PATHOLOGY: Histologically, woven bone is formed within granulation tissue and reactive fibrous tissue (Fig. 22-10B). The center of an early lesion of myositis

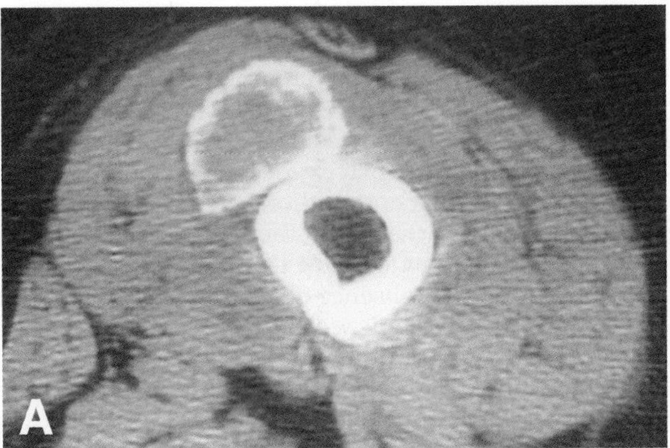

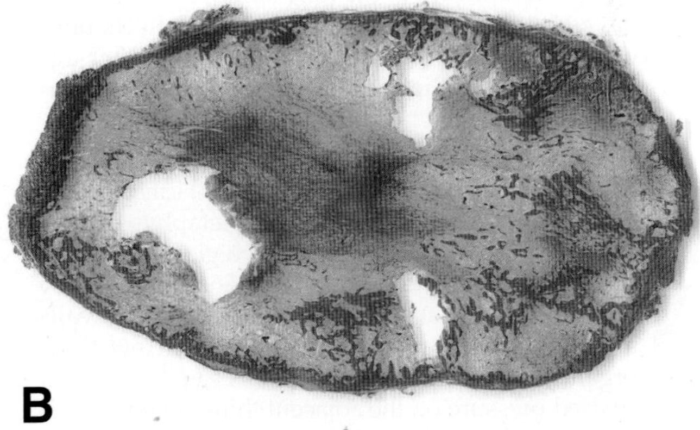

FIGURE 22-10. Myositis ossificans. A. Computed tomography scan of the thigh showing an axial view of an ovoid, intramuscular mass adjacent to the femoral cortex with a radiolucent center and ossification that becomes denser at the periphery. **B.** The mass at low-power magnification with woven bone at the periphery and fibrous tissue in the center.

ossificans is characterized by proliferating fibroblasts and more peripheral osteoblastic cells that begin to form woven bone. The fibroblasts are often cytologically atypical and show abundant mitoses, a histologic appearance that resembles a malignant tumor. ***The key feature that distinguishes myositis ossificans from a neoplasm is that the bone matures peripherally, but in the center of the lesion, it is immature or not formed at all.*** The phenomenon of peripheral maturity with central immaturity, the **zonation effect**, clearly indicates a reactive process. In a well-developed lesion, this phenomenon may be seen radiographically (Fig. 22-10). A neoplasm has an opposite zonation effect; the most mature tissue of the tumor is located centrally.

The growth pattern of myositis ossificans reflects the ingrowth of neovascular tissue from the periphery into the center of the damaged area. In the late stages, the lesion may contain cartilage and even lamellar bone.

INFECTIONS

Osteomyelitis

Any infectious agent may be responsible for involvement of bone, but the most common pathogens are *Staphylococcus* sp. (60% to 80%). Other organisms, such as *Escherichia coli*, *Neisseria gonorrhoeae*, *Haemophilus influenzae*, and *Salmonella* sp., are also seen. The organisms gain entry either via the bloodstream or by direct introduction into the bone.

Direct Penetration

Infection of bone by direct penetration or extension of bacteria is now the most common cause of osteomyelitis in the United States. Bacterial organisms are introduced directly into bone by penetrating wounds, open fractures, or surgery. Although staphylococci and streptococci are still commonly incriminated, in 25% of postoperative infections, anaerobic organisms are detected. Rarely, a Gram-negative organism may seed a hip after urologic or gastrointestinal surgery or instrumentation.

Hematogenous Osteomyelitis

Infectious organisms may reach the bone from a focus elsewhere in the body through the bloodstream. Often, the focus itself (e.g., a skin pustule or infected teeth and gums) poses little threat.

The most common sites affected by hematogenous osteomyelitis are the metaphyses of the long bones, such as in the knee, ankle, and hip. The infection principally affects boys aged 5 to 15 years, but it is occasionally seen in older age groups as well. Drug addicts may develop hematogenous osteomyelitis from infected needles.

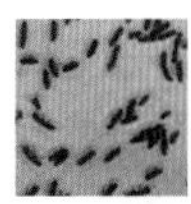

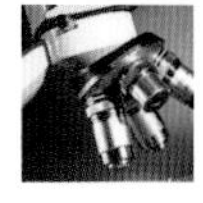

ETIOLOGIC FACTORS AND PATHOLOGY: Hematogenous osteomyelitis primarily affects the metaphyseal area. The unique vascular supply in this region (Fig. 22-11) permits slowing and sludging of blood flow, thereby allowing bacteria to penetrate blood vessel walls and establish infective foci within the marrow. If the organism is virulent and continues to proliferate, it creates increased pressure on the adjacent thin-walled vessels because they lie in the closed marrow cavity. Such pressure further compromises the vascular supply in this region and produces bone necrosis. The necrotic areas coalesce into an avascular zone and so facilitate further bacterial proliferation.

If infection is not contained, pus and bacteria extend into the endosteal vascular channels that supply the cortex and spread throughout the Volkmann and Haversian canals of the cortex. Eventually, pus forms underneath the periosteum, shearing off the perforating arteries of the periosteum and further devitalizing the cortex. Eventually, pus penetrates the periosteum and the skin to form a draining sinus (Fig. 22-11D).

Periosteal new bone formation and reactive bone formation in the marrow tend to wall off the infection. At the same time, osteoclastic activity resorbs bone. If the infection is virulent, this attempt to contain it is overwhelmed and races through the bone, with virtually no bone formation but extensive bone necrosis. More commonly, pluripotent cells modulate into osteoblasts in an attempt to wall off the infection.

In very young children (1-year-old or younger) afflicted with osteomyelitis, the adjacent joint is often involved (septic arthritis). Spread of infection to adjacent joints and subchondral bone regions also occur in adults.

Complications

The complications of osteomyelitis include the following:

- **Septicemia:** Dissemination of organisms through the bloodstream may occur as a result of bone infection. It is unusual for osteomyelitis to result from septicemia.
- **Acute bacterial arthritis:** Joint infection is secondary to osteomyelitis at all ages and represents a medical emergency. Direct digestion of cartilage by inflammatory cells destroys the articular cartilage and produces osteoarthritis. Rapid intervention to prevent this complication is mandatory.
- **Pathologic fractures:** Osteomyelitis may lead to fractures, which heal poorly and may require surgical drainage.
- **Squamous cell carcinoma:** This cancer develops in the bone or the sinus tract of long-standing chronic osteomyelitis, often years after the initial infection. In such cases, squamous tissue arises from the epithelialization of the sinus tract and eventually undergoes malignant transformation.
- **Amyloidosis:** Historically, amyloidosis was a common consequence of chronic osteomyelitis but is now rare in industrialized countries.
- **Chronic osteomyelitis:** Chronic osteomyelitis may follow acute osteomyelitis. It is difficult to treat, especially if it involves the entire bone, because necrotic bone or sequestra function as foreign bodies in avascular areas, and antibiotics do not reach the bacteria. Chronic osteomyelitis is, therefore, treated symptomatically with surgery or antibiotics for the duration of the patient's life.

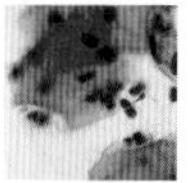

CLINICAL FEATURES: Hematogenous osteomyelitis in children occurs as a sudden illness, with fever and systemic toxicity, or as a subacute illness in which local manifestations predominate. Swelling, erythema, and tenderness over the involved bone are characteristic. The leukocyte count is often conspicuously increased, although the absence of leukocytosis does not rule out the disease. Radiologic workup, including radiography, computed tomography (CT), magnetic resonance imaging (MRI), and bone scan, are very helpful. Bone biopsy is necessary for a definitive diagnosis because it provides material for histologic examination, microbiologic culture, and antibiotic sensitivity.

The treatment of hematogenous osteomyelitis depends on the stage of the infection. Early osteomyelitis is treated with

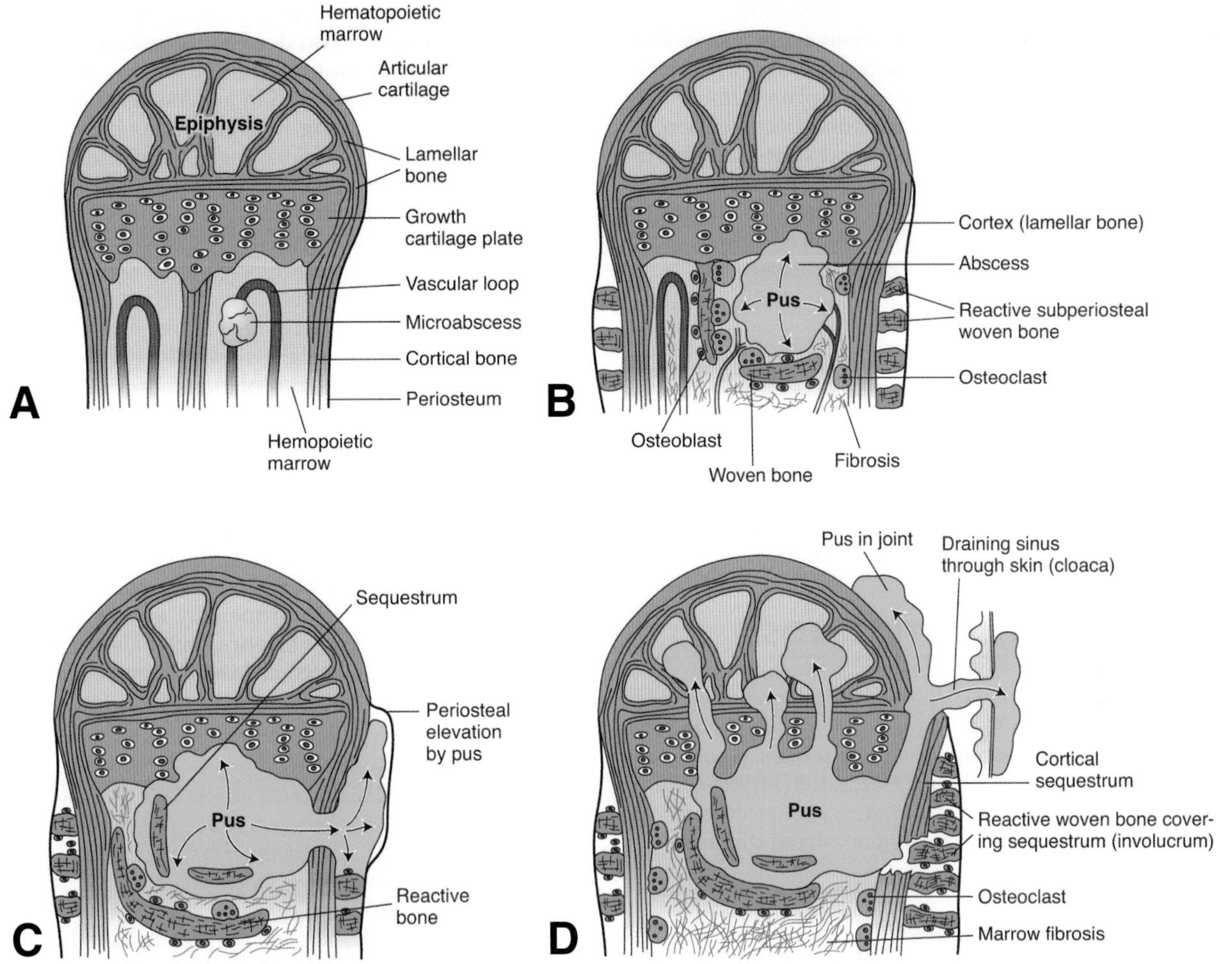

FIGURE 22-11. Pathogenesis of hematogenous osteomyelitis. A. The epiphysis, metaphysis, and growth plate are normal. A small, septic microabscess is forming at the capillary loop. **B.** Expansion of the septic focus stimulates resorption of adjacent bony trabeculae. **Woven bone** begins to surround this focus. The abscess expands into the cartilage and stimulates reactive bone formation by the periosteum. **C.** The **abscess**, which continues to expand through the cortex into the subperiosteal tissue, shears off the perforating arteries that supply the cortex with blood, thereby leading to necrosis of the cortex. **D.** The extension of this process into the joint space, the epiphysis, and the skin produces a **draining sinus**. The necrotic bone is called a **sequestrum**. The viable bone surrounding a sequestrum is termed the **involucrum**.

intravenous antibiotics for 6 weeks or more. Surgery is used to drain and decompress the infection within the bone or to drain abscesses that do not respond to antibiotic therapy. In long-standing, chronic osteomyelitis, antibiotics alone are not curative, and extensive surgical debridement of necrotic bone is often required.

Tuberculosis of Bone

Tuberculosis of bone usually originates in the lungs or lymph nodes (see Chapter 10). The mycobacteria spread to the bone hematogenously, and, only rarely, is there direct spread from the lungs or lymph nodes.

Tuberculous Spondylitis (Pott Disease)

Tuberculous spondylitis (i.e., infection of the spine) is a feared complication of childhood tuberculosis. The disease affects vertebral bodies, sparing the lamina, spines, and adjacent vertebrae (Fig. 22-12). Thoracic vertebrae are usually affected, especially the 11th thoracic vertebra. As a result of currently available effective antibiotic treatment, Pott disease is now rare.

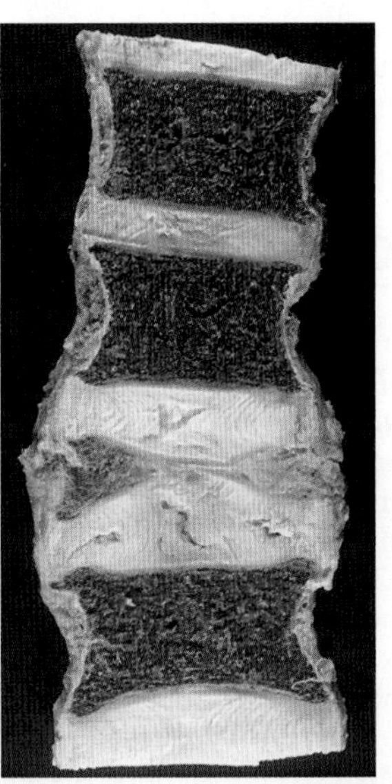

FIGURE 22-12. Tuberculous spondylitis (Pott disease). A vertebral body is almost completely replaced by tuberculous tissue. Note the preservation of the intervertebral disks.

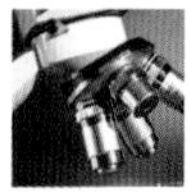

PATHOLOGY: The pathology in tuberculous spondylitis is similar to that of tuberculosis at other sites. The granulomas first produce caseous necrosis of the bone marrow, resulting in slow resorption of bony trabeculae and, occasionally, to cystic spaces in the bone. Because there is little or no reactive bone formation, affected vertebrae tend to collapse, leading to kyphosis and scoliosis. The intervertebral disk is crushed and destroyed by the compression fracture, rather than by invasion of organisms. The typical "hunchback" of bygone days was often the victim of Pott disease.

Syphilis of Bone

Syphilis causes a slowly progressive, chronic, inflammatory disease of bone, characterized by granulomas, necrosis, and marked reactive bone formation. It may be acquired through sexual contact or transmitted transplacentally from mother to fetus (see Chapter 16). The bone changes in syphilis depend on the patient's age and include endosteal and periosteal changes, and the presence or absence of gummas.

LANGERHANS CELL HISTIOCYTOSIS

Langerhans cell histiocytosis (LCH) is a generic term (previously referred to as **histiocytosis X**) for three entities characterized by proliferation of Langerhans cells in various tissues: (1) **eosinophilic granuloma**, a localized form; (2) **Hand–Schüller–Christian disease**, a disseminated variant; and (3) **Letterer–Siwe disease**, a fulminant and often fatal generalized disease (see Chapter 18).

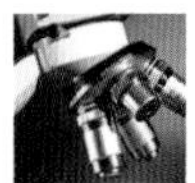

PATHOLOGY: The histologic appearance of the bones in all three variants of LCH is identical and is characterized by collections of large, histiocytic cells with pale, eosinophilic cytoplasm, and convoluted or grooved nuclei (see Fig. 18-45). There are many eosinophils throughout these lesions, occasionally forming collections called "eosinophilic abscesses." Multinucleated **osteoclastic** giant cells are often observed, as are chronic inflammatory cells and neutrophils. Radiologic findings in the bones in all three diseases are identical. The lesions may occur in the metaphysis or diaphysis of long bones, or in a flat bone, especially in the skull. Punched-out lytic defects, with virtually no reactive bone, may precipitate fractures and periosteal callus formation.

OSTEOPOROSIS

Osteoporosis is a metabolic bone disease in which the mass of normally mineralized bone is decreased to the point that it no longer provides adequate mechanical support. The remaining bone has a normal ratio of mineralized and nonmineralized (i.e., osteoid) matrix. Regardless of the underlying causes, bone loss and, eventually, fractures are the hallmarks of osteoporosis (Figs. 22-13 and 22-14). The etiology for bone loss is diverse but includes menopause, smoking, vitamin D deficiency, low body mass index, hypogonadism, a sedentary lifestyle, and glucocorticoid therapy.

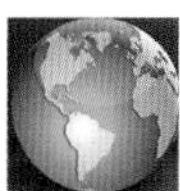

EPIDEMIOLOGY: Osteoporosis and its complications are important public health problems that are expected to expand as life expectancy increases. Bone mass normally peaks between the ages of 25 and 35 and begins to decline in the fifth or sixth decade. Bone loss with age occurs in all races, but because of higher peak bone mass, blacks are less prone to osteoporosis than are Asians and whites. Bone loss during normal aging in women has been divided into two phases: menopause and aging. The latter affects both men and women. At a certain point, the loss of bone suffices to justify the label **osteoporosis** and renders weight-bearing bones susceptible to fractures. The most common fractures occur in the neck and intertrochanteric region of the femur (**hip fracture**; Fig. 22-14), vertebral bodies, and distal radius (**Colles fracture**). In whites in the United States, 15% of people have had a hip fracture by the age of 80 years and 25% by age 90. Women have twice the risk of hip fracture as men, although among blacks and some Asian populations, the incidence is equal among the sexes. Compared with other osteoporotic fractures, hip fractures incur the greatest morbidity, mortality (up to 20% within a year), and direct medical costs. The female predominance of 8:1 is particularly striking for vertebral fractures. A subset of women in the early postmenopausal years is at particular risk of vertebral fractures, which are rare in middle-aged men. The propensity of men to sustain hip fractures as opposed to vertebral ones also reflects factors other than bone mass, such as loss of proprioception.

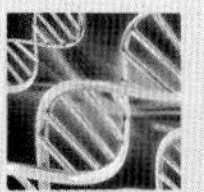

ETIOLOGIC FACTORS AND MOLECULAR PATHOGENESIS: *Regardless of the cause of osteoporosis, it always reflects enhanced bone resorption relative to formation.* Bone resorption and bone formation exist simultaneously. Persons younger than 35 or 40 years completely replace bone resorbed during the remodeling cycle. With age, less bone is replaced in osteoclast associated resorption bays than is removed, leading to a small deficit at each remodeling site. Given the thousands of remodeling sites in the skeleton, net bone loss, even in a short time, can be substantial.

Osteoporosis is classified as either primary or secondary. **Primary osteoporosis**, by far the more common variety, occurs principally in postmenopausal women (type 1) and elderly people of both sexes (type 2). **Secondary osteoporosis** is a disorder associated with a defined cause, including a variety of endocrine and genetic abnormalities.

Type 1 primary osteoporosis is caused by an absolute increase in osteoclast activity. Because osteoclasts initiate bone remodeling, the number of remodeling sites increases, a phenomenon known as **increased activation frequency**.

The increase in osteoclasts in the early postmenopausal skeleton is a direct result of estrogen withdrawal. The lack of estrogen is not targeted directly to the osteoclast, but rather to cells derived from marrow stroma, which secrete cytokines that recruit osteoclasts. These cytokines, which are believed to be estrogen sensitive, include IL-1, IL-6, TNF, and M-CSF.

Type 2 primary osteoporosis, also called **senile osteoporosis**, has a more complex pathogenesis than does type 1. Type 2 osteoporosis generally appears after age 70 and reflects decreased osteoblast function. Thus, although osteoclast activity is no longer increased, the number of osteoblasts and amount of bone produced per cell are insufficient to replace bone removed in the resorptive phase of the remodeling cycle.

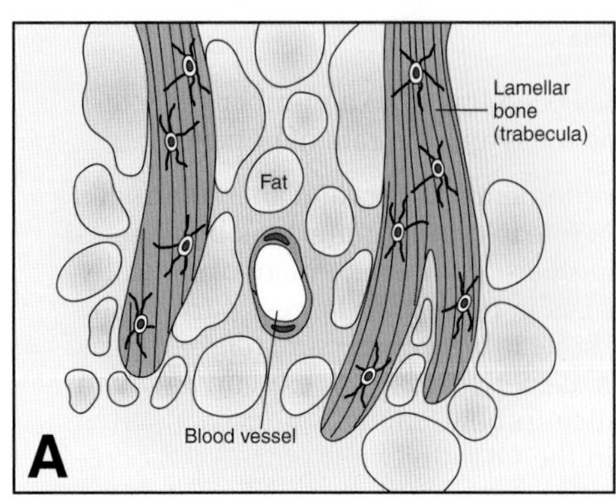

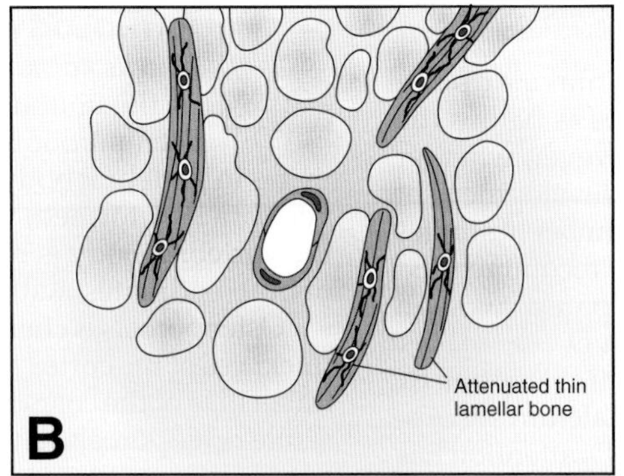

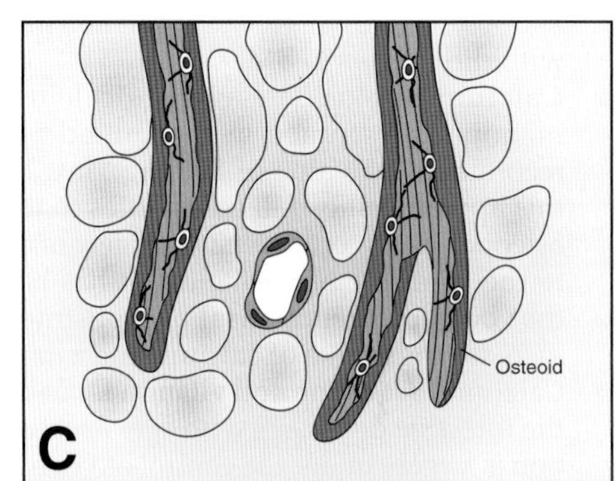

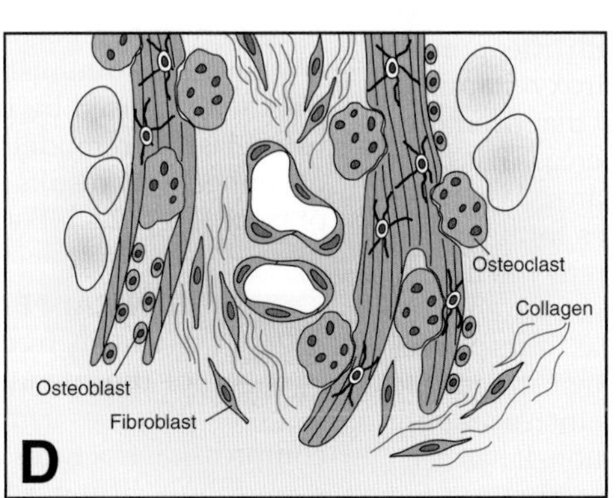

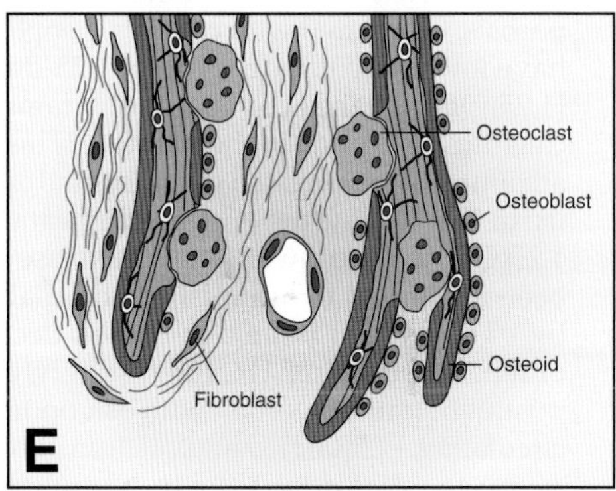

FIGURE 22-13. Metabolic bone diseases. A. Normal trabecular bone and fatty marrow. The trabecular bone is lamellar and contains evenly distributed osteocytes. **B. Osteoporosis.** The lamellar bone trabeculae are discontinuous and thin. **C. Osteomalacia.** The lamellar bone trabeculae have abnormal amounts of nonmineralized bone (osteoid). These osteoid seams are thickened and cover a larger-than-normal area of the trabecular bone surface. **D. Primary hyperparathyroidism.** The lamellar bone trabeculae are actively resorbed by numerous osteoclasts that bore into each trabecula. The appearance of osteoclasts dissecting into the trabeculae, a process termed **dissecting osteitis**, is diagnostic of hyperparathyroidism. Osteoblastic activity also is pronounced. The marrow is replaced by fibrous tissue adjacent to the trabeculae. **E. Renal osteodystrophy.** The morphologic appearance is similar to that of primary hyperparathyroidism, except that prominent osteoid covers the trabeculae. Osteoclasts do not resorb unmineralized bone, and wherever an osteoid seam is lacking, osteoclasts bore into the trabeculae. Osteoblastic activity is also prominent.

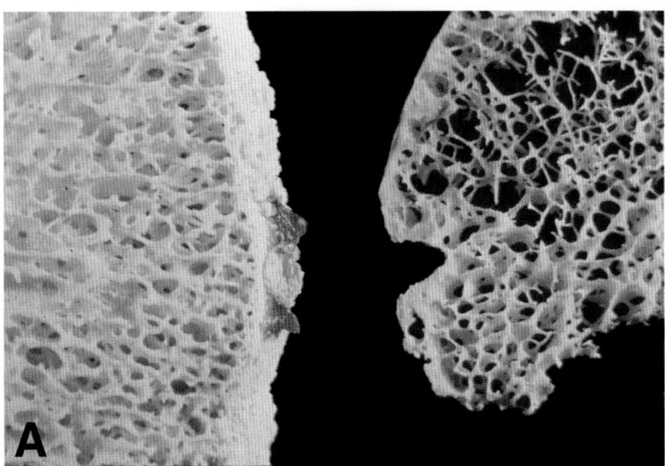

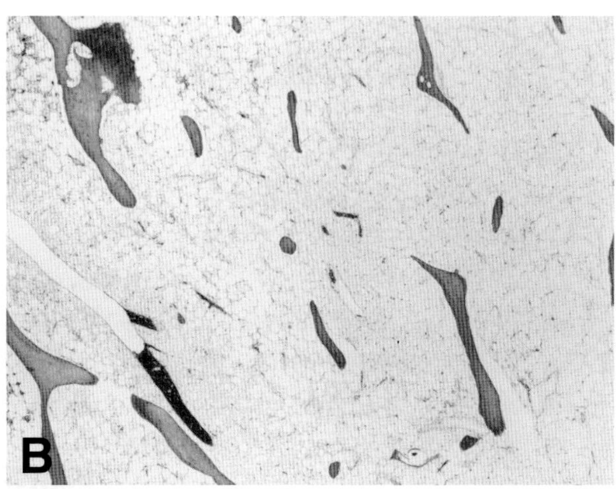

FIGURE 22-14. Osteoporosis. A. Femoral head of an 82-year-old female with osteoporosis and a femoral neck fracture (*right*) compared with a normal control cut to the same thickness (*left*). **B.** Microscopically, there is reduction in the size and thickness of bone trabeculae and loss of connectivity.

Primary Osteoporosis

Primary osteoporosis has been linked to a number of factors that influence peak bone mass and the rate of bone loss:

- **Genetic factors:** Environmental factors and an individual's genotype both play a role in determining peak bone mass and the risk of osteoporosis. The development of clinically significant osteoporosis is related, in largest part, to the maximal amount of bone in a given person, referred to as the **peak bone mass**. Genetic variations explain as much as 70% of the variance in bone mineral density (BMD). Sequence variance in the vitamin D receptor, *Col1A1* collagen gene, estrogen receptor-α, IL-6, and low-density lipoprotein receptor–related protein-5 (LRP5) are associated with differences in BMD.
- **Calcium intake:** The average calcium intake of postmenopausal women in the United States is below the recommended value of 800 mg/day. However, whether this apparent shortfall contributes to the development of osteoporosis is controversial, in view of a number of studies to the contrary. Nevertheless, it has been recommended that both premenopausal and postmenopausal women increase the intake of calcium and vitamin D.
- **Calcium absorption and vitamin D:** Calcium absorption by the intestine decreases with age. Because calcium absorption is largely under the control of vitamin D, attention has been directed to the role of this steroid hormone in osteoporosis. Compared with controls, people with osteoporosis have lower circulating levels of 1,25-dihydroxyvitamin D [$1,25(OH)_2D$], the active form of vitamin D that promotes calcium absorption in the intestine. This decrease has been attributed to age-related decreases in 1α-hydroxylase activity in the kidney, the enzyme that catalyzes formation of $1,25(OH)_2D$. The lower 1α-hydroxylase activity has in turn been attributed to diminished stimulation of the enzyme by PTH, as well as an age-related decrease in responses of renal tubules to PTH. Interestingly, giving estrogens to postmenopausal women with osteoporosis increases both circulating $1,25(OH)_2D$ and calcium absorption. It has been suggested that decreased 1α-hydroxylase activity in the kidney may stimulate PTH secretion and so contribute to bone resorption.
- **Exercise:** Physical activity is necessary to maintain bone mass, and athletes often have increased bone mass. By contrast, immobilization of a bone (e.g., prolonged bed rest, application of a cast) elicits accelerated bone loss.
- **Environmental factors:** Cigarette smoking in women has been correlated with an increased incidence of osteoporosis. It is possible that the decreased level of active estrogens produced by smoking is responsible for this effect.

In summary, the two major determinants of primary osteoporosis are estrogen deficiency in postmenopausal women and the aging process in both sexes. The possible mechanisms for these effects are summarized in Figure 22-15.

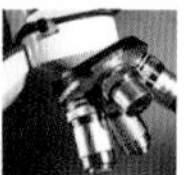

PATHOLOGY: ***The ratio of osteoid and mineralized bone is normal in persons with osteoporosis.*** Because of the abundance of cancellous bone in the spine, osteoporotic changes are generally most conspicuous there. In vertebral body fractures caused by osteoporosis, the vertebra is deformed, with anterior wedging and collapse. If the vertebral body is not fractured, there is a general outline of both endplates, with a virtual absence of cancellous bone.

Osteoporosis is characterized histologically by a decreased thickness of the cortex and reduction in the number and size of trabeculae of the coarse cancellous bone (Fig. 22-14). Although senile osteoporosis tends to feature reduced trabecular thickness, postmenopausal osteoporosis exhibits disrupted connections between trabeculae. The loss of trabecular connectivity is attended by diminished biomechanical strength. Ultimately, fracture is caused by perforation of trabeculae by resorbing osteoclasts in remodeling sites. In histologic sections, the loss of connectivity results in the appearance of "isolated" islands of bone (Figs. 22-13B and 22-14B).

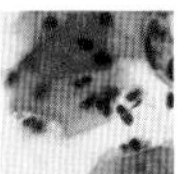

CLINICAL FEATURES: Postmenopausal osteoporosis is usually recognizable within 10 years after the onset of the menopause; senile osteoporosis generally becomes symptomatic after age 70 years. Vertebral compression fractures often occur after trivial trauma or may even follow lifting a heavy object. With each compression fracture, the patient becomes shorter and develops kyphosis (**Dowager hump**).

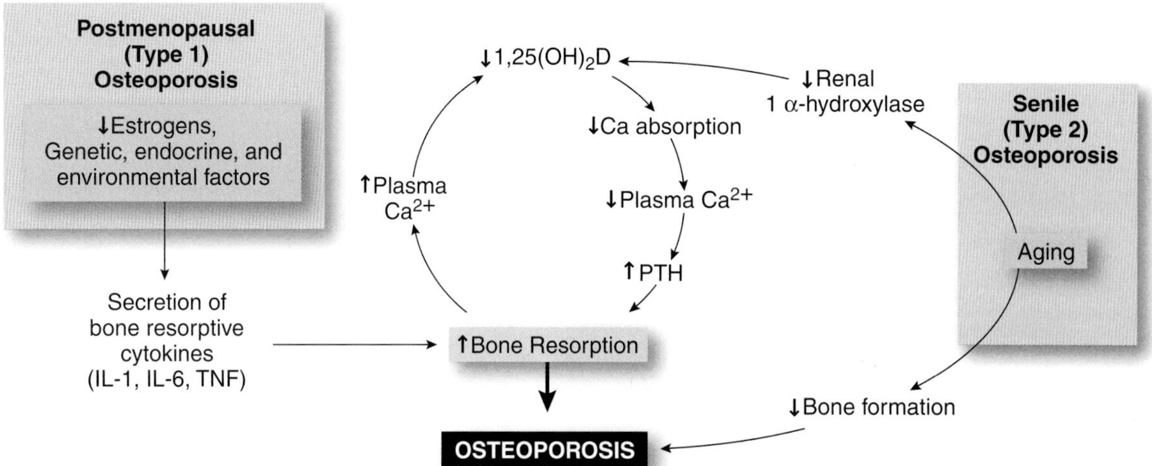

FIGURE 22-15. Pathogenesis of primary osteoporosis. Ca^{2+}, calcium; IL, interleukin; PTH, parathyroid hormone; TNF, tumor necrosis factor.

Estrogen therapy is an effective yet controversial means of preventing postmenopausal osteoporosis. Because hormone treatment carries with it increased risks of breast and endometrial cancers, other bone-specific antiosteoporosis drugs have been developed. **Bisphosphonates** are currently the most popular therapeutic agents used. All successful drugs thus far developed block or slow the rate of bone resorption but do not stimulate bone formation. Thus, treatment may prevent disease progression but cannot cure a patient who already has osteoporosis. Dietary calcium supplementation in elderly patients reduces the risk of osteoporotic fractures by half.

Secondary Osteoporosis

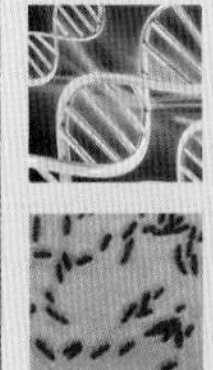

ETIOLOGIC FACTORS AND MOLECULAR PATHOGENESIS: Causes of secondary osteoporosis include adverse effects of drug therapy, endocrine abnormalities, eating disorders, immobilization, marrow-related conditions, diseases of the gastrointestinal or biliary tracts, renal insufficiency, and cancer.

- **Endocrine conditions:** The most common form of secondary osteoporosis is iatrogenic and results from corticosteroid administration. Bone loss may also result from an excess of endogenous glucocorticoids, as in Cushing disease (see Chapter 19). Corticosteroids inhibit osteoblastic activity, thereby reducing bone formation. They also impair vitamin D–dependent, intestinal calcium absorption, an effect that leads to increased secretion of PTH and enhanced bone resorption.
- **Hyperparathyroidism** induces osteoclast recruitment and increased osteoclastic activity, resulting in secondary osteoporosis.
- **Hyperthyroidism** increases osteoclastic activity and causes accelerated turnover of bone. Although thyrotoxicosis is associated with some cases of secondary osteoporosis, bone loss is limited (Fig. 22-13D).
- **Hypogonadism** in both men and women is accompanied by osteoporosis and contributes to bone loss in 25% of elderly males. Decreased bone density follows androgen deprivation therapy for prostatic cancer.
- **Hematologic malignancies:** A variety of hematologic cancers, particularly multiple myeloma, are accompanied by significant bone loss.
- **Malabsorption:** Gastrointestinal and hepatic diseases that cause malabsorption often contribute to osteoporosis, probably because of impaired absorption of calcium, phosphate, and vitamin D.
- **Alcoholism:** Chronic alcohol abuse also has been linked to the development of osteoporosis. Excess alcohol is a direct inhibitor of osteoblasts and may also inhibit calcium absorption.

OSTEOMALACIA AND RICKETS

Osteomalacia (soft bones) *is a disorder of adults characterized by inadequate mineralization of newly formed bone matrix.* **Rickets** *refers to a similar condition in children, in whom the growth plates (physes) are open.* Thus, children with rickets manifest defective mineralization not only of bone (osteomalacia) but also of the cartilaginous matrix of the growth plate. Diverse conditions associated with osteomalacia and rickets include abnormalities in vitamin D metabolism, phosphate deficiency states, and defects in the mineralization process itself (Fig. 22-13C).

Vitamin D Metabolism

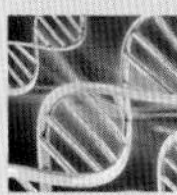

MOLECULAR PATHOGENESIS: Vitamin D is ingested in food or synthesized in the skin from 7-dehydrocholesterol under the influence of ultraviolet light (Fig. 22-16). The vitamin is first hydroxylated in the liver to form its major circulating metabolite, 25-hydroxyvitamin D, then hydroxylated again in proximal renal tubules to produce the active hormone, $1,25(OH)_2D$. Exposure to sunlight provides sufficient vitamin D for bone growth and mineralization, even if there is an inadequate dietary source.

Receptors for $1,25(OH)_2D$ are present not only in classic targets, such as the intestine, bone, and kidney, but also in many other cell types. This hormone is a general inducer of differentiation. For example, it influences maturation of hematopoietic and dermal cells, as well as that of many cancers. In the intestine, $1,25(OH)_2D$ stimulates calcium and phosphate absorption. It is also essential for osteoclast maturation. Regardless of mechanism, $1,25(OH)_2D$, in concert

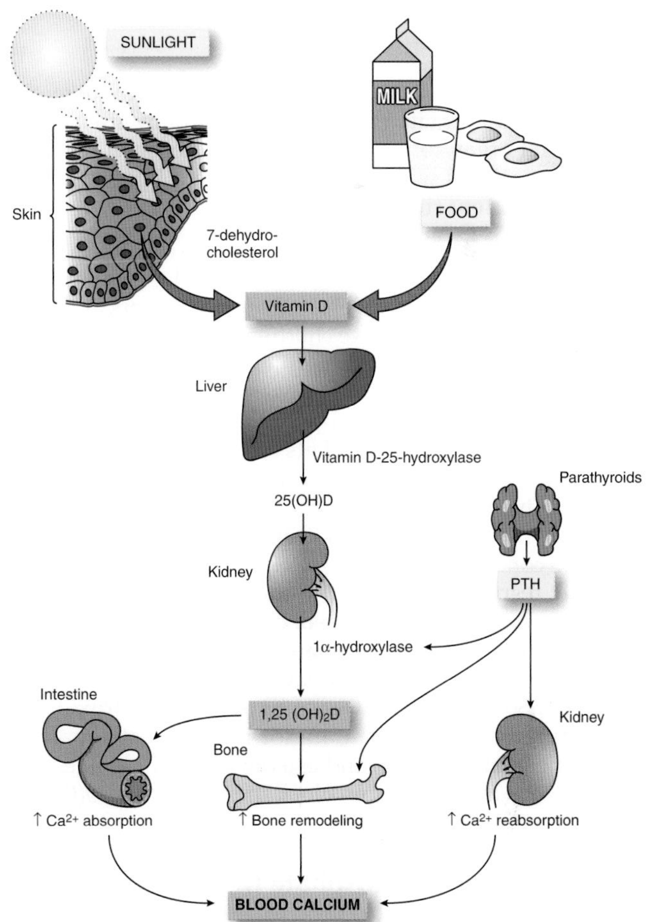

FIGURE 22-16. Metabolism of vitamin D and the regulation of blood calcium. Ca^{2+}, calcium; PTH, parathyroid hormone.

with PTH, maintains blood calcium and phosphate at levels that are required for proper mineralization of bone. ***The key determinant of the formation of 1,25(OH)$_2$D is blood calcium concentration.*** Decreases in blood calcium stimulate the release of PTH, which augments renal synthesis of 1,25(OH)$_2$D.

Hypovitaminosis D can result from (1) inadequate exposure to sunlight; (2) deficient dietary intake, which is now uncommon in Western countries; or (3) defective intestinal absorption. There are also hereditary and acquired disorders of vitamin D metabolism.

Intestinal Malabsorption

In industrialized countries, diseases associated with intestinal malabsorption cause osteomalacia more often than does poor nutrition. ***Intrinsic diseases of the small intestine, cholestatic disorders of the liver, biliary obstruction, and chronic pancreatic insufficiency all impair intestinal absorption and are the most frequent causes of osteomalacia in the United States.***

Malabsorption of vitamin D and calcium complicates a number of inherent small-intestinal diseases, including celiac disease, Crohn disease, scleroderma, and the postsurgical blind-loop syndrome. In obstructive jaundice, the lack of bile salts in the intestine impairs absorption of lipids and lipid-soluble substances, among which is fat-soluble vitamin D.

Disorders of Vitamin D Metabolism

Vitamin D metabolism can be disturbed either by defective 1α-hydroxylation of vitamin D in the kidney or by insensitivity of the target organ to the vitamin. Two autosomal recessive diseases associated with rickets are together known as **vitamin D–dependent rickets**.

- **Vitamin D–dependent rickets type I** results from an inherited deficiency of renal 1α-hydroxylase activity. The clinical and biochemical changes of rickets appear during the first year of life. These children exhibit hypocalcemia, hypophosphatemia, and high levels of serum PTH and alkaline phosphatase. The disease is controlled by the administration of 1,25(OH)$_2$D.
- **Vitamin D–dependent rickets type II** involves inherited mutations of the vitamin D receptor, so that end organs are insensitive to 1,25(OH)$_2$D. The disease usually manifests early in life but may appear at any time up to adolescence. Serum concentrations of 1,25(OH)$_2$D are very high. Patients do not respond to 1,25(OH)$_2$D but are helped by repeated intravenous administration of calcium.
- **Acquired alterations in vitamin D metabolism** include defective renal 1α-hydroxylation and end-organ insensitivity. Some of the causes of impaired α-hydroxylation are hypoparathyroidism, tumor-induced osteomalacia, chronic renal diseases, and osteomalacia of old age. Phenobarbital and phenytoin block the action of 1,25(OH)$_2$D on target organs.

Renal Disorders of Phosphate Metabolism

Both rickets and osteomalacia may result from impaired reabsorption of phosphate by the proximal renal tubules, with resulting hypophosphatemia.

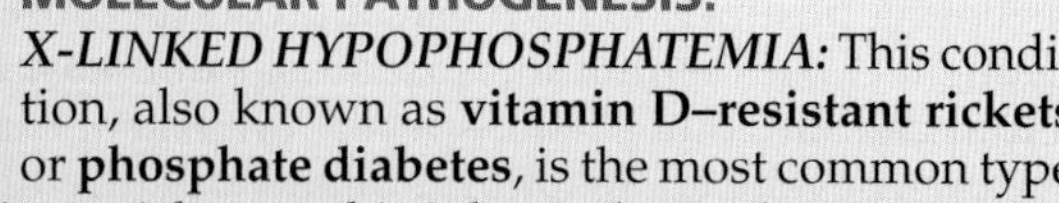

MOLECULAR PATHOGENESIS: *X-LINKED HYPOPHOSPHATEMIA:* This condition, also known as **vitamin D–resistant rickets** or **phosphate diabetes**, is the most common type of hereditary rickets and is inherited as a dominant trait. Inactivating mutations in the *PHEX* (phosphate-regulating) gene on the X chromosome (Xp22) impair transport of phosphate across the luminal membrane of proximal renal tubular cells. The gene product of *PHEX* is a protease that inactivates *FGF23* the gene for fibroblast growth factor 23, critical in plasma phosphate regulation. Thus increased levels of this factor produce renal phosphate wasting. Although renal phosphate wasting is central to the disease, osteoblast function is also impaired. In boys, florid rickets appears during childhood, but girls often suffer only hypophosphatemia. Microscopically, the bones of patients with X-linked hypophosphatemia show severe osteomalacia and wide osteoid seams. They also exhibit characteristic hypomineralized areas surrounding osteocytes, known as **halos**. Treatment consists of lifelong administration of phosphate and 1,25(OH)$_2$D.

FANCONI SYNDROMES: These inborn errors of metabolism are characterized by renal wastage of phosphate, glucose, bicarbonate, and amino acids. They are all characterized by renal tubular acidosis and lead to rickets and osteomalacia. Fanconi syndromes include Wilson disease, tyrosinemia, galactosemia, glycogen storage disease, and cystinosis. Renal tubular damage that leads to phosphate wastage may also be acquired, as in lead or mercury intoxication, amyloidosis, and Bence Jones proteinuria.

TUMOR-ASSOCIATED OSTEOMALACIA: This disorder is a phosphate-wasting syndrome that is associated with predominantly benign and occasionally malignant tumors of soft tissue and bone. The typical laboratory features are hypophosphatemia, hyperphosphaturia, low serum concentrations of 1,25-(OH)$_2$D, and elevated serum alkaline phosphatase. The paraneoplastic phosphaturic factors secreted by the tumor, known as **phosphatonins**, cause renal tubular phosphate wasting and prevent tubular conversion of 25-hydroxyvitamin D into 1,25(OH)$_2$D.

PATHOLOGY: *OSTEOMALACIA:* Osteomalacia, like osteoporosis, causes an osteopenic radiologic pattern. The only findings may be vertebral compression fractures and decreased bone thickness, as in osteoporosis. However, some specific findings may be seen in osteomalacia.

Microscopically, defective mineralization in osteomalacia results in **exaggeration of osteoid seams**, both in thickness and in the proportion of trabecular surface covered (Figs. 22-13C and 22-17). Osteoid seams reflect a time lag between the deposition of collagen and the appearance of the calcium salt.

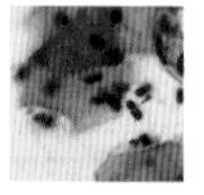

CLINICAL FEATURES: Clinical diagnosis of osteomalacia is often difficult. Patients have nonspecific complaints, such as muscle weakness or diffuse aches and pains. In mild forms of the disease, only slowly progressive changes in bone are seen, and many patients are totally asymptomatic for years. In advanced cases, poorly localized bone pain and tenderness are common, especially in the spine, pelvis, and proximal parts of the extremities.

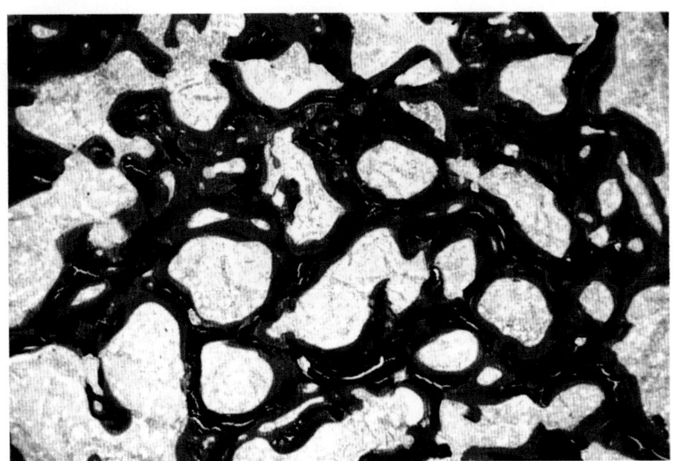

FIGURE 22-17. Osteomalacia. The surfaces of the bony trabeculae (*black*) are covered by a thicker-than-normal layer of osteoid (*red*) with the von Kossa stain, which colors calcified tissue black.

RICKETS: Rickets is a disease of children and thus causes extensive changes at the physeal plate which does not become adequately mineralized. Calcified cartilage and zones of hypertrophy and proliferative cartilage continue to grow because osteoclastic activity does not resorb the poorly mineralized growth plate cartilage. As a consequence, the growth plate is conspicuously thickened, irregular, and lobulated. Endochondral ossification proceeds very slowly and preferentially at the peripheral portions of the metaphysis. The result is a flared, cup-shaped epiphysis.

Microscopically, the growth plate exhibits striking changes. The resting zone is normal, but the zones of proliferating cartilage are greatly distorted. The ordered progression of helix-forming chondrocytes is lost and is replaced by a disorderly profusion of cells separated by small amounts of matrix. The resulting lobulated masses of proliferating and hypertrophied cartilage are associated with increasing width of the growth plate, which may be 5 to 15 times the normal width. Masses of proliferating cartilage extend into the metaphyseal region, without any apparent vascular invasion and with little osteoclastic activity.

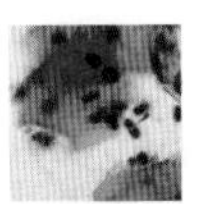

CLINICAL FEATURES: Children with rickets are apathetic and irritable and have short attention spans. They are content to be sedentary, assuming a "Buddha-like" posture. They are short, with characteristic changes of bones and teeth. Flattening of the skull, prominent frontal bones (**frontal bossing**), and conspicuous suture lines are typical. Delayed dentition is associated with severe dental caries and enamel defects. The chest has the classic **rachitic rosary**, which is a grossly beaded appearance of the costochondral junctions as a result of enlargement of the costal cartilages. Patients also display indentations of the lower ribs at the insertion of the diaphragm (Harrison groove). **Pectus carinatum** ("pigeon breast") reflects an outward curvature of the sternum.

The overall musculature is weak, and abdominal weakness generates a "potbelly." The limbs are shortened and deformed, with severe bowing of the arms and forearms and frequent fractures. The femoral head may dislocate from the growth plate (slipped capital femoral epiphysis).

PRIMARY HYPERPARATHYROIDISM

Primary hyperparathyroidism is a metabolic bone disease characterized by generalized bone resorption as a result of inappropriate secretion of PTH. *Some 90% of cases of primary hyperparathyroidism are caused by one or more parathyroid adenomas. Hyperplasia of all four glands accounts for only 10% (see also Chapter 19).* Because PTH promotes phosphate excretion in the urine and stimulates osteoclastic bone resorption, low serum phosphate and high serum calcium levels are characteristic. A familial type of primary hyperparathyroidism is associated with mutations in the calcium-sensing receptor (*CASR*) gene, located on chromosome 3 (3q13.3).

The effects of PTH are mediated by its actions on the bone, kidney, and (indirectly) intestine.

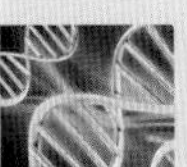

MOLECULAR PATHOGENESIS:

BONE: PTH mobilizes calcium from bone (the major reservoir of calcium in the body) by causing increased osteoclasis. This is accomplished by extant osteoclasts and by recruitment of new osteoclasts from preosteoclastic mesenchymal cells. This action is indirect and is mediated by direct stimulation of osteoblasts by PTH. As a result, osteoblasts secrete RANKL, which then binds to RANK in osteoclasts and osteoclast precursors and results in bone resorption. Under physiologic circumstances, PTH secretion is shut down by increases in ionic calcium. At the same time, the osteoblast stimulation by PTH tends to cause balanced remodeling and does not result in a net loss of bone mass. By contrast, under pathologic conditions, the release of large amounts of PTH and continued RANKL secretion prevent osteoclast apoptosis, prolong osteoclast life and activation, and induce a net loss of bone mass.

KIDNEY: PTH stimulates reabsorption of calcium by the thick ascending and granular portions of the distal renal tubules. It also enhances phosphate excretion in the proximal and distal tubules by directly inhibiting sodium-dependent phosphate transport. PTH also augments the activity of 1α-hydroxylase in the proximal tubules and stimulates production of $1,25(OH)_2D$.

INTESTINE: PTH does not act directly on the intestine, but rather enhances intestinal calcium absorption indirectly by increasing renal synthesis of $1,25(OH)_2D$.

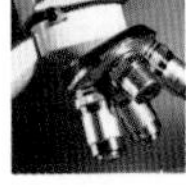

PATHOLOGY: The abnormal histologic appearance of bone in primary hyperparathyroidism is termed osteitis fibrosa. The histogenesis of the condition may be classified into three stages:

- **Early stage:** Initially, osteoclasts are stimulated by the increased PTH levels to resorb bone. From the subperiosteal and endosteal surfaces, osteoclasts bore their way into the cortex. This process is called **dissecting osteitis** because each osteon is continually hollowed out by osteoclastic activity (Figs. 22-13D and 22-18A). At the same time, collagen fibers are laid down in the endosteal marrow, and additional osteoclasts penetrate the bone.
- **Second stage:** In this stage, the trabecular bone is resorbed, and marrow is replaced by (1) loose fibrosis, (2) hemosiderin-laden macrophages, (3) areas of hemorrhage from microfractures, and (4) reactive woven bone. These features constitute the "osteitis fibrosa" portion of the complex.

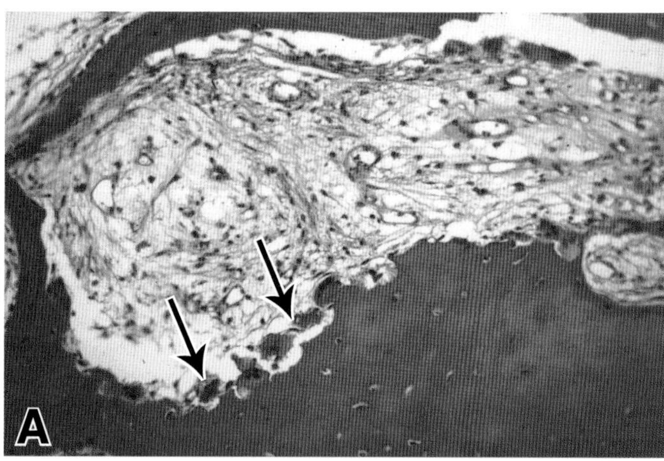

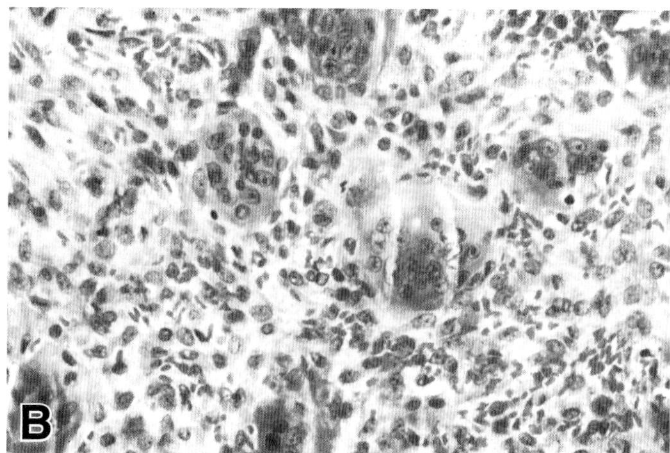

FIGURE 22-18. Primary hyperparathyroidism. A. Section through compact bone showing tunneling resorption of a Haversian canal. Numerous osteoclasts (*arrows*) and stromal fibrosis are evident. **B.** A section of tissue obtained from a "brown tumor" revealing numerous giant cells in a cellular fibrous stroma. Scattered erythrocytes are present throughout the tissue.

- **Osteitis fibrosa cystica:** As primary hyperparathyroidism progresses and hemorrhage continues, cystic degeneration ultimately occurs, evoking the final stage of the disease. The areas of fibrosis that contain reactive woven bone and hemosiderin-laden macrophages often display many osteoclastic giant cells. Because of its macroscopic appearance, this lesion has been dubbed **brown tumor** (Fig. 22-18B). This is not a neoplasm, but rather a repair reaction as an end stage of hyperparathyroidism. A classic feature of osteitis fibrosa cystica is the presence of multiple, localized, lytic lesions, which represent hemorrhagic cysts or masses of fibrous tissue. These eccentric and well-demarcated lesions are separated from the soft tissue by a periosteal shell of bone. The focal, tumorlike, lytic lesions always occur in the context of an abnormal skeleton produced by hyperparathyroidism. If a single lesion is examined in isolation, it may be mistaken for a primary giant cell neoplasm of bone.

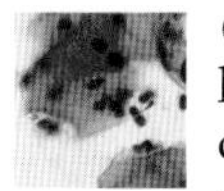

CLINICAL FEATURES: The symptoms of primary hyperparathyroidism are related to the abnormality of calcium homeostasis and have been characterized as "stones, bones, moans and groans." The "stones" refer to kidney stones, and the "bones" to the skeletal changes. The "moans" describe psychiatric depression and other abnormalities associated with hypercalcemia. The "groans" characterize the gastrointestinal irregularities associated with a high serum calcium level (see Chapter 19).

RENAL OSTEODYSTROPHY

Renal osteodystrophy is a complex metabolic bone disease that occurs in the context of chronic renal failure. Severe renal osteodystrophy is most common in patients maintained on long-term dialysis because they live long enough to develop conspicuous bone disease. The pathogenesis of renal osteodystrophy is similar to that of osteomalacia, with secondary hyperparathyroidism exerting its influence by way of osteoclastic bone resorption (Fig. 22-13E).

The **adynamic variant of renal osteodystrophy (ARO)** is characterized by arrested bone remodeling. More than 40% of adults who are treated with hemodialysis and more than 50% of those who are treated with peritoneal dialysis have bone biopsy evidence of ARO. Old bone accumulates because it is not remodeled, thus causing structural compromise of the skeleton and an increased tendency to fractures.

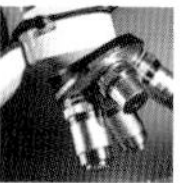 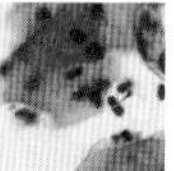

PATHOLOGY AND CLINICAL FEATURES: As a result of these effects of chronic renal failure, renal osteodystrophy is characterized by varying degrees of osteitis fibrosa, osteomalacia, osteosclerosis, and adynamic bone disease (Fig. 22-19).

Management of renal osteodystrophy involves not only treatment of renal failure but also control of phosphate levels by drug therapy and infusions. Occasionally, parathyroidectomy is required to control hyperparathyroidism, and the administration of vitamin D may also be necessary.

PAGET DISEASE OF BONE

Paget disease is a chronic condition characterized by lesions of bone resulting from disordered remodeling. Excessive bone resorption initially results in lytic lesions and is followed by disorganized and excessive bone formation.

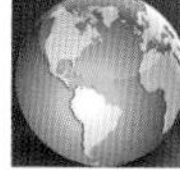

EPIDEMIOLOGY: Paget disease generally affects men and women older than 50 years. In the United States, 3% of the elderly manifest the disease. People of English origin have a high incidence of the disease. The disorder is almost nonexistent in Asia and in the indigenous populations of Africa and South America.

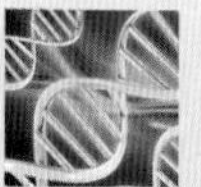

MOLECULAR PATHOGENESIS: Paget disease resembles a metabolic bone disease histologically; there is an increase in bone turnover in affected patients. However, the tendency to involve one or only a few bones does not fulfill the definition of a metabolic disorder.

A hereditary predisposition has been suggested by reports of families in whom Paget disease is transmitted as an autosomal dominant trait with incomplete penetrance that increases with age. There is evidence that Paget disease and

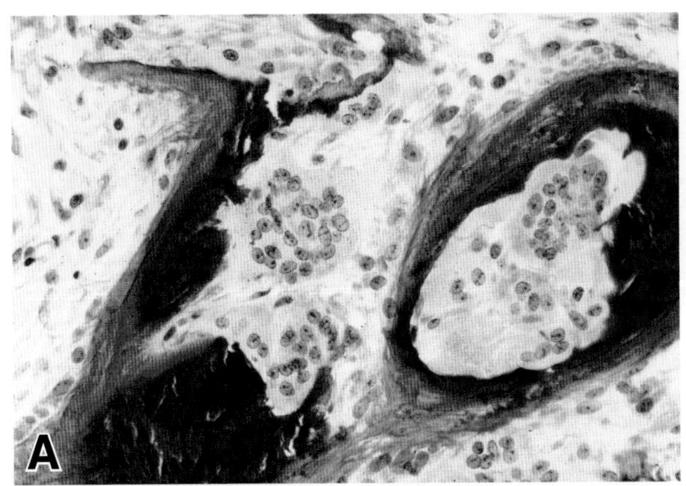

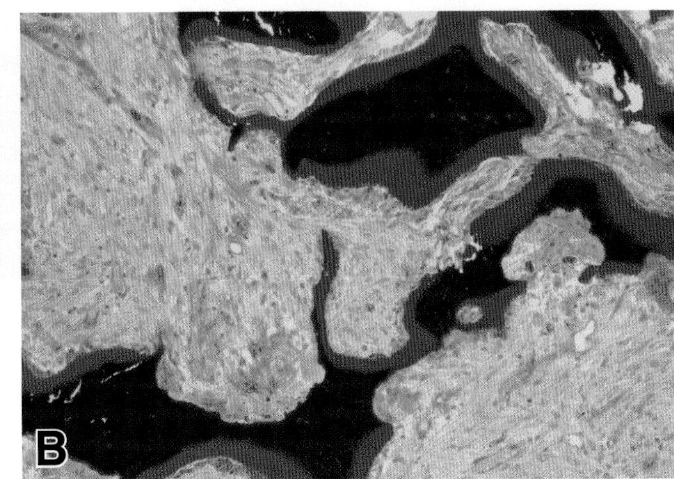

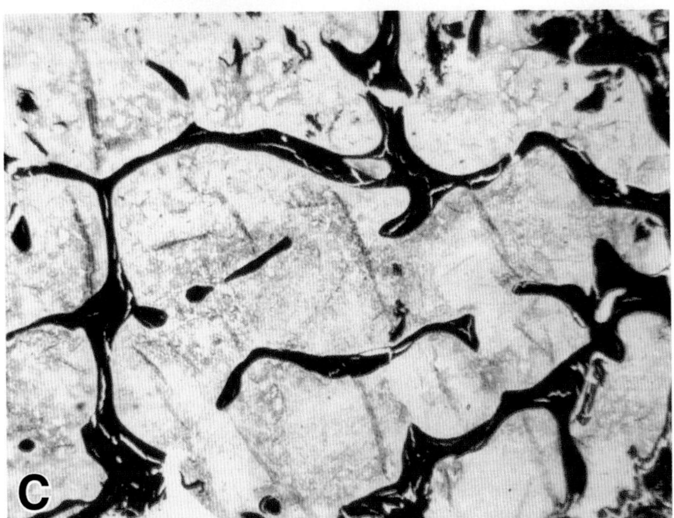

FIGURE 22-19. Renal osteodystrophy. A. Osteitis fibrosa. Several large multinucleated osteoclasts are resorbing these bone spicules, and the paraosseous tissue is fibrotic. Note that the osteoclastic resorption takes place only on the mineralized (*blue*) portions of the trabeculae. In this undecalcified section, the unmineralized bone (osteoid) appears *red*. **B. Osteomalacia.** This is a von Kossa stain prepared on an undecalcified section. The mineralized bone is *black*, and the abundant osteoid appears *magenta*. Osteoid is thick and lines a large proportion of the bone surfaces. Surfaces not covered by the osteoid demonstrate scalloped Howship lacunae and contain abundant osteoclasts. **C. Adynamic bone disease** in which remodeling is attenuated, with a paucity of osteoblasts, osteoclasts, and osteoid (von Kossa stain).

some related diseases are caused by mutations in genes encoding proteins in the RANK signaling pathway. Specifically, mutations in *Sequestosome 1* (*SQSTM1*) have been found in familial and sporadic forms of Paget disease. The *SQSTM1* gene encodes a protein, also known as p62, which may act as a scaffold protein in the RANK signaling pathway.

Some evidence indicates that Paget disease is of viral origin (Fig. 22-21). Virtually, all patients exhibit nuclear inclusions in osteoclasts and osteoclast precursors. These inclusions are not found in any other skeletal disease other than giant cell tumors of bone, suggesting that a virus may be involved. Support for this hypothesis has come from the finding that the marrow of the patients with Paget disease contains paramyxovirus nucleocapsid transcripts. Although a viral etiology seems plausible, actual live viruses have not been isolated from pagetic bone, and it is difficult to explain single bone involvement by a systemic viral infection or a germline mutation.

Overall, Paget disease is characterized by localized increases in osteoclast formation that lead to bone resorption and associated osteoblastic activity. The increased osteoclastogenic nature of the bone microenvironment is mediated by increases in IL-6 and the RANK signaling pathway. The result is uncoupling of the normal osteoclast/osteoblast remodeling unit.

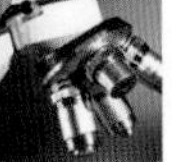

PATHOLOGY: The lesions of Paget disease may be solitary (monostotic) or may involve multiple bones (polyostotic). They tend to localize to the bones of the axial skeleton, including the spine, skull, and pelvis. Solitary Paget disease rarely involves the humerus, but in polyostotic disease, lesions involving this bone are common.

Paget disease is triphasic:

1. **"Hot" or osteoclastic resorptive stage:** Radiologically, there is a characteristic, flame- or wedge-shaped lysis of the cortex, which may mimic a tumor (Fig. 22-20A). Histologically, there is widespread **osteolysis**, with marked osteoclastic resorption, marrow fibrosis, and dilation of marrow sinusoids.
2. **Mixed stage of osteoblastic and osteoclastic activity:** By radiography, the bones are larger than normal. In fact, Paget disease is one of only two diseases that produce **larger-than-normal bones** (the other is fibrous dysplasia, discussed below). The cortex in the mixed phase is thickened, and the accentuation of the coarse cancellous bone makes the bone appear heavy and enlarged (Fig. 22-20B and C). Involvement of vertebral bodies evokes a "picture frame" appearance (Fig. 22-20D), because cortices and endplates become greatly exaggerated, compared to the coarse cancellous bone of the vertebral body. Histologically,

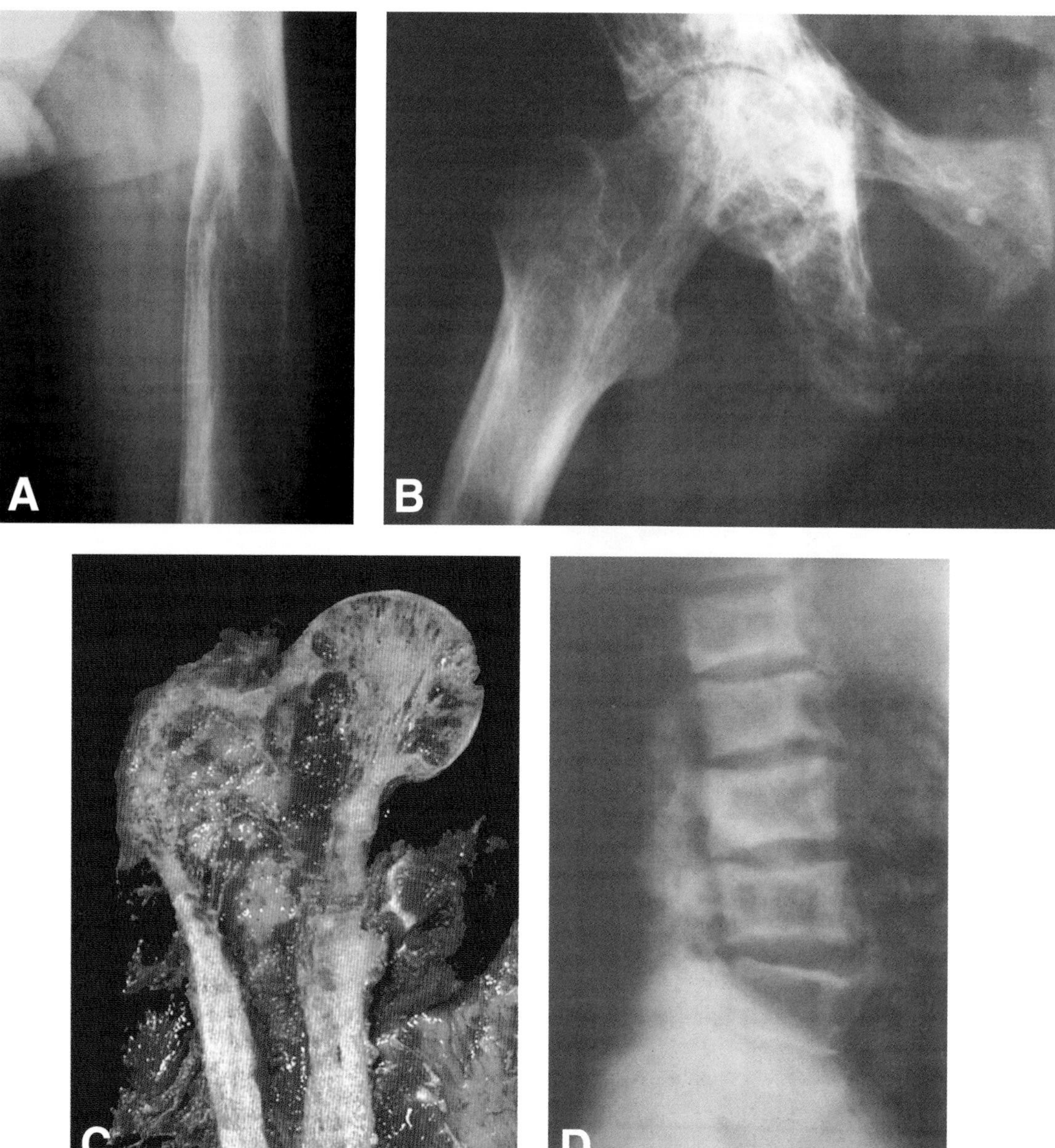

FIGURE 22-20. Paget disease. A. A radiograph of early Paget disease showing cortical dissolution, increased diameter of the diaphysis, and an advancing, wedge-shaped area of cortical resorption ("flame sign"). Proximal to the edge of this wedge, the femur appears entirely normal. **B.** Later, Paget disease of the proximal femur and pelvis showing cortical disorganization and irregular coarse trabeculations. **C.** Gross specimen of proximal femur showing cortical thickening and coarse trabeculations of the femoral head and neck. **D.** Paget disease of the spine showing shortening and widening of the lumbar vertebral bodies. Their cortices and endplates are thickened and have a "picture frame" appearance.

there is evidence of both increased osteoclastic and osteoblastic activity (Figs. 22-21 and 22-22B).

3. **"Cold" or burnt-out stage:** This period is characterized histologically by little cellular activity and radiologically by thickened and disordered bones.

Paget disease need not progress through all three stages, and in polyostotic disease, various foci may appear in different stages.

The osteoclast is the pathologic cell of Paget disease, and its appearance is characteristic. Although normal osteoclasts contain fewer than a dozen nuclei, those of Paget disease are huge and may have over 100 (Fig. 22-22B). Many nuclei contain intranuclear inclusions that contain viruslike particles (Fig. 22-22B and C).

Because active Paget disease is a disorder of accelerated remodeling, its histologic features are those of severe osteitis fibrosa. Numerous large osteoclasts, active osteoblasts, and peritrabecular marrow fibrosis are encountered (Fig. 22-22B). The rapid remodeling creates disruption of the trabecular architecture. Trabeculae are characteristically distorted and irregular, with a high surface to volume ratio. Bone collagen is often arranged in a woven rather than lamellar pattern.

With time, the lesions of Paget disease burn out and become inactive. The diagnostic hallmark of this stage is the abnormal

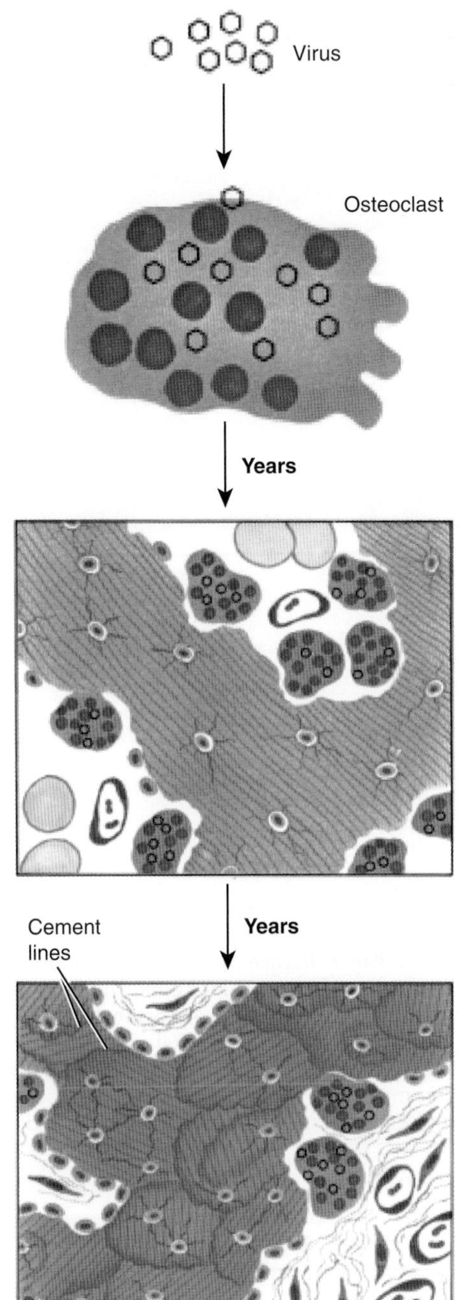

FIGURE 22-21. Hypothetical viral etiology of Paget disease of bone. A virus infects osteoclastic progenitors or osteoclasts in a genetically predisposed individual and stimulates osteoclastic activity, thereby leading to excessive resorption of bone. Over a period of years, the bone develops a characteristic mosaic pattern, produced by chaotically juxtaposed units of lamellar bone that form irregular cement lines. The adjacent marrow is often fibrotic, and there is a mixture of osteoclasts and osteoblasts on the surface of the bone.

arrangement of lamellar bone, in which islands of irregular bone formation resembling pieces of a jigsaw puzzle are separated by prominent irregular **cement lines** (Fig. 22-22A). The result is a **mosaic pattern** in the bone, which can be seen particularly well under polarized light. In the cortex of an affected bone, the osteons tend to be destroyed, and concentric lamellae are incomplete. Although the changes in lamellar bone are diagnostic, it is common to see woven bone as part of the pathologic process. In this situation, the woven bone is a reactive phenomenon, as in a microcallus, and represents a temporary bridge between islands of the mosaic bone of Paget disease.

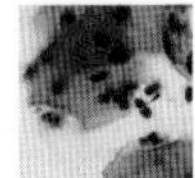

CLINICAL FEATURES: The most common focal symptom of Paget disease is pain in the affected bone, although its cause is not clear. The pain may be related to microfractures, stimulation of free nerve endings by dilated blood vessels adjacent to the bones, or weight bearing in weaker bones. The diagnosis is made primarily by radiologic findings, and bone biopsy is seldom necessary.

SKULL: Involvement of the skull is particularly common. The skull exhibits localized lysis, called **osteoporosis circumscripta**, generally in the frontal and parietal bones. Alternatively, there may be thickening of the outer and inner tables, which is most pronounced in the frontal and occipital bones. The skull becomes very heavy and may collapse over the C1 vertebra, compressing the brain and spinal cord. Hearing loss follows involvement of the middle ear ossicles and bony impingement on the eighth cranial nerve at the foramen. **Platybasia** (flattening of the base of the skull) impinges on the foramen magnum, compressing the medulla and upper spinal cord.

The jaws may be grossly misshapen, and the teeth may fall out. Often, facial bones increase in size, especially the maxillary bones, producing the so-called **leontiasis ossea** (lionlike face).

PAGETIC STEAL: Occasionally, patients feel lightheaded, owing to the so-called pagetic steal. In this situation, blood is shunted from the internal carotid system to the bones rather than directed to the brain.

FRACTURES AND ARTHRITIS: Fractures are common in Paget disease, the bones snapping transversely like a piece of chalk. Incomplete fractures without displacement are called **infractions**. Involvement of the pelvis engenders hip problems. The loss of subchondral bone compliance causes secondary osteoarthritis and destruction of the articular cartilage.

HIGH-OUTPUT CARDIAC FAILURE: With extensive Paget disease, blood flow to the bones and subcutaneous tissue increases remarkably, requiring increased cardiac output. In the presence of underlying cardiac disease, it may be severe enough to result in cardiac failure.

SARCOMATOUS CHANGE: Neoplastic transformation may occur in Paget disease, usually in the femur, humerus, or pelvis. This complication occurs in less than 1% of all cases and usually arises in patients with severe polyostotic disease. However, the incidence of bone sarcoma is 1,000 times higher than that in the general population. Interestingly, the skull and vertebrae, the bones most commonly involved by Paget disease, rarely undergo sarcomatous change. Osteosarcoma is the most common tumor although fibrosarcoma or chondrosarcoma are occasionally encountered.

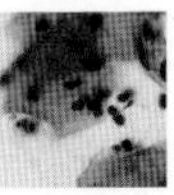

CLINICAL FEATURES: Serum calcium and phosphorus levels in Paget disease are normal, even though bone turnover increases more than 20-fold. The serum alkaline phosphatase level is the most useful laboratory test in diagnosing Paget disease. It increases enormously and correlates with osteoblastic activity. The alkaline phosphatase levels are disproportionately high with skull involvement but tend to be lower when only the pelvis is affected.

Fortunately, most patients with Paget disease are asymptomatic and require no treatment. Fractures, osteoarthritis,

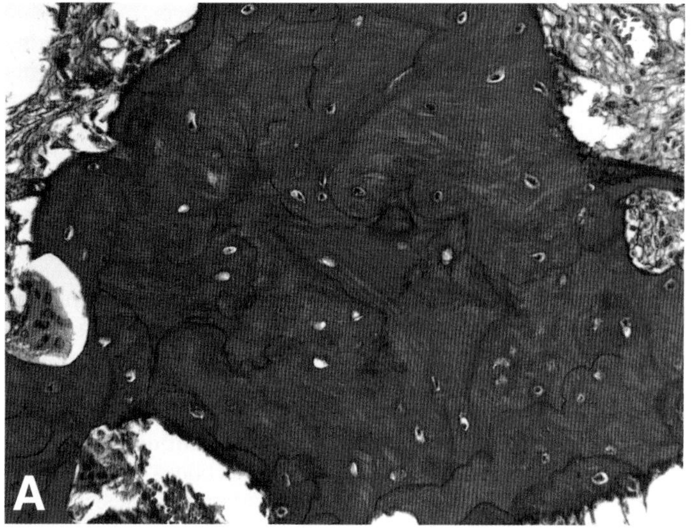

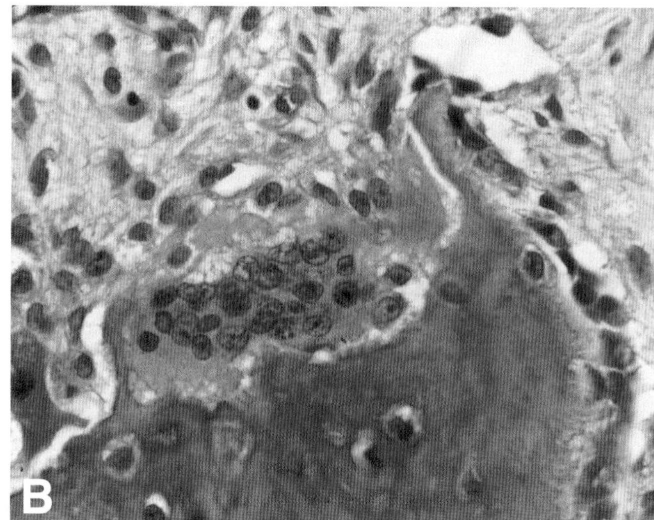

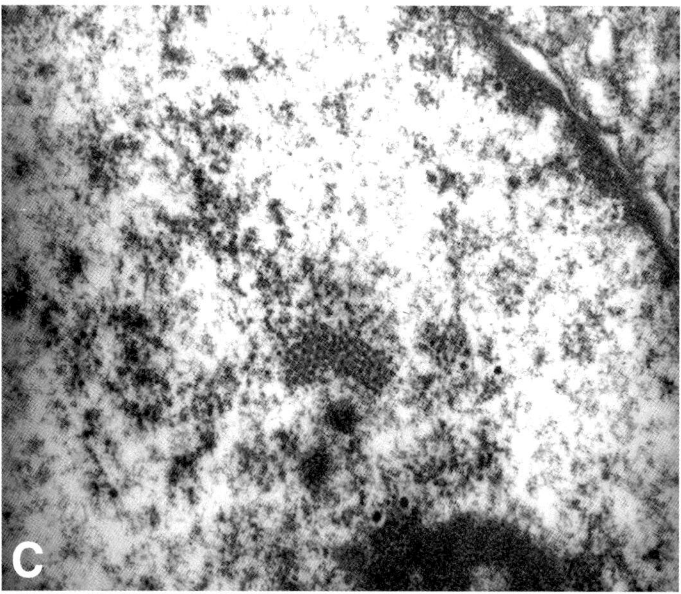

FIGURE 22-22. Paget disease. A. A section of bone showing prominent and irregular basophilic cement lines and numerous lining osteoclasts and osteoblasts. **B.** An osteoclast in pagetic bone contains many more nuclei than a usual osteoclast. A few of the nuclei contain eosinophilic intranuclear inclusion-like particles. **C.** On electron microscopy, the nuclei of the osteoclasts contain particles that resemble paramyxovirus in their shape and orientation.

and other orthopedic complications are treated symptomatically. Drugs directed at hindering the abnormal osteoclast hyperfunction, including calcitonin and bisphosphonates, are useful.

GIANT CELL TUMOR: Giant cell tumor may arise in Paget disease. It is not a neoplasm but rather a reactive phenomenon, similar to the "brown tumor" of hyperparathyroidism. Giant cell tumor is an overshoot of osteoclastic activity, which generates an associated fibroblastic response.

GAUCHER DISEASE

This autosomal recessive hereditary storage disease is discussed in Chapter 5. We consider here only its skeletal manifestations. Failure of remodeling results in skeletal abnormalities, characteristically an Erlenmeyer flask shape of the distal femur and proximal tibia. The more serious consequences of the disease are localized and diffuse bone loss, osteonecrosis, most often involving the femoral head or proximal humerus, pathologic fractures, osteomyelitis, and septic arthritis.

FIBROUS DYSPLASIA

Fibrous dysplasia is viewed as a developmental abnormality, which is characterized by a disorganized mixture of fibrous and osseous elements in the medullary region of affected bones. It occurs in children and young adults and may be monostotic or polyostotic. Fibrous dysplasia may occur as an isolated finding or in combination with endocrine and skin pigment changes (café au lait spots), a triad defining McCune–Albright syndrome.

MOLECULAR PATHOGENESIS: Somatic activating mutations in the *GNAS1* gene encoding the α subunit of the stimulatory $G_S\alpha$ protein, which is linked to adenylyl cyclase, have been described in bone cells from patients with fibrous dysplasia and McCune–Albright syndrome. The resulting increased levels of cAMP and enhanced functions of the affected cells result in the characteristic fibrous dysplasia.

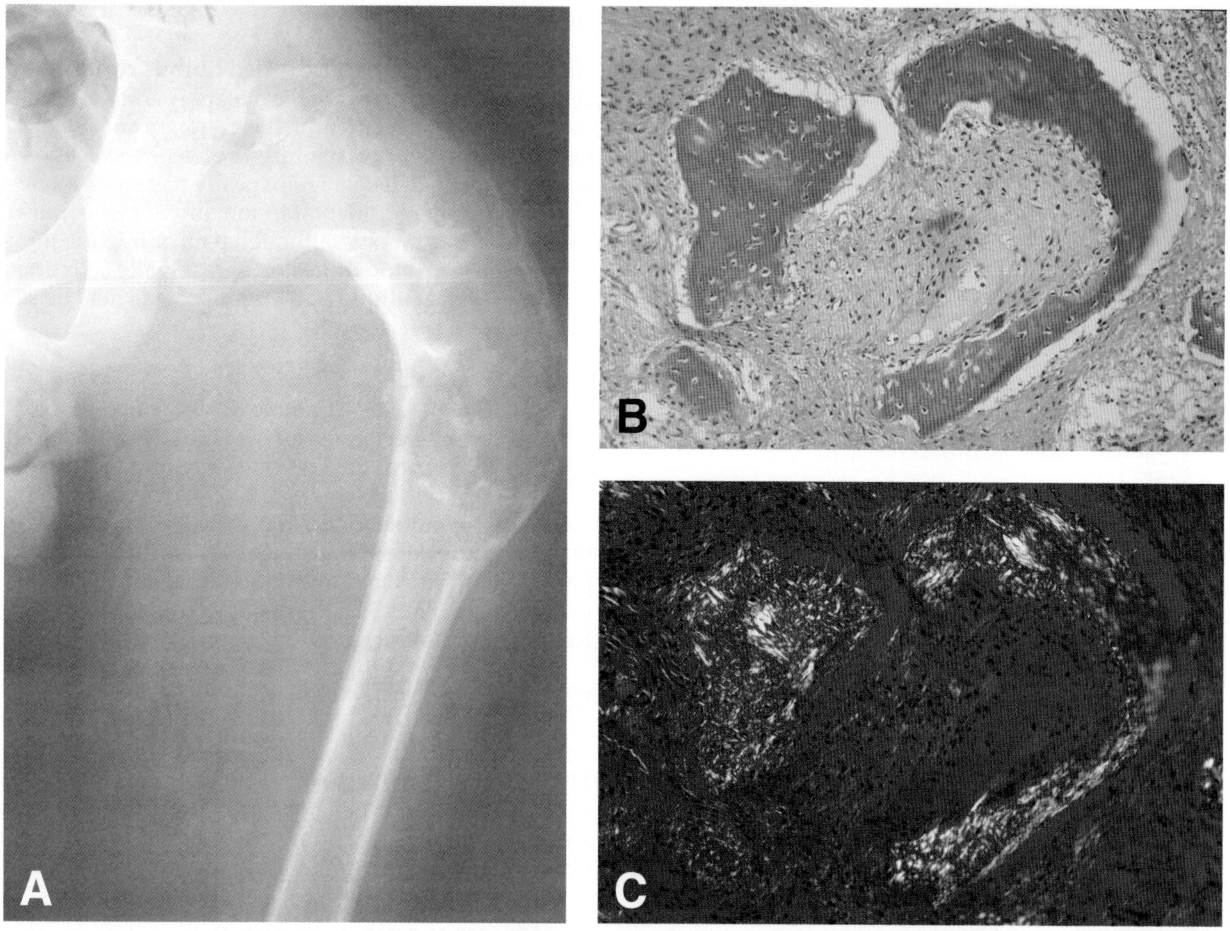

FIGURE 22-23. Fibrous dysplasia. A. A radiograph of the proximal femur showing the "shepherd's crook" deformity caused by fractures sustained over the years. Irregular, marginated, ground-glass lucencies are surrounded by reactive bone. The shaft has an appearance that has been likened to a soap bubble. **B.** Histologically, fibrous dysplasia consists of moderately cellular fibrous tissue in which irregular, curved spicules of woven bone develop without discernible appositional osteoblast activity. **C.** The same section in polarized light demonstrating not only that the spicules are woven but also that their fiber pattern extends imperceptibly into the fiber pattern of the surrounding stroma.

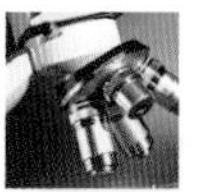

PATHOLOGY AND CLINICAL FEATURES: *MONOSTOTIC FIBROUS DYSPLASIA:* Monostotic fibrous dysplasia is the most common form of the disease and is most often seen in the second and third decades, with no predilection for either sex. The bones commonly involved are the proximal femur, tibia, ribs, and facial bones, although any bone may be affected. The disease may be asymptomatic or it may lead to a pathologic fracture (Fig. 22-32A).

POLYOSTOTIC FIBROUS DYSPLASIA: One fourth of patients with polyostotic fibrous dysplasia exhibit disease in more than half of the skeleton, including the facial bones. Symptoms are usually seen in childhood, and almost all patients have pathologic fractures, limb deformities, or limb-length discrepancies. Polyostotic fibrous dysplasia is more common in females. Sometimes, the disease becomes quiescent at puberty, but pregnancy tends to stimulate the growth of lesions.

Polyostotic fibrous dysplasia may also be associated with soft tissue myxomas (**Mazabraud syndrome**).

All forms of fibrous dysplasia have an identical histologic pattern (Fig. 22-23B and C). Benign fibroblastic tissue is arranged in a loose, whorled pattern. Irregularly arranged, purposeless spicules of woven bone that lack osteoblastic rimming are embedded in the fibrous tissue. In 10% of cases, irregular islands of hyaline cartilage are also present. Occasionally, cystic degeneration occurs, with hemosiderin-laden macrophages, hemorrhage, and osteoclasts congregated about the cyst. Rarely (<1% of cases), malignant transformation (osteosarcoma, chondrosarcoma, and fibrosarcoma) has been reported, but many of these cases involved prior radiation therapy. Treatment of fibrous dysplasia consists of curettage, repair of fractures, and prevention of deformities.

BENIGN TUMORS OF BONE

Although bone tumors of all kinds are uncommon, they are nevertheless important neoplasms because many occur in children and young adults and are potentially lethal. A primary bone tumor may arise from any of the cellular elements of bone. Most neoplasms of bone occur near the metaphyseal area, and more than 80% of primary tumors are found in the distal femur or proximal tibia (Fig. 22-24). In a growing child, these areas show conspicuous growth activity.

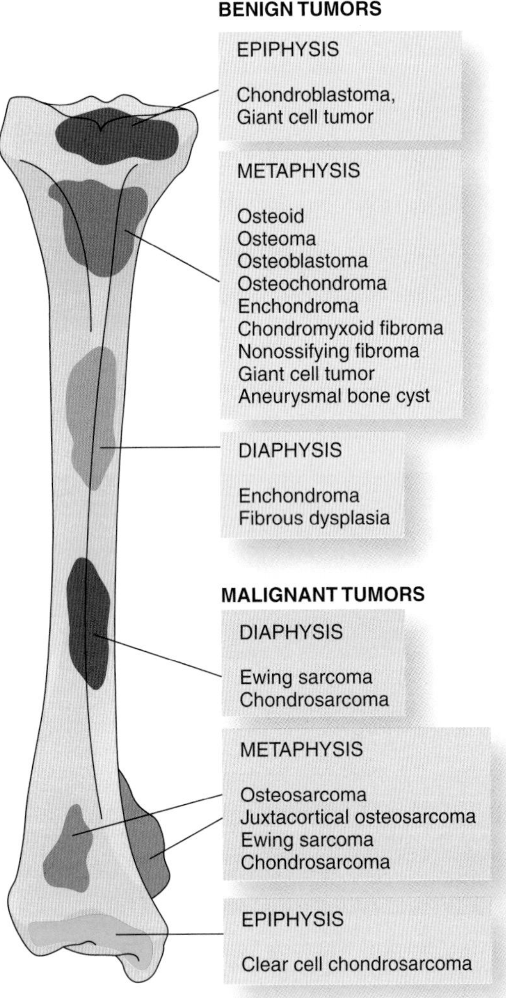

FIGURE 22-24. Location of primary bone tumors in long tubular bones.

Nonossifying Fibroma

Nonossifying fibroma, also called **fibrous cortical defect**, is a benign lesion that occurs in the metaphysis of a long bone, most commonly the tibia or femur. It is common and may be present in as many as 25% of all children between the ages of 4 and 10 years, after which it characteristically regresses. Nonossifying fibroma is a developmental lesion and not a neoplasm. Most cases are asymptomatic, although pain or fracture through the thin cortex overlying the lesion occasionally calls attention to the condition. Multiple ossifying fibromas may be seen with neurofibromatosis type 1.

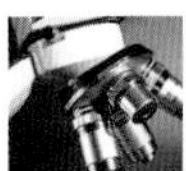

PATHOLOGY: Radiologically, nonossifying fibromas are characterized by a cortical, eccentric position and by central lucent zones surrounded by scalloped, sclerotic margins (Fig. 22-25A). On gross examination, the lesion is granular and dark red to brown. Microscopically, bland spindle cells are arranged in an interlacing, whorled pattern, with scattered multinucleated giant cells and foamy macrophages (Fig. 22-25B). Spontaneous regression is common. Radiologic follow-up is sufficient management in most cases.

Solitary Bone Cyst

Solitary, bone cyst is a benign, fluid-filled, unilocular lesion. There is a male predilection (3:1), and 80% occur in the first two decades of life. More than two thirds of all solitary bone cysts are located in the proximal humerus, proximal femur, or proximal tibia, usually in the metaphysis adjacent to the growth plate.

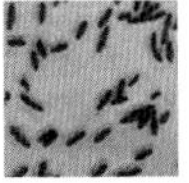

ETIOLOGIC FACTORS: Solitary bone cysts are not neoplasms but rather disturbances of bone growth with superimposed trauma. Secondary organization of a hematoma or some abnormality of the metaphyseal vessels causes accumulation of fluid. The "tumor" then grows by expansion of the fluid cavity. The resulting pressure causes

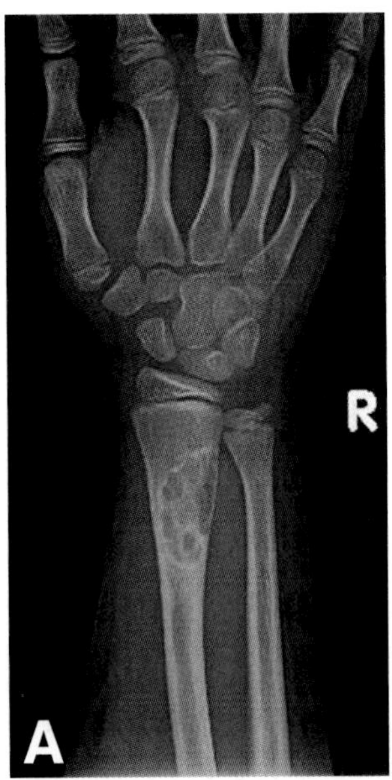

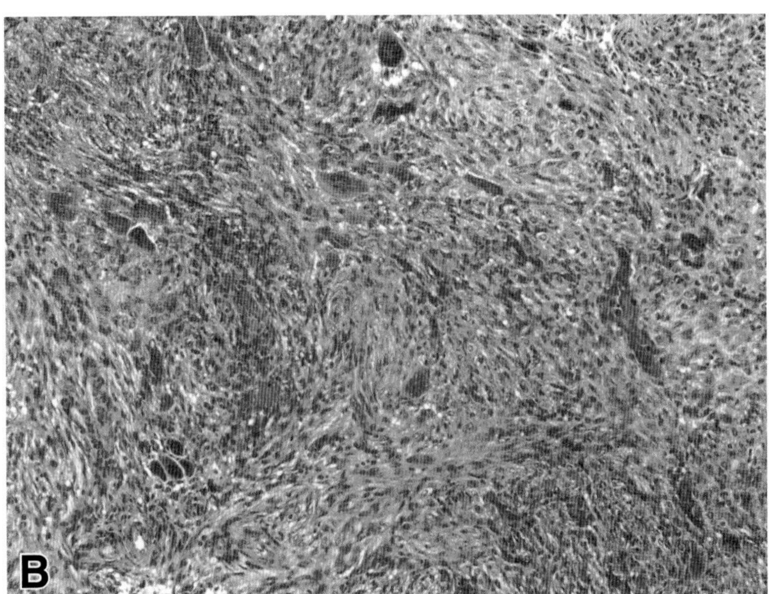

FIGURE 22-25. Nonossifying fibroma. A. A radiograph of the distal radius of a child showing an eccentric, metaphyseal lytic lesion with scalloped and sclerotic margins. **B.** Microscopically, the lesion is composed of bland spindle cells arranged in interlacing fascicles, with scattered, multinucleated, osteoclast-type giant cells.

bone resorption, mediated by neighboring osteoclasts. The process is slow, so that as the endosteal surface of the cortex is resorbed, a thin periosteal shell of new bone is laid down. This sequence results in a thin, well-marginated, radiolucent bone lesion, which is never greater in diameter than the growth plate and is particularly susceptible to pathologic fracture.

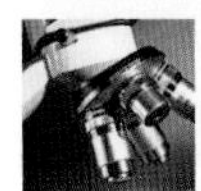

PATHOLOGY: Solitary bone cyst is not a true cyst because there is no distinct cell lining. It is rather lined by fibrous tissue, a few osteoclastic giant cells, hemosiderin-laden macrophages, chronic inflammatory cells, and reactive bone. Osteoclasts are present in the advancing front of the cyst and allow expansion of the lesion. The cyst wall may contain characteristic masses of amorphous, calcified, fibrinous material resembling cementum.

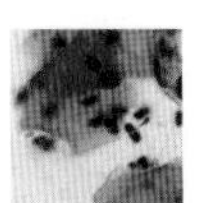

CLINICAL FEATURES: Most solitary bone cysts are entirely asymptomatic until a pathologic fracture calls attention to it. Curettage and bone grafting are the preferred treatments.

Aneurysmal Bone Cyst

ABC is an uncommon, benign, expansive, and often destructive lesion arising within a bone or on its surface. It occurs in children and young adults, with a peak incidence in the second decade. Although the lesion has been observed at every skeletal site, it is most frequent in the metaphysis of long bones and the vertebral column.

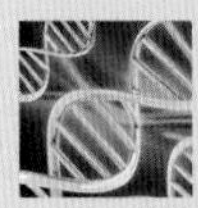

MOLECULAR PATHOGENESIS: The pathogenesis of ABC is controversial. Some cases represent cystic and hemorrhagic transformation of an underlying lesion, most commonly chondroblastoma, osteoblastoma, fibrous dysplasia, giant cell tumor, and osteosarcoma ("secondary ABC"). Other cases of ABC have no detectable associated lesion ("primary ABC") and may be a true neoplasm because it is associated with a recurring chromosomal translocation [t(16;17)(q22;p13)].

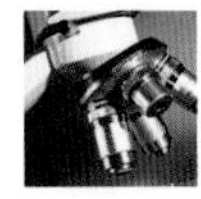

PATHOLOGY: The periosteum around an aneurysmal bone cyst is ballooned but intact. By MRI, fluid–fluid levels may be seen as blood cells separate from plasma (Fig. 22-26A). The cut surface of the cyst resembles a sponge permeated with blood and blood clots (Fig. 22-26B). The walls and septa are composed of moderately cellular fibrous tissue, multinucleated giant cells, and reactive bone (Fig. 22-26C).

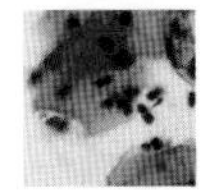

CLINICAL FEATURES: Although some aneurysmal bone cysts tend to grow slowly, most expand rapidly, and some are enormous. They usually manifest with pain and swelling, sometimes in relation to trauma. A bone cyst may "blow out," that is, rupture and produce local hemorrhage. Treatment is usually excision and curettage, with bone grafting. The recurrence rate is variable (20% to 70%). At surgery, incising the cyst decreases its internal pressure, causing brisk bleeding that may be difficult to control.

Osteoma

Osteoma is a benign, slow-growing tumor composed of cortical-type dense bone. Some osteomas are likely developmental or hamartomatous in nature. However, sinonasal osteomas may represent benign osteoblastic neoplasms. Interestingly, multiple osteomas are associated with familial adenomatous polyposis in Gardner syndrome, a form of familial adenomatous polyposis (FAP) (see Chapter 11).

Osteoid Osteoma

Osteoid osteoma is composed of immature osseous tissue surrounded by a halo of dense reactive bone. The typical patient is between the ages of 5 and 25 years. Boys are affected more often than girls (3:1). The lesion frequently arises in the diaphyseal cortex of the tubular bones of the leg, but may occur elsewhere. Osteoid osteomas have limited growth potential and do not metastasize. Chromosomal analysis of a few osteoid osteomas has disclosed structural abnormalities of chromosome 22q13 and loss of part of 17q, suggesting that the lesions are neoplasms.

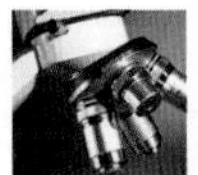

PATHOLOGY: Osteoid osteoma is a spherical, hyperemic tumor, about 1 cm in diameter, which is considerably softer than the surrounding bone (Fig. 22-27A) and easily enucleated at surgery. Microscopically, the center of the tumor is composed of thin, irregular trabeculae of woven bone within a cellular and vascular fibrous stroma, which contains many osteoblasts and osteoclasts (Fig. 22-27B). The trabeculae are more mature in the center, which is often partially calcified. Reactive sclerotic bone surrounds the nidus.

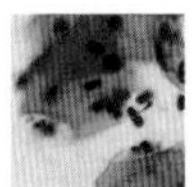

CLINICAL FEATURES: Pain is typically nocturnal and out of proportion to the size of the lesion. Interestingly, the pain is often exacerbated by drinking alcohol and promptly relieved by aspirin or other anti-inflammatory drugs, possibly because of the high prostaglandin content and abundant nerve fibers within the tumor. Surgical excision or radioablation (electric probe inserted into the tumor) is curative.

Osteoblastoma

Osteoblastoma is an uncommon, benign neoplasm that is histologically similar to osteoid osteoma but larger (usually >2 cm) and with a tendency to progressive growth. It is not accompanied by the characteristic nocturnal pain of osteoid osteoma, although dull pain sometimes occurs.

Osteochondroma

Osteochondroma is a benign cartilaginous neoplasm consisting of a bony projection with a cartilaginous cap that arises on the surface of the bone. It occurs in bones formed by endochondral ossification. Most are solitary, but 15% are multiple and hereditary. Mutations in the exostosin (*EXT*) gene in osteochondromas support the neoplastic nature of the tumor. This gene is important in the biosynthesis of heparin sulfate chains, which play a role in cartilage development. Solitary osteochondroma is one of the most common benign bone tumors and is more frequent in young males. Most osteochondromas are asymptomatic, and some may need surgical excision if cosmetically displeasing or if they press upon an artery or a nerve. Recurrence is rare.

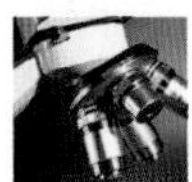

PATHOLOGY: Osteochondromas tend to grow away from the nearest joint. In radiographs, the cartilaginous mass is in direct continuity with the parent

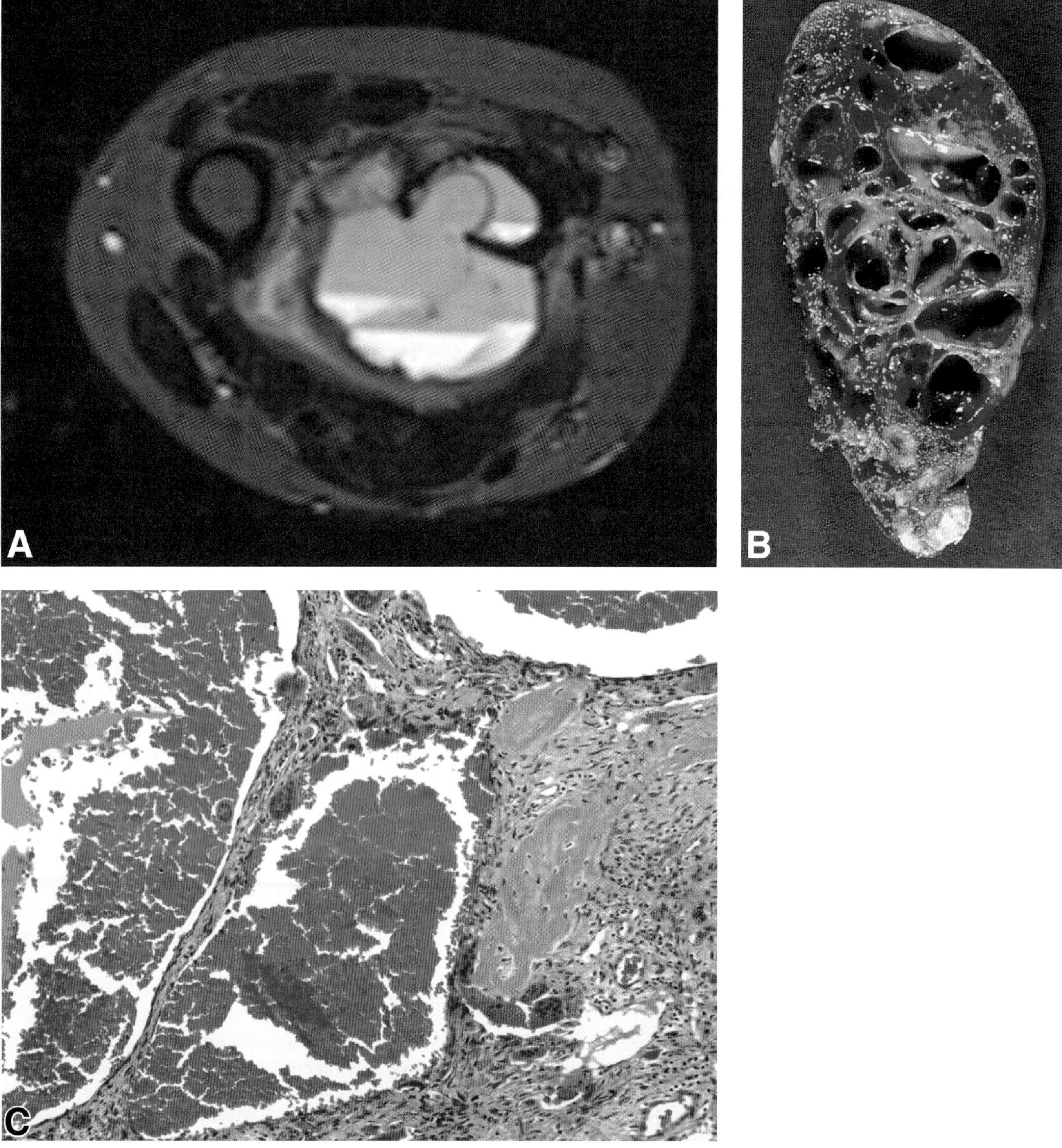

FIGURE 22-26. Aneurysmal bone cyst. A. A magnetic resonance image showing fluid–fluid levels. **B.** In cross section, the lesion consists of a spongy mass containing multiple blood-filled cysts. Some of the septa between the cysts contain bony tissue. **C.** Microscopically, the blood-filled spaces are separated by cellular fibrous septa with scattered osteoclast-type giant cells and reactive bone. From Bullough PG. *Atlas of Orthopaedic Pathology*. 2nd ed. New York, NY: Gower Medical Publishing; 1992. Copyright Lippincott Williams & Wilkins.

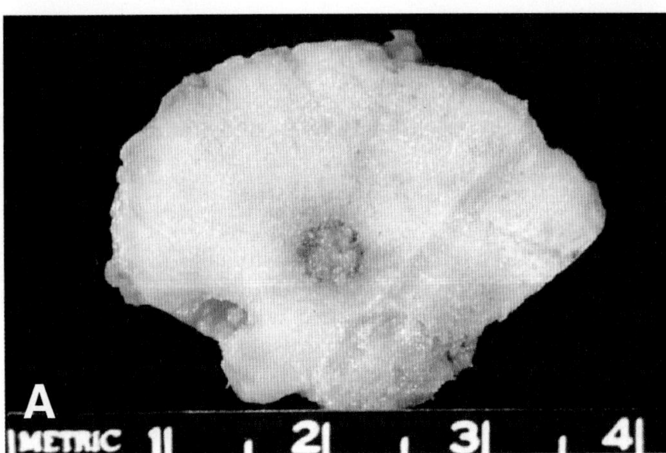

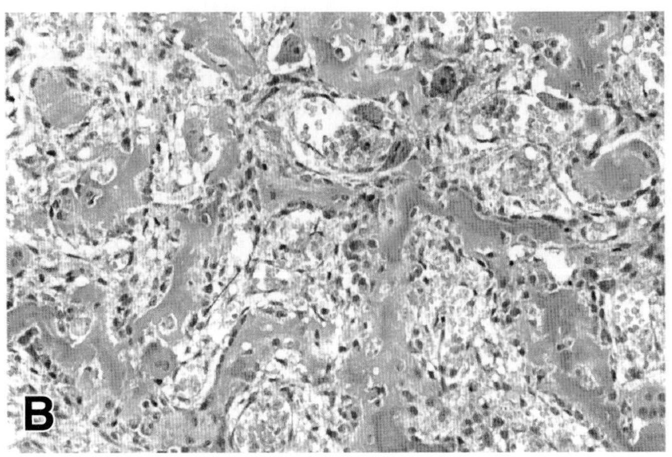

FIGURE 22-27. Osteoid osteoma. A. A gross specimen of an osteoid osteoma showing the central nidus, which is embedded in dense bone. **B.** A photomicrograph of the nidus revealing irregular trabeculae of woven bone surrounded by osteoblasts, osteoclasts, and fibrovascular marrow.

bone and lacks an underlying cortex (Fig. 22-28A). The marrow cavity of the lesion is in continuity with that of the bone where it arose. The cartilage-capped, bony mass is surrounded by a surface fibrous membrane, which is the perichondrium. Histologically, the cap is composed of benign hyaline cartilage with active endochondral ossification, which is morphologically similar to that seen in the epiphyseal growth plate (Fig. 22-28B and C). The bony stalk is composed of cortical lamellar bone, and the medullary cavity contains lamellar bone trabeculae and fatty marrow.

HEREDITARY MULTIPLE OSTEOCHONDROMATOSIS (HMO): This inherited autosomal dominant disorder is characterized by multiple osteochondromas and associated skeletal deformities. HMO is one of the most common inherited musculoskeletal disorders and is caused by loss of *EXT* gene function. The heritable variety is uncommon, with an incidence of about 1 in 50,000. It occurs predominantly in males, but because of its variable expression, an unaffected female from an afflicted family may transmit the disorder to her offspring.

Chondrosarcoma is a rare complication.

Solitary Chondroma

Although their neoplastic nature has been questioned, these benign tumors, also called **enchondromas (because most are intramedullary)**, may be associated with mutations in the *IDH1* and *IDH2* (isocitrate dehydrogenase) genes, suggesting that they are true neoplasms. They occur at any age, and many cases are entirely asymptomatic.

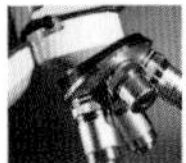

PATHOLOGY: Most solitary enchondromas occur in the metacarpals and phalanges of the hands, the remainder being in almost any other tubular bone. The tumor is usually small and grows slowly.

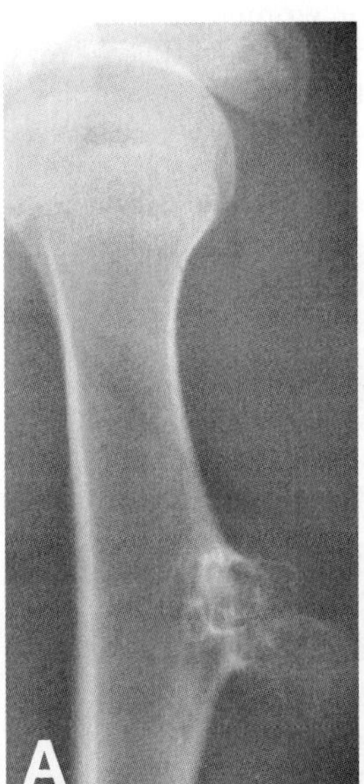

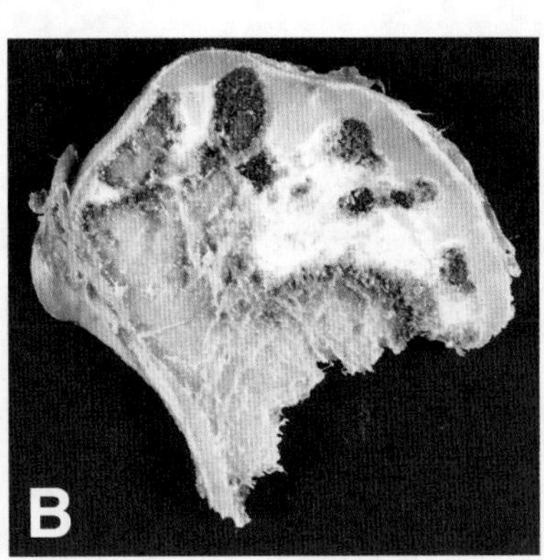

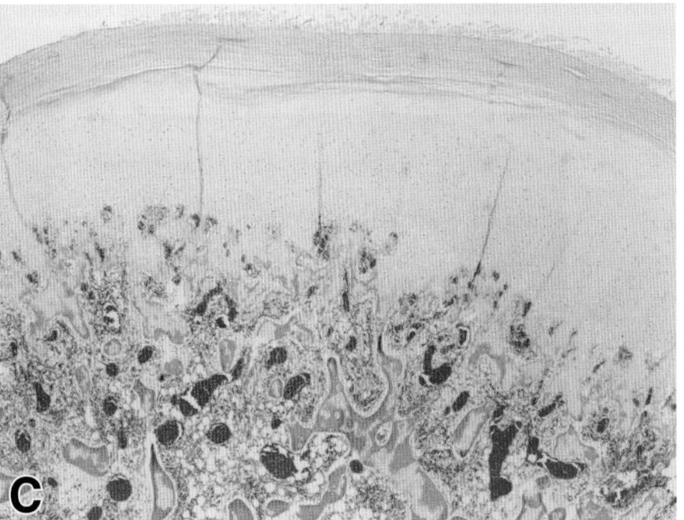

FIGURE 22-28. Osteochondroma. A. A radiograph of an osteochondroma of the humerus showing a lesion that is directly contiguous with the marrow space. **B.** The cross section of an osteochondroma showing the cap of calcified cartilage overlying poorly organized cancellous bone. **C.** Microscopically, the cartilaginous cap is covered by a fibrous membrane (perichondrium) and undergoes endochondral ossification.

Radiologically, it appears as an intramedullary radiolucent area, sometimes containing stippled calcifications. On gross examination, solitary enchondromas have the semitranslucent appearance of hyaline cartilage, often with a few calcified areas. Microscopically, the cartilaginous tissue is well differentiated with sparse chondrocytes, extensive cartilaginous matrix, and a lobular configuration. Asymptomatic enchondromas are best left untreated and followed radiographically. When pain or pathologic fracture occurs, curettage and bone grafting are the treatment of choice. Recurrences are uncommon.

Enchondromatosis

Enchondromatosis, *also termed* **Ollier disease,** ***is characterized by multiple cartilaginous masses that lead to bony deformities.*** Bones show numerous, tumorlike masses of abnormally arranged hyaline cartilage (enchondromas), with zones of proliferative and hypertrophied cartilage. These tumors tend to be located in the metaphyses. As growth continues, the enchondromas settle in the diaphysis of adolescents and adults.

Enchondromatosis is asymmetric and may cause bone deformities. There is a strong tendency for malignant transformation, mostly into chondrosarcoma. Therefore, a patient with enchondromatosis who has increasing pain or a lesion that is actively growing should be evaluated to rule out an underlying sarcoma.

Maffucci syndrome is characterized by multiple enchondromas and cavernous or spindle cell hemangiomas of soft tissue. It usually manifests in early childhood and may lead to significant skeletal deformities. Chondrosarcoma develops in as many as half of all patients with Maffucci syndrome. The incidence of extraskeletal malignant tumors of different types (e.g., carcinomas and gliomas) is also greatly increased in patients with the condition. As is the case with solitary chondromas, the syndrome is associated with *IDH1* and *IDH2* mutations.

Chondroblastoma

Chondroblastoma is an uncommon, benign, chondrogenic tumor with a predilection for epiphyses of the proximal femur, tibia, and humerus. It is more common in males than in females (2:1), and 90% of cases occur in young people between the ages of 5 and 25 years.

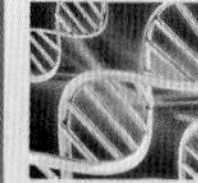

MOLECULAR PATHOGENESIS: Genetic abnormalities suggest a neoplastic origin of chondroblastoma, including aneuploidy, abnormalities involving chromosomes 5 and 8, and mutations in the *p53* gene.

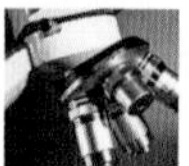

PATHOLOGY: Chondroblastoma grows slowly and, on radiologic examination, displays an eccentric, radiolucent appearance, with sharply defined borders (Fig. 22-29A). On gross examination, the tumor is soft and compact and exhibits scattered gray or hemorrhagic areas. Microscopically, primitive chondroblasts are arranged as sheets of round to polyhedral cells that have well-defined cytoplasmic borders and large, ovoid nuclei, often with prominent nuclear grooves (Fig. 22-29B). Osteoclastic-type giant cells are frequently present. The scanty cartilage matrix is usually variably calcified and appears primitive. The tumor causes bone destruction by stimulating osteoclastic resorption. In fact, these neoplasms may perforate the cortex, although they remain confined by the periosteum.

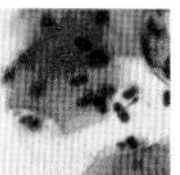

CLINICAL FEATURES: Because of its para-articular location, chondroblastoma tends to cause joint pain, with mild swelling and functional limitation of joint movement. If neglected, it may (rarely) attain a large size, destroy the epiphyseal area, and invade the joint. Curettage is the treatment of choice, although in over 10% of cases, the tumor recurs.

Giant Cell Tumor of Bone

GCT of bone is a benign, locally aggressive neoplasm characterized by the presence of osteoclastic, multinucleated giant cells, randomly distributed in a background of proliferating mononuclear cells. It usually occurs in the third and fourth decades, has a slight predilection for women, and is more common in Asia than in Western countries. Paget disease may produce a giant cell reactive lesion that closely resembles a true GCT.

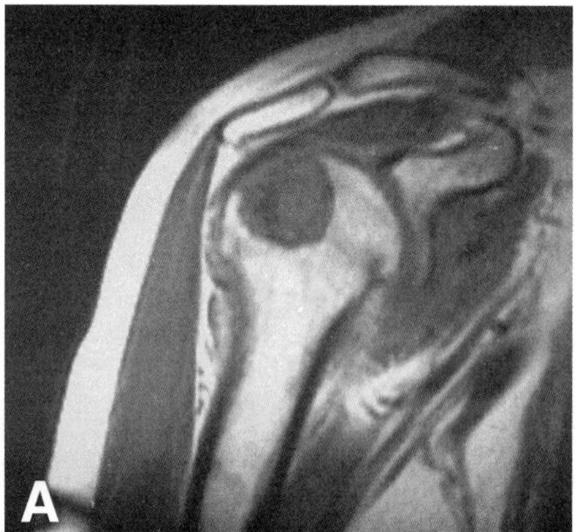

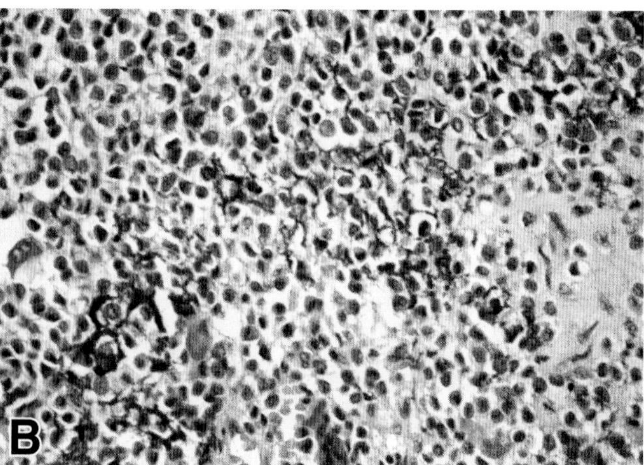

FIGURE 22-29. Chondroblastoma. A. A magnetic resonance image of the shoulder of a child showing a prominent lytic lesion of the head of the humerus that involves the epiphysis and extends across the epiphyseal plate. **B.** The histologic appearance of a chondroblastoma is defined by plump, round cells (chondroblasts) surrounded by a mineralized primitive chondroid matrix.

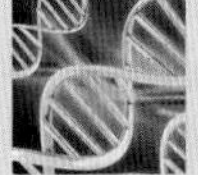

MOLECULAR PATHOGENESIS: GCT is composed of numerous, large osteoclastic giant cells and two lineages of mononuclear cells. One population has a preosteoblastic phenotype. The other population consists of neoplastic cells that are spindle-shaped and of stromal origin. They produce RANKL and induce osteoclast formation (hence the large number of giant cells). GCT is associated with mutations in the gene for a replication-independent histone (H3.3).

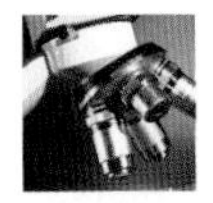

PATHOLOGY: In most cases (90%), GCT of bone originates at the junction between the epiphysis and the metaphysis of a long bone, with more than half being situated in the knee area (distal femur and proximal tibia). The lower end of the radius, humerus, and fibula are also occasionally involved. Radiologically, the tumor presents as an eccentric, expansile, lytic lesion with no matrix formation, which tends to be surrounded by a thin bony shell (Fig. 22-30A). Often, it has a multiloculated or "soap-bubble" appearance, representing endosteal resorption of the bone.

On gross examination, GCT is circumscribed, and its cut surface is soft and light brown, without bone or calcification. Numerous hemorrhagic areas result in the appearance of a sponge full of blood. In some cases, cystic cavities and necrotic areas are present. GCT is often limited by the periosteum, although aggressive forms penetrate the cortex and the periosteum, even reaching the joint capsule and the synovial membrane.

Microscopically, GCT exhibits two types of cells (Fig. 22-31B). The mononuclear ("stromal") cells are plump and oval, with large nuclei and scanty cytoplasm. Large osteoclastic giant cells, some with more than 100 nuclei, are scattered throughout the richly vascularized stroma. Diffuse interstitial hemorrhage is common. Secondary aneurysmal bone cyst may also be seen. It is evident that the mononuclear cells are the neoplastic and proliferative components of GCT. Mitotic activity is common in the mononuclear cells but is not observed in the giant cells.

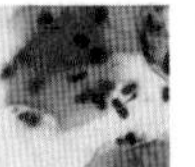

CLINICAL FEATURES: The vast majority of GCTs are considered benign, but locally aggressive tumors have the potential to recur locally after simple curettage and (rarely) metastasize to distant sites, particularly the lungs.

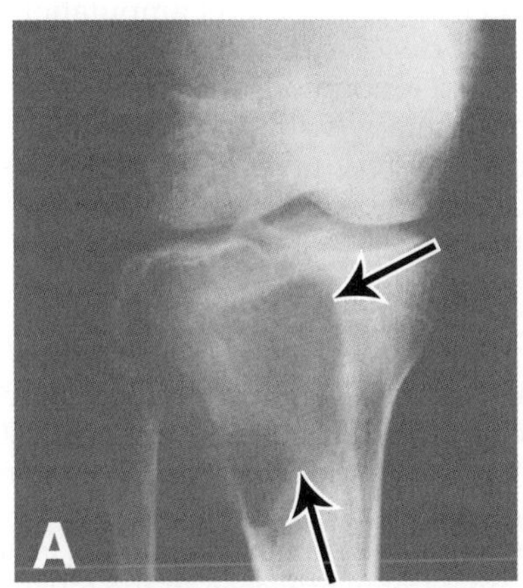

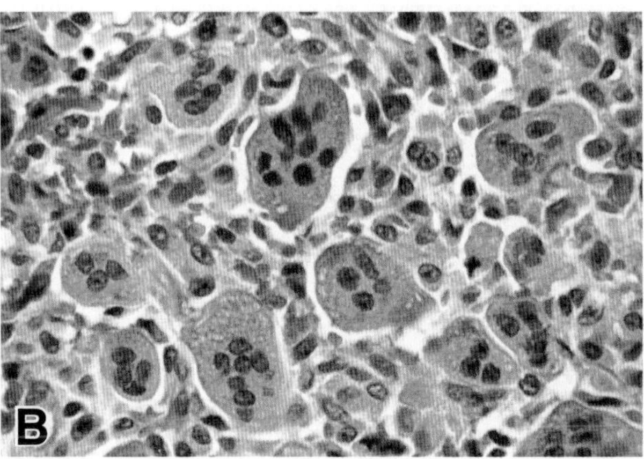

FIGURE 22-30. Giant cell tumor of bone. A. Radiograph of the proximal tibia showing an eccentric lytic lesion with virtually no new bone formation (*arrows*). The tumor extends to the subchondral bone plate and breaks through cortex into the soft tissue. **B.** Photomicrograph showing osteoclast-type giant cells and plump, oval, mononuclear cells. The nuclei of both types of cells are identical.

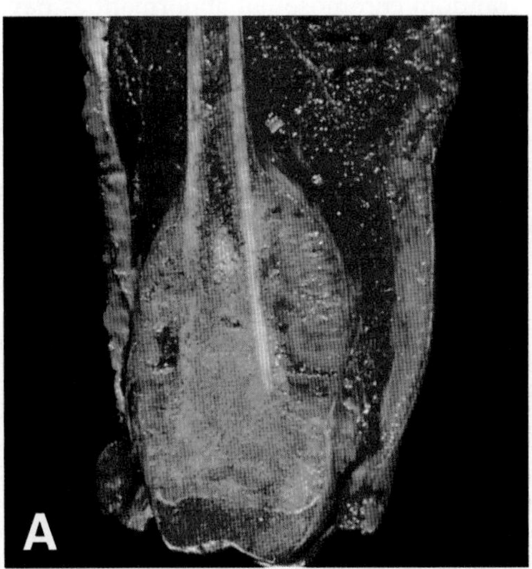

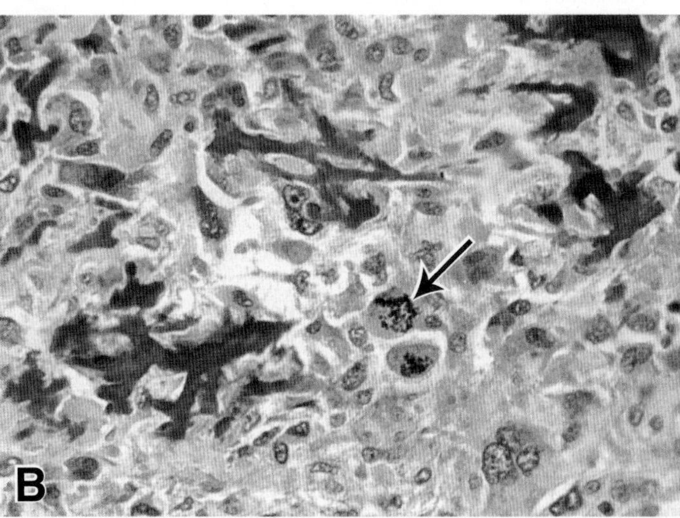

FIGURE 22-31. Osteosarcoma. A. The distal femur contains a dense osteoblastic malignant tumor that extends through the cortex into the soft tissue and the epiphysis. **B.** A photomicrograph revealing pleomorphic malignant cells, tumor giant cells, and mitoses (*arrows*). The tumor cells produce woven bone that is focally calcified.

True malignancy in GCT is observed in 1% of cases as either a sarcomatous lesion arising in a typical GCT or as a sarcoma after a GCT has been curetted.

GCTs manifest with pain, usually in the joint adjacent to the tumor. Microfractures and pathologic fractures are frequent, owing to thinning of the cortex. The tumor is treated with thorough curettage and bone grafting. A monoclonal antibody to RANKL (denosumab) may control tumor growth in recurrent cases and be used as adjunctive therapy. Local recurrence after simple curettage has been reported in one third to one half of cases, and 2% to 5% metastasize to the lungs.

MALIGNANT TUMORS OF BONE

Osteosarcoma

Osteosarcoma, also termed* osteogenic sarcoma, *is a highly malignant bone tumor characterized by formation of bone tissue by tumor cells. It represents one fifth of all bone cancers and is most frequent in adolescents between the ages of 10 and 20 years, affecting boys more often than girls (2:1).

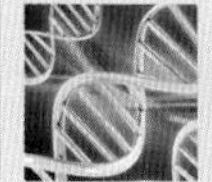

MOLECULAR PATHOGENESIS: Conventional osteosarcoma has complex karyotypes, with multiple numerical and structural chromosomal aberrations. The tumors are associated with mutations in tumor suppressor genes; almost two thirds show mutations in the retinoblastoma (*Rb*) gene (see Chapter 4), and many have mutations in the *p53* gene. There are molecular abnormalities pertaining to apoptosis, replicative potential, insensitivity to growth inhibitory signals, and cell cycle regulation.

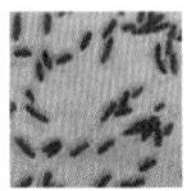

ETIOLOGIC FACTORS: Osteosarcoma is more common in tall people. Interestingly, they occur more frequently in tall breeds of dogs. In older people, they usually occur in the context of Paget disease or radiation exposure. Several preexisting benign bone lesions are associated with an increased risk of developing osteosarcoma, including fibrous dysplasia, osteomyelitis, and bone infarcts. Although trauma may call attention to an existing osteosarcoma, there is no evidence that it ever causes the tumor.

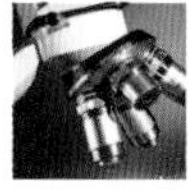

PATHOLOGY: Osteosarcomas often arise near the knee, in the distal femur (Fig. 22-31A), proximal tibia, or fibula, although any metaphyseal area of a long bone may be affected. The proximal humerus is the second most common site; 75% of tumors arise adjacent to the knee or shoulder.

Radiologic evidence of bone destruction and bone formation by osteosarcoma is characteristic. Often, incomplete rim of reactive bone adjacent to the site where the periosteum is lifted from the cortical surface by the tumor is evident. When this appears on a radiograph as a shell of bone intersecting the cortex at one end and open at the other end, it is referred to as **Codman triangle**. A "sunburst" periosteal reaction is also often superimposed (Fig. 22-9).

The gross appearance of osteosarcoma is highly variable, depending on the proportions of bone, cartilage, stroma, and blood vessels. The cut surface may show any combination of hemorrhagic, cystic, soft, and bony areas. The neoplastic tissue may invade and break through the cortex, spread into the marrow cavity, elevate or perforate the periosteum or grow into the epiphysis, and even reach the joint space.

Histologic examination reveals malignant polygonal to spindled cells with osteoblastic differentiation, producing woven bone (Fig. 22-31B). The malignant cells have large hyperchromatic and pleomorphic nuclei, with a high nucleocytoplasmic ratio. Numerous mitoses, including atypical forms, are commonly seen. The tumor cells stain prominently for alkaline phosphatase, osteocalcin, and osteonectin. The tumorous bone is laid down haphazardly and not aligned along stress lines. Often, foci of malignant cartilage or pleomorphic giant cells are intermixed. In areas of osteolysis, non neoplastic osteoclasts are found at the advancing front of the tumor.

Osteosarcoma spreads through the bloodstream to the lungs. In fact, almost all patients (98%) who die of this disease have lung metastases. Less commonly, the tumor metastasizes to other bones (35%), the pleura (33%), and the heart (20%).

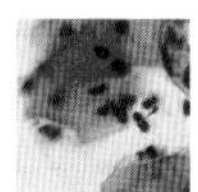

CLINICAL FEATURES: Osteosarcoma presents with mild or intermittent pain around the involved area. As pain intensifies, the area becomes swollen and tender. The adjacent joint becomes functionally limited. Serum alkaline phosphatase is increased in half of patients and may decrease after amputation, only to increase again with recurrence or metastasis. Metastatic disease heralds, rapid clinical deterioration, and death.

Standard therapy with preoperative chemotherapy and limb-sparing surgery gives 5-year disease-free rates from 60% to 80%. Resection of isolated pulmonary metastases may prolong survival.

Chondrosarcoma

Chondrosarcoma is a malignant tumor of cartilage that arises from a preexisting cartilage rest or a preexisting lesion, such as an enchondroma. Most have no known preexisting lesion. ***Chondrosarcoma is the second most common primary malignant bone tumor and is more common in men than in women (2:1).*** It is most frequently seen in the fourth to sixth decade (average age, 45 years).

MOLECULAR PATHOGENESIS: Numerous nonrandom chromosomal abnormalities have been discovered in chondrosarcoma. Central chondrosarcoma may develop by upregulation of *PTHrP* and *Bcl-2* expression in an osteochondroma, along with mutations in other genes, such as *p53*, and nonspecific chromosomal abnormalities. Development of central chondrosarcoma is related, at least in part, to abnormalities of chromosome 9p12-22, which may involve the *CDKN2A* tumor suppressor gene.

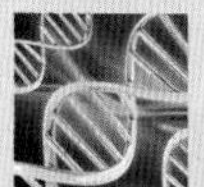

PATHOLOGY: Chondrosarcoma occurs in three anatomic variants:

CENTRAL CHONDROSARCOMA: This form arises in the medullary cavity of pelvic bones, ribs, and long bones, although any site may be affected. Radiologically, poorly defined borders, a thickened shaft, and perforation of the cortex characterize these tumors. There are usually stippled or ringlike radiopacities, representing calcification or endochondral ossification in the tumor (Fig. 22-32A). Although central chondrosarcoma may penetrate the cortex, extension beyond the periosteum is uncommon. On gross

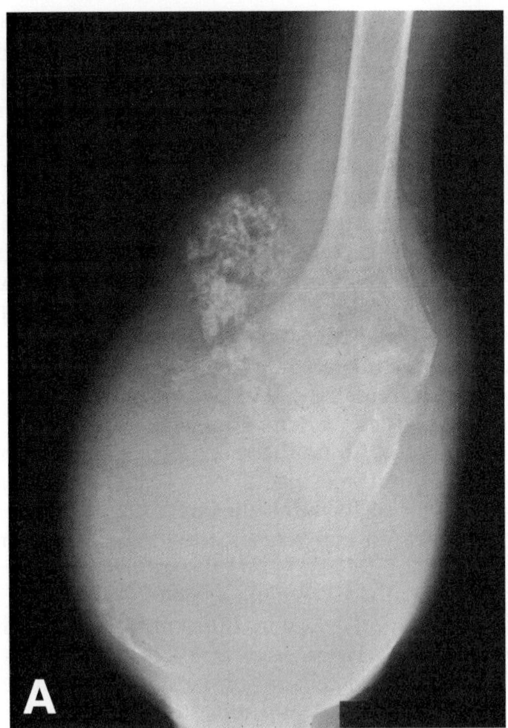

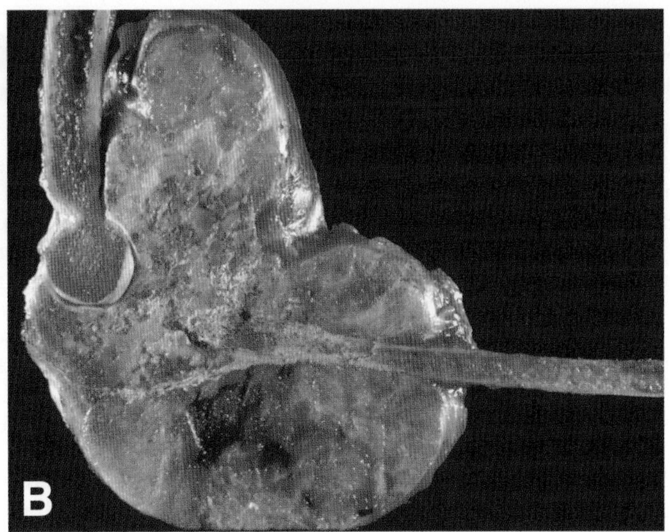

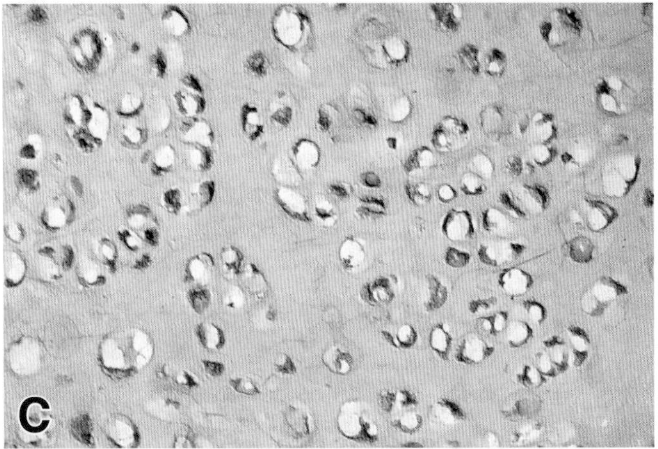

FIGURE 22-32. Chondrosarcoma. A. Radiograph demonstrating a large, destructive mass replacing the proximal ulna. There is a huge soft tissue mass containing aggregates of ring-shaped and popcorn-like calcifications. **B.** Resected gross specimen demonstrating lobulated hyaline cartilage with calcifications, ossification, and focal liquefaction. **C.** A photomicrograph of a chondrosarcoma showing malignant chondrocytes with pronounced atypia.

examination, the neoplastic cartilaginous tissue is compressed inside the bone and exhibits areas of necrosis, cystic change, and hemorrhage (Fig. 22-32B). The cortex of the bone and the intertrabecular spaces of the marrow are infiltrated by the tumor.

Central chondrosarcoma begins with deep pain, which becomes more intense with time. The tumor is only rarely palpable, but in untreated cases, large masses may eventually form.

PERIPHERAL CHONDROSARCOMA: This variant is less common than the central variety of chondrosarcoma and arises outside the bone, almost always in the cartilaginous cap of an osteochondroma. It occurs after the age of 20 years and never before puberty. The most frequent location of peripheral chondrosarcoma is the pelvis, followed by the femur, vertebrae, sacrum, humerus, and other long bones. It arises only rarely distal to the knee or elbow. Radiologically, characteristic radiopacities, representing calcification or ossification of the neoplastic cartilage, are virtually pathognomonic for the lesion. Macroscopically, peripheral chondrosarcoma tends to be a large bosselated mass that surrounds the base of an osteochondroma and invades and destroys the bone.

Expansion of the mass causes pain and local symptoms. In the pelvis, the lumbosacral plexus may be compressed, and tumors in the vertebrae may cause paraplegia.

JUXTACORTICAL CHONDROSARCOMA: This is the least common variety of chondrosarcoma and is similar to central chondrosarcoma in its predilection for middle-aged men. It tends to be situated in the metaphysis of long bones, lying on the outer surface of the cortex. Thus, it is probably periosteal or parosteal in origin. Radiologically, it may be entirely translucent or focally calcified. The symptoms of juxtacortical chondrosarcoma are dominated by swelling, with little accompanying pain.

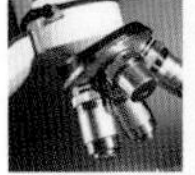

PATHOLOGY: Histologically, chondrosarcomas are composed of malignant cartilage cells in various stages of maturity (Fig. 22-32C). Occasionally, a well-differentiated chondrosarcoma is difficult to distinguish from a benign enchondroma on cytologic grounds alone. Zones of calcification are often conspicuous and are seen radiographically as splotches or bulky masses. Chondrosarcoma expands by stimulating osteoclastic resorption of bone and often breaks through the cortex. Most chondrosarcomas grow slowly, but hematogenous metastases to the lungs are common in poorly differentiated variants.

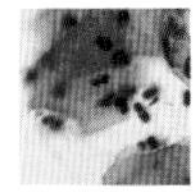

CLINICAL FEATURES: Patients generally present with pain at the affected site. Chondrosarcoma is one of the few tumors in which microscopic grading has a significant prognostic value. The 5-year survival rate for low-grade conventional chondrosarcomas is 80%, for moderate-grade tumors 50%, and for high-grade tumors only 20%. Wide excision is the usual treatment because response to radiation and chemotherapy is poor.

Ewing Sarcoma

EWS is an uncommon malignant bone tumor composed of small, uniform, round cells (blue cells). It represents only 5% of all bone tumors and is found in children and adolescents, with two thirds of cases occurring in patients younger than 20 years. Boys are affected more often than girls (2:1). EWS is very rare in blacks. About 10% to 20% of Ewing sarcomas are extraskeletal.

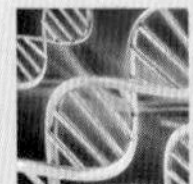

MOLECULAR PATHOGENESIS: EWS is thought to arise from primitive marrow elements or immature mesenchymal cells. Most (90%) of these tumors have a reciprocal translocation between chromosomes 11 and 22 [t(11;22)(q24;q12)], resulting in the fusion of the amino terminus of the *EWS1* gene to the carboxy terminus of the *FLI-1* gene, which encodes a transcription factor. The resulting fusion protein, EWS/FLI-1, is an aberrant transcription factor whose target genes are not yet fully identified.

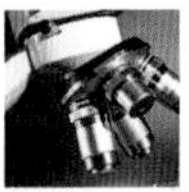

PATHOLOGY: EWS is primarily a tumor of the long bones in childhood, especially the humerus, tibia, and femur, where it occurs as a midshaft or metaphyseal lesion. It tends to parallel the distribution of red marrow, so when it arises in the third decade or later, it affects the pelvis and spine. However, no bone is immune from involvement.

The radiographic findings are variable and depend on the interaction of the tumor with the host bone. There is often a destructive process in which the border between normal bone and the lesion is indistinct. Periosteal reaction and a soft tissue mass are also commonly seen (Fig. 22-33A). Some patients present with fever and weakness as well as bone pain, so their condition may be mistaken for osteomyelitis.

On gross examination, EWS is typically soft and grayish white, often studded by hemorrhagic foci and necrotic areas. The tumor may infiltrate the medullary spaces without destroying the bony trabeculae. It may also diffusely infiltrate the cortical bone or form nodules in which the bone is completely resorbed. In many cases, the tumor mass penetrates the periosteum and extends into the soft tissues.

Microscopically, EWS cells appear as sheets of closely packed, small, round cells with little cytoplasm, which are up to twice the size of a lymphocyte (Fig. 22-33B). Fibrous strands separate the sheets of cells into irregular nests. There is little or no interstitial stroma, and mitoses are frequent. In some areas, the neoplastic cells tend to form rosettes. An important diagnostic feature is the presence of substantial amounts of glycogen in the cytoplasm of the tumor cells, which is well visualized with the PAS stain.

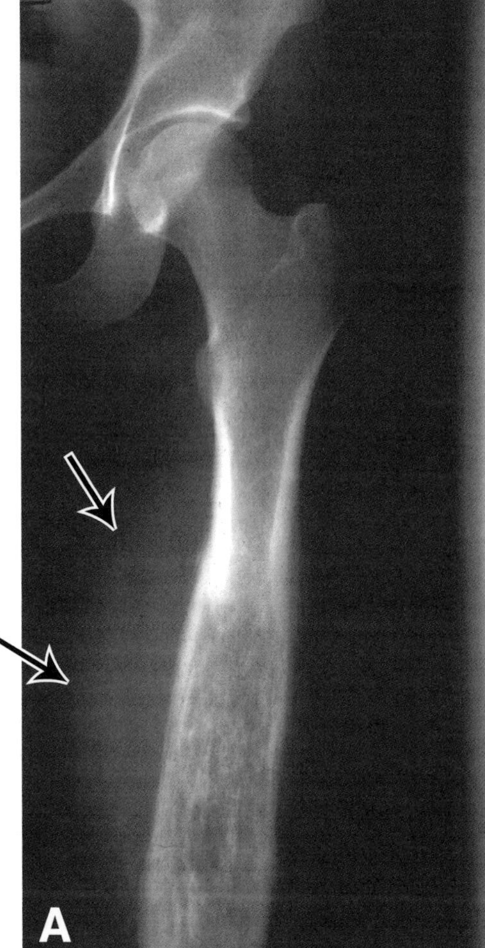

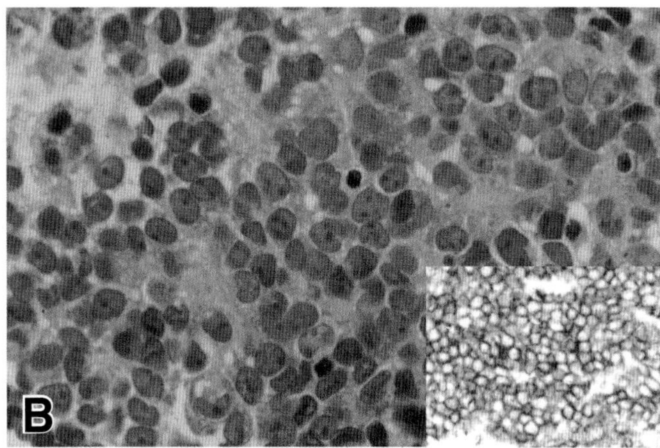

FIGURE 22-33. Ewing sarcoma. A. A clinical radiograph demonstrating expansile cortical destruction with poor circumscription and a delicate interrupted periosteal reaction (*arrows*). **B.** A biopsy specimen showing fairly uniform small cells with round, dark blue nuclei and poorly defined cytoplasm. Immunohistochemical stain for CD99 shows a membranous pattern (*inset*).

EWS metastasizes to many organs, including the lungs and brain. Other bones, especially the skull, are common sites for metastases (50% to 75% of cases).

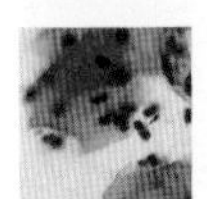

CLINICAL FEATURES: EWS initially presents with mild pain, which becomes more intense and is followed by swelling of the affected area. Nonspecific symptoms, including fever and leukocytosis, commonly follow. In some cases, a soft tissue mass is encountered.

Although EWS prognosis was previously dismal, with current use of chemotherapy plus radiation and limb-sparing surgery, the 5-year disease-free survival is 60% to 75% in the absence of metastases.

Multiple Myeloma

Malignant plasma cell tumors may be either localized (plasmacytoma) or diffuse (see Chapter 18). Multiple myeloma occurs mostly in older people (average age, 65) and affects men twice as often as women. Because myeloma cells secrete cytokines that recruit osteoclasts, the lesions are unique in that they are almost exclusively lytic. The bones most frequently involved are the skull, spine, ribs, pelvis, and femur. Pathologic fractures are common. On microscopic examination, sheets of plasma cells show varying degrees of maturity. Amyloid deposits, in both skeletal and extraskeletal sites, are seen in 10% of patients.

With newer therapeutic agents, the median survival of patients with multiple myeloma now is about 5 years. Death is usually due to infection or renal failure. Solitary plasmacytoma has a better prognosis, with a 60% 5-year survival.

Metastatic Tumors in Bone

In adults, most metastatic lesions to bone are carcinomas, particularly of the prostate, breast, lung, and kidney. In children, the most common bone metastases are from rhabdomyosarcoma, neuroblastoma, Wilms tumor, and clear cell carcinoma of the kidney. Tumor cells usually arrive in the bone via the bloodstream; in the case of spinal metastases, the vertebral veins often transport them. Most deposits of metastatic cancer in the bones have mixtures of both lytic and blastic elements.

Joints

A joint (or articulation) is a union between two or more bones, whose construction varies with the function of that joint. There are two types of joints. A **synovial** or **diarthrodial joint** is a movable joint, such as the knee or elbow, that is lined by a synovial membrane. A **synarthrosis** is a joint that has little movement.

One third of the population of the United States older than 50 years develop some form of clinically significant joint disease.

Once there is an insult to one component of the joint, the resulting dysfunction can lead to degeneration of other components of the joint. For example, knee ligament injuries sustained by athletes, such as a torn anterior cruciate ligament, can result in joint instability. Over time, this situation contributes to degeneration of articular cartilage, owing to changes in movement and load on the joint (secondary osteoarthritis).

ARTHRITIS: Arthritis refers to joint inflammation, usually accompanied by pain, swelling, and sometimes change in structure. Arthritis is divided into two major forms. **Inflammatory arthritis** usually involves the synovium and is mediated by inflammatory cells (e.g., rheumatoid arthritis). **Noninflammatory arthritis**, as featured in primary osteoarthritis, may involve cytokines in its pathogenesis (see below).

STRUCTURES OF THE SYNOVIAL JOINT

Movement plays a major role in joint formation. Lack of movement retards joint development and may be associated with **arthrogryposis**, a group of rare but crippling congenital syndromes characterized by joint contractures.

Synovium

Synovial joints are partially lined on their internal aspects by the synovium. Synovial linings are not true membranes because they lack basement membranes to separate synovial lining cells from subsynovial tissue. The synovium is composed of one to three layers of lining cells and is made up of two cell types. **Type A cells** are macrophages that contain lysosomal enzymes and dense bodies. **Type B cells** secrete hyaluronic acid. Synovial cell membranes are disposed in villi and microvilli, an arrangement that creates an enormous surface area. It is estimated that the knee alone has 100 m^2 of synovial lining.

The synovium controls (1) diffusion in and out of the joint; (2) ingestion of debris; (3) secretion of hyaluronate, immunoglobulins, and lysosomal enzymes; and (4) lubrication of the joints by secreting glycoproteins. Synovial fluid is clear, sticky, and viscous. It is present only in small amounts, not exceeding 1 to 4 mL, and is the main source of nourishment for chondrocytes of the articular cartilage, which lacks a blood supply. Synovial fluid is an ultrafiltrate that does not contain tissue thromboplastin and so cannot clot. Hyaluronate is a very large molecule and, because it is highly charged, has a high affinity for water.

Articular Cartilage

The hyaline cartilage that covers the articular ends of bones does not participate in endochondral ossification and is well suited for its dual role of absorbing shocks and lubricating the surfaces of movable joints. On gross examination, the articular cartilage is glistening, smooth, white, and semirigid and is generally not thicker than 6 mm.

OSTEOARTHRITIS

OA, also known as degenerative joint disease (DJD), is a slowly progressive destruction of articular cartilage that affects weight-bearing joints and fingers of older individuals or the joints of younger people subjected to trauma. OA is the single most common form of joint disease and the major form of noninflammatory arthritis. It is a group of conditions that have in common the mechanical destruction of a joint.

In **primary OA**, destruction of joints results from intrinsic defects in the articular cartilage. The prevalence and severity of primary OA increase with age. About 4% of people aged 18 to 24 are affected, versus 85% of those 75 to 79 years. Before age 45, the disease mainly affects men. After age 55, OA is more common in women. Many cases of primary OA exhibit a familial clustering, suggesting a hereditary predisposition.

In primary OA, progressive degradation of articular cartilage leads to joint narrowing, subchondral bone thickening, and, eventually, a nonfunctioning painful joint. Although OA is not primarily an inflammatory process, a mild inflammatory reaction may occur within the synovium.

Secondary OA has a known underlying cause, including congenital or acquired incongruity of joints, trauma, crystal deposits, infection, metabolic diseases, endocrinopathies, chronic inflammatory diseases, osteonecrosis, and hemarthrosis.

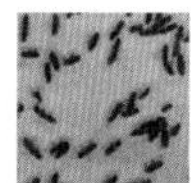

ETIOLOGIC FACTORS: *INCREASED UNIT LOAD:* Abnormal force on the cartilage may have many causes but is often attributable to incongruities of the joint. Thus, in secondary OA associated with congenital hip dysplasia, a fairly common abnormality, less surface area is covered by articular cartilage, which thus bears an increased load. When the critical unit load is exceeded, chondrocyte death causes degradation of articular cartilage.

RESILIENCE OF THE ARTICULAR CARTILAGE: Because articular cartilage binds extensive amounts of water, it normally has a swelling pressure of at least three atmospheres. Disruption in water bonding leads to decreased resilience.

STIFFNESS OF SUBCHONDRAL COARSE CANCELLOUS BONE: The structure of bone adjacent to a joint is important in maintaining articular cartilage. Mechanical forces are not transferred to articular cartilage by normal stress, but rather are dissipated by microfractures of coarse cancellous bone. Damage to this structure results in an increased unit load on the cartilage because of an increase in the stiffness of subchondral bone (e.g., in Paget disease).

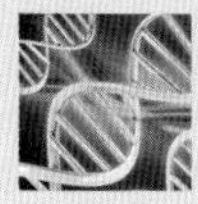

MOLECULAR PATHOGENESIS: *BIOCHEMICAL ABNORMALITIES:* The biochemical changes of OA mainly involve proteoglycans. Proteoglycan content and aggregation decrease, and glycosaminoglycan chain length is reduced. Collagen fibers are thicker than normal, and the water content of osteoarthritic cartilage increases. The reduction in proteoglycans allows more water to be bound to the collagen. Thus, osteoarthritic cartilage, or any cartilage that is fibrillated, swells more than normal cartilage.

Acid cathepsin, which attacks the protein cores of the matrix macromolecules, increases in osteoarthritic cartilage. Collagenase is absent in normal cartilage but is found in osteoarthritic cartilage.

Chondrocyte apoptosis, decreased type II collagen synthesis, and breakdown of extracellular matrix also occur and have been correlated with local increases in IL-1β and TNF-α. In turn, these cytokines increase the production of matrix metalloproteinases (MMPs), nitric oxide, and PGE2. Mechanical stress appears to be the triggering factor for these signaling cascades.

Studies of identical twins have demonstrated genetic contributions to the prevalence of OA. Genetic analysis of patients with a type of familial, early-onset OA revealed a variety of mutations in the gene for type II collagen (*COL2A1*), the major collagen species of articular cartilage.

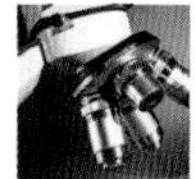

PATHOLOGY: Joints commonly affected by OA are the proximal and distal interphalangeal joints of the fingers, as well as the joints of the arms, knees, hips, and cervical and lumbar spine. Radiologically, OA is characterized by (1) narrowing of the joint space, which represents the loss of articular cartilage; (2) increased thickness of the subchondral bone; (3) subchondral bone cysts; and

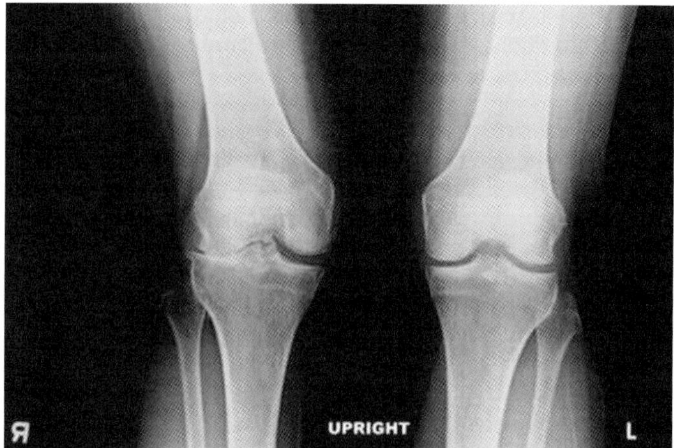

FIGURE 22-34. A radiograph of a patient with osteoarthritis of the right knee demonstrating marked narrowing of the joint space, increased density of subchondral bone, and osteophyte formation laterally.

(4) large peripheral growths of bone and cartilage, called **osteophytes** (Fig. 22-34). Histologic changes follow a well-described sequence (Fig. 22-35).

1. First, loss of proteoglycans from the surface of the articular cartilage is seen histologically as decreased metachromatic staining. At the same time, empty lacunae in articular cartilage indicate that chondrocytes have died (Fig. 22-35A). Viable chondrocytes enlarge, aggregate into groups or clones (Fig. 22-35C), and become surrounded by basophilic staining matrix, called the **territorial matrix**.
2. OA may arrest at this stage for many years before progressing to the next stage, which is characterized by fibrillation (i.e., development of surface cracks parallel to the long axis of the articular surface). These fibrillations may persist for many years before further progression occurs (Fig. 22-35B).
3. As fibrillations propagate, synovial fluid begins to flow into the defects. The cracks are progressively oriented more vertically, parallel to the long axis of the collagen fibrils. Synovial fluid penetrates deeper into the articular cartilage along these cracks. Eventually, pieces of articular cartilage break off and lodge in the synovium, inducing inflammation and a foreign-body giant cell reaction. The result is a hyperemic and hypertrophied synovium.
4. As the crack extends down and crosses the tidemark, the interface between mineralized and unmineralized cartilage, neovascularization from the epiphysis and subchondral bone extends into the area of the crack, inducing subchondral osteoclastic bone resorption (Fig. 22-35C). Adjacent osteoblastic activity also occurs and results in a thickening of the subchondral bone plate in the area of the crack. As neovascularization progressively extends into the area of the crack, mesenchymal cells invade, and fibrocartilage forms as a poor substitute for the articular hyaline cartilage (Figs. 22-35D and 22-36A). These fibrocartilaginous plugs may persist, or they may be swept into the joint. The subchondral bone becomes exposed and burnished as it grinds against the opposite joint surface, which is undergoing the same process. These thick, shiny, smooth areas of subchondral bone are referred to as **eburnated** (ivorylike) bone.

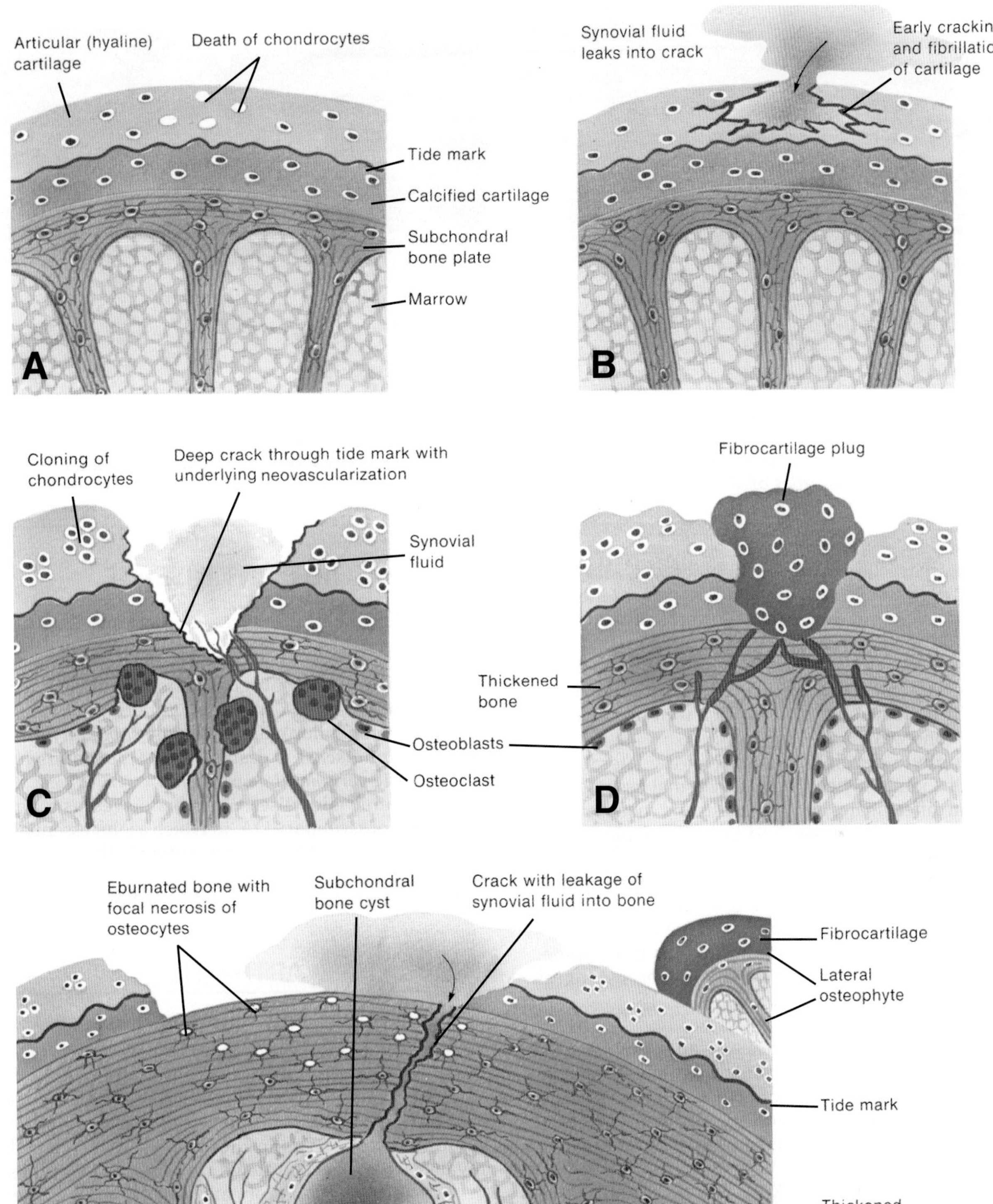

FIGURE 22-35. Histogenesis of osteoarthritis. A, B. The death of chondrocytes leads to a crack in the articular cartilage, followed by an influx of synovial fluid and further loss and degeneration of cartilage. **C.** As a result of this process, cartilage is gradually worn away. Below the tidemark, new vessels grow in from the epiphysis, and fibrocartilage (**D**) is deposited. **E.** The fibrocartilage plug is not mechanically sufficient and may be worn away, thus exposing the subchondral bone plate, which becomes thickened and eburnated. If there is a crack in this region, synovial fluid leaks into the marrow space and produces a subchondral bone cyst. Focal regrowth of the articular surface leads to the formation of osteophytes.

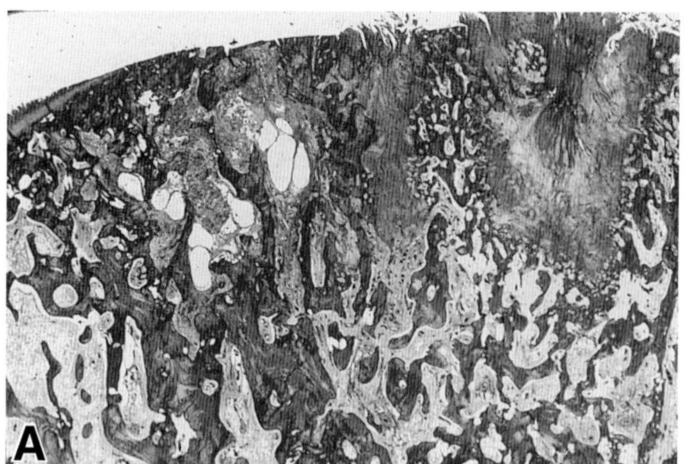

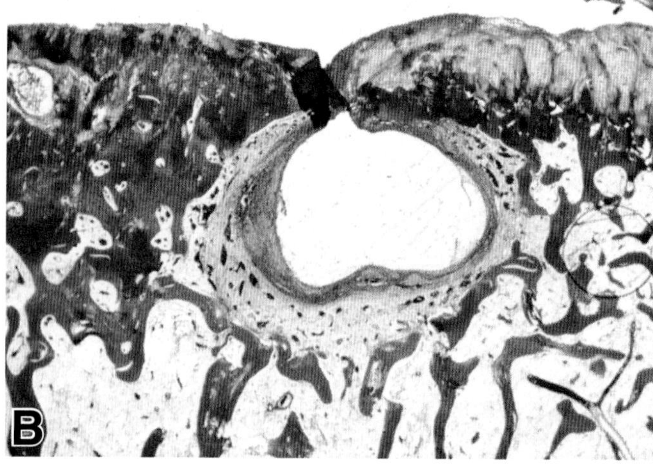

FIGURE 22-36. Osteoarthritis. A. A femoral head with osteoarthritis showing a fibrocartilaginous plug (*far right*) extending from the marrow onto the joint surface. Eburnated bone is present over the remaining surface. **B.** A section through the articular surface of an osteoarthritic joint demonstrating focal absence of the articular cartilage, thickening of subchondral bone (*left*), and a subchondral bone cyst. From Bullough PG. *Atlas of Orthopaedic Pathology*. 2nd ed. New York, NY: Gower Medical Publishing; 1992. Copyright Lippincott Williams & Wilkins.

5. In some areas, the eburnated bone cracks, allowing synovial fluid to extend from the joint surface into the subchondral bone marrow, where it eventually produces a **subchondral bone cyst** (Figs. 22-35E and 22-36B). These cysts increase in size because synovial fluid is forced into the space but cannot exit. The result is a subchondral bone cyst filled with synovial fluid, with a well-marginated, reactive bone wall.
6. An osteophyte develops—usually in the lateral portions of the joint—when the mesenchymal tissue of the synovium differentiates into osteoblasts and chondroblasts to form a mass of cartilage and bone. Osteophytes are pearly grayish bone nodules on the periphery of the joint surface. These osteophytes, or bony spurs, also occur at lateral edges of intervertebral disks, extending from the adjacent vertebral bodies. They produce the "lipping" pattern seen on radiologic studies of OA of the spine. In the fingers, osteophytes at the distal interphalangeal joints are called **Heberden nodes**.

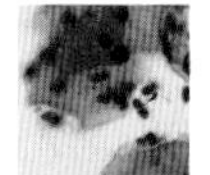

CLINICAL FEATURES: The signs and symptoms of OA are functions of the location of the involved joints and the severity and duration of the joint deterioration. Physical findings vary. The involved joints may be enlarged, tender, and boggy and may demonstrate crepitus. Deep, achy joint pain that follows activity and is relieved by rest is the clinical hallmark of OA. Pain is usually a sign of significant joint destruction and arises in the periarticular structures because articular cartilage lacks a nerve supply. Discomfort also is caused by short periods of stiffness, which is frequently experienced in the morning or after periods of minimal activity. Restricted joint motion indicates severe disease and may result from joint or muscle contractures, intra-articular loose bodies, large osteophytes, and loss of congruity of the joint surfaces.

At present, OA cannot be prevented or arrested. Therapy is directed at specific orthopedic conditions and includes exercise, weight loss, and other supportive measures. In disabling osteoarthritis, joint replacement may be necessary.

NEUROPATHIC JOINT DISEASE (CHARCOT JOINT)

Neuropathic joint disease is a form of noninflammatory arthritis characterized by progressive joint destruction due to a primary neurologic disorder, such as peripheral neuropathy or central motor abnormality. ***The most common form of neuropathic joint disease is destruction of foot joints in people with diabetic peripheral neuropathy.***

Neuropathic joint disease can be viewed as a rapid and severe form of secondary OA, in which a joint essentially fragments. It is likely that loss of innervation to the joint structures brings on a lack of proprioception and pain, abnormal joint mechanics, and ultimately joint destruction.

RHEUMATOID ARTHRITIS

RA is a systemic, chronic inflammatory disease in which chronic polyarthritis involves diarthrodial joints, symmetrically and bilaterally. The proximal interphalangeal and metacarpophalangeal joints, elbows, knees, ankles, and spine are most commonly affected. RA may occur at any age but usually begins in the third or fourth decade, and prevalence increases until age 70. The disease afflicts 1% to 2% of the adult population, and its incidence is greater in women than in men (3:1). Commonly, joints of the extremities are simultaneously affected, often in a symmetric manner. The course of the disease varies and is often punctuated by remissions and exacerbations. The broad spectrum of clinical manifestations ranges from barely discernible to severe, destructive, mutilating disease.

It is now thought that classic RA comprises a heterogeneous group of disorders. Patients who are persistently seronegative for rheumatoid factor probably have disease of a different etiology than those who are seropositive. There are also rheumatoid-like diseases associated with underlying conditions, such as inflammatory bowel disease and cirrhosis.

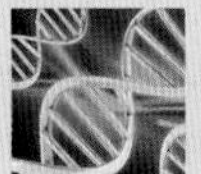

MOLECULAR PATHOGENESIS:
GENETIC FACTORS: A contribution of hereditary factors to RA susceptibility is suggested by the increased frequency of the disease in first-degree relatives of affected patients and by the concordance for the illness in monozygotic twins (15%). In addition, certain major histocompatibility genes are expressed in a nonrandom manner in patients with RA. An important genetic locus that predisposes to RA is present in *HLA II* genes, and a specific set of HLA-DR alleles (DR4, DR1, DR10, and DR14) is consistently increased in these patients. These alleles share a pentapeptide sequence motif (shared epitope) in a hypervariable segment of the *HLA-DRB1* gene, which forms the peptide-binding pocket on the HLA molecule. The binding properties of this pocket influence the type of peptides that can be bound by RA-associated HLA-DR molecules and so affect the immune response to these peptides. Interestingly, seropositive RA (poor prognosis) is associated with a high frequency of an arginine in the shared epitope, whereas seronegative disease (good prognosis) commonly exhibits a lysine in the same position. Several non-HLA loci have been linked to RA, including a region of chromosome 18q21 that encodes the receptor activator of NF-κB, or RANK.

HUMORAL IMMUNITY: Immunologic mechanisms are important in the pathogenesis of RA. Lymphocytes and plasma cells accumulate in the synovium, where they produce immunoglobulins, mainly of the IgG class. In addition, immune complex deposits are present in the articular cartilage and the synovium. Increased serum levels of IgM, IgA, and IgG are also seen.

Some 80% of patients with classic RA are positive for rheumatoid factor (RF). RF represents multiple antibodies, mostly IgM, but sometimes IgG or IgA, directed against the Fc fragment of IgG. Significant titers of RF are also found in patients with related collagen vascular diseases, such as systemic lupus erythematosus, and also in many nonrheumatic disorders, including pulmonary fibrosis, cirrhosis, sarcoidosis, tuberculosis, and others. Even healthy elderly individuals, particularly women, occasionally test positive for RF.

Although patients with classic RA may be seronegative, the presence of RF in high titer is frequently associated with severe and unremitting disease, many systemic complications, and a serious prognosis.

Immune complexes (RF + IgG) and complement components are found in the synovium, synovial fluid, and extra-articular lesions of patients with RA. Furthermore, patients with seropositive RA have lower levels of complement in their synovial fluid than do those who are seronegative.

Anticitrullinated protein antibody (ACPA) is positive in two thirds of cases of RA. The test may be positive even before the onset of clinical disease, suggesting that an autoimmune response to endogenous citrullinated peptides may be involved in disease pathogenesis.

CELLULAR IMMUNITY: It has also been postulated that cell-mediated immunity contributes to RA. Abundant T lymphocytes in rheumatoid synovium are frequently Ia positive ("activated") and of the helper type ($CD4^+$). They are often in close contact with HLA-DR–positive cells, which are either macrophages or dendritic Ia-positive cells.

T cells may directly or indirectly interact with macrophages through production of cytokines that inhibit migration and proliferation of the latter. Hence, joint destruction in RA may reflect local production of cytokines, especially TNF-α and IL-1.

INFECTIOUS AGENTS: Infectious bacteria and viruses are not detected in joints of patients with RA, although structures resembling viruses have been reported early in the disease. Most patients with RA develop antibodies against a nuclear antigen in B cells infected with EBV. Moreover, EBV is a polyclonal B-cell activator that stimulates production of RF.

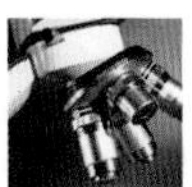

PATHOLOGY: The early synovial changes of RA are edema and accumulation of plasma cells, lymphocytes, and macrophages (Fig. 22-37A). Vascularity increases, with exudation of fibrin into the joint space, which may result in small fibrin nodules that float in the joint (**rice bodies**).

PANNUS FORMATION: Synovial lining cells, normally only one to three layers thick, undergo hyperplasia and form layers 8 to 10 cells deep. Multinucleated giant cells are often found among the synovial cells. The synovial lining is thus thrown into numerous villi and frond-like folds that fill the peripheral recesses of the joint (Figs. 22-37C and 22-38). This inflammatory synovium, which now contains mast cells, creeps over the surface of the articular cartilage and adjacent structures and is termed a **pannus**. Pannus covers the articular cartilage and isolates it from the synovial fluid (Fig. 22-37D). Lymphocytes aggregate and eventually develop follicular centers (Figs. 22-37C and 22-38B and C). The pannus erodes the articular cartilage and adjacent bone, probably through the action of collagenase produced. Because PGE_2 and IL-1 are produced in the rheumatoid synovium, they may mediate bone erosion by stimulating osteoclasts.

The characteristic bone loss of RA is juxta-articular; that is, it is immediately adjacent to both sides of the joint. The pannus penetrates the subchondral bone and may involve tendons and ligaments, leading to deformities and instabilities. Eventually, the joint is destroyed and undergoes fibrous fusion, or **ankylosis** (Figs. 22-37E and 22-39). Long-standing cases feature bony bridging of the joint (**bony ankylosis**).

Changes in synovial fluid include a massive increase in volume, increased turbidity, and decreased viscosity. The protein content and the number of inflammatory cells in the fluid increase, correlating with the activity of the rheumatoid process. In some cases, the leukocyte count in the joint exceeds 50,000/μL, with 95% polymorphonuclear leukocytes.

RHEUMATOID NODULES: RA is a systemic disease that also involves tissues other than joints and tendons. A characteristic lesion, the rheumatoid nodule, is found in extra-articular locations. It has a central core of fibrinoid necrosis, which is a mixture of fibrin and other proteins, such as degraded collagen (Fig. 22-40). A surrounding rim of macrophages is arranged in a radial or palisading manner. Beyond the macrophages is a circle of lymphocytes, plasma cells, and other mononuclear cells. The overall appearance resembles a peculiar granuloma

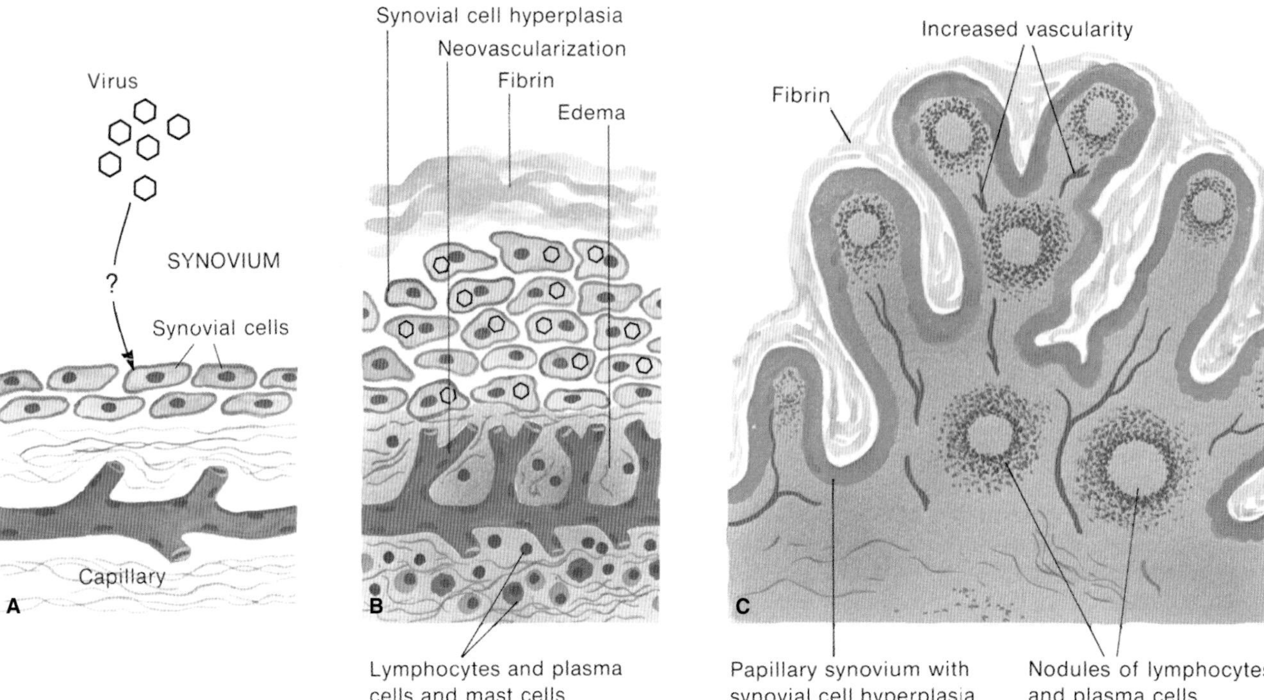

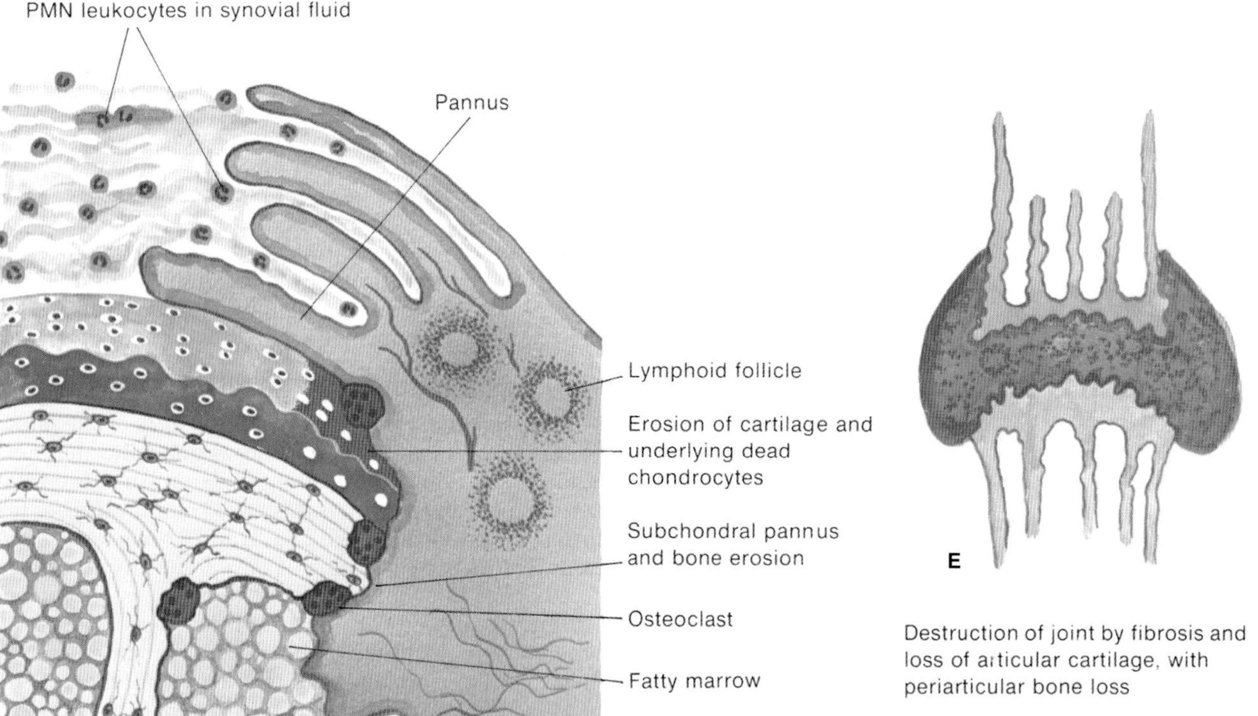

FIGURE 22-37. Histogenesis of rheumatoid arthritis. A. A virus or an unknown stress may stimulate the synovial cells to proliferate. **B.** The influx of lymphocytes, plasma cells, and mast cells, together with neovascularization and edema, leads to hypertrophy and hyperplasia of the synovium. **C.** Lymphoid nodules are prominent. **D.** Proliferating synovium extends into the joint space, burrows into the bone beneath the articular cartilage, and covers the cartilage as a pannus. The articular cartilage is eventually destroyed by direct resorption or deprivation of its nutrient synovial fluid. The synovial tissue continues to proliferate in the subchondral region, as well as in the joint. **E.** Eventually, the joint is destroyed and becomes fused, a condition termed **ankylosis**. PMN, polymorphonuclear neutrophil.

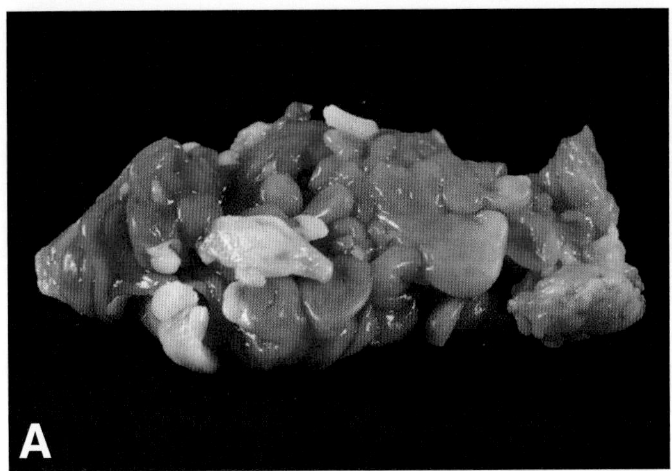

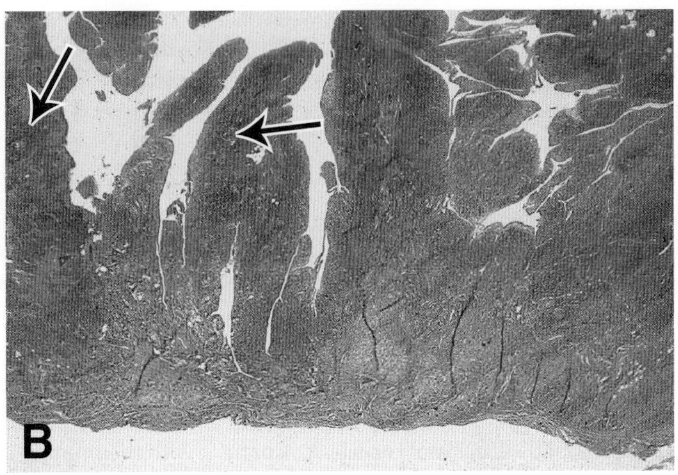

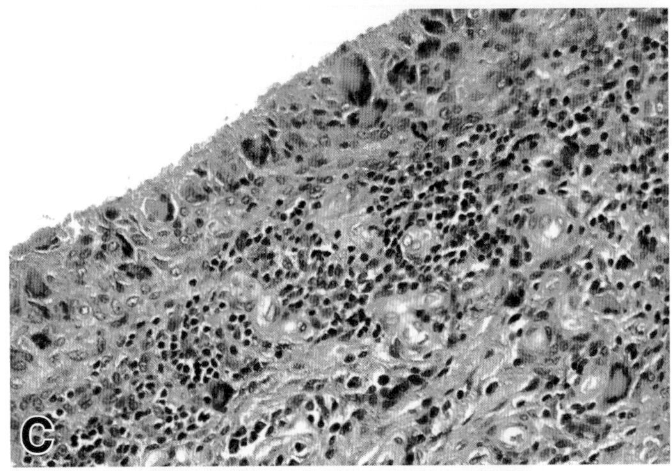

FIGURE 22-38. Rheumatoid arthritis (RA). A. Hyperplastic synovium from a patient with RA showing numerous fingerlike projections, with focal pale areas of fibrin deposition. The brownish color of the synovium reflects hemosiderin accumulation derived from old hemorrhage. **B.** A microscopic view revealing prominent lymphoid follicles (Allison–Ghormley bodies; *arrows*), synovial hyperplasia and hypertrophy, villous folds, and thickening of the synovial membrane by fibrosis and inflammation. **C.** A higher power view of the inflamed synovium demonstrating hyperplasia and hypertrophy of the lining cells. Numerous giant cells are on and below the surface. The stroma is chronically inflamed.

surrounding a core of fibrinoid necrosis. Rheumatoid nodules, which are usually found in areas of pressure (e.g., the skin of elbows and legs), are movable, firm, rubbery, and, occasionally, tender. A large nodule may ulcerate.

Rheumatoid nodules may also be seen in lupus erythematous and rheumatic fever. They are sometimes found in visceral organs, such as the heart, lungs, intestinal tract, and even the dura. Nodules in the bundle of His may cause cardiac arrhythmias; in the lungs, they produce fibrosis and even respiratory failure. RA may also be accompanied by **acute necrotizing vasculitis**, which can affect any organ.

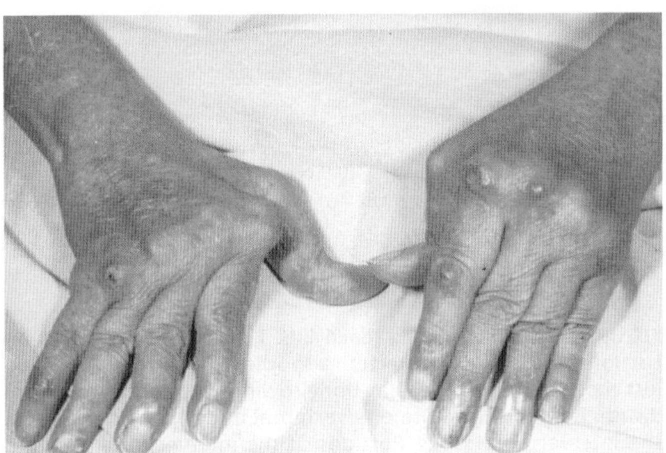

FIGURE 22-39. Rheumatoid arthritis. The hands of a patient with advanced arthritis showing swelling of the metacarpophalangeal joints and the classic ulnar deviation of the fingers.

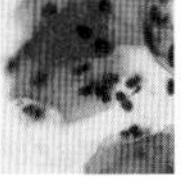

CLINICAL FEATURES: The clinical diagnosis of RA is imprecise and is based on a number of criteria, such as the number and types of joints involved, the presence of rheumatoid nodules and RF, and radiographic characteristic of the disease.

The onset of RA may be acute, slowly progressing, or insidious. In most patients, disease activity waxes and wanes. Diseased joints tend to be warm, swollen, and painful. The pain is heightened by motion and is most severe after periods of disuse. Unabated disease causes progressive destruction of the joint surfaces and periarticular structures. Eventually, patients manifest severe flexion and extension deformities, associated with joint subluxation, which may terminate in joint ankylosis.

The natural history of RA is variable. One fourth of patients seem to recover completely. Another one quarter have only slight functional impairment for many years. However, half develop serious progressive and disabling joint disease. There is increased mortality from infection, gastrointestinal hemorrhage and perforation, vasculitis, heart and lung involvement, amyloidosis, and subluxation of the cervical spine.

Three types of drugs are used to suppress synovial inflammation and to induce a remission. These include nonsteroidal anti-inflammatory agents, corticosteroids, and the so-called **disease-modifying antirheumatic drugs (DMARDs)** which suppress immune response and inhibit cytokines such as TNF.

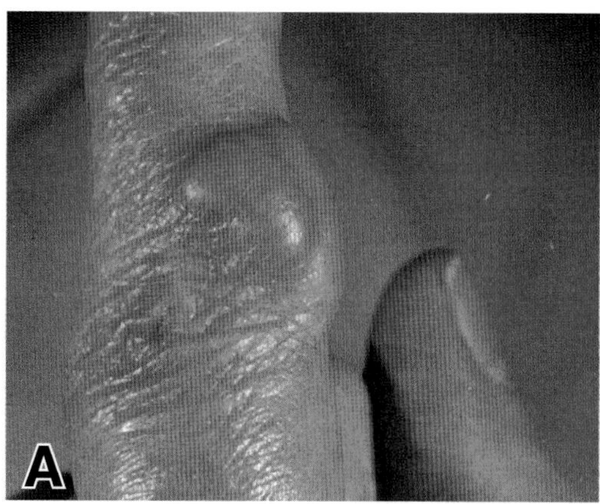

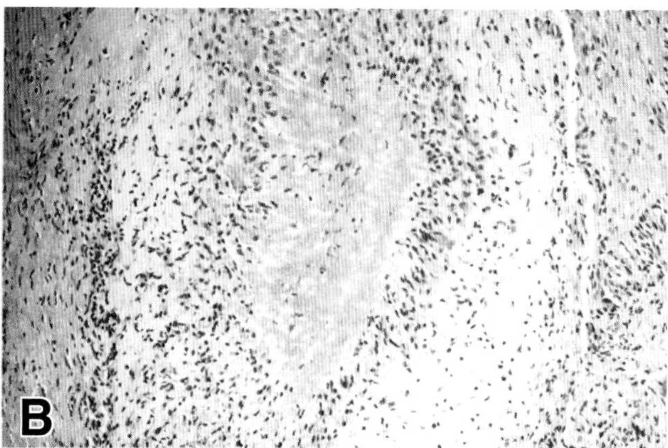

FIGURE 22-40. Rheumatoid nodule. A. A patient with rheumatoid arthritis has a subcutaneous mass on a digit. **B.** Microscopic view of a rheumatoid nodule showing a central area of necrosis surrounded by palisaded macrophages and a chronic inflammatory infiltrate.

SPONDYLOARTHROPATHY

A number of clinical entities were formerly classified as variants of RA but are now recognized to be distinct disorders. These forms of arthritis are now known as **spondyloarthropathies** and include ankylosing spondylitis, Reiter syndrome, psoriatic arthritis, and arthritis associated with inflammatory bowel disease. They share several features:

- Seronegativity for RF and other serologic markers of RA
- Association with class I histocompatibility antigens, particularly HLA-B27
- Sacroiliac and vertebral involvement (spondylitis)
- Asymmetric involvement of only a few peripheral joints
- A tendency to inflammation of periarticular tendons and fascia
- Systemic involvement of other organs, especially uveitis, carditis, and aortitis
- Preferential onset in young men

Ankylosing Spondylitis

Ankylosing spondylitis is an inflammatory arthropathy of the vertebral column and sacroiliac joints. It may be accompanied by asymmetric, peripheral arthritis (30% of patients) and systemic manifestations. It is most common in young men, with a peak incidence at about age 20. Over 90% of patients express HLA-B27 (normal, 4% to 8%), although the disorder affects only 1% of people with this haplotype.

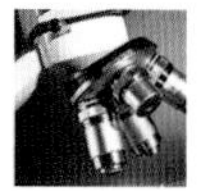

PATHOLOGY: Ankylosing spondylitis begins at the sacroiliac joints bilaterally, then ascends the spinal column by involving the small joints of the posterior elements of the spine. The result is destruction of these joints, after which the spine becomes fused posteriorly (Fig. 22-41).

Although a few patients with ankylosing spondylitis rapidly develop crippling spinal disease, most are able to maintain their employment and live a normal life span. However, up to 5% of patients develop AA amyloidosis and uremia, and a few manifest severe cardiac involvement.

Reactive Arthritis

Reactive arthritis (previously known as Reiter syndrome) is a triad that includes (1) seronegative polyarthritis, (2) conjunctivitis and uveitis, and (3) nonspecific urethritis. It occurs almost exclusively in men and usually follows venereal exposure or an episode of bacillary dysentery. As in ankylosing spondylitis, this syndrome is associated with HLA-B27 in 90% of patients. In fact, after an attack of dysentery, 20% of HLA-B27–positive men develop reactive arthritis.

The pathologic features of this syndrome are comparable to those of RA. More than half of patients develop mucocutaneous lesions similar to those of pustular psoriasis (**keratoderma blennorrhagica**) over the palms, soles, and trunk. In most

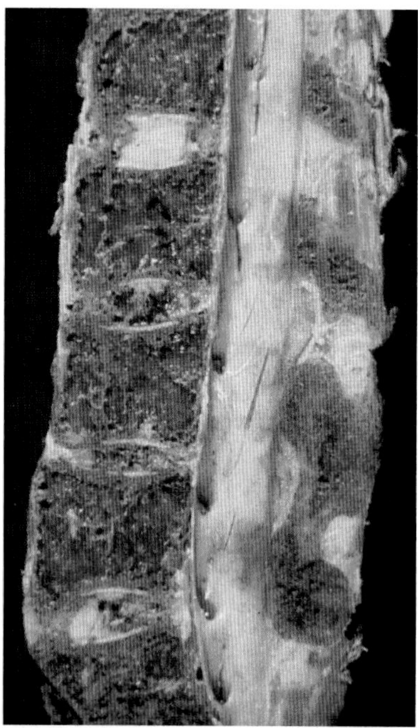

FIGURE 22-41. Ankylosing spondylitis. The vertebrae have been cut longitudinally. The vertebral bodies are square and have lost most of their trabecular bone, owing to osteoporosis from disuse. Bone bridges fuse one vertebral body to the next across the intervertebral disks. Portions of the intervertebral disk are replaced by bone marrow. Bony bridges also fuse the posterior elements (**ankylosis**). From Bullough PG. *Atlas of Orthopaedic Pathology*. 2nd ed. New York, NY: Gower Medical Publishing; 1992. Copyright Lippincott Williams & Wilkins.

patients, the disease remits within a year, but in 20%, progressive arthritis develops, including ankylosing spondylitis.

Psoriatic Arthritis

Of all patients with psoriasis, particularly in those with severe disease, 7% develop an inflammatory seronegative arthritis. HLA-B27 has been linked to psoriatic spondylitis and inflammation of distal interphalangeal joints, and HLA-DR4 has been associated with a rheumatoid pattern of involvement. Joint disease is usually mild and slowly progressive, although a mutilating form is occasionally encountered.

Enteropathic Arthritis

Ulcerative colitis and Crohn disease are accompanied by seronegative peripheral arthritis in 20% of cases and spondylitis in 10%. This form of arthritis is also seen in patients with Whipple disease and after certain bacterial infections of the gut. No particular tissue type is associated with peripheral arthritis, but most patients with spondylitis are HLA-B27 positive. Resection of the affected bowel in ulcerative colitis relieves the arthritis, but in Crohn disease, this complication often does not resolve.

JUVENILE ARTHRITIS

Several different chronic arthritic conditions in children are included in this designation, formerly called **Still disease**.

- **Seropositive arthritis:** Fewer than 10% of children with arthritis are positive for RF and have a polyarticular presentation. Females predominate (80%) among children with seropositive disease, and in most cases (75%), antinuclear antibodies are present. HLA-D4 is often present, and more than half of the children eventually develop severe arthritis.
- **Polyarticular disease without systemic symptoms:** One fourth of juvenile arthritis patients (90% girls) have disease of several joints, are seronegative, and do not manifest systemic symptoms. Fewer than 15% of these patients eventually develop severe arthritis.
- **Polyarticular disease with systemic symptoms:** Twenty percent of children with polyarticular arthritis have prominent systemic symptoms, including high fever, rash, hepatosplenomegaly, lymphadenopathy, pleuritis, pericarditis, anemia, and leukocytosis. Most (60%) are boys who are negative for RF, and one fourth of all of these children are left with severe arthritis.
- **Pauciarticular arthritis:** Children with involvement of only a few large joints, such as the knee, ankle, elbow, or hip girdle, account for half of all cases of juvenile arthritis and fall into two general groups. The larger group (80%) mainly comprises girls who are negative for RF but exhibit antinuclear antibodies and are positive for HLA-DR5, HLA-DRw6, or HLA-DRw8. Of these patients, one third have ocular disease, characterized by chronic iridocyclitis (inflammation of the iris and ciliary body). Only a small minority of these children experience residual polyarthritis or ocular damage. The smaller group of children with a pauciarticular presentation is (1) composed almost exclusively of boys, (2) negative for both RF and antinuclear bodies, and (3) positive for HLA-B27 (75%). A few have acute iridocyclitis, which resolves spontaneously. Some of these boys subsequently develop ankylosing spondylitis.

GOUT

Primary Gout

Gout is a heterogeneous group of diseases collectively characterized by increased serum uric acid and urate crystal deposition in joints and kidneys. All such patients have hyperuricemia, but fewer than 15% of people with hyperuricemia have gout. This disorder is characterized by acute and chronic arthritis. Gout is classified as primary or secondary, depending on the etiology of the hyperuricemia. In **primary gout**, hyperuricemia occurs without any other disease; **secondary gout** occurs in association with another illness that results in hyperuricemia. Of all cases of hyperuricemia, one third are primary, and the remainder secondary.

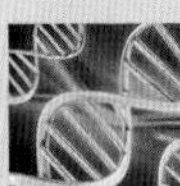

MOLECULAR PATHOGENESIS: Uric acid results from purine catabolism, owing to either a high-purine diet or increased de novo synthesis. In humans, there is a tight balance between uric acid production and tissue deposition of urates. Uric acid is only eliminated in the urine. Thus, the blood uric acid level (normal, <7.0 mg/dL in men, <6.0 mg/dL in women) reflects the difference between the total amount of purines ingested and synthesized and renal excretion. Gout can result from (1) overproduction of purines, (2) increased catabolism of nucleic acids owing to greater cell turnover, (3) decreased salvage of free purine bases, or (4) decreased urinary uric acid excretion (Fig. 22-42). A high dietary intake of purine-rich foods (e.g., meat) by an otherwise normal person does not lead to hyperuricemia and gout.

Most cases (85%) of idiopathic gout result from an as-yet-unexplained impairment of renal uric acid excretion. In the remainder, there is a primary overproduction of uric acid, but the underlying abnormality has been identified in only a minority of cases.

There is a ***familial tendency*** to gout, and hyperuricemia is common among relatives of patients with gout. The consensus today is that multiple genes control the level of serum uric acid.

Lesch–Nyhan syndrome is an inherited, X-linked (Xq26-q27) deficiency of HPRT, a defect that leads to accumulation of PP-ribose-P and, in turn, to enhanced purine synthesis. Children with this syndrome are clinically normal at birth but exhibit delays in development and neurologic dysfunction within the first year. Most are mentally retarded and exhibit self-mutilation. They are hyperuricemic and eventually develop gouty arthritis. In addition, obstructive nephropathy and hematologic abnormalities are often present.

Secondary Gout

As in primary gout, secondary hyperuricemia may reflect overproduction or decreased urinary excretion of uric acid. Increased production is most often associated with increased nucleic acid turnover, as seen in leukemias and lymphomas and after chemotherapy. Reduced urate excretion may result from primary renal disease. Chronic lead nephropathy was historically associated with gout (Saturnine gout). Dehydration

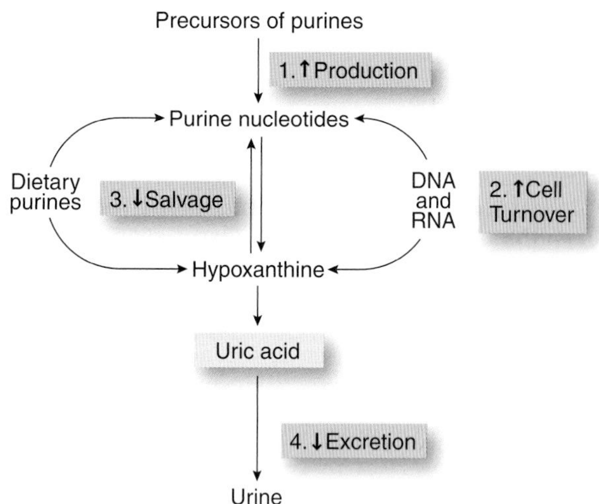

FIGURE 22-42. Pathogenesis of hyperuricemia and gout. Purine nucleotides are synthesized de novo from nonpurine precursors or derived from preformed purines in the diet. Purine nucleotides are catabolized to hypoxanthine or incorporated into nucleic acids. The degradation of nucleic acids and dietary purines also produces hypoxanthine. Hypoxanthine is converted to uric acid, which, in turn, is excreted into the urine. Hyperuricemia and gout result from (*1*) increased de novo purine synthesis, (*2*) increased cell turnover, (*3*) decreased salvage of dietary purines and hypoxanthine, and (*4*) decreased uric acid excretion by the kidneys.

and diuretics increase tubular reabsorption of uric acid and induce hyperuricemia. In fact, various drugs are implicated in 20% of patients with hyperuricemia.

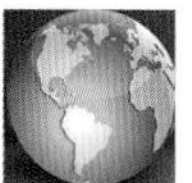

EPIDEMIOLOGY: Primary gout usually afflicts adult men; only 5% of cases occur in women. Many patients have a family history of gout, but environmental factors are also important. Positive correlations exist between the prevalence of hyperuricemia in a population and mean weight, protein intake, alcohol consumption, social class, and intelligence. Thus, gout is a disease that exemplifies the interplay between genetic predisposition and environmental influences.

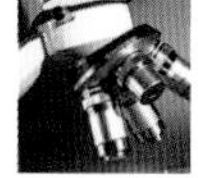

PATHOLOGY: When sodium urate crystals precipitate from supersaturated body fluids, they absorb fibronectin, complement, and a number of other proteins on their surfaces. Neutrophils that have ingested urate crystals release activated oxygen species and lysosomal enzymes, which mediate tissue injury and promote an inflammatory response.

The presence of long, needle-shaped crystals that are negatively birefringent under polarized light is diagnostic of gout (Fig. 22-43). A **tophus** is an extracellular soft tissue deposit of urate crystals, which is surrounded by foreign-body giant cells and an associated inflammatory response of mononuclear cells. These granuloma-like areas are found in cartilage, in any of the soft tissues around joints, and even in the subchondral bone marrow adjacent to joints.

Macroscopically, any chalky-white deposit on intra-articular surfaces, including articular cartilage, suggests gout. Renal urate deposits are between the tubules, especially at the apices of the medulla. These areas are grossly visible as small, shiny, golden yellow, linear streaks in the medulla.

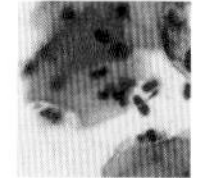

CLINICAL FEATURES: The clinical course of gout is divided into four stages: (1) asymptomatic hyperuricemia, (2) acute gouty arthritis, (3) intercritical gout, and (4) chronic tophaceous gout. Renal urate stones may occur in any stage except the first. In most cases, symptomatic gout appears before renal stones, which usually require 20 to 30 years of sustained hyperuricemia.

- **Asymptomatic hyperuricemia** often precedes clinically evident gout by many years.
- **Acute gouty arthritis** is a painful condition that usually involves one joint, without constitutional symptoms. Later in the course of the disease, polyarticular involvement with fever is common. At least half of patients are first seen with a painful and red first metatarsophalangeal joint (great toe), designated **podagra.** Eventually, 90% of all patients have such an attack. Commonly, a gouty attack begins at night and is exquisitely painful, simulating an acute bacterial infection of the affected joint. Even when untreated, acute attacks of gout are self-limited.
- The **intercritical period** is the asymptomatic interval between the initial acute attack and subsequent episodes. These periods may last up to 10 years, but later attacks tend to be increasingly severe, prolonged, and polyarticular.
- **Tophaceous gout** eventually appears in the untreated patient in the form of tophi in the cartilage, synovial membranes, tendons, and soft tissues.

Renal failure is responsible for 10% of deaths in patients with gout. One third of patients have mild albuminuria, reduced glomerular filtration, and decreased renal concentrating ability. However, the contribution of urate nephropathy to chronic renal dysfunction is unclear, and hypertension, preexisting kidney disease, and the intake of analgesic drugs may be more important.

Treatment of gout is designed to (1) decrease the severity of acute attacks, (2) reduce serum urate, (3) prevent future attacks, (4) promote dissolution of urate deposits, and (5) alkalinize the urine to prevent stone formation. The main drugs used to interrupt the inflammatory process, thereby preventing or controlling the acute attack, are nonsteroidal anti-inflammatory agents. Colchicine has been used for hundreds of years and has been administered prophylactically during the intervals between gouty attacks to prevent recurrent episodes. Uricosuric drugs that interfere with urate reabsorption by the renal tubules are often useful.

Allopurinol is a competitive inhibitor of xanthine oxidase, the enzyme that converts xanthine and hypoxanthine to uric acid. This drug causes a prompt decrease in uricosemia and uricosuria and is used in people with renal insufficiency and those who are resistant to other uricosuric drugs.

CALCIUM PYROPHOSPHATE DIHYDRATE DEPOSITION DISEASE (PSEUDOGOUT)

Calcium pyrophosphate dihydrate (CPPD) deposition disease refers to the accumulation of this compound in synovial membranes (pseudogout), joint cartilage (chondrocalcinosis), ligaments, and tendons. The disease can be (1) idiopathic, (2) associated with trauma, (3) linked to a number of metabolic disorders, or (4) in rare cases, hereditary.

CPPD deposition disease is principally a condition of old age, and half of those over age 85 are afflicted. Most cases in the elderly are asymptomatic. In such cases, punctate or linear

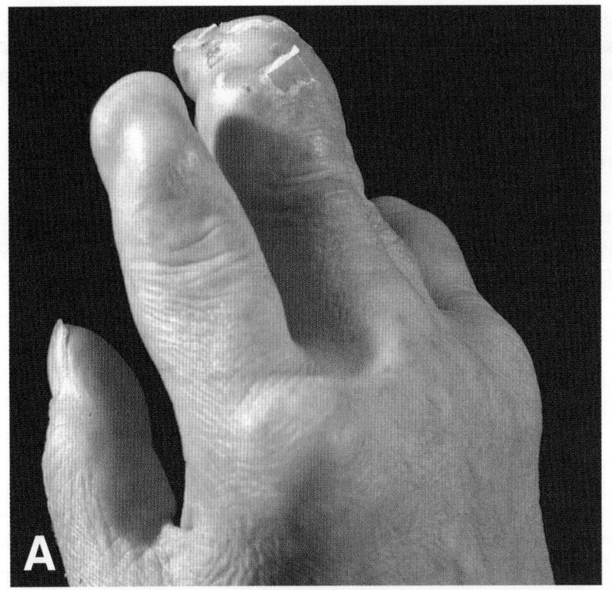

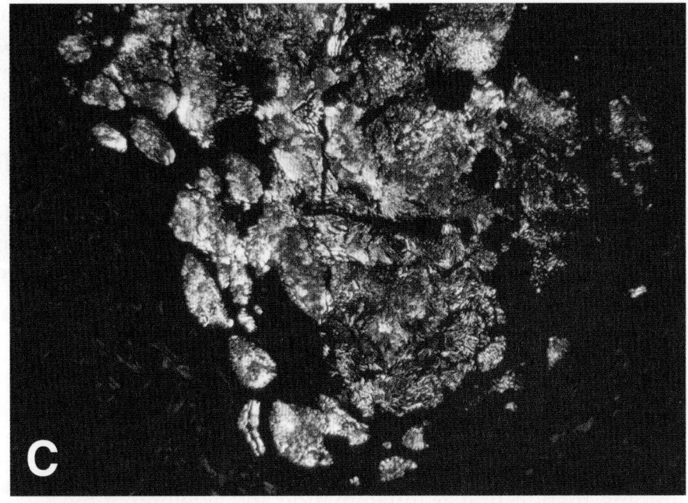

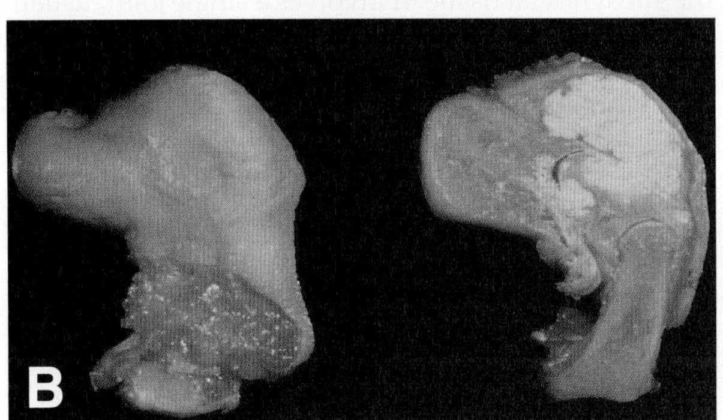

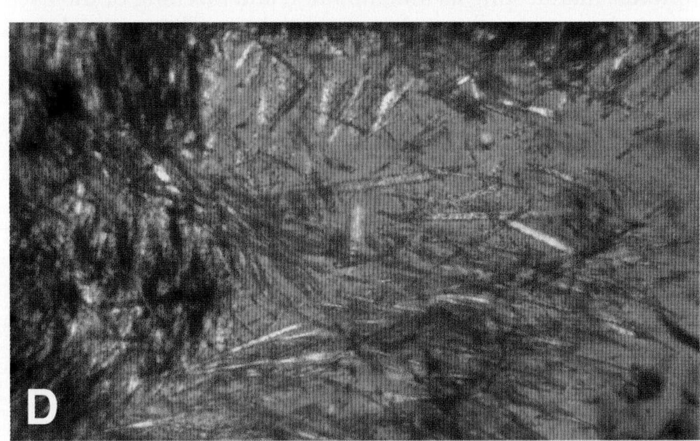

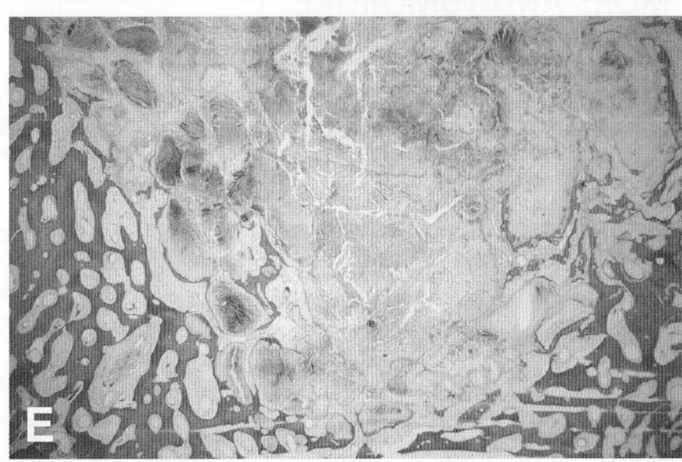

FIGURE 22-43. Gout. A. Gouty tophi of the hands appear as multiple rubbery nodules, one of which is ulcerated. **B.** A cross section of a digit demonstrating a tophaceous collection of toothpaste-like urate crystals. **C.** Histologic section in bright field demonstrating brownish monosodium urate crystals within the bone. **D.** High-power micrograph in polarized light with a quartz compensator plate demonstrating negative birefringence of the crystals (those having their long axes parallel to the slow compensator axis are yellow). **E.** A section through the tophus (if usual aqueous processing is used) demonstrating a foreign-body reaction around a pink, amorphous lesion from which the urate crystals have been dissolved during processing.

calcifications may be present in any fibrocartilage or hyaline cartilage surface. For example, radiography of the knee may disclose linear streaks that outline the menisci.

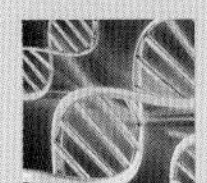

MOLECULAR PATHOGENESIS: The major predisposing abnormality in patients with CPPD deposition disease is an excessive level of inorganic pyrophosphate in the synovial fluid. This material derives from hydrolysis of nucleoside triphosphates in joint chondrocytes. Increased pyrophosphate levels in synovial fluid can result from either increased production or decreased catabolism.

CPPD deposition is commonly found in the knees after trauma and after surgical removal of the meniscus. A number of other disorders are associated with deposition of CPPD crystals, including hyperparathyroidism, hypothyroidism, hemochromatosis, and Wilson disease. Iron and copper are presumed to inhibit pyrophosphatase, accounting for decreased degradation of pyrophosphate.

Mutations in the *ANKH* gene cause familial autosomal dominant CPPD chondrocalcinosis. The *ANKH* gene is thought to encode a membrane pyrophosphate transporter that inhibits mineralization of several tissues, including joints, articular cartilage, and tendons. Mutated ANKH elevates intracellular pyrophosphate and reduces extracellular pyrophosphate.

Hypophosphatasia is a heritable condition in which activity of alkaline phosphatase (the enzyme that hydrolyzes pyrophosphate) in serum and tissue is deficient. As a result, pyrophosphate is not adequately metabolized and accumulates in synovial fluid.

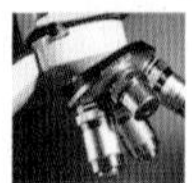

PATHOLOGY AND CLINICAL FEATURES: A minority of patients who are symptomatic with CPPD deposition disease are classified according to the nature of joint involvement.

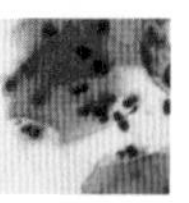

Pseudogout refers to self-limited attacks of acute arthritis lasting from 1 day to 4 weeks and involving one or two joints. Some 25% of patients with CPPD deposition disease have an acute onset of gout-like symptoms, manifesting as inflammation and swelling of the knees, ankles, wrists, elbows, hips, or shoulders. The synovial fluid exhibits abundant leukocytes containing CPPD crystals.

On gross examination, CPPD deposits appear as chalky-white areas on cartilaginous surfaces (Fig. 22-44A). Unlike needle-shaped urate crystals, they are stubby, short, and rhomboid ("coffin-shaped") and display weak birefringence under polarized light. In contrast to urate crystals, CPPD crystals do not dissolve in water and are easily found in tissue sections (Fig. 22-44B). Only a few mononuclear cells and macrophages surround foci of crystal deposition.

The treatment of CPPD is essentially symptomatic (pain control). Nonsteroidal anti-inflammatory drugs and steroids are commonly used.

TUMORS AND TUMORLIKE LESIONS OF JOINTS

True neoplasms of the joints are rare. The most common malignant lesions of the synovium are metastatic carcinomas, particularly adenocarcinoma of the colon, breast, and lung. Lymphoproliferative diseases (e.g., leukemia) may also involve the synovium, mimicking other conditions, such as RA. It is unusual for primary malignant bone tumors to extend into the joint, although they may invade the joint capsule from the soft tissues.

Tenosynovial Giant Cell Tumor

This is the most common benign neoplasm of the synovium and tendon sheath and occurs in a localized and a diffuse form. The lesions may be intra- or extra-articular.

- **Localized tenosynovial giant cell tumor or giant cell tumor of the tendon sheath** involves the hands and feet. In fact, it is the most common soft tissue tumor of the hand. It occurs mostly in young and middle-aged women (30 to 50 years) and involves flexor surfaces of the middle or index fingers. The tumor is usually well circumscribed and grows slowly.
- **Diffuse tenosynovial giant cell tumor or pigmented villonodular synovitis (PVNS)** is characterized by an ill-defined, exuberant proliferation of synovial lining cells arising from periarticular soft tissues, with extension into the subsynovial tissue. It involves a single joint, usually in young adults, and is seen equally in both men and women. The most common site is the knee (80%), but it also occurs in the hip, ankle, calcaneocuboid joint, elbow, and, less frequently, tendon sheaths of the fingers and toes.

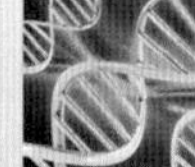

MOLECULAR PATHOGENESIS: In the past, these lesions were regarded as reactive/inflammatory, but recurrent chromosomal aberrations have been described in both forms, supporting a neoplastic nature. Translocations involving the short arm of chromosome 1 have been detected. However, the association of these anomalies with tumor pathogenesis is unclear.

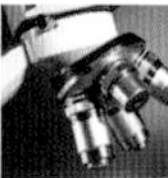

PATHOLOGY: The localized tenosynovial giant cell tumor is characterized by a small (<4 cm), multinodular, smooth-contoured, partially encapsulated, exophytic mass attached to a tendon sheath. The

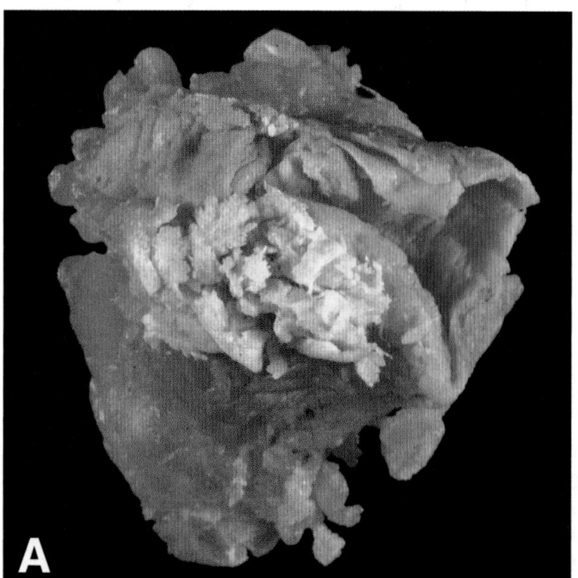

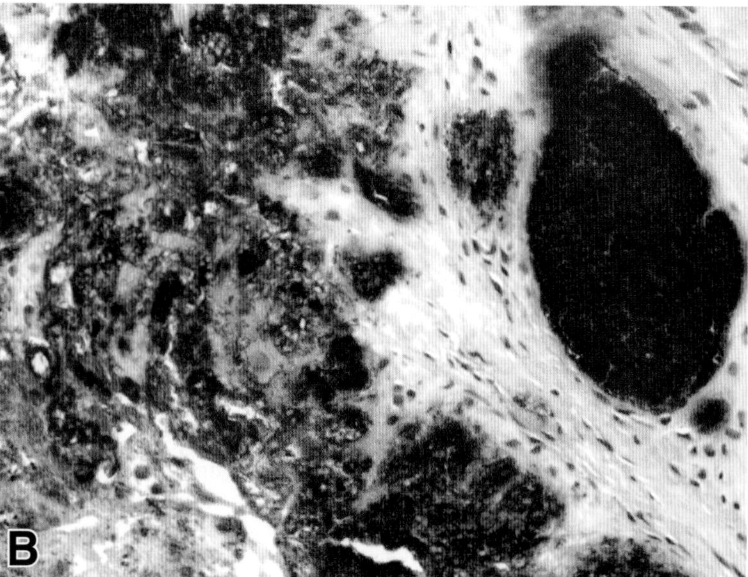

FIGURE 22-44. Calcium pyrophosphate dihydrate (CPPD) deposition disease. A. Gross specimen demonstrating chalky-white calcific material. **B.** Microscopically, the deposits are deep purple with discernible rhomboid-shaped crystals.

diffuse form is usually larger than 5 cm and poorly circumscribed. It invades the joint and erodes the bone (Fig. 22-45A). It may insinuate through joint capsules into soft tissue and encompass nerves and arteries, sometimes necessitating radical surgical excision. The synovium develops enlarged folds and nodular excrescences, which are brown colored owing to their iron pigment content (Fig. 22-45B). Microscopically, both tumors have similar histology. They are composed of bland mononuclear cells resembling macrophages, admixed with scattered multinucleated giant cells, fibroblasts, and foam cells. Hemosiderin-laden macrophages reflect previous hemorrhage (Fig. 22-45C and D). The diffuse form extensively infiltrates the surrounding tissue and frequently displays a villous configuration.

Treatment for these lesions is surgical excision. Amputation is occasionally necessary for local control. Tumors recur in 10% to 20% of cases of localized tenosynovial giant cell tumor, in contrast to 40% to 50% in the diffuse form. Metastases do not occur. A malignant counterpart has been described but is rare.

Soft Tissue Tumors

Soft tissue tumors are mesenchymal neoplasms that may arise anywhere in the body but are most commonly found within skeletal muscle, fat, fibrous tissue, or blood vessels. Tumors of peripheral nerves (see Chapters 23 and 24) and other tumors of neuroectodermal differentiation may be included in the category of soft tissue tumors. Malignant soft tissue tumors are rare, accounting for less than 1% of all malignancies in the United States. Benign soft tissue neoplasms are 100 times more common than malignant ones.

Although soft tissue tumors may show evidence of differentiation toward a particular cell type (e.g., fibroblastic, adipocytic, vascular, and myoid), they are thought to arise from pluripotent mesenchymal stem cells that reside in soft tissues and bone marrow. Not all soft tissue tumors can be readily classified by their line of differentiation. However, many do have characteristic and unique genomic abnormalities that are diagnostically useful.

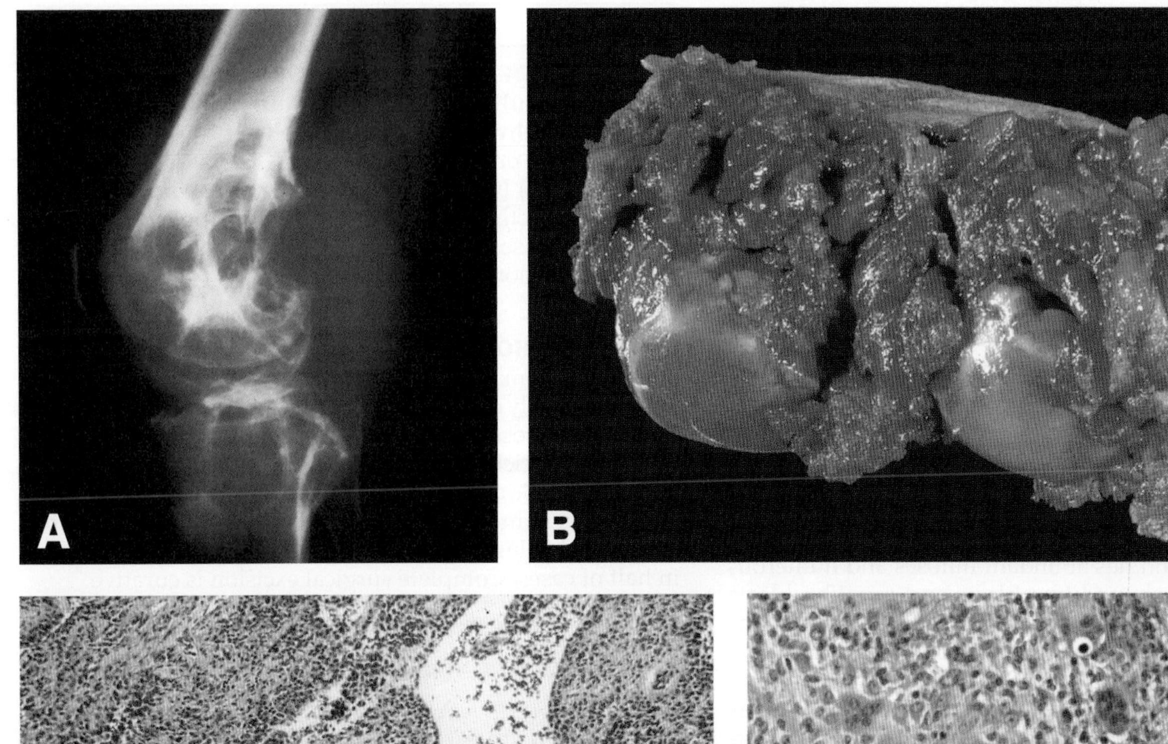

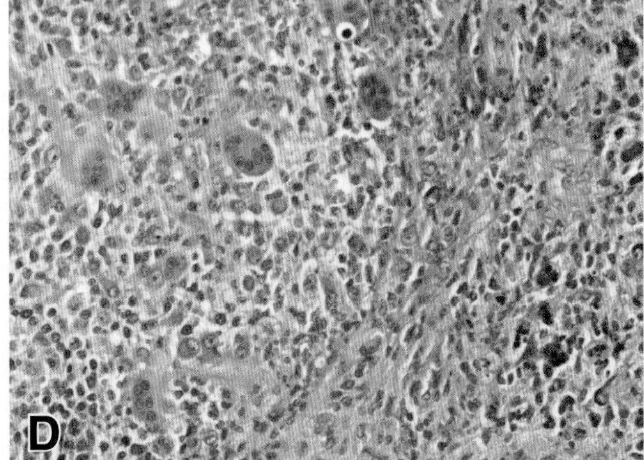

FIGURE 22-45. Tenosynovial giant cell tumor. A. Radiograph of the knee demonstrating confluent erosions of the distal femur and proximal tibia and a soft tissue mass within the joint. **B.** Gross specimen showing massive destruction of the femoral condyles. Note brown color and nodular thickenings. **C.** Low-power microscopy demonstrating thickened villous synovium. **D.** At higher power, the cellular infiltrate mainly consists of mononuclear histiocytic synoviocytes, many of which contain brown hemosiderin pigment, and multinucleated giant cells.

Soft tissue tumors may be benign, locally aggressive, or malignant. Locally aggressive tumors invade and may recur locally (e.g., fibromatosis). Malignant soft tissue tumors (sarcomas) can metastasize via the bloodstream, usually to the lungs or bone. ***Patients generally die of metastatic disease rather than local invasion at the primary tumor site.***

The ability to distinguish malignant sarcoma from benign is predicated upon both tumor grade and stage. Grading is based on cellular phenotype (histologic tumor type and degree of differentiation), mitotic activity, and the presence of tumor necrosis as indicators of aggressive behavior. In addition, tumor size and depth (superficial vs. deep soft tissue) are regarded by some as the most important prognostic criteria in primary tumors. These criteria are combined with grade and metastatic status for overall staging and risk prediction.

A few important general principles relate to soft tissue tumors are as follows:

- Superficial tumors tend to be benign.
- Deep lesions are often malignant.
- Large tumors are more often malignant than small ones.
- Rapidly growing tumors are more likely to be malignant than tumors that develop slowly.
- Calcification may exist in both benign and malignant tumors.
- Benign tumors are relatively avascular, whereas most malignant ones are hypervascular.
- Some soft tissue tumors are classified on the basis of genetic or molecular findings.

TUMORS OF FIBROUS ORIGIN

Nodular Fasciitis

Nodular fasciitis is a rapidly growing but self-limited tumor that commonly affects superficial tissues of the forearm, trunk, and back. It is characterized by a t(17;22)(p13;q13) translocation. Most cases occur in young adults who present to medical attention following the rapid growth of the lesion. Histologically, nodular fasciitis may be mistaken for a sarcoma because it is hypercellular and has abundant mitoses and numerous immature, spindle-shaped fibroblasts and myofibroblasts in a myxoid stroma (Fig. 22-46). While nodular fasciitis was long thought to be a post-traumatic reactive condition, the discovery of a recurrent translocation and associated chimeric fusion gene has resulted in a reclassification of this tumor as a form of neoplasia. *MYH-USP6* gene fusion results in overexpression of USP6, an oncogenic protein with possible roles in inflammation and proliferation. In addition, cytogenetic abnormalities involving chromosome 15 have been reported in some cases. The affected region on chromosome 15 codes for several proteins involved in tissue repair (e.g., FGF7) and oncogenesis. Despite these underlying genetic alterations, nodular fasciitis is self-limited and is cured by surgical excision.

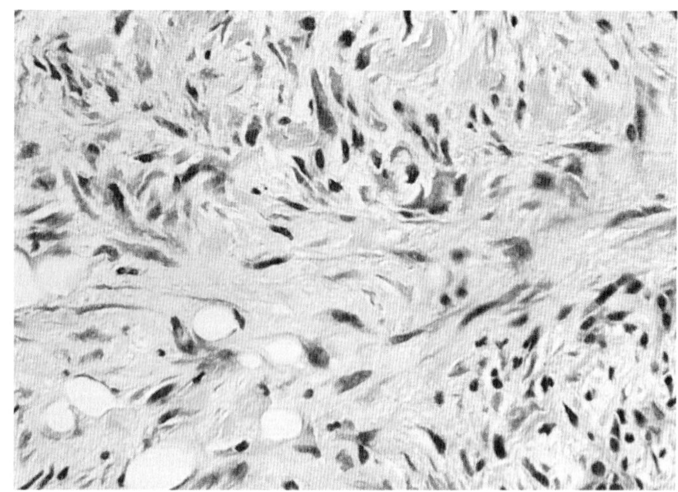

FIGURE 22-46. Nodular fasciitis. This neoplastic lesion contains atypical and bizarre fibroblasts, which may be mistaken for a fibrosarcoma.

Fibromatosis

Fibromatosis is a locally invasive, slowly growing mass that may occur virtually anywhere in the body. Although histologically similar, there are genetic distinctions between superficial and deep "aggressive" variants of fibromatosis. Fibromatosis does not metastasize, but surgical resection of deep tumors is often followed by local recurrence. Diabetics, alcoholics, and epileptics have an increased incidence of fibromatosis, as do patients with familial adenomatous polyposis.

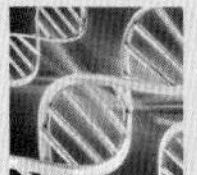

MOLECULAR PATHOGENESIS: Fibromatosis results from signaling alterations in the Wnt pathway. Mutations involving *APC* or *CTNNB1* are present in deep aggressive fibromatosis (desmoid tumor) but have not been identified in superficial variants. Inactivating mutations in the *APC* gene are found mostly in cases of fibromatosis that are associated with familial adenomatous polyposis.

PATHOLOGY: On gross examination, the lesions of fibromatosis tend to be large, firm, and whitish, with poorly demarcated borders and a whorled cut surface. Microscopic examination reveals sheets and interdigitating fascicles of benign-appearing spindle cells (fibroblasts) with little mitotic activity (Fig. 22-47). Because microscopic tongues of tumor extend between preexisting structures, surgical "shelling out" of the lesion is followed by recurrences in half of cases. Complete surgical excision is curative.

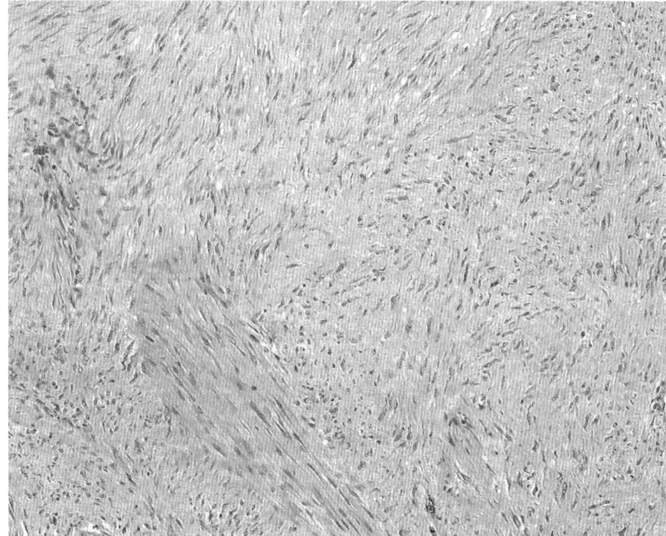

FIGURE 22-47. Fibromatosis. Microscopically, the lesion is composed of fascicles of bland spindle cells arrayed in long sweeping fascicles in a collagenous stroma.

Specific forms of fibromatosis are identified by their characteristic locations:

- **Palmar fibromatosis** (Dupuytren contracture) is the most common form of fibromatosis. It affects 1% to 2% of the general population but as many as 20% of people older than 65 years. Fibrous nodules and cordlike bands in the palmar fascia eventually lead to flexion contractures of the fingers, particularly the fourth and fifth digits.
- **Plantar fibromatosis** is similar to palmar fibromatosis, except that it is less frequent and involves the plantar aponeurosis.
- **Penile fibromatosis** (Peyronie disease) is the least common of the localized fibromatoses. It is characterized by induration of, or a mass in, the penile shaft, causing it to curve toward the affected side (**penile strabismus**). The lesion leads to urethral obstruction and pain on erection.
- **Deep aggressive fibromatosis** (desmoid tumor) frequently involves fascia and muscular aponeuroses of the extremities or abdominal wall musculature. It may also arise in the mesentery. Lesions are highly infiltrative and difficult to resect completely, accounting for the high recurrence rates. Mesenteric fibromatosis is more commonly associated with APC mutations, whereas abdominal fibromatosis shows a predilection for women.

Fibrosarcoma

Many subtypes of sarcoma show evidence of fibroblastic differentiation. Pure adult fibrosarcoma is a diagnosis of exclusion, which shows no characteristic cytogenetic abnormality and accounts for less than 3% of adult sarcomas. Congenital (infantile) fibrosarcoma is characterized by a chromosomal translocation, t(12;15)(p13;q26), that fuses the *ETV6* and *NTRK3* genes. Fibrosarcomas arise from deep connective tissue, such as fascia, scar tissue, periosteum, and tendons. Macroscopically, the tumors are sharply demarcated and frequently exhibit necrosis and hemorrhage. They are characterized histologically by malignant-appearing fibroblasts (Fig. 22-48), which often form densely interlacing bundles and fascicles, producing a "herringbone" pattern.

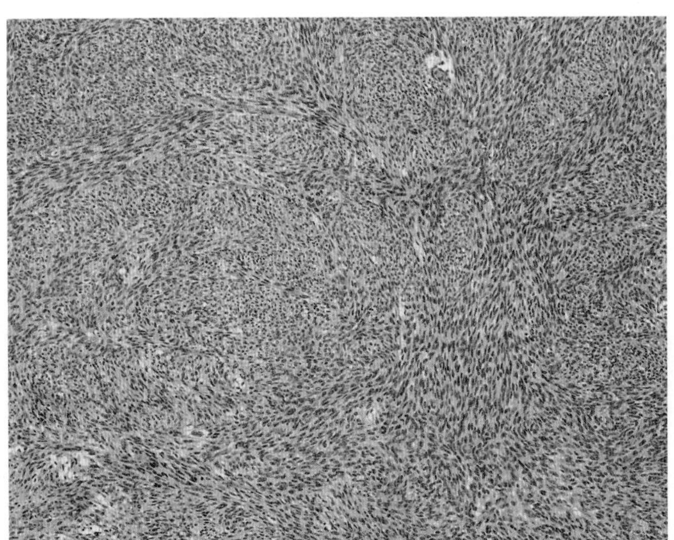

FIGURE 22-48. Fibrosarcoma. A photomicrograph demonstrating irregularly arranged malignant fibroblasts characterized by dark, irregular, and elongated nuclei of varying sizes.

The prognosis for high-grade adult fibrosarcoma is guarded; the survival at 5 years is only 40% and at 10 years is 30%. Infantile fibrosarcoma rarely metastasizes, with a less than 5% mortality rate.

Undifferentiated Pleomorphic Sarcoma

UPS, also termed malignant fibrous histiocytoma, is a phenotypically heterogeneous group of sarcomas. Immunohistochemical, ultrastructural, and, more recently, genomic studies have shown that the large majority of UPS cases represents the pleomorphic variants of liposarcoma, leiomyosarcoma, or rhabdomyosarcoma. If no specific line of differentiation can be demonstrated, then the tumor can be considered to be an **undifferentiated pleomorphic sarcoma**. Collectively, UPS is the most common sarcoma in patients over the age of 40, but cases have been recorded at all ages. In half of the cases, tumors arise in the deep fascia or within skeletal muscle of the lower limbs.

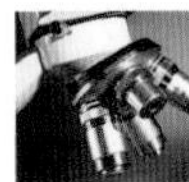

PATHOLOGY: Adult UPS is usually unencapsulated, gray-white, or tan and may have areas of hemorrhage and necrosis. Microscopically, the tumor displays a highly variable morphologic pattern, with areas of spindle-shaped cells arrayed in an irregularly whorled (storiform) pattern adjacent to fields with bizarre pleomorphic cells (Fig. 22-49). The spindle cells tend to be better differentiated and often show focal fibroblastic features. Mitoses are abundant. The extent of collagen deposition varies and sometimes dominates the microscopic pattern. Necrosis is often present and may be extensive. A few tumors reveal a conspicuous myxoid stroma.

The prognosis of adult UPS depends on the degree of cytologic atypia, the extent of mitotic activity, and the degree of necrosis. Almost half of the patients develop a local recurrence after surgery, and a comparable proportion later manifests metastatic disease, particularly in the lungs. The overall 5-year survival range is about 50%.

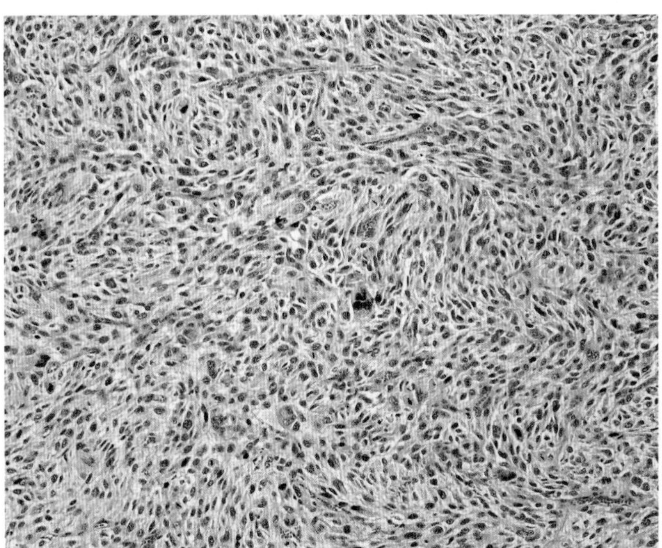

FIGURE 22-49. Undifferentiated pleomorphic sarcoma. An anaplastic tumor exhibits spindle cells, plump polygonal cells, bizarre tumor giant cells, and scattered chronic inflammatory cells. This appearance can be seen in pleomorphic sarcomas with other lines of differentiation (e.g., pleomorphic liposarcoma).

TUMORS OF ADIPOSE TISSUE

Lipoma

Composed of well-differentiated adipocytes, these benign, circumscribed tumors can originate at any site in the body that contains adipose tissue. Most occur in the subcutaneous tissues of the upper half of the body, especially the trunk and neck. Lipomas are seen mainly in adults, and patients with multiple tumors often have relatives with a similar history.

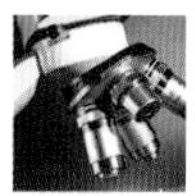

PATHOLOGY: On gross examination, lipomas are encapsulated, soft, yellow lesions that vary in size and may become very large. Deeper tumors are often poorly circumscribed. Histologically, a lipoma is often indistinguishable from normal adipose tissue. Lipomas are adequately treated by simple local excision.

An **angiolipoma** is a small, well-circumscribed, subcutaneous lipoma with extensive vascular proliferation that usually occurs in the upper extremities and trunk of young adults. They are often multiple and painful.

Liposarcoma

Liposarcomas account for 25% of all malignant soft tissue tumors. The neoplasm arises after age 50 and is most common in the deep thigh and retroperitoneum. They tend to grow slowly but may become extremely large.

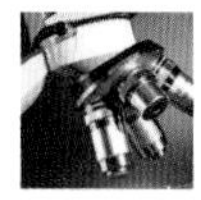

PATHOLOGY: Gross appearances of liposarcoma subtypes vary depending on the proportions of adipose, mucinous, and fibrous tissue. Well-differentiated tumors may resemble normal fat or may show fibrotic or gelatinous cut surfaces. Dedifferentiated or pleomorphic liposarcomas grossly can appear soft and gelatinous, with necrosis, hemorrhage, and cysts. Lipoblasts are early adipocytes with univacuolated or multivacuolated cytoplasmic fat vesicles indenting the nucleus. Although frequently seen in liposarcoma, lipoblasts may also be present in reactive or regenerative conditions and are neither necessary nor sufficient for the diagnosis of liposarcoma.

TUMORS OF STRIATED MUSCLE

Rhabdomyosarcoma

Rhabdomyosarcoma is a malignant tumor that displays features of striated muscle differentiation. It is uncommon in mature adults but is the most frequent soft tissue sarcoma of children and young adults.

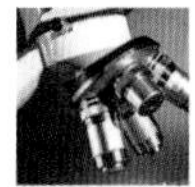

PATHOLOGY: In addition to their light microscopic features, all subtypes of rhabdomyosarcoma show immunohistochemical evidence of skeletal muscle differentiation. Tumors may express nonspecific myoid markers, such as actin and desmin, but most demonstrate at least focal expression of skeletal muscle–specific markers, such as the transcription factors myogenin and MyoD1.

EMBRYONAL RHABDOMYOSARCOMA: This form is most common in children between the ages of 3 and 12 years and frequently involves the head and neck, genitourinary tract, and retroperitoneum. Its appearance varies from that of a highly differentiated tumor containing rhabdomyoblasts (strap cells), with large eosinophilic cytoplasm and cross-striations (Fig. 22-50A and B), to that of a poorly differentiated small cell neoplasm.

BOTRYOID EMBRYONAL RHABDOMYOSARCOMA: This tumor, also known as **sarcoma botryoides**, is distinguished by the formation of polypoid, grapelike tumor masses. Microscopically, the malignant cells are scattered in an abundant myxoid stroma. Botryoid foci may occur in any type of embryonal rhabdomyosarcoma, but they are most common in tumors of hollow visceral organs, including the vagina and urinary bladder.

ALVEOLAR RHABDOMYOSARCOMA: This neoplasm occurs less frequently than the embryonal type and principally affects young people between the ages of 10 and 25 years; rarely, it may be seen in elderly patients. It is most common in the upper and lower extremities, but it can also be distributed in the same sites as the embryonal type. Typically, club-shaped tumor cells are arranged in clumps that are outlined by fibrous septa. The loose arrangement of the cells in the center of the clusters generates an "alveolar" pattern (Fig. 22-50B and C). The tumor cells exhibit intense eosinophilia, and occasional multinucleated giant cells are identified. Malignant rhabdomyoblasts, recognizable by their cross-striations, occur less commonly in the alveolar variant than in embryonal rhabdomyosarcoma, being present in only 25% of cases.

PLEOMORPHIC RHABDOMYOSARCOMA: The least common form of rhabdomyosarcoma is found in the skeletal muscles of older individuals, often in the thigh. This tumor differs from the other types of rhabdomyosarcoma in the pleomorphism of its irregularly arranged cells. It can be categorized as a type of adult undifferentiated pleomorphic sarcoma. Large, granular, eosinophilic rhabdomyoblasts, together with multinucleated giant cells, are common. Cross-striations are virtually nonexistent.

The historically dismal prognosis associated with most rhabdomyosarcomas has improved in the past two decades as a result of the introduction of combined therapeutic modalities, including surgery, radiation therapy, and chemotherapy. Today, more than 80% of patients with localized or regional disease are cured.

TUMORS OF SMOOTH MUSCLE

These tumors are characterized histologically by fascicles of spindle cells with brightly eosinophilic cytoplasm, cylindrical nuclei, and immunohistochemical expression of smooth muscle actin, muscle-specific actin and desmin.

LEIOMYOMA: This benign soft tissue tumor usually arises in sites associated with normal smooth muscle, including erector pili muscles in the dermis, blood vessel walls in subcutaneous or deep somatic tissues, and the muscular wall of the esophagus or uterus (in which location they are commonly referred to as fibroids). Leiomyomas appear as firm, gray-white, well-circumscribed nodules. Dermal or subcutaneous tumors may be painful. Microscopically, they are composed of intersecting fascicles of uniform spindle cells with cigar-shaped nuclei and very low mitotic activity. Some display prominent blood vessels (angiomyoma). Simple excision is curative.

LEIOMYOSARCOMA: This malignant soft tissue neoplasm is an uncommon tumor of adults that typically arises from the wall of blood vessels in the soft tissue of the extremities or in the retroperitoneum. Macroscopically, leiomyosarcomas

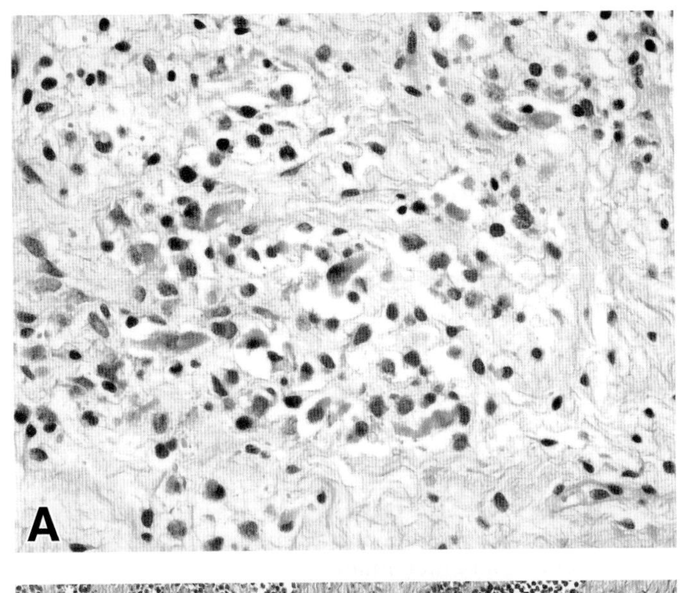

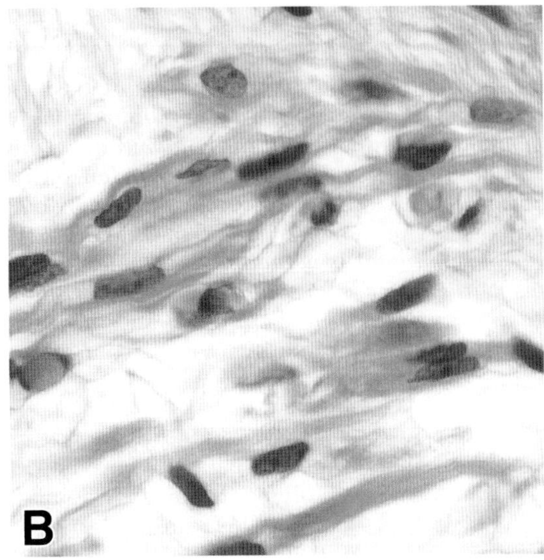

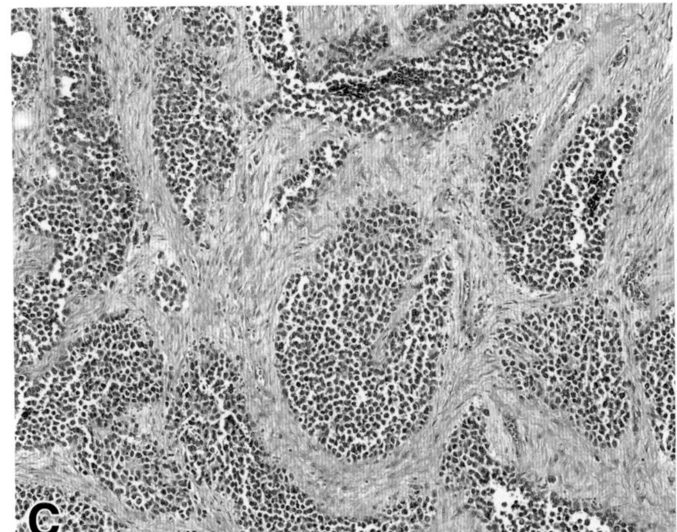

FIGURE 22-50. Rhabdomyosarcoma. A, B. Embryonal rhabdomyosarcoma. Tumors may show a spectrum of differentiation from **(A)** primitive small round cells and polyhedral tumor cells with enlarged, hyperchromatic nuclei and deeply eosinophilic cytoplasm to **(B)** differentiated strap cells with clearly visible cross-striations. **C.** Alveolar rhabdomyosarcoma. Tumors are composed of primitive small round cells, which are arranged in discohesive nests within a fibrous stroma.

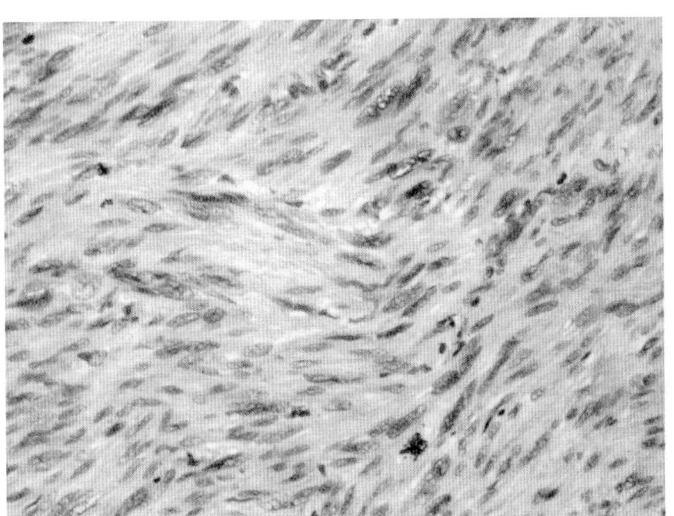

FIGURE 22-51. Leiomyosarcoma. The tumor is composed of spindle cells with elongated, hyperchromatic nuclei; a variable degree of pleomorphism; and frequent mitoses.

tend to be well circumscribed but are larger and softer than leiomyomas and often exhibit necrosis, hemorrhage, and cystic degeneration. Histologically, the tumor cells are arranged in broad, intersecting fascicles. Well-differentiated tumor cells have elongated nuclei and eosinophilic cytoplasm; poorly differentiated ones show marked increased cellularity and severe cytologic atypia (Fig. 22-51). Leiomyosarcoma is differentiated from leiomyoma mainly by cellularity, atypia, mitotic activity, and necrosis, which also indicates the prognosis.

Leiomyosarcomas may develop in a small number of uterine fibroids (0.1% to 0.5%). Because the very common uterine fibroids are often surgically removed, surgical techniques (morcellation) which fragment the fibroid, could potentially spread an undiagnosed leiomyosarcoma contained within a fibroid. Most leiomyosarcomas eventually metastasize, although dissemination may be discovered as late as 15 years or more after resection of the primary tumor.

VASCULAR TUMORS

Vascular tumors are discussed in detail in Chapter 8.

SYNOVIAL SARCOMA

Synovial sarcoma is a highly malignant soft tissue tumor characterized by translocations between chromosomes X and 18. They may arise anywhere in the body but are commonly located in deep soft tissues near joints, tendon sheaths, or joint capsules. Synovial sarcomas occur principally in young adults and usually present as a painful mass in the extremity. ***The name of this tumor is actually a misnomer as synovial sarcomas neither arise from synovial tissues nor show synoviocyte differentiation.*** Dual epithelial and mesenchymal differentiation are often seen in synovial sarcoma.

MOLECULAR PATHOGENESIS: Synovial sarcomas display a specific, balanced chromosomal translocation involving chromosomes X and 18 [t(x;18)(p11.2;q11.2)]. This translocation results in fusion of the *SS18/SYT* (synteny) gene on chromosome 18 to the *SSX* gene (a transcriptional repressor) on the X chromosome, leading to production of a hybrid protein.

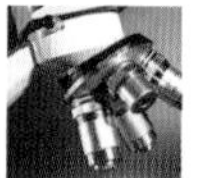

PATHOLOGY: On gross examination, synovial sarcomas are usually circumscribed, round, or multilobular masses attached to tendons, tendon sheaths, or the exterior wall of the joint capsule (Fig. 22-52A). The tumors tend to be surrounded by a glistening pseudocapsule and, in many instances, are cystic. Areas of hemorrhage, necrosis, and calcification may be seen. They range from small nodules to masses of 15 cm or more in diameter, the average being 3 to 5 cm.

Microscopically, synovial sarcoma is described as having a **biphasic pattern** (Fig. 22-52B). Fluid-filled glandular spaces lined by epithelial-like tumor cells are embedded in a sarcomatous, spindle cell background. These elements vary in proportion, distribution, and cellular differentiation, with the spindle cells usually considerably more numerous than the glandular elements. Calcifications may be conspicuous within the tumor. A poorly differentiated morphology imparts a poorer prognosis. Synovial sarcoma usually expresses cytokeratin or epithelial membrane antigen, further evidence of epithelial differentiation.

The recurrence rate of synovial sarcoma is high, and metastases occur in over 60% of cases. The 5-year survival rate is 50%, and those who die usually have extensive lung metastases.

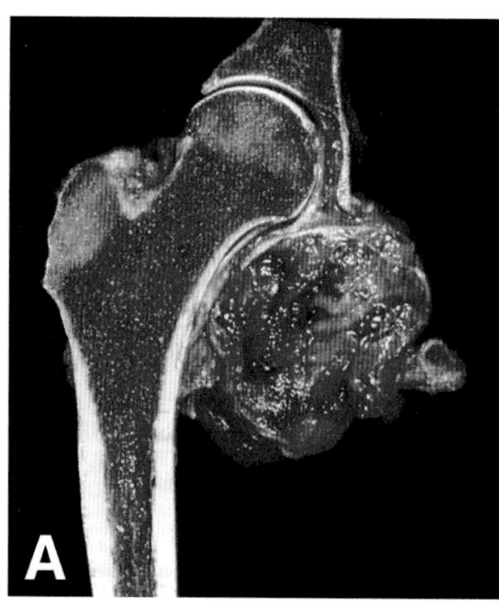

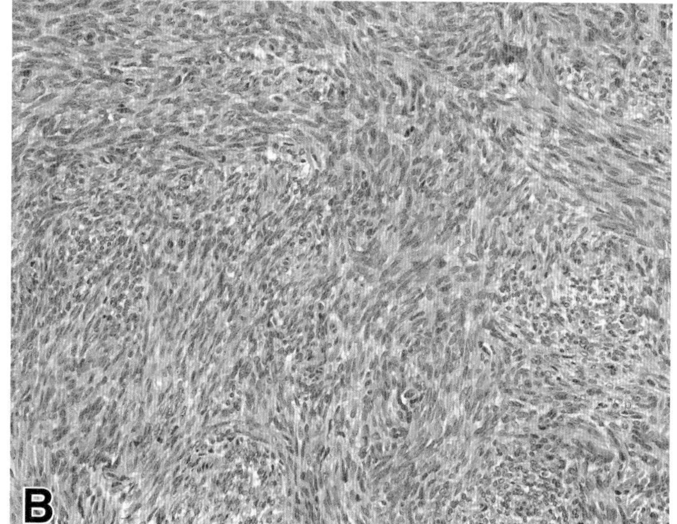

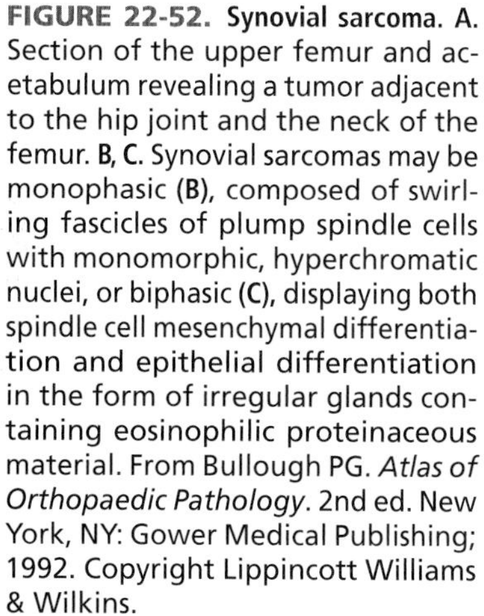

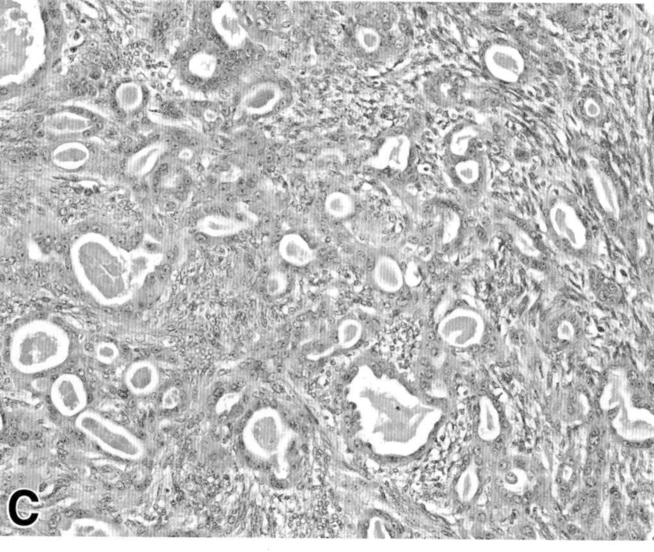

FIGURE 22-52. Synovial sarcoma. A. Section of the upper femur and acetabulum revealing a tumor adjacent to the hip joint and the neck of the femur. **B, C.** Synovial sarcomas may be monophasic (**B**), composed of swirling fascicles of plump spindle cells with monomorphic, hyperchromatic nuclei, or biphasic (**C**), displaying both spindle cell mesenchymal differentiation and epithelial differentiation in the form of irregular glands containing eosinophilic proteinaceous material. From Bullough PG. *Atlas of Orthopaedic Pathology*. 2nd ed. New York, NY: Gower Medical Publishing; 1992. Copyright Lippincott Williams & Wilkins.

23 Skeletal Muscle

Lawrence C. Kenyon ▪ Thomas W. Bouldin

LEARNING OBJECTIVES

- Distinguish between types I, IIA, and IIB fibers in terms of physiology and enzymatic staining properties.
- What is the histopathologic response of myofibers to injury?
- Distinguish between the clinical presentation and molecular pathogenesis of Duchenne and Becker muscular dystrophies.
- Describer the histopathology and clinical features of Duchenne muscular dystrophy.
- Distinguish between limb-girdle muscular dystrophy and congenital muscular dystrophy.
- Discuss the molecular pathogenesis and clinical features of myotonic dystrophy.
- Distinguish between oculopharyngeal and fasicohumeral muscular dystrophies.
- What are common examples of congenital myopathies in infancy?
- Mutations in the ryanodine receptor are associated with which congenital myopathy and what other serious clinical condition?
- Distinguish between dermatomyositis, polymyositis, and inclusion body disease in terms of pathology and clinical presentation.
- What pathophysiologic process is responsible for muscle fatigability in myasthenia gravis? Distinguish myasthenia gravis from Eaton–Lambert syndrome.
- Describe the association between glycogen storage diseases and myopathies.
- Describe the genetics, pathology, and clinical features of mitochondrial myopathies.
- Describe the histopathology of skeletal muscle denervation.
- Define fiber-type groupings associated with skeletal muscle denervation.
- Describe the common variants of spinal muscular atrophy.
- Describe the patterns of injury exhibited by peripheral nerves.
- Define dying-back atrophy, distal axonal degeneration, Wallerian degeneration, and segmental demyelination.
- Describe the histopathology of diabetic neuropathy.
- What clinical syndromes are associated with acute inflammatory demyelinating polyradiculoneuropathy (AIDP)? What are their etiology, pathology, and clinical features?
- Present an overview of Charcot–Marie–Tooth disease.
- Describe the histopathology of traumatic neuromas.
- Distinguish between vestibular, spinal and peripheral schwannomas, and neurofibromas in terms of clinical presentation and histopathology.

Skeletal Muscle

EMBRYOLOGY AND ANATOMY

The myoblast is a primitive cell that fuses with other myoblasts to form a cylindrical multinucleated myotube. The periphery of the myotube rapidly accumulates myofibrils that contain myosin and actin, which become arrayed in the cross-banded pattern characteristic of striated muscle (Fig. 23-1). The myofiber has a distinctive ultrastructural architecture (Fig. 23-2).

The myotube matures completely when it is innervated by the terminal axon of a lower motor neuron. After innervation, the myofiber nuclei move from the center to arrange themselves in a regular pattern beneath the sarcolemma (Fig. 23-3A). Mature skeletal muscle cells are syncytia (multiple nuclei within a single cytoplasm) and can be several centimeters in length.

Muscle fibers responsible for movement are **extrafusal fibers**, whereas those in stretch receptors (muscle spindle organs, Fig. 23-3C) are **intrafusal fibers.** ***In most primary myopathies, the damage affects extrafusal fibers but not intrafusal fibers.*** Thus, muscle spindle organs, which are usually inconspicuous in routine histologic preparations, become more prominent as extrafusal fibers disappear.

Myofibers

After innervation, a characteristic metabolic profile develops for different muscle fibers. Muscle fiber types are

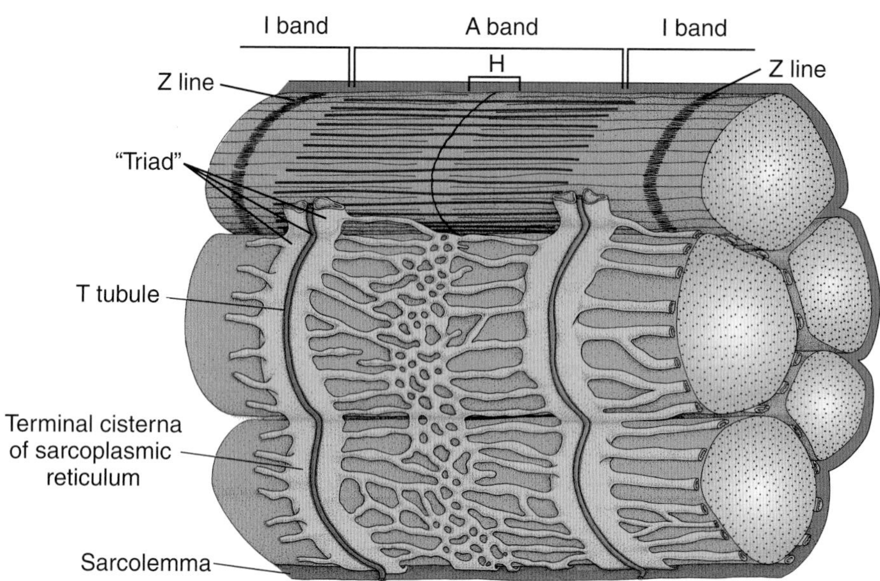

FIGURE 23-1. Normal striated muscle. Cross-striations of striated muscle are created by the arrangement of the myofilaments of the myofibril (compare to Fig. 23-2). The dark A band results from the thick myosin filaments and the thinner, partially overlapping actin filaments. In the middle portion of the myosin filaments where the actin does not overlap, there is a lighter band called the H zone or H band. In the middle of the H band, the center of each myosin filament thickens, forming intermolecular bridging with the adjacent myosin filament and giving rise to the M line (see Fig. 23-2). The finer actin filaments are anchored on the dark Z disk of the lighter I band. With contraction, the myosin filaments pull the actin filaments, causing the H zone to disappear, the I band to shrink, and the A band to remain the same. The mitochondria are scattered throughout the sarcoplasm among the myofibrils. The endoplasmic reticulum (sarcoplasmic reticulum) forms an extensive, complex tubular network with periodic dilations (cisternae) around each myofibril. The cisternae are closely apposed to the transverse tubules, which are derived from the cell membrane (sarcolemma) and form a transverse network, which resembles chicken wire, around each myofibril, giving extensive communication between the internal and external environments. A triad consists of a T tubule and adjacent terminal cisternae of the sarcoplasmic reticulum. From Ross MH, Pawlina W. *Histology: A Text and Atlas*. 5th ed. Philadelphia, PA: Lippincott Williams & Wilkins; 2006.

broadly classified by the rate of contraction and fatigability as follows:

- **Type I** slow-twitch fibers, fatigue resistant
- **Type II** fast-twitch fibers
  - **Type IIA** fatigue resistant
  - **Type IIB** fatigue sensitive
  - **Type IIC** an immature fiber type.

In lower mammals, some muscles are colored deep red (type I), whereas others are pale (type II).

TYPE I FIBERS (RED, SLOW TWITCH): Whenever a nerve stimulates a dark (red) muscle, the resulting contraction is slower and more prolonged than when it excites a pale (white) muscle. For this reason, red muscles have been classified as "slow twitch." Type I fibers tend to have more mitochondria and more myoglobin, the red, oxygen-storing pigment. Krebs cycle enzymes and electron-transport–chain proteins are all more abundant in slow-twitch muscle than in fast-twitch muscle. ***The histochemical reaction for myosin ATPase provides a sharp distinction between the two fiber types. Type I fibers stain poorly at high (alkaline) pH, but type II fibers stain darkly* (Fig. 23-3B).**

Functionally, type I muscles have a greater capacity for long, sustained contractions and resist fatigue. A training program that increases endurance produces little change in the size of type I fibers, but conditioning of these fibers results in mitochondrial proliferation and increased capacity for generating energy.

TYPE II FIBERS (WHITE, FAST TWITCH): Stimulation of type II fibers elicits faster, shorter, and stronger contractions than with type I fibers. Glycogen, phosphorylase, and other enzymes that produce energy by anaerobic glycolysis are present in higher concentrations in white muscle (particularly type IIB). Type II muscle fibers are used for rapid, brief contractions; they hypertrophy during strength training. Type II fibers also hypertrophy in response to androgenic steroids and undergo selective atrophy after disuse.

The lower motor neuron influences fiber type. During embryonic development, early muscle cells begin to express type-specific contractile proteins before muscle is innervated. Thus, the phenotype of a myofiber seems to be a programmed characteristic of the cell, rather than one induced by the nerve supply. However, the kind of innervation can alter the types of myofibers. For example, after denervation injury, reinnervation of a slow-twitch muscle (type I) by a nerve from a fast-twitch muscle (type II) causes the newly innervated type I fibers to resemble type II fibers. It is thought that the pattern or rate of discharge of lower motor neurons plays an important role in this process. Because lower motor neurons can determine fiber type, it follows that all muscle fibers in a given motor unit are

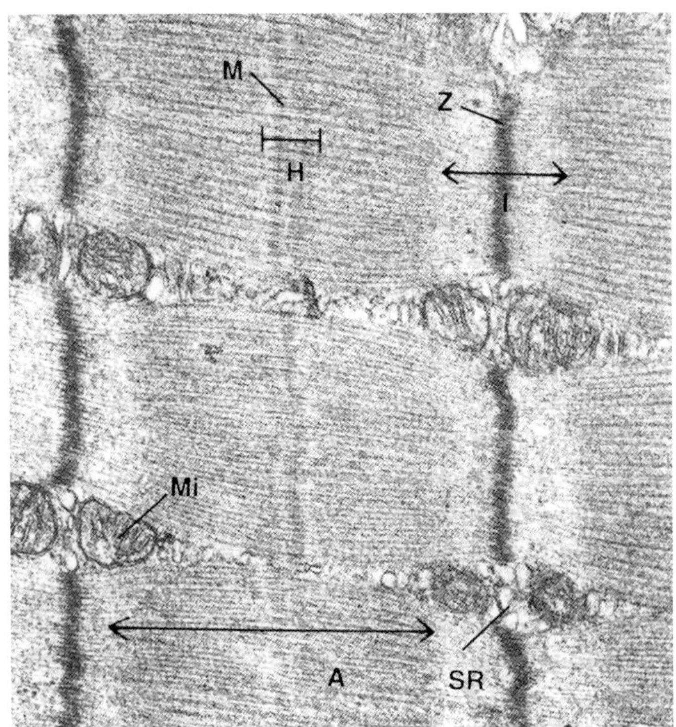

FIGURE 23-2. Normal muscle. An electron micrograph of the biceps muscle demonstrating the ultrastructure of the sarcomere. The thin dark band, the Z disk (*Z*), bisects the broad, pale I band (*I*), a zone composed of the thin actin filaments. The broad, dark band, made up of the thick myosin filaments and overlapping actin filaments, is the A band (*A*). The middle of the A band consists of the pale H zone (*H*), which, in turn, is bisected by a slightly darker M line (*M*), representing a zone of intermolecular bridging of myosin. Small membrane-bound vesicles compose the sarcoplasmic reticulum (*SR*) and the transverse tubules. Pairs of mitochondria (*Mi*) tend to be located between myofibrils at the level of the I bands.

of the same type. A cross section of muscle stained for ATPase (see above) shows a random mixture of fiber types (Fig. 23-3B) because motor units interdigitate extensively with each other.

In humans, no muscles are composed exclusively of one fiber type. However, the proportions of fiber types vary from muscle to muscle. For example, the soleus muscle mainly contains (≥80%) type I fibers.

MUSCLE BIOPSY: Because normal muscle patterns are more constant within a specific muscle, the same muscles are biopsied from case to case. Samples from the quadriceps femoris or biceps brachii are suitable for biopsy diagnosis in most primary muscle diseases (myopathies). Biopsies of the sural nerve and gastrocnemius muscle are often done if a peripheral neuropathy is suspected.

Biopsy sampling of a moderately affected muscle is most informative. Muscles that are uninvolved may show few or no pathologic changes, whereas very weak muscles may be end stage—largely replaced by fat and fibrous connective tissue (Fig. 23-4).

GENERAL PATHOLOGIC REACTIONS

Necrosis is a common response of myofibers to injury in primary muscle diseases (**myopathies**). Widespread acute necrosis of skeletal muscle fibers (***rhabdomyolysis***) releases cytosolic proteins, including myoglobin, into the circulation, which may lead to myoglobinuria and cause acute renal failure (see below). In many human myopathies, segmental necrosis occurs along the length of a fiber, with intact muscle flanking the site of damage (Fig. 23-5). The injury quickly elicits several responses: (1) blood-borne macrophages infiltrate into the necrotic cytoplasm. (2) Satellite cells, a population of dormant myoblasts nearby each fiber, are activated. (3) Macrophages gradually phagocytose necrotic debris and remove it, satellite cells proliferate and become active myoblasts. (4) Within 2 days, myoblasts begin to fuse to each other and to the ends of the intact fiber remnants, to form a joining multinucleated segment. This regenerating fiber is narrower than the parent fiber and has basophilic cytoplasm (owing to increased

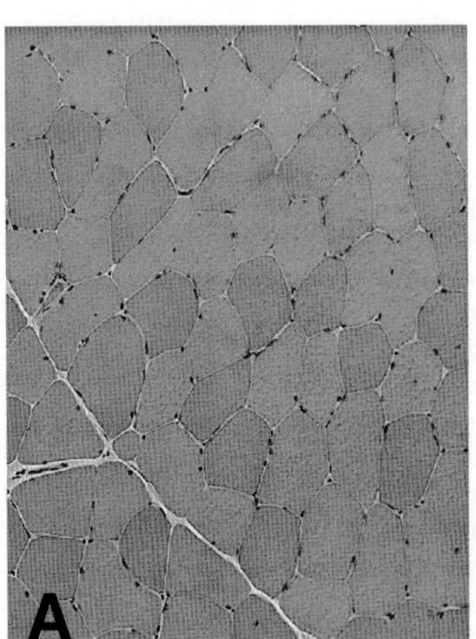

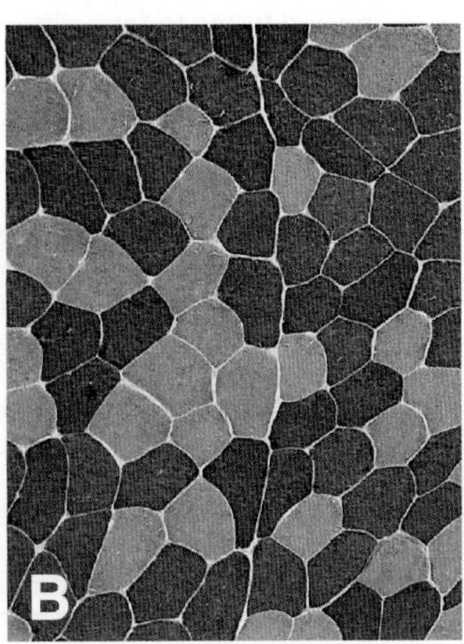

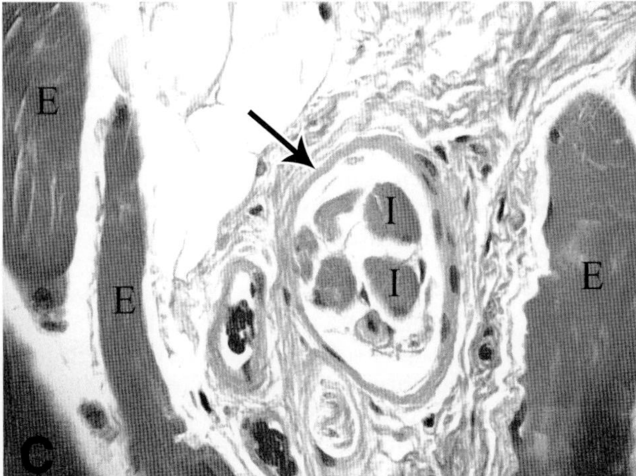

FIGURE 23-3. Normal muscle. A. Hematoxylin and eosin stain. In this transverse frozen section of the vastus lateralis, the polygonal myofibers are separated from each other by an indistinct, thin layer of connective tissue, the endomysium. The thicker band of connective tissue, the perimysium, demarcates a bundle or fascicle of fibers. All of the nuclei in this field are located at the periphery of the cells. Satellite cell nuclei are contained within the basement membrane of the muscle cell and cannot be distinguished from those of the myofibers by light microscopy. **B. Myofibrillar (myosin) ATPase.** Type I fibers are pale, at high (alkaline) pH; type II fibers are dark. Note the intermixture of fiber types. **C. Muscle spindle organ (stretch receptor).** The *arrow* marks the capsule of the muscle spindle organ. E, extrafusal fibers; I, intrafusal fibers.

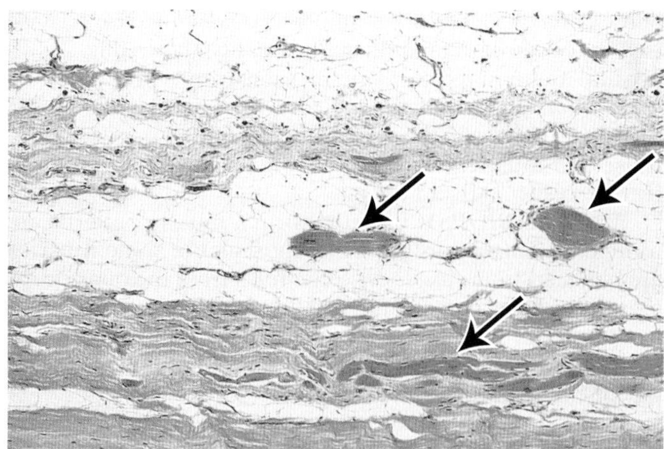

FIGURE 23-4. End-stage neuromuscular disease. In this section of the deltoid muscle stained by hematoxylin and eosin, skeletal muscle has been largely replaced by fibrofatty connective tissue. The few surviving muscle fibers have a deeper eosinophilia than does the abundant collagenous component (*arrows*).

ribosomes). Large, vesicular nuclei, with prominent nucleoli arranged in long chains, are evident.

Regeneration can restore normal structure and function of muscle fibers within a few weeks after a single episode of injury. With subacute or chronic disorders, fiber necrosis proceeds concurrently with fiber regeneration, gradually leading to atrophy of muscle fibers and fibrosis.

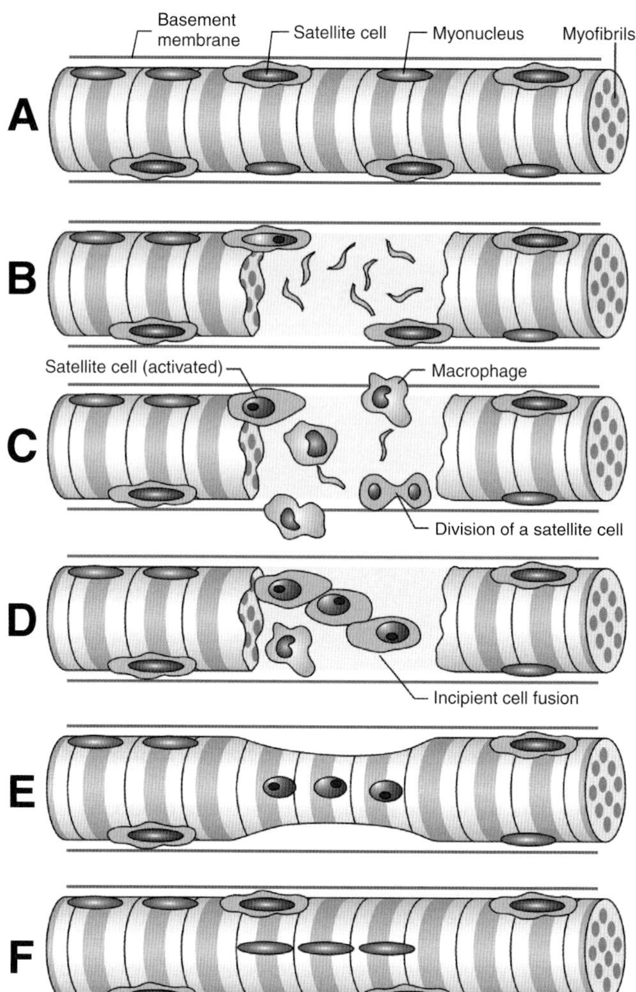

FIGURE 23-5. Segmental necrosis and regeneration of a muscle fiber. A. A normal muscle fiber contains myofibrils and subsarcolemmal nuclei and is covered by a basement membrane. Scattered satellite cells are situated on the surface of the sarcolemma, inside the basement membrane. These cells are dormant myoblasts, capable of proliferating and fusing to form differentiated fibers. They constitute 3% to 5% of the nuclei, as observed in a cross section of skeletal muscle. **B.** In many muscle diseases (e.g., Duchenne muscular dystrophy or polymyositis), injury to the muscle fiber causes segmental necrosis with disintegration of the sarcoplasm, leaving a preserved basement membrane and nerve supply (not shown). **C.** The damaged segment attracts circulating macrophages that penetrate the basement membrane and begin to digest and engulf the sarcoplasmic contents (myophagocytosis). Regenerative processes begin with the activation and proliferation of the satellite cells, forming myoblasts within the basement membrane. Macrophages gradually leave the site of injury with their load of debris. **D.** At a later stage, the myoblasts are aligned in close proximity to each other in the center of the fiber and begin to fuse. **E.** Regeneration of the fiber segment is prominent, as indicated by the large, pale, vesicular, centrally located nuclei. **F.** The fiber is nearly normal except for a few persistent central nuclei. Eventually, the normal state **(A)** is restored.

MUSCULAR DYSTROPHY

Progressive weakness of voluntary muscles can be caused by either a disorder of the nervous system or primary muscle degeneration. The latter is termed **muscular dystrophy**. It is frequently hereditary and relentlessly progressive. Muscles from such patients show fiber necrosis with regeneration, progressive fibrosis, and infiltration by fatty tissue (Fig. 23-4). Little or no inflammation is seen.

Duchenne and Becker Muscular Dystrophies

Duchenne muscular dystrophy (DMD) is characterized by progressive degeneration of muscles, particularly in the pelvic and shoulder girdles. ***It is the most common noninflammatory myopathy in children.*** A milder form of the disease is known as **Becker muscular dystrophy (BMD)**. Serum creatine kinase is usually greatly increased in both conditions.

MOLECULAR PATHOGENESIS: DMD and BMD are caused by several mutations in a large gene on the short arm of the X chromosome (*Xp21*). This gene encodes **dystrophin,** a protein at the inner surface of the sarcolemma. Dystrophin links the subsarcolemmal cytoskeleton to the exterior of the cell via a transmembrane complex of proteins and glycoproteins that binds to laminin (Fig. 23-6). If the complex is absent or greatly decreased, often owing to deletions of the gene, the normal interaction between the sarcolemma and extracellular matrix is absent. This effect causes an increase in osmotic fragility of dystrophic muscle, excessive influx of calcium ions, and release of soluble muscle enzymes (such as creatine kinase) into the serum.

Dystrophin genes may show point mutations, deletions, or duplications, which result in altered, usually truncated, proteins. Some mutated proteins may retain sufficient function to localize correctly to the muscle fiber surface but may distribute abnormally in that location. Such partly active proteins tend to produce the less

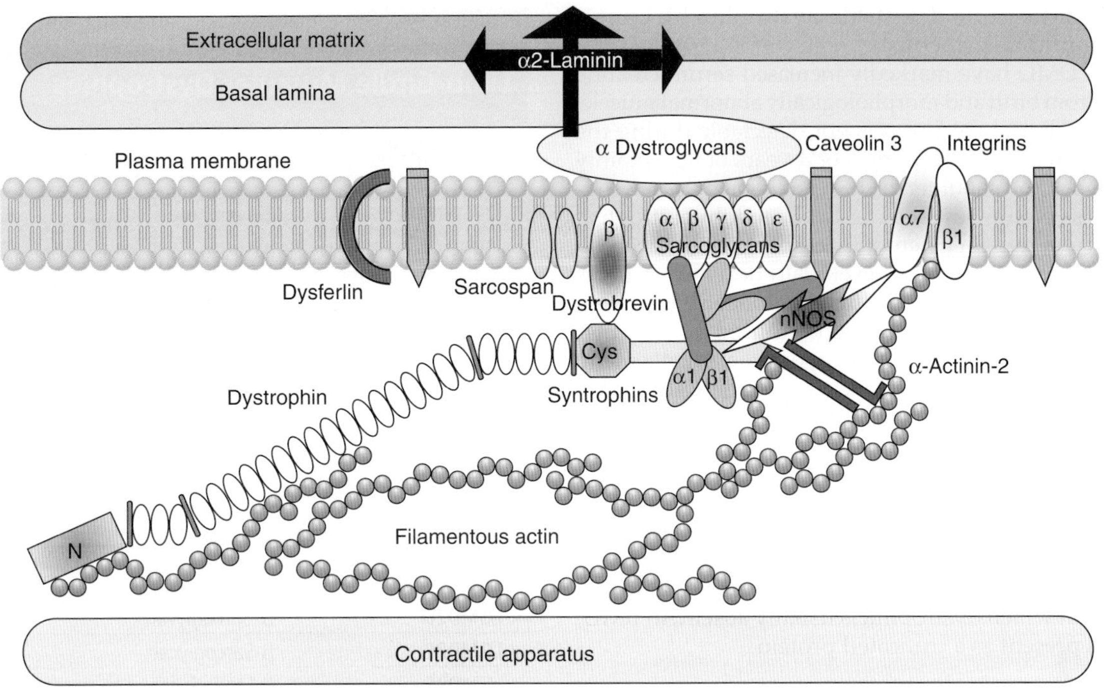

FIGURE 23-6. Diagrammatic representation of proteins linking dystrophin to the plasma membrane and the contractile apparatus. Several of these linking proteins are associated with known myopathies (see Table 23-1). Redrawn from Karpati G. *Structural and Molecular Basis of Skeletal Muscle Diseases*. Basel, Switzerland: ISN Neuropath Press; 2002: 8, Fig. 2. N amino terminus, nNOS neuronal nitric oxide synthetase.

severe disease termed BMD. Some patients have mutations in transmembrane proteins or glycoproteins, which normally link the cytoskeleton and extracellular matrix (Fig. 23-6). In such **limb-girdle muscular dystrophies**, dystrophin may also be decreased or abnormally localized because its binding partners are abnormal, thereby complicating diagnosis (see below).

Because DMD is inherited as an X-linked recessive disease, the abnormal gene is passed from heterozygous carrier mothers. About 30% of cases are caused by spontaneous mutations. Until recently, female carriers were best detected by repeatedly measuring serum creatine kinase, which is moderately increased in 75% of heterozygotes. Expression of the carrier state is variable, probably because of fluctuations in the random inactivation of the X chromosome. Dystrophin immunolocalization on muscle biopsy also identifies some carriers who show a characteristic mosaic pattern of deficient and normal myofibers. Molecular testing can now identify the mutation in about 70% of families in which DMD is inherited. However, carrier detection in some families can still be problematic.

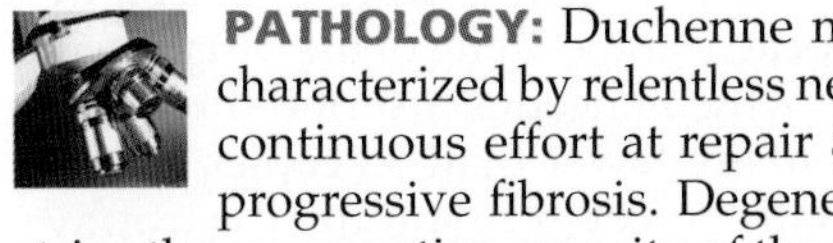

PATHOLOGY: Duchenne muscular dystrophy is characterized by relentless necrosis of muscle fibers, continuous effort at repair and regeneration, and progressive fibrosis. Degeneration eventually outstrips the regenerative capacity of the muscle. The number of muscle fibers then progressively decreases, to be replaced by fibrofatty connective tissue. In the end stage, skeletal muscle fibers disappear almost completely (Fig. 23-4), although muscle spindle fibers (intrafusal fibers) are relatively spared.

Early in the disease, necrotic fibers and regenerating fibers tend to occur in small groups, together with scattered, large, hyalinized dark fibers. The latter are overly contracted and are thought to precede fiber necrosis (Fig. 23-7). Macrophages invade necrotic fibers and reflect a scavenging function rather than an inflammatory process.

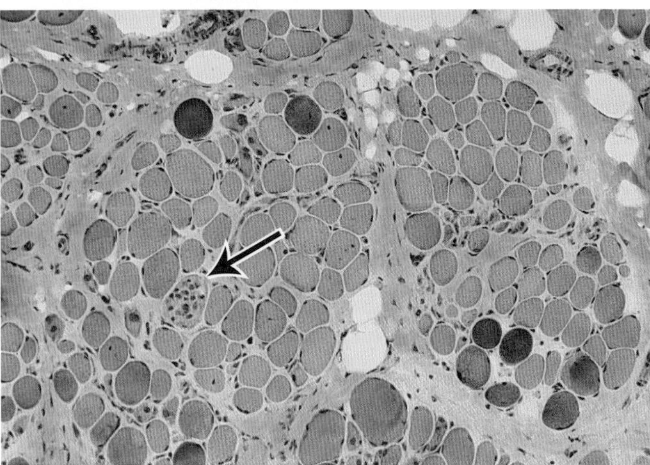

FIGURE 23-7. Duchenne muscular dystrophy. Modified Gomori trichrome stain. A section of vastus lateralis muscle showing necrotic muscle fibers, some of them invaded by macrophages (*arrow*). Dark-staining, enlarged fibers represent overly contracted fibers. Green amorphous material between the fascicles of muscle represents fibrosis. Calcium influx across the defective surface membrane overwhelms mechanisms that maintain a low resting Ca^{2+} concentration and triggers excessive contraction. There is conspicuous perimysial and endomysial fibrosis.

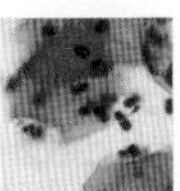

CLINICAL FEATURES: About 30% of patients with DMD have small rearrangements or point mutations which are difficult to detect by DNA analysis. Such patients are evaluated by muscle biopsy, which shows little or no detectable dystrophin by immunoblot or immunohistochemistry.

Boys with DMD have markedly increased serum creatine kinase levels from birth and morphologically abnormal muscle, even in utero. Clinical weakness is not detectable during the first year but is usually evident by 3 or 4 years of age, mainly around the pelvic and shoulder girdles (proximal muscle weakness). Weakness progresses relentlessly. "Pseudohypertrophy" (enlargement of a muscle when muscle fibers are replaced by fibroadipose tissue) of calf muscles eventually develops. Patients are usually wheelchair bound by age 10 and bedridden by 15. Death is usually due to respiratory insufficiency caused by muscular weakness or cardiac arrhythmia from myocardial involvement. Other extraskeletal manifestations include gastrointestinal dysfunction (from degeneration of smooth muscle). Many boys with Duchenne dystrophy show variably severe mental retardation, apparently owing to lack of dystrophin in the brain.

Although the clinical presentation of patients with BMD is typically milder and of later onset than that of DMD, affected individuals often have exercise intolerance with muscle cramping, occasional rhabdomyolysis, and myoglobinuria. Unlike DMD, in which dystrophin is usually absent, in BMD, dystrophin is present as a truncated protein.

Limb-Girdle Muscular Dystrophy

Limb-girdle muscular dystrophies (LGMDs) are a group of disorders with several defective proteins and modes of inheritance (Table 23-1). Defects in many proteins have been implicated, but these patients show similar clinical features, which include pelvic and shoulder girdle weakness. The onset may be in childhood or adulthood, with variable muscle weakness. Patients may have difficulty walking, running, or rising from a sitting position. Cardiac involvement is common. The histologic appearance resembles that of all muscular dystrophies, but some variants show unusual features including inflammation (LGMD2B, Miyoshi myopathy) and rimmed vacuoles (LGMD1A) similar to those seen in inclusion body myositis (see below). As a result, proper diagnosis requires detailed clinical histories, plus immunohistochemical, immunoblotting, and genetic tests. LGMD (2C through 2F) are also known as the sarcoglycanopathies (Fig. 23-6).

Table 23-1

Limb-Girdle Muscular Dystrophies

Limb-Girdle Muscular Dystrophies[a]	Defective Protein	Subcellular Location
LGMD1A	Myotilin	Sarcomere
LGMD1B	Lamin	Nuclear envelope
LGMD1C	Caveolin 3	Sarcolemma
LGMD1D	DNAJB6 protein	?
LGMD1E	Desmin	?
LGMD1F	Transportin 3	?
LGMD1G	HNRPDL	?
LGMD2A	Calpain 3	Sarcoplasm
LGMD2B/Miyoshi	Dysferlin	Sarcolemma
LGMD2C	γ-Sarcoglycan	Sarcolemma
LGMD2D	α-Sarcoglycan	Sarcolemma
LGMD2E	β-Sarcoglycan	Sarcolemma
LGMD2F	δ-Sarcoglycan	Sarcolemma
LGMD2G	Telethion	Sarcomere
LGMD2H	Trim32	Sarcoplasm
LGMD2I	Fukutin-related protein	Golgi
LGMD2J	Titin	Sarcomere
LGMD2K	POMT1	Endoplasmic reticulum
LGMD2L	Eukutin	Golgi
LGMD2M	DOMGnT1	Golgi

[a]LMGD1s show autosomal dominant inheritance, whereas LMGD2s show autosomal recessive inheritance. HNRPDL heterogeneous nuclear nucleoprotein D-like ? Not characterized

Adapted from Sewry CA, Jimenez-Mallebrera C, Brown SC, Muntoni F. Diseases of Muscle. In Love S, Louis DN, Ellison DW, eds. *Greenfield's Neuropathology*. 8th ed. New York, NY: Oxford University Press; 2008.

Congenital Muscular Dystrophies

These diseases are characterized by hypotonia, weakness, and contractures with onset at or near birth.. Depending on the variant, patients may also present with leukoencephalopathy (white matter brain disease), brain malformations, and eye involvement.

Pathologically, congenital muscular dystrophies resemble other muscular dystrophies, with variable fibrosis and fatty infiltration of muscle. Many of these disorders reflect mutations in extracellular matrix proteins (e.g., collagens, laminin, and integrins) or abnormal glycosylation of α-dystroglycan (α-dystroglycanopathies) and sarcoplasmic reticulum (rigid spine muscular dystrophy). Some affected proteins also cause certain limb-girdle muscular dystrophies, albeit with different mutations.

NUCLEOTIDE REPEAT SYNDROMES

Myotonic Dystrophy

Myotonic dystrophy, the most common adult muscular dystrophy, is an autosomal dominant disease characterized by slowed muscle relaxation (myotonia), progressive muscle weakness, and wasting. Its prevalence is about 14 per 100,000, although minimally affected individuals are difficult to diagnose, so this estimate may be low. The age at onset and severity of symptoms vary greatly. Myotonic dystrophy may be either of adult onset or congenital.

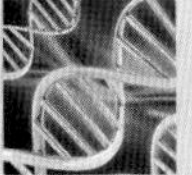

MOLECULAR PATHOGENESIS: The two forms of myotonic dystrophy (DM1 and DM2) both follow autosomal dominant inheritance and reflect mutations in different genes. DM1 is caused by expansion of a CTG repeat near the 3′ end of the DM protein kinase (*DMPK*) gene, which encodes a serine-threonine kinase. Normally, there are fewer than 30 copies of this repeat, but in minimally affected myotonic dystrophy patients, there tend to be 50 or more copies. The greater the number of repeats (sometimes as many as 4,000), the more severe the disorder. The mechanism of injury brought about by expansion of CTG repeats in myotonic dystrophy, as in other trinucleotide repeat disorders, is not understood. DM2 is caused by expansion of the tetranucleotide repeat CCTG in the first intron of the *ZNF9* gene.

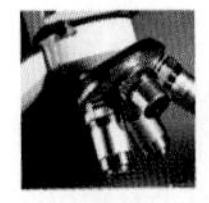

PATHOLOGY: The morphologic changes in adult myotonic dystrophy are highly variable, even in muscles from the same patient. Most patients show type I fiber atrophy and type II fiber hypertrophy. By contrast, most muscle disorders show predominant type II fiber atrophy. Internally situated nuclei are a constant feature. Necrosis and regeneration, although occasionally present, are not as prominent as they are in Duchenne muscular dystrophy.

Muscles in congenital myotonic dystrophy show myofiber atrophy, frequent central nuclei, and failure of fiber differentiation. These features closely resemble those of the X-linked, recessive type of myotubular myopathy (see below).

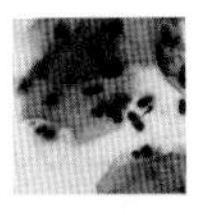

CLINICAL FEATURES: People with DM1 experience slowly progressive muscle weakness and stiffness, principally in the distal limbs (proximal weakness is more common in DM2) . Facial and neck weakness as well as ptosis are typical of DM1 but are less common in DM2. Extraskeletal features that are sometimes present in myotonic dystrophy include frontal balding, gonadal atrophy, cataracts, personality degeneration, and endocrine abnormalities. Cardiac arrhythmias and, less often, cardiomyopathy may occur. A few patients exhibit involvement of smooth muscle, with disorders of the gastrointestinal tract, gallbladder, and uterus.

The diagnosis of myotonic dystrophy is based on clinical features, family history, and characteristic electromyography, which features myotonic discharges. Identifying an expanded CTG repeat (DM1) or CCTG (DM2) is predictive in utero and can be diagnostic in patients.

Congenital myotonic dystrophy is seen only in children of women with DM1 who themselves show symptoms of myotonic dystrophy. Affected infants have severe muscle weakness at birth. Myotonia is inconspicuous or absent but appears in later childhood. Many of these patients suffer mental retardation. Congenital DM2 has not been identified.

Oculopharyngeal Muscular Dystrophy

OPMD is typically diagnosed in middle age (over 45 years) and mostly shows autosomal dominant inheritance. However, an autosomal recessive form does exist. Patients develop slowly progressive eyelid ptosis, dysphagia, and weakness of other muscle groups, including the face and limbs. The autosomal dominant form is prevalent among French Canadians in Quebec and Bukhara Jews (formerly from central Asia), now living in Israel. Both autosomal dominant and recessive forms are caused by abnormally increased numbers of GCG repeats in the poly(A)-binding protein nuclear 1 gene (*PABPN1*) but differ in where these increased repeats are within the gene. Biopsies show intranuclear inclusions, rimmed vacuoles, and filamentous inclusions, similar to those in inclusion body myositis (see below).

Facioscapulohumeral Muscular Dystrophy

FSHD is a common muscular dystrophy, inherited as an autosomal dominant disease that begins in childhood or young adulthood. Patients suffer from facial and shoulder girdle weakness, and scapular winging is prominent. Other muscles may also be affected. Life expectancy is usually normal; extraskeletal involvement includes bundle branch block, hearing loss, and retinal vasculopathy. FSHD is caused by deletion of part of a repetitive DNA fragment in the subtelomeric region of chromosome 4q; affected patients have fewer repeats than normal. Chronic inflammation is prominent, resembling an inflammatory myopathy such as polymyositis (see below), but does not correlate with the disease course. A detailed clinical history is essential to making the proper diagnosis. Otherwise, a patient with muscle weakness and a lymphocytic inflammatory infiltrate could easily be misdiagnosed as suffering from polymyositis.

CONGENITAL MYOPATHIES

A newborn occasionally shows generalized hypotonia, with decreased deep tendon reflexes and muscle bulk. Many of these children have a difficult perinatal period because of pulmonary complications secondary to weak respiration. ***Many of the muscle diseases already described are "congenital" in the sense that they are due to mutations present at birth. However, such disorders are not clinically evident until much later. By contrast, congenital myopathies, as described here, are evident at birth.***

Some infants have progressive "malignant" hypotonia, which often results in death within the first year of life, for example, infantile acid maltase deficiency (Pompe disease) discussed below. In other patients, hypotonia may persist with little or no progression. These people become ambulatory and live a normal life span, although sometimes they suffer secondary skeletal complications of hypotonia, such as severe scoliosis. Muscles from these patients rarely reveal distinctive structurally abnormal myofibers.

However, they all show decreased deep tendon reflexes, decreased muscle bulk, and delayed motor milestones. In the conditions described below, abnormal muscle morphology is usually limited to type I fibers, with type I fiber predominance in some disorders and type I atrophy in others. There is no active myofiber necrosis or fibrosis, and patients have normal serum creatine kinase. The most common examples are as follows:

- **Central core disease:** Affected patients have decreased deep tendon reflexes and delayed motor development. The disease has been traced to a dominant mutation on the long arm of chromosome 19 that codes for the ryanodine receptor, the calcium release channel of the sarcoplasmic reticulum. Mutations in this gene also cause **malignant hyperthermia**, a potentially fatal disorder that is triggered by succinylcholine and some anesthetic agents, particularly halothane. It is characterized by hyperpyrexia and rhabdomyolysis. Central core disease and malignant hyperthermia may coexist in some patients.
  - **Pathology:** There is a striking predominance of type I fibers, often showing a central zone of degeneration with loss of NADH-TR staining and extending the entire length of the fiber. By electron microscopy, mitochondria and other membranous organelles are lost in the central cores, with or without myofibril disorganization. Membranous organelles tend to condense around the margin of the central core. The periphery of the fiber is unremarkable.
- **Rod myopathy (nemaline myopathy)**: This disease is characterized by rodlike inclusions, which accumulate within skeletal muscle sarcoplasm. Autosomal dominant and recessive inheritance are described. Genes responsible for rod myopathy include nebulin (most common), α-actin, α-tropomyosin and β-tropomyosin, and slow troponin T.

Mutations in the ryanodine receptor gene may also lead to rod formation.

- **Pathology:** There is a variable predominance of type I fibers containing rod-shaped structures in their sarcoplasm. Aggregates of these inclusions often occur in subsarcolemmal regions, near nuclei. They are brilliant, red to dark red, using Gomori trichrome stain, or blue on toluidine blue stain (Fig. 23-8A). The rods are often not visible with hematoxylin and eosin stain. The rod-shaped inclusions arise from the Z band, which they resemble ultrastructurally (Fig. 23-8B). Rods are described in several neuromuscular diseases, including denervation atrophy, muscular dystrophy, and inflammatory myopathies. Other abnormalities (inflammation and denervation) are absent.
- **Clinical Features:** In the classic congenital form of rod myopathy, patients show congenital hypotonia, delayed motor milestones of variable clinical severity, and secondary skeletal changes, such as kyphoscoliosis. Some exhibit severe involvement of muscles of the face, pharynx, and neck. Later-onset (childhood and adult) forms tend to be associated with some muscle degeneration, increased serum creatine kinase levels, and a slowly progressive or nonprogressive course.

- **Central tubular and myotubular myopathy:** These conditions are clinically and genetically heterogeneous and display muscle cells that have centrally located nuclei. Autosomal recessive and autosomal dominant varieties are known. *Central tubular myopathy* progresses slowly and, like rod myopathy, resembles the limb-girdle dystrophies (see above). Some patients exhibit a striking involvement of facial and extraocular musculature. Bilateral ptosis is almost always present. The gene responsible, dynamin 2, is involved in endocytosis, membrane trafficking, and centrosome and actin assembly. *Myotubular myopathy* is an X-linked disorder caused by myotubularin gene mutations. Clinically, myotubular myopathy is characterized by marked neonatal hypotonia and respiratory failure at birth, although late-onset forms occur.
    - **Pathology:** Muscle biopsies show predominance of type I fibers, many of which are small and round, with a single central nucleus (hence the name of the disease). They resemble the myotubular stage in skeletal muscle embryogenesis.

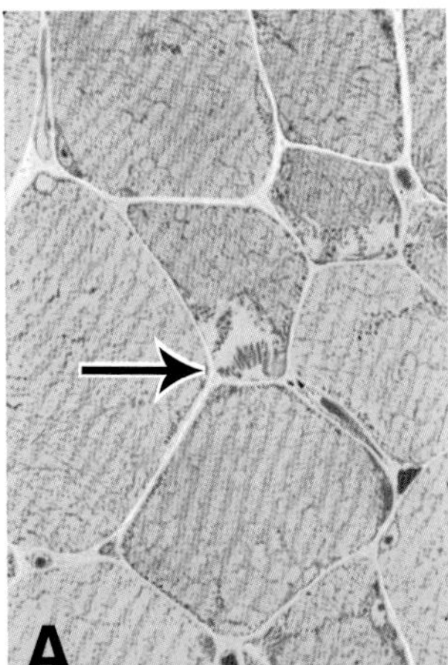

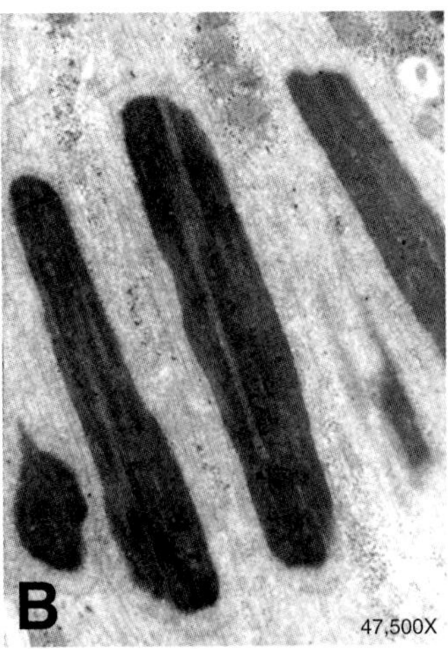

FIGURE 23-8. Rod (nemaline) myopathy. **A.** Muscle fibers contain dark aggregates of rods (*arrow*) (toluidine blue, ×1000). **B.** An electron micrograph of the same biopsy showing that the structures are rod shaped and are derived from the Z disk (×47,500).

INFLAMMATORY MYOPATHIES

Inflammatory myopathies comprise a heterogeneous group of acquired disorders, all of which feature symmetric proximal muscle weakness, increased serum levels of muscle-derived enzymes, and nonsuppurative inflammation of skeletal muscle.

These are uncommon diseases, with the annual incidence being 1 in 100,000. ***Dermatomyositis afflicts children and adults, but polymyositis almost always begins after 20 years of age.*** Both disorders occur more often in females than males. By contrast, inclusion body myositis is usually a disease of men over age 50.

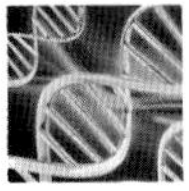

PATHOGENESIS: These myopathies are thought to have an autoimmune origin because (1) they often occur in association with other autoimmune and connective tissues diseases, (2) the pathology suggests autoimmune cellular injury, (3) serum autoantibodies are detected, and (4) polymyositis and dermatomyositis (but not inclusion body myositis) respond to immunosuppressive therapy. No specific target autoantigens in muscle or blood vessels have been identified, but antinuclear and anticytoplasmic antibodies against several different antigens exist in these myopathies. Unlike normal muscle, cells in inflammatory myopathies express MHC I antigens, an aberrant expression that promotes an autoimmune reaction.

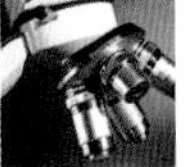

PATHOLOGY: The inflammatory myopathies are characterized by (1) the presence of inflammatory cells, (2) necrosis and phagocytosis of muscle fibers, (3) a mixture of regenerating and atrophic fibers, and (4) fibrosis.

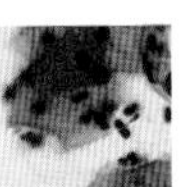

CLINICAL FEATURES: All inflammatory myopathies manifest as insidious proximal and symmetric muscle weakness, gradually increasing over weeks to months. Patients have problems with simple activities that require use of proximal muscles, including lifting objects, climbing steps, or combing hair. The dysphagia and difficulty in holding up the head reflect involvement of pharyngeal and neck-flexor muscles. Some patients with inclusion body myositis have distal muscle weakness of the limbs that equals or exceeds that of proximal muscles. In advanced cases, respiratory muscles may be affected. Interstitial lung disease may also compromise respiratory function in 10% of polymyositis and dermatomyositis patients. Myocardial involvement may also occur. Weakness progresses over weeks or months and leads to severe muscular wasting. Specific characteristics of the inflammatory myopathies are as follows:

- **Polymyositis:** Polymyositis often has detectable anti-Jo-1, an antibody against histidyl-transfer RNA synthetase, with concomitant interstitial lung disease, Raynaud phenomenon, and nonerosive arthritis. However, the role of the antibody in disease pathogenesis is unknown. Viral infections may precede polymyositis, but viral cultures of muscle are negative.

- **Pathology:** In polymyositis, there is no detectable microangiopathy as is seen in dermatomyositis (see below). In this disorder, healthy muscle fibers are initially surrounded by $CD8^+$ T lymphocytes and macrophages, after which the fibers degenerate. Inflammatory cells infiltrate connective tissue, mostly within fascicles (i.e., endomysial inflammation), and invade apparently healthy muscle (Fig. 23-9). Isolated degenerating or regenerating fibers are scattered throughout fascicles. Perifascicular atrophy does not occur in polymyositis.

- **Inclusion body myositis**: This disorder is the most common myoinflammatory condition of the elderly, typically occurring after the age of 50. An autosomal recessive hereditary form of the disease shows similar features but may present in late adolescence or adulthood.
  - **Pathology**: The disease resembles polymyositis pathologically, showing single-fiber necrosis and regeneration, with predominantly endomysial cytotoxic T cells and a slight inflammatory infiltrate. Basophilic granular material is seen at the edge of vacuoles (rimmed vacuoles) within muscle fibers (Fig. 23-10A and B). These inclusions are Congo red positive and contain intracellular β-amyloid protein, the same type of amyloid as in senile plaques in Alzheimer disease (Fig. 23-10C) (see Chapter 24). Other proteins associated with Alzheimer and Parkinson diseases are also present. The pathogenic role of these inclusions is unclear because the accumulation of similar proteins associated with neurodegenerative diseases has been observed in other rare myopathies and chronic denervation. Immunosuppressive therapy does not mitigate the disease, but intravenous immunoglobulin may be therapeutically useful.

- **Dermatomyositis:** Unlike other myopathies, the disease is characterized by a rash on the upper eyelids, face, trunk, and sometimes elsewhere. It may occur alone or together with scleroderma, mixed connective tissue disease, or other autoimmune conditions.
  - **Pathophysiology:** Dermatomyositis is characterized by (1) deposition of immune complexes of IgG and IgM; (2) deposition of complement components, including membrane attack complex, C5b-9, in the walls of capillaries and other blood vessels; (3) microangiopathy with loss of capillaries; (4) signs of injury and atrophy of myofibers; and (5) perivascular infiltrates of B cells and $CD4^+$ helper T cells (Fig. 23-11). Muscle injury in dermatomyositis is mainly mediated by complement-fixing cytotoxic antibodies against skeletal muscle microvasculature. The resultant microangiopathy leads to ischemic injury of individual muscle fibers and eventually to fiber atrophy. True infarcts may result from involvement of larger intramuscular arteries.
  - **Pathology:** The most specific finding is complement deposition in capillary walls preceding inflammation or damage to muscle fibers. B and T lymphocytes infiltrate around blood vessels and in perimysial connective tissue, with a high $CD4^+$ to $CD8^+$ T cell ratio. Immune complexes in the walls of blood vessels (Fig. 23-11, inset) are associated with microangiopathy. Perifascicular atrophy (one or more layers of atrophic fibers at the periphery of fascicles) is pathognomonic.

MYASTHENIA GRAVIS

Myasthenia gravis is an acquired autoimmune disease in which antibodies to the acetylcholine (Ach) receptor at the neuromuscular junction cause abnormal muscular fatigability. It occurs in all races and is twice as common in women as in men. The disease typically begins in young adults, but first presentations may vary from childhood to old age. Patients with myasthenia gravis often suffer other autoimmune diseases.

PATHOPHYSIOLOGY: In myasthenia gravis, antibodies bind to the Ach receptor of the motor endplate but do not directly block Ach receptor binding. Complement activation leads to shedding of the terminal portions of the neuromuscular junctions which are rich in Ach receptors. The IgG antibodies also cross-link receptor proteins that remain in the postsynaptic membrane, thereby accelerating Ach receptor endocytosis. The result is impaired signal transmission, which causes muscle weakness and abnormal fatigability.

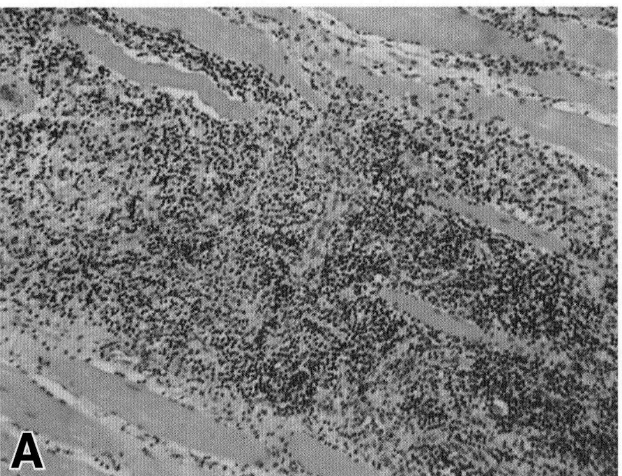

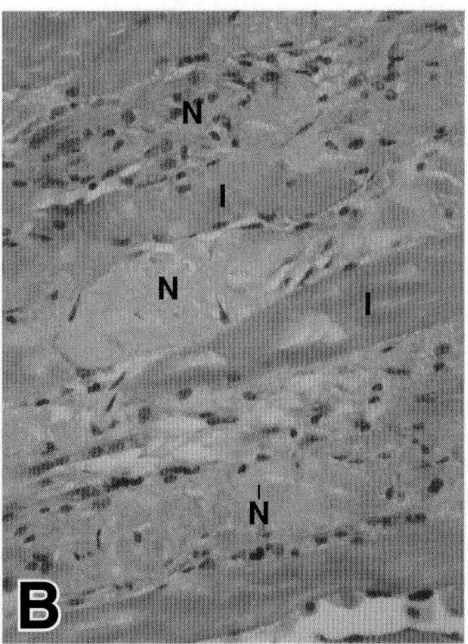

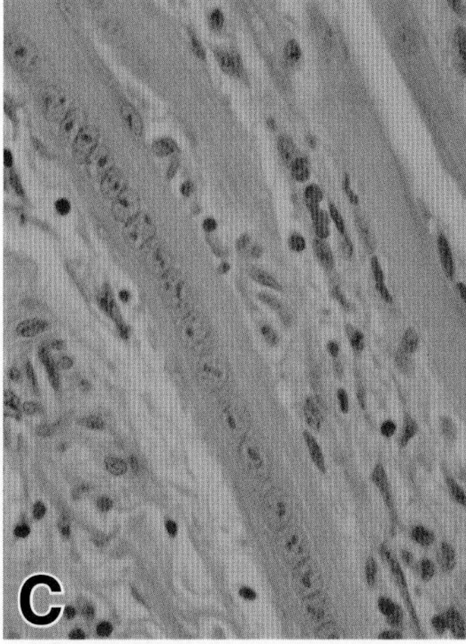

FIGURE 23-9. Polymyositis. A. Hematoxylin and eosin stain. A section of affected muscle showing an inflammatory myopathy. Mononuclear inflammatory cells infiltrate chiefly the endomysium. The field includes single-fiber necrosis. **B.** Region of healing inflammatory myopathy demonstrating intact fibers (*I*) and necrotic fibers (*N*). The uppermost necrotic fiber is heavily infiltrated with macrophages. **C.** Regenerating fiber displaying a linear array of enlarged centrally placed nuclei.

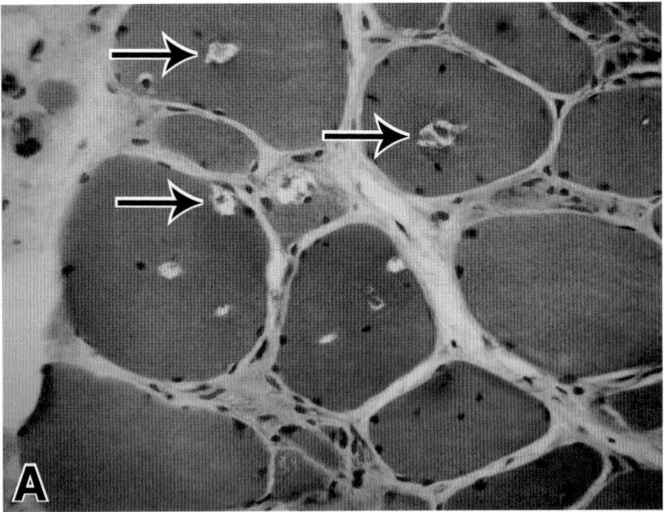

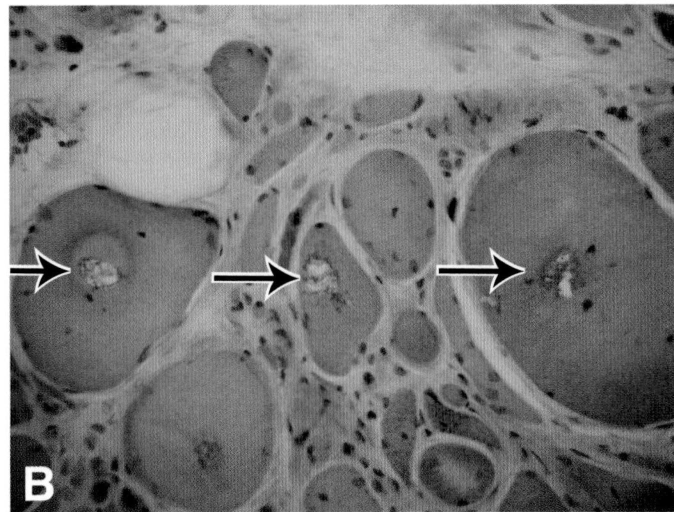

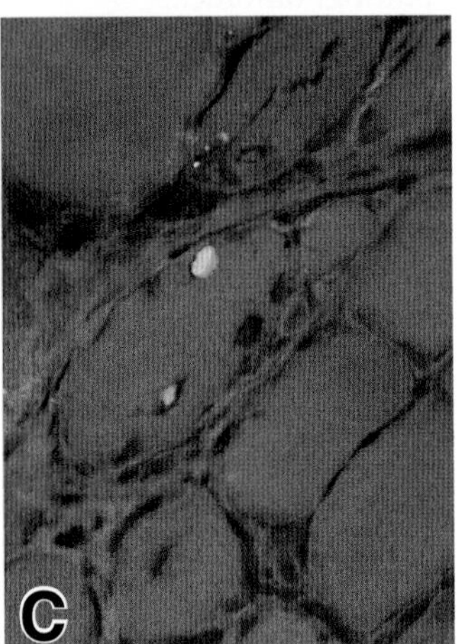

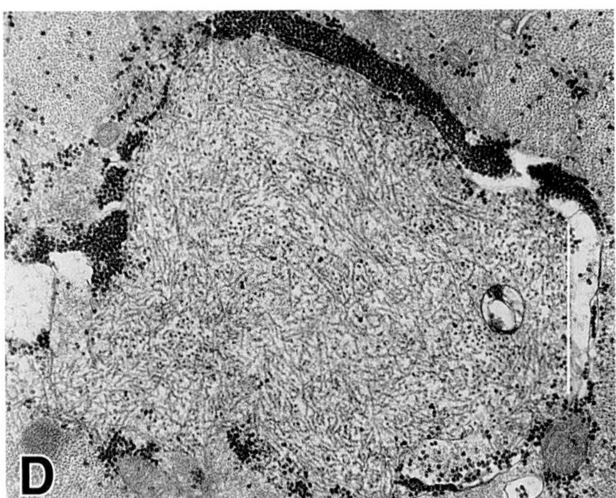

FIGURE 23-10. Inclusion body myositis (IBM). A. Hematoxylin and eosin stain (cryostat section). The features in IBM resemble those of polymyositis, but the muscle fibers also exhibit rimmed vacuoles (*arrows*) corresponding to enlarged lysosomes. **B.** Modified Gomori trichrome stain (cryostat section) showing granular basophilic rimming of vacuoles (*arrows*). **C.** Congo red stain. The inclusion has weak congophilia, but the color signal is strong because it has been enhanced by fluorescence excitation. **D.** An electron micrograph showing the characteristic filaments of the amyloid inclusions.

Most patients with myasthenia gravis have anti–Ach receptor antibodies and thymic hyperplasia. About 15% have an associated thymoma. Surgical removal of the hyperplastic thymic tissue or the thymoma often causes the myasthenia gravis to remit. Ach receptors on the surface of some thymic cells in thymoma and thymic hyperplasia may trigger production of antireceptor antibodies.

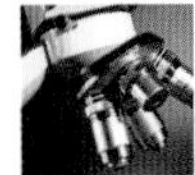

PATHOLOGY: Light microscopy may reveal atrophy of type II muscle fibers and focal collections of lymphocytes within fascicles. Electron microscopy shows that most muscle endplates are abnormal.

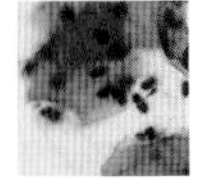

CLINICAL FEATURES: The clinical severity of myasthenia gravis is quite variable, and symptoms tend to wax and wane. Weakness may be limited to the extraocular muscles, in which case it is severe and causes ptosis and diplopia. More commonly, it progresses to other muscles, for example, those associated with swallowing, the trunk, and extremities.

The overall mortality from myasthenia gravis is 10%, often because muscle weakness leads to respiratory insufficiency. In addition to thymectomy, corticosteroids, methotrexate, and anticholinesterase drugs are used. Plasmapheresis provides transient clinical improvement.

INHERITED METABOLIC DISEASES

Skeletal muscle is dramatically affected by many endocrine and metabolic diseases, such as Cushing syndrome, Addison disease, hypothyroidism, hyperthyroidism (see Chapter 19), and conditions associated with hepatic or renal failure. Only primary hereditary abnormalities in metabolism of skeletal muscle that result in abnormal muscular function are discussed here.

Glycogen Storage Diseases

Glycogen storage diseases (glycogenoses) are autosomal recessive, inherited, metabolic disorders characterized by an inability to degrade glycogen (see Chapter 5). There are many glycogenoses, but only some of them affect skeletal muscle.

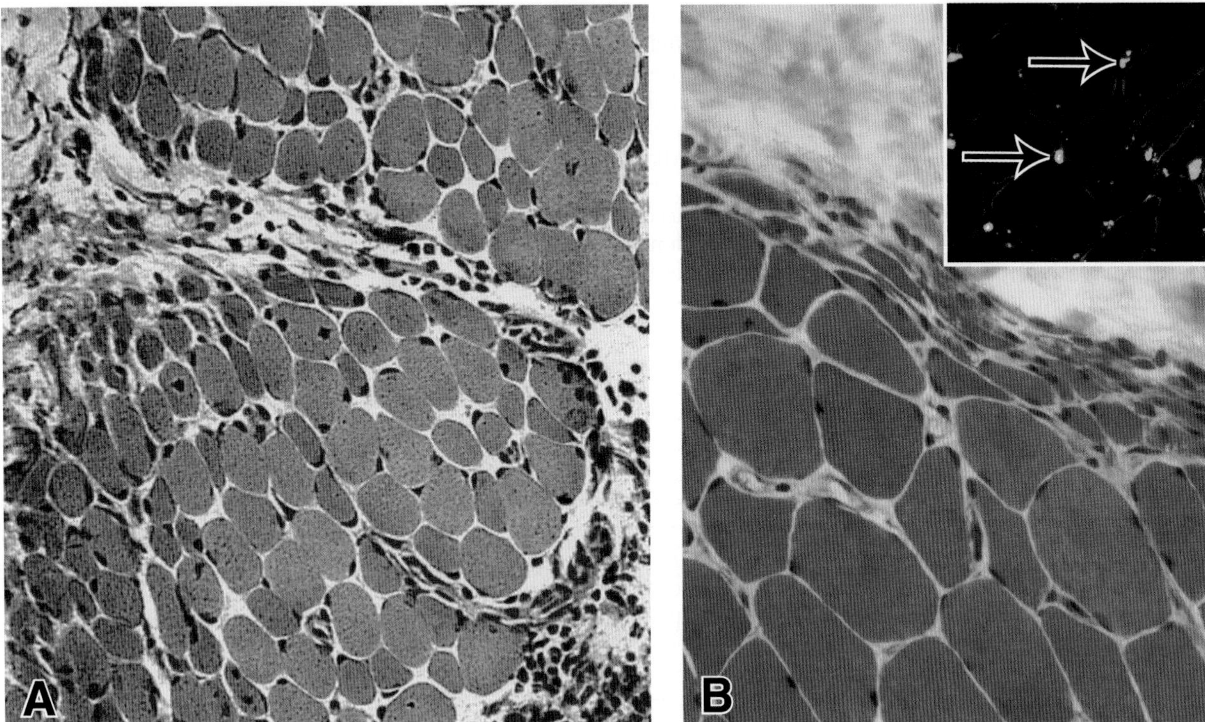

FIGURE 23-11. Dermatomyositis. A. Hematoxylin and eosin stain. The inflammatory cells infiltrate predominantly the perimysium rather than the endomysium. The periphery of muscle fascicles showing most of the muscle fiber atrophy and damage, resulting in a pattern of injury characteristic of dermatomyositis, termed *perifascicular atrophy.* **B.** High-magnification image of perifascicular atrophy demonstrating the flattening and shrinkage of fibers at the periphery of the fascicle. Immunofluorescence (*inset*) revealing that the walls of many capillaries display C5b-9 (membrane attack complex), reflecting the altered microvasculature typical of dermatomyositis.

The most important glycogenoses affecting skeletal muscle include the following:

- **Type II glycogenosis (Pompe disease):** Various mutations affect muscle acid maltase activity and lead to distinctly different clinical syndromes. Acid maltase is a lysosomal enzyme that is expressed in all cells and participates in glycogen degradation. When the enzyme is deficient, glycogen is not broken down, accumulates within lysosomes, and remains membrane bound (Fig. 23-12B).
  - **Pathology:** In all forms of glycogenosis caused by acid maltase deficiency, the morphologic changes are distinctive and almost pathognomonic (Fig. 23-12A). In the severe form, namely, Pompe disease, muscle shows massive accumulation of membrane-bound glycogen. Myofilaments and other sarcoplasmic organelles disappear. There is little regeneration, and apparently inactive satellite cells are present at the surfaces of muscle fibers that have been almost completely destroyed by the disease.

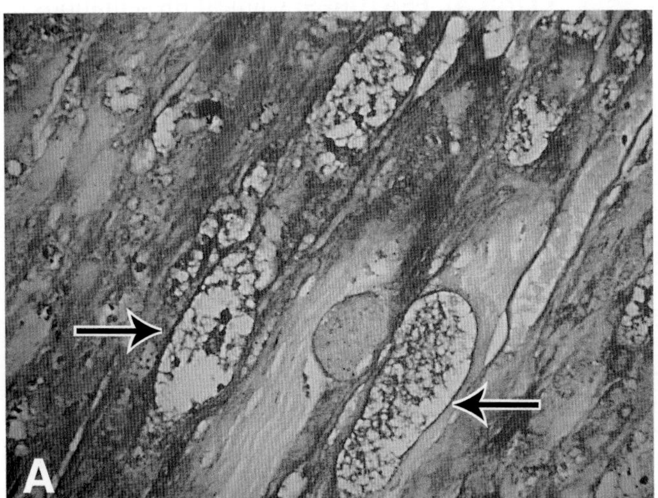

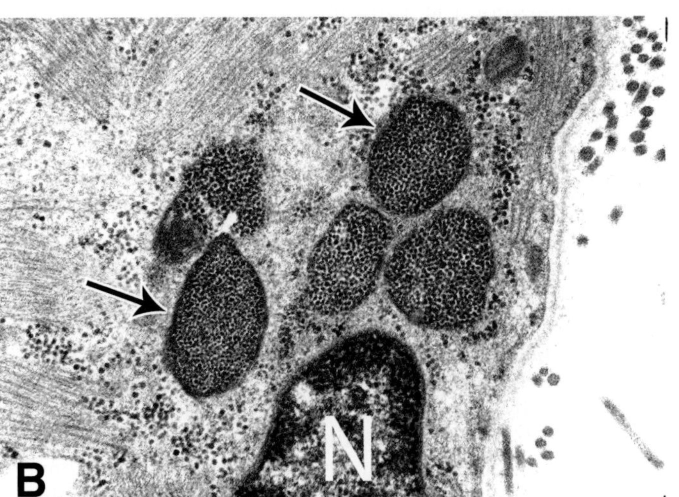

FIGURE 23-12. Acid maltase deficiency—adult onset. A. Periodic acid–Schiff (PAS) stain demonstrating large vacuoles filled with PAS-positive glycogen granules (*arrows*). **B.** Electron micrograph demonstrating membrane-bound glycogen granules (*arrows*). The structure marked *N* is a nucleus.

- **Clinical Features:** *Pompe disease* occurs in neonates or young infants and is the most extreme form of acid maltase deficiency. Patients have severe hypotonia and areflexia. Some have enlarged tongues and cardiomegaly and die of cardiac failure, usually within their first 2 years. Many tissues are affected, but skeletal and cardiac muscle, the CNS, and the liver are most involved. The serum creatine kinase level is only moderately increased. Later-onset forms of the disease entail milder, but relentlessly progressive, myopathy. Glycogen accumulates in other organs, but clinical expression of the disorder is usually limited to muscle.

- **Type V glycogenosis (McArdle disease):** This disorder is a metabolic myopathy that is usually not progressive or severely debilitating. The deficient enzyme, myophosphorylase, is specific for skeletal muscle. Without this enzyme, skeletal muscle glycogen cannot be cleaved at 1,4-glycosidic chains to produce glucose for energy production during physical exertion. Thus, muscles cramp with exercise. Patients also cannot produce lactate during ischemic exercise, which is the basis for a metabolic test for the condition. The disease usually does not interfere with normal life. However, prolonged, vigorous exercise can lead to widespread myofiber necrosis and release of soluble muscle proteins, such as, creatine kinase and myoglobin, into the blood. This complication can cause myoglobinuria and renal failure.
  - **Pathology:** Muscle tissue may appear completely normal, except for the absence of phosphorylase activity. However, there is usually subtle evidence of abnormal accumulation of glycogen granules within the sarcoplasm, mainly in the subsarcolemmal area.
- **Type VII** glycogenosis **(Tarui disease):** Phosphofructokinase (PFK) deficiency is less common than McArdle disease but causes the same syndrome.

Lipid Myopathies

A muscle biopsy from a patient with exercise intolerance or muscle weakness may sometimes show excess neutral lipids (Fig. 23-13). This finding occurs in several metabolic disorders of lipid metabolism, more than a dozen of which are known. Lipid myopathies may involve deficiencies in fatty acid transport into mitochondria (carnitine deficiency syndromes and carnitine palmityl transferase deficiency) and several other metabolic pathways involving lipids.

Mitochondrial Diseases

Inherited defects of mitochondrial metabolism are uncommon but conceptually important disorders. Historically, diseases of muscle were recognized first and designated mitochondrial myopathies. However, others affect both CNS and muscle and are known as **mitochondrial encephalomyopathies**. The nervous system, skeletal muscle, heart, kidney, and other organs can be affected in different combinations as part of a multisystem disease.

Inherited diseases of mitochondria are divided into defects of **nuclear DNA** (nDNA) or **mitochondrial DNA** (mtDNA). Point mutations, deletions, and duplications of mtDNA have been linked to several mitochondrial encephalomyopathies. ***The fraction of mutant mtDNA must exceed a critical value for a mitochondrial disease to be symptomatic.*** This threshold varies in different organs and is related to cellular energy requirements.

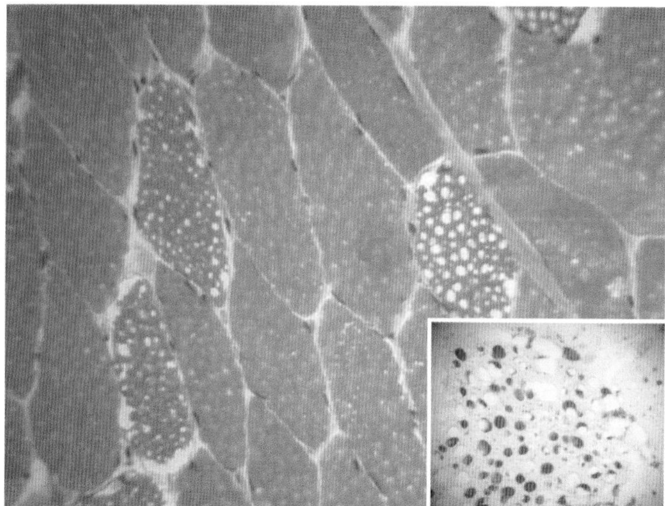

FIGURE 23-13. Lipid storage myopathy. Hematoxylin and eosin–stained frozen section. Numerous cytoplasmic vacuoles are present in the muscle fibers. Oil red-orcein stain (*inset*) demonstrating that the cytoplasmic vacuoles contain neutral lipid.

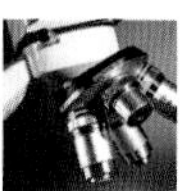

PATHOLOGY: In skeletal muscle, defects of mtDNA lead to the accumulation of mitochondria, excessive numbers of which may appear as aggregates of reddish granular material in a subsarcolemmal location (underneath the myocyte plasma membrane) with the Gomori trichrome stain (Fig. 23-14A). These are called **ragged red fibers** because the deposits have an irregular contour at the fiber periphery. Pathogenic mutations of mtDNA may impair complex IV (cytochrome oxidase) activity, so that ragged red fibers are often deficient in cytochrome oxidase activity (Fig. 23-14B). By contrast, they stain intensely for succinic dehydrogenase (SDH, complex II); this complex is exclusively encoded by nDNA (Fig. 23-14C). The increased SDH reflects mitochondrial proliferation. Such changes cause myofiber atrophy and the accumulation of sarcoplasmic lipid and glycogen owing to impaired mitochondrial energy utilization.

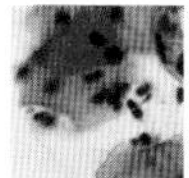

CLINICAL FEATURES: Clinical presentations of encephalomyopathies vary, but diseases may begin in children or adults. Some patients start with muscle weakness and then develop brain disorders. Others present with CNS disease, with or without overt muscle weakness, even though muscle biopsy shows mitochondrial pathology. Other organs, such as the heart (arrhythmias), are often affected as part of a multisystem disorder.

Three well-known neurologic syndromes include (1) **Kearns–Sayre syndrome**, which features progressive ophthalmoplegia, retinitis pigmentosa, cardiac arrhythmias, diabetes mellitus, cerebellar ataxia, multifocal neurodegeneration, and often muscle weakness; (2) **MELAS** (**m**itochondrial myopathy, **e**ncephalopathy, **l**actic acidosis, **a**nd **s**troke-like episodes); and (3) **MERRF** (**m**yoclonic **e**pilepsy and **r**agged **r**ed **f**ibers).

Familial Periodic Paralysis

Familial periodic paralysis encompasses several autosomal dominant disorders in which episodic muscular weakness, or even complete paralysis, is followed by rapid recovery. These

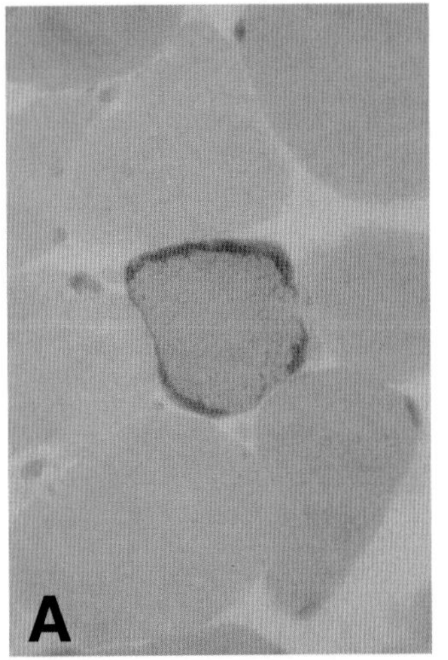

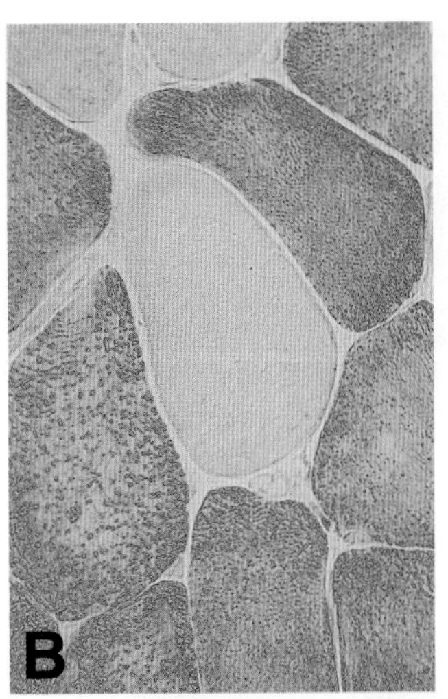

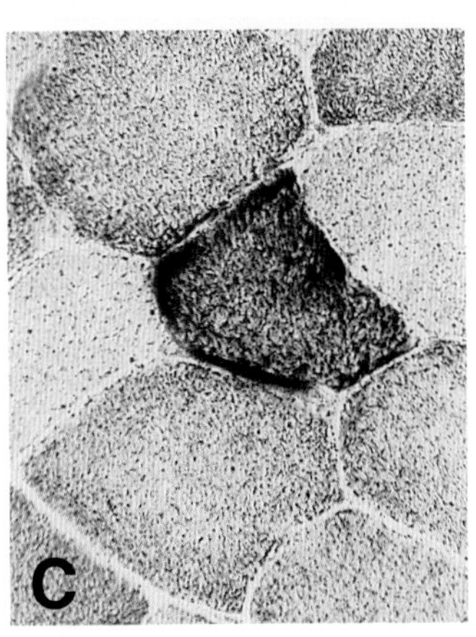

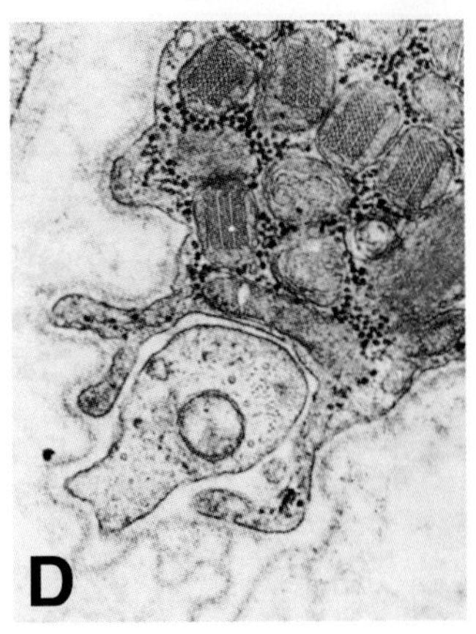

FIGURE 23-14. Mitochondrial myopathy caused by deletions of mitochondrial DNA (mtDNA). A. Modified Gomori trichrome. A ragged red fiber showing prominent proliferation of reddish, granular mitochondria, located chiefly in a subsarcolemmal region. **B.** A ragged red fiber displaying lack of **histochemical staining for cytochrome oxidase** (central pale fiber). Three subunits of this electron-transport carrier are coded by mtDNA, and the mutations have interfered with function in this fiber. **C. Succinate dehydrogenase (SDH) stain.** A ragged red fiber showing overexpression of SDH, an enzyme that is entirely encoded by nuclear DNA (nDNA). **D.** An electron micrograph revealing mitochondria with ultrastructural abnormalities, including paracrystalline inclusions.

symptoms reflect abnormalities in sodium and potassium fluxes into and out of muscle cells. During an attack, muscle fiber surfaces do not propagate action potentials, although calcium entry into the muscle fiber causes contraction.

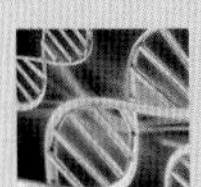

MOLECULAR PATHOGENESIS: These dyskalemic syndromes include hypokalemic and hyperkalemic periodic paralysis. The former type is linked to mutations in several genes, including a calcium channel (*CACNA1S*), a sodium channel (*SCN4A*), and a potassium channel (*KCNE3*). In the hyperkalemic form, the same sodium channel gene (*SCN4A*) is mutated, but the hyperkalemic form reflects a gain-of-function mutation of *SCN4A*. The hypokalemic form is caused by a loss-of-function mutation in the same sodium channel gene.

RHABDOMYOLYSIS

Rhabdomyolysis refers to dissolution of skeletal muscle fibers and release of myoglobin into the blood, which may cause myoglobinuria and acute renal failure. The disorder may be acute, subacute, or chronic. During acute rhabdomyolysis, muscles are swollen, tender, and profoundly weak.

Episodes of rhabdomyolysis are precipitated by diverse stimuli. They may complicate or follow bouts of influenza. Some patients develop rhabdomyolysis with apparently mild exercise and probably have some form of metabolic myopathy. A spectrum of muscle dysfunction, from pain (myalgia) to rhabdomyolysis, is also well known during treatment with statin cholesterol-lowering agents. Rhabdomyolysis may also complicate heat stroke or malignant hyperthermia. Alcoholism is occasionally associated with either acute or chronic rhabdomyolysis.

Pathologically, rhabdomyolysis is an active, noninflammatory myopathy, with scattered muscle fiber necrosis and varying degrees of degeneration and regeneration. Macrophages, but no other inflammatory cells, are present in and around muscle fibers.

DENERVATION

The diagnostic consideration in any patient with muscle weakness is whether the cause is myopathic or neurogenic. Myopathic conditions are those intrinsic to muscle and have been discussed above. Neurogenic causes of muscle weakness feature denervation, which reflects lesions of lower motor neurons or axons. Although muscle biopsy detects lower motor neuron lesions, patterns of denervation do not identify the cause of the lesion. Damage to upper motor neurons, as in multiple sclerosis or stroke, lead to paralysis and atrophy, but leave lower motor neurons intact. Under these conditions, pathologic changes reflect nonspecific atrophy rather than denervation atrophy.

When a skeletal muscle fiber becomes separated from contact with its lower motor neuron, it invariably atrophies, owing to progressive loss of myofibrils. On cross section, atrophic fibers are characteristically angular, as though compressed by surrounding normal muscle fibers (Fig. 23-15). If a fiber is not reinnervated, atrophy progresses to complete loss of myofibrils, with nuclei condensing into aggregates. In the end stage, muscle fibers disappear and are replaced chiefly by adipose tissue.

Early in denervation, fibers are irregularly scattered, angular, and atrophic. As the disease progresses, these fibers are first seen in small clusters of several fibers and then in progressively larger groups (Fig. 23-15B). Groups of denervated fibers include both type I and type II fibers; **denervating conditions are not selective for only one type of motor neuron**.

Denervation is always followed by an effort at reinnervation. The denervated state induces sprouting of new nerve endings from adjacent surviving nerves. If denervation proceeds slowly, reinnervation may keep pace. New sprouting nerve endings make synaptic contact with the muscle fiber at the site of the previous motor endplate. Nicotinic Ach receptors (extrajunctional receptors) cover muscle fibers soon after denervation. With reinnervation, extrajunctional receptors again disappear from the sarcolemma, except at the point of synaptic contact.

In a chronic denervating condition, reinnervation of each surviving motor unit gradually enlarges. ***As a specific type of lower motor neuron takes over innervation of a given field***

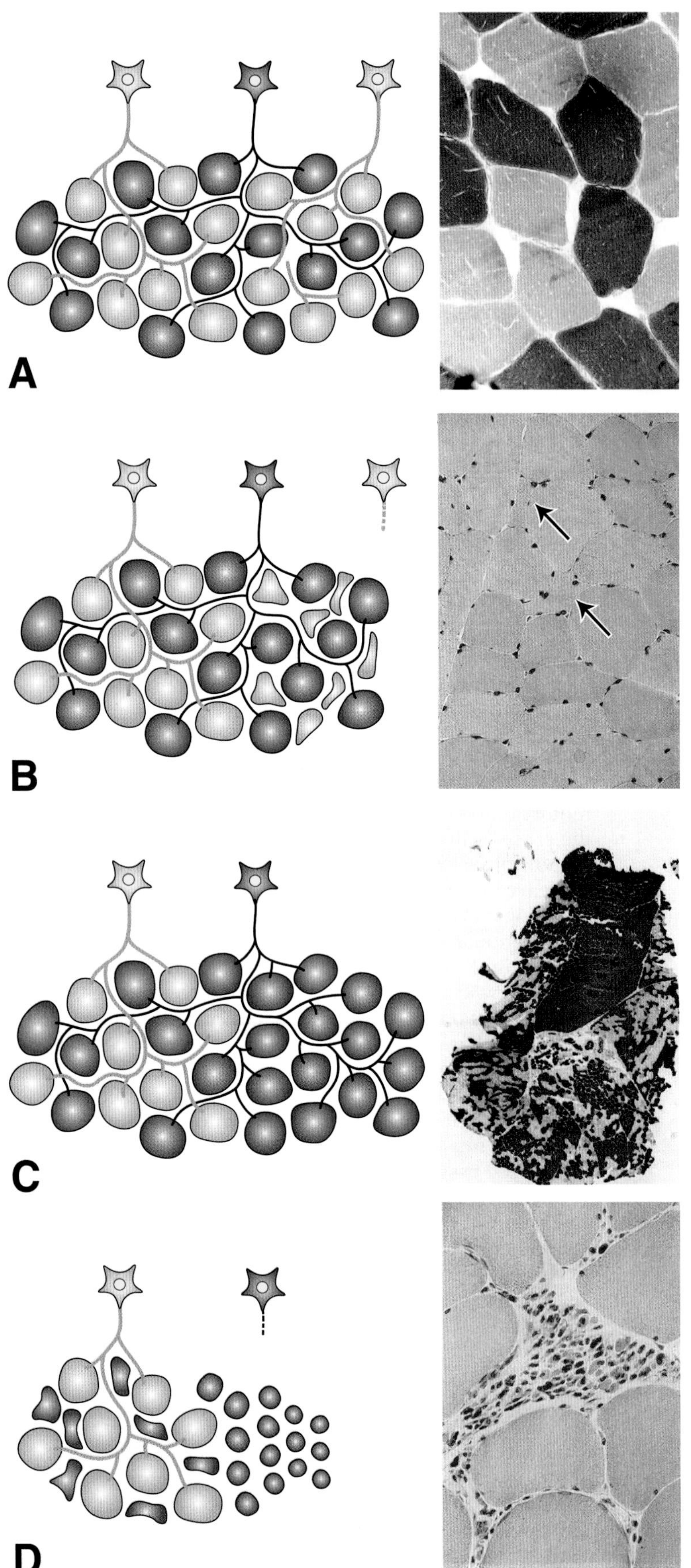

FIGURE 23-15. Denervation/reinnervation. A. As shown in the photomicrograph, the normal intermixed distribution of type I (*pale*) and type II (*dark*) muscle fibers is shown by staining for ATPase. In the drawing, two neurons (*pale*) innervate type I muscle fibers, and two neurons (*dark*) supply type II fibers. **B.** Denervation; hematoxylin and eosin stain. With early (mild) denervation, portions of the axonal tree degenerate, resulting in angular atrophy of scattered type I and II muscle fibers (*arrows*). **C.** Reinnervation; myofibrillar ATPase. As neurons degenerate, surviving neurons sprout more nerve endings and reinnervate some of the denervated fibers. These reinnervated fibers become either type I or type II, according to the type of neuron that reinnervates them. This process results in fewer, but larger, motor units and the appearance of clusters of fibers of one type adjacent to clusters of the other type, a pattern called "type grouping." The photomicrograph demonstrating type grouping. This field would appear normal except for a few atrophic fibers if it were stained with hematoxylin and eosin. **D.** With more advanced (severe, chronic) denervation, entire lower motor neurons or numerous axonal processes degenerate, causing small groups of angular atrophic fibers (grouped atrophy) to appear as illustrated in the photomicrograph.

of fibers, fiber groups of one type are seen adjacent to groups of another type. This pattern, called fiber-type grouping, is pathognomonic of denervation followed by reinnervation (Fig. 23-15C).

If denervation continues after the development of fiber-type grouping, large motor units become atrophic. Such **grouped atrophy** (Fig. 23-15D) is characteristic of chronic denervating disorders, such as amyotrophic lateral sclerosis.

Spinal Muscular Atrophy

This disease is, strictly speaking, not a primary muscle disorder, but it is usually included in discussions of skeletal muscle because it represents a major consideration in the differential diagnosis of childhood or infantile weakness. ***SMA is the second most common lethal autosomal recessive disorder after cystic fibrosis.*** The survival motor neuron gene (5q11.2-13.3) is mutated in SMA, mostly as a result of deletion, a defect that results in premature death of motor nerve cells.

- **Types I and II SMA (Werdnig–Hoffmann disease, infantile SMA):** *Infants show progressive and severe weakness* and seldom survive beyond 1 year of life. Denervation seems to begin in utero after motor units are established. The histology is virtually pathognomonic (Fig. 23-16). Groups of minute, rounded, atrophic fibers are still identifiable with the ATPase reaction as being either type I or type II. There are also fascicles of normal muscle fibers and almost invariably clusters of hypertrophied type I fibers. **Type II disease intermediate SMA** is intermediate in severity.
- **Type III SMA (Kugelberg–Welander disease, juvenile SMA):** This variant is a later-onset form of SMA and is not necessarily progressive.

Type II Fiber Atrophy

A commonly misinterpreted pathologic pattern in muscle biopsy specimens is atrophy from (1) disuse, (2) wasting, (3) upper motor neuron disease, and (4) corticosteroid toxicity. This nonspecific atrophy is a selective angular atrophy of type II fibers (Fig. 23-17). Type II fiber atrophy is common and is often related to a more chronic problem, often a complication of corticosteroid therapy (steroid myopathy).

Critical Illness Myopathy

If patients on high-dose corticosteroids and neuromuscular-blocking agents experience severe weakness despite removal of drugs, they may have **critical illness myopathy**, also known as **myosin heavy-chain depletion syndrome**. These patients show loss of thick myosin filaments from muscle fibers. Myosin thick filaments reappear with discontinuation of corticosteroids, and muscle strength returns.

The Peripheral Nervous System

ANATOMY

The peripheral nervous system (PNS) is external to the brain and spinal cord and includes (1) cranial nerves III to XII, (2) dorsal and ventral spinal roots, (3) spinal nerves and their continuations, and (4) ganglia. Peripheral nerves carry somatic motor, somatic sensory, visceral sensory, and autonomic fibers.

Peripheral nerve axons may be myelinated or unmyelinated. Myelinated axons are 1 to 20 μm in diameter, whereas unmyelinated ones are much smaller at 0.4 to 2.4 μm. Schwann cells surround both myelinated and unmyelinated fibers. The axon determines whether the Schwann cell produces myelin. Myelin sheath thickness, internodal length (distance between two nodes of Ranvier), and conduction velocity are proportional to axonal diameter.

REACTIONS TO INJURY

Peripheral nerve fibers show only a limited number of reactions to injury (Fig. 23-18). The major types of nerve fiber damage are axonal degeneration and segmental demyelination. ***PNS fibers differ from those in the CNS by their ability to regenerate and remyelinate to recover function.***

Axonal Degeneration

Degeneration (necrosis) of the axon occurs in many neuropathies; it may be limited to distal axons or involve both axons and neuronal cell bodies (Fig. 23-19A). Immediately after the axon degenerates, the myelin sheath breaks down, and Schwann cells proliferate. The latter effect initiates myelin degradation, which is completed by macrophages that infiltrate the nerve within 3 days after axonal degeneration. If injury is restricted to the distal axon, regenerating axons may sprout within 1 week from the intact, proximal axonal stump. There are several types of axonal degeneration.

DISTAL AXONAL DEGENERATION: In many neuropathies, axonal degeneration is initially limited to the distal ends of long fibers (**dying-back neuropathy** or **distal axonopathy**) (Fig. 23-18B). Peripheral neuropathies characterized by distal axonal degeneration typically present clinically as distal ("length-dependent" or "glove-and-stocking") neuropathies.

In this setting, neuronal cell bodies and proximal axons remain intact. Axons may thus regenerate, and nerve function may return if the cause of the distal axonal degeneration is removed. This rescue must occur before the dying-back degeneration reaches the proximal axon and causes the neuronal cell body to die.

NEURONOPATHY: Axonal degeneration may result from death of a neuronal cell body, as in autoimmune dorsal root ganglionitis (Fig. 23-18C). Peripheral neuropathies with selective damage to neuronal cell bodies are **neuronopathies** and are much rarer than distal axonopathies. Death of the neuronal cell body precludes axonal regeneration, making recovery impossible.

WALLERIAN DEGENERATION: This term describes axonal degeneration distal to transection or crush of the nerve. If the injury is not too proximal, the nerve may regenerate.

Segmental Demyelination

Loss of myelin from one or more internodes (segments) along a myelinated fiber indicates Schwann cell dysfunction (Fig. 23-18D). This condition may be due either to direct injury to the Schwann cell or to the myelin sheath (**primary demyelination**). In some cases, underlying axonal abnormalities (**secondary demyelination**) are responsible.

Table 23-2

Etiologic Classification of Neuropathies

Etiologic Classification of Neuropathies
Immune-mediated neuropathies
Acute inflammatory demyelinating polyradiculoneuropathy (Guillain–Barré syndrome)
Acute motor (and sensory) axonal neuropathy (axonal form of Guillain–Barré syndrome)
Fisher syndrome
Chronic inflammatory demyelinating polyradiculoneuropathy (CIDP)
Multifocal motor neuropathy
Dorsal root ganglionitis (sensory neuronopathy)
Immunoglobulin M (IgM) paraproteinemia-associated demyelinating neuropathy
Vasculitic neuropathy (systemic vasculitis, connective tissue disease, cryoglobulinemia)
Metabolic neuropathies
Diabetic polyneuropathy and mononeuropathies
Uremic neuropathy
Critical illness polyneuropathy
Hypothyroid neuropathy
Acromegalic neuropathy
Nutritional neuropathies
Neuropathy associated with deficiency of vitamin B_1, B_6, B_{12} or E
Copper deficiency myeloneuropathy
Alcoholic neuropathy
Toxic and drug-induced neuropathies (see Table 23-3)
Amyloid neuropathy (AL amyloidosis and familial amyloid polyneuropathy)
Hereditary neuropathies (see Tables 23-4 and 23-5)
Neuropathies associated with infections
Leprosy
HIV
Cytomegalovirus
Hepatitis B and C (vasculitic neuropathy or CIDP)
Herpes zoster
Lyme disease
Diphtheria (toxic neuropathy)
Paraneoplastic neuropathy
Sarcoid neuropathy
Radiation neuropathy
Traumatic neuropathy
Chronic idiopathic axonal polyneuropathy

Loss of the myelin sheath does not cause the underlying axon to degenerate. Macrophages infiltrate the nerve and clear the myelin debris. Degeneration of the internodal myelin sheath is followed sequentially by (1) Schwann cell proliferation, (2) remyelination of the demyelinated segments, and (3) functional recovery. Remyelinated internodes have shortened internodal lengths (Fig. 23-18E). Repeated episodes of segmental peripheral nerve demyelination and remyelination, as occurs in chronic demyelinating neuropathies, cause supernumerary Schwann cells to appear. They encircle the axons (**onion bulbs**) (Fig. 23-19B) and cause clinically evident nerve enlargement (**hypertrophic neuropathy**).

PERIPHERAL NEUROPATHIES

Peripheral neuropathy is a process that affects the function of one or more peripheral nerves. It may be restricted to the peripheral nervous system (PNS), involve both the PNS and CNS, or affect multiple organ systems. Peripheral neuropathies occur in all age groups and may be hereditary or acquired.

There are many causes of peripheral neuropathy (Table 23-2), but ***diabetes mellitus is the most common cause of generalized peripheral neuropathy in the United States.*** Other common causes include hereditary disorders, alcoholism, chronic renal failure, neurotoxic drugs, autoimmune diseases, paraproteinemia, nutritional deficiencies, infections, cancer, and trauma.

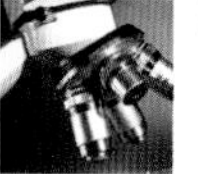

PATHOLOGY: Pathologic findings in most neuropathies are limited to axonal degeneration or segmental demyelination or both. If axonal degeneration predominates, the neuropathy is an **axonal neuropathy**; if segmental demyelination predominates, it is called a **demyelinating neuropathy.** ***Most (80% to 90%) neuropathies are axonal and of the dying-back type (distal axonal neuropathy).*** Electrophysiologic studies often help to distinguish axonal and demyelinating neuropathies. Nerve conduction velocity is typically near normal in axonal neuropathies but is impaired in demyelinating neuropathies. The distinction between axonal and demyelinating neuropathies is useful clinically. Axonal neuropathies have many causes, but demyelinating neuropathies have a limited number of etiologies, which are most likely to be hereditary or immunologically mediated.

The histopathology of many neuropathies does not indicate the underlying cause, so that clinicopathologic correlation is usually needed to establish causation. Less often, a specific etiology may be seen. Examples are necrotizing arteritis

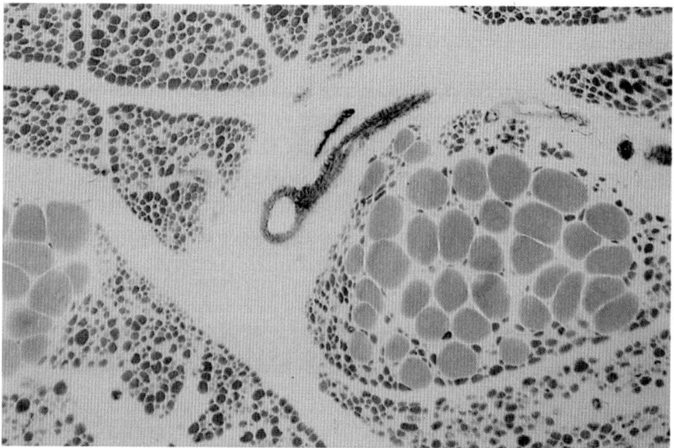

FIGURE 23-16. Werdnig–Hoffman disease (infantile spinal muscular atrophy). This cross section of skeletal muscle stained for myofibrillar ATPase is derived from an infant with severe hypotonia. It shows groups of extremely atrophic, rounded type I and type II fibers, and clusters of markedly hypertrophied pale type I fibers.

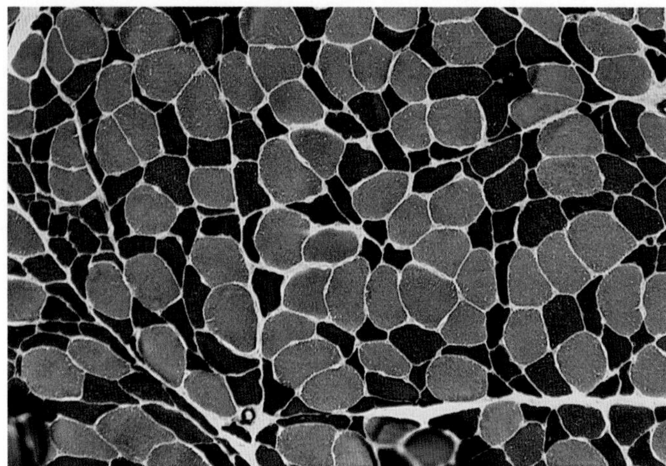

FIGURE 23-17. **Type II fiber atrophy.** This biopsy of the vastus lateralis muscle was taken from a 48-year-old man with proximal muscle weakness because of endogenous corticosteroid toxicity (Cushing syndrome). Virtually, all of the angular atrophic fibers are type II. This form of atrophy closely mimics denervation atrophy when visualized with the hematoxylin and eosin stain.

(vasculitic neuropathy), granulomatous inflammation (leprosy and sarcoid), amyloid deposits (amyloid neuropathy), abnormalities of the myelin sheath (IgM paraproteinemic neuropathy and hereditary neuropathy with liability to pressure palsies), and abnormal accumulations within Schwann cells (leukodystrophy) or axons (giant axonal neuropathy).

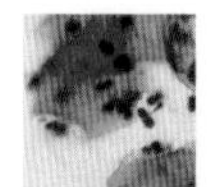

CLINICAL FEATURES: The major clinical manifestations of peripheral neuropathy are muscle weakness and atrophy, sensory loss, paresthesia, pain, and autonomic dysfunction. Motor, sensory, and autonomic functions may be equally or preferentially affected. Predominant involvement of large diameter sensory fibers affects position and vibration sense, whereas injury to small diameter fibers hinders pain and temperature sensation. A neuropathy may be acute (days to weeks), subacute (weeks to months), or chronic (months to years). It may (1) affect one nerve (**mononeuropathy**), (2) several (**mononeuropathy multiplex**), (3) dorsal root ganglia (**sensory neuronopathy**), or (4) nerve roots (**radiculopathy**). The disorder may also affect multiple peripheral nerves (**polyneuropathy**) or both nerve roots and peripheral nerves (**polyradiculoneuropathy**).

Diabetic Neuropathy

Diabetic neuropathy may manifest as (1) distal sensorimotor polyneuropathy, (2) autonomic neuropathy, (3) mononeuropathy, or (4) mononeuropathy multiplex. The mononeuropathies may involve cranial nerves (cranial neuropathy), nerve roots, or proximal peripheral nerves. ***Distal, predominantly sensory, polyneuropathy is the most common form of diabetic neuropathy.***

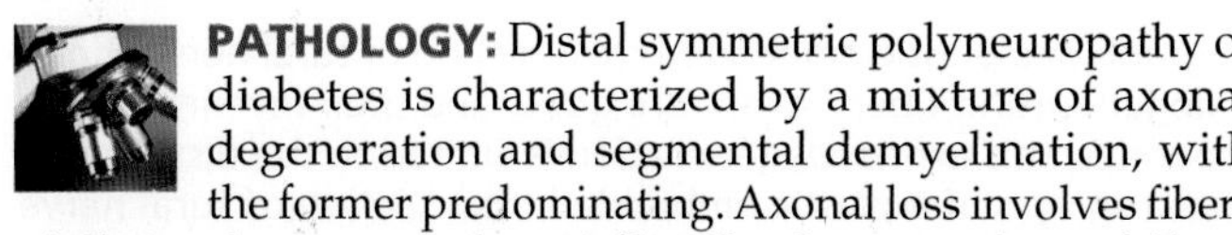

PATHOLOGY: Distal symmetric polyneuropathy of diabetes is characterized by a mixture of axonal degeneration and segmental demyelination, with the former predominating. Axonal loss involves fibers of all sizes but may preferentially affect large myelinated fibers (**large-fiber neuropathy**), small myelinated fibers, or unmyelinated fibers (**small-fiber neuropathy**).

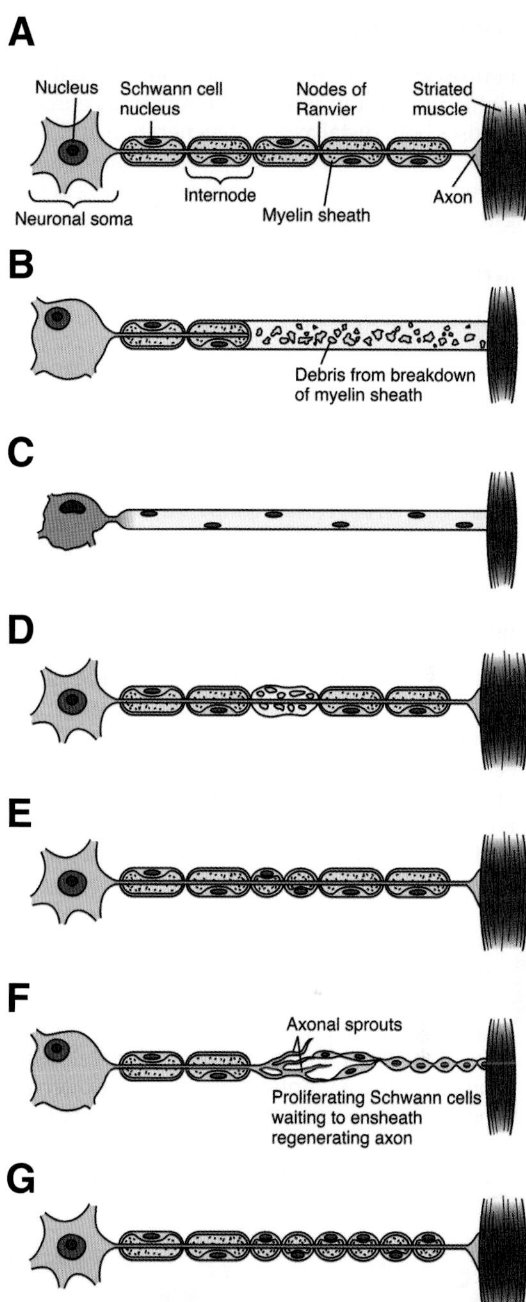

FIGURE 23-18. **Basic responses of peripheral nerve fibers to injury. A. Intact myelinated fiber.** The axon is insulated by the Schwann cell–derived myelin sheaths. **B. Distal axonal degeneration.** The distal axon has degenerated, and myelin sheaths associated with the distal axon have secondarily degenerated. The striated muscle shows denervation atrophy. **C. Degeneration of cell body and axon.** Degeneration involves the neuronal cell body and its entire axon. The myelin sheaths associated with the axon have also degenerated. **D. Segmental demyelination.** The myelin sheath associated with one Schwann cell has degenerated, leaving a segment of axon uncovered by myelin. The underlying axon remains intact. **E. Remyelination.** Proliferating Schwann cells cover the demyelinated segment of the axon and elaborate new myelin sheaths. The remyelinating Schwann cells have short internodal lengths. **F. Regenerating axon.** Regenerating axons sprout from the distal end of the disrupted axon. Ideally, the regenerating axons reinnervate the distal nerve stump, where they will be ensheathed and myelinated by Schwann cells of the distal stump. **G. Regenerated nerve fiber.** The regenerated portion of the axon is myelinated by Schwann cells with short internodal lengths. The striated muscle is reinnervated.

Uremic Neuropathy

Uremic neuropathy is a distal sensorimotor axonal polyneuropathy, which is seen in half of patients with chronic renal failure. It causes both distal axonal degeneration and segmental demyelination. The former predominates and mainly affects large diameter fibers. Uremic neuropathy often stabilizes or improves with long-term dialysis and resolves after renal transplantation.

Acute Inflammatory Demyelinating Polyradiculoneuropathy

AIDP is an acquired, immune-mediated neuropathy that often follows bacterial, viral, or mycoplasmal infections. It may also follow immunization or surgery. Usually, there is an antecedent upper respiratory or gastrointestinal infection. Commonly associated infectious agents include *Campylobacter jejuni*, cytomegalovirus, Epstein–Barr virus, and *Mycoplasma pneumoniae*. AIDP is the most common cause of **Guillain–Barré syndrome** in children and adults. This disorder is an acute symmetric neuromuscular paralysis that often begins distally and ascends proximally. Sensory and autonomic disturbances may also occur in AIDP, and 5% of cases present with ophthalmoplegia, ataxia, and areflexia (**Fisher syndrome**). Muscular paralysis may cause respiratory embarrassment, and autonomic involvement may lead to cardiac arrhythmias, hypotension, or hypertension. AIDP begins to resolve 2 to 4 weeks after onset, and most patients recover. Characteristically, the cerebrospinal fluid has increased protein but few white blood cells (albuminocytologic dissociation), a situation attributable to inflammation of spinal roots.

PATHOLOGY: AIDP may affect all levels of the PNS, including spinal roots (polyradiculoneuropathy), ganglia, craniospinal nerves, and autonomic nerves. Involved regions show endoneurial infiltrates of lymphocytes and macrophages, segmental demyelination, and relative axonal sparing. Lymphoid infiltrates are often perivascular, but there is no true vasculitis. Macrophages are frequently adjacent to degenerating myelin sheaths and can strip off and phagocytose superficial myelin lamellae. Such macrophage-mediated demyelination is rare in other neuropathies.

Guillain–Barré syndrome may also be caused by an immune-mediated axonal neuropathy (**acute motor axonal neuropathy** or **acute motor and sensory axonal neuropathy**). The axonal form often follows *C. jejuni* infection and shows serum antiganglioside antibodies (anti-GM_1 and others).

Chronic inflammatory demyelinating polyradiculoneuropathy (CIDP) is similar to AIDP but has a protracted course, with multiple relapses or slow continuous progression, and usually lacks evidence of antecedent infection. The neuropathy may occur sporadically (idiopathic CIDP) or in association with paraproteinemia, HIV infection, chronic active hepatitis, connective tissue disease, inflammatory bowel disease, or Hodgkin lymphoma. Nerves and nerve roots in CIDP often show many onion bulbs owing to recurring episodes of demyelination, Schwann cell proliferation, and remyelination (Fig. 23-19B).

Monoclonal Gammopathy-Associated Neuropathies

Monoclonal gammopathies may cause (1) amyloid neuropathy, (2) cryoglobulinemia-associated vasculitic neuropathy, or (3) chronic demyelinating polyneuropathy. The last often occurs when the IgM paraprotein binds myelin-associated glycoprotein (MAG) and precipitates demyelination. Anti-MAG neuropathy is characterized by extensive segmental demyelination, a variable number of onion bulbs, axonal loss, and a distinctive widening of myelin lamellae.

Amyloidosis-Associated Neuropathies

In addition to its effects on sensory and motor nerves, amyloid infiltration of the PNS often leads to prominent autonomic dysfunction. The disorder may be hereditary but more often complicates light-chain amyloidosis (AL) in primary systemic amyloidosis or multiple myeloma (see Chapter 7). Amyloid deposits in endoneurial and epineurial extracellular spaces and vascular walls in

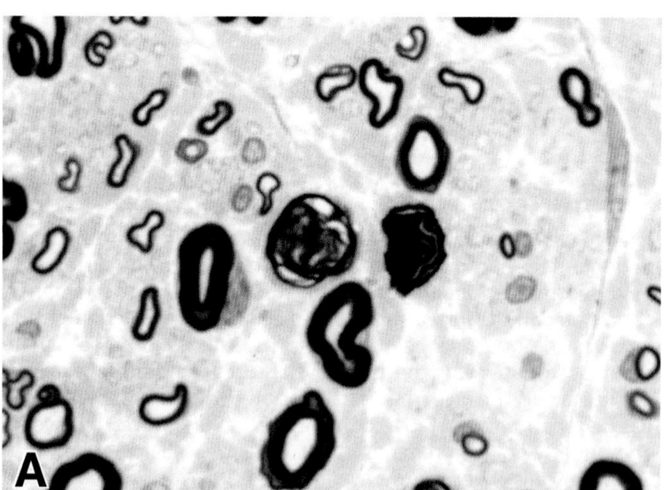

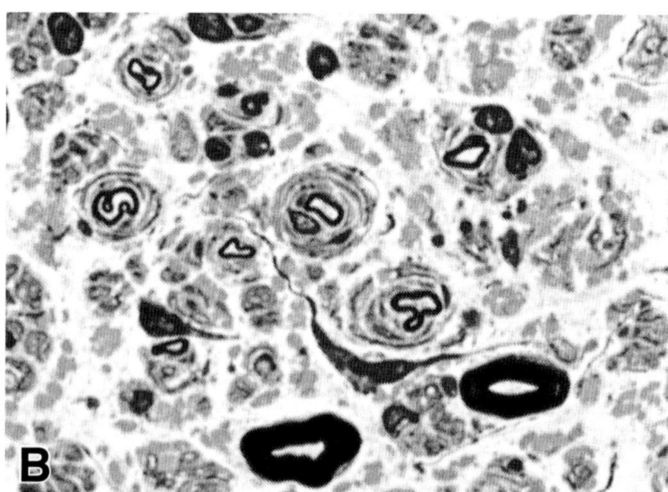

FIGURE 23-19. A. Axonal degeneration in an axonal neuropathy. Photomicrograph of a plastic-embedded cross section of sural nerve showing two degenerating myelinated fibers in the center of the field. The degenerating fibers' axons are gone, and their myelin sheaths are reduced to rounded masses of myelin debris. In most axonal neuropathies, this axonal degeneration is limited to the distal axon. **B. Onion bulbs in chronic inflammatory demyelinating polyneuropathy.** Photomicrograph of a plastic-embedded cross section of sural nerve showing several remyelinating axons with thin myelin sheaths in the center of the field. The remyelinating axons are surrounded by multiple concentric layers of Schwann cell cytoplasm, which resemble the concentric rings of a sectioned onion. Onion bulb formation is common in neuropathies with recurrent episodes of demyelination and remyelination.

peripheral nerves, dorsal root ganglia, and autonomic ganglia. Loss of myelinated or unmyelinated fibers or both ensues.

Toxic Neuropathy Is Often Iatrogenic

A variety of environmental agents and industrial compounds cause peripheral neuropathy (Table 23-3), but most cases of toxic neuropathy result from drugs. Almost all toxic neuropathies are characterized by axonal degeneration, usually of the dying-back type.

Hereditary Chronic Neuropathies

Many inherited diseases manifest as peripheral neuropathies (Tables 23-4 and 23-5); the neuropathy may be the sole manifestation of a hereditary disease or part of a multisystem disease.

Charcot–Marie–Tooth Disease

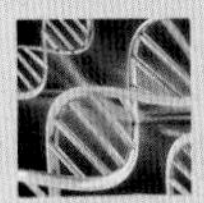

MOLECULAR PATHOGENESIS: CMT disease is a genetically and pathologically heterogeneous group of slowly progressive distal sensorimotor polyneuropathies that manifest in childhood or early adult life. It is the most common inherited neuropathy with a prevalence of 1 in 2,500. CMT is broadly divided into **demyelinating** and **axonal** types. **CMT1**, the most common form, is a chronic demyelinating polyneuropathy with onion bulbs and axonal loss. The less common **CMT2** variety features distal axonal degeneration. Both CMT1 and CMT2 are autosomal dominant diseases. The classification is complex because mutations in diverse genes may produce the same phenotype, and different mutations in the same gene may lead to different phenotypes (Table 23-5).

Table 23-3

Agents Associated With Toxic Neuropathy

Drugs	Environmental and Industrial Agents
Amiodarone	Acrylamide
Bortezomib	Allyl chloride
Colchicine	Arsenic
Dapsone	Buckthorn toxin
Disulfiram	Carbon disulfide
Gold salts	Chlordecone
Isoniazid	Dimethylaminopropionitrile
Metronidazole	Diphtheria toxin
Misonidazole	Ethylene oxide
Nitrofurantoin	n-Hexane (glue sniffing)
Nucleoside analogs (antiretrovirals)	Methyl n-butyl ketone
Paclitaxel (taxanes)	Lead
Phenytoin	Mercury
Platinum compounds	Methyl bromide
Podophyllin	Organophosphates
Pyridoxine (vitamin B_6)	Polychlorinated biphenyls
Suramin	Thallium
Thalidomide	Trichloroethylene
Vincristine	Vacor

Table 23-4

Inherited Diseases Associated With Neuropathy

Ataxia-telangiectasia
Abetalipoproteinemia
Acute intermittent porphyria, hereditary coproporphyria, and variegate porphyria
Cerebrotendinous xanthomatosis
Fabry disease (α-galactosidase A deficiency)
Familial amyloid polyneuropathy (transthyretin, apolipoprotein A1, and gelsolin amyloidosis)
Friedreich ataxia
Giant axonal neuropathy
Hereditary motor and sensory neuropathies (Charcot–Marie–Tooth disease)
Hereditary motor neuropathies
Hereditary neuropathy with liability to pressure palsies
Hereditary sensory and autonomic neuropathies
Infantile neuroaxonal dystrophy
Leukodystrophies (metachromatic, globoid cell, and adrenoleukodystrophy)
Refsum disease (phytanic acid storage disease)
Tangier disease

HIV-1 Infection-Associated Neuropathies

Distal symmetric polyneuropathy is the most common type of neuropathy in HIV-positive patients although other forms may be encountered. It usually occurs during the later stages of AIDS and is characterized by distal axonal degeneration.

TRAUMATIC NEUROMA

Traumatic (amputation) neuromas are masses of regenerating axons and scar tissue that form at the proximal stump of a nerve that has been disrupted physically. Within a week after transection of a peripheral nerve, regenerating axonal sprouts arise from the distal ends of the intact axons in the proximal nerve stump. If the severed ends of the proximal and distal nerve stumps are closely approximated, regenerating axonal sprouts may find and reinnervate the distal stump. However, if the cut nerve ends are not closely apposed, or if there is an impediment (e.g., scar tissue) between the two stumps, regenerating sprouts may not reinnervate the distal stump. In that case, the regenerating axons grow haphazardly into the scar tissue at the end of the proximal stump to form a painful swelling. **Morton neuromas** (plantar interdigital neuromas) are sausage-shaped swellings of the plantar interdigital nerve between the second and third or third and fourth metatarsal bones. It is not a true neuroma but rather is caused by repeated nerve compression. Endoneurial, perineurial, and epineurial fibrosis; fiber loss; and areas of myxoid degeneration are prominent. Morton neuroma is particularly common in women who wear high heels.

Table 23-5

Charcot–Marie–Tooth Disease (CMT) and Related Hereditary Motor and Sensory Neuropathies

Disease	Inheritance	Gene	Pathology
CMT1	Autosomal dominant	Peripheral myelin protein 22 (*PMP22*), myelin protein zero (*MPZ*), and others	Demyelinating neuropathy with onion bulbs; axonal loss also present
CMT2	Autosomal dominant	Mitofusin 2 and others	Axonal neuropathy
CMTX	X linked	Gap junction protein β1 (connexin 32)	Axonal loss, demyelination, and regenerating axons
Dejerine–Sottas syndrome (congenital hypomyelinating neuropathy)	Autosomal dominant or recessive	*PMP22, MPZ,* early growth response 2 (*EGR2*) and others	Demyelinating neuropathy with onion bulbs; axonal loss also present
Hereditary neuropathy with liability to pressure palsies	Autosomal dominant	*PMP22*	Demyelinating neuropathy with tomacula; axonal loss also present

TUMORS

Primary PNS tumors are of neuronal or nerve sheath origin. The former (e.g., neuroblastoma and ganglioneuroma) usually arise from the adrenal medulla or sympathetic ganglia (see Chapter 19). The common nerve sheath tumors are schwannoma and neurofibroma.

Schwannomas

These benign neoplasms of Schwann cells are slowly growing and encapsulated. They originate in cranial nerves, spinal roots, or peripheral nerves (Fig. 23-20A). Schwannomas usually occur in adults and rarely become malignant.

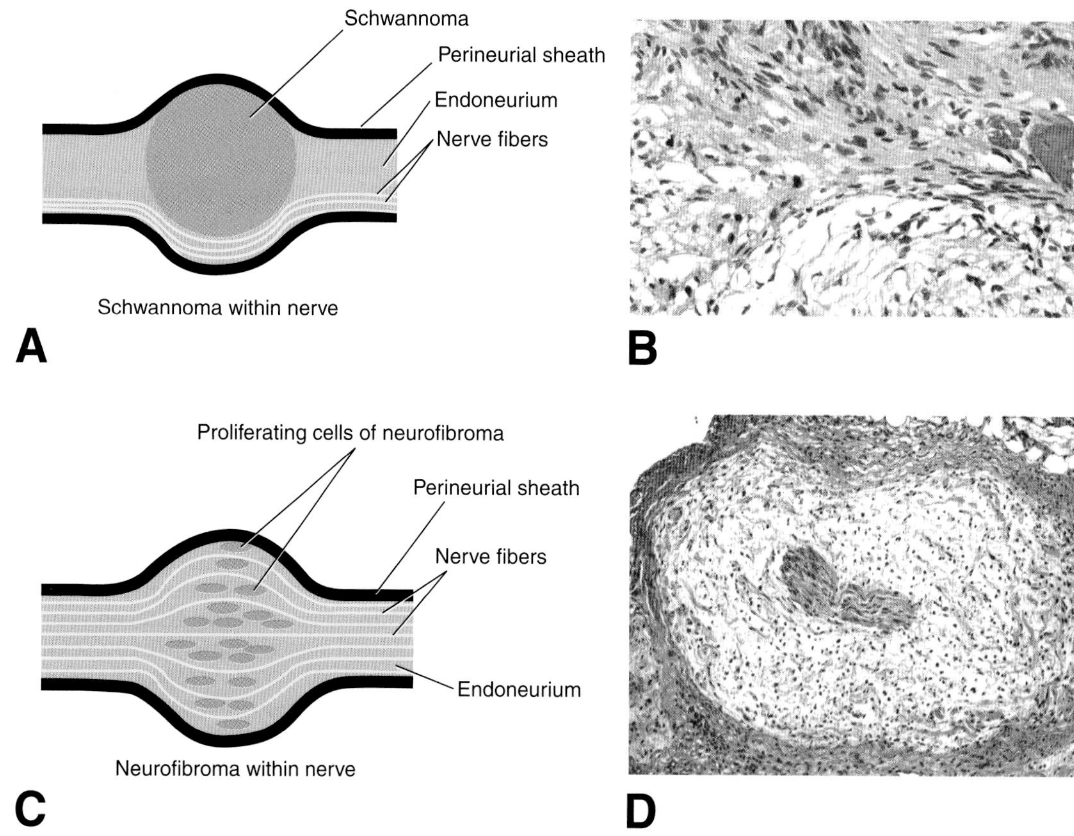

FIGURE 23-20. Growth patterns of schwannoma and neurofibroma within peripheral nerve. **A.** The cellular proliferation of the schwannoma is well circumscribed and pushes surviving nerve fibers to the periphery of the tumor. **B.** A photomicrograph of a schwannoma showing the characteristically abrupt transition between the compact Antoni type A histologic pattern (*top*) and the spongy Antoni type B histologic pattern (*bottom*). **C.** The cellular proliferation of the neurofibroma is interspersed among the surviving nerve fibers. **D.** Photomicrograph of neurofibroma showing that the proliferating spindle-shaped Schwann cells form small strands that course haphazardly through a myxoid matrix. A small cluster of surviving nerve fibers is in the center of the neurofibroma.

VESTIBULAR SCHWANNOMA (ACOUSTIC SCHWANNOMA): Intracranial schwannomas account for 8% of all primary intracranial tumors. Most arise from the vestibular branch of the eighth cranial nerve within the internal auditory canal or at the meatus. They cause unilateral, sensorineural hearing loss, tinnitus, and vestibular dysfunction. The slowly growing tumor enlarges the meatus, extends medially into the subarachnoid space of the cerebellopontine angle (**cerebellopontine angle tumor**), and compresses the fifth and seventh cranial nerves, brainstem, and cerebellum. Most vestibular schwannomas are unilateral and are not associated with neurofibromatosis (see Chapter 5). Bilateral vestibular schwannomas are a defining feature of neurofibromatosis type 2 (NF2).

SPINAL AND PERIPHERAL SCHWANNOMAS: Spinal schwannomas are intradural, extramedullary tumors that arise most often from the dorsal (sensory) spinal roots. They produce radicular (root) pain and spinal cord compression. More peripherally located schwannomas usually arise from nerves of the head, neck, and extremities.

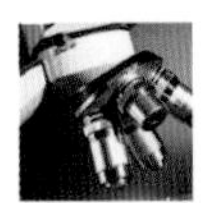

PATHOLOGY: Schwannomas tend to be oval and well demarcated and vary from a few millimeters to several centimeters. The nerve of origin, if large enough, may be identifiable. The cut surface is firm and tan to gray, often with focal hemorrhage, necrosis, xanthomatous change, and cystic degeneration. The proliferating Schwann cells form two distinctive histologic patterns (Fig. 23-20B).

- **Antoni A pattern** is characterized by interwoven fascicles of spindle cells with elongated nuclei, eosinophilic cytoplasm, and indistinct cytoplasmic borders. Nuclei may palisade (a picket fence–like pattern) in areas to form structures known as **Verocay bodies**.
- **Antoni B pattern** features spindle or oval cells with indistinct cytoplasm in a loose, vacuolated matrix.

Degenerative changes in schwannomas are common and include collections of foam cells, recent or old hemorrhage, focal fibrosis, and hyalinized blood vessels. Scattered atypical nuclei are frequently encountered in schwannomas, but mitotic figures are uncommon.

Neurofibroma

Neurofibromas are benign, slowly growing tumors of peripheral nerve, composed of Schwann cells, perineurial-like cells, and fibroblasts. ***The Schwann cells are the neoplastic cells in these tumors.*** Neurofibromas should be distinguished from schwannomas because the former are associated with neurofibromatosis type 1 (NF1) and may become malignant peripheral nerve sheath tumors.

Neurofibromas may be solitary or multiple and may arise on any nerve. They occur in children and adults. The tumors mostly involve skin, subcutis, major nerve plexuses, large deep nerve trunks, retroperitoneum, and gastrointestinal tract. Most **solitary cutaneous neurofibromas** are not part of NF1 and do not degenerate into sarcomas. The presence of multiple neurofibromas or one large plexiform neurofibroma strongly suggests NF1 and should prompt a search for other stigmata of the disease.

PATHOLOGY: Neurofibromas arising in large nerves are poorly circumscribed and fusiform (spindle shaped). A **diffuse**, intrafascicular growth of tumor within multiple nerve fascicles may so enlarge the fascicles that the nerve looks like a multistranded rope (**plexiform neurofibroma**). Cutaneous neurofibromas originate from dermal nerves and are seen as soft nodular or pedunculated skin tumors.

Tumors arising in large nerves are characterized by endoneurial proliferation of spindle cells with elongated nuclei, eosinophilic cytoplasm, and indistinct cell borders (Fig. 23-20D). The proliferating spindle cells include Schwann cells, fibroblasts, and perineurial-like cells. Mast cells are also increased. An extracellular myxoid matrix, wavy bands of collagen, and residual nerve fibers are interspersed among the spindle cells. The nerve fibers coursing through a neurofibroma contrast with the pattern in schwannomas, in which nerve fibers are pushed peripherally into the tumor capsule (compare Fig. 23-20A and C). The neurofibromatous proliferation often extends beyond the nerve fascicle into adjacent tissue.

Some 5% of NF1-associated plexiform neurofibromas become **malignant peripheral nerve sheath tumors**. Increased cellularity, nuclear atypia, and mitotic figures herald malignant transformation. These tumors are prone to local recurrence and blood-borne metastases.

PARANEOPLASTIC SYNDROMES INVOLVING MUSCLE AND PERIPHERAL NERVES

Neurologic disorders are common in cancer patients, usually resulting from metastases or from endocrine or electrolyte disturbances. Vascular, hemorrhagic, and infectious conditions affecting the nervous system are also common. However, additional neurologic complications of malignancies may appear before the underlying tumor is detected. Many of these paraneoplastic syndromes are mediated by autoimmune mechanisms.

Sensory Neuropathy and Encephalomyeloneuritis

Patients afflicted with this paraneoplastic syndrome complain of numbness and paresthesias and, conversely, acute aching and pain. These symptoms may be focal, but often affect all extremities over time, and are often complicated by disorders of gait, confusion, and weakness. This syndrome may occur in patients with small-cell lung cancer (SCLC; see Chapter 10) and is caused by circulating antibodies against Hu, an RNA-binding protein. High titers of anti-Hu antibodies are almost exclusively detected in people with SCLC. Lymphocytic infiltration of dorsal root ganglia is seen. Anti-Hu antibodies may also be associated with autonomic neuropathies, which include those of vascular tone, bowel, and bladder.

Peripheral Neuropathies

An array of peripheral neuropathies may be paraneoplastic in origin. Sensorimotor neuropathy, most likely attendant to lung cancer, is not associated with detectable antibodies. Some types of lymphoproliferative disorders associated with paraproteins, especially the sclerosing variant of plasma cell myeloma, may exhibit peripheral neuropathies.

Neuromuscular Junction Disorders

The most common association is with thymomas (see above).

Eaton–Lambert Syndrome

This syndrome is a paraneoplastic disorder that manifests as muscle weakness, wasting, and fatigability of proximal limbs and trunk. Also called **myasthenic–myopathic syndrome**, it is usually associated with small cell lung carcinoma, but may also occur with other malignancies, and rarely in the absence of an underlying cancer. Pathogenic IgG autoantibodies target voltage-sensitive calcium channels expressed in motor nerve terminals and in the cells of lung cancer. These calcium channels are necessary for Ach release and are greatly reduced in presynaptic membranes in these patients, thereby reducing neuromuscular transmission. Eaton–Lambert syndrome responds to corticosteroid treatment.

24 The Central Nervous System and Eye

Gregory N. Fuller ▪ J. Clay Goodman ▪ Gordon K. Klintworth

LEARNING OBJECTIVES

- Describe the pathophysiologic mechanisms and clinical consequences of brain herniation.
- Differentiate between cytotoxic, vasogenic, and interstitial cerebral edema.
- Differentiate between communicating and noncommunicating hydrocephalus.
- What is the most frequent cause of noncommunicating hydrocephalus?
- Define hydrocephalus ex vacuo.
- Differentiate between the pathophysiologic mechanism, progression, and clinical consequences of epidural and subdural hematomas.
- Discuss the pathophysiologic mechanisms and pathology associated with cerebral contusions.
- Discuss the etiologic factors and pathophysiologic mechanisms of ischemic stroke.
- Define watershed infarcts and laminar necrosis.
- What etiologic factors are involved in hemorrhagic versus ischemic (bland) infarcts?
- Describe the temporal progression of the pathologic changes associated with cerebral edema.
- What etiologic factors are associated with intracranial hemorrhage?
- Define "berry" (saccular) aneurysms. What is the most likely intracerebral location for such aneurysms?
- What are the most common bacterial agents responsible for leptomeningitis? What histopathologic and clinical signs are associated with such diseases?
- What fungal agents are commonly associated with CNS infections?
- What agents and histopathology are commonly associated with viral encephalitis and specifically with arbovirus-mediated infection?
- What etiologic agents and pathology are associated with subacute sclerosing panencephalitis and progressive multifocal leukoencephalopathy?
- What are the unique etiologic and pathophysiologic mechanisms associated with spongiform encephalopathies?
- Differentiate between kuru, Creutzfeldt–Jakob, and new variant Creutzfeldt–Jakob disease in terms of epidemiology and clinical consequences.
- Describe the etiology and pathophysiologic mechanism responsible for multiple sclerosis.
- Define the term "leukodystrophy." Discuss potential mechanisms, clinical consequences, and common etiologies.
- Define the pathophysiology often common to neurodegenerative disorders.
- Differentiate between the pathologic characteristic of Alzheimer, Pick, and Lewy body dementias, concentrating on the abnormal protein accumulations that characterize them.
- Describe the epidemiology, molecular pathogenesis, histopathology, and clinical consequences of Parkinson disease.
- Describe the epidemiology, molecular pathogenesis, histopathology, and clinical consequences of Huntington disease, Friedreich ataxia, and amyotrophic lateral sclerosis.
- What are the genetic factors and pathologic consequences of neural tube defects?
- Differentiate between anencephaly and spina bifida occulta. Discuss meningocele, meningomyelocele, and rachischisis in terms of gross pathology and clinical consequences.
- Describe the abnormal structural pathology associated with the Arnold–Chiari malformation.
- Define the following terms: lissencephaly, schizencephaly, heterotopia, polymicrogyria, and pachygyria.
- Describe the potential etiologies, pathology, and clinical consequences of meningiomas.
- Differentiate between the histopathology of diffuse and circumscribed astrocytomas.
- Describe the histopathology of WHO grades II to IV: astrocytomas low grade, anaplastic, and glioblastoma multiforme.
- Describe the epidemiology, molecular basis, and histopathology of medulloblastoma.
- What are the typical characteristics of metastatic tumors to the CNS? Which are most common?
- Describe the molecular and histopathology associated with tuberous sclerosis.
- What are the histopathologic effects of corneal infection with either primary or reactivation herpes simplex virus?

- Describe the pathologic changes in the lens associated with cataract formation.
- Describe the retinal pathology associated with hypertensive disease.
- What are the pathologic and clinical consequences of diabetic retinopathy?
- What are the pathologic and clinical consequences associated with retinitis pigmentosa?
- Differentiate between primary open and closed-angle glaucoma.
- What is the most common primary intraocular malignancy? Describe the associated histopathology and clinical consequences.
- Review the molecular pathology and describe the histopathology associated with retinoblastoma.

Central Nervous System

CELLS OF THE NERVOUS SYSTEM

GRAY MATTER AND THE NEUROPIL: Gray matter includes all regions of the CNS rich in neurons: cerebral and cerebellar cortices, basal ganglia, and central gray matter of the spinal cord. Gray matter consists of cell bodies (perikarya) of neurons and supporting glial cell nuclei, plus the intervening delicate meshwork of neuronal and glial cell processes, the **neuropil** (Fig. 24-1). Circumscribed collections of neuronal cell bodies that share a common functional task are referred to as "nuclei."

WHITE MATTER: White matter consists of compact bundles (**tracts** and **fascicles**) of myelinated axons with many oligodendrocytes and interspersed astrocytes (Fig. 24-2).

NEURONS: The morphology of neuronal subtypes in the gray matter varies owing to functional subspecialization, ranging from large motor and primary sensory neurons to tiny "granular cell" neurons (Fig. 24-3A). For example, pigmented neurons, which occur only in specific brainstem nuclei, are distinguished by cytoplasmic brown neuromelanin pigment, a by-product of catecholaminergic neurotransmitter synthesis (Fig. 24-3B). These clusters of pigmented neurons are so dense as to be visible to the naked eye in the midbrain (substantia nigra) and pons (locus ceruleus).

ASTROCYTES: Astrocytes outnumber neurons at least 10:1 and play a critical supportive role in regulating the CNS microenvironment. They are also one of two primary CNS cell types that respond to many CNS insults (the other being microglia). Astrocytes responding to acute injury upregulate the synthesis of glial fibrillary acidic protein (GFAP) and assemble it into intracytoplasmic intermediate filaments, resulting in prominent cell bodies and cytoplasmic processes (Fig. 24-4A). With advancing age, astrocyte peripheral processes may accumulate spherical inclusion bodies, termed "corpora amylacea." These are glucose polymers that are especially numerous in subpial, subependymal, and perivascular sites and in olfactory tracts (Fig. 24-4B). Cytoplasmic strap-like densities, namely, Rosenthal fibers (Fig. 24-4C), appear in long-standing astrogliosis as densely compacted glial intermediate filaments with entrapped cytosol proteins.

OLIGODENDROGLIA: Oligodendroglia produce and maintain CNS axon myelin sheaths and so are CNS counterparts of Schwann cells in the peripheral nervous system. Oligodendroglia cell bodies are dominated by uniform round nuclei that, in formalin-fixed, paraffin-embedded, tissue sections, are characteristically surrounded by only a small clear rim of vacuolated cytoplasm ("perinuclear halo") (Fig. 24-5).

MICROGLIA: Microglia are bone marrow–derived mononuclear phagocytes of the CNS. In health, they are inconspicuously distributed throughout the brain and spinal

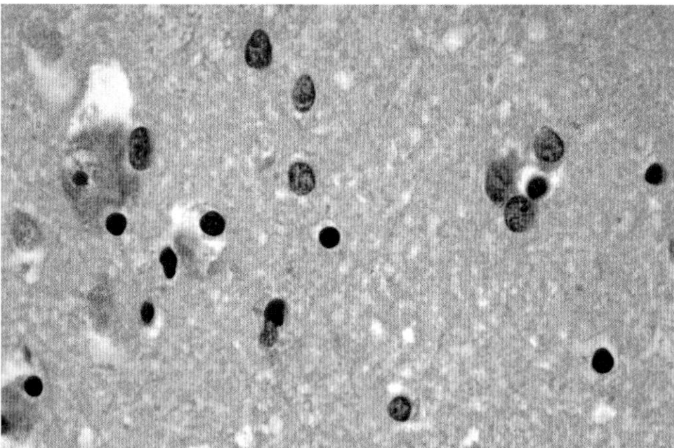

FIGURE 24-1. Gray matter and the neuropil. Gray matter by definition contains neuronal cell bodies. In addition, the nuclei of supporting glial cells, astrocytes, and satellite oligodendroglia are present. The remaining finely fibrillar background meshwork is called the neuropil and consists of intimately intermingled axons, dendrites, and astrocytic cytoplasmic processes.

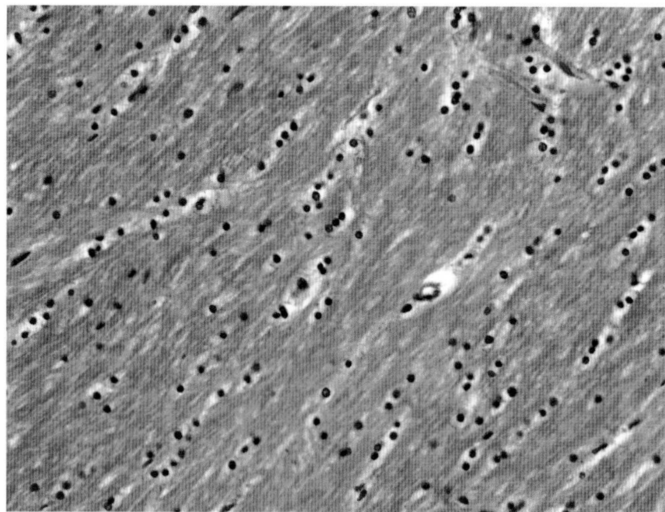

FIGURE 24-2. White matter. In contrast to gray matter, white matter is composed almost entirely of myelinated axons and the cells that produce and maintain their myelin sheaths, the oligodendroglia, whose small round nuclei are seen in between the fiber bundles.

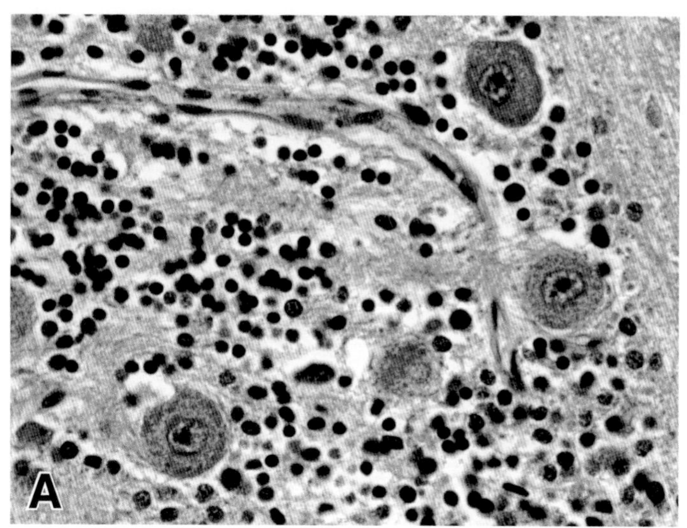

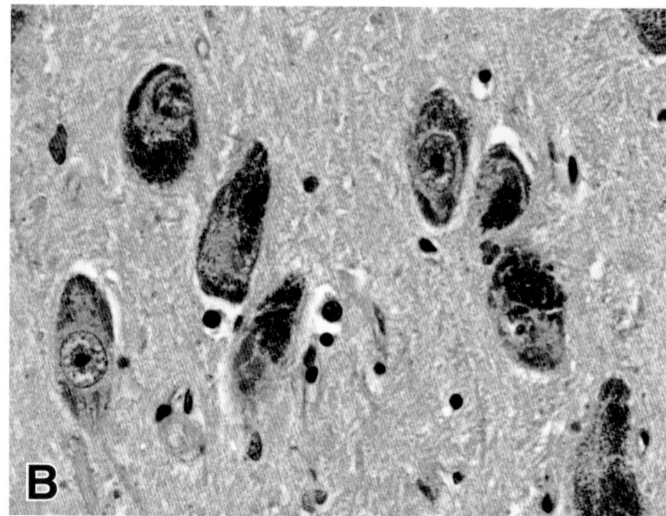

FIGURE 24-3. Neurons. A. The different neuronal populations of the central nervous system (CNS) subserve different functions, and this diversity is reflected in their morphology. Illustrative of the extremes are the large cell bodies of Purkinje cell neurons juxtaposed next to the diminutive granular cell neurons of the cerebellar cortex; the entire granular neuron cell body is not much bigger than the nucleolus of a Purkinje cell neuron! **B.** The pigmented catecholaminergic neurons with their prominent neuromelanin content serve as an additional, striking example of diversity in form and function among CNS neuronal populations.

cord. However, they respond quickly to CNS insults such as ischemia, trauma, or viral infections (1) by developing thin, elongated nuclei; (2) migrating through the CNS; and (3) localizing to the site of injury (Fig. 24-6A and B).

EPENDYMA: The ependymal lining of the ventricular system forms a barrier between cerebrospinal fluid (CSF) and brain parenchyma and regulates fluid transfer between these two compartments. The normal ependyma is lined by ciliated cuboidal-to-columnar simple epithelium (Fig. 24-7).

SPECIALIZED REGIONS OF THE CENTRAL NERVOUS SYSTEM

CHOROID PLEXUS: The choroid plexus produces cerebrospinal fluid (CSF). It resides in the cerebral ventricles, including the temporal horns bilaterally, interventricular foramen of Monro, the roof of the third ventricle, and the roof and lateral recesses of the fourth ventricle. The choroid plexus is composed of cuboidal epithelium (derived from embryologic ependyma) that covers a fibrovascular core (Fig. 24-8A). The highly vascular core is critical to CSF formation. It develops from leptomeninges (pia and arachnoid) and contains scattered nests of arachnoid (meningothelial) cells (Fig. 24-8B), hence the occasional "intraventricular" meningioma that is actually a choroid plexus meningioma.

MENINGES: Three layers of meninges cover and protect the CNS. The **dura** is the tough outer fibrous membrane. It is primarily composed of collagen. Its outer surface is the inner periosteum of the cranial bones, and its inner surface attaches weakly to the subjacent arachnoid via cell junctions. The two dural sheets separate in several sites to form dural venous sinuses, the largest of which is the superior sagittal sinus. The underlying arachnoid is bound to the overlying dura by a loosely cohesive layer of cells, the **dural border cell (DBC) layer**. This covering is the path of least resistance to pathogenic fluids, which easily dissect the weak intercellular junctions to form the so-called subdural hematoma, hygroma, and empyema. The meningeal layer just beneath the DBC layer is the **arachnoid barrier cell (ABC)**. It forms a cohesive outer limiting membrane of the subarachnoid space via abundant intercellular junctions (desmosomes) which weld together elongated, interlacing arachnoid (meningothelial) cell processes. Whorls of arachnoid cells are common in thicker areas of the arachnoid (Fig. 24-9); this feature is often recapitulated in arachnoid tumors (meningiomas).

INCREASED INTRACRANIAL PRESSURE AND HERNIATION

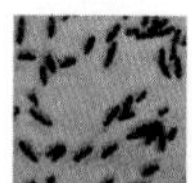

ETIOLOGIC FACTORS: ***The brain, CSF, and blood going to and from the brain occupy the intracranial space. In the adult, this is a rigidly fixed cavity. Any disease that takes up space does so at the expense of brain, CSF, or blood.***

Space-occupying lesions may occur with most diseases, except for degenerative disorders. Examples include brain tumors, abscesses, swollen brain contusions following trauma, and stroke with brain swelling.

Fitting more volume into the fixed space of the intracranial vault increases intracranial pressure (ICP). The normal ICP is less than 200 mm H_2O or 15 mm Hg for a patient in the lateral decubitus position. The pressure can be measured by lumbar puncture or by an intracranial pressure transducer. As ICP increases, patients have headaches, confusion, and drowsiness and may develop edema of the optic nerve (papilledema). To compensate, CSF volume is reduced; hence, the ventricles are compressed to small slits, and sulci are effaced.

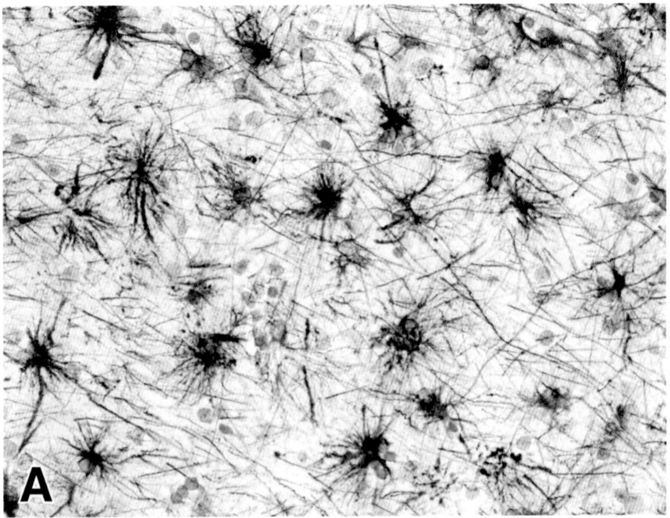

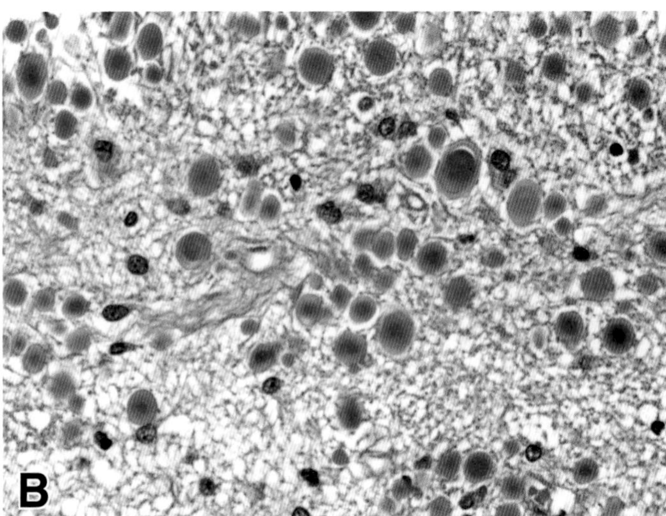

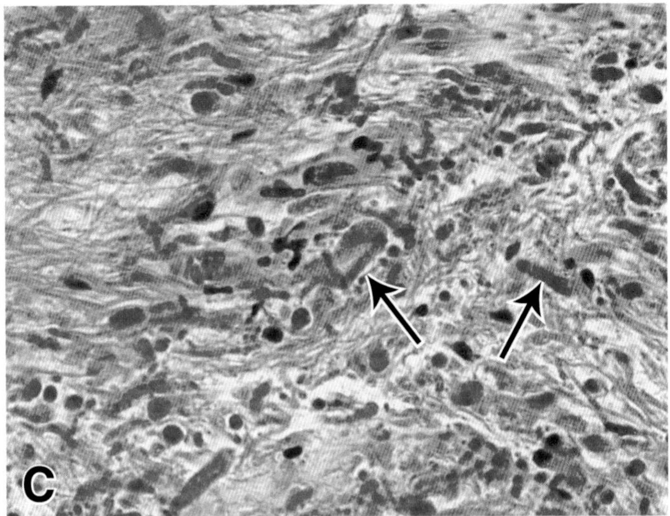

FIGURE 24-4. **Astrocytes. A.** Astrocytes have been called "the fibroblast of the central nervous system," referring to their role as the ubiquitous supporting cell of the brain and spinal cord that reacts to any pathologic insult. As seen in this immunostain directed against glial fibrillary acidic protein, astrocytes occupy adjacent domains and send cytoplasmic process radiating out in all directions to fill their individual fiefdoms. **B.** With advancing age, astrocytes are prone to develop glucose polymer inclusion bodies, called **corpora amylacea**, in the distal distribution of their cell processes, particularly around blood vessels and subjacent to the pia and ependyma. **C. Rosenthal fibers** are another astrocytic inclusion body formed as a response to long-standing astrogliosis; they are composed of densely compacted glial intermediate filaments together with entrapped cytosolic proteins (*arrows*).

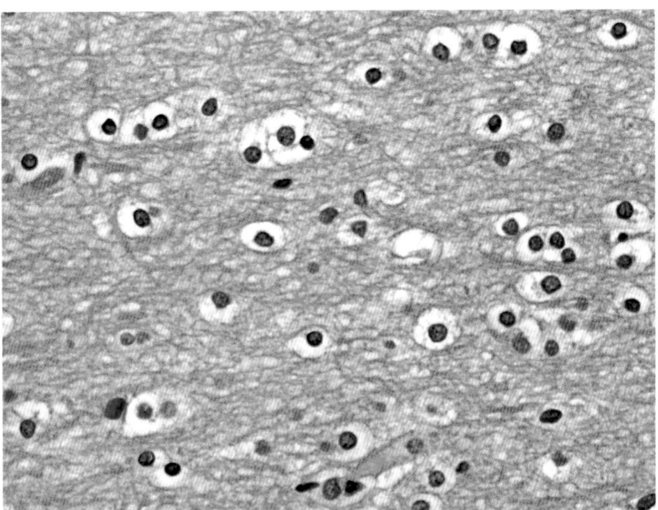

FIGURE 24-5. **Oligodendroglia.** Oligodendroglia are the myelin-forming glia of the central nervous system (CNS; including the optic "nerves," which are actually CNS tracts). On routine histologic imaging, oligodendroglia are easily recognized by their monotonous small dark round nuclei surrounded by a halo of vacuolated cytoplasm ("fried-egg" appearance). This characteristic appearance is recapitulated in neoplastic oligodendrogliomas.

If a lesion takes up more space than a reduction in CSF volume can accommodate, blood flow decreases. Such lower cerebral blood flow may have an immediate adverse impact because the brain is critically dependent on an uninterrupted supply of oxygen and nutrients. If the lesion expands further, the only structure remaining to "give" is the brain itself. The intracranial compartment is subdivided by the dura into supratentorial and infratentorial compartments. The falx divides the supratentorial compartment into right and left compartments. Depending on the location of the space-occupying lesion, the brain may be forced out of one compartment into another. Such shifts are called brain herniations.

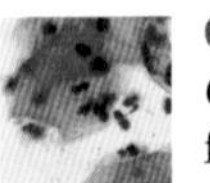

CLINICAL FEATURES:

CINGULATE HERNIATION: If a hemisphere is forced under the falx, the cingulate lobe is the first part of that hemisphere to be displaced. This results in **subfalcine**, or **cingulate, herniations**. Someone experiencing such a herniation becomes confused and drowsy. The anterior cerebral artery is also displaced beneath the falx, so that infarction within this vessel's territory may occur, leading to contralateral lower extremity weakness and urinary incontinence.

UNCAL HERNIATION: If one hemisphere is forced from the supratentorial compartment toward the infratentorial

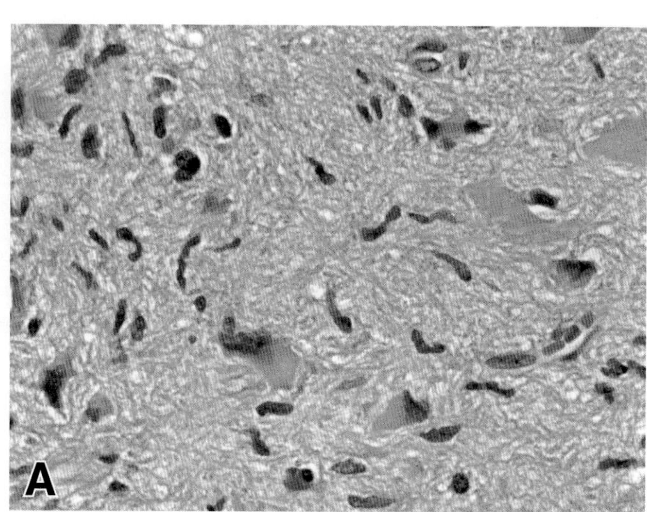

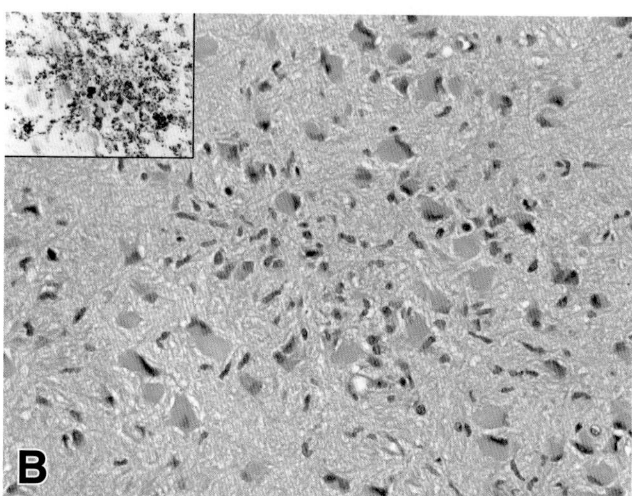

FIGURE 24-6. **Microglia. A.** Microglia are the resident representatives of the monocyte–macrophage system in the brain and spinal cord. While inconspicuous in normal healthy brain ("resting microglial"), they become very prominent when responding to central nervous system (CNS) injury and are easily recognized by their elongated nuclei ("rod cells"), which reflect their infiltrative phenotype. **B.** Actively migrating through CNS parenchyma, they commonly cluster around foci of disease; such collections are known as "microglial nodules." Microglia demonstrate strong immunohistochemical reactivity for the macrophage marker CD68 (*inset*).

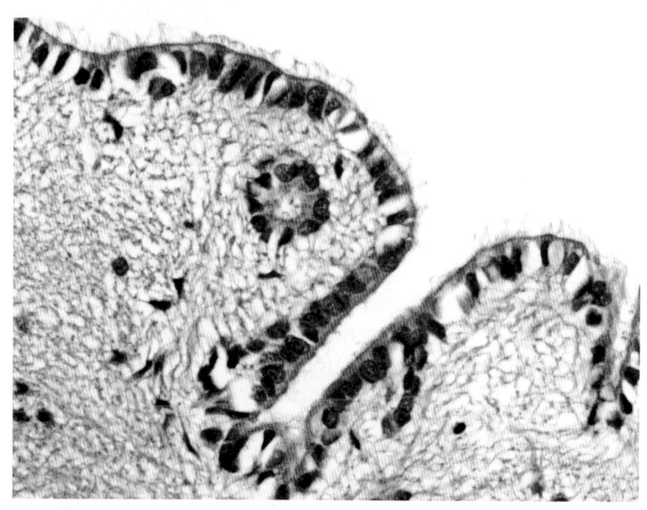

FIGURE 24-7. **Ependyma.** Ependymal cells form a ciliated cuboidal-to-columnar epithelium that lines the cerebral ventricles and spinal cord central canal. Ependymal cell clusters and true rosettes, as seen here, commonly are scattered beneath the ependymal lining.

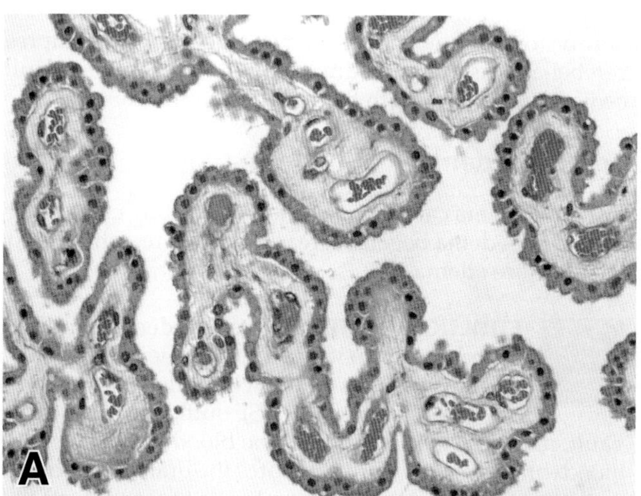

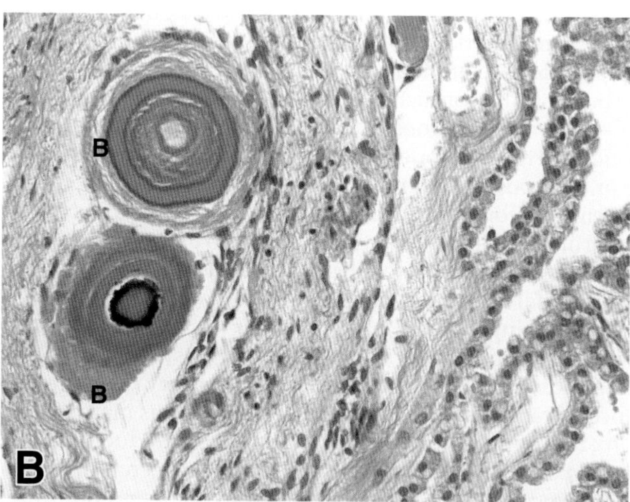

FIGURE 24-8. **Choroid plexus. A.** Choroid plexus is the central nervous system organ responsible for producing cerebrospinal fluid and consists of innumerable papillae with a highly vascular core covered by cuboidal epithelium that is derived embryologically from the ependyma. **B.** The core also contains arachnoid (meningothelial) cell nests (by virtue of its embryologic derivation from the pia-arachnoid) that tend to mineralize with age, forming psammoma bodies (*B*).

FIGURE 24-9. Arachnoid villi. The arachnoid membrane forms the outer boundary of the subarachnoid space and also protrudes into the dural venous sinuses, as seen here, to form arachnoid villi whose function is to return cerebrospinal fluid into the venous circulatory system. The villi are covered by a layer of meningothelial cells, called arachnoid cap cells, that varies in thickness from a single cell to multilayered whorls.

compartment, the medial temporal lobe (the uncus) is the first portion of the hemisphere displaced; thus, this is an **uncal**, or **transtentorial**, **herniation** (Fig. 24-10). The ipsilateral oculomotor nerve (cranial nerve III) is crushed by the displaced temporal lobe and gives rise to ipsilateral pupillary dilation and paresis of all extraocular muscles, except for the lateral rectus (cranial nerve VI) and superior oblique (cranial nerve IV). The unopposed action of the lateral rectus provokes the eye to look laterally. A dilated unresponsive pupil indicates extreme danger and necessitates immediate measures to arrest the herniation.

As medial displacement continues, the midbrain shifts away from the displaced hemisphere, with the contralateral cerebral pedicle driven into the unyielding tentorium. This crushing injury of the cerebral pedicle (**Kernohan notch**) causes hemiparesis on the same side of the body as the offending mass. A hemispheric mass will normally cause hemiparesis on the opposite side of the body; ipsilateral hemiparesis, which may be clinically confusing, is called a "false localizing" sign.

Downward and medial displacement of a hemisphere through the tentorial opening may also lead to compression of one or both posterior cerebral arteries as they travel from the infratentorial compartment to the now crowded supratentorial compartment. This can impair blood flow to the occipital lobes, resulting in infarction with attendant visual field disturbances. This occipital lobe infarction and its attendant signs are also "false localizing."

Uncal herniation syndrome is ominous but reversible with removal of the offending mass. Temporary measures to reduce intracranial pressure include intravenous mannitol to shrink the brain osmotically. Hyperventilation reduces PCO_2-inducing cerebral vasospasm and so decreases cerebral blood volume and pressure. These actions may gain enough time for definitive surgical treatment.

CENTRAL HERNIATION: If both hemispheres herniate transtentorially, **central herniation syndrome** results. Both

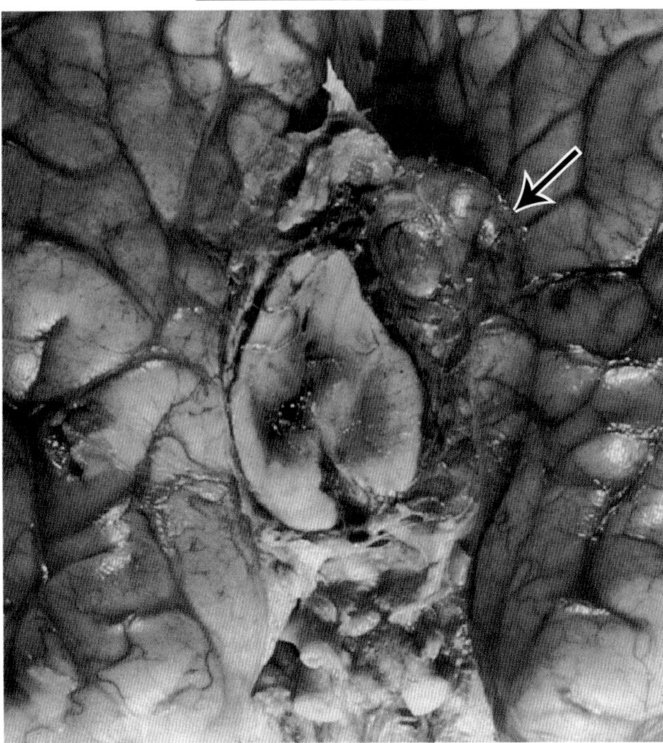

FIGURE 24-10. Transtentorial herniation. The uncus (*arrow*) of the parahippocampal gyrus is herniated downward to displace the midbrain, resulting in distortion of the midbrain with increased anterior-to-posterior and diminished left-to-right dimensions. The oculomotor nerve may be compromised, leading to an ipsilateral third nerve palsy.

pupils dilate; flaccidity and coma ensue. The downward displacement of the brainstem may wrench vessels from their parenchymal beds within the midbrain and pons and cause multiple linear hemorrhages, known as **Duret hemorrhages** or secondary hemorrhages of herniation.

CEREBELLAR TONSILLAR HERNIATION: If the infratentorial compartment becomes crowded either from migrating supratentorial contents or from a mass arising in the infratentorial compartment, the brainstem and cerebellum may be forced through the foramen magnum. The compressed cerebellar tonsils and medulla may compress vital medullary centers and cause death by **tonsillar herniation**.

Cerebral Edema

Cerebral edema can set up a self-perpetuating cycle in which increasing edema begets increasing pressure, which, in turn, begets more edema.

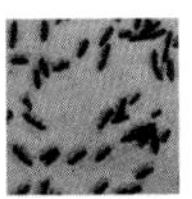

ETIOLOGIC FACTORS: Cerebral edema is an absolute increase in brain water content. The amount of water in brain tissue is tightly controlled by (1) the rates of CSF production, (2) CSF outflow from the cranial vault, and (3) water flux across the blood–brain barrier. The blood–brain barrier (BBB) separates the brain from the blood so that only lipid-soluble molecules, or those that can access specialized transport systems, enter the brain. The structural basis of the BBB is endothelial cell tight junctions lining cerebral vessels. Water can enter the brain uncontrollably if the barrier is disrupted or if osmotic forces across it are sufficient to drive water into cerebral tissues. Three major forms of cerebral edema may occur:

- **Cytotoxic edema:** Water flows across an intact BBB by osmotic forces that arise (1) because cells within the brain fail to maintain osmotic homeostasis or (2) because of systemic water overload. In either case, water is driven down its concentration gradient into cerebral tissues until osmotic equilibrium is reestablished.
- **Vasogenic edema:** The BBB loosens, permitting uncontrolled entry of water into the tissues. ***This is the most common cause of edema*** and occurs with neoplasms, abscesses, meningitis, hemorrhage, contusions, and lead poisoning. A combination of cytotoxic and vasogenic edema is common in infarcts. The above processes may disrupt endothelial barrier activity, or the vessels formed in neoplasms may be defective from their inception. Vasogenic edema often responds dramatically to administration of corticosteroids, which restore barrier integrity, even in tumors.
- **Interstitial edema:** Interstitial edema involves CSF overproduction or its failure to leave the cranial cavity, so that the fluid seeps across the ependymal lining of the ventricles and accumulates within the white matter.

Hydrocephalus

Hydrocephalus refers to accumulation of CSF within the ventricles, causing them to dilate (Fig. 24-11). When ventricular distension is sufficiently advanced, fluid leaks into the white matter, causing interstitial edema. CSF accumulation can arise from (1) ***overproduction of CSF, which is rare,*** occurring only in the context of tumors of the choroid plexus; and (2) ***failure of CSF to leave the cranial vault, which is more common.*** If the blockage occurs within the ventricular system itself, ventricles proximal to the block dilate, whereas those situated downstream from the block are spared. This is termed **obstructive**, or **noncommunicating, hydrocephalus**. The most frequent site of block is at the ventricular system's narrowest strait—the aqueduct of Sylvius connecting the third and fourth ventricles.

A block may occur after the CSF leaves the ventricular system and travels over the cerebral convexities to the arachnoid granulations that usher the fluid into the venous sinuses. As a result, all the ventricles dilate. This is called **communicating hydrocephalus**, meaning that the ventricles are unobstructed in fluid flow. Communicating hydrocephalus may complicate subarachnoid hemorrhage or inflammation, resulting in arachnoid scarring, or may result from thrombosis of the dural venous sinuses themselves.

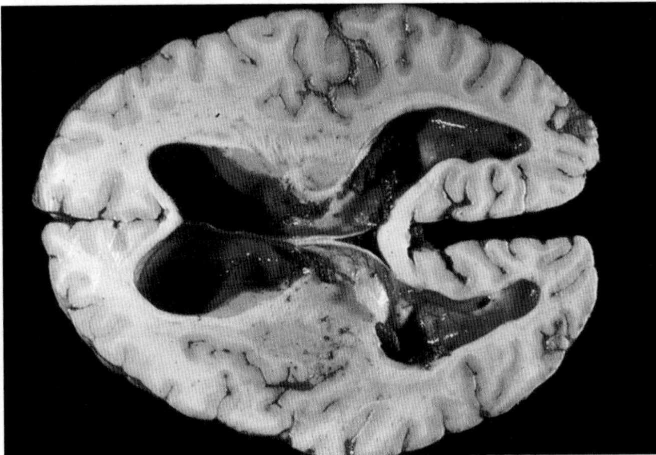

FIGURE 24-11. Hydrocephalus. Horizontal section of the brain from a patient who died of a brain tumor that obstructed the aqueduct of Sylvius shows marked dilation of the lateral ventricles.

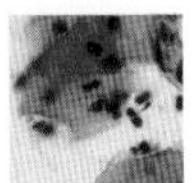

CLINICAL FEATURES: The clinical features of hydrocephalus depend on the patient's age. In infants and children, before cranial sutures have fused, the head enlarges (sometimes to grotesque proportions) as the ventricles dilate. Because hydrocephalus in infants is treatable by shunting, measurement of the head circumference is a fundamental part of the pediatric physical examination.

After sutures fuse, hydrocephalus in adults cannot enlarge the head, but rather increases intracranial pressure. This causes headache, confusion, drowsiness, papilledema, and vomiting. Ventricles enlarge at the expense of brain volume so that in advanced cases, only a thin mantle of cortical tissue remains. Remarkably, such individuals often retain substantial cognitive abilities, although spasticity may cloak the expression of this intelligence.

All of the above forms of hydrocephalus result from disturbance of CSF dynamics unlike **hydrocephalus ex vacuo**, which is compensatory ventricular enlargement owing to loss of CNS tissue from other diseases. This occurs most often in diffuse cortical atrophy, but focal destruction, such as occurs at the site of an old infarct, may lead to focal compensatory ventricular enlargement.

TRAUMA

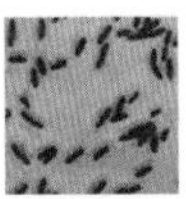

ETIOLOGIC FACTORS: The brain and spinal cord are enclosed in protective bony cases that dissipate forces delivered to these delicate structures. The degree of injury to the nervous system correlates with the quantity of energy delivered and the time over which it was delivered. This energy transfer may directly disrupt tissues in penetrating injuries, or the energy may be translated into movement and compression of neural structures within the skull or spinal canal in a closed injury. Extreme injury of the brain and cord is possible with minimal disruption of overlying tissues. Conversely, superficial tissues can sustain dramatic injury while the nervous system underneath remains unaltered.

Epidural Hematoma

Epidural hematomas usually result from blows to the head with skull fracture. Unless treated promptly, they can be fatal. The middle meningeal arteries reside in grooves in the inner table of the bone between the dura and the calvaria, and their branches splay across the temporal–parietal area. The temporal bone, being one of the thinnest bones of the skull, is particularly vulnerable to fracture. Seemingly, minor trauma may fracture it, which may, in turn, lacerate branches of the middle meningeal artery, causing life-threatening epidural hemorrhage (Fig. 24-12).

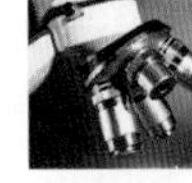

PATHOLOGY: Transection of the middle meningeal artery allows blood under arterial pressure to escape into the epidural space that separates the dura from the calvaria. The dura is tightly bound to the calvarium at the coronal sutures. Thus, epidural

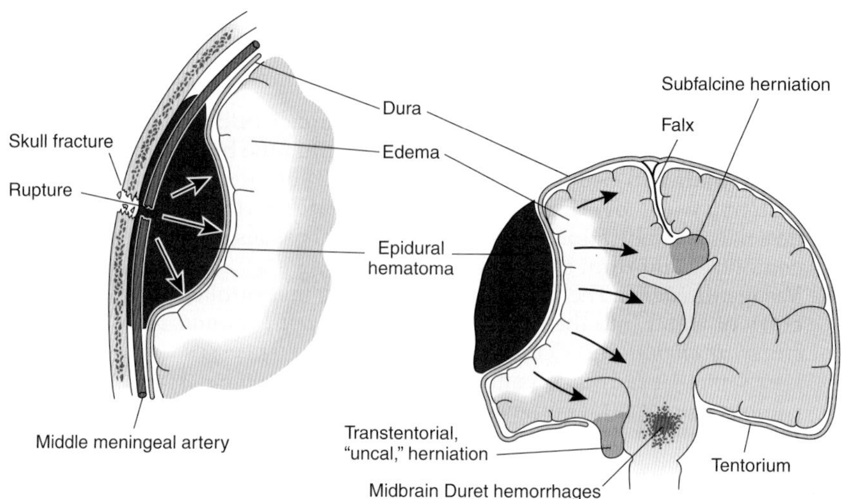

FIGURE 24-12. Development of an epidural hematoma. Laceration of a branch of the middle meningeal artery by the sharp bony edges of a skull fracture initiates bleeding under arterial pressure that dissects the dura from the calvaria and produces an expanding hematoma. After an asymptomatic interval of several hours, subfalcine and transtentorial herniation occur, and if the hematoma is not evacuated, lethal Duret hemorrhages will occur.

bleeding will not extend beyond the suture lines. This leads to a lens-shaped accumulation of fresh blood that stops at the coronal suture lines.

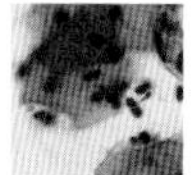

CLINICAL FEATURES: Up one third of patients do not lose consciousness at the time of the precipitating injury and may have a "lucid interval" of unimpaired consciousness for several hours while epidural blood accumulates under arterial pressure. When the hematoma reaches 30 to 50 mL, symptoms of a space-occupying lesion appear. Epidural hematomas are invariably progressive and, when not recognized and evacuated, may be fatal in 24 to 48 hours.

Subdural Hematoma

Subdural hematomas are a significant cause of death after head injuries from falls, assaults, vehicular accidents, and sporting accidents. The hematomas expand more slowly than do epidural hematomas, so their clinical tempo is slower. However, once critically increased intracranial pressure is attained, clinical deterioration and death can occur rapidly.

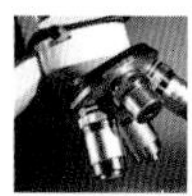

PATHOLOGY: The cerebral hemispheres float in the CSF, tethered loosely by blood vessels and cranial nerves. Blood drains from cerebral hemispheres through veins that cross the subarachnoid space and arachnoid to breach the dura and enter the dural sinus. There is no true subdural space per se, but the inner layer of meningothelial cells of the dura has fewer tight junctions than those in the outer layers of the dura. Shearing forces will separate these cells, allowing blood to seep between them. Because bleeding in this situation is under low venous pressure, it is slow and may stop spontaneously from a local tamponade effect. The bleeding is within the dura itself and readily extends beyond the coronal sutures, causing a hematoma that can extend along the entire anterior-to-posterior dimensions of the calvarium (Fig. 24-13). Granulation tissue forms in reaction to the blood, and the delicate capillaries of this tissue may themselves leak. This leads to gradual accumulation of an ever-enlarging subacute, and ultimately chronic, subdural hematoma.

A subdural hematoma may evolve in three ways. It may (1) be reabsorbed and leave only a small amount of telltale hemosiderin; (2) remain static, and perhaps calcify; or (3) enlarge as a result of recurrent microhemorrhages in the granulation tissue.

Expansion of the hematoma and the onset of symptom commonly result from rebleeding, usually within 6 months. Granulation tissue is fragile and so vulnerable to minor trauma, even that caused by shaking the head. Thus, subdural hematomas can rebleed and create a new hematoma subjacent to the outer membrane.

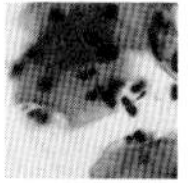

CLINICAL FEATURES: Symptoms and signs of subdural hematomas are diverse: (1) stretching of meninges leads to headaches; (2) pressure on the motor cortex produces contralateral weakness; and (3) focal cortical irritation can initiate seizures. Subdural hematomas are bilateral in 15% to 20% of cases, and these may impair cognitive function and lead to a mistaken diagnosis of dementia. Rebleeding with expansion sometimes causes lethal transtentorial herniation (Fig. 24-13A).

Parenchymal Injuries

Traumatic brain and spinal cord injuries range in severity from temporary loss of function, with little or no discernible structural damage in concussion, to intermediate damage with hemorrhage and necrosis of the tissue in contusions, to profound disruption of structure and function in lacerations.

Concussion

Concussion refers to transient loss of consciousness owing to biomechanical forces acting on the CNS. A blow that causes an epidural hematoma does not necessarily produce a concussion. Consciousness depends on a functional brainstem reticular formation interacting with the cerebral hemispheres and is lost if either the reticular formation or both hemispheres are damaged. A classic example of concussion occurs in boxing, from a blow that deflects the head upward and posteriorly, often with a rotatory component. These motions impart quick rotational acceleration to the brainstem and cause dysfunction of reticular formation neurons. By contrast, a blow to the temporal–parietal area may cause a skull fracture and lethal epidural hematoma but may not induce loss of consciousness because lateral movement of the cerebral hemispheres does not occur.

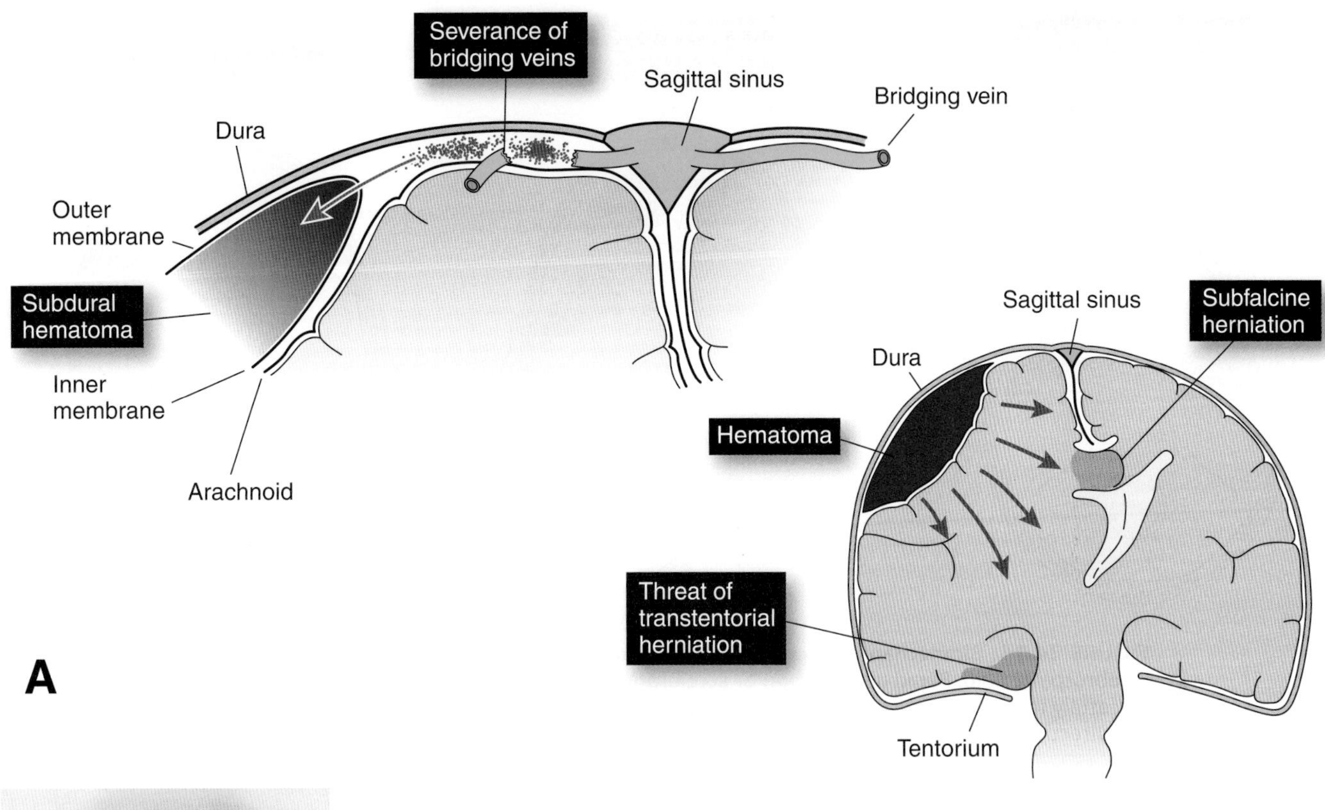

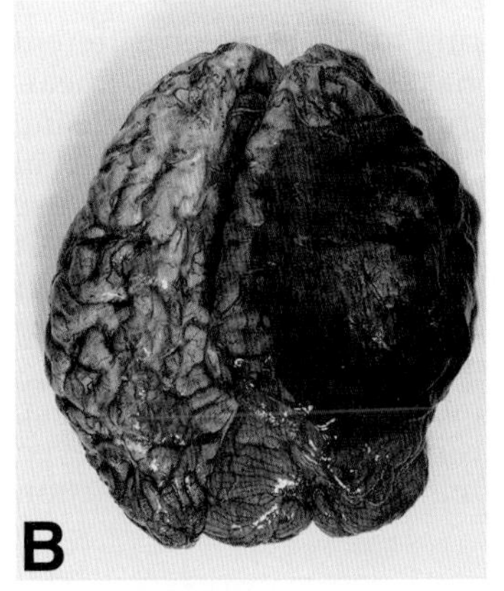

FIGURE 24-13. Development of a subdural hematoma. A. With head trauma, the dura moves with the skull, and the arachnoid moves with the cerebrum. As a result, the bridging veins are sheared as they cross between the dura and the arachnoid. Venous bleeding creates a hematoma in the expansile subdural space. Subsequent transtentorial herniation is life-threatening. **B.** The right hemisphere exhibits a large collection of blood in the "subdural space," owing to rupture of the bridging veins.

Classically, concussion is not associated with gross neuropathology, and because the condition is not lethal, microscopic examination is not possible.

Cerebral Contusion

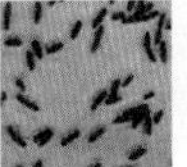

ETIOLOGIC FACTORS: A cerebral contusion is a brain bruise, that is, an area of tissue disruption and blood seepage. It usually occurs when the brain strikes the irregular bony contours of the skull because of abrupt acceleration or deceleration. When a moving object strikes the head, acceleration is imparted to the skull and the brain. By contrast, a fall results in an abrupt deceleration. When a contusion occurs at a point of impact, the lesion is a **coup** injury (French, *coup* = "blow") (Fig. 24-14). If the side of the brain opposite the impact site strikes the skull, the resulting contusion is contralateral to the point of initial contact and termed **contrecoup**. Coup injuries are maximal when the head is stationary and struck by an object, whereas contrecoup contusions are more severe when the head is in motion and abruptly stops.

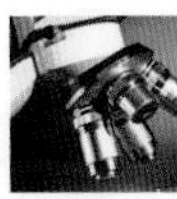

PATHOLOGY: If the force of impact is mild, cerebral contusion is limited to the cortex and the crowns of gyri (Fig. 24-15A). Greater force destroys larger expanses of cortex, creating cavitary lesions that may extend into the white matter or lacerate the cortex, causing intraparenchymal hemorrhage (Fig. 24-15B). Together, edema and hemorrhage in a contusion may cause the contusion to expand over several days, which can become life-threatening as a result of increased intracranial pressure.

Contusions leave permanent marks on the brain. Bruised, necrotic tissue is phagocytosed by macrophages and eliminated in large part via the bloodstream. Astrocytosis then leads to local scar formation, which persists as telltale evidence of a prior contusion. Usually, some residual hemosiderin imparts an orange-brown hue to the old contusion.

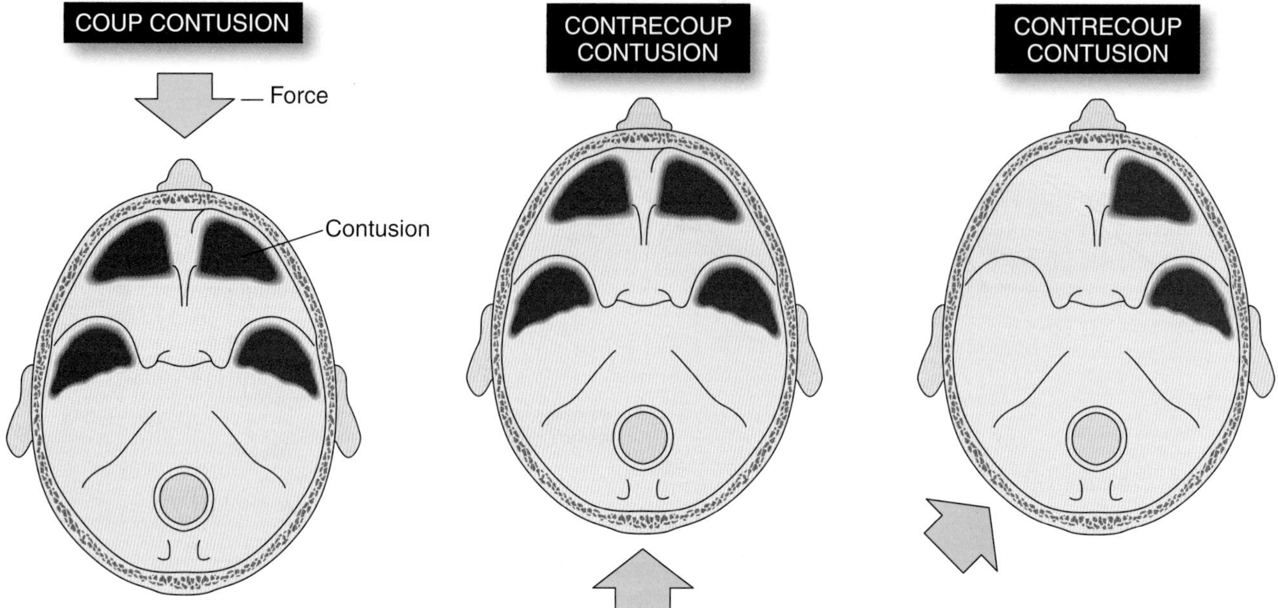

FIGURE 24-14. Biomechanics of cerebral contusion. The cerebral hemispheres float in the cerebrospinal fluid. Rapid deceleration or acceleration of the skull causes the cortex to impact forcefully into the anterior and middle fossae. The position of a contusion is determined by the direction of the force and the intracranial anatomy.

Diffuse Axonal Injury

DAI is a common result of traumatic brain injury and may create severe neurologic deficits and coma in patients without gross hematomas, contusions, or lacerations. There is also increased interest in DAI as part of blast injuries.

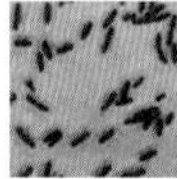

ETIOLOGIC FACTORS: The parasagittal cerebral hemispheres are anchored to arachnoid villi (**pacchionian granulations**), whereas the lateral aspects of the cerebrum move more freely. This anatomic feature, together with the differential density of gray and white matter, allows for shearing forces between different brain regions, leading to axonal shearing injuries. Shearing injuries can distort or disrupt axons, thereby causing immediate loss of function. Physical separation results in axons to form axonal retraction spheroids. Because diffuse axonal injury evolves over time, it may be possible to arrest its progression and preserve axonal structural integrity. If an injury is severe, the functional loss of axonal activity may immediately render the patient comatose, but imaging may show only small hemorrhages and focal edema, particularly in the corpus callosum and midbrain. However, more widely distributed axonal swelling and retraction

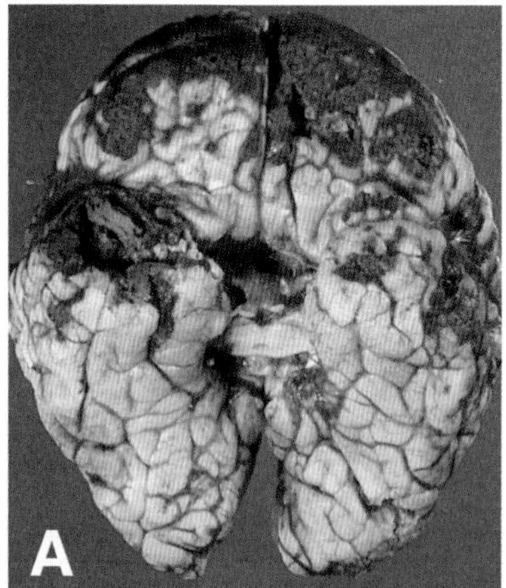

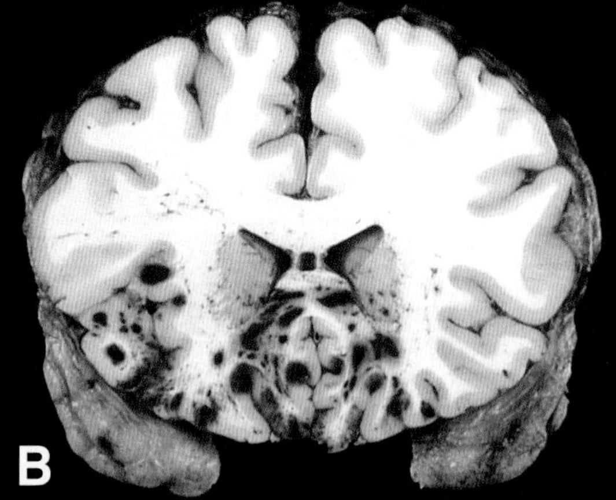

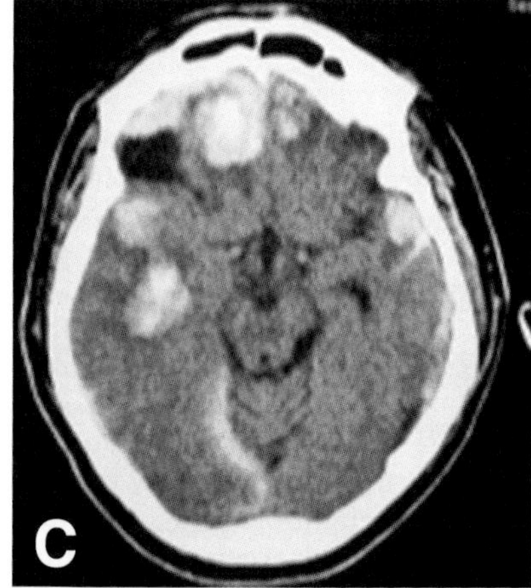

FIGURE 24-15. Acute contusions of the brain. A. After an automobile accident, the brain exhibits necrosis and hemorrhage involving the frontal and temporal lobes. **B.** In addition, there are some underlying white matter hemorrhages. **C.** Axial noncontrast computed tomography showing acute contusions in the basal frontal and temporal tips regions. The hemorrhage is the white signal in the frontal and temporal regions. (15A and 15B Courtesy of Dr. F. Stephen Vogel, Duke University.)

spheroids may be seen in cerebral white matter, corpus callosum, and brainstem.

Chronic Traumatic Encephalopathy

Acute traumatic brain injury has long been the primary focus of neurotrauma research, but long-term effects are now receiving considerable attention as large numbers of military service members return from Iraq and Afghanistan. In addition, major concern has been raised in professional and amateur athletics. For example, boxers with repetitive head injury develop dementia; their brains show neuronal loss and neurofibrillary tangles. CTE occurs in persons with varying degrees of repetitive head injury. Younger people (ages 20 to 40) tend to have a rapidly progressive course, primarily involving behavioral and mood changes. Older persons (ages 50 to 70) have slower disease, usually characterized by cognitive difficulties.

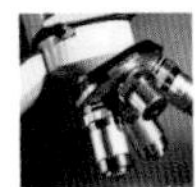

PATHOLOGY: The most distinctive finding in CTE is deposition of tau protein in neurons at the depths of sulci and around blood vessels. Abnormal tau accumulation occurs in many neurodegenerative diseases, including Alzheimer disease, frontotemporal lobar degeneration, and progressive supranuclear palsy. However, it is the distribution of neurofibrillary tangles in CTE that is unique.

Penetrating Traumatic Brain Injury

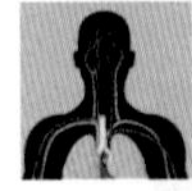

PATHOPHYSIOLOGY: Penetrating objects like bullets and knives enter the cranium and traverse the brain with variable velocities. If there is no direct damage to vital brain centers, hemorrhage is the immediate threat to life. However, a high-velocity bullet can cause an explosive increase in intracranial pressure, which forcefully herniates the cerebellar tonsils into the foramen magnum, causing immediate death.

Spinal Cord Injury

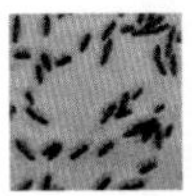

ETIOLOGIC FACTORS: Traumatic lesions of the spinal cord may result from direct injury by penetrating wounds (e.g., stab wounds and bullets) or indirect injury from vertebral fractures or displacement. The spinal cord may be contused not only at the site of injury but also above and below the point of trauma. In some instances, compromised arterial supply to the cord, with resulting infarction, complicates traumatic injury.

The consequences of a spinal cord injury depend on the severity of the trauma. **Spinal cord concussion** is the mildest injury, with transient, reversible functional disturbance. **Contusion of the spinal cord** results from more severe trauma, varying from minor transient bruises to hemorrhagic spinal cord necrosis. Spinal cord necrosis and edema due to severe contusion is termed **myelomalacia**. A hematoma within the cord is a **hematomyelia**. **Lacerations and transections of the spinal cord** are usually caused by penetrating wounds or severely displaced spinal fractures. The lesions are irreversible and lead to complete loss of function below the spinal level of the injury. Whether paralysis affects only the legs (**paraplegia**) or all four extremities (**quadriplegia**) depends on the spinal level and extent of the injury. If even as little as 10% to 15% of the cross-sectional diameter of the spinal cord is spared, functional recovery is much better than with complete transection.

CEREBROVASCULAR DISORDERS

Stroke is the third leading cause of death in the United States, after myocardial infarction and cancer. As elsewhere, vascular disease can result from either vessel obstruction, causing ischemia, or vascular leakage that results in hemorrhage. Vascular disorders of the nervous system lead to (1) inadequate blood flow (ischemia), which, if sufficiently protracted, produces infarction; or (2) rupture of vascular structures that causes either intraparenchymal hemorrhage or subarachnoid hemorrhage.

Ischemic Stroke

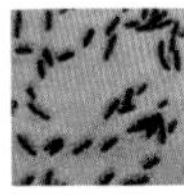

ETIOLOGIC FACTORS: The brain receives about 20% of basal cardiac output with aerobic glycolysis being virtually the sole source of energy. CNS glycogen reserves are meager, and oxygen reserves are nil; hence, uninterrupted supply of oxygenated blood is essential for brain integrity. The brain's blood supply comes via paired internal carotid and vertebral arteries. The carotids comprise the "anterior circulation" and supply most superficial and deep cerebral hemisphere structures. The vertebral arteries make up the "posterior circulation," which feeds the brainstem, cerebellum, and territory of the posterior cerebral arteries. The posterior and anterior circuits anastomose via the circle of Willis. This anastomotic network at the base of the brain is variable, but in some fortunate individuals, the blood supply of the brain is sufficiently redundant that complete blockage of two carotids and one vertebral can be asymptomatic.

Global ischemia, which is usually caused by cardiopulmonary arrest or extreme hypotension in severe shock, leads to widespread tissue injury, resulting in ischemic encephalopathy. Hemodynamic factors cause **watershed** or **borderzone infarcts**, which occur at the precarious distal regions of arterial supply. If perfusion pressure drops, these are the first areas affected. The classic border zone lies between the distal territories of the anterior and middle cerebral arteries (Fig. 24-16). With global ischemia, this area in both hemispheres may be characterized by symmetric, wedge-shaped, parasagittal infarcts.

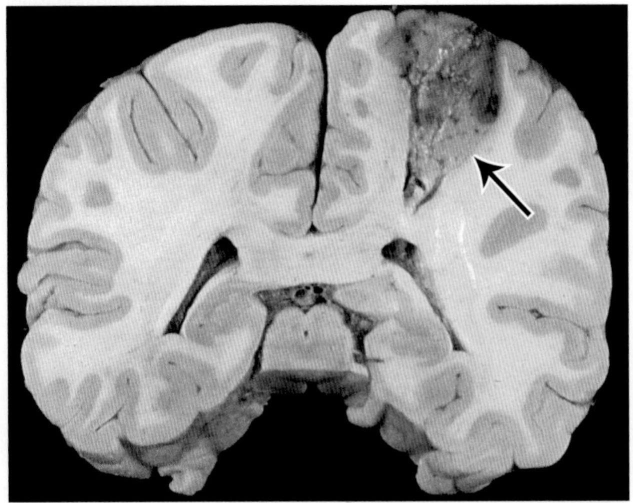

FIGURE 24-16. Watershed infarct. In global hypoperfusion, the most precarious perfusion zones are at the distal overlapping portions of the major cerebral vessels. Here, an acute infarct is seen at the watershed of the anterior and middle cerebral arteries (*arrow*). (Courtesy of Dr. F. Stephen Vogel, Duke University.)

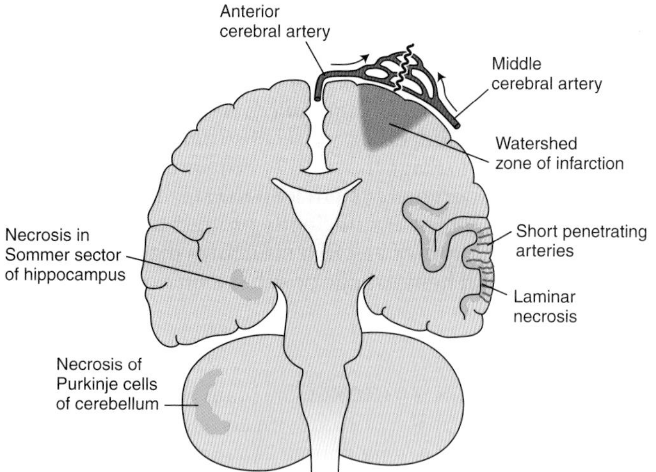

FIGURE 24-17. Mechanisms of injury in global ischemia. A global insult induces lesions that reflect the vascular architecture (watershed infarcts and laminar necrosis) and the selective vulnerability of individual neuronal systems (pyramidal cells of the Sommer sector, Purkinje cells, and laminar necrosis). Both rheologic (blood flow) and neurochemical (excitotoxicity) factors may be operational in laminar necrosis.

If perfusion failure is brief (minutes), neurologic functions may quickly be restored. If the ischemic period is protracted, the patient (1) does not regain consciousness, (2) shows decorticate posturing and seizures, and (3) remains in a coma indefinitely.

When the entire brain is inadequately perfused, there is surprising focality to the pathologic alterations. Cell populations most vulnerable to ischemic injury include the (1) large neurons in the Sommer sector of the hippocampus, (2) Purkinje cells of the cerebellum, and (3) neurons of layers 3 and 5 of the cerebral cortex (Fig. 24-17).

The basis of this selective vulnerability is not clear. It may be related to local metabolic requirements, hemodynamic factors, and local neurotransmitters. Injury produced by abnormally released neurotransmitters is termed **excitotoxicity**. As infarcted tissue is infiltrated by macrophages, it becomes grossly conspicuous as **laminar necrosis**.

Regional Ischemia

Cerebrovascular occlusive disease remains a major cause of morbidity and death because atherosclerosis is ubiquitous and progressive. ***Atherosclerosis predisposes to vascular thrombosis and embolism, both of which result in localized ischemia and subsequent cerebral infarction.***

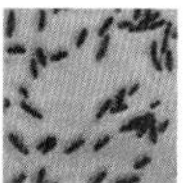

ETIOLOGIC FACTORS: Cerebral infarcts are usually designated **hemorrhagic** or **bland (ischemic).** *In general, infarcts caused by emboli are hemorrhagic, whereas those due to local thrombosis are ischemic.* Emboli occlude vascular flow abruptly, after which the distal segments of affected blood vessels lose integrity and leak blood into the region during reperfusion (Fig. 24-18A). Atherosclerotic plaques in the common and internal carotid arteries may give

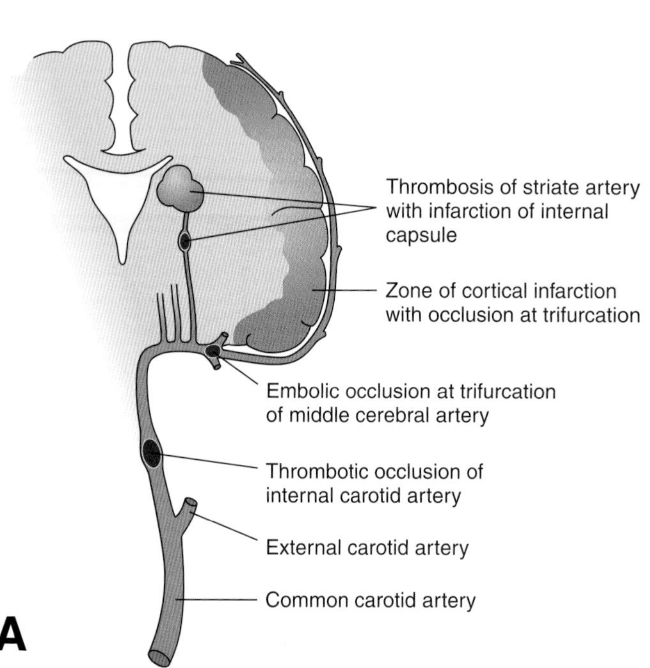

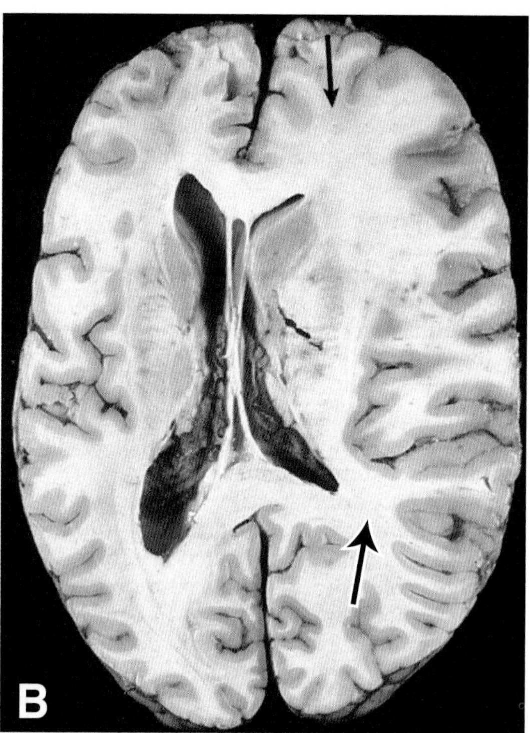

FIGURE 24-18. Distribution of cerebral infarcts. A. The normal distribution of the cerebral vasculature defines the pattern and size of infarcts and, consequently, their symptoms. Occlusion at the trifurcation causes cortical infarcts with motor and sensory loss and often aphasia. Occlusion of a striate branch transects the internal capsule and causes a motor deficit. **B. Acute middle cerebral artery distribution infarct.** An axial section of the brain of a patient who suffered thrombosis of the middle cerebral artery reveals a large infarct of the right hemisphere (*between arrows*) with swelling and focal dusky discoloration. (18B Courtesy of Dr. F. Stephen Vogel, Duke University.)

rise to emboli, although the heart is also a rich source of such (see Chapters 8 and 9).

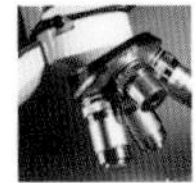

PATHOLOGY: As in other tissues, an orderly procession of pathologic changes allows estimation of an infarct's age. Most infarcts caused by thrombosis are anemic or bland and are difficult to see grossly for several hours. However, if blood flow is restored to a bland infarct, blood seeps into the softened tissues. This hemorrhagic infarct is readily discernible grossly and radiologically. During the first 6 to 24 hours, the ischemic infarct is slightly discolored and softened, with blurring of the border between gray and white matter. Shrunken eosinophilic neurons ("red neurons") with nuclear pyknosis are present in the infarct (Fig. 24-19). By 24 to 72 hours, neutrophils infiltrate the tissue, and blood vessels are prominent. The tissue is soft and edematous and may be sufficiently swollen to cause a lethal mass effect (Fig. 24-18B). By 3 to 4 days, macrophages replace neutrophils and clear debris in the infarct at a rate of about 1 mL per month. The infarct then evolves over weeks to months into a glial-lined cystic space (Fig. 24-20), sometimes accompanied by compensatory ventricular enlargement.

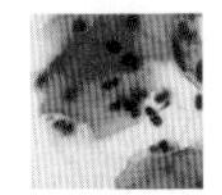

CLINICAL FEATURES: The lengthy and slender striate arteries, which take origin from the proximal middle cerebral artery, are commonly occluded by atherosclerosis and thrombosis. The resultant infarcts often impact the internal capsule to produce hemiplegia (Fig. 24-18A). Similarly, trifurcation of the middle cerebral artery is a favored site for lodgment of emboli and for thrombosis due to atherosclerosis. Occlusion at this site deprives much of the lateral hemispheric cortex of blood, producing motor and sensory deficits. If the dominant hemisphere is involved, aphasia may develop.

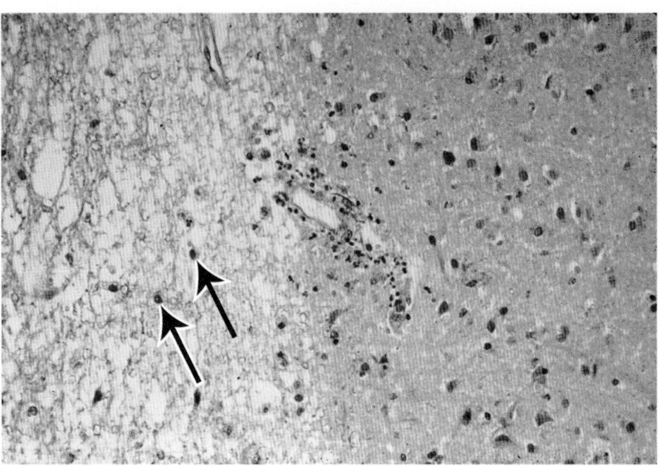

FIGURE 24-19. Acute cerebral infarct histopathology. An 18-hour-old cerebral infarct (*left*) shows edema, hypereosinophilic neurons, and perivascular polymorphonuclear leukocytes. Pyknotic nuclei of dying neurons are shown (*arrows*).

Localized ischemia is associated with three distinct clinical syndromes:

- **Transient ischemic attack (TIA)** is focal cerebral dysfunction, lasting under 24 hours, and often only a few minutes. Although complete neurologic recovery follows, TIA heralds an increased risk of cerebral infarction. ***TIAs are often harbingers of a stroke, but many people (50% to 85%) who develop cerebral infarcts never have a preceding TIA.***
- **Stroke in evolution** describes the often-stuttering progression of neurologic symptoms as a patient is being observed.

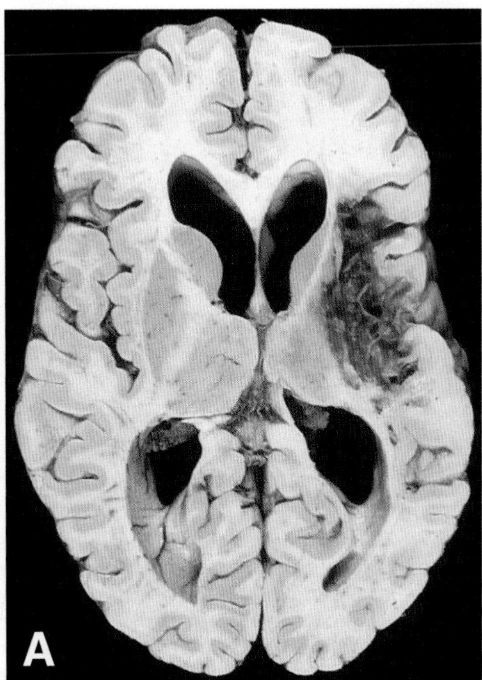

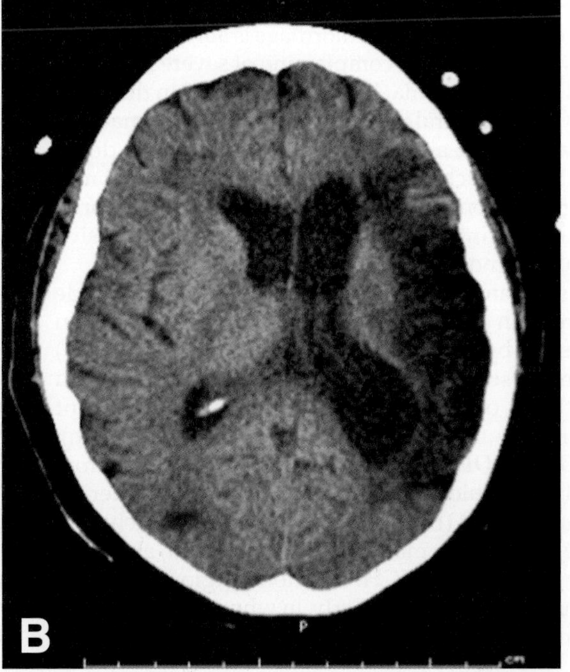

FIGURE 24-20. Remote middle cerebral artery distribution infarct. A. An axial section of the brain showing a remote middle cerebral artery distribution cystic infarct. The brain in Figure 20-17B would transform to this state as a result of clearing out of the large infarct by macrophages. **B.** Axial noncontrast computed tomography showing a remote middle cerebral artery distribution infarct resulting from a cardiogenic embolus. Note the low signal in the middle cerebral artery territory and the compensatory enlargement of the ventricles. (20A Courtesy of Dr. F. Stephen Vogel, Duke University.)

This clinically unstable situation reflects propagation of a thrombus in the carotid or basilar arteries and necessitates urgent treatment.

- **Completed stroke** describes a stable or fixed neurologic deficit caused by a cerebral infarct. Two to three days after a completed stroke, there can be sufficient cerebral cytotoxic and vasogenic edema in the infarct to increase intracranial pressure and cause herniation.

Intracranial Hemorrhage

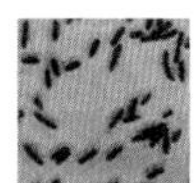

ETIOLOGIC FACTORS: Intraparenchymal hemorrhage (intracerebral hemorrhage) usually results from rupture of small fragile vessels or vascular malformations. Subarachnoid hemorrhage is mostly caused by rupture of aneurysms or vascular malformations.

Intracerebral Hemorrhage

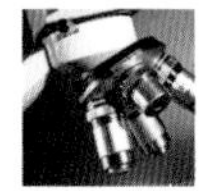

PATHOLOGY: Cerebral hemorrhages that occur without trauma are usually caused by vascular malformations or are due to long-standing hypertension. **Hypertensive intracerebral hemorrhage (ICH)** occurs at preferential sites, which in order of frequency are (1) basal ganglia–thalamus (65%), (2) pons (15%), and (3) cerebellum (8%). Hypertensive ICH also occurs in the white matter of cerebral hemispheres, where it is called **lobar ICH**. Lobar ICH suggests possible amyloid angiopathy, vascular malformation, coagulopathy, or bleeding into a tumor, as well as simple hypertensive hemorrhage.

Hypertension compromises the integrity of cerebral arterioles by causing lipid and hyaline material to deposit in their walls, a change called **lipohyalinosis**. Weakening of the wall leads to formation of **Charcot–Bouchard aneurysms**, which occur mainly along the trunk of an arteriole rather than sites where it bifurcates (Fig. 24-21).

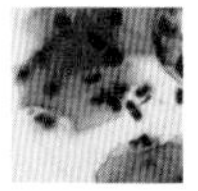

CLINICAL FEATURES: The onset of symptoms of a hypertensive cerebral hemorrhage is abrupt. A patient may clutch his head complaining of severe headache and lapse into coma. Hypertensive ICH in the basal ganglion may cause contralateral hemiparesis. If a hematoma progressively expands, as is common in the first day, death may occur when it reaches a critical volume of about 30 mL. An enlarging hematoma may cause death by transtentorial herniation. Rupture into a lateral ventricle results in massive intraventricular hemorrhage.

Causes of spontaneous ICH other than hypertension include (1) leakage from an arteriovenous malformation, (2) erosion of a blood vessel by a primary or secondary neoplasm, (3) endothelial injury such as occurs in rickettsial infections, (4) a bleeding diathesis, or (5) embolic infarction with consequent hemorrhage into the area of necrosis (hemorrhagic conversion).

AMYLOID ANGIOPATHY: This vascular change results from deposition of β-amyloid protein in vascular walls, rendering them weak and friable (Fig. 24-22). Small intraparenchymal vessels in the lobar white matter are most affected, and their rupture may lead to lobar ICH. Amyloid angiopathy is an important cause of ICH in the elderly, in whom it may coexist with Alzheimer disease.

Subarachnoid Hemorrhage

Intravascular pressure and weakness in arterial walls give rise to cerebral aneurysms that may rupture and result in subarachnoid hemorrhage (SAH). Ruptured aneurysms cause about 85% of SAH, whereas vascular malformations account for 15%.

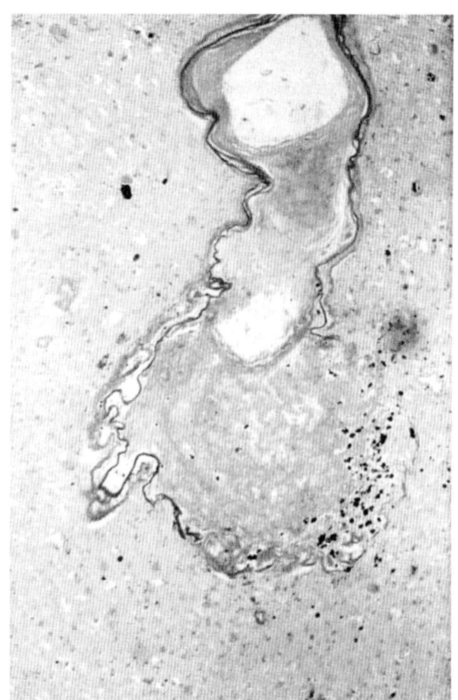

FIGURE 24-21. Charcot–Bouchard aneurysm. The combination of small penetrating cerebral vessels and high perfusion pressure leads to small microaneurysms that may rupture, leading to intracerebral hemorrhage. Effective treatment of hypertension reduces the formation of microaneurysms and the frequency of intracerebral hemorrhage. (Courtesy of Dr. F. Stephen Vogel, Duke University.)

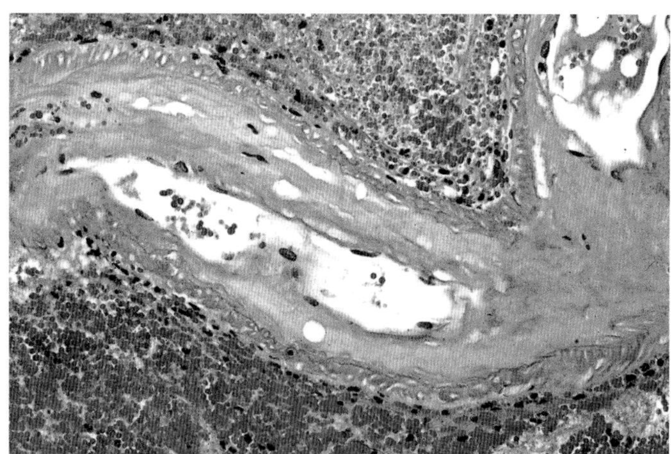

FIGURE 24-22. Amyloid angiopathy. While hypertension is the most common cause of intracerebral hemorrhage in the classic locations—basal ganglia and thalamus, pons, and cerebellum—hemorrhage in the white matter of the cerebral hemispheres has a broader range of possible etiologies. These hemorrhages, called lobar hemorrhages, may be caused by amyloid angiopathy in which β-amyloid protein is deposited in the walls of vessels, rendering them weak and friable. This is the same protein as is involved in plaque formation in Alzheimer disease; amyloid angiopathy and Alzheimer disease frequently coexist.

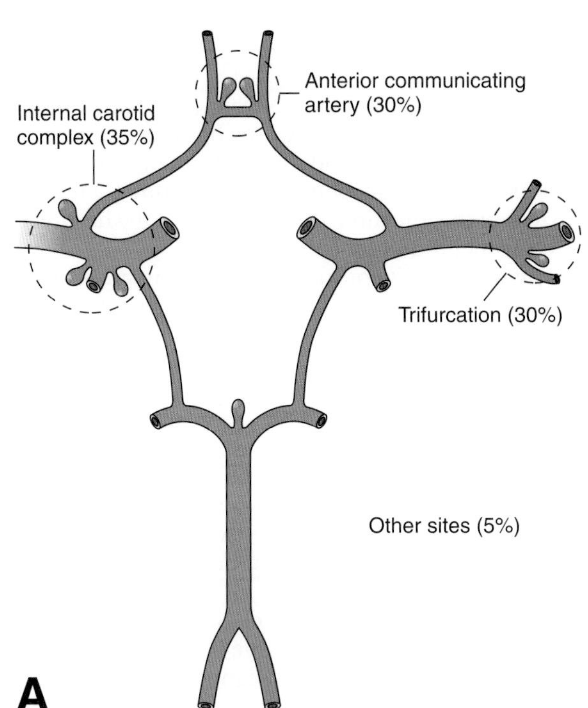

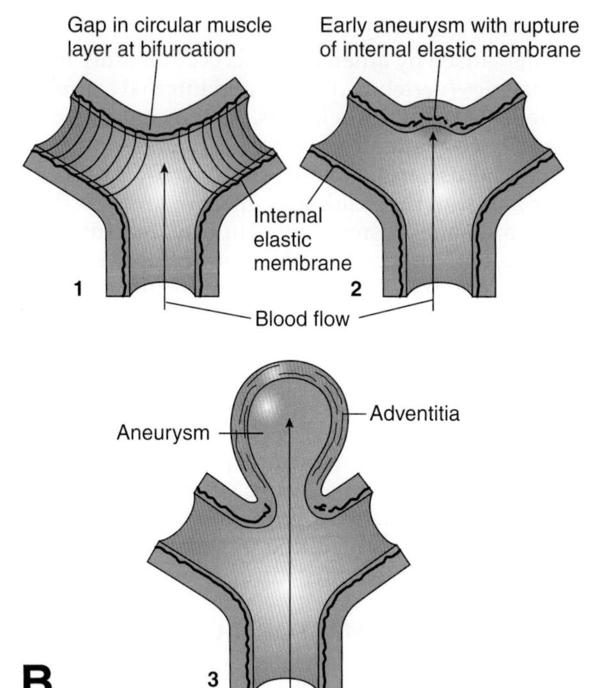

FIGURE 24-23. Pathophysiology of saccular aneurysm. A. The incidence of saccular aneurysms (berry aneurysms), which preferentially involve the proximal carotid tributaries, is shown. **B.** The lesion evolves as a result of blood under pressure acting on an early embryonic defect of the vascular wall at bifurcations.

Saccular (Berry) Aneurysms

Saccular aneurysms are balloon-like outpouchings of cerebral arteries that may rupture to cause catastrophic subarachnoid hemorrhage. They tend to occur at branch points of the cerebral vasculature in or near the circle of Willis (Fig. 24-23).

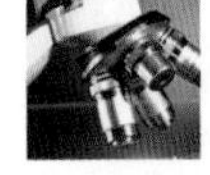

PATHOLOGY: When a developing blood vessel bifurcates into two branches, the muscularis layer may not adequately span the branch point. This situation leaves an area of congenital muscularis thinning, covered only by endothelium, the internal elastic membrane, and a thin adventitia. Over time, pressure from the pulsatile blood flow in the parent vessel enlarges the defect. The internal elastic membrane fragments, after which a saccular aneurysm evolves, which is covered only by a layer of adventitia.

More than 90% of saccular aneurysms occur at proximal branch points in the anterior circulation fed by the carotid system; however, some may arise on branches of the posterior circulation, particularly on the posterior communicating and posterior cerebral arteries (Fig. 24-24). Multiple aneurysms are encountered in 15% to 20% of cases. The incidence of cerebral aneurysms is increased in polycystic kidney disease, coarctation of the aorta, and Ehlers–Danlos syndrome.

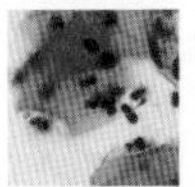

CLINICAL FEATURES: Rupture of a saccular aneurysm leads to life-threatening SAH, with 35% mortality due to the initial hemorrhage. Blood may jet under arterial pressure to produce intracerebral or intraventricular hemorrhage in up to one third of patients. The subarachnoid blood irritates pain-sensitive vessels and dura, thereby resulting in "the worst headache in my life" and subsequent coma. Survivors of the initial episode often rebleed within 21 days, and half of those who rebleed will perish. Therapy is directed at isolating the aneurysm from the circulation by surgical occlusion of the vasculature that connects the sac of the aneurysm to the parent vessel. A metallic clip across the neck of the aneurysm renders the aneurysm bloodless. An endovascular approach can also be taken: a catheter inserted through the femoral artery is guided to the cerebral circulation. Thin thrombogenic metallic coils are then threaded into the aneurysm sac, causing the blood in the aneurysm to clot.

At times, rather than rupturing, a saccular aneurysm enlarges to form a mass that may compress cranial nerves and produce palsies or impinge on parenchymal structures and induce neurologic symptoms.

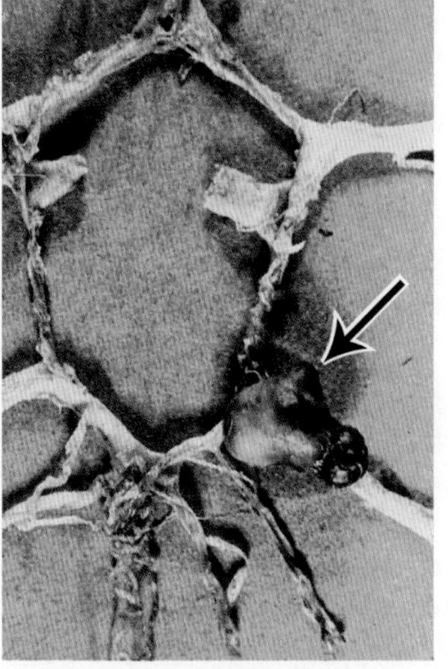

FIGURE 24-24. Berry aneurysm. A saccular aneurysm (*arrow*) arises from the posterior cerebral artery. The dark color is a result of subarachnoid blood from this aneurysm that ruptured.

Atherosclerotic Aneurysms

Aneurysms caused by atherosclerosis occur mainly in major cerebral arteries (vertebral, basilar, and internal carotid) that are favored sites of atherosclerosis. As they enlarge, atherosclerotic aneurysms tend to be fusiform and elongate. An enlarging atherosclerotic aneurysm may compress cranial nerves or parenchyma, leading to focal neurologic deficits. Atherosclerotic aneurysms rarely rupture, but intraplaque hemorrhage may proceed to vascular occlusion or a complicated plaque may proceed to arterial thrombosis and ischemic stroke.

Vascular Malformations

Vascular malformations arise during embryogenesis but evolve during angiogenesis, vascular remodeling, and recruitment of vessels from normal parenchyma. Vascular malformations may bleed to cause subarachnoid or intraparenchymal hemorrhage or both. They may also irritate normal cerebral cortex, resulting in seizures; diversion of blood flow from adjacent structures may cause focal neurologic deficits.

ARTERIOVENOUS MALFORMATION: An arteriovenous malformation (AVM) is a tangle of arteries and veins of varying caliber and wall thickness, separated by abnormal gliotic parenchyma (Fig. 24-25). The abnormal vessels form in embryogenesis from focal communications between cerebral arteries and veins, without intervening capillaries. The resulting congeries of abnormal vessels are typically located in the cerebral cortex and the contiguous underlying white matter. AVMs enlarge with time and recruit vessels from adjacent tissue.

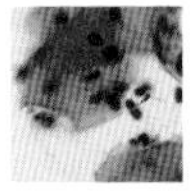

CLINICAL FEATURES: Seizure disorders result from irritation of neural tissue by AVMs. Focal neurologic deficits are caused by vascular steal. Intracranial hemorrhages, usually subarachnoid or intracerebral, commonly arise in the second or third decade. The hemorrhage is not usually catastrophic but may be recurring.

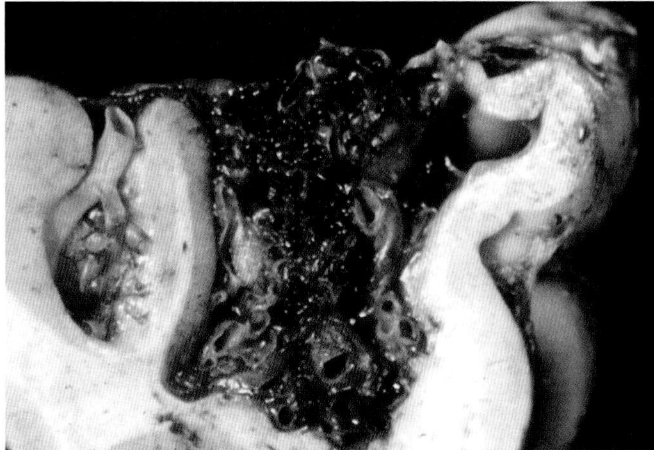

FIGURE 24-25. Arteriovenous malformation (AVM). A disorganized collection of arteries and veins is seen within the substance of the brain extending to the surface. AVMs may result in subarachnoid hemorrhage if they bleed on the surface or intraparenchymal hemorrhage if deeper vascular channels rupture. The hemorrhage is usually not as catastrophic as that seen in aneurysm subarachnoid hemorrhage or hypertensive intracerebral hemorrhage.

CENTRAL NERVOUS SYSTEM INFECTIONS

Many of the infections of the CNS are devastating or lethal if untreated. Their clinical course may be swift and ferocious or indolent and progressive and can mimic many other disorders. Evaluation of CNS infections should include (1) the location and extent of the infection, (2) the nature of the host response, and (3) the inciting organism.

Empyema in the epidural or subdural space is usually related to trauma or spread from contiguous infection—usually bacterial—in the sinuses or ear.

In **meningitis** (leptomeningitis), the inflammatory response and most of the inciting organisms are in the subarachnoid space, floating in the CSF. The vigor of the inflammatory response may lead to parenchymal involvement, including cerebral edema and vasculitis, with thrombosis, hemorrhage, infarction, and **cerebritis**. Long-term complications include effusions, obstruction of CSF flow with hydrocephalus, and cranial neuropathies, particularly deafness from VIII nerve involvement.

Cerebritis is a purulent parenchymal infection that is usually bacterial or fungal. Brain tissue becomes soft and soupy, and the borders of the infection cannot be easily discerned. If a host can contain the process, the cerebritis is walled off to form a brain abscess. Abscesses have many neutrophils within a necrotic core, surrounded by granulation tissue, a dense fibrovascular capsule and a gliotic rind.

Encephalitis, like cerebritis, is a parenchymal infection, but the term is usually reserved for viral infections that exhibit necrosis, perivascular lymphocytic cuffing, and microglial nodules. Intranuclear or cytoplasmic viral inclusions are common as are gliosis, demyelination, and status spongiosus.

Bacterial Infections

Leptomeningitis is located between the pia and arachnoid layers of the meninges. The CSF filling this compartment is an excellent culture medium for most bacteria. The inflammatory response in the CSF to infections varies with the virulence of the organism and the tempo of the infection. Changes are detectable in the cellular constituents of the CSF as well as glucose and protein concentrations. Organisms are sometimes visible microscopically in the CSF and can be definitively characterized by culture, antigenicity, and, in some cases, polymerase chain reaction (PCR).

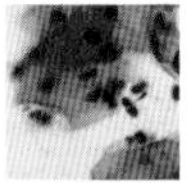

CLINICAL FEATURES: The signs and symptoms of meningitis include headache, vomiting, fever, altered mental status, and seizures. Classic signs of meningeal inflammation are neck rigidity, knee pain with hip flexion (Kernig sign), and knee/hip flexion when the neck is flexed (Brudzinski sign). At the extremes of age—newborn and senescence—clinical manifestations vary more widely. A newborn may have autonomic instability and fragmentary seizures, whereas the elderly may have altered mental status without fever or headache.

Bacterial Meningitis

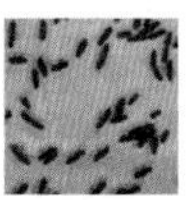

ETIOLOGIC FACTORS: Because most bacteria initiate purulent responses, the presence of neutrophils in the CSF is strong evidence of meningitis. CSF glucose will often be decreased, and protein elevated. The causes of bacterial meningitis depend on the age of the patient.

Gram-negative *Escherichia coli* and β-hemolytic *Streptococcus* sp. predominate in neonates. In unvaccinated young children, *Haemophilus influenzae* dominates, but vaccination programs against the organism have changed the epidemiology, so that *Streptococcus pneumoniae* and *Neisseria meningitidis* are becoming more prevalent. *N. meningitidis* is most common in adolescence and early adult life. *S. pneumoniae* is most common thereafter. Routes of entry to the intracranial vault are shown in Figure 24-26A.

ESCHERICHIA COLI: In newborns, whose resistance to Gram-negative bacteria has not yet fully developed, *E. coli* is a major cause of meningitis. Transplacental transfer of maternal IgG protects newborns from many bacteria. However, *E. coli* and similar Gram-negative organisms require IgM for neutralization, and IgM does not cross the placenta. Thus, in infancy, Gram-negative organisms quickly produce purulent meningitis with a high mortality.

HAEMOPHILUS INFLUENZAE: Environmental exposure to *H. influenzae* is somewhat delayed. Thus, the incidence of meningitis peaks from 3 months to 3 years. *H. influenzae* meningitis has decreased in recent years (see above).

STREPTOCOCCUS PNEUMONIAE: Later in life, *Pneumococcus* is the main cause of meningitis. Patients with a history of basilar skull fracture with CSF leak have a high incidence of pneumococcal meningitis, which often recurs after treatment. Alcoholics and patients who are asplenic are highly susceptible.

NEISSERIA MENINGITIDIS: The meningococcus resides in the nasopharynx, and airborne transmission in crowded places (e.g., schools or barracks) causes "epidemic meningitis." Initially, bacteremia is accompanied by fever, malaise, and petechial rash, but intravascular coagulopathy may cause lethal adrenal hemorrhage (**Waterhouse–Friderichsen syndrome**). Untreated meningococcal bacteremia can trigger acute fulminant meningitis. An available polyvalent vaccine is recommended for all young people, but there are strains of *N. meningitidis* that are not covered by the vaccine.

LISTERIA MONOCYTOGENES: Listerial meningitis is increasing at all ages and accounts for up to 10% of bacterial meningitis. Its course is less fulminant than other bacterial meningitides, and CSF cellular responses may be lymphocyte predominant.

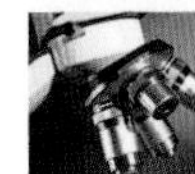

PATHOLOGY: In bacterial meningitis, an exudate of leukocytes and fibrin opacifies the arachnoid. This exudate varies from mild and equivocal to the naked eye to prominent enough to obscure blood vessels. Purulent exudates are most conspicuous over the cerebral hemispheres (Fig. 24-26B) but may extend to the base of the brain and from intracranial to intraspinal and subarachnoid spaces. Cerebral abscesses rarely complicate meningitis. The pia forms sleeves around blood vessels that penetrate the brain (**Virchow–Robin spaces**) in continuity with the subarachnoid space, which is usually packed with neutrophils and organisms (Fig. 24-27). A vigorous host response is essential to clear the infection, but significant vascular and neuropil damage results from cytotoxic substances, such as free radicals and cytokines released by inflammatory cells. Low CSF glucose in bacterial meningitis mostly reflects glucose consumption by inflammatory cells. Corticosteroids may be given with antibiotics to mitigate host response–induced damage.

Cerebral Abscess

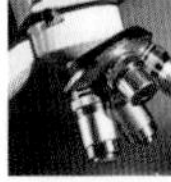

PATHOLOGY: A localized intraparenchymal abscess begins when bacteria or fungi lodge in the neuropil and incite an acute inflammatory and edematous reaction, called **cerebritis**. Within days, liquefactive necrosis causes an expanding mass that may threaten life by herniation or rupture into a ventricle (Fig. 24-28).

Choroid plexus
Parenchymal vessels
Penetrating wound
Osteomyelitis
Otitis media
Skull fracture
Meningeal vessels
A

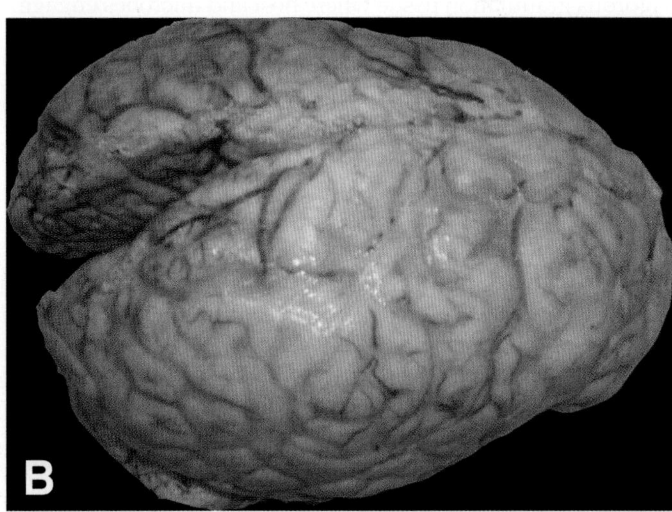

FIGURE 24-26. Purulent meningitis. A. Routes of entry of infectious organisms into the cranial cavity. B. A creamy exudate opacifies the leptomeninges in bacterial meningitis. The superficial veins are engorged and may develop thrombosis, and the arteries on the surface of the brain may also develop thrombosis, leading to infarcts.

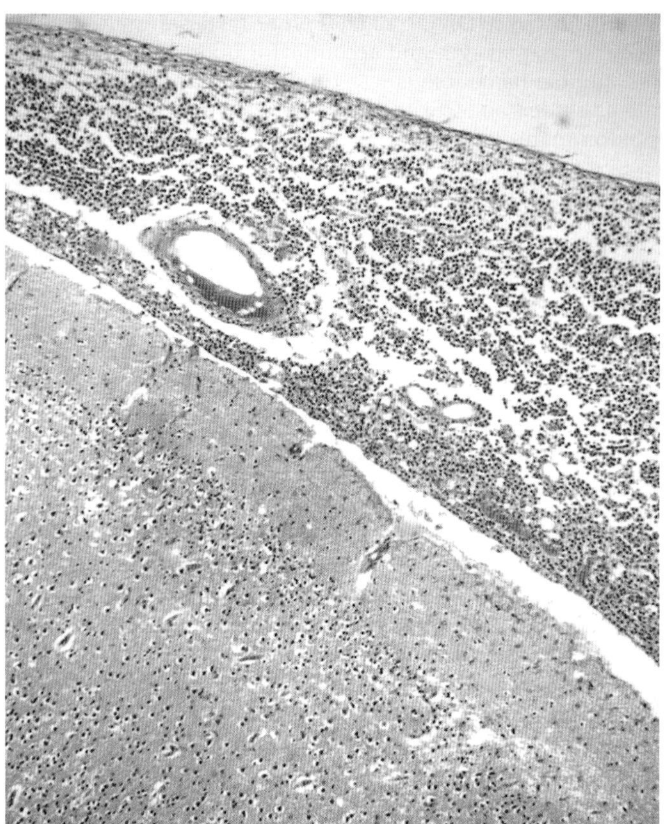

FIGURE 24-27. Bacterial meningitis. A microscopic section shows the accumulation of numerous neutrophils in the subarachnoid space.

As the abscess matures over days to weeks, three layers surround a central core of purulent debris: (1) an inner layer of vigorous granulation tissue where host and microbes engage in open warfare; (2) a second layer of a dense meshwork of fibroblasts and collagen that forms a tough rind around the core and granulation tissue; and (3) finally, a zone of intense astrogliosis, microglial activation, and edema (Fig. 24-29). The granulation tissue layer lacks a blood–brain barrier and during radiography leaks contrast material, thereby causing a smooth ring of radiographic enhancement.

Neurosyphilis

Secondary syphilis is heralded by a maculopapular rash on the skin and mucous membranes. A few lymphocytes and plasma cells and increased protein in the CSF reflect entry of blood-borne spirochetes. The organisms sometimes initiate a meningeal fibroblastic response, accompanied by obliterative endarteritis that induces multiple, small infarcts of the cerebral cortex or brainstem. Plasma cells, the inflammatory hallmark of syphilis, surround arterioles of the cerebral cortex in meningovascular syphilis.

Tabes dorsalis, which can accompany tertiary syphilis, is impairment of spinal dorsal column function, as manifested by loss of joint position sense and fine touch. Fibrous tissue triggered by the inflammation constricts nerve roots, causing axonal (Wallerian) degeneration. The patient loses position sense in the legs and comes to rely on visual cues for the position of his feet and legs in space. In darkness, or with his eyes closed, the patient becomes unsteady and may even fall, a situation that reflects severe posterior column dysfunction.

Luetic dementia results from spirochetes that replicate sluggishly and escape eradication, producing dementia and psychosis years after the initial infection. The morphologic features include (1) focal loss of cortical neurons, (2) disfigurement of residual nerve cells ("wind-blown appearance"), (3) marked gliosis, and (4) conversion of microglia into elongated forms encrusted with iron ("rod cells") associated with nodular ependymitis.

Fungal Infections

Fungal infections of the CNS are often opportunistic, reflecting the indolent saprophytic lifestyle of these organisms, although a few fungi are sufficiently virulent to cause disease in immunocompetent people. Fungi invading tissue may be round to oval, often budding, yeast forms, or branching hyphae. In some infections, yeast and hyphae both appear in infected tissues, facilitating tentative identification of fungi in tissue sections. However, ultimate speciation requires antigenic, PCR, or culture confirmation.

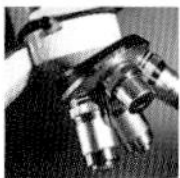

PATHOLOGY: Fungal infections progress more slowly than bacterial infections. Multinucleated giant cells are admixed with lymphocytes and plasma cells. Exudate tends to accumulate at the base of the brain, around the brainstem, rather than over the convexities as in bacterial meningitis.

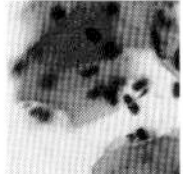

CLINICAL FEATURES: This chronic basilar meningitis may block CSF flow through the foramina of Magendie and Luschka, leading to hydrocephalus, headache, nausea, and vomiting. Cranial nerve palsies can occur because these nerves traverse the exudate where they emerge from the brainstem.

Cryptococcus

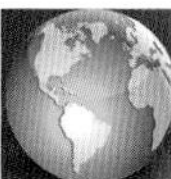

EPIDEMIOLOGY: Cryptococci are the most common fungal causes of meningitis. *Cryptococcus* often acts opportunistically in immunocompromised patients, but it can also establish meningitis in an immunologically competent host. *Cryptococcus neoformans* enters the host by inhalation. Birds are the major reservoir, and their inhaled fungus-laden excreta initiate a lung infection that may remain confined to the lungs or may disseminate to involve other organs, including the brain.

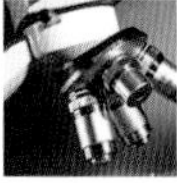

PATHOLOGY: *C. neoformans* typically elicits granulomatous responses, with infectious foci appearing as discrete white meningeal nodules. The organism may remain confined to the subarachnoid space, but infection sometimes spreads to the brain parenchyma. The gelatinous fungal capsule appears clear and glistening, so that microabscesses resemble soap bubbles (Fig. 24-30).

C. neoformans may be abundant, particularly in the Virchow–Robin spaces. An occasional multinucleated giant cell, sometimes with phagocytosed organisms, accompanies scant epithelioid cells and a few lymphocytes. The organisms are encapsulated, budding yeast forms that are large by fungal standards (5 to 15 μ) and have an external gelatinous capsule that resembles a clear halo. Its capsule shields the organism from host immune responses and accounts for the usually feeble inflammatory reaction. The capsule sheds specific antigens that can be detected in the CSF by the latex cryptococcal antigen test.

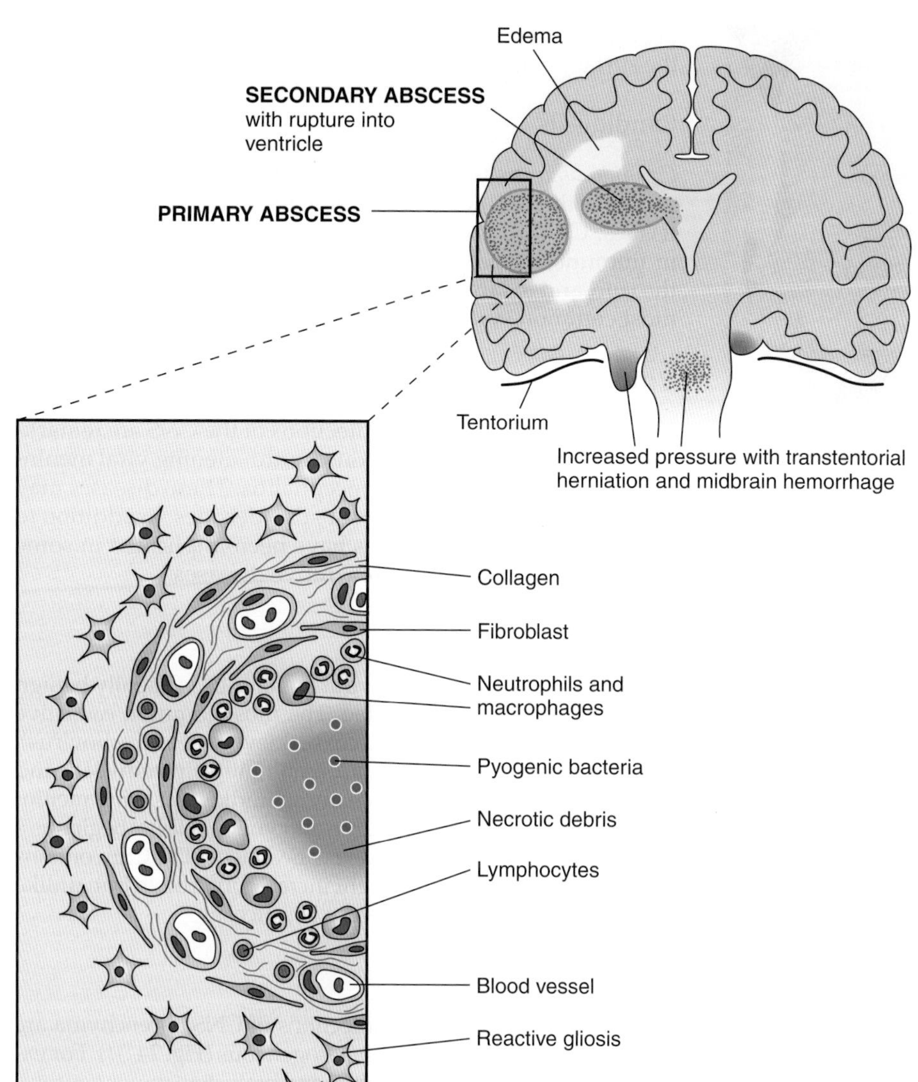

FIGURE 24-28. Brain abscess development and its complications. A cerebral abscess may cause death through the production of secondary abscesses with intraventricular rupture; alternatively, death may result from transtentorial herniation. The abscess consists of a necrotic purulent core, a layer of granulation tissue, and a layer of fibrosis, and finally, the abscess is surrounded by gliosis.

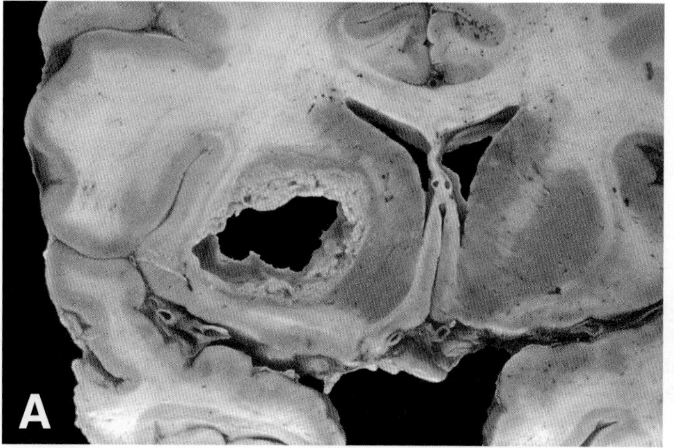

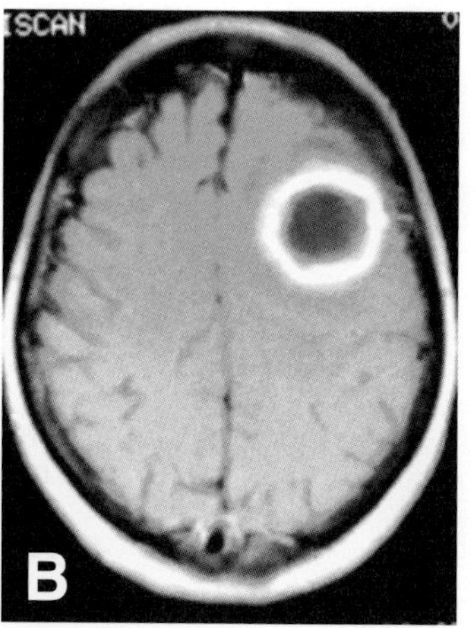

FIGURE 24-29. Cerebral abscess. A. A young man with bacterial endocarditis developed an abscess in the left basal ganglia. **B.** Axial contrast-enhanced computed tomography showing a smooth uniform ring of enhancement around a necrotic core of a brain abscess. A smooth ring-enhancing lesion is very suggestive of a brain abscess but may be seen with primary or secondary neoplasms of the brain.

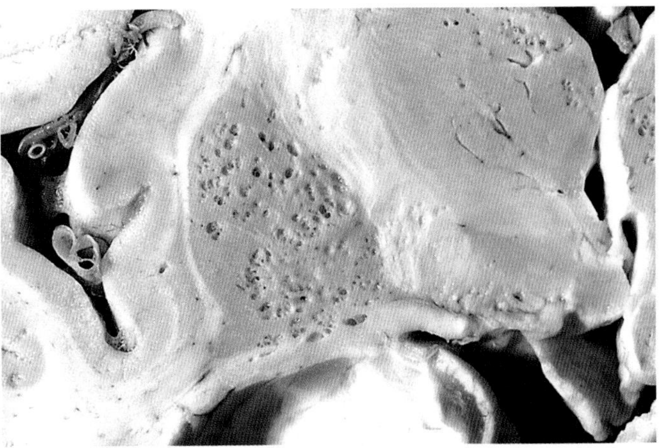

FIGURE 24-30. Cryptococcal "soap-bubble" abscesses. The encapsulated organisms occur in great abundance in the Virchow–Robin space and in microabscesses within the parenchyma. The microbial capsule imparts a glistening clear appearance to these collections that has been likened to soap bubbles. (Courtesy of Dr. F. Stephen Vogel, Duke University.)

Coccidioidomycosis

Coccidioides immitis is endemic in arid regions of the Southwest and San Joaquin Valley in California. The initial pulmonary infection is usually asymptomatic and rarely spreads. It causes suppurative and granulomatous inflammation, which sometimes includes an arteritis that may be complicated by infarction. The organism appears in tissue as an eye-catching refractile endosporulating spherule.

Histoplasmosis

Histoplasma capsulatum is endemic in the Mississippi basin and usually causes asymptomatic pulmonary infections. Rare CNS dissemination of this tiny, intracytoplasmic yeast form residing in macrophages may occur. A chronic meningitis ensues in which the surface of the brain may be studded by small granulomas.

Candidiasis

Candida albicans is a ubiquitous opportunistic fungus that shows both yeast and pseudohyphae morphology in infected tissues. *Candida* produces many microabscesses, most often in immunocompromised patients. Systemic involvement is the rule, and in large hospital-based autopsy series, this is the most common systemic fungal infection.

Viral Infections

The manifestations of viral infections of the CNS are remarkably diverse, ranging from non–life-threatening viral meningitis to more ominous viral encephalitis. These diseases may unfold over a period of hours or span decades. In addition to producing infections, viruses have been implicated in some autoimmune and neurodegenerative diseases.

Viral Meningitis

Unlike bacterial meningitis, viral meningitis is usually benign and resolves without sequelae. The most common causative agents are enteroviruses (e.g., coxsackievirus B and echovirus), but mumps, lymphocytic choriomeningitis, Epstein–Barr and herpes simplex viruses cause many sporadic cases. Viral meningitis (mainly a disease of children and young adults) begins as a sudden febrile illness with a severe headache. The CSF contains excess lymphocytes and a slight increase in protein but, unlike bacterial meningitis, no decrease in glucose.

Viral Encephalitis

The manifestations of viral infections of CNS parenchyma are clinically and pathologically heterogeneous (Fig. 24-31). For example, poliomyelitis affects spinal and brainstem motor neurons, whereas herpes simplex targets the temporal lobes. Subacute

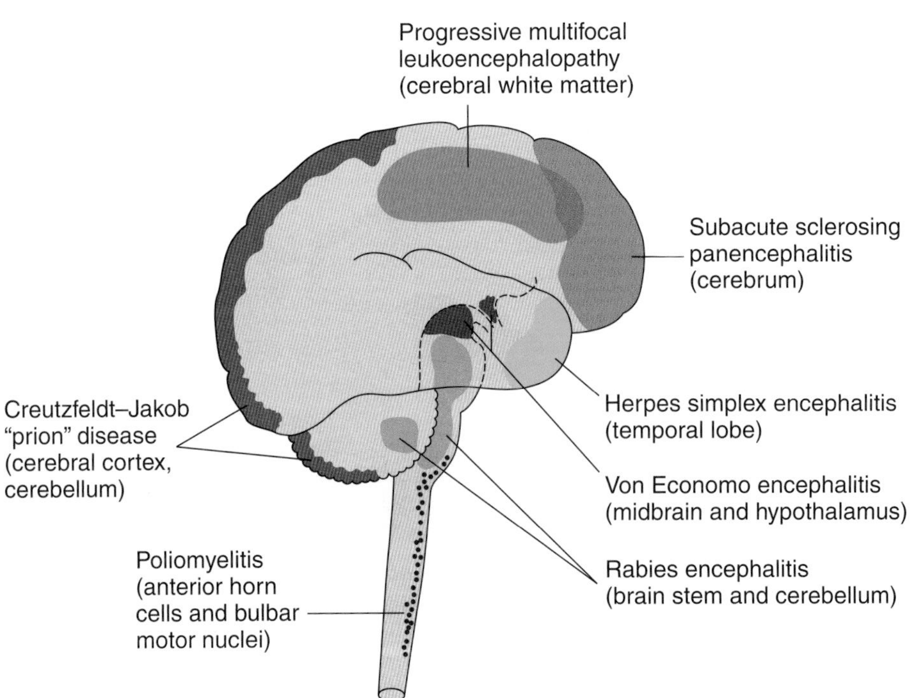

FIGURE 24-31. Distribution of the lesions of viral encephalitides.

sclerosing panencephalitis involves the gray matter, whereas progressive multifocal leukoencephalopathy is a white matter disorder. The mechanisms of viral tropism may reflect binding of viruses to plasma membrane structure on specific CNS cells, the ability of viruses to remain latent, or selective replication in specific intracellular microenvironments. Viruses may exploit axonal transport to travel to sites far distant from their point of entry, as exemplified by rabies and herpes viruses.

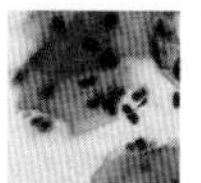

PATHOLOGY: Most CNS viral infections elicit perivascular lymphocytes, macrophage and microglial activation, and gliosis (Fig. 24-32). Although these changes are not specific for viral infections, the presence of viral inclusions strongly suggests a viral infection (Fig. 24-33). Such inclusion bodies do not occur with all viral infections. In situ hybridization, PCR, and immunochemistry are most often used to establish a diagnosis.

CLINICAL FEATURES: Most viral encephalitides begin abruptly. Specific neurologic deficits (e.g., paralysis of poliomyelitis and difficulty in swallowing in rabies) reflect the localization of the infection. Most encephalitides run a rapid course, but the tempo can vary. For example, the clinical course of subacute sclerosing panencephalitis may last years. Herpes simplex and varicella-zoster viruses tend to be latent in sensory ganglia for years, only to be reactivated decades after initial infection.

Poliomyelitis

The term **poliomyelitis** describes any inflammation of the gray matter of the spinal cord. In common usage, it implies an infection by poliovirus, which is one of the single-stranded RNA enteroviruses. Affected people shed large amounts of virus in their stools, and spread is by the fecal–oral route.

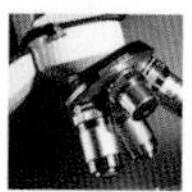

PATHOLOGY: Polio virus enters motor neurons via binding sites on their plasma membranes and replicates there. Infected cells may undergo chromatolysis (distinctive changes to the nissl bodies within the neuron indicative of nerve injury), after which they are phagocytosed by macrophages (neuronophagia). Initial inflammatory responses briefly include neutrophils. Lymphocytes follow and surround blood vessels in the spinal cord and brainstem. The motor cortex usually shows no inflammation but may contain microglial nodules, which are focal collections of microglia and lymphocytes. Sections of spinal cord in cases of healed poliomyelitis show loss of neurons, with secondary degeneration of corresponding ventral roots and peripheral nerves.

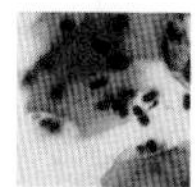

CLINICAL FEATURES: Nonspecific symptoms, such as fever, malaise, and headache, are followed in several days by signs of meningitis and then by paralysis.

Improvement begins in about a week, and only some of the muscles affected at the outset may remain permanently paralyzed. Mortality is 5% to 25%, with death usually caused by respiratory failure. Development of effective vaccines in the 1950s has largely eliminated polio in most of the world.

Rabies

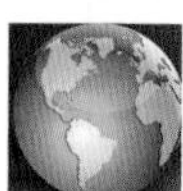

EPIDEMIOLOGY: Rabies is an encephalitis caused by a, single-stranded RNA virus of the rhabdovirus group. Dogs, wolves, foxes, and skunks are the main reservoirs, but bats and domestic animals, including

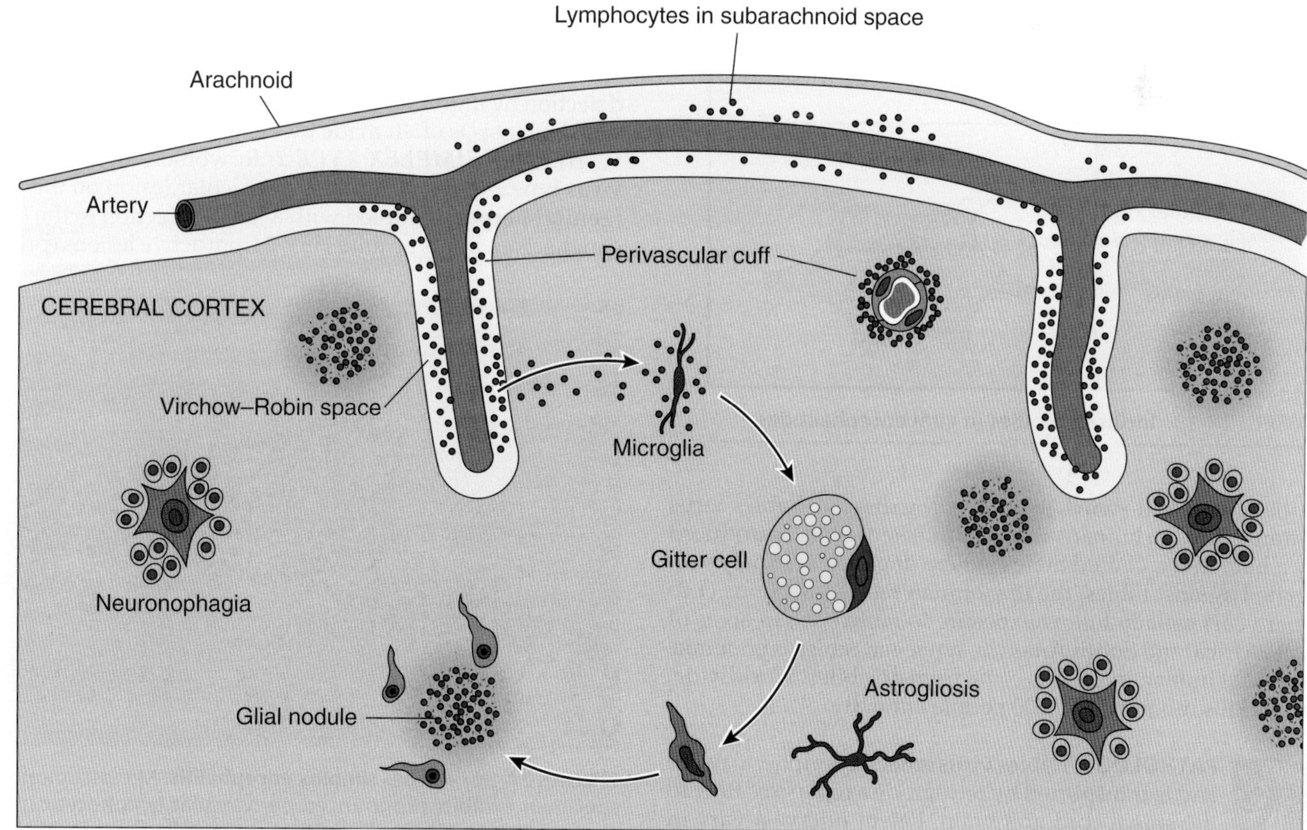

FIGURE 24-32. The lesions of viral encephalitis.

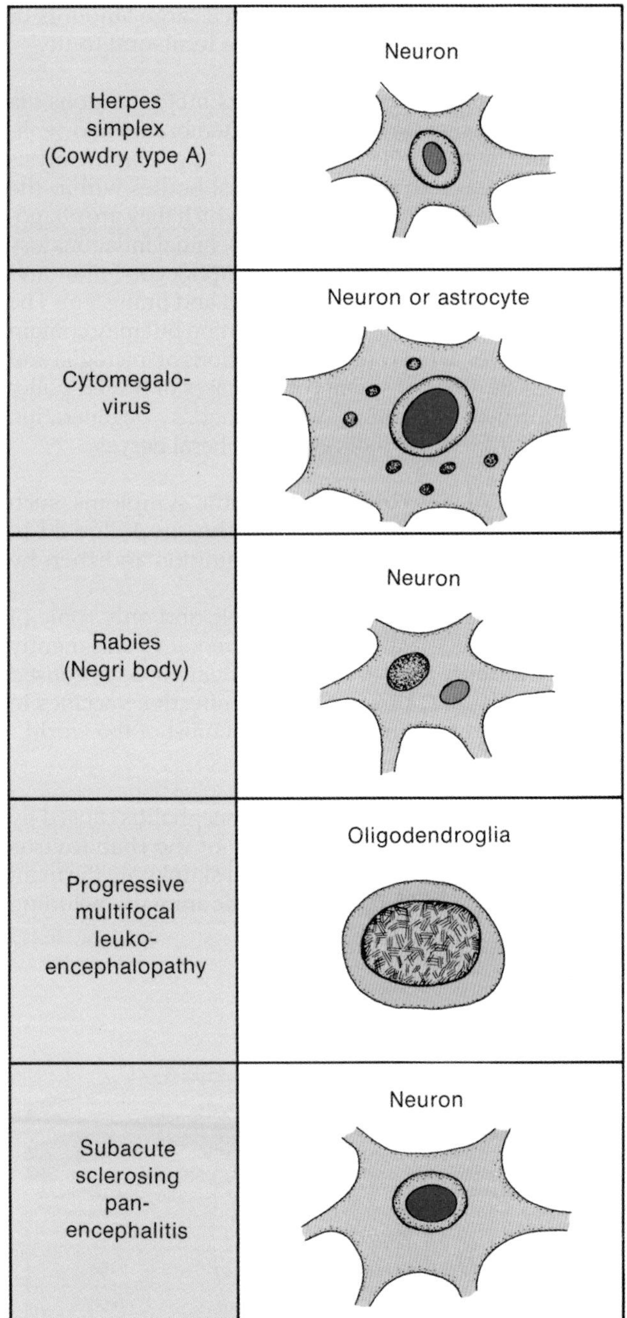

FIGURE 24-33. Inclusion bodies in viral encephalitides.

cattle, goats, and swine, also carry the disease. Rabies virus is transmitted to humans via contaminated saliva, introduced by a bite. In the United States, where dogs are routinely vaccinated against rabies, the few human rabies infections (1 to 5 per year) usually follow exposure to rabid bats. In areas of Asia, Africa, and South America, however, rabies is endemic, and most human infections come from dog bites. Worldwide, rabies kills more than 50,000 people annually.

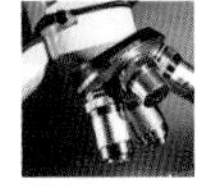

PATHOLOGY: Rabies virus enters a peripheral nerve and is transported by retrograde axoplasmic flow to the spinal cord and brain. Latent intervals vary in proportion to the distance of transport, from 10 days to as long as 3 months.

Perivascular lymphocytes, scattered neurons with chromatolysis and neuronophagia, and microglial nodules are seen. Inflammation is mainly in the brainstem and affects the cerebellum and hypothalamus. Eosinophilic cytoplasmic viral inclusion bodies in the hippocampus, brainstem, and cerebellar Purkinje cells (**Negri bodies**) confirm the diagnosis (Fig. 24-33).

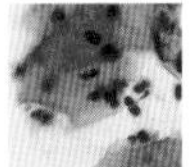

CLINICAL FEATURES: Destruction of brainstem neurons by rabies virus initiates painful spasms of the throat, difficulty swallowing, and a tendency to aspirate fluids (which prompted the original name, "hydrophobia"). Clinical symptoms also reflect a general encephalopathy, with irritability, agitation, seizures, and delirium. In up to 15% of cases, rabies may present in the paralytic form resembling Guillain–Barré syndrome rather than the encephalopathic form. Once symptoms develop, the illness relentlessly progresses to death within one to several weeks. Urgent rabies vaccination and hyperimmune globulin are administered for postexposure prophylaxis.

Herpes Viruses

Herpes viruses include herpes simplex (types 1 and 2), varicella-zoster virus, cytomegalovirus (CMV), Epstein–Barr virus (EBV), and simian B virus.

HERPES SIMPLEX TYPE 1: Reactivation and spread of HSV-1 to the CNS results in herpes encephalitis, which is the most common sporadic (i.e., nonepidemic) viral encephalitis.

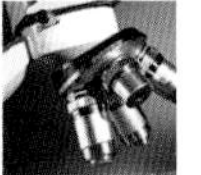

PATHOLOGY: Herpes encephalitis is a fulminant infection that localizes mainly in one or both temporal lobes. The temporal lobes become swollen, hemorrhagic, and necrotic. Inflammation is mainly lymphocytic, with perivascular cuffing (Fig. 24-34). The small arteries and arterioles become hemorrhagic and edematous. Intranuclear eosinophilic inclusions, usually surrounded by a halo (Cowdry A), occur in neurons and glial cells (Fig. 24-35). Viral protein detection by immunohistochemistry is diagnostically reliable. The diagnosis is often made by PCR of CSF and viral culture.

HERPES SIMPLEX TYPE 2: In women, herpes simplex virus type 2 (HSV-2) initiates a vesicular lesion on the vulva (**genital herpes**), coupled with a latent infection in the pelvic ganglia. Newborns acquire HSV-2 from active lesions (primary

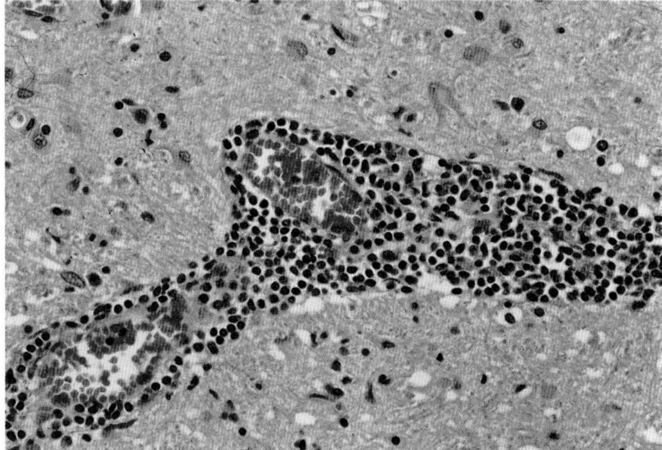

FIGURE 24-34. Herpes simplex encephalitis. Microscopically, the specimen exhibits pronounced perivascular lymphocytic inflammation. This finding indicates that active inflammation is present but is not etiologically specific.

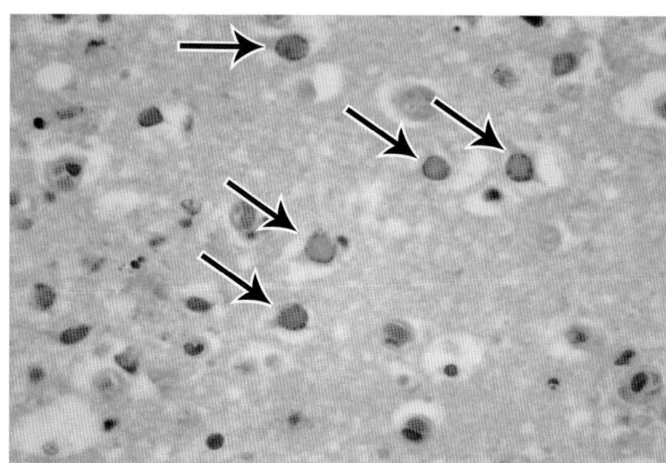

FIGURE 24-35. Herpes simplex encephalitis. The infected neurons display intranuclear, eosinophilic viral inclusions (Cowdry A inclusions) that fill the nuclei (*arrows*). The presence of these findings is extremely valuable in guiding diagnostic evaluation because a limited number of viruses produce Cowdry A inclusions.

or recurrent) as they pass through the birth canal. Thereafter, they may develop fulminant encephalitis with extensive liquefactive necrosis in the cerebrum and cerebellum.

CYTOMEGALOVIRUS: CMV crosses the placenta to induce encephalitis in utero. Lesions in the embryonic CNS are characterized by periventricular necrosis and calcification. Because of the proximity of these lesions to the third ventricle and the aqueduct, they may cause obstructive hydrocephalus. In adults, CMV encephalitis occurs in immunocompromised hosts. Eosinophilic nuclear and cytoplasmic viral inclusions are present in astrocytes and neurons, most conspicuously in enlarged nuclei, where they are sharply defined and surrounded by a halo (Fig. 24-33).

Arthropod-Borne Viral Encephalitis

EPIDEMIOLOGY: Arthropod-borne viruses, or **arboviruses**, are transmitted between vertebrates by blood-sucking vectors (e.g., mosquitoes and ticks). The Togaviridae, Bunyaviridae, and Flaviviridae include most of the arboviruses that cause human encephalitis. Arbovirus infections are zoonoses of animals; humans are infected when bitten by virus-harboring arthropods. Humans are not generally reservoirs, nor do they continue viral propagation. The various encephalitides caused by arboviruses are named principally for the location where they were first noted (Table 24-1), for example, Eastern, Western, and Venezuelan equine encephalitis; St. Louis encephalitis; Japanese B encephalitis; California encephalitis; and West Nile encephalitis. The last has numerically eclipsed all other arbovirus encephalitides in the United States since it first appeared in 1999. West Nile encephalitis epidemics continue to occur, underscoring the importance of mosquito control. Most cases of West Nile infection are asymptomatic, so most infections are unrecognized. Because infection can be transmitted by blood transfusion, it is now necessary to screen blood for West Nile virus. Recently, maternal infection during pregnancy with Zika virus, an arbovirus member of the Flaviviridae family, has been associated with congenital malformations of the developing fetal brain especially microcephaly. Diffuse white and gray matter involvement, accompanied by dystrophic calcification and gliosis, results from neurotropic viral infection.

Table 24-1

Insect-Borne Viral Encephalitis

Virus	Insect Vector	Distribution
St. Louis encephalitis	Mosquito	North and South America
Western equine encephalitis	Mosquito	North and South America
Venezuelan equine encephalitis	Mosquito	North and South America
Eastern equine encephalitis	Mosquito	North America
California encephalitis	Mosquito	North America
Murray Valley encephalitis	Mosquito	Australia, New Papua
Japanese B encephalitis	Mosquito	Eastern and southeastern Asia
Tick-borne encephalitis	Tick	Eastern Europe, Scandinavia
West Nile encephalitis	Mosquito	Global

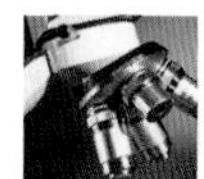

PATHOLOGY: The lesions of the several arbovirus encephalitides resemble each other and vary from mild meningitis with scattered lymphocytes to severe inflammation of gray matter, thrombosis of small blood vessels, and prominent necrosis. There are no inclusions in infected neurons. In necrotic foci, neuronophagia is evident, and if the patient survives, demyelination and gliosis often develop. West Nile encephalitis has a tropism for the spinal cord and may produce a syndrome clinically indistinguishable from classic poliomyelitis.

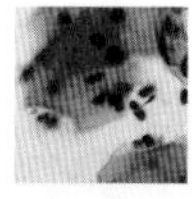

CLINICAL FEATURES: Arthropod-borne encephalitides share many features, but each has a different course. For example, Eastern equine encephalitis is commonly a more fulminant potentially lethal disease, but Venezuelan equine encephalitis tends to pursue a more benign course. Mild cases of arbovirus encephalitis may entail only a flu-like syndrome and may not be diagnosed as encephalitis. In more severe cases, the onset is abrupt, often with high fever, headache, vomiting, and meningeal signs, followed by lethargy and coma. Death is more likely at the extremes of age, and those who survive may be left with cognitive impairment and seizures. As noted above, congenital malformations of the CNS are associated with Zika virus infection during pregnancy.

Subacute Sclerosing Panencephalitis

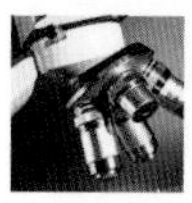

PATHOLOGY: SSPE is a consequence of infection with the measles virus, and most patients have a history of measles. The disease develops 6 to 8 years after the initial infection and is caused by a measles virus with defective expression of viral M (Matrix) protein. Nuclear inclusions that are basophilic and rimmed by a prominent halo occur in neurons and oligodendroglia. Marked gliosis affects gray and white matter, accompanied by patchy loss of myelin and ubiquitous perivascular lymphocytes and macrophages. Intranuclear inclusions occur in neurons and oligodendroglia. Affected neurons may have neurofibrillary tangles.

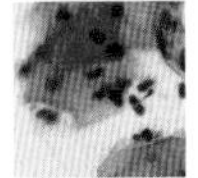

CLINICAL FEATURES: SSPE is a chronic viral infection of the brain that has an insidious onset, mainly in childhood, with cognitive and behavioral decline over months to years, ultimately leading to death. The CSF typically has increased antibodies to measles virus. The course is protracted, and inflammation occurs mainly in cerebral gray matter. In adults, SSPE may follow a more rapid course.

Progressive Multifocal Leukoencephalopathy

PML is an increasingly common, infectious, demyelinating disease. It is caused by a ubiquitous polyoma virus that infects oligodendrocytes and leads to cytolysis and patchy multifocal demyelination. Astrocytes are also infected, but instead of dying, they show extreme pleomorphism.

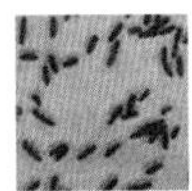

ETIOLOGIC FACTORS: JC virus is a polyoma virus, closely related to simian virus 40 (SV40). Over 50% of people harbor JC virus, which resides in a latent state in the bone marrow after asymptomatic acquisition earlier in life. If the host becomes immunosuppressed, viremia ensues with specific neurovirulent viral strains.

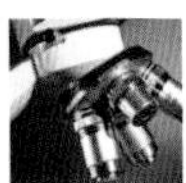

PATHOLOGY: Lesions typical of PML appear as widely scattered discrete foci of demyelination near the gray–white junction in the cerebral hemispheres and brainstem (Figs. 24-36 and 24-37). They are several millimeters in diameter and spherical, with a central area largely devoid of myelin. Axons are retained, a few oligodendrocytes are seen, and the lesion is infiltrated by macrophages. At the edge of the demyelinated area, there are oligodendrocytes with enlarged nuclei that display hyperchromatic, "ground-glass" inclusions lacking a halo.

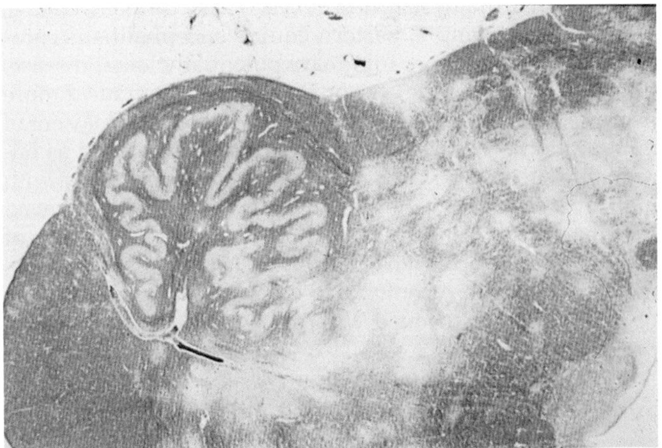

FIGURE 24-36. Progressive multifocal leukoencephalopathy. A Luxol fast blue stain of the medulla reveals severe patchy loss of myelin.

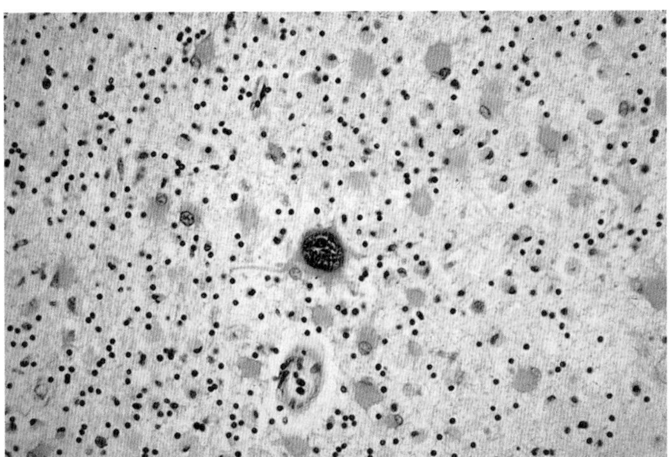

FIGURE 24-37. Progressive multifocal leukoencephalopathy (PML). A bizarre astrocyte is present (*center*) and may mimic neoplasia. The presence of macrophages and ground-glass inclusions should direct diagnostic consideration away from neoplasia and toward PML.

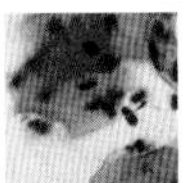

CLINICAL FEATURES: PML occurs mostly in immunocompromised patients and manifests as dementia, weakness, visual loss, and ataxia, usually leading to death within 6 months. It is a terminal complication in immunosuppressed patients, such as those treated for cancer or lupus erythematosus, organ transplant recipients, and especially people with AIDS. PML may complicate the use of drugs that inhibit T-cell adherence to endothelial cells as a treatment of immunologic disorders.

Human Immunodeficiency Virus

There are many opportunistic nervous system infections that may complicate AIDS, and it is important to remember that the clinical presentation may be more fulminant or atypical than in immunocompetent individuals.

HIV Encephalopathy

Many AIDS patients have diffuse encephalopathy directly attributable to active CNS infection by HIV-1 retrovirus itself. This is variously called HIV encephalopathy (HIVE) or HIV-associated neurologic disease (HAND). CNS macrophages and microglial cells are productively infected by HIV-1. Although infection of neurons and astrocytes is probably not clinically significant, these cells are injured indirectly by neurotoxic viral proteins produced by infected cells or various cytokines that cause oxidant-mediated cell injury. Frank dementia has become less common, but a combination of sensory, motor, and other defects causing minor cognitive motor disease (MCMD) affects as many as 30% of HIV-1–positive patients.

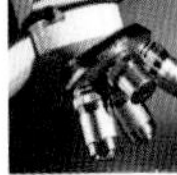

PATHOLOGY: HAND is characterized by mild cerebral atrophy, dilation of the lateral ventricles, and slight prominence of gyri and sulci. Histologic changes are usually in the subcortical gray and white matter. Multinucleated giant cells of monocyte/macrophage lineage are associated with microglial nodules (Fig. 24-38). In addition, myelin pallor, reflecting diffuse

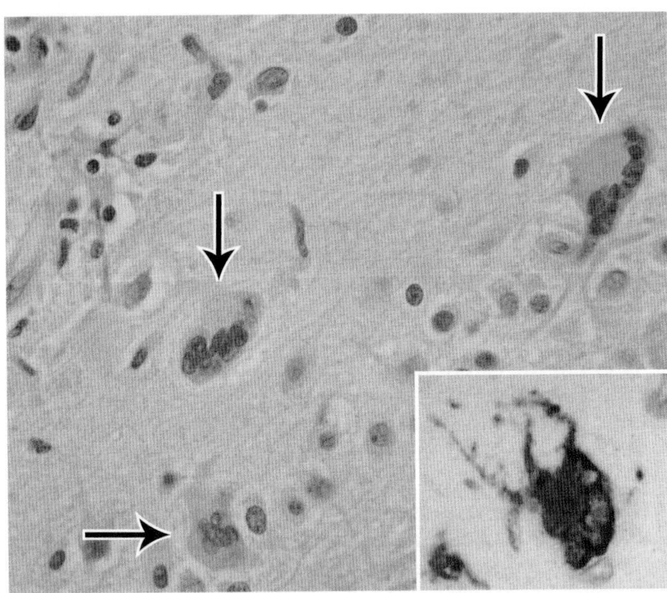

FIGURE 24-38. **HIV encephalitis or encephalopathy.** Multinucleated giant cells (*arrows*) often in a perivascular location are characteristic of HIV encephalitis. *Inset.* Immunohistochemical stain for HIV anti-p24.

demyelination, intense astrogliosis, and loss of neurons, is common (Fig. 24-39).

Protozoan and Metazoan Parasites

Protozoan Infections

- **Toxoplasmosis** is a ubiquitous protozoan to which most persons have protective immunity. However, immunocompromised patients lose the ability to contain these organisms. Small comma-like tachyzoites and large polyorganismal cysts (bradyzoites) are seen in association with chronic inflammation, tissue necrosis, and vasculitis. Toxoplasmosis is the most common cause of multiple intracranial masses in AIDS patients (Fig. 24-40).
- ***Naegleria* spp.,** especially *Naegleria fowleri*, cause primary amebic meningoencephalitis, a fulminant, and rapidly fatal disease with diffuse brain swelling. The ameba infects the nasal cavities of people who swim in stagnant warm freshwater ponds or who irrigate their sinus passages with inadequately decontaminated water. The organisms enter the brain by migrating up the olfactory bulb, through the cribriform plate. *Naegleria* trophozoites resemble macrophages.
- ***Acanthamoeba*** produces granulomatous amebic encephalitis, a subacute, usually fatal illness characterized by multiple granulomatous abscesses. This condition is usually seen in immunocompromised hosts.
- ***Entamoeba histolytica*** leads to amebic brain abscess by spread from a gastrointestinal or hepatic locus. Amebae in tissue sections can be difficult to distinguish from foamy macrophages.
- **CNS malaria** is most commonly caused by *Plasmodium falciparum*. During attacks of cerebral malaria, the CSF

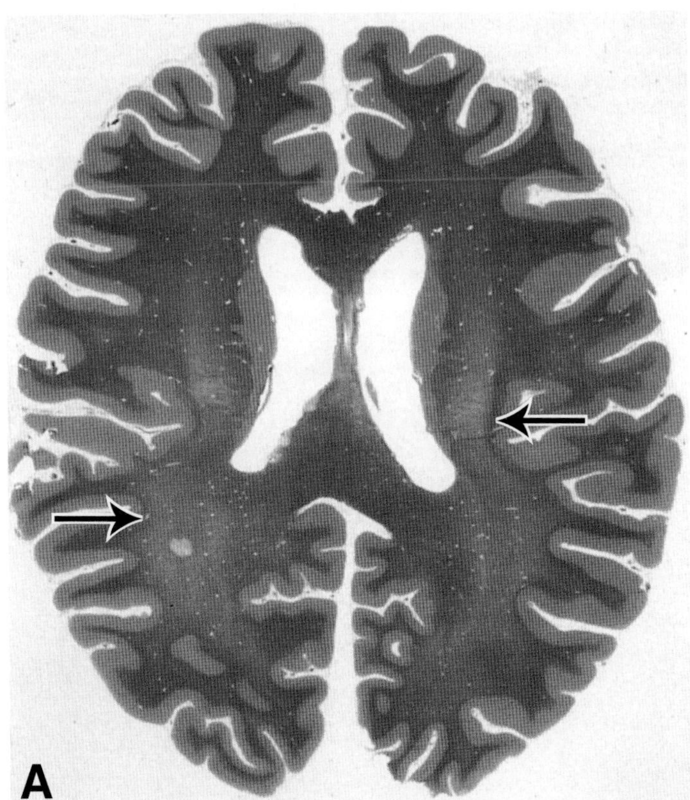

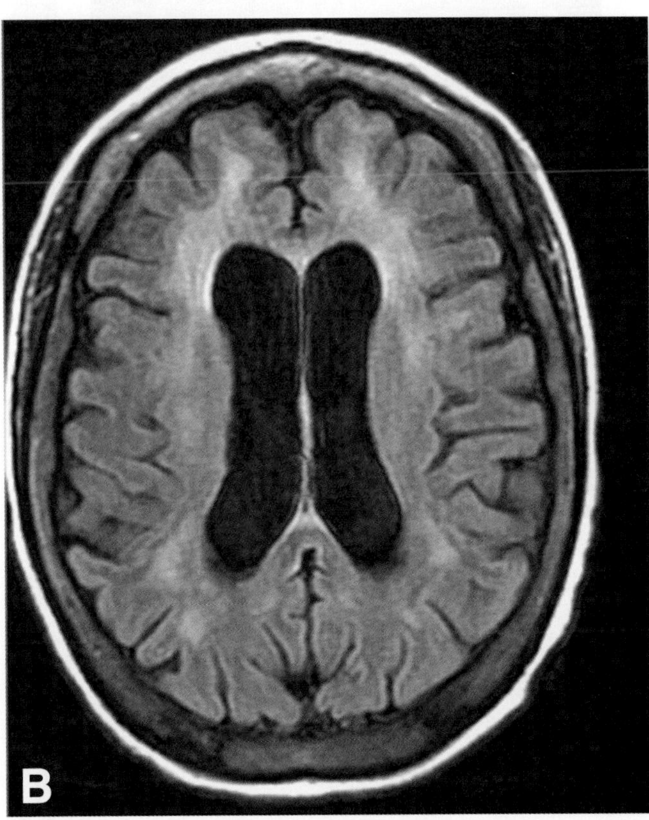

FIGURE 24-39. **HIV encephalitis or encephalopathy (HIVE). A.** An axial whole brain section in HIVE showing symmetric myelin pallor (*arrows*) caused by HIV-1. Demyelination caused by progressive multifocal leukoencephalopathy (PML) would be less symmetric and patchy. **B.** Axial magnetic resonance image showing bilateral white matter signal abnormalities in HIVE. The primary differential diagnosis is HIVE versus PML. (39A Courtesy of Dr. F. Stephen Vogel, Duke University.)

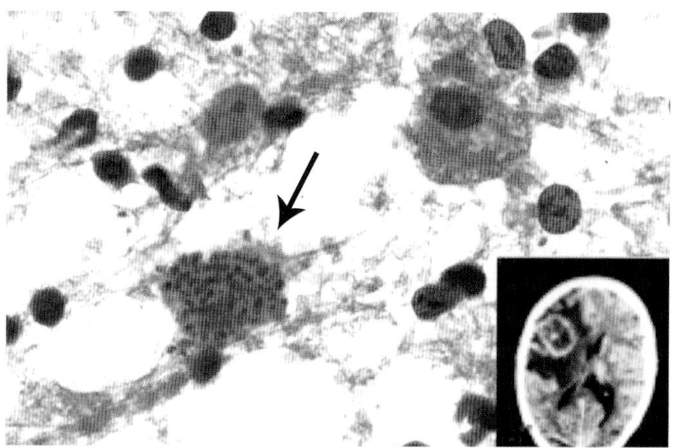

FIGURE 24-40. Toxoplasmosis in an HIV patient. This previously asymptomatic patient presented with an irregularly enhancing mass with surrounding edema that was initially thought to be a high-grade neoplasm. *Toxoplasma gondii* bradyzoites (*arrow*) are present in a necrotic inflammatory background. Toxoplasmosis is the most common mass lesion in patients with AIDS and is an indicator disease of HIV infection. Inset shows radiographic appearance of intracranial mass associated with toxoplasmosis infection.

shows elevated protein and high pressure. In fatal cases, the brain is diffusely swollen and may be otherwise unremarkable. However, one may see microinfarcts with gliosis (Dürck granulomas) in white matter or many small hemorrhages.

- **Trypanosomal infections** of the CNS include African sleeping sickness and American trypanosomiasis (Chagas disease). Insect vectors transmit the disease. A meningoencephalitis may occur during the primary phase of infection.
- **Metazoan infections** set as Protozoan infections above.
- **Cysticercosis** caused by infection by *Taenia solium*, the pig tapeworm, may lead to multiple parasitic cysts up to 1 cm in the cerebral parenchyma, intraventricularly or in the basal cisternae. The intraparenchymal disease usually becomes symptomatic when the organism dies and is recognized immunologically by the host (Fig. 24-41). Treatment of neurocysticercosis may result in massive cerebral edema caused by host immune responses to the suddenly necrotic metazoan tissue. From a global health perspective, neurocysticercosis is one of the most common causes of epilepsy and intracranial mass lesions.
- **Echinococcosis** results from *Taenia echinococcus* or *Echinococcus granulosus*, the dog tapeworm, and produces cerebral cysts. The cysts are usually solitary and may be huge, in

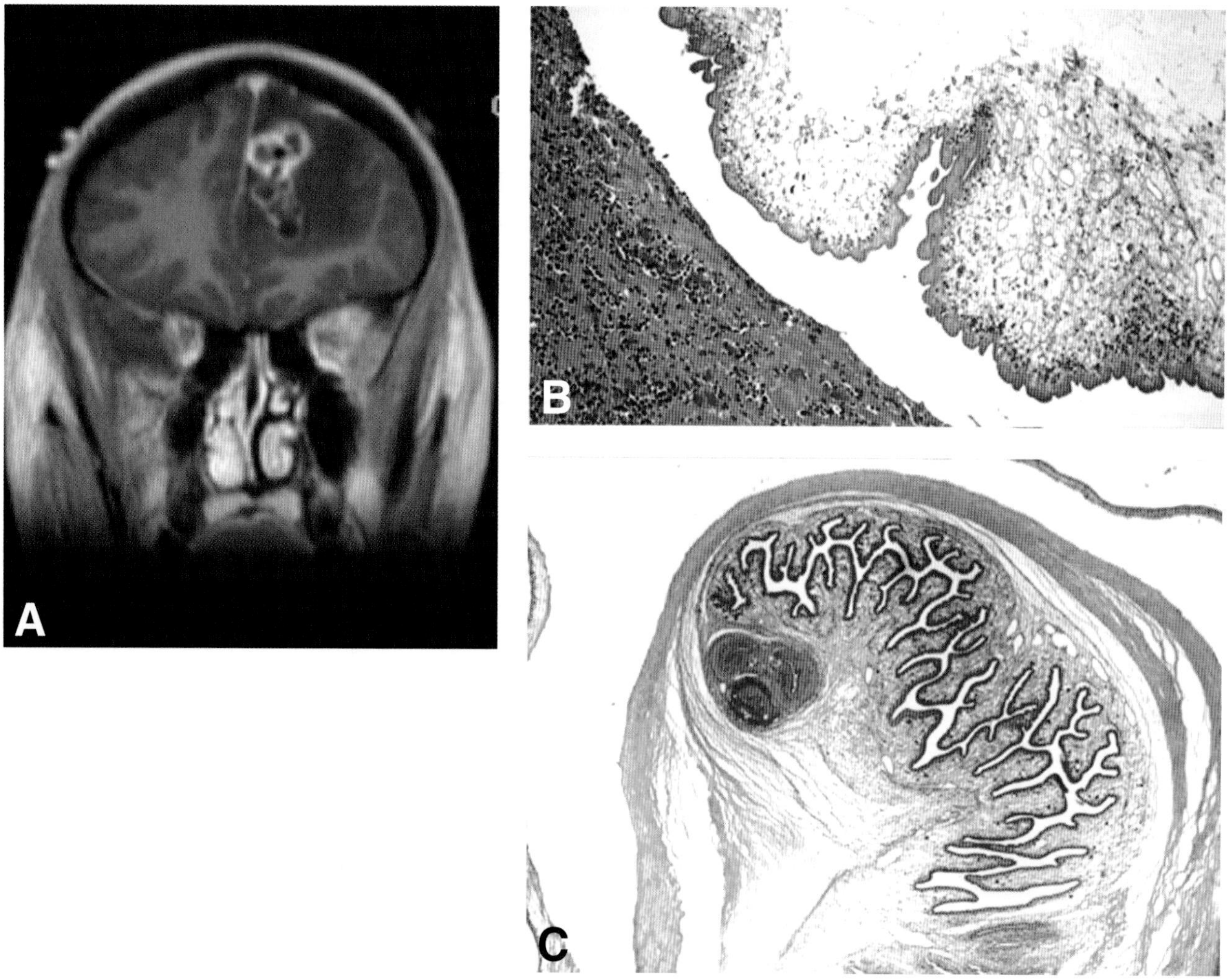

FIGURE 24-41. Neurocysticercosis. A. Radiographic appearance. Brain involvement by *Taenia solium* may result in solitary or multiple contrast-enhancing masses with surrounding edema. **B.** As the parasite begins to die and is detected by the host immune response, the lesions may become symptomatic. The corrugated cuticular surface forms an eosinophilic interface with inflamed adjacent brain. **C.** At low magnification, the worm scolex and gastrointestinal tract can sometimes be seen.

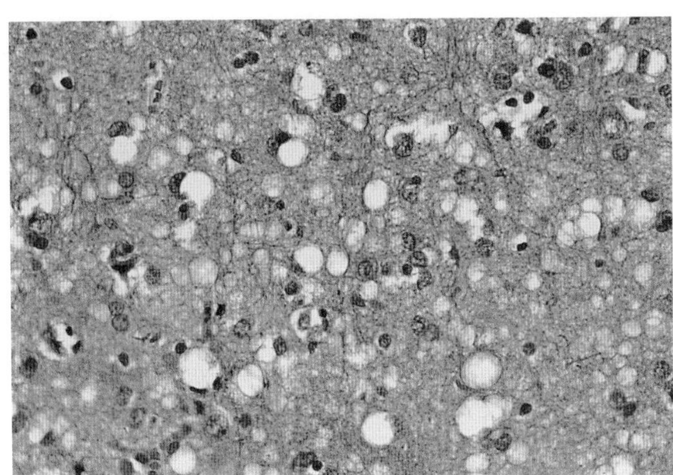

FIGURE 24-42. Creutzfeldt–Jakob disease. Spongiform degeneration of the gray matter is characterized by individual and clustered vacuoles, with no evidence of inflammation. (Courtesy of Dr. F. Stephen Vogel, Duke University.)

contrast to the smaller multiple cysts of cysticercosis. The brain lesion is frequently accompanied by hepatic cysts.

- **Trichinosis (Trichinellosis)** is caused by *Trichinella spiralis* infection of skeletal and cardiac muscle, producing an acute eosinophilic myositis during the invasive phase. Larvae may then die and calcify, resulting in fibrosis and low-grade inflammation. On rare occasions, infection encroaches on the CNS, producing lymphocytic–eosinophilic aseptic meningitis.

Prion Diseases (Spongiform Encephalopathies)

Prion diseases are characterized clinically by rapidly progressive ataxia and dementia. Pathologically, they feature (1) accumulations of fibrillar or insoluble prion proteins, (2) neuronal degeneration, and (3) vacuolization called **spongiform encephalopathy** (Fig. 24-42). The spongiform encephalopathies are biologically remarkable because the causative infectious agents, called **prions** (proteinaceous infectious particles), lack nucleic acids.

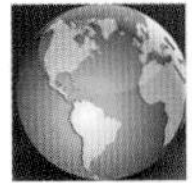

EPIDEMIOLOGY: The classic spongiform encephalopathies in humans include kuru, Creutzfeldt–Jakob disease (CJD), Gerstmann–Sträussler–Scheinker (GSS) syndrome, and fatal familial insomnia (Table 24-2). Similar diseases occur in animals, including scrapie in sheep and goats, bovine spongiform encephalopathy (BSE; mad cow disease), transmissible mink encephalopathy, and chronic wasting disease in mule deer and elk. BSE is of particular interest because it resulted from inadvertent introduction of prion-contaminated feed to cattle, thereby establishing that prions can be transmitted by the oral route. It decimated the cattle industry in the United Kingdom and spread to other regions of the world and to other species, including zoo animals, pets, and humans.

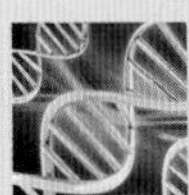

MOLECULAR PATHOGENESIS: The signal molecular event in prion disorders is conversion of a native α-helix–rich protein into a pathogenic β-sheet–rich isoform that tends to polymerize with subsequent fibril formation (Fig. 24-43). Uniquely, conversion of the native protein to the pathogenic form is autocatalyzed by the latter itself. The pathogenic protein forms more of the same from the limitless supply of native protein. The normal protein is coded by a human prion gene (*PRNP*) on the short arm of chromosome 20. The normal gene product, prion protein (PrP), is a constitutively expressed cell surface glycoprotein that binds neuronal plasmalemma via a glycolipid anchor. PrP is made widely throughout the body, but the highest levels of PrP mRNA are in CNS neurons. Its function is unknown. Defects produced by ablation of the gene in transgenic animal, if any, are subtle. The normal cellular prion protein, cellular PrP or PrP^{C}, and the pathogenic (infectious) prion protein, known as scrapie PrP or PrP^{SC}, have the same primary amino acid sequence but

Table 24-2

Prion Diseases

- **I. Human**
  - A. Creutzfeldt–Jakob disease (CJD)
    - 1. Sporadic (85% of all CJD cases; incidence 1 per million worldwide)
    - 2. Inherited mutation of the prion gene, autosomal dominant transmission (15% of all CJD cases)
    - 3. Iatrogenic
      - a. Hormone injection: human growth hormone, human pituitary gonadotropin
      - b. Tissue grafts: dura mater, cornea, pericardium
      - c. Medical devices: depth electrodes, surgical instruments (none definitely proven)
    - 4. New variant CJD
  - B. Gerstmann–Sträussler–Scheinker disease (inherited prion gene mutation, autosomal dominant transmission)
  - C. Fatal familial insomnia (inherited prion gene mutation, autosomal dominant transmission)
  - D. Kuru (confined to the Fore people of Papua New Guinea, formerly transmitted by cannibalistic funeral ritual)
- **II. Animal**
  - A. Scrapie (sheep and goats)
  - B. Bovine spongiform encephalopathy ("mad cow disease")
  - C. Transmissible mink encephalopathy
  - D. Feline spongiform encephalopathy
  - E. Captive exotic ungulate spongiform encephalopathy (nyala, gemsbok, eland, Arabian oryx, greater kudu)
  - F. Chronic wasting disease of deer and elk
  - G. Experimental transmission to many species, including primates and transgenic mice

different tertiary structures and patterns of glycosylation. Specifically, PrP^C is rich in α-helix configuration, but the β-pleated sheet configuration predominates in PrP^{SC}. The pathogenic conformation is extremely stable, so that PrP^{SC} strongly resists conventional microbial decontamination methods. If PrP^{SC} enters the brain either through infectious transmission or by spontaneous misfolding of native protein, it changes other PrP^C proteins into pathogenic PrP^{SC}, leading to autocatalytic, exponentially expanding accretion of abnormal PrP^{SC}. The masses of PrP^{SC} compromise cell function and cause neurodegeneration by mechanisms that remain to be elucidated.

All spongiform encephalopathies are transmissible, and inadvertent human transmission of CJD may follow administration of contaminated human pituitary growth hormone, corneal transplantation from a diseased donor, poorly sterilized neurosurgical instruments, and surgical implantation of contaminated dura (Table 24-2).

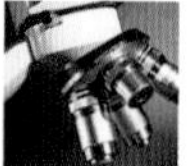

PATHOLOGY: Prion diseases entail neuronal degeneration, gliosis, spongiform degeneration, and accumulations of insoluble prions that form extracellular plaques. There are many small, clear, often confluent microcysts in the neuropil (Fig. 24-43). Lesions occur mostly in cortical gray matter, but also involve deeper nuclei of the basal ganglia, thalamus, hypothalamus, and cerebellum.

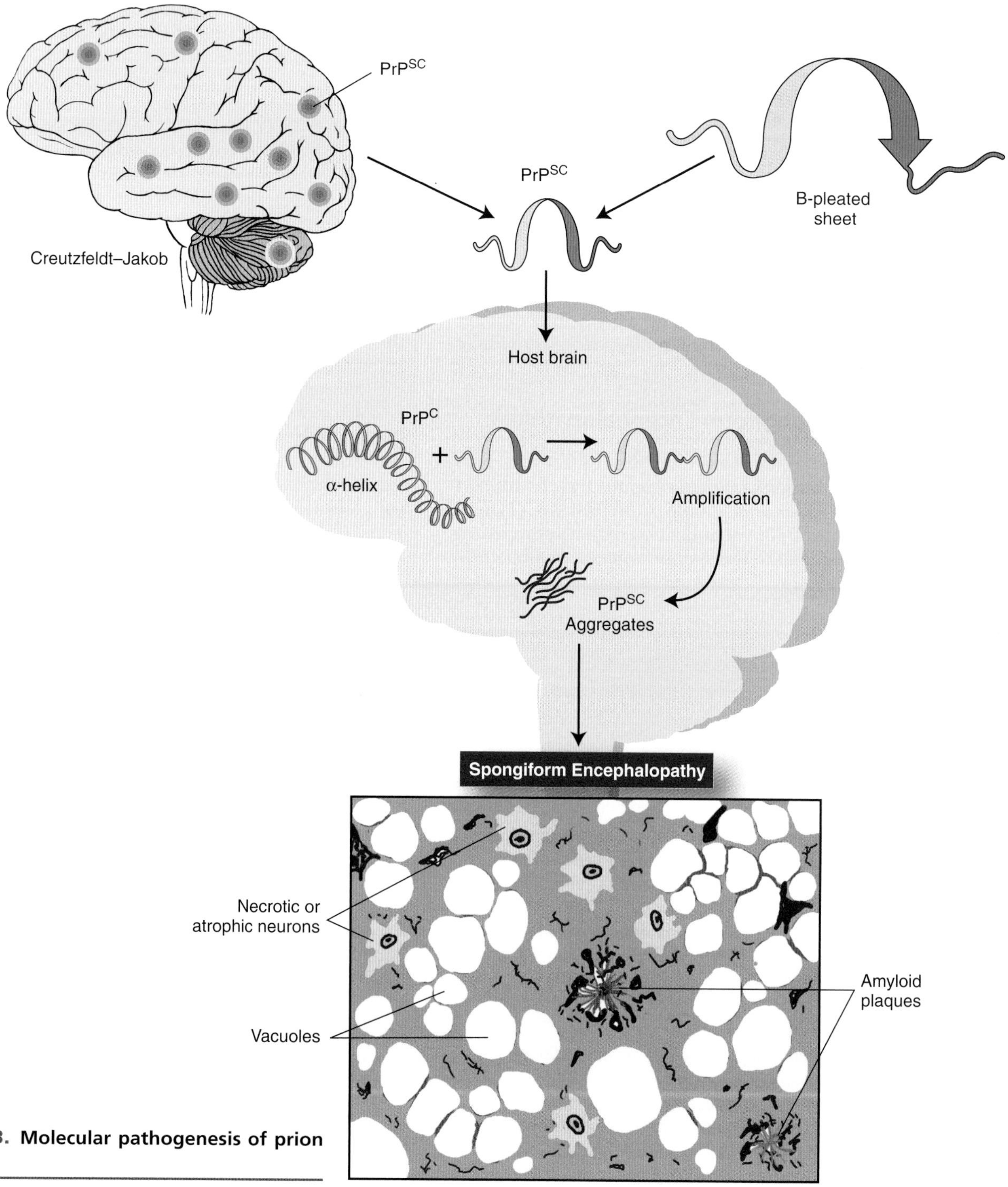

FIGURE 24-43. Molecular pathogenesis of prion disorders.

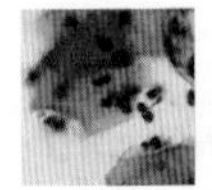

CLINICAL FEATURES:
KURU: Kuru was the first human prion disease shown to be transmissible. It attained epidemic proportions in the Fore people of New Guinea but was eliminated when cannibalism involving the brain ceased. The initial and most prominent clinical feature of kuru is ataxia of the limbs and trunk, as a result of severe cerebellar involvement. In 70% of cases, insoluble, fibrillar prion proteins accumulate extracellularly in plaques. Spongiform change is present in both the cerebral hemispheres and cerebellum.

CREUTZFELDT–JAKOB DISEASE: CJD is the most common form of spongiform encephalopathy. Symptoms begin insidiously, but usually within 6 months to 3 years, patients exhibit severe dementia, leading to death. Cerebellar involvement produces ataxia, which helps to distinguish CJD from Alzheimer disease. Myoclonus often occurs for some weeks to months during the afflicted person's decline. CJD is classified based on etiology: sporadic, familial, iatrogenic, and new variant:

- **Sporadic CJD:** The sporadic form occurs worldwide, with an incidence of one per million, and accounts for 75% of cases. The mode of acquisition is unknown; patients do not have the mutations associated with inherited forms of CJD or other prion diseases, and there is no history of iatrogenic exposure. A polymorphism in PRNP codon 129 confers differential susceptibility to CJD: homozygosity for either methionine (M) or valine (V) at this codon leads to disproportionate susceptibility to prion disorders, whereas heterozygotes (M/V) are resistant. Codon frequencies for the white population are 51% M/V, 37% M/M, and 12% V/V.
- **Inherited CJD: Familial CJD** accounts for 15% of prion diseases, with an incidence of 1 in 10 million. Several different PRNP mutations are documented in various kindreds. In those cases, PrP^C has a greater tendency to misfold into the pathogenic isoform. The mutated PRNP causes familial CJD, fatal familial insomnia, and Gerstmann–Sträussler–Scheinker disease.
- **Iatrogenic CJD:** As listed in Table 24-2, several iatrogenic causes of CJD are known, but most agents now have been eliminated. Conventional autoclaving and most standard disinfectants do not eradicate this hardy infectious agent.
- **New variant CJD (vCJD or nvCJD):** This form was identified by a surveillance program in the United Kingdom after the BSE epidemic (see above) between 1980 and 1996. The mean age at the onset of symptoms for sporadic CJD is 65 years, but for vCJD, it is 26. Also, vCJD patients had a longer duration of illness (median, 12 months vs. 4 months) and an atypical clinical presentation, including various behavioral changes or sensory disturbances (dysesthesias) and none of the usual electroencephalographic (EEG) findings of sporadic CJD. At autopsy, vCJD is characterized by prominent spongiform change in the basal ganglia and thalamus, and extensive PrP plaques in the cerebrum and cerebellum. The plaques are distinctive in that they resemble those of kuru. Finally, brains from vCJD patients contain much more PrP than do brains of sporadic CJD patients. Bovine spongiform encephalopathy is considered to be the source of nvCJD. Current evidence suggests that the incidence of vCJD cases has peaked and is now declining. In all, 231 cases have been reported through 2016. Of these, four cases have occurred in the United States with evidence suggesting infection occurred elsewhere (the Middle East and United Kingdom).

DEMYELINATING DISEASES

Demyelinating diseases include flawed manufacture of myelin (**dysmyelination**), destruction of myelin (**demyelination**), or disruption of myelin metabolism (**leukodystrophies**). Central myelin is made by oligodendrocytes, whereas peripheral myelin is made by Schwann cells (see Chapter 23). These two types of myelin differ biochemically. Myelin disorders affect central or peripheral myelin or both.

Multiple Sclerosis

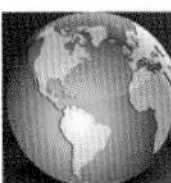

EPIDEMIOLOGY: MS is a chronic demyelinating disease. With a prevalence of 1 per 1,000, it is the most common chronic CNS disease of young adults in the United States. The disease is characterized by exacerbations and remissions over many years. It becomes symptomatic at a mean age of 30, and women are afflicted almost twice as often as men.

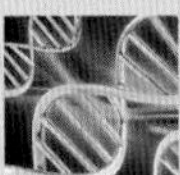

MOLECULAR PATHOGENESIS: The etiology of MS is obscure, but genetic predisposition and immune dysfunction are probably involved. MS is mainly a disease of temperate climates. People who emigrate before age 15 from areas with a low prevalence to more temperate endemic areas assume the increased risk associated with their destinations, suggesting that environmental factors are important.

There are familial aggregates of the disease, with increased risk in second- and third-degree relatives of MS patients, and 25% concordance for MS in monozygotic twins. Susceptibility is also linked to certain MHC alleles (HLA-DR2), implying that immune mechanisms are involved in the pathogenesis.

The microscopic appearance of MS also suggests immune involvement. For example, chronic MS lesions show perivascular lymphocytes, macrophages, and many $CD4^+$ and $CD8^+$ T cells. Although no target antigen is established, data suggest an immune response to a specific CNS protein.

An assortment of viruses has been implicated in the etiology of MS, but to date, there is no compelling evidence for the involvement of any infectious agent.

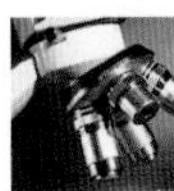

PATHOLOGY: The demyelinated plaque is the hallmark of MS (Fig. 24-44). Plaques, rarely more than 2 cm in diameter, accumulate in great numbers in the brain and spinal cord (Fig. 24-45). They are discrete, with smoothly rounded contours, and are usually in white matter, although they may breach the gray matter. The lesions preferentially affect the optic nerves, chiasm, paraventricular white matter, and spinal cord, but any part of the CNS may be involved.

Evolving plaques are marked by selective loss of myelin in regions of relative axonal preservation. Lymphocytes clustering about small veins and arteries with an influx of macrophages and considerable edema occurs.

Neuronal bodies within plaques are remarkably spared, but axons may degenerate. The number of oligodendrocytes is moderately decreased. As plaques age, they become more discrete and less edematous. This sequence emphasizes the focal nature of the injury and its selectivity and severity because demyelination is total within a plaque. Axons that

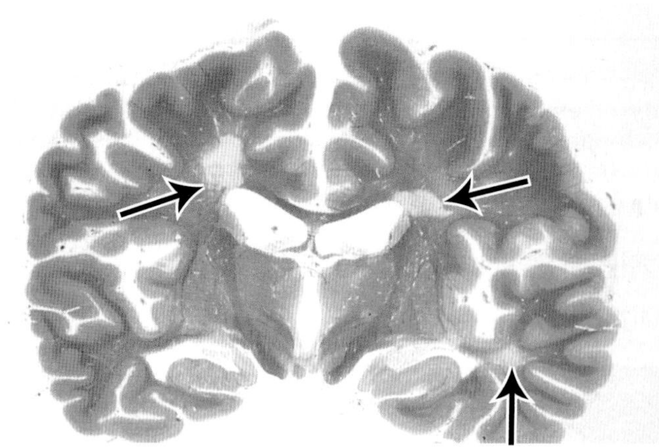

FIGURE 24-44. Multiple sclerosis. This myelin-stained coronal whole brain section of the brain of a patient with long-standing multiple sclerosis shows many areas of myelin loss—plaques (*arrows*)—with characteristic periventricular demyelination especially prominent at the superior angles of the lateral ventricles. (Courtesy of Dr. F. Stephen Vogel, Duke University.)

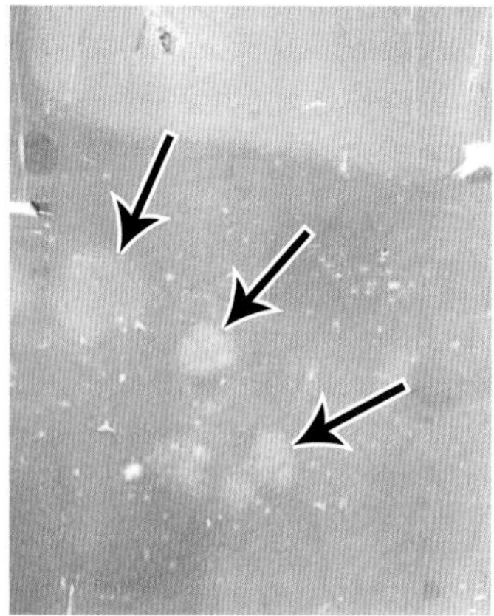

FIGURE 24-45. Multiple sclerosis. The subcortical white matter of a patient with multiple sclerosis shows multiple small irregular, partially confluent areas of demyelination (*arrows*). Normal intact myelin stains blue in this Luxol fast blue–stained section.

traverse the plaques tend to lose their myelin abruptly. Old MS plaques are dense and gliotic.

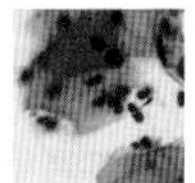

CLINICAL FEATURES: Most commonly, MS begins in the third or fourth decade, after which patients experience abrupt episodes of clinical progression, separated by periods of relative stability. The essential clinical criterion for MS is dissemination of lesions in space and time; that is, multiple separate areas of the CNS are affected at differing times. Serial MRI studies show ongoing disease activity despite apparent clinical quiescence. New plaques emerge and regress, only occasionally causing clinical manifestations. Contemporary diagnostic criteria for MS strongly incorporate periodic imaging to visualize plaques. Thus, the disease is an ongoing active process even between clinical exacerbations. The therapeutic focus is now suppression of ongoing disease activity using a variety of immune system modulators, such as β-interferon, and MRI efficacy is an endpoint in drug trials and clinical management.

Many patients with MS pursue a relapsing and remitting clinical course, but some suffer a relentless progression without remissions. MS typically begins with symptoms relating to lesions in the optic nerves, brainstem, or spinal cord. Blurred vision or loss of vision in one eye as a result of optic neuritis is often the presenting complaint. When the initial lesion is in the brainstem, double vision and vertigo occur. In particular, internuclear ophthalmoplegia, caused by disruption of the medial longitudinal fasciculus, strongly suggests demyelinating disease when it occurs in a young person. Acute demyelination within the spinal cord is called **transverse myelitis** and produces weakness of one or both legs and sensory symptoms in the form of numbness in the lower extremities. Many of the initial symptoms are partially reversible within a few months.

Despite the fact that most patients have a chronic relapsing and remitting course, neurologic deficits accumulate gradually and relentlessly. Even in relatively quiescent plaques, axonal attrition often leads to irreversible lesions. In established cases, the degree of functional impairment is highly variable, ranging from minor disability to severe incapacity, with widespread paralysis, dysarthria, ataxia, severe visual defects, incontinence, and dementia. The latter usually die of respiratory paralysis or urinary tract infections. Most patients survive 20 to 30 years after the onset of symptoms.

Neuromyelitis Optica

NMO is a demyelinating disorder with a striking predilection for the optic nerves and spinal cord. Once regarded as a variant of MS, NMO is now recognized as the action of autoantibodies against a water channel, aquaporin 4, and is thus quite distinct from MS. It responds poorly to conventional MS therapy.

Leukodystrophies

Leukodystrophies often impact both central and peripheral myelin and usually manifest in infancy or childhood, although milder adult phenotypes may occur. Disruption of central myelin gives rise to blindness, spasticity, and loss of developmental milestones, whereas loss of peripheral myelin results in weakness and loss of reflexes.

Metachromatic Leukodystrophy

Metachromatic leukodystrophy, the most common leukodystrophy, is an autosomal recessive disorder characterized by accumulation of a cerebroside (galactosyl sulfatide) in the white matter of the brain and peripheral nerves. The disorder most commonly occurs in infancy, although rare juvenile or adult cases are described. It is lethal within several years. A clinical trial using gene-corrected, bone marrow transplantation has shown promise in preventing MLD progression.

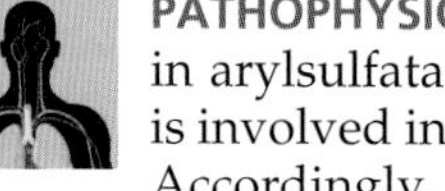

PATHOPHYSIOLOGY: MLD is caused by a deficiency in arylsulfatase A activity. This lysosomal enzyme is involved in the degradation of myelin sulfatides. Accordingly, there is progressive accumulation of sulfatides within the lysosomes of myelin-forming Schwann cells and oligodendrocytes.

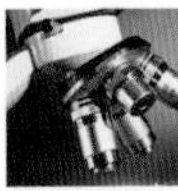

PATHOLOGY: In MLD, the accumulated sulfatides form cytoplasmic spherical granules, 15 to 20 μ in diameter, which stain metachromatically with cresyl violet and toluidine blue. Cresyl violet or toluidine blue ordinarily stains tissue violet or blue. In metachromasia, tissue stained with cresyl violet or toluidine blue looks rusty brown to red. The brain shows diffuse myelin loss, accumulation of metachromatic material in white matter, and astrogliosis. Demyelination of peripheral nerves is less severe.

Krabbe Disease (Globoid Cell Leukodystrophy)

Krabbe disease is a rapidly progressive, fatal, autosomal recessive neurologic disorder caused by a deficiency of galactocerebroside β-galactosidase.

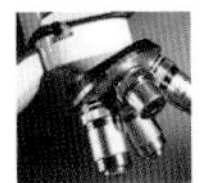

PATHOLOGY: The brain is small, with widespread loss of myelin and preservation of the cerebral cortex. Astrogliosis is severe. Multinucleated "globoid cells" develop in the white matter and cluster around blood vessels, leading to the alternative name, **globoid cell leukodystrophy**. The globoid cells are multinucleated macrophages full of undigested galactocerebroside (galactosylceramide). These cells are up to 50 μ in diameter, with up to 20 peripheral nuclei. In end-stage disease, the numbers of globoid cells decline, and in areas of severe myelin loss, only scattered globoid cells remain. Marbled areas of partial and total demyelination are present. By electron microscopy, the globoid cells contain crystalloid-like inclusions with straight or tubular profiles.

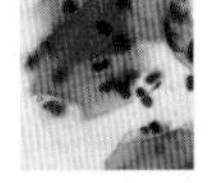

CLINICAL FEATURES: Krabbe disease appears in infancy and progresses to death within 1 to 2 years. Severe motor, sensory, and cognitive defects reflect diffuse involvement of the nervous system.

Adrenoleukodystrophy

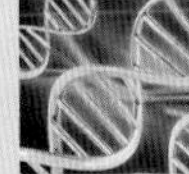

MOLECULAR PATHOGENESIS: ALD is an X-linked (Xq28) inherited disorder in which dysfunction of the adrenal cortex and nervous system demyelination are associated with high levels of saturated, very–long-chain fatty acids (VLCFAs) in tissue and body fluids. The enzyme mutation in ALD impairs degradation of VLCFAs by preventing normal activation of free VLCFAs by the addition of coenzyme A (CoA). The disease reflects accumulation of abnormal cholesterol esters and VLCFA toxicity.

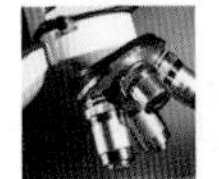

PATHOLOGY: In the brain, there is confluent, bilaterally symmetric demyelination. The most severe lesions are in the subcortical white matter of the parieto-occipital region, which then extend rostrally (while sparing cortex) to result in severe loss of myelinated axons and oligodendrocytes. Gliosis and perivascular infiltrates of mononuclear cells (mostly lymphocytes) are prominent in affected areas. Scattered macrophages contain PAS-positive and sudanophilic material. Peripheral nerves are affected, but to a lesser degree than is the brain. The adrenal glands are atrophic. Electron microscopy of cortical cells shows pathognomonic cytoplasmic, membrane-bound, curvilinear inclusions, or clefts (lamellae) containing VLCFAs. Similar inclusions occur in Schwann cells and CNS macrophages.

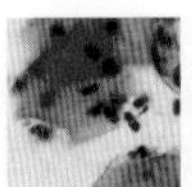

CLINICAL FEATURES: ALD occurs in children aged 3 to 10 years, in whom neurologic symptoms precede signs of adrenal insufficiency. The disease progresses rapidly for 2 to 4 years, and the patient is quickly reduced to a vegetative state, which may persist for several years before death. Allogeneic bone marrow transplantation and trial using genetically modified autologous bone marrow improve prognosis but are not curative.

TOXIC AND METABOLIC DISORDERS

Given the enormous appetite of the brain for oxygen, amino acids, and other metabolites, it is not surprising that the brain is subject to malfunction as a result of (1) lack or malutilization of essential substances, (2) intoxication, and (3) hereditary metabolic diseases. These disorders are particularly important because correction of underlying metabolic derangements restores function. In most cases, these dysfunctions may be functionally profound but have no morphologic correlate; however, in some instances, pathologic changes occur.

Metabolic Storage Diseases

Neuronal storage diseases are inherited enzyme defects in which normal metabolic products accumulate in lysosomes. Unlike leukodystrophies, which produce blindness and spasticity, these disorders affect neurons to cause seizures and cognitive decline (see also Chapter 5).

Tay–Sachs Disease

Tay–Sachs disease is a lethal, autosomal recessive disorder caused by deficiency of hexosaminidase A. Because a ganglioside accumulates in CNS neurons, the disease is fatal in infancy and early childhood. Retinal involvement increases macular transparency and causes a **cherry-red spot** in the macula.

The brain is the major site of ganglioside storage, and it progressively enlarges in infancy. Lipid droplets in the cytoplasm distend CNS and peripheral neurons (Fig. 24-46A). Electron microscopy demonstrates the lipid within lysosomes as whorled "myelin figures" (Fig. 24-46B). The neural tissues develop diffuse astrogliosis. An affected infant appears normal at birth but by age 6 months shows delayed motor development. Thereafter, progressive deterioration leads to flaccid weakness, blindness, and severe mental impairment. Death usually supervenes before the end of the second year.

Hurler Syndrome

Hurler syndrome is an autosomal recessive disturbance in glycosaminoglycan metabolism that results in intraneuronal accumulation of mucopolysaccharides. Clinical variants of this syndrome are distinguished by variable involvement of visceral organs and the nervous system. The disease is typically expressed in infancy or early childhood as reduced stature, corneal opacities, skeletal deformities, and hepatosplenomegaly. The intraneuronal storage distends the cytoplasmic compartment and is accompanied by astrogliosis and progressive mental deterioration.

Gaucher Disease

Gaucher disease is an autosomal recessive genetic deficiency of glucocerebrosidase, leading to glucocerebroside accumulation,

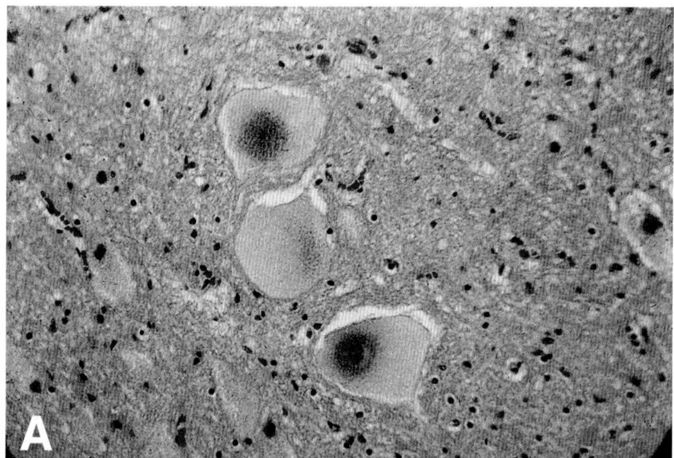

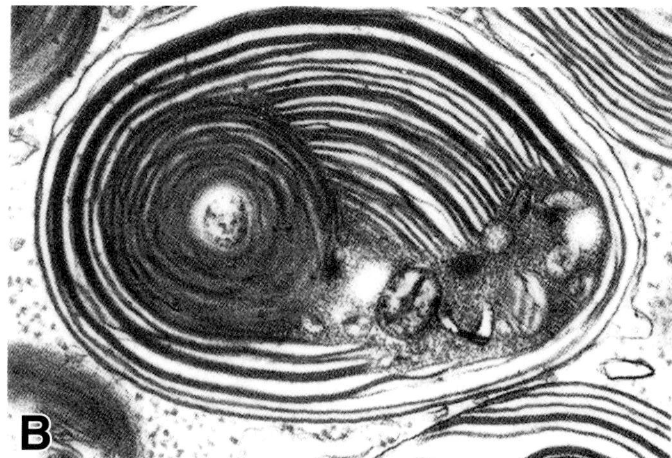

FIGURE 24-46. Tay–Sachs disease. A. The cytoplasm of the neurons is distended by the accumulation of eosinophilic storage material. **B.** Ultrastructurally, whorled "myelin bodies" composed of accumulated gangliosides are present within the cytoplasm.

principally in macrophages. The CNS is most severely involved in infantile (type II) Gaucher disease. Although intraneuronal accumulation of glucocerebroside is not conspicuous, neuronal loss is severe and is accompanied by diffuse astrogliosis. These infants fail to thrive and die at an early age.

Niemann–Pick Disease

Niemann–Pick disease is an autosomal recessive disorder in which a deficiency of sphingomyelinase results in intraneuronal storage of sphingomyelin. Symptoms occur early, with failure of the infant to develop and thrive. The mononuclear phagocyte system is targeted for storage, but the nervous system may predominate symptomatically during infancy. The brain becomes atrophic, with marked astrogliosis. Retinal degeneration may produce a cherry-red spot, like that in Tay–Sachs disease.

Wilson Disease

Wilson disease, or **hepatolenticular degeneration**, affects the brain and the liver and is caused by mutations of the *WD* gene (see Chapter 12). Defective excretion of copper in the bile gives rise to copper deposition in the brain.

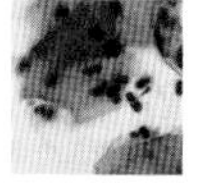

CLINICAL FEATURES: Symptoms of cerebral involvement appear as a movement disorder with a tendency to choreoathetosis, usually in the second decade, although the disease may not become apparent until as late as the eighth decade. The movement disorder may be associated with psychosis. Before, during, or after the appearance of neurologic symptoms, an insidiously developing cirrhosis may result in hepatic failure. Copper deposition in the limbus of the cornea produces a visible golden brown band, the **Kayser–Fleischer ring**.

The lenticular nuclei of the brain show a light golden discoloration, and 25% of cases have small cysts or clefts in the putamen or in deep layers of the neocortex. Mild neuronal loss and gliosis are characteristic.

Some patients are "presymptomatic," never developing high enough levels of copper to accumulate in the brain or eyes or developing cirrhosis. The diagnosis is critical because Wilson disease is treatable, and failure to treat can lead to irreversible hepatic and CNS damage. Anyone presenting with a hyperkinetic movement disorder, particularly with the onset in early adult life, in association with psychiatric or hepatic manifestations must be evaluated for Wilson disease.

Vitamin Deficiencies

Vitamin deficiencies are discussed in Chapter 19.

Intoxication

Neurotoxicology is a major aspect of contemporary neuropathology. The breadth of this area far exceeds the scope of this chapter, so we concentrate on the more common and better-understood toxic injuries to the brain.

ETHANOL: The signs and symptoms of acute alcohol intoxication correspond to dose-related blood level. A blood alcohol level (BAC) of 0.05 to 0.1 mg/dL is associated with disinhibition and motor impairment; 0.1 to 0.3 mg/dL with frank inebriation and ataxia; and 0.3 to 0.35 mg/dL with extreme intoxication and sleepiness, nausea, and vomiting. A BAC of over 0.35 mg/dL is potentially lethal owing to respiratory depression and inability to protect the airway from aspiration.

Chronic alcohol use is associated with neurologic complications caused by (1) nutritional deficiencies, including Wernicke–Korsakoff syndrome; (2) possibly peripheral neuropathy; (3) liver failure with hepatic encephalopathy; (4) cerebral lesions; and (5) metabolic derangements, including central pontine myelinolysis from rapid correction of hyponatremia (Fig. 24-47).

METHANOL: In their quest for ethanol, alcoholics may substitute methanol, which is oxidized to formaldehyde and formic acid. Severe cerebral edema with hemorrhagic necrosis of the lateral putamen may ensue. Retinal edema and ganglion cell degeneration account for the blindness that afflicts these patients. Blindness may result from ingestion of as little as 4 mL of methanol, whereas a lethal dose is in the range of 8 to 10 mL.

CARBON MONOXIDE (CO): This colorless, odorless, tasteless gas is formed by incomplete combustion. Severe intoxication causes almost pathognomonic bilateral liquefactive necrosis of the globus pallidus. Other areas of CNS ischemic injury may be seen.

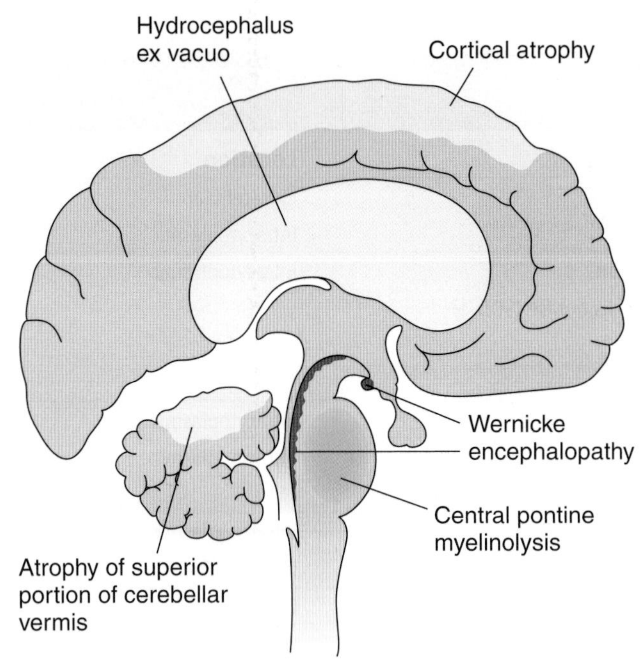

FIGURE 24-47. Regions of the brain with lesions associated with chronic ethanol abuse.

METAL INTOXICATION OR DEFICIENCY: Many metals employed in industry and medicine can cause neurologic disease; additionally, the biocidal properties of some of these substances, such as arsenic and thallium, have made them favorite tools of murderers, suicidal individuals, and pesticide users.

- **Lead:** Acute lead intoxication produces an edema-based encephalopathy, especially in childhood. An amorphous exudate around microvessels may be seen, as may some vascular proliferation. Chronic exposure in children from ingestion of lead-based paint, fishing sinkers, and lead alloy-based children's jewelry results in intellectual deficits. In adults, lead poisoning more commonly presents as a neuropathy, rather than as an encephalopathy.
- **Mercury:** Although now rare, chronic inorganic mercury intoxication may present with dementia, delirium, tremor, irritability, and insomnia. Cerebellar atrophy with loss of Purkinje cells is seen. Organomercurial poisoning is more prevalent. Congenital methylmercury neurotoxicity (seen most notably in the Minamata Bay environmental release in Japan) from in utero exposure results in severe mental retardation, athetosis, ataxia, and spastic quadriparesis. Severe atrophy of the cerebrum with milder cerebellar atrophy is evident, with loss of the cortical lamellar organization.
- **Arsenic and thallium:** Intoxication with these elements manifests with gastrointestinal complaints, including nausea, vomiting, and diarrhea. Swelling and petechiae may be present in the brain. Long-term exposure has other risks.

NEURODEGENERATIVE DISORDERS

Neurodegenerative disorders involve death of functionally related neurons; hence, these disorders can be classified by the primary functional system involved: (1) **cortical** degeneration leads to dementia, (2) **basal ganglia** loss to movement disorders, (3) **spinocerebellar** lesions to ataxia, and (4) **motor neuron** loss to upper and lower motor neuron weakness. ***Neuropathologically, loss of neurons in these systems is characteristic. There are often cellular inclusions and extracellular protein accumulations in these conditions and variable glial and microglial activation.*** Neurodegenerative disorders often begin focally and then spread in reasonably predictable ways throughout the CNS. This stereotypical dissemination likely involves abnormally folded pathogenic proteins that recruit and transform native proteins. ***This phenomenon is reminiscent of the molecular pathogenesis of prion diseases and is called "prion-like" protein misfolding or "templating."***

PATHOPHYSIOLOGY: At their core, the neurodegenerative diseases are largely disorders of proteostasis involving impaired cellular pathways that control protein synthesis, folding, trafficking, aggregation, disaggregation, and degradation. Because of this unifying theme, fundamental pathogenetic insights derived from one neurodegenerative disease may be generalizable to others.

Neurodegenerative disorders are classified according to which neuronal systems are most involved and the proteins that accumulate in those cells.

Intracellular, and particularly intracytoplasmic, inclusions are inextricably bound to neurodegenerative disorders. These protein aggregates may cause disease (Fig. 24-48; Table 24-3) by several routes. Sequestering protein or other macromolecules makes them unavailable for their normal functions. As aggregates enlarge, they may physically obstruct axons, dendrites, or movement of material within the cytoplasm. As these proteins aggregate, they initially form ultrastructural fibrils that may be extremely cytotoxic. Thus, it appears that cellular stresses from a variety of causes may disrupt proteostasis and generate toxic fibrils that themselves can perpetuate and amplify the cellular stress.

Major Cerebral Neurodegenerative Diseases

The clinical and pathologic features of these disorders are distinctive because different polymerized proteins accumulate

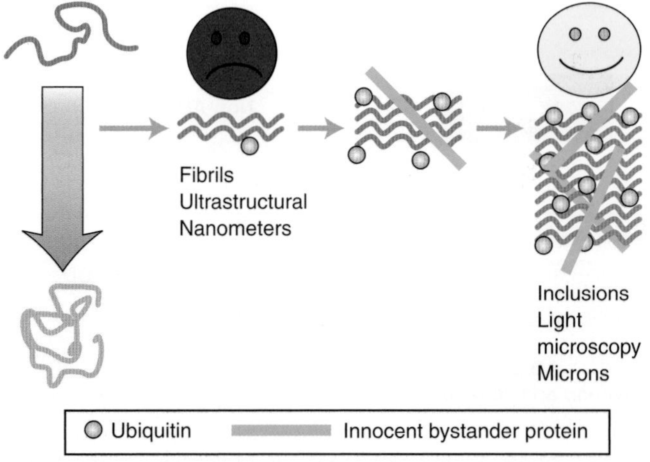

FIGURE 24-48. Fibrillogenesis and inclusions. Misfolded proteins with a tendency toward polymerization may form extremely cytoxic fibrils that are only visible by electron microscopy. The cellular stress response may facilitate hyperaggregation to inclusions that are visible by light microscopy. Such inclusions may be considered "toxic landfills" and may be protective.

Table 24-3

Representative Neurodegenerative Diseases With Fibrillogenesis

Disease	Lesion	Components	Location
Alzheimer disease	Senile plaques	β-Amyloid	Extracellular
	Neurofibrillary tangles	Tau	Intracytoplasmic
Amyotrophic lateral sclerosis	Spheroids	Neurofilament	Intracytoplasmic
		Superoxide dismutase (SOD-1)	
		TDP43	
		FUS	
Dementia with Lewy bodies	Lewy bodies	α-Synuclein	Intracytoplasmic
Frontotemporal dementias	Neurofibrillary tangles	Tau	Intracytoplasmic
		TDP43, progranulin, and other proteins	
Multiple system atrophy	Glial inclusions	α-Synuclein	Intracytoplasmic
Parkinson disease	Lewy bodies	α-Synuclein	Intracytoplasmic
Prion diseases	Prion deposits	Prions	Extracellular
Trinucleotide repeat diseases	Inclusions	Polyglutamine tracts	Intranuclear and cytoplasmic

(Fig. 24-49). These cortical degenerations ultimately lead to dementia.

- **Alzheimer disease (AD)** accounts for most cases of neurodegenerative dementia. It is characterized by abnormal accumulation of two proteins: β-amyloid and tau.
- **Pick disease** is the prototypical frontotemporal lobar dementia and is characterized by the accumulation of abnormal tau without β-amyloid.
- **Lewy body dementia** features accumulation of α-synuclein.

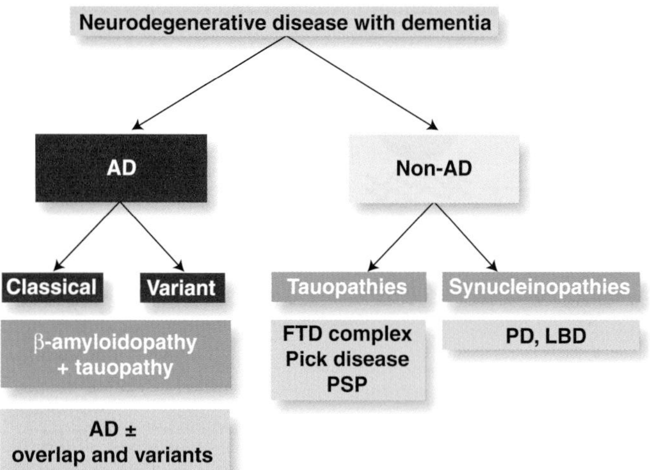

FIGURE 24-49. Protein fibrillogenesis. Molecular classification of the dementias and other neurodegenerative diseases now recognizes disorders based on the proteins that undergo fibrillogenesis. Alzheimer disease (AD) is a combination of a β-amyloidopathy and a tauopathy. Most of the frontotemporal lobar degenerations (FTLDs) such as Pick disease and progressive supranuclear palsy (PSP) are pure tauopathies. Lewy body dementia (LBD) and Parkinson disease (PD) complex are α-synucleinopathies.

Alzheimer Disease

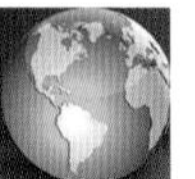

EPIDEMIOLOGY: AD is an insidious progressive neurologic disorder characterized clinically by loss of memory, cognitive impairment, and, eventually, dementia. Although Alzheimer's origin patients were younger than 65 and suffered "presenile dementia," the term is now used for dementia at any age that features characteristic pathologic changes. ***It is the most common dementia in the elderly, accounting for over half of cases.*** The prevalence of the condition is closely related to age. In patients younger than 65, Alzheimer disease affects at most 1% to 2%, but it occurs in 40% or more of patients older than 85. Women are affected twice as often as men. Most cases are sporadic, but familial variants occur.

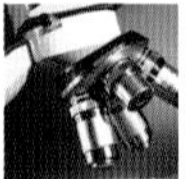

PATHOLOGY: AD brains show cortical atrophy with hydrocephalus ex vacuo (Figs. 24-50 and 24-51). Gyri narrow, sulci widen, and cortical atrophy are especially apparent in the parahippocampal regions. However, as the disease progresses, atrophy of temporal, frontal, and parietal cortex becomes more severe.

Senile plaques and neurofibrillary tangles (NFTs) dominate the histology. Small numbers of plaques and tangles are common in elderly patients with mild forgetfulness and mild cognitive impairment, which in half of cases is a prodrome of AD.

NEURITIC PLAQUES: The most conspicuous histologic lesions are senile or neuritic plaques. These lesions are ***extracellular*** spherical deposits of β-amyloid, several hundred microns in diameter. In end-stage disease, senile plaques occupy large volumes of affected cerebral gray matter (Fig. 24-52). They (1) bind planar amyloid-binding dyes such as Congo red and thioflavin S, and silver-containing dyes (argentophilic); (2) and are immunoreactive for β-amyloid protein (Aβ) at the core and periphery. The plaques are surrounded by reactive astrocytes and microglia and display swollen distorted neuronal processes (dystrophic neurites). The number and distribution of plaques do not correlate well with the severity of clinical disease.

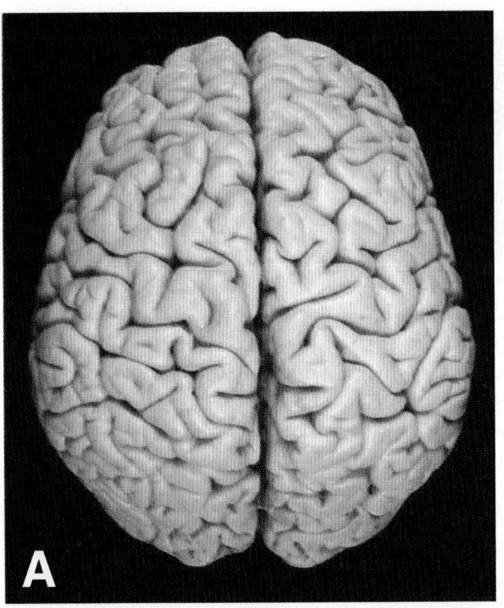

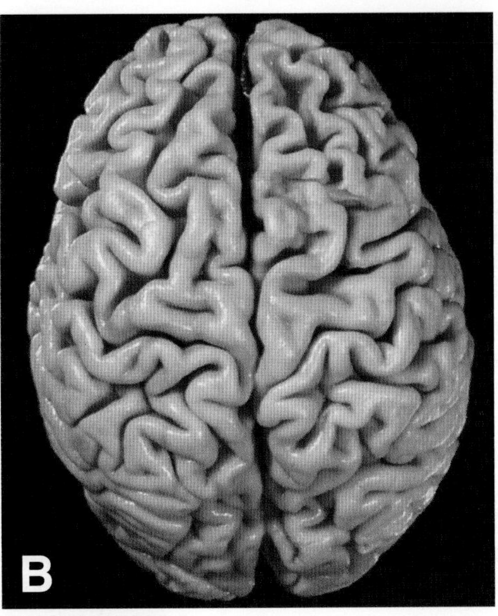

FIGURE 24-50. Cortical atrophy. A normal brain is shown on the left **(A)** and a brain with cortical atrophy caused by Alzheimer disease is shown on the right **(B)** with thinning of the gyri and prominent sulci. (Courtesy of Dr. F. Stephen Vogel, Duke University.)

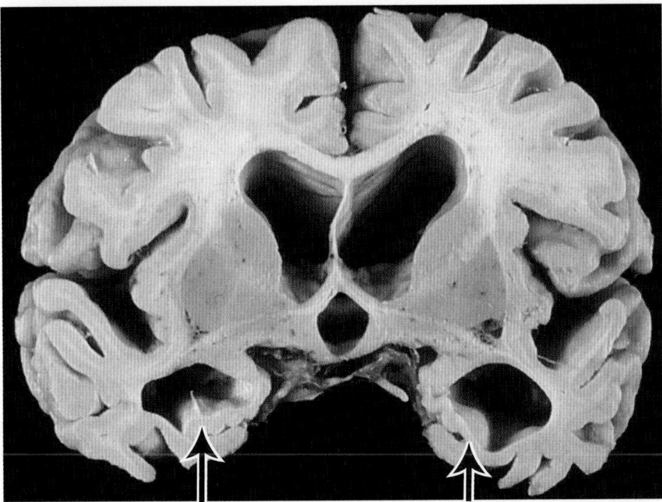

FIGURE 24-51. Cerebral atrophy with hydrocephalus ex vacuo in Alzheimer disease. Note also the severe atrophy of the hippocampus (*arrows*) leading to early memory disturbances in this disease. (Courtesy of Dr. F. Stephen Vogel, Duke University.)

NEUROFIBRILLARY TANGLES: NFTs are ***intracytoplasmic*** collections of polymerized tau filaments (Fig. 24-53). They contain irregular bundles of fibrils that are positive by Congo red and thioflavin S and immunoreactive for tau. The tangles are paired, 10-nm-thick, helical filaments with abundant insoluble tau proteins. Their distribution correlates with the clinical severity of AD. Tangles in the entorhinal cortex and parahippocampal gyrus can be seen in asymptomatic people decades before the usual age of onset of AD and may represent the earliest phases of the condition. As more temporal neocortex comes to possess tangles, mild cognitive impairment

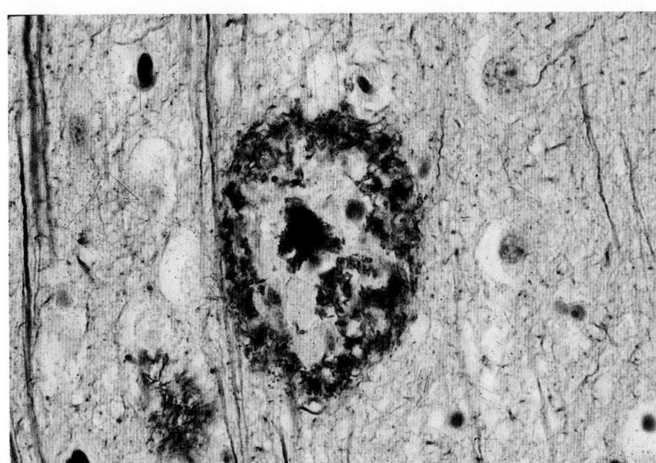

FIGURE 24-52. Neuritic plaques are extracellular accumulations of polymerized β-amyloid centrally with a rim of dystrophic neuritic processes. The number of plaques in the cerebral cortex does not correlate well with the severity of dementia in Alzheimer disease.

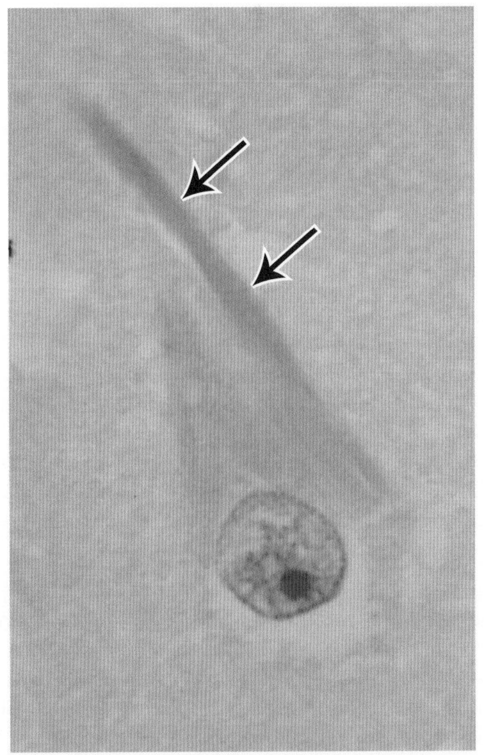

FIGURE 24-53. Neurofibrillary tangles are intracytoplasmic intraneuronal accumulations of polymerized hyperphosphorylated tau protein (*arrows*). The sites and degree of distribution of neurofibrillary tangles correlate with clinical symptoms.

may develop. Finally, when large swaths of neocortex, deep nuclei, and brainstem are involved, full-blown AD is present.

NFTs are not unique to AD. They also occur in other neurodegenerative diseases, including dementia pugilistica (punch drunk syndrome in boxers), postencephalitic parkinsonism, Guam ALS/parkinsonism dementia complex, Pick disease, corticobasal degeneration, and sporadic and hereditary frontotemporal dementias. Collectively, these neurodegenerative diseases that show abnormal tau aggregation are called **tauopathies** and may share common mechanisms of brain degeneration. ***Alzheimer disease is both a tauopathy and a β-amyloidopathy, leading to intracellular and extracellular tangles and plaques, respectively.***

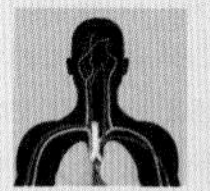
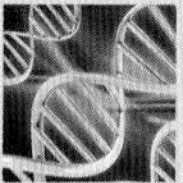

PATHOPHYSIOLOGY AND MOLECULAR PATHOGENESIS: The cause of AD is not known, but the origins of associated amyloid and NFTs are increasingly understood.

β-Amyloid protein (Aβ): Increasing evidence points to the importance of deposition of Aβ protein in **neuritic plaques** of Alzheimer disease. The core of these plaques contains a distinct form of Aβ peptide, which is mainly 42 amino acids long. Aβ is derived by proteolysis from a much larger (695 amino acids), membrane-spanning amyloid β-protien precursor (APP). Full-length APP has an extracellular region, a transmembrane sequence, and a cytoplasmic domain. The region comprising Aβ anchors the amino-terminal portion of APP to the membrane. The physiologic functions of APP and Aβ remain obscure.

The normal degradation of APP involves proteolytic cleavage in the middle of the Aβ domain; a non amyloidogenic fragment from the middle of the Aβ domain to the amino end of APP is released. Proteolysis at either end of the Aβ domain then detaches intact and highly amyloidogenic Aβ, which accumulates in senile plaques as amyloid fibrils.

Aβ deposition may be required for Alzheimer disease to develop because of the following:

- Patients with **Down syndrome** (trisomy 21) develop clinical and pathologic features of Alzheimer disease, including deposition of Aβ in neuritic plaques, generally by age 40. The gene for APP is on chromosome 21, and the additional dose of the gene product in trisomy 21 predisposes to precocious accumulation of Aβ.
- Some patients with familial AD carry mutant *APP* genes or mutant presenilin genes. These mutations lead to increased production of Aβ, the amyloidogenic part of APP.
- Transgenic mice expressing mutant human *APP* genes develop senile plaques in the brain similar to those of AD. However, these mice lack other critical features of AD, such as NFTs, and evidence of neurodegeneration, such as significant loss of neurons.

Neurofibrillary tangles: NFTs are paired helical filaments that contain tau that is abnormally phosphorylated at aberrant sites. The resultant protein does not associate with microtubules but instead aggregates to form paired helical filaments. Release of tau from microtubules may deprive cells of tau's microtubule-stabilizing effects, thereby impairing axonal transport and compromising neuronal function. Alternatively, fibril formation occurring as the hyperphosphorylated tau aggregates may itself be cytotoxic.

There are several genetic risk factors for Alzheimer disease. Mutations in the *APP* gene have been associated with early-onset familial variants of AD. Additional genetic associations (Table 24-4) involve apolipoprotein E (apoE) genotype and the genes for presenilin 1 and 2.

Proposed mechanisms leading to development of AD are shown in Figure 24-54.

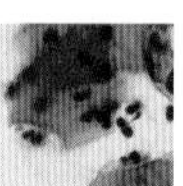

CLINICAL FEATURES: Patients with AD come to medical attention because of gradual loss of memory and cognitive function, difficulty with language, and changes in behavior. Those with mild cognitive impairment are increasingly being recognized because they move on to full-blown dementia at a rate of about 15% per year. Alzheimer disease progresses inexorably, so that previously intelligent and productive people become demented, mute, incontinent, and bedridden. Bronchopneumonia, urinary tract infections, and pressure decubiti are common medical complications that lead to death.

Frontotemporal Lobar Degeneration

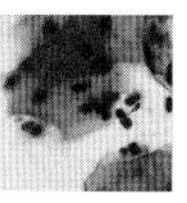

CLINICAL FEATURES: The frontotemporal lobar degenerations (FTLDs) are mainly tauopathies in which the frontal and temporal lobes bear the early brunt of the disease. The prototype eponymic disorder of the FTLDs is **Pick disease**, which manifests clinically as loss of frontal executive function causing disinhibition, loss of judgment about social propriety, and inability to plan or foresee the consequences of one's actions. Most cases are sporadic, although Pick disease kindreds have been described. Sporadic Pick disease becomes symptomatic in midadult life and progresses relentlessly to death in 3 to 10 years. A respected pillar of the community may be reduced to a vulgar, disheveled derelict as this tragedy unfolds. Unlike AD, which generally begins with memory difficulties, FTLD starts with disruptive, inappropriate behavior. At the end, these dementias converge clinically.

Table 24-4

Genetic Factors in Alzheimer Disease

Gene	Chromosome	Disease Association
Amyloid precursor protein (*APP*)	21	Mutations of the *APP* gene are associated with early-onset familial Alzheimer disease
Presenilin 1 (*PS1*)	14	Mutations of the *PS1* gene are associated with early-onset familial Alzheimer disease
Presenilin 2 (*PS2*)	1	Mutations of the *PS2* gene are associated with Volga German familial Alzheimer disease
Apolipoprotein E (*apoE*)	19	Presence of the ε4 allele is associated with increased risk and younger age of onset of both inherited and sporadic forms of late-onset Alzheimer disease

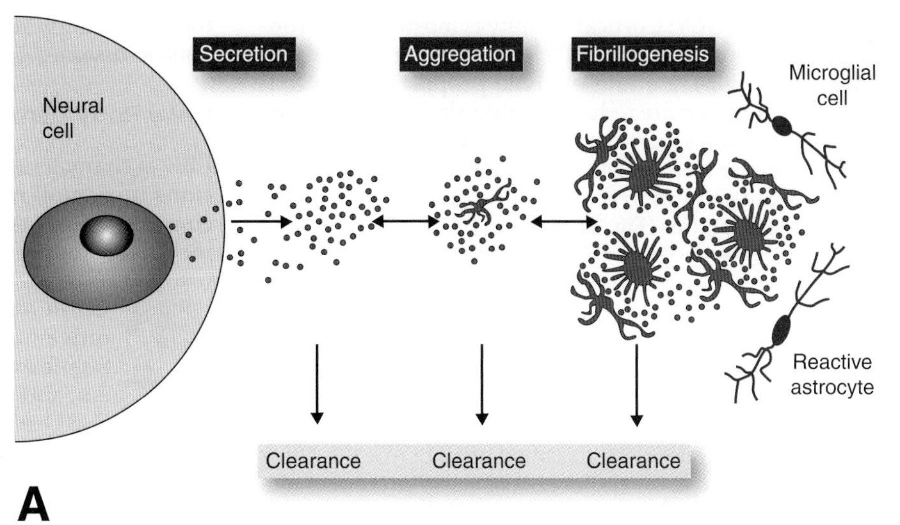

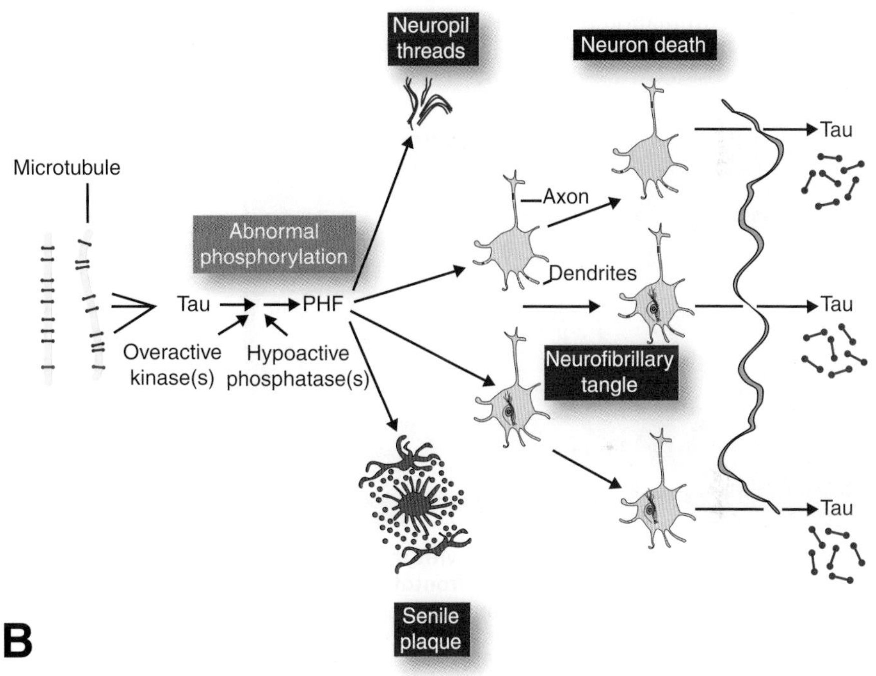

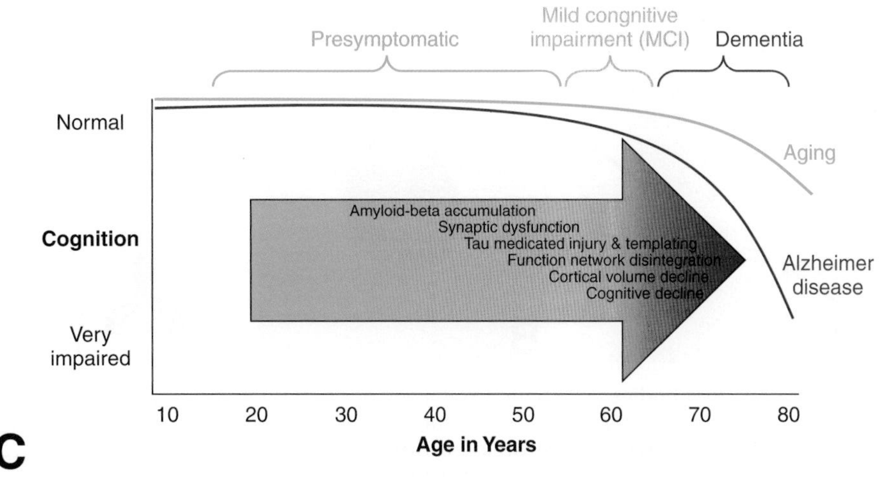

FIGURE 24-54. Mechanisms of amyloidosis and brain degeneration in Alzheimer disease. **A.** A schematic illustrating a hypothetical mechanism for the formation of senile plaques (SPs) from soluble Aβ peptides produced inside cells and secreted into the extracellular space. Amyloidogenic Aβ may encounter fibril-inducing cofactors and go on to form A fibrils to deposit in SPs (*far right*). SPs are surrounded by reactive astrocytes and microglial cells, which secrete cytokines that may contribute to the toxicity of the SPs. These steps may be reversible. Increasing Aβ clearance or reducing its production, as well as modulating the inflammatory response, may be effective therapeutic interventions for Alzheimer disease, in combination with therapies that target brain degeneration caused by neurofibrillary tangles (NFTs). **B.** A schematic illustrating a hypothetical mechanism leading to the conversion of normal human central nervous system (CNS) tau overlying two microtubules into paired helical filaments (PHFs). PHFs are generated in neuronal perikarya and their processes. Overactive kinase(s) or hypoactive phosphatase(s) may contribute to this effect. Abnormally phosphorylated tau forms PHFs in neuronal processes (neuropil threads) and neuronal perikarya (NFTs). Tau in PHFs loses the ability to bind microtubules, thus causing their depolymerization, disruption of axonal transport, and degeneration of neurons. Accumulation of PHFs in neurons could exacerbate this process by physically blocking transport in neurons. The death of affected neurons would release tau and increase the levels of tau in the cerebrospinal fluid of patients with Alzheimer disease. NFT formation may be reversible, and drugs that block NFT formation, reverse it or stabilize microtubules may be effective therapeutic interventions for Alzheimer disease. **C.** The National Institute on Aging/Alzheimer Association (NIA/AA) 2011 formulation on Alzheimer disease formally recognizes the temporal evolution of the disease from a long presymptomatic phase in which β-amyloid is accumulated and the pathophysiologic cascade is initiated. The pathogenic mechanisms interact to move the disease to mild cognitive impairment (MCI) and finally to frank dementia. Interventions during the symptomatic phase may be too late to fundamentally change the trajectory of the disease, and increased attention is being directed at the presymptomatic phase of the illness. This would be a primary prevention approach not unlike the highly successful presymptomatic intervention in myocardial infarction and stroke by exercise and control of hypertension and hyperlipidemia.

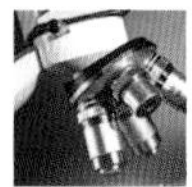

PATHOLOGY: Cortical atrophy is mostly in the frontotemporal regions in Pick disease (Fig. 24-55). The atrophy may attain extreme proportions, so that affected gyri are reduced to thin slivers (**knife-edge atrophy**). The involved cortex is severely depleted of neurons and shows intense astrogliosis. Residual neurons have argentophilic and tau-immunoreactive, round, cytoplasmic inclusions called **Pick bodies** (Fig. 24-56A and B). These are formed by densely aggregated straight tau filaments.

Pick disease is the prototypical FTLD, but there are others that only recently have begun to reveal their molecular secrets. In any cohort of patients with clinical FTLD, many have Pick disease, but a significant number do not. Often, their neurons are immunoreactive for ubiquitin, implying an as yet unidentified protein triggering an unfulfilled degradative response. These are classified at FTLD-U, the U for ubiquitin immunoreactivity. Several of these proteins have recently been identified.

The protein TDP43 bears brief consideration because its abnormal accumulation occurs in both FTLD and motor neuron disease. This molecular commonality coincides with the increasingly recognized coexistence of FTLD and motor neuron disease.

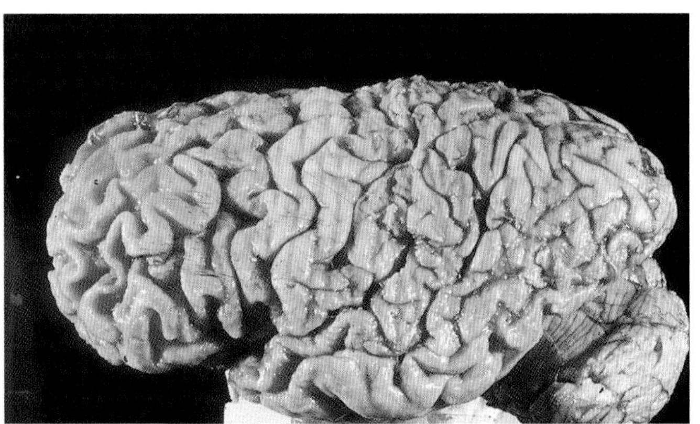

FIGURE 24-55. Severe cortical atrophy with marked frontotemporal atrophy is characteristic of the frontotemporal lobar degenerations, such as Pick disease, but may be seen in Alzheimer disease. Frontal atrophy correlates with loss of executive function, impaired judgment, and disinhibition.

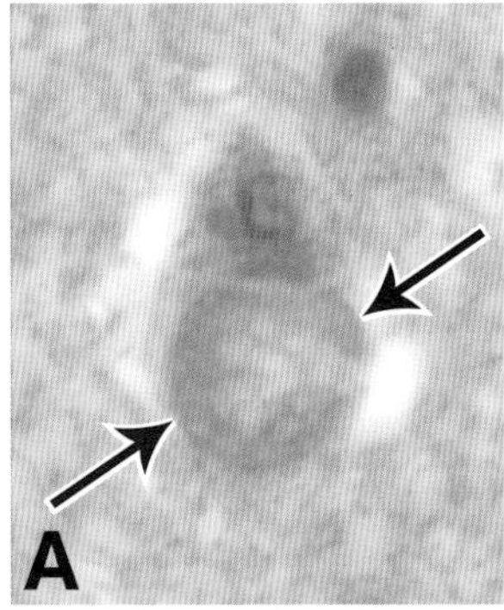

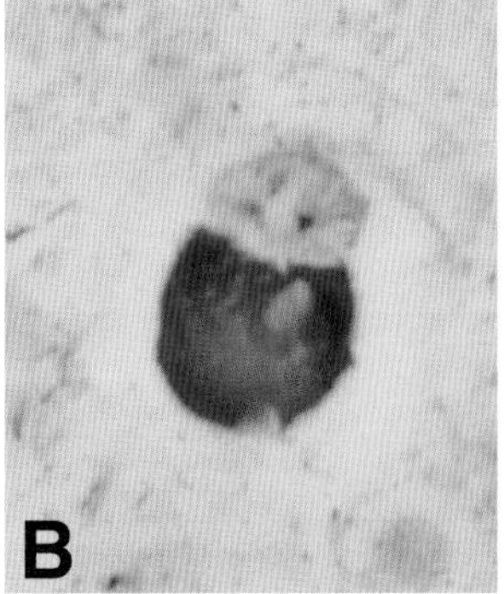

FIGURE 24-56. Pick bodies. A. In hematoxylin and eosin–stained sections, Pick bodies are basophilic, spherical, intracytoplasmic, intraneuronal aggregates of tau protein (*arrows*). They tend to be round rather than angular like the neurofibrillary tangles (NFTs) in Alzheimer disease, but like NFTs, they are argentophilic (silver impregnation) **(B)**.

Lewy Body Dementia

LBD is characterized by intracytoplasmic α-synuclein inclusions in a small number of cortical neurons, mostly in the cingulate cortex. AD pathology may coexist with Lewy body inclusions at the end stage of the disease.

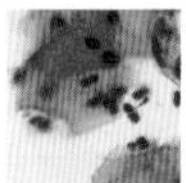

CLINICAL FEATURES: LBD is distinctive in that cognitive function fluctuates greatly from day to day. Subtle extrapyramidal manifestations may be present, and the patient may experience visual hallucinations. LBD exists on a continuum with the other α-synucleinopathies, which include Parkinson disease and multiple system atrophy.

Neurodegeneration of the Basal Ganglia

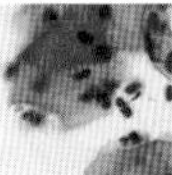

CLINICAL FEATURES: Movement disorders may result in too little (**bradykinetic**) or too much **(hyperkinetic)** involuntary movement. Parkinson disease is the prototypical bradykinetic movement disorder, characterized by (1) difficulty initiating and sustaining voluntary movement, (2) resting tremor, and (3) postural instability. This clinical triad is **parkinsonism,** and whereas the most common cause is Parkinson disease, other disorders such as progressive supranuclear palsy, multiple system atrophy, and even neuro-AIDS may result in parkinsonism.

The prototypical hyperkinetic movement disorder is Huntington disease, with progressive development of involuntary rapid twitching movements (chorea) and writhing dance–like movements (athetosis), which may conflate as choreoathetosis.

Parkinson Disease

PD is characterized clinically by tremors at rest, cogwheel rigidity (stop and go tremor during movement), expressionless countenance, postural instability, and, less often, cognitive impairment. Pathologically, neurons are lost, largely in the substantia nigra; Lewy bodies, which are filamentous aggregates of α-synuclein, accumulate. Dopaminergic neurons that project from the substantia nigra to the striatum are diminished.

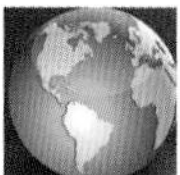

EPIDEMIOLOGY: PD typically appears in the sixth to eighth decades. It is common: 1% to 2% of the population in North America eventually develops the disorder. The prevalence of PD has remained unchanged for at least the past 40 years. No racial differences are apparent, but men are more affected than women.

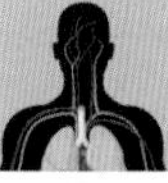

PATHOPHYSIOLOGY: Most cases of PD are sporadic, but missense mutations in the α-synuclein gene cause rare autosomal dominant, early-onset, familial PD. The finding that wild-type α-synuclein is the major polymerized protein in Lewy bodies led to consideration of fibrillogenesis as a major contributor to the pathogenesis of neurodegenerative diseases. Accumulating evidence suggests that oxidative stress as a result of auto-oxidation of catecholamines during melanin formation injures neurons in the substantia nigra. Such stress promotes misfolding of α-synuclein and the formation of filamentous inclusions.

In addition to PD, the accumulation of filamentous α-synuclein inclusions is seen in other diseases, including multiple system atrophy, Lewy body disease, progressive autonomic failure, and rapid eye movement (REM) sleep behavior disorder. These disorders are now called **α-synucleinopathies** and, like the tauopathies, are considered brain-specific amyloidoses.

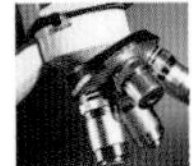

PATHOLOGY: Brains of PD patients show loss of pigmentation in the substantia nigra and locus ceruleus (Fig. 24-57). Other brain regions are less affected. Pigmented neurons are scarce, and small extracellular deposits of melanin are derived from dying neurons. Some residual neurons are atrophic, and a few contain Lewy bodies, which are spherical, eosinophilic cytoplasmic inclusions (Fig. 24-58). By electron microscopy, Lewy bodies show amyloid-like filaments of insoluble α-synuclein.

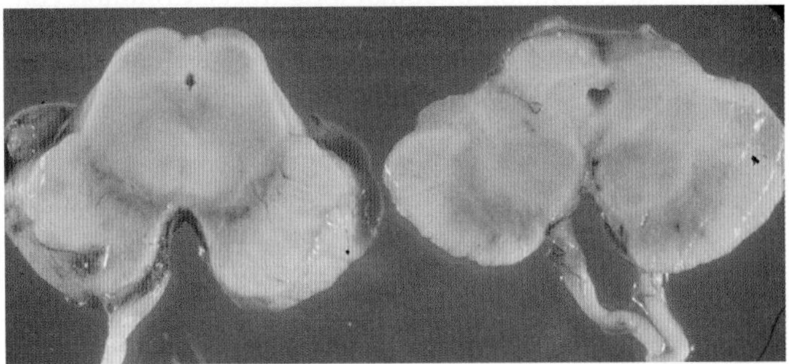

FIGURE 24-57. Parkinson disease. The normal substantia nigra on the left in an adult is heavily pigmented, whereas the substantia nigra in a patient with Parkinson disease has lost pigmented neurons and the nucleus now blends inconspicuously with the rest of the midbrain. The locus ceruleus in the pons is also depigmented (not shown). (Courtesy of Dr. F. Stephen Vogel, Duke University.)

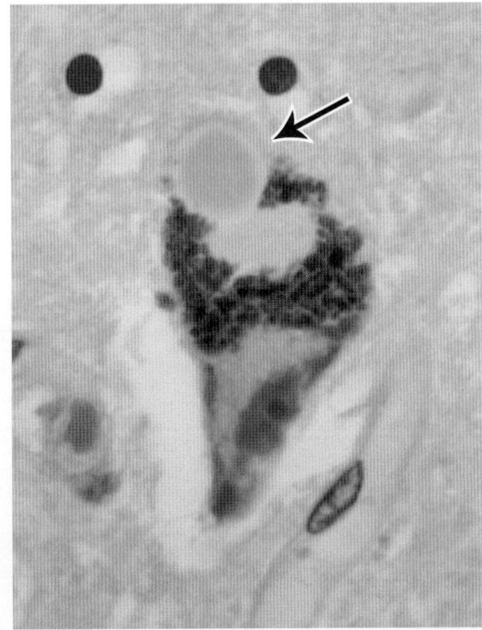

FIGURE 24-58. Lewy body in Parkinson disease. Examination of residual neurons in the substantia nigra show intracytoplasmic, intraneuronal, spherical eosinophilic inclusions composed of polymerized α-synuclein called Lewy bodies (*arrow*). These inclusions often have a thin clear halo.

Other Disorders Causing Parkinsonism

PD is not the sole cause of parkinsonism. Other disorders share a common theme of loss of pigmented dopaminergic neurons in the substantia nigra. Normal aging is associated with some neuron loss in the substantia nigra and reduced dopamine levels, but these features are exaggerated in PD and other causes of parkinsonism.

- **Striatonigral degeneration** is a rare disorder that closely mimics PD. At autopsy, the striatum (caudate and putamen) is visibly atrophied, with severe loss of neurons in this region. Changes in the substantia nigra and locus ceruleus are less severe. This condition may coexist with Shy–Drager disease (dysautonomia) and olivopontocerebellar atrophy (OPCA). These conditions are part of a unified disorder of **multiple system atrophy (MSA)**, in which filamentous α-synuclein inclusions, known as **glial cytoplasmic inclusions**, accumulate primarily in oligodendroglia. They also occur to a lesser extent in neurons, where they resemble the Lewy bodies of Parkinson disease and Lewy body dementia.
- **Progressive supranuclear palsy (PSP)** is an uncommon disorder characterized by parkinsonism, severe postural instability with falls, and progressive paralysis of vertical eye movements. Pathologic changes in the brain are more widespread than in PD, but the hallmark is atrophy of the midbrain tegmentum. Because the midbrain, as well as the substantia nigra, is the locus of integration of vertical eye movement, the combination of parkinsonism and vertical gaze dysfunction makes anatomic sense. PSP is a **tauopathy:** the sole inclusions are tau-rich NFTs. PSP spreads throughout the nervous system, and cognitive impairment complicates the disease course.

Huntington Disease

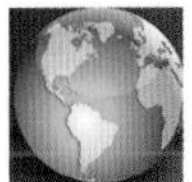

EPIDEMIOLOGY: HD is an autosomal dominant genetic disorder characterized by (1) involuntary movements, (2) deterioration of cognitive function, and (3) often severe emotional disturbances. It mainly affects whites of northwestern European ancestry, with an incidence of 1 in 20,000. Genealogic studies indicate that all cases derive from an original founder in northern Europe; the disease is very rare in Asia and Africa.

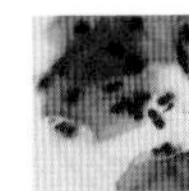

CLINICAL FEATURES: Symptoms of HD usually begin by age 40, but 5% of patients with the disorder develop neurologic signs before age 20, and a similar proportion first present after age 60. Cognitive and emotional disturbances precede the onset of abnormal movements by several years in over half of patients. Once it develops, choreoathetosis may be incapacitating. Cortical involvement leads to a severe loss of cognitive function and intellectual deterioration, often accompanied by paranoia and delusions. The interval from the onset of symptoms to death averages 15 years.

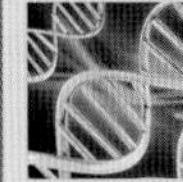

MOLECULAR PATHOGENESIS: The *HD* gene, on chromosome 4 (4p16.3), codes for the protein **huntingtin**. The aberration at this locus is expansion of a trinucleotide (CAG) repeat (see Chapter 5). The repeat is within a coding region of the gene and yields an altered protein, with a polyglutamine tract near the N-terminus. In agreement with the dominant mode of inheritance, the triplet expansion causes a toxic gain of function.

Huntingtin is widely expressed in tissues throughout the body and in all regions of the CNS by neurons and glia, but its function is unknown. As with other CAG repeat expansion diseases, the longer the CAG repeat, the more severe the disease phenotype and the earlier the age of clinical onset. In HD, CAG length is more unstable and tends to be longer when inherited from the father than in maternal transmission. As a result, transmission of the *HD* mutation from the father results in clinical disease some 3 years earlier than when it is passed on from the mother. Of children with juvenile-onset HD, the ratio of those who inherit the expanded CAG allele from their father and those who inherit it from their mother is 10:1.

PATHOLOGY: The frontal cortex is symmetrically and moderately atrophic, whereas the lateral ventricles are disproportionately large, owing to loss of the normal convex curvature of the caudate nuclei (Fig. 24-59). There is symmetric atrophy of the caudate nuclei, with lesser involvement of the putamen. Neuronal populations of the caudate and putamen, especially the small neurons, are severely depleted, with accompanying astrogliosis. The cerebral cortical neurons are similarly, but less severely, lost. Huntingtin aggregates in neurons, mainly in nuclei, but also in neuronal processes, potentially impairing axodendritic transport. γ-Aminobutyric acid (GABA) and glutamic acid decarboxylase are markedly decreased.

Spinocerebellar Neurodegeneration

Cerebellar dysfunction leads to ataxia—the inability to execute motor tasks smoothly, particularly those requiring rapid alternating movement or precise motor control. Ataxia results from defects in the major cerebellar input pathways, including the middle cerebellar peduncle. These circuits convey motor execution commands from the cerebral motor and premotor cortex, together with the inferior cerebellar peduncle, which receives proprioceptive data from the spinal cord via the spinocerebellar tracts. If the cerebellar parenchyma itself degenerates, ataxia will reflect a distribution congruent to the functional portion of the cerebellum involved. For example, vermal degeneration leads to truncal ataxia, whereas cerebellar hemispheric degeneration causes appendicular ataxia. Finally, the cerebral outflow—the dentatorubrothalamic pathway—may degenerate, resulting in a peculiarly high-amplitude ataxia called "wing-beating ataxia."

Friedreich Ataxia

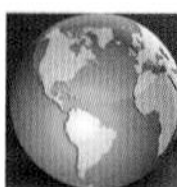

EPIDEMIOLOGY: Friedreich ataxia is the most common inherited ataxia. Its prevalence in European populations is 1 in 50,000. Inheritance is autosomal recessive, but many cases arise sporadically without a prior family history.

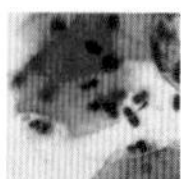

CLINICAL FEATURES: Symptoms of Friedreich ataxia usually begin before age 25, followed by an unremittingly progressive course of about 30 years to death. The condition reflects a cerebellar inflow disorder with ataxia of both the upper and lower limbs, dysarthria, lower limb areflexia, extensor plantar reflexes, and sensory loss reflecting degeneration of spinal long tracts. Common concomitants include deformities of the skeletal system (e.g., scoliosis and pes cavus), hypertrophic cardiomyopathy (which commonly causes death), and diabetes mellitus.

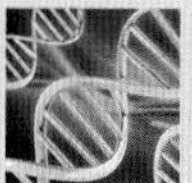

MOLECULAR PATHOGENESIS: The genetic defect in Friedreich ataxia is an autosomal recessive loss of function of the genes encoding a mitochondrial protein (**frataxin**), which is involved in iron transport into mitochondria. In most cases, the mutation is an unstable expansion of a trinucleotide (GAA) repeat in the first intron of this gene (9q13.3–21.1). The expansion mutation may impede transcription or RNA processing. Lack of frataxin is probably responsible for both neurologic and cardiac manifestations of Friedreich ataxia. The longer the repeat, the earlier the age of disease onset, the faster the rate of progression, and the greater the frequency of hypertrophic cardiomyopathy.

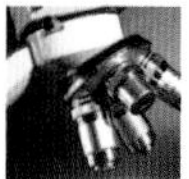

PATHOLOGY: The most prominent postmortem findings in Friedreich ataxia are in the spinal cord, which shows degeneration of the posterior columns, corticospinal pathways, and spinocerebellar tracts. Posterior column degeneration accounts for the sensory loss

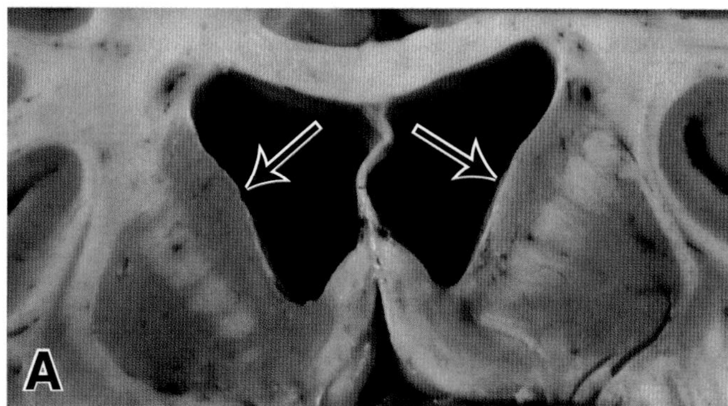

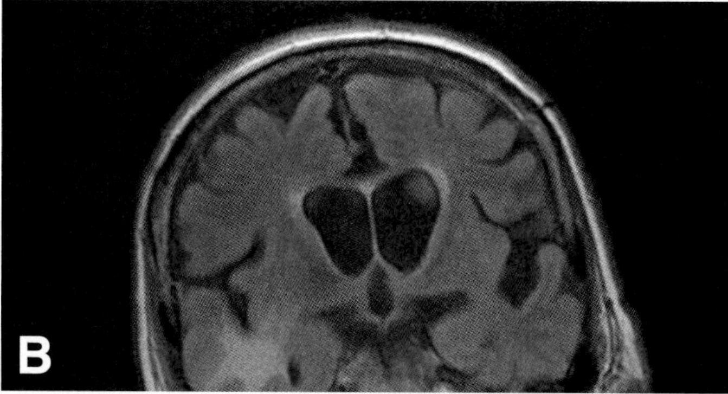

FIGURE 24-59. Huntington disease. A. The caudate nuclei (*arrows*) bilaterally are atrophic, leading to enlarged lateral ventricles. Some cortical atrophy is also seen, but it is usually not as severe as that seen in the primary cortical dementias, such as Alzheimer and Pick disease. **B.** Axial magnetic resonance image showing the enlarged lateral ventricles accompanied by modest cortical atrophy. The square-shaped lateral ventricles of Huntington disease are sometimes called "box-car ventricles."

experienced by these patients and results from disappearance of the parent neuronal cell bodies in the dorsal root ganglia. In advanced cases, this degeneration appears grossly as shrinkage of dorsal spinal roots and posterior funiculi.

Amyotrophic Lateral Sclerosis

ALS is a degenerative disease of upper and lower motor neurons of the brain and spinal cord. The disease is characterized by (1) progressive weakness and wasting of extremities and tongue, (2) a sometimes-confusing combination of hyper-reflexia and hyporeflexia, and (3) eventual impairment of respiratory muscles.

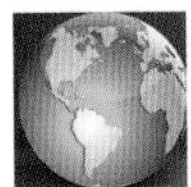

EPIDEMIOLOGY: It is a worldwide disease with an incidence of 1 in 100,000. It peaks in the fifth decade, and it is rare in people before age 35. There is a 1.5- to 2-fold excess of ALS in men.

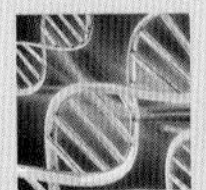

MOLECULAR PATHOGENESIS: Familial ALS cases, with an autosomal dominant pattern, account for 5% of ALS. One form of the disease has been associated with missense mutations in the gene that codes for the cytosolic form of the antioxidant enzyme superoxide dismutase. Loss of enzyme activity does not appear to be associated with disease, but mutant SOD1 is more prone to aggregation than wild-type SOD1, so familial ALS may be a **protein conformational disorder**.

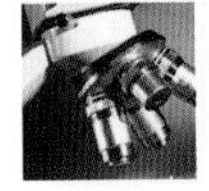

PATHOLOGY: ALS affects lower motor neurons, including anterior horn cells of the spinal cord and the motor nuclei of the brainstem, especially the hypoglossal nuclei. The upper motor neurons of the cerebral cortex also degenerate. Loss of the upper motor neurons leads to degeneration of their axons, with secondary demyelination. These changes are visualized in myelin-stained axial sections of the spinal cord as loss of the lateral and anterior corticospinal pathways (Fig. 24-60).

The main histologic change in ALS is loss of large motor neurons, with mild gliosis. This is most apparent in the anterior horns of the lumbar and cervical enlargements of the spinal cord, and the hypoglossal nuclei. There is also a loss of the giant pyramidal Betz cells in the cerebral motor cortex. The anterior nerve roots bearing the few remaining axons of the dying lower motor neurons become atrophic, and affected muscles are pale and shrunken, reflecting severe neurogenic atrophy.

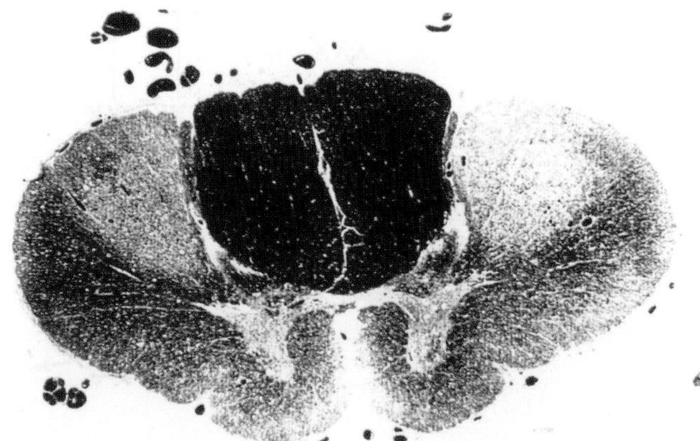

FIGURE 24-60. Amyotrophic lateral sclerosis spinal cord showing upper motor neuron loss. Myelin-stained sections show degeneration of the lateral corticospinal tracts reflecting degeneration of the axons of the upper motor neurons originating in the motor strip of the cerebral cortex. Note the preservation of the dorsal columns, spinothalamic tracts, and spinocerebellar pathways.

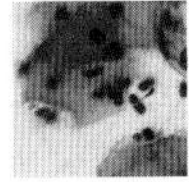

CLINICAL FEATURES: ALS often begins asymmetrically as weakness and wasting of the muscles of one hand. Irregular, rapid, involuntary contractions of small muscle groups (fasciculations) are characteristic and arise from hyperirritability of terminal arborizations of dying lower motor neurons. The disease is inexorably progressive, with increasing weakness of the limbs leading to total disability. Speech may become unintelligible, and respiratory weakness supervenes. Despite the dramatic wasting of the body, intellectual capacity is preserved to the end, although some patients with ALS also suffer dementia of the frontotemporal lobar type. The clinical course does not usually exceed a decade.

Spinal muscular atrophy (Werdnig–Hoffman disease) is the second most common lethal, autosomal recessive condition in white populations. It usually presents in infancy with extreme muscle weakness and atrophy, owing to severe loss of anterior horn cells. Death from respiratory failure or aspiration pneumonia usually occurs within a few months of diagnosis. This disorder results from a loss-of-function mutation of a neuronal apoptosis inhibitor protein. As a result, the neurons have an extremely low threshold for initiating programmed cell death.

Several neurodegenerative, infectious, and vitamin deficiency disorders impact the spinal long tracts and are summarized in Figure 24-61.

DEVELOPMENTAL MALFORMATIONS

Neural Tube Defects

Anencephaly

Anencephaly is the congenital absence of all or part of the brain as a result of unsuccessful closure of the cephalad (anterior neuropore) portion of the neural tube.

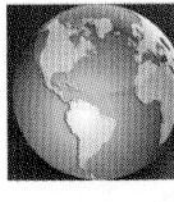

EPIDEMIOLOGY: Anencephaly is the second most common CNS malformation after spina bifida and is the most common lethal CNS malformation. Anencephalic fetuses are stillborn or die in the first few days of life.

Anencephaly is a multifactorial birth defect exhibiting geographic variation in incidence. In the United States, it occurs in 0.3 per 1,000 live births and stillbirths. In Ireland, the frequency is 20-fold greater (5 to 6 per 1,000). The incidence declines to 2 to 3 per 1,000 among Irish immigrants to North America. It is rare among blacks.

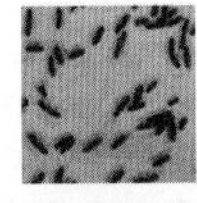

ETIOLOGIC FACTORS: Anencephaly is a dysraphic defect of neural tube closure (Fig. 24-62). Its concurrence with other neural tube defects (NTDs), such as spina bifida, suggests shared pathogenic mechanisms. During development, the neural plate invaginates and is transformed into the neural tube by fusion of the posterior surfaces. Mesenchymal tissue overlying the primitive neural

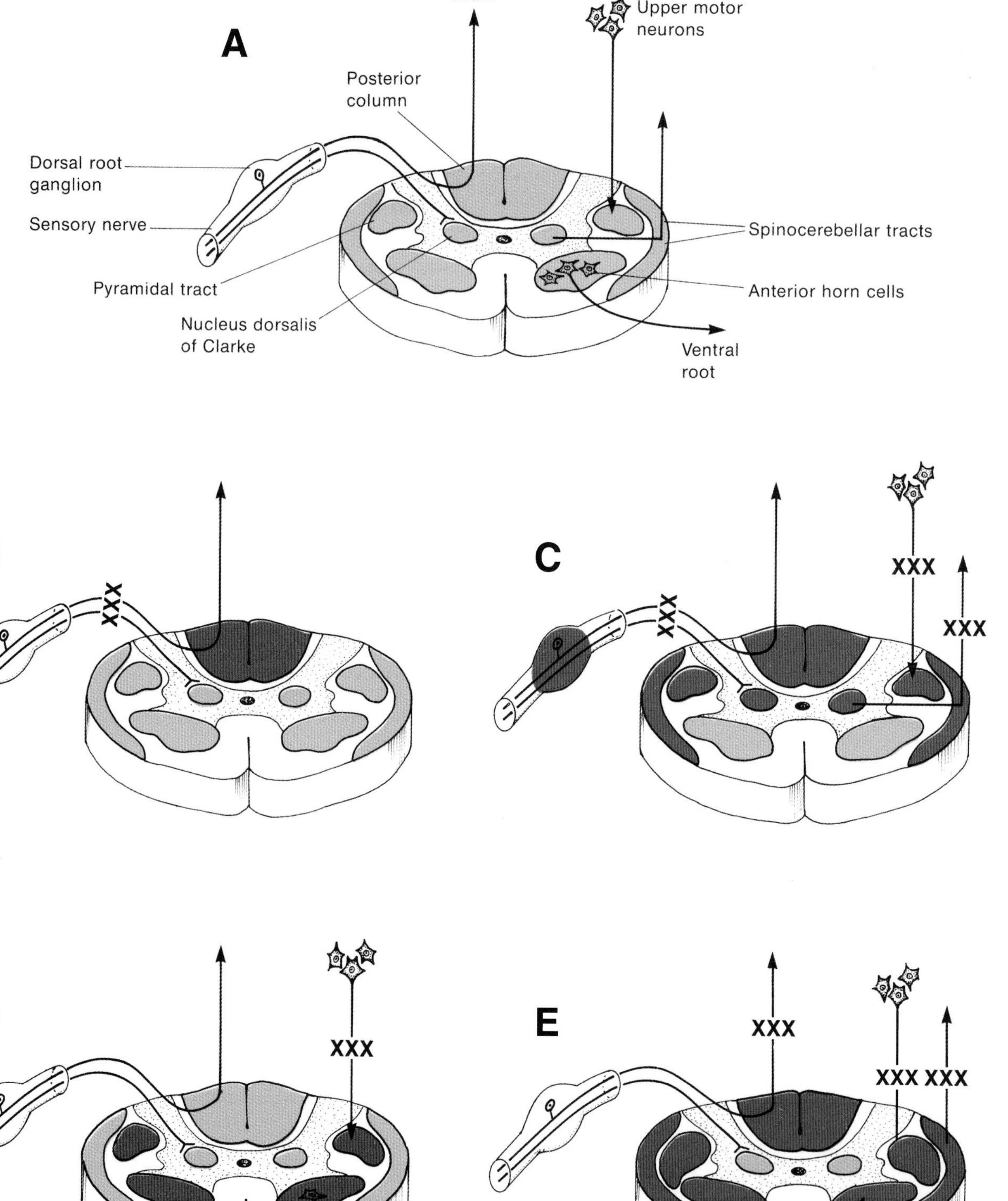

FIGURE 24-61. Tract degeneration in diseases of the spinal cord. Ascending (*blue*) sensory and descending (*green*) pathways travel through the spinal cord. These tracts may be differentially affected (*red*) depending on the nature of the underlying disease, as shown in this example of four diseases that we have considered. **A.** Normal. **B.** Tabes dorsalis. **C.** Friedreich ataxia. **D.** Amyotrophic lateral sclerosis. **E.** Subacute combined degeneration.

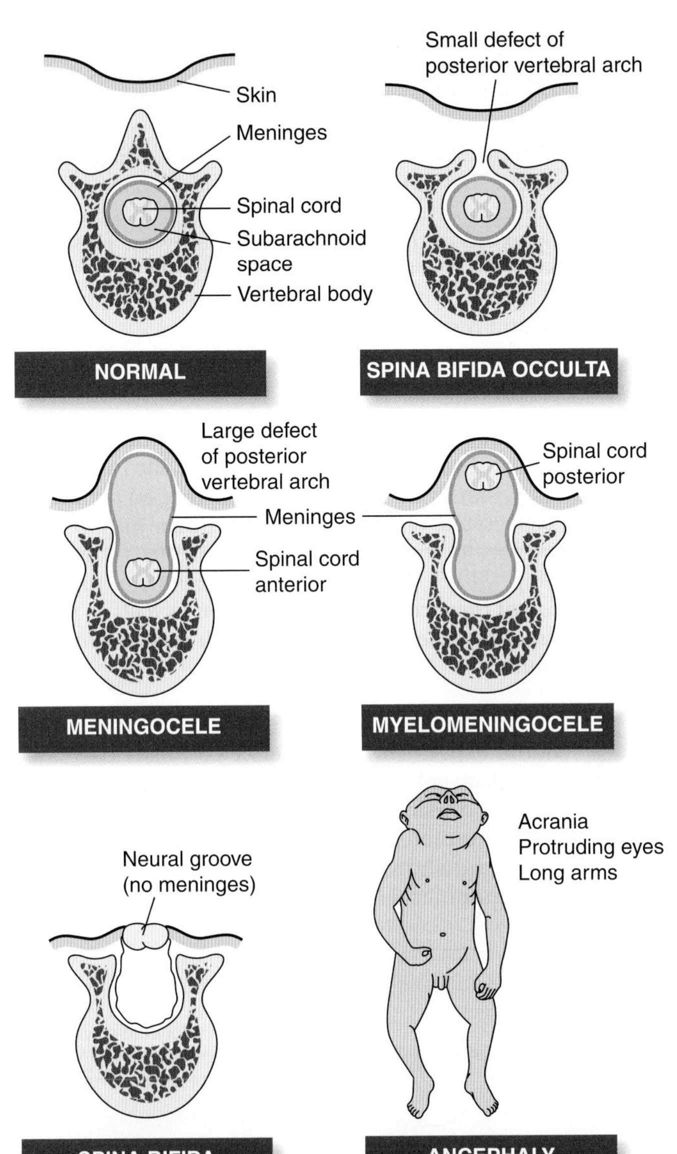

FIGURE 24-62. Defects of the neural tube. The first critical step in neural development is neurulation—formation and closure of the neural tube. Incomplete fusion of the neural tube and overlying bone, soft tissues, or skin leads to several defects, varying from mild anomalies (e.g., spina bifida occulta) to severe anomalies (e.g., anencephaly).

tube then forms the skull and vertebral arches posterior to the spinal cord, whereas ectoderm forms the overlying skin. If the neural tube does not close, the overlying bony structures of the cranium do not form. The calvarium, skin, and subcutaneous tissues will be absent in this region. The exposed brain is incomplete or even entirely absent. Most often, the base of the skull has only bits of neural and ependymal tissue and residues of meninges.

Genetic factors contribute to the pathogenesis of anencephaly. The anomaly is twice as common in female as in male fetuses, and it occurs with higher frequency in certain families. The risk of a second anencephalic fetus is 2% to 5%. After two anencephalic fetuses, the risk reaches 25% for each subsequent pregnancy.

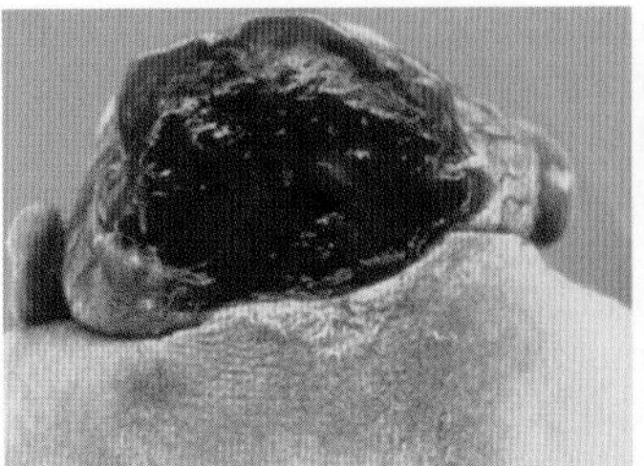
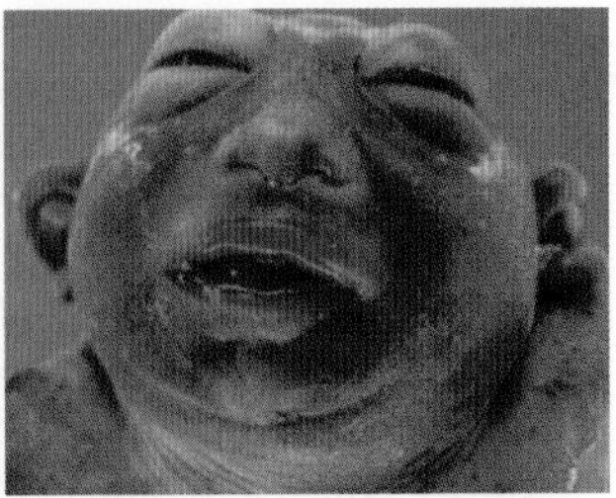

FIGURE 24-63. Anencephaly is the most severe defect of neurulation. The cerebral vault is absent (*right panel*), and the absence of a calvarium exposes a mass of vascularized tissue (cerebrovasculosa, *left panel*), in which there are rudimentary neuroectodermal structures. The lesion is bounded anteriorly by normally formed eyes and posteriorly by the brainstem.

Folic acid supplied in the periconceptional period lowers the incidence of NTDs. In 1998, the U.S. Food and Drug Administration began requiring supplemental folate to be added to enriched flour, bread, cereals, and some other products. This led to a significant decrease in the incidence of NTDs of all types.

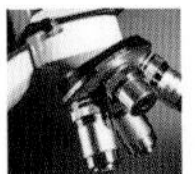

PATHOLOGY: The cranial vault is absent. The cerebral hemispheres are replaced by a highly vascularized, disorganized neuroglial tissue, the **cerebrovasculosa** (Fig. 24-63), on the flattened base of the skull. Two well-formed eyes with well-differentiated retinas mark the anterior margin of disturbed organogenesis. Short segments of optic nerves extend posteriorly. The posterior aspect of the malformation forms a variable transitional zone with a recognizable midbrain, but the brainstem and cerebellum are usually rudimentary. The upper spinal cord is hypoplastic, and a dysraphic bony posterior spinal column defect (**rachischisis**) may affect the cervical area.

Two thirds of anencephalic fetuses die in utero; those that are alive at birth rarely survive more than a week. Screening of pregnant women for serum α-fetoprotein and ultrasonography detect virtually all anencephalic fetuses.

Spina Bifida

Spina bifida refers to a group of NTDs that are due to failure of neural tube closure in the more caudal regions (Fig. 24-62). These anomalies are usually in the lumbar region and vary in severity from asymptomatic to disabling. They are not usually lethal. Spina bifida results from an insult between the 25th and 30th days of gestation, reflecting the timing of neural tube closure. These anomalies are classified by the severity of the defect:

- **Spina bifida occulta:** This defect is restricted to the vertebral arches and is usually asymptomatic. It frequently manifests externally only by a dimple or small tuft of hair on the lower back.
- **Meningocele:** This condition features a greater bone and soft tissue defect that permits the meninges to protrude as a fluid-filled sac visible on the external surface of the back, in the midline. The sides of the sac are usually covered by a thin layer of skin. Its apex may be ulcerated, allowing microorganisms to enter the CSF.
- **Meningomyelocele:** This is an even more extensive defect that exposes the spinal canal and causes nerve roots

(particularly those of the cauda equina) and spinal cord to be entrapped in an externally visible, protruding, CSF-filled sac (Fig. 24-64). Usually, the spinal cord is a flattened, ribbon-like structure. Severe neurologic consequences include motor and sensory defects of the lower extremities and compromise of bowel and bladder neurogenic control.

- **Rachischisis:** In this extreme defect, the spinal column is a gaping canal, often without a recognizable spinal cord. Rachischisis is usually lethal and seen in abortuses.

Some drugs, notably retinoids used for acne and valproic acid administered to manage seizures, must be avoided by women of childbearing age because of their association with NTDs.

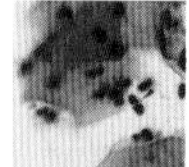

CLINICAL FEATURES: Clinical neurologic deficits in NTDs range from no symptoms in spina bifida occulta to lower limb paralysis, sensory loss, and incontinence in meningomyelocele. Associated malformations include Arnold–Chiari malformation, hydrocephalus, polymicrogyria, and hydromyelia of the spinal central canal (see below).

Syringomyelia

Syringomyelia is a congenital tubular cavitation (syrinx), which may or may not communicate with the central canal, which extends for variable distances within the spinal cord. Many cases represent congenital malformations, but the condition progresses slowly and usually first presents clinically in adults. Some cases of syringomyelia are not congenital but are caused by trauma, ischemia, or tumors. The syrinx is filled with a clear fluid similar to CSF.

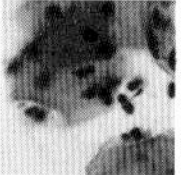

CLINICAL FEATURES: The symptoms of syringomyelia are present at the spinal level of the syrinx. At that point, the centrally located syrinx disrupts the crossing axons of the spinothalamic pathway. This leads to loss of pain and thermal sensation bilaterally at the spinal level of the syrinx, with relative sparing of fine touch, proprioception, and motor pathways.

Arnold–Chiari Malformation

Arnold–Chiari malformation is a complex condition in which the brainstem and cerebellum are compacted into a shallow, bowl-shaped posterior fossa with a low-positioned tentorium. It is often associated with syringomyelia or a lumbosacral meningomyelocele. Symptoms depend on the severity of the defect (Fig. 24-65). ***Because this malformation involves segmentation of the medulla and cerebellum as well as neural tube closure, it represents a defect of both neurulation and segmentation.***

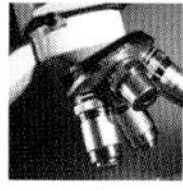

PATHOLOGY: In Arnold–Chiari malformation, the caudal aspect of the cerebellar vermis is herniated through an enlarged foramen magnum and protrudes onto the dorsal cervical cord, often reaching C3–C5 (Fig. 24-66). The herniated tissue is held in position by thickened meninges and shows pressure atrophy (i.e., depletion of Purkinje and granular cells). The brainstem is also displaced

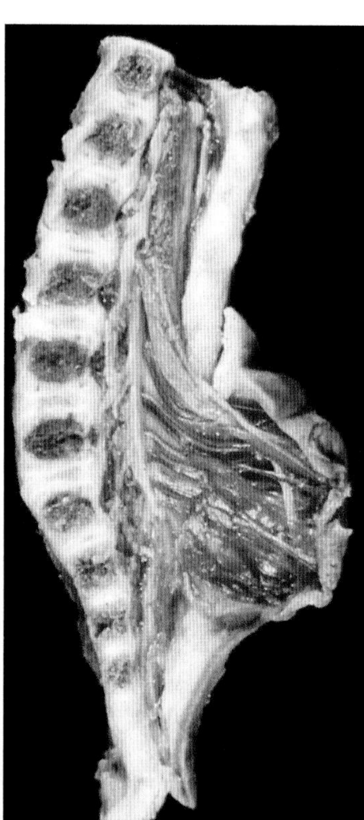

FIGURE 24-64. Meningomyelocele. This dysraphic defect, which is caused by lack of fusion of the spinal canal usually in the lumbar region, reveals disorganized spinal cord tissue with entrapment of nerve roots in a cerebrospinal fluid–filled sac. (Courtesy of Dr. F. Stephen Vogel, Duke University.)

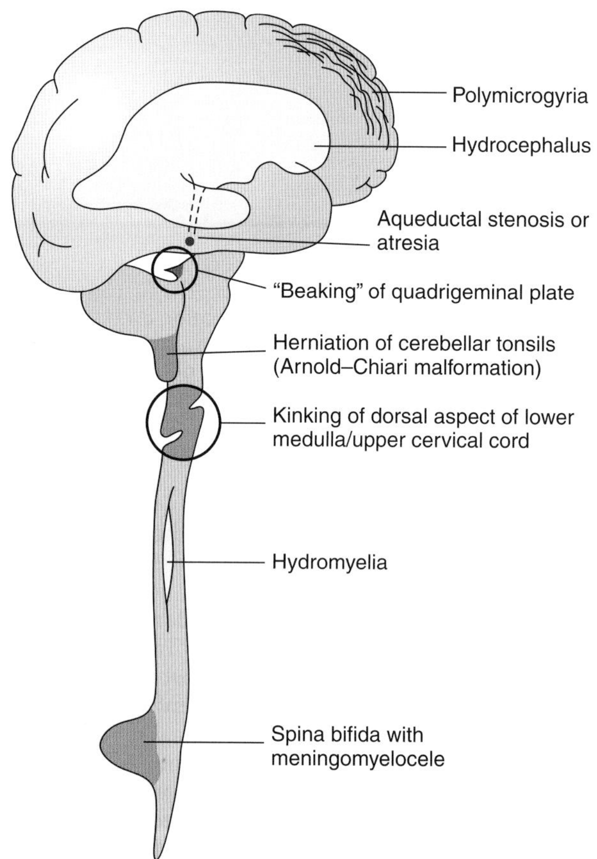

FIGURE 24-65. Arnold–Chiari malformation and associated lesions.

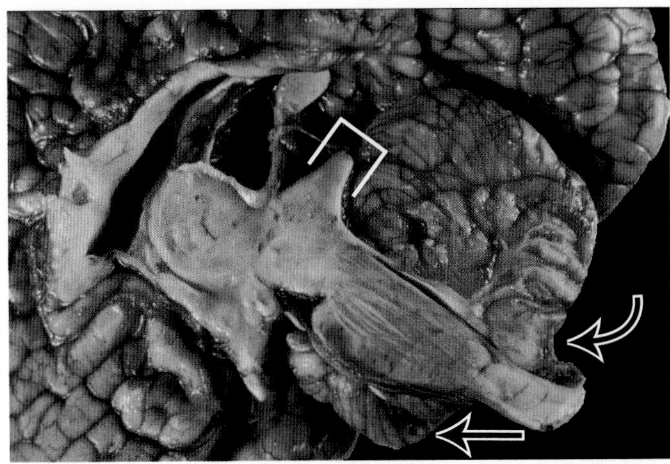

FIGURE 24-66. Arnold–Chiari malformation. The cerebellar vermis is herniated below the level of the foramen magnum (*arrow*). The downward displacement of the dorsal portion of the cord causes the obex of the fourth ventricle to occupy a position below the foramen magnum (*curved arrow*). The midbrain shows extreme "beaking" of the tectum with the four colliculi being replaced by a single pyramidal-shaped structure (*bracket*).

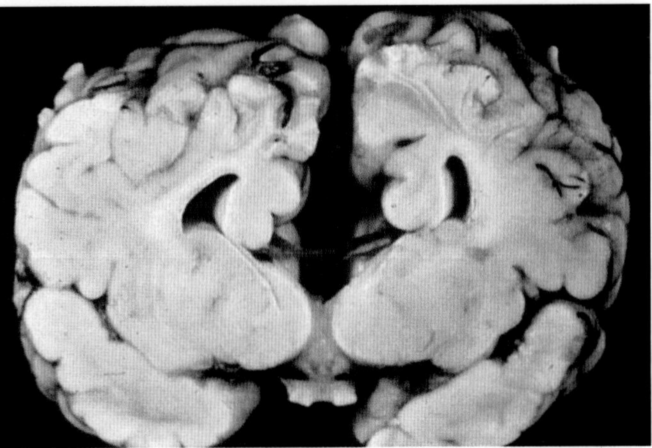

FIGURE 24-67. Congenital absence of the corpus callosum. A coronal section of the brain at the level of the thalamus reveals absence of the corpus callosum and "bat-wing" shape of the lateral ventricles. (Courtesy of Dr. F. Stephen Vogel, Duke University.)

caudally. From a lateral perspective, the lower medulla is angulated in its midsegment, creating a dorsal protrusion. The foramina of Magendie and Luschka are compressed by the bony ridge of the foramen magnum, causing hydrocephalus. The cerebellum is flattened to a discoid contour, and the quadrigeminal plate is often deformed by a "beak-shaped" dorsal protrusion of the inferior colliculi.

Defects of Segmentation and Cleavage

Holoprosencephaly

This condition represents a series of defects in which the interhemispheric fissure is absent, or partly formed, owing to a failure of the telencephalon to divide into the two hemispheres. Holoprosencephaly is rarely compatible with life beyond a few weeks or months, and survival is associated with severe mental retardation and seizures.

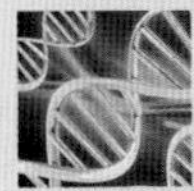

MOLECULAR PATHOGENESIS: Some 25% to 50% of patients with holoprosencephaly have numerical or structural chromosomal abnormalities. Monogenic holoprosencephaly is sometimes associated with mutations in *sonic hedgehog*, an important signaling molecule.

Agenesis of the Corpus Callosum

This anomaly is a regular feature of holoprosencephaly but can also be a solitary lesion. Lack of a corpus callosum does not entail significant loss of interhemispheric functional coordination, but it is associated with seizures. The corpus callosum physically tethers and functionally interconnects the hemispheres, so its absence permits the lateral ventricles to drift outward and upward, radiographically termed "bat-wing" ventricles (Fig. 24-67).

Congenital Atresia of the Aqueduct of Sylvius

This is the most common cause of congenital obstructive hydrocephalus. It may result from deranged mesencephalic (midbrain) development and occurs in 1 in 1,000 live births. The brain is enlarged owing to grotesque ventricular enlargement, with thinning of the cerebral cortex and stretching of white matter tracts. The midbrain may show multiple atretic channels or an aqueduct narrowed by gliosis. These defects may result from developmental failure during segmentation or later in gestation as a result of transplacental transmission of infections that induce ependymitis.

Cortical Malformations

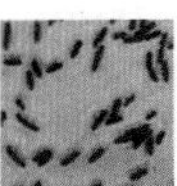

ETIOLOGIC FACTORS: The disorders of cortical development reflect the nature and severity of disruption of gyral patterning and may be global or focal. Portions of the germinal matrix induce formation of specific overlying portions of the cerebral cortex; there is a spatial destiny of neuroglial cells in a given region of germinal matrix. **Schizencephaly** is an example of a localized failure of focal cortical development, characterized by a patch of cortex that is "missing." More global, often genetically determined defects of neuroglial proliferation and migration result in a more widespread and severe cortical defect, called lissencephaly, meaning "smooth brain."

- **Lissencephaly** is the most severe congenital disorder of cortical development. The cortical surface of the cerebral hemispheres is smooth or has imperfectly formed gyri. Some 60% of patients with lissencephaly show deletions in the region of the *LIS1* gene on chromosome 17p13.3. This gene encodes a protein involved in cytoskeletal dynamics that affects cell proliferation and motility. The white matter contains clusters of neurons that failed to reach the cortex.
- **Heterotopias** are focal disturbances in neuronal migration that lead to nodules of ectopic neurons and glia, usually in white matter. They are often associated with mental retardation and seizures and may be caused by maternal alcoholism.

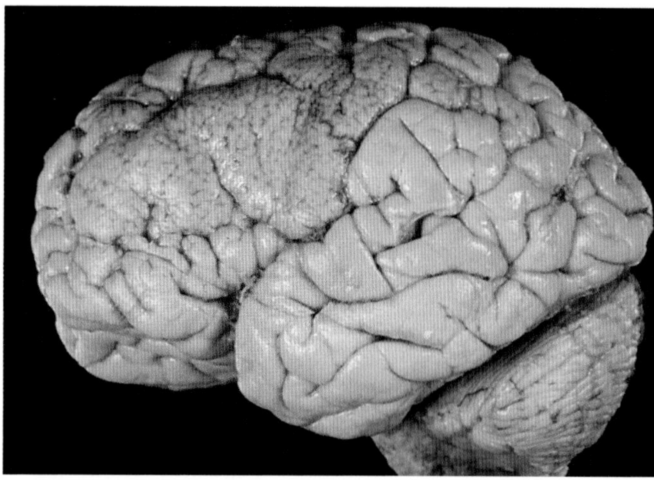

FIGURE 24-68. Pachygyria. Broad textured gyri are seen here in the superior frontal region, indicating a defect in cortical formation. (Courtesy of Dr. F. Stephen Vogel, Duke University.)

- **Polymicrogyria** describes the presence of small and excessive gyri. The brain surface appears to be textured with many small bumps.
- **Pachygyria** is a condition in which the gyri are reduced in number and unusually broad (Fig. 24-68).

CENTRAL NERVOUS SYSTEM NEOPLASIA

Primary CNS cancers represent 1.5% of all primary malignant tumors. Metastatic tumors to the CNS are far more common than are primary tumors and are a major problem in clinical management. By far, the most common primary CNS neoplasms are meningiomas and gliomas, each of which accounts for one third of CNS tumors (Table 24-5). Whereas most brain tumors arise in adults, some are more common in childhood. Together, primary brain tumors are second only to leukemia as the most common childhood malignancy and are the most common pediatric solid tumors.

Meningioma

Meningiomas are derived from the middle layer of arachnoid (meningothelial) cells that form the outer boundary of the subarachnoid space. These tumors can arise at any CNS site where arachnoid cells are present.

Table 24-5

Major Types of Primary Central Nervous System (CNS) Tumors
Meningioma
Gliomas (including diffuse and circumscribed astrocytomas, oligodendroglioma, ependymoma, choroid plexus tumors, several rare glioma subtypes)
Medulloblastoma and other primitive neuroectodermal tumors
Craniopharyngioma
Germ cell tumors
Hemangioblastoma
Neuronal and mixed glioneuronal tumors
Pineal tumors
Primary CNS lymphoma

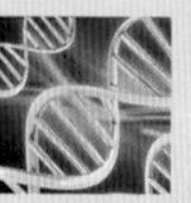

MOLECULAR PATHOGENESIS: Meningiomas typically arise in one of three settings:

- **Sporadic:** ***The vast majority of meningiomas arise sporadically.*** Many show loss, partial deletion or mutation of the *NF2* locus (22q12). Disturbances of this tumor suppressor gene may thus be involved not only in neurofibromatosis type 2 (NF2)-associated tumors but also in the origin of many sporadic meningiomas (and schwannomas).
- **Iatrogenic:** Induction of meningiomas by radiation therapy generally involves a latent period of a decade or more and is directly related to radiation dosage. With higher radiation doses, such as are used for head and neck cancers, the interval may be as short as 5 years.
- **Tumor predisposition syndromes:** Meningiomas also occur in conjunction with several genetic syndromes, most importantly NF2 (Table 24-6).

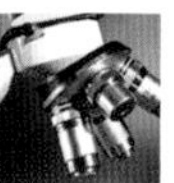

PATHOLOGY: On MRI and gross examination, most meningiomas are well-circumscribed dura-based masses of variable size, which compress, but do not invade, the underlying brain (Fig. 24-69A and B). The cut surface is fleshy and tan. The classic histologic hallmark of meningiomas is a whorled pattern, often in association with psammoma bodies (laminated, spherical calcospherites) (Fig. 24-69C and D). However, these tumors can show diverse morphologic patterns. Meningiomas typically express epithelial membrane antigen (EMA) focally (Fig. 24-69C). They have many intercellular junctions, owing to their origin from the cohesive arachnoid barrier cell layer (Fig. 24-69E).

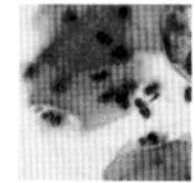

CLINICAL FEATURES: The indolent growth of most meningiomas enables them to enlarge slowly for years before becoming symptomatic. During that time, they displace the brain but do not infiltrate it (Fig. 24-70A and B). Patients often have seizures, particularly with tumors at parasagittal sites over the convexity of the hemispheres. In other locations, meningiomas compress a variety of functional structures. Invasion of cranial bone, often accompanied by hyperostosis on CT scans, is relatively common, and growth through the calvarium may create a tumor mass beneath the scalp. By contrast, meningiomas rarely invade the underlying brain. Tumors that are not completely excised tend to recur, and some may undergo anaplastic progression over time. On rare occasions, anaplastic (malignant) meningiomas may also arise de novo.

Astrocytoma

Astrocytomas can be divided into two major categories based on how diffusely they infiltrate the brain parenchyma. ***Diffuse astrocytoma*** infiltrate the brain widely and includes low-grade fibrillary astrocytoma, anaplastic astrocytoma, ***and the most malignant astrocytic tumor, glioblastoma.*** Members of the other major category of astrocytomas, including pilocytic astrocytoma, typically do not infiltrate the CNS but rather

Table 24-6

Major Nervous System Tumor Predisposition Syndromes

Syndrome	Chromosome Locus	Gene (Protein)	Associated Nervous System Tumors
Neurofibromatosis type 1 (NF1)	17q11.2	*NF1* (neurofibromin)	Neurofibromas (dermal and plexiform) Malignant peripheral nerve sheath tumor Pilocytic astrocytoma ("optic glioma") Diffuse astrocytoma Glioblastoma
Neurofibromatosis type 2 (NF2)	22q12	*NF2* (merlin/ schwanomin)	Vestibular schwannomas (bilateral) Other schwannomas Meningiomas (multiple) Meningioangiomatosis Ependymoma of spinal cord Diffuse astrocytoma
Schwannomatosis (sometimes referred to as "NF3")	Unknown	Unknown	Schwannomas (multiple, spinal roots, cranial nerves, skin, not vestibular)
von Hippel–Lindau (vHL)	3p25–26	*VHL* (pVHL)	Hemangioblastomas (multiple) of cerebellum, spinal cord, brainstem, retina, spinal peripheral nerve roots Endolymphatic sac tumor
Tuberous sclerosis complex	9q34 16p13.3	*TSC1* (hamartin) *TSC2* (tuberin)	Subependymal giant cell astrocytoma
Li–Fraumeni syndrome	17p13	*TP53* (TP53 protein)	Diffuse astrocytomas, including glioblastoma Medulloblastoma Choroid plexus papilloma Ependymoma Oligodendroglioma Meningioma
Cowden disease	10q23	*PTENIMMAC1* (PTEN protein)	Dysplastic gangliocytoma of the cerebellum (Lhermitte–Duclos disease)
Turcot type 1 syndrome (mismatch repair [MMR]/hereditary nonpolyposis colon cancer [HNPCC]–associated Turcot)	3p21.3 2p16 5q11–q13 2q32 7p22	*MLH1* *MSH2* and *MSH6 MSH3* *PMS1* *PMS2* *APC* (APC protein)	Glioblastoma
Turcot type 2 syndrome (familial adenomatous polyposis [FAP]–associated Turcot)	5q21		Medulloblastoma
Nevoid basal cell carcinoma (Gorlin) syndrome	9q22.3	*PTCH* (Ptch protein)	Medulloblastoma
Rhabdoid tumor predisposition syndrome	22q11.2	*INI1* (INI1 protein)	Atypical teratoid/rhabdoid tumor

are slowly enlarging, compact masses that cause symptoms by compressing adjacent structures.

Diffuse Astrocytoma

The most salient biologic characteristic of diffuse astrocytomas, as the name implies, is the ability of individual tumor cells to infiltrate widely through brain and spinal cord parenchyma (Fig. 24-71). This property reaches its extreme in **gliomatosis cerebri**, in which infiltrating glioma cells (usually astrocytes but occasionally oligodendroglia) involve at least three cerebral lobes, and often more. Infiltration often extends into both hemispheres, the brainstem, the cerebellum, and even the spinal cord.

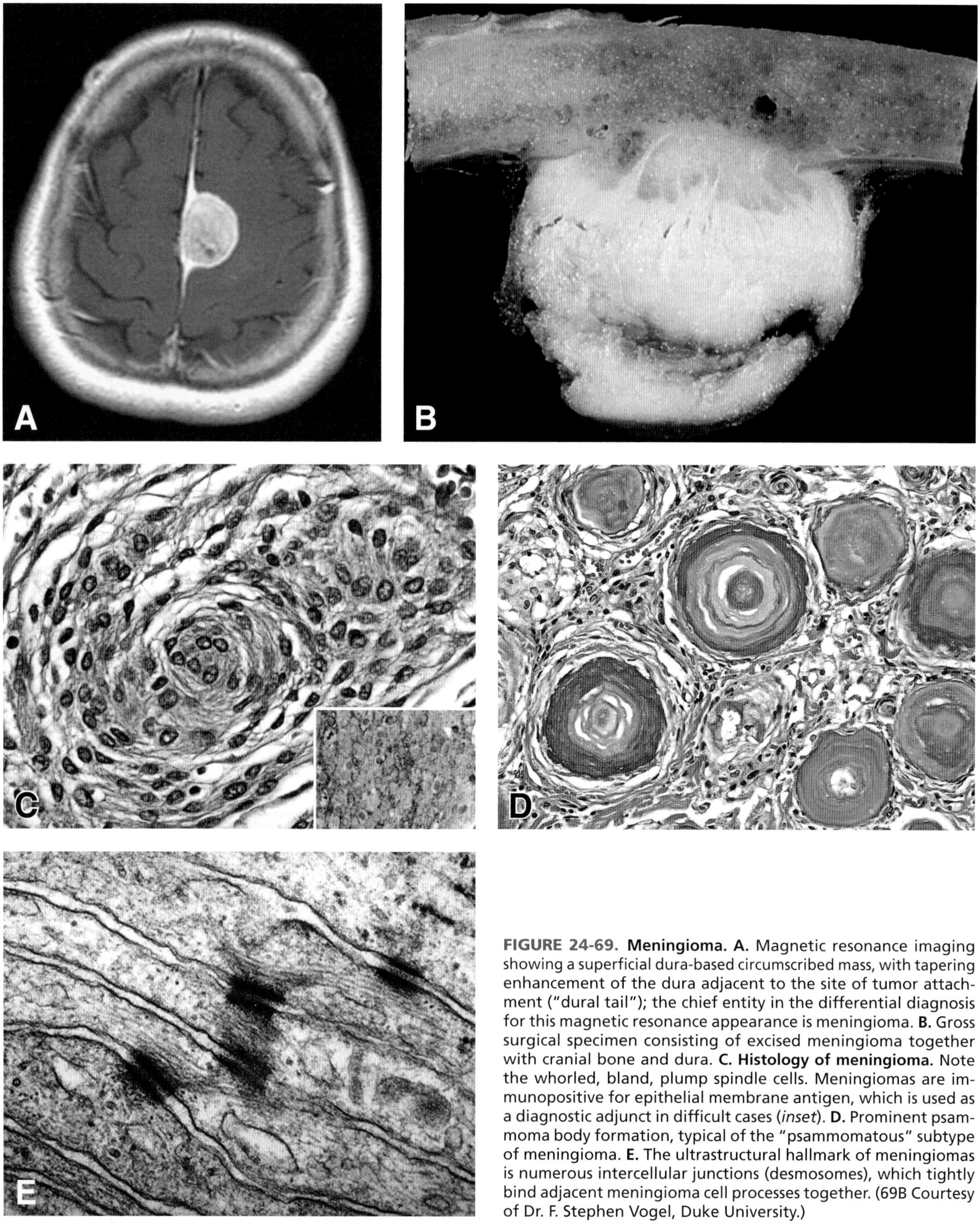

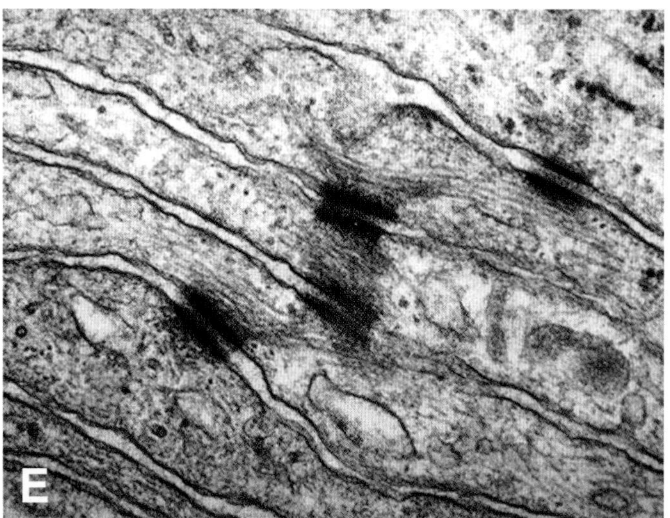

FIGURE 24-69. Meningioma. A. Magnetic resonance imaging showing a superficial dura-based circumscribed mass, with tapering enhancement of the dura adjacent to the site of tumor attachment ("dural tail"); the chief entity in the differential diagnosis for this magnetic resonance appearance is meningioma. **B.** Gross surgical specimen consisting of excised meningioma together with cranial bone and dura. **C. Histology of meningioma.** Note the whorled, bland, plump spindle cells. Meningiomas are immunopositive for epithelial membrane antigen, which is used as a diagnostic adjunct in difficult cases (*inset*). **D.** Prominent psammoma body formation, typical of the "psammomatous" subtype of meningioma. **E.** The ultrastructural hallmark of meningiomas is numerous intercellular junctions (desmosomes), which tightly bind adjacent meningioma cell processes together. (69B Courtesy of Dr. F. Stephen Vogel, Duke University.)

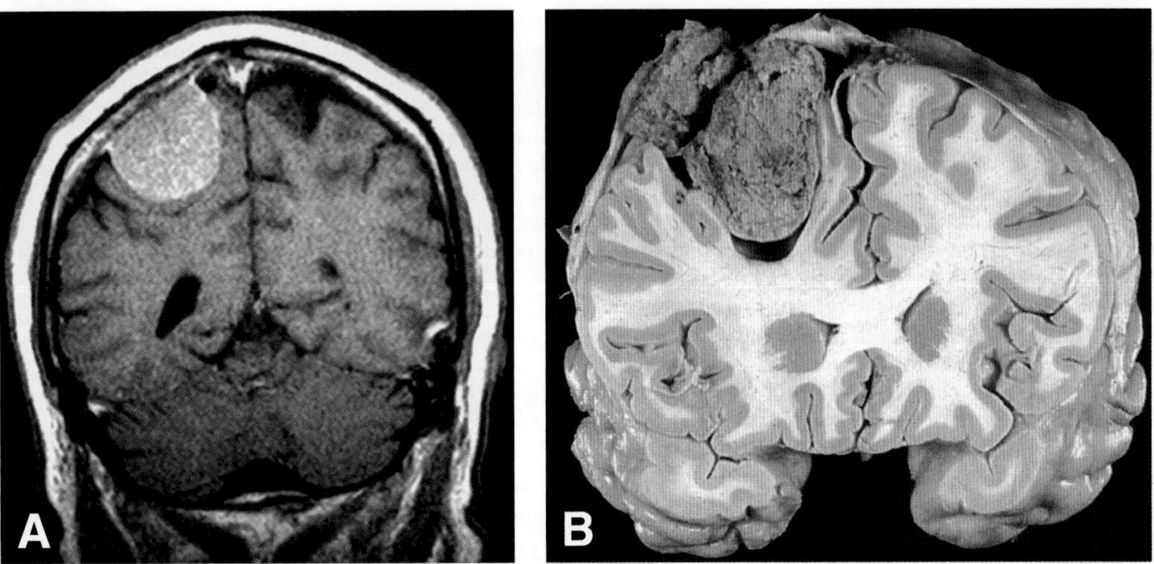

FIGURE 24-70. Meningioma. Meningiomas compress, but do not usually invade, the underlying brain. **A.** Magnetic resonance image. **B.** Gross specimen. (70B Courtesy of Dr. F. Stephen Vogel, Duke University.)

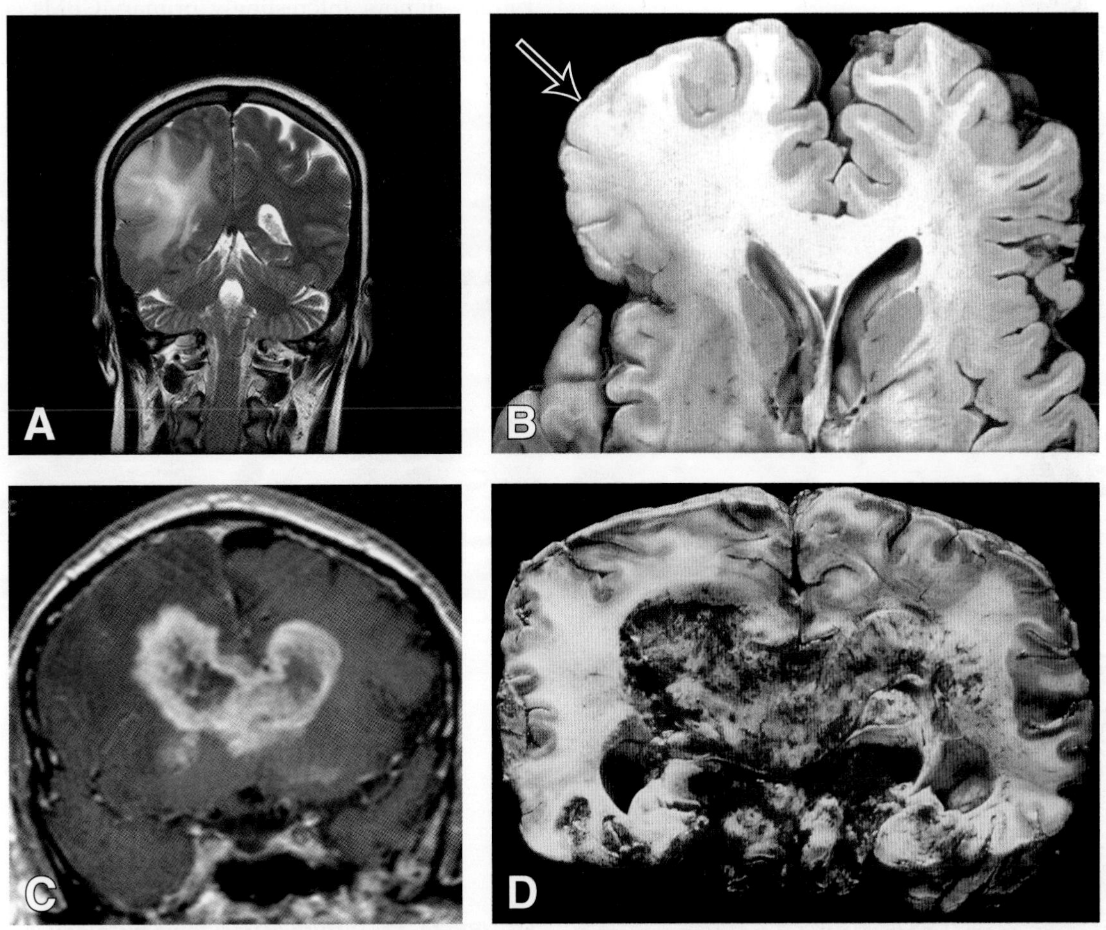

FIGURE 24-71. Gliomas. A. Infiltrating astrocytomas exhibit a diffuse, fuzzy interface with the adjacent brain tissue that is being invaded on magnetic resonance imaging. **B.** One manifestation of diffuse infiltration is "blurring" of the normally sharp interface between the gray matter and white matter as astrocytoma cells overrun the cortex, as seen (*arrow*) in this gross specimen. **C.** In contrast to low-grade diffuse astrocytomas, **glioblastomas** show prominent irregular ring contrast enhancement and often infiltrate across the corpus callosum to involve the contralateral hemisphere ("butterfly" glioblastoma), as seen in this preoperative magnetic resonance image. **D.** Autopsy gross specimen. (71B, 71D Courtesy of Dr. F. Stephen Vogel, Duke University.)

Glioblastoma typically presents as a large, ring-enhancing mass with an irregular central area of necrosis and prominent edema of surrounding white matter. The infiltrating component of glioblastomas often crosses to contralateral hemispheres via the corpus callosum; such cases are referred to as "butterfly" glioblastomas based on their appearance on coronal MRI (Fig. 24-71).

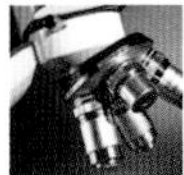

PATHOLOGY: **Low-grade fibrillary astrocytomas (WHO grade II)** have well-differentiated astrocytic tumor cells with little nuclear atypia or cell proliferation. **Gemistocytic astrocytoma** is a distinctive subtype of low-grade astrocytoma in which the main population of cells has prominent globular cytoplasm filled with glial intermediate filaments (Fig. 24-72). Diffuse astrocytomas often undergo anaplastic progression, usually over several years, into high-grade astrocytoma (anaplastic astrocytoma, WHO grade III) and, ultimately, into glioblastoma (WHO grade IV). This tendency for anaplastic progression is even more pronounced with the gemistocytic variant. **Anaplastic astrocytoma (WHO grade III)** is more cellular than low-grade fibrillary astrocytoma, and individual tumor cells are more pleomorphic (Fig. 24-72). Mitotic rates are elevated. Anaplastic astrocytomas typically progress to glioblastoma within a few years.

Glioblastoma multiforme (GBM; WHO grade IV) is the single most common primary malignant brain tumor. It accounts for about 20% of all CNS tumors. GBMs are cytologically highly pleomorphic, and constituent cells vary greatly in size and shape, with large bizarre nuclei and multinucleated cells. They may arise by anaplastic progression from lower-grade diffuse astrocytomas or, much more commonly, de novo (primary glioblastoma; 95% of GBMs). Mitotic activity in GBMs is high; vascular proliferation and foci of tumor necrosis, surrounded by a densely cellular cuff of tumor cells ("pseudopalisading necrosis"), are characteristic (Fig. 24-72C).

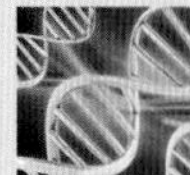

MOLECULAR PATHOGENESIS: *The vast majority of GBMs are sporadic,* but a minority arise in the setting of a genetic tumor predisposition syndrome (Table 24-6). Primary GBMs often show amplification of the epidermal growth factor receptor (*EGFR*) gene and mutation of the *PTEN* gene; *TP53* is more often mutated in secondary GBMs. More recent molecular and genomic profiling studies have identified mutation of the isocitrate-dehydrogenase genes 1 or 2 (*IDH1* or *IDH2*), especially *IDH1*. This is a very common signature of low-grade (grade II) and anaplastic (grade III) diffuse gliomas and also of a majority of secondary GBMs that arise from these lower-grade tumors. Interestingly, primary GBMs generally do not show *IDH* mutations.

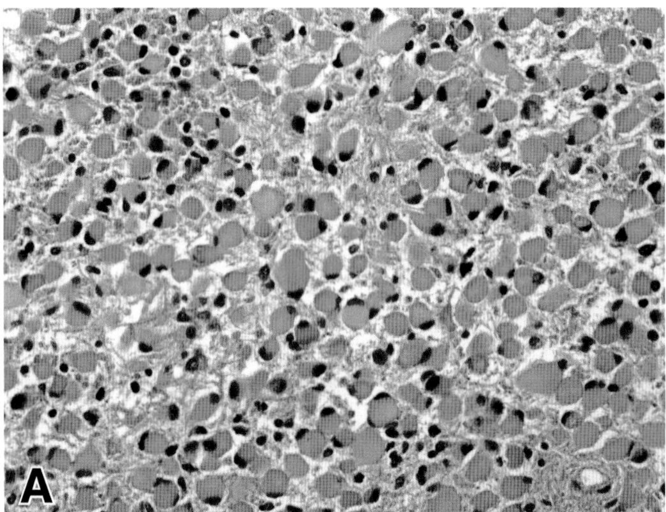

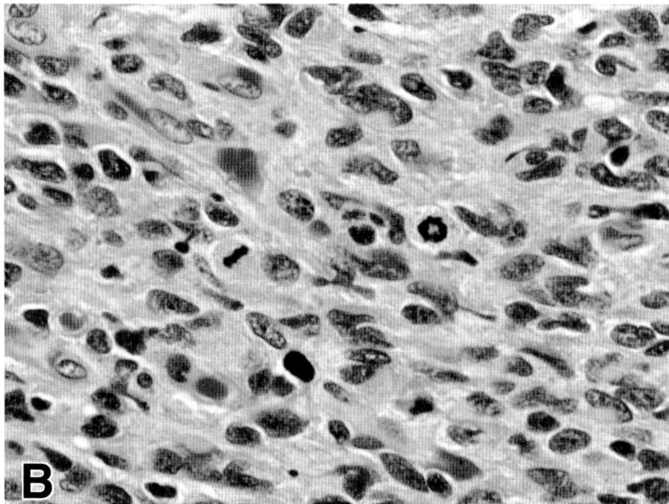

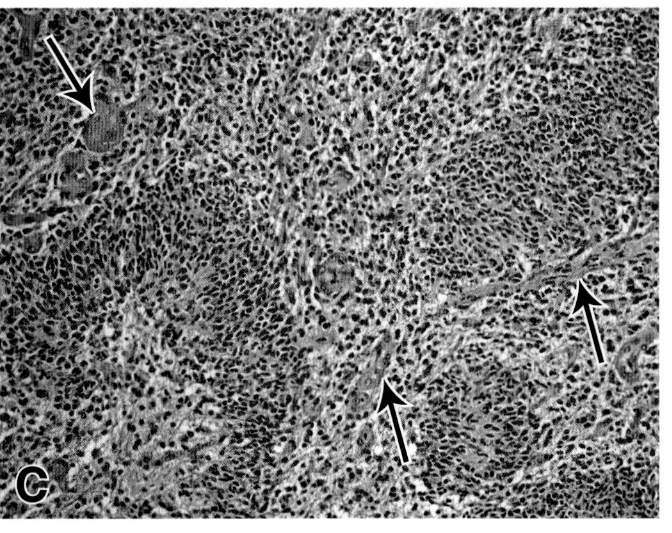

FIGURE 24-72. **Diffuse astrocytoma histology. A. Gemistocytic astrocytomas** are low-grade (World Health Organization [WHO] grade II) diffuse astrocytomas characterized by prominent globular cytoplasm. **B. Anaplastic astrocytoma (WHO grade III)**, in contrast, is more cellular and more pleomorphic, in addition to having a higher proliferation rate. **C. Glioblastoma (WHO grade IV)** displays foci of tumor necrosis surrounded by hypercellular cuffs of tumor cells ("pseudopalisading necrosis") as well as vascular proliferation (*arrows*).

GBMs can be stratified into two groups based on whether (1) the promotor for the DNA repair gene *MGMT* is methylated, and hence inactivated, or (2) unmethylated, and so capable of repairing damage caused by alkylating agents used in chemotherapy. Patients with *MGMT* promotor methylation (inactivation) respond significantly better to treatment.

Pilocytic Astrocytoma

Pilocytic astrocytomas (PAs) are circumscribed gliomas that typically arise in children and young adults and expand very slowly. Unlike diffuse astrocytomas, PAs do not infiltrate brain or spinal cord parenchyma diffusely and rarely progress to higher grade tumors. Common locations include the cerebellum, brainstem, optic nerves, and third ventricular region. PAs are contrast enhancing, may be associated with a cystic component, and are well circumscribed on preoperative imaging studies (Fig. 24-73).

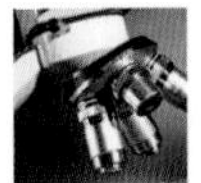

PATHOLOGY: PAs consist of compact areas of tumor cells with elongated bipolar cytoplasmic processes (pilocytes), which are separated by prominent microcysts. The compact areas frequently have prominent **Rosenthal fibers**, a histologic hallmark of pilocytic astrocytoma. Vascular proliferation is typical and correlates with the contrast enhancement seen on preoperative MRI studies. In favorable anatomic locations, such as the cerebellum, surgical resection may be curative.

Subependymal Giant Cell Astrocytoma

SEGA is an indolent, low-grade glioma that arises from the wall of the lateral ventricle. It grows slowly within the ventricular cavity until it causes obstructive hydrocephalus by encroaching on the interventricular foramen of Monro. SEGAs are associated with **tuberous sclerosis** and may be the presenting feature in a child with otherwise inconspicuous stigmata of that disease. Pharmacologic inhibitors of the mTOR pathway can shrink SEGAs and provide a medical approach in the management of these patients.

Oligodendroglioma

Like diffuse astrocytomas, ODGs are highly infiltrative. However, their response to treatment and overall survival are much more favorable than for diffuse astrocytomas of similar grade.

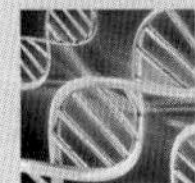

MOLECULAR PATHOGENESIS: Translocation between chromosomes 1 and 19 is a characteristic ODG molecular signature. This translocation causes complete loss of the short arm of chromosome 1 (1p) and the long arm of chromosome 19 (19q). ***Combined whole arm deletion of 1p and 19q is a favorable genetic signature in diffuse gliomas and correlates closely with classic ODG morphologic features.***

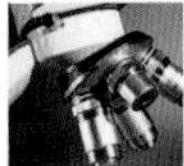

PATHOLOGY: Most ODGs arise in adults in the fourth and fifth decades, largely in the white matter of cerebral hemispheres. They commonly infiltrate into overlying cerebral cortex. ODGs show a monotonous population of cells with regular round nuclei surrounded by a small rim of clear cytoplasm ("perinuclear halo" or "fried-egg" appearance); the appearance is similar to normal oligodendroglia (Fig. 24-74A). This halo is a diagnostically useful artifact of specimen processing. Other characteristic features of ODGs include a network of delicate, branching blood vessels ("chicken-wire" pattern), and scattered microcalcifications. In areas of cortical infiltration, ODG cells tend to cluster around neuron cell bodies (perineuronal satellitosis) and blood vessels (perivascular satellitosis). They also form an infiltrating layer just beneath the pia (subpial growth). Mitotic activity is inconspicuous in low-grade ODG (WHO grade II), but these tumors recur and ultimately undergo anaplastic progression. **Anaplastic oligodendroglioma** differs from WHO grade II ODG by showing increased mitotic activity and microvascular proliferation. These may sometimes be accompanied by foci of tumor necrosis (Fig. 24-74B).

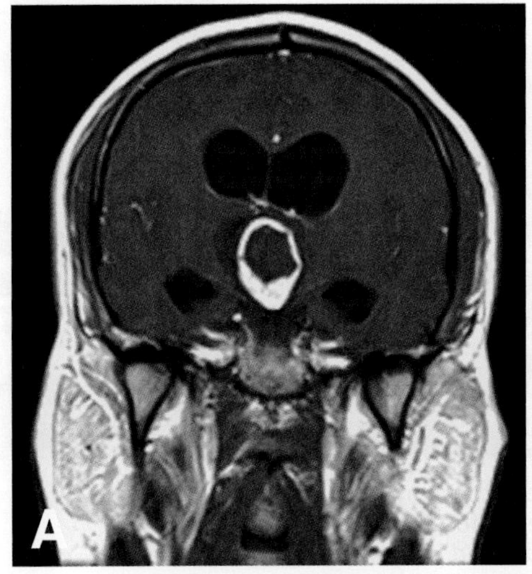

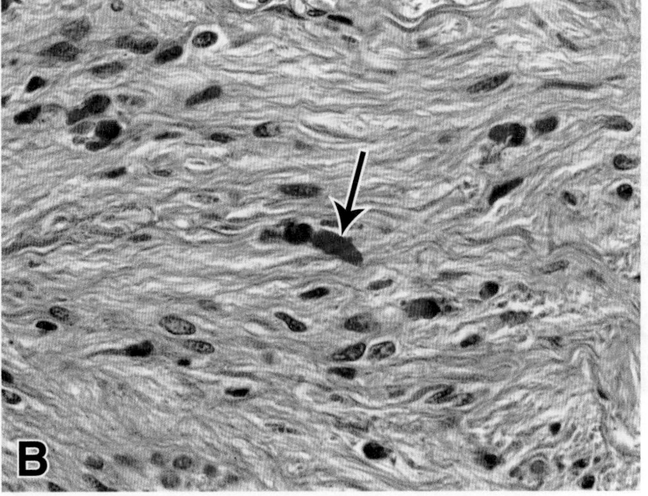

FIGURE 24-73. Pilocytic astrocytoma (World Health Organization grade I). A. Pilocytic astrocytomas are very low-grade circumscribed contrast-enhancing gliomas. **B.** Histologically, the neoplastic pilocytes ("hair cells") exhibit greatly elongated bipolar cytoplasmic processes that are prone to Rosenthal fiber formation (*arrow*).

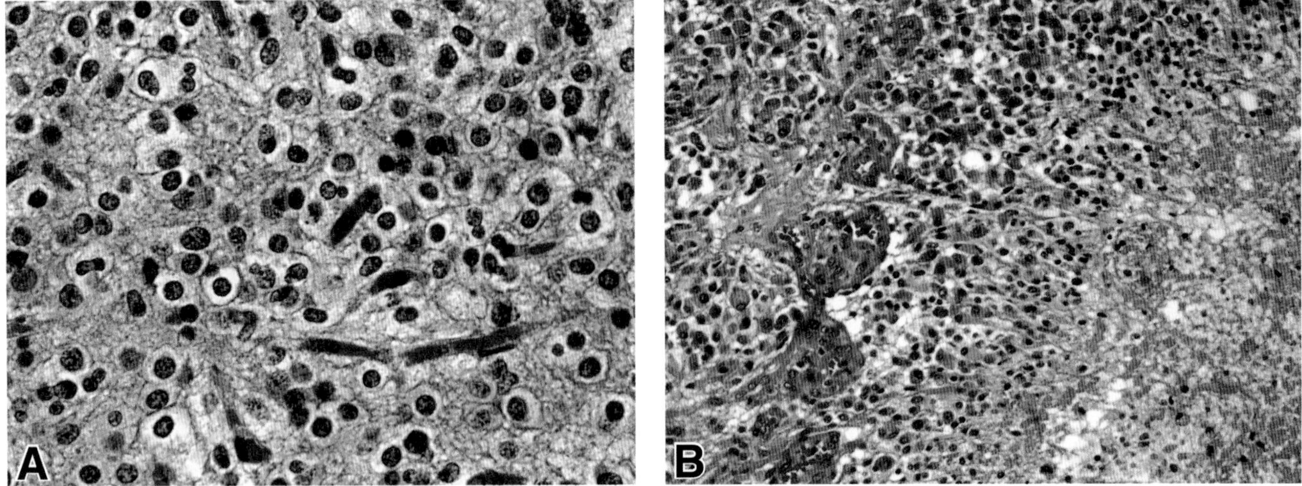

FIGURE 24-74. Oligodendroglioma. A. The cells of **low-grade oligodendroglioma** (World Health Organization grade II) closely resemble normal oligodendrocytes, with regular round nuclei surrounded by perinuclear halos. **B. Anaplastic oligodendroglioma** (AO) displays increased cellularity and brisk mitotic activity, with some tumors also developing foci of necrosis with tumor cell pseudopalisading.

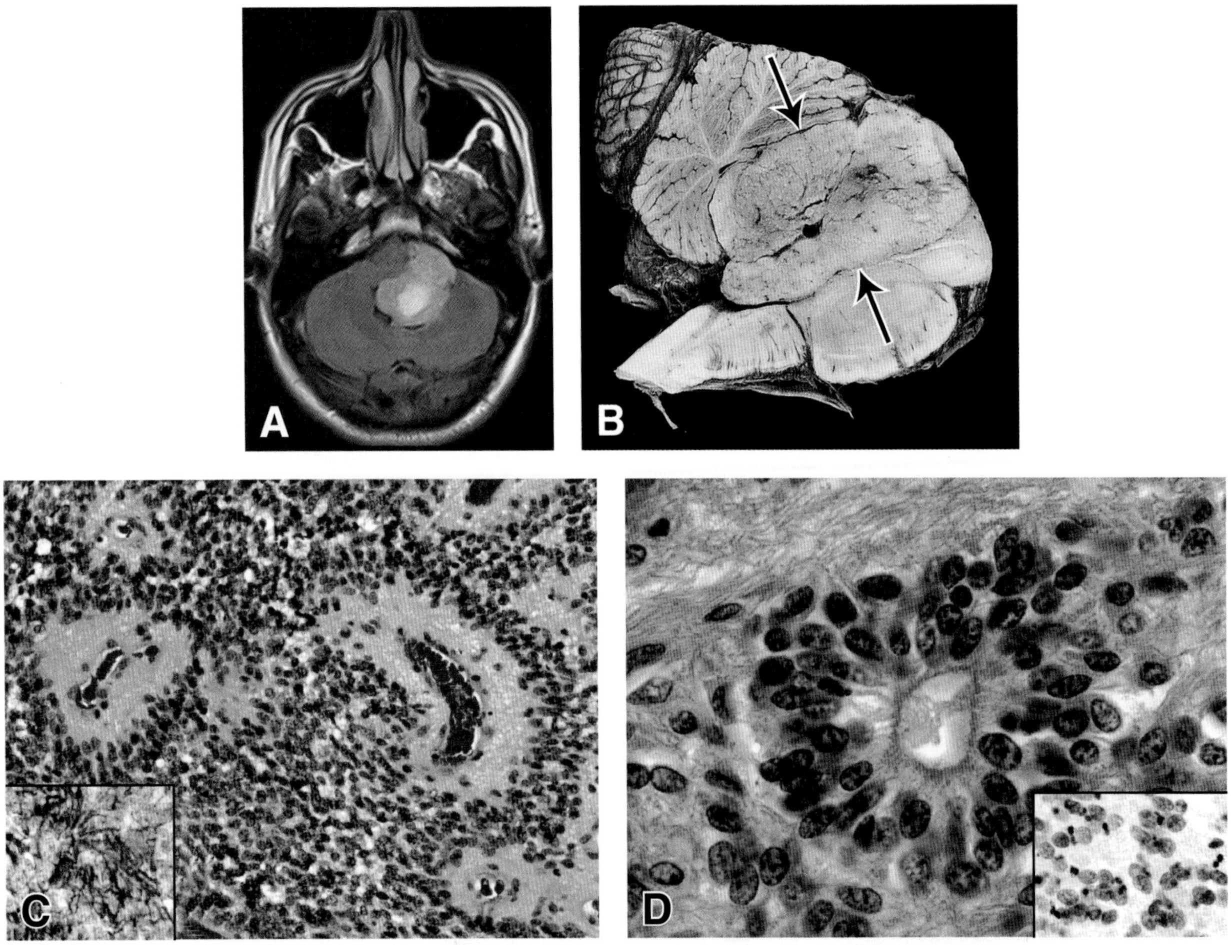

FIGURE 24-75. Ependymoma. A. Ependymomas can arise in the ventricles, the cerebral hemisphere, or the spinal cord. Those located within the posterior fossa tend to grow through the ventricular outlet foramina (median foramen of Magendie and lateral foramina of Luschka) into the subarachnoid space, as seen in this magnetic resonance image. **B.** Autopsy gross specimen. Tumor is identified between the arrows. **C.** Microscopically, the hallmark of ependymomas is the perivascular pseudorosette. The immunophenotype of ependymoma includes dot-like and ring-like positivity for epithelial membrane antigen (*inset*). **D.** Well-formed true ependymal rosette with immunoreactivity of the glial marker glial fibrillary acidic protein (*inset*). (75B Courtesy of Dr. F. Stephen Vogel, Duke University.)

Ependymoma

Ependymomas are typically slow-growing tumors of children and young adults that originate in the cerebral ventricles or central canal of the spinal cord. In children, the posterior fossa fourth ventricle is the preferred location, whereas in adults, most are in the supratentorial compartment. They may arise in either the ventricle or in the cerebral hemisphere white matter. Ependymomas of the fourth ventricle tend to fill the ventricle and grow into the lateral recesses, occasionally even flowing through the lateral foramina of Luschka into the subarachnoid space (Fig. 24-75A and B). In the spinal cord, ependymomas are the most common intra-axial tumors, followed by diffuse astrocytoma.

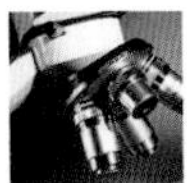

PATHOLOGY: Ependymomas grow as circumscribed masses and so are amenable to surgical resection. Their histologic hallmark is perivascular pseudorosettes, cuffs of radiating tumor cell cytoplasmic processes around vessels (Fig. 24-75C). True ependymal rosettes, in which tumor cells surround a central lumen, can also be seen but are less common. Ependymomas express epithelial membrane antigen (EMA; Fig. 24-75C, *inset*) and GFAP (Fig. 24-75D, *inset*). EMA staining in ependymomas is characteristically in a cytoplasmic dot-like and ring-like distribution unlike the membranous pattern of EMA expression in meningiomas. **Anaplastic ependymoma (WHO grade III)** shows increased mitotic activity and microvascular proliferation.

Choroid Plexus Papilloma

Unlike other common childhood brain tumors, which favor the posterior fossa (cerebellum, fourth ventricle, and brainstem), **CPPs (WHO grade I)** in children most commonly arise in the lateral ventricles (Fig. 24-76A). In adults, the fourth ventricle is preferred. CPPs are benign and, given their location within ventricles, are potentially curable by surgery. However, CSF dissemination can occur, significantly worsening the prognosis in such cases.

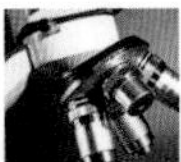

PATHOLOGY: CPP closely recapitulates the papillary architecture of the normal choroid plexus, but the tumor cells tend to be more crowded together and commonly assume a columnar rather than cuboidal architecture (Fig. 24-76B). Their immunophenotype includes reactivity for glial markers (S-100, GFAP) and transthyretin (prealbumin). There are two higher grade choroid plexus tumors: **atypical CPP (WHO grade II)**, which has increased mitotic activity compared to grade I tumors, and **choroid plexus carcinoma (WHO grade III)**, which shows increased

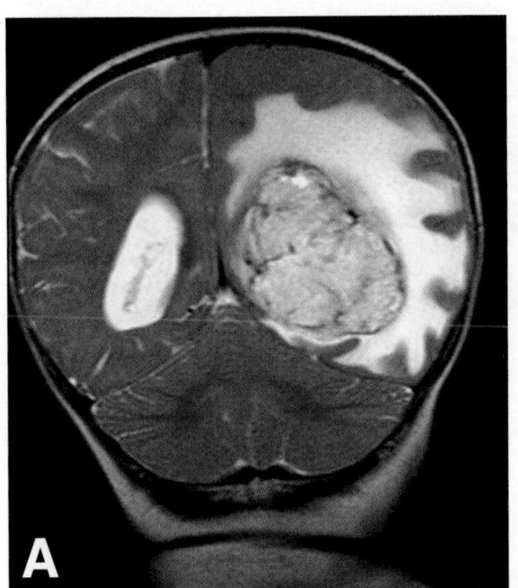

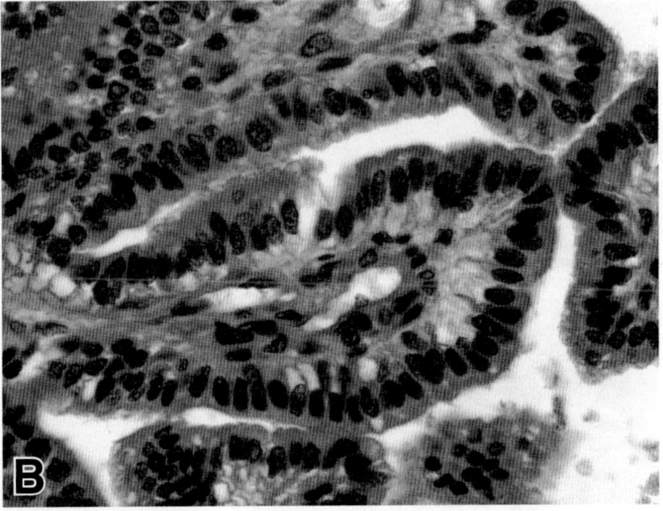

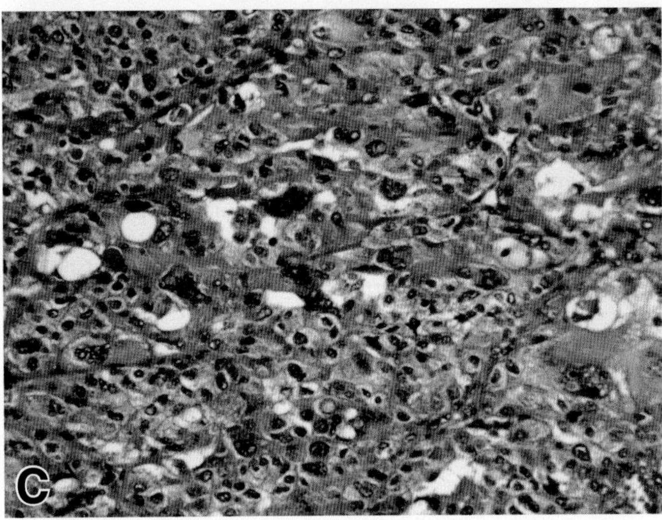

FIGURE 24-76. Choroid plexus papilloma (CPP) and carcinoma (CPC). A. CPP is a low-grade intraventricular tumor that arises from the fourth ventricular choroid plexus in adults and the lateral ventricular choroid plexus in children. **B.** Histologically, **CPP** retains the papillary architecture of choroid plexus, but the cells are more crowded and columnar rather than cuboidal. **C. CPC** is a high-grade tumor that differs from CPP in showing loss of papillary architecture, marked cellular pleomorphism, an increased proliferation rate, and a more aggressive clinical course.

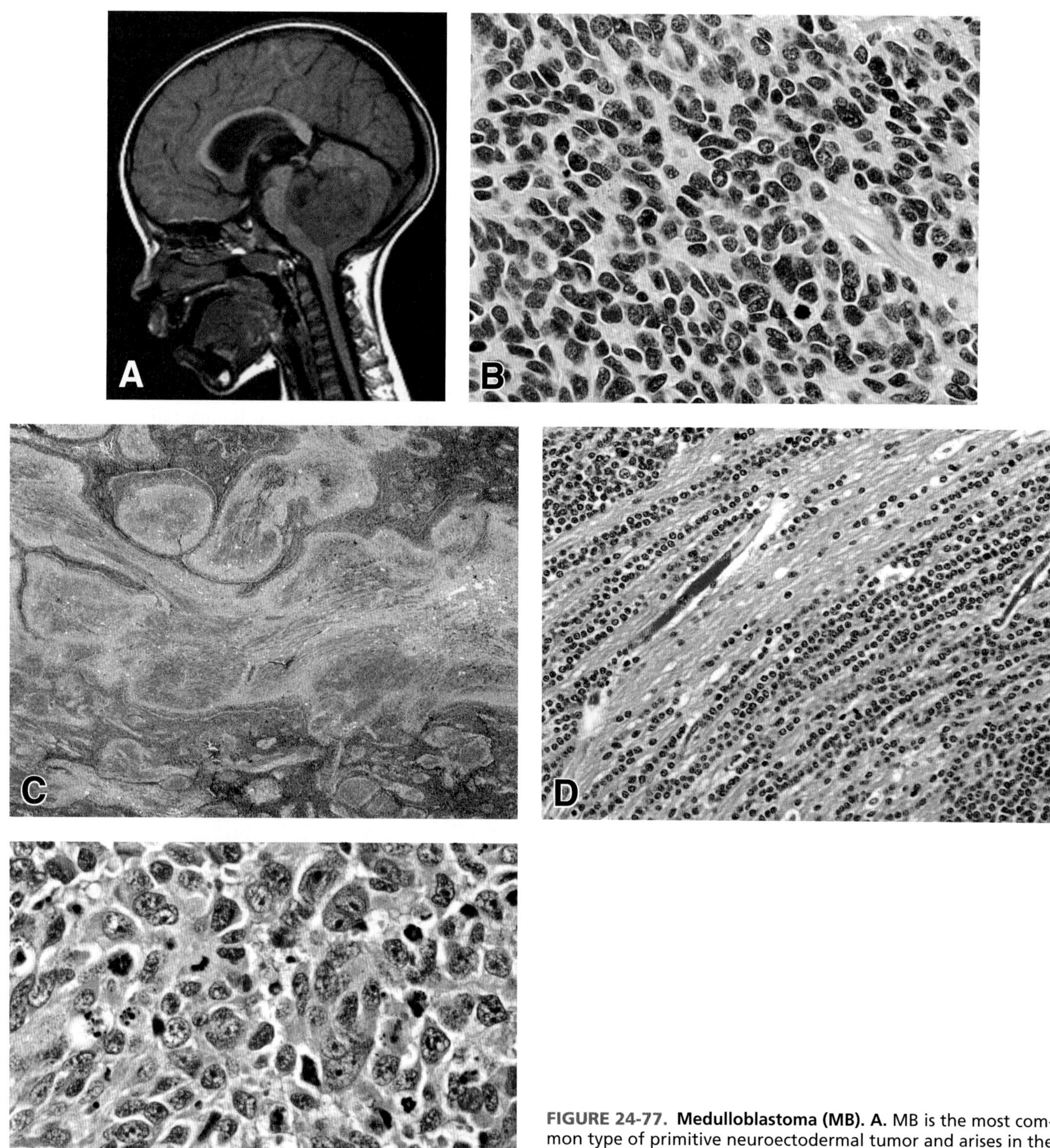

FIGURE 24-77. Medulloblastoma (MB). A. MB is the most common type of primitive neuroectodermal tumor and arises in the cerebellum. **B.** By light microscopy, MB is a "small blue cell" tumor. **C, D.** Two MB variants, desmoplastic/nodular MB and MB with extensive nodularity, have a better prognosis. **E.** Variants with large, anaplastic cells pursue a more aggressive clinical course.

mitotic activity, loss of papillary architecture, a solid growth pattern, and often nuclear atypia and cellular pleomorphism (Fig. 24-76C). The latter tumors can invade adjacent brain parenchyma and can also disseminate via the CSF.

Medulloblastoma and Other Primitive Neuroectodermal Tumors

MB is by far the most common of the primitive neuroectodermal tumors (PNETs). By definition, MBs arise in the cerebellum. Their peak incidence is at 7 years, but they also occur in 20- to 45-year-old adults. Childhood MBs commonly arise in the midline vermis, often expanding to fill the fourth ventricle (Fig. 24-77A). The adult versions prefer the cerebellar hemispheres. There are, however, many exceptions in both children and adults. About one third of patients have leptomeningeal spread, a negative prognostic factor, at the time of presentation. Partial surgical resection, large cell, or anaplastic morphology and amplification of the *MYCN* oncogene all portends poor prognosis. MB arises from stem cells of the fetal external granular layer or the periventricular germinal matrix. Molecular studies have implicated the *Wnt* and *sonic hedgehog* (*SHH*) signaling in tumor genesis.

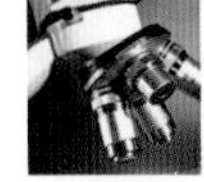

PATHOLOGY: MBs are composed of sheets of densely packed malignant small cells with a high nucleus to cytoplasm ratio (Fig. 24-77B). Neuroblastic (Homer Wright–type) rosettes are present in 40% of cases. Mitotic activity is high. Desmoplastic/nodular MB superficially resembles lymph node tissue, with reticulin-free neurocytic islands ("pale islands") that resemble germinal centers (Fig. 24-77D). Most MBs show neuronal differentiation, in the form of immunoreactivity for synaptophysin; some also express GFAP, like glial cells. **Anaplastic MB and large cell MB** are aggressive variants with overlapping morphologies (Fig. 24-77E). The former shows marked nuclear pleomorphism, nuclear molding, and cell–cell wrapping. By contrast, the large cell variant has a monomorphous population of large cells, whose nuclei display prominent nucleoli. Both variants have high proliferative rates and abundant apoptosis.

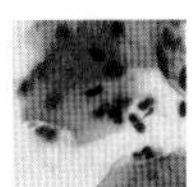

CLINICAL FEATURES: CSF dissemination is common and may be a presenting feature of the tumor. MBs sometimes metastasize to regional lymph nodes, lungs, or bone.

Craniopharyngioma

Craniopharyngioma (CP) is a circumscribed epithelial tumor, presumptively derived from Rathke cleft remnants. It arises mainly in children but also occurs in adults. These tumors typically show complex, heterogeneous solid and cystic areas on imaging (Fig. 24-78A). Given the origin and expansile growth in the sellar/suprasellar region, CPs typically present with mixed endocrine and visual disturbances, owing to compression of the pituitary below and optic chiasm above. Surgical resection is the preferred treatment; however, encroachment on the many vital structures in this area, including cranial

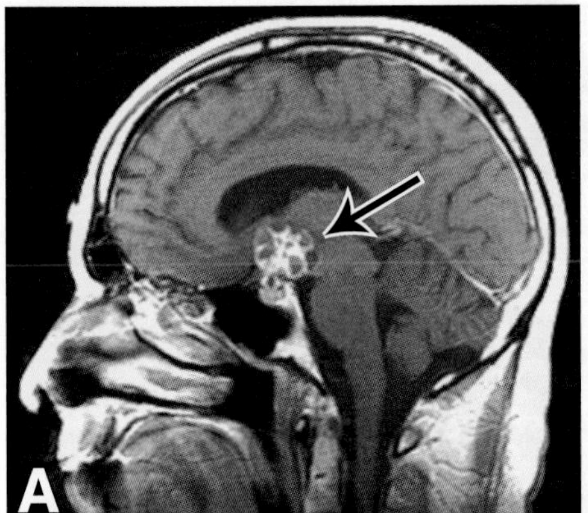

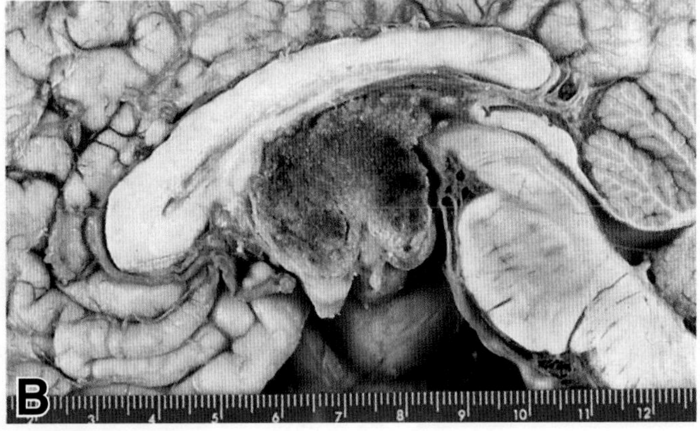

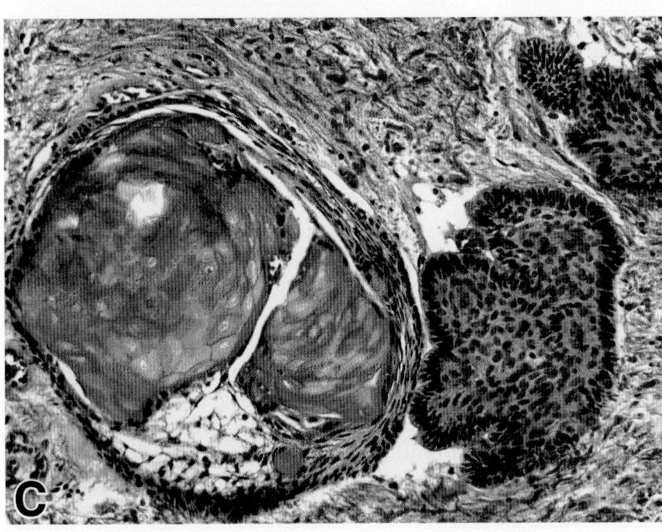

FIGURE 24-78. Craniopharyngioma. A. Craniopharyngiomas arise in the sellar/suprasellar region (*arrow*). **B.** Craniopharyngioma, gross photograph. **C.** Histologically, craniopharyngiomas are composed of squamous epithelium that displays a number of distinctive morphologic features, including peripheral palisaded nuclei and nodules of plump keratinocytes ("wet keratin") that are prone to calcify. (78B Courtesy of Dr. F. Stephen Vogel, Duke University.)

nerves and blood vessels, often limits resectability, and residual tumor inexorably recurs.

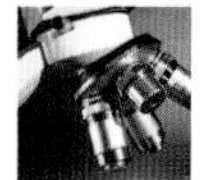

PATHOLOGY: There are two morphologic subtypes of CP: **adamantinomatous** (by far the more common), which arises in children and adults, and the rarer **papillary**, which occurs almost exclusively in adults. The former has distinctive morphology, including (1) sheets of squamous epithelium with prominent peripheral palisading, (2) hydropic degeneration of central areas of the epithelium ("stellate reticulum"), and (3) nodular aggregates of plump keratinocytes ("wet keratin"), which tend to calcify (Fig. 24-78C). Papillary CP contains exclusively nonkeratinizing squamous epithelium. Its histologic appearance is very bland compared to the variegated morphology of the adamantinomatous subtype.

Germinoma

Germ cell tumors (GCTs) of the CNS most often arise in midline structures, especially the pineal gland and third ventricular region (Fig. 24-79A). **Germinomas** tend to have a biphasic cell composition: large malignant cells are interspersed with swarms of small reactive lymphocytes (Fig. 24-79B). In some cases, β-human chorionic gonadotropin (β-HCG) expression identifies isolated syncytiotrophoblastic cells. Pure germinomas are highly radiosensitive, and patients may receive radiation therapy, chemotherapy, or a combination of both. Other germ cell tumors from the pineal region and at other CNS sites include **teratoma** (mature and immature), **yolk sac tumor**, **embryonal carcinoma**, and **choriocarcinoma**.

After germinomas, teratomas are the most common of this group to occur as pure (nonmixed) tumors. The remaining GCTs are mostly **mixed germ cell tumors**. The prognosis for nongerminomatous GCTs is less favorable than that for pure germinoma and largely depends on the extent of surgical resection.

Primary Central Nervous System Lymphomas

Systemic lymphomas often spread to the CNS, but lymphomas may also originate in the CNS. PCNSLs are tumors of adults and have increased in incidence in the past several decades. They may present with a wide variety of MRI patterns, including in superficial cortical, deep periventricular, or cerebellar locations, and may be solitary or multiple.

The vast majority are large cell B-cell tumors and express CD20 and other B-cell markers. In immunocompromised individuals, PCNSL may be driven by Epstein–Barr virus, which can be detected by immunohistochemistry. They are highly sensitive to steroids, often shrinking dramatically after glucocorticoid treatment. However, this response is temporary.

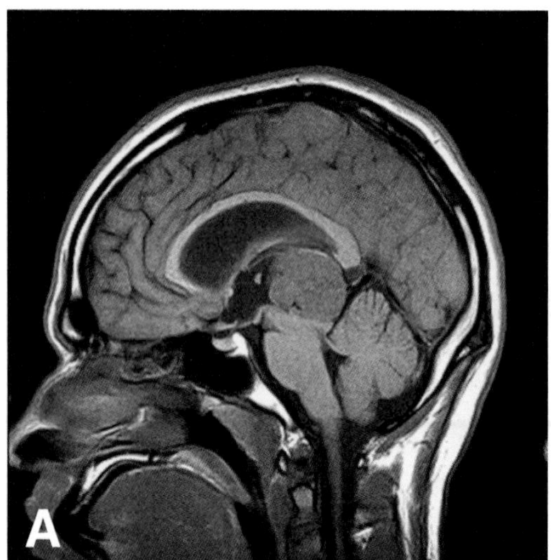

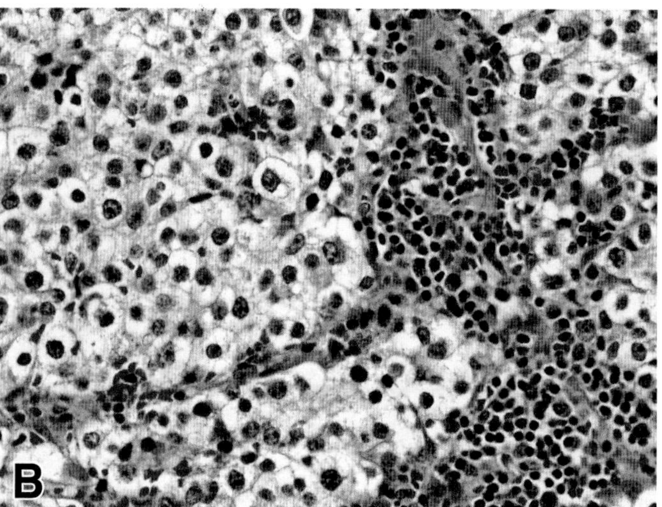

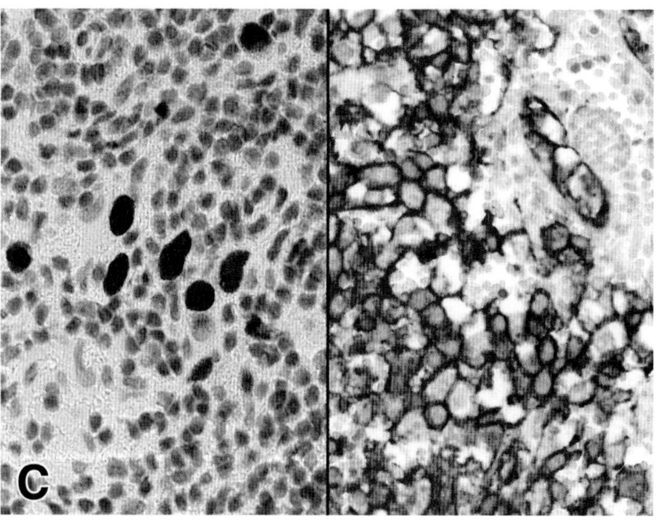

FIGURE 24-79. Germinoma. A. Germ cell tumors most commonly arise in the midline, such as in the pineal gland, as illustrated here. **B.** Microscopically, germinoma, the most common central nervous system germ cell tumor, exhibits a biphasic population of cells: very large germinoma tumor cells and small reactive lymphocytes. **C.** The germinoma immunophenotype includes diagnostically useful nuclear positivity for OCT3/4 (*left panel*) and cytoplasmic positivity for placental alkaline phosphatase (*right panel*).

Table 24-7

Central Nervous System Cysts
Choroid plexus cyst
Pineal cyst
Epidermoid cyst
Dermoid cyst
Arachnoid cyst
Ependymal cyst
Neurenteric (enterogenous) cyst
Rathke cyst
Colloid cyst

Radiation or chemotherapy gives a median survival of 70% at 2 years and up to 45% at 5 years in immunocompetent patients.

Benign Cysts

These tumors are listed in Table 24-7. Some are degenerative in nature and are usually incidental findings on neuroimaging studies done for other reasons, or at autopsy. **Choroid plexus cysts** and **pineal gland cysts** only rarely cause clinical symptoms. Others, such as **arachnoid cysts** and **ependymal cysts**, are largely asymptomatic but may occasionally require surgical fenestration of the cyst wall to release pressure and relieve mass effects on surrounding structures. Members of the remaining group are primarily of developmental origin and often cause mass effects that only require simple surgery.

Metastases

Metastatic tumors far surpass primary CNS tumors in numbers. Autopsy series show that up to 25% of patients with systemic cancers have CNS metastases. The most common site for brain metastasis is at the gray–white junction of the cerebral cortex, but any CNS region may be affected, including the choroid plexus, pineal gland, and pituitary gland.

The most common primary tumors that involve the CNS are derived from the lung (most frequent for both men and women), breast, melanoma, kidney, and gastrointestinal tract. Over half of all metastatic disease cases involve multiple metastases (Fig. 24-80A). For example, CNS metastases from cancers of gastrointestinal, breast, prostate, and uterine origin are frequently solitary, but those from lung carcinomas and melanomas are usually multiple. For some very common cancers, such as carcinoma of the uterine cervix, CNS metastases are rare.

Injury to surrounding CNS parenchyma by metastatic tumors entails (1) tumor growth itself, (2) vasogenic edema in surrounding brain tissue, (3) hemorrhage in the tumor (especially with melanomas, renal cell carcinomas, and choriocarcinomas), and (4) depending on the location of metastasis, obstructive hydrocephalus (e.g., when metastases to the midbrain cause occlusion of the cerebral aqueduct).

Hereditary Intracranial Neoplasms

Several hereditary disorders associated with CNS tumors and the genetic bases of the major syndromes are listed in Table 24-6. In some, neoplasms of systemic organs are most prominent, but nervous system tumors also occur. Thus, malignant gliomas occur in Li–Fraumeni syndrome, and medulloblastomas are associated with gastrointestinal tumors in Turcot syndrome.

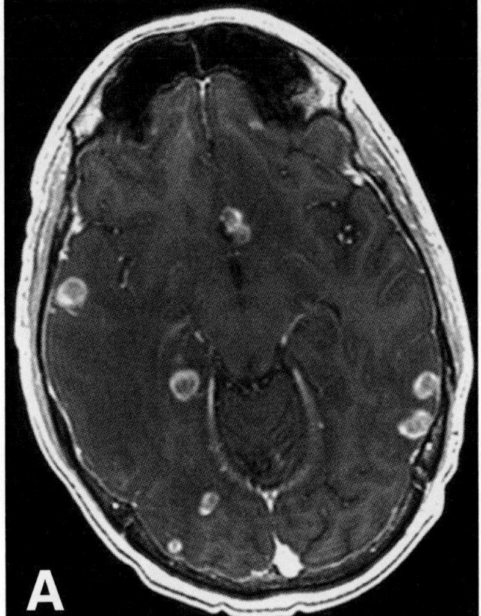

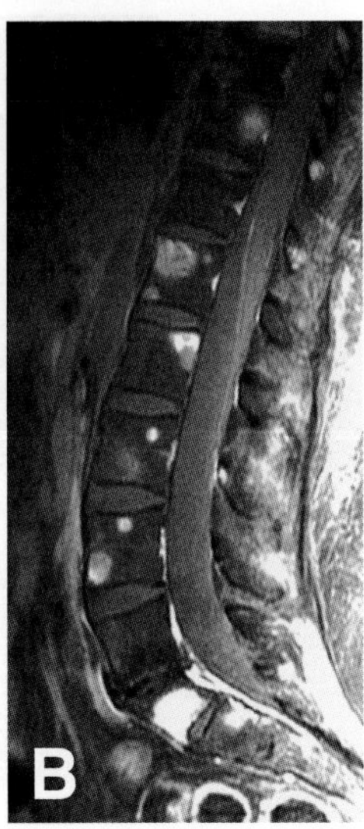

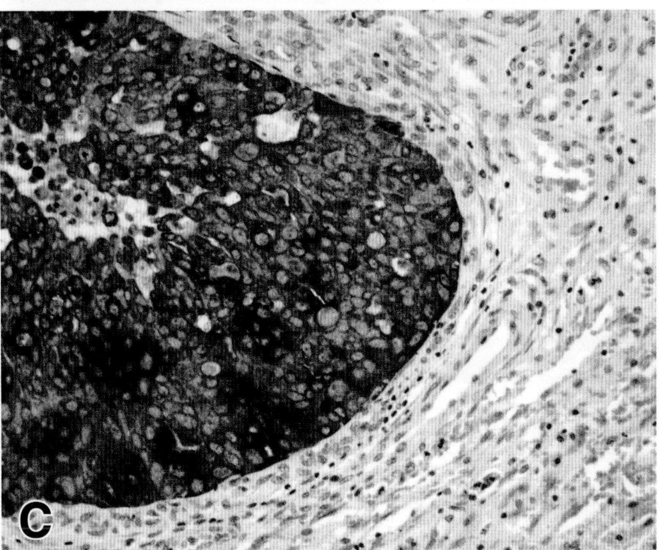

FIGURE 24-80. Metastatic disease. Metastases to the central nervous system commonly produce multiple lesions in both the brain **(A)** and spine **(B)**. **C.** Metastatic tumor masses typically show very sharp "pushing" borders with the adjacent brain tissue, as illustrated here with metastatic carcinoma immunostained for keratin.

Tuberous Sclerosis (Bourneville Disease)

Tuberous sclerosis is an autosomal dominant disease characterized by hamartomas (tubers) of the brain, retina, and viscera, as well as various neoplasms. It reflects disordered migration and arrested maturation of neuroectoderm, leading to formation of "tubers" in the cerebral cortex and of subependymal giant cell astrocytomas (Fig. 24-81). The tubers are discrete cortical areas with bizarre cells that exhibit neuronal and glial features. The subependymal giant cell astrocytomas resemble "candle drippings."

In addition to intracranial lesions, tuberous sclerosis includes (1) facial angiofibromas (adenoma sebaceum), (2) cardiac rhabdomyomas, and (3) mesenchymal tumors of

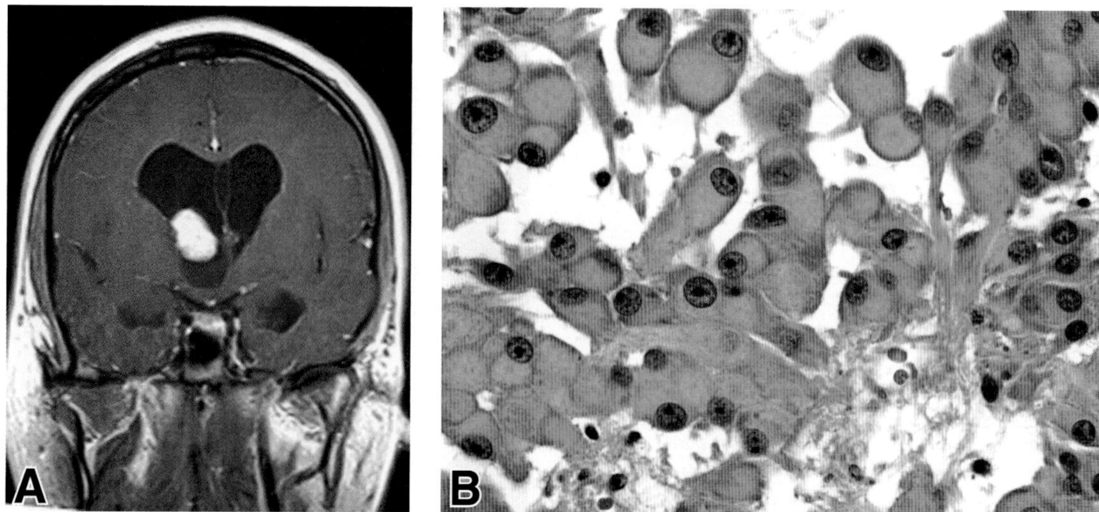

FIGURE 24-81. Subependymal giant cell astrocytoma (SEGA). A. This World Health Organization grade I astrocytoma arises within the lateral ventricle, often obstructing the interventricular foramen of Monro, resulting in obstructive hydrocephalus. **B.** Microscopically, SEGAs have globular eosinophilic cytoplasm, and the nuclei often display single prominent nucleoli, thus mimicking gemistocytic astrocytoma or ganglion cell tumor. However, the anatomic location within the cerebral ventricle should preclude misdiagnosis.

the kidney (angiomyolipomas). Most patients have seizures and are mentally retarded. Mutations in *TSC1* and *TSC2* are responsible. *TSC1* (9q34) encodes a protein called hamartin, and *TSC2* (16p13) encodes tuberin, which is homologous to a GTPase-activating protein. Both are tumor suppressors.

The Eye

THE CONJUNCTIVA

Conjunctivitis

Microorganisms lodging on the surface of the eye frequently cause conjunctivitis, keratitis (corneal inflammation), or a corneal ulcer. The conjunctiva, as well as other parts of the eye, may also become infected by hematogenous spread from a focus of infection elsewhere. Iatrogenic eye infections (e.g., with adenovirus) may follow ophthalmic manipulations, such as corneal grafts, intraocular implantation of lens prostheses, or the use of infected eyedrops or diagnostic instruments (Fig. 24-82).

At some stage in life, virtually everyone has viral or bacterial conjunctivitis. This extremely common eye disease is characterized by hyperemic conjunctival blood vessels (pink eye). The inflammatory exudate that accumulates in the conjunctival sac commonly crusts, causing the eyelids to stick together in the morning. The conjunctival discharge may be purulent, fibrinous, serous, or hemorrhagic. Participating inflammatory cells vary with the etiologic agent. Because many allergens are seasonal, the allergic conjunctivitis they elicit tends to occur

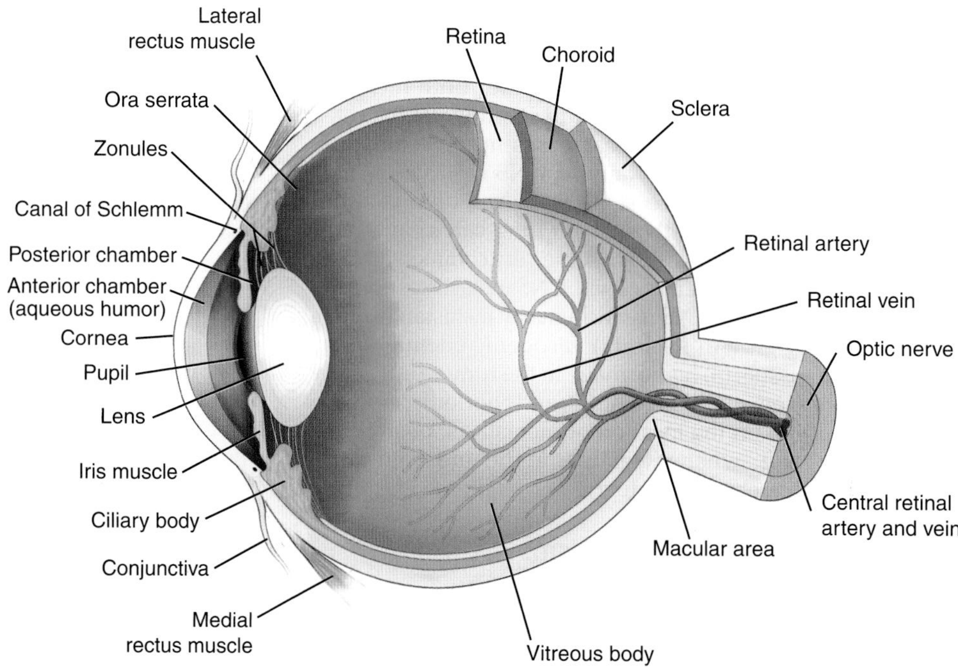

FIGURE 24-82. Diagram of the eye. Hinkle JL, Cheever KH. *Brunner & Suddarth's Textbook of Medical-Surgical Nursing*. 14th ed. Baltimore, MD: Wolters Kluwer; 2017.

only at particular times of the year. **Trachoma**, a chronic, contagious conjunctivitis caused by *Chlamydia trachomatis*, is discussed in Chapter 6.

THE CORNEA

Herpes Simplex Virus

HSV has a predilection for corneal epithelium, where it causes keratitis, but it can invade corneal stroma and, occasionally, other ocular tissues.

PRIMARY INFECTION BY HSV-1: Subclinical or undiagnosed localized ocular lesions are caused by HSV-1 in childhood. These infections are accompanied by regional lymphadenopathy, systemic infection, and fever. Except in newborns infected during passage through an infected mother's birth canal, HSV-2 rarely causes ocular infection. When it does, it may produce widespread lesions of the cornea and retina. Most corneal lesions due to HSV are asymptomatic plaques of diseased epithelial cells that contain replicating virus. These usually heal without ulceration, but an acute unilateral follicular conjunctivitis may occur. Corneal ulcers appear after serum antibody levels increase.

REACTIVATION OF HSV INFECTION: Latent in the trigeminal ganglion, HSV may pass down the nerves and reactivate the infection. Unlike primary HSV infection, reactivation disease is characterized by corneal ulceration and a more severe inflammatory reaction. Recurrence of corneal ulcers due to HSV may be precipitated by ultraviolet light, trauma, menstruation, emotional and physical stress, exposure to light or sunlight, vaccination, and other factors.

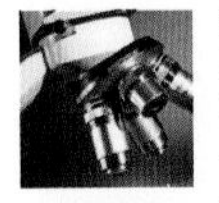

PATHOLOGY: HSV causes multiple, minute, discrete, intraepithelial corneal ulcers (superficial punctate keratopathy). Although some of these lesions heal, others enlarge and eventually coalesce to form linear or branching fissures (dendritic ulcers). The epithelium between the fissures desquamates, leading to sharply demarcated, irregular geographical ulcers. The corneal ulcers are readily visualized after the cornea is stained with fluorescein. Affected epithelial cells, which may become multinucleated, contain eosinophilic, intranuclear inclusion bodies (Lipschütz bodies).

The lesions of the corneal stroma vary in reactivated HSV infection. Typically, a central disc-shaped corneal opacity develops beneath the epithelium, owing to edema and minimal inflammation (**disciform keratitis**). The corneal stroma may become markedly thinned, and the Descemet membrane may bulge into it (descemetocele). Corneal perforation can also occur.

THE LENS

Cataracts

Cataracts are a major cause of visual impairment and blindness throughout the world and are the outcome of numerous conditions.

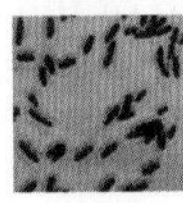

ETIOLOGIC FACTORS: The most common cause of lens cataracts in the United States is advancing age (age-related cataract). Other causes of cataracts include (1) diabetes, (2) nutritional deficiencies (e.g., deficiencies in riboflavin or tryptophan), (3) toxins (e.g., dinitrophenol, naphthalene, and ergot), (4) drugs (e.g., corticosteroids, topical phospholine iodide, and phenothiazines), or (5) physical agents (e.g., heat, ultraviolet light, trauma, intraocular surgery, and ultrasound).

Cataracts may develop in ocular diseases, such as uveitis, intraocular neoplasms, glaucoma, retinitis pigmentosa, and retinal detachment. Cataracts are also associated with congenital rubella virus infection, some skin diseases (e.g., atopic dermatitis and scleroderma), and various systemic diseases.

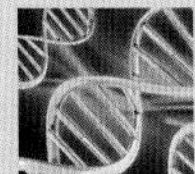

MOLECULAR PATHOGENESIS: A wide variety of cataracts result from genetic disorders, and some of them are associated with other ocular or systemic abnormalities.

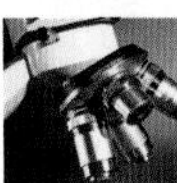

PATHOLOGY: In the development of cataracts, clefts appear between the lens fibers, and degenerated lens material accumulates in these spaces (morgagnian corpuscles, incipient cataract). Degenerated lens material exerts osmotic pressure, causing the damaged lens to imbibe water and swell. The swollen lens may obstruct the pupil and cause glaucoma (phacomorphic glaucoma).

In a *mature cataract* (Fig. 24-83), the entire lens degenerates, and the lenticular debris escapes into the aqueous humor through the lens capsule, diminishing the volume of the lens (hypermature cataract). After becoming engulfed by macrophages, the extruded lenticular material may obstruct aqueous outflow and produce glaucoma (phacolytic glaucoma). The compressed lens fibers in the center of the lens normally harden with aging (simple nuclear sclerotic cataract) and may become brown or black. If the peripheral part of the lens (lens cortex) becomes liquefied (morgagnian cataract), the sclerotic nucleus may sink within the lens by gravity.

Fortunately, cataractous lenses can be surgically removed, and optical devices can be provided to permit focusing of light on the retina (spectacles, contact lenses, and implantation of prosthetic lenses).

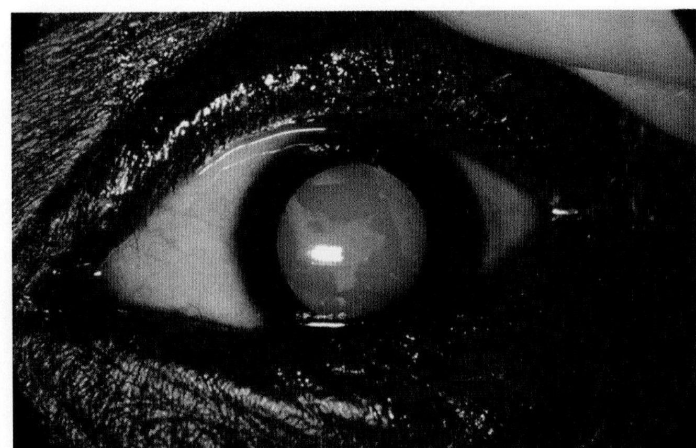

FIGURE 24-83. Cataract. The white appearance of the pupil in this eye is caused by complete opacification of the lens ("mature cataract").

THE UVEA

Inflammatory Conditions

Inflammation of the uvea (**uveitis**) also encompasses inflammation of the iris (**iritis**), the ciliary body (**cyclitis**) and the iris plus the ciliary body (**iridocyclitis**). Inflammation of the iris and ciliary body typically causes a red eye, photophobia, moderate ocular pain, blurred vision, a pericorneal halo, ciliary flush, and slight miosis. A flare is common in the anterior chamber on slit-lamp biomicroscopy, and keratic precipitates or a **hypopyon** (leukocytic exudate in the anterior chamber) also develops.

In sympathetic ophthalmitis, the entire uvea develops granulomatous inflammation after a latent period, in response to an injury in the other eye. Perforating ocular injury and prolapse of uveal tissue often lead to a progressive, bilateral, diffuse, granulomatous inflammation of the uvea. This uveitis develops in the originally injured eye (exciting eye) after a latent period of 4 to 8 weeks. The latent period may, however, be as short as 10 days or as long as many years. The uninjured eye (sympathizing eye) becomes affected at the same time as the injured eye, or shortly thereafter. Experimental studies suggest that the antigen responsible for sympathetic ophthalmitis resides in the photoreceptors of the retina (**arrestin**).

THE RETINA

Retinal Hemorrhage

The important causes of retinal hemorrhages are hypertension, diabetes mellitus, central retinal vein occlusion, bleeding diatheses, and trauma, including the "shaken baby syndrome." The appearance varies with the cause and location. Hemorrhages in the nerve fiber layer spread between axons and cause a flame-shaped appearance on funduscopy, whereas deep retinal hemorrhages tend to be round. When located between the retinal pigment epithelium and Bruch membrane, blood appears as a dark mass, which may resemble a melanoma.

After accidental or surgical perforation of the globe, choroidal hemorrhages may detach the choroid and displace the retina, vitreous body, and lens through the wound.

Retinal Occlusive Vascular Disease

Vascular occlusion results from thrombosis, embolism, stenosis (as in atherosclerosis), vascular compression, intravascular sludging or coagulation, and vasoconstriction (e.g., in hypertensive retinopathy or migraine). Thrombosis of ocular vessels may accompany primary disease of these vessels, as in giant cell arteritis.

Certain disorders of the heart and major vessels, such as the carotid arteries, predispose to emboli that may lodge in the retina and are evident on funduscopic examination at points of vascular bifurcation. Within the optic nerve, emboli in the central retinal artery frequently lodge in the vessel where it passes though the scleral perforations (**lamina cribrosa**). ***Permanent blindness follows central retinal artery obstruction unless the ischemia is of short duration.*** Unilateral blurred vision, lasting a few minutes (**amaurosis fugax**), occurs with small retinal emboli.

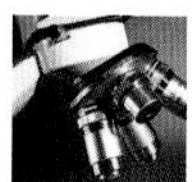

PATHOLOGY: The effect of vascular occlusion depends on the size of the vessel involved, the degree of resultant ischemia, and the nature of the embolus. Small emboli often do not interfere with retinal function, whereas septic emboli may cause foci of ocular infection. Retinal ischemia due to any cause frequently leads to white fluffy patches that resemble cotton on ophthalmoscopic examination (**cotton-wool spots**). These round spots, which are seldom wider than the optic nerve head, consist of aggregates of swollen axons in the nerve fiber layer of the retina. Affected axons contain numerous degenerated mitochondria and dense bodies related to the lysosomal system, which accumulate because of impaired axoplasmic flow. Histologically, in cross section, individual swollen axons resemble cells (cytoid bodies). Cotton-wool spots are reversible if circulation is restored in time.

Hypertensive Retinopathy

Increased blood pressure commonly affects the retina, causing changes that can readily be seen with the ophthalmoscope (Figs. 24-84 and 24-85).

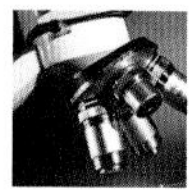

PATHOLOGY: Features of hypertensive retinopathy include:

- **Arteriolar narrowing**
- **Hemorrhages** in the retinal nerve fiber layer (flame-shaped hemorrhages)
- **Exudates**, including some that radiate from the center of the macula (macular star)
- **Cotton-wool spots**, fluffy white bodies in the superficial retina
- **Microaneurysms**

In the eye, arteriolosclerosis accompanies long-standing hypertension and commonly affects the retinal and choroidal vessels. Lumina of the thickened retinal arterioles become narrowed, increasingly tortuous and of irregular caliber. At sites where arterioles cross veins, the latter appear kinked (**arteriovenous nicking**). The kinked appearance of the vein reflects sclerosis within the venous walls because retinal arteries and veins share a common adventitia at sites of arteriovenous crossings, rather than compression by a taut sclerotic artery.

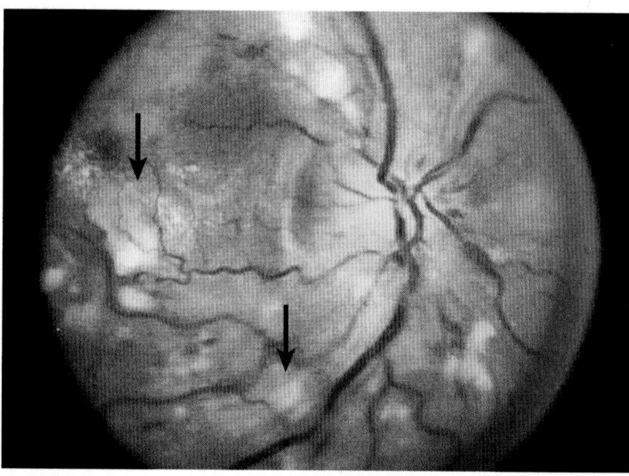

FIGURE 24-84. Hypertensive retinopathy. A photograph of the ocular fundus in a patient with extensive retinopathy. The optic nerve head is edematous; the retina contains numerous "cotton-wool spots" (*arrows*).

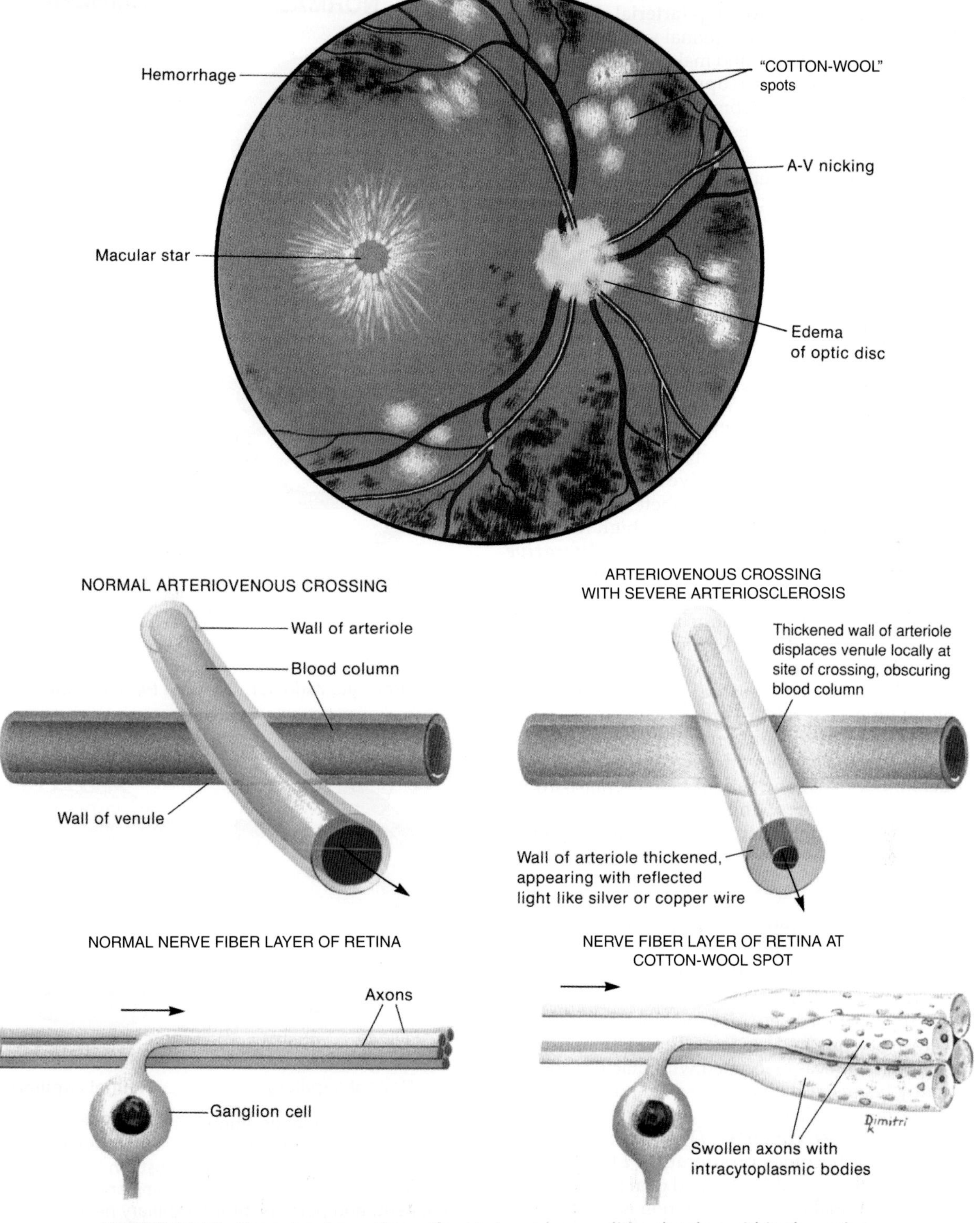

FIGURE 24-85. Hypertensive retinopathy. Various abnormalities develop within the retina in hypertension. The commonly associated arteriolosclerosis affects the appearance of the retinal microvasculature. Light reflected from the thickened arteriolar walls mimics silver or copper wire. Blood flow through the retinal venules is not well visualized at the sites of arteriolar–venular crossings. This effect is due to a thickening of the venular wall rather than to an impediment to blood flow caused by compression; the column of blood proximal to the compression is not wider than the part distal to the crossing. Impaired axoplasmic flow within the nerve fiber layer, caused by ischemia, results in swollen axons with cytoplasmic bodies. Such structures resemble cotton on funduscopy ("cotton-wool spots"). Hemorrhages are common in the retina, and exudates frequently form a star around the macula.

By funduscopy, abnormal retinal arterioles appear as parallel white lines at sites of vascular crossings (**arterial sheathing**). Initially, the narrowed lumen of the retinal vessels decreases the visibility of the blood column and makes it appear orange on ophthalmoscopic examination (**copper wiring**). However, as the blood column eventually becomes completely obscured, light reflected from the sclerotic vessels appears as threads of silver wire (**silver wiring**).

Small superficial or deep retinal hemorrhages often accompany retinal arteriolosclerosis. **Malignant hypertension** is characterized by necrotizing arteriolitis, with fibrinoid necrosis and thrombosis of precapillary retinal arterioles.

Diabetic Retinopathy

Ocular symptoms occur in 20% to 40% of diabetics and may even be evident at the time diabetes is diagnosed. Virtually, all patients with type 1 (insulin-dependent) diabetes and many of those with type 2 (non–insulin-dependent) diabetes develop some background retinopathy (see below) within 5 to 15 years of the onset of diabetes (Figs. 24-86 and 24-87). The more dangerous **proliferative retinopathy** does not appear until at least 10 years of diabetes, after which its incidence increases rapidly and remains high for many years. ***In type 1 diabetes, the frequency of proliferative retinopathy correlates with the degree of glycemic control; patients whose diabetes is better controlled develop retinopathy less frequently.*** The relationship between retinal microvascular disease and blood glucose levels in type 2 diabetes is less clear, and other parameters (e.g., blood cholesterol levels and blood pressure) may play more of a role than blood glucose levels.

Retinal ischemia can account for most features of diabetic retinopathy, including the cotton-wool spots, capillary closure, microaneurysms, and retinal neovascularization. Ischemia results from narrowing or occlusion of retinal arterioles (as from arteriolosclerosis or platelet and lipid thrombi) or from atherosclerosis of the central retinal or ophthalmic arteries.

PATHOLOGY: The retinopathy of diabetes is characterized by background and proliferative stages.

BACKGROUND (NONPROLIFERATIVE) DIABETIC RETINOPATHY: This stage exhibits venous engorgement, small hemorrhages (dot and blot hemorrhages), capillary microaneurysms, and exudates. These lesions usually do not impair vision unless associated with macular edema. The retinopathy begins at the posterior pole but eventually may involve the entire retina.

PROLIFERATIVE RETINOPATHY: After many years, diabetic retinopathy becomes proliferative. Delicate new blood vessels grow along with fibrous and glial tissue toward the vitreous body. Retinal neovascularization is a prominent feature of diabetic retinopathy and of other conditions caused by retinal ischemia. Tortuous new vessels first appear on the surface of the retina and optic nerve head and then grow into the vitreous cavity. The newly formed friable vessels bleed easily, and the resultant vitreal hemorrhages obscure vision. Neovascularization is associated with proliferation and immigration of astrocytes, which grow around the new vessels to form delicate white veils (gliosis). The proliferating fibrovascular and glial tissue contracts, often causing retinal detachment and blindness.

Diabetic retinopathy, glaucoma, and age-related maculopathy are the leading causes of irreversible blindness in the United States. Blindness in diabetic retinopathy results when the macula is involved, but it also follows vitreous hemorrhage, retinal detachment, and glaucoma. Laser phototherapy and strict glycemic control early in the course of proliferative retinopathy have proved effective in controlling this complication.

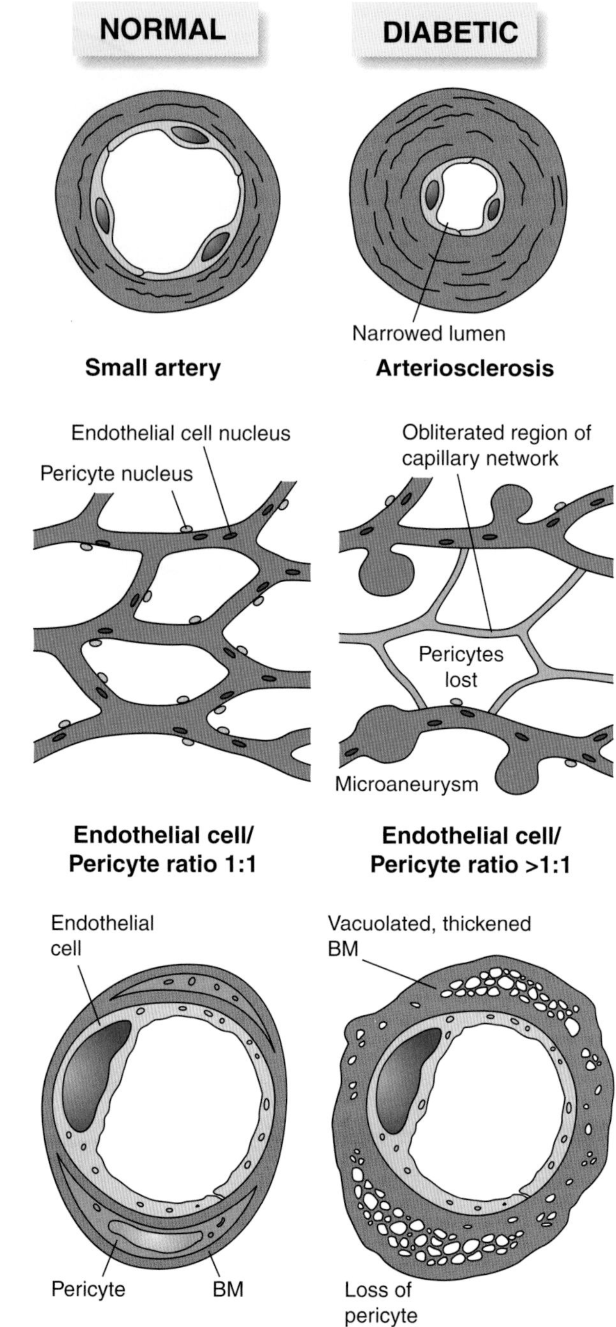

FIGURE 24-86. Diabetic retinopathy. In diabetic retinopathy, the microvasculature is abnormal. Arteriosclerosis narrows the lumen of the small arteries. Pericytes are lost, and the endothelial cell to pericyte ratio is greater than 1. Capillary microaneurysms are prominent, and portions of the capillary network become acellular and show no blood flow. The basement membrane (BM) of the retinal capillaries is thickened and vacuolated.

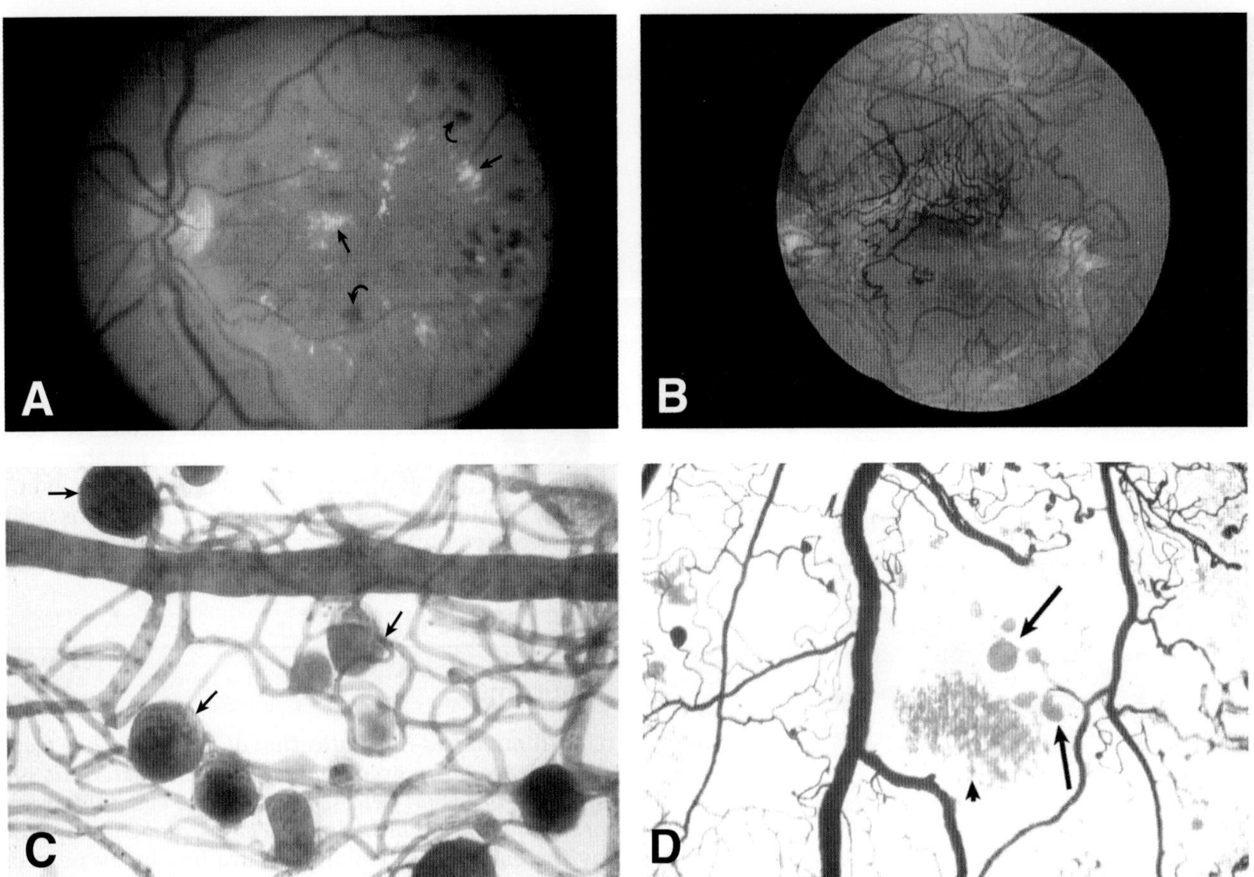

FIGURE 24-87. Diabetic retinopathy. A. The ocular fundus in a patient with background diabetic retinopathy. Several yellowish "hard" exudates (*straight arrows*), which are rich in lipids, are evident, together with several relatively small retinal hemorrhages (*curved arrows*). **B.** A vascular frond (*top half*) has extended anteriorly to the retina in the eye with proliferative diabetic retinopathy. **C.** Numerous microaneurysms (*arrows*) are present in this flat preparation of a diabetic retina. **D.** This flat preparation from a diabetic was stained with periodic acid–Schiff after the retinal vessels had been perfused with India ink. Microaneurysms (*arrows*) and an exudate (*arrowhead*) are evident in a region of retinal nonperfusion.

Retinal Detachment

During fetal development, the space between the sensory retina and the retinal pigment epithelium is obliterated when these two layers become apposed. However, the sensory retina readily separates from the retinal pigment epithelium when fluid (liquid vitreous, hemorrhage, or exudate) accumulates within the potential space between these structures. Such a separation is a common cause of visual impairment and blindness. Laser therapy and surgical approaches have greatly improved the prognosis for patients with detached retina.

ETIOLOGIC FACTORS: Retinal detachment follows intraocular hemorrhage (e.g., after trauma) and is a potential complication of cataract extractions and several other ocular operations. Factors predisposing to retinal detachment include retinal defects (due to trauma or certain retinal degenerations), vitreous traction, diminished pressure on the retina (e.g., after vitreous loss), and weakening of the fixation of the retina.

After they separate in a retinal detachment, oxygen and nutrients that normally reach the outer retina from the choroid must diffuse across a greater distance. This situation causes the photoreceptors to degenerate, after which cyst-like extracellular spaces appear within the retina.

Retinitis Pigmentosa

Retinitis pigmentosa (pigmentary retinopathy) is a generic term that refers to a variety of bilateral, progressive, degenerative retinopathies. These disorders are characterized clinically by night blindness and constriction of peripheral visual fields and pathologically by loss of retinal photoreceptors (rods and cones) and pigment accumulation within the retina.

The term "retinitis" is a misnomer because inflammation of the retina is not a feature of this disease.

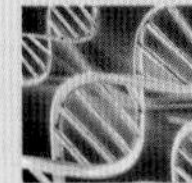

MOLECULAR PATHOGENESIS: Mutations in at least 48 different genes and loci are associated with nonsyndromic retinitis pigmentosa. Some are isolated ocular disorders, with autosomal dominant, autosomal recessive, or X-linked recessive inheritance. Some pigmentary retinopathies are associated with neurologic and systemic disorders.

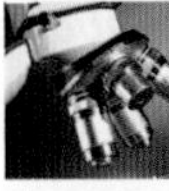

PATHOLOGY: In retinitis pigmentosa, destruction of rods, and subsequently cones, is followed by migration of retinal pigment epithelial cells into the sensory retina (Fig. 24-88). Melanin appears within slender processes of spidery cells and accumulates mainly around

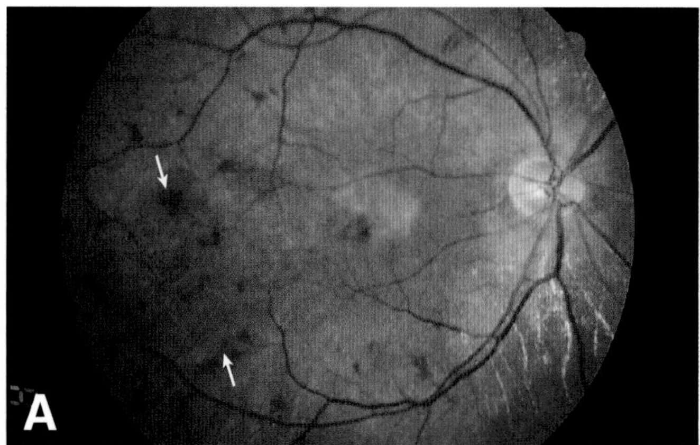

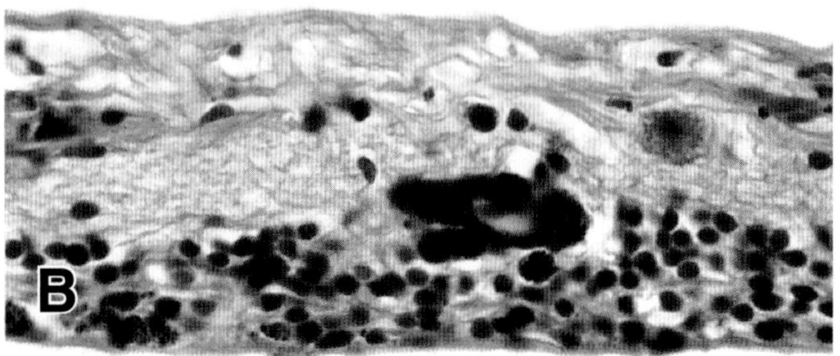

FIGURE 24-88. Retinitis pigmentosa. A. Fundus photograph of the retina of a patient with pigmentary retinopathy (retinitis pigmentosa) showing attenuated retinal vessels and foci of retinal pigmentation (*arrows*). **B.** Microscopic appearance of a severely degenerated retina in pigmentary retinopathy. Note the focal accumulations of pigmented, brown cells (derived from retinal pigmented epithelium) within the retina.

small branching retinal blood vessels (especially in the equatorial portion of the retina). The retinal blood vessels then gradually attenuate, and the optic nerve head acquires a characteristic waxy pallor.

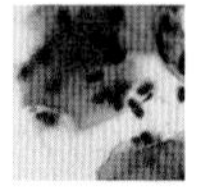

CLINICAL FEATURES: The clinical manifestations of retinitis pigmentosa, including the appearance and distribution of the retinal pigmentation, vary with the causes of the retinopathy. Half of these patients have a family history of the disease. As the condition progresses, contraction of visual fields eventually leads to tunnel vision. Central vision is usually preserved until late in the course of the disease. In some cases, blindness follows macular involvement.

Macular Degeneration

The center of the macula, the foveola, is the point of greatest visual acuity. In this area, a high concentration of cones rests on the retinal pigment epithelium. Surrounding the macula, the retina has a multilayered concentration of ganglion cells. With aging, in certain drug toxicities (e.g., chloroquine) and in several inherited disorders, the macula degenerates, causing central vision to be impaired.

Age-related macular degeneration currently affects about 15 million people in the United States and is the most common cause of blindness among individuals of European descent older than 65. Dry and wet forms of age-related macular degeneration are recognized. The wet variety of this disease accounts for 20% of cases and is associated with subretinal fibrovascular tissue and, sometimes, bleeding into the subretinal space. Laser photocoagulation and other intraocular antiangiogenic therapies are beneficial in this type of the disorder.

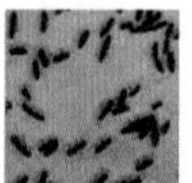

ETIOLOGIC FACTORS: There is general agreement that age-related maculopathy is a multifactorial disease to which environmental and genetic factors contribute. Risk factors include advancing age, smoking, carotid/cardiovascular disease, and elevated serum cholesterol levels.

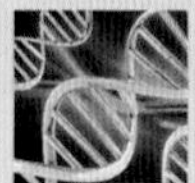

MOLECULAR PATHOGENESIS: A common missense variant of the *CFH* gene that encodes for complement factor H is a risk factor for about 50% of cases of age-related macular degeneration. Susceptibility has also been associated with mutations or single-nucleotide polymorphisms in a number of genes.

THE OPTIC NERVE

Glaucoma

Glaucoma refers to a collection of disorders that feature an optic neuropathy accompanied by a characteristic progressive loss of visual field sensitivity and eventual excavation of the optic nerve head. In most cases, glaucoma is produced by increased intraocular pressure (**ocular hypertension**); however, increased intraocular pressure does not necessarily cause glaucoma, and not all patients with glaucoma have elevated intraocular pressure.

After being produced by the ciliary body, the aqueous humor enters the posterior chamber (the space between the iris and the zonules) before passing through the pupil to the anterior chamber (between the iris and the cornea). From that site, it drains into veins by way of the trabecular meshwork and the canal of Schlemm (Fig. 24-89). A delicate balance between production and drainage of the aqueous humor maintains intraocular pressure within its physiologic range (10 to 20 mm Hg). In certain pathologic states, the drainage of aqueous humor from the eye becomes impaired, and intraocular pressure increases. Temporary or permanent impairment of vision results from pressure-induced degenerative changes in the retina and optic nerve head (Fig. 24-90) and from edema and opacification of the cornea.

Glaucoma, one of the most common causes of preventable blindness in the United States, almost always follows a congenital or acquired lesion of the anterior segment of the eye, which mechanically obstructs the aqueous drainage. The obstruction may be located between the iris and lens, in the angle of the anterior chamber, in the trabecular meshwork, in the canal of Schlemm, or in the venous drainage of the eye.

Adult-Onset Primary Glaucoma

Adult-onset primary glaucoma develops in a person with no apparent underlying eye disease. It is subdivided into **primary open-angle glaucoma** (in which the anterior chamber angle is open and appears normal) and **primary closed-angle glaucoma** (in which the anterior chamber is shallower than normal, and the angle is abnormally narrow) (Fig. 24-89).

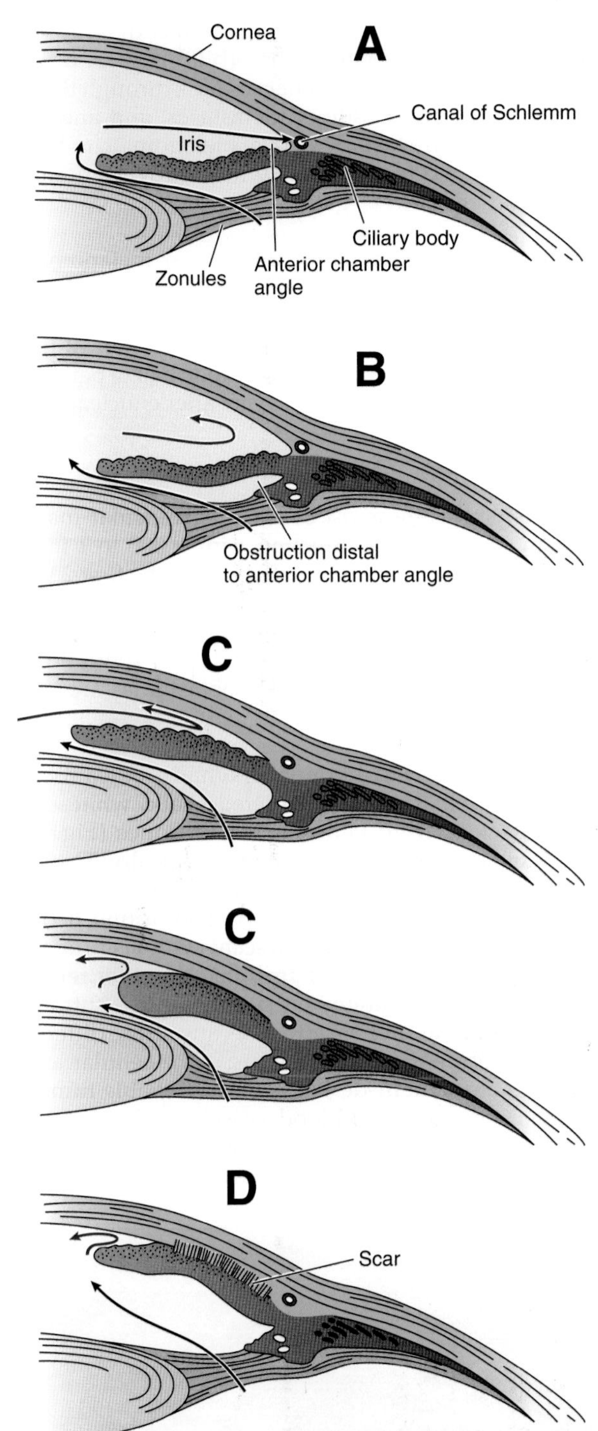

FIGURE 24-89. Pathogenesis of glaucoma. The anterior segment of the eye is affected differently in various forms of glaucoma. **A.** Structure of the normal eye. **B.** In primary open-angle glaucoma, the obstruction to the aqueous outflow is distal to the anterior chamber angle, and the anterior segment resembles that of the normal eye. **C.** In primary narrow-angle glaucoma, the anterior chamber angle is open, but narrower than normal when the pupil is constricted **(C1)**. When the pupil becomes dilated in such an eye, the thickened iris obstructs the anterior chamber angle **(C2)**, causing increased intraocular pressure. **D.** The anterior chamber angle can become obstructed by a variety of pathologic processes, including an adhesion between the iris and the posterior surface of the cornea **(peripheral anterior synechiae)**.

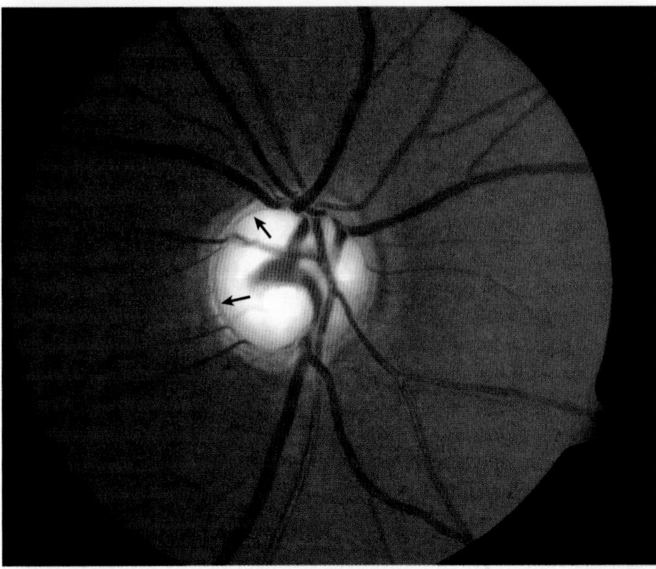

FIGURE 24-90. Optic nerve head in glaucoma. The anterior part of the optic nerve is depressed ("optic cupping"; *arrows*), and the blood vessels crossing the margin of the optic nerve head are displaced to the nasal side. The fundus appears dark because this eye of a black patient contains numerous pigmented melanocytes in the choroid.

Primary Open-Angle Glaucoma

Primary open-angle glaucoma is the most frequent type of glaucoma and a major cause of blindness in the United States. It affects 1% to 3% of the population older than 40 years and occurs principally in the sixth decade. The angle of the anterior chamber is open and appears normal, but there is increased resistance to the outflow of the aqueous humor in the vicinity of the canal of Schlemm. The intraocular pressure increases insidiously and asymptomatically, and although almost always bilateral, one eye may be affected more severely than the other. With time, damage to the retina and optic nerve causes irreversible loss of vision.

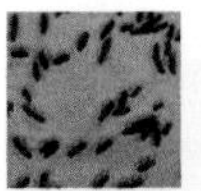

ETIOLOGIC FACTORS: Persons with diabetes mellitus and myopia have an increased risk of primary open-angle glaucoma.

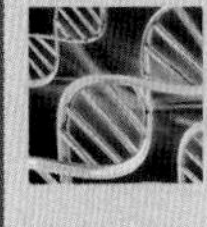

MOLECULAR PATHOGENESIS: Primary open-angle glaucoma has been mapped to at least 13 loci on multiple chromosomes, and three genes have been identified.

Primary Closed-Angle Glaucoma

Primary closed-angle glaucoma, differentiated from open-angle glaucoma above, occurs after age 40 years. ***It is the predominant form of primary glaucoma in adults living in Asia.*** The disorder afflicts persons whose peripheral iris is displaced anteriorly toward the trabecular meshwork, thereby creating an abnormally narrow anterior chamber angle.

The disease has a familial predisposition, but in contrast to primary open-angle glaucoma, genetic loci have not yet been identified. Acute closed-angle glaucoma is an ocular emergency, and it is essential to start ocular hypotensive treatment within the first 24 to 48 hours if vision is to be maintained.

OCULAR NEOPLASMS

The eye and adjacent structures contain a large number of cell types, and as one might expect, benign and malignant neoplasms arise from them. ***Intraocular neoplasms arise mostly from immature retinal neurons (retinoblastoma) and uveal melanocytes (melanoma).*** Although the retinal pigment epithelium often undergoes reactive proliferation, it seldom becomes neoplastic.

Malignant Melanoma

Malignant melanoma is the most common primary intraocular malignancy. It may arise from melanocytes in any part of the eye, the choroid being the most common site.

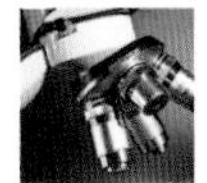

PATHOLOGY: Choroidal melanomas are mostly circumscribed and commonly invade the Bruch membrane, causing a mushroom-shaped mass (Fig. 24-91). By contrast, some tumors are flat (diffuse melanoma) and cause a gradual deterioration of vision over many years. Some do not become apparent until extraocular dissemination has occurred. Orange lipofuscin pigment is sometimes evident over the surface of some choroidal melanomas.

Microscopically, uveal melanomas may be composed mainly of (1) variable numbers of spindle-shaped cells without nucleoli (spindle A cells), (2) spindle-shaped cells with prominent nucleoli (spindle B cells), (3) polygonal cells with distinct cell borders and prominent nucleoli (epithelioid cells), or (4) a cell type that is similar to epithelioid cells but smaller with indistinct cell borders.

Melanomas of the ciliary body and iris may extend circumferentially around the globe (ring melanoma). Melanomas in the iris are usually diagnosed clinically one to two decades earlier than those in the choroid and ciliary body, perhaps because they are more easily seen and are often first observed by the patient.

Lymphatic spread of ocular melanoma does not occur because the eye has no lymphatic vessels. Aside from hematogenous spread, uveal melanomas disseminate by traversing the sclera to enter the orbital tissues, usually at sites where blood vessels and nerves pass through the sclera. The liver is a common site of metastases, and anecdotally, the diagnosis of metastatic ocular melanoma can be made intuitively by astute clinicians who discover an enlarged liver in a patient with a "glass eye."

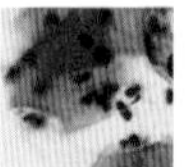

CLINICAL FEATURES: Intraocular melanomas may cause cataract, glaucoma, retinal detachment, inflammation, and hemorrhage. The options for treating uveal melanomas include enucleation of the eye, radiotherapy, and local excision. More than half of patients with uveal melanomas survive for 15 years after enucleation.

Retinoblastoma

Retinoblastoma is the most common intraocular malignant neoplasm of childhood, affecting 1 in 20,000 to 1 in 34,000 children. It occurs most frequently within the first 2 years of life and may even be found at birth. Most retinoblastomas occur sporadically and are unilateral. Some 6% to 8% of retinoblastomas are inherited. Up to 25% of sporadic retinoblastomas and most inherited retinoblastomas are bilateral (see Chapter 5 for details).

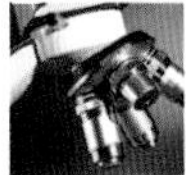

PATHOLOGY: Retinoblastoma is a cream-colored tumor that contains scattered, chalky white, calcified flecks within yellow necrotic zones (Fig. 24-92), which may be detected radiologically. The tumors are intensely cellular and display several morphologic patterns. In some instances, densely packed, round neoplastic cells with hyperchromatic nuclei, scant cytoplasm, and abundant mitoses are randomly distributed. In other retinoblastomas, the cells are arranged radially around a central cavity (**Flexner–Wintersteiner rosettes**) because they differentiate toward photoreceptors. In some cases, the cellular arrangement resembles a fleur-de-lis (**fleurette**). Viable tumor cells align themselves around blood vessels, and necrotic areas with calcification are seen a short distance from the vascularized regions.

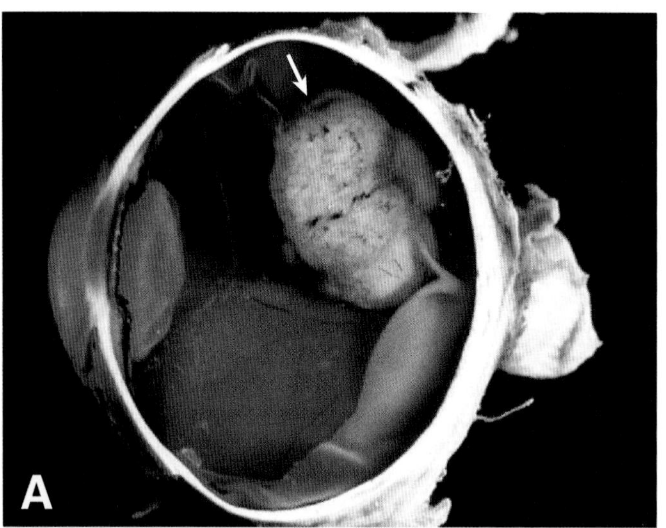

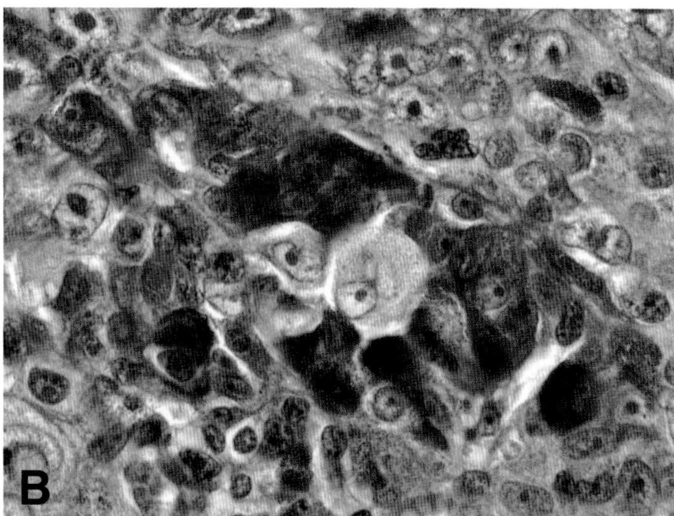

FIGURE 24-91. Malignant melanoma. A. A mushroom-shaped melanoma of the choroid is present in this eye (*arrow*). Choroidal melanomas commonly invade through the Bruch membrane and result in this appearance. **B.** Photomicrograph of a heavily pigmented melanoma of the choroid depicting epithelioid tumor cells with prominent nucleoli.

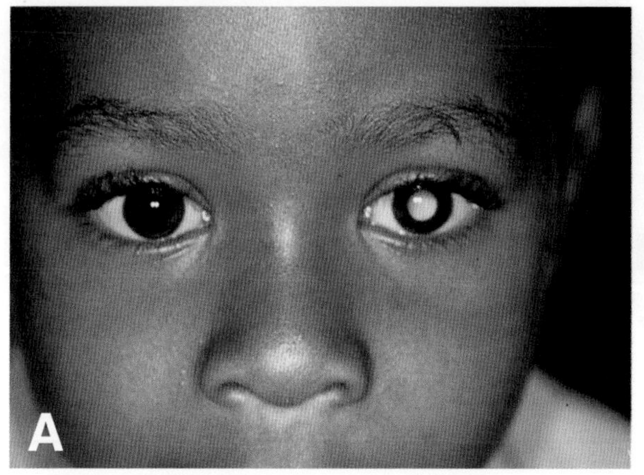

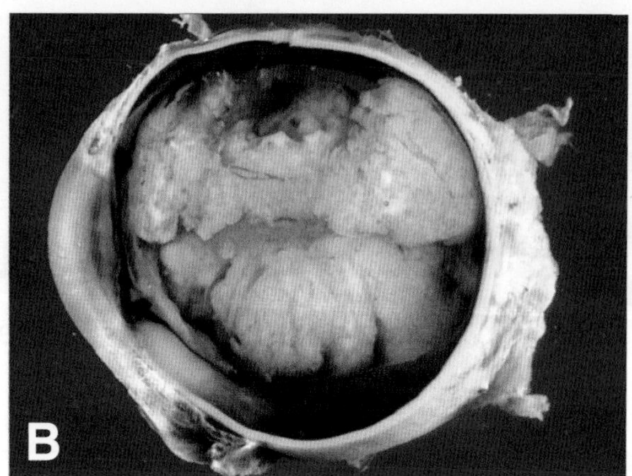

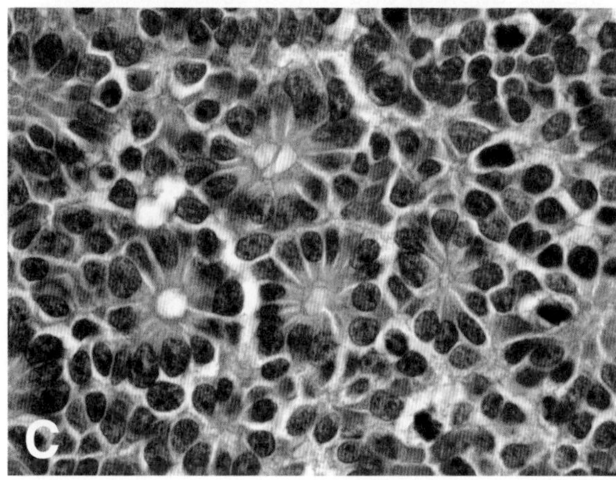

FIGURE 24-92. Retinoblastoma. A. The white pupil (leukocoria) in the left eye is the result of an intraocular retinoblastoma. **B.** This surgically excised eye is almost filled by a cream-colored intraocular retinoblastoma with calcified flecks. **C.** Light microscopic view of a retinoblastoma showing Flexner–Wintersteiner rosettes characterized by cells that are arranged around a central cavity.

Retinoblastomas disseminate by several routes. They commonly extend into the optic nerve, from where they spread intracranially. They also invade blood vessels, especially in the highly vascular choroid, before metastasizing hematogenously throughout the body. Bone marrow is a common site of blood-borne metastases, but surprisingly, the lung is rarely involved.

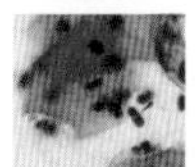

CLINICAL FEATURES: Presenting signs include a white pupil (leukocoria), squint (strabismus), poor vision, spontaneous hyphema, or a red, painful eye. Secondary glaucoma is a frequent complication. Light entering the eye commonly reflects a yellowish color similar to that from the tapetum of a cat (cat's eye reflex).

Retinoblastomas are almost always fatal if left untreated. However, with early diagnosis and modern therapy, survival is high (about 90%). Rarely, spontaneous regression occurs for reasons that remain unknown. Patients with inherited retinoblastomas, presumably as a consequence of the loss of *Rb* gene function, show increased susceptibility to other malignant tumors, including osteogenic sarcoma, Ewing sarcoma, and pinealoblastoma.

25 Traumatic and Environmental Injury

Marc S. Micozzi ▪ David S. Strayer ▪ Emanuel Rubin

LEARNING OBJECTIVES

- Differentiate between the cause and manner of death.
- How do caliber and range affect tissue injury resulting from gunshot wounds?
- Define contusion. How may it be used to assist in timing an injury?
- Describe the pathophysiology of strangulation.
- Differentiate between generalized and focal hypothermia. Describe the pathophysiology of tissue injury in both cases.
- Define the potential causes and effects of systemic hyperthermia.
- What are the etiology and clinical consequence of heat stroke?
- Differentiate between partial-thickness and full-thickness cutaneous burns.
- By what mechanisms may electrical energy produce injury?
- What classes of agents/drugs are most likely to result in abuse?
- What complications are associated with intravenous drug abuse?
- What industrial chemicals are most likely to result in poisoning and in cancer risk?

THE MANNER OF DEATH

The causes of death are multiple, and the manner is classified into five categories: (1) accident, (2) homicide, (3) suicide, (4) natural, and (5) undetermined/unclassified.

Most of the cases that fall under medical examiner jurisdiction actually support areas beyond or outside public safety. Only about 20% of cases are **homicides**. A rule of thumb is that the rate of **suicide** is double the rate of homicide (except in excessively violent, crime-ridden jurisdictions). In most locations, about one half of **accidents** relate to motor vehicle accidents and traffic fatalities, whereas the other half are industrial accidents and those in the home or in recreational settings. In terms of **natural** causes of death occurring outside the presence of a treating physician, these investigations are often important in identifying acute or chronic threats to public health, such as infectious disease outbreaks, contaminated water supplies, accidental poisonings, or other toxic exposures.

Cause of Death Versus Mechanism of Death

Both resident and practicing physicians frequently complete a death certification incorrectly stating "cardiopulmonary" arrest as the cause of death. Cardiopulmonary arrest is not a cause of death but a final common pathway in which the underlying disease process finally leads to cessation of vital signs. The mechanism of cardiopulmonary arrest may be precipitated by (1) an event that causes respiratory arrest, evolving rapidly to cardiac arrest; (2) a fatal occurrence causing cardiac arrest, leading rapidly to respiratory arrest; or (3) a fatal central nervous system (CNS) injury that rapidly causes cessation of vital functions in both the heart and the lungs. Through the intervention of respiratory ventilation therapy and cardiac electroversion, an otherwise fatal CNS event leading to "brain death" may not immediately cause physiologic death.

Causes of true sudden death, whereby an otherwise healthy ambulatory person suddenly "drops dead in his tracks," are few.

TRAUMATIC INJURIES

Traumatic injuries result from incidents such as violent assaults upon one person by another, by encounters with machinery at high velocity, or by random physical forces and gravity. Fatal assaults are usually carried out with weapons such as (1) firearms, knives, and other bladed weapons; (2) blunt objects of various kinds; or (3) fists and other hard bodily surfaces such as feet, knees, elbows, or even the forehead. Forceful contact against a hard surface, such as concrete, is occasionally fatal.

Gunshot Wounds

In densely populated areas, most fatal assaults with firearms involve handguns or small arms. Such weapons are really useful only at shorter ranges, and much of the forensic work involves identifying the distance between the muzzle of the firearm and the entrance wound. There are basically two types of gunshot wounds, namely, (1) penetrating wounds in which the projectile enters the body but does not exit and (2) perforating wounds in which the projectile passes through the body, creating both entrance and exit wounds (Fig. 25-1).

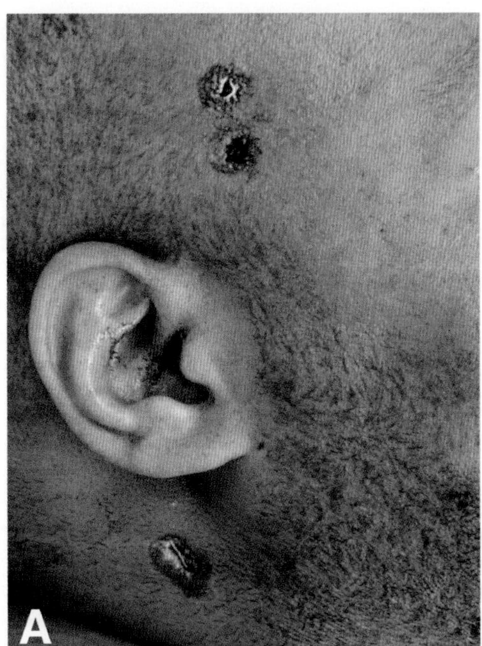

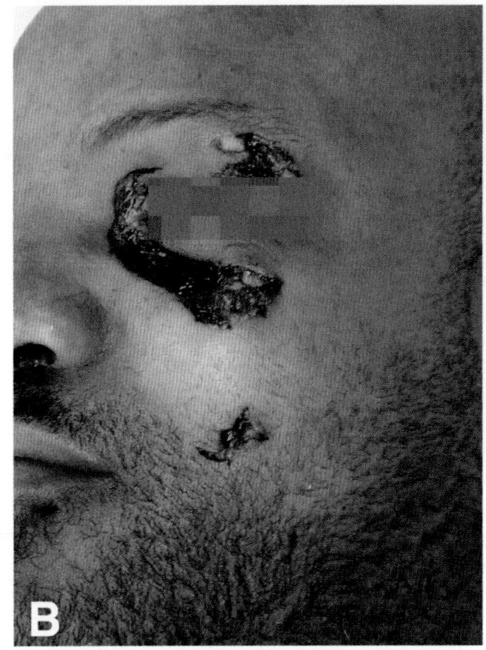

FIGURE 25-1. Entrance wounds (A) and exit wounds (B) on the right and left sides of the face, respectively, of a 39-year-old man with multiple gunshot wounds. The smaller entrances show a round to oval skin defect surrounded by abrasion rings. The exits are irregular lacerations, generally larger than the entrances, and lack a surrounding abrasion. From Troncoso JC, Rubio A, Fowler DR. *Essential Forensic Neuropathy*. Baltimore, MD: Lippincott Williams & Wilkins; 2010.

Caliber

Small caliber wounds (e.g., .22 caliber) can be fatal, especially in the case of head wounds. A small caliber projectile frequently penetrates the skull, but without the force to perforate the back of the skull, it may ricochet or "rattle around" within the skull, causing extensive brain damage. Likewise, the ability of a projectile to traverse and exit a body partially depends on whether or not it encounters bone, especially dense cortical bone, as in the mandible.

Notwithstanding the above considerations, the amount of damage caused by a projectile is directly related to its caliber (mass) and its velocity, thus momentum. The larger and heavier the projectile, the larger its momentum. Traveling at high velocity, a bullet transfers the force to the tissues of the body, causing tissue disruption. In the head, in addition to the focal injury in the path of the projectile, there is diffuse injury throughout the brain because of compression, stretching, and tearing at the microscopic level, owing to the "shock wave" within an enclosed space. With penetrating wounds, exit wounds are larger and more irregular than the smaller and rounder entrance wounds.

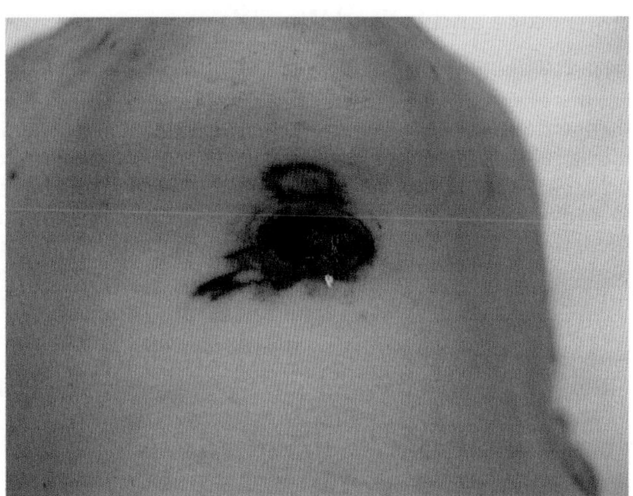

FIGURE 25-2. A muzzle imprint surrounds the entrance wound under the chin in a self-inflicted gunshot wound to the head. From Troncoso JC, Rubio A, Fowler DR. *Essential Forensic Neuropathy*. Baltimore, MD: Lippincott Williams & Wilkins; 2010.

Range

At extremely close range (contact wound), with the muzzle pressed against the skin, there may be stellate lesions, with star-shaped defects extending from the borders of the wound, owing to expansion of hot gases from the barrel trapped in the enclosed space. There may also be a muzzle burn mark around the perimeter of the wound from the heat of the metal (Fig. 25-2).

At close range, where the muzzle is separated from the surface of the skin, there tends to be stippling in a perimeter around the wound (Fig. 25-3). In this situation, the heated detritus that exits from the barrel along with the projectile reaches the surface of the skin. These particles expand out of the barrel of the firearm following the inverse square law for expanding particles from a point source; the perimeter of the stippling increases as the square of the distance from the gun barrel increases. Ultimately, there comes a point where the particles do not reach the surface of the skin at all in a long- or midrange wound.

The wounds caused by a shotgun (especially with a "sawed-off" or intentionally shortened barrel) also follow

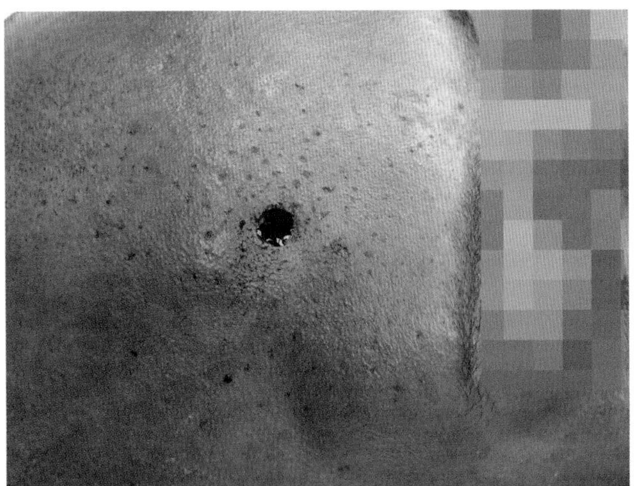

FIGURE 25-3. A close-range gunshot wound of entrance with surrounding stippling. From Troncoso JC, Rubio A, Fowler DR. *Essential Forensic Neuropathy*. Baltimore, MD: Lippincott Williams & Wilkins; 2010.

a pattern dictated by the inverse square law. The shotgun pellets describe a larger perimeter of entrance wounds as the distance from the barrel increases, owing to the dispersal of the pellets from the barrel of the shotgun.

Sharp Force and Incised Wounds

Incised wounds are caused by bladed objects such as knives. Features of entry wounds made by a knife are distinguished by whether there is a single- or double-edged blade. The former is distinguished by a sharp incision at one border of the wound and a blunt border at the opposite edge. If the knife enters the body up to the hilt, a mark may be left behind on the skin where the hilt impacted the skin. When a blade is inserted at an oblique angle, it causes a wound whose dimensions are wider than the maximum width of the blade.

A sharp force wound also includes incised wounds that result from sharp, round, pointed objects, such as an ice pick, knitting needle, sharp stick, or bone, or even an icicle (which has the feature of making the evidence rapidly disappear). Although small in diameter, such wounds can be deadly.

Blunt Force Injuries

Blunt force trauma can be inflicted by any object with enough hardness, mass, and momentum to damage tissues. Such assaults cause blunt force injuries, which may or may not break the surface of the skin, and which may cause external or internal bleeding. Because of the strength and resilience of the skin, sufficient force may be transmitted to the underlying tissues and organs to cause extensive injury, even when the skin remains unbroken.

When the skin surface is broken by blunt trauma, it may manifest as a puncture, abrasion, laceration, maceration, or avulsion. If the surface of the skin is not broken, internal bleeding may still be extensive. Exsanguination can be caused either by bleeding out from the body or into internal body cavities.

Other blunt force injuries may result from the encounter of the body with hard surfaces of machinery, with surfaces of a motor vehicle, or with the ground.

When they break the surface of the skin, such wounds may include punctures, avulsions, abrasions, and incisions.

Contusions

Whether or not the skin is broken from blunt force contact, a contusion (bruise) may develop in the underlying tissues. Contusions result from bleeding into the surrounding tissues by ruptured blood vessels. As the bleeding occurs into any enclosed space (e.g., a muscle or joint compartment, or connective tissues), swelling occurs, pressure increases, and the back pressure helps to staunch further blood flow while clotting takes place. Because hemoglobin in red blood cells breaks down over time, contusions manifest various pigment colorations of black-blue, purple, green, and yellow (Fig. 25-4). These variations assist in the timing of the bruise in a victim who survives the injury.

Exsanguination

Where the surface of the skin and the underlying blood vessels are broken, the body may exsanguinate quickly because the heart continues to pump large quantities of blood through the wounds. Deeper injuries involving the arteries at high blood pressure are also capable of causing exsanguination. More superficial injuries involving only veins at lower blood pressure are not likely to cause exsanguination unless the injury covers extensive surfaces or blood loss is prolonged.

Internal Bleeding

If the skin surface is not broken, internal bleeding may still occur. Even at a relatively "bloodless" scene of the death, body cavities may contain copious quantities of blood, resulting in exsanguination.

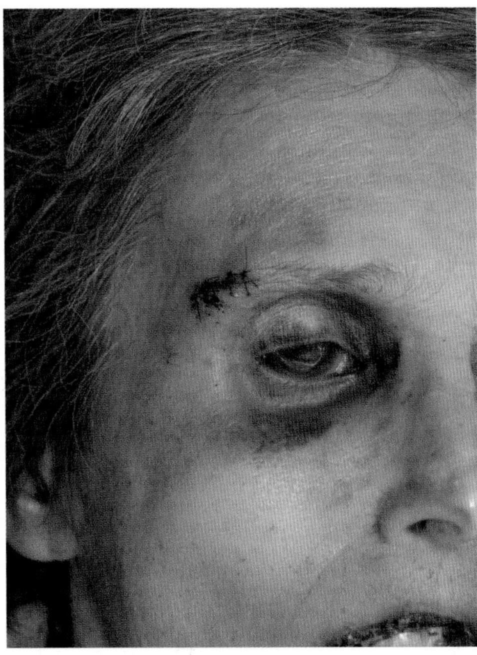

FIGURE 25-4. A sutured laceration present on the orbital ridge is surrounded by a healing contusion (with red, blue, yellow, and green hues) in a patient with multiple sclerosis who suffered a fall 10 days before being pronounced dead. From Troncoso JC, Rubio A, Fowler DR. *Essential Forensic Neuropathy*. Baltimore, MD: Lippincott Williams & Wilkins; 2010.

Asphyxiation

Death by asphyxiation is a relatively slow process. During asphyxiation, the brain maintains consciousness for 2 to 3 minutes, at which point the victim may be expected to cease struggling. After an additional 2 to 3 minutes of asphyxiation, the brain dies from anoxia.

Strangulation: Ligature and Manual

The neck is a narrow structure that carries about one third of the total blood volume at any given time to meet the high metabolic demands of the brain. Thus, it represents a convenient and efficient location for inducing asphyxiation by strangulation, either forcefully using the hands (manual) or by a ligature around the neck. In a homicidal assault by strangulation, there may be ligature marks around the neck; the hyoid bone, thyroid cartilage, cricoid cartilage, and tracheal rings may (or may not) be broken. Petechial hemorrhages may occur in the eyes and elsewhere.

In addition to closing off the airway and causing asphyxiation, strangulation may compress the carotid arteries, directly cutting off blood flow to the brain. Extensive stress and stimulation to the carotid artery may also result in a reflex that induces cardiac arrhythmia.

To strangulate the neck structures, about 7 lb (3.2 kg) of pressure is required. Against a normal blood pressure of 120/80 mm Hg, the carotid artery is compressed by about 11 to 13 lb (5.0 to 5.9 kg) of pressure. The larynx is crushed by about 30 lb (13.6 kg) of pressure. These forces can be delivered by the hands (to a lean person) or by the elbow, knee, or foot.

If a single blunt injury is applied by striking the neck with sufficient power to crush and collapse the larynx, suffocation and asphyxia will inexorably progress, whether or not any continued force is applied, because the airway has been cut off.

Asphyxiation by strangulation of the neck also occurs in judicial, suicidal, and accidental hangings in autoerotic asphyxia. In a judicial hanging, the neck may be broken, causing instantaneous death because of injury to the cervical spine and CNS. If the hanging is not carried out "humanely," the neck may remain intact, and death eventually ensues from asphyxiation.

THERMAL REGULATORY DYSFUNCTION

Hypothermia

Hypothermia can result in systemic or focal injury, the latter exemplified by **trench foot** or **immersion foot**. In localized hypothermia of these types, actual tissue freezing does not occur. **Frostbite**, by contrast, involves the crystallization of tissue water.

Generalized Hypothermia

Generalized hypothermia may occur in a number of settings, including drowning and immersion in cold water and exposure to extremely cold air temperatures, especially after taking agents that impair thermoregulation, such as alcohol and some drugs.

Drowning

In water, the body rapidly loses heat, causing death from hypothermia in minutes in freezing water and in up to a few hours in water at 40°F to 50°F (4°C to 10°C). Death may also result in water as warm as 70°F to 80°F (21°C to 27°C) when exposure is sufficiently prolonged.

A normal human body immersed in cold water will go through the following stages of reaction:

- 0 to 2 minutes:
  Cold shock: Initial reaction, most likely to recover rapidly
- 5 to 15 minutes:
  Motor incapacitation: Normal muscle movements maintained
- Greater than 30 minutes:
  Onset of hypothermia: Perceptions and sensations remain
- Greater than 1 hour; up to 2 hours or more: Loss of consciousness

The ability to maintain consciousness, to survive, and to maintain body functions in hypothermia is related to the time of immersion and the temperature of the water.

In cases of fatal drowning, water is usually present in the lungs. However, there are a minority of cases in which "dry drowning" occurs, owing to laryngeal spasm that closes off the lower respiratory system, causing asphyxiation with dry lungs. Water enters the sinuses, and the presence of water in the sphenoid sinus is a typical sign of drowning.

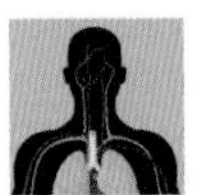

PATHOPHYSIOLOGY: Acute immersion in water at 4°C to 10°C (39.2°F to 50°F) reduces central blood flow. Coupled with decreased core body temperature and cooling of the blood perfusing the brain, this results in mental confusion. Attempting to increase heat production, the immersed body immediately responds by increasing muscle activity and oxygen consumption. As the core temperature approaches 35°C, there is an increased sympathetic neural discharge, resulting in increased heart and basal metabolic rates and shivering. This activity may be three to six times above normal. Below 35°C, respiratory rate, heart rate, and blood pressure decline because the functional reserve is reduced. If hypothermia is prolonged, decreased body temperature alters cerebrovascular function. When body core temperature reaches 32°C (89.6°F), the person becomes lethargic, apathetic, and withdrawn. If temperature falls further, intermittent "stupor," and eventually coma, supervene. If core temperature goes below 28°C (82.4°F), pulse and breathing weaken.

Although there are no specific morphologic changes in those who die from hypothermia, the skin shows red and purple discolorations, ears and hands swell, and there is irregular vasoconstriction and vasodilation. Areas of cardiac myocytolysis are seen. Lungs may display pulmonary edema and intra-alveolar, intrabronchial, and interstitial hemorrhage.

Focal Hypothermia

Local reduction in tissue temperature, particularly in the skin, is associated with local vasoconstriction. Tissue water crystallizes if blood circulation is insufficient to counter persistent thermal loss. The most biologically significant cell injury appears in the endothelial lining of the capillaries and venules, which alters small vessel permeability. This injury initiates extravasation of plasma, formation of localized edema and blisters, and an inflammatory reaction. Whereas **frostbite** results from the actual freezing of water, **immersion foot (trench foot)** is caused by a prolonged reduction in tissue temperature to a point not low enough to freeze tissue. This cooling causes cellular disruption. Endothelial cell damage leads to local thrombosis, and changes caused by altered permeability are prominent. Vascular occlusion often leads to gangrene.

Hyperthermia

Tissue responses to hyperthermia are similar in some respects to those caused by freezing injuries. In both instances, injury to the vascular endothelium results in altered vascular permeability, edema, and blisters. The degree of injury depends on the extent of temperature elevation and how quickly it is reached. Small increases in body temperature increase the metabolic rate. However, above a certain limit, enzymes denature, other proteins precipitate, and "melting" of lipid bilayers of cell membranes takes place.

Systemic Hyperthermia

Systemic hyperthermia, or **fever**, is an elevation of body core temperature. It occurs because of (1) increased heat production, (2) decreased elimination of heat from the body (reflecting an aberrant response of the thermal regulatory center), or (3) a disturbance of the thermal regulatory center itself. Hyperthermia can also occur because heat is conducted into the body faster than the system can clear it.

A body temperature above 42.5°C (108.5°F) leads to profound functional disturbances, including general vasodilation, inefficient cardiac function, and altered respiration. Isolated heart–lung preparations fail at about the same temperature, suggesting an inherent limitation in the cardiovascular system and perhaps in the myocardial cells themselves. ***In general, systemic temperature elevations above 42°C (107.6°F) are not compatible with life.***

Heat stroke is a form of hyperthermia that occurs under conditions of very high ambient temperatures and is not mediated by endogenous pyrogens. It reflects impaired thermal regulatory cooling responses and characteristically occurs in infants, young children, and the very aged. Lactic acidosis, hypocalcemia, and rhabdomyolysis may be severe problems, and one third of patients with exertional heat stroke develop myoglobinuric acute renal failure. Heat stroke is amenable to external cooling and fluid and electrolyte replacement.

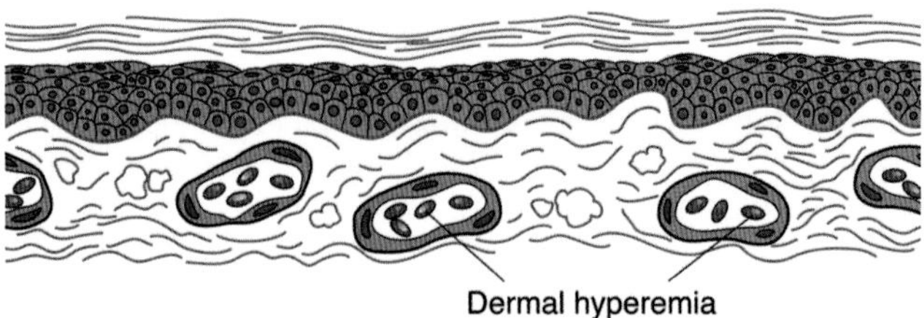

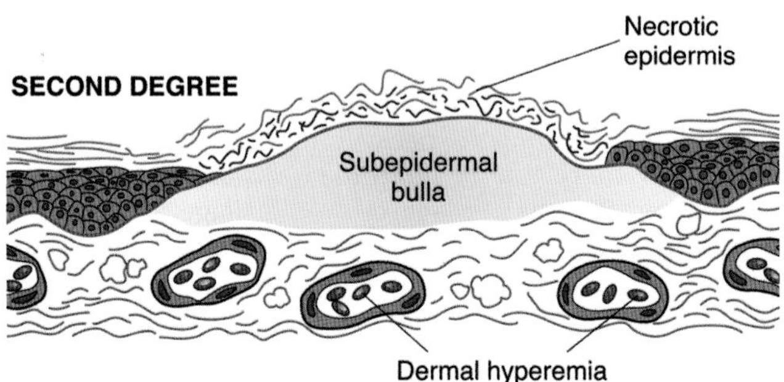

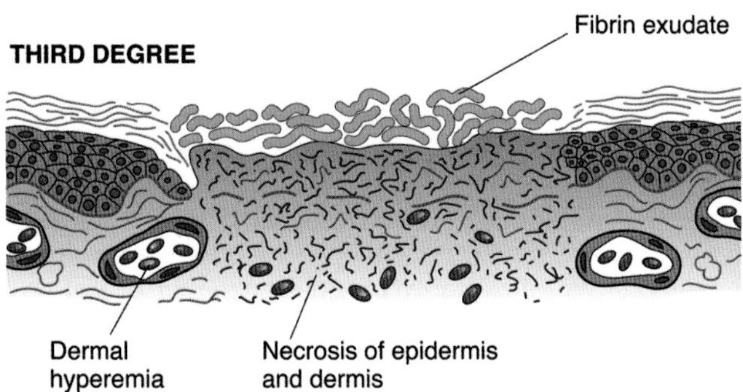

FIGURE 25-5. The pathology of cutaneous burns. A first-degree skin burn exhibits only dilation of the dermal blood vessels. In a second-degree burn, there is necrosis of the epidermis, and subepidermal edema collects under the necrotic epidermis to form a bulla. In a third-degree burn, both the epidermis and the dermis are necrotic.

Cutaneous Burns

Cutaneous burns are the most common form of localized hyperthermia. Both the elevated temperature and the rate of temperature change are important in determining the tissue response. A temperature of 50°C (120°F) may be sustained for 10 minutes or more without cell death, whereas a temperature of 70°C (158°F) or higher for even several seconds causes necrosis of the entire epidermis.

Cutaneous burns have been separated into full thickness (previously, third-degree) and partial thickness (previously, first- and second-degree) (Fig. 25-5).

- **Full-thickness burns** char both epidermis and dermis. Histologically, they are carbonized and cellular structure is lost.

One of the most serious systemic disturbances caused by extensive cutaneous burns is fluid loss. Patients with full-thickness burns can lose about 0.3 mL of body water/cm^2 of burned area per day. The resulting hemoconcentration and poor vascular perfusion of the skin and other viscera complicate the recovery of these patients. Many severely burned people, particularly those with more than 70% of their body surface involved with full-thickness burns, develop shock and acute tubular necrosis of the kidneys; mortality is very high. Severely burned patients who survive longer are at great risk of lethal surface infections and sepsis. Even normal skin saprophytes may cause infection of charred tissue and pose another difficulty for healing.

Healing of cutaneous burns is related to the extent of tissue destruction. Mild partial-thickness burns, by definition, have little if any cell loss, and healing requires only repair or replacement of injured endothelial cells. More severe partial-thickness burns also heal without a scar because epidermal basal cells remain and are a source of regenerating cells for the epithelium. Full-thickness burns, in which the entire thickness of the epidermis is destroyed, pose a separate set of problems. If the skin appendages are spared, reepithelialization can arise from them. Initially, islands of proliferation at the orifices of these glands grow and coalesce to cover the surface. Deeper burns that destroy the skin appendages require new epidermis to be grafted to the debrided area to establish a functional covering. Burned skin that is not replaced by a graft heals with dense scarring. Because this scar tissue lacks the elasticity of normal skin, contractures that limit motion may eventually result.

Electrical Injury

Electrical injury produces damage through (1) electrical dysfunction of cardiovascular conduction and the nervous system and (2) conversion of electrical energy to heat energy when the current encounters the resistance of the tissues. ***Because electrical energy can potentially disrupt the electrical system within the heart, it frequently causes death through ventricular fibrillation.*** The amount of current necessary for such a disruption depends in part on its pathway through the body and its ease in penetrating the skin. Someone who inadvertently touches a 120-volt line in a living room may suffer burns on the hand because the skin that contacts the wire has substantial resistance to the flow of electrical current. If that resistance is decreased, as when a person inadvertently touches the same line in a bathtub, the lower resistance increases transmitted current, leading to disordered cardiac electrical activity.

Electrical burns of the skin reflect the voltage, the area of electrical conductance, and the duration of current flow. Very–high-voltage current chars tissue and produces a third-degree burn. On the other hand, broad, moist surfaces exposed to the same flow exhibit less-severe change. With exposure to very–high-voltage currents, the force may be almost "explosive," in which case vaporization of tissue water produces extensive damage.

Fire-Related Death

Asphyxiation is a frequent cause of death in fire victims owing to inhalation of carbon monoxide (Table 25-1) and other noxious combustion gases. Death from smoke inhalation usually occurs before thermal injuries occur or become fatal. The presence of soot in the airway of an outwardly burned body is a sign that the victim was alive and breathing at the time of the fire. The level of carbon monoxide in the blood is also a measure of smoke inhalation (Table 25-1).

When bodies are extensively damaged by fire, the tissues contract, and the body assumes a "pugilistic" or defensive posture, drawing inward. This is not a conscious defensive pose but a postmortem artifact. Fire also sterilizes the body, resulting in reduced or absent postmortem decomposition and preservation of the remaining, albeit burned, tissues of the body.

Table 25-1

Effects of Carbon Monoxide Poisoning

Blood Level of CO (Hemoglobin Concentrations)	Exposure	Effects
<10%	Tobacco smoking	None
10%–30%	Smoke/exhaust	Headache, dyspnea
30%–50%		Confusion, lethargy
50%–60%		Convulsions, coma
>60%		Death

Carbon monoxide (CO) binds preferentially to hemoglobin, displacing oxygen and causing chemical asphyxia.

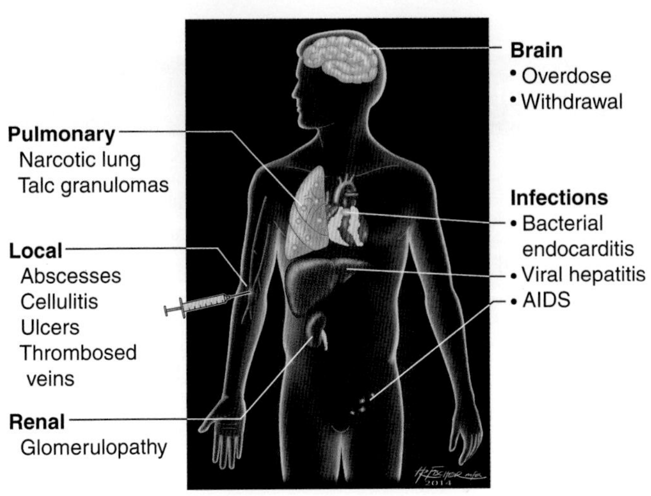

FIGURE 25-6. Complications of intravenous drug abuse.

DRUG ABUSE

Drug abuse has been defined as "the use of any substance in a manner that deviates from the accepted medical, social, or legal patterns within a given society." For the most part, drug abuse involves agents that are used to alter mood and perception. These include (1) derivatives of opium (heroin, morphine); (2) synthetic opiates; (3) depressants (barbiturates, tranquilizers, alcohol); (4) stimulants (cocaine, amphetamines), marijuana, and psychedelic drugs (PCP, lysergic acid diethylamide [LSD]); and (5) inhalants (amyl nitrite, organic solvents such as those in glue). The rate of illicit drug deaths in the US has doubled in the last decade to 64,000 deaths per year. Much of this increase is a result of the abuse of synthetic opiates and, in particular, fentanyl and its derivatives.

Complications of Intravenous Drug Abuse

Apart from reactions related to pharmacologic or physiologic effects of substance abuse, including overdose-related deaths,

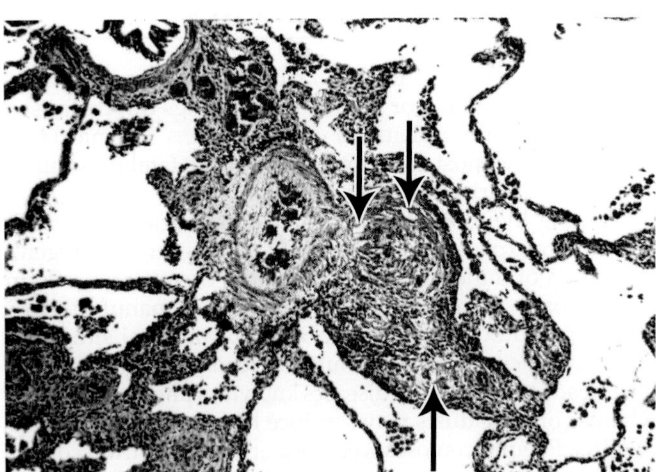

FIGURE 25-7. Talc granulomas in the lung. A section of lung from an intravenous drug abuser viewed under polarized light reveals a granuloma adjacent to a pulmonary artery. The refractile material (*arrows*) is talc that was used to dilute the drug prior to its intravenous injection.

Table 25-2

Acute Fatal Chemical Poisonings

Chemical	Exposures	Toxicity
Benzene	Occupational—industrial, chemical manufacturing, solvent use, gasoline (3%)	Acute CNS and respiratory failure
Chloroform and carbon tetrachloride	Cleaning solvents	Depressant effects on CNS and heart Hepatic necrosis, fatty liver, liver failure
Cyanide/prussic acid	Trace amounts in nuts and fruit seeds as natural pesticides (e.g., bitter almond [*Prunus amygdalus*])	Acute global anoxia; binds to mitochondrial cytochrome oxidase, arrests cellular respiration
Ethylene glycol	Antifreeze (ethanol substitute)	CNS depression and metabolic acidosis Oxalate urinary crystals and renal failure
Gasoline and kerosene	Accidental ingestion Inhalation of combustion products	Gastrointestinal Asphyxiation, CO poisoning (see Table 25-1)
Methanol	Ethanol substitute	Metabolism to formaldehyde, then formic acid; blindness, seizures, coma
Trichloroethylene	Industrial solvent	CNS depression; minimal liver toxicity

CNS, central nervous system.

the most common complications are caused by introducing infectious organisms by a parenteral route. Most occur at the site of injection: cutaneous abscesses, cellulitis, and ulcers (Fig. 25-6). Thrombophlebitis of the veins draining sites of injection is common. Intravenous introduction of bacteria may lead to septic complications in internal organs. Bacterial endocarditis, often involving *Staphylococcus aureus*, occurs on both sides of the heart and may cause pulmonary, renal, and intracranial abscesses; meningitis; osteomyelitis; and mycotic aneurysms.

Intravenous drug abusers are at very high risk for AIDS, as well as hepatitis B and C. Intravenous injection of talc, which is used to dilute pure drug, is associated with the appearance of foreign body granulomas in the lung (Fig. 25-7). These may be severe enough to lead to interstitial pulmonary fibrosis.

ENVIRONMENTAL CHEMICALS

There are many natural and manufactured substances that may cause poisoning, fatal or nonfatal. Poisonings can be caused by chemicals, drugs, plants, or other biotoxins. Chemical poisonings are the most common form of acute fatal poisonings and are summarized in Table 25-2.

Among the most important chemical hazards to which humans are exposed are environmental dusts and carcinogens. Inhalation of mineral and organic dusts occurs primarily in occupational settings (e.g., mining, industrial manufacturing, farming) and occasionally as a result of unusual situations (e.g., bird fanciers, pituitary snuff inhalation). Inhaling mineral dusts leads to pulmonary diseases known as **pneumoconioses**, whereas organic dusts may produce **hypersensitivity pneumonitis**. Pneumoconioses were formerly common, but control of dust exposure in the workplace through modifications of manufacturing techniques, improvements in air handling, and use of masks has substantially reduced the incidence of these diseases. Because of their importance, pneumoconioses and hypersensitivity pneumonitis are discussed in detail in Chapter 10.

Table 25-3

Cancers Associated With Exposure to Occupational Carcinogens

Agent or Occupation	Site of Cancer
Arsenic	Lung cancer
Asbestos	Mesothelioma (pleura and peritoneum) Lung cancer (in smokers)
Aromatic amines	Bladder cancer
Benzene	Leukemia, multiple myeloma
bis(Chloromethyl)ether	Lung cancer
Chromium	Lung cancer
Furniture and shoe manufacturing	Nasal carcinoma
Hematite mining	Lung cancer
Nickel	Lung cancer, paranasal sinus cancer
Tars and oils	Cancers of lung, gastrointestinal tract, bladder, and skin
Vinyl chloride	Angiosarcoma of liver

Chemical carcinogens are ubiquitous in the environment. Their potential for causing disease has elicited widespread concern. In particular, exposure to carcinogens in the workplace has been associated epidemiologically with a number of cancers (Table 25-3).

INDEX

Note: Locators followed by the letter 'f' and 't' refers to figures and tables.

B

H

J

K

L

M

N

O

Q

R

T

W

X

Y

Z